Hutchison's

Atlas of Paediatric PHYSICAL DIAGNOSIS

Hutchison's

Atlas of Paediatric PHYSICAL DIAGNOSIS

Second Edition

Editors

Krishna M. Goel MD DCH FRCP (Lond, Edin & Glas) Hon FRCPCH
Formerly
Honorary Senior Lecturer of Child Health
University of Glasgow
Consultant Paediatrician
Royal Hospital for Sick Children
Glasgow, Scotland, UK

Robert Carachi MBE MD PhD FRCS (Glas) FRCS (Eng) FEBPS
Emeritus Professor of Surgical Paediatrics
University of Glasgow
Royal Hospital for Sick Children
Glasgow, Scotland, UK

Foreword

Neena Modi

JAYPEE

JAYPEE BROTHERS MEDICAL PUBLISHERS
The Health Sciences Publisher
New Delhi | London

JAYPEE Jaypee Brothers Medical Publishers (P) Ltd.

Headquarters
EMCA House
23/23-B, Ansari Road, Daryaganj
New Delhi 110 002, India
Landline: +91-11-23272143, +91-11-23272703
+91-11-23282021, +91-11-23245672
E-mail: jaypee@jaypeebrothers.com

Corporate Office
4838/24, Ansari Road, Daryaganj
New Delhi 110 002, India
Phone: +91-11-43574357
Fax: +91-11-43574314
E-mail: jaypee@jaypeebrothers.com

Overseas Office
J.P. Medical Ltd.
83, Victoria Street, London
SW1H 0HW (UK)
Phone: +44 20 3170 8910
E-mail: info@jpmedpub.com

EU GPSR Authorised Representative
Logos Europe, 9 rue Nicolas Poussin
17000, La Rochelle, France
Phone: +33 (0) 6 67 93 73 78
E-mail: contact@logoseurope.eu

Website: www.jaypeebrothers.com
Website: www.jaypeedigital.com

Inquiries for bulk sales may be solicited at: jaypee@jaypeebrothers.com

Hutchison's Atlas of Paediatric Physical Diagnosis

First Edition: 2014
Second Edition: **2019**

Reprint 2026

ISBN: 978-93-5270-159-9

Printed at Replika Press Pvt. Ltd.

Dedication

All the children in the world.

Contributors

Alison E. Balfour
MBChB BSc FRCPath
Consultant Microbiologist
Queen Elizabeth University Hospital
Glasgow, Scotland, UK

Elaine M. Balmer
MBChB MRCPCH
Consultant Neonatologist
Wishaw General Hospital
Wishaw, Scotland, UK

Mona Basker
MD DCH PGDAP Clin Fellowship Adolescent Medicine
Professor, Adolescent Medicine Unit
Department of Paediatrics
Christian Medical College
Vellore, Tamil Nadu, India

Richard Bowman
MA MD FRCOphth
Consultant Ophthalmologist
Great Ormond Street Hospital, London
Senior Lecturer
International Centre for Eye Health
London
School of Hygiene and Tropical Medicine
London, UK

Sandra J. Butler
BSc (Hons) MBChB MRCPCH FRCR
Consultant Paediatric Radiologist
Royal Hospital for Sick Children
Glasgow, Scotland, UK

Alison M. Cairns
BDS MSc MFDS RCSEd M Paed Dent FDS (Paed Dent) RCPSG Dip Ac Prac FHEA
Senior Clinical University Teacher
Honorary Consultant
Paediatric Dentistry
University of Glasgow
Dental Hospital and School
Glasgow, Scotland, UK

Andrew Carachi
MB ChB BSc Hons (Med Sci) MRCEM CT2 ACCS EM
Royal Victoria Infirmary
Newcastle, England, UK

Robert Carachi
MBE MD PhD FRCS (Glas) FRCS (Eng) FEBPS
Emeritus Professor of Surgical Paediatrics
University of Glasgow
Royal Hospital for Sick Children
Glasgow, Scotland, UK

Salvatore Cascio
MS FRCSI FRCS (Paed Surg) FEBPS
Consultant Paediatric Surgeon and Urologist
Children's University Hospital
Dublin, Ireland, UK

Elizabeth A. Chalmers
MBChB MD MRCP (UK) FRCPath
Consultant Paediatric Haematologist
Royal Hospital for Sick Children
Glasgow, Scotland, UK

Jugesh Chhatwal
MD DCH
Professor and Head
Department of Paediatrics
Vice-Principal (Postgraduate)
Christian Medical College
Ludhiana, Punjab, India

W. Andrew Clement
FRCS (Edin) FRCS - ORL (UK)
Consultant Paediatric Otolaryngologist
Royal Hospital for Sick Children
Glasgow, Scotland, UK

Sarah Coles
MBChB MRCPCH
ST3 Paediatric Registrar
Royal Victoria Infirmary
Newcastle, England, UK

Sarada David
MS DO
Professor and Head
Department of Ophthalmology
Christian Medical College
Vellore, Tamil Nadu, India

Anne Margaret Devenny
FRCPCH
Consultant
Paediatric Respiratory Medicine
Royal Hospital for Sick Children
Glasgow, Scotland, UK

Gordon N. Dutton
MD FRCS FRCOphth
Emeritus Professor of Visual Science
Department of Optometry and Visual Science
Glasgow Caledonian University
Glasgow, Scotland, UK

Paul Galea
MD DCH FRCP (Glas) FRCPCH
Formerly, Consultant Paediatrician
Royal Hospital for Sick Children
Glasgow, Scotland, UK

Peter Galloway
DCH FRCP FRC Path
Consultant Medical Biochemist
New South Glasgow Biochemistry Laboratory
Glasgow, Scotland, UK

Krishna M. Goel
MD DCH FRCP (Lond, Edin & Glas) Hon FRCPCH
Formerly, Honorary Senior Lecturer of Child Health
University of Glasgow
Consultant Paediatrician
Royal Hospital for Sick Children
Glasgow, Scotland, UK

Ram Gulati
MBBS MD (Dermatology & Venereology) MRCPCH (UK)
Formerly, Locum Consultant Dermatologist
Royal Hospital for Sick Children
Glasgow, Scotland, UK

Rosemary Anne Hague
MD MRCP (UK) FRCPCH
Consultant
Paediatric Infectious Diseases and Immunology
Honorary Senior Lecturer
University of Glasgow
Lecturer
University of the Highlands and Islands
Royal Hospital for Sick Children
Glasgow, Scotland, UK

Christina Halsey
BM BCh BA (Hons) MRCP MRCPath PhD
Honorary Consultant
Paediatric Haematologist and
Scottish Senior Clinical Fellow
Department of Paediatric Haematology
Royal Hospital for Sick Children
Glasgow, Scotland, UK

Philip Hammond
FRCS (Paed Surg)
Consultant Paediatric and Neonatal Surgeon
Royal Hospital for Sick Children
Edinburgh, Scotland, UK

Kevin P. Hanretty
MD FRCOG
Formerly, Consultant Obstetrician and Gynaecologist
Southern General Hospital
Glasgow, Scotland, UK

Jean Herbison
MBChB MRCP FRCPCH DCCH MFFLM
Professor, Child Health and Protecting Children
University of West of Scotland
Consultant Paediatrician and Clinical Director
Child Protection Services
Greater Glasgow and Clyde Health Board
Child Protection Unit
Royal Hospital for Sick Children
Glasgow, Scotland, UK

David James
MBChB Dip Ed DCH DPM FRCPsych FRCP (Glas)
Retired Child Psychiatrist
Department of Child and Family Psychiatry
Royal Hospital for Sick Children
Glasgow, Scotland, UK

Judy Ann John
MD DipNB (PMR)
Associate Professor
Department of Physical Medicine and Rehabilitation
Christian Medical College
Vellore, Tamil Nadu, India

Benjamin Joseph
MS Orth MCh Orth
Professor of Orthopaedics and
Head of Paediatric Orthopaedic Service
Kasturba Medical College
Manipal, Karnataka, India

Catherine Jury
MBChB MRCP (Glas)
Consultant Dermatologist
Royal Hospital for Sick Children
Glasgow, Scotland, UK

Phyllis Kilbourn
International Director
Crisis Care Training International
International Office
South Carolina, USA

Ameet Kishore
MBBS (AFMC) FRCS (Glas) FRCS (Edin) FRCS-ORL (UK)
Senior Consultant ENT Surgeon
Indraprastha Apollo Hospitals
New Delhi, India
Director and Chief Consultant
ADVENTIS (Advanced ENT Service)
Gurugram, Haryana, India

Maya Kommer
MBBS BA(Hons) OXON MRCS
Specialist Registrar Neurosurgery
Royal Hospital for Sick Children
Glasgow, Scotland, UK

B. Koshy
MBBS MD (Paed) PDFDP
Professor
Developmental Paediatric Unit
Christian Medical College
Vellore, Tamil Nadu, India

Louis C.K. Low
BSc (Hons) MBChB FRCP (Glas, Edin & Lond) FRCPCH FHKAM (Paediatrics) FHKCPaed
Honorary Clinical Professor
Department of Paediatrics and Adolescent Medicine
The University of Hong Kong
Paediatric Specialist
Hong Kong Sanatorium and Hospital
Hong Kong, China

Helen Mactier
MD MRCP UK (Paed) FRCPCH
Consultant Neonatologist
Honorary Clinical Associate Professor
University of Glasgow
Princess Royal Maternity
Glasgow, Scotland, UK

N.V. Mahendri
MSc MPhil MHRM & RD
Retired Head HOD
Department of Dietetics
Christian Medical College
Vellore, Tamil Nadu, India

Sanjay V. Maroo
MBChB M-Med FRCR
Staff Paediatric and Interventional Radiologist
BC Children's Hospital
Vancouver British Columbia, Canada

Mary Mealyea
MBChB Diploma in Dermatology
Formerly, Associate Specialist
Paediatric Dermatology
Royal Hospital for Sick Children
Glasgow, Scotland, UK

Khursheed F. Moos
OBE MBBS (Lond) BDS (Lond) FRCS (Edin) FDS RCS (Eng and Edin) FDS RCPS (Glasg) FRCPS (Glasg) Honorary FCPS (Pakistan) Honorary
Honorary Professor of Oral and Maxillofacial Surgery
Glasgow University
Consultant Oral and Maxillofacial Surgeon
West of Scotland Plastic and Maxillofacial Unit
Canniesburn Hospital, Glasgow
Civilian Consultant to the Royal Navy
Glasgow, Scotland, UK

Stewart C. Morrison
PhD SFHEA MChS
Senior Lecturer in Podiatry
University of Brighton
Brighton, England, UK

Michael Morton
MPhil MA MBChB FRCPsych FRCPCH
Formerly, Consultant Child and Adolescent Psychiatrist
In-patient, Liaison Child and Adolescent Psychiatry with Neuropsychiatry
Department of Child and Family Psychiatry
Royal Hospital for Sick Children
Glasgow, Scotland, UK

P.D. Moses
MBBS MD (Paed) MRCP (UK) FRCP (Edin) FCAMS
Consultant in Paediatrics
Wellcome Research Unit
Christian Medical College
Vellore, Tamil Nadu, India

S. Muthusamy
MD(Paeds) DM (Neuro) DNB (Neuro)
Associate Professor
Paediatric Neurology Unit
Department of Neurological Sciences
Christian Medical College
Vellore, Tamil Nadu, India

Roddy O'Kane
MBChB BSc FRCS (SN) MEd
Consultant Paediatric Neurosurgeon
Royal Hospital for Sick Children
Glasgow, Scotland, Uk

Ian W. Pinkerton
OBE TD FRCP (Edin) FRCP (Glas)
Formerly, Consultant Physician
Department of Infectious Diseases
Ruchill Hospital, Glasgow
Honorary Lecturer in Infectious Diseases
University of Glasgow
Glasgow, Scotland, UK

Lydia Edward Raj
MSOT
Reader (In-Charge OT Education)
Department of Physical Medicine and Rehabilitation
Christian Medical College
Vellore, Tamil Nadu, India

Daniel Reid
OBE MD FRCP (Edin and Glas) Hon FFTM FFPHM DPH FRS (Edin)
Professor
Formerly, Director
Scottish Centre for Infection and Environmental Health
Honorary Lecturer
University Department of Infectious Diseases
Ruchill Hospital
Glasgow, Scotland, UK

Trevor Richens
MBBS BSc (Hons) MRCP (Lond)
Consultant Paediatric Cardiologist
University Hospital Southampton
Southampton, England, UK

Rosemary Sabatino
Trainer and Educator
Crisis Care Training International
International Office
South Carolina, USA

R. Cameron Shepherd
BA MBChB FRCP(G) FRCPCH DCH
Formerly, Consultant General and Community Paediatrician
Royal Alexandra Hospital Paisley and Inverclyde Royal Hospital
Greenock, Scotland, UK

Debbie Skeil
BM BCh FRCP DM
Volunteer Consultant
Department of Physical Medicine and Rehabilitation
Christian Medical College
Vellore, Tamil Nadu, India

Rajeev Srivastava
MBBS FRCS FRCPath Eur Clin Chem
Consultant
Clinical Biochemist and
Senior Clinical Lecturer
Southern General Hospital
Glasgow, Scotland, UK

Mairi Steven
MB ChB BSc (Medi Sci) Hons MRCS
Consultant in Paediatric Surgery (ST7)
Royal Hospital for Sick Children
Glasgow, Scotland, UK

M. Thomas
DCH MD (Paeds) DM (Neuro)
Professor
Paediatric Neurology Unit
Department of Neurological Sciences
Christian Medical College
Vellore, Tamil Nadu, India

Kirsteen J. Thompson
MSc FRCS (Edin)
Consultant Ophthalmologist
Inverclyde Royal Hospital
Greenock, Scotland, UK

Alastair Turner
BSc Med Sci MBChB MRCPCH
Consultant
Paediatric Intensive Care
Honorary Senior Clinical Lecturer
University of Glasgow
Royal Hospital for Sick Children
Glasgow, Scotland, UK

James Wallace
BSc MR PharmS FRCPCH (Hon)
Formerly, Chief Pharmacist
Royal Hospital for Sick Children
Glasgow, Scotland, UK

Gordon F. Watt
FFPM RCPS (Glasg) FCPM MChS DPod M Cert FE
Formerly, Lecturer in Podiatry
Glasgow Caledonian University
Consultant Podiatrist
Royal Hospital for Sick Children
Glasgow, Scotland, UK

Martyn H.C. Webster
MBChB FRCS (Glas & Edin)
Formerly, Consultant and Senior Lecturer
Glasgow University
Canniesburn Plastic Surgical Unit
Glasgow, Scotland, UK

Richard Welbury
MBBS BDS PhD FDSRCS FDSRCPS FRCPCH
Professor, Paediatric Dentistry
University of Glasgow Dental School
Glasgow, Scotland, UK

Margo L. Whiteford
CBE BSc FRCP (Glas)
Consultant Clinical Geneticist
Southern General Hospital
Glasgow, Scotland, UK

Suzie Wills
MBChB MRCPCH
Locum Consultant Neonatologist
Royal Hospital for Children
Glasgow, Scotland, UK

Paul L. Wood
MD FRCOG
Consultant Obstetrician and Gynaecologist
Kettering General Hospital
Kettering, UK

S. Yoganathan
MD(Paeds) DNB(Paeds) DM(Paed Neuro)
Associate Professor
Paediatric Neurology Unit
Deapartment of Neurological Sciences
Christian Medical College
Vellore, Tamil Nadu, India

Foreword to the Second Edition

Pictorial recognition can be very important in making a correct diagnosis. I am delighted that the editors Krishna M. Goel and Robert Carachi have produced a second edition of their marvellous *Hutchison's Atlas of Paediatric Physical Diagnosis*. This Atlas is a visual encyclopaedia of paediatrics with an ideal mix of material to maximise learning. In this comprehensive work of thirty-nine chapters, every paediatric subspeciality is included.

This text will be of great value to all who use it, whether students, those preparing for professional examinations, or paediatricians seeking insights into difficult clinical problems in daily practice.

Neena Modi
President
Royal College of Paediatrics and Child Health
London, UK

Foreword to the First Edition

There are many different reasons for buying a medical textbook; these range from "it might look good on the coffee table" through "I am interested in this topic and rate these authors" to "the examination is next week". The impending examination is a potent driver for such a spending spree, and I remember only too well as a medical student the exponential textbook-purchasing curve that shot up steeply as the fateful day approached. Many of these books, which can only be described as a product of panic-buying, remained pristine and unread before being sold on to the next unfortunate. So what distinguishes a textbook that is likely to be of more value? As you stand in the bookstore flicking through a range of options, which should you buy? The short answer is the one that will help you acquire and embed knowledge most effectively.

One of the oft-quoted sources on learning techniques is Edgar Dale's Cone of Learning.[1] This describes a hierarchy of what we remember, with a progressive increase through just reading, just hearing, just seeing, to various combinations of reading, seeing and hearing, and ultimately direct experience. Some authors have criticised the way in which Edgar Dale's Cone has been portrayed, with hard percentages applied at each level in the absence of any data to support this. However, the essential principle—that multimodal learning is superior to monomodal learning—remains unchallenged. What we do know about successful learning is that we have to be able to process information effectively in our short-term memory in order to lay down longer-term memories. However, one of the limitations of our short-term memory is that there are separate buffers for verbal/text elements and visual/spatial elements. This means that in order to avoid overloading one or other buffer, the best way to present information is by using textual and pictorial elements in tandem. Couple that with the much quoted maxim "a picture is worth a thousand words" and you arrive at the raison d'être of this book.

By combining the dual elements of authoritative text, alongside an excellent range of images covering the full breadth of paediatric medicine, the editors and chapter authors have produced the ideal mix of material to maximise learning. This book may well sit on the coffee table, but only because it is in regular use, and it will certainly not be passed on in pristine condition.

Hilary Cass
Neurodisability Consultant
Evelina London Children's Hospital
President
Royal College of Paediatrics and Child Health
London, UK

1. Edgar Dale, Audiovisual Methods in Technology, Holt, Rinehart and Wonston.

Preface to the Second Edition

The aim of this Atlas is to widen the visual experience of clinical paediatrics for medical undergraduates, postgraduates specialising in paediatrics and for general practitioners whose daily work is concerned with care of children in health and disease. For many paediatric conditions, pictorial recognition is the most important factor in making a correct diagnosis. A concise text clearly integrated with high-quality colour clinical photographs. The diverse authorship of chapters in this Atlas reflects the growing dependence upon co-operative interests of colleagues in paediatrics. In clinical practice, such collaborative work can only be accomplished within a large hospital or a unit devoted to children. The experienced paediatricians who have seen a broad spectrum of different paediatric disorders carries a great wealth of knowledge for diagnosis and teaching. They have contributed in countless ways to this Atlas. We seek to give advice about the diagnosis and investigations of the full spectrum of childhood disorders, both medical and surgical.

However, an encouraging response to the first edition of the Atlas led us to produce the second edition. Every chapter has been revised, reviewed and updated. One new chapter on Paediatric Podiatry has been included and sections on surgical urology and neurosurgery have been incorporated. The chapter on surgical oncology has been completely rewritten. Also the new images have been added. Additional contributors have added greater depth and knowledge to the Atlas. It is hoped that this Atlas will continue to provide an essential and practical visual recognition to those who care for children.

We are especially grateful to the parents and to children and their families who contributed to our knowledge and understanding of paediatrics and willingly gave permission to reproduce these photographs. A book such as this cannot be written without reproducing material reported in the medical literature. We acknowledge here, with gratitude the permission granted free of charge by publishers to reproduce material for which they hold the copyright.

Finally, we should like to acknowledge our gratitude to the various contributors to this Atlas for their co-operation in its production. We could not have succeeded without their help.

Krishna M. Goel
Robert Carachi

Preface to the First Edition

The pattern of childhood disease throughout the world is changing with advancing knowledge, altering standards of living, life style and rising levels of medical care. The origins of physical and mental health and disease lie predominantly in the early development of the child. Most of the abnormalities affecting the health and behaviour of children are determined prenatally or in the first few years of life by genetic and environmental factors.

The aim of this Atlas is to widen the visual experience of clinical paediatrics for medical undergraduates, postgraduates specialising in paediatrics and for general practitioners whose daily work is concerned with care of children in health and disease. For many paediatric conditions, pictorial recognition is the most important factor in making a correct diagnosis. A concise text clearly integrated with high-quality colour clinical photographs. The diverse authorship of chapters in this Atlas reflects the growing dependence upon co-operative interests of colleagues in paediatrics. In clinical practice, such collaborative work can only be accomplished within a large hospital or a unit devoted to children. The experienced paediatricians who have seen a broad spectrum of different paediatric disorders carries a great wealth of knowledge for diagnosis and teaching. They have contributed in countless ways to this Atlas. In the Atlas we seek to give advice about the diagnosis and investigations of the full spectrum of childhood disorders, both medical and surgical.

We are especially grateful to the parents and to the many children and their families who contributed to our knowledge and understanding of paediatrics and willingly gave permission to reproduce these photographs. A book such as this cannot be written without reproducing material reported in the medical literature. We acknowledge here, with gratitude the permission granted free of charge by individual publishers to reproduce material for which they hold the copyright.

Finally, we are extremely grateful to the various contributors to this Atlas for their co-operation in its production. We could not have succeeded without their help.

Krishna M. Goel
Robert Carachi

Acknowledgements

We would like to thank Shri Jitendar P Vij (Group Chairman), Mr Ankit Vij (Group President) and Ms Chetna Malhotra Vohra (Associate Director–Content Strategy) of Jaypee Brothers Medical Publishers (P) Ltd, New Delhi, India, for enabling us to publish this book. We would also like to thank Ms Kritika Dua (Senior Development Editor), and the complete Production Team for helping us in the whole process.

Contents

CHAPTER 1

Paediatric History and Examination

Krishna M. Goel, Robert Carachi

INTRODUCTION

At all times, the physician must show genuine concern and interest when speaking with parents of child patients. The parents and the child must feel that the doctor has the time, interest and competence to help them. A physician who greets the child by name, irrespective of age, will convey an attitude of concern and interest. Parents tell us about the child's signs and symptoms, although children contribute more as they grow older.

The doctor–patient relationship gradually develops during history taking and physical examination. Considerable tact and discretion are required when taking the history, especially in the presence of the child: questioning on sensitive subjects should best be reserved for a time when the parents can be interviewed alone. It may, therefore, be necessary to separate the parent and the child (patient) when taking the history, especially when the problems are related to behaviour, school difficulties and socioeconomic disturbances in the home environment.

The medical student, having been instructed in the history taking and physical examination of adults, needs to appreciate the modifications necessary when dealing with a child patient. A basic template for history taking is useful and serves as a reminder of the ground to be covered **(Box 1.1)**. Initially, the medical student may be confused because of the need to obtain information from someone other than the patient, usually the mother. Useful information may be obtained by observing infants and young children during the history taking. Older children should be given an opportunity to talk, to present their symptoms and to tell how they interfere with school and play activities.

The simple act of offering a toy, picture book or pen torch is often an effective step towards establishing rapport. Rigid adherence to routine is both unnecessary and counterproductive. A lot may be learned of the family constellation and the parent–child relationship by simply observing the parent(s) and child during the history taking and physical examination. Therefore, watching, listening and talking are of paramount importance in paediatric practice and are invaluable in arriving at a working diagnosis.

> **KEY LEARNING POINT**
>
> Useful information may be obtained by observing infants and young children during the history taking.

HISTORY OF PRESENT COMPLAINT

Even before language develops in the infant (from the Latin word *infans*, meaning without speech), parents can detect altered behaviour and observe abnormal physical signs. It is sensible to commence with the history of the presenting observations because that is what the parents have come to talk about. In the newborn infant, the history from the attending nurse and medical staff is important.

Every endeavour should be made to ask appropriate questions and discuss relevant points in the history in order to identify the nature of the child's problems and come to a tentative diagnosis. Ask what the child is called at home and address the child with this name, since otherwise he/she may be less forthcoming. Let the parents give the history in their own way and then ask specific questions. Ask the parents the following: how severe are the symptoms; have the symptoms changed during the past days, weeks or months; has there been any change recently in the child's appetite, energy or activities; has the child been absent from school; has anyone who cares for the child been ill; has the child been thriving or losing weight; what change in behaviour has there been; has there been a change in appetite, micturition or bowel habits? An articulate older child can describe feelings and symptoms more accurately, as the child's memory for the time and sequence of events may be more precise than the parents.

BOX 1.1 History taking—the paediatric patient.

Disease

Presenting problem
History of the presenting problem
Previous history
Pregnancy and delivery
Neonatal period and infancy
Subsequent development
Other disorders or diseases
Dietary
Immunisation
Family history
Parents
Siblings
Others
Draw a family tree if indicated

KEY LEARNING POINT

Establishing rapport: The paediatrician should start the interview by welcoming and establishing rapport with the parent(s) and the child. Always refer to the infant or child by name rather than by 'him', 'her' or 'the baby'. Also ask children about their clothes, siblings' name, friends' name, their toys and what book, games or TV programs they enjoy. Thus, spending sometime at the start of the interview would put both the child and the parents at ease.

PAST MEDICAL HISTORY

The past history is the documentation of significant events that have happened in the child's life and that may be of relevance in coming to a diagnosis. Therefore, the doctor should try to obtain relevant information concerning the past from the family and any other sources that are available. It is useful if the events are recorded in the sequence of their occurrence. A careful history should contain details of pregnancy, delivery, neonatal period, early feeding, the child's achievement of developmental milestones and details of admissions to hospital, with date, place and reason for admission. A complete list of current medication including vitamins and other supplements should be obtained. An enquiry should be made of any drug or other sensitivity, which should always be prominently recorded. Details of immunisation and all previous infectious diseases should be elicited.

KEY LEARNING POINT

Dietary history is of vital importance in paediatric history taking, especially if the child is neither thriving nor has vomiting, diarrhoea, constipation or anaemia.

Mother's Pregnancy, Labour, Delivery and the Neonatal Period

The younger the child, the more important is the information about the period of intrauterine life. The history of pregnancy includes obstetric complications during the pregnancy; history of illness, infection or injury and social habits, e.g. smoking by the mother, are important. Drug or alcohol ingestion and poor diet during pregnancy may have an adverse effect on the foetus and lead to problems. The estimated length of gestation and the birth weight of the baby should be recorded. Details of any intrapartum or perinatal problems should be recorded.

Dietary History

The duration of breastfeeding or the type of artificial feed and any weaning problems should be recorded. The dietary history can be of major importance in paediatric history taking. If the patient is neither thriving nor has vomiting, diarrhoea, constipation or anaemia, then the physician must obtain a detailed dietary history. The dietary history should include not only solid foods, but also the consumption of liquid foods and any other supplements such as vitamins. In this way, the quality of the diet and the quantity of nutrients can be assessed and compared to the recommended intake. Any discrepancy between the actual and recommended intake may have a possible bearing on the diagnosis.

Developmental History

Inquiries about the age at which major developmental milestones in infancy and early childhood were achieved are necessary when faced with an infant or child who is suspected of developmental delay. However, for a child who is doing well at school and whose physical and social activities are normal, less emphasis on the minutiae of development is needed. Some parents are vague about the time of developmental achievements, unless very recently acquired, but many have clear recall of the important events such as smiling, sitting and walking independently. It can be helpful to enquire whether this child's development paralleled to that of other children.

Family and Social History

The health and educational progress of a child is directly related to the home and the environment. Medical, financial and social stresses within the family sometimes have a direct or indirect bearing on the child's presenting problem. It is, therefore, essential to know about the housing conditions and some information of parental income and working hours, as well as the child's performance in school and adjustment to playmates.

The family history should be thoroughly evaluated. The age and health of the close relatives are important to record.

Height and weight of parents and siblings may be helpful, especially when dealing with children of short stature, obesity or failure to thrive, or an infant with an enlarged head. Consanguinity is common in some cultures, and offspring of consanguineous marriages have an increased chance of receiving the same recessive gene from each parent and thus developing a genetically determined disease. Therefore, it is important to draw a family tree and to identify children at high risk of genetic disease and to make appropriate referrals.

KEY LEARNING POINT

A history of recent travel abroad, particularly in tropical areas, is important as the child may have a disorder uncommon in his/her own country, but having been contracted in another country where the disease may be endemic.

PHYSICAL EXAMINATION

The physical examination of the paediatric patient requires a careful and gentle approach. It should be carried out in an appropriate environment with a selection of books or toys around, which can be used to allay the apprehension and anxiety of the child. More can be learned by careful inspection than by any other single examination method. The baby should be examined in a warm environment in good light. Nappies must be removed to examine the baby fully. The doctor must look first at the baby as a whole, noting specially the colour, posture and movements, and then should proceed to a more detailed examination starting at the head and working down to the feet ('top to toe').

It is important to realise that the child may be apprehensive with a stranger, especially when faced with the unfamiliar surroundings of a surgery or hospital outpatient department. It is essential that the doctor be truthful with the child regarding what is going to be done. The child should never be made to face sudden unexpected manoeuvres and should be allowed to play with objects such as the stethoscope. It may be useful to let him or her examine a toy animal or doll to facilitate gaining confidence. Infants and young children are often best examined on the mother's lap where they feel more secure. The doctor should ensure that his/her hands and instruments used to examine the child are suitably warmed. It is not always mandatory to remove all the child's clothes, although it is often essential in the examination of the acutely ill child. Procedures that may produce discomfort, such as examination of the throat, ears or rectum, should be left until towards the end of the examination. The order of the examination may be varied to suit the particular child's needs. Awareness of the normal variations at different ages is important.

A thorough physical examination is a powerful therapeutic tool, especially if the problem is one primarily of inappropriate parental anxiety. Understandably, parents do not usually accept reassurance if the doctor has not examined the child properly. Examination of the infant or child is often preceded by recording the patient's height, weight and head circumference on the growth chart. This may be done by a nurse before the doctor sees the family. These measurements are plotted on graphs or charts, which indicate the percentiles or standard deviations at the various ages throughout childhood. If these measurements are out with the 3rd to 97th centile for children of that sex and age, further study is indicated. If previous records of height, weight or head circumference are available for comparison with the current measurements, this may provide considerable help towards diagnosis and management. Inquiry of parental height, weight or head size may also be important, e.g. in familial macrocephaly or constitutional short stature.

KEY LEARNING POINT

Allow the child patient to see and touch the stethoscope, auriscope, ophthalmoscope and other tools, which are going to be used during examination. Ask the child which ear or which part of the body the child would like to be examined first. It is vital to use the reassuring voice throughout the examination of the child.

General Inspection

The general appearance of the child may suggest a particular syndrome. Does the child look like the rest of the family? The facies may be characteristic in Down syndrome and other chromosomal disorders or in mucopolysaccharidoses. Peculiar odours from an infant may provide a clue to diagnosis of aminoacidurias, such as maple syrup disease (maple syrup-like odour), phenylketonuria (mousy odour) and trimethylaminuria (fishy odour) **(Table 1.1)**. The statements by mothers about peculiar odours of the infants should be taken seriously, and in addition, the paediatrician will do well to take a deep sniff of each infant he/she examines. A more detailed examination should then be performed. The most valuable of the physician's senses are his/her eyes, as more can be learned by careful inspection and also on watching the patient's reactions than by any other single procedure.

Colour

The colour should be pink with the exception of the periphery, which may be slightly blue. Congenital heart disease is only suggested if the baby has central cyanosis. A pale baby may be anaemic or ill and requires careful investigation to find the cause. A blue baby may have either a cardiac anomaly or respiratory problems and rarely methaemoglobinaemia.

TABLE 1.1 Some diseases associated with an unusual odour.

Disease	*Characteristic odour*
Disorders of amino acid metabolism	
Phenylketonuria	In sweat and urine: musty, 'wolf-like' barny or like the odour of 'stale sweaty locker-room towels'
Maple syrup urine disease	In urine, sweat and earwax: 'caramel-like', 'malty', or like 'maple syrup'
Oasthouse syndrome	In urine: 'dried malt or hops'
Hypermethioninemia	In urine, sweat and breath: 'fishy', 'sweet and fruity', like 'rancid butter' or boiled cabbage'
Isovaleric acidaemia syndrome	The patient smells 'cheesy' or like 'sweaty feet'
Disorders of fatty acid metabolism	
Odour-sweaty-feet syndrome	The urine, sweat and breath: 'sweaty feet'

KEY LEARNING POINT

Central cyanosis: Central cyanosis in a child of any age should always raise the possibility of congenital heart disease. Ideally, the best areas to look for central cyanosis are the tongue and buccal mucosa, not the limbs and the nails.

Posture and Movements

A term baby lies supine for the first day or two and has vigorous, often asymmetric movements of all limbs. In contrast, a sick baby adopts the frog position with legs abducted and externally rotated and is inactive. Older infants and children should be observed for abnormal movements, posture and gait.

KEY LEARNING POINT

Always leave the most upsetting parts of the examination until the end, such as inspection of the throat or taking the blood pressure. If epiglottitis is a possibility, do not examine the throat because obstruction may be precipitated.

Skin

The skin is a major body organ which, because of the larger surface area in relationship to weight of the young, means that the skin is relatively more important in the immature. It forms a barrier against environmental attack, and its structure and function reflect the general health of the child, that is, in states of malnutrition and dehydration. The presence of any skin rash, its colour and whether there are macules, papules, vesicles, bullae, petechiae or pustules should be recorded (Table 1.2). The skin texture, elasticity, tone and subcutaneous thickness should be assessed by picking up the skin between the fingers. Pigmented naevi, strawberry naevi, haemangiomata or lymphangiomata may be present and may vary in size and number. They may be absent or small at birth and grow in subsequent days or weeks.

TABLE 1.2 Dermatological terminology.

Terminology	*Definition*
Macule	Area of discoloration, any size, not raised—flat with skin
Papule	Small raised lesion (<5 mm)
Petechiae	Haemorrhage in skin, nonblanching (<1 mm)
Purpura	Haemorrhage in skin, nonblanching (2–10 mm in diameter)
Ecchymoses	Large bruise, nonblanching
Vesicle	Small blister, elevated, fluid-filled (<5 mm)
Bullae	Large blister, elevated, fluid-filled (>5 mm)
Weal	Elevation in skin, due to acute oedema in dermis, surrounding erythematous macule
Pustule	Elevated, pus-filled
Lichenification	Thickened skin, normal lines in skin more apparent

KEY LEARNING POINT

Port-wine stain: Unilateral port-wine stain over the distribution of the ophthalmic division of the trigeminal nerve is usually a manifestation of Sturge–Weber syndrome. It may be associated with seizures, glaucoma, hemiparesis and mental retardation.

Head

The head should be inspected for size, shape and symmetry. Measurement of the head circumference [occipitofrontal circumference (OFC)] with a nonelastic tape by placing it to encircle the head just above the eyebrows around maximum protuberance of the occipital bone should be performed and charted. In the infant, the skull should be palpated to determine the size and tension in the fontanelles and assess the skull sutures (Fig. 1.1).

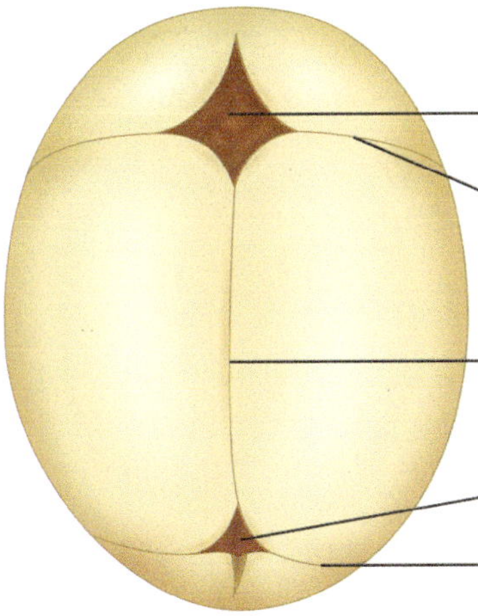

Figure 1.1 Top head anterior fontanelle and cranial sutures.

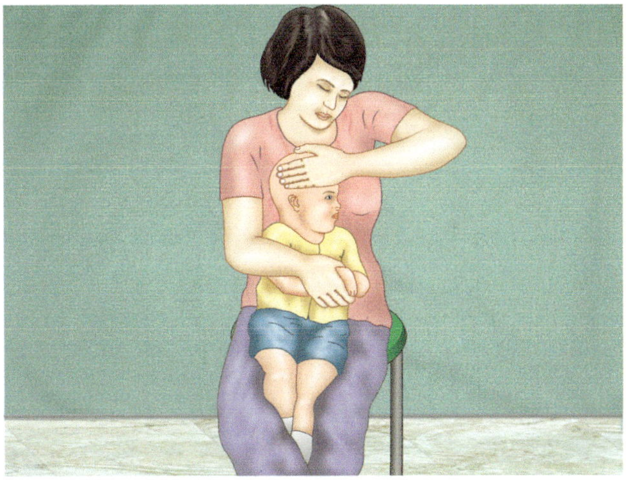

Figure 1.2 Method of restraining a child for examination of the ear.

Premature fusion of sutures suggests craniostenosis. In the neonate, the posterior fontanelle may be very small and subsequently closes by 3 months of age, but the anterior fontanelle is larger, only closing at around 18 months. A tense and bulging fontanelle suggests raised intracranial pressure and a deeply sunken one suggests dehydration.

Large fontanelles, separation of sutures and delayed closure of the fontanelles may be associated with raised intracranial pressure or other systemic disorders such as hypothyroidism and rickets.

> **KEY LEARNING POINT**
>
> Occipitofrontal circumference: An abnormally 'large head' [> 97th centile or 2 SD (standard deviation) above the mean] is due to macrocephaly, which may be due to hydrocephalus, subdural haematoma or inherited syndromes. Familial macrocephaly (autosomal dominant) is a benign familial condition with normal brain growth.

Ears

Position and configuration of the ears should be observed. While abnormalities such as low setting of the ears are frequently associated with renal tract anomalies, absence of an ear or nondevelopment of the auricle will require early referral to an otolaryngologist. It often requires the parent to hold the child on his/her lap and provide reassurance during the examination. Methods of doing this are illustrated in **Figure 1.2**. Parents are usually very competent in detecting hearing impairment. The exception to this is where the child has intellectual disability. All infants should be given a screening test for hearing at 6 months of age. Simple testing materials are required, e.g. a cup and spoon, high- and low-pitched rattles and devices to imitate bird or animal sounds, or even snapping of finger tips is usually effective if hearing is normal. The sounds should be made quietly at a distance of 2–3 feet out of view of the child. By 6 months of age, a child should be able to localise sound. To pass the screening test, the child should turn and look directly at the source of the sound.

> **KEY LEARNING POINT**
>
> Hearing deficit: A number of children with hearing deficits may not be diagnosed until they are 2 years of age. The main pointers to hearing deficits include parental concern about their child's hearing, speech delay and lack of developmental markers of hearing.

Eyes

These should be inspected for subconjunctival haemorrhages, which are usually of little importance, and also for cataracts, for papilloedema, and congenital abnormalities, such as colobomata **(Figs. 1.3A and B)**. 'Rocking' the baby from the supine to vertical position often results in the eyes opening, so they can be inspected. Squint is a condition in which early diagnosis and treatment is important. There are two simple tests which can be carried out to determine whether or not a squint is present.

The position of the 'corneal light reflection' should normally be in the centre of each pupil if the eyes are both aligned on a bright source of light, usually a pen torch. Should one eye be squinting, then the reflection of the light from the cornea will not be centred in the pupil of that eye. It will be displaced outwards if the eye is convergent and inwards towards the nose if the eye is divergent. It may be displaced by such a large amount that it is seen over the iris or even over the sclera, where of course it may be rather more difficult to identify, but with such obvious squints, the diagnosis is usually not in doubt.

In the 'cover test', one chooses an object of interest for the child, e.g. a brightly coloured toy with moving components. When the child is looking at the object of interest, the eye thought to be straight is covered with an opaque card and the uncovered eye is observed to see whether it

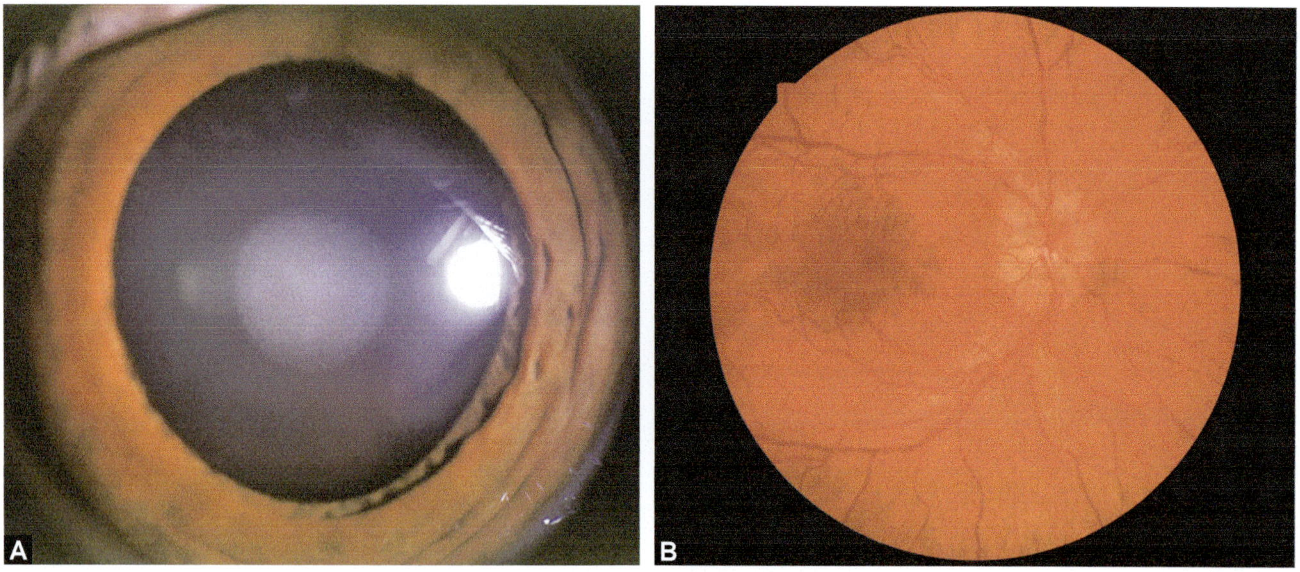

Figures 1.3A and B (A) Congenital cataract and (B) papilloedema.

moves to take up fixation on the object of interest. If the child has a convergent squint, then the eye will move laterally to take up fixation, and this is the usual situation, since convergent squints are four times more common than divergent squints. If the eye was divergent, it would move medially.

The most common cause for apparent blindness in young children is developmental delay. Assessment of whether a young baby can see is notoriously difficult; fixation should develop in the first week of life, but an early negative response is of no value, as the absence of convincing evidence of fixation is not synonymous with blindness. The failure to develop a fixation reflex results in ocular nystagmus, but these roving eye movements do not appear until the age of 3 months.

A misleading response may be obtained when a bright light stimulus is applied to a child, preferably in a dimly lit room. The normal response is a blinking or 'screwing up' the eyes, occasionally by withdrawing the head. This is a subcortical reflex response and may be present in babies, despite them having cortical blindness. The absence of this response increases the probability of blindness.

KEY LEARNING POINT

Distraction and play: If the doctor cannot distract the infant or make the awake 'infant' attend to an object or look at the paediatrician's face or a source of sound, consider a possible visual or hearing deficit.

Face

Abnormalities of facial development are usually obvious, and an example is the infant with cleft lip. Associated with this, there may be a cleft palate, but full visual examination of the palate including the uvula is necessary to ensure that the palate is intact and there is no submucous cleft of the soft palate or a posterior cleft. Submucous and soft palate clefts cannot be felt on palpation.

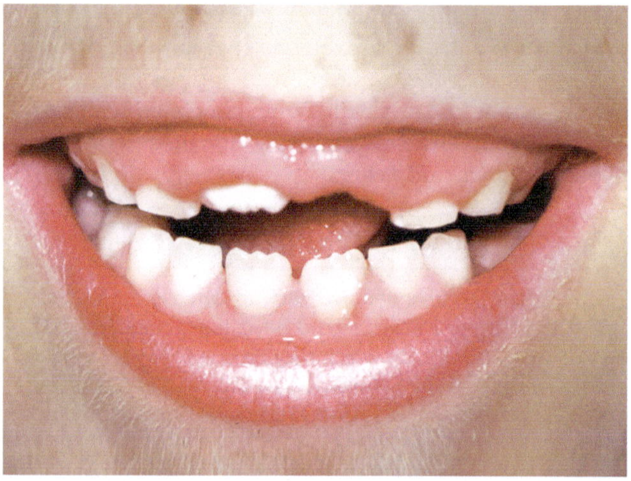

Figure 1.4 Gingival hyperplasia caused by phenytoin.

Mouth

Inspection of the mouth should include visualisation of the palate, fauces, gum disease and the dentition **(Fig. 1.4)**. A cleft lip is obvious, but the palate must be visualised to exclude a cleft. The mouth is best opened by pressing down in the middle of the lower jaw. A baby is rarely born with teeth, but if present, these are almost always the lower central incisors. The soft palate should be inspected to exclude the possibility of a submucous cleft, which could be suggested by a bifid uvula. Small fibromata are sometimes seen in the gums. They are white and seldom require treatment. These are normal. The lower jaw should be seen in profile, as a receding chin (micrognathia) may be the cause of tongue swallowing or glossoptosis (Pierre Robin syndrome) and it may be associated with a cleft palate.

Neck

Examination of the neck may reveal congenital goitre, midline cysts, which may be thyroglossal or dermoid in origin, or lateral cysts, which may be of branchial origin, or sometimes, there may be extensive swellings, which may be cystic hygroma or lymphangiomata. In early infancy, a sternomastoid tumour may be palpable in the midregion of the sternomastoid muscle. Associated with this, there may be significant limitation of rotation and lateral flexion of the neck. Palpation along the clavicle will define any tenderness or swelling suggestive of recent or older fractures.

Chest

The shape, chest wall movement and the nature and rate of the breathing (30–40 per minute) as well as the presence of any indrawing of the sternum and rib cage should be noted. In a normal baby without respiratory or abdominal problems, the abdomen moves freely during breathing and there is very little chest movement. Most of the movements of the breathing cycle are carried out by the movement of the diaphragm. The nipples and axillary folds should be assessed to exclude conditions such as absent pectoral muscle. In Poland syndrome, there is amastia, associated with ipsilateral absence of sternal head of pectoralis major. Ten percent may have dextrocardia, dextroversion or syndactyly. Anterior chest wall deformities, such as pectus excavatum (funnel chest) and pectus carinatum (pigeon chest), should be recorded (Fig. 1.5).

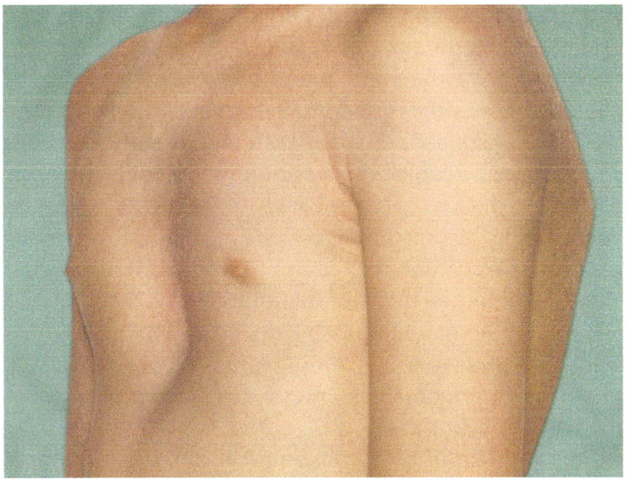

Figure 1.5 Pectus excavatum (funnel chest).

Cardiovascular

Examination of the cardiovascular system of infants and children is carried out in a similar manner to that of adults. The examiner should always feel for femoral pulses and ascertain whether there is any radiofemoral or brachiofemoral delay, as this would suggest the possibility of coarctation of the aorta. The most important factor in recording the blood pressure of children is to use a cuff of the correct size. The cuff should cover at least two-thirds of the upper arm. If the cuff size is less than this, a falsely high blood pressure reading may be obtained. In small infants, relatively accurate systolic and diastolic pressures as well as mean arterial pressure can be obtained by use of the Doppler method. The apex should be visible and palpable and the position noted. The precordial areas should be palpated for the presence of thrills. If the apex beat is not obvious, look for it on the right side of the chest as there could be dextrocardia or a left-sided congenital diaphragmatic hernia with the heart pushed to the right or collapse of the right lung. All areas should be auscultated while the baby is quiet; systolic murmurs may be very harsh and can be confused with breath sounds.

Lungs

Small children frequently cry when the chest is percussed and when a cold stethoscope is applied. If the mother holds the child over her shoulder and soothes him/her, it is often easier to perform a thorough chest examination. Light percussion can be more valuable than auscultation in some situations, but the basic signs are similar to those found in an adult. Breath sounds are usually harsh, high-pitched and rapid. Any adventitious sounds present are pathological. Percussion of the chest may be helpful to pick up the presence of a pleural effusion (stony dull), collapse, consolidation of a lung (dull) or a pneumothorax (hyperresonant). These pathological states are usually associated with an increase in the respiratory rate as well as clinical signs of respiratory distress.

Abdomen

In the infant, the abdomen and umbilicus are inspected and attention should be paid to the presence of either a scaphoid abdomen, which in a neonate may be one of the signs of diaphragmatic hernia or duodenal atresia or a distended abdomen, which suggests intestinal obstruction, especially if visible peristalsis can be seen. Peristalsis from left to right suggests a high intestinal obstruction, whereas the one from the right to the left would be more in keeping with low intestinal obstruction. Any asymmetry of the abdomen may indicate the presence of an underlying mass. Abdominal movement should be assessed and abdominal palpation should be performed with warm hands.

Palpation of the abdomen should include palpation for the liver, the edge of which is normally felt in the newborn baby; the spleen, which can only be felt if it is pathological; and the kidneys, which can be felt in the first 24 hours with the fingers and thumb palpating in the renal angle and abdomen on each side. The lower abdomen should be palpated for the bladder and an enlargement can be confirmed by percussion from a resonant zone, progressing to a dull zone. In the baby with abdominal distension where there is suspicion of perforation and free gas in the abdomen, the loss of superficial liver dullness on percussion may be the only physical sign present early on. Areas of tenderness can be elicited by watching the baby's reaction to gentle palpation of the abdomen. There may be areas of erythema, cellulitis and oedema of the abdominal wall, and on deeper palpation, crepitus can occasionally be felt from pneumatosis intestinalis (intramural gas in the wall of the bowel).

Auscultation of the abdomen in the younger patients gives rather different signs than in the adult. The infant even in the presence of peritonitis may have some bowel sounds present. However, in the presence of ileus or peritonitis, breath sounds become conducted down over the abdomen to the suprapubic area, and in even more severe disorders, the heart sounds similarly can be heard extending down over the abdomen to the suprapubic area.

Perineal examination is important in both sexes. Examination of the anus should never be omitted. Occasionally, the anus is ectopic (e.g., placed more anteriorly than it should be), stenotic or even absent. The rectal examination is an invasive procedure and should be carried out in a comfortable warm environment, preferably with the child in the left lateral position and the mother holding the hand of the child at the top end of the bed.

The testes in boys born at term should be in the scrotum. The prepuce cannot be and should not be retracted. The prepuce can be retracted after several months or years, and stretching is both harmful and unnecessary. In girls, the labia should be separated and genitalia examined.

The presence of a swelling in the scrotum or high in the groin may suggest torsion of a testis and requires urgent attention. The testis that cannot be palpated in the scrotum and cannot be manipulated into the sac indicates the presence of an undescended testis, which needs to be explored and corrected before the age of 2 years. A swelling in the scrotum which has a bluish hue to it suggests the presence of a hydrocele due to a patent processus vaginalis and one can get above such a swelling in most children. Palpation of the scrotum is initially for testes, but if gonads are not present, then palpation in the inguinal, femoral and perineal regions to determine presence of undescended or ectopic testes should be carried out.

Conditions such as hypospadias, epispadias, labial adhesions or imperforate hymen or ambiguous genitalia should be diagnosed on inspection (Fig. 1.6).

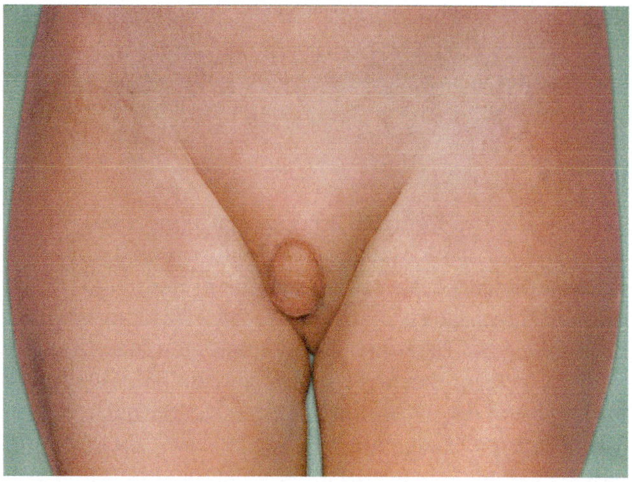

Figure 1.6 Ambiguous genitalia in a 10-year-old girl (clitromegaly, labial fusion and empty scrotal folds of virilised female).

Limbs

Upper and lower limbs are examined in detail. Hands and feet should be examined for signs, and those experienced in dermatoglyphics may define a finger print pattern that is consistent in various syndromes. The presence of a simian palmar crease may suggest trisomy 21 (Down syndrome) and thumb clenching may suggest neurological disease. The feet, ankles and knees should be examined for the range of movement in the joints and tone of the muscles. The femoral head may be outside the acetabulum at birth in true dislocation of the hip or it may be dislocated over the posterior lip of the acetabulum by manipulation, in which case the hip is described as unstable, dislocatable or lax. There are conditions in which the acetabulum is hypoplastic and shallow and the femoral head itself is distorted. Congenital dislocation of the hip is more common after breech deliveries in girls and in certain parts of the world. All newborn infants should be screened shortly after birth. The infant is placed supine with the legs towards the examiner and each hip is examined separately. The knee and hip of the baby are flexed to 90% and the hip fully abducted by placing the middle finger over the greater trochanter and the thumb on the inner side of the thigh opposite to the position of the lesser trochanter. When the thigh is in the midabducted position, forward pressure is exerted behind the greater trochanter by the middle finger. The other hand holds the opposite femur and pelvis steady. A dislocated femoral head is felt to slip over the acetabular ridge and back into the acetabulum as a definite movement. This part of the test is called the Ortolani manoeuvre. The second part of the test is the Barlow procedure. With the infant still on his back and the legs and hands in the same position, the hip is brought into the position of midabduction with the thumb exerting gentle pressure laterally and posteriorly; at the same time, the palm exerts posterior and medial pressure. If a hip is dislocatable, the femur can be felt to dislocate over the posterior lip of the acetabulum. There is need for caution in performing this test and no force should be employed. Caution is particularly required in infants born with neural tube defects and paralysis of the lower limbs.

Dorsiflexion of the feet should allow the lateral border to come in contact with the peroneal compartment of the leg. Failure indicates a degree of talipes equinovarus, which is of concern to the parents, although, with simple physiotherapy, there are seldom long-term problems in the absence of underlying neurological abnormality.

Spine

With the baby held face downwards, fingers should be run along the spine excluding spinal defects, such as spina bifida occulta, and noting the presence of the common postanal dimple, a tuft of hair, a pad of fat, and haemangioma. A Mongolian blue spot is commonly seen over the sacrum in Asian babies. The presence of a posterior coccygeal dimple or a sacral pit is common in babies and is due to tethering of the skin to the coccyx. When one stretches the skin and the base of the pit can be seen, then nothing needs to be done about it. Very rarely, there is communication with the spinal canal, which could be the source of infection and cause meningitis.

Stool and Urine Examination

Examination of a stool which is preferably fresh is often informative. The colour, consistency and smell are noted as well as the presence of blood or mucus. Urine examination is also important in children, since symptoms related to the urinary tract may be nonspecific.

Neurological Examination

The neurological examination of the young infant and child is different from that routinely carried out in the adult. Muscle tone and strength are important parts of the examination. In infants, muscle tone may be influenced by the child's state of relaxation. An agitated hungry infant may appear to be hypertonic, but when examined in a cheerful postprandial state, the tone reverts to being normal. The examination of the neurological system cannot be complete without the evaluation of the child's development level relating to gross motor, fine motor and vision, hearing and speech and social skills. All older children should be observed for gait to detect abnormal coordination and balance.

Older children may be tested for sense of touch and proprioception as in adults. Tests of sensation as well as motor power must be performed in the paediatric patient, but are difficult to assess in the very young child. The normal newborn has a large number of primitive reflexes (Moro, asymmetric tonic neck, glabellar tap, sucking and rooting process). The 'Moro reflex' is a mass reflex, which is present in the early weeks after birth. Its absence suggests cerebral damage. It consists of throwing out of the arms followed by bringing them together in an embracing movement. It can be demonstrated by making a loud noise near the child. The 'sucking reflex' is present at birth in the normal baby as is the 'swallowing reflex'. If the angle of the baby's mouth is touched by the finger or teat, the baby will turn his head towards it and search for it. It is looking for its mother's nipple and is known as the 'rooting or searching reflex'.

The grasp reflex is illustrated by gently stroking the back of the hand so that the fingers extend, and on placing a finger on the palm of the baby, it takes a firm grip. Similar reflexes are present in the toes. If the baby is held up under the arms so that his/her feet are touching a firm surface, he/she will raise one leg and hesitatingly put it down in front of the other leg, taking giant strides forwards. This is the 'primitive walking reflex'.

Tendon reflexes, such as the biceps and knee jerks, are easily obtainable but the ankle and triceps jerks are not readily elicited. Important as an indication of nervous system malfunction are muscle tone, posture, movement and the primitive reflexes of the newborn that have been described. Plantar reflex is usually extensor and is of little diagnostic importance in the first year. Delay in disappearance of the primitive reflexes suggests cerebral damage.

A GUIDE TO EXAMINATION OF A CHILD PATIENT

Checklist of Bodily Systems

General Examination

- Is the child unwell, breathless or distressed?
- Level of consciousness
- Is the child cyanosed, pale or jaundiced? (In carotenaemia, the sclerae are not yellow.)
- ENT examination: child's ears, nose and throat
- Is the child dehydrated? Skin turgor, sunken eyes, sunken fontanelle
- Nutritional state
- Peripheral perfusion: capillary refill time should occur within 2 seconds
- Does the child have any dysmorphic features, that is, an obvious syndrome?
- Check blood pressure, temperature and pulses, that is, radial and femoral
- Hands: for clubbing (look at all fingers), peripheral cyanosis, absent nails (ectodermal dysplasia), pitted nails (psoriasis), splinter haemorrhages **(Fig. 1.7)**
- Height, weight and head circumference (OFC): plot these on a percentile chart
- Rash: generalised or localised, bruises, petechiae, purpura, birth marks (learn dermatological terminology; **Table 1.1**)
- Abnormal pigmentation: café au lait spots, Mongolian blue spots, elasticity of skin and hypermobility of joints **(Figs. 1.8A and B)**
- Palpate for lymph nodes in the neck (from behind), axillare and groins
- Teeth: any dental caries, a torn lip frenulum (physical abuse)

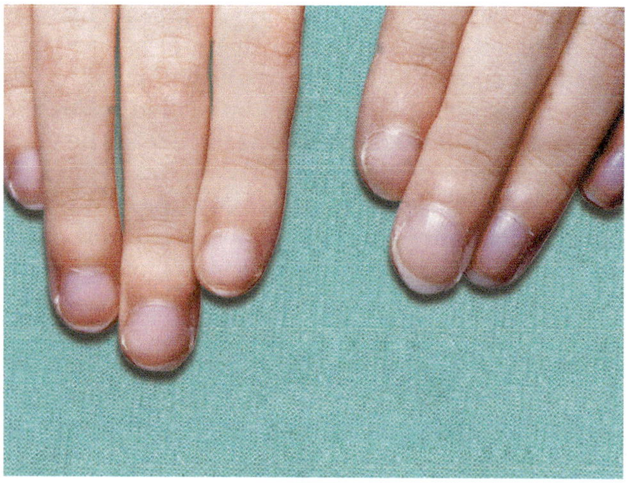

Figure 1.7 Finger clubbing in cystic fibrosis.

- Genitalia: injuries to genitalia or anus—sexual abuse
- Head shape: normal, small (microcephaly), large (macrocephaly), plagiocephaly, brachycephaly, oxycephaly (turricephaly). Feel the sutures. Is there evidence of craniostenosis?
- Hair: alopecia, seborrhoea of the scalp
- Eyes: subconjunctival haemorrhage, ptosis, proptosis, squint, nystagmus, cataract, aniridia, optic fundi
- Mouth: thrush, fauces, tonsils, teeth, palate
- Ears: normal, low-set, shape, preauricular skin tags
- Anterior fontanelle: diamond-shaped, open, closed, sunken, bulging, tense
- Head circumference: measure the child's OFC and plot it on a growth chart (if not done under general examination)

Neck

- Short, webbed (Turner syndrome), torticollis
- Thyroid: enlarged, bruit
- Swellings
- Midline: thyroglossal cyst, goitre **(Figs. 1.9A and B)**
- Lateral: lymph nodes, branchial cyst, cystic hygroma, sternomastoid tumour

Respiratory System

Inspection

- Use of accessory muscles of respiration
- Intercostal recession, any stridor, audible wheeze
- Shape: normal, pectus carinatum (undue prominence of the sternum—pigeon chest), pectus excavatum (funnel chest), Harrison sulci, hyperinflation (increased anteroposterior diameter)
- Count the respiratory rate
- Scars of past surgery (look at the front and the back of the chest)

Palpation

- Chest wall movement: is it symmetrical?
- Feel the trachea: central or deviated
- Tactile vocal fremitus (over 5 years of age—ask the child to say 99)

Percussion

- Percuss all areas: normal, resonant, hyperresonant, dull (collapse, consolidation), stony dull (pleural effusion)

Auscultation

- Air entry, vesicular (normal), absent breath sounds (pleural effusion) and bronchial (consolidation)
- Added sounds: wheeze, inspiratory or expiratory, crackles (fine vs. coarse), pleural friction rub
- Vocal resonance

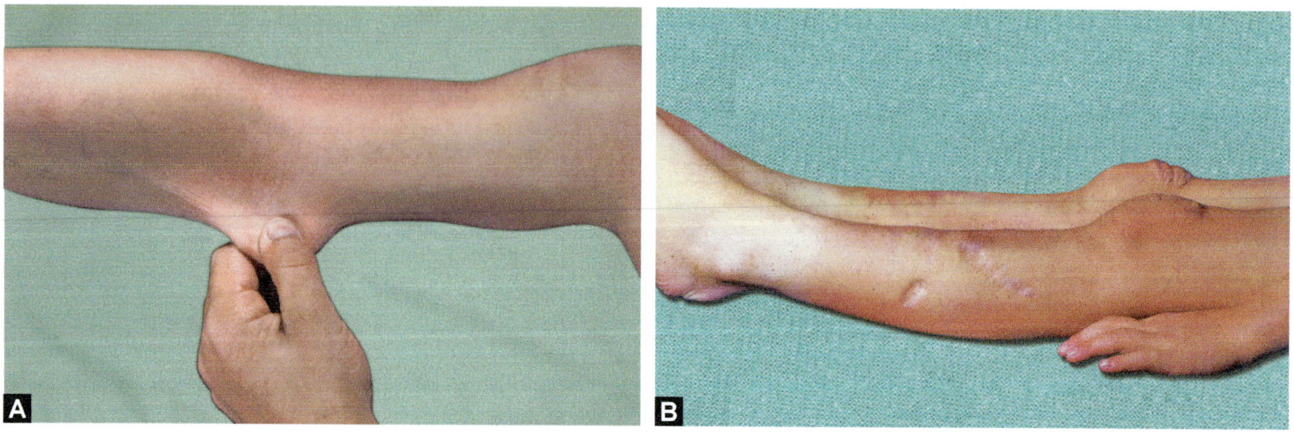

Figures 1.8A and B (A) Hyperextensible skin and (B) genu recurvatum in Ehlers–Danlos syndrome.

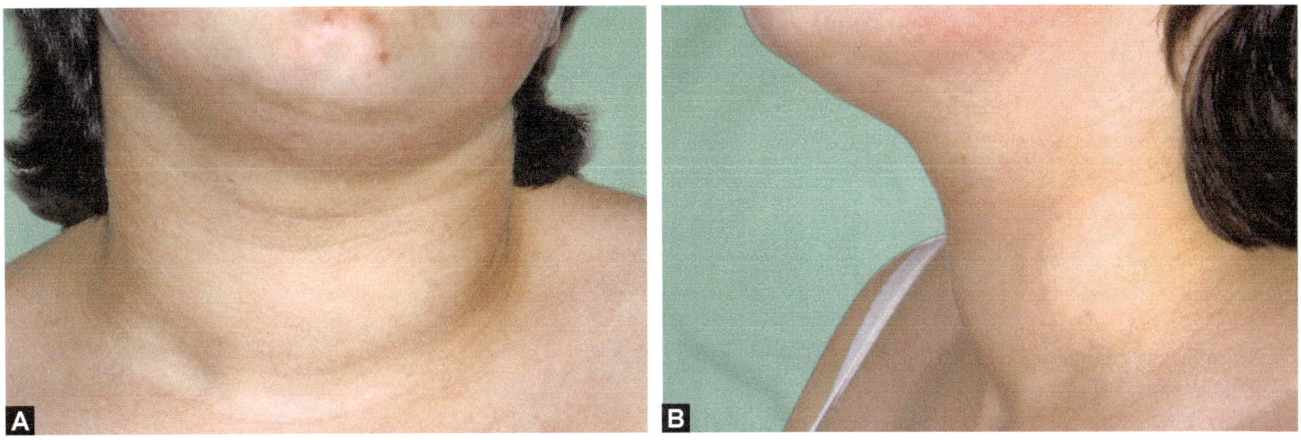

Figures 1.9A and B Goitre in Hashimoto's thyroiditis: (A) anteroposterior neck and (B) lateral view neck.

Cardiovascular System

Inspection

- Are there features of Down [atrial septal defect (ASD) and ventricular septal defect (VSD)], Turner (coarctation of the aorta) or Marfan (aortic incompetence) syndrome?
- Cyanosis: peripheral and central
- Hands: clubbing and splinter haemorrhages (endocarditis)
- Oedema: precordium, ankles and sacrum
- Precordium for scars of past surgery

Palpation

- Pulses: radial/brachial/femoral—radiofemoral delay (synchrony of the two pulses), rate
- Character of pulse: collapsing, volume
- Heart rate: rhythm
- Apex beat: position (normal position in children, fourth to fifth left intercostal space in the midclavicular line), beware of dextrocardia
- Palpate for a parasternal heave and for precordial thrills

Percussion

Percussion of the heart is not normally undertaken in children.

Auscultation

- Listen to all four valve areas (apex, lower L sternal edge, upper L sternal edge and upper R sternal edge)
- Quality of heart sounds
- Additional sounds, that is, clicks, murmur (timing of the murmur)
- Blood pressure: use a cuff that covers at least two-thirds of the upper arm or use Doppler

Gastrointestinal System

Inspection

- General distension
- Superficial veins: direction of flow, striae, umbilicus
- Masses, scars, visible peristalsis

Palpation and Percussion

- First, lightly palpate the entire abdomen; keep looking at the child's face all the time
- Localised tenderness, rebound tenderness and rigidity
- Masses
- Ascites: percuss for the shifting dullness
- Spleen, liver and kidneys
- Hernial orifices
- Genitalia (testes) and anus (site)

Auscultation

- *Bowel sounds:* absence implies ileus

Nervous System

- Level of consciousness
- Right or left handed
- Orientation, memory (past and present)
- Speech
- Posture

Cranial Nerves

I	Smell ability of each nostril to different smells
II	Visual acuity, visual fields, pupils (size, shape, reaction to light and consensual); fundoscopy: papilloedema, optic atrophy, cataract

III	Palsy: unilateral ptosis, fixed dilated pupil, eye down and out
IV	Palsy: diplopia on looking down and away from the affected side
V	Palsy: motor-jaw deviates to the side of lesion
	Sensory: corneal reflex lost
VI	Palsy: convergent squint
VII	Facial nerve lesions: weakness

Only the lower two-thirds are affected in upper motor neuron lesions, but all of one side of the face is affected in lower motor neuron lesions. Ask the child to screw-up eyes, raise eyebrows, blow out cheeks and show teeth.

VIII	Hearing, balance and posture
IX and X	Gag reflex: look at palatal movement
XI	Trapezii: shrug your shoulders
XII	Tongue movement: deviates to the side of lesion

Cerebellar Function

- Jerk nystagmus (worse on gaze away from midline)
- Truncal ataxia (if worse when eyes closed, then lesion is of dorsal columns; not cerebellum)
- Intention tremor: ask the child to pick up a small object and watch for tremor
- Past pointing: ask the child to cover one eye with one hand and with the index finger of the other hand ask him to touch his nose and then touch your finger
- Gait: ask the child to walk normally and then walk heel-to-toe, look for ataxic gait

Locomotor System

Arms

- Tone, muscle bulk, muscle power: oppose each movement
- Joints: hands swollen/tender metacarpophalangeal/proximal interphalangeal joints, test joints for hypermobility
- Reflexes: biceps (C5, C6) and triceps (C7, C8)—compare both sides
- Hand: ask child to squeeze fingers or spread fingers
- Coordination: finger-nose touching
- Sensation: test light touch

Legs

- Tone, quadriceps or gastrocnemius bulk
- Power: oppose each movement
- Coordination: rub heel up and down shin ('heel-shin test')
- Joints: swollen, tender, patella tap test (effusion in knee)
- Reflexes: knee (L3, L4), ankle (S1, S2), plantar reflex—the plantar is normally up-going in infants until they begin to walk
- Feet: any deformity in arches high or low

Sensation

- Joint position sense
- Fine touch discrimination

Gait

- Ask the child to walk normally across the room

Gower Sign

Ask the child to stand from supine. A child will normally sit up from lying, and then stand. In Duchenne muscular dystrophy, the child will have to roll over onto their front and then climb up their legs.

DEVELOPMENTAL ASSESSMENT

This should be carried out under four headings: (1) gross motor, (2) fine motor and vision, (3) hearing and (4) speech and social behaviour. These milestones are based for a child who is aged 6 weeks to 5 years.

Birth to 6 Weeks

Gross Motor

- Marked head lag at birth on pulling to sit. By 6 weeks, moderate head lag on pull to sit prone, brings chin momentarily off couch

KEY LEARNING POINT

Delayed walking could be due to the fact that the child is a bottom shuffler. There is a family history of bottom shuffling. It is autosomal dominant in inheritance. Rest of the developmental milestones is within the normal range.

Fine Motor and Vision

- Can see at birth
- By 6 weeks, can fix and follow across to 90°

Hearing and Speech

- Can hear at birth
- Startles and becomes quiet to a soothing voice

Social Behaviour

- Stops crying when picked up
- By 6 weeks, smiling to familiar noises and faces

Three to Six Months

Gross Motor

- By 3 months, on ventral suspension brings head above level of back
- Prone lifts head and upper chest off couch
- By 6 months, sits with support or tripod sits
- Beginning to weight bear. Rises to stand when supported

Fine Motor and Vision

- By 3 months, holds hands loosely open and has hand regard
- By 6 months, reaches for toys with palmar grasp
- Transfers hand-to-hand and hand-to-mouth

Hearing and Speech

- Can laugh, gurgle and coo
- Starts to babble around 6 months. Will turn when called

Social Behaviour

- Holds on to bottle or feeding cup when fed
- Frolics when played with
- Examines and plays with hands and places feet in mouth

Six to Nine Months

Gross Motor

- By 6 months can roll from front to back
- Sits unsupported with a straight back
- Begins to pivot around on arms and legs into the crawling position

Fine Motor and Vision

- Small objects picked up between index finger and thumb in a pincer grasp
- Transfers from hand-to-hand

Hearing and Speech

- By 9 months, shouts to gain attention
- Vocalises nonspecific syllables such as 'dada' and 'mama'

Social Behaviour

- Turns when talked to
- Resists when objects taken away
- Tries to reach for objects out of reach
- Likes to feed with fingers

Nine to Twelve Months

Gross Motor

- By 9–10 months, most infants are crawling
- Around 10% of normal infants never crawl, but move around by rolling, padding or bottom shuffling. These children are often late walkers and may not walk alone until 2 years of age
- By 9–12 months, begins to pull to standing and cruise

Fine Motor and Vision

- Will bang two cubes together
- Looks for fallen objects

Hearing and Speech

- By 9–12 months, usually have one or two recognisable words in addition to 'mama' and 'dada'

Social Behaviour

- Enjoys imitative games, such as clapping hands and waving goodbye
- Shy with strangers until the end of the first year

Twelve to Eighteen Months

Gross Motor

- By 12 months, can walk with hands held and begins to stand alone
- By 18 months, climbs onto chair and upstairs. Holds on to toys while walking

Fine Motor and Vision

- Pincer grip refined. Tiny objects can be picked up delicately
- Points at objects with index finger
- Can be persuaded to give objects to another on request
- Builds a tower of two or three bricks

Hearing and Speech

- Vocabulary of several words
- Comprehension is more advanced than speech at this age
- Enjoys looking at pictures on a book and points and babbles while doing this

Social Behaviour

- By 12 months indicates, wants, usually by pointing
- Drinks from a cup and helps to feed themselves
- Begins to help with dressing
- Learns to throw
- Enjoys simple games such as peekaboo

Two Years

Gross Motor

- Can walk, run, squat and climb stairs 2 feet per step

Fine Motor and Vision

- Builds tower of six or seven cubes
- Spontaneous scribbling
- Hand preference
- Holds pencil with thumb and first two fingers
- Imitates vertical lines

Hearing and Speech

- Uses 50 or more recognisable words and understands many more
- Forms simple sentences
- Carry out simple instructions

Social Behaviour

- Feeds with a spoon, drinks from a cup
- Usually dry through day (variable)
- Demands mother's attention
- Tantrums when frustrated
- Instant gratification

Three Years

Gross Motor

- Climbs stairs 1 foot per step
- Pedals a tricycle
- Kicks a ball

Fine Motor and Vision

- Copies a circle, imitates a cross
- Builds a tower of nine cubes
- Threads beads

Hearing and Speech

- Speaks in sentences and may know a few colours
- Recites nursery rhymes
- Counts to 10

Social Behaviour

- Eats with fork and spoon
- Dry through night
- Likes to help in adult activities
- Vivid imaginary play
- Joins in play with others

Four Years

Gross Motor

- Walks up and down stairs, one foot per step
- May hop

Fine Motor and Vision

- Copies cross
- Draws a man with head, legs and trunks
- Picks up very small objects and threads beads
- Knows four primary colours

Hearing and Speech

- Intelligible speech
- Knows name, address and usually age
- Listens to and tells stories
- Enjoys jokes

Social Behaviour

- May wash, dress, undress, but not yet manage laces
- Understand taking turns, as well as sharing
- Appreciates past, present and future time

Five Years

Gross Motor

- Catches a ball

Fine Motor and Vision

- Draws triangle and detailed man

Hearing and Speech

- Clear speech

Social Behaviour

- Comforts others
- Group play

Primitive Reflexes

- Rooting reflex: appears at birth, disappears at 4 months
- Palmar/plantar reflex: appears at birth, disappears at 4 months
- Stepping reflex: appears at birth, disappears at 4 months
- Moro reflex: appears at birth, disappears at 4 months
- Tonic neck reflex: appears at 1 month, disappears at 6 months
- Delay in disappearance of the primitive reflexes suggests cerebral damage

ADDITIONAL ILLUSTRATIONS

Illustrations of some conditions of the face, the neck, the chest, the back, the skin, the genitalia, the limb and the placenta are shown below **(Figs. 1.10 to 1.65)**.

FACE

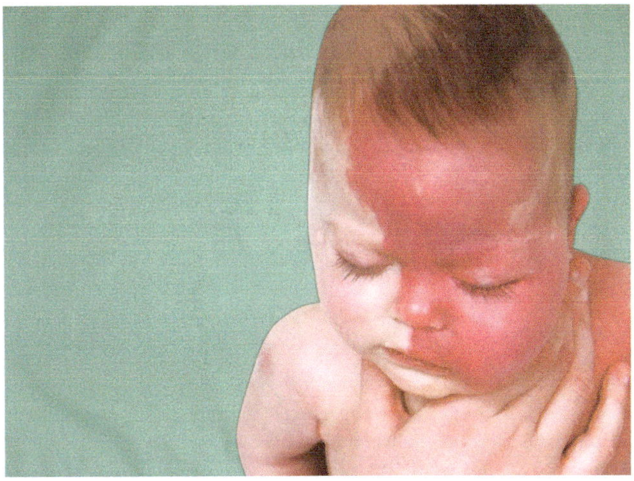

Figure 1.10 Sturge–Weber syndrome: port-wine stain.

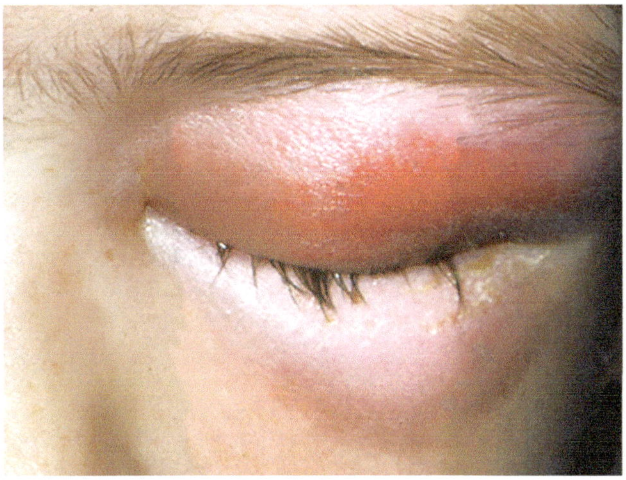

Figure 1.11 Orbital cellulitis.

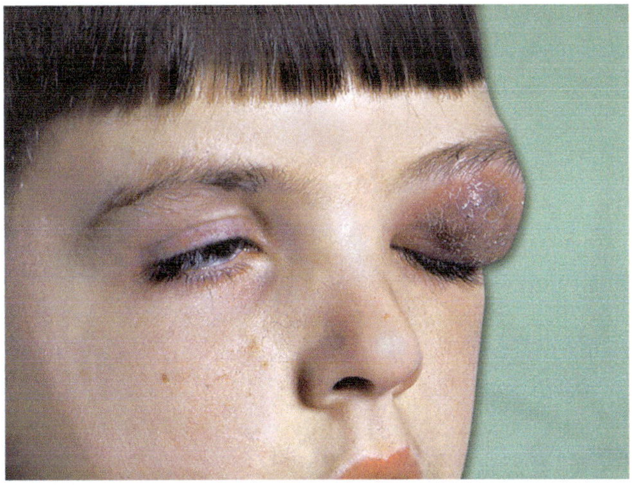

Figure 1.12 Langerhans cell histiocytosis (eosinophilic granuloma): orbital disease showing marked proptosis.

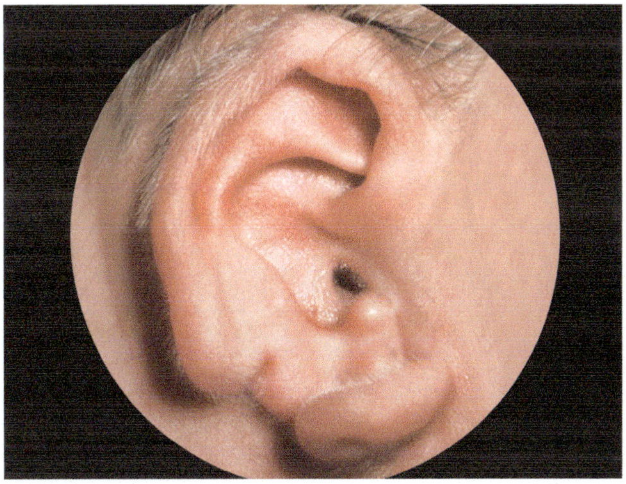

Figure 1.13 Malformed auricle.

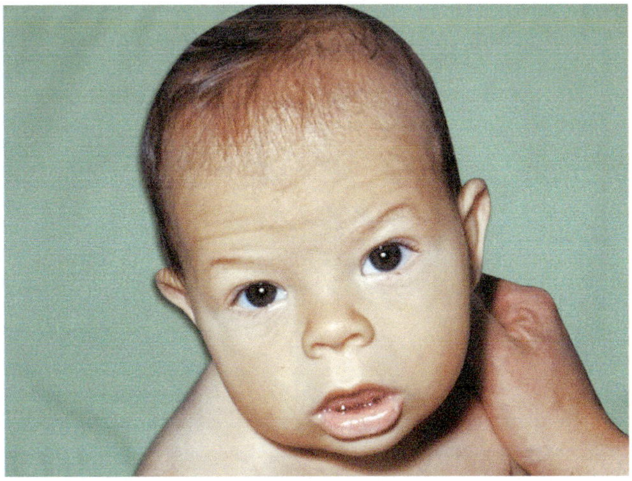

Figure 1.14 Congenital hypothyroidism.

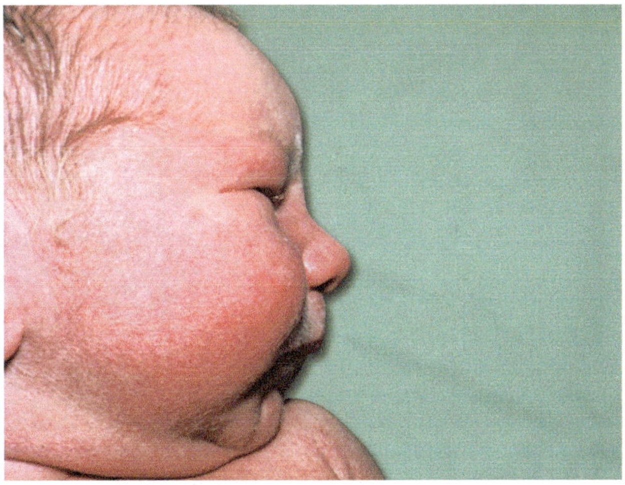

Figure 1.15 Pierre Robin syndrome. note micrognathia.

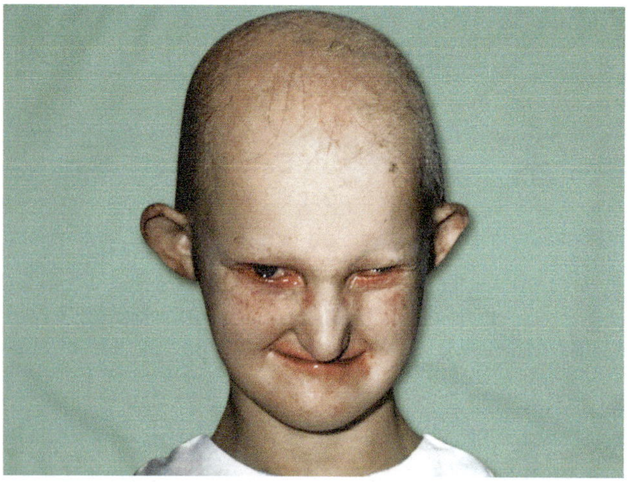

Figure 1.16 Ectodermal dysplasia: hypohidrotic ectodermal dysplasia is characterised by pointed ears, fine hair, periorbital hyperpigmentation and midfacial hypoplasia.

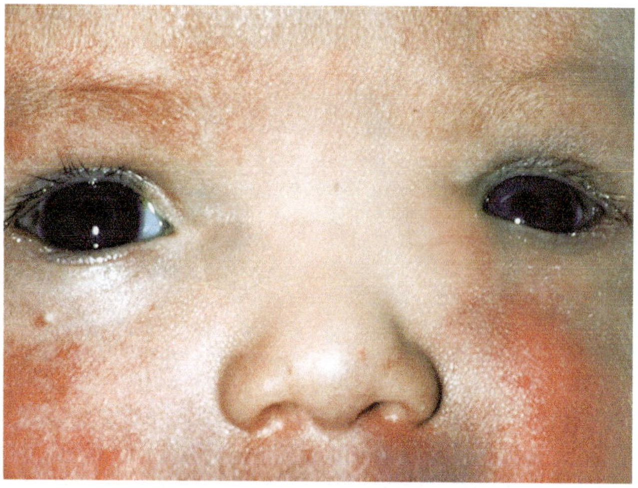

Figure 1.17 Dacryocystitis: an infection of the lacrimal sac. *Note* redness and swelling over the region of the left lacrimal sac.

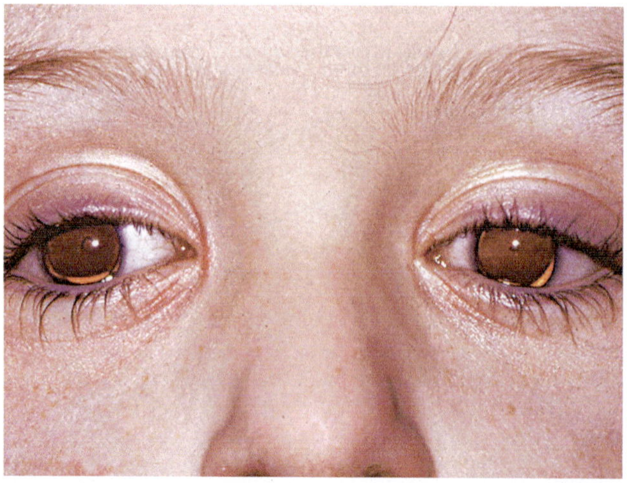

Figure 1.18 Aniridia: sporadic aniridia is associated with Wilms' tumour.

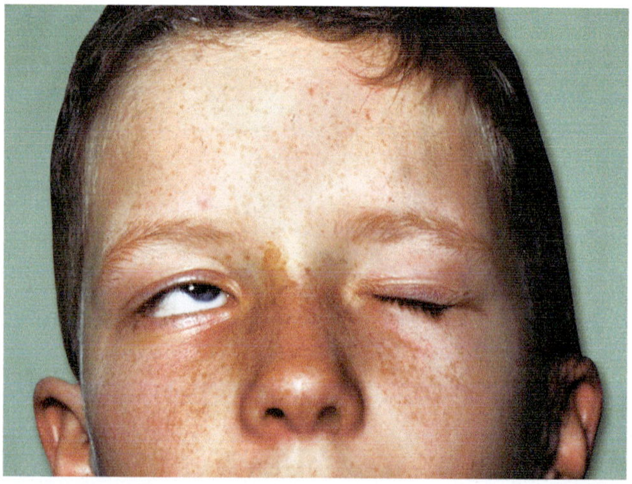

Figure 1.19 Bell palsy (right), eyes closed.

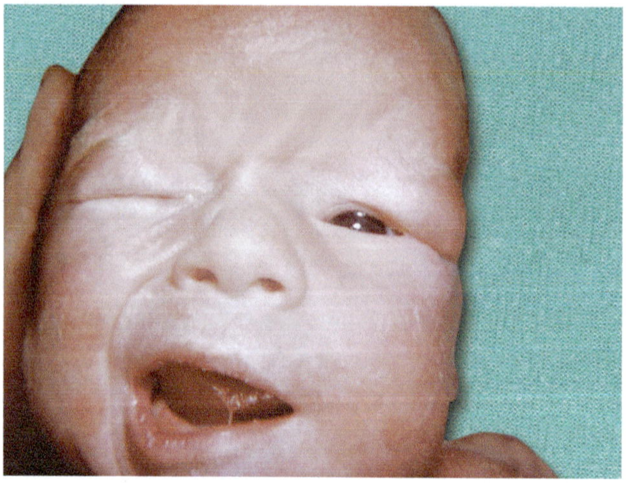

Figure 1.20 Facial palsy (left).

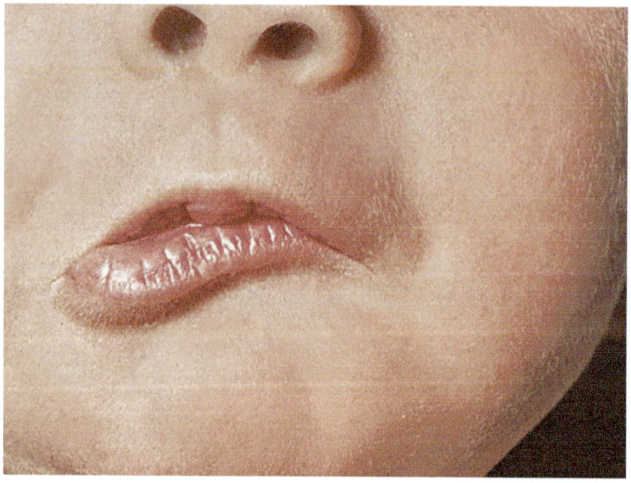

Figure 1.21 Depressor anguli oris muscle hypoplasia should not be confused with facial palsy.

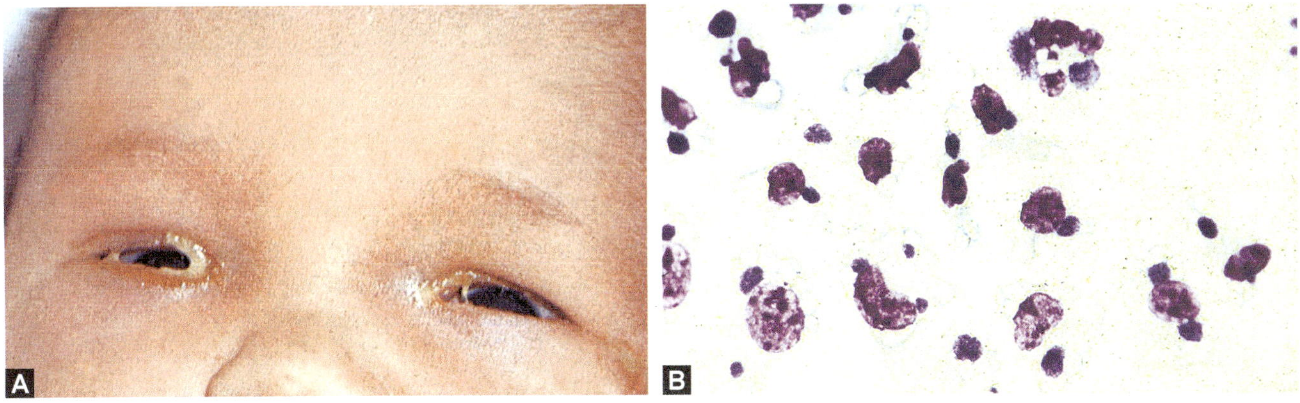

Figures 1.22A and B (A) Neonatal chlamydial conjunctivitis and (B) *Chlamydia trachomatis*, epithelial cells with semilunar inclusion bodies (Giemsa stain).

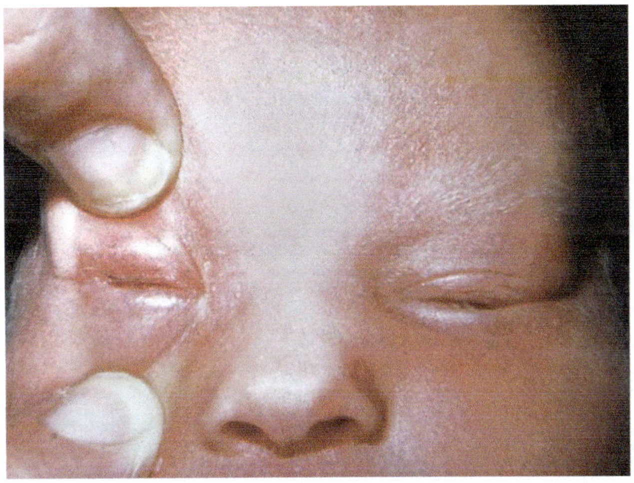

Figure 1.23 Microphthalmia.

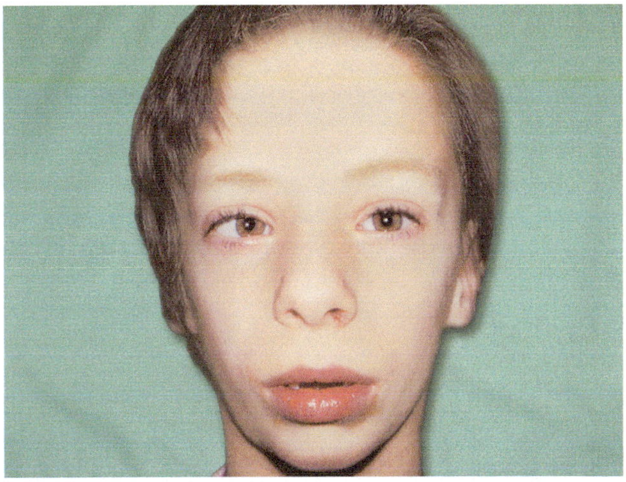

Figure 1.24 Partial lipodystrophy. *Note* the loss of fat from the face.

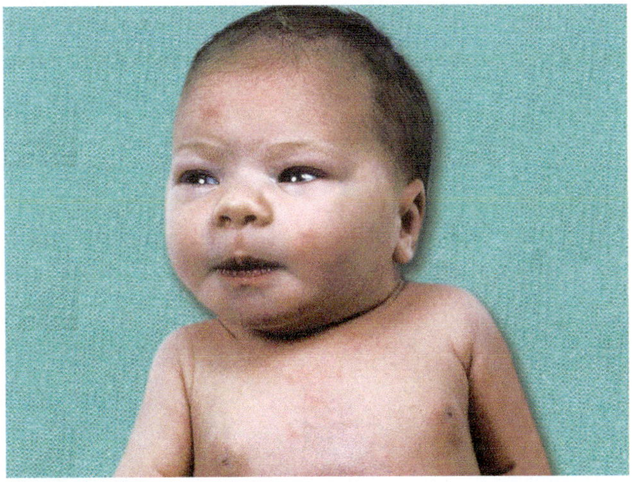

Figure 1.25 A cyanosed infant.

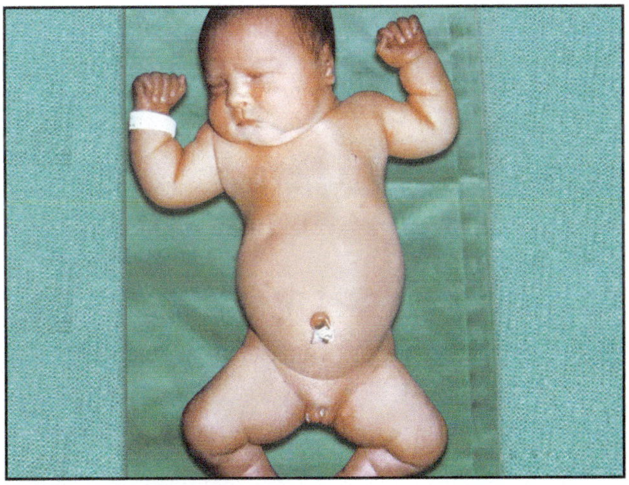

Figure 1.26 Maternal diabetes: infant of diabetic mother is born large and obese.

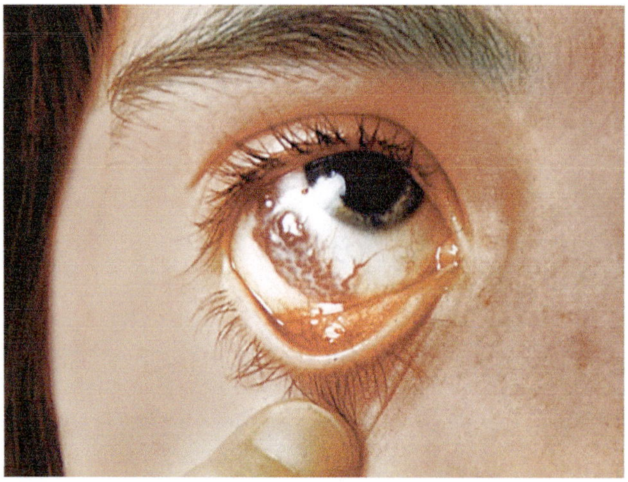

Figure 1.27 Ocular haemangioma.

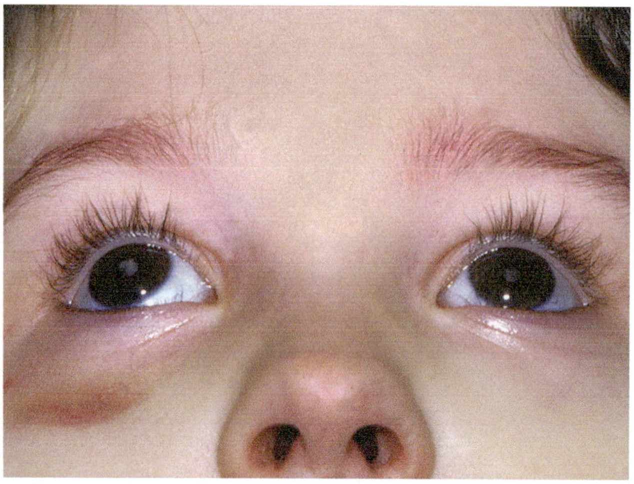

Figure 1.28 Bilateral cataracts.

NECK

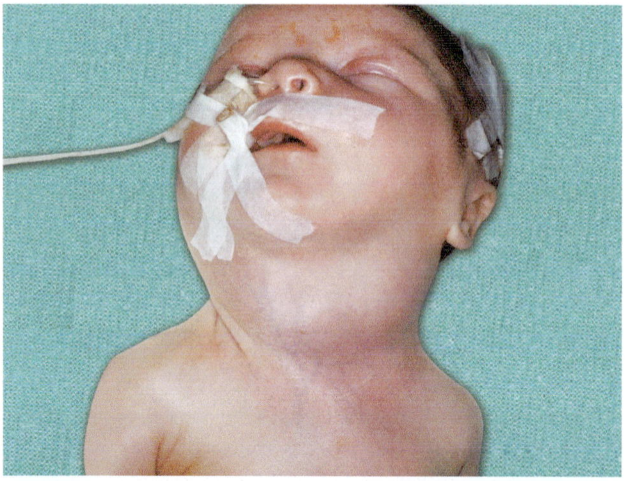

Figure 1.29 Newborn with goitre.

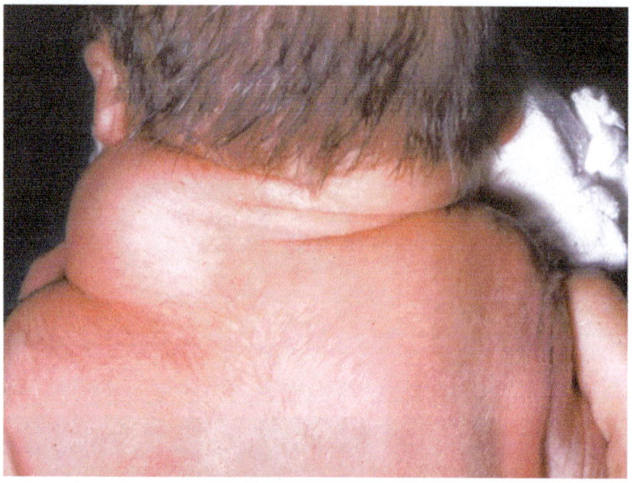

Figure 1.30 Cervical cystic hygroma.

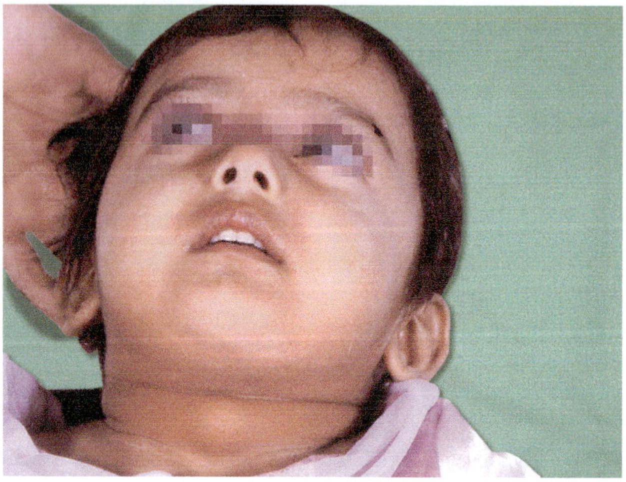

Figure 1.31 Thyroglossal cyst.

CHEST

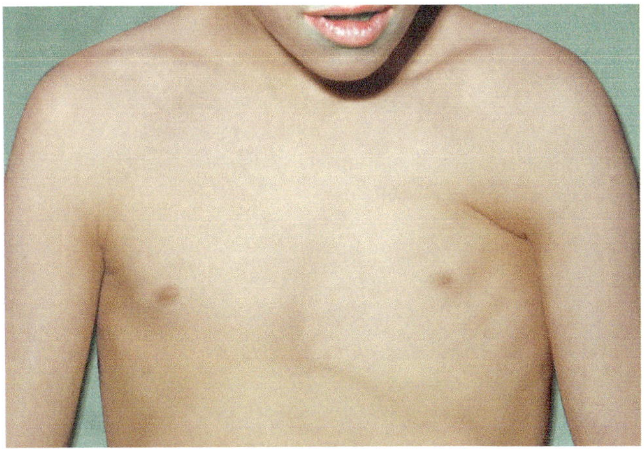

Figure 1.32 Poland syndrome: aplasia of the sternal portion of the pectoralis major muscle. *Note* the muscle defect is unilateral (left).

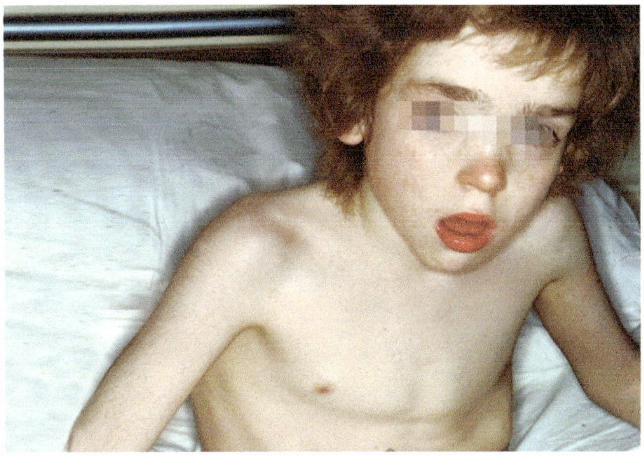

Figure 1.33 Pigeon chest deformity.

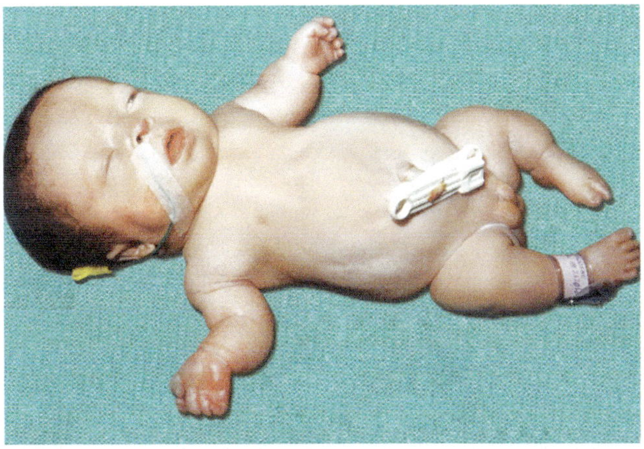

Figure 1.34 Asphyxiating thoracic dysplasia.

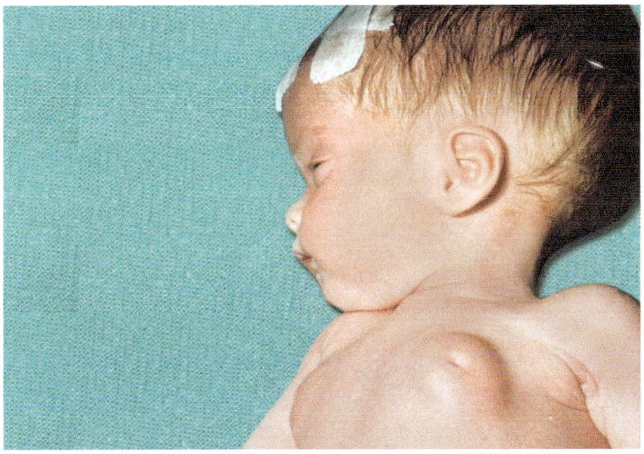

Figure 1.35 Physiologic gynaecomastia—due to normal stimulation by maternal estrogen.

UMBILICUS

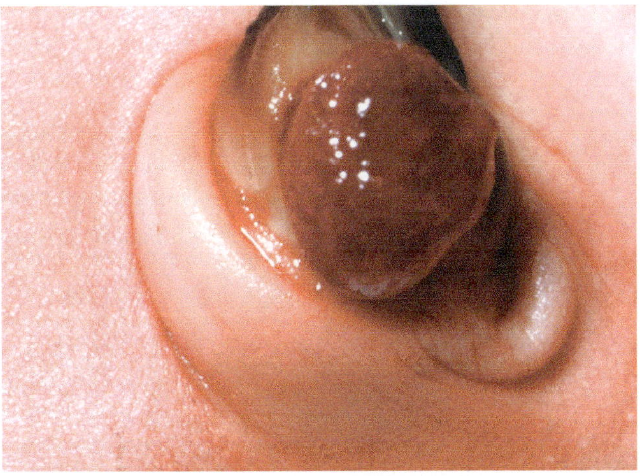

Figure 1.36 Vitello-intestinal remnant in a neonate. *Note* nodule attached to the umbilicus; it comprises small intestinal mucosa.

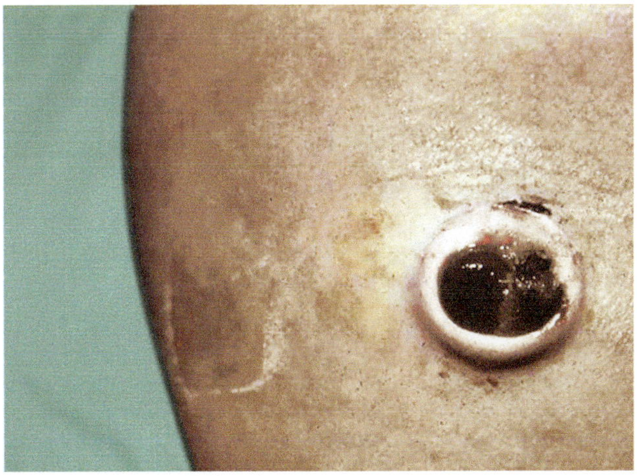

Figure 1.37 Umbilical granuloma.

BACK

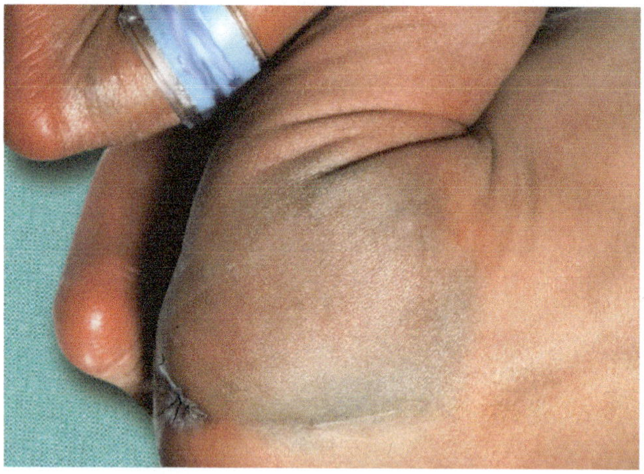

Figure 1.38 Mongolian blue spot: the Mongolian spot is found on the sacrum or low back at birth and often disappearing completely within a few years.

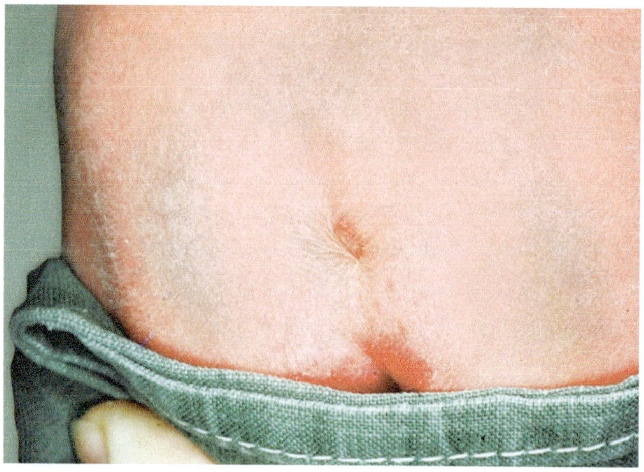

Figure 1.39 Midline dimple: simple midline dimple at the level of coccyx is seen relatively commonly in normal infants.

SKIN

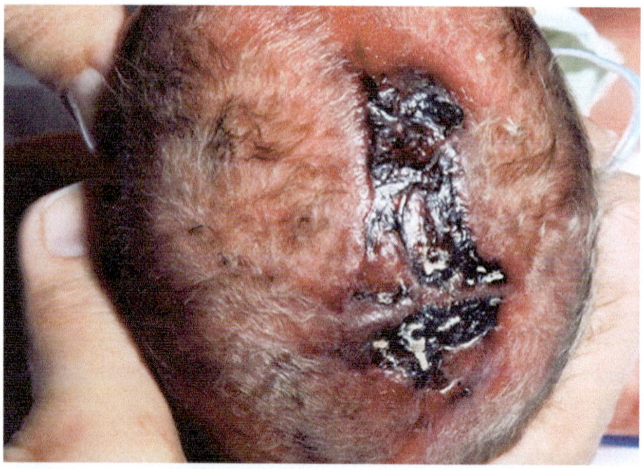

Figure 1.40 Cutis aplasia.

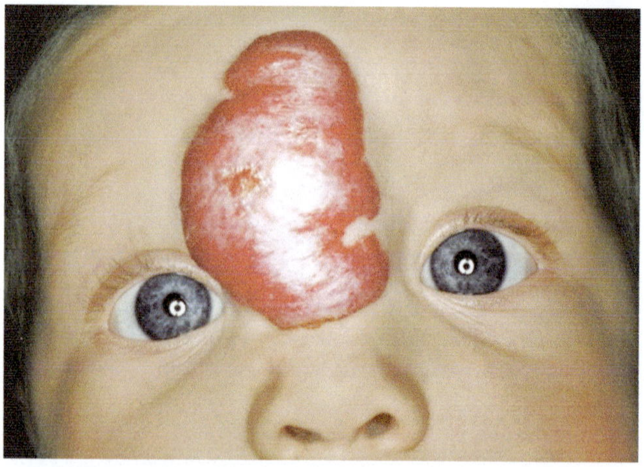

Figure 1.41 Strawberry naevus.

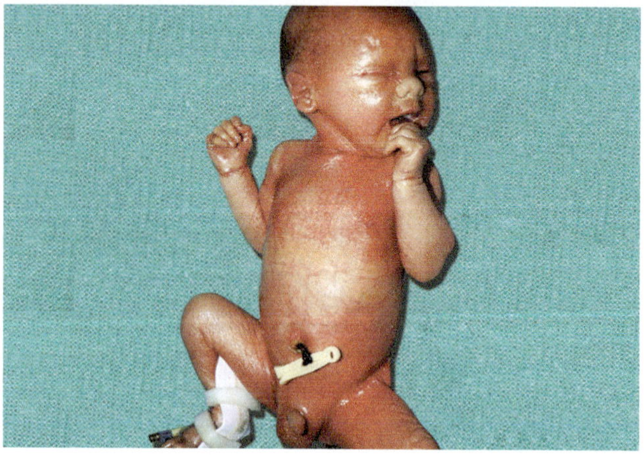

Figure 1.42 Collodion baby: a newborn infant covered with oiled parchment-like shiny skin is characteristic. The thick membrane encases skin.

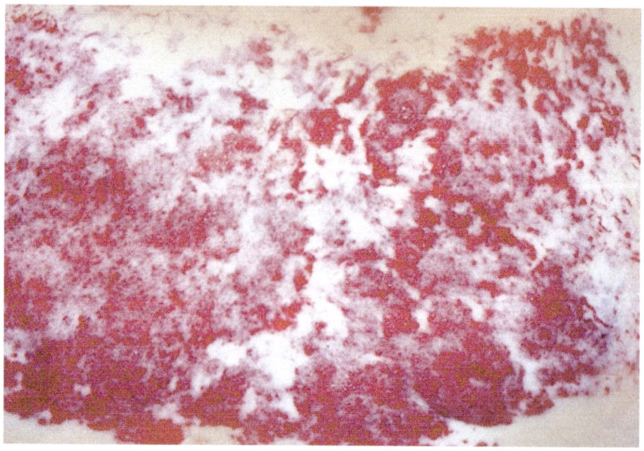

Figure 1.43 Cavernous haemangioma.

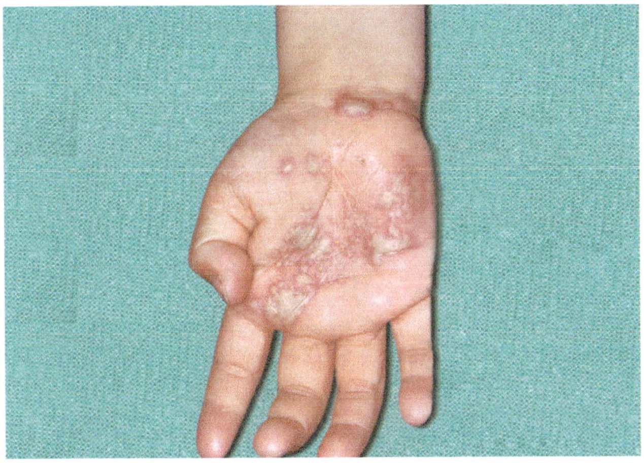

Figure 1.44 Herpes simplex of palm of the hand.

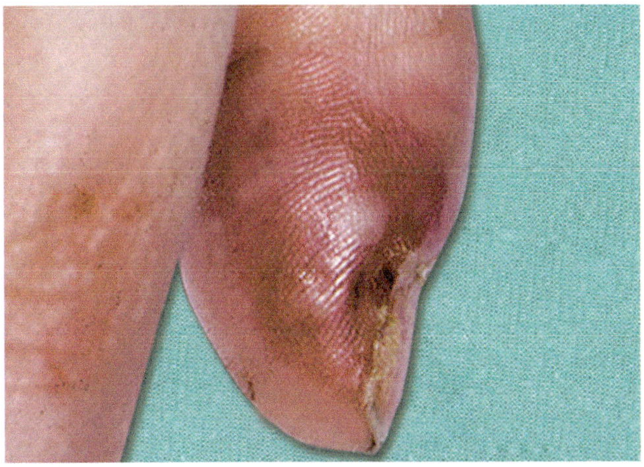

Figure 1.45 Whitlow: infection about the nail and under the nail due to thumb sucking.

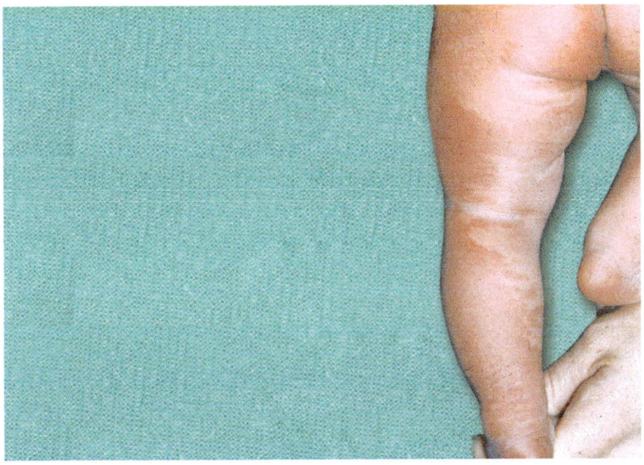

Figure 1.46 Capillary haemangioma.

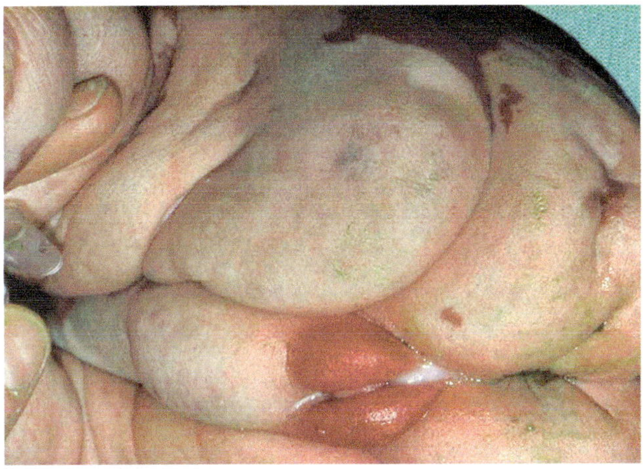

Figure 1.47 Kasabach–Merritt syndrome.

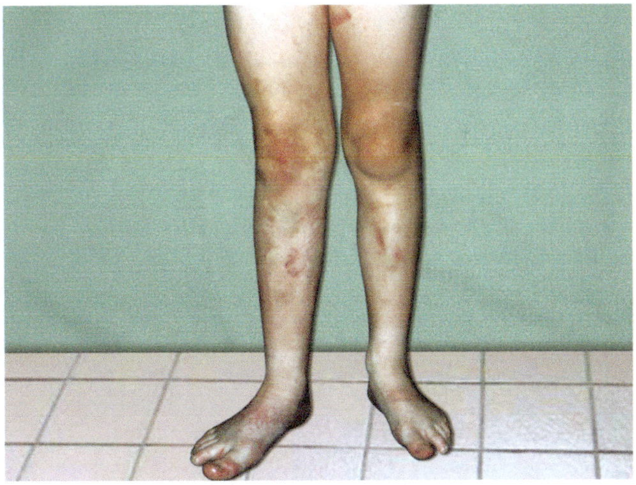

Figure 1.48 Klippel–Trénaunay syndrome: unusual leg lengths, with ipsilateral hypertrophy of bones.

GENITALIA

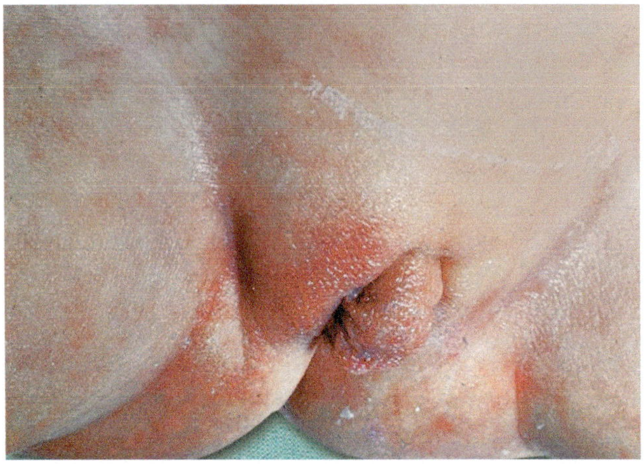

Figure 1.49 Congenital adrenal hyperplasia. *Note* enlarged clitoris and a urogenital sinus are present.

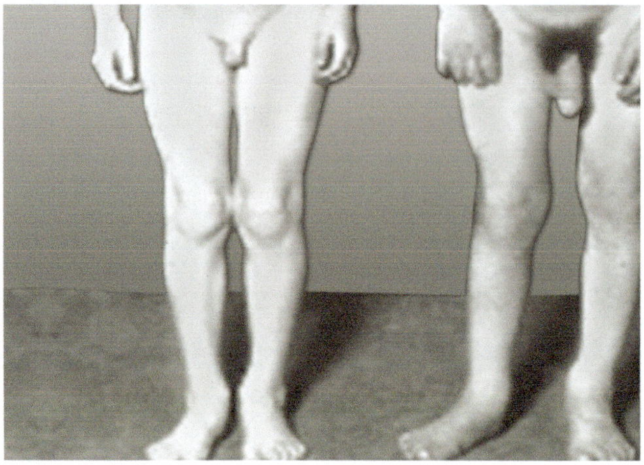

Figure 1.50 Precocious puberty: A 10-year-old boy with precocious puberty, caused by tuberculous meningitis. Pubertal development began at 5 years of age with control on the left.

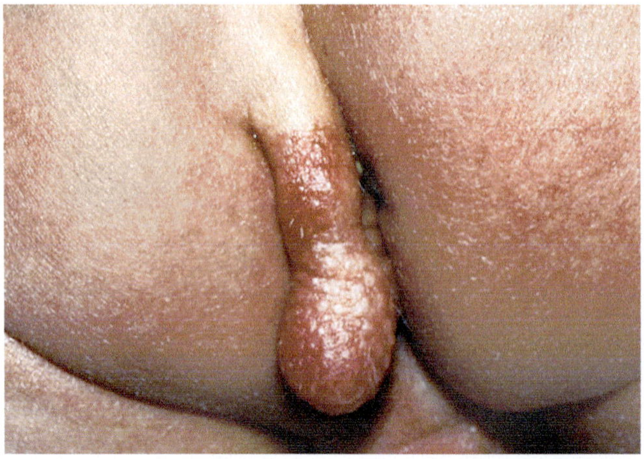

Figure 1.51 Perineal skin tag.

LIMBS

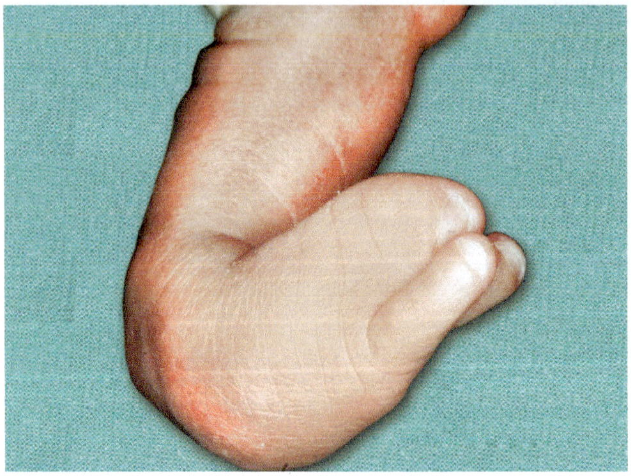

Figure 1.52 Lobster-claw hand: a thumb and a little finger only, results from a central defect of the intervening fingers.

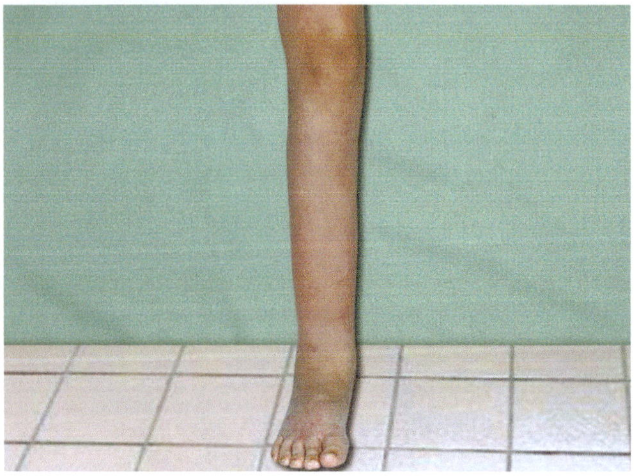

Figure 1.53 Lymphoedema. *Note* swelling of the whole of one leg; lymphangioscintigraphy should help establish the diagnosis.

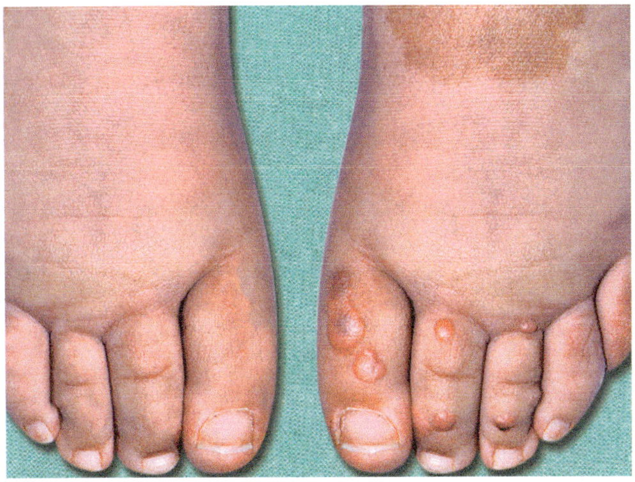

Figure 1.54 Lymphangioma: these lesions represent dilated lymphatic vessels.

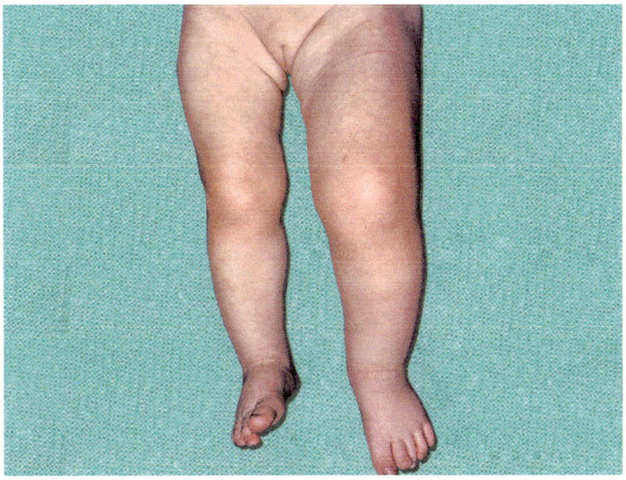

Figure 1.55 Local gigantism: overgrowth of the left limb or part of a limb in the presence of normal arteries, veins and lymphatics is called gigantism.

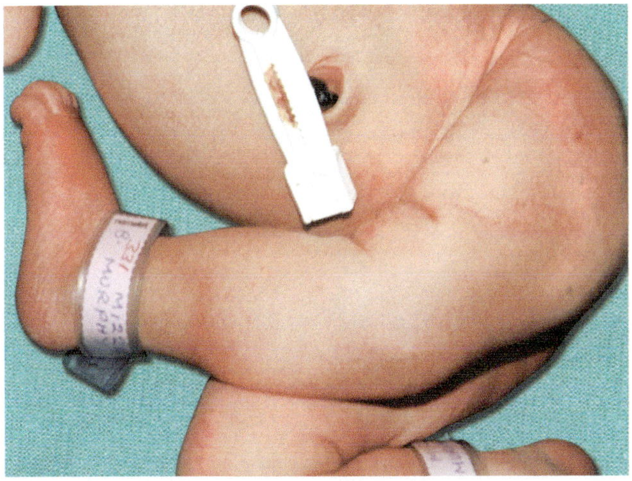

Figure 1.56 Dislocation of the left knee: congenital dislocation of the knee in a newborn infant, demonstrating the severe hyperextension deformity.

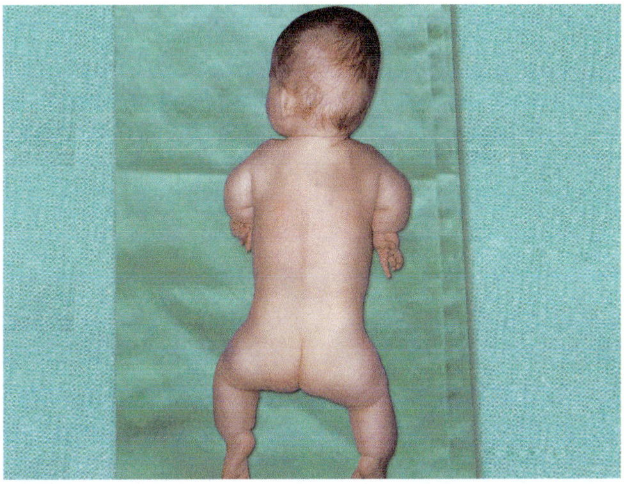

Figure 1.57 Phocomelia.

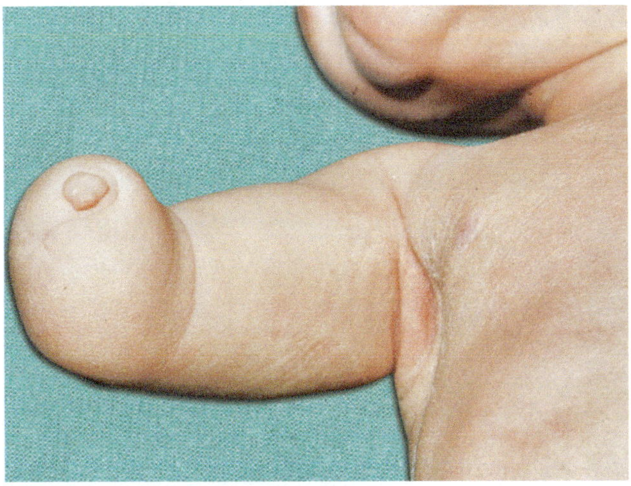

Figure 1.58 Amniotic band syndrome: causes absence of hand.

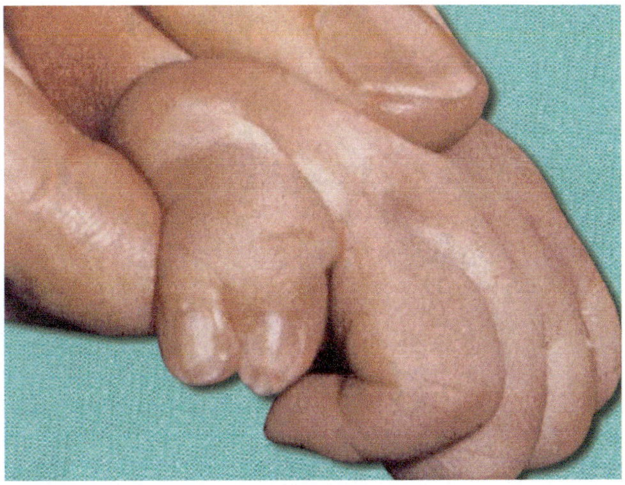

Figure 1.59 Bifid thumb.

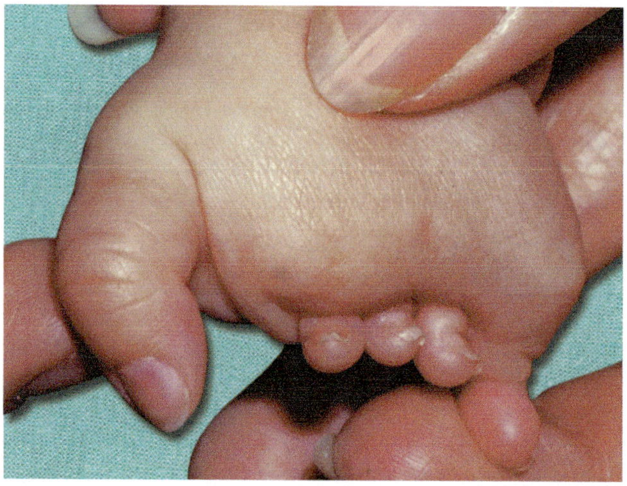

Figure 1.60 Absence of three digits: transverse arrest of development. *Note* spherical remnants of fingers.

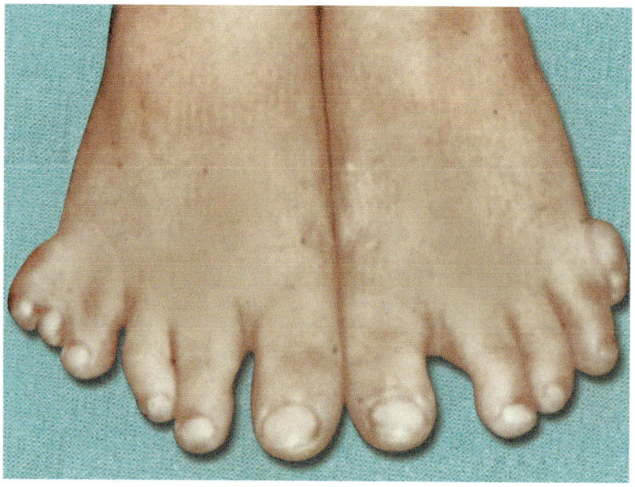

Figure 1.61 Polydactyly and syndactyly.

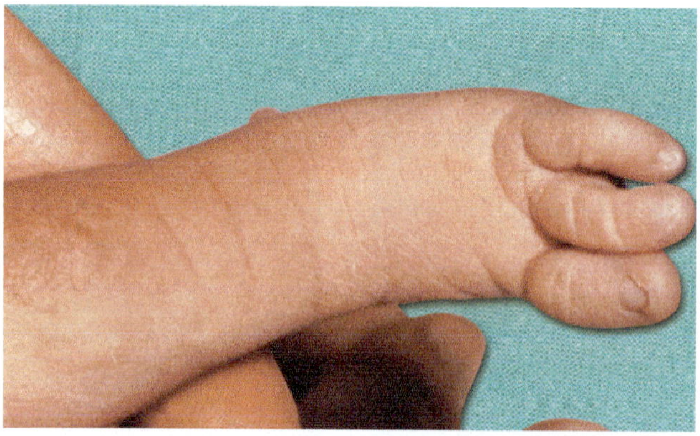

Figure 1.62 Oligodactyly.

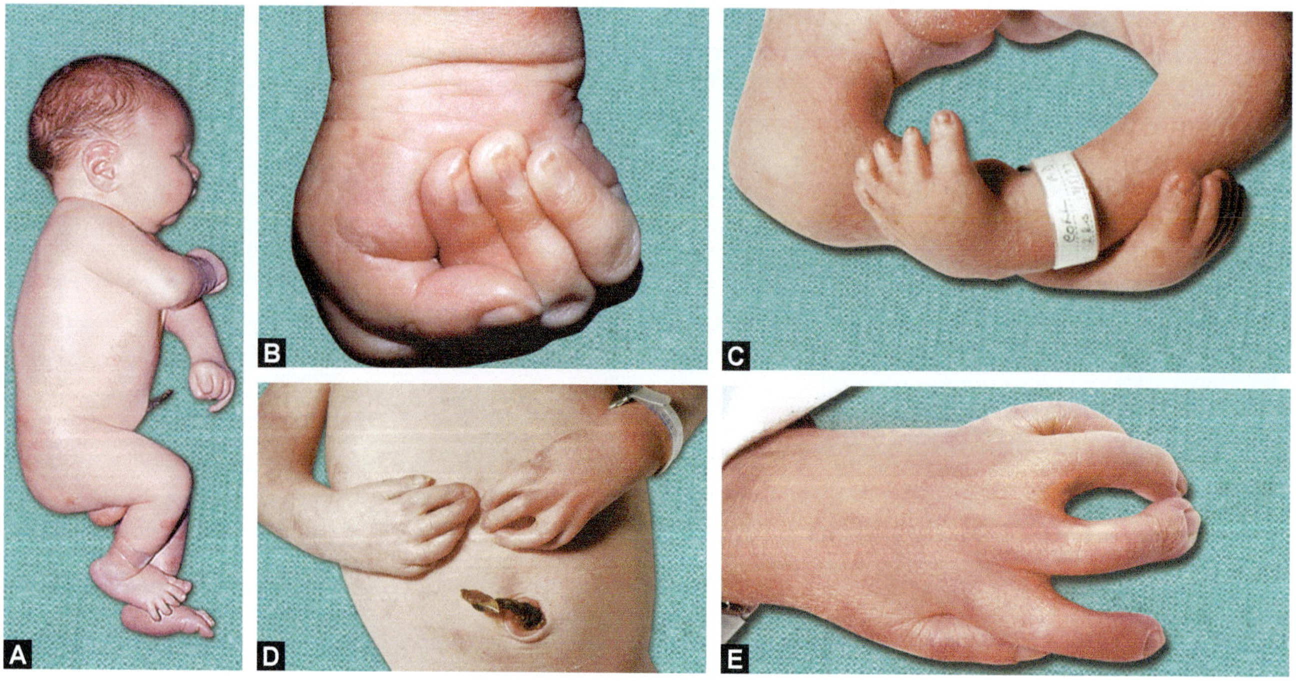

Figures 1.63A to E Arthrogryposis multiplex congenital. *Note* multiple congenital contractures.

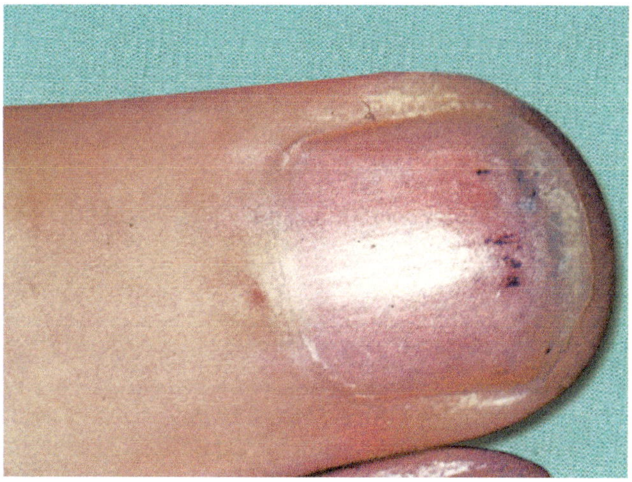

Figure 1.64 Splinter haemorrhages.

PLACENTA

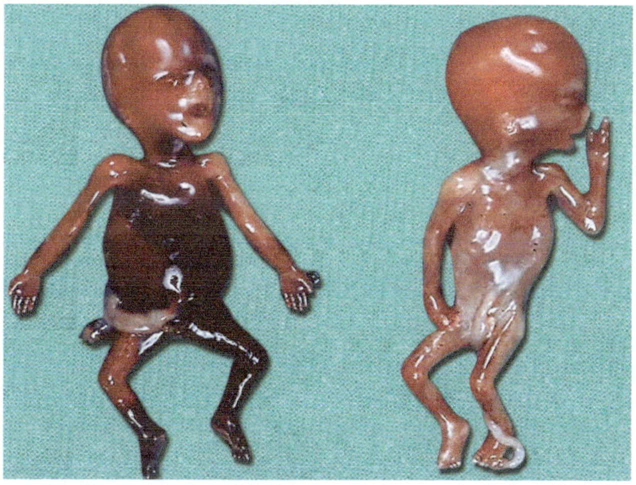

Figure 1.65 Twins with monochorionic placentae showing antepartum twin–twin transfusion (ATTT). The twin on the right is paler (donor) and the twin on the left is plethoric (recipient)—both died.

SUGGESTED READING

1. EL-Naggar M. Short Atlas in Pediatrics, 2nd edition. New Delhi: Jaypee Brothers Medical Publishers (P) Ltd; 2009.
2. Kulkarni ML. An Atlas of Neonatology. New Delhi: Jaypee Brothers Medical Publishers (P) Ltd; 2005.
3. Parthasarathy A. IAP Color Atlas of Pediatrics (A Publication of Indian Academy of Pediatrics). New Delhi: Jaypee Brothers Medical Publishers (P) Ltd; 2012.
4. Zitelli MD, Davis HW. Atlas of Pediatric Physical Diagnosis. Philadelphia: Mosby; 2002.

CHAPTER 2

Growth and Development

Louis C.K. Low

NORMAL GROWTH

Human growth is determined by an interaction of genetic and environmental factors. The infancy-childhood-puberty (ICP) growth model breaks down the human linear growth curve into three additive and partly superimposed components **(Fig. 2.1)**.[1] There are different growth promotion systems for each component. The infancy phase describes the period of rapid growth in utero and in infancy, and this phase of growth is predominantly nutritionally dependent. Maternal nutrition before and during pregnancy is an important determinant of foetal growth, and low prepregnancy weight increases the risk of intrauterine growth retardation (odds ratio, 2.55). An additional intake of 300 kcal and 15 g of protein per day is recommended for pregnant mothers above the recommended intake for nonpregnant women. Nutrient supply to the growing foetus is the dominant determinant in foetal growth, which is also dependent on placental function. Multiple approaches of nutritional intervention, control of infection, and improved antenatal care to pregnant women are more effective than any single intervention. Nutritional deprivation during pregnancy can have an epigenetic effect on foetal growth extending over many generations. Studies from the Netherlands have shown that maternal smoking and *Cannabis* use in pregnancy result in significant foetal growth retardation, which is progressive through gestation. Cytokines are essential for implantation and insulin-like growth factor 2 (IGF-2) is important for placental growth. Apart from nutrition, hormones and growth factors have an important role in the control of foetal growth. Foetal insulin secretion is dependent on the placental nutrition supply and foetal hyperinsulinaemia, which stimulates cell proliferation and foetal fat accumulation from 28 weeks gestation onwards. Thyroid hormone, which affects cell differentiation and brain development, is also regulated by nutrition. Cortisol is essential for the prepartum maturation of different organs including the liver, lung, gut and pituitary gland. Although growth hormone (GH) is important in postnatal growth, it plays an insignificant role in foetal growth except for an effect on foetal fat content. Animal knockout studies and human observations have shown that IGFs are most important for metabolic, mitogenic and differentiative activities of the foetus. IGF-2 is more important in early embryogenesis. In humans, foetal body weight is more closely correlated with the concentration of foetal serum IGF-1 than IGF-2.

In the childhood phase of growth, hormones such as GH, thyroid hormone and growth factors, such as IGF, begin to exert their influence from the end of the first year of life. A delay in the onset of the childhood phase of growth results in faltering of growth during this critical period. The growth faltering commonly observed between 6 and 18 months of life in children from developing countries is due to nutritional and socioeconomic factors rather than ethnic differences. The importance of the GH and IGF-1 axis and other hormones in the childhood phase of growth is described in a subsequent section of this chapter. Short-lived growth acceleration between 7 and 8 years of age can be observed in two-thirds of healthy children, followed by a fall in growth velocity before the onset of puberty. The pubertal phase of growth is controlled by nutrition, health, GH–IGF-1 axis and pubertal secretion of adrenal androgens and sex steroids. The onset of the childhood component has been known to be positively associated with the magnitude of the foetal or infancy component. The height at onset of puberty is an important determinant of the final adult height. The onset of puberty component is negatively correlated with the height at onset of puberty.

The United Nations Children's Fund (UNICEF) has identified access to nutritionally adequate diet, health care for mothers and children, and environmental health factors as conditioning factors of child growth worldwide. The care required includes care of women in the reproductive age, breastfeeding and feeding practices, psychological care, food preparation, hygiene and home health practices. Low food intake and the burden of common

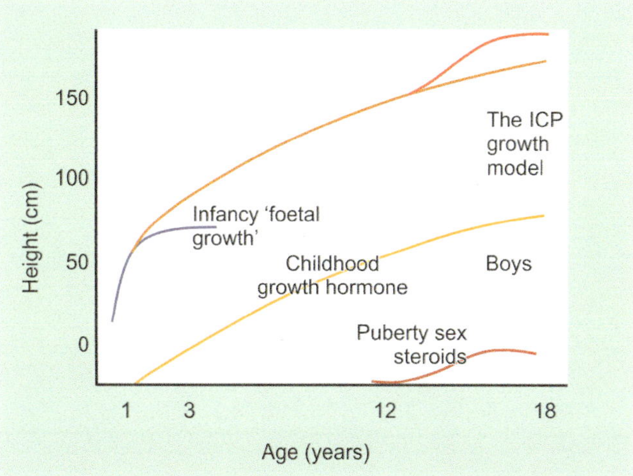

Figure 2.1 Analysis of linear growth using a mathematical model.
(*Courtesy:* Karlberg J, Engström I, Karlberg P, et al. Analysis of linear growth using a mathematical model I. From birth to three years. Acta Paediatr Scand. 1987;76(3):478-88.)

childhood infectious diseases, diarrhoea, respiratory infections and infestations limit the full realisation of the genetic potential in children from developing countries. As more and more women join the workforce, their duration of time spent in childcare and income generation determines whether child care is compromised. Quality child care is not affordable or accessible to low-income working mothers. Environmental pollution (air, heavy metals and smoking) can affect the growth of children, especially those living in developing countries undergoing rapid economic transition. The negative effects of active and passive smoking in mothers on foetal growth and growth in early life have been well characterised. Environmental exposure to lead in children has been linked to impaired physical and neurodevelopment growth and delayed puberty. Mercury poisoning from industrial pollution and teething powder and drugs are less common. There are claims of association of increased mercury exposure with neurodevelopment deficits. No significant association of prenatal and postnatal exposure to methyl mercury from fish consumption with childhood neurodevelopment has been found in populations with high fish consumption. A negative association between environmental sulphur dioxide, total suspended particulates, exposure to herbicide, and birth weight has been consistently reported in the literature. Impaired growth in infancy and childhood is associated with short adult stature and impaired cognitive development. The World Health Organization (WHO) global database on child growth and malnutrition provides information on growth and nutrition worldwide[2] based on the National Center for Health Statistics (NCHS)/WHO international growth reference. The prevalence of wasting in preschool children in Cambodia, Indonesia, Indian subcontinent, some island states in the Indian Ocean and some countries in Africa, and the Middle East has remained above 10%. According to WHO, 110 million stunted children lived in Asia in 2005. With the improvement in socioeconomic conditions and health care in most countries, there is a dramatic secular increase in mean stature of populations from Asia and other developing countries, while the positive secular trends in growth have slowed or even plateaued in developed countries in Europe and North America.

Although malnutrition remains a problem in some parts of the world, there is now a worldwide obesity epidemic in both developing and developed countries. The reason for the increase in body weight in children in the community is multifactorial, including genetic, cultural differences and dietary changes, especially increase in intake of high-fat energy-dense foods, but, most importantly, the increasing sedentary lifestyle adopted by different sectors of the population. The decrease in daily physical activity is due to mechanisation and computerisation. Time spent in watching television and playing or working on the computer is now regarded as a surrogate marker of inactivity in children. The health burden of excessive weight gain in childhood will be amplified in the years to come, and urgent action by international organisations, governments and all national and region stakeholders is needed.

ASSESSMENT AND MONITORING OF GROWTH

A clinician should take the opportunity to assess the growth of each child at each clinical encounter. The head circumference should be measured as the biggest circumference between the frontal region and the occipital prominence using a nonstretchable measuring tape. The body weight should be measured with a calibrated electronic scale, without shoes or socks and the child wearing light clothing. In infants and young children, the supine length should be measured with an infant stadiometer **(Fig. 2.2)**. Children older than 2 years should be measured while standing using a wall-mounted stadiometer **(Fig. 2.3)**, without shoes or socks, with the eyes and external auditory meatus held in the same plane and a slight upward pressure exerted on the jaw and occiput. The anthropometric measurements should be plotted accurately on the appropriate chart.

Growth in children and adolescents has been widely used by paediatricians as a marker of their general well-being. The normal pattern of growth in children is traditionally described in an up-to-date ethnic-specific growth chart. Growth references are valuable tools for accessing the health of individuals and for health planner to assess the well-being of populations. A survey involving 178 countries found growth monitoring in the first 6 years of life to be an integral part of paediatric care. Two-thirds of these countries use the NCHS or WHO growth reference, while more developed countries use their own national

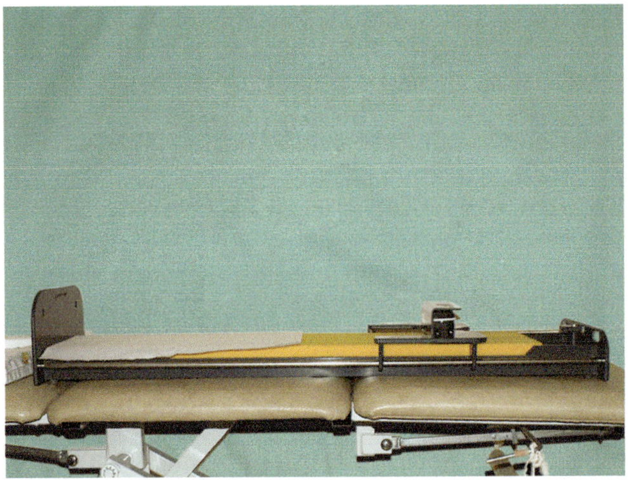

Figure 2.2 Stadiometer for measurement of supine length.

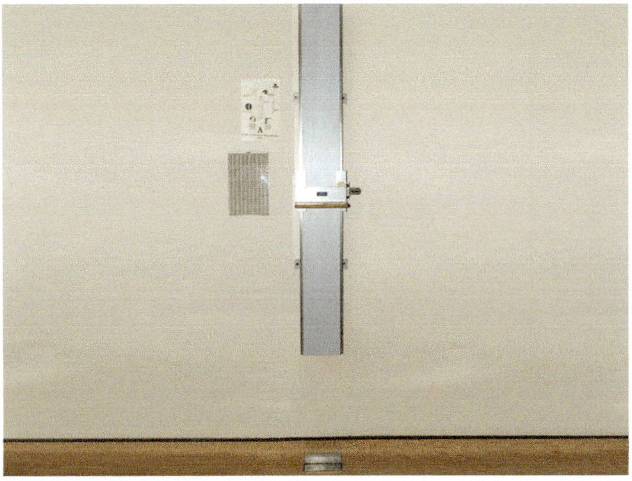

Figure 2.3 Wall-mounted stadiometer for height measurement.

growth reference. In developing countries, healthcare workers monitor growth to detect and intervene when children have growth faltering. In developed countries, growth monitoring has been regarded as a useful tool for detecting unrecognised organic diseases, as the provision of reassurance to parents, and for monitoring the health of children in the population. Understanding the ethnic differences in childhood and pubertal growth helps doctor in interpretation of results of surveillance of child growth based on the NCHS or WHO growth standard, which has a number of limitations. A WHO multicentre growth reference has been developed, based on a longitudinal study of exclusively breastfed children from birth to 24 months and a cross-sectional study of children from 18 to 71 months from 6 countries (Brazil, Ghana, India, Norway, Oman and the United States). Babies in the Euro-Growth study who were breastfed according to the WHO recommendations showed higher weight gain in the first 3 months of life and were lower in weight and length between 6 months and 12 months as compared to the NCHS or WHO growth reference. No significant differences in growth from the NCHS reference in these children were noted between 12 and 36 months. The finding was similar to that of the WHO multicentre growth reference. The WHO multicentre growth reference was completed[3] and is considered as the gold standard for assessing growth of children worldwide.

Despite widespread acceptance of routine growth monitoring of children as the standard of care, a recent meta-analysis questioned the benefits of growth monitoring in childhood, as there have been very few trials that evaluated the impact of this practice on child health. Infants should be weighed at birth and at times of their immunisation. Surveillance of children's weight for more than 1 year is only recommended in children whose growth causes clinical concerns. Clinicians should pay more attention to growth parameters collected during clinical consultations. Length measurement should only be done in children younger than 2 years if there is a concern in their growth or weight gain.

In a normal population, less than 5% of the infants will drop their weight through two centile lines and less than 1% of infants will have a fall in weight across three centile lines in the first year of life. A baby would be regarded as failing to thrive if there is a fall in weight across more than two centile lines in infancy. In the United Kingdom, it has been recommended that primary care physicians should refer children for assessment if their heights fall below the 0.4th percentile [–2.67 standard deviation (SD)], and a single height measurement at school entry using this criteria has been found to be a sensitive marker for undiagnosed organic disease. The sensitivity of this recommended height screening test can be improved by making a correction for the height of the parents. Height measurements taken during other clinical encounters during childhood are further opportunities for referral using the 0.4th percentile as the cutoff for action. Clinicians have long placed a lot of emphasis on growth assessment using height velocity, which is calculated from the difference between two height measurements, thereby combining the imprecision of the two readings. Successive measurements of height over time in an individual are highly correlated, whereas successive annual growth velocities are not. This suggests that growth velocity estimates are not reliable and do not have a useful role in routine growth monitoring. Despite its imprecision, a grossly abnormal growth velocity can still be regarded as an indicator of disease. Whether routine height screening every 2–3 years between 5 and 12 years of age will be cost-effective in detecting silent disease without the capacity to cause harm within the paediatric population remains to be proven. However, routine monitoring of the height and weight in both developing and developed countries is likely to continue in the years to come.

In the monitoring of overweight and underweight, both the WHO and the International Obesity Task Force (IOTF) have suggested the use of different body mass index (BMI) [derived from weight (in kilograms)/height^2 (in metres)] cutoffs for identifying these problems in the clinical and public health setting. The WHO has adopted the updated BMI reference based on the US NHANES I data collected from 1971 to 1974,[4] while IOTF has adopted an international BMI reference derived from six population growth studies[5] as the gold standard for international comparison. The WHO proposed a BMI below the 5th percentile, above 85th percentile and above 95th percentile as cutoffs for underweight, overweight and obesity, respectively. The IOTF established BMI percentile cutoffs at different ages based on extrapolation of adult BMI cutoffs of 25 and 30 kg/m^2 for overweight and obesity, respectively. In addition, national BMI references are now available in many developed countries. The cutoffs based on the US reference data are related to some measures of morbidity, but the newly developed IOTF BMI cutoff points for children still require validation with data on morbidity measures such as blood pressure, serum lipids, insulin resistance and diabetes. In a meeting organised by WHO or International Association for the Study of Obesity (IASO)/IOTF in Hong Kong in 1999, the experts were of the opinion that lower BMI cutoffs might need to be set for adult Asian populations because of their predisposition to deposit abdominal fat. The proposed revised BMI cutoff is 23 and 25 kg/m^2 for overweight and obesity, respectively.

GROWTH HORMONE: IGF-1 AXIS

The pulsatile secretion of GH from the pituitary gland is under the control of the stimulatory action of growth hormone-releasing hormone (GHRH) and the suppressive effect of somatostatin. Multiple neurotransmitters and neuropeptides are involved in the hypothalamic release of these hormones. GH is essential for normal human growth in childhood and adolescence. The liver is the organ with the highest GH receptor concentrations and is the main source of GH-binding protein (cleaved extracellular portion of the GH receptor) found in the circulation. After binding to its receptor and inducing dimerisation, GH activates the JAK2/STAT pathway to bring about the stimulation of epiphyseal growth, osteoclast differentiation, lipolysis and amino acid uptake into muscles. The more important growth promotion action of GH is mediated by IGF-1. Circulating IGF-1 comes predominantly from the liver and is associated with IGF binding protein-3 (IGFBP-3) and the acid labile submit (ALS) to form a ternary complex. The action of IGF-1 is modified by six binding proteins in the circulation. Although IGF-1 is important in foetal growth, serum concentration of IGF-1 is low in foetal life and in early infancy. A significant rise in IGF-1 and IGFBP-3 concentrations is observed in normal children from 10 months onward. There is further progressive rise of serum IGF-1 to two to three times of the adult serum concentrations as the children progress through puberty. The serum IGF-1 level in childhood is also dependent on nutrients availability. It has now been shown that the local generation of IGF-1 in tissues in response to GH rather than the circulating IGF-1 is essential for normal growth; liver-specific IGF-1 knockout mice have low circulating IGF-1 levels and yet they have near-normal growth. Short stature has been reported in humans with mutations in the genes of GHRH, GH, GH receptor, STAT5B, IGF-1, ALS and IGF-1 receptor.

GENETICS OF STATURE

Fisher proposed in 1918 that many genetic factors, each having a small effect, explain the heritability of height.[6] This is still true in the genome era. From five genome-wide association studies (GWASs) using analysis of single nucleotide polymorphisms, investigators have identified over 50 chromosome locations (implicating nearby genes) that appear to be partially responsible for the regulation of adult stature in humans. Collectively, these genes account for about 4% of adult stature. One gene LIN28B on chromosome 6q21 which is shown to be important in the determination of stature is also found to be associated with the age at menarche (AAM). Heterozygous carriers of mutations of natriuretic peptide receptor B (NPR2) have a mean height of -1.1 ± 0.8 SD and the carrier frequency is 1 in 5–700, and some short children may be NPR2 mutation carriers. Heterozygous IGF acid labile subunit (IGFALS) gene mutation carriers have -0.9 ± 1.51 SD loss in height compared with the normal population. It is possible that carriers of some of these single gene defects can be the cause of some short children in the population. It is likely that more and more height determining genes will be described in future.

PUBERTY

Puberty is defined as the maturational transition of an individual from the sexually immature state to adulthood with the capacity to reproduce. The hypothalamic-pituitary-gonadal axis is active in utero and at birth. After this period of activation, the axis undergoes a long period of relative quiescence from 3 to 6 months after birth until late childhood when pubertal development occurs. The onset of puberty is the result of decreasing sensitivity of the regulatory system of gonadotropin secretion (gonadostat) in the hypothalamus to the negative feedback of the small amounts of gonadal steroids secreted by the prepubertal gonads, as well as a decrease in the central neural inhibition of gonadotropin-releasing hormone (GnRH) release. Disruption of genes controlling the migration of GnRH neurons from the olfactory epithelium to the forebrain can result in delayed puberty. The initiation of puberty is associated with a decrease in transsynaptic inhibition by GABAergic neurons and an activation of excitatory glutamatergic neurotransmission in the control of GnRH secretion. There is also evidence that glial to neuron signalling through growth factors is important in the neuroendocrine control of puberty. Evidence for genetic regulation of the timing of puberty is suggested by the correlation of the age of onset of puberty in mother and their offspring. It has been suggested that 50–80% of the variance in pubertal onset may be genetically controlled. Kisspeptin, which is encoded by the KISS1 gene on chromosome 1q31, is cloned as a tumour metastasis suppressor gene. Kisspeptin/G protein-coupled receptor 54 (GPR54) signalling complex is important in the control of puberty. Inactivating GPR54 mutations leads to hypogonadotropic hypogonadism and an activating mutation of GPR54 has been described in a girl with slowly progressive precocious puberty. GWASs and AAM identified a significant association of LIN28B and AAM. A meta-analysis of 32 GWAS identified 30 loci associated with AAM, and these genetic loci explained 3.6–6.1% of the variance in the AAM, equivalent to 7.2–12.2% of its heritability.

Light-dark rhythm and climatic conditions have little effect on the AAM. Children adopted from developing countries to live in a developed country have early puberty as a general rule. Exposure to endocrine-disrupting chemicals can affect timing of puberty and, e.g. isomers of dichlorodiphenyltrichloroethane (DDT) have oestrogen agonistic and androgen antagonistic effect. Mycoestrogenic zearalenone was reported to be elevated in 35% of girls with central precocious puberty in a study from Italy. Zearalenone is a nonsteroidal mycotoxin produced by *Fusarium* species on grains and causes contamination of grains and animal feeds. Brominated flame retardant and dichlorodiphenyldichloroethylene (DDE) have been found to have an association with earlier puberty in girls. The timing of puberty is also influenced by nutrition and metabolic cues. A direct relationship between a particular ratio of fat to lean body mass and onset of puberty has been described. Leptin plays a role in informing the brain of peripheral energy stores and body composition and may act as a permissive signal for the onset of puberty.

With the onset of puberty, there is increasing pulsatile secretion of luteinising hormone (LH) and, to a lesser extent, follicle-stimulating hormone (FSH), mainly at night through gradual amplification of GnRH pulse frequency and amplitude. In pubertal boys and girls, sleep-entrained pulsatile GnRH is secreted every 60–90 minutes, progressing to become more regular throughout the day. In boys, the pulsatile gonadotropin secretion stimulates the testes to develop and the Leydig cells to produce testosterone. Testosterone production increases progressively and is responsible for the metabolic changes and the development of secondary sexual characteristics. Both LH and FSH are required for the development and maintenance of testicular function. In early puberty, in girls, circulating FSH level increases disproportionately to the LH level in response to GnRH stimulation. Gonadotropin stimulation leads to a rapid rise in ovarian oestrogen production before menarche. When the concentration of oestradiol rises above 200 pg/mL for a few days, the negative feedback on GnRH and gonadotropin release turns to positive feedback leading to the ovulatory LH surge. In humans, the ability of the hypothalamus to stimulate gonadotropin secretion in response to positive feedback effects of oestrogen does not occur until after menarche. In adult females, the GnRH pulse frequency starts at 90 minutes in early follicular phase, increases to one pulse every 60 minutes in midfollicular phase and slows to one pulse every 4–6 hours in the lateral phase.

From the age of 6–8 years onwards, there is a progressive rise in adrenal androgens secretion up to 20 years of age. This process of maturation of the adrenal gland, referred to as adrenarche, is responsible for pubic and axillary hair development and this event occurs independent of the maturation of the hypothalamic-pituitary-gonadal axis, although the timing of the two processes are usually related in normal puberty. Adrenarche is coincident with the mid-childhood adiposity rebound and there is evidence that nutritional status measured as a change in the BMI is an important physiological regulator of adrenarche.

The progressive changes in the secondary sexual characteristics have been described in a standardised format by Tanner (**Figs. 2.4 and 2.5**).[7] There is considerable variation in the age of onset and the tempo of progression of puberty among normal children. Over the last century, children have tended to be taller in stature and reach sexual maturity at an earlier age. In a recent population study from the United States, 5 and 15% of the white and African American girls had breast development before the age of 7 years. Since the mean age of menarche in these American girls have not changed significantly over time, puberty in American girls is associated with earlier onset of breast development, but with a slower tempo of pubertal progression. An age of onset of puberty before the age of 9 years in boys and before 7 years in girls is regarded as premature. Girls and boy without signs of puberty by the age of 13 years and 14 years should be monitored carefully and considered for evaluation of delayed puberty. The mean age of onset on menarche can vary: 11.2 years in African Americans, 11.27 years in China and 13.4 years in Denmark.

CHILD DEVELOPMENT

Development in children is predominantly determined by genetic factors, but a significant contribution comes from environmental factors (maternal nutrition during pregnancy, birth, socioeconomic factors, nutrition and health after birth). Intellectual development in childhood and adolescence is a complex and dynamic process with

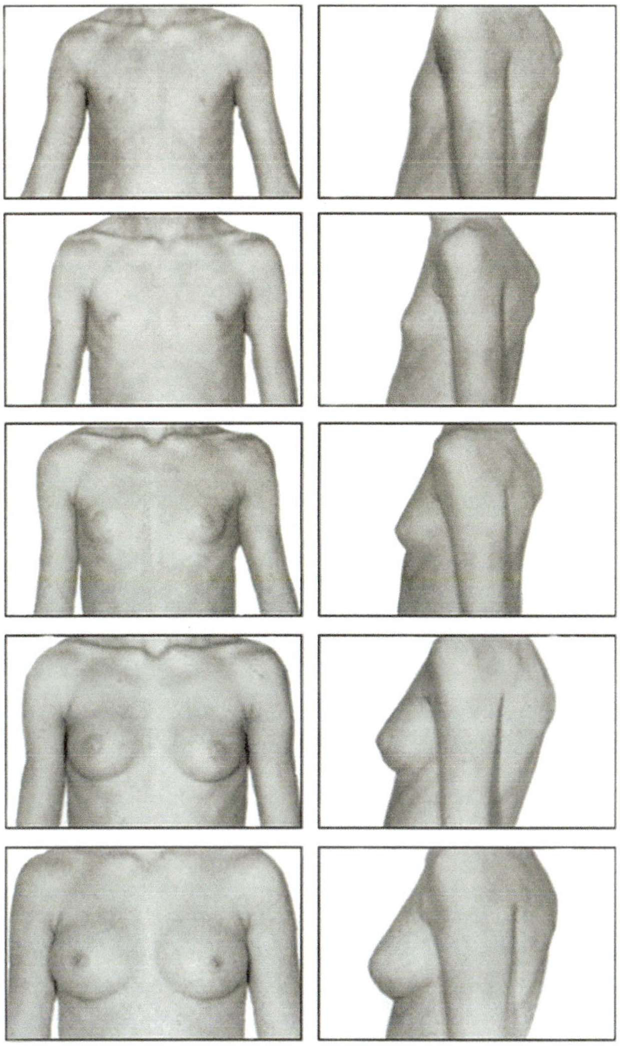

Figure 2.4 Standards for breast development. (From Tanner JM. Growth and endocrinology of the adolescent. In: Gardner L (Ed). Endocrine and Genetic Diseases of Childhood, 2nd edition. Philadelphia: Saunders; 1975.)

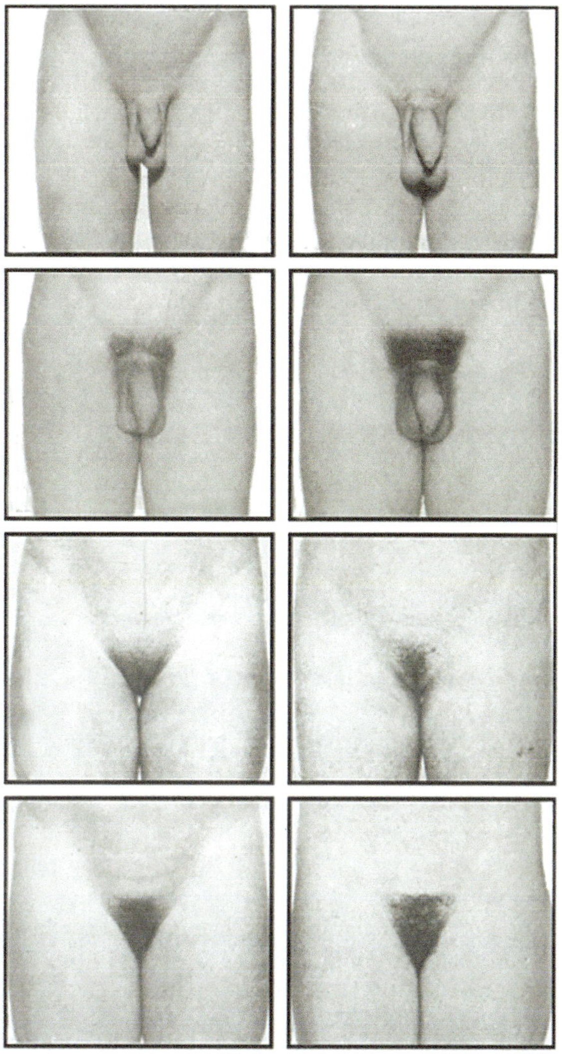

Figure 2.5 Standards of pubic hair ratings in boys and girls development. (From Tanner JM. Growth and endocrinology of the adolescent. In: Gardner L (Ed). Endocrine and Genetic Diseases of Childhood, 2nd edition. Philadelphia: Saunders; 1975.)

the interaction between genes and the environment continuously changing over time. Antenatal and postnatal depression, maternal malnutrition, maternal smoking during pregnancy, antenatal exposure to organic pollutants and adverse child care practice can disrupt the development of different psychomotor domains in infancy and childhood. Home environment, parent–child relationship, parenting style and discipline practices, and school environment can have a major influence on the socioemotional and cognitive growth of an individual in childhood and adolescence. Traditionally, early childhood development can be described in stages in four functional skill areas: gross motor, fine motor, language and speech, and social and emotional development. It is also important for paediatricians to be familiar with the development of the special senses, such as hearing, vision, taste, smell, sensation and proprioception. Timing of achievement of major milestones in the various domains of development can vary enormously in normal children. Sound knowledge of development in childhood and adolescence allow us to recognise global or specific developmental delay beyond the normal acceptable age, disordered developmental sequence or developmental regression.

Gross Motor Development

Motor development progresses in a cephalocaudal direction with suppression of primitive reflexes and development of postural tone and secondary protective reflexes. The primitive reflexes including the Moro, grasp, stepping and asymmetric tonic neck reflexes must have disappeared by 3–6 months of age before head control (4 months) and independent sitting at 6–8 months can occur. Prior to walking, an infant can crawl on all four limbs, bottom shuffle, commando creep or roll along the ground. Shufflers, creepers and rollers tend to attain independent walking at a later age than infants who crawl on all fours. Thus, early locomotor patterns can result in significant variation in the age of achieving independent walking. A delay in walking beyond 18 months of age is a warning sign in children who have been crawling as the early locomotor pattern. An infant stands holding on furniture by 9 months of age, cruises round furniture by 12 months and walks independently by 13–15 months. At 18 months of age, a child can climb onto a chair and walks up and down stairs 2 feet per step by 24 months of age. By 2.5 years of age, a child should be able to stand on tiptoes, jump on both feet, and kick a ball. A 3-year-old child can walk backwards and can ride a tricycle. There is further development of gross motor skill and balance with age, and most children can participate in a variety of activities such as swimming, skating, gymnastics and ball games by 6–7 years of age.

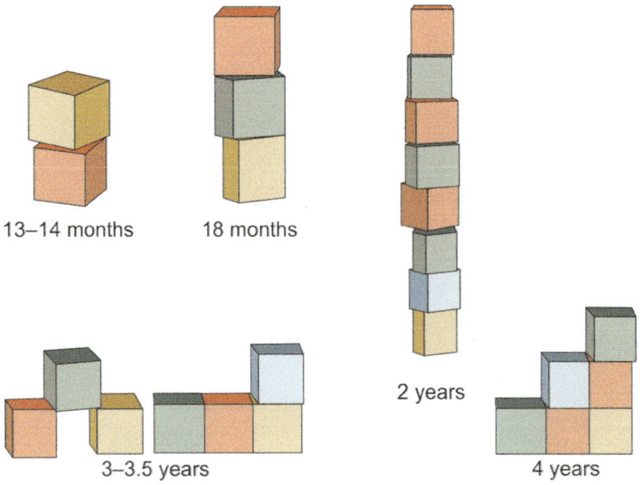

Figure 2.6 Build cubes.

Fine Motor Development in Early Childhood

The development of fine motor skills in childhood is conditional upon the development of normal vision. Voluntary movements and fine motor manipulations require the coordinated development of nervous system and visuomotor coordination. Visual fixation can be demonstrated in babies by 4–6 weeks of life. The grasp reflex is usually inhibited by 3 months of age, and babies can be seen opening their hands and clasping and unclasping their hands at the midline of the body. Between 3 and 5 months, babies find their hands interesting, but persistence of 'hand regard' beyond 5 months is unusual. By 6 months of age, babies can reach and grasp an object (1-inch cube) with the palm of their hands (palmar grasp). Putting objects in the mouth is a common activity at this age. Transfer of objects from one hand to the other can be seen at 6 months. By 9 months of age, babies can hold a cube in each hand and bring them together for comparison. Grasping of small objects with the thumb and index finger (pincer grasp) can be achieved between 9 and 12 months. Casting of objects is frequently observed towards the end of the first year of life, but voluntary release of an object on command only takes place at 15 months. By 15 months of age, a child can hold a pen in his/her palm and scribble. The child can build a tower of two to three cubes between 15 and 18 months. At 2 years of age, a child's ability to manipulate small objects continues to improve (**Fig. 2.6**). Hand dominance can be observed at 2.5 years of age and the child can scribble and draw a line or circle with a tripod pen grip. At 3 years of age, a child can build a tower of eight to nine cubes and copy building patterns using three to four cubes. A child can eat with a fork or spoon. By 4 years, a child can draw a man showing body parts and copy some alphabets. Between 5 and 6 years, a child can write well and eat properly with knife and fork.

Language and Speech Development in Childhood

Language can be defined as an arbitrary set of symbols, which, when combined in a particular sequence, allows an individual to convey a specific message or conceptualisation and transmit them to another individual. When the transmission of messages between individuals is performed verbally, the action is referred to as speech. Language acquisition is a complex process integrating interaction between many factors. Genetic factors possibly play an important role early in the developmental process, but neurological (cerebral palsy, neuromuscular disorders, hearing impairment, autism), cognitive (mental retardation, specific learning disabilities and specific developmental language impairment) and environmental (psychosocial deprivation, bilingual or multilingual environments, cultural differences, maternal depression and large sibship) factors are important determinants of speech development. Impaired hearing is associated with impairment in language and speech development and the prevalence of severe hearing loss has been estimated to be between 1:900 and 1:2,500 in newborn infants. It has been shown that universal newborn hearing screening, using auditory brainstem response (ABR) or two-step screening (ABR–ABR) and otoacoustic emissions, enables the early identification of infants with moderate to severe hearing impairment. There is evidence that early diagnosis of impaired hearing and intervention can be associated with a better-improved language and communication skills by 2–5 years of age. Cochlear implant is an alternative for children with severe sensorineural hearing loss who do not benefit from conventional hearing aids. Early cochlear implantation before 3 years of age has been associated with a better outcome in terms of speech and language development as compared to children receiving cochlear implants in later life.

A 1-month-old baby startles to sound, but a baby can localise the source of sound presented at ear level at 6 months of age. At 3 months, they respond to the call of their names, smile and laugh, or are comfortable in response to the sound of the mother's voice. Babies can make consonant sounds at 3 months of age (e.g., ba, ka, da), and deaf infants are usually referred to as quiet babies at this stage. Babbling in strings usually occur after 6 months of age. At 12 months of age, the baby understands some simple commands and uses increasing variety of intonation when babbling. At 1 year of age, an infant understands simple commands such as 'blow a kiss' or 'wave bye-bye.' They are able to say a few words with meaning and have at least six recognisable words with meaning by 18 months. At 18 months of age, they can name body parts on request and start to use word combinations. By 2 years of age, children have a vocabulary of many words and can speak in simple sentences. A 9-month-old child can look for an object after being hidden, demonstrating their grasp of the concept of object permanence. Before the development of expressive speech, infants of 1 year age can indicate their desire by pointing or gesture. They demonstrate definition by use of common objects such as cup, brush, comb and spoon. Symbolisation occurs at 18 months with the child imitating the mother's household chore or feeding a doll. Between 18 and 22 months, children can engage in constructive symbolic play with toys of miniature.

Both expressive and receptive language involves three important aspects, namely, phonology and articulation, semantics and syntax. The coordinated neuromuscular mechanisms, which produce the desire sequence of phonemes, constitute expressive phonology. The neurological process involved in the identification of the phonemes in a spoken message is referred to as receptive phonology. Semantics refers to the process involved in relating a spoken word to its meaning. In most cases, a thought cannot be expressed simply by a single word. In constructing a spoken message, syntax governs the particular order of words as they appear sequentially in speech. It also governs the use of tense, plurality, grammar and the relationship between the different words. Syntactic process works in conjunction with the semantic process in deriving the meaning conveyed by a sequence of words. The use of two to three word combinations in young children involves the omission of function words, which are used in the more complex adult speech. The simple word combinations also reflect the reduced memory capacity of young children. By 3 years of age, a child can use plurals, pronouns and prepositions (e.g., under, behind, in front of) in their speech. Most young children are disfluent, but a child should be wholly intelligible and have few infantile substitutions or consonant substitutions at the age of 4 years. As children become older and with experience, they incorporate new rules and expand rules already acquired, in such a fashion that their speech becomes progressively a close approximation to the syntactic structure characteristic of adult speech. After the age of 6 years, children are able to engage in a long conversation with family members and their peers. They can perform simple tasks in command. At 7 years of age, children are able to express their thoughts in speech and writing.

As the number of children raised in bilingual or multilingual families increases, paediatricians should have some knowledge of the normal patterns of bilingual language acquisition. A child may acquire two languages simultaneously with an initial undifferentiated simple language composed of elements from both languages. By 2–3 years of age, the child begins to differentiate the two languages. The child can use the appropriate language when speaking to a particular person or in a particular environment (e.g., home or school). Normal children in bilingual families can also acquire the two languages in a sequential manner. In this situation, the first or dominant language is acquired first in the usual manner and then the children develop an understanding of the second language drawing on the experience with the first language. There may be a period of selective mutism before the child can switch from one language to the other proficiently. Bilingualism may contribute to delay in language development, but it is not a cause of disorder of language or cognitive development. Parents should be consistent in setting the boundaries for where each language is spoken.

Social Development

By 4 weeks of age, babies show social smile in response to the caregiver and enjoyment to cuddling, bathing and the voice of the mother. At 6 months of age, a baby is able to finger-feed and is more wary of strangers. A child can drink from a cup with help and enjoy songs and nursery rhymes at 9 months of age. They also desire a comfort object (such as a soft toy, cloth or blanket) and become anxious when they are separated from their caregivers (separation anxiety). Babies can play pat-a-cake or wave bye-bye and show affection to family members towards the end of the first year. At 18 months, they can feed themselves with a spoon and they can feed themselves properly using knife and fork at 4 years. The age of achievement of bladder and bowel control is variable, but is usually towards the end of the second year of life, but bedwetting at night can persist into mid- or late childhood. Beyond 2 years of age, children are increasingly mobile and are curious and interested in exploring their environment. They can help with dressing and bathing. They can manage to use the toilet independently by age of 3 years. At the age of 4 years, they can groom and dress themselves and brush their teeth. At age of 18 months, children are contented to play by themselves; at 2 years of age, they still play alone or alongside other children (parallel play). At 3 years of age, they start playing with other children and start making friends. They share toys and develop the concept of being helpful to others.

Emotional and Cognitive Development

Soon after birth, a baby demonstrates a keen interest in human faces and voices. They also become aware of other sensations such as hunger and noxious stimuli and respond to unpleasant sensations by crying. Even at 1 month, a baby exhibits different dimensions of behaviour such as activity, placidity, irritability, excitability and anger regulation that is commonly referred to as temperament. Infants with different temperament are at increased risk of behavioural problems in later life. The bonding of a baby with the parents depends on the baby's temperament and the personality, sensitivity and caring nature of the parents. At 6 months of age, a baby already becomes aware of the emotional state of the parents or caregiver through their actions and their voices. Secure attachment relationship between infant and mother, and to a certain extent with fathers and caregivers, is established towards the end of the first year of life. Secure mother–infant bonding buffers a baby against the short-term influence of adverse psychosocial effects in childhood development. By 1 year of age, infants start to develop their own sense of identity. They have fluctuating moods and occasionally throw temper tantrums, but also show affection towards familiar people. In the next 2–3 years, young children become increasingly aware of other people's intention, desires and emotions. They begin to show empathy (comfort a crying baby). They are inquisitive and constantly ask questions. They recognise primary colours (30 months) and begin to grasp the concept of numbers and time. They play and communicate with other children. They have increased memory capacity and reasoning and problem-solving skills. They can remember and give an account of past events. Children learn by observing and experiencing repeated stimuli and social situations, imitating and experimenting with speech and actions. They apply a set of concrete rules for exploring and interacting with the outside world. Their ability to appreciate logical arguments improves with age. They become aware of their body image and develop self-esteem. Their self-concept becomes differentiated and they begin to realize that they are not always competent in different developmental domains. During middle childhood, children further develop their fundamental skills of reading, writing, mathematics, long-term memory and recall. They are able to comprehend complex instructions. Significant amount of learning is acquired during the school hours. Adolescence is the period of transition from childhood to mature adulthood with physical maturation and acquisition of reproductive capability, and socioeconomic independence from the family. With the increasing number of young people entering into tertiary education, this period of adolescent development has been lengthened in the developed world. Adolescents become increasingly competent in logical and scientific reasoning, and these abilities are reflected in their ability to analyse and solve problems in mathematics and science, and formulate arguments and opinions in different fields of study. They are able to think in abstract terms and develop an understanding of issues such as responsibility, morality, peer relationships and sexuality.

DEVELOPMENT ASSESSMENT

A comprehensive child health assessment would not be complete without a proper developmental history, examination and assessment of emotion and mental well-being of the child. To obtain a developmental history of children, ask the parents open-ended questions and to elaborate on developmental concerns, if any, and provide them examples of their concerns. A paediatrician should be able to identify 'developmental red flags' (**Box 2.1**), developmental delay, disordered developmental sequence and developmental regression. Observations and interactive assessment in different developmental domains (gross motor, fine motor, visuospatial coordination, language and speech, emotion and social behaviour, cognition, hearing and vision) should be carried out. After assessment, a profile of developmental abilities and difficulties should form the basis for the necessity of referral for multidisciplinary specialist assessments by developmental paediatrician, psychologist and speech, physiological and occupational therapists.

Intelligence tests have been used to assess the innate cognitive ability and to indicate deficiencies of different domains of development in a child who is struggling and underachieving in school. The Wechsler Intelligence Scale for Children (WISC III and IV) is one of the most widely used intelligence quotient (IQ) tests and has been translated into many languages and validated. Some Wechsler

BOX 2.1 Developmental 'red flags' in infancy and early childhood.

- No visual following by 8 weeks and poor eye contact
- Uncoordinated eye movements with head turning after 3 months
- Persistent fisting (especially with thumbs adducted across the palms beyond 3 months)
- No head control by 6 months
- Not sitting independently by 10 months
- Unable to walk alone at 18 months
- No pointing to show demand or interest by 14 months
- No words with meaning by 18 months
- Not joining two words by 30 months
- Features of pervasive developmental disorders (compulsive and ritualistic activities, severe language delay, poorly developed social relationship, abnormal attachment to inanimate objects, inappropriate affect and tantrums, developmental delay)

subtests do not require skills in English and may be used to address referrals of non-English speaking children for certain developmental problems. The tests provide four index scores reflecting verbal comprehension, perceptual reasoning, working memory and processing speed. An IQ test is the first step towards the assessment of specific learning disabilities and the provision of support and intervention for children with difficulties in schools. A high IQ score, however, does not guarantee future success in life. Children with an uneven developmental profile on IQ testing require further specialist neuropsychological assessment using specialised test instruments for memory, visuospatial skills, language, attention, motor skills, social cognitive and planning and execution of tasks.

In recent years, there has been an increasing demand for paediatricians to develop skills in dealing with children with behavioural and emotional disorders. Measurements of behavioural and emotional well-being, and adjustment in children and their family members can be achieved using the child behaviour checklist for parents, teachers and older children. Paediatricians should be aware of common presentations of such disorders and have some knowledge of neuropsychological test instruments for the assessment of childhood depression, anxiety, obsessive-compulsive, attention deficit hyperactivity disorders, eating disorders and conduct disorders. These conditions have been discussed in greater details under the different chapters of this book.

REFERENCES

1. Karlberg J, Engström I, Karlberg P, Fryer JG. Analysis of linear growth using a mathematical model. I. From birth to three years. Acta Paediatr Scand. 1987;76(3):478-88.
2. World Health Organization. WHO global database on child growth and malnutrition. [online]. Available from http://www.who.int/nutgrowthdb/en/ [Accessed July 2013].
3. WHO Child Growth Standards. Acta Paediatrica Scandinavica. 2006;(Supp 450):1-106.
4. Centers for Disease Control and Prevention. (2010). Growth Charts. [online] Available from www.cdc.gov/growth charts [Accessed July 2013].
5. Cole TJ, Bellizzi MC, Flegal, KM, Dietz WH. Establishing a standard definition for child overweight and obesity worldwide: international survey. Br Med J. 2000;320(7244):1240-3.
6. Fisher RA. The correlation between relatives on the supposition of Mendelian Inheritance. Transactions of the Royal Society of Edinburgh. 1918;52:399-433.
7. Gardner LI (Ed). Endocrine and genetic diseases of childhood and adolescence. Philadelphia: WB Saunders Company; 1975.

CHAPTER 3

Neonatal Medicine

Elaine M. Balmer, Suzie Wills, Helen Mactier

INTRODUCTION

The neonatal period covers birth through the first 28 days of life. Conditions presenting in the neonatal period may conveniently be divided into those conditions affecting all infants regardless of gestation and complications specific to preterm birth. The relative importance of each category for the workload of a neonatal unit will depend on geographical location and local (or national) arrangements for provision of neonatal care.

Preterm birth is defined as birth before 37 completed weeks of gestation, with gestation defined traditionally from the first date of the last menstrual period and thus more strictly described as menstrual age.[1] With advent of near-universal ultrasound dating of early and/or mid-pregnancy, gestation is fairly certain for the vast majority of women, at least in developed countries; when gestation is in doubt, reasonably accurate clinical assessment of gestation may be made by a combination of external appearance and muscular tone and positioning, according to predefined criteria **(Fig. 3.1)**.[2]

Neonatal mortality and morbidity follow a U-shaped curve and are increased for both preterm and post-mature

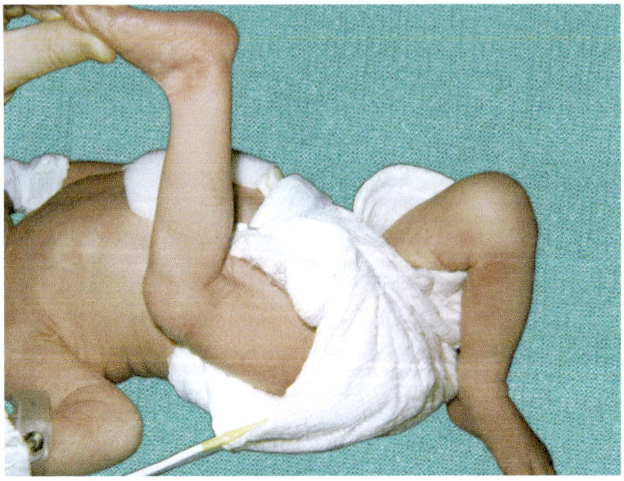

Figure 3.1 Clinical assessment of gestation.

(delivered after 42 completed weeks' gestation) babies.[3] Induction of labour after 40 weeks' gestation reduces the risk of perinatal death, although the absolute risk is very low [number needed to treat, 410].[4] Both preterm and post-term birth are associated with behavioural and emotional problems in early childhood, especially attention deficit/hyperactivity problem behaviour but the mechanism of this, particularly for post-mature infants, remains to be elucidated.[5]

Several terms are used to describe pregnancy outcome, national health and the outcome of neonatal care:

Infant mortality = number of deaths before 1 year of age per 1,000 liveborn children

Perinatal mortality = number of still births and deaths within the first 7 days per 1,000 total births

Neonatal mortality = number of deaths in the first 28 days of life per 1,000 live births. Neonatal mortality can be divided into early (≤7 days) and late (8–28 days) mortality, but these differences have become blurred which promotes longer survival of the sickest and most pre-term infants.

In utero growth is determined by many factors, including maternal health and nutritional status as well as hypertension, cigarette smoking and/or substance misuse. Foetal growth can be compromised by intrauterine infection, e.g. rubella or toxoplasmosis, chromosomal abnormality and multiple pregnancy. Low birth weight is defined by the World Health Organization as less than 2,500 g at birth regardless of gestation, and needs to be distinguished from intrauterine growth restriction (IUGR) (failure to achieve genetic growth potential) and small for gestational age (birth weight below the 10th percentile for gestational age). Since birth weight is influenced by maternal stature and ethnicity, foetal growth is best assessed by use of customised birth weight charts.[6] Postnatal growth should be assessed by use of the WHO growth charts, which were updated in 2006 following the WHO Multicentre Growth Reference

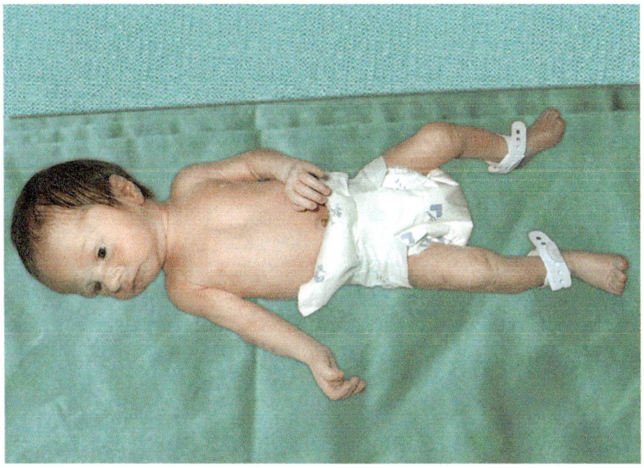

Figure 3.2 Symmetrical intrauterine growth restriction.

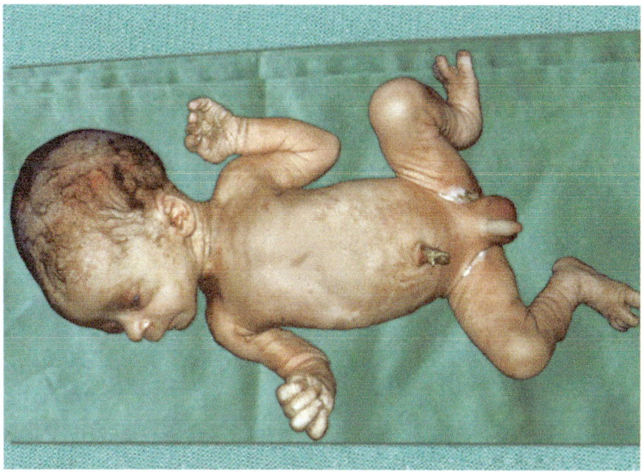

Figure 3.3 Asymmetrical intrauterine growth restriction.

Study implemented between 1997 and 2003.[7] For infants born before completing 37 weeks' gestation, birth weight and subsequent growth should be plotted on a preterm growth chart, such as the UK-WHO Neonatal and Infant Close Monitoring Chart, appropriate to the infant's sex (Figs. 3.2 to 3.4).[8]

GENERAL ASSESSMENT OF THE NEWBORN

Examination of a newborn infant can conveniently be divided into immediate post-birth assessment and the routine examination of the newborn.

Post-birth Examination

Examination of the infant immediately after delivery should assess if resuscitation is required and ascertain if there are any factors likely to have immediate consequences for the infant such as significant prematurity or major congenital abnormality. The eponym Apgar score was first described in 1953 as an objective means of assessing the condition of the newborn[9]; although now commonly replaced by a simplified assessment of heart rate, breathing, tone and colour,[10] the Apgar score remains useful in indicating the severity of distress at birth and in predicting longer-term outcome.[11] On an individual basis, however, the infant's condition at birth is of limited prognostic value and outcome is more related to response to resuscitation and the subsequent neonatal course (Table 3.1).

Heart rate at birth can be assessed either with a stethoscope or by palpating for a pulse at the base of the umbilical cord; absence of a palpable pulse should be confirmed by auscultation. Infants who are pink with a heart rate above 100 beats per minute and who are breathing regularly do not need active intervention, nor suctioning of the airway. They should be dried and, whenever possible, given to their mother for skin-to-skin contact and initiation of breastfeeding. If the infant has not established spontaneous respiration, or if the infant remains blue and/or bradycardia persists, then basic resuscitation should be commenced (vide infra).

Routine Examination of the Newborn

This clinical assessment should include top-to-toe physical examination, with particular emphasis on auscultation of the heart, palpation of the abdomen and examination of the eyes, genitalia and hips. Routine examination of the newborn may be undertaken by any suitably trained person, including midwife or doctor, and affords an opportunity to enquire about familial conditions likely to have implications for the newborn and to offer support to new parents. It is ideally conducted before 72 hours of life.[12]

TABLE 3.1 The Apgar scoring system.[6]

Score	*0*	*1*	*2*
Heart rate (beats per minute)	0	<100	>100
Respiratory rate	Absent	Slow, irregular, weak cry	Good, vigorous cry
Muscle tone	Flaccid, limp	Some flexion of extremities	Good flexion, active motion
Reflex irritability	No response	Weak cry and grimace	Vigorous cry, cough, sneeze
Skin colour	Blue	Acrocyanosis	Pink

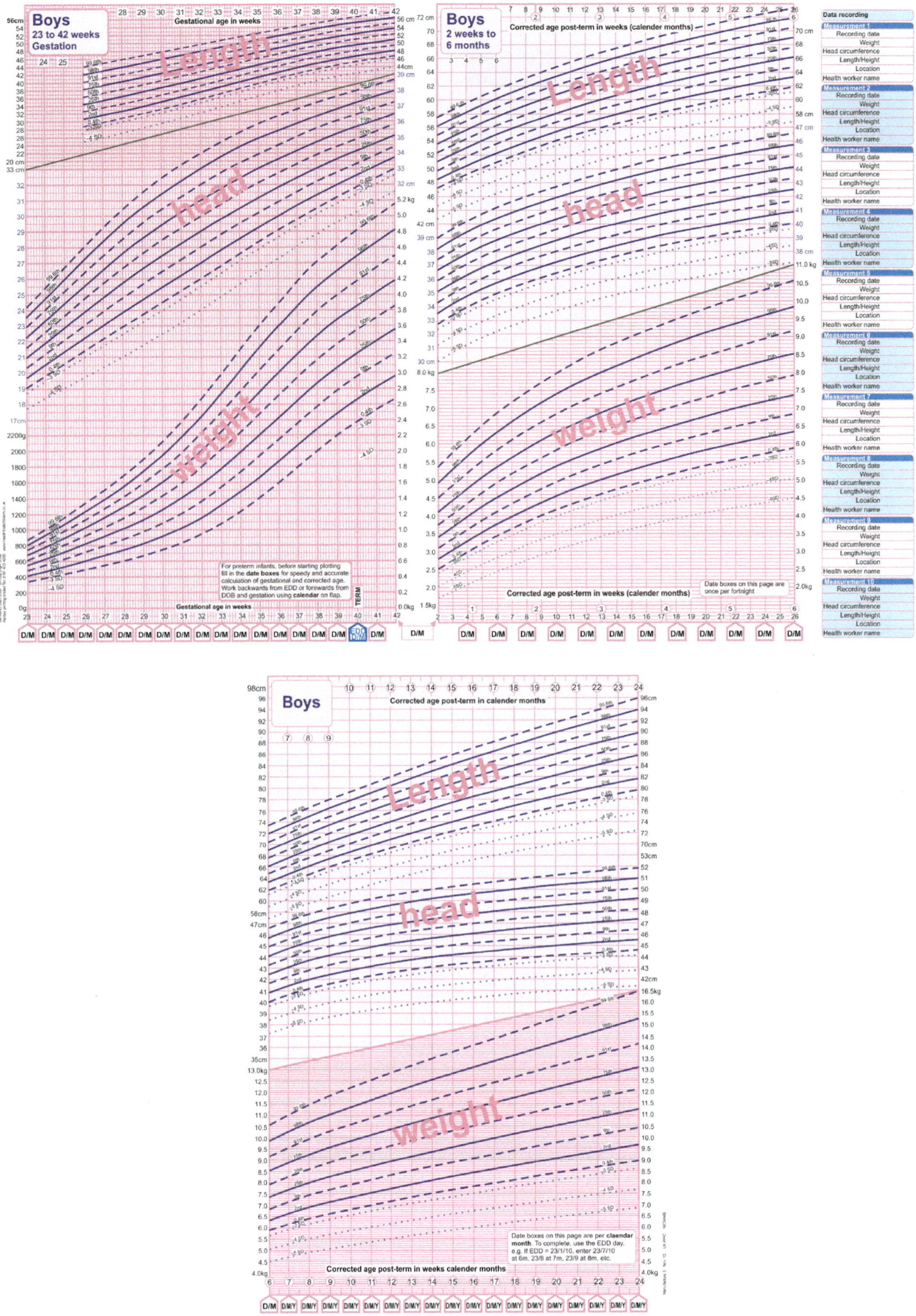

Figure 3.4 Growth chart—UK-WHO Neonatal and Infant Close Monitoring Chart.

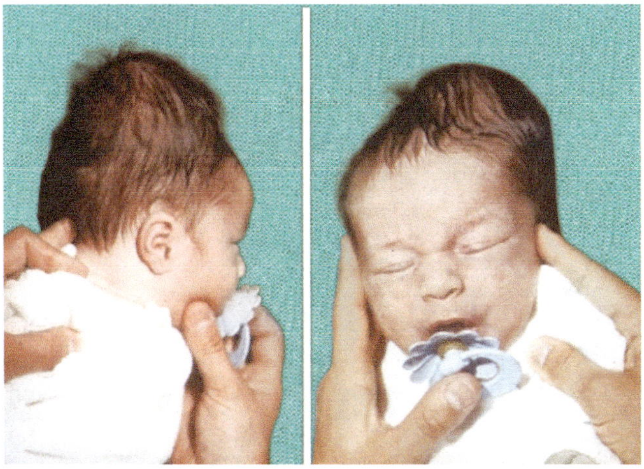

Figure 3.5 Caput succedaneum.

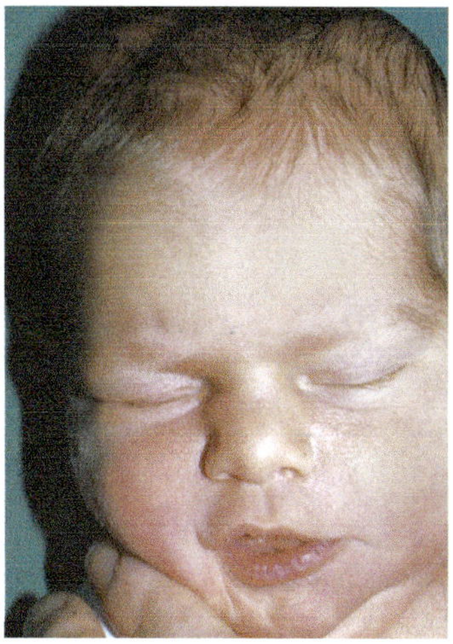

Figure 3.6 Bilateral cephalhaematoma.

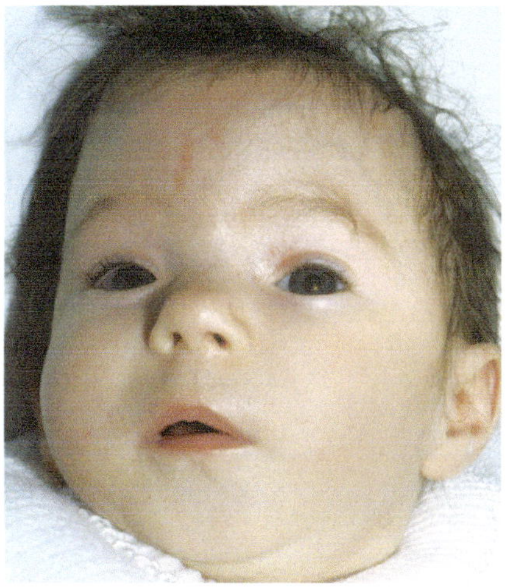

Figure 3.7 Foetal alcohol syndrome.

Although full clinical examination will require that the infant is naked, it is important that the infant is as quiet as possible, and so it is often useful to auscultate the heart sounds and check the red reflexes before the infant is disturbed by being fully undressed.

Scalp

Head shape should be noted, and the head circumference measured and plotted on a standardised, sex-specific growth chart. The anterior fontanelle should be patent; the posterior fontanelle is also commonly palpable in the newborn. Some skull moulding is usual after a vaginal delivery; caput succedaneum is a serosanguinous, subcutaneous, extraperiosteal fluid collection with poorly defined margins caused by pressure of the presenting part of the scalp against the dilating cervix. Caput succedaneum extends across the midline, crossing over suture lines, and usually resolves within a few days **(Fig. 3.5)**.

Cephalhaematoma results from bleeding between the skull and the periosteum, generally in the parietal region and usually associated with prolonged or instrumental delivery. Cephalhaematoma may be bilateral; the swelling does not cross the suture lines **(Fig. 3.6)**. An underlying associated skull fracture is rare. Resolution of a cephalhaematoma may take several weeks as the blood clot is absorbed from the periphery towards the centre, and parents should be counselled that the swelling will harden, leaving a slightly softer area in the centre. Early and exaggerated neonatal jaundice is a common consequence.

A chignon may be evident in infants delivered by vacuum extraction. This should resolve within a few hours to several days. Rarely, vacuum extraction may be complicated by subaponeurotic haemorrhage.

Face and Mouth

The overall appearance of the face may be indicative of congenital abnormality, and this should be described in terms of the specific features, e.g. hypertelorism, low set ears, long thin philtrum. Sometimes, a constellation of features will point to a specific diagnosis, such as Down or Alpert syndrome, or may suggest exposure to a single teratogen such as alcohol or sodium valproate **(Fig. 3.7)**. When the appearance of the infant is unusual and no immediate diagnosis comes to mind, comparison should be made with both parents.

Cleft lip (cheiloschisis) will be immediately evident; cleft palate (palatoschisis) can only be excluded after direct visual inspection of the palate **(Fig. 3.8)**.

Epstein pearls, or palatal cysts of the newborn, are small (1–3 mm) white or yellow cystic vesicles commonly seen in the median palatal raphe of the mouth. They will resolve spontaneously over the first few weeks of life.

Natal teeth may be present and will require to be removed; if not securely fixed within the gum, this should be undertaken as soon as possible **(Fig. 3.9)**.

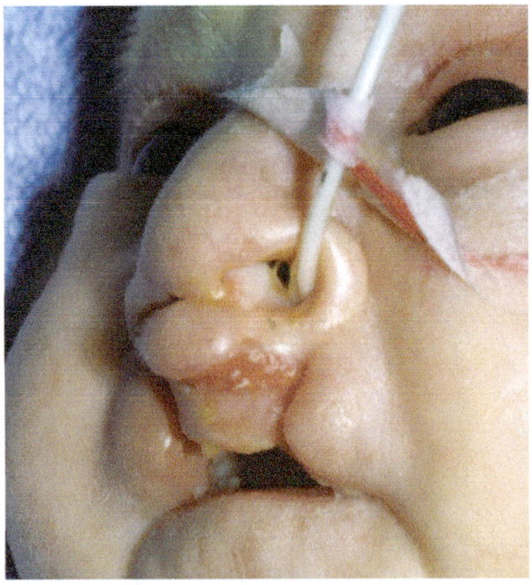

Figure 3.8 Bilateral cleft lip.

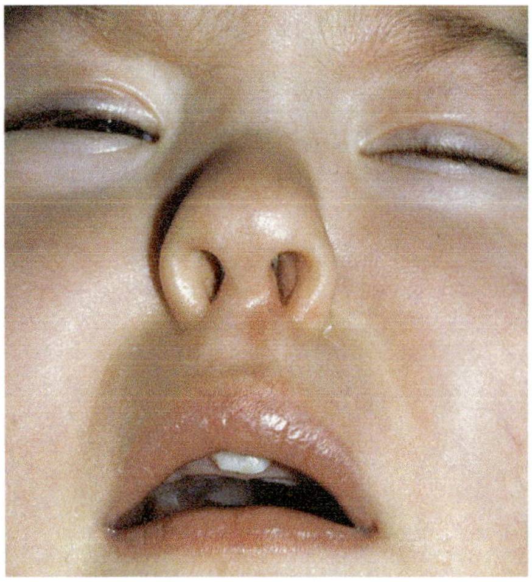

Figure 3.9 Natal teeth.

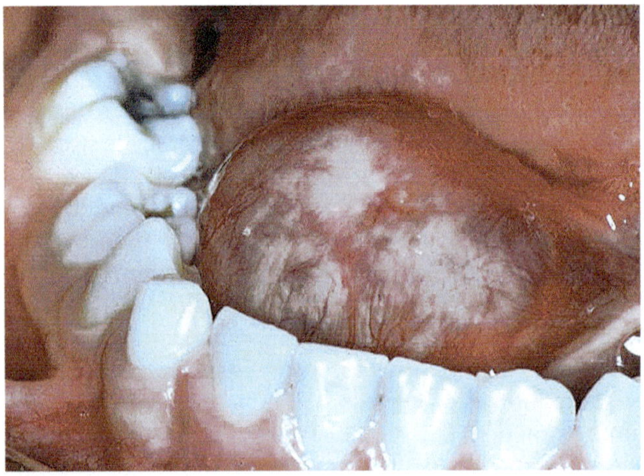

Figure 3.10 Ranula. (*See* Fig. 19.52.)

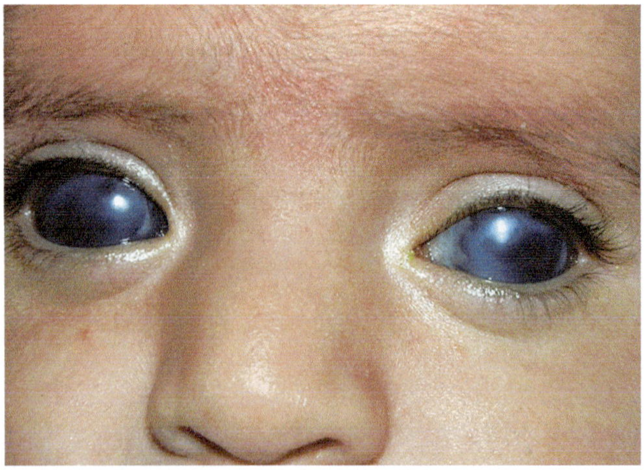

Figure 3.11 Cloudy corneas.

(*Source:* Baiyeroju A, Bowman R, Gilbert C, et al. Managing eye health in young children. Community Eye Health. 2010;23(72):4-11.)

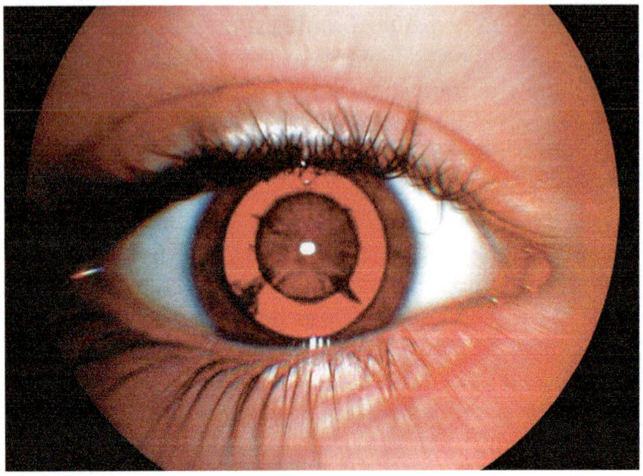

Figure 3.12 Dilated pupil with cataract visible as a black shadow obstructing the red reflex.

(*Source:* Baiyeroju A, Bowman R, Gilbert C, et al. Managing eye health in young children. Community Eye Health. 2010;23(72):4-11.)

A ranula is a mucocele which is usually confined to the floor of the mouth. This swelling is benign, but will require surgical excision **(Fig. 3.10)**.

Eyes

Subconjunctival haemorrhage is common and self-resolving; blue discolouration is associated with osteogenesis imperfecta. Yellow sclerae are indicative of significant neonatal jaundice (which may be difficult to assess in a dark-skinned infant) and should prompt measurement of serum bilirubin. Cloudy corneas suggest congenital glaucoma or inherited metabolic disorder **(Fig. 3.11)**.

It is essential that a red reflex is demonstrated in each eye to exclude cataract or retinoblastoma. Both of these conditions require prompt ophthalmology referral **(Fig. 3.12)**.

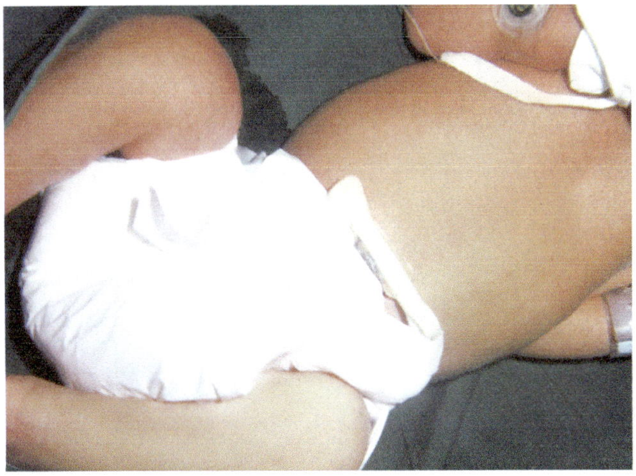

Figure 3.13 Harlequin colour change.

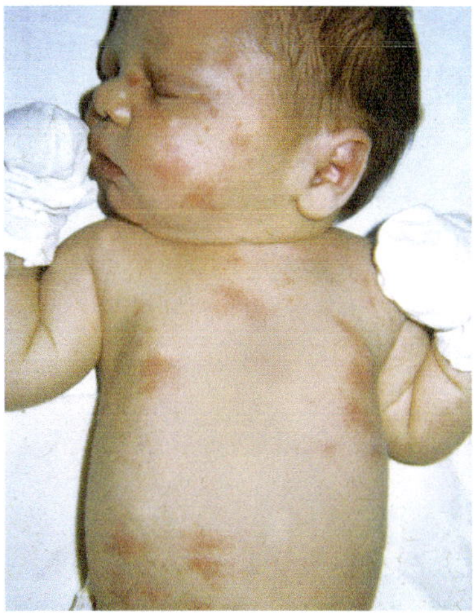

Figure 3.14 Erythema toxicum.

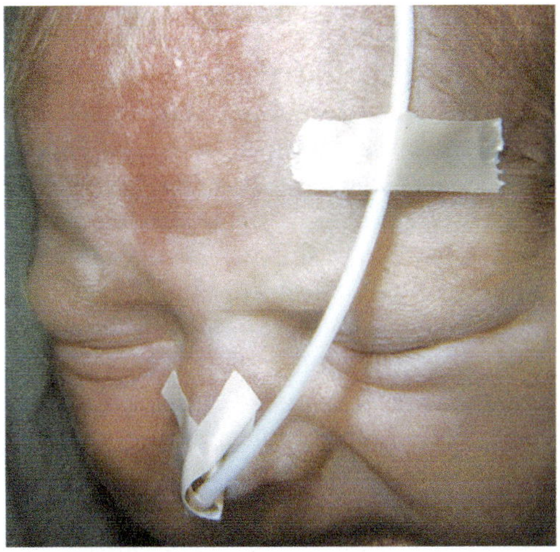

Figure 3.15 Salmon patch.

Skin

Physiological skin changes are commonly seen in the newborn, and may cause unnecessary alarm. Cutis marmorata describes a normal physiological response to cold with a characteristic bluish mottling seen on the extremities and trunk. Harlequin colour change is seen as a transient erythema involving one half of the infant's body with simultaneous blanching of the other side, strictly demarcated in the midline. This unusual vascular phenomenon is thought to be due to immaturity of the hypothalamic centre controlling dilation of peripheral blood vessels; it resolves with crying or movement and does not require treatment **(Fig. 3.13)**.

Milia are tiny white spots that occur on the faces of around 50% of newborn babies, most often on the nose and cheeks. They represent collections of secretions from immature sweat glands and will resolve spontaneously, usually by 1–2 months of age. Erythema toxicum is an extremely common rash that appears within the first few days of life, presenting as erythematous macules with white/yellow coloured vesicles. The vesicles contain eosinophils. Parents should be reassured that the rash will disappear and that no treatment is required **(Fig. 3.14)**.

Neonatal pustular melanosis presents at birth with small, flaccid, superficial fragile pustules. Commonly, some of the pustules will already have ruptured in utero, leaving pigmented macules. The macules tend to fade over 3–4 weeks. All areas of the body may be affected. This benign condition is more common in black-skinned infants; recognition is important to avoid unnecessary investigation and treatment.

Vascular naevi are due to abnormal blood vessels in the skin. They vary in severity and permanence; hence, accurate diagnosis is important. The most common of the vascular birthmarks, occurring in around 50% of newborns, are salmon patches or stork bites. These fine capillary haemangiomas are visible as flat, deep red areas on the eyelids, bridge of nose, upper lip and nape of neck, and tend to darken in colour when the baby cries. Most fade during the first 6–12 months, although areas on the nape of the neck may persist. No treatment is required **(Fig. 3.15)**.

Port-wine stains are large, flat, deep purple/red lesions, which may occur on any part of the body. The incidence is about 3 per 1,000 births; males and females and all racial groups are equally affected. The lesions are due to lack of small nerves that normally control constriction of blood vessels. Lesions appear dark pink, smooth and flat in the neonatal period, but become darker with thickening of the overlying skin as the child ages. Port-wine stains tend to affect only one side of the body, most commonly on the face and upper trunk **(Fig. 3.16)**. Lesions in the distribution of the trigeminal nerve may be associated with retinal and intracranial haemorrhages, and ophthalmological assessment is required. Associated vascular malformations of the ipsilateral meninges and cerebral cortex occur in Sturge-Weber syndrome, which may be complicated

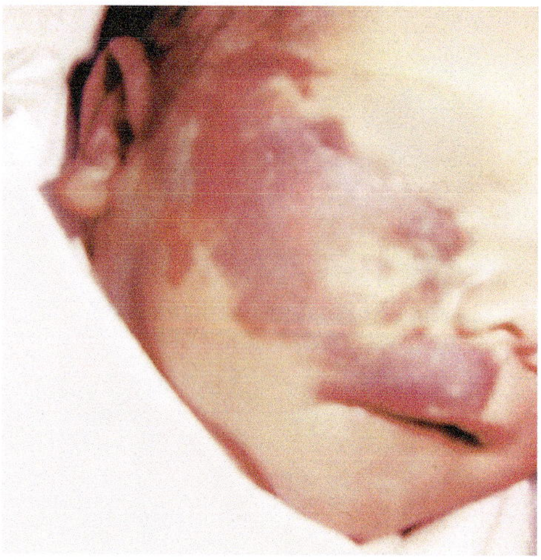

Figure 3.16 Port-wine stain.

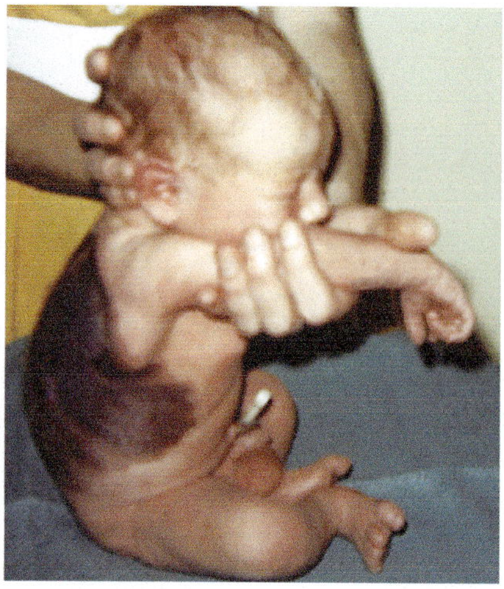

Figure 3.17 Congenital melanocytic naevus.

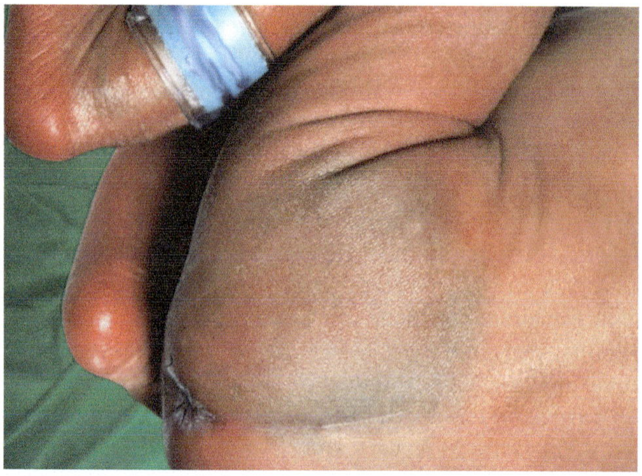

Figure 3.18 Mongolian blue spot. (*See* Fig. 1.38.)

by seizures and neurological disability. Port-wine stains may be improved with laser treatment as an alternative to camouflage make-up.

Pigmented birthmarks include congenital melanocytic naevi, which occur in 1–6% of newborns.[13] These naevi can be present on any part of the body as circumscribed, light brown to black patches, heterogeneous in size and consistency. They may be hairy and tend to grow in proportion to the infant's growth. Larger melanocytic naevi have the potential to become malignant, and require regular dermatological review **(Fig. 3.17)**.

Mongolian blue spots are flat, bluish-coloured lesions representing a collection of melanocytes in the dermis. They are most commonly seen in the lumbosacral area in oriental and black infants and can be single or multiple. Mongolian blue spots tend to fade as the infant gets older; accurate documentation at birth can be useful if concerns are raised later regarding bruising injury. No treatment is necessary **(Fig. 3.18)**.

Cardiovascular System

Examination of the cardiovascular system begins with inspection, looking for respiratory distress and/or cyanosis. The apical impulse is normally felt in the fifth intercostal space in the mid-clavicular line, and both brachial and femoral pulses should be palpable. Difficulty feeling the femoral pulses should prompt urgent exclusion of coarctation of the aorta. The normal predominance of the right ventricle in the neonatal period may be evident as mild parasternal heave during the early hours of life, particularly if there is clinical evidence of persisting pulmonary hypertension. Thrills are unusual, and will be accompanied by a loud murmur. Murmurs are common in the first day or two of life, often reflecting delayed closure of the ductus arteriosus, and significant cardiac pathology may be present without a murmur. Oxygen saturation in a healthy term infant breathing room air should be greater than 90% by 10 minutes of age and above 94% by 24 hours of age; since lower saturations may not be clinically evident, routine post-ductal oxygen saturation monitoring as a means of early detection of congenital heart disease is becoming a recommended standard of care.[14] It should be noted that this test is considerably more costly than clinical examination alone, and that the cost effectiveness for an individual facility will depend, among other factors, on the rate of antenatal detection.

Respiratory System

The healthy newborn is an obligate nasal breather, and relies on diaphragmatic excursion for effective respiration. Normal respiration should be quiet, at a rate of 40to 60 breaths per minute. Tachypnoea may reflect respiratory disease, sepsis or systemic illness, and should never be ignored.

Abdomen

The abdomen should be soft, with no palpable masses. The liver is normally palpable 1 cm below the liver edge;

hepatomegaly may be isolated or associated with splenomegaly (e.g. severe haemolysis, congenital infection, metabolic disease). Autosomal recessive polycystic kidney disease may present as bilateral masses. Divarication of the rectus abdominal muscles is a benign condition, which should improve with age; similarly, umbilical herniae will generally resolve spontaneously within the first year **(Fig. 3.19)**. Careful inspection of the anus is important, as rarely meconium may be passed through a rectovaginal fistula in female children with imperforate anus **(Figs. 3.20A and B)**.

Genitalia

In males, the scrotum may be enlarged due to a hydrocoele or inguinal hernia. The former will transilluminate (more easily visible in a darkened room) and is expected to resolve within the first few weeks **(Fig. 3.21)**.

An inguinal hernia should be reducible with gentle pressure; a tender and non-reducible groin swelling requires urgent surgical attention **(Fig. 3.22)**.

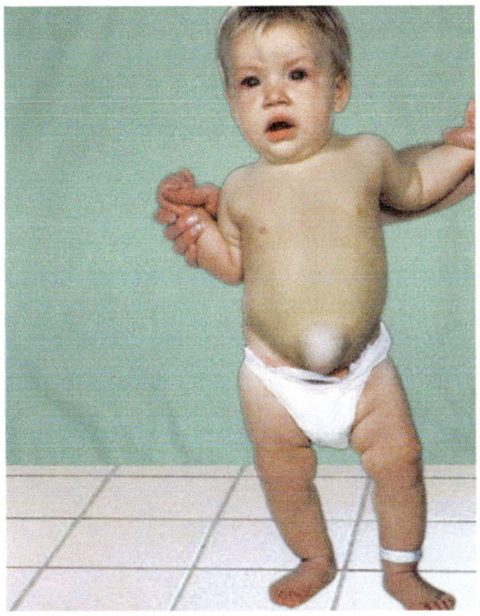

Figure 3.19 Umbilical hernia.

If neither testis can be felt in the scrotum or groin (and particularly if the penis is small or there is apparent hypospadias), urgent sex chromosomal analysis is indicated. Parents should be counselled not to name the child until the results are known **(Figs. 3.23A and B)**.

Unilateral undescended testis is not uncommon, particularly in preterm infants; the family should be advised to seek medical advice if both testes have not descended to the scrotum by 1 year of age. Pigmentation of the scrotum or labia is normal in babies whose parents are not white, but may be an early sign of congenital adrenal hyperplasia.

Hips

An important part of the newborn examination is screening for developmental dysplasia of the hip. Hips should abduct equally **(Fig. 3.24A)**, buttock and thigh creases **(Fig. 3.24B)** and leg length should be symmetrical. Leg length is best assessed by flexing the knees and placing the feet on a flat surface; the knees should be at an equal height. Ortolani manoeuvre will detect a congenitally dislocated hip; with the knees flexed at right angles, the hips should be slowly abducted from the midline position through 90° **(Fig. 3.24C)**. A dislocated hip will clunk back into place. If Ortolani test is negative, Barlow test should be performed to check for stability of the hip; with the hips and knees held flexed, gentle pressure is applied to front of the knee in an attempt to slide the femur backwards **(Fig. 3.24D)**. An unstable hip will dislocate out of the acetabulum. Babies with unstable hips should be referred for prompt orthopaedic assessment; the investigation of choice is ultrasound of the hips **(Figs. 3.25A and B)**.

Spine

The spine should be carefully examined to exclude any obvious deformity; hairy tufts or pits may be indicative of underlying spinal deficits. Spina bifida may present as either a closed or an open lesion; the clinical effects will depend on the site and extent of the lesion. Spina bifida

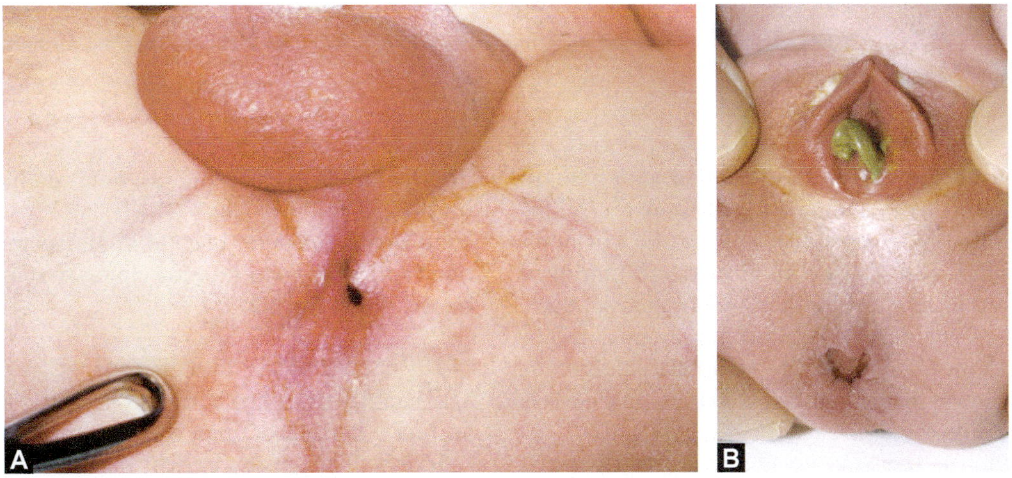

Figures 3.20A and B (A) Imperforate anus; (B) Imperforate anus with rectovaginal fistula.

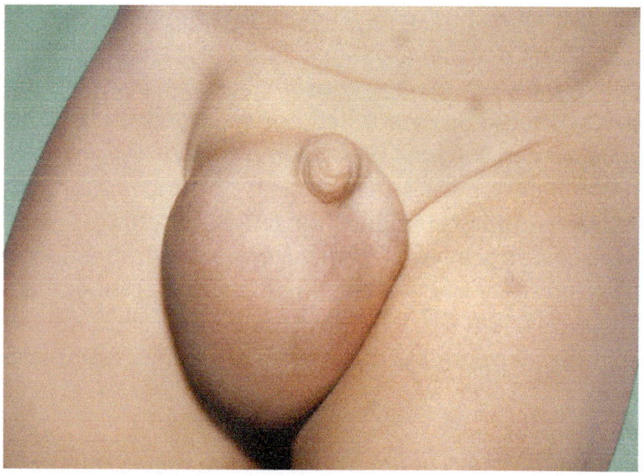

Figure 3.21 Hydrocoele.

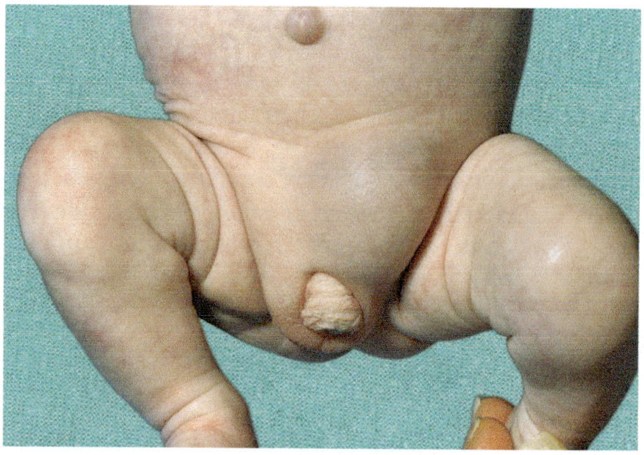

Figure 3.22 Inguinal hernia.

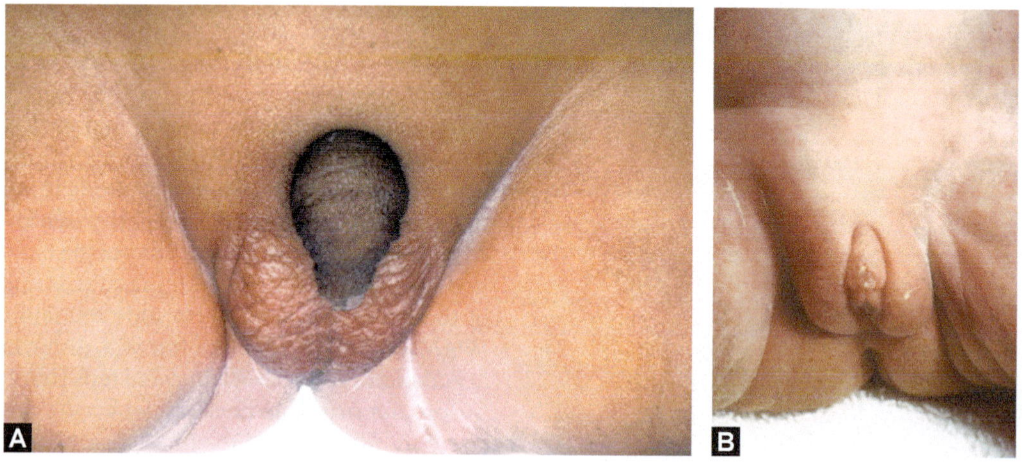

Figures 3.23A and B Ambiguous genitalia.

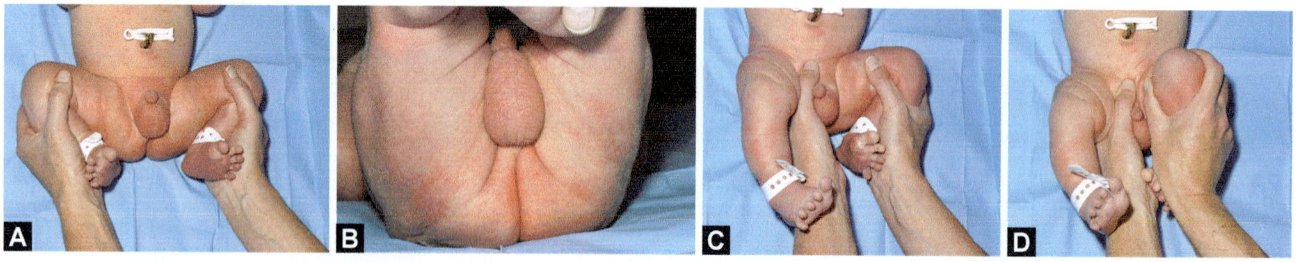

Figures 3.24A to D Clinical examination of hips.

occulta indicates a defect in the vertebral arch with an intact spinal cord and meninges. More extensive lesions may be indicated by an overlying patch of hair or other skin abnormality, and can be complicated by tethering of the spinal cord during childhood. In meningocele, there is herniation of the meninges through the bony defect in the spine and the lesion is covered with skin. Surgery is required but, since the spinal cord is spared, prognosis is usually good **(Fig. 3.26)**.

The situation is worse in myelomeningocele—spinal cord involvement leads to complications including lower limb paralysis, hydrocephalus, neuropathic bladder and bowel and kyphoscoliosis. The lesion is usually closed as soon as possible after birth to minimise the risk of infection, and long-term multidisciplinary management will be required **(Fig. 3.27)**.

Primitive Reflexes

The healthy term newborn will exhibit a flexed posture, and have periods of quiet wakefulness. Several primitive reflexes will be present from birth, gradually disappearing with the progress of normal development.

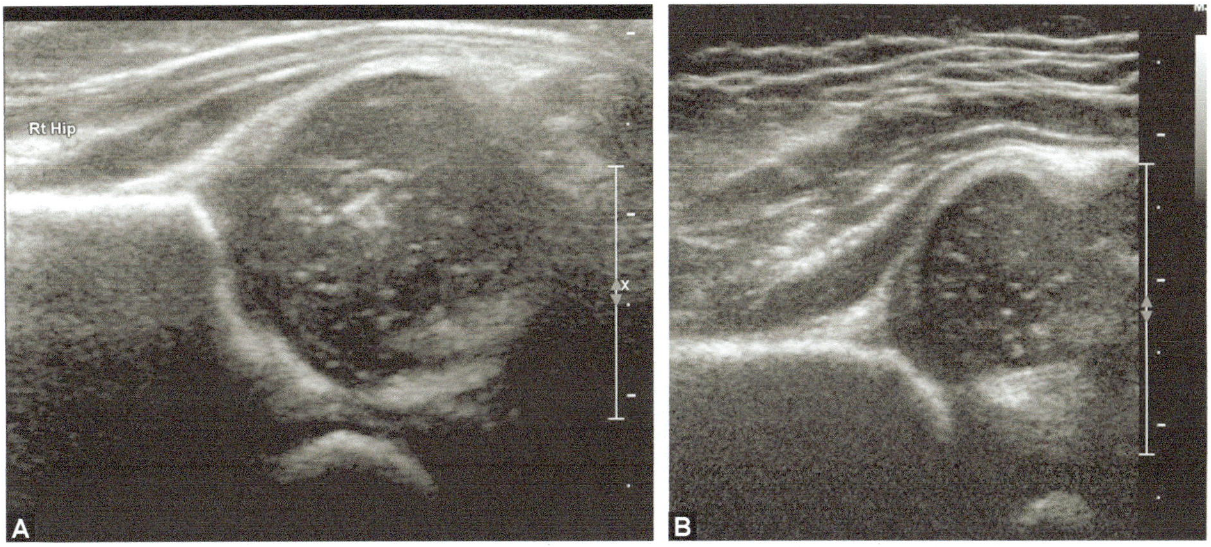

Figures 25A and B Hip ultrasound. (A) Normal right hip; (B) Decentred right hip.

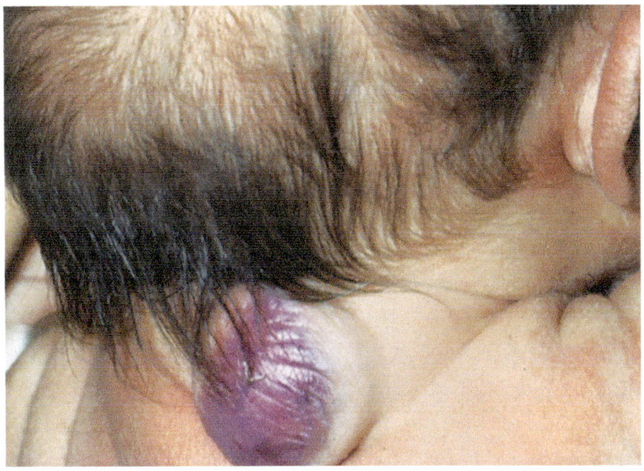

Figure 3.26 Meningocele.

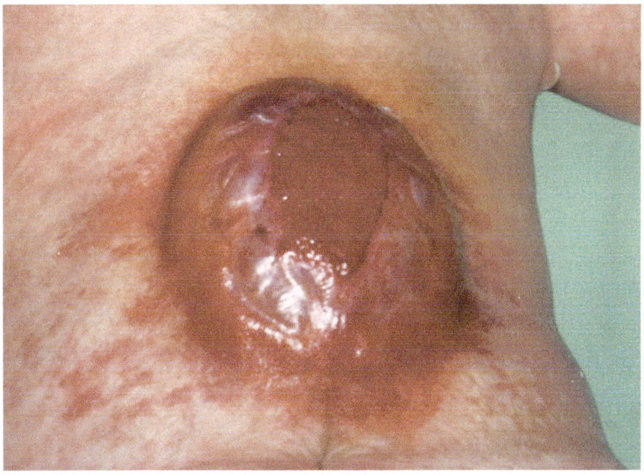

Figure 3.27 Myelomeningocele.

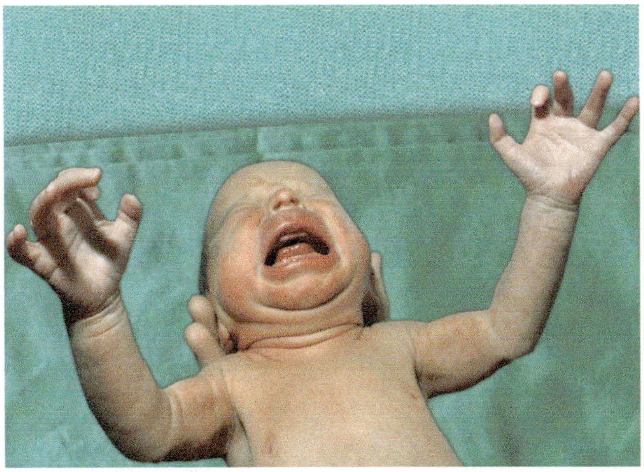

Figure 3.28 Moro response.

The Moro response, or embracing reflex, was described by Ernst Moro in 1918.[15] This reflex is present at birth, peaks in the first month of life, and generally disappears around 3 months of age. It is elicited by a sudden shift in position of the infant's head, generally by allowing the head to fall backwards while supporting the body. The legs and head extend and the arms jerk up and out with palms up and thumbs flexed before being brought together. The infant will then generally clench his hands and cry. Bilateral absence of the Moro response indicates damage to the central nervous system, while a unilateral absence suggests either a fractured clavicle or injury to the brachial plexus. It is postulated that in human evolution, the Moro reflex helped the infant cling to his mother while she carried him around all day by providing a reflex grasping onto his mother if the infant slipped **(Fig. 3.28)**.

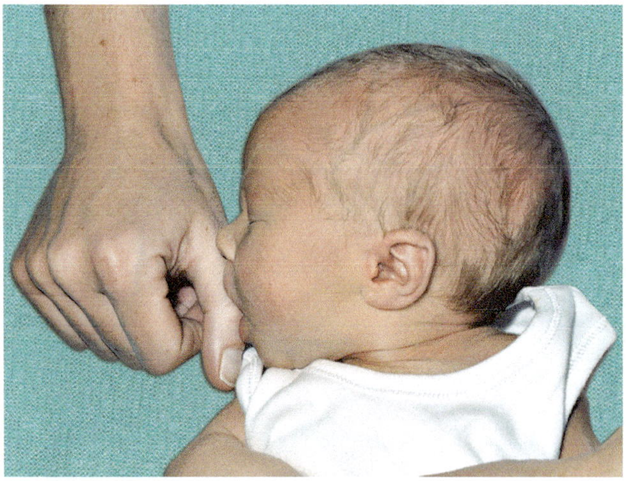

Figure 3.29 Rooting reflex.

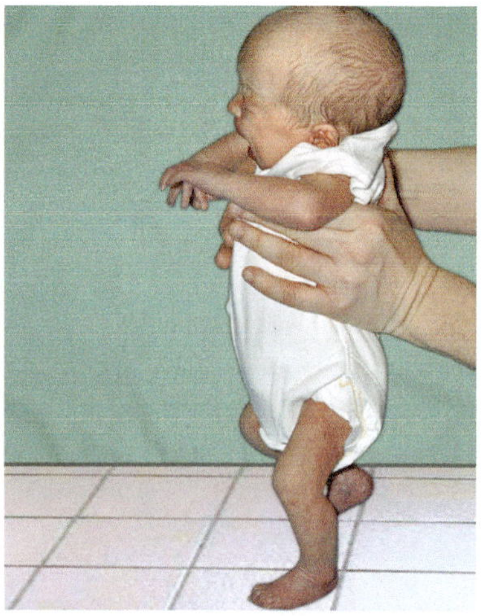

Figure 3.30 Stepping reflex.

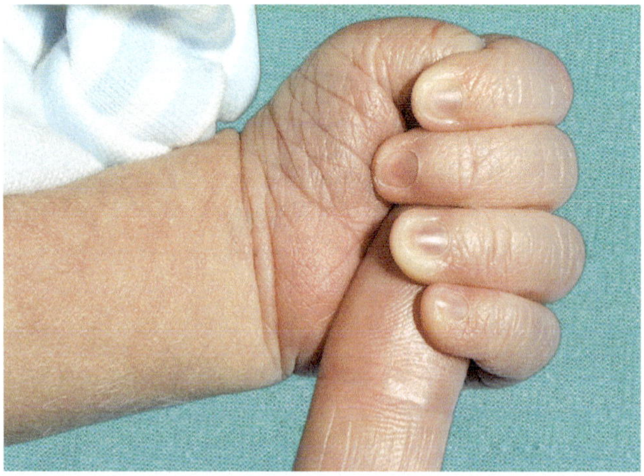

Figure 3.31 Palmar grasp.

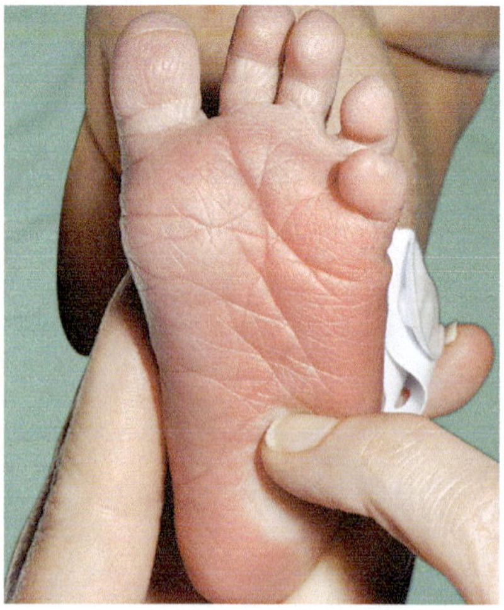

Figure 3.32 Positive Babinski sign.

The sucking and rooting reflexes also help the infant to survive by facilitating breastfeeding. The rooting reflex causes the newborn infant to turn his head towards anything that strokes his cheek or mouth; it disappears by 4 months of age, long after the breastfed infant has learned how to find his mother's nipple (Fig. 3.29).

When a newborn baby's feet are placed on a flat surface, he/she will instinctively put one foot in front of the other, thus appearing to walk, even though he cannot support his/her own weight. This primitive stepping reflex is short-lived, disappearing by around 6 weeks of age. It subsequently reappears as a voluntary action towards 1 year of age, prior to independent walking (Fig. 3.30).

The palmar grasp reflex is also present at birth and persists until 5 or 6 months of age. Grasping is elicited by either stroking the palm or placing an object into the infant's palm. The grasp is strong, but unpredictable in that it may be suddenly released. Stroking the back of the infant's clenched fist will induce opening of the hand (Fig. 3.31).

Reflecting immaturity of the corticospinal tracts, stroking the plantar surface of the foot in a newborn will elicit an extensor response or positive Babinski sign. This will be replaced by a flexor response by the age of 2 years (Fig. 3.32).

The other primitive reflex present at birth is the Galant reflex. This is elicited by stroking the skin along the side of the infant's back, following which he/she will swing towards the side that was stroked. This reflex disappears by 6 months of age. The tonic (or asymmetric) neck reflex is usually present between 1 and 4 months of age. When the child's head is turned to the side, the arm on that side will straighten and the opposite arm will bend, in the position of a fencer. Persistence of the reflex beyond 6 months suggests upper motor neuron dysfunction. The tonic neck reflex is thought to have an evolutionary function in preparing the infant for voluntary reaching (Fig. 3.33).

CONGENITAL ABNORMALITIES

Congenital abnormalities may result from a multitude of causes. Chromosomal non-disjunction during meiosis may result in either too many or too few chromosomes; common examples include trisomy 21 (Down syndrome)

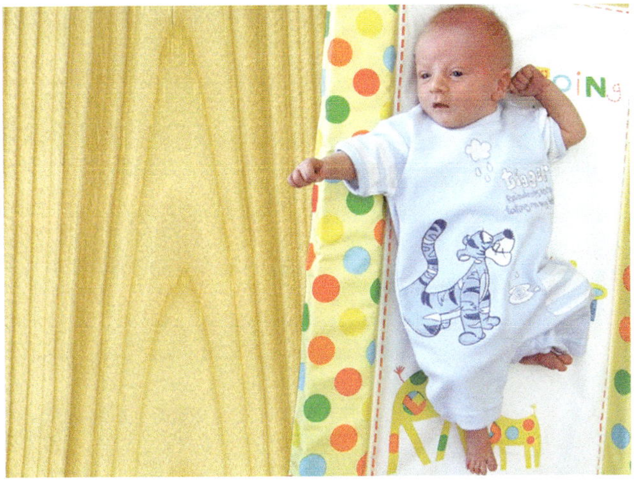

Figure 3.33 Tonic neck reflex.

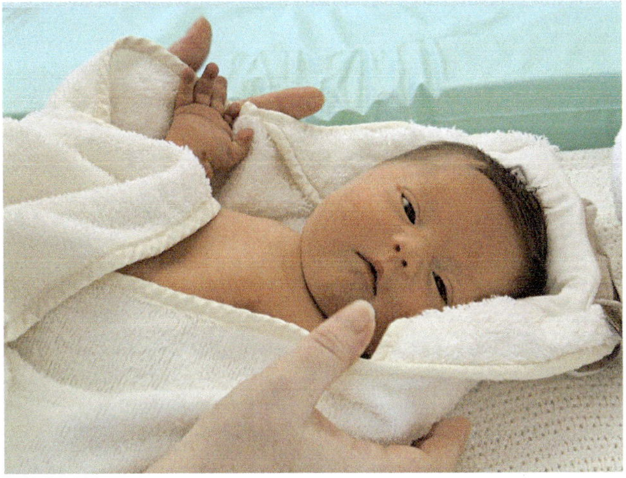

Figure 3.34 Down syndrome.

(*Courtesy:* Image courtesy of Down Syndrome, Scotland.)

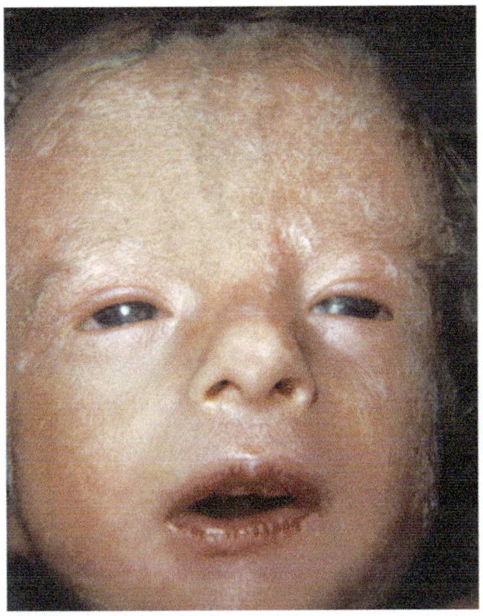

Figure 3.35 Edward syndrome facies.

and 45,XO (Turner syndrome). Partial deletion of a chromosome may occur (e.g. 1q21.1 deletion syndrome or 7q11 deletion William syndrome) or additional chromosomal material may be inherited (e.g. 22q11 duplication). Damage may occur to the developing embryo, either unexplained or as a result of vascular accident (e.g. transposition of the great arteries, holoprosencephaly, isolated limb abnormalities), or the developing embryo or foetus may be affected by an infectious organism [e.g. *Cytomegalovirus* (CMV)] or by toxins such as alcohol or prescription drugs (e.g. retinoic acid, sodium valproate). Single gene defects will manifest in one in four children born to apparently healthy parents who are asymptomatic carriers; the homozygous state occurs more commonly with consanguineous parents. Generally speaking, the earlier in pregnancy the insult occurs, the more devastating the consequences in terms of structural abnormality.

Whole Chromosomal Addition or Deletion

The most common three trisomies presenting at birth are 21 (Down syndrome), 18 (Edward syndrome), and 13 (Patau syndrome). These conditions are more common in older mothers, and are increasingly diagnosed by antenatal screening, with termination of pregnancy an option for affected pregnancies. The prognosis varies, being worse for trisomy 13 and 18, the majority of whom die within the first year.

Down Syndrome

Described by John Langdon Down in 1866, trisomy 21 is the most common genetic condition in human. Affected individuals have a typical facies, with epicanthic folds, flat nasal bridge, protruding tongue and low set ears with brachycephaly. Other common features include hypotonia, clinodactyly, sandal gap, and Brushfield spots. The incidence of congenital heart disease is up to 50%, with atrioventricular or ventricular septal defects most common. Learning disability is universal, ranging from mild to moderate and is reflected in delayed gross motor and speech development. Weight gain may be problematic in the neonatal period because of poor feeding, but obesity is common in later life. All children with Down syndrome will manifest stunted longitudinal growth, with final adult height averaging 154 cm for males and 144 cm for females. Specialised growth charts are available for children with Down syndrome and for some other genetic conditions **(Fig. 3.34)**.[16]

Edward Syndrome

The association of IUGR, congenital heart disease (most commonly septal defects with or without patent ductus arteriosus), micrognathia, cleft lip and/or cleft palate, hypertelorism, webbed toes, rocker bottom feet and cryptorchidism is suggestive of trisomy 18 **(Fig. 3.35)**. Affected children show a typical clenching of the hand

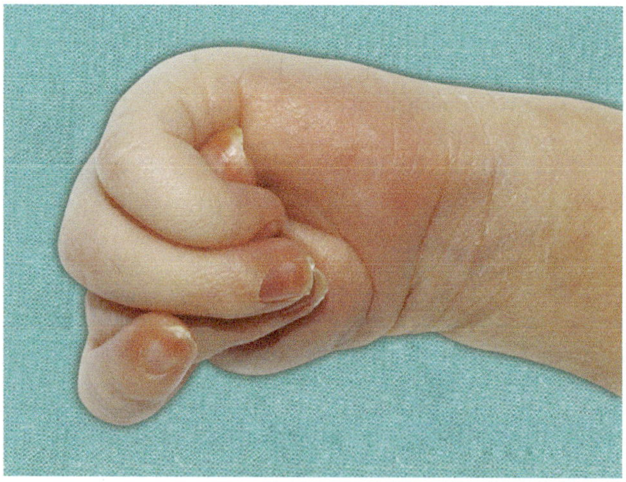

Figure 3.36 Edward syndrome: Clenched overlapping fingers on hands.

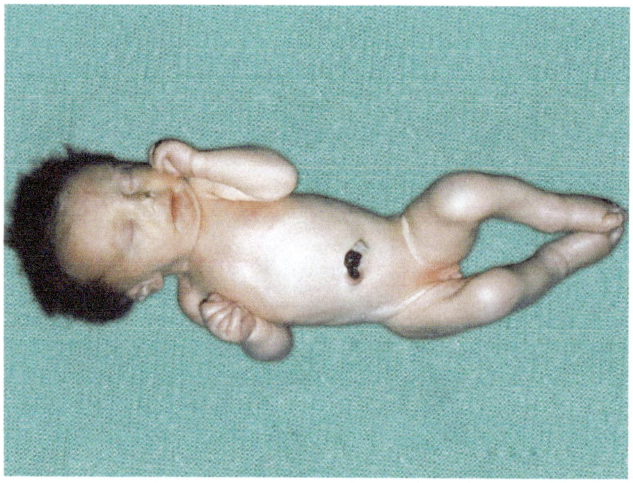

Figure 3.37 Patau syndrome.

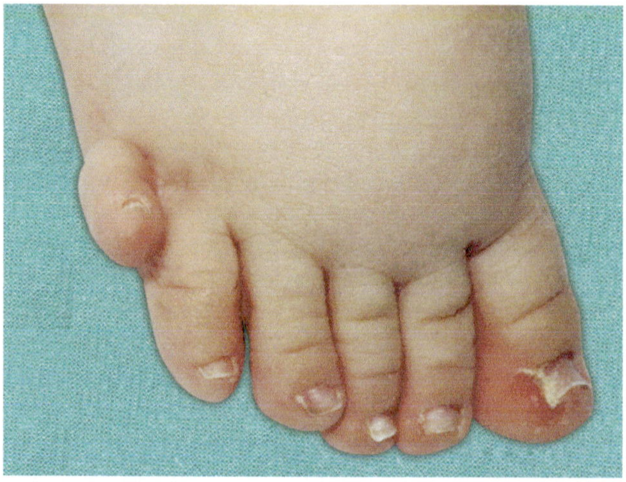

Figure 3.38 Polydactyly.

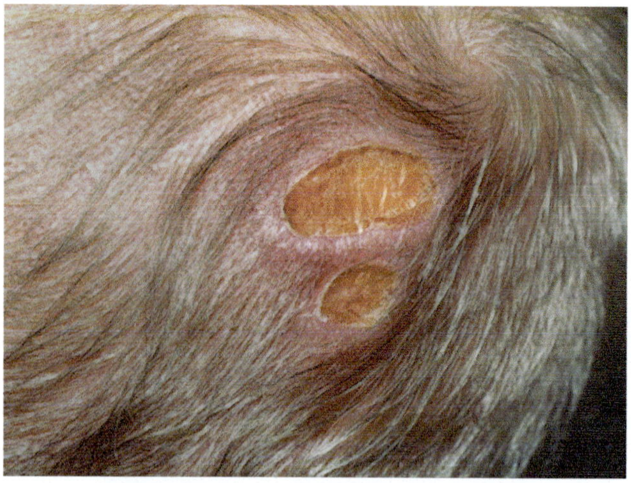

Figure 3.39 Cutis aplasia.

with overlapping of the index and fifth finger **(Fig. 3.36)** and frequently have respiratory difficulties including hypoventilation and apnoea. The majority of foetuses conceived with trisomy 18 abort spontaneously; when pregnancy continues, polyhydramnios is a common complication. Survival beyond the second week is unusual, and severe learning difficulties are present in the few children who survive the neonatal period.

Patau Syndrome

Features of trisomy 13 include cleft lip and palate, microcephaly with hypotelorism and low set ears, scalp defects (cutis aplasia), cryptorchidism and polydactyly with overriding fingers. Cardiac abnormalities are common, and severe intellectual disability is evident in those rare children who survive beyond infancy **(Figs. 3.37 to 3.39)**.

Turner Syndrome (45,X)

Signs of Turner syndrome (gonadal dysgenesis) presenting in the neonatal period include cardiac abnormalities (coarctation of the aorta, bicuspid aortic valve), shield chest with widely spaced nipples, shortened fourth finger, low set ears and lymphoedema. The latter sign in a female child should prompt chromosomal analysis **(Fig. 3.40)**. Cystic hygroma **(Figs. 3.41 and 3.42)** may have been noted on antenatal ultrasound, and explains the webbed neck typical of girls with Turner syndrome. Cardiac abnormalities occur more commonly in pure 45,XO monosomy. No immediate treatment is required, but early consultation with an endocrinologist experienced in the management of Turner syndrome is recommended. Long-term issues to be considered include hormonal replacement therapy and hypothyroidism. Without growth hormone replacement, typical final adult height is around 140 cm.

Klinefelter Syndrome (47,XXY)

47,XXY is the most common sex aneuploidy occurring in human males, with an estimated incidence of 1 in 500 to 1 in 1,000. It is likely to present in the newborn only if diagnosed incidentally by amniocentesis prior to delivery.

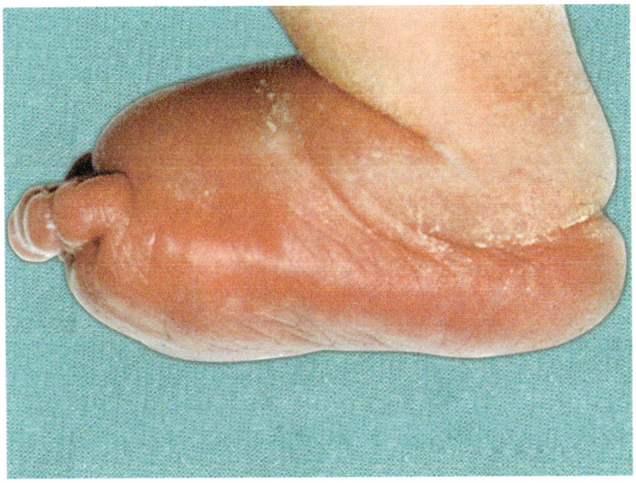

Figure 3.40 Lymphoedema in Turner syndrome.

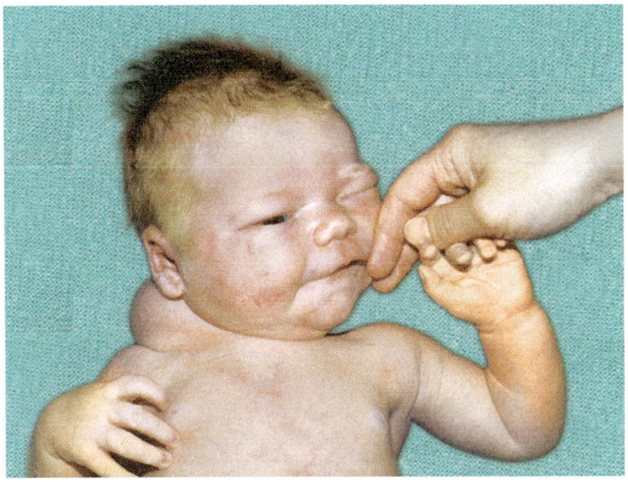

Figure 3.41 Cystic hygroma.

Figure 3.42 Transilluminated cystic hygroma.

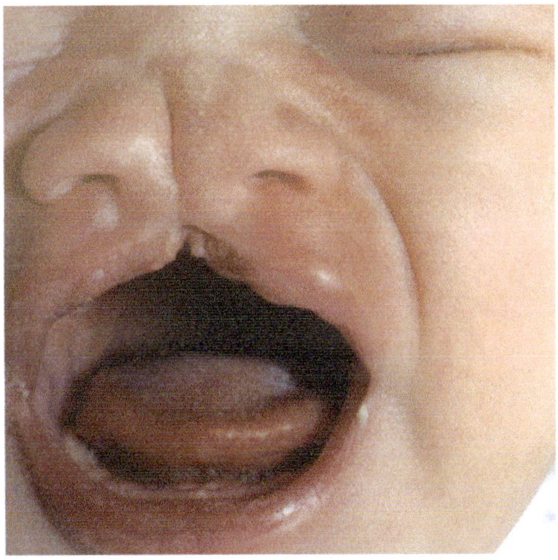

Figure 3.43 Severe facial cleft.

Single Gene Defects

A full description of single gene defect presenting in the newborn is out of scope of this textbook, but some more common conditions include: haemophilia A and B (X-linked recessive deficiencies of factors VIII and IX, respectively); Stickler syndrome, an autosomal dominantly inherited disorder of collagen metabolism with features including myopia, arthritis and hearing loss; and Holt-Oram syndrome.

Multifactorial

Cleft lip and/or palate (or orofacial clefts) are among the most common congenital anomalies, occurring in approximately 1 in 700 live births (Fig. 3.43). Cleft lip and/or palate may be present in isolation or (less commonly) in association with other anomalies and result from failure of closure of the palatal ridges between 4 and 9 weeks' gestation. The cause is multifactorial in a majority of cases, although some are associated with heritable conditions, including Stickler syndrome (cleft palate, myopia, hearing loss and arthritis) and Treacher Collins syndrome (mandibulofacial dysostosis) (Fig. 3.44). Pierre Robin sequence occurs when an abnormally small jaw prevents the tongue from descending and thus the palatal ridges from fusing (Fig. 3.45). Postnatally, the posteriorly displaced tongue may obstruct the airway, particularly when the infant is supine (glossoptosis). Cleft lip is not associated with Pierre Robin sequence, but up to 30–40% will have Stickler syndrome.

Amniotic Bands

Amniotic band syndrome is a congenital disorder caused by entrapment of foetal parts, most commonly a limb or digits, in fibrous amniotic bands. The cause of the amnion tearing is not known and there are no preventative measures that can be taken. The amniotic bands may result in constriction rings around the affected parts, oedema of the extremities distal to the point of constriction, or amputation of the affected parts (Fig. 3.46).

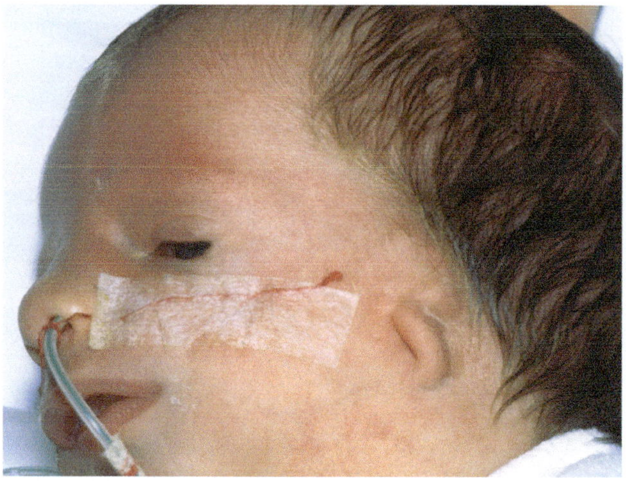

Figure 3.44 Treacher Collins syndrome.

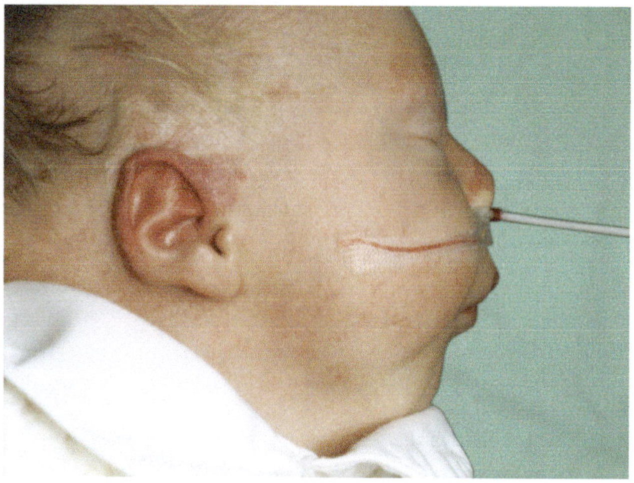

Figure 3.45 Pierre Robin syndrome.

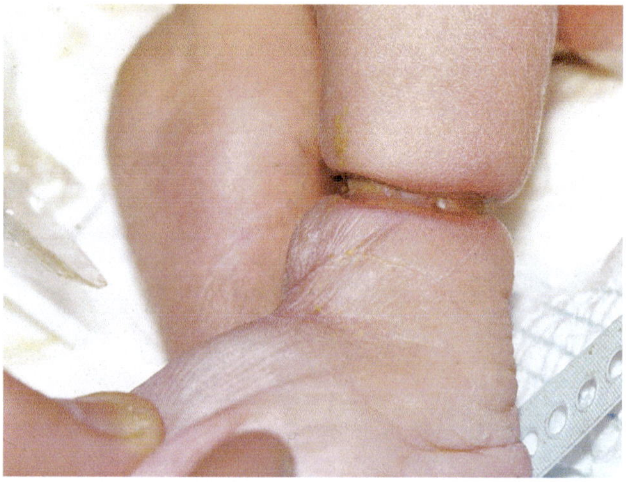

Figure 3.46 Amniotic bands.

The frequency of amniotic band syndrome is approximately 1 per 3,000 pregnancies but only 1 per 10,000-15,000 live births.[17] Around half of the cases have other anomalies including cleft lip and palate, talipes and/or hand and finger anomalies. The likelihood of recurrence in a future pregnancy is low.

TRANSITION TO EXTRAUTERINE LIFE

Globally, approximately four million newborn infants die per annum in the neonatal period; depending on the locale, as many as one-quarter of these deaths occur as a result of birth asphyxia.[18] The majority of healthy, term foetuses manage the transition to extrauterine life without help, but a significant number of newly born babies (and the majority of very-low-birth-weight babies) require some assistance in the critical first few minutes of life, and for a few, respiratory and metabolic adaptation is significantly delayed. Immediate post-birth stabilisation has become much better with improved understanding of basic physiology, widespread teaching of basic newborn resuscitation and greater consideration given to thermal stability. Although there is little scientific evidence, it is widely held that basic neonatal resuscitation training has the potential to reduce term intrapartum-related deaths by 30%.[19]

Factors increasing the risk of birth asphyxia include maternal illness, antepartum or intrapartum bleeding, abnormal foetal presentation, prolapsed umbilical cord, meconium staining of the liquor and prematurity. Even with sophisticated monitoring in labour (which is, of course, available to only a tiny number of births worldwide), compromise at birth can only be predicted in around 50% of cases. Therapeutic hypothermia can improve developmental outcome in cases of birth asphyxia but this treatment is only available in specialised neonatal centres.[20]

Establishment of Respiration

A mature, well-grown foetus will usually gasp and cry within the first 90 seconds of birth. The first breath is facilitated by several factors, including cold, touch, hypoxia and increased pCO_2; following the first breath, increased oxygen tension stimulates formation of prostaglandins and release of nitric oxide, facilitating reduction in pulmonary vascular resistance and constriction of the ductus arteriosus. Suctioning of the airway is not required for those babies who are crying at birth; indeed, over-vigorous stimulation of the airway can result in vagal stimulation with resultant bradycardia and laryngeal spasm. Respiration is impaired initially by foetal lung fluid, which is mostly resorbed by pulmonary lymphatics, facilitated by intrathoracic pressures of up to 100 cm H_2O generated by the infant's first breath.[21] Resorption of foetal lung fluid normally commences prior to onset of labour, as a consequence of maternal-foetal hormonal changes; this accounts for the increased incidence of

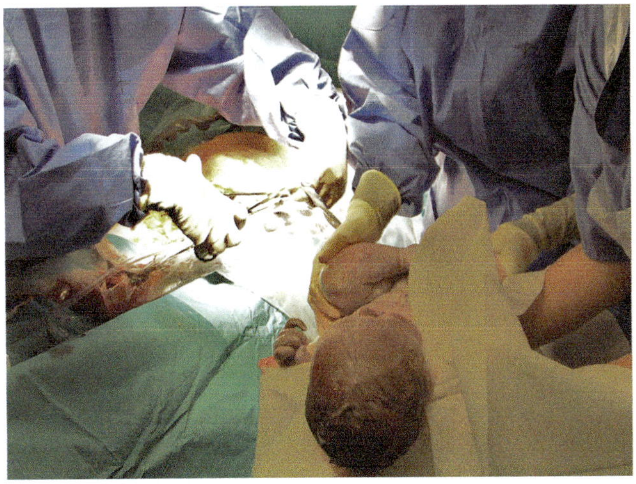

Figure 3.47 Delayed cord clamping.

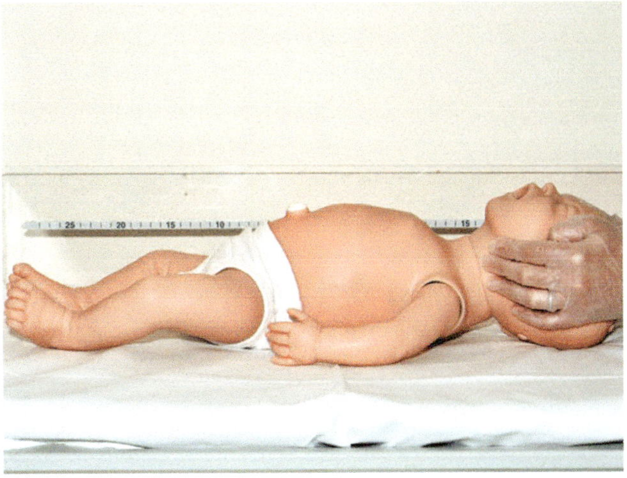

Figure 3.48 Head in the neutral position.

transient tachypnoea of the newborn (TTN) after delivery by elective pre-labour caesarean section.

Cord Clamping

Delayed (at least 1 minute after birth or after cessation of cord pulsation) versus immediate (less than 1 minute) cord clamping has advantages for baby in terms of higher haemoglobin at birth and improved iron status at 6 months of age.[22] Although delayed cord clamping increases the need for phototherapy in the neonatal period, it does not affect Apgar score or umbilical cord pH, nor does it increases the risk of postpartum haemorrhage. Studies in preterm infants have shown reduced need for blood transfusion and significantly reduced incidence of intraventricular haemorrhage (IVH) [relative risk, 1.74; 95% confidence interval, 1.08–2.81], with delayed (up to 120 seconds) versus immediate cord clamping.[23] Thus, unless there is a need for immediate resuscitation of either mother or baby, cord clamping should be delayed for 2–3 minutes in term infants, and for at least 40 seconds in preterm infants. Skin-to-skin contact may be initiated prior to cord clamping, but the infant should be kept as low as reasonably practical (Fig. 3.47).

Keeping Warm

It is essential that the newborn infant is kept warm. Term-born infants allowed to become cool in the immediate post-birth period are at risk of hypoglycaemia, as well as hypoxia and metabolic acidosis. In animal models, hypothermia reduces surfactant production. Hypothermia on admission to the neonatal unit is associated with increased mortality in preterm infants. Heat loss occurs via four mechanisms, namely evaporation, convection, conduction and radiation, and can be greatly reduced by drying the infant at delivery, ensuring that the delivery room is warm and draught-free and that the baby is received into warm towels. If the infant is clinically stable, heat is best maintained by skin-to-skin contact with the mother; otherwise, the infant should be swaddled unless he/she is to be nursed in an incubator. Use of food grade plastic bags for preterm infants less than 28 weeks' gestation reduces the incidence of hypothermia and should be the standard of care.[24] This simple measure can easily be achieved in even the most resource-poor setting. Early bathing of babies is unnecessary, and unless there is a pressing need to clean off maternal blood and secretions (e.g. HIV positive mothers), bathing should be deferred for at least a few hours and preferably until the second or third day.

Basic Resuscitation

Appropriate and effective resuscitation of the newborn is based on an understanding of basic respiratory physiology and the transition from foetal to infant circulation. As for older children and adults, resuscitation of the newborn should follow the ABCD acronym (airway, breathing, circulation, drugs). Basic resuscitation of the newborn, including clearing of the airway, head positioning and positive pressure ventilation via bag and mask, will be described here; for more advanced resuscitation, the reader is referred to other texts.[10,25] All persons attending women in labour should be trained in basic resuscitation of the newborn.

Patency of the newborn airway depends on head positioning and (to a much lesser extent) absence of secretions or blood clots. The relatively larger occiput of infancy means that the neck tends naturally to flexion, which can compromise the airway. Similarly, overextension of the head (as may occur on a sloping surface) is to be avoided. If the infant does not begin to breathe shortly after birth despite gentle stimulation, he/she should be placed supine on a level surface (preferably with an overhead heat source) and the head placed in the neutral position (Fig. 3.48). For many babies, this will be sufficient to initiate respiration. If the baby remains floppy

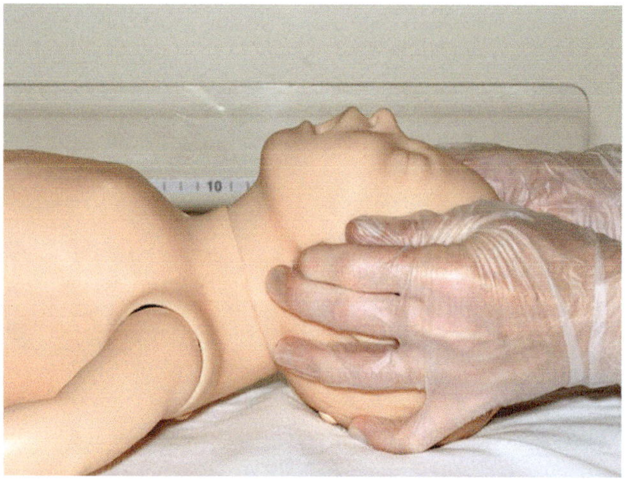

Figure 3.49 Jaw thrust.

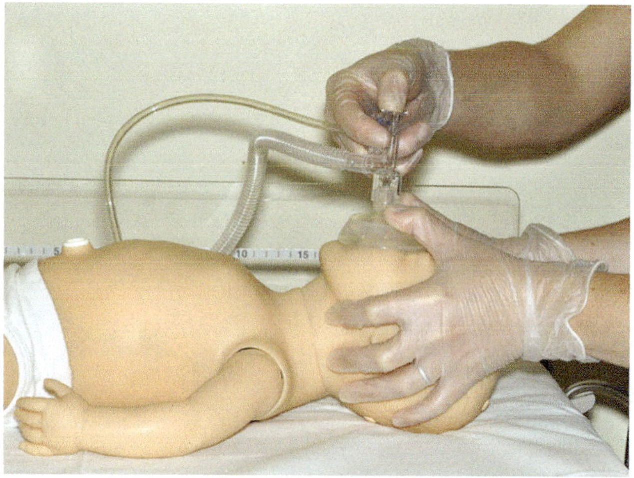

Figure 3.50 Two-person ventilation via T-piece with jaw thrust.

and apnoeic, the chin should be gently supported by a finger placed under the bony part, or by two fingers placed under the angle of the jaw. If this manoeuvre does not elicit gasping, then the lungs should be inflated, using a face mask and either a self-inflating bag or a T-piece. The latter is commonly used on modern hospital resuscitation platforms, but requires a source of pressurised gas and is not applicable to community or resource-poor settings. It is essential that the face mask used is of the correct size with a broad, soft deformable surface; it should sit comfortably over the baby's nose and mouth, but not squash the eyes. In order to overcome the presence of pulmonary fluid, an initial five inflation breaths at 30 cm H_2O, each sustained over 3 seconds, should be given. Adequate response to this will be either visible chest wall movement or increase in heart rate. If neither of these occurs, it should be assumed that inflation of the lungs has not occurred, and the airway should be rechecked. The baby should be repositioned in the neutral position, jaw thrust applied and the airway gently inspected for blood clot or other debris **(Fig. 3.49)**. When establishing and maintaining the airway proves problematic, consideration should be given to use of a Guedel airway or to endotracheal intubation. If spontaneous respiration does not occur after adequate lung inflation, ventilation breaths should be continued at a rate of 60 breaths per minute, with an inflation pressure sufficient to inflate the lungs (generally around 20–24 cm H_2O) **(Fig. 3.50)**. The vast majority of term infants who require intervention at birth will establish spontaneous respiration in response to one or more inflation breaths, with or without a brief period of intermittent positive pressure ventilation, and can then be left with their mother to initiate breastfeeding. Rarely, even with adequate lung inflation and ventilation breaths, the infant's heart rate will not increase; in this scenario, it can be assumed that significant hypoxia has occurred. Chest compressions are indicated if the heart rate does not respond to adequate ventilation and can be delivered either by encircling the thorax or by the two-finger method. A second person will be required. The rationale for chest compressions is to move oxygenated blood from the lungs to the coronary arteries and thus 'kick start' the heart; chest compressions are thus pointless if the baby's lungs are not being inflated. Further resuscitation may include administration of adrenaline and/or sodium bicarbonate and intravenous fluids (dextrose, blood or saline), which should be given via an umbilical venous catheter.

Evidence for Oxygen

There is now good evidence that room air is preferable to oxygen for initial resuscitation of term infants.[26] The situation is less clear for the preterm infant, but hyperoxia is certainly to be avoided. Based on available evidence, infants born before 32 weeks' gestation should be resuscitated initially with supplemental oxygen, but this should be weaned as soon as the infant's oxygen saturation has improved.[27] It should also be borne in mind that the normal healthy term infant may not achieve an oxygen saturation of 90% until 10 minutes of age.[28]

Early Feeding

The healthy, appropriately grown term infant is designed to withstand relative starvation for the first few days of life, until lactation is established. The rooting and sucking reflexes ensure that if the infant is held close to his mother's breast in skin-to-skin contact, he/she will begin to suckle soon after birth; this suckling will gradually become more rhythmical and sustained over the following few days as milk is produced. Early and exclusive breastfeeding is recommended for almost all infants; when safe formula milk is available, rare exceptions to this rule include infants born to HIV positive mothers and mothers treated with a few specific drugs, including radioactive iodine and lithium. Unless the infant is at risk of hypoglycaemia, breastfeeding should be offered on demand, and neither supplementary feeds nor blood sugar monitoring is indicated. Intervals between feeds may be very variable in the first few days, but so long as the infant is alert and appears well, this is not a problem. A physiological fall in blood glucose levels occurs in the first 4 hours after birth before the counter-regulatory hormones of glucagon, adrenaline, growth hormone and cortisol induce endogenous glucose production. During this period, normal healthy term infants will use alternative cerebral fuels such as ketone bodies and lactate and so hypoglycaemia should not be screened for routinely in the healthy term newborn.

More caution must be exercised in those infants with potentially impaired postnatal metabolic adaptation, including preterm and unwell infants, infants with poor hepatic stores of glycogen (IUGR, birth asphyxia), and infants with increased circulating levels of insulin (diabetic mothers). It is particularly important that these at-risk babies are kept warm and offered an early feed; since the majority of babies with moderate hypoglycaemia will be asymptomatic, blood sugar monitoring should be undertaken before the second feed (at around 4–6 hours of life) to indicate whether the infant can cope with a 3- to 4-hour period of fasting. Most at-risk babies can be managed with regular oral feeds, but when blood glucose cannot be reliably sustained above 2.5 mmol/L, intravenous glucose will be required. Symptoms that should alert staff to the possibility of hypoglycaemia include lethargy, hypotonia, abnormal neurological behaviour, and seizures. Prolonged symptomatic hypoglycaemia has adverse implications for neurodevelopmental outcome.

Breastfeeding

Exclusive breastfeeding is recommended for the first 6 months of a baby's life (Fig. 3.51). Rates of breastfeeding vary across the world, being lowest in some industrial countries, particularly among young mothers and disadvantaged socioeconomic groups, thus potentially widening existing health inequalities. Breastfeeding has many advantages for baby, including: optimal nutritional content; immune factors; reduced incidence of gastroenteritis, respiratory infections and ear infections; better tolerance than formula milk; reduced incidence of allergic diseases such as eczema and asthma and of both type 1 diabetes and inflammatory bowel disease; and less obesity. There are also modest benefits in terms of improved visual development and higher IQ, and in preterm infants, breast milk lowers the risk of necrotising enterocolitis. As well as improved mother–child bonding, breast feeding offers advantages to mother, including earlier return to pre-pregnancy weight and reduced risk of osteoporosis and both breast and ovarian cancer. Furthermore, although not a reliable contraceptive, breastfeeding prolongs the time to return of ovulation, thus increasing the interval between pregnancies. Regular weighing of breastfeeding infants is important in helping to detect poorly established lactation and resultant hypernatraemic dehydration. When postnatal weight loss exceeds 12.5%, active management of breastfeeding should be instigated, to include expressing of milk and consideration of supplemental feeds.

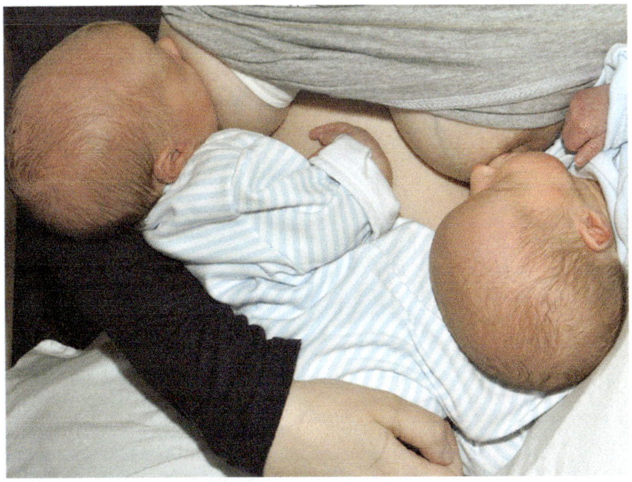

Figure 3.51 Breastfeeding twins.

The 'Ten steps to successful breastfeeding' were developed by WHO and UNICEF to ensure that maternity services provide the right start for every infant and the necessary support for mothers to breastfeed. Today, this checklist is used by hospitals in more than 150 countries (Box 3.1).[29]

BOX 3.1 Ten steps to successful breastfeeding.

Step 1: Have a written breastfeeding policy that is routinely communicated to all healthcare staff.

Step 2: Train all healthcare staff in the skills necessary to implement this policy.

Step 3: Inform all pregnant women about the benefits and management of breastfeeding.

Step 4: Help mothers initiate breastfeeding within half an hour of birth.

Step 5: Show mothers how to breastfeed and how to maintain lactation even if they should be separated from their infants.

Step 6: Give newborn infants no food or drink other than breast milk unless medically indicated.

Step 7: Practise 'rooming in'—allowing mothers and infants to remain together 24 hours a day.

Step 8: Encourage breastfeeding on demand—whenever the baby is hungry.

Step 9: Give no artificial teats or pacifiers (also called dummies or soothers) to breastfeeding infants.

Step 10: Foster the establishment of breastfeeding support groups and refer mothers to them on discharge from the hospital or clinic.

Infant Formula

Although manufactured to resemble human milk, infant formula does not contain the anti-infective and other benefits of human milk, and in developing countries, infant formula poses a significant health risk if reconstituted with contaminated water. Formula milk does, however, have benefits as a complementary feed when lactation fails, in helping to prevent perinatal transmission of HIV and as an alternate feed for infants diagnosed with an inborn error of metabolism such as galactosaemia or phenylketonuria. There are also instances where maternal medication will contraindicate breastfeeding; up-to-date advice should be sought from pharmacy monographs.

BIRTH INJURY

The incidence of trauma associated with vaginal birth has decreased dramatically in the last 50 years, reflecting, at least in part, increase in availability and safety of delivery by caesarean section. Nevertheless, birth injuries still occur, most commonly in infants requiring instrumental delivery, or in those whose delivery is complicated by shoulder dystocia or breech presentation.

Subaponeurotic Haemorrhage

Subaponeurotic haemorrhage occurs between the skull periosteum and the galea aponeurosis, and is generally associated with vacuum delivery. Prematurity is a risk factor, and underlying coagulopathy should be considered. Diagnosis is clinical, with a fluctuant boggy mass found over the scalp, particularly in the occipital region. The swelling commonly develops gradually over 12–72 hours following delivery, but in severe cases it may be apparent shortly after delivery. As the bleeding is not contained by the sutures, up to 50% of the newborn's blood volume may leak into the subaponeurotic space, leading to haemorrhagic shock and even death. Treatment is with replacement of blood, fresh-frozen plasma and coagulation factors as required. Affected infants require close observation in the first 2–3 days, and may develop significant jaundice.

Skull Fractures

Skull fractures are uncommon. They are usually associated with forceps delivery but can occur with non-instrumental delivery. The parietal bone is most often affected; the occipital bone may be affected in breech deliveries. Fractures may be linear or depressed; depressed fractures may rarely require surgery **(Figs. 3.52A to C)**.

Fractured Clavicle

Fractured clavicle is most commonly associated with shoulder dystocia or breech delivery. Tenderness may be evident, with crepitation, oedema or bruising, and there will be decreased active movement of the arm and an asymmetrical Moro reflex. An X-ray will confirm the diagnosis. Clavicular fractures heal spontaneously; oral paracetamol may be indicated if the infant is in pain, but is not generally required for more than a couple of days. For a significant number of cases, presentation is towards the end of the first week with a clavicular lump due to callus formation at the fracture site **(Fig. 3.53)**.

Facial Nerve Palsy

The seventh nerve may be damaged by pressure from either obstetric forceps at delivery or prolonged contact with the maternal sacral promontory. This lower motor neuron palsy is generally unilateral, with facial weakness most evident when the infant cries **(Fig. 3.54**, also *see* **Figs. 34.15A to C)**. Facial nerve palsy should be distinguished from asymmetrical crying facies, which results from absence of the depressor anguli oris muscle. In the latter condition, the eye will close normally, but there is

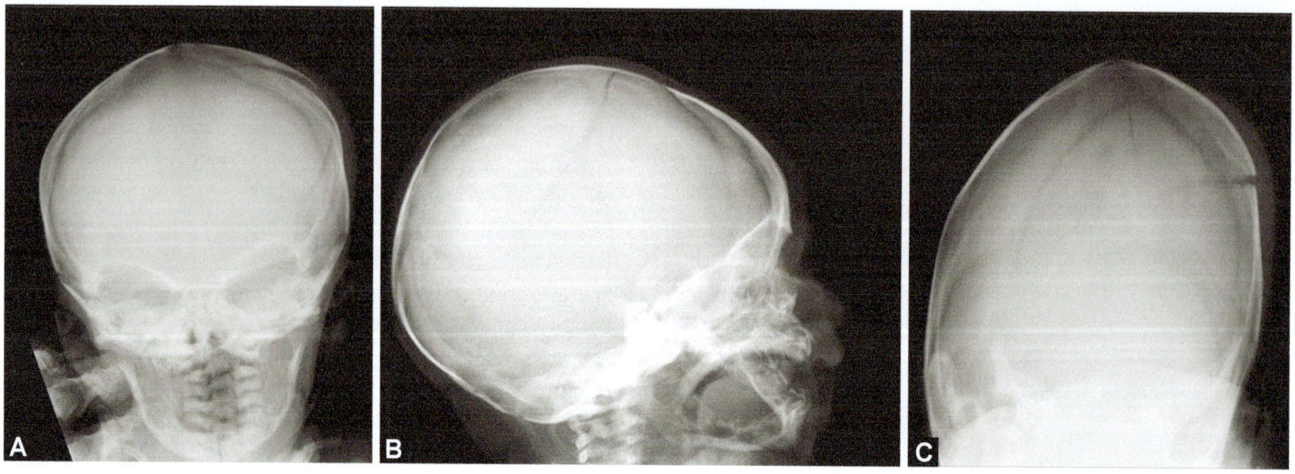

Figures 3.52A to C Skull fracture.

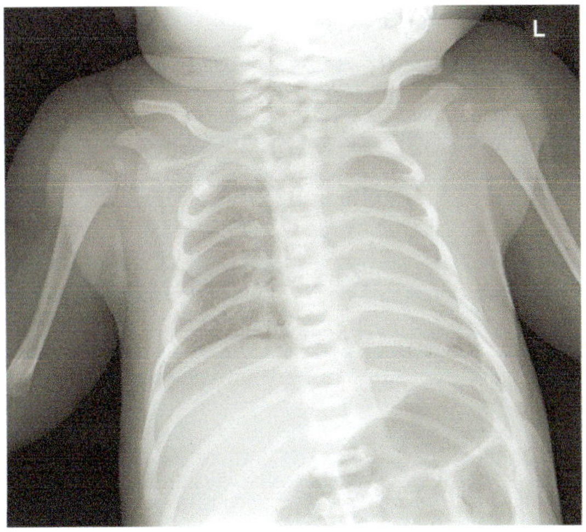

Figure 3.53 Clavicular fracture.

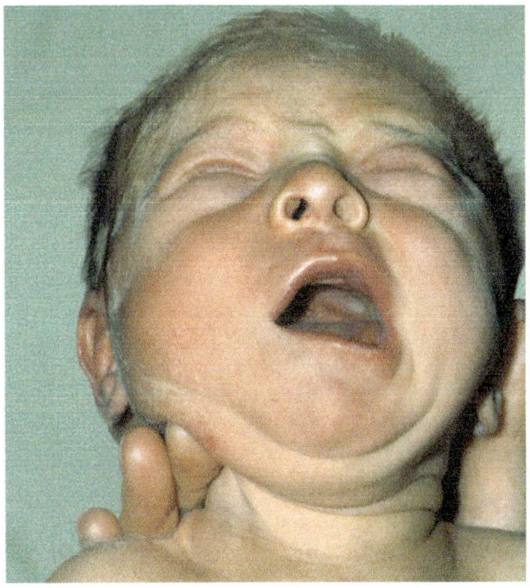

Figure 3.54 Right-sided facial palsy.

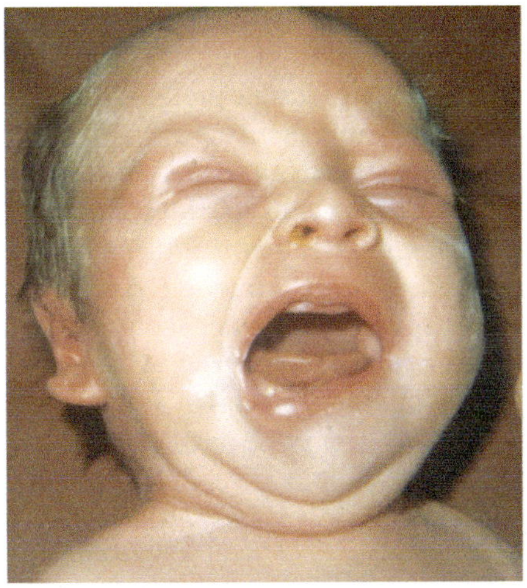

Figure 3.55 Asymmetrical crying facies (depressor anguli oris muscle hypoplasia (DAOM)).

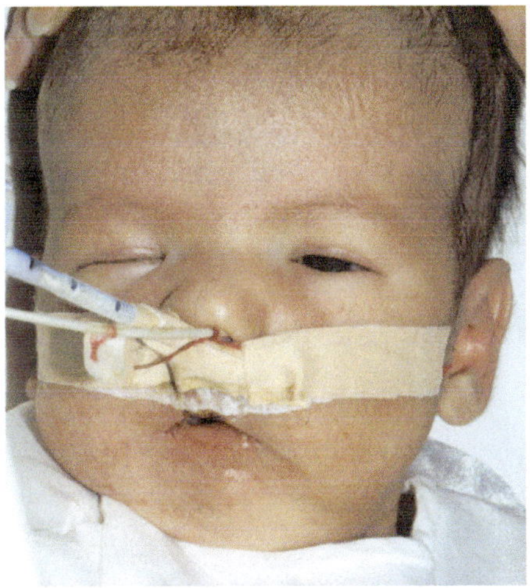

Figure 3.56 Moebius syndrome.

failure of the mouth to move downwards and outwards when the infant is crying **(Fig. 3.55)**.

Asymmetrical crying facies persist into adult life but becomes less apparent over time. Facial nerve palsy resolves completely in the majority of cases and requires no treatment; if the eye cannot be closed, then patching and artificial tears should be used to prevent corneal abrasion. Rarely, facial nerve palsy will be associated with other anomalies, including hemifacial microsomia and CHARGE syndrome. Bilateral facial nerve palsy is present in Moebius syndrome in association with unilateral or bilateral palsy of the abducens nerve and/or involvement of the hypoglossal nerve **(Fig. 3.56)**.

Brachial Plexus Injury

Brachial plexus injury can occur at delivery from excessive lateral flexion, rotation or traction on the neck. It is most commonly seen after breech delivery or vaginal delivery complicated by shoulder dystocia, but has been documented after delivery by caesarean section. There are two main types of brachial plexus injury: (1) Erb palsy, and (2) Klumpke paralysis.

Erb Palsy

This is the most common type of injury, accounting for more than 90% of brachial plexus injuries. Injury to the fifth and sixth cervical nerve roots results in loss of shoulder abduction. The arm is held in adduction, with the elbow extended and the forearm pronated with the wrist flexed. It is commonly referred to as the 'waiter's tip' position **(Fig. 3.57)**.

Klumpke Paralysis

Less commonly, the seventh and eighth cervical and first thoracic nerve roots are injured. Clinically, this presents as wrist drop with flaccid paralysis of the hand, but sparing of shoulder abduction. The grasp reflex will be absent.

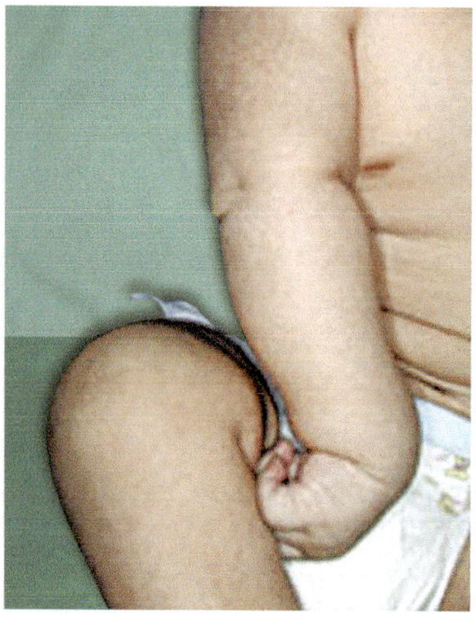

Figure 3.57 Erb palsy.

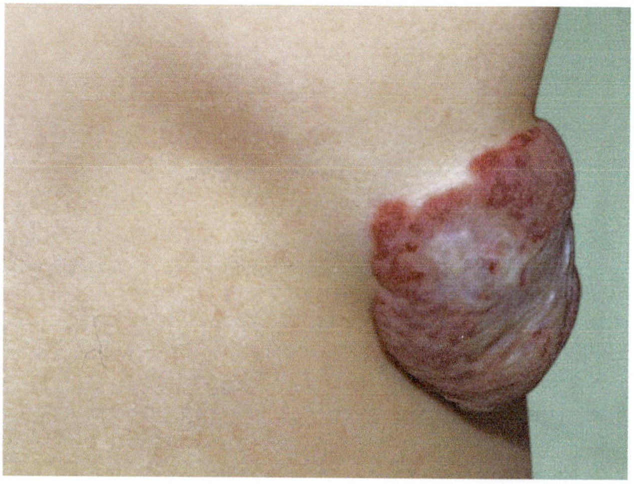

Figure 3.58 Infantile haemangioma.

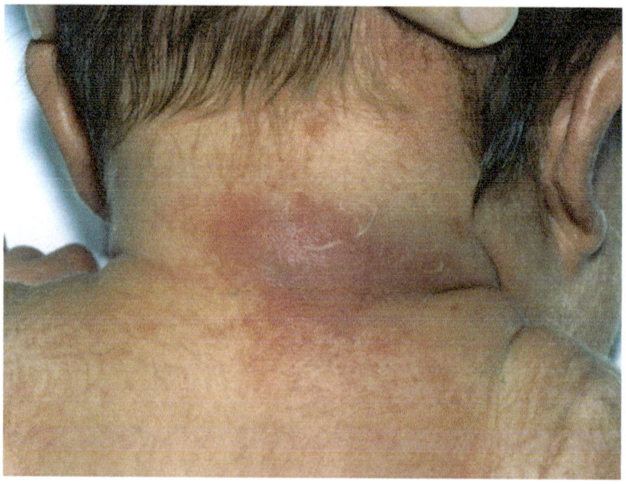

Figure 3.59 Subcutaneous fat necrosis.

Treatment

Active treatment of brachial plexus injuries is not required, but passive movement of the joints is necessary to prevent contractures. Mild injuries will resolve within a few days, but more severe injuries may take several months to resolve. The prognosis depends on the severity of the injury, the time of onset, and initial (early) rate of improvement. Most infants recover spontaneously with complete or almost complete return of function, but if there is no evidence of spontaneous recovery at 4 months of age, surgical treatment options should be considered.[30]

DERMATOLOGY

Infantile Haemangioma

Simple vascular naevi presenting at birth have been described under the examination of the newborn. Another common vascular naevus is the infantile haemangioma or strawberry mark. This is occasionally present in the first few days of life, but usually appears after birth. Infantile haemangiomas are more common in Caucasian babies (affecting up to 10%) and in ex-preterm infants, and generally grow quickly to reach their final size in around 3–9 months before starting to shrink slowly. The majority will be resolved by 7 years of age. Most infantile haemangiomas do not require treatment and any bleeding resultant upon trauma is usually minor. If a lesion is growing extremely rapidly on the face and potentially interfering with vision, breathing or feeding, or if there are concerns that a haemangioma in the napkin area is causing problems with the passage of urine or stools, then treatment is indicated. Oral propranolol is very effective, and the incidence of side effects is low **(Fig. 3.58)**.[31]

Subcutaneous Fat Necrosis

Subcutaneous fat necrosis is a rare, temporary and self-limiting condition which affects the adipose tissue of full-term or post-mature infants, usually within the first 4 weeks of life and more commonly after a complex delivery. It presents with painless, subcutaneous, indurated mobile nodules or well-defined inflammatory plaques. The overlying skin may be violaceous, erythematous or normal in colour. The most common sites are the back, buttocks, thighs, arms and cheeks. Resolution is normally within several weeks but may take up to 6 months. Extracutaneous manifestations can occur, including hypertriglyceridaemia, anaemia, thrombocytopenia and, most importantly, hypercalcaemia. No treatment is required but infants should be tested for hypercalcaemia **(Fig. 3.59)**.

Ichthyotic Disorders

Ichthyotic skin disorders present with dry, scaling skin at birth. There are several varieties, but the most severe and problematic is the collodion baby. At birth, the skin appears to have a dry scaly plastic covering which cracks easily. These infants may develop lamellar ichthyosis but

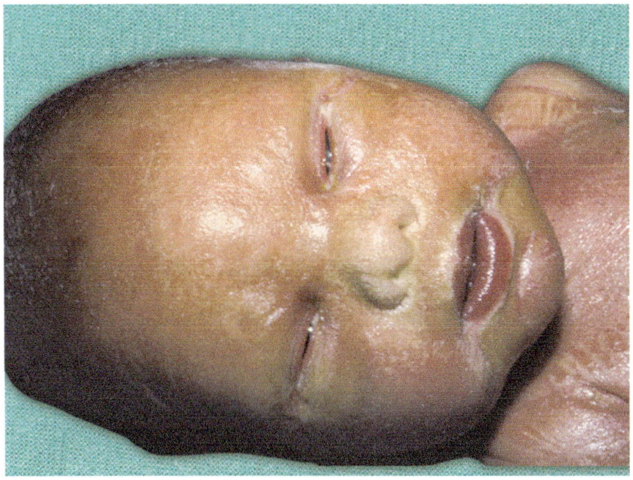

Figure 3.60 Collodion baby.

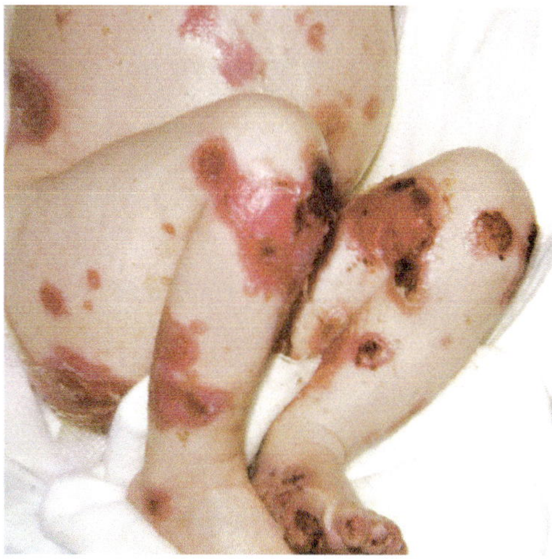

Figure 3.61 Epidermolysis bullosa.

some have no persistent skin abnormality. Treatment at birth involves intensive moisturisation of the skin and careful fluid balance management (Fig. 3.60).

Epidermolysis Bullosa

Epidermolysis bullosa describes a rare collection of skin disorders in which blistering or bullous eruptions occur at birth or later in childhood in response to mechanical trauma. The three main types of epidermolysis bullosa are classified according to the location within the skin of the blistering. Inheritance can be autosomal dominant or autosomal recessive; diagnosis is by biopsy of the skin.

Epidermolysis Bullosa Simplex

In this condition, blistering occurs in the epidermis. This is the mildest and most common type, accounting for 70% of cases.

Dystrophic Epidermolysis Bullosa

In this condition, blistering occurs below the basement membrane zone in the upper part of the dermis. Some cases of dystrophic epidermolysis bullosa are mild and cause no serious complications, while others are severe and can lead to skin cancer in later life.

Junctional Epidermolysis Bullosa

In this most severe type of epidermolysis bullosa, blistering occurs in the basement membrane zone, at the junction between the epidermis and the dermis (Fig. 3.61). Up to 90% of affected children will die within the first 2 years of life. Treatment is aimed at relieving painful symptoms and preventing complications such as infection. There is no cure.

Skin Infection

Candida

This rash is most commonly present in the napkin area involving the skin creases. Satellite lesions are generally present. Diagnosis can be confirmed by swabbing the area for hyphae. Treatment should be with both a topical and an oral antifungal agent, to eradicate oral disease and prevent reinfection. Consideration should also be given to whether mother's nipples are colonised.

Staphylococcal Skin Sepsis

Staphylococcal skin sepsis presents with red blistering skin that looks like a burn or scald, hence the colloquial term staphylococcal scalded skin syndrome. It is caused by the release of epidermolytic toxins A and B from the bacteria *Staphylococcus aureus*. Infants usually present with fever, irritability and widespread erythema of the skin. Fluid-filled blisters rupture easily and the rash may spread quickly to other areas of the body. Treatment is with intravenous antibiotics and attention to fluid and electrolyte balance, with analgesia as required. Most infants will recover fully if the condition is promptly diagnosed and appropriately treated but overwhelming sepsis, pneumonia, and even death may occur. The infection is highly contagious (Figs. 3.62A and B).

NEONATAL INFECTION

The foetus and newborn infant are susceptible to many infectious agents, which can be acquired before or after birth, resulting in a wide variety of clinical presentation. The manifest effects will depend on the causative agent and the route and timing of infection.

Transplacentally Acquired Infection

Infections that may be acquired by haematogenous spread across the placenta include CMV, toxoplasmosis, syphilis, rubella, varicella and *Listeria*. Such congenital infections may cause miscarriage, stillbirth or preterm delivery. Earlier infection is more likely to be teratogenic.

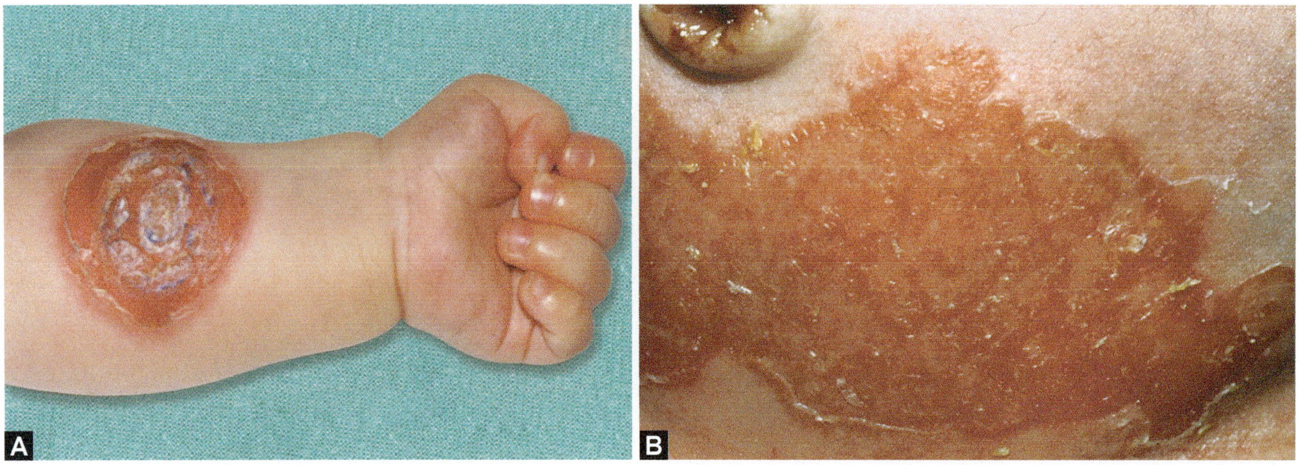

Figures 3.62A and B Staphylococcal skin infection.

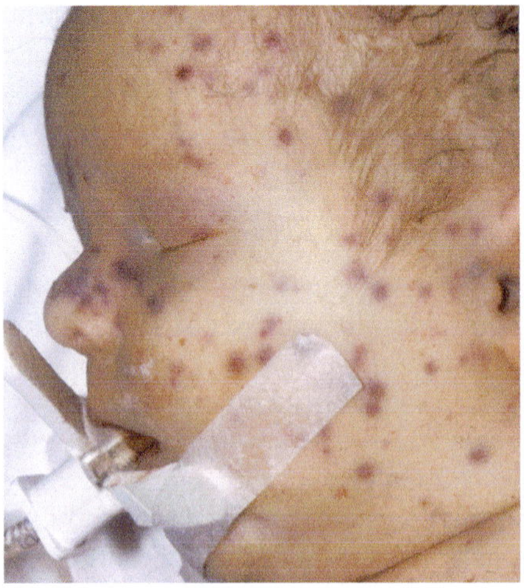

Figure 3.63 Blueberry muffin rash.

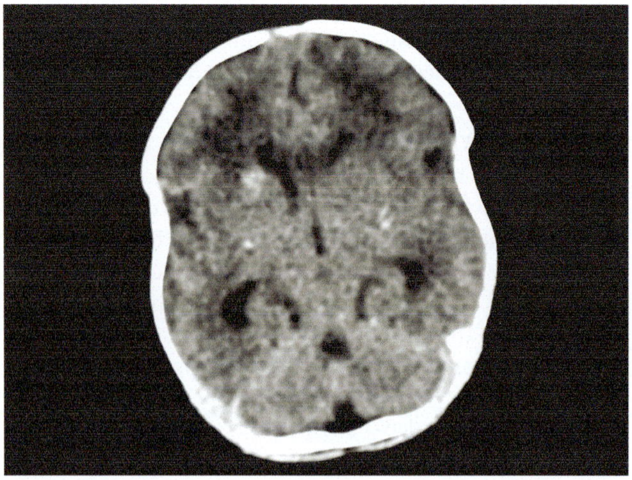

Figure 3.64 Intracerebral calcification due to congenital CMV.

Cytomegalovirus

Cytomegalovirus is the most common congenital infection in the UK and the USA, affecting approximately 0.5–1 per 1,000 live births. Most CMV infection in pregnancy is due to reactivation of the virus; primary infection occurs in around 1–2% of pregnancies, and carries much greater risk to the foetus. The overall mother to foetus transmission is 40% with approximately 5–10% of infants severely affected. The affected infant is characteristically born with a rash, splenomegaly and/or hepatomegaly, jaundice, inflammation of the retina and microcephaly **(Fig. 3.63)**. This may be accompanied by intracerebral calcification visualised on ultrasound or CT/MRI. Sensorineural hearing loss will develop in up to 10% of asymptomatic cases. Diagnosis is usually by viral isolation from urine or saliva. There is some evidence that treatment with ganciclovir will improve outcome, in particular with regard to hearing deficit **(Fig. 3.64)**.[32]

Toxoplasmosis

Seronegative mothers are most at risk from poorly cooked meat; there is also a risk of infection from handling faeces of recently infected cats. The transmission rate from mother to foetus in the first trimester is 15%—of such affected infants, 35% will die before birth and 40% will be severely affected. The majority of foetuses (60%) become infected in the third trimester, of which only 10% will have signs of infection at birth. Signs of congenital toxoplasmosis include fever, jaundice, microcephaly, rash, anaemia, hepatosplenomegaly and seizures. Hearing and visual loss may also occur **(Fig. 3.65)**.

Syphilis

Syphilis is caused by the bacterium *Treponema pallidum*. Without treatment of an infected mother, one-third of pregnancies will abort and the majority of surviving foetuses will become infected. Signs in the newborn include fever, irritability, no bridge to the nose (saddle nose),

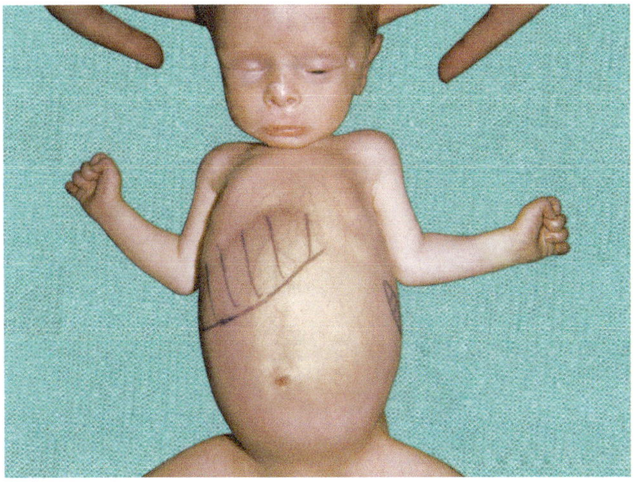

Figure 3.65 Congenital toxoplasmosis.

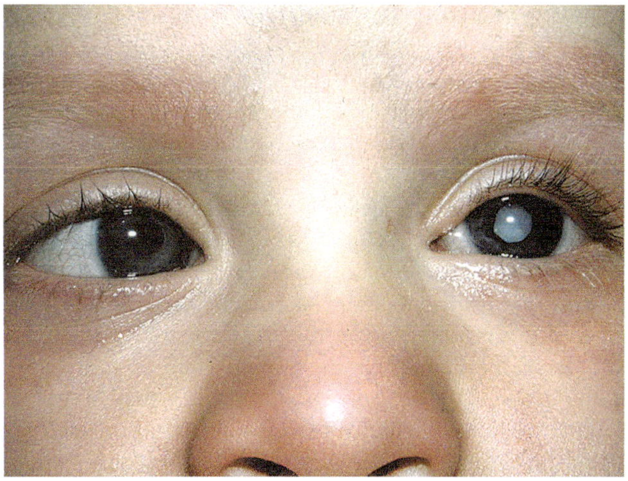

Figure 3.66 Rubella cataract. (*See* Fig. 22.11.)

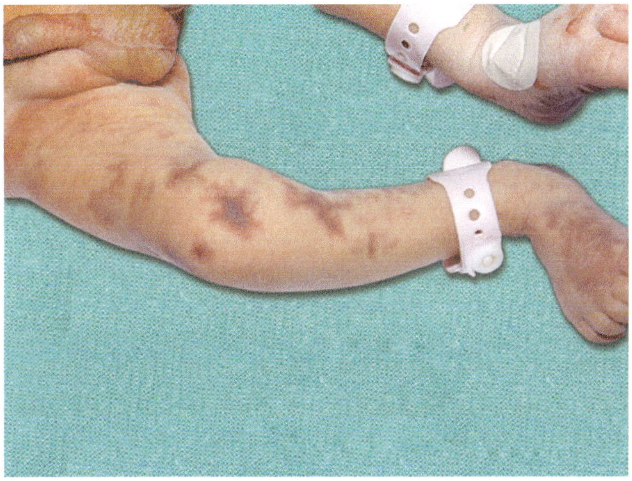

Figure 3.67 Congenital varicella.

rhinitis and failure to thrive. Rashes are typical: an early blistering rash on the palms and soles and a later copper-coloured rash affecting the face, palms and soles. Signs in older children may include abnormal notched and peg-shaped 'Hutchinson' teeth, corneal clouding, sensorineural hearing loss and abnormal shins. All pregnant women infected with syphilis should be treated with penicillin and infants should receive 10 days' treatment with intravenous benzylpenicillin, commenced immediately after birth.

Rubella

Congenital rubella syndrome occurs more likely the earlier in pregnancy when the maternal primary infection occurs. The risk is 90% during the first 10 weeks of pregnancy, reducing to around 10–20% between 11th week and 16th week of pregnancy. Teratogenicity is rare after the 16th week, but sensorineural hearing loss remains a risk. Widespread rubella immunisation means that the classic triad of deafness, ocular abnormalities (retinopathy, cataracts and microphthalmia) and congenital heart disease is rarely seen **(Fig. 3.66)**.

Varicella

Contraction of the virus during weeks 8–12 of pregnancy carries a 2% risk of congenital varicella syndrome. The most common manifestation of this syndrome is skin scarring; other signs include microcephaly, eye problems, low birth weight, small limbs and developmental delay. Perinatal varicella infection can be problematic; if a mother develops chickenpox in the 5 days prior to delivery or the 48 hours after delivery, then the infant is at risk of disseminated varicella infection. At-risk infants should be given prophylactic varicella zoster immunoglobulin and infected infants should be treated with acyclovir. Disseminated varicella infection carries a fatality rate of 25% **(Fig. 3.67)**.

Listeria

Listeria monocytogenes is a gram-positive coccobacillus. Pregnant woman are more susceptible to infection and can become infected through the consumption of unpasteurised milk, soft cheeses and pate. *Listeria* can result in miscarriage, stillbirth and either early-onset or late-onset infection. *Listeria* infection should be suspected if a preterm baby is reported to have passed meconium in utero. There may be abscesses on the surface of the placenta, pinkish-grey granulomas on the skin or a non-specific rash. Late-onset infection may occur between the first week and third week of life, usually presenting as meningitis. *Listeria* infection is commonly treated with ampicillin and gentamicin.

Postnatally Acquired Infection

The relative immaturity of the neonatal immune system increases susceptibility to infection. This may be acquired during delivery from organisms present in the maternal gut or the birth canal, or after birth. When infection is a known risk at delivery, e.g. Group B streptococcus, there may be an opportunity to reduce the risk of infection by administration of antibiotics during labour. Prolonged rupture of membranes (PROM) increases the risk of ascending infection. For the preterm foetus, even in the absence of overt infection, PROM may initiate a chain of inflammatory processes which result in chronic lung disease.

The risk of postnatal infection is increased in the premature infant due to reduced transplacental passage of maternal antibody during the third trimester. Potential routes of infection include broken skin or indwelling catheters (*Staphylococcus epidermidis*), translocation of organisms from an inflamed or immature gut (*Escherichia coli*) and droplet spread (pertussis). Good hand hygiene and adherence to strict aseptic techniques in the management of indwelling lines are vitally important within the neonatal unit.

Early-onset Neonatal Sepsis

It presents within 72 hours of birth and is caused by exposure to organisms before or during birth. Infants commonly become colonised with Group B streptococcus from the maternal gut or birth canal at delivery. Most of these infants will not come to any harm, but a small number may become infected; most will show signs of being unwell within the first 12 hours. Risk factors include preterm birth, PROM (>24 hours) and maternal pyrexia in labour. Features of major illness include septicaemia, pneumonia and/or meningitis. Treatment is with high-dose intravenous benzylpenicillin. Even with good supportive management, consequences may include death, hearing or vision loss or cerebral palsy. Although fulminant infection is rare, intrapartum antibiotics are recommended for women who have had a previous baby affected with Group B streptococcus, or if there are risk factors including preterm labour and PROM.[33]

Late-onset Sepsis

It presents after 72 hours of age and is usually caused by organisms acquired from nosocomial transmission. By altering the bacterial milieu of the infant skin and gut, injudicious use of antibiotics is a risk factor for severe late-onset sepsis.

The early signs of infection in a newborn may be non-specific and include: temperature instability; bradycardia and apnoea; increased ventilatory requirements; feed intolerance; and early jaundice. Laboratory indices suggestive of infection include hypo- or hyperglycaemia, neutropenia, thrombocytopenia and increased C-reactive protein. It should be remembered that elevation of C-reactive protein may be delayed for up to 24 hours after initial presentation. Management of suspected infection should be supportive; empiric antibiotic treatment guided by the clinical features, timing of onset of infection and level patterns of infection.

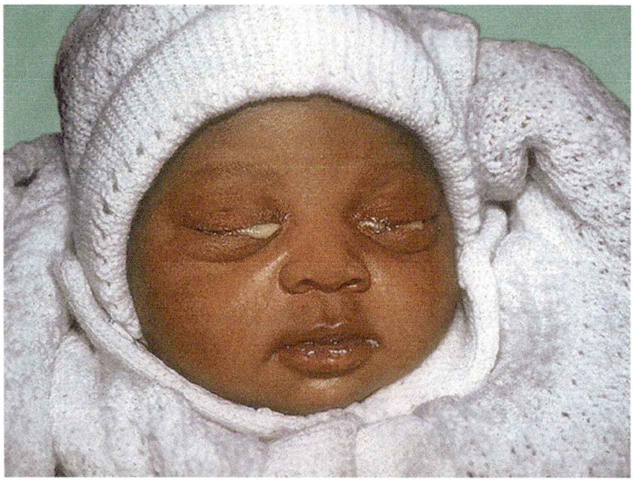

Figure 3.68 Ophthalmia neonatorum. (*See* Fig. 22.14.)

Conjunctivitis

Many infants suffer from sticky eyes, most commonly 3–5 days after birth. Initial management should be to cleanse the eyes regularly with sterile water. If the ocular discharge continues, or if there is associated conjunctival inflammation, swabs should be taken and consideration given to topical antibiotic treatment. An on-going weepy eye suggests failure of the nasolacrimal duct to open; in most cases, this will resolve spontaneously by 1 year of age and no treatment is required.

Purulent conjunctivitis with swelling of the eyelids within 48 hours of birth should raise suspicion of gonococcal infection (ophthalmia neonatorum). Prompt investigation and treatment must be initiated as visual impairment may occur. The discharge should be sent for urgent microscopy and systemic antibiotic treatment commenced in addition to regular irrigation of the eye with sterile water **(Fig. 3.68)**.

Chlamydia trachomatis may also cause purulent discharge, normally towards the end of the first week of life. The discharge should be swabbed and sent in appropriate medium for culture and treatment with erythromycin commenced. There may also be associated respiratory signs, which suggest associated pneumonia.

VIRAL INFECTIONS

Herpes Simplex

Neonatal herpes simplex virus (HSV) infection is a rare but potentially devastating condition. Type 1 infection is common and involves 'cold sores' on the lips and mouth. Type 2 infection is due to sexual contact and involves lesions in the genital area. With type 1 infection, simple hand washing and advising parents not to kiss their babies while lesions are present are all that is required to prevent transmission. With type 2 infection, infants are at risk of infection if contact with an active lesion occurs

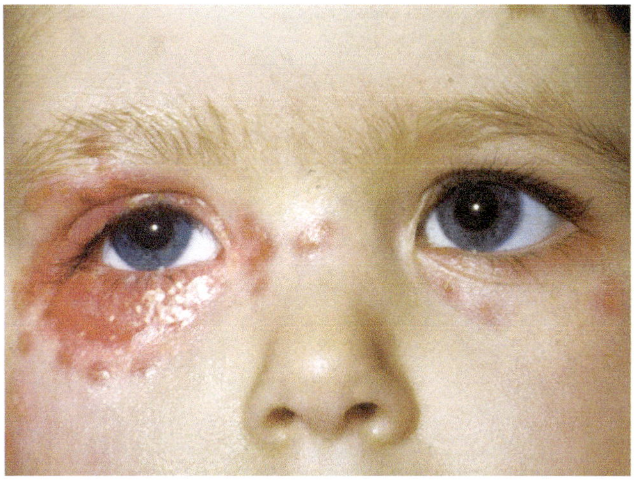

Figure 3.69 Herpetic lesions.

during passage through the genital tract. The risk of infection to the infant of a mother with a primary infection who delivers vaginally is 50%; with recurrent maternal infection, the risk of transmission to the infant is much lower. Congenital (intrauterine acquired) infection is very rare. Caesarean section is the preferred mode of delivery in women with a primary infection, although this does not eliminate the risk of transmission.

Infection may present soon after birth, or within the first few days, with or without a vesicular rash. The herpes virus affects multiple organs, especially the lungs and liver, and there may be central nervous system involvement. Infants may rapidly become extremely unwell with purpura, jaundice and systemic collapse. Features of congenital infection include microcephaly, chorioretinitis, purpura and vesicular rash **(Fig. 3.69)**.

Babies who are thought to have HSV infection must be nursed in isolation and urgent confirmation of diagnosis sought by culture of vesicle fluid. Treatment should be commenced with intravenous acyclovir, continued for at least 14 days; infants with disseminated disease will require full intensive care support.

Hepatitis B

Over 350 million people worldwide are chronically infected with hepatitis B virus, and in high prevalence areas including sub-Saharan Africa, Asia and the Pacific islands, rates of chronic maternal infection can be up to 10%. Without immunoprophylaxis, the risk of the baby becoming infected at birth is around 90%, of whom 90% will become chronic carriers of the virus. One in ten of these babies will ultimately develop liver cirrhosis or hepatocellular carcinoma. All pregnant women should be offered screening for hepatitis B infection, and infants of hepatitis B antigen-positive mothers should be offered immunisation at birth. Active immunisation with hepatitis B vaccine combined with hepatitis B immunoglobulin at birth for infants of the most infectious mothers prevents hepatitis B virus infection in 90% of cases.[34]

Hepatitis C

Mother-to-baby transmission of hepatitis C virus is around 4% if the mother has active disease [both antibody and PCR (polymerase chain reaction) positive]; the rate of transmission is higher if there is coexistent HIV infection.[35] Infants who become carriers are at risk of chronic liver disease and hepatocellular carcinoma. There is no evidence that breastfeeding increases the risk of transmission, nor is there a vaccine currently available for hepatitis C virus.

Human Immunodeficiency Virus

Mother-to-infant transmission of human immunodeficiency virus (HIV) rarely occurs in utero. Most cases of perinatal infection happen at birth or during breastfeeding. Without medical intervention, the risk of viral transmission is 25–40% in a breastfed infant. Factors increasing the rate of mother-to-child transmission include: high maternal viral load; lower maternal CD4 count; primary HIV infection occurring during pregnancy or breastfeeding; co-existing sexually transmitted diseases; rupture of membranes for greater than 4 hours prior to delivery; instrumental delivery; and preterm birth. With appropriate antiretroviral treatment of mother and baby and avoidance of breastfeeding, the risk of mother-to-child transmission can be reduced to less than 1%.[36]

HAEMATOLOGY

The average blood volume at birth is around 85–90 mL/kg. For term infants, haemoglobin concentration is normally 150–200 g/L, rising slightly within the first few hours after birth and then gradually falling to a nadir of 100–110 g/L at 3 months of age. In the preterm infant, physiological anaemia occurs earlier and results in a lower haemoglobin nadir of around 70–80 g/L; contributing factors include lower haemoglobin at birth, reduced erythropoietin production and (sometimes) repeated blood sampling in the neonatal unit. Preterm infants should be supplemented with iron from around 4 weeks of age, to prevent exhaustion of already depleted iron stores.

Polycythaemia

Defined as a venous haematocrit of greater than 0.65, polycythaemia may be caused by increased erythropoietin production or increased blood volume. The former may be associated with intrauterine hypoxia, IUGR, and maternal diabetes; increased blood volume is usually the result of delayed cord clamping and rarely twin-to-twin transfusion syndrome. Although a high haematocrit results in hyperviscosity of the blood, significant clinical complications, including renal vein thrombosis, are very rare. More common features include hypoglycaemia,

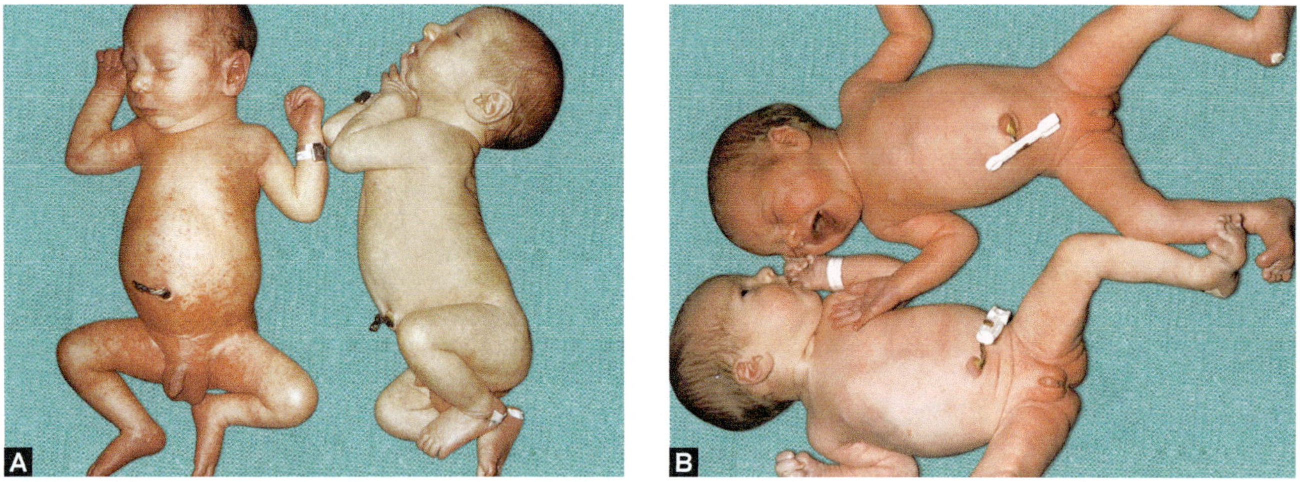

Figures 3.70A and B Polycythaemic infant in twin-to-twin transfusion syndrome. (*See* Figs. 11.22A and B.)

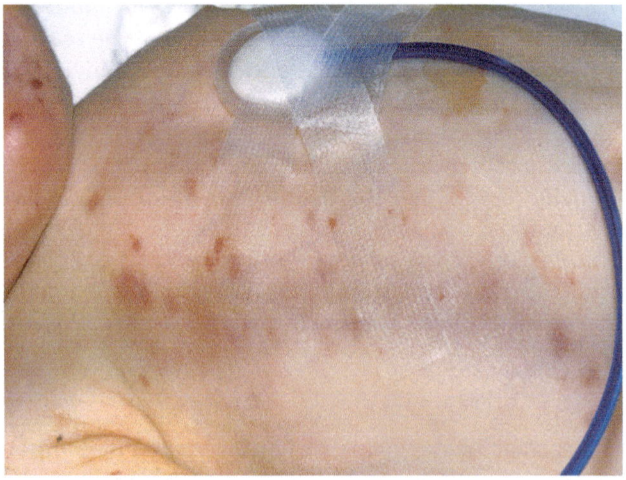

Figure 3.71 Purpuric rash.

hypocalcaemia, thrombocytopenia, hyperbilirubinaemia and respiratory distress. In symptomatic infants, partial exchange transfusion with 0.9% saline may be undertaken **(Fig. 3.70)**.

Thrombocytopenia

Thrombocytopenia is defined as a platelet count less than 150,000/mm^3; severe thrombocytopenia will be accompanied by petechiae, purpura or bleeding. Causes of thrombocytopenia include neonatal alloimmune thrombocytopenia, maternal autoimmune thrombocytopenia (idiopathic thrombocytopenic purpura, systemic lupus erythematosus SLE, congenital infection (CMV, rubella, herpes, syphilis) and severe rhesus disease. Thrombocytopenia may also be associated with trisomies 21, 18 and 13. In the first 72 hours of life, thrombocytopenia is also commonly seen with placental insufficiency. After 72 hours of age, thrombocytopenia is most commonly caused by late-onset bacterial or fungal infections, necrotising enterocolitis, and giant haemangiomata (Kasabach-Merritt syndrome is a rare cause). Treatment is directed towards the underlying cause, with platelet transfusion in more severe cases **(Fig. 3.71)**.

Coagulation Disorders

Coagulation problems can occur as a result of an inherited bleeding disorder, or as a result of coagulation cascade and poor liver reserve of clotting factors in a preterm, sick or septic infant. Coagulation studies are indicated when there is a family history of a bleeding disorder and in cases of abnormal bleeding or sepsis. Coagulation studies are also indicated in extremely preterm babies, bearing in mind that the parameters of normal are different from those in term infants.

Haemorrhagic Disease of the Newborn

Haemorrhagic disease of the newborn is caused by a lack of the vitamin K-dependent clotting factors. It is entirely preventable by routine administration of intramuscular vitamin K at birth. Vitamin K is naturally produced by the bacterial flora of the gut; production is therefore delayed pending postnatal colonisation of the gut. The breastfed baby is most at risk of haemorrhagic disease of the newborn which presents with spontaneous bleeding late in the first week of life, usually either haematemesis, melaena, or bleeding from the umbilicus. Intracranial bleeding may be fatal. Coagulation screen will show a prolonged prothrombin time (PT) but a normal activated partial thromboplastin time (APTT); treatment is with intramuscular or intravenous vitamin K.

Disseminated Intravascular Coagulation

Disseminated intravascular coagulation (DIC) is an acquired coagulation disorder in which intravascular consumption of platelets and clotting factors II, V, VIII, and fibrinogen results from the deposition of thrombi in small vessels. It may occur in association with septicaemia, shock, birth asphyxia or severe rhesus disease. Investigations will show thrombocytopenia, prolonged PT, APTT and thrombin time, and low fibrinogen together with fragmented and distorted red cells. Treatment should be focused on treating the underlying cause; the disordered coagulation is treated with replacement of clotting factors and circulatory support.

Inherited Disorders of Coagulation

Coagulation factors are not transferred from the maternal circulation to the foetus and so factor VIII and factor IX deficiency (haemophilia A and B, respectively) may present in the newborn period, typically following intramuscular injection. The diagnosis is confirmed by prolonged APTT, normal PT, and decreased factor VIII assay. Diagnosis at birth can be difficult as clotting factor assays may be low even in healthy newborns.

JAUNDICE

Many neonates become visibly jaundiced in the first week of life. In the vast majority, this resolves spontaneously and causes no harm. Typically, jaundice is visible first on the face and eyes and then the trunk followed by the extremities; it fades in the opposite direction (Fig. 3.72).

Such 'physiological jaundice' occurs as a result of two mechanisms:

- The shorter lifespan of foetal red cells and the relatively higher haematocrit at birth means that red blood cells are broken down in large numbers, producing unconjugated bilirubin.
- In utero only unconjugated bilirubin passes across the placenta, so the foetal liver downregulates the conjugation process by reducing levels of the binding protein ligandin and activity of the enzyme glucuronyltransferase. Hepatic conjugation of bilirubin remains reduced in the early days of life and thus unconjugated bilirubin accumulates.

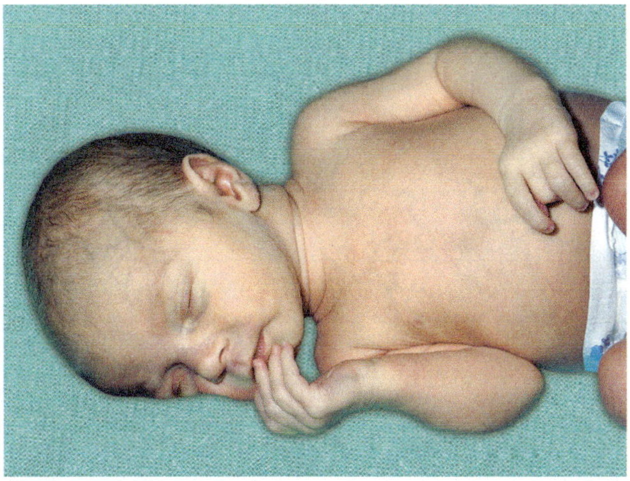

Figure 3.72 Jaundiced baby.

TABLE 3.2 Pathological aetiologies of jaundice.

Increased bilirubin production	*Decreased bilirubin clearance*
Polycythaemia	Gilbert syndrome
Extensive bruising	Crigler–Najjar syndrome
Cephalhaematoma, subaponeurotic haemorrhage	Lucey–Driscoll syndrome Hypothyroidism
Immune haemolytic anaemia	
Rh, D, c, Kell, Duffy, ABO incompatibility	
Non-immune haemolytic anaemia, e.g. G6PD deficiency, hereditary spherocytosis	

Around 60% of full-term and 80% of preterm babies become jaundiced in the first 2 weeks of life. Breastfed babies are more likely to become jaundiced and for this to extend beyond 14 days but jaundice is not an indication to discontinue breastfeeding.

Causes of excessive neonatal jaundice are given in Table 3.2. Jaundice visible before 24 hours of age is commonly pathological.

Haemolytic disease of the newborn caused by RhD isoimmunisation is now rare, thanks to the introduction of prophylactic anti-D for Rh-negative mothers. Cases due to other antibodies such as c, Kell and Duffy are not amenable to antenatal prophylaxis. Rarely ABO incompatibility can cause significant haemolytic disease of the newborn. Haemolysis does not commence at birth but will have been on-going in utero; although excess bilirubin will be removed by the placenta, the affected foetus may become anaemic. Severe anaemia leads to high-output cardiac failure and hydrops fetalis. In utero blood transfusion is effective in reducing morbidity and mortality in haemolysing foetuses.

Treatment of Neonatal Jaundice

The aim of treatment of neonatal jaundice is to anticipate and prevents neurotoxic bilirubin levels. Gestation-specific charts exist to guide when treatment is indicated, taking into account the age of the baby and the rate of bilirubin accumulation (Fig. 3.73).

Phototherapy

Light containing wavelengths between 430 and 490 nm converts bilirubin into photoisomers which are excreted in bile and urine, thus bypassing the overloaded hepatic excretory mechanisms. In most cases, phototherapy can be delivered on the postnatal wards without separating mother and infant, allowing brief breaks in phototherapy for feeding, changing and handling.[37] Response to treatment should be monitored by repeated serum bilirubin

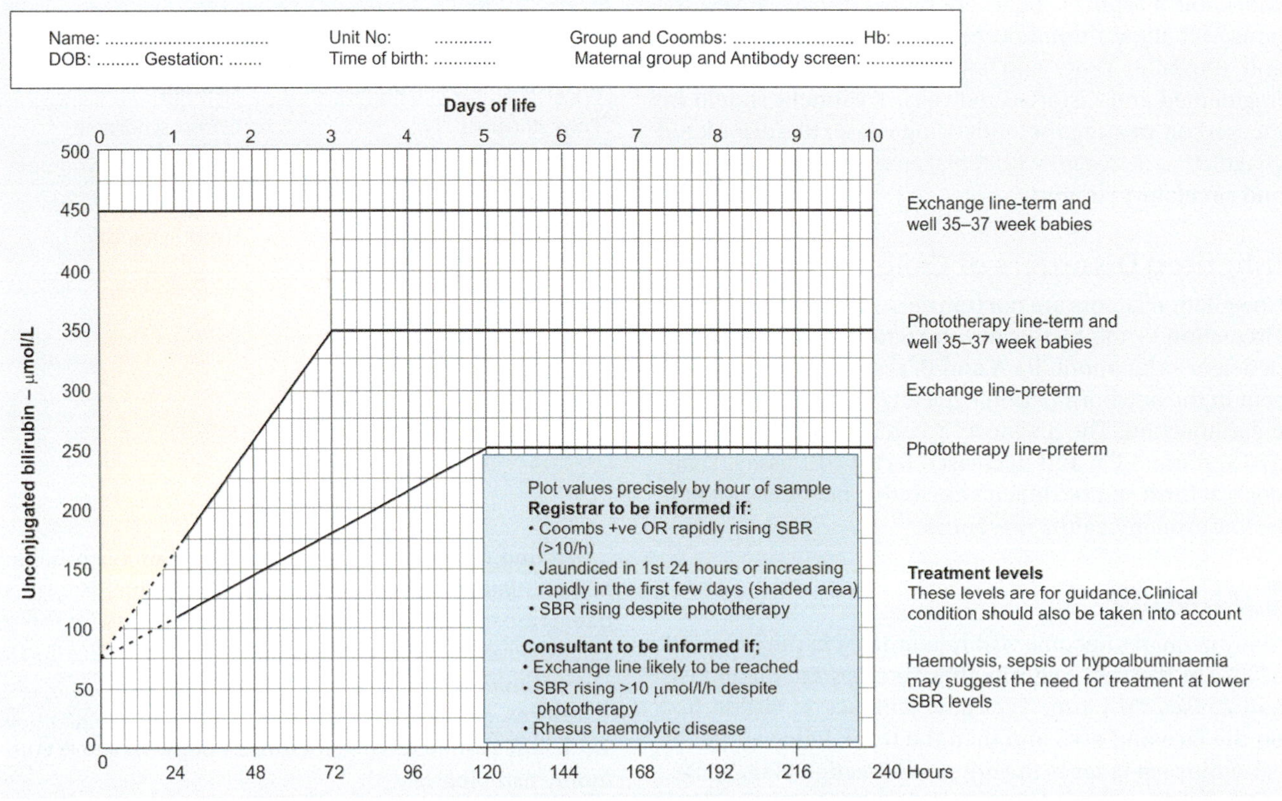

Figure 3.73 Treatment threshold charts: NICE phototherapy chart for infants >38 weeks. Gestation specific charts must be used (treatment threshold charts available at http://www.nice.org.uk/guidance/cg98/evidence/treatment-threshold-graphs-245372941).

measurements; visual estimation of the severity of jaundice should never be relied on during phototherapy.

Intravenous immunoglobulin: Intravenous immunoglobulin infusion may be used in cases of immune haemolysis where phototherapy alone is not controlling serum bilirubin levels. The number needed to treat to avoid one exchange transfusion has been estimated between two (for rhesus disease) and five (for ABO in compatibility).[38]

Exchange transfusion: Double-volume exchange transfusion is an effective but highly invasive treatment of incipient bilirubin toxicity. Central venous access is required (usually obtained via the umbilical vessels) for the incremental removal and replacement of aliquots of blood until double the infant's blood volume has been exchanged. The procedure generally takes around 2–3 hours to complete and carries risks of electrolyte and coagulation disturbances, thrombosis and infection. Exchange transfusion remains, however, a valuable tool in the treatment of extreme hyperbilirubinaemia and profound anaemia secondary to haemolytic disease.

Bilirubin Encephalopathy

Excessive amounts of unconjugated bilirubin can cause permanent neurological damage and even death. The risk increases at bilirubin levels greater than 350 μmol/L, but in a well-term baby, bilirubin encephalopathy is generally not seen with serum bilirubin levels below 450 μmol/L. The integrity of the blood–brain barrier is important in a baby's susceptibility to bilirubin encephalopathy at any given bilirubin level. Prematurity, sepsis, hypoxia, acidosis and seizures all render the infant more vulnerable to the harmful effects of hyperbilirubinaemia. Acute presentation of bilirubin encephalopathy can include poor feeding, irritability, reduced level of consciousness, high-pitched cry and extensor posturing (retrocollis and opisthotonus); long-term sequelae in survivors include deafness and athetoid cerebral palsy. Kernicterus describes the postmortem yellow staining of the basal ganglia following acute bilirubin encephalopathy (Fig. 3.74).

RESPIRATORY DISEASES OF THE NEWBORN

Respiratory distress is one of the most common presentations of illness in the newborn. Tachypnoea is commonly associated with intercostal, subcostal and sternal recession, nasal flaring, expiratory grunt and/or cyanosis. Respiratory distress can be due to a variety of conditions; history, clinical assessment, blood tests and X-ray examination will all help to narrow the differential diagnosis. Significant respiratory distress precludes effective suck

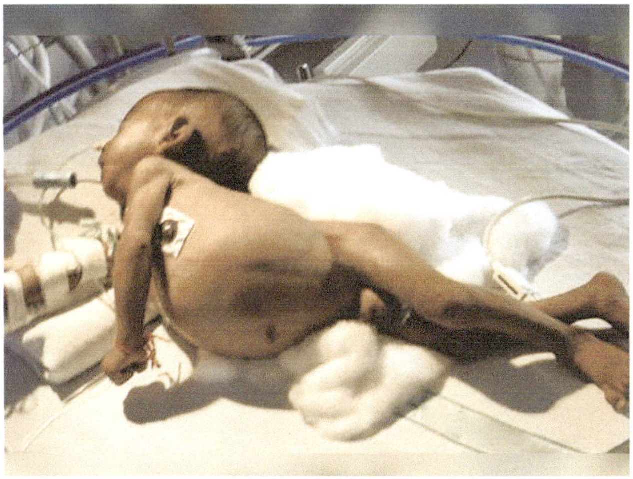

Figure 3.74 Opisthotonos. (*See* Fig. 21.3.)

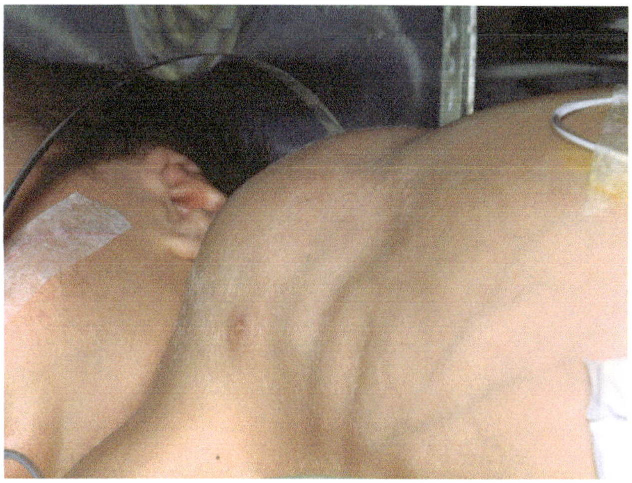

Figure 3.75 Intercostal recession.

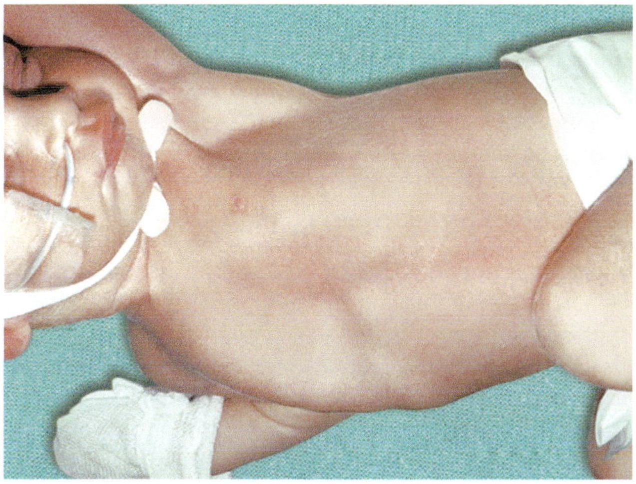

Figure 3.76 Sternal recession.

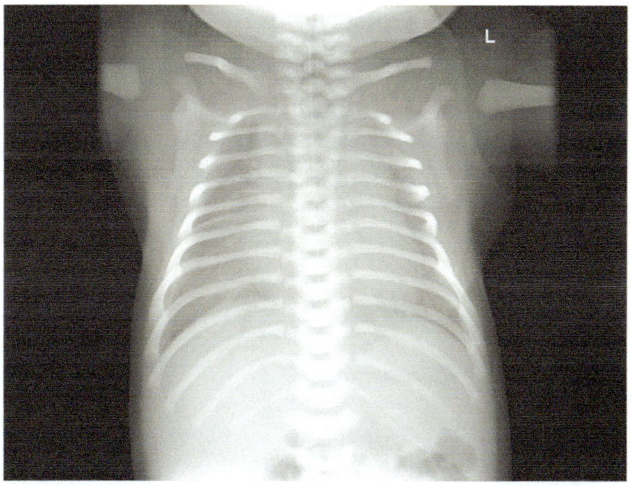

Figure 3.77 Transient tachypnoea of the newborn.

feeding and so gastric tube feeding or parenteral nutrition may be required **(Figs. 3.75 and 3.76)**.

Transient Tachypnoea of the Newborn

TTN primarily affects term and near-term babies delivered by pre-labour caesarean section. In the absence of the onset of spontaneous labour, the normal catecholamine and glucocorticoid surge initiating active resorption of alveolar lung fluid does not occur. Inadequate clearance of lung fluid increases airway resistance and reduces lung compliance. Infants with TTN develop respiratory distress shortly after birth and may require supplemental oxygen or respiratory support, usually in the form of continuous positive airway pressure (CPAP), until resolution of symptoms. Most infants improve within 24–72 hours of birth but TTN can persist for up to 5 days. Blood gases typically show mild hypoxia; hypercarbia may occur in an infant who is tiring. Chest X-ray shows mild hyperinflation with perihilar streakiness, a haze of interstitial fluid, fluid in the transverse fissure and sometimes small pleural effusions. Radiographic changes are diffuse and symmetrical but can mimic other causes of neonatal respiratory distress. Both symptoms and chest X-ray appearances should resolve within 1–3 days **(Fig. 3.77)**.

MECONIUM ASPIRATION SYNDROME

Meconium is the sterile viscous green/black contents of the foetal gut consisting of cellular debris, bile, lanugo and mucus **(Fig. 3.78)**. It may be expelled in utero in response to hypoxia; the latter can also induce deep agonal gasping, resulting in aspiration of the meconium. Thus, conditions causing foetal hypoxia during or prior to labour can result in meconium aspiration, including post-maturity, preeclampsia, cord compression and placental insufficiency. Meconium aspiration syndrome is rare before 34 weeks' gestation and increasingly common with advancing gestation. Thankfully, only a minority of infants born through meconium develop meconium aspiration syndrome;

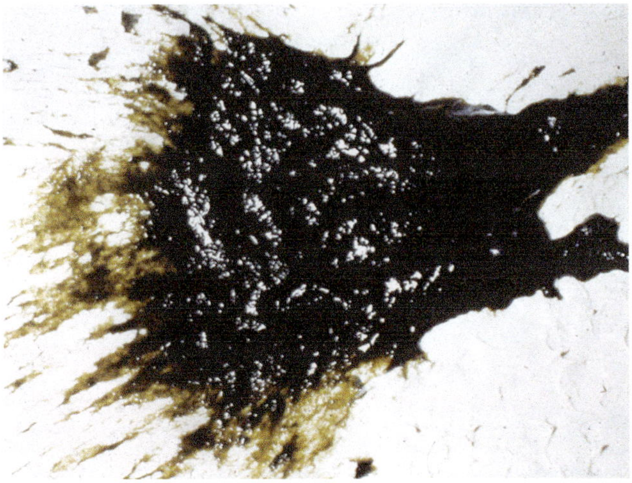

Figure 3.78 Meconium.

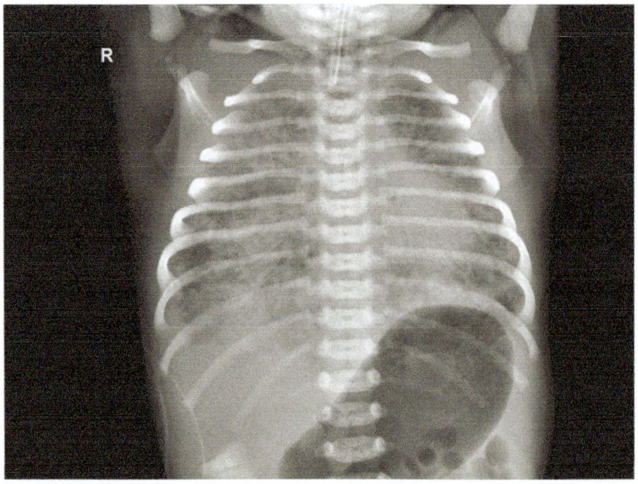

Figure 3.79 Meconium aspiration.

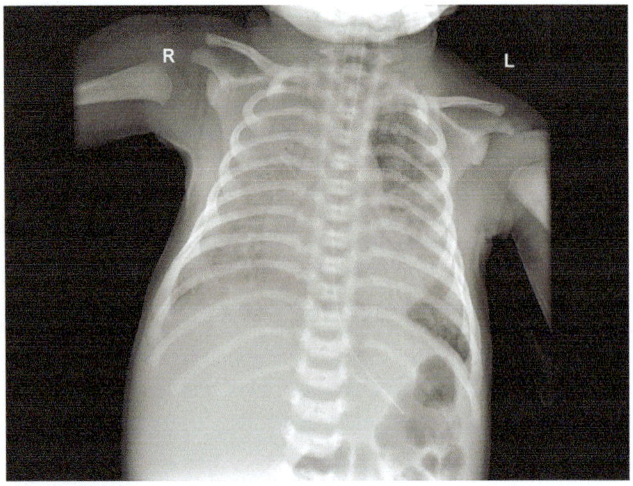

Figure 3.80 X-ray congenital pneumonia.

such infants may be depressed at birth from the preceding hypoxia. Thus, if the infant does not establish spontaneous respiration at birth, opportunity should be taken to remove meconium from the airways by suction under direct vision prior to inflating the lungs. Meconium affects the respiratory system in several ways, including airway obstruction, surfactant dysfunction, pulmonary hypertension and chemical pneumonitis. Patchy atelectasis and hyperinflation are typical findings on chest X-ray and render the infant at risk of pneumothorax or pneumomediastinum (Fig. 3.79).

Treatment is aimed at maximising oxygenation while reducing lung trauma and air leaks, and includes surfactant replacement. Antibiotics should be given since meconium predisposes to secondary infection. Critically ill infants may require inotropic support and treatment of co-existing hypoxic ischaemic encephalopathy and/or multi-organ dysfunction. Minimal handling, adequate sedation and sometimes muscle relaxation of ventilated infants are required to reduce the incidence of both air leak and pulmonary hypertensive crises. Inhaled nitric oxide may be used to treat established pulmonary hypertension. Extracorporeal membrane oxygenation significantly improves outcome in severe cases when conventional management is failing.[39]

CONGENITAL PNEUMONIA

Congenital pneumonia can be acquired transplacentally as part of a systemic congenital sepsis (e.g. CMV, *Listeria*, syphilis), or more commonly secondary to chorioamnionitis and inhalation of infected amniotic fluid (usually due to ascending infection after membrane rupture), or directly from the birth canal and perineum during delivery (e.g. Group B streptococcus, *E. coli*, HSV). The clinical course varies in severity with the infecting organism (Fig. 3.80).

PERSISTENT PULMONARY HYPERTENSION OF THE NEWBORN

The process of transition from foetal to neonatal circulation may be interrupted by various factors, including congenital pneumonia, meconium aspiration or perinatal asphyxia, resulting in persistent pulmonary hypertension of the newborn. Failure of reduction of the pulmonary arterial pressure restricts pulmonary blood flow, and a variable proportion of right heart output instead flows through the ductus arteriosus into the systemic circulation, resulting in severe cyanosis with relatively little respiratory distress. Oxygen saturation measured from the right arm, which is supplied from vessels branching off before the insertion of the ductus arteriosus into aorta, will be 6–10% higher than oxygen saturation measured from the other limbs. Severe persistent pulmonary hypertension of the newborn is a life-threatening condition which must be distinguished from cyanotic congenital heart disease. Echocardiography is useful in differentiating the two; in persistent pulmonary hypertension of the newborn, the heart is structurally

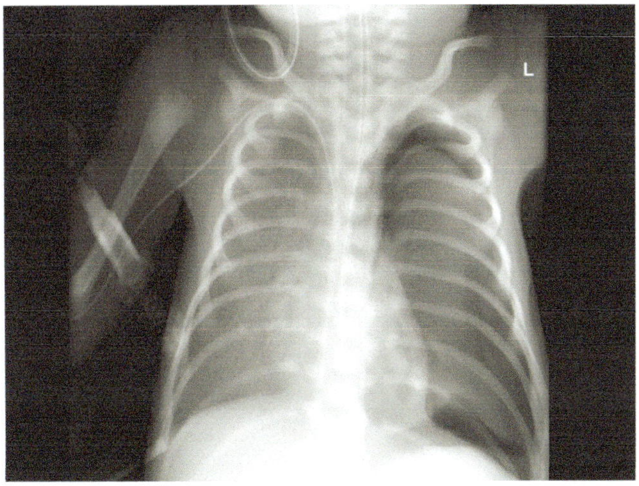

Figure 3.81 Left pneumothorax.

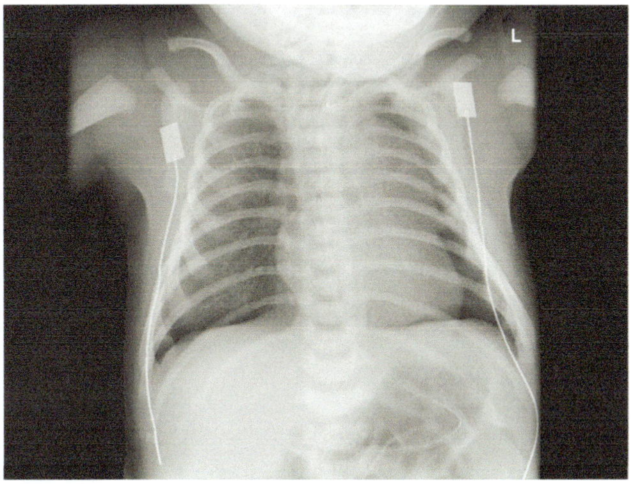

Figure 3.82 Bilateral pneumothoraces.

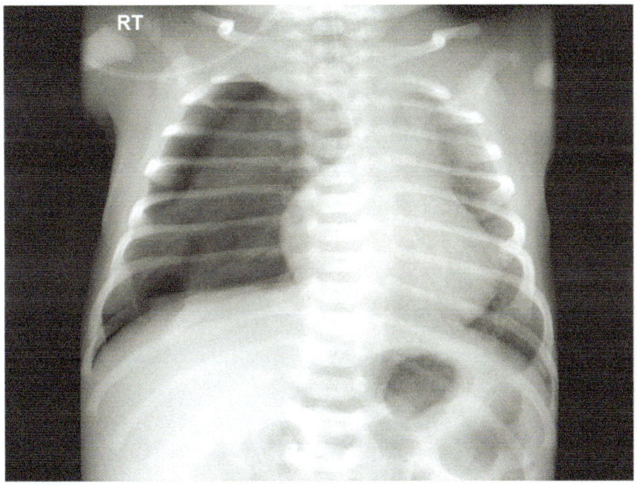

Figure 3.83 Right tension pneumothorax.

normal with right to left flow through a patent ductus arteriosus and tricuspid regurgitation reflecting high pulmonary pressures. Poor myocardial function is often seen.

Persistent pulmonary hypertension of the newborn can be idiopathic, or primary, or may complicate other conditions including congenital diaphragmatic hernia, congenital cystic adenomatous malformation or pulmonary hypoplasia. It is associated with chronic foetal hypoxia, maternal diabetes and Down syndrome. It may also be idiopathic (primary), unassociated with other pathologies.

Treatment

Pulmonary hypertension is exacerbated by hypoxia, acidosis, hypercarbia, hypoglycaemia and hypocalcaemia, and so prompt management is important. Oxygen is a potent pulmonary vasodilator and liberal use to maintain saturations above 95% with normalisation of blood glucose and temperature may be all that is required to reverse mild persistent pulmonary hypertension in a maladapted term infant. In unstable infants in whom persistent pulmonary hypertension is well established, more aggressive treatment will be required, including assisted ventilation and specific treatments such as inhaled nitric oxide and inotropic support to alter pulmonary and systemic pressures. Extracorporeal membrane support may be life-saving when conventional management fails.

AIR LEAKS

A spontaneous pneumothorax is present shortly after birth in 1–2% of all infants, of whom approximately half will be symptomatic. Only a minority will have received positive pressure ventilation at delivery. Pneumothorax and pneumomediastinum are associated with meconium aspiration syndrome, respiratory distress syndrome (RDS), assisted ventilation, CPAP and male sex. Larger collections of air will result in significant respiratory distress, with or without haemodynamic compromise and will require to be drained **(Figs. 3.81 to 3.83)**.

PROBLEMS OF PREMATURITY

Respiratory

Respiratory Distress Syndrome

Affecting structurally immature and surfactant deficient lungs, RDS is typically evident soon after birth with increasing respiratory distress. Chest X-ray shows a ground-glass appearance with air bronchograms. In milder cases, X-ray changes may take a few hours to develop. Antenatal corticosteroids reduce the risk of RDS; the strongest effect is seen when corticosteroids are given between 48 hours and 7 days prior to delivery.[40] CPAP reduces work of breathing and should be given in conjunction with supplemental oxygen to maintain pre-ductal saturations between 91 and 95%. Infants who require more than 40% inspired oxygen to maintain saturations are likely to require assisted ventilation. Surfactant

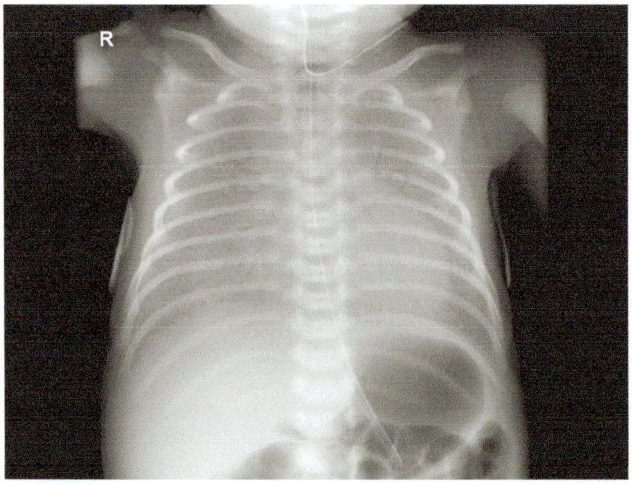

Figure 3.84 Respiratory distress syndrome (X-ray).

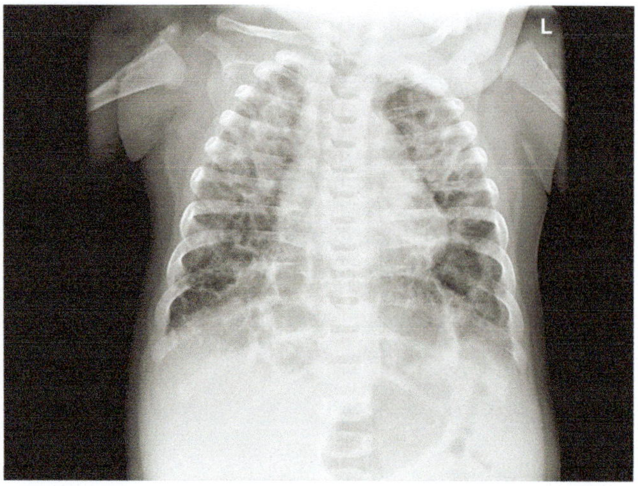

Figure 3.85 X-ray of chronic lung disease.

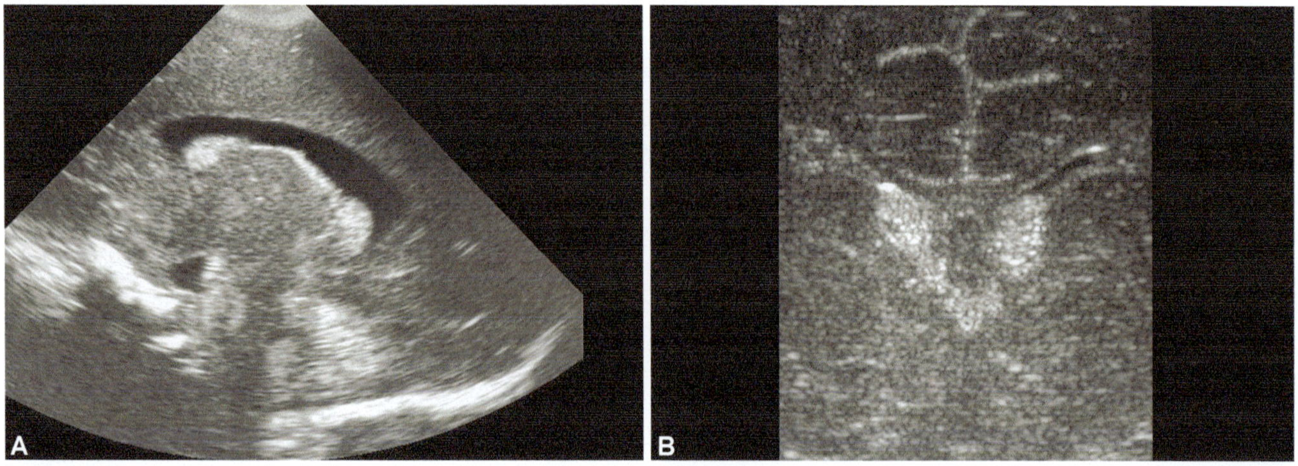

Figures 3.86A and B Grade I intraventricular haemorrhage.

replacement should be given to all preterm infants who require endotracheal intubation, but many can be managed with early use of CPAP alone.[41] Without surfactant, the natural course is of worsening RDS before gradual improvement from 48 hours of age **(Fig. 3.84)**.

Chronic Lung Disease

Chronic lung disease is defined as an on-going oxygen requirement at 28 days or 36 weeks corrected gestational age in a preterm infant. Risk factors include prematurity, low birth weight, mechanical ventilation (particularly volutrauma), patent ductus arteriosus, chorioamnionitis and postnatal infection which combine to result in poor septation of alveoli and disordered angiogenesis in the developing preterm lung. Affected infants have poorly compliant lungs with reduced area for gas exchange and may require an extended period of respiratory support and subsequent home oxygen therapy. Infants with severe chronic lung disease are at increased risk of lower respiratory tract infection, airway hyper-reactivity, pulmonary hypertension and adverse neurodevelopmental outcome. Respiratory status improves with age and growth, although abnormal pulmonary function is demonstrable into adulthood **(Fig. 3.85)**.

INTRACEREBRAL HAEMORRHAGE

Cerebral haemorrhage occurs in 25–30% of infants weighing less than 1,000 g, usually within 72 hours of birth.[42] Bleeding is more likely in unstable infants and generally occurs from fragile vessels in the germinal matrix which overlies the caudate nucleus and is more likely in unstable infants. Haemorrhages may be confined to germinal matrix (grade I), extend into the ventricle, without (grade II) or with (grade III) ventricular dilatation, or extend into the brain parenchyma (grade IV). At-risk infants should have regular cranial ultrasound imaging during the first week of life, with follow-up scans at day 28 and at term-corrected age **(Figs. 3.86 to 3.89)**.

Clinical features are related to the severity of the IVH and include apnoea and bradycardia, increased

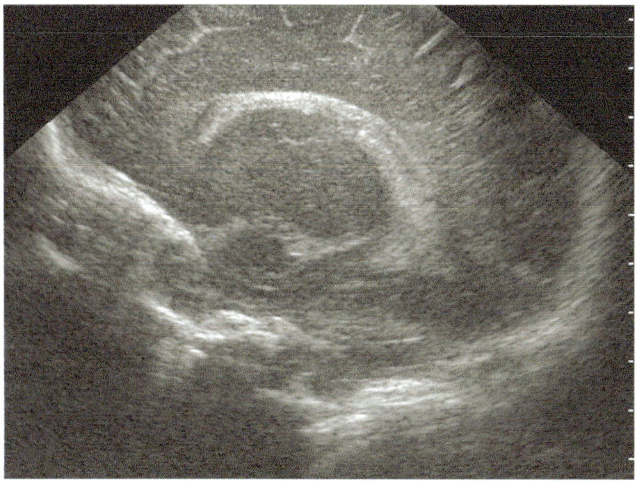

Figure 3.87 Grade II intraventricular haemorrhage.

ventilatory requirements, hypotension secondary to anaemia and abnormal neurology (decreased activity, poor muscle tone, seizures, bulging fontanelle). Most IVH are mild (Grade I or II), and resolve with little or no developmental problems. Grade III and grade IV haemorrhages are more likely to have longer-term sequelae, including cerebral palsy, hearing loss, vision problems and learning disabilities. Up to 90% of children who survive a grade IV IVH will have significant long-term disabilities.

Periventricular Leukomalacia

Periventricular leukomalacia (PVL) is the loss of periventricular white matter in watershed areas around the lateral ventricles. Damage becomes evident as cystic lesions on serial ultrasound examinations, generally from about 3 weeks after the insult. PVL is thought to be due primarily

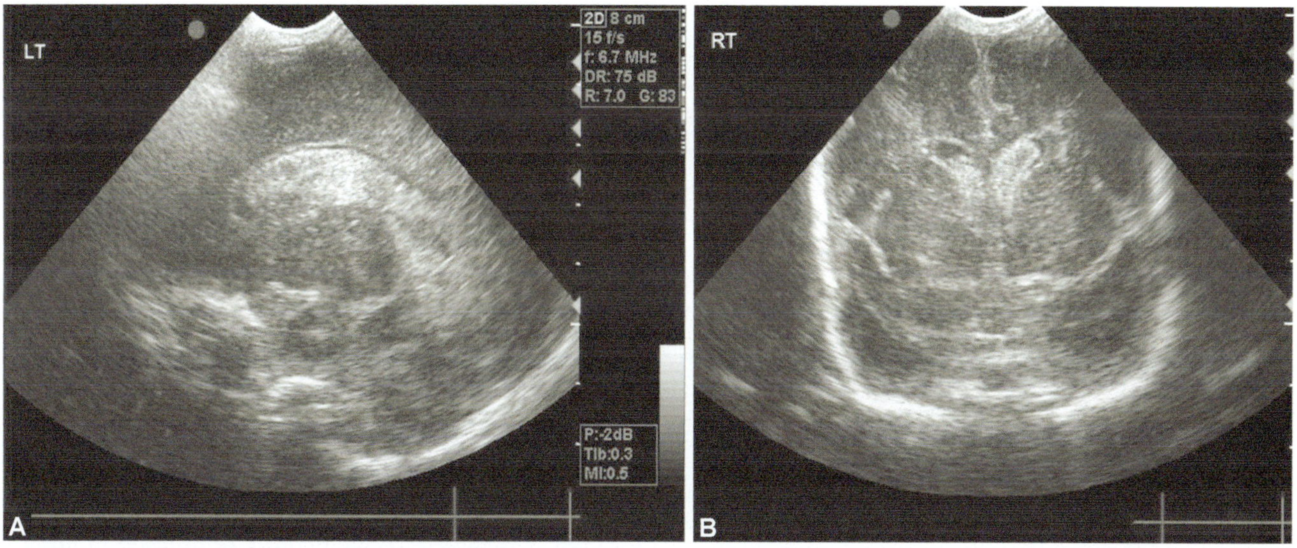

Figures 3.88A and B Grade III intraventricular haemorrhage.

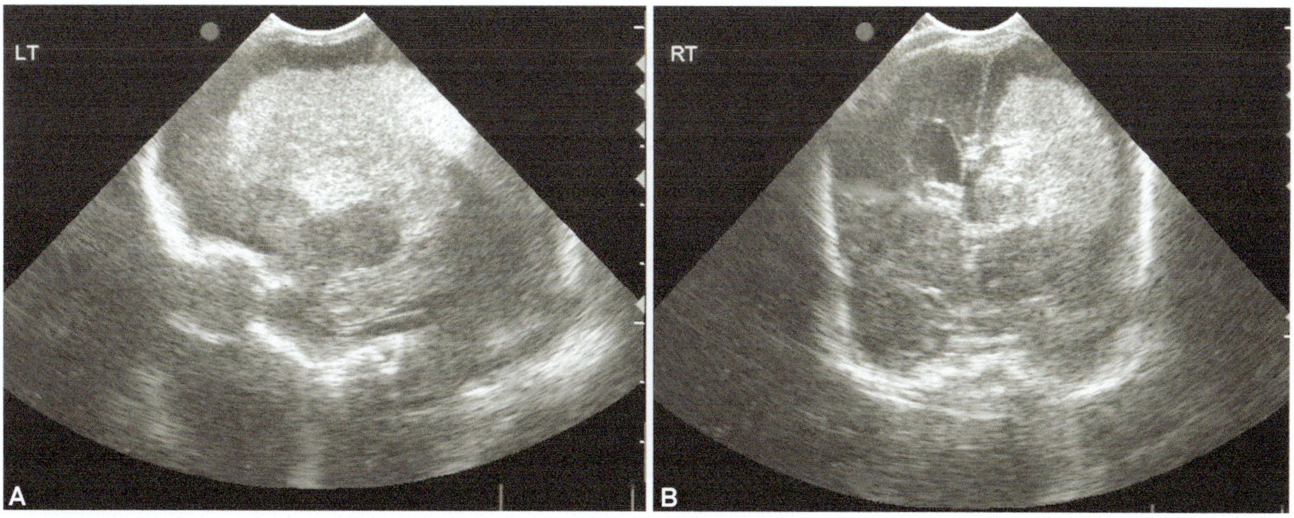

Figures 3.89A and B Grade IV intraventricular haemorrhage.

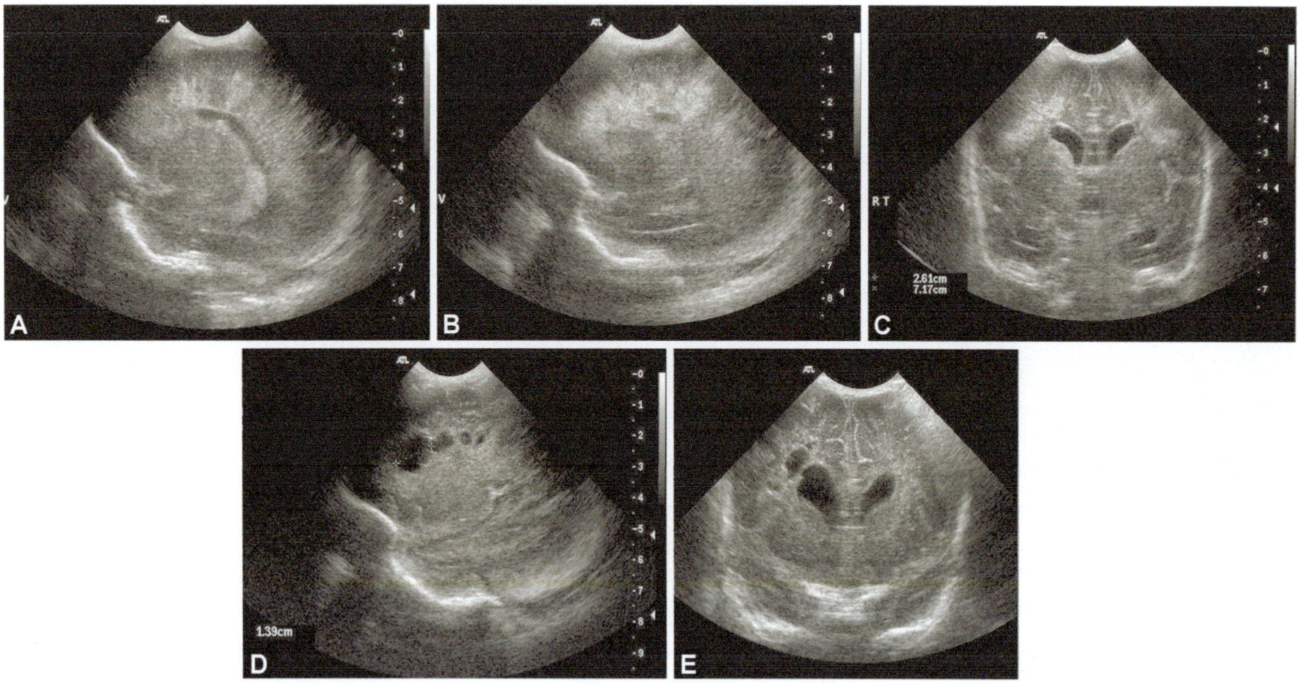

Figures 3.90A to E Periventricular leukomalacia.

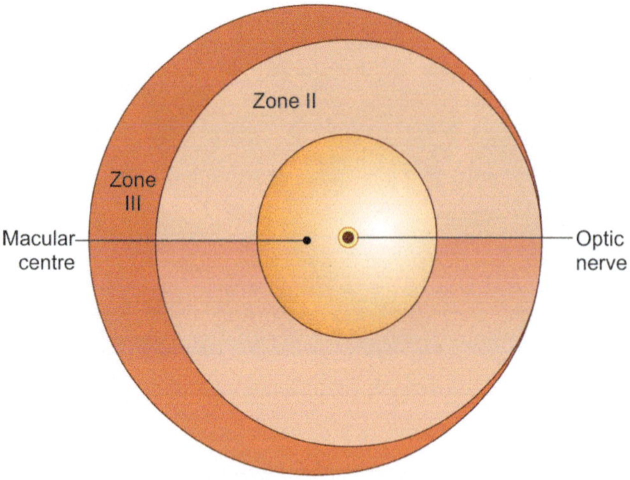

Figure 3.91 Zones of the retina.

to changes in blood flow to the area around the ventricles of the brain. Other contributing factors include perinatal infection and severe neonatal illness. Developmental problems are to be expected in preterm infants who develop PVL (Fig. 3.90).

RETINOPATHY OF PREMATURITY

Retinopathy of prematurity (ROP) is a potentially preventable cause of childhood visual loss most commonly associated with preterm birth at less than 32 weeks' gestation and/or birth weight below 1,500 g. In developed countries, severe ROP is usually seen only in infants of less than 26 weeks' gestation but it may affect more mature preterm infants in resource-poor settings, particularly if supplemental oxygen therapy cannot be accurately monitored. ROP affects the developing vessels within the retina which should normally grow from the optic disc to the peripheral retina between the fourth month of gestation and term.[43] The pathophysiology of ROP involves hyperoxia and then hypoxia, causing production of vascular endothelial growth factor (VEGF), which triggers abnormal vessel growth. Clinical instability including periods of hypotension, episodes of sepsis and excess exogenous oxygen administration increase the risk of ROP. Abnormal vessels may regress spontaneously or proceed to fibrous tissue formation and ultimately retinal detachment. The classification of retinal vascularisation and ROP staging is complex, reflecting the fact that both the location and severity of abnormal vessel growth are important. The location of ROP is described by zone, with each zone centred on the optic disc (Fig. 3.91):

- Zone I: A circle of radius twice the distance from the optic disc centre to the centre of the macula.
- Zone II: From the edge of zone I to the nasal ora serrate.
- Zone III: The residual crescent of retina anterior to zone II.

Staging reflects severity from stage 1, which is mild, to stage 5, when retinal detachment occurs. Ophthalmological screening of all at-risk babies should be undertaken twice weekly from 28 days of life or 31 postmenstrual weeks (whichever is later) until the retinae are vascularised into zone 3 or until disease has regressed.[44] Obliteration of the peripheral retina by laser photocoagulation

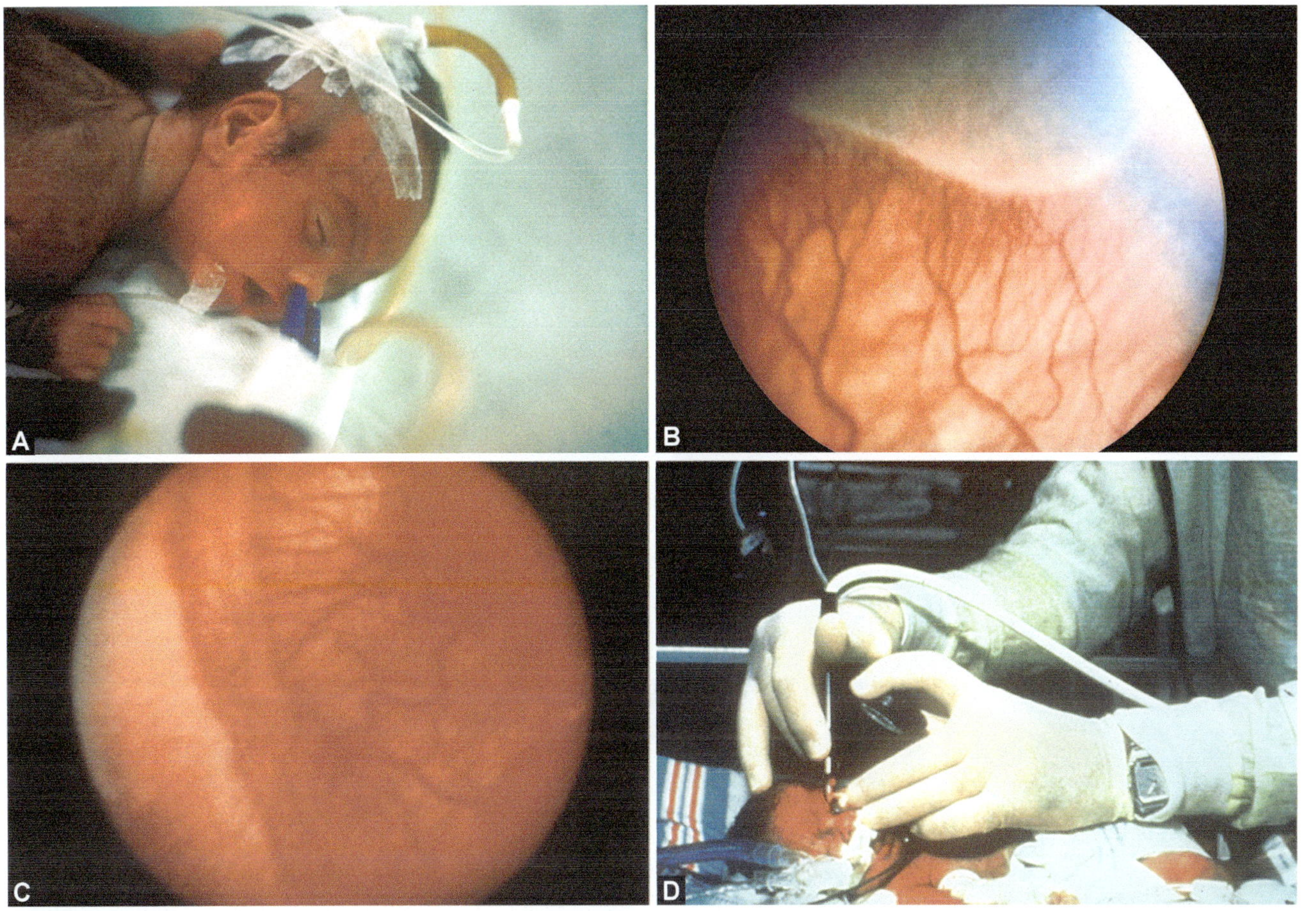

Figures 3.92A to D (A) Supplemental oxygen being given to premature or low-birth-weight baby; (B) Stage 1 disease is shown with a clearly visible boundary between central, vascularised retina, and peripheral, avascular retina; (C) Stage 3 'plus' disease with extensive fibrovascular proliferation (new vessels), and dilated, tortuous retinal blood vessels; (D) A baby with Stage 3 'plus' disease is being given gentle cryotherapy to the avascular retinal periphery under general anaesthesia.

(*Source:* Zin A. The increasing problem of retinopathy of prematurity. Community Eye Health. 2001;14(40)58-9.)

reduces the likelihood of progression of ROP and is indicated for severe disease. Novel approaches to treatment of ROP may include intravitreal anti-VEGF therapy.[45] Infants who have required treatment for ROP may be left with impaired visual acuity and are at increased risk of strabismus and myopia. Follow-up should continue into childhood **(Figs. 3.92A to D)**.

NECROTIZING ENTEROCOLITIS

Necrotizing enterocolitis (NEC) is an inflammatory condition of the bowel of uncertain cause which affects primarily preterm infants. Serious intestinal injury follows a combination of vascular, mucosal and toxic insults to a relatively immature gut. Genetic predisposition may be a contributing factor, and epidemic clusters have pointed towards an infective aetiology, although many infants with NEC will have negative blood cultures. Organisms isolated from infants with NEC may also be found in healthy infants, suggesting that damage to the intestinal mucosa is the main underlying problem which allows spread of commensal organisms beyond their normal location. Inflammation of the bowel starts from the mucosal surface and progresses to haemorrhagic and coagulative necrosis with the ensuing loss of mucosal integrity and transmural necrosis. Although NEC can affect any part of the large or small bowel, the most common location is the terminal ileum. The incidence is very variable, but is positively associated with increasing prematurity and decreasing birth weight. Mortality ranges between 20 and 30%, with the highest mortality in infants requiring surgery.[46] Risk factors additional to prematurity include IUGR, particularly with absent or reversed end-diastolic flow of umbilical and foetal arteries, congenital heart disease and perinatal asphyxia. In preterm infants, the risk is reduced by feeds of expressed breast milk rather than infant formula.

Presentation

Presentation may be non-specific or include poor feed tolerance, bile-stained vomiting, abdominal distension, bloody stools, respiratory distress and general clinical

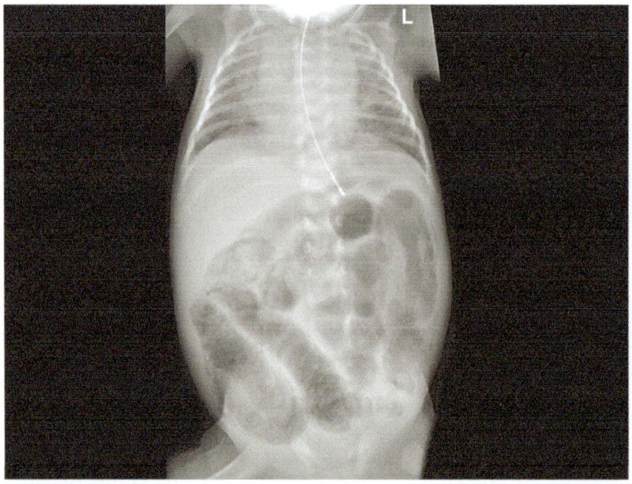

Figure 3.93 Pneumatosis intestinalis.

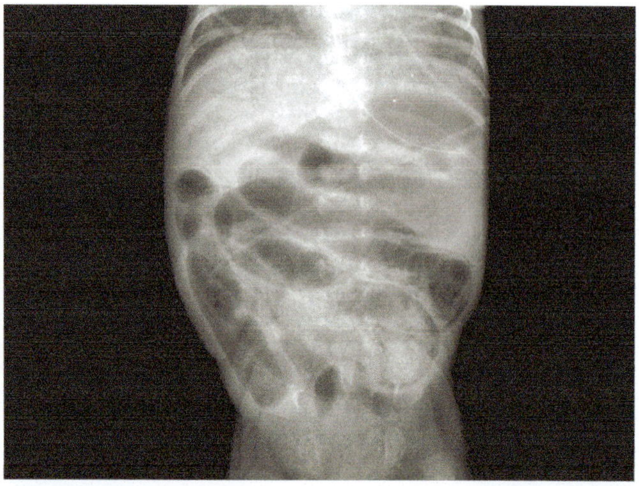

Figure 3.94 Portal venous gas.

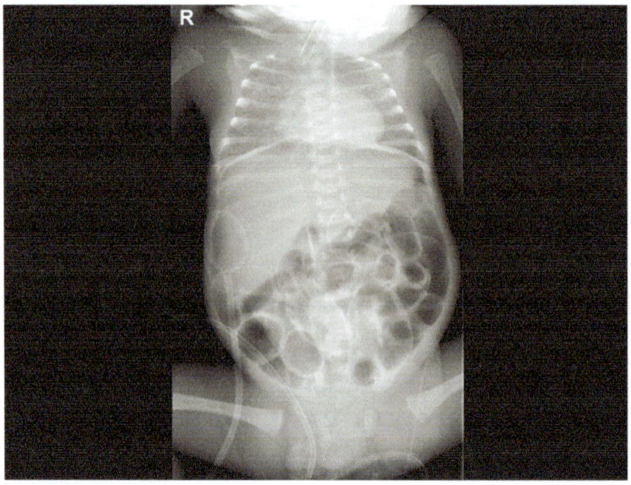

Figure 3.95 Perforation with Rigler sign.

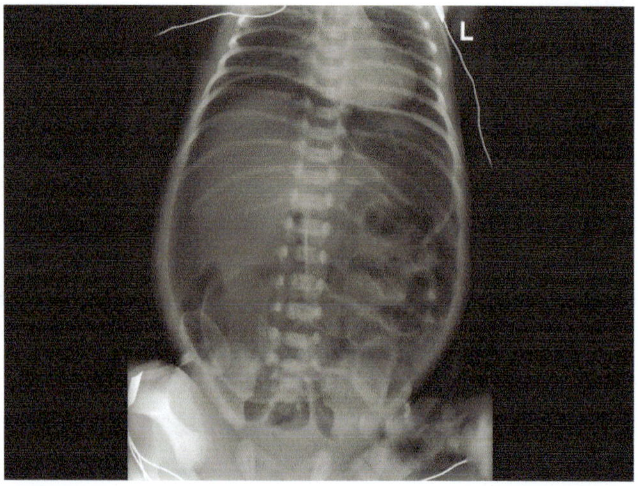

Figure 3.96 Perforation with football sign.

deterioration. Bowel perforation may occur and is likely to be associated with abdominal tenderness, a tense and discoloured abdominal wall, and possibly a palpable mass in the abdomen. Radiographic features include: dilated bowel loops—thickened intestinal wall, bowel wall oedema with thumb printing—pneumatosis intestinalis (intramural gas) and portal venous gas. Pneumoperitoneum indicates perforation; this may be evident as air on both sides of the bowel ('Rigler sign') or air outlining the falciform ligament ('football sign') **(Figs. 3.93 to 3.96 and Table 3.3)**.[47]

Management

Management is primarily supportive. Respiration may be compromised by increasing abdominal distension, and infants may require assisted ventilation. Oral feeding should be stopped and broad spectrum antibiotics administered, with fluid resuscitation as required. Surgery is usually reserved for patients with evidence of perforation, and entails resection of clearly necrotic bowel and the creation of a proximal enterostomy. Other relative indications for surgery include portal venous gas, a fixed dilated loop on serial X-rays and abdominal wall erythema. In the short term, infants are at risk of the complications of prolonged parenteral nutrition including infection, electrolyte derangement and conjugated hyperbilirubinaemia. In the longer term, children may suffer the effects of short bowel syndrome if extensive portions of the bowel are removed. Stricture formation may also occur.

ACKNOWLEDGEMENTS

All X-rays and ultrasound images courtesy of Royal Hospital for Sick Children, Glasgow, Scotland, Radiology Department, with thanks to Dr Sandra Butler. Thanks

TABLE 3.3 Modified Bell staging criteria for necrotizing enterocolitis.[47]

Stage	*Systemic signs*	*Abdominal signs*	*Radiographic signs*
IA Suspected	Temperature instability, apnoea, bradycardia, lethargy	Gastric retention, abdominal distension, vomiting, FOB-positive stool	Normal or intestinal dilation, mild ileus
IB Suspected	As per IA	Grossly bloody stool	Same as above
IIA Definite, mildly ill	As per IA	As above, plus absent bowel sounds with or without abdominal tenderness	Intestinal dilatation, ileus, pneumatosis intestinalis
IIB Definite, moderately ill	As per IA, plus mild metabolic acidosis and thrombocytopenia	As above, plus absent bowel sounds, definite tenderness, with or without abdominal cellulitis or right lower quadrant mass	As per IIA, plus ascites
IIIA Advanced, severely ill, intact bowel	As per IIB, plus hypotension, bradycardia, severe apnoea, combined respiratory and metabolic acidosis, DIC and neutropenia	As above, plus signs of peritonitis, marked tenderness, and abdominal distension	As per IIA, plus ascites
IIIB Advanced, severely ill, perforated bowel	As per IIIA	As per IIIA	As per IIA, plus pneumoperitoneum

Abbreviations: DIC, disseminated intravascular coagulation; FOB, faecal occult blood.

to Dr Richard Bowman, Great Ormond Street Hospital, London, UK, for **Figures 3.11, 3.12 and 3.92**.

REFERENCES

1. Hadlock FP, Shah YP, Kanon DJ, Lindsey JV. Fetal crown-rump length: reevaluation of relation to menstrual age (5-18 weeks) with high-resolution real-time US. Radiology. 1992;182(2):501-5.
2. Dubowitz LM, Dubowitz V, Goldberg C. Clinical assessment of gestational age in the newborn infant. J Pediatr. 1970;77(1):1-10.
3. De Los Santos-Garate AM, Villa-Guillen M, Villanueva-García D, Vallejos-Ruíz ML, Murguía-Peniche MT; NEOSANO's Network. Perinatal morbidity and mortality in late-term and post-term pregnancy. NEOSANO perinatal network's experience in Mexico. J Perinatol. 2011;31(12):789-93.
4. Gülmezoglu AM, Crowther CA, Middleton P, Heatley E. Induction of labour for improving birth outcomes for women at or beyond term. Cochrane Database Syst Rev. 2012;6:CD004945.
5. El Marroun H, Zeegers M, Steegers EA, et al. Post-term birth and the risk of behavioural and emotional problems in early childhood. Int J Epidemiol. 2012;41(3):773-81.
6. McCowan LM, Harding JE, Stewart AW. Customized birth-weight centiles predict SGA pregnancies with perinatal morbidity. BJOG. 2005;112(8):1026-33.
7. World Health Organization. WHO child growth standards: methods and development [online]. 2013. Available from: http://www.who.int/childgrowth/publications/technical_report_velocity/en/index.html [accessed August 2013].
8. RCPCH. Available from: http://www.rcpch.ac.uk/system/files/protected/page/GIRLS%20NICM%20(4th%20Jan%20 2013.pdf. Accessed April 19, 2013.
9. Apgar V. A proposal for a new method of evaluation of the newborn infant. Curr Res Anesth Analg. 1953;32(4):260-7.
10. Newborn life support – resuscitation at birth. 3rd ed. Oxford: Blackwell Publishers; 2011.
11. Laptook AR, Shankaran S, Ambalavanan N, et al. Outcome of term infants using Apgar scores at 10 minutes following hypoxic-ischemic encephalopathy. Pediatrics. 2009;124(6):1619-26.
12. National Institute for Health and Care Excellence. Routine postnatal care of women and their babies. CG37. London: National Institute for Health and Care Excellence; 2006.
13. Price HN, Schaffer JV. Congenital melanocytic nevi-when to worry and how to treat: Facts and controversies. Clin Dermatol. 2010;28(3):293-302.
14. Ewer AK, Middleton LJ, Furmston AT, et al.; PulseOx Study Group. Pulse oximetry screening for congenital heart defects in newborn infants (PulseOx): a test accuracy study. Lancet. 2011;378:785-94.
15. Moro E. Das erste Trimenon. Münchener Medizinische Wochenschrift. 1918;65:1147-50.
16. Cronk C, Crocker AC, Pueschel SM, et al. Growth charts for children with Down syndrome: 1 month to 18 years of age. Pediatrics. 1988;81(1):102-10.
17. Cignini P, Giarlandino C, Padula F, Dugo N, Cafà EV, Spata A. Epidemiology and risk factors of amniotic band syndrome, or ADAM sequence. J Prenat Med. 2012;6(4):59-63.
18. Adamson SL. Regulation of breathing at birth. J Dev Physiol. 1991;15(1):45-52.
19. McDonald SJ, Middleton P. Effect of timing of umbilical cord clamping of term infants on maternal and neonatal outcomes. Cochrane Database Syst Rev. 2008;(2).CD004074.
20. Rabe H, Diaz-Rossello JL, Duley L, Dowswell T. Effect of timing of umbilical cord clamping and other strategies to influence placental transfusion at preterm birth on maternal and infant outcomes. Cochrane Database Syst Rev. 2012;8:CD003248.

21. McCall EM, Alderdice FA, Halliday HL, Jenkins JG, Vohra S. Interventions to prevent hypothermia at birth in preterm and/or low birthweight babies. Cochrane Database Syst Rev. 2005;(1):CD004210.
22. American Academy of Pediatrics, American Heart Association. Advanced neonatal life support. Textbook of Neonatal Resuscitation. Washington, DC: American Academy of Pediatrics; 2011.
23. Saugstad OD. Resuscitation of newborn infants: from oxygen to room air. Lancet. 2010;376:1970-1.
24. Rabi Y, Singhal N, Nettel-Aguirre A. Room-air versus oxygen administration for resuscitation of preterm infants: the ROAR study. Pediatrics. 2011;128(2):e374-81.
25. Dawson JA, Kamlin CO, VentoM, et al. Defining the reference range for oxygen saturation for infants after birth. Pediatrics. 2010;125(6):e1340-7.
26. Cramton R, Zain-Ul-Abideen M, Whalen B. Optimizing successful breastfeeding in the newborn. Curr Opin Pediatr. 2009;21(3)386-96.
27. Lawn JE, Cousens S, Zupan J; Lancet Neonatal Survival Steering Team. 4 million neonatal deaths: when? Where? Why? Lancet. 2005;365:891-900.
28. Lee AC, Cousens S, Wall SN, et al. Neonatal resuscitation and immediate newborn assessment and stimulation for the prevention of neonatal deaths: a systematic review, meta-analysis and Delphi estimation of mortality effect. BMC Public Health. 2011;11(Suppl 3):S12.
29. Azzopardi DV, Strohm B, Edwards AD, et al.; TOBY Study Group. Moderate hypothermia to treat perinatal asphyxial encephalopathy. N Engl J Med. 2009;361(14):1349-58.
30. Ruchelsman DE, Pettrone S, Price AE, Grossman JA. Brachial plexus birth palsy: an overview of early treatment considerations. Bull NYU Hosp Jt Dis. 2009;67(1):83-9.
31. Menezes MD, McCarter R, Greene EA, Bauman NM. Status of propranolol for treatment of infantile hemangioma and description of a randomized clinical trial. Ann Otol Rhinol Laryngol. 2011; 120(10):686-95.
32. Kadambari S, Williams EJ, Luck S, Griffiths PD, Sharland M. Evidence based management guidelines for the detection and treatment of congenital CMV. Early Hum Dev. 2011;87(11):723-8.
33. National Institute for Health and Care Excellence. Antibiotics for the prevention and treatment of early-onset neonatal infection. CG149. London: National Institute for Health and Care Excellence; 2012.
34. Yahyapour Y, Karimi M, Molaei HR, Khoddami E, Mahmoudi M. Active-passive immunization effectiveness against hepatitis B virus in children born to HBsAg positive mothers in Amol, North of Iran. Oman Med J. 2011;26(6):399-403.
35. Mohsen AH, Easterbrook P, Taylor CB, Norris S. Hepatitis C and HIV-1 coinfection. Gut. 2002;51(4):601-8.
36. Paintsil E, Andiman WA. Update on successes and challenges regarding mother-to-child transmission of HIV. Curr Opin Pediatr. 2009;21(1):94-101.
37. National Institute for Health and Care Excellence Recognition and treatment of neonatal jaundice. CG98. London: National Institute for Health and Care Excellence; 2010.
38. Alcock GS, Liley H. Immunoglobulin infusion for isoimmune haemolytic jaundice in neonates. Cochrane Database Syst Rev. 2002;(3):CD003313.
39. UK collaborative randomised trial of neonatal extracorporeal membrane oxygenation. UK collaborative ECMO trial group. Lancet. 1996;348(9020):75-82.
40. Robert D, Dalziel S. Antenatal corticosteroids for accelerating fetal lung maturation for women at risk of preterm birth. Cochrane Database Syst Rev. 2006;(3) CD004454.
41. Morley CJ, Davis PG, Doyle LW, Brion LP, Hascoet JM, Carlin JB; COIN Trial Investigators. Nasal CPAP or intubation at birth for very preterm infants. N Engl J Med. 2008;358(7):700-8.
42. Papille LA, Burstein J, Burstein R, Koffler H. Incidence and evolution of subependymal and intraventricular haemorrhage: a study of infants with birth weights less than 1,500 gm. J Pediatr. 1978; 92:529-34.
43. Pierce EA, Foley ED, Smith LE. Regulation of vascular endothelial growth factor by oxygen in a model of retinopathy of prematurity. Arch Ophthalmol. 1996;114(10):1219-28.
44. Royal College of Ophthalmologists and Royal College of Paediatrics and Child Health. Guideline for the screening and treatment of retinopathy of prematurity. Available from: http://www.rcpch.ac.uk/system/files/protected/page/ROP%20gUIDELINE%20-%20Jul08%20final.pdf. Accessed April 19, 2013.
45. Mintz-Hittner HA, Best LM. Antivascular endothelial growth factor for retinopathy of prematurity. Curr Opin Pediatr. 2009;21(2):182-7.
46. Fitzgibbons SC, Ching Y, Yu D, et al. Mortality of necrotizing enterocolitis expressed by birth weight categories. J Pediatr Surg. 2009;44(6):1072-5.
47. Kliegman RM, Welsh MC. Neonatal necrotising enterocolitis: pathogenesis, classification and spectrum of illness. Curr Probl Pediatr. 1987;17(4):213-88.

CHAPTER 4

Paediatric Genetics

Margo L. Whiteford

INTRODUCTION

With the improvements in treatment of infectious diseases in the developed world, conditions that are either wholly or partially genetic in their aetiology have become more prominent as a cause of childhood morbidity and mortality. It is estimated that around one-third of admissions to paediatric wards are due to conditions with some genetic component, and therefore, an understanding of basic genetic principles is becoming increasingly important.

The field of medical genetics is an ever-expanding one, and within the context of this text, it is not possible to cover all areas of the speciality in detail. Instead, this chapter tries to provide enough basic genetic information to allow understanding of the aspects of medical genetics encountered during day-to-day paediatric practice.

In practice, clinical genetics does not differ from any other speciality, in that the clinician's ability to make a diagnosis relies on the same skills, i.e. the ability to take a detailed history, including pregnancy and family history, perform a physical examination, arrange appropriate investigations and interpret the results. However, the emphasis may be slightly different, with more time being taken over the family history, and the physical examination may extend to other members of the family as well as the child who is the patient.

HISTORY

A detailed history of a child's illness is always required when a child is seen as an outpatient or admitted to hospital. Obviously, if a child is admitted acutely unwell, then treating the current illness is paramount, but if a genetic cause for the illness is suspected, it is important, once the child's condition is stable, to return to asking questions about the child's previous health, growth and development in much more detail.

In addition to trying to ascertain genetic factors that may have contributed to the child's illness, it is equally important to look for non-genetic factors that may offer an explanation and allow a genetic cause to be excluded: for instance, a history of significant perinatal asphyxia in a child with severe microcephaly and seizures or the ingestion of teratogens such as alcohol and antiepileptic medication during pregnancy if a child has multiple congenital anomalies.

Care has to be taken when drawing family trees in order to get the correct information without causing offence or distress to the family. For instance, many parents feel guilty if their child has been diagnosed with a genetically inherited condition and worry that it may have been inherited from their side of the family. In the developed world, it is not unusual for a woman to have had children by several different partners, and sensitivity must be used while obtaining this information. Similarly, in other populations, asking questions about consanguineous (related) marriages may also cause concern.

Within the genetics clinic, family trees or 'pedigrees' are usually drawn to at least three generations. An example of various family trees is shown in **Figure 4.1**. The child who brings the family to medical attention is usually known as the 'proband', with the parents being referred to as 'consultands'. By convention, males are represented by squares and are drawn to the left of a couple and females are represented by circles. 'Affected' individuals are shaded in, while carriers of recessive disorders and chromosome translocations are half-shaded and female carriers of X-linked disorders are indicated by a central dot. Other commonly used family tree symbols are listed in **Figure 4.1**.

Well before people were interested in human genetics, patterns of inheritance had been recognised in both animal breeding and plant crossing experiments. In the 19th century, Gregor Mendel was the first person to propose the idea of 'recessive' genes to explain why some traits appeared to 'skip generations'. Nowadays, many patterns of inheritance are recognised, and often by drawing a family tree, it is possible to predict the 'risk' to offspring of subsequent generations even in situations where no specific genetic diagnosis has been made.

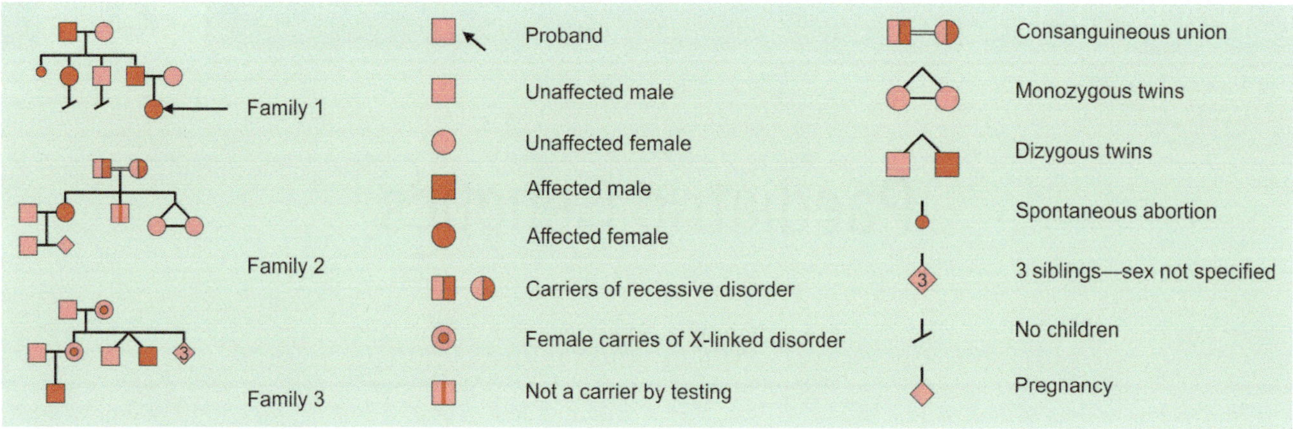

Figure 4.1 Patterns of inheritance.

PATTERNS OF INHERITANCE

Autosomal Dominant Inheritance

With conditions that are autosomal dominantly inherited, the condition typically appears to occur in all generations of a family, and males and females are equally affected [Fig. 4.1 (Family 1)]. The important point to note with dominantly inherited conditions is that males can pass the condition to their sons, and this can be a useful feature for distinguishing an autosomal dominant condition from an X-linked condition in which females are sometimes 'affected.'

The clinical status of an individual is usually referred to as 'phenotype,' whereas their genetic constitution is the 'genotype.' Some autosomal dominant conditions are not fully penetrant, which means that not all individuals who inherit the mutant gene will be clinically affected and others may be so mildly affected that the condition is not immediately noticed. For this reason, an autosomal dominant condition may appear to 'skip' a generation and then return. Thus, when a condition is known to have a variable penetrance, it is important to exercise caution when determining the risk to the next generation, even when an individual has a normal phenotype.

Males and females affected by an autosomal dominant condition will transmit the condition to 50% of their sons and 50% of their daughters.

Autosomal Recessive Inheritance

Typically, autosomal recessive conditions only affect individuals in one generation of a family [Fig. 4.1 (Family 2)], but exceptions to this will occur when the carrier frequency of the gene in a population is high, e.g. 1 in 10 people of Caucasian origin is a carrier of a hemochromatosis gene mutation, and therefore, it is not uncommon for a person who is affected by hemochromatosis to have a partner who is also a carrier of the condition, resulting in the possibility of their offspring also being affected. This phenomenon is known as 'pseudodominance.' Autosomal recessive conditions may also occur in more than one generation of a family if there are many consanguineous marriages within the family.

When both parents are carriers of an autosomal recessive condition, they will transmit the condition to 25% of their children, whether they are male or female, and 50% of their children will be carriers. A person affected by an autosomal recessive condition will have a low risk of having an affected child, provided that their partner is not a relative and that the carrier frequency of the condition in the population is low.

X-linked Recessive Inheritance

X-linked recessive conditions generally only affect males and never pass from father to son [Fig. 4.1 (Family 3)]. However, occasionally a female may be affected by an X-linked recessive condition if she only has one X chromosome (as a result of also having Turner syndrome), if she has a skewed X-inactivation pattern (discussed later), or if she has inherited a mutant gene on both of her X chromosomes, which may occur if (1) her father is affected by the condition and her mother is a carrier or (2) a new mutation arises in the gene on one X chromosome and her other X chromosome is inherited from a parent who is affected or a carrier.

Female carriers of an X-linked recessive condition will have a 25% chance of having an affected son and a 25% chance of having a carrier daughter. All of the daughters of a male affected by an X-linked recessive condition will be carriers and none of his sons will be affected.

X-linked Dominant Inheritance

X-linked dominant conditions also affect both males and females and occur in several generations of a family but their distinguishing feature is that they never pass from father to son.

A female affected by an X-linked dominant condition will transmit the condition to 50% of her sons and 50% of her daughters. A male affected by an X-linked dominant condition will transmit the condition to all of his daughters and none of his sons.

Mitochondrial Inheritance

Although the majority of deoxyribonucleic acid (DNA) inherited from parents occurs within the chromosomes in the nucleus of cells, a small amount of DNA also occurs within the mitochondria, which are the organelles responsible for cell energy production. As sperm do not contain any mitochondria, conditions that occur as a result of mutations in mitochondrial DNA are always maternally transmitted.

The proportion of mitochondria containing the mutant gene varies from cell to cell in all tissues of the body, and therefore, an individual's phenotype will also vary depending on the proportion of mutant mitochondria in relation to normal or 'wild-type' mitochondria. It can be extremely difficult to predict the chance of a woman having an affected child if she is either affected by or a carrier of a mitochondrial condition. The various possibilities arising in this situation are illustrated in **Figure 4.2**.

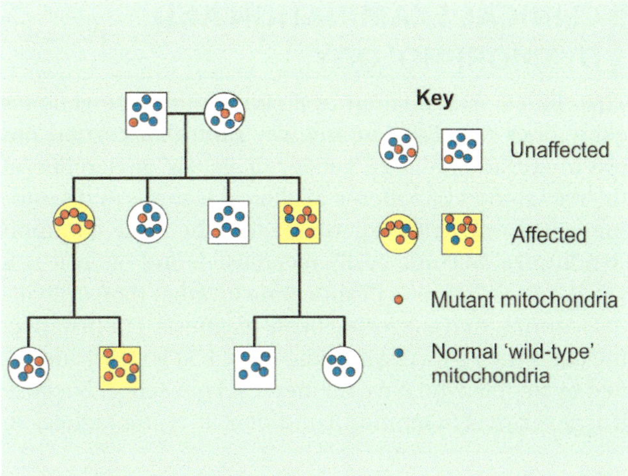

Figure 4.2 Mitochondrial inheritance.

Polygenic Inheritance

Many congenital anomalies and later-onset diseases, e.g. diabetes and hypertension, occur more commonly in some families than would be predicted from the population incidence of the disorder, but do not follow the patterns of single gene inheritance, described earlier. Such conditions are referred to as 'polygenic' or 'multifactorial,' and their aetiology involves both genetic and environmental factors. In this situation, the disorder only occurs if an individual inherits a sufficient quantity of 'susceptibility' genes and is also exposed to specific environmental factors. Many of these multifactorial conditions exhibit a threshold effect **(Fig. 4.3)**, and it is only when this threshold is exceeded that the condition occurs.

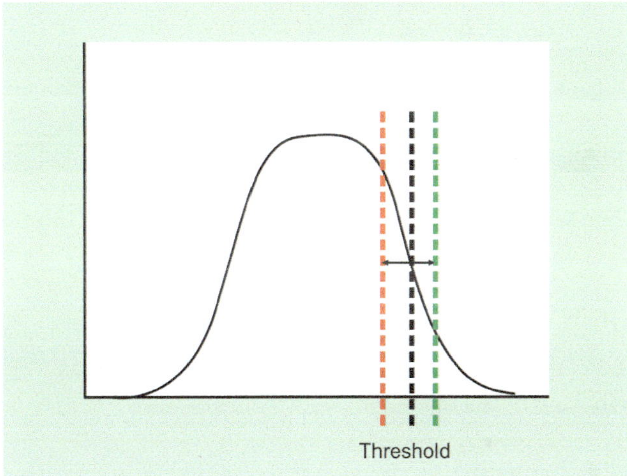

Figure 4.3 Threshold effect.

For the majority of multifactorial disorders, neither the susceptibility genes nor the specific causative environmental factors are known. The exception to this is perhaps illustrated with neural tube defects where the result of the Medical Research Council multivitamin trial, published in 1991, concluded that the risk of neural tube defects occurring could be reduced by 60–70% with periconceptual folic acid supplementation. This in effect moved the 'threshold' to the right of the curve. Conversely, it is well recognised that taking folic acid antagonists, such as some antiepileptic drugs, during pregnancy increases the risk of neural tube defect, and in this case, the threshold is shifted to the left of the curve **(Figs. 4.4A and B)**.

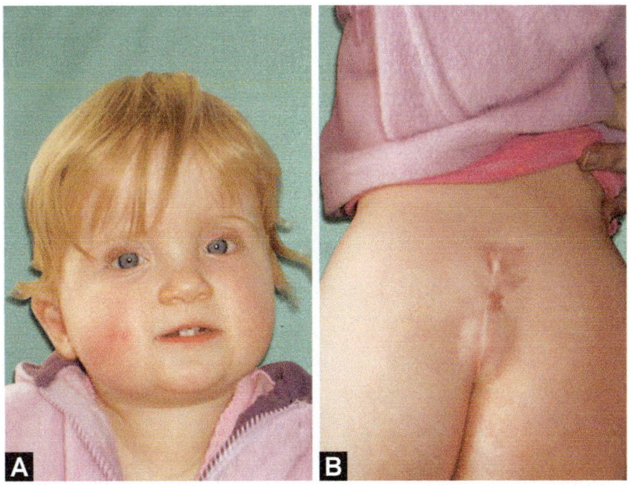

Figures 4.4A and B Repaired neural tube defect in a girl who also has facial features of 'foetal valproate syndrome' (flat nasal bridge, hypertelorism, infraorbital crease, long smooth philtrum).

In order to predict the recurrence risk for multifactorial conditions, geneticists rely on population studies which provide 'empiric' recurrence risks. For most of the congenital anomalies, the risk figures lie between 2 and 5%. If a couple have a second affected child, the risk increases, since it is more likely that for this particular family, genetic factors are involved.

CLINICAL EXAMINATION AND DYSMORPHOLOGY

The clinical examination of a child within the genetics clinic does not differ in any way from that carried out elsewhere, but making a 'genetic diagnosis' often relies on the recognition of patterns of clinical features and symptoms. It is only with experience that the more common 'syndromes' become easily recognised, and often it is a facial 'gestalt', i.e. overall appearance, rather than individual features, that suggests a likely diagnosis. For instance, the child with Down syndrome **(Fig. 4.5)** is easily identified by people who have no medical knowledge, because it is a relatively common condition. It is impractical to memorise the features of hundreds of genetic syndromes, and modern-day geneticists frequently use computerised dysmorphology databases to aid diagnosis. These databases contain information on the clinical features of syndromes compiled from the published literature, and by searching on a patient's key clinical features, it is possible to obtain a list of suggested diagnoses, which aids the direction of further investigations in order to confirm or exclude a particular diagnosis. Clinical features may be regarded as 'hard handles' if they only occur with a small number of conditions, e.g. ectrodactyly **(Fig. 4.6)**, whereas features such as single palmar creases and hypoplastic nails **(Figs. 4.7A and B)** are 'soft signs', which occur with many different genetic diagnoses. Features such as

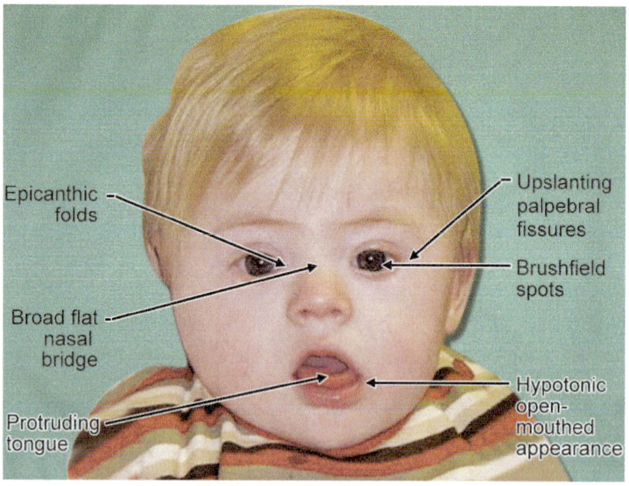

Figure 4.5 Down syndrome (trisomy 21) facial appearance.

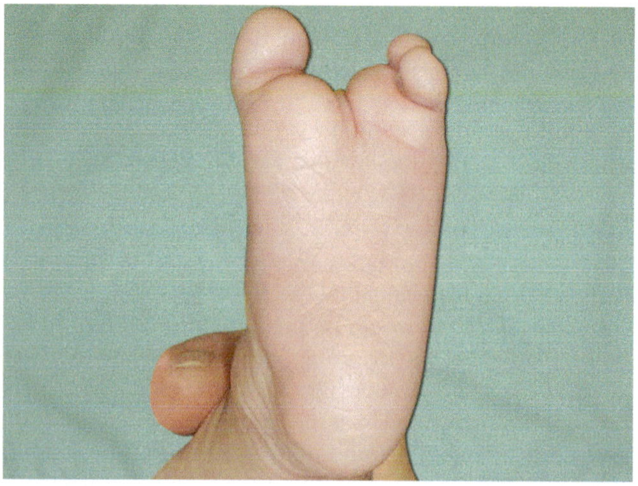

Figure 4.6 Ectrodactyly (split-foot).

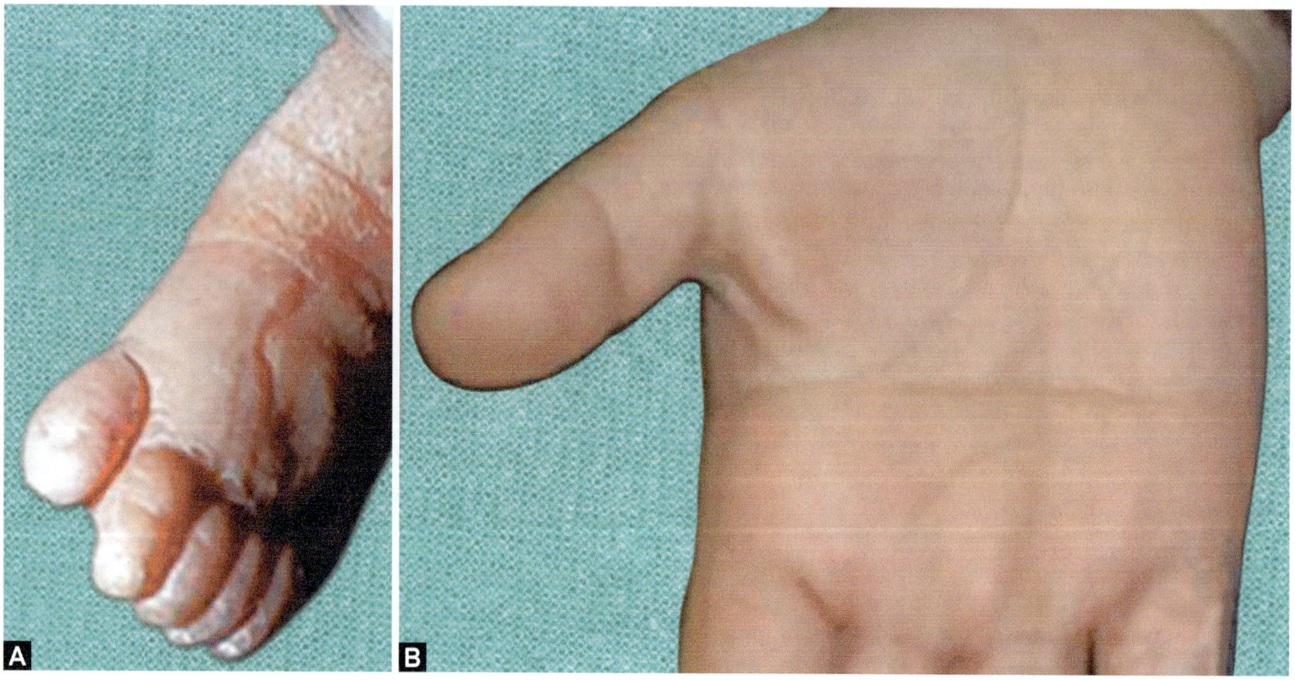

Figures 4.7A and B (A) Hypoplastic nails; (B) Single palmar crease.

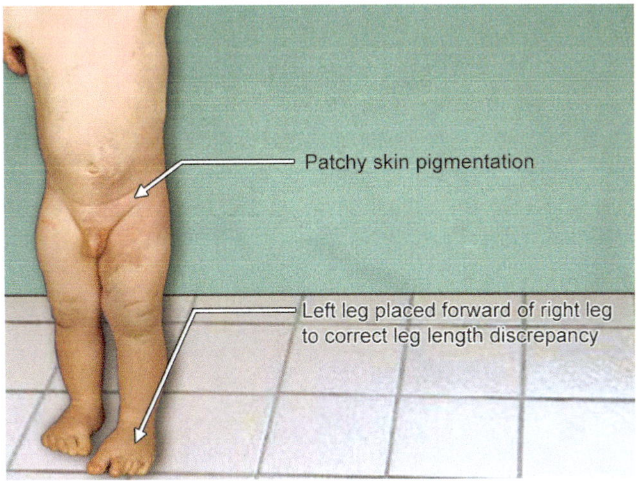

Figure 4.8 Asymmetry.

marked asymmetry of any part of the body (Fig. 4.8) and patchy abnormalities of skin pigmentation are suggestive of 'mosaicism, and a skin biopsy should be considered.

INVESTIGATIONS

The diagnosis of many genetic disorders can be made on the basis of biochemistry results, e.g. sweat electrolytes in the case of cystic fibrosis or urinary glycosaminoglycans in the case of the mucopolysaccharidoses. Similarly, radiographs are an essential tool for the diagnosis of inherited skeletal dysplasias (discussed in Chapter 29). However, the investigations specific to the field of genetics are chromosome tests (cytogenetics) and DNA analysis (molecular genetics), which are discussed in more detail in the following.

Cytogenetics

The study of chromosomes was perhaps the earliest branch of medical genetics to develop, with Hsu and Levan being the first to accurately observe human chromosomes in 1952 and the correct human chromosome number being recorded, in 1956, by Tjio and Levan.

Chromosomes are the structures in the nucleus of the cell into which DNA is packaged. In humans, there are 46 chromosomes in all nucleated cells except the gametes. The 46 chromosomes occur as 23 pairs, with one copy of each pair being inherited from the mother and the other from the father. The first 22 pairs of chromosomes are the same whether an individual is male or female and are known as 'autosomes' and the remaining pair are the 'sex chromosomes'. Females have two X sex chromosomes, while males have one X and one Y sex chromosome. The chromosome constitution of an individual is usually referred to as their karyotype and the normal karyotype for a female is denoted 46,XX and for a male 46,XY.

The chromosomes can only be examined in dividing cells and are best seen during the metaphase stage of mitosis. For this reason, it usually takes around 1 week to get the result of a chromosome test. Various staining techniques can be used to examine chromosomes with the light microscope in order to show the 'banding pattern' along the length of each chromosome. The stain most commonly used is Giemsa, which reveals dark and light regions of chromosomes like a bar code (Fig. 4.9), and by searching for variations in the pattern created by these bands, trained cytogeneticists are able to identify structural abnormalities along the length of any chromosome. The chromosomes are photographed and then arranged in their pairs starting with the largest autosome to the smallest and finally the sex chromosomes. The diagrammatic representation of a chromosome (Fig. 4.10) shows that the chromosome is divided into two arms, (1) the 'p' short arm and (2) the 'q' long arm, by the narrowed centromere region. With the larger chromosomes, the 'short arms' are almost as long as the 'long arms'.

Numerical Chromosome Abnormalities

Soon after the correct number of human chromosomes was determined, it was recognised that numerical abnormalities of chromosomes were associated with clinical disorders. Numerical abnormalities can arise with both the autosomes and sex chromosomes.

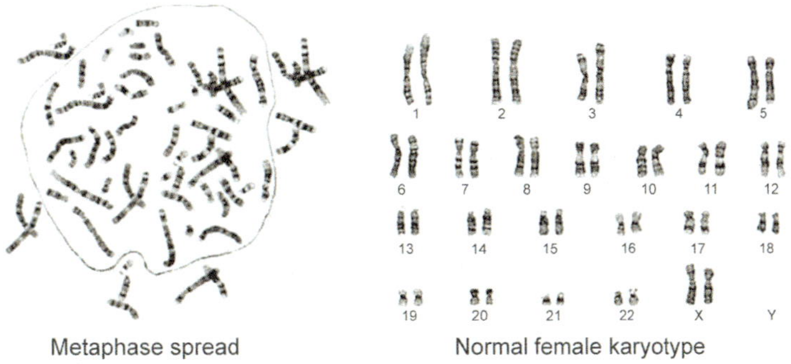

Figure 4.9 Giemsa-banded chromosomes.

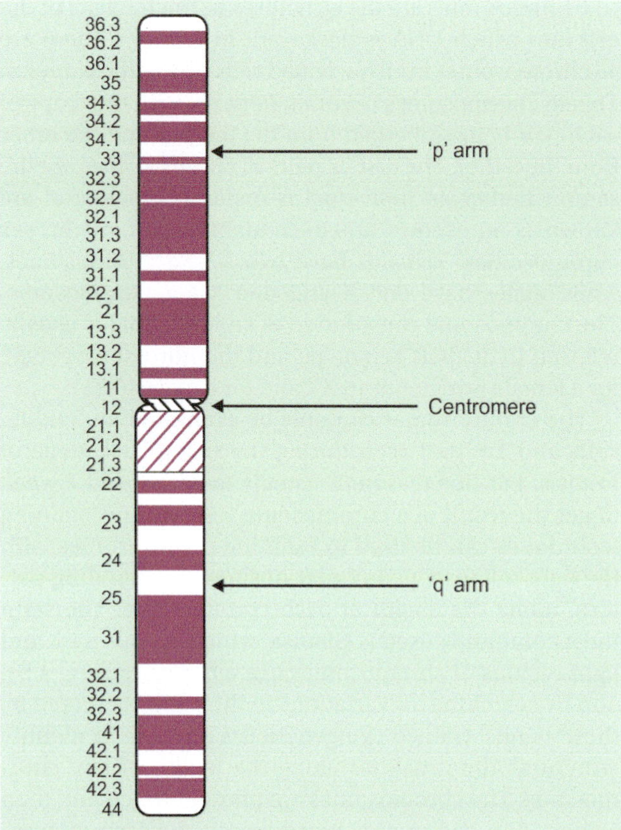

Figure 4.10 Chromosome diagram.

Numerical Abnormalities of Autosomes

Extra or missing copies of any of the autosomes can arise as a result of non-disjunction occurring during meiosis, which is the process by which the total chromosome number is halved during gamete formation. Numerical abnormalities of chromosomes are known as 'aneuploidy,' and most autosome aneuploidies are incompatible with survival, leading to spontaneous abortions of affected pregnancies. The exceptions to this are trisomies of chromosomes 13, 18 and 21, and the clinical features of these conditions are summarised in **Table 4.1**.

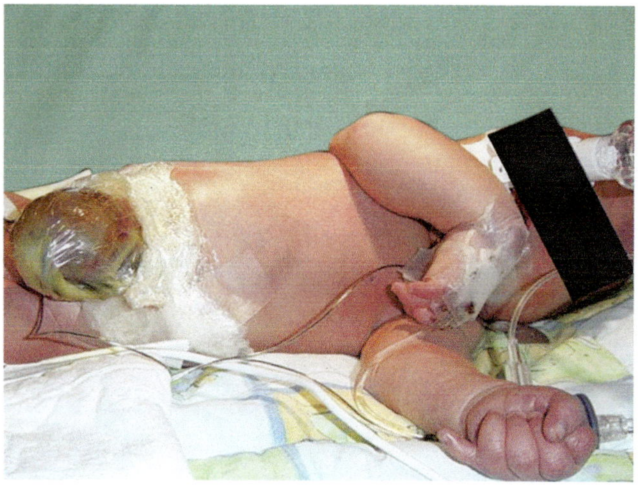

Figure 4.11 Trisomy 13—*note* exomphalos and polydactyly.

Trisomy 13 **(Fig. 4.11)** and trisomy 18 **(Fig. 4.12)** are both associated with multiple congenital anomalies, and the majority of babies born with these conditions die within the first year of life. These autosomal trisomies occur with increased frequency with increasing maternal age, and tables are available for advising women of their age-related risk of having a liveborn baby with an autosomal trisomy. After a couple have had a child with an autosomal trisomy, the risk of recurrence for future pregnancies is around 1% and prenatal diagnosis could be offered in the form of chorionic villus sampling or amniocentesis.

The most frequent autosomal trisomies found in tissue from spontaneous abortions are trisomy 16 and trisomy 22, but these are generally only found in liveborn babies in the mosaic state, i.e. the situation where only a proportion of the patient's cells have the chromosome abnormality **(Fig. 4.13)**. Such mosaic aneuploidies are often only identified by carrying out chromosome analysis of a fibroblast

TABLE 4.1 Autosomal trisomies.

Trisomy	*Name*	*Approximate birth incidence*	*Main clinical features*
13	Patau syndrome	1:5,000	Cleft lip and palate, microcephaly, holoprosencephaly, seizures, severe learning disability, scalp defects, colobomata, microphthalmia, cardiac defects, exomphalos, polydactyly
18	Edwards syndrome	1:3,000	Low birth weight, female preponderance, small facial features, prominent occiput, severe learning disability, low set malformed ears, cardiac defects, renal anomalies, flexion deformities of fingers, rocker-bottom feet
21	Down syndrome	1:700	Hypotonia, flat occiput, up-slanting palpebral fissures, epicanthic folds, Brushfield spots, flat nasal bridge, protruding tongue, learning disability, cardiac defects, intestinal atresia, imperforate anus, Hirschsprung disease

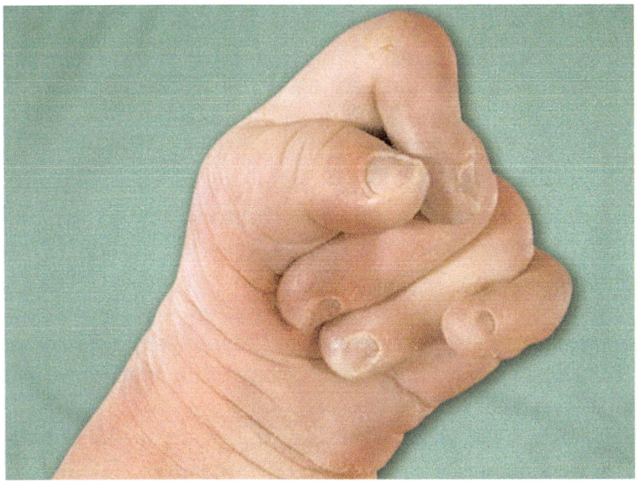

Figure 4.12 Trisomy 18—typical overlapping fingers.

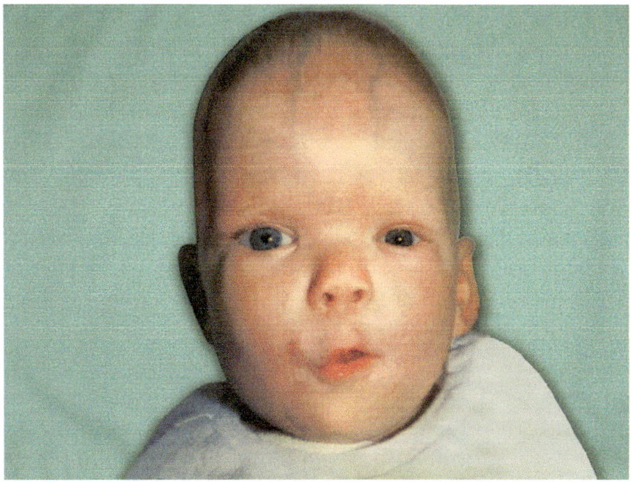

Figure 4.13 Mosaic trisomy 22—*note* marked facial asymmetry.

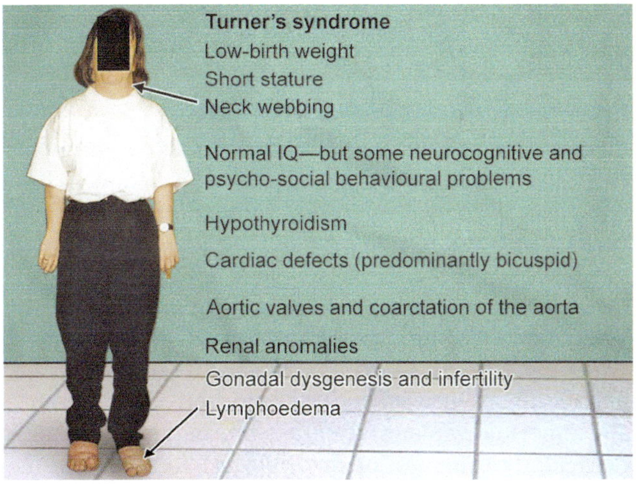

Figure 4.14 Clinical features of Turner syndrome.

culture from a skin biopsy. Analysis of skin chromosomes should always be considered if a patient has marked asymmetry or if a diagnosis of Pallister-Killian syndrome is being considered. Pallister-Killian syndrome arises as a result of mosaic tetrasomy 12p, i.e. some cells have two additional copies of the short arms of chromosome 12 joined together to form an additional chromosome. The clinical features of Pallister-Killian syndrome are summarised in Table 4.2.

Numerical Abnormalities of Sex Chromosomes

It is unusual for abnormalities of the sex chromosome number to be detected in newborn babies as they are not usually associated with physical abnormalities. The exception to this may be girls affected by Turner syndrome, who have only one X chromosome (i.e., a 45,XO karyotype) and who may have congenital malformations (Fig. 4.14). Even in the absence of structural malformations, a diagnosis of Turner syndrome may be suspected in a newborn infant because of intrauterine growth retardation and the presence of lymphedema. This can, on occasions, persist into adulthood (Fig. 4.14).

A 47,XYY karyotype is often detected by chance when chromosomes are being checked for an unrelated reason, e.g. a family history of a structural chromosome abnormality, as this chromosome abnormality is not usually associated with any phenotypic effect. There are some studies that suggest that behaviour abnormalities are more common in boys with 47,XYY karyotypes, but this probably just reflects the fact that boys with behavioural abnormalities are more likely to have their chromosomes checked. An additional X chromosome present in a male (i.e., 47,XXY karyotype) is generally referred to as Klinefelter syndrome and in a female (i.e., 47,XXX karyotype) is called triple X syndrome.

In females, with normal karyotypes, only one X chromosome is active in each cell and the other is condensed into a structure called a 'Barr body'. The X chromosome

TABLE 4.2 Pallister–Killian syndrome—clinical features.

Clinical features	*Description*
Neurological features	Profound learning disability, seizures profound hypotonia
Dysmorphic facial features	General 'coarse' appearance, high forehead, sparseness of hair in frontal region in infancy, hypertelorism, epicanthic folds, flat nasal bridge, large mouth with down turned corners, macroglossia, abnormal ears
Other features	Pigmentary skin anomalies, short neck, diaphragmatic hernia, supernumerary nipples

which is active varies from cell to cell, usually with the maternal X being active in 50% of cells and the paternal X being active in the remaining 50%. If this is not the case, it is referred to as 'skewed X-inactivation'. In children with additional copies of the X chromosome, only one X chromosome remains activated and the additional copies are inactivated to form extra Barr bodies.

Males with Klinefelter syndrome are usually diagnosed in adulthood as they are taller than would be predicted from their parental heights and have hypogonadism, resulting in infertility.

Females with triple X syndrome are also taller than average, and some may experience fertility problems. Around 30% of girls with triple X syndrome have significant learning difficulties, and mild learning difficulties may occur in a small proportion of males with 47,XXY or 47,XYY karyotypes. Multiple extra copies of the sex chromosomes can also occur, e.g. 48,XXYY, 48,XXXX or even 49,XXXXY karyotypes. In general, higher numbers of additional X chromosomes are associated with significant learning difficulties.

The frequency of Turner syndrome is around 1:3,000 female births, while the frequency of Klinefelter syndrome, triple X syndrome and 47,XYY is around 1:1,000 live births.

Sex chromosome aneuploidies are not associated with increased maternal age and the recurrence risk for future pregnancies is not increased.

Structural Chromosome Abnormalities

Structural chromosome abnormalities are termed 'unbalanced' if there is loss or gain of chromosomal material and 'balanced' if the overall amount of chromosomal material remains unchanged. Generally speaking, balanced chromosome abnormalities are unlikely to cause any adverse effect. The main categories of structural chromosome abnormalities are listed in the following and illustrated in **Figure 4.15**.

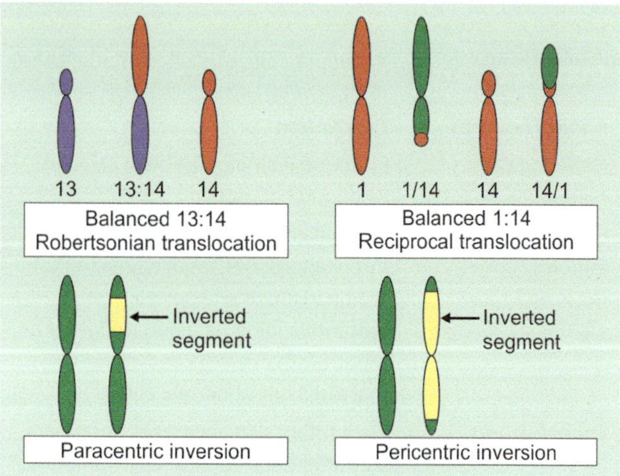

Figure 4.15 Structural chromosome rearrangements.

Robertsonian Translocations

A robertsonian translocation is the fusion of two of the smaller chromosomes at their centromeres. During this process, the short arms of the chromosomes are lost, but as these contain no essential genetic material, no harmful effect occurs. A carrier of a balanced robertsonian translocation will have a total of 45 chromosomes as the two fused chromosomes are counted as one. Similarly, the correct cytogenetic nomenclature for a person with an unbalanced robertsonian translocation describes them as having 46 chromosomes, but they will of course have three copies of the long arms of one of the chromosomes involved in the translocation.

Carriers of balanced translocations are at risk of having children with unbalanced chromosomes. The actual risk varies depending on: (1) The chromosomes involved in the translocation—highest when chromosome 21 is involved, and (2) the sex of the parent who is a carrier—higher when it is the mother. It is important to recognise that all of the children of a carrier of a 21:21 robertsonian translocation will be affected by Down syndrome.

Reciprocal Translocations

A reciprocal translocation is the exchange of segments of chromosomal material between non-identical chromosomes; usually two chromosomes are involved but complicated exchanges between several chromosomes can occasionally occur. This is detected by the presence of a disruption to the normal banding pattern along the length of the chromosomes involved.

Carriers of balanced reciprocal translocations are healthy, but as they produce a proportion of chromosomally abnormal gametes, they may present with infertility, particularly in males, or recurrent miscarriages. Sometimes an individual will be identified as being a carrier of balanced reciprocal translocation following the birth of child with congenital malformations, dysmorphism or learning disability, if investigations reveal the unbalanced form of the translocation in the child. The birth of a liveborn child with chromosomal imbalance arising from a reciprocal translocation is more likely to occur if the length of the chromosomal segments involved in the translocation represents less than 5% of the overall length of all 46 chromosomes.

Inversions

An inversion is the term used to describe a segment of chromosome that has broken away and then rejoined in the same position but rotated through 180°. If the inverted segment is confined to one arm of the chromosome, it is termed a 'paracentric inversion', and if the segment spans the centromere, it is termed a 'pericentric inversion'. Chromosomal inversions usually have no phenotypic effect, but they interfere with meiosis and again may result in chromosomally abnormal gametes being produced. The chromosome abnormalities arising from paracentric inversions are unlikely to be compatible with survival and are, therefore, more likely to result in recurrent early miscarriages. Pericentric inversions, on the other hand, may result in small chromosomal deletions or duplications and can result in liveborn children with malformations or learning disability arising from chromosomal imbalance.

Chromosomal Deletions and Duplications

Deletions or duplications of chromosomal segments may arise, and most of these are unique to the individuals in whom they are identified. However, there are some regions of chromosomes which are more prone to deletions or other rearrangements. These are termed 'subtelomeric' if they occur at the ends of the chromosomes and 'interstitial' if they occur elsewhere. It is now clear that many of these recurrent rearrangements give rise to recognisable dysmorphic syndromes **(Table 4.3 and Fig. 4.16)** and that some of the variability in the features of these syndromes is due to the size of the deletion and the number of genes that are missing as a result.

Many chromosomal deletions are visible when observing chromosomes with the light microscope but others are too small to be seen and require a specialised technique, called fluorescent in situ hybridisation (FISH), to be detected. FISH is basically a molecular genetic technique (discussed later) whereby a fluorescent probe is attached to the region of interest of the chromosome. In the normal setting, two fluorescent signals should be seen, i.e. one on each of the chromosome pair, but if that particular region of chromosome is deleted, only one signal will be seen. In practice, two different probes of different colours are used—one purely to identify the particular chromosome of interest and the other for the specific region **(Fig. 4.17)**.

TABLE 4.3 Chromosomal deletion syndromes.

Chromosome segment	*Syndrome*
4p16.3	Wolf–Hirschhorn syndrome
5p15.2	Cri-du-Chat syndrome
5q35	Sotos syndrome
7q11.23	Williams syndrome
11p15.5	Beckwith–Wiedemann syndrome
13q14.11	Retinoblastoma
15q12	Angelman and Prader–Willi syndromes
16p13.3	Rubinstein–Taybi syndrome
17p11.2	Smith–Magenis syndrome
22q11.2	DiGeorge/Velocardiofacial syndrome

UNIPARENTAL DISOMY AND IMPRINTING

Uniparental disomy (UPD) is a relatively recently recognised form of chromosome abnormality. It is defined as the 'inheritance of a pair of homologous chromosomes from one parent', with no copy of that chromosome being inherited from the other parent. There are various mechanisms by which UPD can arise but it is thought that it most commonly occurs as a result of 'trisomic rescue', i.e. the

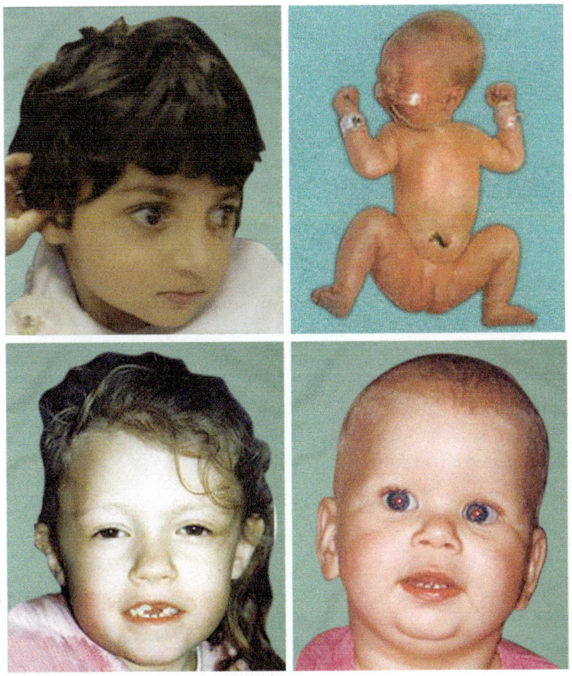

Angelman's Syndrome

Severe learning disability, happy disposition, virtually absent speech, seizures, hypotonia, ataxic gait, microcephaly, prominent jaw, large open mouth, protruding tongue

Prader–Willi Syndrome

Mild-moderate learning disability, severe neonatal hypotonia, poor suck and weak cry, hypogonadism, hyperphagia and obesity in childhood, short stature, small hands and feet, bitemporal narrowing of the skull, 'almond' shaped eyes, upslanting palpebral fissures, stabismus

Velocardiofacial Syndrome

Mild-moderate learning disability, cardiac defects, palatal anomalies, hypocalcaemia, thymic aplasia, myopathic facies, short palpebral fissures, long nose, broad nasal tip, ear anomalies, long slender fingers

Williams Syndrome

Moderate learning disability, characteristic outgoing personality, heart defects (supravalvular aortic stenosis most commonly), renal anomalies, hypercalcaemia, hyperacusis, short stature, 'elfin' facies, full cheeks, thick lips, stellate irides, features coarsen with increasing age

Figure 4.16 Clinical features of some chromosome microdeletion syndromes.

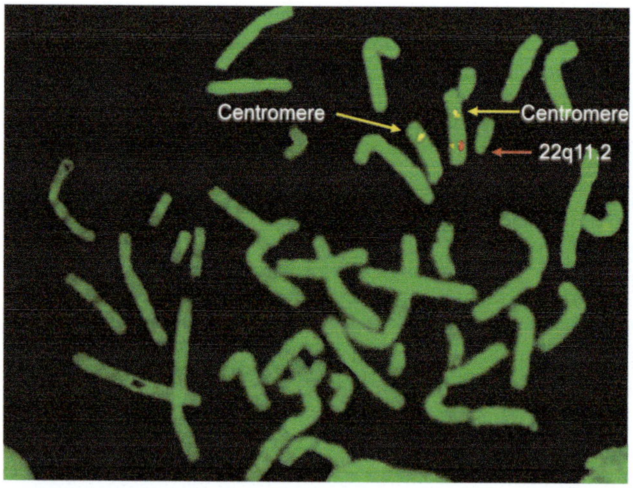

Figure 4.17 FISH technique used to detect the 22q11.2 deletion associated with velocardiofacial syndrome.

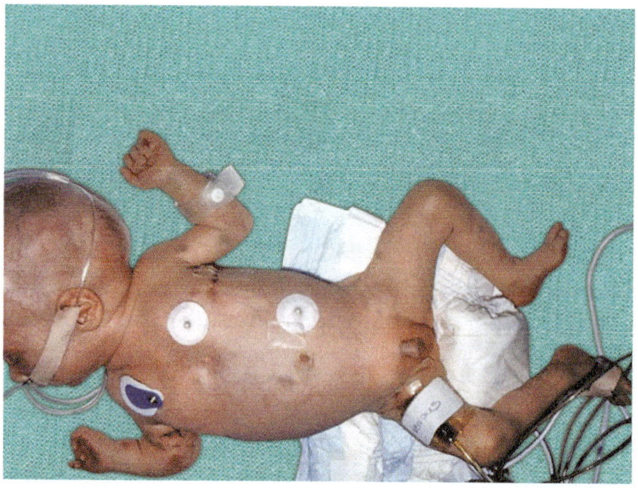

Figure 4.18 Infant with multiple congenital anomalies due to maternal uniparental disomy 16.

loss of one copy of a chromosome during early cell division in an embryo which was originally destined to be trisomic for that chromosome.

With most autosomal genes, both the paternal and maternal copies of the gene are expressed, but a small number of genes are 'imprinted', which means that only the maternal or paternal (depending on the particular gene) copy is expressed. Therefore, although UPD can occur without clinical effect, for certain chromosomes it can mimic a deletion of an imprinted gene, e.g. Angelman syndrome can arise as a result of a deletion of the maternal copy of the chromosome region 15q12, but it will also occur if a child has paternal UPD of chromosome 15, since there will be no maternal copy of 15q12 present. Other conditions arising as the result of abnormalities of imprinted genes are summarised in **Box 4.1**. 'Isodisomy' is a form of UPD where a child inherits two identical copies of the same chromosome from one parent and 'heterodisomy' is the inheritance of a homologous pair of chromosomes from one parent. Thus, another consequence of UPD may be the occurrence of an autosomal recessive disorder in a child, when only one of the parents is a carrier of the disorder. The first case of UPD reported was in fact a child with short stature and cystic fibrosis, which occurred as a result of maternal isodisomy of chromosome 7.

BOX 4.1	Syndromes due to abnormalities in the expression of imprinted genes.
Angelman syndrome	
Prader–Willi syndrome	
Beckwith–Wiedemann syndrome	
Russell–Silver syndrome	
Transient neonatal diabetes	

Another consequence of UPD of certain chromosomes is a recognisable pattern of congenital malformations, e.g. UPD of chromosome 16 can give rise to intrauterine growth retardation, cardiac defects, imperforate anus, scoliosis, hypospadias and hernia **(Fig. 4.18)**.

Molecular Genetics

Before discussing the more clinical aspects of molecular genetics, it is useful to review some basic genetic principles. DNA is the genetic template required to construct all the enzymes and proteins, which are necessary for the formation and function of the human body. DNA consists of strands of nucleic acids, containing the bases, adenosine, guanine, cytosine and thymine, held together by a sugar-phosphate backbone **(Fig. 4.19)**. Each DNA molecule exists as two of these strands wrapped around each other to form

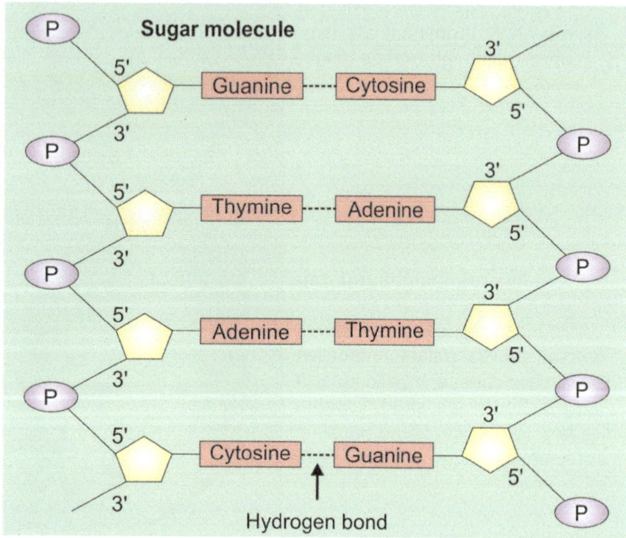

Figure 4.19 DNA structure.

a 'double helix'. The variable part of the DNA chain is the order of the bases along the backbone and the two strands of DNA are linked by hydrogen bonds between these bases. As a result of their shapes, adenine always pairs with thymine and cytosine always pairs with guanine.

It is the order of the DNA bases that form the 'genetic code' required for the production of amino acids and subsequently proteins. The code is a triplet code, as each of the three bases codes for an amino acid or provides the instruction 'stop' at the end of a peptide chain. As there are 43, i.e. 64 possible combinations of these bases and only 20 amino acids, the code is said to be 'redundant' and more than one triplet may code for the same amino acid. This can obviously be useful when it comes to DNA mutations arising since not all base substitutions will alter the sequence of amino acids in a protein, and therefore the protein function will not be lost. Such harmless substitutions are referred to as 'harmless' or 'benign' polymorphisms.

In order to understand how this system works, it is necessary to look at the DNA molecule, shown in **Figure 4.19**, more closely. The deoxyribose sugars of the DNA backbone each have two hydroxyl groups, which occur at the 3 prime and 5 prime positions (denoted 3' and 5', respectively). The phosphate molecules join the sugar molecules together by forming a phosphodiester bond between the 3' hydroxyl group of one deoxyribose molecule and the 5' hydroxyl group of another. This gives the DNA strand a direction, running from the free 5' hydroxyl group of the first deoxyribose molecule to the free 3' hydroxyl group of the last. The two strands of DNA will of course be 'complementary' in view of the base pairing, with one strand running in one direction and the other in the opposite direction.

DNA replication is an extremely complicated process, whereby the strands of DNA are separated and copied to produce new daughter strands. The process is initiated by the enzyme DNA polymerase, and as the initial strands are separated, new deoxyribonucleoside triphosphates are added in a 5' to 3' direction. The process is said to be semiconservative as each new DNA molecule will consist of one of the initial 'parent' strands bound to a new 'daughter' strand.

It was originally thought that genes consisted of a length of DNA providing the triplet code for the necessary amino acids to form a peptide chain. However, it is now recognised that this is not the case and the DNA sequence of each gene contains regions in between its protein coding sequence, known as intervening sequences (IVS). The nomenclature generally used is 'exons' (protein coding sequences) and 'introns' (IVS). There are particular DNA codes which herald the start (TAG) and end of protein synthesis (TAA, TAG or TGA). Similarly, the dinucleotides GT and AG are found at the start and end of introns, respectively. Other particular nucleotide codes, which may be some distance away from the first exon of a gene, are also important for protein synthesis and are known as promoter regions.

The first stage of protein synthesis is known as transcription and involves the processing of messenger ribonucleic acid (mRNA). DNA acts as a template for the production of mRNA and is read in a 5' to 3' direction. The process is initiated by enzymes known as RNA polymerases, which separate the strands of DNA. As with DNA replication, the order of bases along the strand of mRNA, which is produced, is complementary to the original DNA bases. The only difference between DNA and RNA is that the backbone sugar is ribose rather than deoxyribose and in RNA the base thymine is replaced by the base uracil. The primary transcript of mRNA, which is produced, contains the entire DNA coding region, including introns and exons. The mRNA then undergoes a number of processing steps, which result in the introns being cleaved out and the exons being spliced together **(Fig. 4.20)**. Finally, the

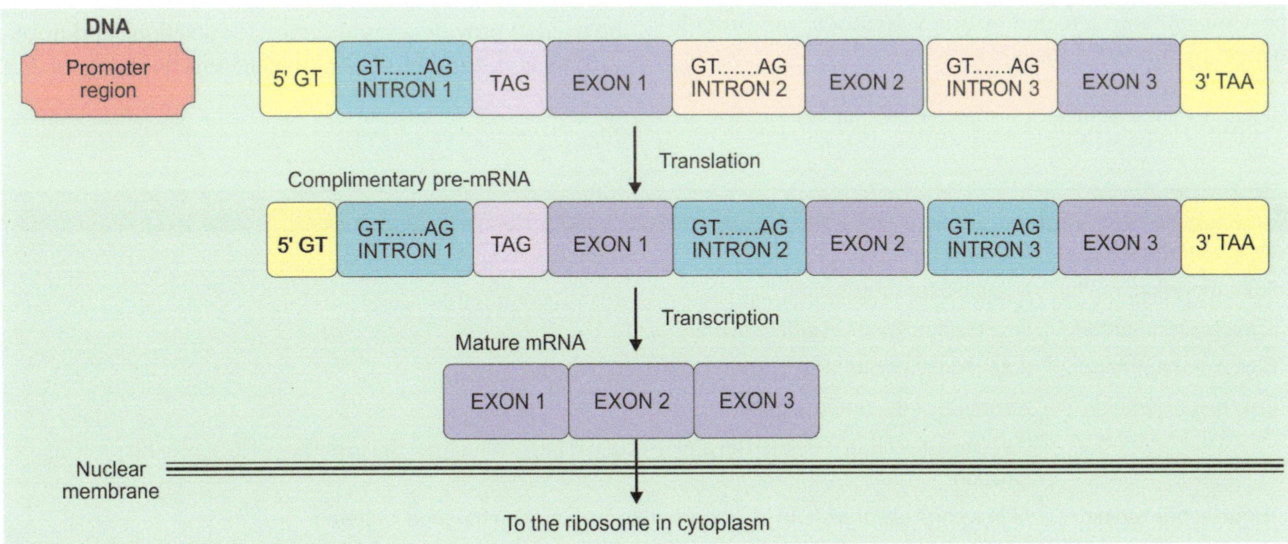

Figure 4.20 DNA translation and transcription.

mRNA is modified by the attachment of various adenylic acids and protein molecules, which serve to protect the mRNA as it passes from the nucleus into the cytoplasm, in preparation for protein synthesis.

The process of protein synthesis also involves several different steps, namely: 'initiation', whereby the ribosome is assembled on the mRNA; 'elongation', where complementary transfer RNA molecules attach to each codon in turn, resulting in the addition of amino acids to the growing peptide chain; and finally, 'termination', when the polypeptide is released into the cytoplasm.

Not surprisingly, with such a complicated process, errors (mutations) can arise and this results in the genetically inherited single gene disorders. There are various different types of mutation and these are summarised in Table 4.4.

MOLECULAR GENETIC INVESTIGATIONS

Southern Blotting

This is one of the older techniques used for DNA analysis, but it is still sometimes needed for detecting large genomic rearrangements, such as the large trinucleotide repeats, which can occur in patients with myotonic dystrophy. The Southern blotting technique is labour intensive and it can take several weeks to obtain results when this process is used.

Polymerase Chain Reaction

For many single gene disorders, 'polymerase chain reaction' (PCR) is now the method of choice for DNA analysis. This process allows the analysis of short sequences of DNA which have been selectively amplified, and tests looking for common recurring mutations, such as in cystic fibrosis, or known familial mutations which have previously been detected by other methods, can provide results within 48 hours.

DNA Sequencing

This type of testing reveals the specific sequence of bases within a region of DNA and compares them to reference sequence data in order to determine if any substitutions, deletions, etc., have occurred. Although much of this type of DNA testing has been computerised, it initially only allowed the testing of one specific gene at a time and was fairly slow to produce results. However, in the 1990s advances in technology allowed the analysis of several genes in parallel, so-called 'next-generation sequencing', now known as high-throughput sequencing, and currently hundreds of thousands of DNA sequences can be run concurrently. This allows 'panels' of genes associated with causing a particular genetically inherited condition, such as hypertrophic cardiomyopathy and neurological movement disorders, to be analysed simultaneously and thus a diagnosis can be made more rapidly.

With these advances in technology, it is now also possible to perform whole exome sequencing and whole genome sequencing, where the sequence of an individual's entire genome can be determined with relative ease in a short period of time. However, the interpretation of the data produced by this methodology is laborious and can result in many unanswered questions, since not all DNA sequence variants are associated with disease, the so-called variants of uncertain significance.

Molecular Cytogenetics

With advancing technology, the distinction between cytogenetic tests and molecular genetic tests is disappearing, and more frequently, molecular genetic techniques are being used to detect chromosome abnormalities. The main techniques used are: (1) multiple ligand probe amplification (MLPA); (2) array comparative genomic hybridisation (array CGH); and (3) single nucleotide polymorphism (SNP) array. MLPA technique is a high-resolution technique for detecting copy number variation of a large number of DNA segments simultaneously and it can, therefore, be used to provide a rapid screen for deletions and duplications at a number of sites throughout the genome. For

TABLE 4.4 Types of mutation.

Type of mutation	*Outcome*
Point mutation:	A single base substitution
a. Missense mutation	Base change results in different amino acid
b. Nonsense mutation	Base change results in 'stop' and a shortened protein
Insertion or deletion	Alteration of the reading frame
	If a complete codon is deleted an amino acid will be missing from the protein, which may or may not affect function
Trinucleotide repeat	After a particular threshold in expansion reached protein function is altered
	Severity of the disorder is generally related to the size of the expansion

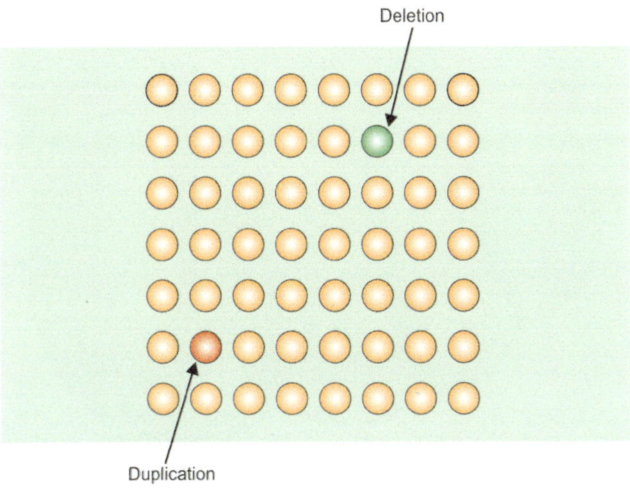

Figure 4.21 Array comparative genomic hybridisation.

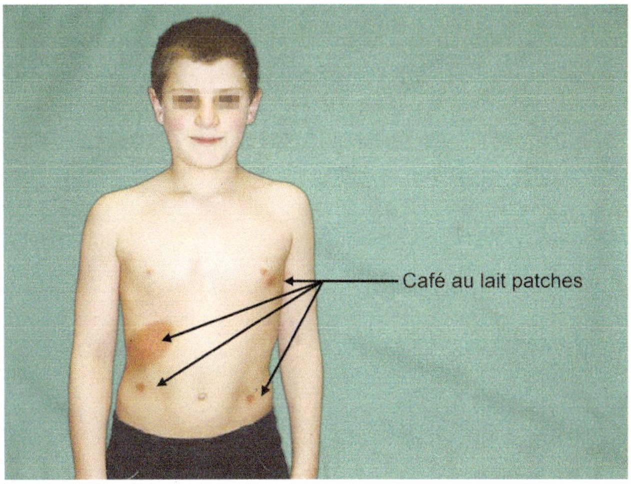

Figure 4.22 Boy with neurofibromatosis type 1.

instance, it can be used to screen for very small chromosomal deletions or duplications in children with learning disability and dysmorphism, in whom conventional cytogenetic testing has failed to reveal any abnormality. With array CGH technique, a DNA sample from the patient and a 'normal control' DNA sample are labelled with different coloured fluorescent dyes (usually red and green) and spread onto a solid surface, which has previously been spotted with short stretches of DNA. The samples bind to these areas of DNA, and the 'spots' look yellow where there is no difference between the patient and control samples, red where the patient has additional chromosomal material (i.e. a duplication) and green where chromosomal material is missing (i.e. a deletion) **(Fig. 4.21)**. These spots are subsequently scanned, and a computerised analysis is carried out to determine the specific regions of chromosomal imbalance and assess which genes are likely be affected by the loss or gain of chromosomal material.

It is now also possible to perform SNP arrays, which means that no control sample is required. With this technique, any 'copy number variants' in an individual's DNA sequence are identified by the amplitudes of the signals produced by probes which are designed to adhere to the A, T, C and G bases in the DNA sequence. One of the advantages of this method over array CGH is that it can detect loss of heterozygosity, which can arise in the presence of consanguinity and UPD.

Single Gene Disorders

The clinical features of many of the single gene disorders have been discussed in other chapters throughout this book, but it may be useful to look at a few specific disorders from a genetics perspective.

Neurofibromatosis Type 1

Neurofibromatosis type 1 (NF1) (von Recklinghausen disease) is one of the most common genetically inherited disorders, having an incidence of approximately 1:3,000. It occurs as a result of mutations in the NF1 gene on chromosome 17 and is essentially fully penetrant, although the phenotype can be extremely variable. In around half of the affected individuals, there is a family history of the condition and in the remainder the condition has occurred as a result of new mutations. The main clinical features are: café au lait patches **(Fig. 4.22)**, which are usually present by 5 years of age, cutaneous neurofibromata, iris Lisch nodules and axillary and groin freckling. Most affected individuals are shorter than average and have larger than average head circumferences. Mild to moderate learning difficulties are common. Regular follow-up is required as a small proportion of people with NF1 develop more severe complications such as pseudoarthroses (present from birth), plexiform neurofibromata of the head and neck (usually present within the first year of life), optic gliomata (usually present by 6 years of age), plexiform neurofibromata of other parts of the body as seen in **Figure 4.23** (usually present before puberty) and scoliosis (usually present between age 6 years to puberty).

In adulthood, other complications such as hypertension (both essential and secondary to renal artery stenosis or phaeochromocytoma) and malignant peripheral nerve sheath tumours may also occur, so follow-up is generally lifelong.

The NF1 gene is a very large gene and mutation analysis is possible, but as NF1 can usually be easily diagnosed on clinical grounds, genetic testing is rarely necessary.

Neurofibromatosis type 1 should not be confused with neurofibromatosis type 2 (NF2), which is a completely separate disorder due to a gene on chromosome 22. Although patients affected by NF2 may have café au lait patches, they seldom have six or more, and they do not have the axillary and groin freckling found in NF1. The most common presenting feature is bilateral vestibular schwannomas.

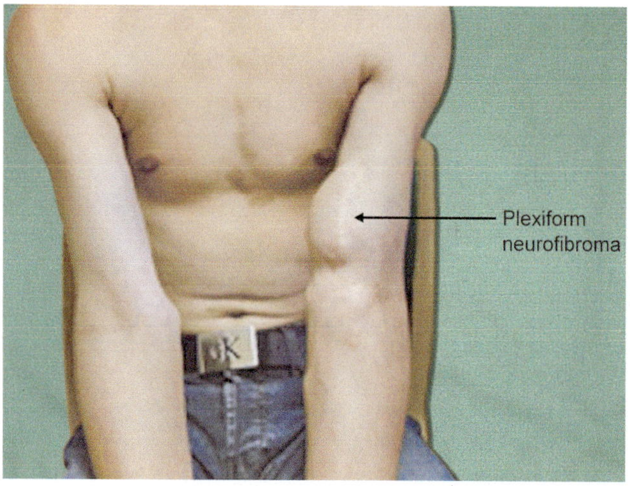

Figure 4.23 Plexiform neurofibroma.

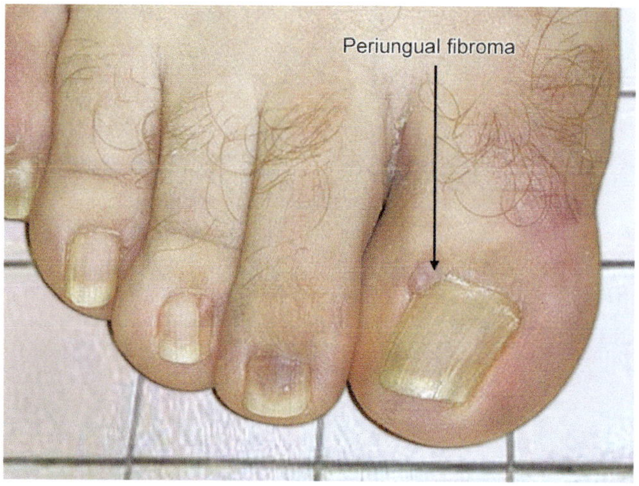

Figure 4.24 Periungual fibroma in patient with tuberous sclerosis.

Tuberous Sclerosis

Tuberous sclerosis complex (TSC) occurs with an incidence of 1:5,000–1:6,000. It can occur as a result of mutations in two different genes, TSC1 (located on chromosome 9) and TSC2 (located on chromosome 16). The condition is now thought to be fully penetrant and recurrences that have occurred when parents are apparently unaffected are now recognised to be due to one of the parents having minimal clinical features such as periungual fibromata **(Fig. 4.24)** and the phenomenon of 'gonadal mosaicism', whereby one of the parents is a carrier of the mutation only in their gametes.

TSC is a multisystem disorder with extreme variability in the phenotype, even within one family. The clinical features are divided into major features (facial angiofibromata, ungual and periungual fibromata, forehead plaques, hypomelanotic macules, shagreen patches (connective tissue naevi), multiple retinal hamartomata, cortical tubers, subependymal nodules, subependymal giant cell astrocytomata, cardiac rhabdomyomata, lymphangiomyomatosis and renal angiomyolipomata) and minor features (dental enamel pits, hamartomatous rectal polyps, bone cysts, cerebral white matter radial migration lines, gingival fibromata, non-renal hamartomata, retinal achromic patches, 'confetti' skin lesions and multiple renal cysts). The clinical diagnosis is based on the presence of two major or one major plus two minor features. In the most severe cases, tuberous sclerosis can present with infantile spasms and such children can remain profoundly handicapped with difficult-to-control seizures throughout their lives. In milder cases, mild to moderate learning disability may be present but some individuals affected by TS have completely normal intelligence. Regular follow-up is again important particularly with regard to the possibility of renal complications.

Mutation analysis is available for both TSC1 and TSC2 and prenatal diagnosis is possible if a mutation is identified.

Marfan Syndrome

Marfan syndrome has an incidence of 1:5,000–1:10,000 and in the majority of affected individuals, the condition is due to mutations in fibrillin 1 on chromosome 15. It is a disorder of collagen and is, therefore, also a multisystem disorder affecting primarily the eye, the skeletal system and cardiovascular system. Individuals affected by Marfan syndrome are usually disproportionately tall with long limbs and arachnodactyly (long fingers and toes) **(Fig. 4.25)**. However, as many people who are tall with long arms and legs do not have Marfan syndrome, it is necessary that patients meet strict clinical criteria, known as the Ghent criteria, before the diagnosis can be made. The main clinical features included in the Ghent criteria are: disproportionate stature, pectus excavatum or carinatum, long fingers, flat feet, protrusion acetabulae (an abnormality of the hip identified by X-rays), dental crowding, joint hypermobility, flat cheek bones, ectopia lentis and other eye abnormalities, dissection or dilatation of the ascending aorta, mitral valve prolapse and spontaneous pneumothoraces.

Although the ocular complications and aortic root dilatation and dissection, associated with this condition, are more common in adulthood, long-term follow-up is required from the time of diagnosis. The diagnosis of Marfan syndrome in the past was mainly based on clinical features but mutation analysis can now be used in combination with clinical features, and in families where a mutation is identified, prenatal diagnosis is possible.

Myotonic Dystrophy

Myotonic dystrophy (dystrophia myotonica) has an incidence of around 1:8,000 and, as the name suggests, is a muscle wasting disease. However, it, too, is a multisystem disorder and can be of very variable severity. The majority of people affected by myotonic dystrophy have

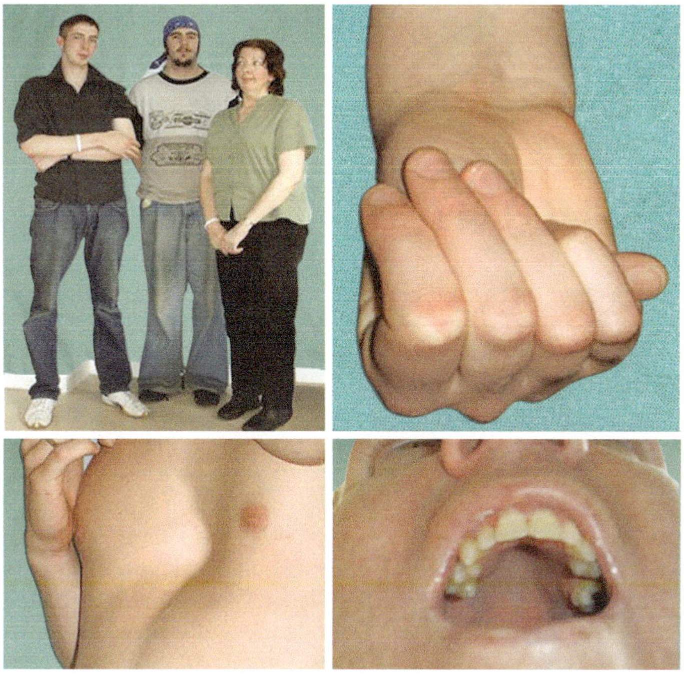

Figure 4.25 Clinical features of Marfan syndrome.

myotonic dystrophy type 1 (DM1) due to abnormalities of the DMPK gene on chromosome 19. Myotonic dystrophy type 2 (DM2) is due to abnormalities of the ZNF9 gene on chromosome 3 and is much rarer. DM1 is an example of a condition due to a 'triplet repeat expansion.' Other trinucleotide repeat disorders which may be encountered in paediatric practice are fragile X syndrome, Friedreich ataxia and juvenile-onset Huntington disease.

In the case of myotonic dystrophy, the repeated trinucleotide is CTG and the normal size is 5–35 repeats. In very general terms, the age of onset and severity of symptoms relate to the size of the expansion of this repeat, although it is not possible to predict with accuracy an individual's prognosis from their expansion size. Like other triplet repeat disorders, myotonic dystrophy exhibits the phenomenon of anticipation. Anticipation is seen because the expanded trinucleotide region is unstable and, therefore, expands further as it passes from one generation to the next, resulting in symptoms occurring earlier and with greater severity in each successive generation. For this reason, it is particularly important to take a detailed three-generation family history as the older, more mildly affected relatives may only have single symptoms, such as cataracts or diabetes, which may otherwise be overlooked.

The clinical features of DM1 are: muscle disease [muscle weakness and myotonia (difficulty in relaxing the muscles after contraction)], gastrointestinal tract symptoms (as smooth muscle is also affected; patients often complain of constipation, colicky abdominal pain and problems with bowel control), cardiovascular disease (conduction defects may lead to sudden death), respiratory problems (alveolar hypoventilation due to diaphragmatic and probably also a central component, post-anaesthetic respiratory depression can be significant and care should be taken), ocular problems (subcapsular cataracts and retinal abnormalities), central nervous system (major cognitive dysfunction is unusual with adult onset disease but personality traits such as apathy, with marked daytime sleepiness and stubbornness, are well-recognised) and endocrine problems (testicular atrophy—sometimes resulting in male infertility, recurrent miscarriages, diabetes mellitus and frontal balding).

Congenital myotonic dystrophy is a severe form of the disorder and almost always occurs when the condition is transmitted by the mother and generally only if the mother has symptomatic disease. Affected neonates have profound hypotonia and usually require prolonged ventilatory assistance. Survivors have learning disabilities in addition to the physical features of the disease.

SUGGESTED READING

1. Clarke A. Harper's Practical Genetic Counselling, 8th edition. Boca Raton: CRC Press; September 2017.
2. Rimoin DL, Pyeritz RE, Korf BR (Eds). Principles and Practice of Medical Genetics, 6th edition. Edinburgh: Churchill Livingstone; 2013.

CHAPTER 5

Disturbances of Nutrition

Krishna M. Goel

VITAMIN D DEFICIENCY

Rickets is a metabolic disturbance of growth, which affects bone, skeletal muscles and sometimes the nervous system. The disorder is due primarily to an insufficiency of vitamin D_3 (cholecalciferol), which is a naturally occurring steroid. It can be formed in the skin from 7-dehydrocholesterol by irradiation with ultraviolet (UV) light in the wavelengths 280–305 nm; or it can be ingested in the form of fish liver oils, eggs, butter, margarine and meat. The most important natural source of vitamin D is that formed from solar irradiation of the skin. UV irradiation of ergosterol produces vitamin D_2 (ergocalciferol), which, in humans, is a potent antirachitic substance. It is, however, not a natural animal vitamin and may have some adverse effects. Less vitamin D is made in the skin of dark-skinned people than white-skinned people.

KEY LEARNING POINT

The term vitamin D (calciferol) is used for a range of compounds including ergocalciferol (vitamin D_2), cholecalciferol (vitamin D_3), dihydrotachysterol, alfacalcidol (1-alpha-hydroxycholecalciferol) and calcitriol (1,25-dihydroxycholecalciferol).

Vitamin D Metabolism

Cholecalciferol is converted in the liver to 25-hydroxyvitamin D_3 (25-OHD_3) by means of enzymatic hydroxylation in the C25 position. This metabolite circulates in the plasma with a transport protein, which migrates with the alpha globulins. It is then 1α-hydroxylated in the kidney to 1,25-dihydroxyvitamin D_3 (1, 25$(OH)_2D_3$) by the action of 25-hydroxyvitamin D hydroxylase. Its production appears to be regulated by several factors, including the phosphate concentration in the plasma, the renal intracellular calcium and phosphate concentrations, and parathyroid hormone. It acts on the cells of the gastrointestinal tract to increase calcium absorption and on bone to increase calcium resorption. In the kidney, it improves the reabsorption of calcium while causing a phosphate diuresis. It also acts on muscle, with the ability to correct the muscle weakness often associated with rickets **(Flow chart 5.1)**.

Vitamin D deficiency causes a fall in the concentration of calcium in extracellular fluid, which in turn stimulates parathormone production. The phosphate diuresis effect of a raised parathyroid hormone level results in lowering of the plasma phosphate. This produces the low calcium (Ca) × phosphate (P) product, which is such a characteristic feature of active rickets. This stage is quickly followed by an increase in the plasma alkaline phosphatase concentration and then by radiological and clinical features of rickets.

Aetiology

Deficiency of vitamin D, which once resulted in so much infantile rickets, with its toll of permanent deformities and death during childbirth, arose principally due to the limited amount of sunshine and skyshine in northern latitudes. Furthermore, in large industrial cities, the skyshine contained very little UV light after filtering through dust, smoke and fog. The need in a cold climate for heat-retaining clothing and the tendency to remain indoors in inclement weather further deprived infants of UV radiation. The natural diet of the human infant contains little vitamin D, especially if fed artificially on cow's milk. Cereals, which are commonly used, have a rachitogenic effect because the phosphorus in cereals is in an unavailable form, phytic acid (inositol hexaphosphoric acid), that combines with calcium and magnesium in the gut to form the complex compound, phytin. It is essential to fortify the infant's diet with vitamin D if rickets is to be avoided. This would not be necessary in the wholly breastfed infant living in a sunny land.

Another important causative factor, necessary for the development of rickets, is growth. The marasmic infant does not develop rickets when vitamin D deficient until re-fed and growth commences. The preterm

Flow chart 5.1 Vitamin D metabolism.

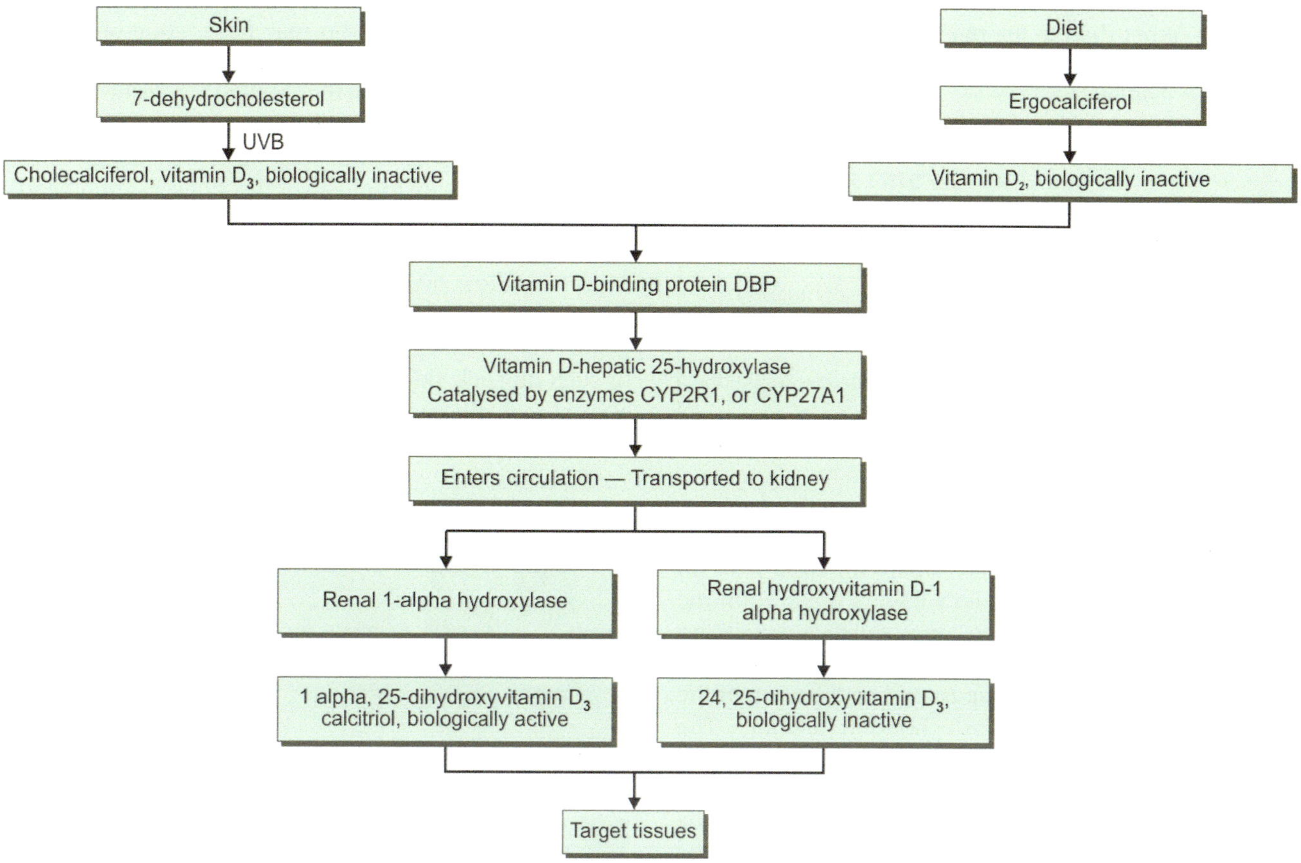

low-birth-weight (LBW) infant who grows rapidly is particularly prone to develop rickets. There is evidence that hydroxylation of vitamin D in the liver of preterm infants is impaired, and this together with dietary phosphate deficiency is an important factor in the osteopenia of preterm infants.

Pathology

In the normal infant, there is a zone of cartilage between the diaphysis and the epiphysis, the epiphyseal plate. At the epiphyseal end, this cartilage is actively growing (proliferative zone), whereas at the diaphyseal end, where mature cartilage cells are arranged in orderly columns, osteoblasts lay down calcium phosphate to form new bone. In rickets, the cartilage near the diaphysis (resting zone) shows a disordered arrangement of capillaries, and although osteoblasts are numerous normal calcification, they do not take place. This is called osteoid tissue. In the meantime, active growth of the proliferative zone continues, so that the epiphyseal plate is enlarged and swollen. Osteoid tissue instead of normal bone is also formed under the periosteum. There is also, in severe cases, a general decalcification of the skeleton, so that curvatures and deformities readily develop.

The diagnosis of infantile rickets is not difficult but its rarity in developed countries has resulted in its being unfamiliar to many doctors. A careful dietary history with special reference to the ingestion of vitamin D-fortified milks and cereals and of vitamin supplements will reveal the child who is at risk. In the case of mothers with osteomalacia from their own malnutrition, rickets has been present in their infants at birth, as the foetal requirements of 25-OHD_3 are obtained directly from the maternal pool. In congenital rickets, the presenting feature is usually a hypocalcaemic convulsion, although typical bone changes are to be expected in radiographs. Subclinical maternal and foetal vitamin D deficiency has also been found in white mothers and infants, particularly in infants born in early spring. It causes compensatory maternal hyperparathyroidism and dental enamel defects in the infant's primary dentition. Such infants are predisposed to neonatal tetany if fed on unmodified cow's milk.

There are few subjective signs of rickets. Head sweating is probably one. General muscular hypotonia encourages abdominal protuberance; this can be increased by flaring out of the rib margins and by fermentation of the excess carbohydrate so commonly included in the diets of nutritionally ignorant people. The rachitic child commonly suffers from concomitant iron-deficiency anaemia.

The child's frequent susceptibility to respiratory infections is related more to the poor environment and overcrowding rather than to the rickets. The same applies to the unhappy irritable behaviour which rachitic children sometimes exhibit.

KEY LEARNING POINTS

- Vitamin D deficiency leads to rickets in children, which is due to undermineralisation of bone.
- There are few rich sources of vitamin D, and it is unlikely that requirements of infants can be met without the use of supplements or food enrichment.
- Some infants are especially sensitive to hypercalcaemia due to vitamin D toxicity.

The objective signs of rickets are found in the skeleton. The earliest physical sign is craniotabes. This is due to softening of the occipital bones where the head rubs on the pillow. When the examiner's fingers press upon the occipital area, the bone can be depressed in and out like a piece of old parchment or table tennis ball. Another common early sign is the 'rachitic rosary' or 'beading of the ribs' due to swelling of the costochondral junctions. The appearance is of a row of swellings, both visible and palpable, passing downwards and backwards on both sides of the thorax at costochondral junctions. Swelling of the epiphyses is also seen at an early stage, especially at the wrists, knees and ankles **(Figs. 5.1A to F)**.

In severe cases, the shafts of the long bones may develop various curvatures, leading to genu varum, genu valgum and coxa vara **(Figs. 5.2A to F)**. A particularly common deformity, shown in **Figure 5.3A**, is curvature at the junction of the middle and lower thirds of the tibiae. This is often due to the child, who may have 'gone off his/her feet', being sat on a chair with his feet projecting over the edge in such a fashion that their weight bends the softened tibial shafts. Bossing over the frontal and parietal bones, due to the subperiosteal deposition of osteoid, gives the child a broad square forehead or the 'hot cross bun head'. The anterior fontanelle may not close until well past the age of 18 months, although this delay can also occur in hypothyroidism, hydrocephalus and even in some healthy children. Another deformity affecting the bony thorax results in Harrison grooves. These are seen as depressions or sulci on each side of the chest running parallel to but above the diaphragmatic attachment. This sign, however,

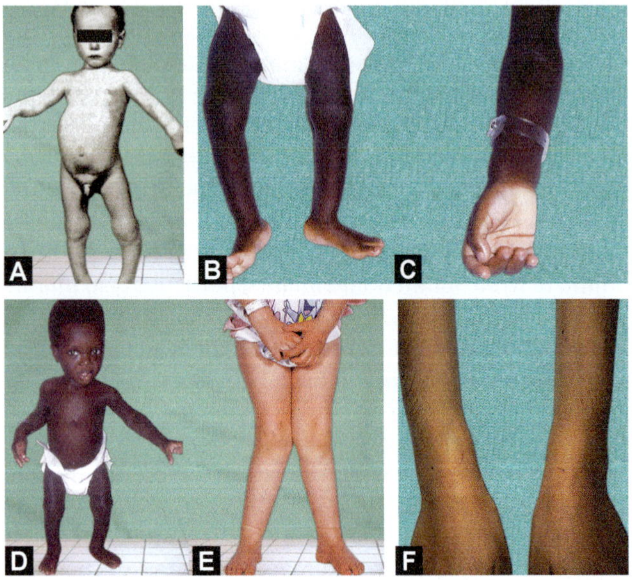

Figures 5.1A to F Children with rickets: *Note* swelling of wrists, knees and ankles.

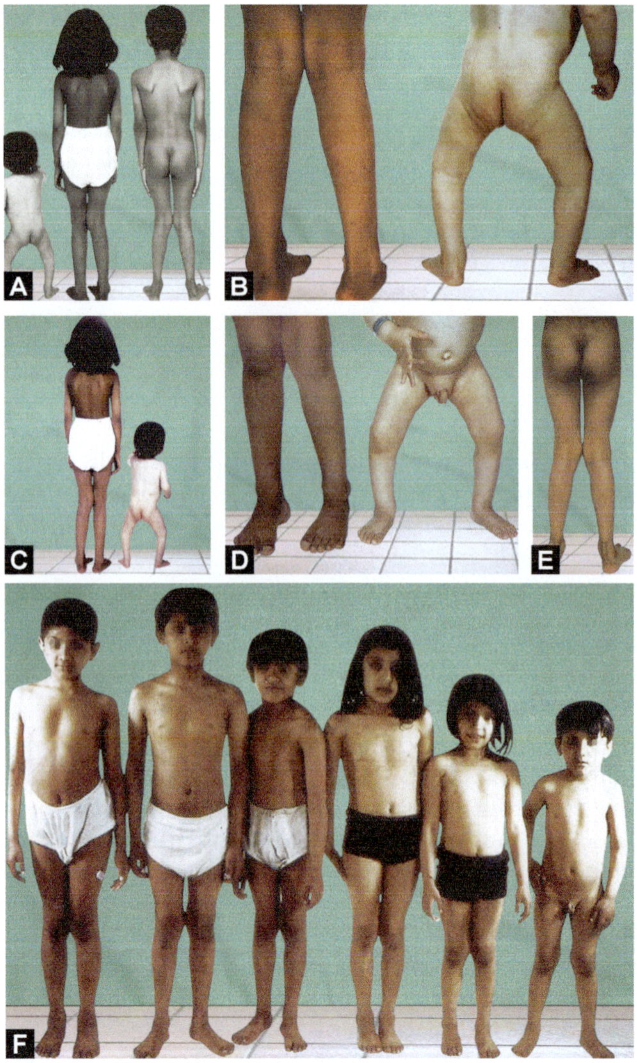

Figures 5.2A to F (A to E) Rickets showing genu valgum (knock knees) and genu varum (bow leg). (F) All these six Pakistani children, four boys and two girls, from one family and aged (left to right) 9, 10, 7, 8, 6 and 5 years, were found to have severe late rickets. All had knock knees (genu valgum). The rickets completely healed after a single intramuscular dose of 60,000 IU of calciferol.

may also develop in cases of congenital heart disease, asthma and chronic respiratory infections. Laxity of the spinal ligaments can also allow the development of various spinal deformities such as dorsolumbar kyphoscoliosis. In children who have learned to stand, there may be an exaggerated lumbar lordosis. The severely rachitic child will also be considerably dwarfed. Pelvic deformities are not readily appreciated in young children but, in the case of girls, they can lead to severe difficulty during childbirth in later years. The pelvic inlet may be narrowed by forward displacement of the sacral promontory, or the outlet may be narrowed by forward movement of the lower parts of the sacrum and of the coccyx.

Radiological Features

The normally smooth and slightly convex ends of the long bones become splayed out with the appearance of fraying or 'cupping' of the edges. The distance between the diaphysis and the epiphysis is increased because the metaphysis consists largely of non-radiopaque osteoid tissue. Periosteum may be raised due to the laying down of osteoid tissue, and the shafts may appear decalcified and curved. In the worst cases, greenstick fractures with poor callus formation may occur. The earliest sign of healing is a thin line of preparatory calcification near the diaphysis **(Figs. 5.3A and B)** followed by calcification in the osteoid just distal to the frayed ends of the diaphysis. In time, both the ends and shafts of the bone usually return to normal.

Biochemical Findings

Typical findings are a normal plasma calcium concentration (2.25–2.75 mmol/L; 9–11 mg/100 mL), whereas the plasma phosphate (normally 1.6–2.26 mmol/L; 5–7 mg/100 mL) is markedly reduced to between 0.64 and 1 mmol/L (2–3 mg/100 mL). The normal plasma calcium in the presence of diminished intestinal absorption of calcium is best explained on the basis of increased parathyroid activity, which mobilises calcium from the bones. Plasma phosphate diminishes due to the phosphaturia, which results from the effects of parathyroid hormone on the renal tubules. A plasma calcium × phosphorus product (mg per 100 mL) above 40 excludes rickets, while a figure below 30 indicates active rickets. This formula is useful in clinical practice but it has no real meaning in terms of physical chemistry. The plasma alkaline phosphatase activity (normal 56–190 IU/L) is markedly increased in rickets and only returns to normal with effective treatment. It is, in fact, a very sensitive and early reflection of rachitic activity but can be raised in a variety of unrelated disease states such as hyperparathyroidism, obstructive jaundice, fractures, malignant disease of bone and the 'battered baby' syndrome. The mean 25-OHD_3 level in healthy British children is 30 nmol/L (12.5 mg/L), although considerably greater concentrations are reported from the USA. In children with active rickets, the level of 25-OHD_3 may fall below 7.5 nmol/L (3 mg/L). However, it is not possible to equate the presence of rickets with particular absolute values for 25-OHD_3, although its measurement can provide the most sensitive index of the vitamin D status of a population. Plasma 1,25$(OH)_2D_3$ can also be measured but is a specialised investigation.

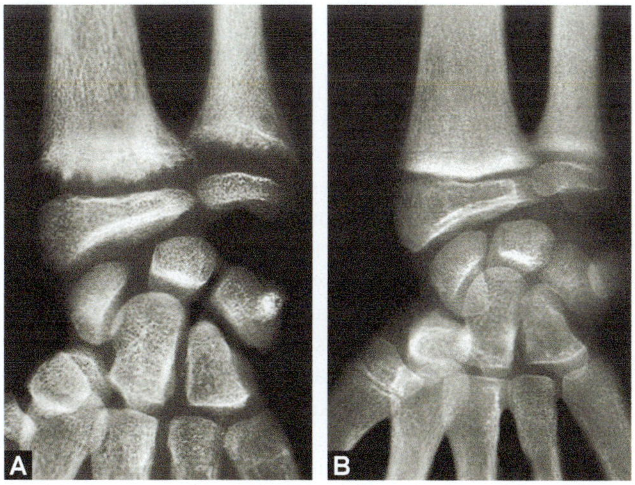

Figures 5.3A and B (A) Florid rickets showing splaying and fraying of ends of the long bones and (B) radiograph of the same case in healed rickets.

Differential Diagnosis

Few diseases can simulate infantile rickets. In hypophosphatasia, some of the clinical and radiological features resemble those seen in rickets, but their presence in the early weeks of life exclude vitamin D deficiency. Other features such as defective calcification of the membranous bones of the skull, low plasma alkaline phosphatase and hypercalcaemia are never found in rickets. The characteristic features of achondroplasia—short upper limb segments, large head with relatively small face and retroussé nose, trident arrangement of the fingers, lordosis, waddling gait and X-ray evidence of endochondral ossification—are unmistakably different from anything seen in rickets. The globular enlargement of the hydrocephalic skull is quite distinct from the square bossed head of severe rickets. The bone lesions of congenital syphilis are present in the early months of life and are associated with other characteristic clinical signs such as rashes, bloody snuffles, hepatosplenomegaly and lymphadenopathy. In later childhood, the sabre-blade tibia of syphilis shows anterior bowing and thickening which is different from rachitic bowing. Some healthy toddlers show an apparent bowing of the legs due to the normal deposition of fat over the outer aspects; this is unimportant and temporary, and there are no other signs of skeletal abnormality. Other normal young children have a mild and physiological degree of genu valgum due to a mild valgus position of the feet; in rachitic genu valgum, there will be other rickety deformities. Other types of rickets due to coeliac disease and renal disease must be excluded by appropriate investigations. Their existence is almost always indicated in a carefully taken history.

KEY LEARNING POINT

Children receiving pharmacological doses of vitamin D or its analogues should have their plasma calcium level checked at intervals of once or twice a week because excessive supplementation may cause hypercalcaemia.

Late Neonatal Hypocalcaemia (Neonatal Tetany)

Late neonatal tetany usually occurs from the second half of the first week up to several weeks in infants artificially fed, being exposed to high phosphorus intake. Although affected infants may have appeared a little jittery or tremulous with increasing tactile irritability of muscles, usually they have been otherwise well, feeding normally, responding normally and with a normal cry, before the sudden onset of convulsions. Jitteriness is evident on stimulation. And increased muscle tone with extension in the legs particularly is usual. Trousseau sign and Chvostek sign may be positive **(Figs. 5.4A and B)**. The diagnosis is based on low serum calcium, less than 1.8 mmol/L, and a high serum phosphorus, more than 2.6 mmol/L. There is usually an associated hypomagnesaemia **(Figs. 5.4A and B)**.

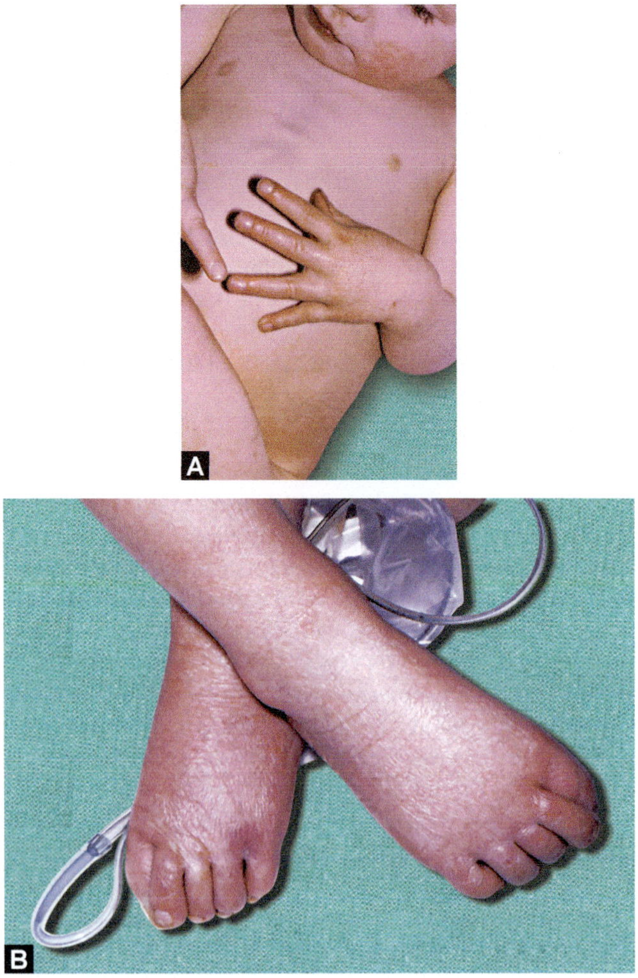

Figures 5.4A and B Hypocalcaemia: The classical signs of peripheral hyperexcitability of motor nerves: Spasm of the muscles of the wrists and ankles (carpopedal spasm).

VITAMIN C (ASCORBIC ACID) DEFICIENCY

Aetiology

The primary cause is an inadequate intake of vitamin C (ascorbic acid), a vitamin that the human, unlike most other animals, is unable to synthesise within his/her own body. It is rare in the breastfed infant unless the mother has subclinical avitaminosis C. Cow's milk contains only about a quarter of the vitamin C content of human milk, and this is further reduced by boiling, drying or evaporating. Scurvy is particularly common in infants who receive a high carbohydrate diet. The suggested recommended dietary allowance is 35 mg/day.

Pathology

Vitamin C deficiency results in faulty collagen, which affects many tissues including bone, cartilage and teeth. The intercellular substance of the capillaries is also defective. This results in spontaneous haemorrhages and defective ossification affecting both the shafts and the metaphyseo-epiphyseal junctions. The periosteum becomes detached from the cortex and extensive subperiosteal haemorrhages occur; these explain the intense pain and tenderness, especially of the lower extremities.

Clinical Features

Increasing irritability, anorexia, malaise and low-grade fever develop between the ages of 7 and 15 months. A most striking feature is the obvious pain and tenderness, which the infant exhibits when handled, e.g. during napkin changing. The legs are most severely affected and they characteristically assume a position ('frog position') in which the hips and knees are flexed and the feet are rotated outwards. Gums become swollen and discoloured and may bleed; this is seen only after teeth have erupted, and the teeth may become loose in the jaws. Periorbital ecchymosis ('black eye') or proptosis due to retro-orbital haemorrhage is common but haemorrhages into the skin, epistaxis or gastrointestinal haemorrhages are not commonly seen in infantile scurvy. The anterior ends of the ribs frequently become visibly and palpably swollen but this does not affect the costal cartilages as in rickets; the sternum has the appearance of having been displaced backwards. Microscopic haematuria is frequently present.

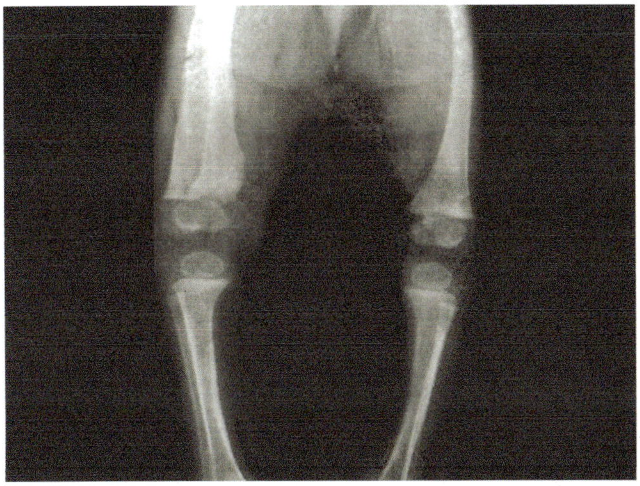

Figure 5.5 Radiograph from a case of infantile scurvy in the healing stage with calcified subperiosteal haematoma. *Note* also 'ringing of epiphyses', Frankel white lines and proximal zone of translucency.

Radiological Features

The diagnosis is most reliably confirmed by X-rays. The shafts of the long bones have a 'ground-glass' appearance due to loss of normal trabeculation. A dense white line of calcification (Fraenkel line) forms proximal to the epiphyseal plate and there is often a zone of translucency due to an incomplete transverse fracture immediately proximal to Fraenkel line. A small spur of bone may project from the end of the shaft at this point ('the corner sign'). The epiphyses, especially at the knees, have the appearance of being 'ringed' by white ink. Subperiosteal haemorrhages only become visible when they are undergoing calcification, but a striking X-ray appearance is then seen (**Fig. 5.5**).

Diagnosis

Measurement of vitamin C in serum and leukocytes is the common means of assessing vitamin C status. For practical purposes, measurement of vitamin C in serum is preferred over leukocyte measurement. Measurement of urinary vitamin C in patients suspected of scurvy can provide supportive diagnostic information. There are no reliable functional tests of vitamin C.

KEY LEARNING POINT

- Vitamin C deficiency manifests as scurvy.
- Vitamin C status is assessed by plasma and leukocyte concentrations.
- At intakes above 100 mg/day, the vitamin is excreted quantitatively with intake in the urine.
- There is little evidence that high intakes have any beneficial effects, but equally there is no evidence of any hazard from high intakes.

VITAMIN B DEFICIENCIES

The B vitamins are widely distributed in animal and vegetable foods. Deficiency of one of the B group vitamins is commonly associated with deficiencies of the others. The main functions of B vitamins are as cofactors for metabolic processes or as precursors of essential metabolites. Deficiencies occur when there is severe famine, where there are dietary fads, where diets are severely restricted or where there has been inappropriate preparation of the food. Many B vitamins are destroyed by cooking.

Thiamine (Vitamin B_1) Deficiency

Thiamine, as are all the B vitamins, is water soluble and readily destroyed by heat and alkali. It is necessary for mitochondrial function and for the synthesis of acetylcholine. It is present in a wide variety of foods but deficiency states have been particularly common in communities where polishing rice and refining flour remove the vitamin B-containing husks. Beriberi is now rare in the countries where it was originally described—Japan, Indonesia and Malaysia.

Clinical Features

Deficiency of thiamine (beriberi) causes clinical manifestations in the nervous and cardiovascular systems predominantly, although all tissues are affected. There is degeneration of peripheral nerve fibres and haemorrhage and vascular dilatation in the brain (Wernicke encephalopathy). There can be high-output cardiac failure and erythemas. Signs of the disease develop in infants born to thiamine-deficient mothers at the age of 2–3 months. They appear restless with vasodilatation, anorexia, vomiting and constipation and pale with a waxy skin, hypertonia and dyspnoea. There is peripheral vasodilatation and bounding pulses with later development of hepatomegaly and evidence of cardiac failure. This is due to a combination of the peripheral vasodilatation and decreased renal flow. This is known as the 'wet' form of beriberi. There is reduction of the phasic reflexes at knee and ankle.

In older children, 'dry' beriberi or the neurological complication of thiamine deficiency results in paraesthesia and burning sensations particularly affecting the feet. There is generalised muscle weakness, and calf muscles are tender. Tendon reflexes may be absent, a stocking and glove peripheral neuritis develops and sensory loss accompanies the motor weakness. Increased intracranial pressure, meningism and coma may follow.

Diagnosis

There are few useful laboratory tests, although in severe deficiency states the red blood cell transketolase is reduced and lactate and pyruvate may be increased in the blood, particularly after exercise.

KEY LEARNING POINTS

- The classical thiamine deficiency disease beriberi, affecting the peripheral nervous system, is now rare.
- Thiamine status is assessed by erythrocyte transketolase activation coefficient.

Riboflavin (Vitamin B_2) Deficiency

Clinical Features

Deficiency is usually secondary to inadequate intake, although in biliary atresia and chronic hepatitis there may be malabsorption. Clinical features are those common to a number of B group deficiency states, namely cheilosis, glossitis, keratitis, conjunctivitis, photophobia and lacrimation. Cheilosis begins with pallor, thinning and maceration of the skin at the angles of the mouth and then extends laterally. The whole mouth may become reddened and swollen, and there is loss of papillae of the tongue. A normochromic, normocytic anaemia is secondary to bone marrow hypoplasia. There may be associated seborrhoeic dermatitis involving the nasolabial folds and forehead. Conjunctival suffusion may proceed to proliferation of blood vessels onto the cornea.

Diagnosis

Urinary riboflavin excretion of less than 30 mg per day is characteristic of a deficiency state. There is reduction of red cell glutathione reductase activity.

KEY LEARNING POINTS

- Riboflavin deficiency is relatively common.
- Phototherapy for neonatal hyperbilirubinaemia can cause iatrogenic riboflavin deficiency.

Pellagra (Niacin Deficiency)

Niacin is the precursor of nicotinamide adenine dinucleotide and its reduced form nicotinamide adenine dinucleotide phosphate. It can be synthesised from tryptophan, and pellagra tends to occur when maize, which is a poor source tryptophan and niacin, is the staple diet. Niacin is lost in the milling process. Communities where millet, which has a high leucine content, is consumed also have a high incidence of pellagra.

Clinical Features

The classical triad for pellagra is diarrhoea, dermatitis and dementia, although in children the diarrhoea and dementia are less obvious than in the adolescent and adult. There is light-sensitive dermatitis on exposed areas, which can result in blistering and desquamation of the skin.

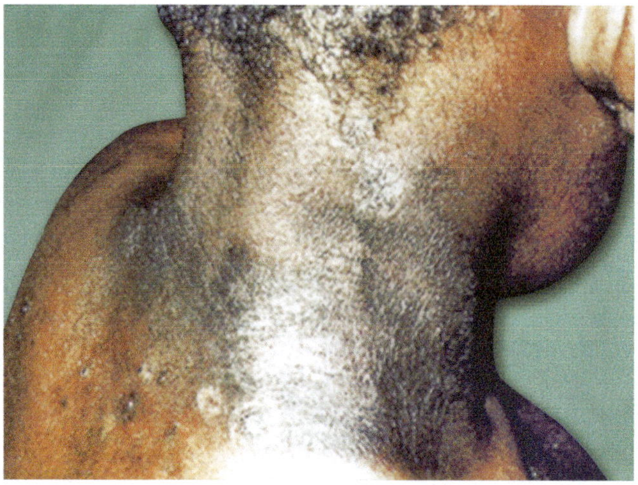

Figure 5.6 Pellagra: 'Casal necklace' on the neck.

On healing, the skin becomes pigmented **(Fig. 5.6)**. The children are apathetic and disinterested and feed poorly due to an associated glossitis and stomatitis.

Diagnosis

The two methods of assessing niacin deficiency are measurement of blood nicotinamide nucleotides and the urinary excretion of niacin metabolites, neither of which is wholly satisfactory.

Vitamin B_6 (Pyridoxine) Deficiency

Vitamin B_6 occurs in nature in three forms: (1) pyridoxine, (2) pyridoxal and (3) pyridoxamine, which are interconvertible within the body. The principal one in the body and in food is pyridoxal.

There may be inadequate intake of dietary pyridoxine when there is prolonged heat processing of milk and cereals or when unsupplemented milk formulae or elemental diets are used. There can be inadequate absorption in coeliac disease, and drug treatment with isoniazid, penicillamine and oral contraceptives will aggravate deficiency states.

The disorder has to be differentiated from pyridoxine dependency in which pyridoxine-dependent convulsions and anaemia are secondary to a genetic disorder of the apoenzyme. Deficiency on its own is rare; it is most often seen with deficiencies of other vitamins or with protein deficiency.

Clinical Features

Pyridoxine deficiency states result in convulsions, peripheral neuritis, cheilosis, glossitis (as in riboflavin deficiency), seborrhoea and anaemia and impaired immunity. The anaemia is microcytic and is aggravated when intercurrent infections complicate the clinical picture. There may be oxaluria with bladder stones, hyperglycinaemia, lymphopaenia and decreased antibody production.

Diagnosis

There is increased xanthurenic acid in the urine after an oral dose of the amino acid tryptophan. Glutamine-oxaloacetic acid transaminase is reduced in the red cells.

Vitamin B_{12} Deficiency

If maternal vitamin B_{12} status is satisfactory, the reserves of B_{12} in the term newborn infant should last throughout the first year of life, especially if the infant is breastfed. Dietary deficiency of vitamin B_{12} is unusual except amongst the strict vegans who consume neither milk nor eggs. Absorption of B_{12} requires a gastric intrinsic factor (IF), which promotes absorption in the terminal ileum. Deficiency of IF, secondary to gastric achlorhydria, is rare in childhood. It has been reported secondarily to the development of gastric parietal cell antibody but this is extremely rare. Familial pernicious anaemia is secondary to a series of autosomal recessively inherited defects in B_{12} metabolism or in the function of B_{12}-binding proteins. Resection of the terminal ileum or Crohn disease will predispose children to B_{12} deficiency unless B_{12} supplementation is given.

Clinical Features

Pallor, anorexia and glossitis are common features. Paraesthesia with loss of position and vibration sense is a disorder of adolescence rather than childhood. There is a megaloblastic anaemia with neutropaenia, thrombocytopaenia and hypersegmentation of polymorphonuclear leukocytes. The bone marrow shows a megaloblastic, erythroid picture with giant metamyelocytes.

The neurological signs of subacute combined degeneration of the cord with peripheral neuritis; degeneration of the dorsal columns and corticospinal tract is a late phenomenon as is retrobulbar neuropathy.

Diagnosis

Normal levels of serum vitamin B_{12} range from 200 to 900 pg/mL or over 150 pmol/L. Deficiency is indicated by values below this. Elevated serum or urinary excretion of methylmalonate and raised plasma homocysteine are the other biochemical tests indicating low B_{12} status. Schilling test is used to confirm the diagnosis of pernicious anaemia. It measures oral absorption of vitamin B_{12} labelled with radioactive cobalt on two occasions, the first without and the second test with IF.

> **KEY LEARNING POINT**
>
> Dietary deficiency of vitamin B_{12} occurs only in strict vegans; there are no plant sources of the vitamin B_{12}.

Folate Deficiency

The word folic is from the Latin 'folia' (leaf), coined in 1941 for an early preparation of this vitamin from spinach leaves.

Deficiency of folic acid is widespread in many communities and is a known factor in the aetiology of neural tube defects. Although found widely in plant and animal tissues, the vitamin is easily destroyed by cooking and storage processes. Requirements for growth during foetal and neonatal life and childhood are high. Deficiency states are likely to occur during childhood particularly when there is excessive cell turnover such as occurs in the haemolytic anaemias and in exfoliative skin conditions such as eczema. Folic acid is the precursor of tetrahydrofolate, which is intimately involved in a series of enzyme reactions of amino acid, purine and intermediary metabolism. Folate is absorbed in the duodenum, and in malabsorptive states including coeliac disease, folate deficiency is common. In some situations where the small intestine is colonised by bacteria (blind loop syndrome), folate is diverted into bacterial metabolism. Some anticonvulsants and antibacterial agents either increase the metabolism of folate or compete with folate.

Clinical Features

Megaloblastic anaemia and pancytopaenia together with poor growth are the result of the cessation of cell division, which comes about when nucleoprotein formation is interrupted because of the lack of synthesis of purines and pyrimidines.

Diagnosis

The blood picture is one of a megaloblastic anaemia with neutropaenia and thrombocytopaenia. The neutrophils contain large hypersegmented nuclei and bone marrow is hypercellular because of erythroid hyperplasia. Although the reticulocyte count is low, nucleated red cells appear in the peripheral blood. Red cell folate measurements are less than 75 ng/mL, and it gives a better idea of cellular status. There is a close interaction of B_{12} and folic acid in the synthesis of tetrahydrofolate and formyltetrahydrofolate, which are required for purine ring formation. With isolated folate deficiency, there are none of the neuropathies associated with the megaloblastic anaemia of B_{12} deficiency.

> **KEY LEARNING POINTS**
>
> - Dietary folate deficiency is not uncommon; deficiency results in megaloblastic anaemia.
> - Low folate status is associated with neural tube defects, and periconceptional supplements reduce the incidence.
> - Folate status can be assessed by measuring plasma or erythrocyte concentrations.

VITAMIN E (TOCOPHEROL) DEFICIENCY

Vitamin E deficiency, except in the preterm infant, is rare. In the preterm, vitamin E deficiency is occasionally associated with haemolytic anaemia and may contribute to the membrane damage associated with intraventricular haemorrhage and bronchopulmonary dysplasia. Vitamin E is essential for the insertion and maintenance of long-chain polyunsaturated fatty acids in the phospholipid bilayer of cell membranes by counteracting the effect of free radicals on these fatty acids. When the essential fatty acid content of the diet is high, vitamin E is required in increased amounts. Plant foods high in fat, particularly polyunsaturated fat, are the best sources of vitamin E. Natural sources of vitamin E are oily fish, milk, cereal, seed oils, peanuts and soya beans. Children with abetalipoproteinaemia have steatorrhoea and low circulating levels of vitamin E associated with neurological signs. More recently, older children and adults with cystic fibrosis have developed neurological signs similar to those in abetalipoproteinaemia due to vitamin E deficiency. In any child with fat malabsorption such as cystic fibrosis and cholestatic liver disease, it would be important to give supplementary vitamin E in addition to correcting the underlying fat malabsorption where possible. The most commonly used index of vitamin E nutritional status is the plasma concentration of alpha-tocopherol. From the plasma concentration of alpha-tocopherol required to prevent haemolysis in vitro, the average requirement is 12 mg/day. Some neonatal units still give a single intramuscular dose of vitamin E at birth to preterm neonates to reduce the risk of complications; however, no trials of long-term outcome have been carried out. The intramuscular route should also be considered in children with severe liver disease when response to oral therapy is inadequate.

KEY LEARNING POINT

Premature infants have inadequate vitamin E status and are susceptible to haemolytic anaemia.

VITAMIN K DEFICIENCY

Vitamin K is necessary for the production of blood-clotting factors and proteins necessary for the normal calcification of bone. Osteocalcin synthesis is similarly impaired, and there is evidence that undercarboxylated osteocalcin is formed in people with marginal intakes of vitamin K who show impairment of blood clotting. Treatment with warfarin or other anticoagulants during pregnancy can lead to bone abnormalities in the foetus, the so-called foetal warfarin syndrome, which is due to impaired synthesis of osteocalcin.

Because vitamin K is fat soluble, children with fat malabsorption, especially in biliary obstruction or hepatic disease, may become deficient. Neonates are relatively deficient in vitamin K and those who do not receive supplements are at risk of serious bleeds including intracranial bleeding. Therefore, newborn babies should receive vitamin K to prevent vitamin K deficiency bleeding (haemorrhagic disease of the newborn). Also babies born to mothers with liver disease or taking enzyme-inducing anticonvulsant drugs (carbamazepine, phenobarbital and phenytoin), rifampicin or warfarin should receive vitamin K because they are at particular risk of vitamin K deficiency.

KEY LEARNING POINTS

- Dietary deficiency of vitamin K is rare.
- Newborn infants have low vitamin K status and are at risk of severe bleeding unless given prophylactic vitamin K.
- Vitamin K status is assessed by estimation of prothrombin time.

BIOTIN AND PANTOTHENIC ACID

Biotin is a coenzyme (CoA) for several carboxylase enzymes. Biotin deficiency is very rare as biotin is found in a wide range of foods, and bacterial production in the large intestine appears to supplement dietary intake.

Pantothenic acid is part of CoA and of acyl carrier protein. Spontaneous human deficiency has never been described. As pantothenic acid is so widely distributed in foods, any dietary deficiency in humans is usually associated with other nutrient deficiencies.

COPPER DEFICIENCY

Copper is the third most abundant dietary trace metal after iron and zinc and is found at high levels in shellfish, liver, kidney, nuts and whole grain cereals. In 1962, copper deficiency was reported in humans.

Copper is also an important constituent of many enzyme systems such as cytochrome oxidase and dismutase, yet clinical copper deficiency states are rare except in very LBW infants, in states of severe protein energy malnutrition and during prolonged parenteral nutrition. The term infant is born with substantial stores of liver copper largely laid down in the last trimester of pregnancy bound to metallothionein. Preterm infants will, therefore, be born with inadequate liver stores of copper and may develop deficiency in the newborn period unless fed foods supplemented with copper. No estimated average requirement or recommended dietary intake has been estimated for copper. Other trace elements such as iron, zinc, cadmium, calcium, copper, sulphur and molybdenum interfere with copper absorption. After absorption, the copper is bound to albumin in the portal circulation. Caeruloplasmin is formed in the liver and is the major transport protein for copper. Frank copper deficiency can be determined by the measurement of plasma copper concentrations or plasma caeruloplasmin, or by determination of the activities of copper-dependent enzymes such as superoxide dismutase. Therefore, plasma copper has been used as a measure of copper deficiency but caeruloplasmin also acts as an acute-phase reactant and will increase in stress situations particularly during infections. The normal plasma copper concentration is 11–25 mmol/L (0.7–1.6 mg/L) and caeruloplasmin 0.1–0.7 g/L. These values are decreased in deficiency states.

Clinical Features

In preterm infants, there may be severe osteoporosis with cupping and flaring of the bone ends with periosteal reaction and submetaphyseal fractures (Fig. 5.7). Severe bone disease has been reported in older infants on bizarre diets. It has been argued that subclinical copper deficiency may account for some of the fractures in suspected non-accidental injury. It is most unlikely that copper deficiency in an otherwise healthy child could result in unexplained fracture. Suggesting that copper deficiency develops without obvious cause and results in bone fractures without other evidence of copper deficiency is at best unwise.

Menkes syndrome, also called steely hair or kinky hair syndrome, is a rare X-linked disorder associated with disturbed copper metabolism. There is gross osteoporosis and progressive neurological impairment. Scalp hair is sparse and brittle with pili torti on microscopic examination (Fig. 5.8). The disorder does not respond to copper therapy.

SELENIUM DEFICIENCY

Muscular dystrophy in lambs and calves has been reported in parts of the world where there is deficiency of selenium in the soil. In humans, Keshan disease has been reported in China. Selenium is essential for glutathione peroxidase activity, which catalyses the reduction of fatty acid hydroperoxides and protects tissues from peroxidation. Thus, selenium is important in maintaining the fatty acid integrity of phospholipid membranes and reducing free radical damage. It is found in fish, meat and whole grain and reflects the soil selenium content of the region. Vitamin C improves the absorption of selenium.

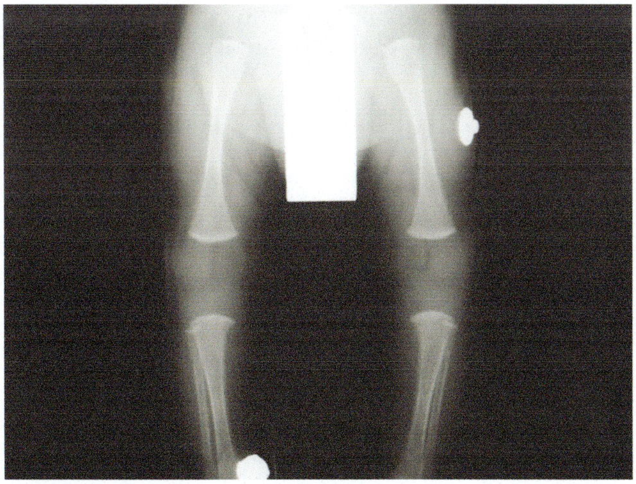

Figure 5.7 X-ray of leg showing osteoporosis with subperiosteal new bone, metaphyseal fraying and widening of the trabecular pattern in the long bones, consistent with copper deficiency.

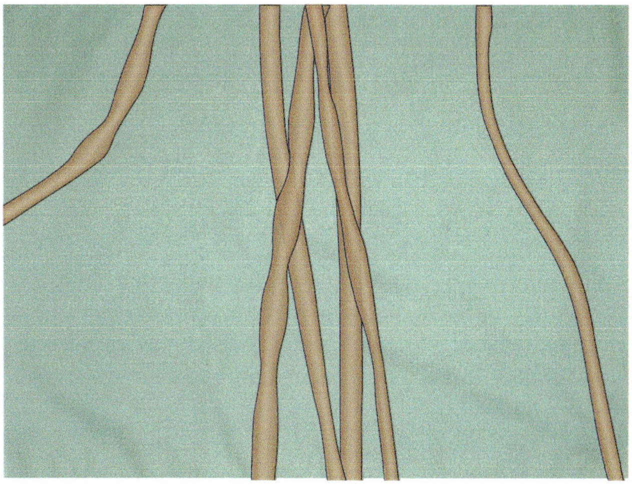

Figure 5.8 Pili torti: Children with pili torti present with spangled, brittle coarse hair of different lengths over cuplike abnormality – the hair shaft is grooved and flattened at irregular intervals. Syndromes in which the hair shaft abnormalities of pili torti are seen in association with other cutaneous and systemic abnormalities include Menkes kinky hair syndrome and ectodermal dysplasia syndromes.

Clinical Features

In China, an endemic cardiomyopathy affecting women of childbearing age and children, known as Keshan disease, has been reported. The condition responds to selenium supplementation. In New Zealand, low selenium concentrations in the soil result in low plasma levels, and in children with phenylketonuria (PKU) on a low phenylalanine diet, low plasma levels of selenium have been reported. There is no obvious clinical abnormality in the New Zealand population, although poor growth and dry skin have been reported in the selenium-deficient PKU children.

Increasingly, epidemiological evidence as well as data from animal studies points to a role for selenium in reducing cancer incidence. However, it should be noted that while selenium is an essential micronutrient and supplementation or fortification of foods may in many cases be advantageous, in excess selenium is exceedingly toxic. The margin between an adequate and a toxic intake of selenium is quite narrow. Symptoms of selenium excess include brittle hair and nails, skin lesions and garlic odour on the breath due to expiration of dimethyl selenide. Lack of dietary selenium has also been implicated in the aetiology of cardiovascular diseases, but the evidence is less convincing than for cancer.

CHROMIUM DEFICIENCY

Chromium may be involved in nucleic acid metabolism and is recognised as a cofactor for insulin. It is poorly absorbed, and there is some evidence that in the elderly, glucose tolerance can be improved by chromium supplementation. Chromium deficiency has been reported in severely malnourished children and in children on prolonged parenteral nutrition. Weight gain and glucose tolerance in such children has been reported to improve after chromium supplementation. In long-term parenteral nutrition, peripheral neuropathy and encephalopathy have also been reported to respond to chromium administration.

IODINE DEFICIENCY

Endemic goitre has been recognised for many centuries in mountainous regions of the world. The Andes, Himalayas, mountains of Central Africa and Papua, New Guinea, and Derbyshire in the United Kingdom are areas where the condition has been recognised. Minimal requirements are probably less than 20 mg/day in infants and young children, increasing to 50 mg/day during adolescence. Breast milk contains up to 90 mg/L. Goitre occurs when the iodine intake is less than 15 mg/day and results in a reduced serum thyroxine (T_4) and a decreased triiodothyronine (T_3). Thyroid-stimulating hormone values increase. The introduction of iodised salt to areas of endemic goitrous and cretinism has largely eradicated goitre cretinism in these regions. Thus, at present this is best achieved through iodine fortification of foods. Some plants including *Brassicas* and bamboo shoots act as goitrogens by inhibiting iodine uptake by the thyroid gland.

KEY LEARNING POINT

Iodisation of salt is the preferred way and most of the families in affected regions now have access to fortified salt.

FLUORIDE

Fluoride is present in most foods at varying levels and also in drinking water, either naturally occurring or added deliberately. Fluoride content of teeth and bones is directly proportional to the amount ingested and absorbed from the diet. Fluoride has been recognised as an important factor in the prevention of caries. Where the fluoride content of the drinking water is less than 700 μg/L (0.7 parts per million), daily administration of fluoride tablets or drops is a suitable means of supplementation. It is now considered that the topical action of fluoride on enamel and plaque is more important than the systemic effect. Systemic fluoride supplements should not be prescribed without reference to the fluoride content of the local water supply. Infants need not receive fluoride supplements until the age of 6 months. Toothpaste or tooth powder, which incorporates sodium fluoride or monofluorophosphate, is also a convenient source of fluoride.

Higher intakes of fluoride (10 mg/L) are toxic and lead to fluorosis. However, fluorosis is common in parts of Southern Africa, the Indian subcontinent and China, where there is a high fluoride content in the subsoil water, which enters the food chain either directly or via plants.

KEY LEARNING POINTS

- It is now considered that the topical action of fluoride on enamel and plaque is more important than the systemic effect. Also, systemic fluoride supplements should not be prescribed without reference to the fluoride content of the local water supply.
- Infants need not receive fluoride supplements until the age of 6 months.

OTHER TRACE MINERALS

Manganese, molybdenum and cadmium are known to be necessary for health in animals but no clear human evidence of deficiency states is known to man. Following recent experience with zinc, copper and chromium, it seems likely that future research will lead to the identification of specific deficiencies of some of these other trace elements in infants and children.

CHILDHOOD OBESITY

The rising prevalence of childhood obesity in most populations around the world is a matter of grave concern because the physical, psychological and social consequences of obesity in childhood are substantial. The causes of childhood and adolescent obesity are multiple and are still being elucidated. The consequences of obesity are: increased blood pressure, increased total cholesterol and decreased high-density lipoprotein concentrations. In addition, obesity in childhood is predictive of adult obesity **(Figs. 5.9A and B)**.

PROTEIN-ENERGY MALNUTRITION

Protein energy malnutrition is the term most frequently used to embrace the severe forms of malnutrition seen in childhood, marasmus and kwashiorkor, and the nutritionally determined growth failure that precedes these clinical syndromes.

Marasmus is severe undernutrition with weight less than 60% of that expected for age **(Figs. 5.10A to D)**. In developed countries, many children are described as clinically marasmic when they are severely wasted, even though their degree of underweight may not be as extreme as that defined above. In developed countries, where underweight is due to a wide variety of factors other than undernutrition, it is vital to distinguish children

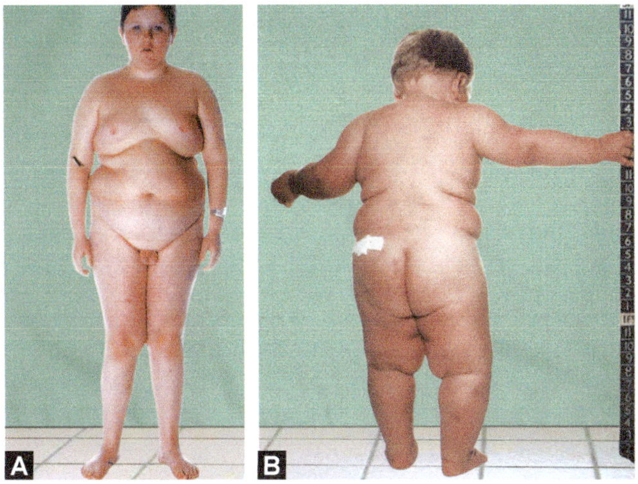

Figures 5.9A and B Children with dietary obesity. Obesity results from an imbalance in energy intake and energy expenditure.

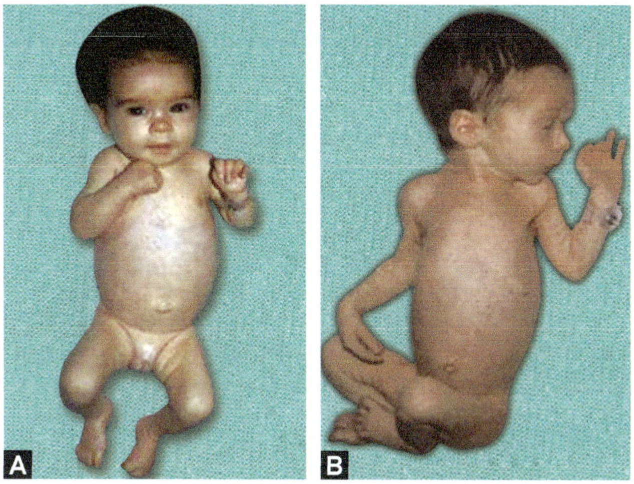

Figures 5.11A and B Two-month-old infants with failure to thrive. Failure to thrive is secondary to inadequate breast milk production. Test weighings over a period of 24 hours would help confirm the diagnosis.

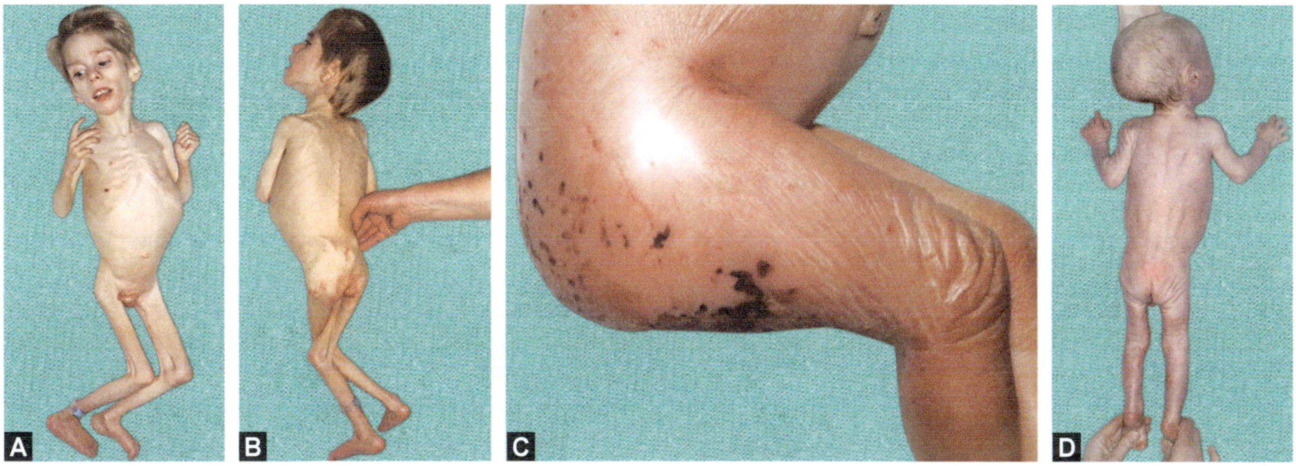

Figures 5.10A to D Children with marasmus.

whose predominant problem is mainly short stature with associated low weight from those who are significantly underweight for their low height. The aetiology of the two conditions is distinct and the former situation may have little to do with nutrition. Nevertheless, distinction between those who are short for age and underweight, and those who are normal stature for age but severely underweight is vital since those who are short are likely to have suffered more prolonged malnutrition or may have other causes for their poor growth.

Marasmus is the usual clinical presentation of severe childhood malnutrition during famine or as a result of starvation from—for example breastfeeding failure **(Figs. 5.11A and B)**. Children are thin with loss of fat and muscle. Wasting is obvious and typically these children are miserable but hungry and often feed well when food is offered. They have distended abdomen secondary to poor muscle tone, abdominal muscle wasting and/or disaccharide intolerance with excessive intestinal gas formation.

CHAPTER 6

Respiratory Disorders

Anne Margaret Devenny

INTRODUCTION

Respiratory disorders are extremely common in paediatrics. In this chapter, radiological and clinical images illustrate congenital and acquired respiratory disorders.

A thorough history and careful examination are vital in paediatrics. With respect to acute and chronic respiratory conditions, there are a number of indicators that should raise significant concerns—so called "red flags." These indicate that either a patient is acutely unwell and needs resuscitation or that there is a significant chronic respiratory problem.

Acute "Red Flag Warning Points"

Too breathless to feed or parents noticing difficulty breathing and/or poor colour

Lethargic

Pyrexia

Apnoeas

Haemoptysis

Increased work of breathing with increased respiratory rate and/or use of accessory muscles of respiration

Pallor, cyanosis or prolonged capillary refill time (>2 seconds)

Stridor

Poorly responsive children

Air entry poor with wheeze and/or crepitations evident.

Chronic "Red Flag Warning Points"

Chronic productive or "wet" cough

Known contact with tuberculosis (TB) or travel to TB endemic area

Recurrent significant respiratory infections

Family history of chronic respiratory disease

Other conditions, e.g. prematurity, congenital heart disease, chronic gastrointestinal symptoms, e.g. steatorrhoea

Frequent other infections suggesting immunodeficiency

Poor growth

Presence of finger clubbing **(Fig. 6.1)**, chest deformity **(Figs. 6.2A and B)**, e.g. Harrison sulci or skeletal dysplasia **(Figs. 6.3 and 6.4)**.

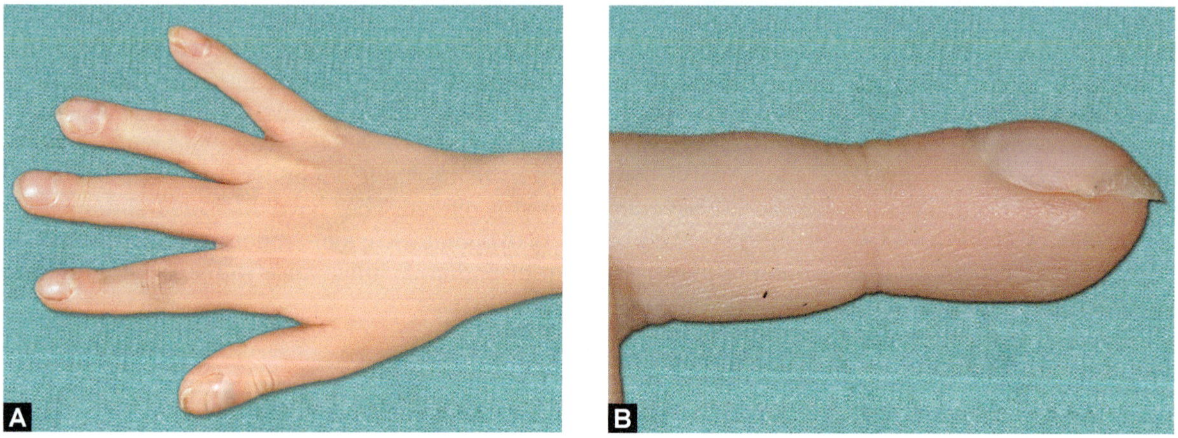

Figures 6.1A and B Moderate finger clubbing in a patient with cystic fibrosis—*note* the extreme curvature of the fingertip and nails with significant increase in the angle made by the proximal nail fold and nail plate (Lovibond angle), which normally is less than or equal to 160°. The distal part of the finger is bulbous in shape.

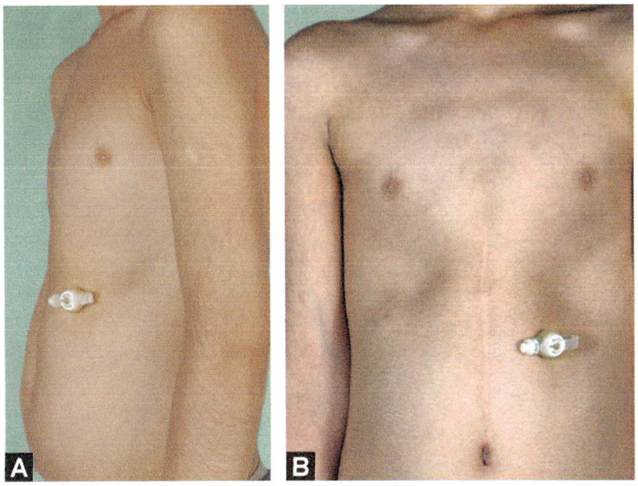

Figures 6.2A and B Chest deformity in a patient with chronic lung disease of prematurity. *Note* gastrostomy tube and scan from Nissen fundoplication.

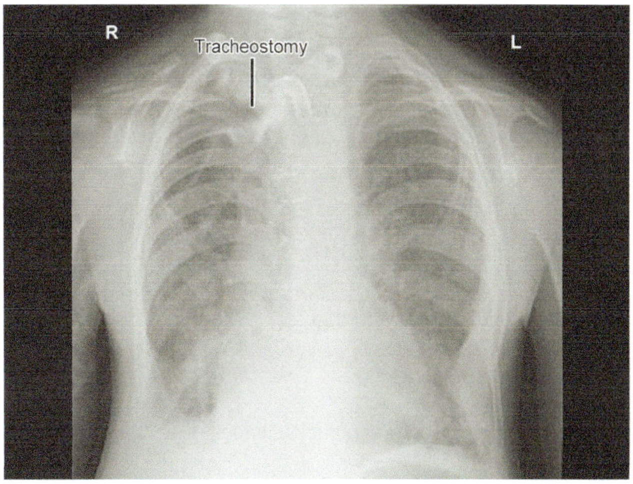

Figure 6.3 Chest X-ray of a 6-year-old child with skeletal dysplasia due to Ellis–van Creveld syndrome. There was significant respiratory compromise needing invasive ventilation. *Note* very small abnormally shaped chest.

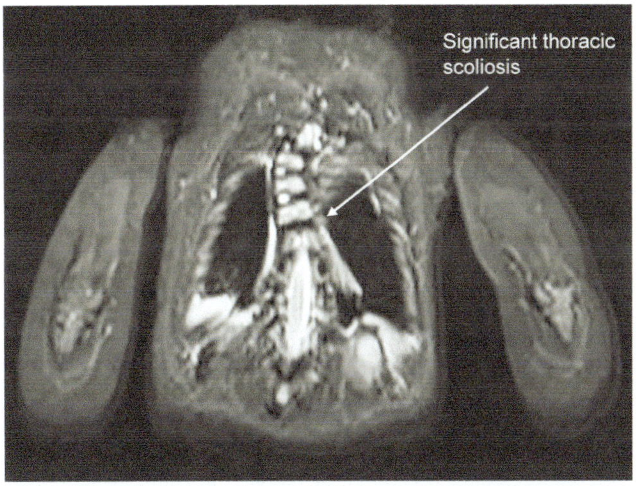

Figure 6.4 MRI of a patient with acampomelic campomelic dysplasia showing small chest with significant thoracic kyphoscoliosis.

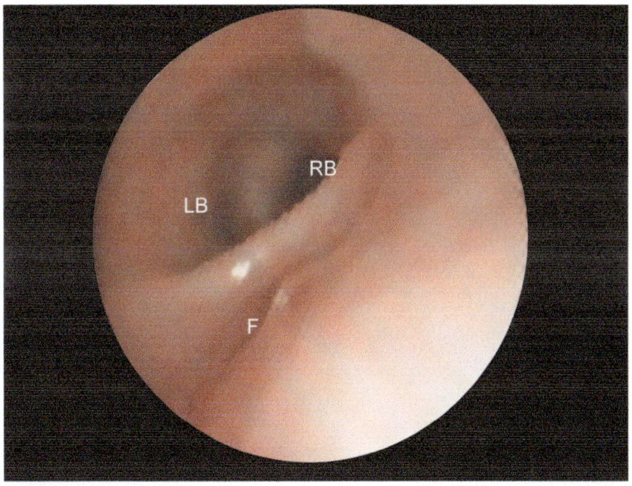

Figure 6.5 Bronchoscopic image of tracheomalacia post-trachea oesophageal fistula repair. Image shows movement of the anterior tracheal wall towards the posterior wall, during inspiration at the site of the repaired tracheo-oesophageal fistula causing an elliptical appearance to the airway.

Abbreviations: RB, right main bronchus; LB, left main bronchus; F, repaired fistula (*Source:* Image courtesy of Dr Jonathan Coutts, Neonatal Consultant, Royal Hospital for Sick Children, Glasgow. Ref. 1 Copyright Elsevier)

DEVELOPMENT OF THE RESPIRATORY TRACT IN CHILDREN

Term newborns lungs have the same number of conducting airways as adults do although they are much smaller. This makes them vulnerable to obstruction from either bronchospasm or respiratory secretions. The number of alveoli present at birth is only one-third to one-half of the total adult number. Lung growth occurs by increasing the number of alveoli and their size and by increasing the size of the airways. Premature infants are particularly at risk of respiratory difficulties as they have physiologically immature lungs—the more premature being more at risk. These difficulties are covered in Chapter 3: Neonatal medicine.

Infants predominantly use diaphragmatic breathing rather than using their intercostal muscles as these develop as children age. Children's ribs lie more horizontally and do not contribute as much to the expansion of their chests. Their ribs have more cartilage and less bone, making the chest wall compliant and also therefore more vulnerable to respiratory difficulties.

Congenital abnormalities of the respiratory tract are rare. They can be divided into abnormalities of the upper airways, e.g. larynx and above, and the lower airways. Congenital abnormalities of the upper airways will mostly be covered in Chapter 26: Paediatric otolaryngology.

Tracheal Oesophageal Fistula with Oesophageal Atresia

A tracheo-oesophageal fistula (TOF) **(Fig. 6.5)**[1] is an abnormal connection between the trachea and oesophagus,

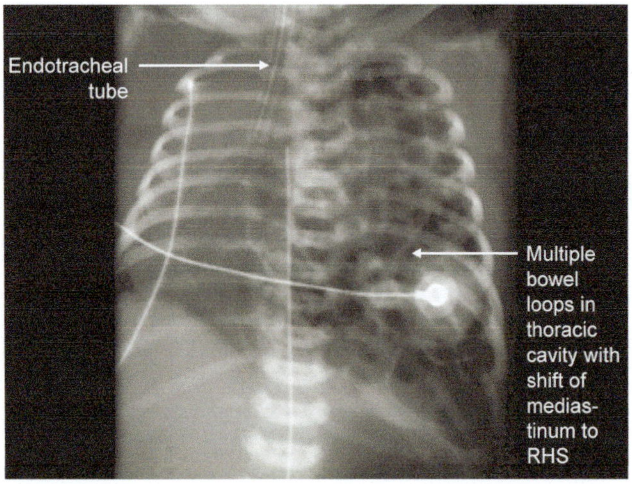

Figure 6.6 Chest X-ray showing large left-sided diaphragmatic hernia in a newborn. *Note* gross mediastinal displacement to the right hand side.

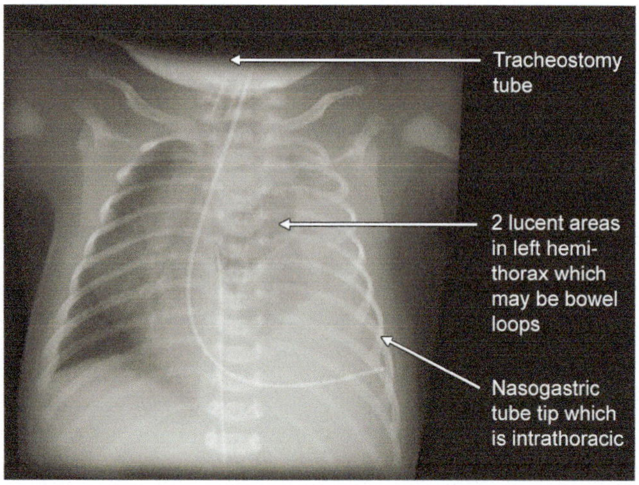

Figure 6.7 Chest X-ray showing large left-sided diaphragmatic hernia. *Note* the position of the NG tube suggesting that the stomach is in the thorax and also the two lucent areas that may be bowel loops.

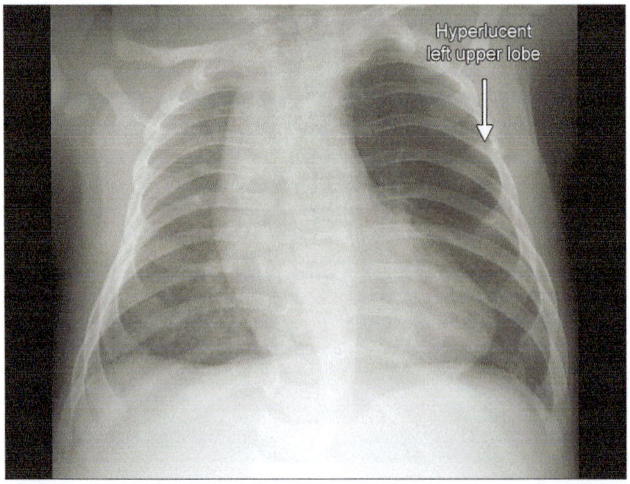

Figure 6.8 Chest X-ray of a 2-month-old infant who presented with fast breathing from birth. His chest computed tomography (CT) scan confirmed congenital lobar emphysema of the left upper lobe. The abnormal lobe was surgically removed and the infant made a complete recovery.

which commonly occurs with oesophageal atresia where the oesophagus is a blind ending pouch. A TOF usually presents as recurrent choking with feeds and oxygen desaturations or with recurrent pneumonias. There can often be malacia of the airway where the fistula occurred. In 25% of cases of TOF, there are other congenital abnormalities, e.g. imperforate anus. The treatment is surgical repair.

Congenital Diaphragmatic Hernia

This is a condition caused by embryonic failure of the closure of the pleural-peritoneal canal. The three types include the posterolateral Bochdalek hernia, the anterior Morgagni hernia and the hiatus hernia. The left-sided Bochdalek hernia occurs in approximately 85% of cases. The defects cause herniation of the abdominal contents into the thoracic cavity compressing the intrathoracic structures (**Figs. 6.6 and 6.7**). Significant pulmonary hypoplasia ensues along with pulmonary hypertension. The mortality rate is about 40%. This condition is usually diagnosed antenatally and may be associated with other congenital abnormalities. An infant with a large diaphragmatic hernia usually presents within the first few hours after birth with breathing difficulties and cyanosis. Treatment involves ideally delivering the infant in a unit with a paediatric surgical team, resuscitation and stabilisation with intubation and ventilation and passage of a nasogastric tube. Surgical repair of the defect in the diaphragm can then be performed. Some infants may also be placed on Extra Corporeal Membrane Oxygenation (ECMO) peri-operatively if they fail to stabilise with ventilation alone.

Congenital Lobar Emphysema

This is a rare condition where there is an abnormally narrowed bronchus or bronchi with weak or absent cartilage. The part of the lung that bronchus supplies becomes over-expanded and compresses on the unaffected lung. This condition is commonly unilateral (**Fig. 6.8**) but can occasionally be bilateral (**Fig. 6.9**). This can present with breathing or feeding difficulties that worsen with intercurrent respiratory infection. The treatment is surgical excision of the affected lobe.

Congenital Pulmonary Airway Malformations (CPAM)

These are the commonest congenital lung malformations. They were previously called Congenital Cystic Adenomatoid Malformations (CCAM). Here, there is an abnormal cystic development of lung tissues during 7–35 weeks of gestation. Large CPAMS may be associated with hydrops fetalis.

Pressure from the CPAM on the unaffected lung from the cystic areas can cause pulmonary hypoplasia. Many of these cysts are picked up antentally by detailed ultrasound. The first image here shows a typical CPAM that was treated surgically with the follow-up film demonstrating mild abnormality of the ribs on the right side postoperative **(Figs. 6.10A and B)**. **Figure 6.11** shows a CPAM affecting the right middle lobe. These lesions can present with significant respiratory difficulties or with recurrent infections. There have been rare cases of malignant transformation in CCAMs, and in the past, the vast majority were removed but many are not opting for conservative management and monitoring if they are asymptomatic.[2]

Foregut Duplication Cyst

Gut duplication cysts are rare. They can occur anywhere in the gastrointestinal tract. One-third of all duplications are foregut duplications (oesophagus, stomach and first and second part of duodenum) and usually present with respiratory symptoms and are more common in girls. **Figure 6.12** shows a chest CT scan of a 2-year-old boy who presented with recurrent significant chest infections with persistently abnormal chest X-rays with a hyperlucent left lung. His chest CT showed a large cystic mediastinal mass that was removed surgically and confirmed as an oesophageal duplication cyst.

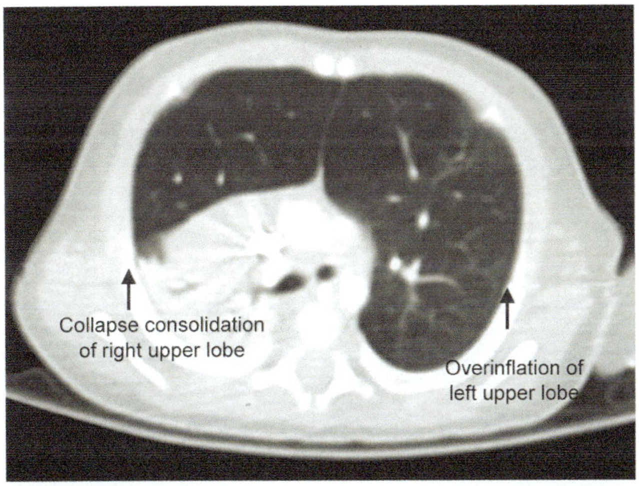

Figure 6.9 Chest CT scan demonstrating emphysema of left upper and right middle lobe causing collapse of right upper lobe.

Abnormalities of the Thoracic Skeleton

There are common abnormalities of the thoracic skeleton like pectus excavatum, where there is an abnormal development of the skeleton leading to the anterior art of the chest having a "caved in" appearance **(Figs. 6.13A and B)**. It rarely affects respiratory function and surgery can be done if there are cosmetic concerns. **Figure 6.14** demonstrates a thoracolumbar scoliosis that can either be idiopathic or in association with neurological disorders such as cerebral palsy or as part of a congenital skeletal dysplasia. Treatment of thoracic scoliosis can include thoracic bracing or spinal fusion. This will be covered in the Chapter 18: Paediatric orthopaedics. In the severe forms of this, respiratory function can be impaired so much that ventilatory support is needed along with corrective surgery, if this is clinically indicated.

ACQUIRED LOWER RESPIRATORY TRACT DISORDERS

Viral Pneumonia

Respiratory syncytial virus (RSV) is the single most important cause of viral lower respiratory tract infection in infancy and childhood worldwide. During 1997–2006, estimated 132,000–172,000 children aged less than 5 years

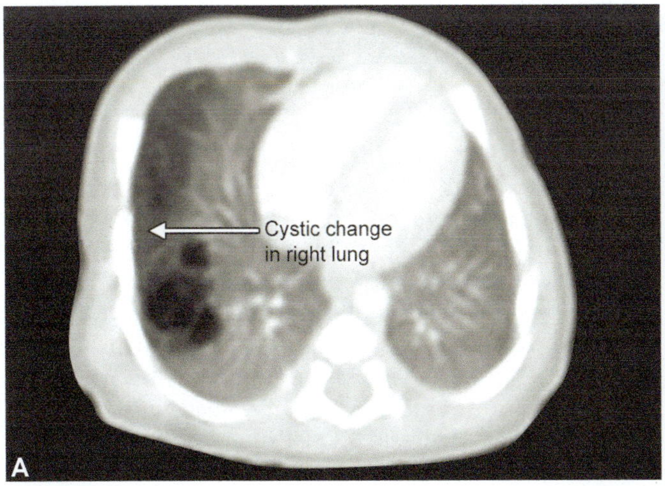

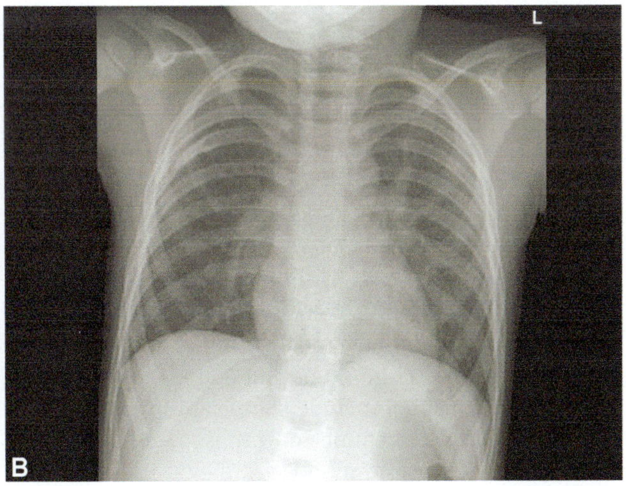

Figures 6.10A and B Chest computed tomography (CT) scan of a 3-day-old baby who had an antenatal diagnosis of possible cystic malformation of right lung. This was removed soon after birth and confirmed as a cystic adenomatoid malformation. The chest X-ray shows the appearance postoperative several years later.

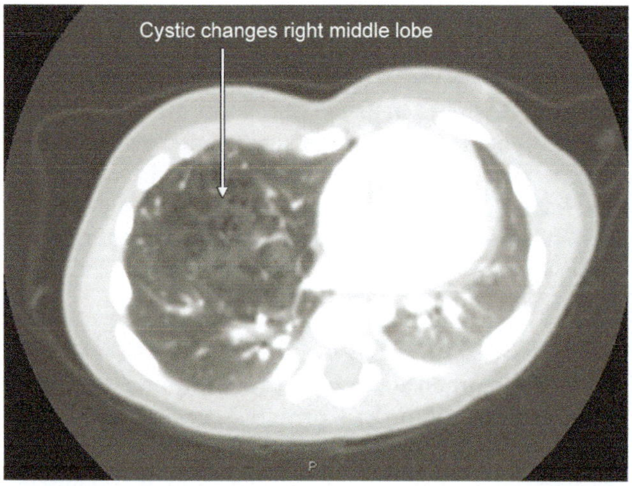

Figure 6.11 Chest CT scan showing abnormal right middle lobe with cystic lesions, pectus excavatum also present consistent with right-sided pulmonary airway malformation type 2.

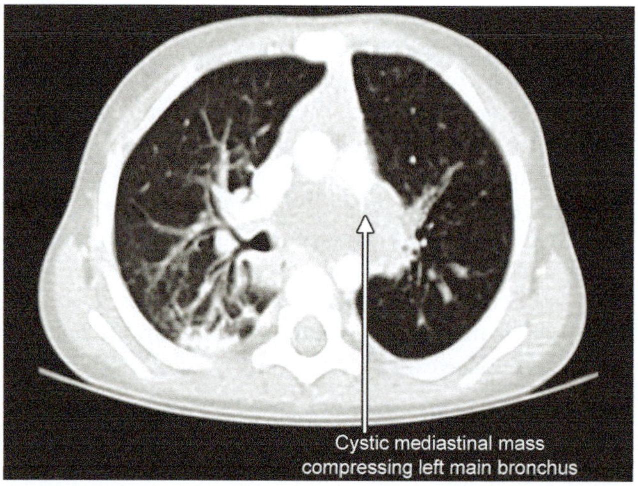

Figure 6.12 Chest computed tomography (CT) scan showing cystic mediastinal mass that was surgically removed and confirmed as a gut duplication cyst.

(*Source:* Image courtesy of Dr Phil Davies, Consultant Respiratory Paediatrician, Royal Hospital for Sick Children, Glasgow)

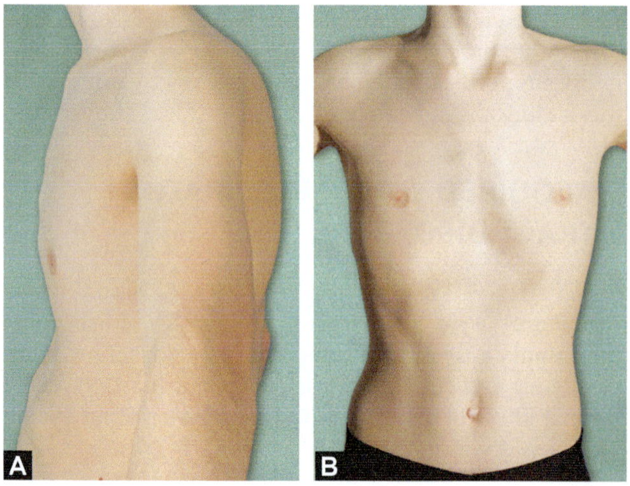

Figures 6.13A and B Lateral and AP views of patient with asymmetric pectus excavatum.

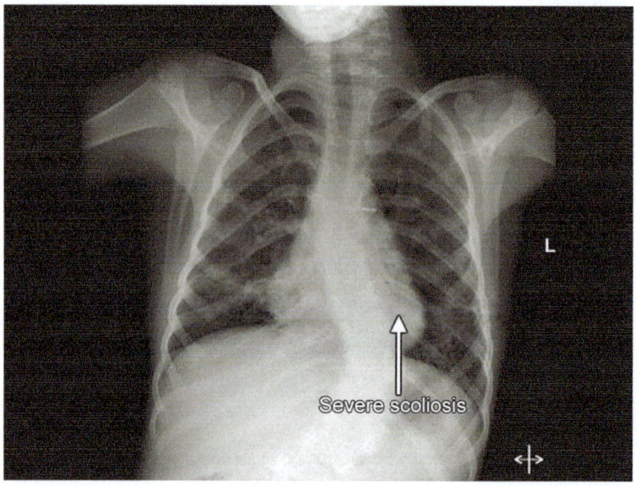

Figure 6.14 Chest X-ray of a severe thoracolumbar scoliosis convex to the patient's left in an 11-year-old girl.

were hospitalised for RSV infection annually in the United States.[3] It typically causes bronchiolitis and is most common in winter. There is significant inflammation and destruction of the airways leading to airway obstruction and air trapping and ensuing respiratory difficulties. Babies affected by RSV often have coryza, cough, fever and difficulty breathing and feeding. There are often crackles and or wheeze on auscultation. Indications for admission to hospital include significant breathing difficulties, dehydration, apnoea and those needing oxygen. In total, 90% of those admitted are infants.

Chest radiographs are not clinically indicated in most cases of bronchiolitis—they typically show bilateral hyperinflation with increased lung markings bilaterally. In infants with worsening respiratory distress and indeed those who require ventilation, they can show consolidation of one or more lobes of the lungs such as where the right upper lobe is consolidated **(Fig. 6.15)**. Premature infants, those with neuromuscular disease or those with haemodynamically significant congenital heart disease, are more at risk of severe disease.[4] It can result in an acute severe respiratory distress syndrome picture where the infant requires ventilation and may need chest drains for air leaks **(Figs. 6.16 and 6.17)**. Extracorporeal membrane oxygenation has also been used successfully. Despite this mortality from RSV is rare.[5]

Vaccines have been developed for RSV but as yet none have been shown to be safe and effective enough for use

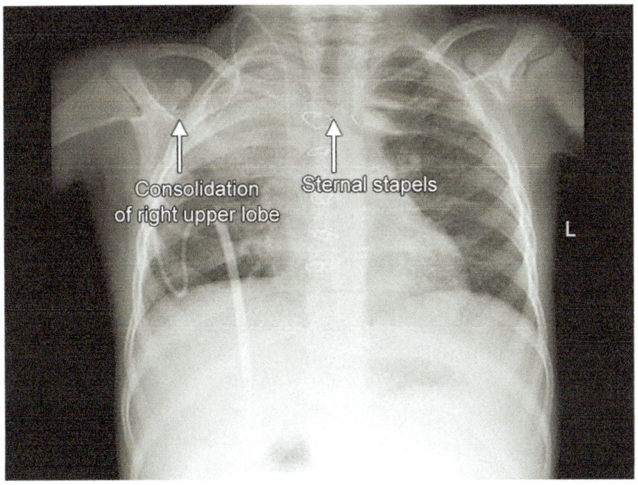

Figure 6.15 Chest X-ray showing consolidation of the right upper lobe due to respiratory syncytial virus infection in a postoperative cardiac patient.

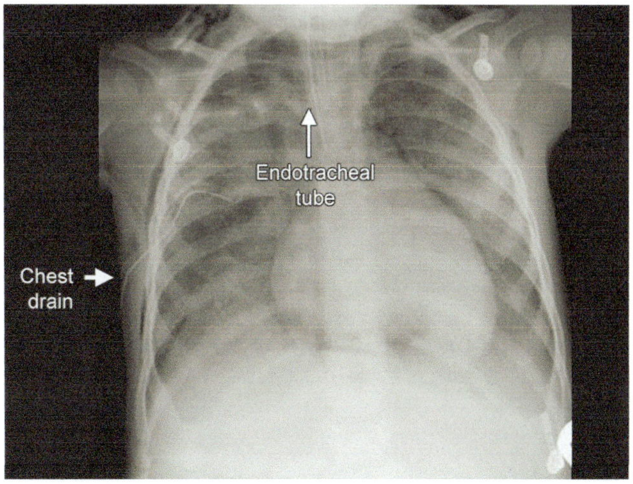

Figure 6.16 Chest X-ray of an infant with severe acute respiratory distress syndrome in an infant with respiratory syncytial virus infection. He had an air leak in the right lung that needed chest drain insertion. *Note* almost confluent areas of infiltrates bilaterally.

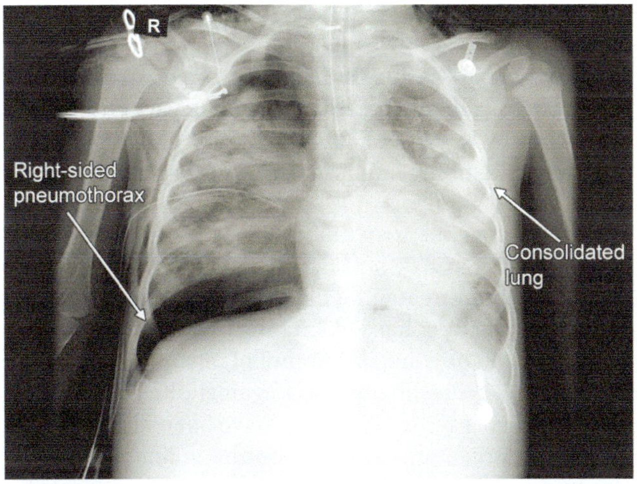

Figure 6.17 Chest X-ray of a right-sided pneumothorax in ventilated child with respiratory syncytial virus infection. *Note* chest drains.

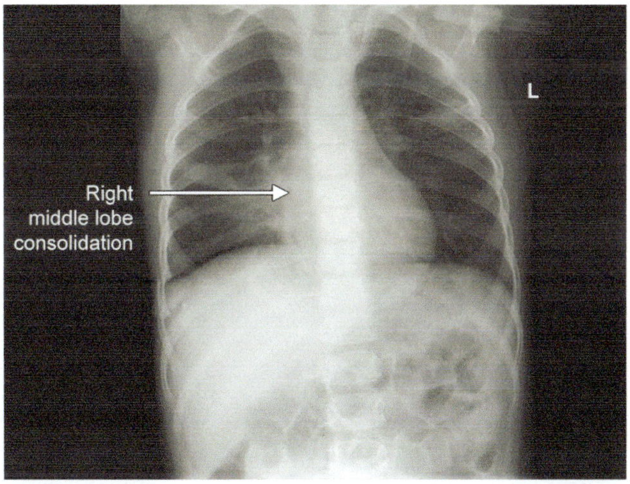

Figure 6.18 Chest X-ray (CXR) showing consolidation of right middle lobe secondary to pneumonia.

at present. Palivizumab is a monoclonal antibody preparation that has been shown to reduce hospitalisation in children from certain "at risk" groups. These are infants less than 6 months of age who were born at 35 weeks of gestation or less, those less than 2 years with chronic lung disease of prematurity and those with congenital heart disease. In some centres, Palivizumab is given to babies in those high-risk groups with the hope that it will prevent severe RSV infection.[6]

Bacterial Pneumonia

Bacterial pneumonias are an extremely common cause of death in the developing world. Causal organisms include *Streptococcus pneumonia* and *Haemophilus influenzae*. Elsewhere they cause significant morbidity and can be fatal.[7] In developing countries, these infections account for almost a half million deaths among children less than 5 years of age.[8] These pathogens cause inflammation inside the lungs with purulent secretions in the bronchi and alveoli. Affected children usually present with a high fever, cough and difficulty breathing.

Clinical signs include crackles, decreased air entry and or wheeze in the affected areas. If there is significant consolidation and or collapse, bronchial breathing may also be evident. Many cases of childhood pneumonia are managed in the community and they respond to oral antibiotics such as amoxicillin. Failure to respond to treatment could indicate either a different pathogen such as *Mycoplasma pneumoniae* or severe disease that requires investigation and treatment.

Figure 6.18 demonstrates consolidation in the right middle lobe secondary to pneumonia, **Figure 6.19** demonstrates complete collapse of the left lower lobe and **Figure 6.20** demonstrates collapse/consolidation

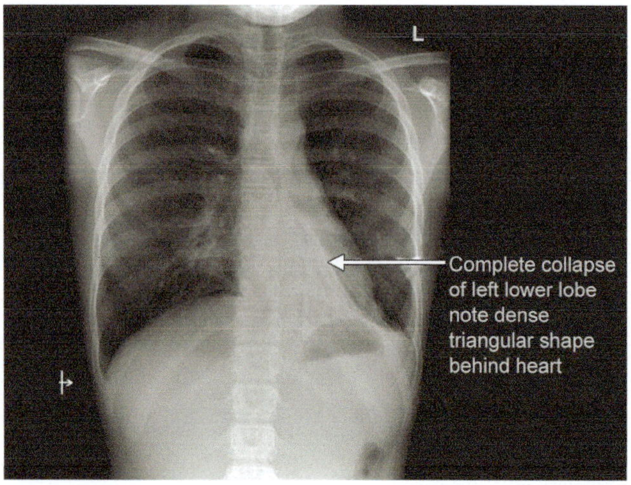

Figure 6.19 Chest X-ray (CXR) demonstrating left lower lobe collapse due to an infective exacerbation in an 8-year-old girl with primary ciliary dyskinesia.

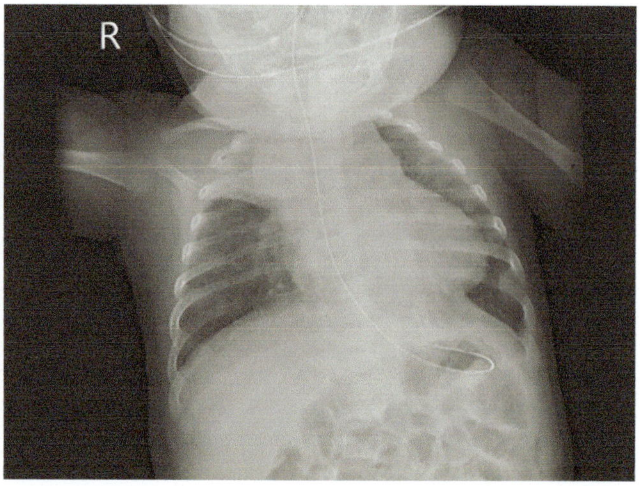

Figure 6.20 Chest X-ray showing collapse/consolidation of right upper lobe due to infection in a child with bronchomalacia.

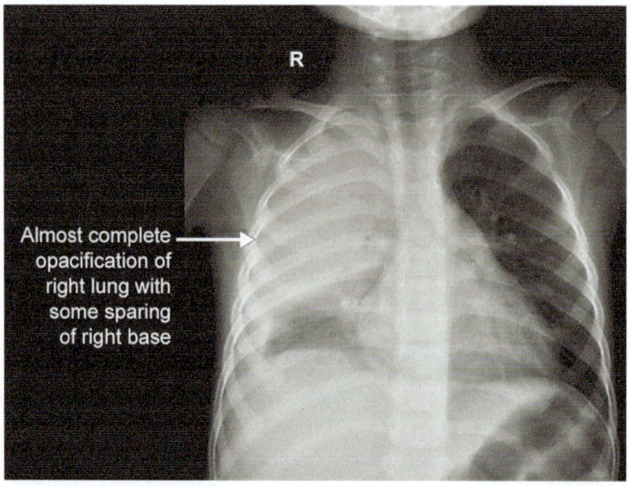

Figure 6.21 Chest X-ray (CXR) showing a complex right-sided empyema.

of right upper lobe due to infection in a child with bronchomalacia.

Other investigations include a full blood count, nasopharyngeal aspirate for viral culture for those less than 2 years. A throat swab can be done for viral polymerase chain reaction (PCR) testing. Children rarely produce sputum but if they do a sample could be sent for bacterial culture.

Indications for admission include those who have failed to respond to current antibiotics, signs of respiratory distress with low oxygen saturation levels and those who are dehydrated and cannot feed. Children with severe disease needing oxygen and intravenous fluids need to be admitted in the hospital. They may require intravenous antibiotics, oxygen and fluids. Children with persistent collapse of a lobe may need further investigations such as bronchoscopy and investigation for underlying immune deficiency or cystic fibrosis (CF).

Those with atypical or severe consolidative changes on their chest X-rays, e.g. **Figure 6.21** where there is extensive consolidation in an unusual pattern in the right lung need further imaging to assess whether there is a lung abscess, empyema or an underlying congenital lung cyst. **Figures 6.22A and B** show the chest X-rays from a patient who had a life-threatening bilateral pneumonia and who has a chronically collapsed left lung as a result.

There is an ongoing development of conjugated pneumococcal vaccines that protect against different types of pneumococcal serotypes. These have been introduced in many countries as part of the routine infant vaccination programme. They have been shown to reduce bacterial pneumonias secondary to pneumococcal disease.[9,10]

PLEURAL EFFUSION IN CHILDREN

Pleural effusion in childhood is usually due to pneumonia. Other causes include congestive heart failure, malignancy and lymphatic abnormalities. The fluid can be a transudate such as in heart failure or in a parapneumonic effusion. It can also be an exudate as occurs in empyema where the pleural fluid is infected, or it can be chylous. Effusions are usually evident on chest radiography; however, chest ultrasound is a very useful measure to confirm the presence of an effusion, its size, and whether there are fibrin stands present which would suggest an empyema. Small effusions usually need no treatment apart from treating the underlying condition; however, large effusions **(Fig. 6.23)** often need a chest drain inserted and the fluid drained, as they usually cause respiratory compromise. Chest drains can be either large bore chest drains or smaller "pig tail" chest drains **(Fig. 6.24)**. All chest tubes

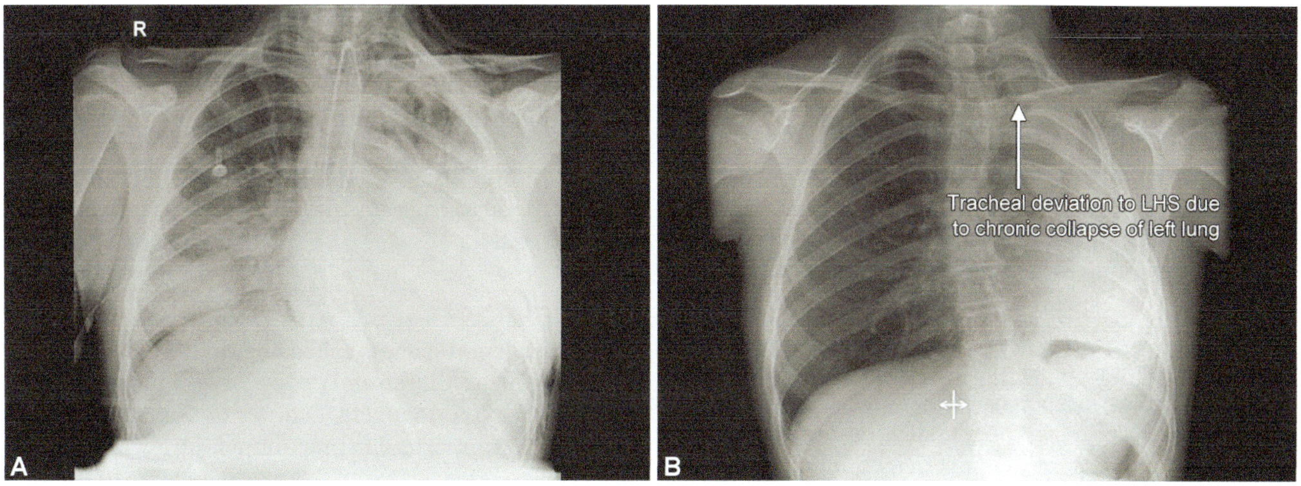

Figures 6.22A and B Chest X-rays from a teenager who presented with severe bilateral staphylococcal pneumonia secondary to influenza. The patient required ventilation for several weeks and made a partial recovery but was left with significant damage bilaterally—the left lung worse than the right with chronic collapse as demonstrated in the second chest X-ray.

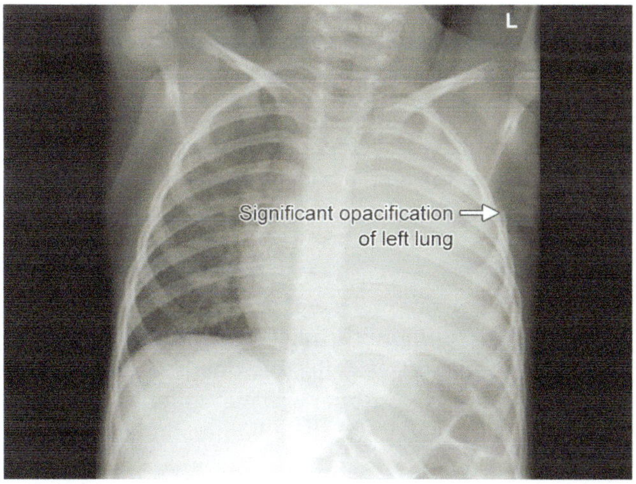

Figure 6.23 Chest X-ray showing almost complete opacification of left lung due to a pleural effusion secondary to pneumonia.

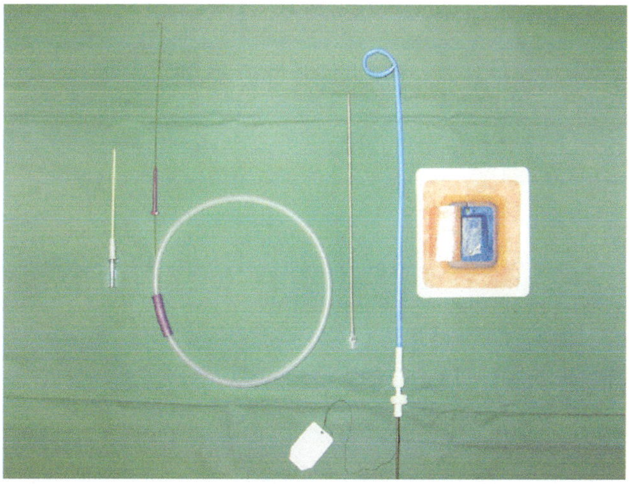

Figure 6.24 Pigtail chest drain insertion set.

should be connected to a unidirectional flow drainage system such as an underwater seal system, which often also has measurements on it so that the amount of fluid drained can be assessed. The drain collecting system needs to be at a lower level than the patient. The pleural fluid is usually sent for gram stain, bacterial culture and pneumococcal antigen testing. Biochemical analysis is performed in suspected chylothorax. Cytology is indicated where there are concerns about malignancy such as lymphoma.

Empyema

This occurs as a complication of bacterial pneumonia. It is infection in a pleural effusion with pus in the pleural space. They are rare but the incidence is increasing. *Streptococcus pneumoniae* is the most common organism responsible with serotype 1 being the most common; however, there are concerns about other serotypes becoming increasingly common, e.g. 19A.[11] Empyema presents with cough, persistent fever, cough and difficulty breathing. Clinical signs can include signs of respiratory distress and dullness to percussion on the affected side. **Figure 6.25** shows a left lower lobe pneumonia and left lower lobe collapse with a left-sided empyema.

Other investigations include a chest ultrasound, white cell count and C-reactive protein. Management includes intravenous antibiotics that will cover *S. pneumoniae*, e.g. amoxicillin or cefotaxime, antipyretics and oxygen therapy when needed. Large collections causing difficulty breathing and those with loculated effusions often need drainage. Intrapleural fibrinolytics can be used if there are loculations present or if there is overt pus evident.[12]

If the above treatments are not effective further imaging, e.g. CT of the chest and more invasive thoracic procedures, e.g. thoracotomy and decortication are indicated. Video-assisted thoracoscopic techniques have also been used. Children should have a follow-up CXR at approximately 6 weeks to ensure radiographic resolution. The majority of children make a complete recovery.

Pneumonectomy

Pneumonectomy is rarely performed in paediatrics with indications being pulmonary malignancy either primary or secondary, complex congenital lung abnormalities, intractable pulmonary haemorrhage and previously severe bronchiectasis or necrotising pneumonia.[13] Primary lung tumours in children are rare **(Fig. 6.26)**. **Figure 6.27** shows a typical appearance postpneumonectomy where the left lung was congenitally abnormal and the child was having severe respiratory infections. Postoperatively, the side of the thorax where the lung has been removed fills with fluid and over time a scoliosis often develops as the thoracic cage on the affected side fails to grow appropriately.

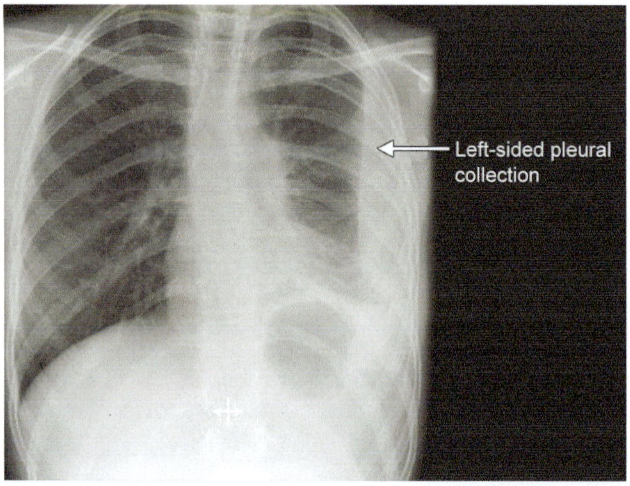

Figure 6.25 Chest X-ray showing empyema of the left lung with left lower lobe collapse and consolidation.

Pneumothorax

Air in the pleural space is called pneumothorax. These are uncommon in children and can occur spontaneously with no identifiable underlying disorder or secondary to diseases, e.g. asthma, severe pneumonia, CF and congenital lung bullae **(Figs. 6.28 and 6.29)** or secondary to trauma. There is also an association with Marfan syndrome[14] and it is important to exclude this. Small pneumothoraces need no treatment and will resolve spontaneously or with treatment of the underlying condition. A tension pneumothorax is one where the air collection gets larger with each breath and causes mediastinal shift to the opposite side of the chest. Clinical signs of this are hyper-resonance and decreased air entry on the affected side with tracheal shift to the opposite side. This requires immediate resuscitation and needle decompression by placement of an intravenous cannula in the second intercostal space in the mid-clavicular line on the affected side followed by chest drain insertion.

Asthma

Asthma is a common chronic recurrent inflammatory condition of the airways affecting one in 11 children. A child is admitted to hospital every 20 minutes in the UK due to an asthma attack.[15] The inflammation is mediated

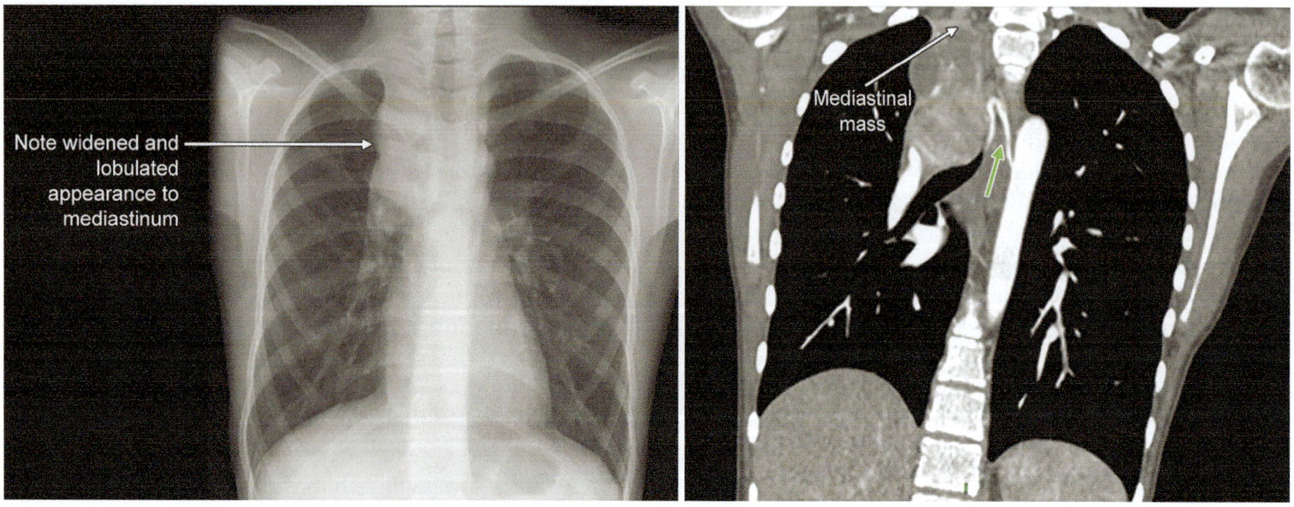

Figure 6.26 Chest X-ray and chest CT scan of a 14-year-old teenager whose mediastinal mass was detected during TB contact tracing. Biopsy demonstrated a rare mucoepidermoid tumour and she required a right-sided pneumonectomy. The green arrow shows compression of the right upper lobe bronchus by the mass above this.

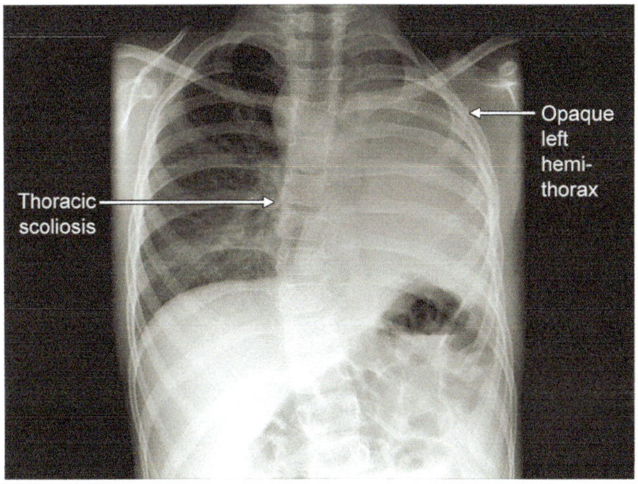

Figure 6.27 Chest X-ray of a patient who had a left-sided pneumonectomy—the left hemithorax is partly filled with fluid making it opaque, there is shift of the mediastinum to the left and a thoracic scoliosis.

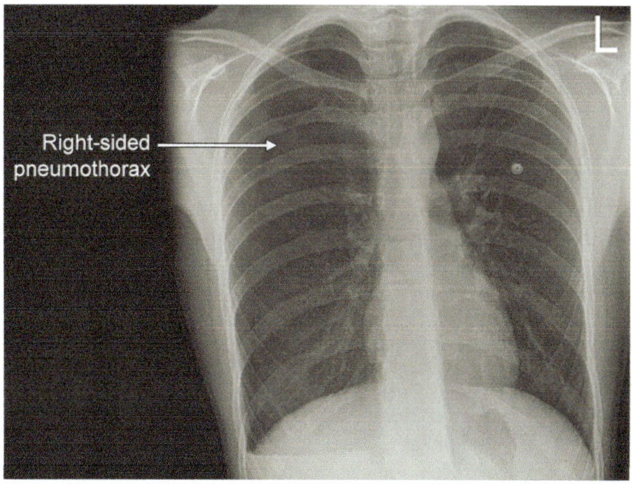

Figure 6.28 Chest X-ray showing-a right-sided pneumothorax in a child who presented with sudden right sided chest pain.

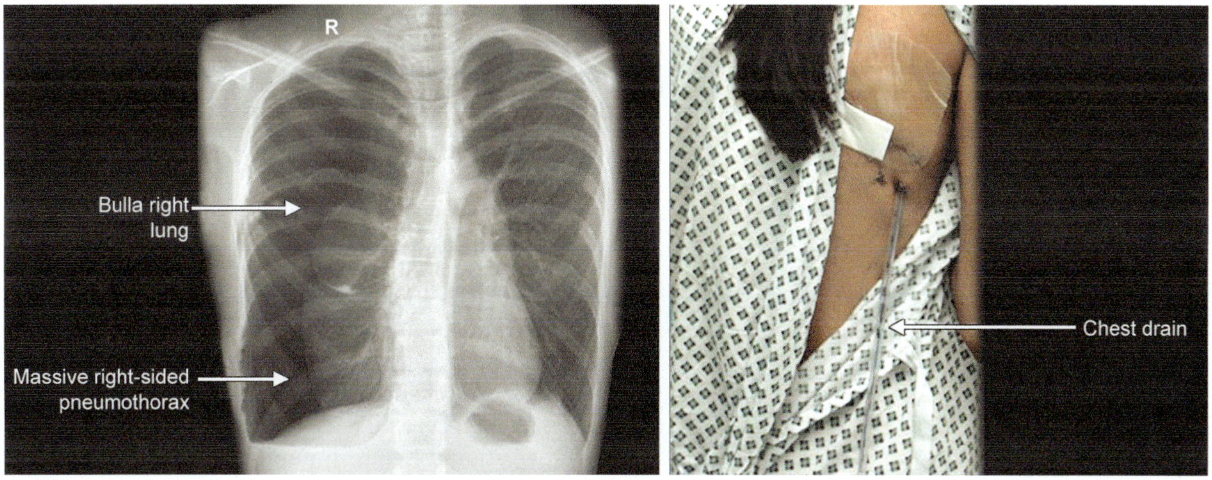

Figure 6.29 Chest X-ray showing a massive right-sided pneumothorax due to lung bullae. This was initially drained with a chest drain but needed thoracotomy and surgical repair of bulla. Clinical image shows patient post-thoracotomy.

by a number of inflammatory cells including mast cells, neutrophilic granulocytes and eosinophils. These infiltrate the mucosa of the airways and cause oedema of the airways, disruption of the epithelium, mucus hypersecretion and bronchial hyper-responsiveness. This reversible airways obstruction can be triggered by a number of factors the most common in children being upper-respiratory tract infection.

Other common precipitating factors include exercise, emotion, cold weather and smoking. Children with asthma may have other atopic conditions such as hay fever and eczema. Persistent asthma is commonly associated with atopy and with elevated Immunoglobulin E levels.[16]

Airways obstruction leads to the clinical symptoms of wheeze, nocturnal cough and difficulty breathing—a child sometimes will complain of chest tightness or chest pains. On examination during an acute attack signs of respiratory distress include tachypnoea, hyperinflation and subcostal recession and use of accessory muscles of respiration. If severe, the child may be hypoxic or confused. On auscultation, there is usually wheeze, which is often bilateral, and reduced air entry. The child with severe acute asthma may have a silent chest. Routine chest radiographs are usually not needed in asthma; however, they usually show marked hyperinflation **(Fig. 6.30)**.

Severe chronic asthma can lead to chest deformity of the lower part of the chest, that is, Harrison sulci and/or a barrel-shaped chest. There is no gold standard diagnostic test for asthma in children, and it can be difficult to diagnose in the young child. Usually the diagnosis is made on the

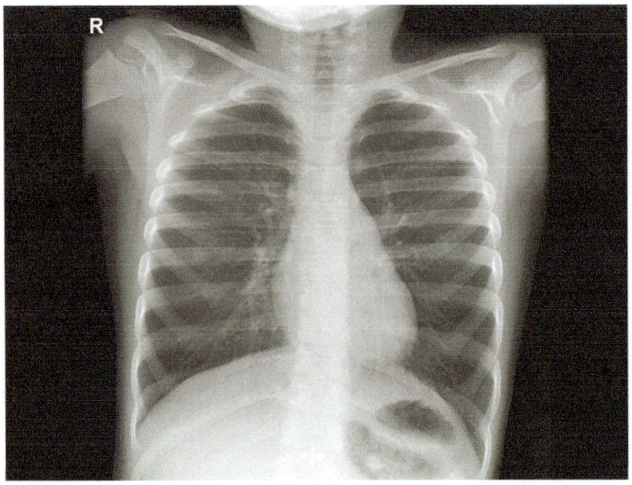

Figure 6.30 Chest X-ray showing moderate bilateral hyperinflation secondary to acute asthma.

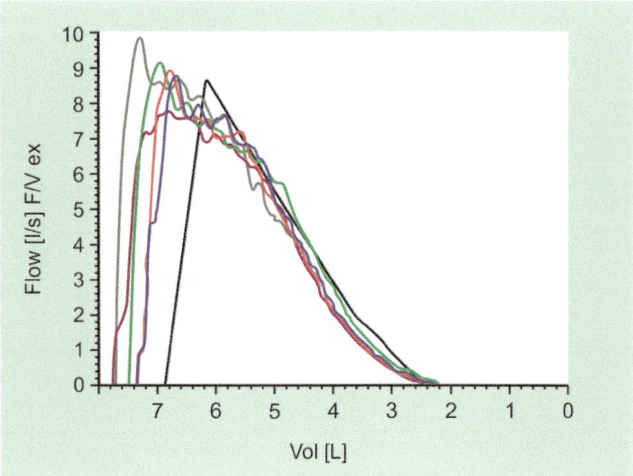

Figure 6.31 Normal flow volume loop.

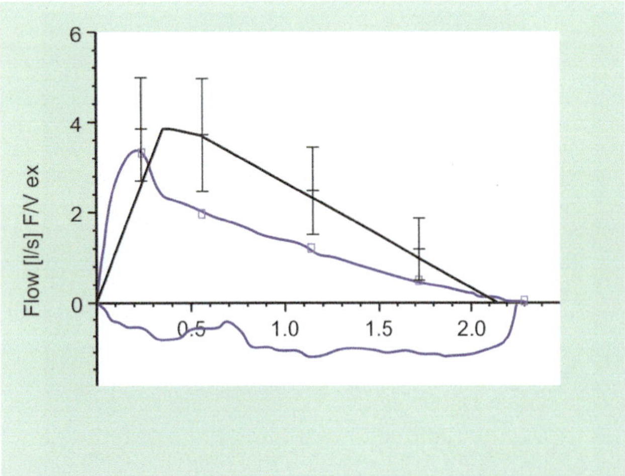

Figure 6.32 Obstructive flow volume loop.

basis of a suggestive history and/or examination findings. The lung function tests can be done only in children over 5 years—often these show normal spirometry (Fig. 6.31); severe or persistent asthma can show airways obstruction (Fig. 6.32) and classically shows reversibility of this obstruction when a bronchodilator is given (Fig. 6.33). If the asthma is induced by exercise, this can be seen by doing an exercise stimulation test.

Some children can have recurrent wheeze that appears to be only precipitated by viruses and there is often discussion as to whether this is asthma and how it should be treated. The acute management of both is similar with the use of bronchodilators via spacer devices. There have been various studies examining whether virus-induced wheeze and multi-trigger wheeze should have the same long-term therapy but the ideal therapy has not been agreed on.[17]

Asthma Management

The goal of asthma management is for the child to have well-controlled asthma and not to need frequent rescue medication. They would hope to have normal lung function. Detailed guidelines for acute and chronic asthma management are available from the British Thoracic Society (BTS).[18] The management of acute asthma will be covered in Chapter 25: Paediatric emergencies.

Education and Management Plans

The key to good asthma management is education. This includes education of the parents and of the child as well as healthcare professionals. The majority of asthma management occurs in general practice. Parents who smoke should be given guidance on smoking cessation and advice about reducing allergen exposure, e.g. to the house dust mite. Asthma management plans are very useful. They document a child's individual symptoms and signs of their asthma, what their medication is, when to give it and when to call for help.

Drug Treatment of Asthma

Inhalers are the main form of treatment for asthma. In children, these are usually metered dose inhalers given using a spacer device that can either be a small volume spacer (Fig. 6.34) or a large volume one (Fig. 6.35). Dry powder devices, activated by sucking, e.g. turbohalers and accuhalers can be useful in children over 8 years of age. Inhaler technique needs to be checked. There are clinical videos on the asthma United Kingdom website that demonstrate the correct use of spacers and inhalers.

Mild intermittent asthma symptoms should be managed with a short-acting inhaled beta agonists, given as required (step 1 of BTS guidelines).

Children with more persistent asthma symptoms require an inhaled steroid, at as low a dose as possible to

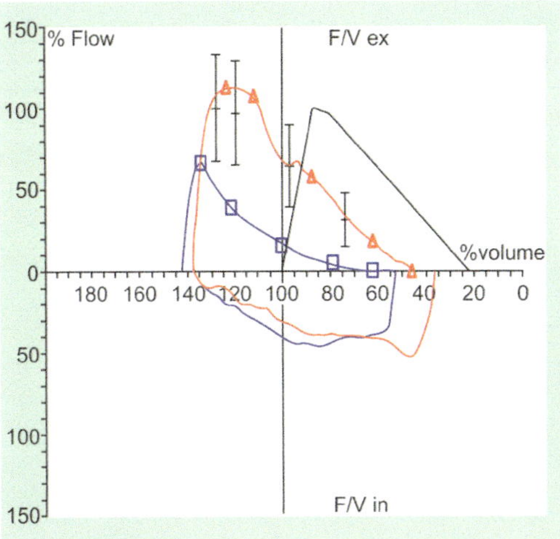

Test date: 31/03/2011		Predicted	Baseline	Baseline SDS	Post Bronchodilator	Post BD SDS	Post BD % change
Spirometry				(% Pred)			
Forced exp Vol 1.0 sec	L	1.72	1.21	–2.19	1.96	1.01	62.0%
Forced vital capacity	L	1.95	1.82	–0.50	2.39	1.60	31.3%
FEV, NC	%	90.8%	66.48%	–3.35	82.01%	-1.21	23.4%
Max mid-exp flow	L/s						#DIV/0
Max flow @ 75% VC	L/s		1.77		3.33		88.1%
Max flow @ 50% VC	L/s	2.48	0.96	-2.55	2.63	0.25	174.0%
Max flow @ 25% VC	L/s	1.21	0.30	-2.36	0.89	-0.83	196.7%
PEFR	L/min	230	187	-0.93	261	0.68	39.6%
PIFR	L/min	184	111	-1.84	108	-1.92	-2.7%

Figure 6.33 Flow volume loop and accompanying table of results from spirometry. Patient's baseline flow volume loop is in blue with the squares. The pink loop shows the flow volume loop post bronchodilator. The table clearly shows the forced expiratory volume in 1 second (FEV_1) at baseline being significantly reduced in comparison to the forced expiratory ratio (FVC) that is within the normal range giving a FEV_1/FVC of 66%. The FEV_1 improves to above the predicted level post bronchodilator.

(*Image courtesy*: Mr Andrew Morley, Chief Respiratory Physiologist, Royal Hospital for Sick Children, Glasgow)

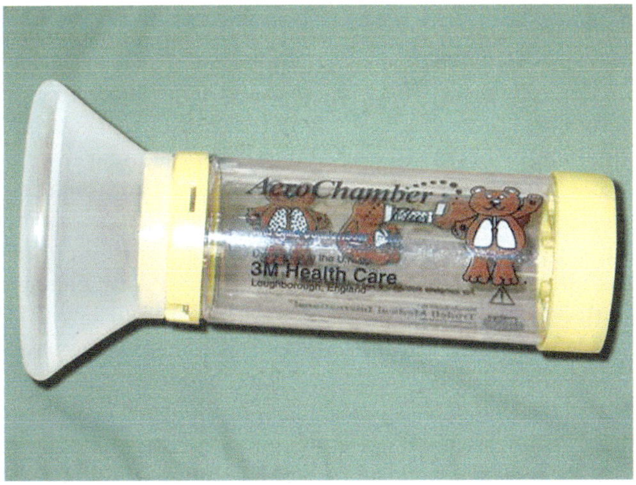

Figure 6.34 Paediatric aerochamber.

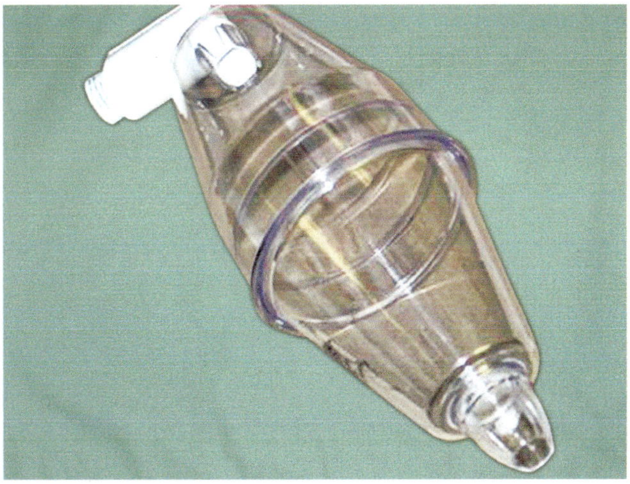

Figure 6.35 Volumatic device with metered dose inhaler.

maintain symptom control, e.g. 100 μg twice daily of Clenil Modulite or equivalent. Children less than 5 years who are unable to take inhaled steroids can have a trial of a leukotriene receptor antagonist (LRTA) (step 2).

Children with moderate asthma symptoms, not controlled on the above therapy, can have their dose of inhaled steroids increased to 200 μg twice daily of Clenil Modulite or equivalent. A long-acting beta 2 agonist (LABA) or an LRTA can also be tried (step 3).

Step 4 of the guidelines suggests that if asthma control is still not achieved with inhaled steroids (children: 400 μg/day) as well as an LABA, then the inhaled steroid dose can be increased to 800 μg/day, adding an LRTA and/or theophylline. If asthma symptoms persist, then the child should be referred on to specialist care as they require further investigations and management. Children under 5 years should be referred earlier if there are persistent symptoms.

Bronchiectasis

Bronchiectasis is a condition where the bronchi are irregularly shaped and dilated (**Fig. 6.36**). Pulmonary secretions do not drain properly, and the lungs are prone to infection. This causes further inflammation and scarring, with airways obstruction, chest infections and a chronically productive cough. This can lead to decreased lung function and potential respiratory failure.

In many patients with bronchiectasis no underlying cause can be found; however, it can occur due to the following—CF, post severe chest infection, recurrent aspiration, primary ciliary dyskinesia, foreign body aspiration and congenital and acquired immunodeficiency

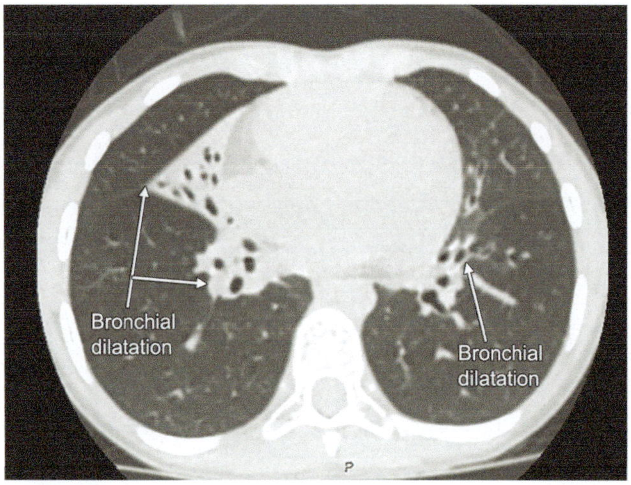

Figure 6.36 Chest computed tomography (CT) slice showing bronchiectasis in the right middle lobe and lingula.

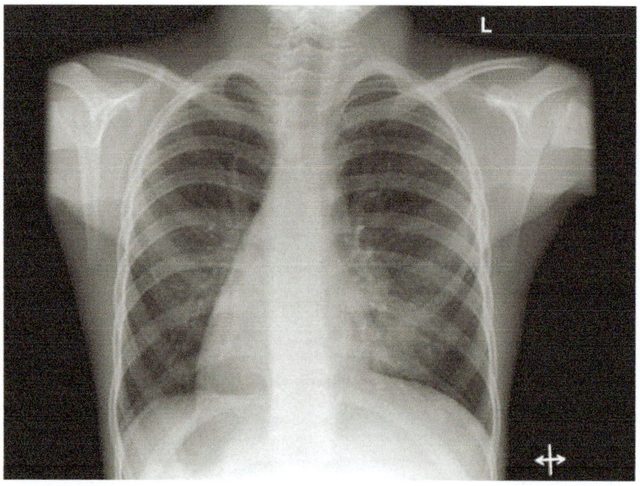

Figure 6.37 Chest X-ray of a 4-year-old boy with primary ciliary dyskinesia demonstrating dextrocardia.

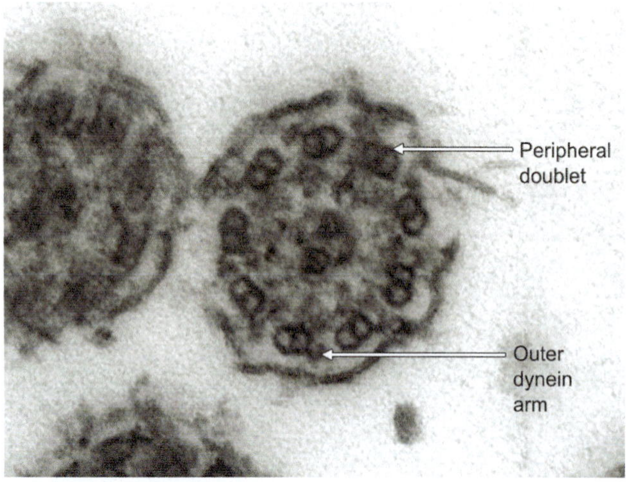

Figure 6.38 Electron micrograph of cilia.

syndromes. It is important to look for these conditions and treat them. The clinical features of bronchiectasis include finger clubbing and chest deformity. During infections there are often crackles heard in the affected areas. Children with bronchiectasis need to be referred to a chest physiotherapist and then later the child to learn chest physiotherapy techniques. Lung function tests should be done to monitor their condition. They also need early antibiotic therapy if there are signs of an exacerbation. Patients with frequent exacerbations may benefit from prophylactic antibiotics. Sputum cultures and/or cough swabs can guide antibiotic therapy but usually antibiotics such as co-amoxiclav and erythromycin are used.[19]

Primary Ciliary Dyskinesia

Kartagener first described the syndrome of bronchiectasis, situs inversus (where the heart and abdominal organs are located on the opposite sides of the body to normal) and sinusitis in the 1930s (Fig. 6.37). Later this was found to be due to defective cilia in the respiratory tract and throughout the body. Primary ciliary dyskinesia is a rare autosomal recessive condition, in which the cilia are structurally defective and beat abnormally. There are different mutations leading to PCD that cause defects in different parts of the cilia e.g. the outer or the inner dynein arms. The abnormality of the cilia results in abnormal mucus clearance with recurrent chest infections, serous otitis media and acute otitis media and persistent nasal symptoms. There is airways obstruction and damage with chronic cough and bronchiectasis. The diagnosis is made by a brush biopsy of the nasal cilia and the material obtained is analysed for cilia movement and ultrastructure (Fig. 6.38). Genetic testing is also available for the common mutations. Many patients with PCD have a reduced nasal nitric oxide level. Treatment of this condition includes chest physiotherapy, prompt treatment of infections with antibiotics and review by ear, nose and throat (ENT).

CYSTIC FIBROSIS

This is a common genetic autosomal recessive life-shortening condition in Caucasians. In the UK, the carrier rate is approximately 1 in 25 and carriers are asymptomatic. It is caused by mutations in the CF gene, which is located on the long arm of chromosome 7. The mutations are found in the gene that codes for the CF transmembrane regulator (CFTR) protein, which is made up of 1,480 amino acids.

This protein is a chloride channel regulator, an adenosine triphosphate (ATP)-binding cassette (ABC) transporter. It is involved in the transportation of molecules such as chloride across the membranes of cells in the lungs, liver, pancreas, digestive tract, reproductive tract and skin. Mutations in it cause defects in chloride and water absorption across cells and resulting disease.

There are over 1,500 mutations in the CF gene, but the Delta F508 mutation is the most common. The mutations are divided into six classes of severity. In Class 1 mutations, there is significant impairment of CFTR function, e.g. mutation G542X where there is almost no CFTR produced and Classes 4 to 6 are the milder F mutations which do have some functioning CFTR. The Delta F508 mutation is a Class 2 mutation where there is abnormal folding of the protein and it does not reach the apical surface of the cell membrane, and those patients who are homozygous for this mutation usually have severe disease and are pancreatic insufficient.

Carriers of one CF mutation are usually asymptomatic. Affected individuals with two severe mutations are likely to have severe classical CF disease with bronchiectasis and less than 1% of normal CFTR function.[20]

Presentation of Cystic Fibrosis

In many countries, CF is now diagnosed on newborn screening. It is based on checking the immunoreactive trypsin (IRT) level in the newborn blood spot, which is obtained at 5 days of age. If the IRT level is significantly elevated then the blood is sent for screening for CF mutations. It has been shown that children diagnosed after newborn screening have better growth and better lung function than those diagnosed clinically.[21]

"Classic CF" presents in childhood with recurrent chest infections, malabsorption and failure to thrive due to exocrine pancreatic insufficiency. Clinical signs include finger clubbing, chest deformity, crackles and wheeze and abdominal distension.

CF can also present as neonatal gut obstruction, where the bowel is obstructed by inspissated meconium. This causes small bowel obstruction and can be associated with large bowel abnormalities, e.g. microcolon and other small bowel abnormalities (Figs. 6.39 and 6.40). The affected bowel can be necrotic and frequently major bowel surgery is required with resection of affected areas and stoma creation. Bowel dysfunction is common and requires specialist input from dieticians and gastroenterology.

The small bowel distension can be detected on antenatal ultrasound and if it is found then the prospective parents should be offered genetic counselling and testing to see whether they are CF carriers. "Mild CF" may only present in adulthood with male infertility.

Cystic Fibrosis Diagnosis

The gold standard for the diagnosis of CF is the sweat test. This involves obtaining a sample of sweat, induced by pilocarpine iontophoresis and measuring the amount of chloride present (Figs. 6.41A and B). This shows a common method of performing this test called the Macroduct System.[22] In children, a sweat chloride concentration over 60 mmol/kg is considered diagnostic of CF. However, false-positive and false-negative sweat tests do occur. Borderline sweat tests between 40 and 60 require further investigation.

If a newborn screening of an infant has been found to have two CF mutations, a sweat test is performed to confirm the diagnosis. If the sweat test is done as there are clinical concerns, the child may be affected and the result is borderline or positive, bloods should be sent for CF mutation analysis. There are different CF mutation kits available that check for varying number of CF mutations and are often specific to the country where the genetic test is being done, that is, will contain the common mutations found in that population.

Additional tests that can help include tests for malabsorption that are faecal chymotrypsin and elastase levels that are reduced in patients with CF, who are pancreatic insufficient.[23]

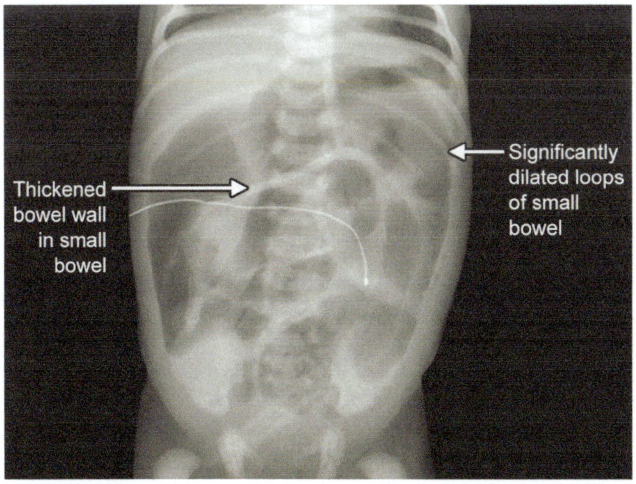

Figure 6.39 Abdominal X-ray from a newborn term infant who presented with abdominal distension and vomiting. Here meconium ileus, secondary to cystic fibrosis, has caused small bowel obstruction.

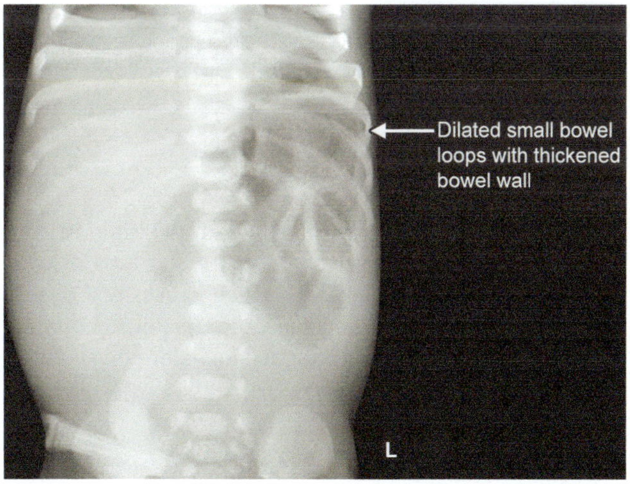

Figure 6.40 Abdominal X-ray of a newborn with abdominal distension and vomiting due to a segmental volvulus and meconium ileus secondary to cystic fibrosis.

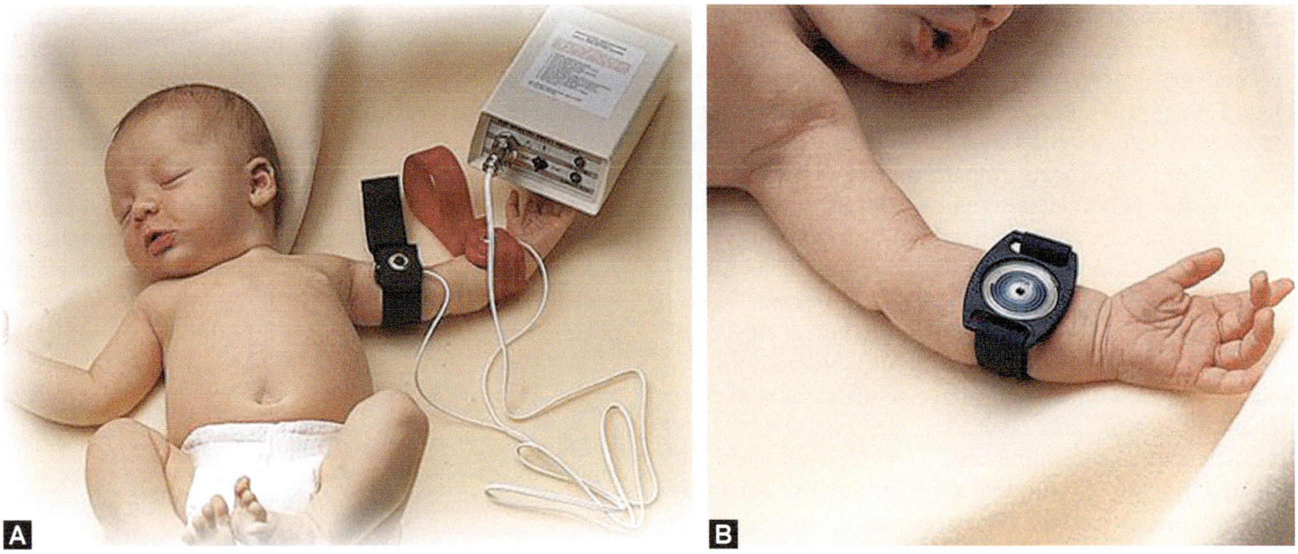

Figures 6.41A and B Infants with equipment in situ of one method of performing a sweat test for cystic fibrosis. The "Webster Sweat Inducer" (A) and the "Macroduct Collecting System" (B), which collects the sweat which is then analysed for chloride levels.

(*Source:* Images courtesy of the ELITech Group)

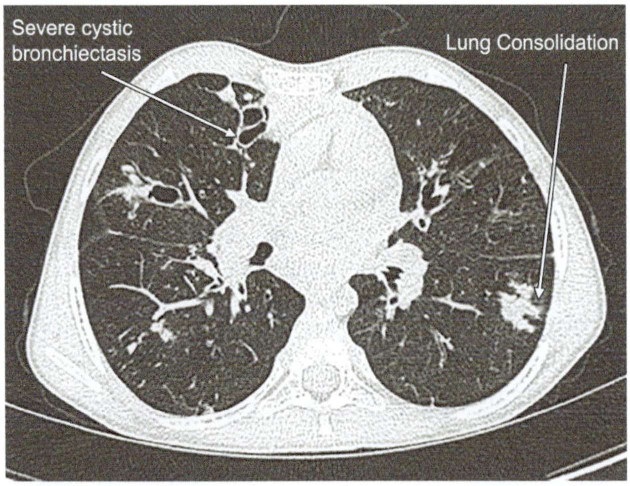

Figure 6.42 Chest computed tomography (CT) slices showing severe bilateral bronchiectasis with cystic lung destruction and additional consolidative changes due to infection and mucus trapping in a patient with cystic fibrosis.

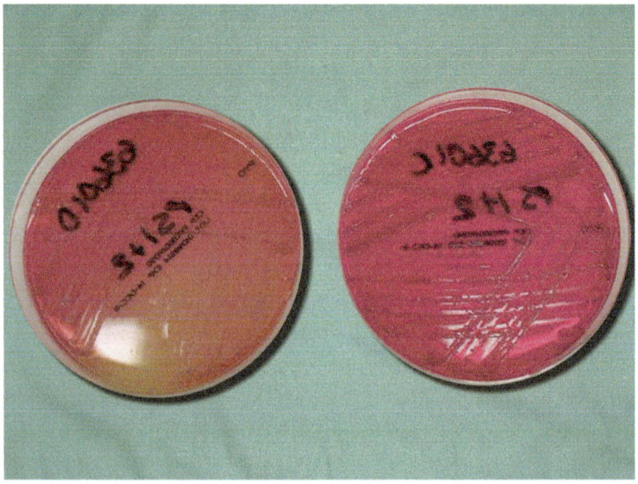

Figure 6.43 Pink colonies of Burkholderia Cepacia Complex (BCC) stains grown on selective cepacia agar.

Disease Progression

The abnormal mucus composition, inflammation and recurrent lung infections lead to obstructive lung disease and bronchiectasis **(Fig. 6.42)** which causes respiratory failure. The average life expectancy is approximately 40 years—however, many patients die before this.

Common Respiratory Pathogens in Cystic Fibrosis

The CF lung is susceptible to infection and damage from a number of organisms. These include *Staphylococcus aureus, Pseudomonas aeruginosa, Haemophilus influenzae* and *Burkholderia cepacia* **(Fig. 6.43)**. Chronic colonisation with *P. aeruginosa* has been shown to adversely affect survival with CF. Epidemic subtypes of *B. cepacia* can cause the "Cepacia" syndrome where patients rapidly decline with high fevers and severe respiratory infections which have a significant mortality. Segregation of inpatients and outpatients with such organisms is now commonly practiced to reduce chances of patient to patient transfer of unwanted bacteria.

Management of Cystic Fibrosis

This is multidisciplinary and involves specialist physiotherapists, dieticians, dedicated nursing, medical and surgical staff, social workers, psychologists, pulmonary physiologists and geneticists. Key aspects to therapy are chest physiotherapy, regular cough swabs and or sputum cultures to monitor what organisms are present, nutritional input, prophylactic antibiotics primarily against *S. aureus* in children and prompt antibiotic treatment of increased respiratory symptoms.

If *P. aeruginosa* is isolated, even if a child is well, eradication measures, including oral, nebulised and intravenous anti-pseudomonal antibiotics are used in an attempt to prevent colonisation with *P. aeruginosa.*

Physiotherapy

Physiotherapy is vital for clearing the abnormal mucus present in the airways of a patient with CF. Also physiotherapists have important roles in promoting physical fitness. There are various airway clearance techniques available and they depend on the age of the child and their clinical condition. Techniques involve using positive expiratory pressure (PEP) masks, flutter devices, space hoppers to bounce parents and child on and activated cycle of breathing techniques.[24]

Chest physiotherapy ideally should be performed once to three times daily depending on the individual and whether they have an exacerbation or not. There are however many issues with adherence to therapy particularly physiotherapy. Daily activity is encouraged in children and aimed at being fun including trampoline use and full participation in games. Also it is often the physiotherapist in the team who obtains either the cough swab or the sputum culture from the patient, when they are at clinic, or an inpatient.

Nutrition

The vast majority of children with CF are pancreatic insufficient and therefore have malabsorption. CF leads to an increased metabolic rate as a result of the chronic inflammatory state, recurrent chest infections and malabsorption. This means that they usually require a higher caloric intake than children of the same age. Pancreatic enzyme replacement therapy (PERT) containing primarily lipase is used to combat the pancreatic insufficiency. These are given with all meals and snacks containing fat and need to be taken within 20 minutes of the food. Fat-soluble vitamins, e.g. vitamins A, D and E are given daily usually in multivitamin preparations to those who are pancreatic insufficient.

Children may need calorie supplements and also occasionally gastrostomy feeding.

Antibiotics

Mild pulmonary exacerbations are treated with additional oral antibiotics and extra chest physiotherapy. Moderate to severe exacerbations **(Fig. 6.44)** are treated with intravenous antibiotic. Policies vary between centres but most would use two different antibiotics, e.g. ceftazidime and tobramycin. The reason why two antibiotics are used is to try to reduce antibiotic resistance. The patients sputum culture or cough swab microbiology is used to guide antibiotic choice. **Figure 6.45** shows antibiotic disc testing of *P. aeruginosa* to try to see what antibiotics the organism is sensitive to and **Figure 6.46** shows minimal inhibitory concentration (MIC) testing of a strain of *P. aeruginosa.*

Semi-permanent subcutaneous central venous access, e.g. "Port-a-Cath" is used for patients with difficult intravenous access or needle phobia. **Figure 6.47** shows the "Port-a-Cath" with the gripper needle in situ and the radiological appearance of a "Port-a-Cath" is shown in **Figure 6.48**. Nebulised antibiotics, e.g. "colomycin" and "TOBI" (nebuliser solution, tobramycin) are also used in eradication protocols for *P. aeruginosa* and in the treatment of patients who are chronically colonised with *P. aeruginosa.*

Azithromycin is also used in patients with CF who are chronically colonised with *P. aeruginosa* or those with significant bronchiectasis. It has been shown in several studies[25] to reduce the number of exacerbations.

Lung Transplantation

Children with end-stage pulmonary disease should be considered for double lung transplant. They are referred

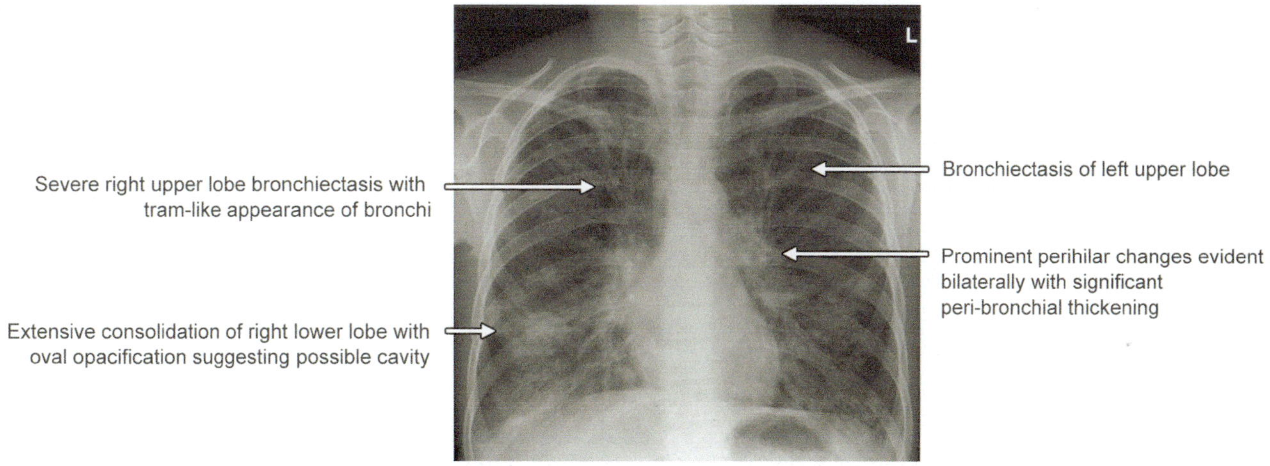

Figure 6.44 Chest X-ray of a 13-year-old girl with cystic fibrosis. There are severe chronic changes throughout.

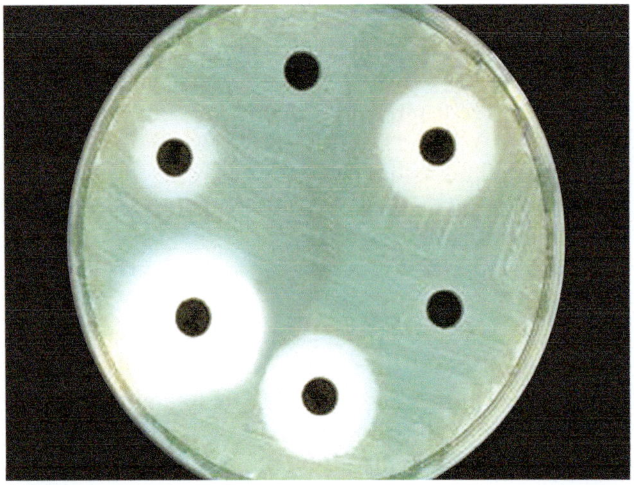

Figure 6.45 Antibiotic disc sensitivity testing of *Pseudomonas aeruginosa*, demonstrating the characteristic green pigmentation produced by many strains of this organism.

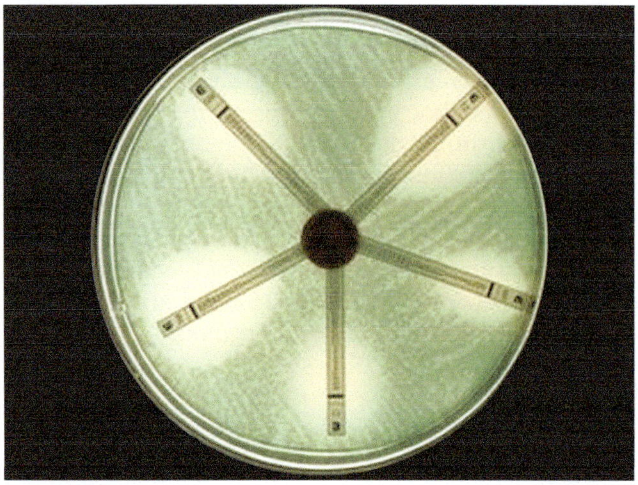

Figure 6.46 Measurement of the minimum inhibitory concentration (MIC) of anti-pseudomonal drugs using Etest strips.

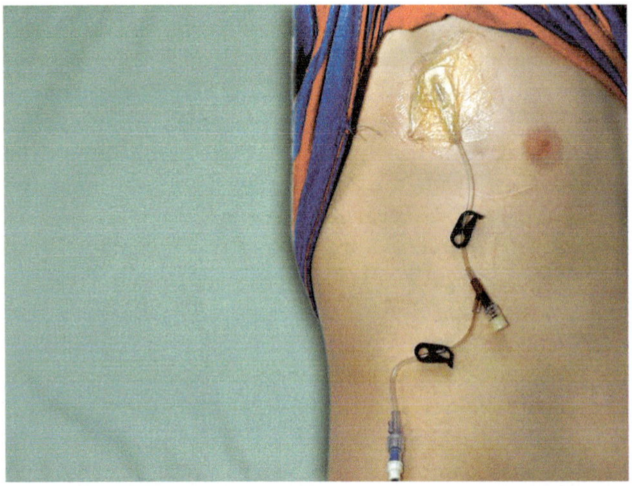

Figure 6.47 Patient with Port-a-Cath and Gripper needle in place.

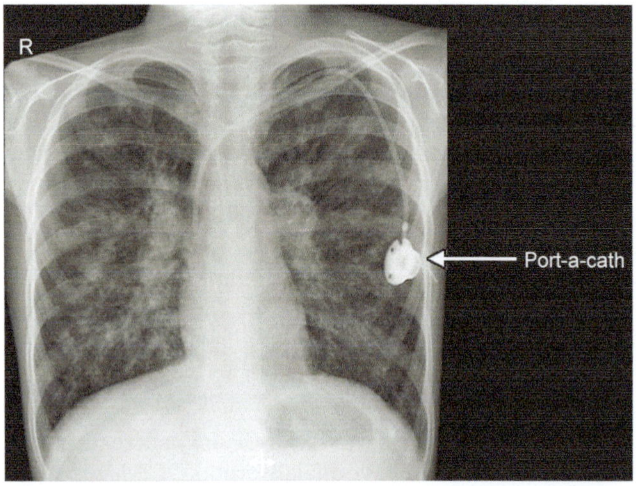

Figure 6.48 Chest X-ray showing cystic fibrosis lung disease—*note* significant hyperinflation, increased perihelia markings and patchy opacification that is worse in the right lung. A Port-a-Cath has been inserted for injection of intravenous antibiotics.

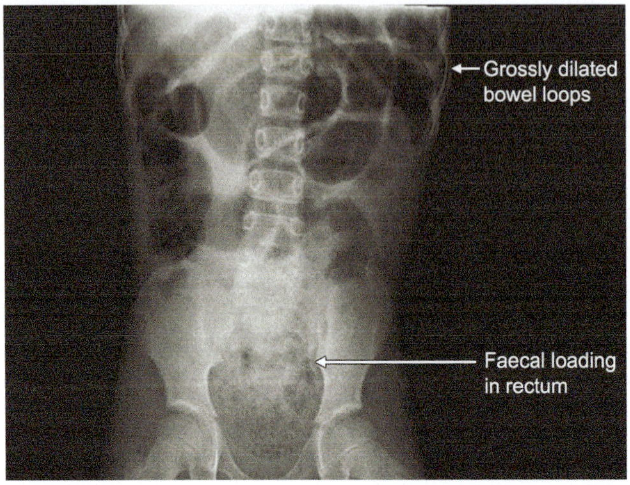

Figure 6.49 Abdominal X-ray showing distal intestinal obstruction syndrome in a patient with cystic fibrosis.

to specialist centres where they are evaluated by a multidisciplinary team with both an evaluation of their physical health, bacterial colonisation as well as psychological and social factors such as adherence to treatment. Unfortunately, there is a significant shortage of organs, particularly for children so there is a chance that patients may die on the transplant list. Transplantation carries significant risks of death and further ill-health, although outcomes are improving.

Cystic Fibrosis Complications

The abnormal bowel secretions can lead to constipation, and bowel obstruction, which is called distal intestinal obstruction syndrome (DIOS—**Fig. 6.49**), CF can affect the liver and cause focal biliary cirrhosis and rarely cirrhosis and portal hypertension **(Fig. 6.50)**. It can also

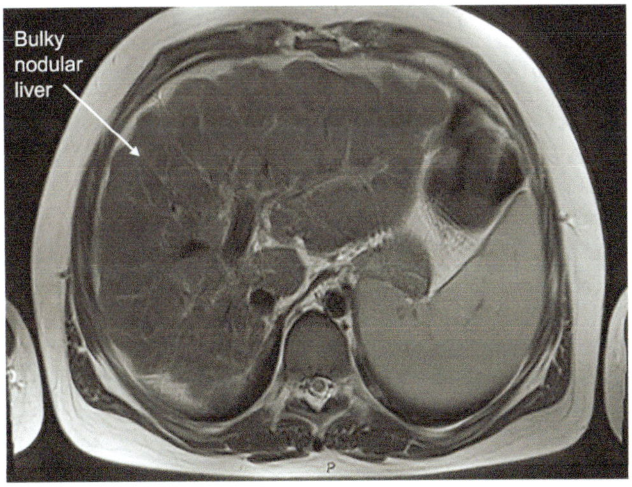

Figure 6.50 MRI of the abdomen showing nodular disease of the liver due to cirrhosis in cystic fibrosis.

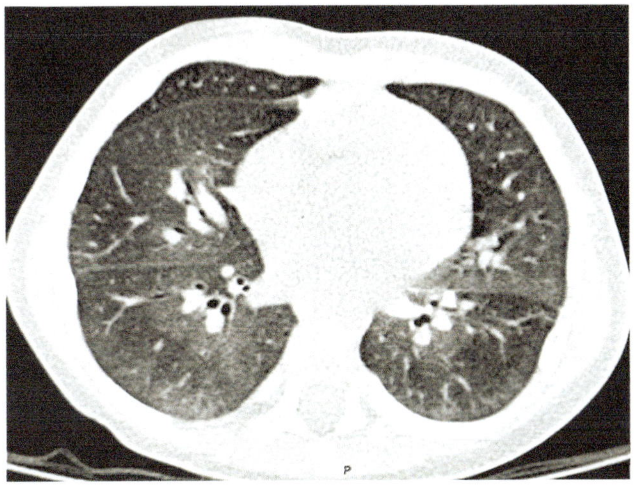

Figure 6.51 High-resolution chest computed tomography (HRCT) slice showing infant with bronchiolitis obliterans. *Note* the areas of mosaic attenuation—that is, a patchwork of areas of different lung attenuation with some areas being more opaque than others.

cause diabetes mellitus due to pancreatic endocrine dysfunction, as there is fibrosis and fatty infiltration of the pancreas.

The Future

There is and has been extensive research into the underlying defect in CF, this has led to the development of mutation specific therapies such as "Kalydeco" that has been shown to be beneficial to patients who carry the G551D mutation.[26]

BRONCHIOLITIS OBLITERANS

Bronchiolitis obliterans is a rare chronic obstructive disease caused by a significant insult to the airways. In children, it is usually post infectious; following infections with, e.g. adenovirus but it can also be seen in lung, heart and stem cell transplant patients. The injury to the bronchioles and smaller airways causes inflammation and fibrosis and this in turn causes airway narrowing or complete obliteration.

Clinical symptoms are persistent cough, wheeze and breathlessness following a viral like illness. There is often wheeze and crackles on auscultation with an increased respiratory rate and oxygen requirement. Bronchiectasis and chronic respiratory failure can occur.

The chest radiograph findings vary from normal to areas of hyperlucency, hyperinflation, to bronchial wall thickening consolidation and bronchiectasis. The changes may be bilateral or unilateral. The diagnosis of bronchiolitis obliterans relies on high-resolution chest CT scan where areas of hyperaeration, mosaic ground glass appearance and bronchial wall thickening are seen **(Fig. 6.51)**. Lung function tests show fixed obstruction.[27] The treatment of bronchiolitis obliterans in children is difficult and often supportive.

Post-transplant Lymphoproliferative Disorder

This is a rare complication of solid organ and bone marrow transplants. It is a neoplastic abnormal proliferation of usually B cells associated with Epstein Barr Virus (EBV) infection. This is either due to reactivation or primary post-transplant infection. The main risk factor is when a positive EBV or cytomegalovirus (CMV) donor is used with an EBV or CMV negative recipient.[28] The disease severity varies depending on the kind of neoplastic process the B cells undergo and whether more than one site is affected.

Presentation in the lungs is rare. It can present with recurrent respiratory infections and persistently abnormal CXRs as seen in **Figures 6.52A and B**. These images are from a 10-year-old renal transplant patient who presented with a productive cough and fever that initially responded to intravenous antibiotics. His symptoms recurred and his CXR showed some improvement; however, there were persistent right-sided abnormalities with nodular change. This was confirmed on his chest CT scan. His bronchoscopy showed normal anatomy but his bronchoalveolar lavage fluid grew *Stenotrophomonas maltophilia* and he had significantly elevated EBV titres. His lung biopsy confirmed post-transplant lymphoproliferative disorder (PTLD). Treatment methods include reduction of immunosuppression, rituximab, a chimeric monoclonal antibody against the protein CD20, which is primarily found on the surface of B cells,[29] low-dose cyclophosphamide and steroids.

Plastic Bronchitis

This is a rare condition where casts **(Figs. 6.52A and B)** develop in the trachea and bronchi and cause life-threatening airways obstruction with consolidation and or collapse of

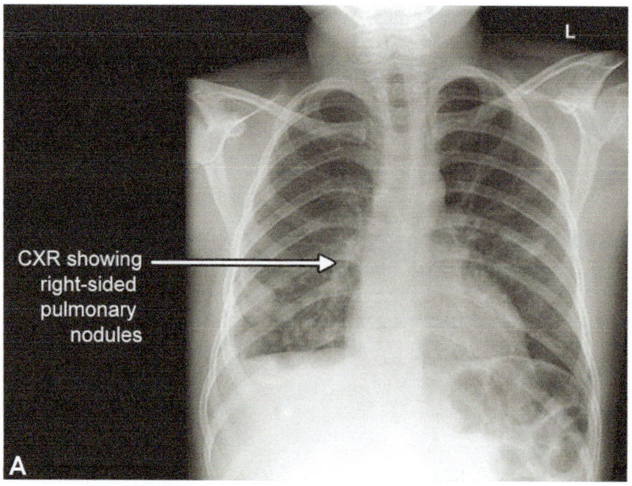

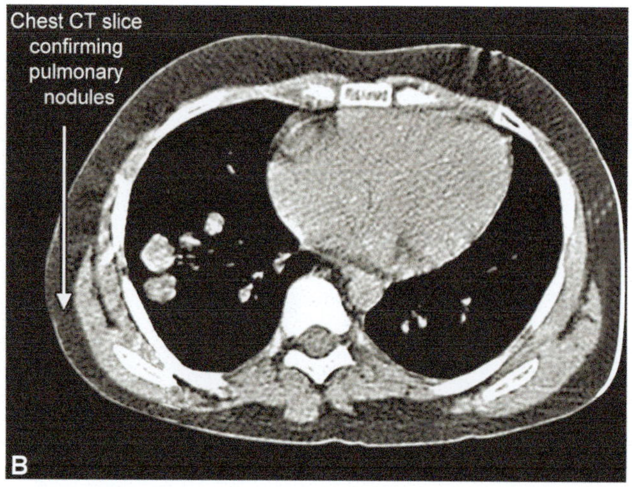

Figures 6.52A and B Chest X-ray and computed tomography (CT) slice from showing right-sided pulmonary nodules due to post-transplant lymphoproliferative disorder (PTLD) in a post-renal transplant patient.

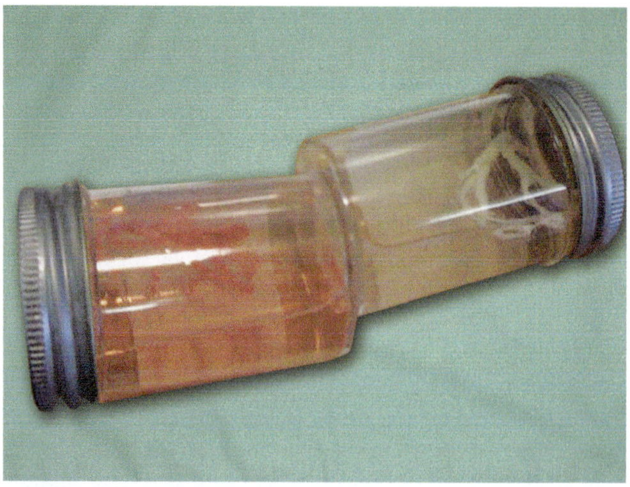

Figure 6.53 Bronchial casts expectorated by a patient with plastic bronchitis.

affected lung segments or indeed the whole lung. In children, it has been reported following surgery, e.g. Fontan procedure, but also has appeared secondary to asthma and infections such as viral pneumonia.[30] There are two types of casts seen type 1 are inflammatory and type 2 hypocellular that are composed of mucin—these tend to be the kind seen in association with severe congenital heart disease. The aims of treatment are to first of all remove the casts using a combination of rigid and flexible bronchoscopy. Instillation of tissue plasminogen activator or dornase alfa can also be done at this time. Then, to try to prevent cast formation using chest physiotherapy, mucolytics and azithromycin. This can prove difficult and the patient whose casts are in the image shown had recurrent episodes of this condition, which meant frequent bronchoscopic procedures for cast removal.

SLEEP-DISORDERED BREATHING IN CHILDREN

When asleep the normal child's breathing control changes. There is reduced muscle tone in the intercostal muscles and the pharyngeal dilator muscles. This increases upper airways resistance. There is also a reduction in minute volume, in functional residual capacity and in respiratory rate. In rapid-eye-movement (REM), sleep respiratory drive is reduced.[31] Not only are there specific sleep related breathing disorders but most forms of chronic lung disease worsen when asleep. Sleep disordered breathing is usually divided into two main groups dependent on the pattern of apnoea seen but there is overlap between both. Obstructive sleep apnoea (OSA) is where there is obstruction to air flow from whatever cause and central sleep apnoea where there is a respiratory drive problem. Clinical history and examination as well as polysomnography are used to determine whether there are obstructive **(Fig. 6.53)** or central apnoeas or whether there is a mixture of both.

Obstructive Sleep Apnoea

This affects approximately 0.7–3% of children, the majority being under 5 years. It is thought to result from a combination of problems with respiratory drive, neuromuscular control and anatomical factors. Children with OSA can often breathe satisfactorily when awake but not when asleep. Occasionally, if the problem is severe, the child's breathing can sound obstructed even when awake. Parents usually report that the child has loud snoring and pauses in breathing with gasping breaths. Children with OSA are often restless during sleep, as they can partially waken during periods of airways obstruction. However, they have also been shown to have an increased tolerance to hypercapnia. Severe OSA in a young child can cause failure to thrive. Untreated OSA in children is also related to reduce intellectual function. It can also cause pulmonary hypertension and cor pulmonale although this is rarely seen due to early recognition and treatment. OSA in young children is often associated with adenotonsillar hypertrophy and often responds to adenotonsillectomy.

Upper airway congenital abnormalities, e.g. cranial and facial abnormalities can also cause OSA. These will be covered in the Chapter 26: Paediatric otolaryngology. Unlike younger children, older children with OSA can be morbidly obese. Conditions that cause hypotonia, e.g. cerebral palsy can also lead to airways collapse and obstruction during sleep.

If there are persisting obstructive symptoms, then treatment involves respiratory support at night with non-invasive ventilation using either a nasal or face mask and a ventilator providing bilateral positive airway pressure (BIPAP) **(Figs. 6.54 to 6.56)**. This method supports

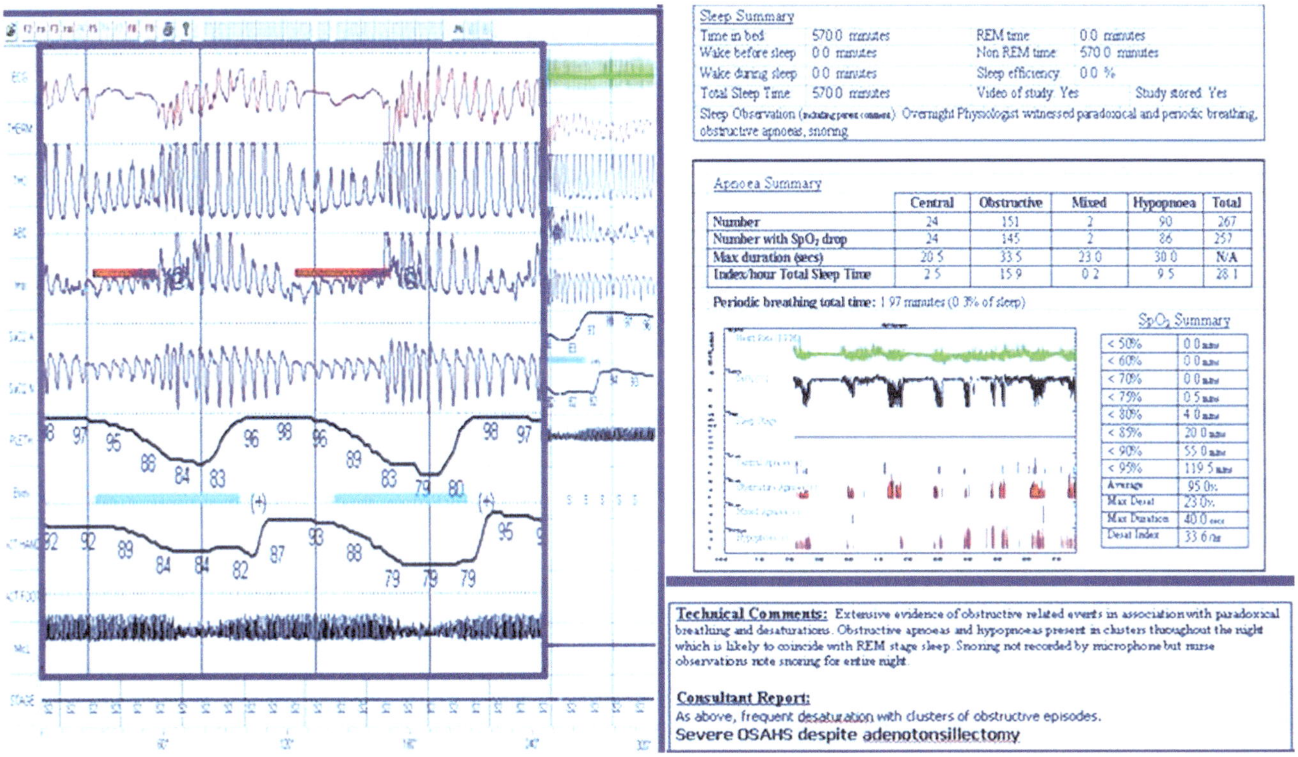

Figure 6.54 Polysomnography report showing obstructive sleep apnoea changes.
(*Image courtesy*: Mr Andrew Morley, Chief Respiratory Physiologist, Royal Hospital for Sick Children, Glasgow)

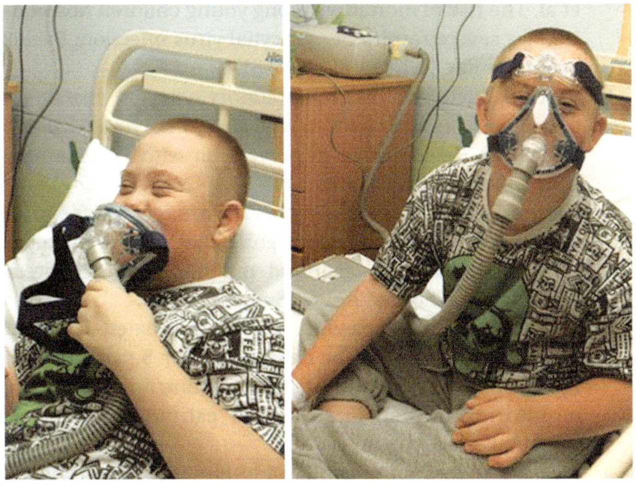

Figure 6.55 Thirteen-year-old boy with Down syndrome and obstructive sleep apnoea. He requires non-invasive ventilation at night with a "variable or bilevel positive airway pressure (VPAP)" machine.

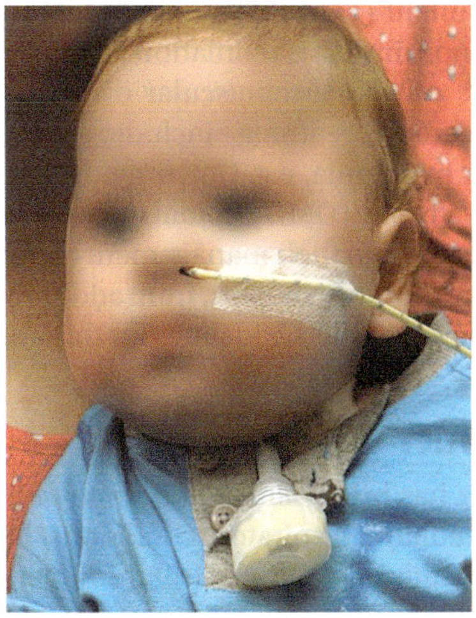

Figure 6.56 Infant with tracheostomy tube and nasogastric tube.

CHAPTER 7

Gastroenterology and Hepatology

Krishna M. Goel, Robert Carachi

GASTROINTESTINAL AND LIVER DISEASE

Introduction

The alimentary tract is a complicated viscous extending from the mouth to the anus with structural differentiation and adaptation according to the specific function needed. The oesophagus is a passage from the pharynx to the stomach, where digestion begins. Food then moves into the small intestine, where further digestion and absorption occur. The large intestine reabsorbs 95% of water and completes absorption of digested products leaving the residue to be expelled intermittently from the rectum.

The most common signs of alimentary tract disorders are vomiting, abdominal distension and disorders of defaecation. In the older infant and child, abdominal pain becomes the most common symptom indicating dysfunction of the gut and requires investigation of its cause. An adequate history from the parents and child is most helpful in arriving at the correct diagnosis, and this may be followed by examination and investigations. Many of the causes of abdominal pain are discussed later in the differential diagnosis of acute appendicitis. Most newborn babies vomit a few times in the first week of life. A small quantity of milk is often regurgitated when wind is "broken" during or after feeding. Persistent vomiting in newborn babies and vomiting in the older child are usually a significant sign and may be associated with a wide variety of pathological conditions. Infections of the alimentary tract such as gastroenteritis result in the infant or child presenting with vomiting, which is also a common non-specific sign in other infections, e.g. meningitis, urinary tract infection or septicaemia. Vomiting is the most consistent sign of intestinal obstruction in the newborn. It usually starts on the first day of life and becomes progressively more frequent. The vomit usually contains bile, as it is rare for the obstruction to be above the ampulla of Vater. Bile-stained vomiting in the absence of an organic cause is rare, and infants and children with bile-stained vomit should be investigated in hospital.

Normal infants should pass meconium within 24 hours of birth. Delay to do so or failure to pass meconium is an important sign, which should not be overlooked. Failure to pass meconium may be due to an organic obstruction but subsequent passage may be a sign of disease such as hypothyroidism or Hirschsprung disease.

The infant normally settles into a pattern of having one, two or more bowel actions daily, but in diarrhoea, increased frequency of passage of stools that become more liquid or constipation is the presenting signs of a variety of disorders. In the early stages of intestinal obstruction, there may be little abdominal distension, and any such distension may be difficult to distinguish from the naturally protuberant abdomen of the newborn. Visible loops of bowel and peristalsis are abnormal in the term or older infant, but in the thin-walled premature infant may not be indicative of obstruction. Surgical paediatric problems are discussed in Chapter 9.

> **KEY LEARNING POINT**
>
> Bile-stained vomiting in the absence of an organic cause is a rare symptom, and infants and children with bile-stained vomit should be investigated in hospital.

Gastro-oesophageal Reflux Disease

Reflux of gastric contents is a physiologic occurrence that takes place more often during infancy and decreases with advancing age. The vast majority of infants with gastro-oesophageal reflux (GOR) who are symptomatic of vomiting during the first year of life resolve their overt symptoms between the ages of 12 months and 18 months. Because most infants with symptoms of GOR are thriving and healthy, they require no diagnostic or therapeutic measures other than a careful history and physical examination, with appropriate reassurance to the parents if they are worried. An increase in the frequency and a decrease in the volume of feeds may reduce symptoms. Also a feed thickener or pre-thickened formula feed can be used. If necessary, a suitable alginate-containing preparation can be used instead of thickened feeds. However, infants and older children who have significant neurological deficits or psychomotor retardation often have significant GOR and may suffer from serious sequelae secondary to GOR. Oesophageal inflammation (oesophagitis), ulceration or stricture formation may develop in early childhood; GOR disease may also be associated with chronic respiratory disorders including asthma. Abnormal posturing with the tilting of the head to one side and bizarre contortions of the trunk has been noted in some children with GOR. These symptoms are often referred to as Sandifer syndrome.

The barium swallow is a sensitive way of detecting reflux but has a very low specificity rate because many infants who have little or no clinical symptoms of GOR experience reflux of some barium into their oesophagus. However, a 24-hour pH probe study can give fairly reproducible information on the amount of reflux that is occurring in an infant. Now pH monitor can be done on children as outpatients with the ambulatory device being read by an automatic system at a later date.

KEY LEARNING POINT

Parents of neonates and infants should be reassured that most symptoms of uncomplicated GOR resolve without treatment.

BOX 7.1 Causes of gastrointestinal bleeding in children.

- Haemorrhagic disease of the newborn
- Swallowed maternal blood (neonate)
- Infectious diarrhoea
- Oesophageal varices
- Mallory–Weiss tear
- Gastric and duodenal ulcers
- Meckel diverticulum
- Intussusception
- Duplication cysts
- Ulcerative colitis
- Crohn disease
- Nonsteroidal anti-inflammatory drugs (NSAIDs)
- Vascular malformations
- Anal fissure
- Haemorrhoids
- Henoch–Schönlein purpura
- Unexplained causes

Gastrointestinal Haemorrhage

The paediatrician who is confronted with a child with gastrointestinal (GI) haemorrhage faces one of the most difficult diagnostic and management problems in clinical practice of paediatrics. In spite of the availability of sophisticated diagnostic tools, many paediatric patients with GI haemorrhage remain undiagnosed. However, differentiating upper GI from lower GI bleeding will guide the sequence of diagnostic tests.

Hematemesis is obviously a marker of upper GI haemorrhage and melena a marker of lower GI bleeding. The term melena signifies the passage of dark stools stained with blood pigments or with altered blood. It is vital that only after exclusion of upper GI bleeding one should consider a colonic lesion in the case of melena. On the other hand, the passage of bloody stools (not dark or maroon) points to a colonic source of blood. Small intestinal bleeding may manifest as either melena or fresh blood. The causes of GI haemorrhage are shown in Box 7.1.

Diagnosis

A history of hematemesis is suggestive of an upper GI bleeding lesion. Therefore, upper GI endoscopy should be carried out and it may lead to the diagnosis. Massive lower GI bleeding in children is uncommon. The presence of leucocytes in the stool suggests an infectious or inflammatory diagnosis. Thus, a stool specimen should be sent for culture and identification of parasites. After anal inspection (digital rectal examination), a flexible sigmoidoscopy is indicated. If this is negative, a colonoscopy should be done to visualise the entire colon and the terminal ileum. If melena (dark stool) is the presenting feature and upper GI endoscopy is negative, colonoscopy should be the next step. However, if the diagnosis remains unclear, a Meckel scan may suggest a bleeding site.

Oesophageal Varices

Bleeding from oesophageal varices (Fig. 7.1) may be sudden and profuse and cause exsanguination of the patient. Rapid and adequate transfusion is necessary. Emergency endoscopy should be undertaken in an attempt to establish this diagnosis and injection of varices with sclerosing agents (sclerosants) may be commenced. If this is impossible, then control of the bleeding may be achieved by giving intravenous infusions of vasopressin or somatostatin. Tamponading of the oesophageal and gastric varices may be possible with the Sengstaken tube. Someone experienced in proper positioning of the balloons should do insertion of this tube, and it should be done under imaging control. The oesophageal balloon is blown up to a pressure of 40 mmHg. This pressure will have to be released intermittently to prevent pressure necrosis. This measure should only be undertaken in an attempt to resuscitate

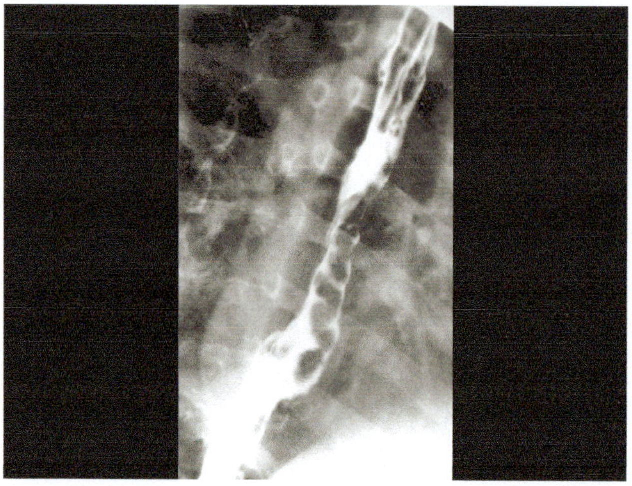

Figure 7.1 Barium swallow demonstrating oesophageal and gastric varices.

the patient prior to more definitive treatment, which may include surgical transection of the oesophagus or hemitransection of the stomach (Tanner operation). Emergency portacaval or splenorenal shunting is rarely necessary in children. Most patients with portal hypertension and variceal bleeding can be managed by repeated injections of sclerosants into the varices, thus allowing collaterals to develop and improve the drainage from the portal venous system.

Peptic Ulcer

Although rare in infancy and childhood, gastric and duodenal ulcers may occur. Secondary ulcers (Curling ulcers) associated with severe infections or extensive burns have become rare.

Clinical Features

Some of the vague abdominal pains, which are so common in childhood, may be due to undiagnosed peptic ulcer. Indeed, many of these patients may have paid several visits to the hospital and seen several consultants, and eventually referred to the psychiatric department before an underlying peptic ulcer may be diagnosed. While the disease may run a silent course in infancy, in the older child, the clinical picture is similar to that in adult life. There is epigastric pain or discomfort relieved by eating; pain at night is common. Vomiting an hour or two after food may follow pylorospasm or actual scarring of the pylorus. There may be evidence of malnutrition. The disease may present with recurrent or severe haemorrhage or with perforation into the peritoneal cavity, which is very rare. Endoscopy is usually diagnostic although barium meal is less invasive and if indicated may not always reveal a peptic ulcer. During endoscopy, biopsies of the pyloric antrum and the duodenal mucosa are examined to establish the presence of *Helicobacter pylori*.

The typical appearance of nodular gastritis is highly suggestive of *H. pylori* infection, especially in the paediatric population. The urea breath test is the most reliable of the non-invasive tests for *H. pylori* infection.

KEY LEARNING POINTS

Long-term healing of gastric and duodenal ulcers can be achieved rapidly by eradicating *H. pylori*.

Antacids have been used for many years in the treatment of ulcer disease in infants and children. H_2-receptor antagonists have made substantial impact on the clinical practice of treating peptic ulcer disease.

Blood Per Rectum

Passage of blood from the rectum is common in paediatric practice. The diagnosis may be straightforward and the cause obvious, but in many, the cause of bleeding is never found even after a full investigation. Serious underlying causes have to be excluded as outlined in **Box 7.1**.

Most children, seen in the outpatient department with rectal bleeding, pass only small quantities of blood after defaecation. Anal fissure is the most common cause, but it may be due to rectal prolapse and proctitis. Acute anal fissure is the most common cause of rectal bleeding. There is usually a history of constipation and generally pain on defaecation. The bleeding is usually small in amount, bright red, streaked on the outside of the stool and occurs during or just after defaecation. The fissure is usually in the midline posteriorly. Perianal redness and shallow fissures may be the first sign of a granulomatous proctitis sometimes associated with Crohn disease. Most fissures are easily seen, and digital rectal examination without anaesthesia, which may be very painful, is unnecessary and should be avoided.

Moderate or extensive bleeding is infrequent, but the common lesions are rectal polyps, enteritis or enterocolitis, intussusception, Meckel diverticulum, volvulus, duplication of the alimentary tract, haemangiomas in the bowel, systemic haemorrhagic disease and in the neonate, necrotising enterocolitis (NEC) and haemorrhagic disease of the newborn.

Digital rectal examination, proctoscopy, sigmoidoscopy, colonoscopy and barium enema may show up the lesion which can then be treated appropriately. A technetium scan may be necessary to demonstrate a Meckel diverticulum or a duplication of the bowel but a negative scan does not exclude either, as it is dependent on the presence of ectopic gastric mucosa.

KEY LEARNING POINT

Acute anal fissure is the most common cause of rectal bleeding.

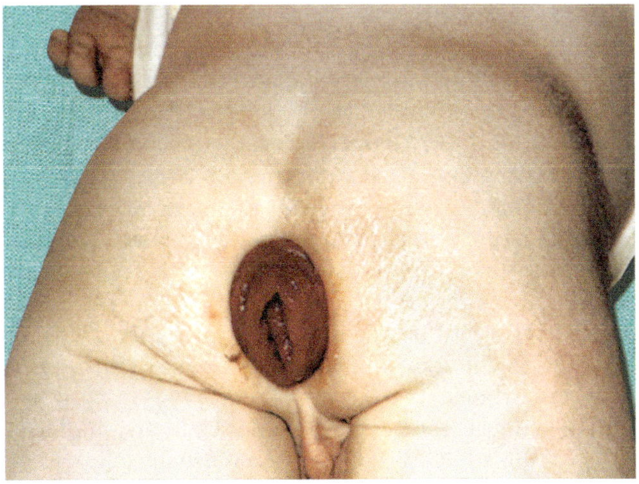

Figure 7.2 Rectal prolapse in a child subsequently confirmed as having cystic fibrosis.

Rectal Prolapse

Rectal prolapse may be partial when the mucous membrane only is prolapsed or complete when there is protrusion of the entire rectal wall **(Fig. 7.2)**. The age group of 1–3 years is the usual age. Mucosal prolapse is more common and occurs in children with chronic constipation and is usually initiated by prolonged straining. Prolapse is sometimes the presenting sign of cystic fibrosis (CF). Complete prolapse occurs in debilitated or malnourished children. It is also seen in children with paralysed pelvic floor muscles as in myelomeningocele.

Parents usually notice the red mucosa coming out of the anus after defaecation. The prolapse has usually reduced before the physician sees the patient. On rectal examination, the anal sphincter is found to be very lax and redundant folds of rectal mucosa often follow the withdrawn finger. The child presenting for the first time with a rectal prolapse should have a sweat test performed to exclude CF.

KEY LEARNING POINT

A child presenting for the first time with a rectal prolapse should have a sweat test to exclude CF.

Intestinal Polyps

A solitary rectal polyp is a common cause of bleeding from the rectum. This low polyp is easily felt on digital rectal examination. The polyp is a granulomatous hamartoma of the mucous membrane, which becomes pedunculated and may protrude at the anus like rectal mucosa prolapse. Polyps high in the rectum and lower colon require sigmoidoscopy under general anaesthesia and may be removed by snaring. Occasionally, juvenile polyps are multiple and may be demonstrated by double contrast studies. True familial polyposis is very rare under the age of 12 years, but the rectum and colon can be carpeted with polyps, which histologically are papillomas or adenomas of the adult type. This disease is usually carried as a Mendelian dominant and cancer of the colon develops in young adult life. Peutz-Jeghers syndrome is a familial condition in which polyps of the small intestine are accompanied by brown pigmentation of the lips and buccal mucosa. Symptoms and signs include repeated episodes of abdominal pain due to transient intussusceptions, blood loss from the intestinal tract and anaemia.

Infantile Colic

Infantile colic is defined as excessive crying in an otherwise healthy infant. The crying usually starts in the first few weeks of life and ends by 4–5 months. The cause is unclear. It may represent part of the normal pattern of infantile crying. Other possible explanations are painful intestinal contractions, lactose intolerance, gas or parental misinterpretation of normal crying. Infantile colic improves with time.

Recurrent Abdominal Pain in Children

Recurring and unexplained abdominal pain often presents a difficult problem to the family physician and to both the paediatric physician and surgeon. Most of these patients do not have underlying disease; however, they often require evaluation and treatment to allay fears and improve their quality of life. The pain may amount to little more than discomfort. It may be accompanied by nausea and vomiting. Physical examination should be complete and not only directed towards the abdomen. It is unusual to find any definite signs on abdominal examination and it may be difficult to assess the severity of the pain. Questions, which should be asked, of the pain are as follows:

- What is the duration of each attack?
- Is the child ever been sent home from school due to the pain?
- Does it interfere with games or does it become worse when there are household chores to be done or errands collected?
- Does the pain ever wake up the child from sleep?

Constipation should always be eliminated in these cases and the presence of dysuria, increased frequency of micturition, pyuria or haematuria call for urological investigation. Plain X-rays of abdomen may be useful to reveal a faecalith in an appendix, calcification in mesenteric glands, or calculus formation in the renal tract. Barium meal or barium enema examination may reveal such lesions such as polyps, peptic ulceration or malrotation, which can be a cause of chronic abdominal pain. In the female, recurrent abdominal pain may precede by many months the onset of the first menstrual period (menarche). When organic disease has been reasonably excluded, the proportion of patients who are found to be suffering from emotional disorders is related to the degree of skill and experience in the diagnosis. The term abdominal migraine covers a group of patients who suffer from recurrent attacks of acute, midline abdominal pain, vomiting and headache, photophobia during episodes, family history of migraine with intervening symptom-free intervals lasting weeks to months.

Appendicitis

Acute appendicitis is the most common lesion requiring intra-abdominal surgery in childhood. The disease runs a more rapid course in children and the criteria for establishing a diagnosis and for treatment are different. Under the age of four, the diagnosis is difficult, and in 90% of the children, the infection has spread transmurally to the peritoneal cavity or the appendix has ruptured.

Pathology

There is marked variation in the anatomy of the appendix. The appendix is attached to the posterior medial quadrant of the caecum. In childhood, the appendix lies in a retrocaecal position in 70% of patients. Obstructive appendicitis is common in childhood, the obstruction being caused by a kink, a faecalith or the scar of a previous attack of inflammation. When inflammation occurs, there is an accumulation of purulent exudate within the lumen and a closed loop obstruction is established. Blood supply to the organ is diminished by distension or by thrombosis of the vessels and gangrene occurs early in children. Fluid is poured into the peritoneal cavity as a result of irritation, and within a few hours this fluid is invaded by bacteria from the perforated appendix or from organisms translocating the inflamed but still intact appendix. Peritoneal infection may remain localised by adhesions between loops of intestine, caecal wall and parietal peritoneum. There is danger in administering a purgative in these children because it increases intestinal and appendicular peristalsis and perforation and dissemination of infection are more likely to occur.

Appendicitis may present as:

- Uncomplicated acute appendicitis
- Appendicitis with local peritonitis
- An appendix abscess or diffuse peritonitis.

The onset of symptoms is vague and initially may be of a general nature. Only one-third of younger patients are seen in hospital within 24 hours of onset of abdominal symptoms, and the appendix has ruptured in a high percentage of these young patients before admission. The diagnosis is made late in many cases. One reason for delay in diagnosis is failure to suspect appendicitis in a child less than 4 years of age and the other is the poor localisation of pain by the younger child. Although often not severe, the pain appears to come intermittently and irritability, vomiting and diarrhoea may result in the mistaken diagnosis of gastroenteritis. Psoas spasm from irritation of the muscle by the inflamed appendix may cause flexion of the hip resulting in a limp, thus distracting attention from the abdomen and directing it to the hip joint. Vomiting occurs in most patients. The child is usually pyrexial, but the temperature is only moderately elevated to between 37°C and 38.5°C. Temperatures higher than this usually suggest upper respiratory tract infections or occasionally diffuse peritonitis from appendicitis. A history of constipation is uncommon and in many patients there is a history of diarrhoea.

The clinical features in the older child are similar to those in the adult. Abdominal pain is usually followed by nausea and vomiting. The pain begins centrally and later shifts to the right iliac fossa. If the appendix is retrocaecal, abdominal pain and tenderness may be slight. If the child has a pelvic appendix then tenderness may again be slight or absent, or elicited only on rectal examination. Anorexia is a common accompanying sign.

Clinical Examination

The child with acute appendicitis is usually anorexic, listless and does not wish to be disturbed. There is often a characteristic fetid odour from the tongue, which is furred.

The child is usually irritable, crying and uncooperative. Low-grade pyrexia is usual but the temperature seldom exceeds 38.5°C. Inspection alone may be very informative while attempting to gain the child's confidence. The most important physical sign on abdominal examination is the area of maximum tenderness located in the right iliac fossa and the presence of rebound tenderness. If this is not defined, then a gentle digital rectal examination should be made and tenderness may be elicited or a mass felt in the pelvis in patients with a pelvic appendix.

Urine should be checked for presence of bacteria or white cells and also to exclude glycosuria or significant proteinuria. Leucocytosis is usually present in children with acute appendicitis but a normal white cell count does not exclude the diagnosis. The child with diffuse peritonitis may have a low white cell count. Plain X-ray of the abdomen often gives useful signs of acute appendicitis **(Fig. 7.3)**.

The sensitivity and specificity of ultrasound examination for appendicitis can be quite variable. The examination must be the part of the whole clinical picture in deciding upon operative intervention. Also a negative ultrasound examination does not exclude appendicitis. Use of computed tomography (CT) scan of abdomen in the evaluation of difficult cases of abdominal pain has been reported. The CT findings suggestive of appendicitis include appendiceal wall thickening, presence of inflammatory changes in the periappendiceal fat or the presence of an abscess.

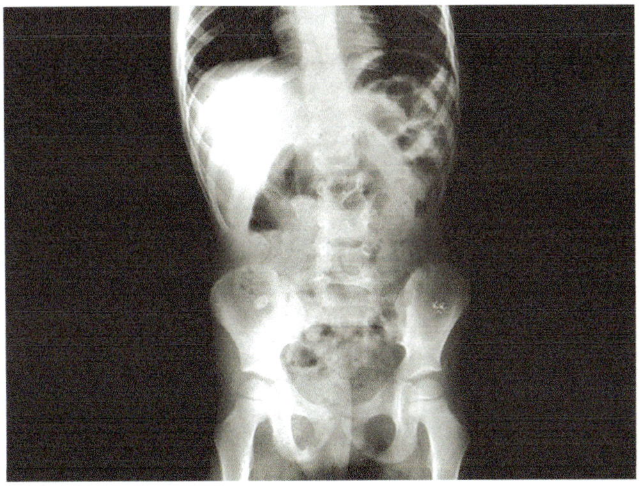

Figure 7.3 X-ray of abdomen showing faecalith, scoliosis with psoas spasm, dilated loops of bowel with fluid level and loss of fat line.

Differential Diagnosis

The differential diagnosis includes numerous other disorders the most common of which is upper respiratory tract infection. Presence of a common cold, sinusitis, acute tonsillitis or pharyngitis may all be associated with acute non-specific mesenteric lymphadenitis. This is the most common condition to be differentiated from acute appendicitis. The presence of enlarged glands elsewhere in the body accompanied with an upper respiratory tract infection may suggest this condition. Fever may be absent but temperature can be very high. The presence of abdominal tenderness is not as acute as that in appendicitis. It is usually more generalised and not localised to the right iliac fossa and there is no rebound tenderness. The presence of a cough increased respiratory rate and runny nose may suggest a respiratory infection. Examination of the chest is mandatory to pick-up any signs of consolidation as right lower lobe pneumonia may result in referred pain occurring in the right lower quadrant of the abdomen. Constipation can cause abdominal pain, nausea and vomiting, with tenderness over the distended caecum. It can be easily mistaken for acute appendicitis. Faecal masses may be felt per abdomen or on digital rectal examination. Usually following a suppository, satisfactory evacuation of the colon and rectum will bring rapid relief in patients whose symptoms are caused by constipation.

Urinary tract infection can usually be differentiated by a higher temperature, pus cells in the urine and tenderness over one or other kidney in the renal angle.

Abdominal trauma, accidental or non-accidental may cause injury to the abdominal viscera. A plain X-ray of the abdomen and a serum amylase should be done to exclude the presence of traumatic or idiopathic pancreatitis and a pneumoperitoneum.

In gastroenteritis and dysentery, there may be severe cramping and abdominal pain. The pain and tenderness may be more marked over the distended caecum. Other members of the family may have similar symptoms or diarrhoea. Rectal examination can help differentiate between a pelvic appendicitis and appendicitis with pelvic peritonitis from gastroenteritis.

Infective hepatitis may occur in epidemic form, but in an isolated case may simulate appendicitis. The temperature is usually elevated and the child complains of a headache with nausea, vomiting, abdominal pain and tenderness. On examination, the liver is enlarged and tender. The child may or may not be jaundiced depending on whether he is seen in the prodromal phase of the disease. Examination of the urine usually reveals the presence of bile salts, but urobilinogen may be present.

Intestinal obstruction may be due to incarceration of a hernia, secondary to anomalies, e.g. a volvulus around a vitellointestinal remnant, or adhesions following previous abdominal operations. Vomiting, abdominal colic, abdominal distension and constipation are the usual signs. After a thorough clinical examination, plain X-ray of the abdomen in the erect and supine positions should be carried out to differentiate intestinal obstruction from appendicitis.

Primary peritonitis is an uncommon diagnosis and almost always affects the female. There is a diffuse infection of the visceral and parietal peritoneum usually due to a pneumococcus. With the peritonitis there is exudation of fluid to the peritoneal cavity. Mesenteric lymph nodes are swollen. Diffuse abdominal pain, vomiting, dehydration and a high fever are the main features and diarrhoea may be present initially, but is usually followed by constipation. Rectal examination usually is suggestive of a pelvic appendicitis as there is diffuse tenderness and heat present. The white blood cell count is usually grossly elevated from 20,000 per cu mm to 50,000 per cu mm. The diagnosis is usually made at laparotomy when peritonitis is found but the appendix is normal.

Severe abdominal pain and vomiting may occur during the passage of a renal calculus. Hydronephrosis due to blockage of the pelviureteric junction by stricture, stone or aberrant vessel may present with abdominal pain and nausea. The pain and tenderness are maximal in the flank. Red or white blood cells may be found in the urine.

Haemolytic uraemic syndrome may present with acute abdominal pain and may be confused with acute appendicitis. The presence of fragmented red blood cells on a blood film and also the presence of oliguria are suggestive of this disease.

Crohn disease is an uncommon diagnosis in childhood but the incidence is increasing in Western countries. It can present with all the symptoms of acute appendicitis and at operation the terminal ileum is found to be acutely inflamed and thickened. A biopsy reveals the diagnosis and barium meal and follow-through very often indicates the presence of other areas of the affected gut.

In torsion of the right cord or testis, confusion with acute appendicitis may occur whereas this is less likely with torsion of the left testis. Routine examination should always include the inguinal regions and the scrotum.

Inflammation of Meckel diverticulum and intussusception in older children may simulate acute appendicitis. Other medical conditions, which should be considered, are those of diabetes mellitus, cyclical vomiting and Addison disease. The onset of menstruation may simulate appendicitis and many girls have recurring attacks of lower abdominal pain, sometimes for a year before menstruation actually begins. Pain associated with torsion of an ovary or an ovarian cyst may also present with signs similar to those of acute appendicitis.

It is not uncommon for children to harbour threadworms (pinworms) without noticeable symptoms. Many symptoms and signs have been ascribed to the presence of threadworms including weight loss, poor appetite, nausea, vomiting and chronic abdominal pain.

Carcinoid tumour in the appendix is rare in childhood, but the tumour may obstruct the lumen of the appendix and lead to obstructive appendicitis. It is far more common to find this as an incidental finding on histopathology of the removed appendix. When it is present in the tip of the appendix, no further follow-up is necessary in these cases. In older children, if a carcinoid exists in the caecal region there is a chance of invasive disease with subsequent evidence of the carcinoid syndrome.

Foreign Bodies

Children frequently place objects in their mouth and occasionally accidentally swallow them. Most pass down the alimentary tract and out of the anus in 24–48 hours, but occasionally the coin, pin or toy may stick in the oesophagus. This causes discomfort and inability to swallow freely. The offending foreign body may be removed by passing a catheter beyond the foreign body, inflating a balloon on the distal end of the catheter, prior to withdrawing the catheter and the object proximal to it. If this fails, removal under direct vision through an endoscope under anaesthesia is the preferred method.

Most foreign bodies, which reach the stomach ultimately, pass spontaneously. Two exceptions to the "wait and see" approach are the hairball and batteries. The formation of a hairball (trichobezoar) may be followed by poor health and vague abdominal pain as the gastric lumen becomes partially occluded by a dense mass. The history of hair eating (trichotillomania) is rarely given spontaneously by the child or the parents. A mass may be palpated in the epigastrium. Diagnosis is confirmed by endoscopy or X-ray after a barium swallow. The hairball may be passed spontaneously but gastrostomy may be required. Children swallow small alkaline batteries and the gastric juice may interact with them and if left may cause severe ulceration. These should not be allowed to remain in the stomach for more than 48 hours and may be removed endoscopically or by gastrotomy under anaesthesia. All other swallowed foreign bodies pass uneventfully through the GI tract once they have reached the stomach.

KEY LEARNING POINTS

Ingested foreign bodies: "Wait and See."

Most ingested foreign bodies, which reach the stomach ultimately, pass uneventfully through the GI tract.

Necrotising Enterocolitis

Necrotising enterocolitis (NEC) is a severe disease of the GI tract. Prematurity or low birth weight is the most commonly associated factor and occurs in 90% of the babies with this disease. Term infants are affected to a lesser extent and constitute about 10% of the affected group. Hypovolaemia and hypoxia result in damage within the mucosa cells initiating the NEC. It is often multifactorial in origin, resulting in loss of integrity of the gut mucosal barrier with passage of bacteria into the wall of the bowel.

Prematurity, respiratory distress syndrome (RDS), congenital cardiac malformations, umbilical vessel catheterisation, exchange transfusions, hypoglycaemia, polycythaemia, postoperative stress and hyperosmolar feeds have all been implicated in the aetiology. Bacterial infection has been implicated in NEC and from time to time one sees some confirmation of this due to the clustering of the disease in neonatal units. There are protective antibodies in breast milk, which decreases but does not completely protect babies at risk from NEC.

The incidence of this disease varies from country to country. There is a very low incidence in Japan and a high incidence in the United States. The severity of the disease is variable from a minor form seen in many cases, which are managed entirely in the neonatal units, to a fulminating type of the disease with perforation, peritonitis and death.

Initially, one sees a preterm infant with signs of sepsis, vomiting of feeds, abdominal distension and frequently the passage of blood or mucus in the stools. Clostridial infections have been associated with some outbreaks of NEC. If the disease continues to progress peritonism develops and this is often appreciated first by nursing staff observing abdominal distension.

Examination of the abdomen may show signs of inflammation, redness, oedema of the abdominal wall with localised or generalised tenderness, and if the baby has a patent processus vaginalis, free fluid or even gas or meconium is occasionally seen in the scrotum. If a perforation has occurred then one loses the area of superficial dullness of the liver on percussion of the abdomen. Palpation may reveal crepitus from the intramural gas, which can be palpated among the coils of distended loops of bowel, and this is an important sign of NEC.

A plain X-ray of abdomen **(Figs. 7.4A to C)** may show pneumatosis intestinalis (gas within the bowel wall) and

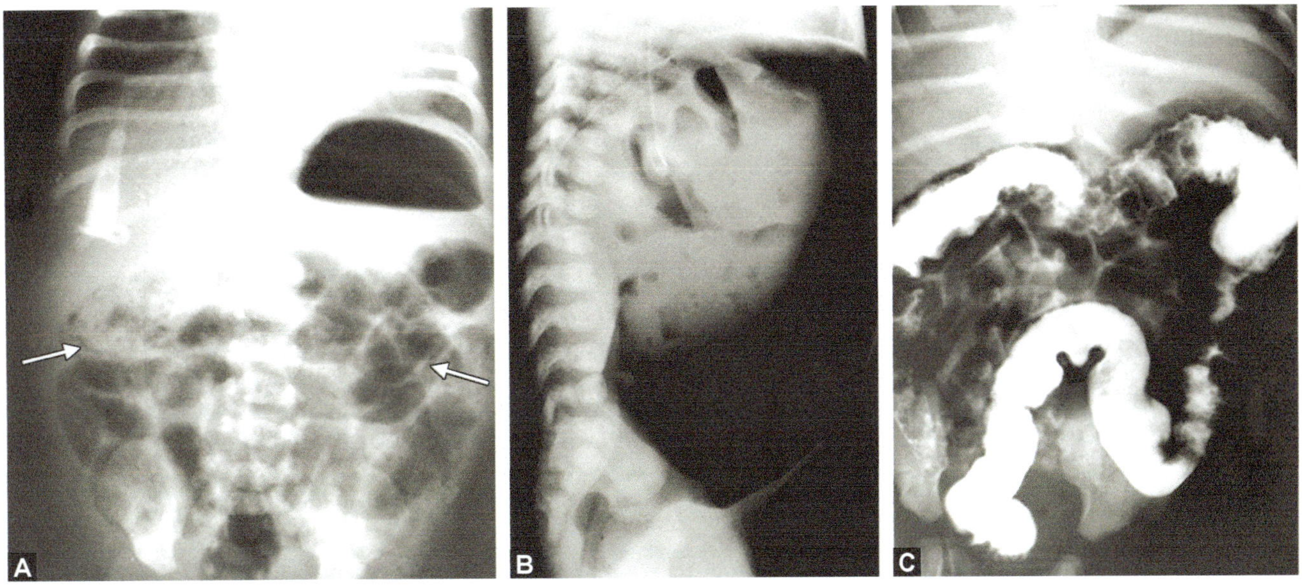

Figures 7.4A to C (A) Abdominal X-ray of premature infant showing pneumatosis (see arrows); (B) The free air in the peritoneal cavity indicates perforation; (C) Barium enema showing extensive pneumatosis coli.

gas in the portal vein and liver. This sign is often an ominous one with a very high mortality. The extent of the NEC may be localised to an area of the bowel, very often the colon, but in extensive disease the whole of the GI tract may be involved.

The differential diagnosis early in this disease may be difficult and one should consider the following diagnoses:

- Septicaemia from other causes
- Volvulus neonatorum
- Hirschsprung enteritis
- Infarction of the bowel

Toddler's Diarrhoea

Toddler's diarrhoea is the most common cause of chronic diarrhoea without failure to thrive in childhood, but its pathogenesis remains unclear. Stool in children with toddler's diarrhoea classically contains undigested food materials due to rapid transit and often is referred to as "peas and carrots" stool.

Diagnosis is based on the history and the clinical criteria; age of onset between 6 months and 36 months, diarrhoea during waking hours and no failure to thrive.

Infectious Diarrhoea in Childhood

This has been discussed later in this chapter.

Fermentative Diarrhoea (Disaccharide Intolerance)

In the healthy child, the disaccharide sucrose is split into the monosaccharides, glucose and fructose by small intestinal sucrase-isomaltase enzyme and the disaccharide lactose into the monosaccharides glucose and galactose by the enzyme lactase. Failure of any of these enzyme systems will result in excess of disaccharide in the intestine where bacteria will ferment the sugars to produce acid and increased osmotic bowel content. This results in fermentative diarrhoea with the passage of highly acid watery stools. Symptoms are relieved when the offending disaccharide is removed from the diet. Lactase deficiency inherited as an autosomal recessive disorder causes persistent diarrhoea from birth because both human and cows' milk contains lactose. When there is a delay in the onset of symptoms this suggests a sucrase-isomaltase deficiency, as sucrose and starch are not usually added to the diet in the first week after birth. In addition to the autosomal recessive inheritance of the deficiency, there can be transient disaccharide intolerance acquired secondarily to gastroenteritis or other intestinal mucosal insult. Investigations which help to confirm disaccharide intolerance include the pH of the fresh stool less than 5.5 and the presence of reducing sugars revealed by the Clinitest and by the identification of faecal sugars on thin-layer chromatography. Removal of all disaccharide from the diet and replacement with monosaccharide will result in a resolution of the diarrhoea. Reintroduction of the disaccharide will result in the return of the diarrhoea and there will be a failure of the normal increase in blood glucose of at least 2.8 mmol/L (50 mg per 100 mL) expected in the normal subject. Rarely, a monosaccharide malabsorption syndrome (glucose-galactose malabsorption) can occur. Jejunal biopsy will allow direct measurement of enzyme activity in the jejunal mucosa. The diarrhoea in infants with the hereditary forms of the disorder can be

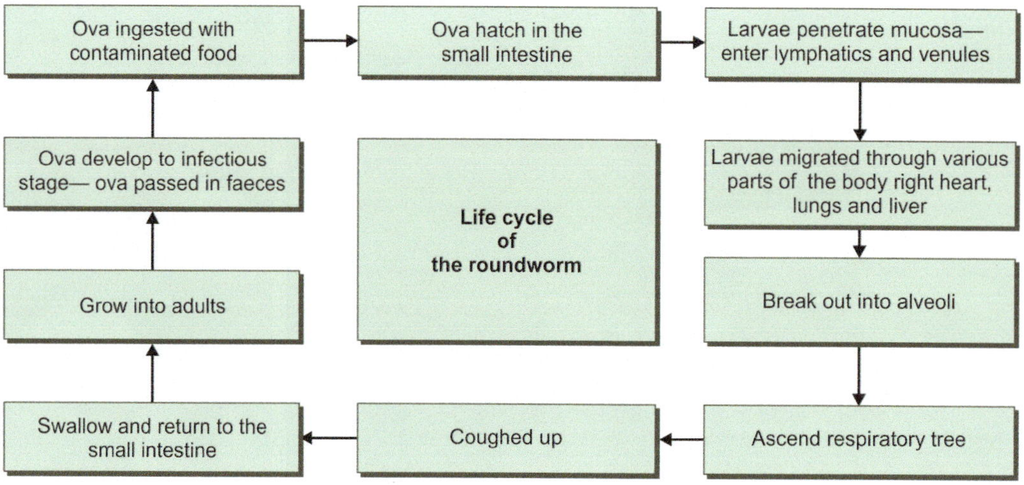

Figure 7.5 Life cycle of the roundworm.

abolished by total exclusion from the diet of the offending carbohydrate.

Systemic Illness

In addition to the acute diarrhoea caused by food poisoning from food toxins or bacterial toxins, viral, bacterial and protozoal bowel infections there are a number of systemic illnesses, which are complicated by acute diarrhoea and vomiting. Septicaemia, meningitis, pneumonia and infectious hepatitis may be accompanied by diarrhoea and vomiting. Abdominal distension with bloody diarrhoea may suggest an acute surgical condition or the haemolytic uraemic syndrome. Hospital admission is indicated if significant dehydration (>5%) is present, when there is doubt about the diagnosis, when hypernatraemia is suspected, when an underlying medical condition such as adrenogenital syndrome or chronic renal insufficiency is present or when outpatient management has failed or is thought to be inappropriate due to adverse social or other circumstances.

Parasitic Intestinal Infection

It is estimated that between 800 million and 1,000 million people in the world are suffering from at least one type of worm infection. The most important intestinal worms are nematodes and cestodes.

Nematodes

These are round, elongated, non-segmented worms with differentiation of the sexes.

Roundworm (*Ascaris lumbricoides*)

Mode of Infection

Infection arises from swallowing ova from soil contaminated with human excreta. The ova are not embryonated when passed in the faeces but they become infective in soil or water. When swallowed by man, the hatched larvae penetrate the intestinal wall and pass via the liver and lungs to the trachea, oesophagus, stomach and intestine where they grow into mature worms (Fig. 7.5).

Clinical Effects

A few roundworms in a well-fed patient usually produce no ill effects and are not noticed until a worm is either vomited or passed in the stool. Typical clinical features include: a protuberant abdomen, intermittent intestinal colic, digestive disturbance, general debility, loss of appetite and insomnia. In heavy infections, worms may migrate into and block the bile duct producing jaundice while similar blocking of the appendix can cause appendicitis. In very heavy infections, intestinal obstruction can occur from a tangled ball of roundworms. The presence and extent of roundworm infection is readily detected by microscopical examination of the stools for ova.

Hookworms (*Ancylostoma duodenale* and *Necator americanus*)

There are two types of hookworms: (1) *Ancylostoma duodenale* being most commonly found in Egypt, Africa, India, Queensland and also in the Southern USA and (2) *Necator americanus*, which is found in the Americas, the Philippines and India. These two species differ in small anatomical details but their life cycles are identical (Fig. 7.6). The male and female worms live chiefly in the jejunum. The worm attaches itself to the intestinal mucosa by its teeth and sucks blood. The ova, passed in the faeces, hatch out in water or damp soil, and larvae penetrate the skin of the buttocks or feet. They reach the heart and lungs by the lymph vessels and bloodstream, penetrate into the bronchi, are coughed up into the trachea and then pass down the oesophagus to mature in the small intestine.

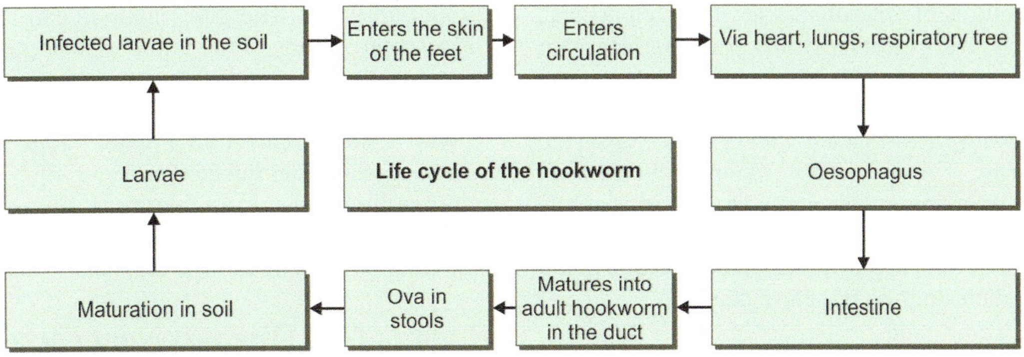

Figure 7.6 Life cycle of the hookworm.

Clinical Effects

The main clinical picture of disease is caused by prolonged loss of blood. Therefore, the clinical manifestations of infection depend on the number of worms present and the nutritional state of the patient. A few hookworms in a fairly well-fed person produce no disease as the small blood loss is constantly being replaced. In children whose diet is inadequate and the worm load heavy, severe anaemia may stunt growth, retard mental development and in very severe cases, result in death through heart failure. Infection is diagnosed by microscopical examination of the stools for eggs, the number of which indicates the severity of infection (72,000 ova/g = significant infection).

Strongyloidiasis (Strongyloides stercoralis)

These worms are fairly widespread in warmer climates and may be found concurrently with hookworm infection. Incidence is often highest in children and the usual mode of infection is penetration of the skin by infective larvae present in the soil. Migration through the lungs also occurs and can produce respiratory signs and there may be abdominal distension, bloody diarrhoea and anaemia. Creeping eruptions, particularly around the buttocks, can develop as a result of the reinfection. Diagnosis is made by identification of larvae in the faeces.

Threadworm (*Enterobius vermicularis, Oxyuriasis, Pinworm or Seatworm*)

The male worm is about 3 mm in length and the female, which looks like a small piece of thread, is about 10 mm. The female lives in the colon. Eggs are deposited on the perianal skin by the female contaminating the fingers of the child who may then reinfect himself/herself. The ova after ingestion hatch in the small intestine. The male worm also fertilises the female in the small intestine, after which the male dies while the female migrates to the caecum. It is common for this infestation to affect all members of a family because the ova can be found on many household objects. The initial infection may also be acquired from contaminated water or uncooked foodstuffs (**Fig. 7.7**).

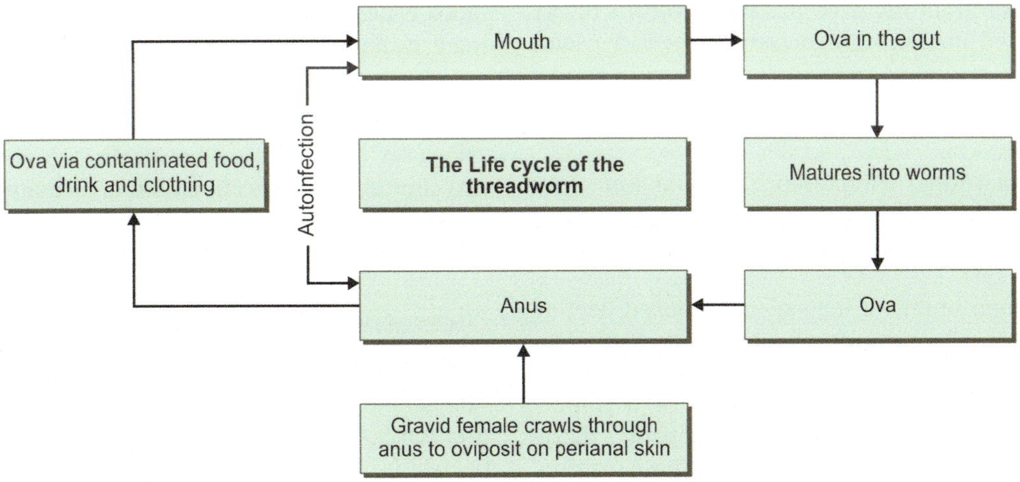

Figure 7.7 Life cycle of threadworm.

Clinical features of enterobiasis are mainly perianal, perineal and vulval pruritus, which can interfere with sleep. Scratching leads to secondarily infected dermatitis and to reinfection through contaminated fingers. Heavy infestations could be associated with episodes of severe abdominal pain. The association of appendicitis with threadworms is exceptionally rare. Diagnosis is made by direct examination of the worms or ova trapped by "sellotape" applied sticky side to the anal skin early in the morning and then stuck on to a glass slide.

Larva Migrans

Cutaneous Variety (Creeping Eruption)

Cutaneous larva migrans is caused by the infective larvae of various dog and cat hookworms. These larvae can penetrate the human skin and finding themselves in an unsuitable habitat wander around in the epidermis for several weeks. Their progress is marked by a characteristic itching and a serpiginous urticarial track. The infection is more common in children than in adults and is occasionally seen in people recently returned from tropical countries.

Visceral Variety

This is caused by various species of the nematode *Toxocara*, usually *Toxocara canis* the common roundworm of the dog. The larvae may penetrate the intestinal wall but are unable to migrate to the lungs of their unnatural host and pass through or become encysted in liver, lungs, kidneys, heart, muscle, brain or eye, causing an intense local tissue reaction. The child may fail to thrive, develop anaemia and become pyrexial with a cough, wheeze and hepatosplenomegaly. There is usually a marked eosinophilia and there can be CNS involvement. In addition to this generalised form of the disorder, there may in the older child (7–9 years old), isolated loss of sight in one eye associated with ocular toxocariasis. The diagnosis can only be established with certainty from a tissue biopsy; generally taken from the liver and the *Toxocara* ELISA (enzyme-linked immunosorbent assay) test is a useful screen.

Cestodes

Cestodes (tapeworms) of importance to humans are *Taenia saginata* (beef tapeworm), *T. solium* (pork tapeworm), *Hymenolepis species* (dwarf tapeworm) and *T. echinococcus* (hydatid cyst).

The ingestion of raw or inadequately cooked beef or pork can result in human infection. Man is the definitive host for both the beef (*T. saginata*) and pork (*T. solium*) tapeworms. Although the infections may be asymptomatic, epigastric discomfort, increased appetite, dizziness and loss of weight sometimes occur. These features may be more marked in children and debilitated persons. Diagnosis is based on the passage of gravid segments through the anus. The differentiation can be made by a microscopical study of the number of lateral branches in the gravid uterus of each segment, the uterus of *T. solium* having about 10 branches and that of *T. saginata* about 20.

With *T. solium* infection a major danger is the ingestion of eggs from an infected person (heteroinfection) or self-ingestion of eggs (autoinfection). This can give rise to cysticercosis where cysticerci develop almost anywhere including brain, skin, muscle and eye.

Hydatid Cyst (*Taenia echinococcus*)

The definitive host of *T. echinococcus* is the dog, wolf, fox or jackal. Man and sheep may become the intermediate host by swallowing the ova from the dog and this is especially likely in sheep-rearing countries. The adult worm in the dog is very small (0.5 cm) but the ingested ovum when swallowed by man liberates a 6-hooked oncosphere into the small intestine. This penetrates to the tissues, usually the liver but sometimes lung, bones, kidneys or brain to form a hydatid cyst. This has a 3-layered wall—an outer layer of host fibrous tissue, a laminated middle layer and an inner germinal layer that produces many daughter and granddaughter cysts.

Clinical Effects

These are largely due to local pressure effects. The liver may be greatly enlarged and there may be a palpable rounded swelling over which the classical "hydatid thrill" can be elicited. Ultrasound and CT scanning can reveal the cystic nature of the lesions. Eosinophilia may be marked. The diagnosis may be confirmed by complement fixation, haemagglutination or latex-slide agglutination tests but the hydatid ELISA test and improved immunoelectrophoresis tests are likely to prove more specific.

Hymenolepis (Dwarf Tapeworm)

Mild infestations due to Hymenolepis (dwarf tapeworm) cause no symptoms, but heavy infestations can sometimes cause diarrhoea, irritability and fits. Diagnosis is made by finding the typical ova in the faeces.

Inflammatory Bowel Disease

The term inflammatory bowel disease (IBD) includes two clinical conditions in children, ulcerative colitis and Crohn disease **(Table 7.1 and Box 7.2)**. On the whole, the prognosis of chronic IBD in childhood is good.

Ulcerative Colitis

Aetiology

The aetiology is unknown. It is fortunately rare in children. Over the past decade, it would appear that there has been little change in the incidence of ulcerative colitis but Crohn disease has increased. The reason for the change is not clear.

TABLE 7.1 Clinical features of ulcerative colitis and Crohn disease.

Clinical features	*Ulcerative colitis*	*Crohn disease*
Location	Rectum and colon (variable)	Ileum and right colon
Diarrhoea	Severe	Moderate
Mucous blood	Frequent	Infrequent
Rectal involvement	Always	Infrequent
Fistula in ano	Absent	Infrequent
Perirectal abscess	Absent	Infrequent
Abdominal wall fistula	Absent	Infrequent
Toxic megacolon	Infrequent	Absent
Arthritis	Rare	Common
Eye pathology	Rare	Iridocyclitis, granuloma
Proctoscopic appearance	Diffuse, ulceration	Cobblestone
Small bowel involvement	Absent	Frequent
Microscopic appearance	Mucosal ulceration	Transmural granulomas

BOX 7.2 Key points to remember in inflammatory bowel diseases.

Ulcerative colitis

- Affects only the colon
- Can be cured by surgery
- Is potentially fatal in a severe attack
- Carries an increased risk of colon cancer in extensive colitis of 8 years duration or more
- Typically has a relapsing course

Crohn disease

- Can affect any part of gastrointestinal tract
- Cannot be cured by surgery
- Is an important cause of growth retardation
- Does not carry the same cancer risk as ulcerative colitis

Severe behavioural problems in some of the affected children and their families have sometimes led physicians to regard the disease as a psychosomatic disorder, but the evidence in support of this hypothesis is extremely slender. Food allergy has been suspected, but only a small group of patients respond to withdrawal of milk. Boys and girls are equally affected. The mean age of onset is about 10 years. There is no clear-cut inheritance pattern but ulcerative colitis is more common in first-degree relatives than in the general population.

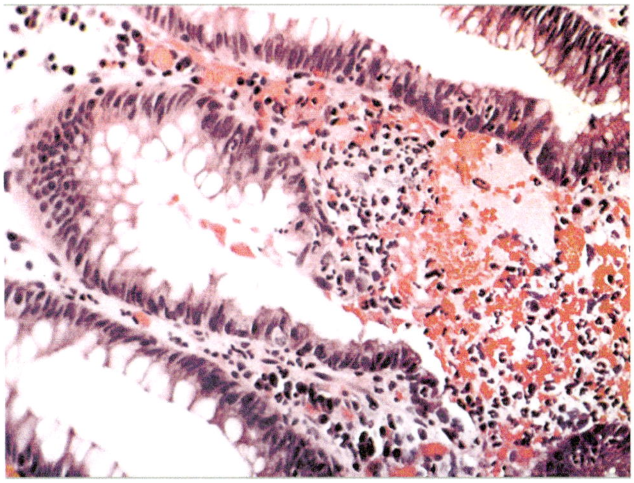

Figure 7.8 Ulcerative colitis. Rectal biopsy with crypt abscesses formation (obj × 25).

Pathology

The mucous membrane of part or all of the colon and sometimes of the terminal ileum becomes hyperaemic, oedematous and ulcerated. The lesion is continuous rather than patchy and usually involves only the mucosal and submucosal layers. The earliest lesion in many cases is a crypt abscess (Fig. 7.8). Granuloma formation is rare. In some cases, oedema may give rise to pseudopolypoid nodules. Ulceration may extend through the muscularis and perforation of the colon can occur. Usually perforation is preceded by toxic megacolon with dilatation of an ulcerated segment of the large bowel. Carcinoma is a common late complication. Hepatic complications such as sclerosing cholangitis and chronic active hepatitis can occur with ulcerative colitis in childhood.

Clinical Features

The onset is sudden with diarrhoea and the frequent passage of small stools containing blood and mucus. This tends to be most severe during the early morning but may also be nocturnal. There may be abdominal pain, anorexia, weight loss or poor weight gain. Tenesmus is common.

Hypochromic anaemia due to chronic blood loss is almost invariably present. Hypoproteinaemic oedema may develop. Associated extraintestinal manifestations of the disease are more common in children than in adults. They may include erythema nodosum, aphthous stomatitis, conjunctivitis, iridocyclitis, haemolytic anaemia, arthralgia or arthritis, pyoderma gangrenosum and finger-clubbing.

After exclusion of infective causes of bloody diarrhoea the diagnosis should be confirmed by rectosigmoidoscopy, mucosal biopsy and barium enema. The last shows loss of normal haustrations in the colon and the so-called "lead-pipe" appearance (Fig. 7.9). Colonoscopy may

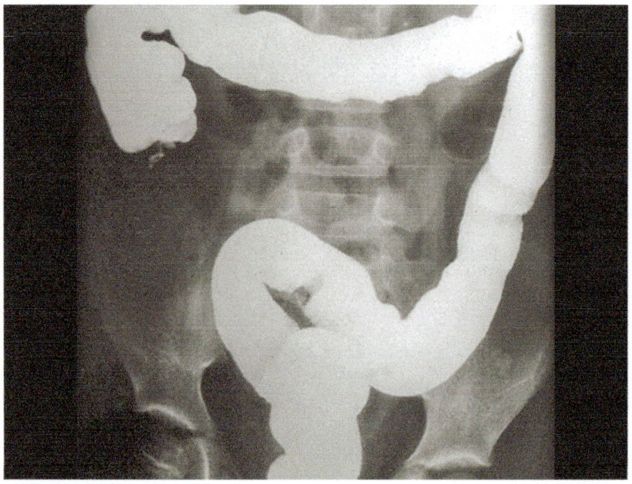

Figure 7.9 Barium enema showing loss of normal haustrations (lead-pipe appearance in the colon) in ulcerative colitis.

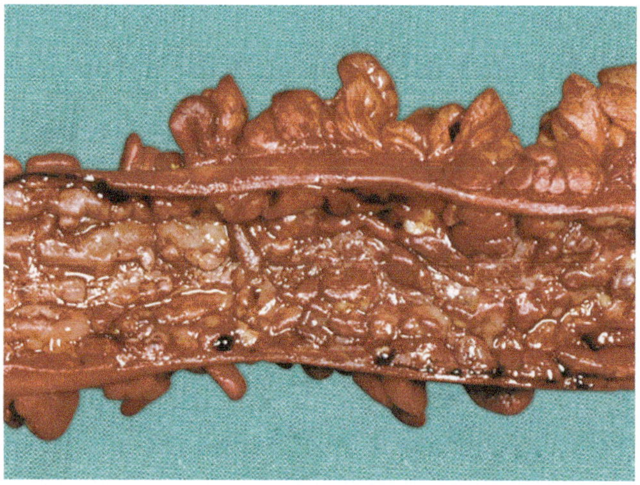

Figure 7.10 Crohn disease. Open loop of ileum showing typical cobblestone appearance of the mucosa.

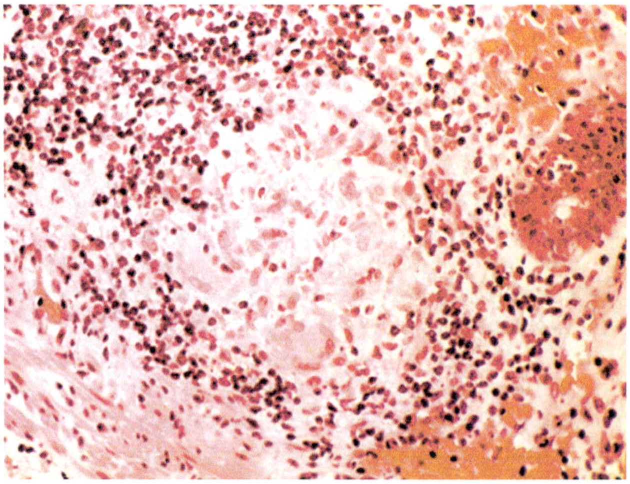

Figure 7.11 Crohn disease showing a diagnostic granuloma in the lamina propria of a colonic biopsy with a central collection of epithelioid and multinucleate cells surrounded by a cuff of lymphocytes and plasma cells (obj × 25).

allow the examination of the whole colonic mucosa and thus the extent of the disease. Radiologically, differentiation of Crohn disease from ulcerative colitis can be made on the basis that Crohn disease can affect any part of the GI tract and is patchy in distribution, whereas ulcerative colitis is a continuous lesion affecting only the rectum, colon and occasionally the terminal ileum (backwash ileitis). It is worth remembering that early in the course of disease no X-ray abnormality may be found.

Ulcerative colitis frequently runs an acute course in the child. The cumulative risk of carcinoma of the colon is 20% per decade after the first decade of the illness. Dysplastic changes in the colonic epithelium are considered to be premalignant.

Crohn Disease

Aetiology

This disorder like ulcerative colitis is not common in children and it is of unknown cause.

Pathology

Crohn disease may affect any part of the GI tract but most commonly the terminal ileum and proximal colon. Although any part of the GI tract from mouth to anus may be affected. The lesions are basically chronic granulomatous and inflammatory with a tendency toward remissions and relapses. The histological changes are transmural, i.e. affecting all layers of the bowel wall with oedema and ulceration of the mucosa, fissures, submucosal fibrosis and many inflammatory foci of mononuclear and giant cells **(Figs. 7.10 and 7.11)**. Perforation, haemorrhage and fistula formation are uncommon complications in childhood.

Clinical Features

In Crohn disease, the diarrhoea is much less severe than in ulcerative colitis; it is often intermittent and there may be little or no obvious blood or mucus in the stools. Crohn disease presents with less specific signs and symptoms than ulcerative colitis hence the delay in diagnosis often found in Crohn disease.

General manifestations commonly include anaemia, loss of weight, growth failure, pubertal delay, erythematous rashes and a low-grade fever. Other associated features are: erythema nodosum, pyoderma, iridocyclitis, arthralgia or arthritis, spondylitis, finger-clubbing, anal skin tags, fissures and fistulae. Quite frequently, the disease presents with oral ulceration and this may progress to extensive involvement of the buccal mucosa, which becomes oedematous and granulomatous sometimes years before there is evidence of intestinal involvement

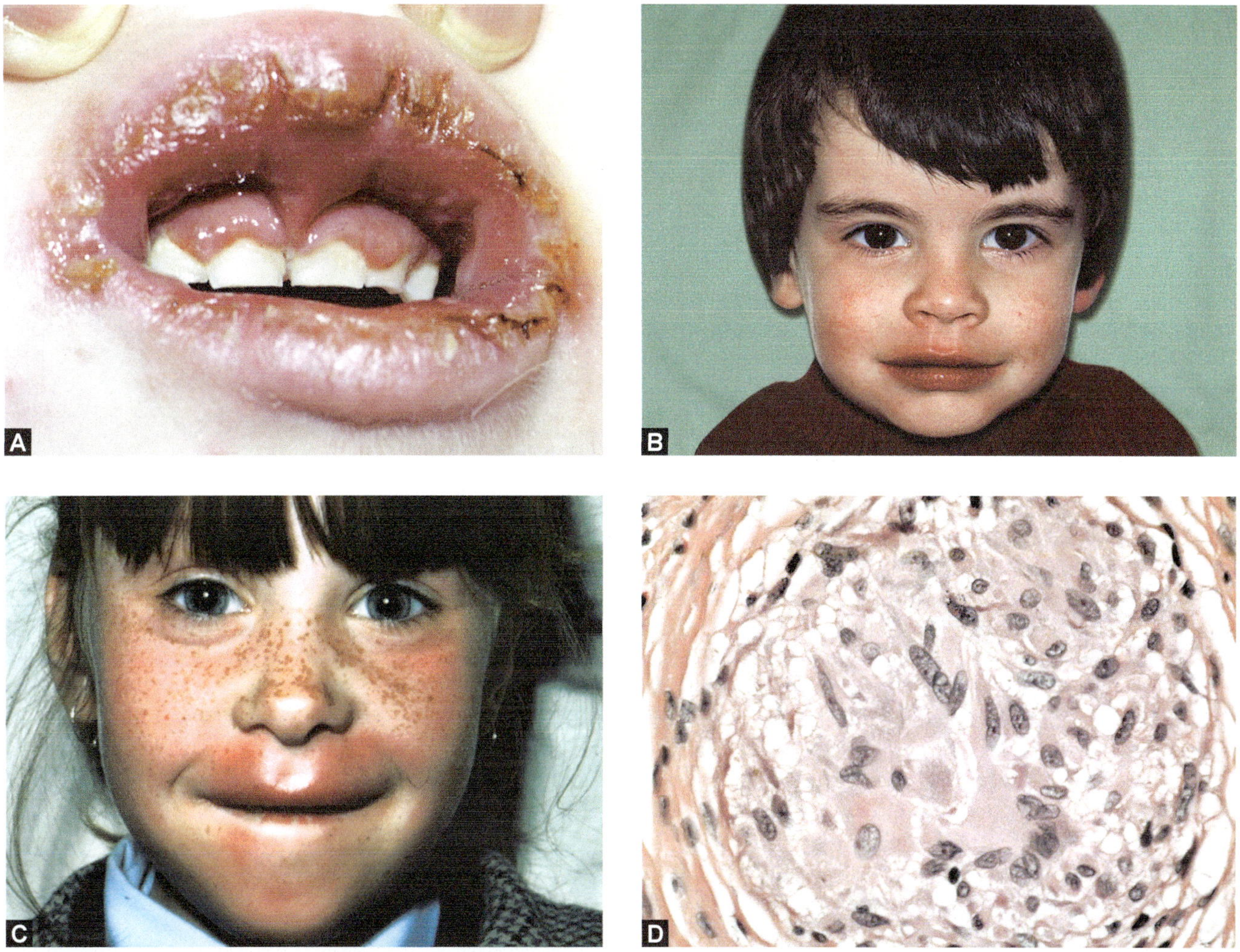

Figures 7.12A to D Oral Crohn disease. (A to C) "aphthoid ulcers," an early feature of Crohn disease. The mucosa is reddish and it may show pinpoint erosions known as "aphthoid ulcers"; (D) Buccal mucosal biopsy showing non-caseating epithelioid cell granuloma with a multinucleate giant cell just below centre (stained with haematoxylin and eosin × 250).

(*Courtesy*: Dr Allan McPhaden).

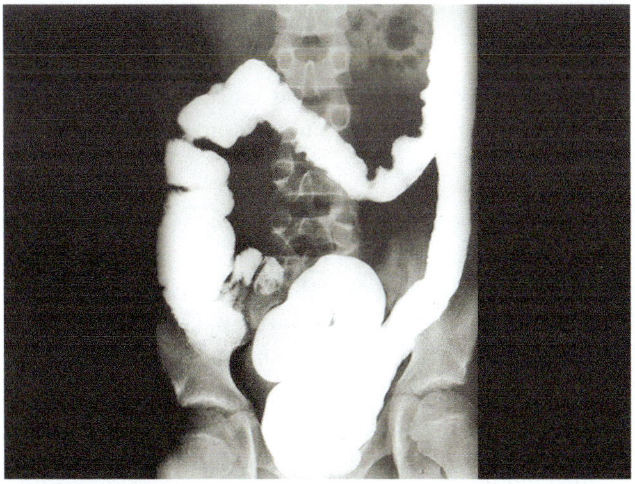

Figure 7.13 Barium meal and follow through illustrating segmental involvement of the same bowel (Crohn disease).

(Figs. 7.12A to D). There is no single gold standard for the diagnosis of Crohn disease. The diagnosis is made by clinical evaluation and a combination of endoscopic, histological, radiological and biochemical investigations. Sigmoidoscopy is only helpful when the left side of the colon is involved. A barium meal or enema typically shows segmental involvement of the small bowel and/or colon, sometimes with intervening areas of normal bowel **(Fig. 7.13)**. Crohn disease shows a segmental lesion while ulcerative colitis is diffuse. The appearances vary from a "cobblestone appearance" due to thickened oedematous mucosa to narrowing of the lumen with the so-called "string sign." There may be fistulous tracts to adjacent loops of bowel. Biopsy of a perirectal lesion or even of the involved buccal mucosa may reveal diagnostic granulomatous changes. Colonoscopy and biopsy may provide an immediate diagnosis.

Case Study

A 10-year-old Asian girl presented with a 10-month history of abdominal pain. The pain was coloicky in nature, occurred most days and usually after meals leading to a desire to defaecate. She usually passed between 2 and 4 stools per day with occasional small quantities of fresh blood. There was no vomiting. Sometimes the pain was severe enough for her to be sent home from school. She also had some mouth ulcers and non-specific joint pains. She had been previously healthy. Further questioning revealed that she had been seen by her general physician 1 year previously because of pallor and treated with iron supplements. She was doing well at school but her attendance had recently deteriorated. There was a family history of peptic ulcer. Her mother had noted that she had not grown much over the last 20 months and seemed easily upset and withdrawn. Otherwise she herself had no concerns about her size and weight.

On examination, she was on the 25th centile for height and 10th centile for weight. There were no signs of puberty. Both parental heights were on the 50th centile.

Systemic examination was unremarkable apart from aphthous ulcers in the mouth and an anal fissure at 4 o'clock which appeared to be painless. There was no evidence of sexual abuse. Urine contained neither protein nor glucose and was normal on microscopy. Blood haemoglobin 10.1 g/dL, white cell count 7.3 × 109/L, platelet count 285 × 109/L, autoantibody profile negative, immunoglobulin A (IgA) anti-tissue transglutaminase (anti-tTG) antibodies negative. Barium meal and follow through showed segmental involvement of the small bowel.

The most likely diagnosis is Crohn disease.

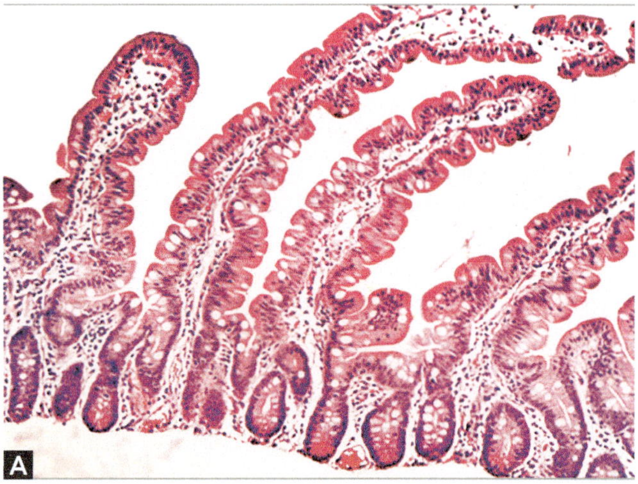

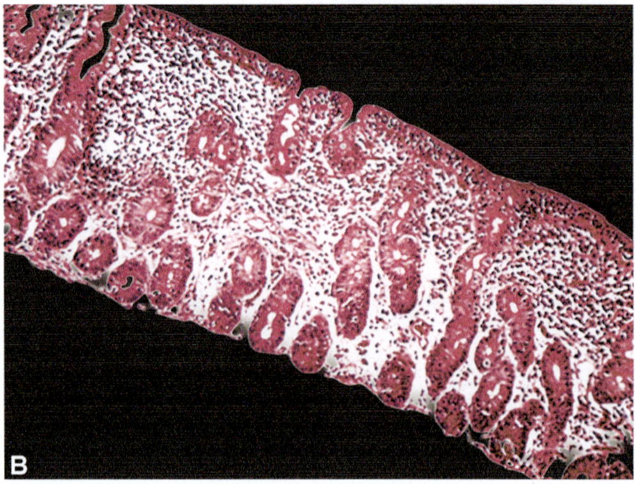

Figures 7.14A and B Total villous atrophy with loss of villi, elongated hyperplastic crypts dense plasmacytic infiltrate in the lamina propria and increased number of surface intra-epithelial lymphocytes (obj × 10).

Coeliac Disease (Gluten-sensitive Enteropathy)

Aetiology

Coeliac disease (CD) is now regarded as an autoimmune type of chronic inflammatory condition and may have its onset at all ages. It is apparent that the harmful substance is in the gliadin fraction of gluten in wheat, barley and rye flour. The immune-mediated enteropathy is triggered by the ingestion of gluten in genetically susceptible individuals. Gluten is a mixture of structurally similar proteins contained in the cereals, wheat, rye and barley. CD is associated strongly with human leucocyte antigen class 11 antigens DQ2 and DQ8 located on chromosome 6p21. CD is frequent in developed world and increasingly found in some areas of the developing world, e.g. North Africa and India.

Pathology

Histological features have been defined mainly from study of jejunal biopsy specimens. The most characteristic appearance is called total villous atrophy in which the mucosa is flat and devoid of normal villi but the underlying glandular layer is thickened and shows marked plasmacell infiltration **(Figs. 7.14A and B)**. Absence of villi has been confirmed by electron microscopy. In other cases, however, there is subtotal villous atrophy in which short, broad and thickened villi are seen. Children with dermatitis herpetiformis also have an intestinal lesion similar to that of CD.

Clinical Features

These do not develop until gluten-containing foods are introduced into the infant's diet. In many cases, the first signs are noted in the last 3 months of the first year of life, but the child may not be brought to the physician until the second year. Delayed introduction of wheat containing cereals into the diet of infants in recent years has resulted in the later onset of CD.

Affected children become fractious and miserable with anorexia and failure to gain weight. Stools are characteristically of porridgy consistency, pale, bulky and foul

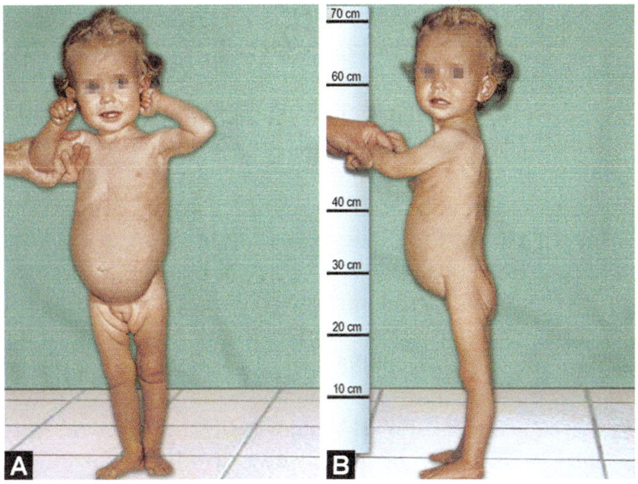

Figures 7.15A and B (A) 14-month-old girl with untreated coeliac disease. *Note* abdominal distension and gross tissue wasting; (B) Lateral view of the same patient.

smelling, but in some children this feature is not very marked. In others, however, the illness may start with vomiting and watery diarrhoea. The abdomen becomes distended as a result of poor musculature, altered peristaltic activity and the accumulation of intestinal secretions and gas. This contrasts with the child's wasted buttocks and thighs and produces the so-called coeliac profile **(Figs. 7.15A and B)**. A small number of children may be desperately ill with profuse diarrhoea leading to dehydration, acidosis and shock (coeliac crisis). In the worst cases, malabsorption of protein can lead to hypoproteinaemic oedema. Some children may present with prolonged fatigue ("tired all the time"), recurrent abdominal pain, cramping or distension.

Various other defects in absorption may become clinically manifest. Iron deficiency anaemia is common. There is usually diminished absorption of folic acid as revealed by a reduced red cell folate concentration. If there is ileal involvement, serum B_{12} may be decreased. Although deficiency of vitamins A and D is probably always present, rickets is quite rare (due to lack of growth) and xerophthalmia is almost unknown. However, rickets may develop after starting treatment with a gluten free diet if supplements of vitamin D are omitted while active growth continues. Hypoprothrombinaemia is often present.

There has been a change in the clinical presentation of the disease since a large fraction of affected patients mainly adults remain undiagnosed due to atypical or vague symptoms, or even the absence of symptoms. We should be especially aware of the disease in certain risk groups, i.e. first-degree relatives of patients with diagnosed disease, patients with autoimmune diseases such as type 1 insulin dependent diabetes, autoimmune thyroid disease, dermatitis herpetiformis and child with Down syndrome.

Diagnostic Tests

While the definitive diagnosis of CD must rest upon jejunal biopsy, the procedure is unpleasant and requires admission to hospital. A variety of screening tests have been developed. The use of serological markers, i.e. serum antigliadin, antiendomysial (IgA-EmA) and anti-tissue transglutaminase (IgA-tTGA) antibodies of IgA isotype for case finding and epidemiological studies is mandatory. However, IgA deficiency must be excluded. Patients with IgA deficiency will have a false negative result if IgA based serological tests are used. However, IgG-tTGA and/or IgG-EmA serological tests should be carried out in patients with confirmed IgA deficiency. The testing for CD is accurate only if the child continues to follow a gluten-containing diet during the diagnostic process (serological tests and jejunal biopsy).

A barium meal and follow-through examination will reveal an abnormal coarsening of the mucosal pattern of the small bowel, jejunal dilatation and possibly delay in the passage of barium to the colon. The bones may become osteoporotic and ossification delayed.

No investigation apart from small intestinal biopsy is 100% diagnostic of children who have CD.

KEY LEARNING POINTS

Diagnosis of coeliac disease.

The only diagnostic test for CD at present is small intestinal biopsy while the child is on a gluten-containing diet. "The Gold Standard for Diagnosis." Serological tests do not diagnose CD, but indicate whether further testing is needed.

Cystic Fibrosis

Aetiology

Cystic fibrosis is an autosomal recessive hereditary multi-organ disease caused by mutations in the CF transmembrane conductance regulator gene. The gene, which codes for this protein is located on chromosome 7 and the most common so far described is at the DF 508 locus and accounts for about 74% of cases in Caucasians. Although the incidence varies considerably between ethnic groups and populations, CF seems to be present in every population studied. CF is much less common in native African and native Asian populations.

Pathology

Although the gene defect is present in all nucleated body cells it is only in those cells where the gene requires to be activated for normal cell function that abnormalities are recognised. It is not surprising that the disease has variable clinical manifestations given the range of gene defects. The pancreas is abnormal in over 90% of the cases. A constant change is fibrosis with atrophy of the exocrine parenchyma. Cystic dilatation of acini and ducts is common but not invariable. Islet tissue, however, is rarely involved until later childhood or adolescence. Mucous glands throughout the body are grossly distended and they secrete abnormal viscid mucus. Stagnation of mucus in the smaller bronchioles usually leads to infection, which in turn stimulates further mucus secretion. The non-resolving neutrophilic inflammatory response to chronic infection in turn causes progressive and permanent airway damage, such that bronchiectasis and respiratory failure are the common findings in end-stage CF lung disease. The liver shows a focal type of biliary cirrhosis, most marked under the capsule, which may progress to produce portal hypertension.

Clinical Features

While most CF patients present disease symptoms at birth or in early infancy, some may not be diagnosed until adulthood.

The symptoms tend to occur in a more or less ordered fashion and the diagnosis is not often unduly difficult. In about 10% of the patients, the illness presents in the neonatal period in the form of meconium ileus in which inspissated meconium causes intestinal obstruction. The most common presentation, however, is in the form of an intractable respiratory infection dating from the early weeks or months of life. Indeed, CF of the pancreas should always be suspected when a respiratory infection in infancy fails to respond promptly to adequate antibiotic therapy. In the early stages of the disease, radiographs of the chest may show only increased translucency of the lung fields; later heavy interstitial markings appear; then multiple soft shadows representing small lung abscesses. In other cases, there may be lobar consolidation, empyema or pyopneumothorax. In children who survive the early months of life, the respiratory picture may become that of bronchiectasis, increasing emphysema, and clubbing of the fingers. Sputum culture in such cases will most often show the predominant organisms to be *Staphylococcus aureus* and *Pseudomonas aeruginosa* and other gram-negative bacteria (e.g. *Burkholderia cepacia complex*, *Stenotrophomonas maltophilia* and *Achromobacter xylosoxidans*) often dominate the clinical picture.

In a minority of cases, the respiratory infection is less prominent than the presence of semi-formed, greasy, bulky and excessively foul smelling stools. These features coincide with the introduction of mixed feeding. After the first year of life, the history of abnormal and frequent stools occurring in association with abdominal distension and generalised tissue wasting may simulate CD. The differential diagnosis can, however, almost always be made on clinical grounds alone. In CF, a careful history will elicit that signs first appeared in the early weeks of life, whereas CD rarely presents before the age of 6 months. The excellent, often voracious appetite in CF contrasts sharply with the unhappy anorexia of the coeliac child. Chronic respiratory infection of some degree, often severe, is an invariable accompaniment of CF but it is not a feature of CD. Furthermore, the diagnosis of CF may be suggested by a history that previous siblings have the disease.

If the affected infant survives the first year, childhood seems often to bring a period of improvement in the chest condition. All too frequently, however, the approach to puberty is associated with cor pulmonale. Less commonly, in about 10% of the patients, during the second decade, biliary cirrhosis and portal hypertension develop and may lead to massive GI haemorrhage. In recent years as an increasing proportion of sufferers from CF survive insulin dependent diabetes mellitus has been found in some as they approach puberty. A further important manifestation, which seems to present in a majority of male survivors into adulthood is aspermia and sterility. This has been shown to be due to absence of the vas deferens. Women have only slightly reduced fertility associated with abnormal tubal ciliary movement and cervical mucus.

Some children with CF can develop distal small bowel obstruction. This disorder is due to viscid mucofaeculent material obstructing the bowel causing recurring episodes of abdominal pain, constipation and acute or sub-acute intestinal obstruction. The cardinal sign is a soft, mobile, non-tender mass palpable in the right iliac fossa. Mild cases can be treated by increasing the intake of pancreatic enzyme. If the condition is not improved oral N-acetylcysteine 10 mL four times a day or one or two doses of oral gastrografin 50–100 mL taken with 200–400 mL of water may relieve the patient discomfort and obstruction. Toddlers with CF may sometimes present with rectal prolapse. Also the incidence of nasal polyps in patients with CF is about 70%.

KEY LEARNING POINT

The vast majority of men with CF (98%) are infertile due to abnormalities in the development of structure derived from the Wolffian duct.

Diagnostic Tests

The sweat test is still sufficient to confirm the diagnosis in typical cases but gene screening for known mutations is now becoming routine in many centres. The sweat test can be carried out from the third week of life on, provided the infant weighs more than 3 kg, is normally hydrated and without significant illness. There are various methods of obtaining sweat for analysis but the most accurate and widely used technique is stimulation of local sweating by pilocarpine iontophoresis. One should try to achieve the collection of at least 100 mg of sweat. To minimise diagnostic errors, two reliable sweat tests confirmed in a laboratory used to performing the test should be obtained. Diagnostic levels of sodium and chloride are 60 mmol/kg. In patients with atypical disease manifestations, the sweat test is often equivocal. Additional diagnostic tests will be necessary to substantiate the diagnosis: Cystic fibrosis transmembrane conductance regulator (CFTR) mutation analysis and, at times, CFTR bioassays.

In neonates, there is a reliable method of screening which is based on the serum concentration of immunoreactive trypsin (IRT). Serum IRT levels are abnormally high (>80 ng/mL) during the first few months of life, although in older children they fall to subnormal values. Prenatal diagnosis by chorionic villus biopsy obtained at 9–12 weeks postconception will allow termination of affected foetuses. As there is still no curative treatment for CF the introduction of screening has to be considered regionally, in close cooperation with CF centres.

KEY LEARNING POINTS

A sweat chloride concentration of greater than 60 mmol/L confirms the clinically suspected diagnosis of CF.

Most patients with CF die from end-stage pulmonary disease; therefore, emphasis is on prevention and treatment of pulmonary infections. Most patients would benefit from improved nutrition, including refined pancreatic supplementation therapy and essential fatty acid status.

Idiopathic Childhood Constipation

Terminology is a problem, which causes confusion in communication between physicians and patients. It is important that the physician be sure of the patient's understanding of the terms used. Constipation may be defined as a difficulty or delay in defaecation that causes distress to the child and the parents. An infrequent passage of stools with no distress does not fall into this category. Encopresis or faecal soiling is the frequent passage of faecal matter at socially unacceptable times. This has been discussed in Chapter 28 (Disorders of Emotion and Behaviour). Psychogenic causes are the most frequent. Faecal continence is the ability to retain faeces until delivery is convenient. Ingestion of fluid or food stimulates the gastrocolic reflex and results in two or three mass colonic propulsive activities per day. This process delivers faecal material to a normally empty rectum. On distension of the rectum, stretch receptors start a rectal contraction and a reflex inhibition is sent to the anal canal. This is mediated via the myenteric plexus of nerves in the submucosa and the plexus of nerves between the outer longitudinal and inner circular smooth muscle layers. The process produces sensation since the upper part of the anal canal has sensitive sensory receptors as well as stretch receptors. The motor element of the external sphincter and the puborectalis muscle make up the striated sphincter together with the smooth muscle of the internal sphincter. The striated sphincter is able to contract strongly to prevent the passage of a stool at an inconvenient time. This, however, can only function for 30 seconds, i.e. long enough to contain a rectal contraction wave till it passes. The internal sphincter can maintain persistent tonic activity so preventing leakage of stool between periods of rectal activity by maintaining closure of a resting anal canal. Clinical experience suggests that the external sphincters are of much less importance than the puborectalis sling and the internal sphincter. Defaecation occurs by inhibiting the activity of the puborectalis sling and the sphincter mechanism of the anus, thus allowing faeces to pass from the rectum into the anal canal. This is augmented by voluntarily increasing intra-abdominal pressure using the abdominal wall musculature as well as the diaphragm as accessory muscles for defaecation. There are two main clinical states, the acute and the chronic state, which must be differentiated. Some children with physical disabilities, such as cerebral palsy are more prone to idiopathic constipation as a result of impaired mobility. Children with Down syndrome and autism are also more prone to the condition.

KEY LEARNING POINT

Hirschsprung disease, CF, anorectal anomalies and metabolic conditions such as hypothyroidism are rare organic causes of childhood constipation.

Acute Constipation

Acute constipation usually occurs in a child after a febrile illness with a reduced fluid intake. This situation arises when convalescing after an illness or in the immediate postoperative period. There is a danger that this acute state of constipation may progress to a chronic state if it is not identified early enough. Treatment with a laxative, suppositories or an enema usually corrects the problem initially but the child must be encouraged to return to a good diet and adequate fluid intake.

Chronic Constipation

Chronic constipation is distressing to the child and the parents. An early diagnosis is essential to prevent a prolonged and persistent problem. In chronic constipation, the rectum is overstretched and ballooned. The sensory receptors are inactive and the bowel is flaccid and unable to contract effectively. A greater amount of water is absorbed from the faecal stream. The stool becomes harder, more solid and more difficult and painful to pass. The faecal mass increases in size and spurious diarrhoea can also occur from stercoral ulceration of the distended rectal mucosa.

History is important as failure to pass meconium within 24 hours of birth in the term infant born normally, makes it likely that there may be some underlying problem. Infants, for whom childbirth has been abnormal, take longer to establish a normal defaecation pattern. The delay in establishing normal stooling may be a sign of other disorders, not only Hirschsprung disease or anal stenosis, but systemic disorders such as hypothyroidism. Psychogenic causes are the commonest origin of constipation in childhood often due to inappropriate toilet training and this aspect has also been discussed in Chapter 28 (Disorders of Emotion and Behaviour).

In older infants and children, the distress caused by constipation may be related to pain. There may be abdominal discomfort, usually a dull ache, which may or may not be related to defaecation. Occasionally, the pain may be localised to the right iliac fossa due to a distended caecum filled with stool. The pain may be in the anal region, particularly when an anal fissure has occurred and bleeding may result from the mucosal tear.

There are occasions when there is no complaint of constipation but the parents may notice a distended abdomen, and may even at times feel a mass arising out of the pelvis.

A full dietary history must be obtained. This should include a detailed account of a typical day's breakfast, lunch, supper and any in-between snacks, noting the amount of fluid taken, any dietary fads and the amount of fruits, vegetables and cereals ingested.

An accurate account of drugs given and other remedies tried by the parents before presenting at the clinic is documented.

Examination

A full examination of the child is important noting the presence of any dysmorphic features, height and weight as well as any signs of failure to thrive. Inspection of the abdomen noting any abdominal distension or the presence of localised swelling. The abdomen is then palpated in routine fashion, feeling for any abdominal mass. A faecal mass can usually be indented through the abdomen, although at times the impacted mass may be so hard as to make it quite impossible to indent, and may mislead one into thinking it is a malignant mass. A loaded, impacted colon with a megarectum can in turn cause retention of urine resulting in a full bladder, which may or may not distress the child if this is a chronic situation.

Digital rectal examination must be carefully explained to the parents and the child before proceeding, explaining the importance of deciding whether constipation is a problem especially in the presence of diarrhoea, which may be spurious in nature. It is helpful to have a nurse in attendance to position the child in the left lateral position with knees bent in the foetal position. It is useful to carry on conversation during this investigation to relax an otherwise tense atmosphere and also explaining to the parent and the child what is being done. While the child is in this position, it is important to examine the spine and the sacrum for any sign of spina bifida occulta. The position of the anus as well as its size should be noted to exclude the possibility of an anterior ectopic anus or an anal stenosis. The skin around the anus should look normal. Erythema may indicate the presence of candida or streptococcal infection or may be due to topical applications by the parents. The presence of puckering of the anus as well as the presence of a skin tag may indicate an underlying anal fissure, which could be the result of the vicious cycle of retention of stool, chronic constipation and painful defaecation. The presence of soiling should be noted and the consistency and volume of stool, if it is hard or soft or liquid in form, as well as whether there is any blood present.

KEY LEARNING POINTS

May not be idiopathic constipation—diagnostic clues are as follows:

- If constipation has occurred from birth or first 2 weeks of life.
- If there is history of failure to pass meconium/delay of greater than 48 hours after birth.
- If there is undiagnosed weakness in legs, locomotor delay.
- If there is abdominal distension with vomiting.
- If lower limb reflexes are abnormal.
- If spine, lumbosacral region/gluteal examination shows sacral agenesis, naevi, hairy patch, asymmetry or flattening of gluteal muscles.

Investigations

A plain abdominal radiograph is only indicated in the ongoing management of intractable idiopathic constipation. A plain X-ray of the abdomen in a child with a distended abdomen and constipation may indicate the degree of constipation and may also detect underlying bony abnormalities such as spina bifida occulta or sacral abnormalities. Barium enema (**Fig. 7.16**) may be carried out in a few children with chronic constipation where there is a suspicion of Hirschsprung disease but in most children radiological investigations are not required if

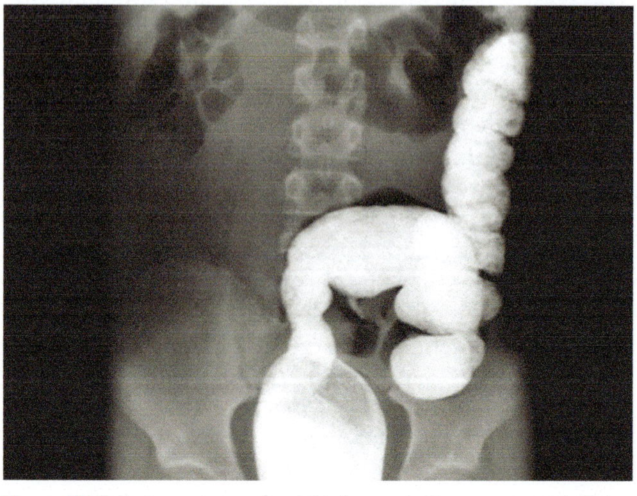

Figure 7.16 Barium enema of a child demonstrating gross rectal dilatation and obstruction with mass of faeces ("terminal reservoir").

an adequate history is taken. These children must not be prepared by bowel washout prior to the barium enema because this will obscure the X-ray appearance. Transit studies are not required to make a diagnosis of idiopathic constipation. However, consider transit studies and abdominal ultrasound in the ongoing management of intractable idiopathic constipation.

Protein-losing Enteropathy

The intestinal loss of proteins may be greatly increased in many diseases, not only diseases which primarily affect the GI tract but many other more generalised disorders such as CF, CD and Henoch–Schönlein purpura.

Little is known about the mechanisms by which the plasma proteins reach the lumen of the gut. In inflammatory and ulcerative conditions, local exudation of protein seems the obvious explanation. In other conditions such as lymphangiectasia, retroperitoneal fibrosis and congestive cardiac failure, the loss may be accounted for by disturbance of lymphatic drainage. For the most part, the mechanism remains obscure. The classification in Box 7.3 includes those found in children.

Gastrointestinal protein loss is non-selective. Serum proteins are lost "in bulk" irrespective of molecular size. Although all serum proteins may be reduced, the abnormality is most obvious in the reduction in concentration of albumin, IgG, IgA and IgM. Abnormal intestinal protein loss may occur without any clinical manifestations.

However, at serum levels below 4 g per 100 mL there is an increasing risk of peripheral oedema, which may then become a major or even the presenting complaint.

Protein-losing enteropathy may be suspected in any case of unexplained hypoproteinaemia or oedema especially in the presence of GI symptoms. Suspicion is strengthened by the demonstration of particularly low levels of albumin and Igs. The diagnosis is proved by the use of such tests as the use of ^{51}Cr-labelled serum proteins. The measurement of faecal a-1 antitrypsin can be used to document protein loss and to potentially localise the site of loss. Diagnosis is not complete without the demonstration of excess intestinal protein loss. It is necessary to determine the nature of the causative disease.

BOX 7.3 Diseases associated with protein-losing enteropathy.

- Invasive bacterial infection (e.g. *Salmonella*, *Shigella*)
- Crohn disease
- Ulcerative colitis
- Intestinal tuberculosis
- Sarcoidosis
- Intestinal lymphangiectasia
- Retroperitoneal fibrosis
- Neoplasia affecting mesenteric lymphatics
- Thoracic duct obstruction
- Congestive cardiac failure
- Menetrier disease
- Cystic fibrosis
- Milk and Soy-induced enteropathy
- Henoch–Schönlein purpura
- Giardiasis
- Kwashiorkor
- Veno-occlusive disease
- Necrotising enterocolitis
- Tropical sprue
- Graft-versus-host disease

Wilson Disease (Hepatolenticular Degeneration)

Caeruloplasmin is a copper-containing a-2 globulin, which functions as a transport mechanism for copper in the plasma. Deficiency of caeruloplasmin is associated with copper deposition in many tissues resulting in Wilson disease.

Clinical Features

Wilson disease may present any time from early childhood to the fifth decade. In early childhood, hepatosplenomegaly, jaundice and acute hepatitis or nodular cirrhosis of the liver are the most common findings. This disease should always be considered in such cases. A brown or green ring around the corneal limbus—the Kayser–Fleischer (K-F) ring—is caused by copper deposited in Descemet's membrane. It is only found in this disease. The ring is often not present under the age of 7 years.

Urine, plasma and tissue concentrations of copper are high and serum caeruloplasmin (or copper oxidase activity) is usually low, although rare families with normal caeruloplasmin levels have been reported. Plasma caeruloplasmin levels are very low in the normal newborn, rising to normal by about 2 years of age.

Diagnosis

Tissue copper is high but serum copper and caeruloplasmin are low, although rare forms are known in which the caeruloplasmin level may be normal although its functional activity is impaired. In these cases, liver biopsy or radioactive copper uptake may be required to make the diagnosis. Some heterozygotes have reduced caeruloplasmin levels; others can be distinguished by measuring caeruloplasmin uptake of radioactive copper. Slit lamp examination may be needed to see the K–F rings.

> **KEY LEARNING POINT**
>
> The diagnosis of Wilson disease may be made readily when the classic triad of hepatic disease, neurologic involvement and K–F rings are present.

Jaundice

Bile Pigment Metabolism

The initial steps in the transformation of haemoglobin to bilirubin occur in the reticuloendothelial cells of the bone marrow, the spleen and the liver. The first step is the formation of water-insoluble free bilirubin. Bilirubin at this stage is transported in the plasma attached to protein, mainly albumin. Bilirubin can be displaced from this albumin binding by several drugs. The liver normally conjugates free bilirubin to form water-soluble bilirubin glucuronide, which is excreted in the bile. Unconjugated and conjugated bilirubins are roughly synonymous with indirect and direct reacting bilirubin, respectively. The conversion of bilirubin to water-soluble glucuronide occurs in the hepatic parenchymal cells. Glucuronyl transferase, the enzyme that catalyses this reaction is relatively deficient in newborn infants especially premature ones, and in children with familial nonhaemolytic jaundice (Crigler–Najjar syndrome). This deficiency leads to an elevated serum level of unconjugated bilirubin. Bilirubin is excreted into the bile capillaries and the intestinal tract. In the newborn infant, some of the conjugated bilirubin is converted to its unconjugated form, reabsorbed into the enterohepatic circulation and presented to the liver for reprocessing.

Two types of jaundice, retention and regurgitation, can be distinguished. Retention jaundice results from failure of the liver cells to convert bilirubin to bilirubin glucuronide at a rate that will prevent accumulation of the unconjugated pigment in the blood. Bile is not present in the urine. Regurgitation jaundice results from the return of bilirubin to the blood stream after conversion to bilirubin glucuronide. Bile is present in the urine.

Regurgitation jaundice may occur secondary to necrosis of liver cells or obstruction of the bile ducts **(Fig. 7.17)**. Retention jaundice may occur in the presence of excessive haemolysis and/or pigment production, impaired liver uptake or defective conjugation.

Therefore, jaundice occurs either when there is excess haemolysis increasing the load of bilirubin, when the diseased liver is not able to cope with the normal load or when there is obstruction to excretion of bilirubin. Jaundice can be classified into haemolytic (prehepatic), hepatocellular (hepatic) and obstructive (posthepatic) varieties. Acquired liver diseases that are seen in adults are rare in children. More commonly seen in children

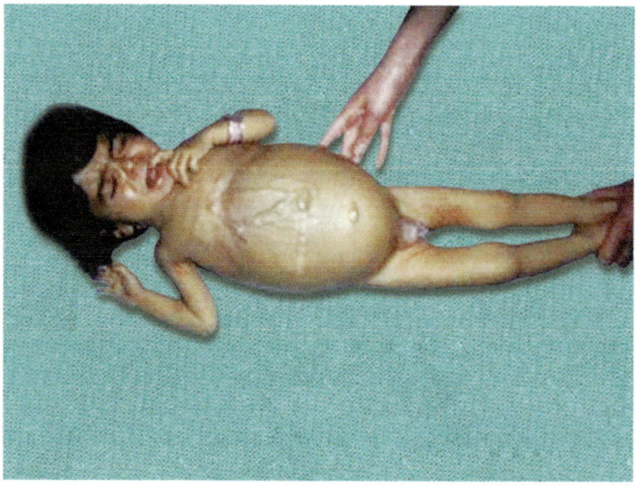

Figure 7.17 Clinical photograph of an infant with biliary atresia. Over 80% of infants are jaundiced from birth. The abdomen is distended due to an enlarged firm liver, ascites due to portal hypertension. *Note* failure to thrive.

are congenital or metabolic disorders. In this chapter, the authors have discussed only virus hepatitis, chronic active hepatitis and cirrhosis of the liver.

Carotenoderma (Carotenaemia)

It is characterised by yellow skin pigmentation ("carroty") usually as a result of excessive dietary intake of foods rich in β-carotene. The pigmentation is marked on the nasolabial folds, forehead, axillae and groin and keratinised surfaces such as the palms and soles **(Figs. 7.18A and B)**. Constitutional symptoms seldom appear in carotenoderma. The sclerae and buccal membranes are not icteric and this helps to distinguish carotenoderma from jaundice in which these tissues are yellowed. Also serum bilirubin is within the normal range but plasma carotene level is raised. No toxicity is apparent and the discolouration gradually disappears with reduction of intake of carotenoids.

> **KEY LEARNING POINT**
>
> Jaundice versus carotenoderma (carotenaemia): There is no scleral icterus in carotenoderma, and this helps clinically to distinguish it from jaundice.

VIRAL INFECTIONS OF THE LIVER

Hepatitis A

Hepatitis A virus (HAV) is present in the blood and stool of a patient for 2–3 weeks before clinical symptoms occur

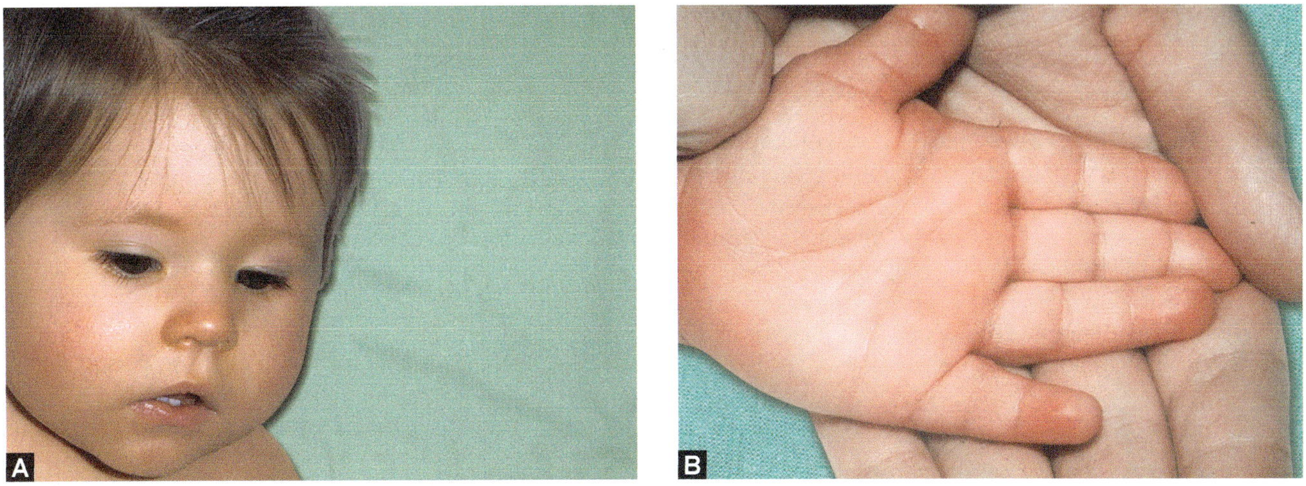

Figures 7.18A and B Carotenaemia and carotenoderma. Clinical photographs showing lemon-yellow colouration of the skin along nasolabial folds, on the palms and soles, around nails and over pressure areas. The sclerae and mucous membranes are not pigmented. (A) Face; (B) Palm of hand.

and it persists in stool for up to 2 weeks after disease onset. The primary mode of transmission is faecal-oral route. Common source outbreaks occur with contamination of water or food. In developing countries with inadequate hygiene and poor sanitation HAV infection is endemic and most children are infected in the first year of life.

Clinical Features

Hepatitis A virus infection is usually an acute self-limiting illness. The mean incubation period is 30 days. In infants and young children, the infection could be entirely asymptomatic. Jaundice is rare in this age group. In older children, there may be a prodromal period of several days in which fever, headache and malaise predominate, followed by the onset of jaundice, abdominal pain, nausea, vomiting and anorexia. Pruritus may accompany the jaundice.

Clinical examination may reveal a mildly enlarged tender liver and occasionally splenomegaly is noted.

Serum aminotransferase values usually are often 20–100 times the upper limit of normal and they decrease rapidly within the first 2–3 weeks.

Diagnosis

The diagnosis of HAV infection is made by detection of the IgM antibody to HAV (IgM and anti-HAV).

Hepatitis B

Hepatitis B virus (HBV) is relatively uncommon in Caucasians but has a high prevalence in Southeast Asia and parts of Africa where highly infective carriage of HBV is common. The incubation period is 90–120 days. HBV is found in high concentration in the blood of infected individuals and in moderate concentrations in semen, vaginal fluid and saliva. Risk factors for acquisition of HBV infection include parenteral exposure to blood or blood products. Risk factors in children include perinatal exposure (vertical) being born to a hepatitis B surface antigen (HBsAg) seropositive mother. Horizontal spread is by living in a household with a chronic HBV carrier.

The hepatic injury that occurs with HBV infection is mediated by the host immune response. Most instances of HBV infection are acute and self-limited. In some individuals, HBV is not cleared by the host immunologic response, and chronic infection results.

Clinical Features

After an incubation period of 30–180 days, patients with HBV infection may develop a prodrome that consists of malaise, fatigue, nausea, low-grade fever or even a serum sickness like illness. Papular acrodermatitis of childhood may be the major or only manifestation of HBV in infants and young children. Patients who manifest these prodromal symptoms are already seropositive for HBsAg.

Within a week or two of the prodrome, clinical hepatitis is seen with jaundice, pruritus, nausea and vomiting. Clinical examination reveals mild hepatomegaly and liver tenderness, and mild splenomegaly may also be noted. Serum bilirubin and aminotransferase levels decrease over several weeks to normal. However, in those children who will develop fulminant hepatitis, the typical features of coagulopathy and encephalopathy will appear. In patients who develop chronic HBV infection, jaundice clears up, but alanine transaminase (ALT) and aspartate transaminase (AST) may or may not return to normal.

Chronic HBV infection is often completely asymptomatic and may not be diagnosed if the patient has not had an acute icteric illness. Chronic hepatitis may manifest as a complication of cirrhosis or portal hypertension.

Chronic HBV infection is highly associated with the risk of developing hepatocellular carcinoma.

Diagnosis

The diagnosis of acute HBV infection is made by detection of HBsAg and IgM anti-HB core; although hepatitis B "e" antigen (HBeAg) confirms active replication, its presence is not essential to confirm the diagnosis. Chronic HBV infection is defined by the presence of HBsAg for more than 6 months; typically it persists for many years. In chronic HBV infection, HBeAg persists, often for many years, indicating ongoing viral infection.

Hepatitis C

Hepatitis C virus (HCV) was discovered in sera from patients with post-transfusion hepatitis and is now the predominant cause of transfusion associated non-A, non-B hepatitis in the world. However, since the institution of screening donors for antibody to HCV (anti-HCV) and thus eliminating positive blood/blood products, the risk of HCV from transfusion has diminished. On the other hand, the proportion of cases associated with intravenous drug abuse has increased. However, exposure to blood products and perinatal exposure have been the most consistent risk factors for HCV acquisition in children. The incubation period for post-transfusion HCV infection ranges from 2 weeks to 26 weeks.

Clinical Features

Many acute HCV infections are clinically asymptomatic but those who become icteric show a modest rise in aminotransferase levels. Some patients have symptoms of acute hepatitis, such as anorexia, malaise, fatigue and abdominal pain. In most instances, chronic HCV infection is asymptomatic.

Hepatitis D (Delta Hepatitis)

Delta hepatitis is caused by the hepatitis D virus (HDV). It occurs only in conjunction with hepatitis B infection. In general, HDV infection does not have specific features to distinguish it from ordinary HBV infection. Testing for HDV infection is recommended in any child with chronic HBV and unusually severe liver disease.

Hepatitis E

Hepatitis E virus (HEV) infection is also called enterically transmitted non-A, non-B hepatitis. The symptoms and signs are similar to those of hepatitis A. At present, the diagnosis depends on the detection of anti-HEV IgM.

Hepatitis G

The clinical significance of hepatitis G virus (HGV) remains uncertain. This virus has not been implicated in acute non-A, non-E hepatitis or fulminant hepatic failure in children.

Hepatitis Caused by Other Viral Agents

Hepatitis viruses A, B, C, D and E are the agents of most viral hepatitis. Other viruses that can cause hepatitis as part of a generalised illness (Cytomegalovirus, herpes virus, Epstein-Barr virus, human parvovirus B 19, rubella, coxsackie B and yellow fever hepatitis and dengue haemorrhagic fever) will not be discussed here.

Cirrhosis of the Liver

Aetiology

Hepatic cirrhosis is uncommon in children in the United Kingdom and the histological differentiation into "portal" and "biliary" types tend to be less well-defined than in adults. A pathological picture similar to that of Laënnec portal cirrhosis may follow neonatal hepatitis, blood group incompatibility, the de Toni–Fanconi syndrome and it may be the form of presentation of Wilson hepatolenticular cirrhosis. Infective hepatitis B may also lead to hepatic cirrhosis. Other rare causes of cirrhosis of the liver include galactosaemia, Gaucher disease, Niemann-Pick disease and xanthomatosis. Pure biliary cirrhosis is seen invariably in congenital biliary atresia and a focal type is very common in CF of the pancreas.

Indian childhood cirrhosis (ICC) is a common and fatal disease, which appears to be restricted to India. There is a positive family history in about 30% of cases. It is not found in Indian expatriates in other parts of the world. It usually presents between the ages of 9 months and 5 years and has characteristic histological features in liver biopsy material. These have been called "micro-micronodular cirrhosis" which includes necrosis and vacuolation of liver cells, aggressive fibrosis both intralobular and perilobular and a variable inflammatory infiltrate. The liver contains an exceedingly high copper content and the hepatocytes contain multiple, coarse, dark brown orcein-staining granules, which represent copper-associated protein. The pathogenic role of chronic ingestion of copper was supported by the finding of a much greater use of copper utensils to heat and store milk by families of affected than unaffected children. Since then, the use of copper pots has reduced, and the disease has largely disappeared from many parts of India. Recently, a copper-binding factor has been identified in ICC, liver cytosol. This factor may play a role in hepatic intracellular copper accumulation. In Jamaica, a form of cirrhosis called veno-occlusive disease of the liver, in which there is occlusion of the small hepatic veins, is due to the toxic effects of an alkaloid in bush tea compared from plants such as *Senecio* and *Crotalaria*.

Chronic Active Hepatitis

Chronic active hepatitis is an autoimmune disorder characterised by hepatic necrosis, fibrosis, plasma cell infiltration and disorganisation of the lobular architecture. In the young adult, often female, associated disorders include thyroiditis, fibrosing alveolitis and glomerulonephritis. Some cases are related to chronic virus B hepatitis (positive HBsAg). In chronic active hepatitis smooth muscle antibodies are found in the serum in two-thirds of cases, antinuclear factor in about 50%, and the gamma globulin level is markedly elevated.

Clinical Features

The child usually presents with abdominal swelling due to enlargement of the liver, which has a firm edge, sometimes smooth, often nodular. Anorexia, lack of energy and slowing of growth are common complaints. Splenomegaly develops if there is portal hypertension. In most cases jaundice makes its appearance sooner rather than later. Spontaneous bleeding is usually due to hypoprothrombinaemia. Orthochromic anaemia is common. When ascites develop the outlook is grave; it is usually associated with hypoproteinaemia and portal hypertension. The latter may result in massive GI haemorrhage. In other cases, death occurs from hepatic encephalopathy with flapping tremor, mental confusion, extensor plantar responses and coma. Spider naevi and "liver palms" are uncommon in children, but clubbing of the fingers may develop. Hypersplenism may produce leucopaenia and thrombocytopenia. Various derangements of liver function can be demonstrated biochemically, e.g. raised direct bilirubin levels, hypoalbuminaemia, and raised serum gamma globulin. In hepatic encephalopathy, the blood ammonia level is high. Diagnosis should be confirmed by liver biopsy.

Cholecystitis

Cholecystitis is uncommon in childhood and rarely presents as an acute emergency. Cholelithiasis is less common in infancy and childhood. It presents with recurrent upper abdominal pain, nausea and vomiting. It is often associated with congenital spherocytosis. The stones are usually bile pigment stones and should be looked for whenever laparotomy is carried out for removal of the spleen in this condition. Most gallstones are clinically silent. Ultrasonography is the most sensitive and specific method to detect gallstones.

Pancreas

Pancreatic disorders are uncommon in childhood except that which is part of the generalised disease of CF. Pancreatitis presents as an acute abdominal emergency but the signs and symptoms are less dramatic than in adults. Single, self-limited attacks, or recurrent attacks of acute pancreatitis are, by far the most frequent feature of this disease in childhood. Chronic pancreatitis is quite rare in children. Based largely upon clinical and epidemiological observations, a broad spectrum of underlying conditions has been associated with acute pancreatitis. According to one series, trauma, structural disease, systemic diseases, drugs and toxins are the major etiological factors. A variety of systemic infectious agents have been implicated in the aetiology of acute pancreatitis. The mumps virus is an important cause of acute pancreatitis in children. Acute pancreatitis has been reported in association with a variety of connective tissue disorders. Abdominal pain and vomiting are the most consistent signs. Abdominal tenderness is more marked in the upper abdomen. There is a lack of a "gold standard" diagnostic test for acute pancreatitis. However, considerable diagnostic importance has been placed on the total serum levels of amylase or lipase, but the specificity and sensitivity of these tests is unsatisfactory. Ultrasonography is now the most commonly used test in the preliminary evaluation of children with abdominal pain when pancreatitis is suspected. Abdominal CT should be reserved where ultrasound examination is technically unsatisfactory.

Juvenile Tropical Pancreatitis

The syndrome of chronic pancreatitis with pancreatic calculi and diabetes has been reported from many countries such as Uganda, Nigeria, Sri Lanka, Malaysia, India and Bangladesh. The exact aetiology has not yet been established; malnutrition is an important epidemiologic association.

The cardinal manifestations of juvenile tropical pancreatitis are recurrent abdominal pain, followed by diabetes mellitus, pancreatic calculi and death in the prime of life.

Abdominal pain followed by diabetes in an emaciated teenager and the radiologic demonstration of calculi in the pancreatic duct are the hallmark of the disease.

Liver Transplantation

Paediatric liver transplantation should be considered at an early stage in babies and children dying of end-stage liver failure. With increasing experience, there are fewer contraindications to liver transplantation. Liver transplantation for children with life-threatening acute or chronic liver disease has proven to be durable with high success rates. The majority of paediatric liver recipients can now expect to enjoy a good quality of life with normal growth and development. Life-long immunosuppressive therapy is required. The circumstances in which liver transplantation should be considered are:

Chronic Liver Disease

- Liver based metabolic disorders
- Acute liver failure
- Unresectable hepatic tumours
- Poor quality of life due to chronic liver disorders.
- Infectious Diarrhoea in Childhood.

Diarrhoea is a common manifestation of infection of the GI tract and can be caused by a variety of pathogens

TABLE 7.2 Common pathogens causing diarrhoea in children.

Bacteria producing inflammatory diarrhoea	*Bacteria producing non-inflammatory diarrhoea*	*Viruses*	*Parasites*
Aeromonas	Enterotoxigenic *E. coli*	Rotavirus	*G. lamblia*
Campylobacter jejuni	*Vibrio cholerae* 01 and 0139	Enteric adenovirus	*E. histolytica*
Clostridium difficile	Enteropathogenic *E. coli*	Astrovirus	*Balantidium coli*
Enteroinvasive *E. coli*	Enterotoxigenic *E. coli*	Norwalk agent-like virus	*C. parvum*
E. coli O157:H7	*V. parahaemolyticus*	Calicivirus	*Strongyloides stercoralis*
Salmonella	*S. aureus*		*Trichuris trichiura*
Shigella			
Y. enterocolitica			
V. parahaemolyticus			
C. perfringens			

including viruses, parasites and bacteria. The most common manifestations of such infections are diarrhoea and vomiting, which may also be associated with systemic features such as abdominal pain, fever, etc. Although several non-infectious causes of diarrhoea are well recognised, the bulk of childhood diarrhoea relates to infectious disorders.

Epidemiology of Childhood Diarrhoea

Despite considerable advances in the understanding and management of diarrhoeal disorders in childhood, these still account for a large proportion of childhood deaths globally. Although the global mortality of diarrhoea has reduced, the overall incidence remains unchanged with many children in developing countries averaging about 3.2 episodes per child year.

Although information on aetiology specific diarrhoea mortality is limited, it is recognised that rotavirus infections account for at least one-third of severe and potentially fatal watery diarrhoea episodes, with an estimated 4,40,000 deaths in developing countries. A similar number may also succumb to *Shigella* infections especially *S. dysenteriae* type 1 infections. In other parts of the world, periodic outbreaks of cholera also account for a large number of adult and child deaths. The peak incidence of diarrhoea as well as mortality is among 6–11 months old infants.

Although there is very little information on the long-term consequences of diarrhoeal diseases, recent data suggest that diarrhoeal illnesses especially, if prolonged, may significantly impair psychomotor and cognitive development in young children.

Aetiology of Diarrhoea

The major factor leading to infectious diarrhoea is infection acquired through the faeco-oral route or by ingestion of contaminated food or water. Hence, this is a disease largely associated with poverty, poor environmental hygiene and development indices. **Table 7.2** lists the common pathogens associated with diarrhoea among children. Enteropathogens that are infectious in a small inoculum (*Shigella, Escherichia coli, enteric viruses, Giardia lamblia, Cryptosporidium parvum* and *Entamoeba histolytica*) may be transmitted from person-to-person contact, whereas others such as cholera are usually a consequence of contamination of food or water supply. In developed countries, episodes of infectious diarrhoea may occur by seasonal exposure to organisms such as rotavirus or by exposure to pathogens in settings of close contact, e.g. in day care centres.

Table 7.3 details the incubation period and common clinical features associated with infection with various organisms causing diarrhoea. Globally, *E. coli* is the most common organism causing diarrhoea followed by *Rotavirus, Shigella* species and non-typhoidal *Salmonella* species.

Clinical Manifestation of Diarrhoea

Most of the clinical manifestations and clinical syndromes of diarrhoea are related to the infecting pathogen and the dose/inoculum. A number of additional manifestations depend upon the development of complications (such as dehydration and electrolyte imbalance) and the nature of the infecting pathogen. Usually, the ingestion of pre-formed toxins (such as those of *S. aureus*) is associated with the rapid onset of nausea and vomiting within 6 hours with possible fever, abdominal cramps and diarrhoea within 8–72 hours. Watery diarrhoea and abdominal cramps after an 8–16 hour incubation period are associated with enterotoxin-producing *Clostridium perfringens* and *Bacillus cereus*. Abdominal cramps and watery diarrhoea after a 16–48 hour incubation period can be associated with calicivirus, several enterotoxin-producing bacteria, *Cryptosporidium* and *Cyclospora*.

TABLE 7.3 Diarrhoea pathogens and clinical syndromes in children.

Pathogen	*Incubation period*	*Clinical features*
Enteropathogenic *E. coli* (EPEC)	6–48 hours	Self-limiting watery diarrhoea, occasional fever and vomiting
Enteroinvasive *E. coli* (EIEC)	1–3 days	Watery diarrhoea, occasionally bloody diarrhoea
Enteroaggregative *E. coli* (EAEC)	8–18 hours	Watery, mucoid diarrhoea. Bloody diarrhoea in a third of cases
Enterohemorrhagic *E. coli* (EHEC)	3–9 days	Abdominal pain, vomiting, bloody diarrhoea, haemolytic uraemic syndrome in 10% of cases
Enterotoxigenic *E. coli* (ETEC)	14–30 hours	Watery diarrhoea, fever, abdominal pain and vomiting
Diffusely adherent *E. coli*	6–48 hours	Mild watery diarrhoea
Shigella	16–72 hours	Mucoid and bloody diarrhoea (may be watery initially), fever, toxicity, tenesmus
Y. enterocolitica	4–6 days	Watery or mucoid diarrhoea (bloody in <10%) with abdominal pain, fever, bacteraemia in young infants
Campylobacter	2–4 days	Abdominal pain (frequently right sided), watery diarrhoea (occasionally mucoid and bloody), fever
Rotavirus	1–3 days	Mostly in young children. Typically watery diarrhoea with upper respiratory symptoms in some children. May cause severe dehydrating diarrhoea

Several organisms including *Salmonella*, *Shigella*, *Campylobacter jejuni*, *Yersinia enterocolitica*, *enteroinvasive E. coli* and *Vibrio parahaemolyticus* are associated with diarrhoea that may contain foecal leucocytes, abdominal cramps and fever, although these organisms can cause watery diarrhoea without fever. Bloody diarrhoea and abdominal cramps after a 72–120 hour incubation period are associated with infections due to *Shigella* and also Shiga toxin-producing *E. coli* such as *E. coli* O157:H7.

Although many of the manifestations of acute gastroenteritis in children are non-specific, some clinical features may help to identify major categories of diarrhoea and could facilitate rapid triage for specific therapy **(Table 7.3)**. However, it must be underscored that there is considerable overlap in the symptomatology and if facilities and resources permit, the syndromic diagnosis must be verified by appropriate laboratory investigations. **Table 7.4** indicates some of the features that help to characterise diarrhoea severity and associated dehydration.

Complications

Most of the complications associated with gastroenteritis are related to the rapidity of diagnosis and of institution of appropriate therapy. Thus unless early and appropriate rehydration is provided, most children with acute diarrhoea would develop dehydration with associated complications. In young children, such episodes can be life-threatening. In other instances, inappropriate therapy can lead to prolongation of the diarrhoeal episodes with consequent malnutrition and complications such as secondary infections and micronutrient deficiencies such as those with iron and zinc.

Diagnosis

The diagnosis of gastroenteritis is largely based on clinical recognition of the disorder, an evaluation of its severity by rapid assessment and confirmation by appropriate laboratory investigations.

Clinical Evaluation of Diarrhoea

The most common manifestation of GI tract infection in children is with diarrhoea, abdominal cramps and vomiting. Systemic manifestations are varied and associated with a variety of causes. The following system of evaluation in a child with acute diarrhoea may allow a reasonably rapid assessment of the nature and severity of the disorder.

Assess the degree of dehydration and acidosis and provide rapid resuscitation and rehydration with oral or intravenous fluids as required.

Obtain appropriate contact or exposure history to determine cause. This can include information on exposure to contacts with similar symptoms, and intake of contaminated foods or water, childcare centre attendance, recent travel to a diarrhoea endemic area and use of antimicrobial agents.

Clinically determine the aetiology of diarrhoea for institution of prompt antibiotic therapy. Although nausea and vomiting are non-specific symptoms, they are indicative of infection in the upper intestine. Fever is suggestive of an inflammatory process and also occurs as a result of dehydration. Fever is common in patients with inflammatory diarrhoea, severe abdominal pain and tenesmus and is indicative of involvement of the large intestine. Features such as nausea and vomiting, absent or low grade fever with mild to moderate periumbilical pain and

TABLE 7.4 Clinical features associated with dehydration.

	Minimal or none (<3% loss of body weight)	***Mild to moderate (3–9% loss of body weight)***	***Severe (>9% loss of body weight)***
Mucous membrane	Moist	Dry	Parched
Eyes/Fontanelle	Normal	Sunken	Deeply sunken
Skin pinch	Normal	Skin pinch goes back slowly 1–2 sec	Skin pinch goes back very slowly >2 second
Tears	Present	Decreased	Absent
Extremities	Perfused	± delayed cap. Refill	Delayed cap. refill >2 second cold, mottled
Mental status	Well, alert	Normal, irritable, iethargic	Lethargic, apathetic, unconscious
Pulse volume/ Heart rate	Normal	Rapid	Thready, weak, impalpable
Blood pressure	Normal	Decreased	Hypotensive or unrecordable (in shock)
Urine output	Normal	Decreased	Absent for >8 hours
Breathing	Normal	Fast	Rapid/Deep

watery diarrhoea are indicative of upper intestinal tract involvement.

Stool Examination

Microscopic examination of the stool and cultures can yield important information on the aetiology of diarrhoea. Stool specimens should be examined for mucus, blood and leucocytes. Foecal leucocytes are indicative of bacterial invasion of colonic mucosa, although some patients with shigellosis may have minimal leucocytes at an early stage of infection, as do patients infected with Shiga toxin-producing *E. coli* and *E. histolytica*. In endemic areas, stool microscopy must include examination for parasites causing diarrhoea such as *G. lamblia* and *E. histolytica*.

Stool cultures should be obtained as early in the course of disease as possible from children with bloody diarrhoea, in whom stool microscopy indicates foecal leucocytes, in outbreaks, with suspected haemolytic uraemic syndrome (HUS), and in immunosuppressed children with diarrhoea. Stool specimens for culture need to be transported and plated quickly and if the latter is not quickly available, may need to be transported in special media. The yield and diagnosis of bacterial diarrhoea can be significantly improved by using molecular diagnostic procedures such as polymerase chain reaction techniques and probes.

CHAPTER 8

Paediatric Cardiology

Trevor Richens

INTRODUCTION

Disorders affecting the cardiovascular system in childhood can be either congenital or acquired in aetiology. Over the last 50 years, the congenital forms of heart disease have evolved from a group of conditions for which no treatment was available to a set of abnormalities, the vast majority of which are treatable if recognised early.

As a group, heart disorders constitute the most common congenital abnormality with incidences quoted between 6/1,000 and 9/1,000. In the developed world, the incidence seems to be declining largely as a result of increased foetal diagnosis and subsequent termination of pregnancy. This effect, however, appears less marked in Asia.

The aetiology of congenital heart disease remains poorly understood. It is well-known that many syndromic abnormalities have been associated with heart defects and that the exposure to certain drugs or toxic agents in utero can result in malformations of the heart (**Table 8.1**). The incidence of congenital heart disease is also known to be higher in siblings or offsprings of those already affected. The incidence rate rises from 6–9/1,000 to 30–40/1,000 for siblings of affected children. Unfortunately, the genetic basis for this remains largely unknown despite intense ongoing research.

Of the acquired forms of heart disease in childhood, those resulting from rheumatic fever remain the most common in Asia. Conversely, rheumatic heart disease is now rare in the developed world, where viral infections and endocarditis are the most common types of acquired heart disease.

Congenital heart disease can be classified in a number of ways. From a clinical view, they are usually split into acyanotic and cyanotic groups before further subdividing on the basis of precise anatomical diagnosis (**Table 8.2**). Acyanotic congenital heart disease is by far the most common group, comprising ventricular septal defect (VSD), atrial septal defect (ASD), atrioventricular septal defect (AVSD), arterial duct, coarctation of the aorta, pulmonary stenosis and aortic stenosis. Together this group accounts for about 90% of congenital heart disease. The principal cyanotic lesions are tetralogy of Fallot (TOF), transposition of the great arteries (TGA), pulmonary atresia (PAt), tricuspid atresia and Ebstein anomaly, altogether comprising about 5% of congenital heart disease. Other rare conditions such as total anomalous pulmonary venous drainage (TAPVD), hypoplastic left heart syndrome (HLHS) and other forms of univentricular heart constitute the remaining 5%. Conveniently, it is this classification that author will use to discuss the individual lesions.

GENERAL PRINCIPLES OF DIAGNOSIS

Despite the huge improvements in echocardiography (echo), there remains no substitute for accurate clinical assessment possibly aided by a 12-lead electrocardiogram (ECG). Echo should be used to confirm and refine the clinical diagnosis and then for follow-up assessment of abnormalities. The ECG remains an extremely important adjunct to the history and clinical examination. It is a simple, cheap, noninvasive tool that can often confirm or refute a diagnosis. The routine use of a chest X-ray is more controversial. Whilst more widely available than echo, it does involve a radiation dose and should probably be confined to children where the suspicion of heart disease is high, and the availability of echo low.

EXAMINATION

Inspection

A complete cardiovascular examination should start with careful inspection of the child asking five questions.

1. Is the child breathless? If a child is breathless as a result of a cardiac abnormality, it suggests pulmonary vascular engorgement, usually caused by heart failure (**Table 8.3**). This may result from increased

TABLE 8.1 Conditions associated with congenital heart disease.

Association	*Defect(s)*
Chromosomal abnormality:	
Trisomy 21	VSD, AVSD (in 50%)
Trisomy 18	VSD, PDA, pulmonary stenosis (in 99%)
Trisomy 13	VSD, PDA, dextrocardia (in 90%)
5p–/Cri-du-chat	VSD, PDA, ASD (in 25%)
XO (Turner)	Coarctation, aortic stenosis, ASD (in 35%)
XXXXY (Klinefelters)	PDA, ASD (in 15%)
Syndrome:	
Noonan	Dysplastic pulmonary stenosis
Williams	Supravalve aortic stenosis, branch pulmonary stenosis
DiGeorge	VSD, tetralogy, truncus, aortic arch abnormality
CHARGE	VSD, tetralogy
VACTERL	VSD, tetralogy
Holt-Oram	ASD
Friedreich ataxia	Hypertrophic cardiomyopathy, heart block
Apert	VSD, tetralogy
Ellis-van Creveld	Common atrium
Pompe's (GSD II)	Hypertrophic cardiomyopathy
Leopard	Pulmonary stenosis, cardiomyopathy, long PR interval
Muscular dystrophy	Dilated cardiomyopathy
Tuberous sclerosis	Cardiac rhabdomyomata
Pierre Robin	VSD, PDA, ASD, coarctation, tetralogy
Long QT syndrome	Long QT interval and torsades de pointes
Maternal conditions:	
Rubella	PDA, branch pulmonary stenosis
Diabetes	VSD, hypertrophic cardiomyopathy (transient)
SLE (anti-Ro/La positive)	Congenital heart block
Phenylketonuria	VSD
Lithium	Ebstein anomaly
Sodium valproate	Coarctation, HLHS
Phenytoin	VSD, coarctation, mitral stenosis
Alcohol	VSD

Abbreviations: VSD, ventricular septal defect; AVSD, atrioventricular septal defect; PDA, patent ductus arteriosus; ASD, atrial septal defect; SLE, systemic lupus erythematosus; HLHS, hypoplastic left heart syndrome.

TABLE 8.2 Classification of congenital heart disease in childhood.

Acyanotic defects
Increased pulmonary blood flow:
Atrial septal defect
Ventricular septal defect
Atrioventricular septal defect
Patent arterial duct
Normal or reduced pulmonary blood flow:
Pulmonary stenosis
Aortic stenosis
Coarctation of the aorta
Cyanotic defects
Normal or reduced pulmonary blood flow:
Tetralogy of Fallot
Transposition of the great arteries
Critical pulmonary stenosis
Ebstein anomaly
Pulmonary atresia
Tricuspid atresia
Single ventricle with pulmonary stenosis
Increased pulmonary blood flow:
Total anomalous pulmonary venous drainage
Hypoplastic left heart syndrome
Truncus arteriosus
Single ventricle without pulmonary stenosis

TABLE 8.3 Causes of heart failure by age.

First week	Left heart obstruction (HLHS, aortic stenosis, coarctation), arrhythmia
First month	Left to right shunt (VSD, AVSD, PDA, truncus arteriosus), arrhythmia
Thereafter	Rheumatic fever, dilated cardiomyopathy, myocarditis, endocarditis, arrhythmia

Abbreviations: VSD, ventricular septal defect; AVSD, atrioventricular septal defect; PDA, patent ductus arteriosus; HLHS, hypoplastic left heart syndrome.

pulmonary blood flow as in the case of a left to right intracardiac shunt, VSD, patent ductus arteriosus (PDA) and AVSD or due to pulmonary venous engorgement—mitral regurgitation, dilated cardiomyopathy, obstructed total anomalous pulmonary venous return and pericardial effusion.

2. Is the child cyanotic? Although the absence of clinical cyanosis does not exclude cyanotic congenital heart

disease, if it is present, it limits the potential diagnoses to a relatively small group of abnormalities. In the newborn, most commonly it would suggest TGA or severely obstructed pulmonary blood flow (TOF, critical pulmonary stenosis, pulmonary atresia (PAt) and tricuspid atresia). In infancy, tetralogy is the most common cause, although transposition with VSD and other rare forms of complex congenital heart disease can also present at this age. In older children, a presentation with cyanosis would suggest pulmonary vascular disease complicating a VSD or PDA. Untreated, the high pulmonary pressures ultimately irreversibly damage the pulmonary vasculature resulting in high pulmonary resistance and a reversal of the intracardiac shunt (right to left) with subsequent cyanosis. This is known as Eisenmenger syndrome. Rarely tetralogy and other complex forms of congenital heart disease can present in later life.

3. Is the child dysmorphic? Many children with congenital syndromes have cardiac abnormalities, the principal ones of which are outlined in **Table 8.1**. Prompt recognition of a syndrome may alert the clinician to search for a particular abnormality.
4. Is the child failing to thrive? There are many causes of failure to thrive in infancy of which heart disease is a relatively minor one. The predominant groups of cardiac disorders causing poor weight gain are those resulting in breathlessness and poor feeding. These include VSD, AVSD and PDA. Whilst some children with cyanotic abnormalities also fail to grow, this is far less common.
5. Does the child have any thoracic scars? If the child has had previous heart surgery, the type of scar may give clues to its nature. A median sternotomy scar suggests an open-heart procedure during which the heart would have been stopped and opened. All major intracardiac abnormalities requiring a surgical repair are corrected in this manner. A right lateral thoracotomy scar is usually only used for a right modified Blalock-Taussig shunt. During this procedure, a tube is interposed between the right subclavian artery and the right pulmonary artery, providing an alternative source of pulmonary blood flow in children who have an obstructed native pulmonary blood flow [TOF, pulmonary atresia (PAt), tricuspid atresia]. A left thoracotomy scar is used in the repair of aortic coarctation, ligation of patent arterial ducts, a left Blalock-Taussig shunt and occasionally a pulmonary artery band (a ligature placed around the main pulmonary artery to protect the lungs from high pressures in children with large VSDs).

Palpation

Always start the examination by feeling the femoral and brachial pulses simultaneously. A reduction in volume or absence of the femoral pulse is strongly suggestive of coarctation of the aorta and should prompt closer examination and investigation. Although classically textbooks talk of radiofemoral delay this really only becomes appreciable as the child reaches adult size. Some children who have had previous procedures have an absent femoral pulse on one side only. It is, therefore, advisable to examine both femoral pulses.

Palpation for an enlarged liver should then be undertaken. The liver enlarges in heart failure and can reach below the umbilicus in some children. The liver is often quite soft and difficult to feel in infants, particularly if the child is struggling so great care must be taken.

The heart enlarges in response to any chronic volume load. This may arise because of a right to left shunt, ASD, VSD, PDA and AVSD, because of valve dysfunction, mitral regurgitation, aortic regurgitation and pulmonary regurgitation or because of a primary myocardial abnormality, viral myocarditis and dilated cardiomyopathy. In younger children, this can be felt as a sub-xyphoid heave by palpating just below the inferior end of the sternum. Children of all ages with a volume loaded heart may have a parasternal heave felt with the palm of the hand on the left side.

Finish off palpation by carefully placing your index finger in the suprasternal notch feeling for a thrill. If one is present, it is strongly suggestive of aortic stenosis, although rarely pulmonary stenosis and a PDA can produce this sign.

Auscultation

Auscultation is often difficult in children. The combination of fast heart rate, noisy breathing and a poorly cooperative child make it the most challenging part of the examination. To ensure that nothing is missed you should follow a fixed pattern when listening to a child's heart. I would suggest listening with the diaphragm at all points over the left side of the praecordium, followed by the right upper sternal edge and at the back. At each point, it is important to listen to systole, diastole and the heart sounds in turn. All can provide vital diagnostic information that is easy to miss when distracted by a loud, obvious systolic murmur. Murmurs are classically graded to permit easy comparison, systolic murmurs out of 6 and diastolic out of 4 **(Table 8.4)**.

A full discussion of the auscultatory findings associated with different abnormalities will follow under the specific conditions.

Innocent Murmurs

By definition, an innocent murmur has no association with the heart disease; however, it is an extremely common finding, reason for referral and some clarification is needed. Innocent murmurs can be heard in up to 80% of children at some point. They can cause considerable diagnostic confusion so if you are in doubt get a more

TABLE 8.4 Grading of heart murmurs.

Murmur	*1*	*2*	*3*	*4*	*5*	*6*
Systolic	Barely audible	Quiet	Easily audible	Associated with thrill	Audible without stethoscope	Audible from end of bed
Diastolic	Quiet	Easily audible	Associated with thrill	Audible without stethoscope		

experienced opinion. Innocent murmurs, all have an otherwise normal cardiovascular examination, are always systolic, often vary with posture and usually have a characteristic quality. Some murmurs are soft, short and heard only at the left sternal edge; others have a typical vibratory quality much like humming and can be quite loud. These are known as Still murmurs. A venous hum is also common, particularly when a child is examined standing up. It is heard beneath either clavicle and extends through systole into diastole sometimes sounding like an arterial duct. Unlike a duct, however, a venous hum disappears as a child rotates his head or is supine.

A positive diagnosis of an innocent murmur enables the examining doctor to be very reassuring with the family that the heart is structurally normal.

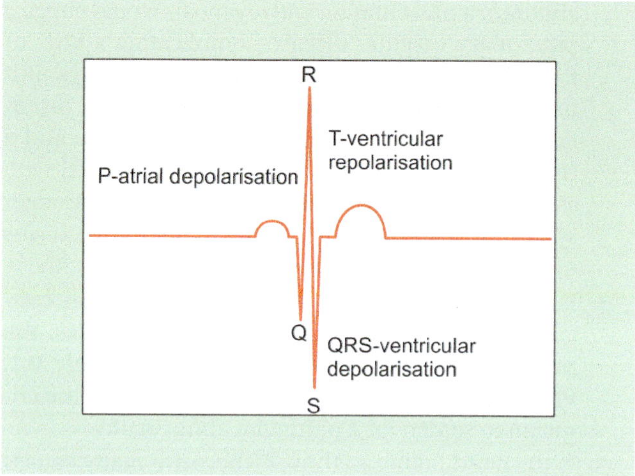

Figure 8.1 ECG complex diagram.

Investigations

Many heart conditions result in failure to thrive in infancy; therefore, height and weight should always be measured and plotted on a centile chart. Where possible, to complete the examination, the child's saturation should be measured using a pulse oximeter. When using this equipment, care should be taken to ensure that the child's peripheries are warm, well-perfused and the oximeter should be left in place on the child for at least 30 seconds to allow stabilisation of the reading. Measurement of the right brachial blood pressure should be made using the correctly sized cuff for the child. If coarctation is a possibility, many advocate the comparison of blood pressure measurements between arm and leg. In author's experience, he has found that this comparison is misleading and does not place great emphasis on its importance. If there is any suspicion of endocarditis, a urine sample should be analysed for haemolysed blood and proteinuria.

Electrocardiography

Electrocardiography is a simple noninvasive tool that records the electrical activity of the heart. A study is performed by attaching recording electrodes to specific sites on the skin to obtain raw recordings of cardiac electrical activity. These recordings are then processed to produce recognised "leads" that are printed out for examination. The electrical activity associated with each heart beat can be seen as a sequence of waves denoted as P, Q, R, S and T **(Fig. 8.1)**. These different leads look at the heart from different aspects allowing information to be obtained from most areas. By analysing the electrical activity of the heart, the precise heart rate and rhythm can be identified; the electrical axis can be measured, as can the heights and durations of the various waves. These measurements give information about the size and thickness of the various heart chambers, areas of ischaemic or infarction, and about abnormalities of conduction that might predispose the child to arrhythmias.

Chest X-ray

Where echo is available, a chest X-ray is not needed to make a diagnosis. However, it remains useful in assessing the severity of an abnormality and monitoring response to treatment. From a cardiac point of view, a chest X-ray provides information about the size of the heart, the pulmonary blood flow and about associated lung abnormalities.

An increased cardiothoracic ratio (over 0.6 in infancy and 0.55 in childhood) suggests enlargement of one or more chambers of the heart indicating volume loading or reduced function. Serial assessments of the cardiothoracic ratio may, therefore, provide information regarding change in severity of the problem over time or the effect of treatment.

Assessment of the pulmonary vasculature may provide information on the volume of pulmonary blood flow. This may be useful when assessing the significance of a moderate sized left to right cardiac shunt in a child; plethoric lung fields would indicate excessive pulmonary

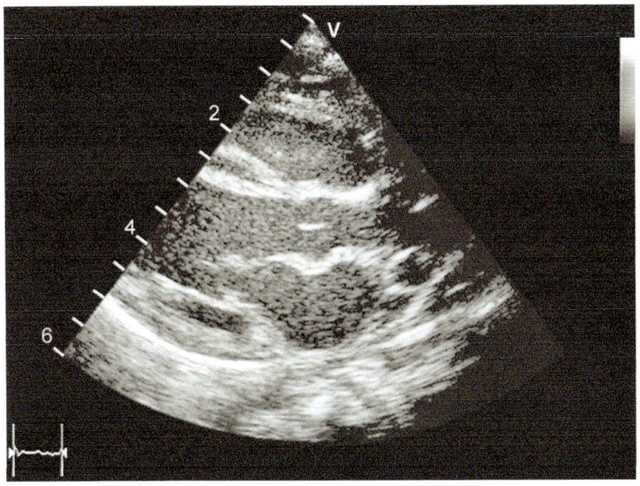

Figure 8.2 Normal parasternal long-axis echocardiogram.

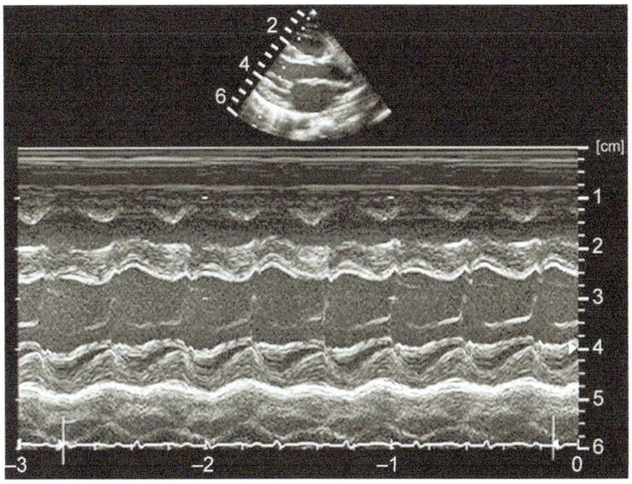

Figure 8.3 Normal M-mode echocardiogram through left ventricle.

blood flow and, therefore, a haemodynamically significant abnormality. In a cyanosed newborn infant, oligaemic lung fields might suggest a cardiac lesion resulting in reduced pulmonary blood flow such as TOF or pulmonary atresia (PAt).

The finding of associated lung abnormalities can give useful information about the significance of the heart lesion or otherwise. Collapse of the left lower lobe is particularly common in children with left atrial enlargement, aspiration due to gastro-oesophageal reflux disease is more common in breathless infants with cardiac problems and the finding of vertebral or rib abnormalities may suggest a generalised syndromic abnormality rather than an isolated cardiac problem.

Echocardiography

Echocardiography is essentially ultrasound of the heart. The differences compared with conventional ultrasound are the hardware and software settings that are configured to view the rapidly moving structures within the heart. Four main types of imaging are used that look at various aspects of cardiac function.

1. Two-dimensional or cross-sectional echo produces conventional ultrasound-type images of the heart structures moving in real time (Fig. 8.2). This modality facilitates accurate anatomical diagnosis of heart conditions by imaging how the various structures relate to each other.
2. M-mode echo takes a single line through the heart and plots all the information obtained against a time axis (Fig. 8.3). This mode is used for measurements and calculations particularly concerning ventricular function.
3. Doppler ultrasound measures the velocity of blood moving through the heart and great vessels. Using this data, it is possible to estimate pressure differences at various points in the heart such as across the aortic, pulmonary, mitral and tricuspid valves, a VSD or PDA and thus measure the severity of any narrowing or estimate the absolute pressure in a particular chamber.
4. Colour Doppler imaging superimposes Doppler information on blood flow on the moving two-dimensional image of the heart. The technique uses different colours to represent both the direction of blood flow and its velocity (Fig. 8.4). This mode allows the identification of valve leaks or heart defects that might not be seen on two-dimensional imaging alone.

Echocardiography is now the mainstay of paediatric cardiac diagnosis. The availability of high-quality machines at relatively low cost has expanded the routine use of this valuable technique such that it is now often undertaken by specialists in neonatology and general paediatrics as well as paediatric cardiologists.

Cardiac Catheter

Cardiac catheterisation is both a diagnostic and treatment tool. Long thin plastic tubes (catheters) are introduced into a vein or artery and threaded though the various chambers of the heart. Direct pressure and oxygen saturation measurements are taken, and radio-opaque contrast is injected into the heart to outline various structures and abnormalities. This technique has evolved over recent years to permit many common cardiac anomalies to be treated using this minimally invasive approach. Suitable ASDs, patent arterial ducts, VSDs, stenotic pulmonary and aortic valves as well as aortic coarctation can all be treated by the transcatheter route using specialised techniques.

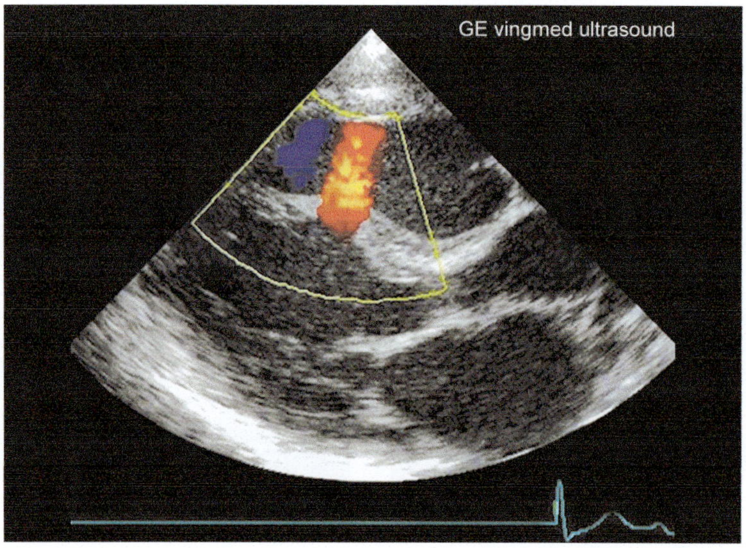

Figure 8.4 Colour flow Doppler echocardiogram demonstrating small mid-septal muscular ventricular septal defect.

CONGENITAL HEART ABNORMALITIES

Acyanotic Congenital Heart Disease

Ventricular Septal Defect

Ventricular septal defect is the most common congenital heart abnormality accounting for a fifth of all lesions. It is caused by a defect in the septum that divides the two ventricles. Defects can exist in the muscular septum (muscular defects) or in the membranous septum (perimembranous defects). The symptoms and signs result from the flow of blood between the two ventricles through the defect. At birth, the resistance to flow through the lungs is equal to the resistance to flow to the body, that is, the pulmonary vascular resistance (PVR) is equal to the systemic vascular resistance (SVR). Consequently, little blood will pass through the VSD and no murmur will be audible. Over the first few days of life, the PVR falls resulting in a drop in right ventricular pressure encouraging flow through a VSD and into the pulmonary circulation. When a VSD is present, blood can exit the left ventricle through both aorta and VSD increasing the required output of the left ventricle. The VSD flow will increase the overall pulmonary arterial flow and thus venous return to the left atrium **(Fig. 8.5)**. The left heart, therefore, has to cope with increased volumes and enlarges producing a characteristic heave. Defects vary widely in size and position, as do the clinical features.

The majority of defects are small communications between the two ventricles through the perimembranous or muscular septum. These usually present as asymptomatic murmurs and require only reassurance as most will close spontaneously and it is unlikely the remainder would ever need to be closed. Clinically small muscular defects can be recognised by the typical high-pitched, harsh, pansystolic murmur, often well localised over the left precordium. The exact position of the murmur is dependent on the location of the defect within the septum. The absence of a precordial or sub-xyphoid heave confirms the lack of a significant left to right shunt, and normal intensity of the second heart sound demonstrates normal pulmonary artery pressure. Small perimembranous defects can be indistinguishable from muscular defects, although the murmur tends to be higher on the left parasternal border. When a perimembranous defect is suspected the early diastolic murmur of aortic regurgitation must be excluded, as this would constitute an indication for repair.

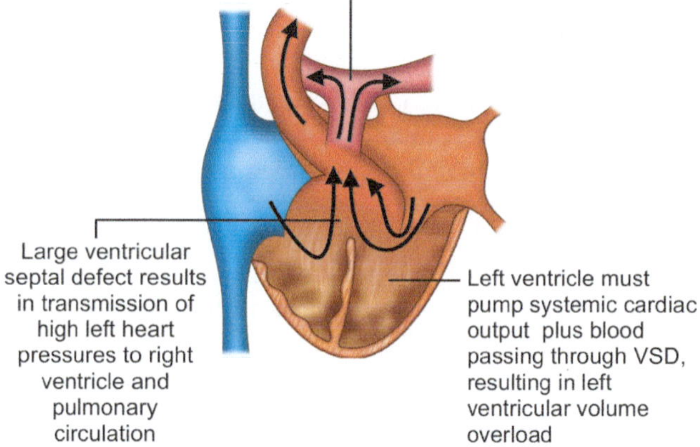

Figure 8.5 Ventricular septal (VSD): left heart volume overload.

Moderate-sized defects, either muscular or perimembranous, usually have a louder murmur. With an increase in the volume of blood flowing through the defect, there is a corresponding increase in the stroke volume of the left ventricle producing a parasternal and sub-xiphoid heave. In large defects, blood flow through the VSD is less turbulent and the murmur will be quieter or even absent in completely unrestrictive defects. In these large defects, the heave is usually marked unless the PVR is elevated. With increasing size of defect, there is a proportional increase in the pulmonary artery pressure resulting in a loud pulmonary component of the second heart sound.

Infants with moderate to large defects develop the classical signs of heart failure as the PVR falls and the shunt increases. Typically, they fail to thrive and feed poorly due to breathlessness and gut oedema. On examination, they are tachypnoeic, tachycardic and sweaty have hepatomegaly a marked heave, variable systolic murmur, loud second heart sound and a summation gallop (combined third and fourth heart sounds producing a noise similar to a horse galloping).

With a significant VSD, the ECG may show the evidence of biventricular hypertrophy and a sinus tachycardia. The chest X-ray will show cardiomegaly and plethoric lung fields. Diagnosis can be confirmed by echocardiogram that will demonstrate the position and size of the defect exclude or confirm additional lesions, measure the size of the left ventricle which will reflect the degree of left to right shunt, and using Doppler estimate the right ventricular pressures to demonstrate any pulmonary hypertension.

Management *Large defects*: Treatment is aimed at stabilisation of the infant and encouragement of growth prior to surgical repair. The mainstays of therapy include nasogastric feeding to maximise caloric intake and minimise the energy expended during feeding. Medical therapy can be used to treat the symptoms of the intracardiac shunt and include diuretics treat the compensatory salt and water retention that is a consequence of heart failure, angiotensin-converting enzyme (ACE) inhibitors such as captopril reduce left ventricular afterload and encourage systemic flow. Digoxin can be used to combat excessive tachycardia and maximise myocardial efficiency. Caution should be exercised when using oxygen as it can cause pulmonary vasodilatation effectively worsening heart failure. Where infants have respiratory distress in the presence of a significant VSD, continuous positive airway pressure (CPAP) with high flow air may be of benefit by increasing the intra-alveolar pressure to avoid end-expiratory collapse whilst avoiding excessive pulmonary vasodilation and subsequent increase in intracardiac shunt.

Ultimately, the majority of children with large defects will require surgical closure of the defect. Where open cardiac surgery is available, repair will usually be undertaken within 6 months to prevent the development of pulmonary vascular disease. Where only closed procedures are possible a pulmonary artery band can be applied to protect the lungs from excessive blood flow and high pressure, permitting later closure.

Children with small to moderate defects may need no therapy at all, if the haemodynamic shunt is small. Others may slowly develop left heart overload and require repair later in life, a number of these being suitable for transcatheter closure using one of the growing number of catheter deployable devices. A small number of children with subaortic defects will develop aortic regurgitation, which is an indication for repair.

Untreated infants with large defects may die, usually from concomitant respiratory infections. Alternatively, the symptoms may resolve from 6 months onwards as PVR increases due to inflammation and thickening of the pulmonary arterioles. These changes usually become irreversible at approximately 6–12 months, tending to slowly worsen thereafter. When the effective PVR becomes greater than the SVR, the haemodynamic shunt through the VSD will reverse and the child will become cyanosed. This situation is known as Eisenmenger syndrome and will not improve with correction of the original cardiac defect.

Patent Ductus Arteriosus

The arterial duct is a vital foetal structure that connects the main pulmonary artery to the aorta. In utero, it allows blood to pass directly to the aorta from the pulmonary artery avoiding the high resistance pulmonary circulation. This "right to left" shunt exists because the PVR exceeds the SVR. At birth, the rise in blood oxygen concentration together with a reduction in circulating prostaglandins usually causes spasm of the duct with eventual permanent closure. Ongoing patency of the duct beyond the immediate neonatal period results in the development of a "left to right" shunt from aorta to pulmonary artery as the PVR drops (Fig. 8.6). The significance of this varies depending upon the size of the child and size of the duct.

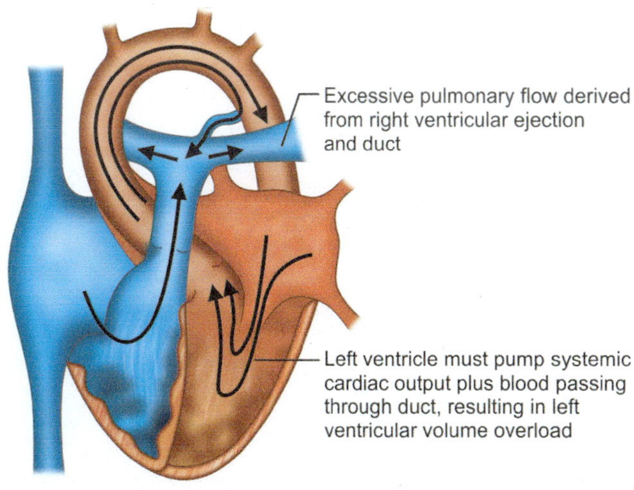

Figure 8.6 Patent ductus arteriosus: left heart volume overload.

Preterm infants have an increased risk of PDA. In this group, the flow of blood through the duct results in excessive pulmonary blood flow, increased pulmonary venous return to the left heart, with subsequent chamber enlargement.

The infant is often breathless and may have high ventilation requirements that can result in ventilator induced lung disease. They will have high volume pulses, a left precordial heave and a systolic or continuous murmur. Term infants with a significant PDA may present with failure to thrive, together with signs of left heart overload and a murmur. The murmur is continuous (extends throughout systole and into diastole), heard best below the left clavicle and has a "machinery" character. Usually older children have small, asymptomatic ducts that are detected either during routine auscultation at a medical check or during an echocardiogram undertaken for an unrelated problem.

Because the haemodynamic effects are similar to those seen in a child with a VSD, the ECG and chest X-ray findings are similar. Echocardiogram allows an appreciation of the size of the duct **(Fig. 8.7)**, as well as assessment of the shunt by the left heart chamber size (often comparing the left atrium to the aorta) and the pulmonary artery pressure using Doppler.

Management Preterm infants with large ducts require duct closure. This can often be accomplished using non-steroidal anti-inflammatory drugs, the most frequently used of which is intravenous indomethacin (three to six doses, 0.1–0.2 mg/kg, 12–24 hours apart). Intravenous ibuprofen has also been used recently with similar success rates and a lower adverse effect rate. If these drugs fail to achieve permanent closure, surgical ligation can be used with a high success rate and low complication rate. In symptomatic children beyond term the duct can be closed either surgically or more commonly by the transcatheter route. Prior to closure symptomatic improvement can be achieved by the use of diuretics with or without digoxin. In the asymptomatic child, closure is only indicated where a murmur is heard. In most cases, this is done to reduce the risk of endocarditis, as the possibility of left heart enlargement is small. In children where there is no murmur and the PDA is only detected by echocardiogram, no treatment (including antibiotic prophylaxis) is indicated.

Atrial Septal Defect

Isolated ASDs rarely cause symptoms in childhood. The most common type of ASD is the secundum defect, which is formed by a gap in the centre of the atrial septum. Less common is the primum type [also called a partial or incomplete AVSD (see below)], where a gap exists low down in the atrial septum adjacent to the mitral and tricuspid valves. In some primum defects, there is also a gap or cleft in the anterior mitral valve leaflet which can result in valve regurgitation. The left to right shunt at atrial level seen in ASD produces enlargement of the right heart **(Fig. 8.8)**.

An ASD may produce no detectable signs; however, with a significant haemodynamic shunt, a heave can be present along with flow murmurs across the pulmonary (systolic) and rarely tricuspid (diastolic) valves. In addition, a characteristic fixed widely split second heart sound may be heard.

The ECG in a secundum defect will show right axis deviation, whereas it will be leftward or superior with a primum defect. As the right ventricle enlarges, a partial right bundle branch block pattern will develop (RSR' in V4R and V1). The chest X-ray will reveal cardiomegaly resulting from enlargement of the right heart structures. Echo confirms size and position of the defect, excludes associated anomalies such as pulmonary valve stenosis and allows assessment of the shunt size by measuring the right ventricular size.

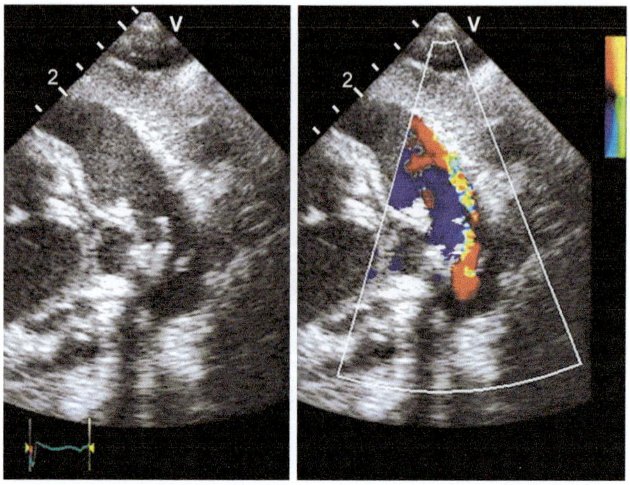

Figure 8.7 Patent ductus arteriosus: Colour Doppler echocardiogram.

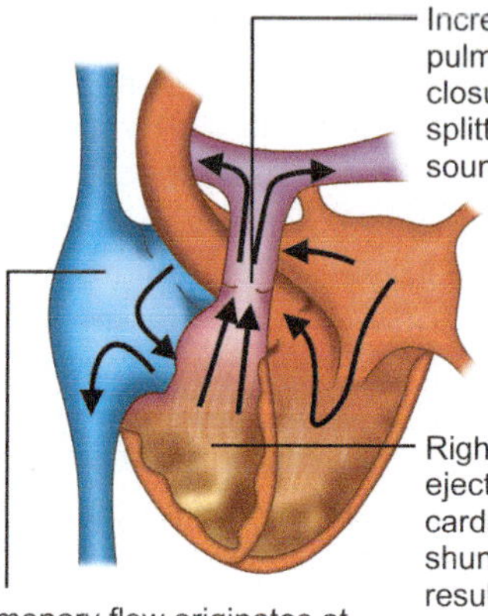

Figure 8.8 Atrial septal defect (ASD): right heart volume overload.

Management It is unusual for an ASD to produce symptoms in childhood and medical therapy is rarely required. Untreated a significant ASD will cause enlargement of the right ventricle with reduction in function and symptoms of reduced stamina and exertional dyspnoea. Chronic atrial enlargement can cause arrhythmias in adulthood. Unlike VSDs, spontaneous closure is rare and therefore closure is indicated where the ASD is felt to be haemodynamically significant as suggested by an increase in the right ventricular size. Interventional catheter techniques can now be used to close many secundum ASDs, although open surgery remains the only treatment for primum defects.

Atrioventricular Septal Defect

Atrioventricular septal defect results from a failure of fusion of the endocardial cushions in the centre of the heart. Defects are said to be complete where a ventricular defect is present and incomplete where the defect is restricted to the atria (**Fig. 8.9**). The inlet valves (tricuspid and mitral) are abnormal and usually composed partly of common (bridging) leaflets that sit across the septal defects. AVSDs are particularly common in Down syndrome where they may be associated with TOF.

Incomplete AVSD, as with all types of ASD, usually presents as an asymptomatic murmur. An isolated atrial defect will cause right ventricular enlargement detectable as a precordial heave. The systolic and diastolic murmurs are similar to other forms of ASD; however, if there is significant mitral regurgitation through a cleft in the anterior mitral valve leaflet, left ventricular enlargement is likely together with an apical systolic murmur.

The presentation of complete AVSD will vary according to the size of the ventricular component. Small ventricular component defects present in a very similar way to incomplete AVSDs; however, it is more common for there to be a large ventricular component which will present with symptoms of heart failure in a similar way to large VSDs. It is not surprising that it can often be difficult to distinguish clinically between VSD and AVSD.

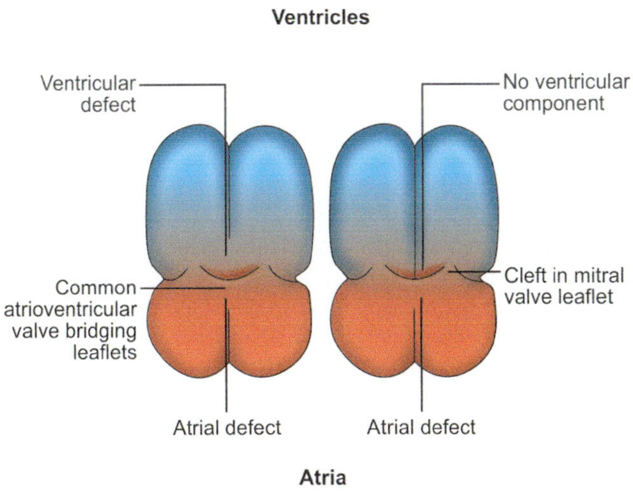

Figure 8.9 Atrioventricular septal defect (AVSD): complete versus incomplete AVSD.

The characteristic finding on electrocardiography is leftward or superior deviation of the QRS axis. This permits distinction from secundum ASD and VSD. Chest X-ray findings depend largely on the size of ventricular defect present and effective left to right shunt. Typically, it will show an enlarged cardiac silhouette and plethoric lung fields.

Management

No AVSD will resolve spontaneously and all need surgical repair. Where a child presents with heart failure due to a large ventricular component, the medical management is as described for VSD. The timing of surgery depends on the lesion; large ventricular components need repair within the first 6 months whereas if the pulmonary artery pressures are normal, providing the mitral leak is not severe, surgery can often be deferred many years.

Coarctation of the Aorta

A coarctation is an area of narrowing in the distal aortic arch that restricts flow to the lower half of the body. A coarctation occurs at the point at which the arterial duct inserts into the aorta, and it is likely that extension of ductal tissue into the aortic wall is responsible for the narrowing. Broadly speaking children with coarctation comprise two groups: (1) those that present in heart failure in infancy and (2) those that present as asymptomatic children or adults with a murmur or hypertension.

Infants

The more severe forms of coarctation present within the first few weeks of life. In these, children closure of the duct results in subtotal or even complete obstruction to the aorta (**Fig. 8.10**). The left heart fails due to the sudden increase in afterload, the lower half of the body including liver, kidneys and gut become ischaemic and a severe metabolic acidosis rapidly ensues. There is a very short history of poor feeding, breathlessness and poor colour. The infant will be grey, peripherally shut down, poorly responsive, cold, tachypnoeic, tachycardic, sweaty, have absent femoral pulses, hepatomegaly, a summation gallop and may or may not have a murmur.

Management This situation constitutes a medical emergency. The child should be resuscitated and vascular access obtained by whatever means possible. As a priority the child should be started on a prostaglandin E (0.01–0.1 μg/kg per minute) infusion as well as an intravenous inotrope (e.g. dopamine 5–20 μg/kg per minute). Prostaglandin E is used to open the arterial duct

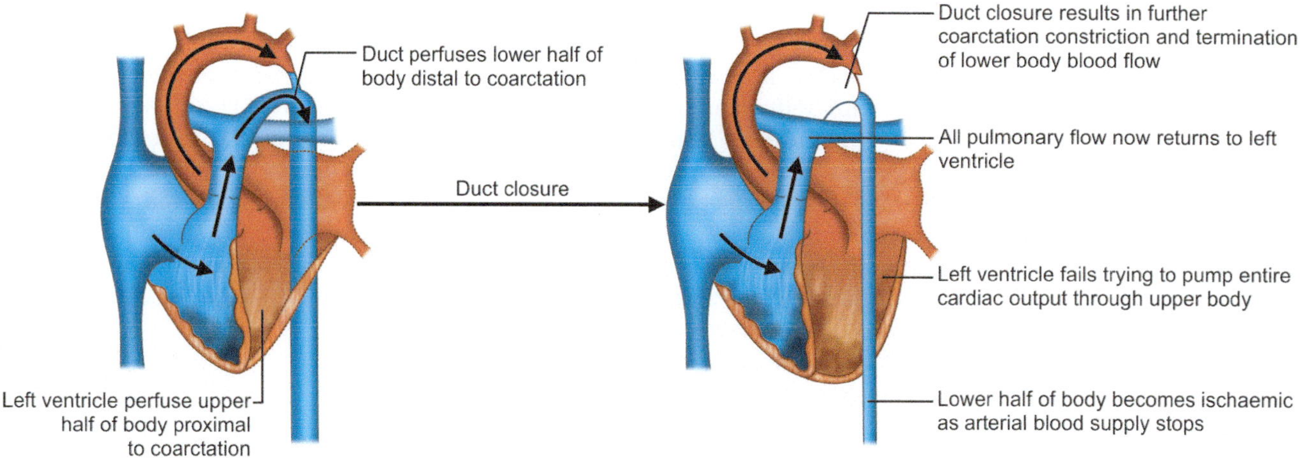

Figure 8.10 Aortic coarctation: effect of duct closure.

and also reduce the severity of the coarctation by relaxing the ductal tissue that may extend into the aortic wall. An unfortunate effect of prostaglandin E is that it can cause apnoea at therapeutic doses and the child may need intubation and ventilation.

Once the child has been resuscitated, a detailed assessment can be made including ECG, chest X-ray and echo to both confirm the clinical diagnosis and exclude any associated lesion. At this age, surgical repair is the only option and should take place as soon as the child is stable. Prostaglandin should not be discontinued until time of repair.

Older Child

Older children, or adults with coarctation, usually present at routine examination with either reduced femoral pulses or hypertension. The narrowing is usually milder and will have progressed over a longer period of time allowing the child's circulation to adjust by developing collateral arteries around the obstruction. In some smaller children, there may be a history of failure to thrive but usually they are symptom free. Examination will show a well, pink child with reduced or absent femoral pulses, a loud second heart sound and a systolic murmur heard over the back at the left hand side of the spine. In teenagers and adults, there may be a delay in the timing of the femoral compared to the radial pulse, so-called radiofemoral delay. Hypertension may be present and four-limb blood pressure recording may reveal an arm/leg gradient, although its absence does not exclude the diagnosis.

The ECG will show evidence of left ventricular hypertrophy, particularly if the coarctation is longstanding and chest X-ray may show characteristic features such as double aortic knuckle and rib notching **(Fig. 8.11)**. An echocardiogram will confirm the diagnosis, allows assessment of the severity and also excludes associated abnormalities such as a bicuspid aortic valve or a VSD.

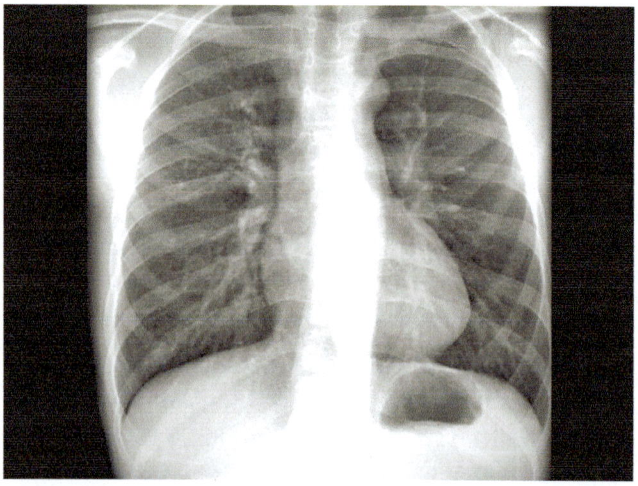

Figure 8.11 Aortic coarctation chest X-ray showing double aortic knuckle and rib notching.

Management Hypertension should be treated carefully, taking care not to reduce the blood pressure excessively as this may precipitate renal failure. Classically coarctation has always been repaired surgically; however, in teenagers and adults, balloon angioplasty with insertion of a Goretex Covered metal stent has become the treatment of choice in many large centres.

Following repair, long-term surveillance is required to watch for restenosis and aneurysm formation at the site of repair. In the long-term patients with coarctation are at risk of hypertension and also intracerebral aneurysms.

Aortic Stenosis

Obstruction of the left ventricular outlet usually occurs at the level of the valve. Less commonly a fibrous ring or membrane can cause sub-valve obstruction, and rarely the obstruction can occur above the valve (e.g. Williams syndrome associated with branch pulmonary stenosis,

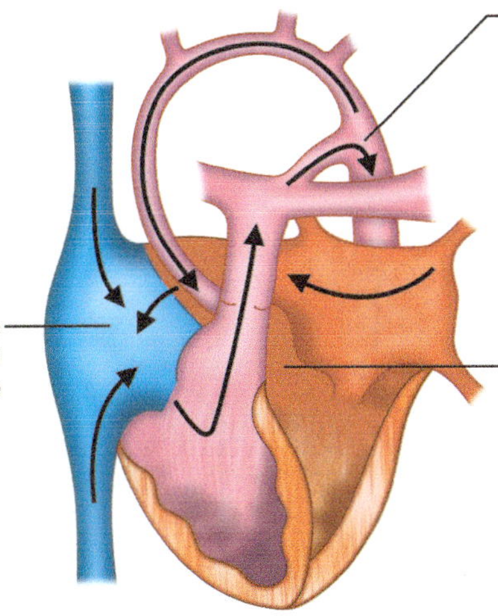

Figure 8.12 Duct-dependent systemic circulation.

hypercalcaemia, mental retardation and elfin facies). Valve obstruction is more common in boys and results from either a bicuspid valve or fusion of the valve cusps with or without dysplasia of the valve tissue. Whilst it is often an isolated lesion, severe aortic stenosis is a key feature of HLHS.

As with most lesions presentation depends on severity. Mild aortic stenosis is usually due to a bicuspid valve and produces no symptoms. It will only be detected in childhood as an asymptomatic murmur, usually preceded by a characteristic ejection click that helps to distinguish it from sub-aortic stenosis. The murmur is heard at the upper left sternal edge, radiates to the neck and is often associated with a thrill in the suprasternal notch. If severe obstruction occurs early in foetal life, it may progress to HLHS by the time of birth; however, more commonly severe aortic stenosis presents in the newborn period as a duct-dependent lesion (in such children the arterial duct permits blood to flow from right to left effectively providing or augmenting the systemic cardiac output) **(Fig. 8.12)**. The child will be cyanosed, possibly with a drop in saturations between upper and lower limbs, and have the characteristic ejection systolic murmur and ejection click (short sharp sound heard immediately before the murmur). Upon closure of the duct, the child may develop a low cardiac output state with poor pulses, cool peripheries, tachypnoea, tachycardia and hepatomegaly.

Children with moderate aortic stenosis usually present with an asymptomatic murmur. The degree of stenosis gradually progresses as the child grows causing exertional dyspnoea when severe angina or syncope. These late symptoms are associated with a risk of sudden death and require urgent investigation and treatment.

Although the chest X-ray may be normal even in quite severe aortic stenosis, the ECG will usually show evidence of left ventricular hypertrophy often with the characteristic ST changes of left ventricular strain **(Fig. 8.13)**. ECG will confirm the diagnosis and also estimate its severity using Doppler. In addition, it will demonstrate any associated aortic regurgitation.

Management

The indications for treating aortic valve stenosis are either symptoms (angina or syncope) or evidence of left ventricular hypertrophy and strain. Where a patient has symptoms directly attributable to the aortic stenosis they should be advised to restrict physical activity and avoid exertion. There is no form of medical treatment indicated and relief of obstruction can be achieved by balloon valvuloplasty, surgical valvotomy or valve replacement. Valvuloplasty and valvotomy are palliative procedures designed to relieve the obstruction temporarily to allow the child to reach adult size before they require a valve replacement. The uncontrolled nature of both techniques produces the risk of aortic valve regurgitation which although well tolerated will in time produce enlargement of the left ventricle requiring a valve replacement. Transcatheter aortic valve replacement is not yet a possibility in childhood.

Sub-aortic stenosis should be treated where there are symptoms and/or evidence of left ventricular strain on the ECG or aortic regurgitation on the echo. Surgical resection is the only treatment option currently available and unfortunately there is a risk of recurrence of the stenosis soon after repair.

Pulmonary Stenosis

As with aortic stenosis, pulmonary stenosis most commonly occurs at the valve itself but can be seen below the valve (e.g. TOF), above the valve or in the pulmonary branches. Valve stenosis results from fusion or dysplasia of the valve cusps and in isolation is a relatively common abnormality.

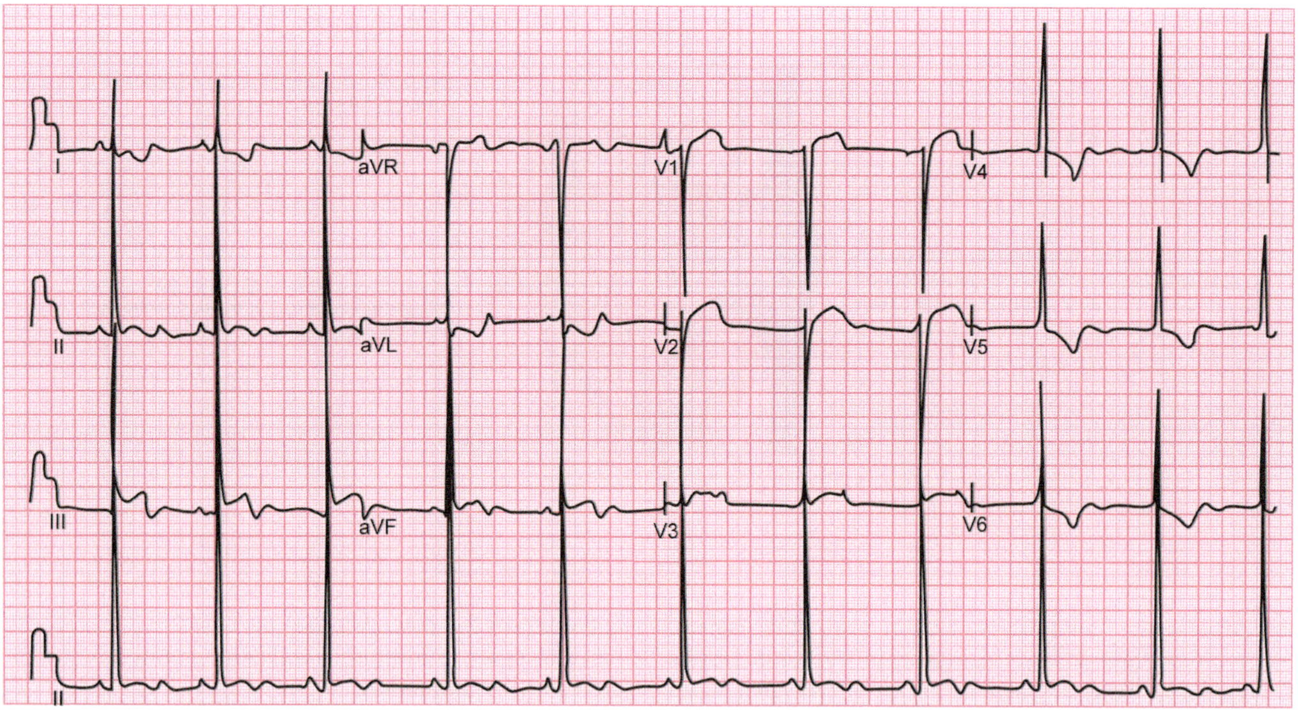

Figure 8.13 ECG showing left ventricular hypertrophy.

Mild pulmonary valve stenosis presents with an asymptomatic ejection systolic murmur and click. The murmur tends to be heard more to the left than with aortic stenosis, may radiate to the back and is not usually associated with a suprasternal thrill. The second heart sound is often quiet and a heave will only be present in the more severe lesions. Mild or even moderately severe pulmonary stenosis can improve in childhood, thus a "wait and see" approach is often appropriate at presentation.

Severe pulmonary stenosis will present in the newborn, lesion, as a duct-dependent lesion. Whereas in aortic stenosis, the arterial duct allows the systemic circulation to be augmented by the pulmonary side, in pulmonary stenosis the converse is true and pulmonary blood flow is derived largely from the aorta **(Fig. 8.14)**. Prior to the duct closure, the infants will be cyanosed (due to a right to left shunt at atrial level), have a characteristic systolic murmur but be otherwise well. Duct closure will herald hypoxia, acidosis and an abrupt deterioration in the child.

The ECG will demonstrate right axis deviation and right ventricular hypertrophy. In more severe cases, *P. pulmonale* and partial right bundle branch block will be present. Chest X-ray may show poststenotic dilation of the pulmonary artery as a bulge around the left hilum together with oligaemic lung fields. As with aortic stenosis, echo will confirm the diagnosis and estimate severity using Doppler. It will also confirm that the right ventricle has grown to a size that will support a normal biventricular circulation.

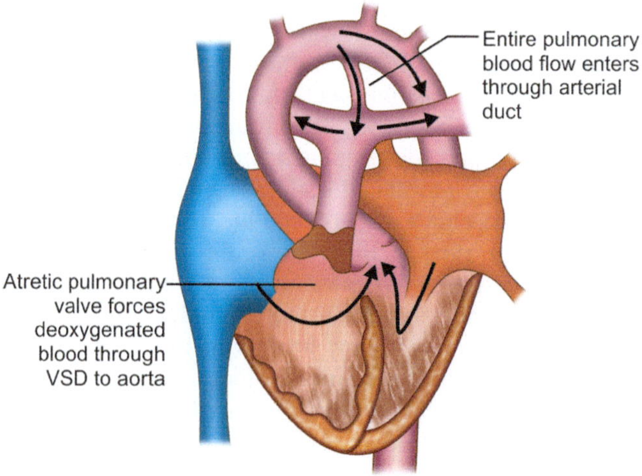

Figure 8.14 Duct-dependent pulmonary circulation.

Management

Transcatheter balloon valvuloplasty is now the treatment of choice for this lesion, producing good results with a very low requirement for re-intervention. The exception to this is in Noonan syndrome where the pulmonary valve is often severely thickened and classically unresponsive to valvuloplasty. In such cases, open surgical valvotomy is still indicated. Balloon valvotomy is generally a very effective treatment for this problem, although in newborns with severe obstruction, relief of the stenosis can precipitate dynamic sub-pulmonary obstruction which will usually resolve over a period of a few weeks.

CYANOTIC CONGENITAL HEART DISEASE

Tetralogy of Fallot

Tetralogy is the most common form of cyanotic congenital heart disease comprising up to 10% of all lesions. It is associated with Down syndrome, deletions of chromosome 22 (DiGeorge syndrome) and VACTERL (vertebral defects, anal atresia, tracheo-oesophageal atresia, sacral aplasia, renal and limb abnormalities), although it usually occurs in isolation. Classically it was described as the tetrad of VSD, right ventricular outflow tract obstruction, aorta overriding the crest of the ventricular septum and right ventricular hypertrophy. In effect only two of these factors are important in the pathogenesis; a completely unrestrictive VSD and significant obstruction to pulmonary blood flow **(Fig. 8.15)**.

Presentation depends on the degree of obstruction to pulmonary blood flow. The level of obstruction varies but usually comprises a degree of muscular sub-valve (infundibular) obstruction together with either valve or supravalve stenosis. Because the VSD is large and does not restrict flow, if there is mild to moderate pulmonary obstruction, there will be no net flow through the VSD and the child will be in a balanced state, sometimes called a "pink tetralogy." With more severe obstruction deoxygenated blood will flow right to left across the defect resulting in cyanosis. The obstruction tends to progress as the infundibular muscle hypertrophy increases culminating in a behaviour known as "spelling." During a hypercyanotic spell without warning the cyanosis becomes acutely worse. This may occur when the child has just been fed, is falling asleep, waking up or when upset. It is likely a reduction in the SVR causes an increase in right to left shunt. This leaves the right ventricle underfilled permitting increased systolic contraction and worsening of the muscular sub-pulmonary stenosis. The cycle is self-perpetuating and may result in hypoxic syncope and convulsions. Children with this problem often develop a behaviour known as squatting, during which they crouch down; effectively increasing the SVR as well as increasing venous return.

On examination infants with tetralogy have a characteristic ejection systolic murmur of pulmonary stenosis radiating through to the back with no ejection click. A right ventricular heave is invariably present. The degree of cyanosis varies in newborns, but tends to worsen as the child grows and if prolonged will result in clubbing of the digits and the plethoric facies of polycythaemia. The child's growth may be affected, although in isolated tetralogy weight gain is often normal. ECG demonstrates right axis deviation and right ventricular hypertrophy. Chest X-ray typically shows a "boot-shaped" heart with upturned apex and oligaemic lung fields **(Fig. 8.16)**. The diagnosis together with the level and severity of the pulmonary obstruction can be determined by transthoracic echo, which can help to exclude associated anomalies such as an AVSD or right aortic arch.

Untreated tetralogy has a poor prognosis. Progressive sub-pulmonary obstruction results in increasing cyanosis, poor exercise tolerance, increasingly frequent hypercyanotic spells and syncope. The obligatory right to left shunt also causes an increased susceptibility to brain abscesses.

Management

The degree of cyanosis determines the timing of intervention. If a child is pink or only mildly desaturated at presentation, it is appropriate to keep them under observation

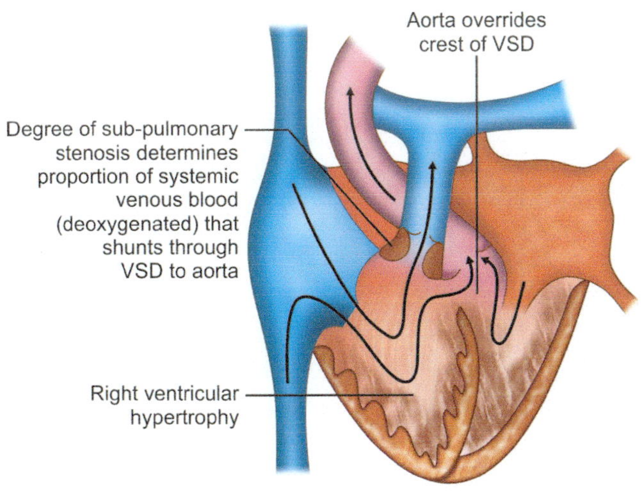

Figure 8.15 Tetralogy of Fallot diagram.

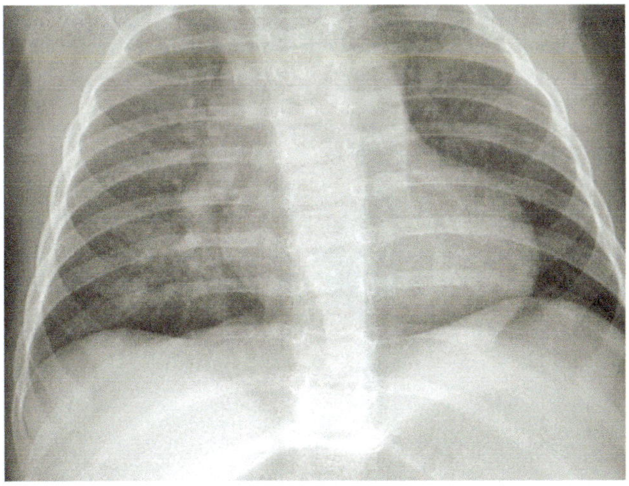

Figure 8.16 Chest X-ray, tetralogy of Fallot showing a "boot-shaped" heart with upturned apex and oligaemic lung fields.

and this can be at a regular out-patient review once the arterial duct closure is confirmed. The timing of repair in a well child with only mild to moderate cyanosis (oxygen saturations of 75% or above) is controversial. Many centres would now opt to repair at 6 months of age to minimise the amount of infundibular muscle that needs to be resected. Other centres prefer to defer elective surgery until a year of age by which time the child will be significantly larger.

Where a child presents with either more than moderate cyanosis (oxygen saturation of less than 75%) or hypercyanotic spells, surgical intervention is required. If the child has not reached the age at which that centre would opt for complete repair, a palliative procedure would be undertaken most commonly in the form of a modified Blalock-Taussig shunt. This procedure involves placing a Gore-Tex tube between the subclavian artery and the pulmonary artery, usually on the right side, allowing blood to flow into the pulmonary circulation irrespective of any intracardiac obstruction. Full repair requires closure of the VSD, resection of the sub-pulmonary muscle and enlargement of the pulmonary valve orifice. Where the pulmonary valve annulus is small a patch is required to enlarge it, unfortunately rendering it regurgitant and introducing the possibility that a pulmonary valve replacement will be required later in life. Although the repair can be complex and requires full cardiopulmonary bypass, it now usually carries an operative mortality of less than 5%.

Hypercyanotic Spells

When a child presents with a hypercyanotic spell, it is important not to panic in front of the mother or child. Calmly tuck the child's knees up to their chest and place them on the parent's chest in this tucked position. Waft oxygen into the child's face but try not to upset them. If this is ineffective then venous access must be obtained and the child given intravenous volume (10 mL/kg), morphine (100 μg/kg) and propanolol (10 μg/kg) intravenously. Once stabilised, they can be commenced on propanolol 1 mg/kg three to four times per day until surgical repair or palliation can be undertaken.

Transposition of the Great Arteries

Transposition of the great arteries is the most common cause of cardiac cyanosis in newborns. It is more common in male infants and is not usually associated with any noncardiac abnormality.

In TGA, the pulmonary artery is connected to the left ventricle and the aorta to the right. Consequently deoxygenated blood circulates around the systemic circulation and oxygenated blood around the pulmonary circulation with mixing between the two circulations occurring through the foramen ovale and the arterial duct (Fig. 8.17). Following birth mixing continues and the child is usually well but cyanotic with an otherwise normal cardiovascular examination. When the duct shuts, mixing between the two circulations is only possible through the persistent foramen ovale (PFO), which is usually inadequate and so the child becomes hypoxic and acidotic. In this situation, the infant is unlikely to survive without urgent medical intervention.

When a VSD is present, this may permit more than adequate mixing to the extent that the child may have oxygen saturations in the low nineties even after the duct has shut. The natural history of TGA/VSD differs from that of isolated TGA. Untreated the children may develop heart failure as the PVR drops but will develop severe hypoxia and so are unlikely to die in the newborn period.

Chest X-ray demonstrates a typical egg-on-side appearance with a narrow mediastinum and usually increased pulmonary vascularity, although oligaemia can be present (Fig. 8.18). ECG shows right axis deviation and right ventricular hypertrophy. Echocardiogram confirms the diagnosis in addition to showing patency of the arterial

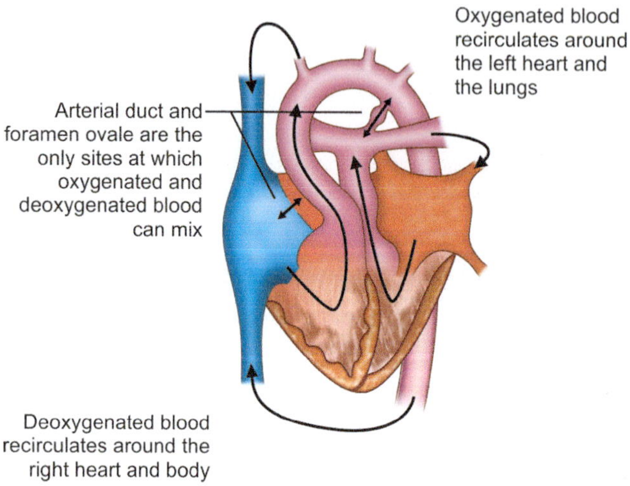

Figure 8.17 Transposition of the great arteries diagram.

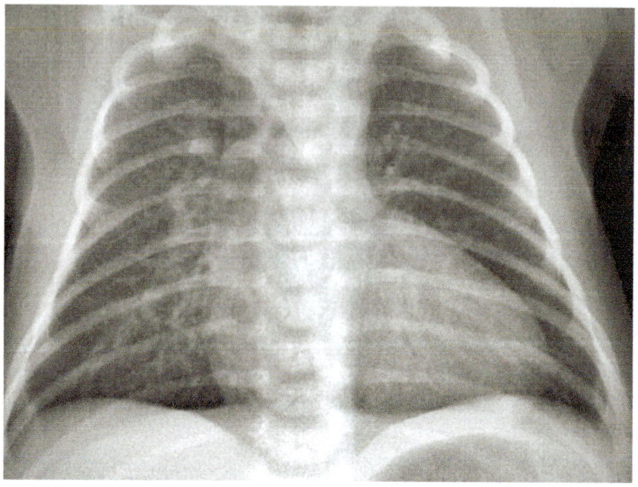

Figure 8.18 Chest X-ray showing transposition of the great arteries.

duct, adequacy of the foramen ovale, coronary artery positions and also any defects in the ventricular septum.

Management

If the infant is unwell, it is likely the arterial duct is narrow or closed. An infusion of prostaglandin E should be started urgently at a dose of 50–100 ng/kg per minute, accepting that the child may become apnoeic and require intubation. If the child improves at this dose, it can be reduced to 5–10 ng/kg per minute facilitating extubation. In addition to prostaglandin E, most infants will require augmentation of the foramen ovale by balloon atrial septostomy. This can be performed either through the umbilical vein or the femoral vein. A specialised balloon septostomy catheter is introduced into the right atrium and manipulated across into left atrium using echo guidance. Once in position the balloon is inflated with up to 4 mL of normal saline and jerked back across the septum using a sharp but controlled tug. The "jump" as the septum tears is usually palpable. Although the pullback may be repeated several times in practice once is often sufficient.

Surgical repair of transposition usually takes place at 1–2 weeks of life. This allows the infant to gain a little maturity, but does not permit the left ventricle to "detrain" by pumping to the low resistance pulmonary circulation for too long. The vast majority of infants with TGA now undergo an arterial switch procedure. This affords a complete anatomical repair by detaching the aorta, coronary arteries and pulmonary artery above the valve and reanastomosing them to the anatomically appropriate ventricles. Where the coronary artery positions are favourable, this produces an excellent repair with a risk of less than 5% in most centres.

Although they may remain deeply cyanosed, many children will survive into infancy without an arterial switch providing an adequate septostomy has been performed.

Tricuspid Atresia

This rare form of cyanotic congenital heart disease comprises less than 2% of all infants with a cardiac anomaly. Absence of normal RV filling in utero results in poor development of the right ventricular cavity, although most infants have a moderate-sized VSD allowing the pulmonary valve to develop reasonably well. Systemic venous return passes through the foramen ovale to mix with the pulmonary venous return before entering the left ventricle. The mixed blood then passes through the aortic valve to the systemic circulation where a proportion will pass to the pulmonary artery via a VSD or PDA (Fig. 8.19). In 30%, the great arteries are transposed and the aorta arises from the hypoplastic right ventricle. Some children, including all without a VSD, have significant obstruction to pulmonary blood flow and are duct dependent. Others have adequate flow through the VSD to the pulmonary circulation at birth; however, obstruction may develop rapidly in the first few weeks of life either at VSD level or in the sub-pulmonary area such that cyanosis becomes a major problem. A small number never develop obstruction and progress to heart failure when the PVR drops.

Usually cyanosis is obvious from birth and deepens with time. Such infants may fail to thrive, develop finger-clubbing and untreated are unlikely to survive more than 12 months. A systolic murmur at the mid left sternal edge may be present from the VSD or sub-pulmonary obstruction and the second heart sound will be single. Electrocardiography shows left axis deviation, which in a cyanotic child is virtually diagnostic of tricuspid atresia. Chest X-ray typically shows a "box" like cardiac silhouette with pulmonary oligaemia (Fig. 8.20). Echo will confirm the diagnosis and show with great detail the VSD and sub-pulmonary area. This allows a tentative prediction to be made regarding the development of obstruction to pulmonary flow.

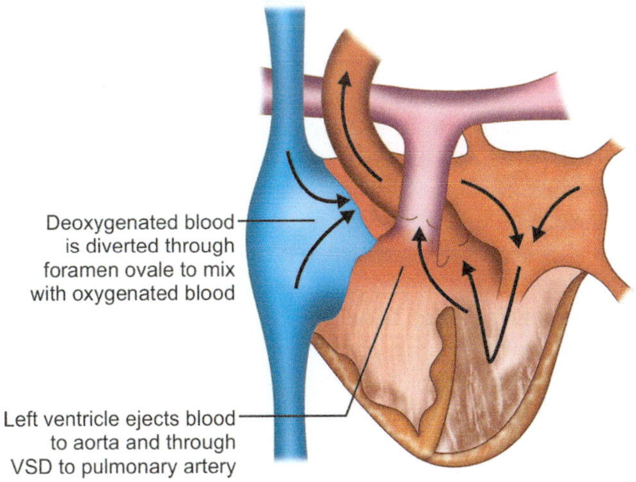

Figure 8.19 Tricuspid atresia.

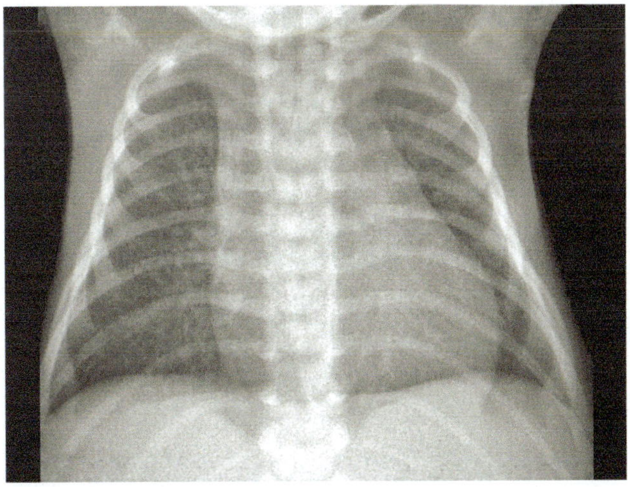

Figure 8.20 Chest X-ray tricuspid atresia.

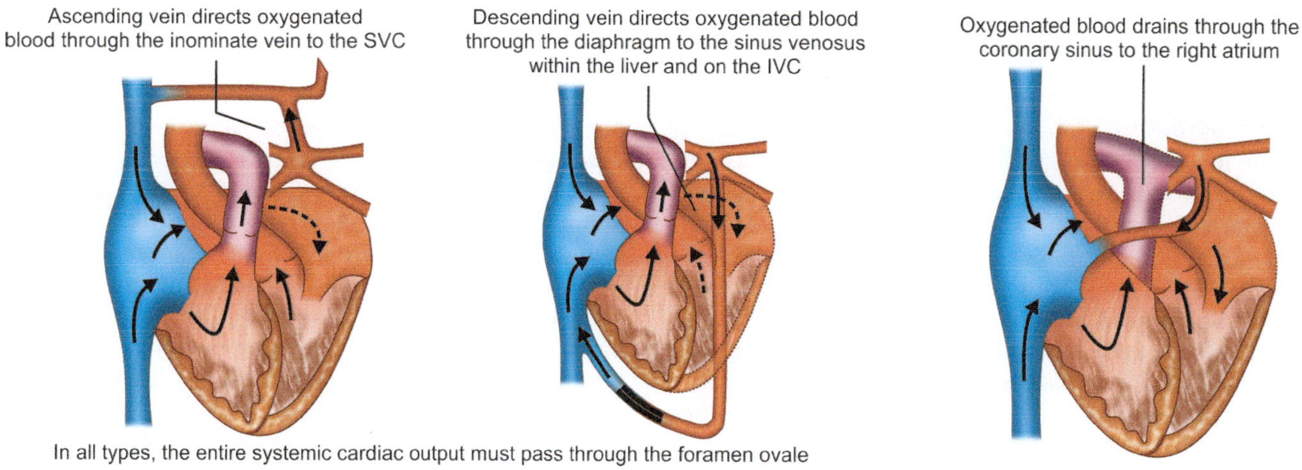

Figure 8.21 Total anomalous pulmonary venous drainage.

Management

Early palliation in excessively cyanotic infants is by a modified Blalock-Taussig shunt as described under TOF. Further palliation follows the Fontan-type pattern and will be summarised later in the univentricular heart section.

Total Anomalous Pulmonary Venous Drainage

This rare cyanotic abnormality accounts for less than 1% of all congenital heart disease; however, with recognition and early surgical repair, it is curable. Although there are three main forms, each with their own peculiarities, all share a common pathophysiology. In foetal life, the pulmonary venous confluence fails to fuse with the left atrium. The pulmonary veins drain to the heart, through either an ascending vein to the superior vena cava, a descending vein to the inferior cava or directly to the coronary sinus and right atrium **(Fig. 8.21)**. As both pulmonary and systemic venous return enters the right atrium, these children are dependent on adequacy of the foramen ovale for the entire systemic cardiac output. Obstruction at this level or any other impairs venous return causing a rise in pulmonary venous pressure with accompanying pulmonary hypertension and pulmonary oedema. Obstruction may be present in the first few hours of life (particularly in infracardiac TAPVD or TAPVC), can develop in the first few weeks as the PVR drops or may take many months to develop as the PFO becomes restrictive. If venous return is unobstructed, these infants have mild cyanosis, are slow to grow but often have no other physical signs. As obstruction develops, cyanosis deepens and the child becomes acidotic causing tachypnoea and tachycardia. The infant will have hepatomegaly, a gallop rhythm and a right ventricular heave.

The ECG demonstrates right axis deviation, right ventricular hypertrophy and P pulmonale. Chest X-ray shows pulmonary venous congestion and in chronic supracardiac TAPVD, the widened superior mediastinum gives the mediastinal silhouette a "figure of eight" appearance. Echo is usually diagnostic confirming the pattern of pulmonary venous drainage and demonstrating any area of obstruction.

Management

There is no effective medical therapy and all children with this condition will eventually die without repair. A small percentage of children will go on to develop pulmonary vein obstruction even after successful early repair.

Pulmonary Atresia

Pulmonary atresia is a widely varying condition; however, all infants are cyanosed and most are duct dependent. There are three main groups: (1) PAt/intact ventricular septum (IVS), (2) PAt/VSD and confluent pulmonary arteries and (3) PAt/VSD and major aortopulmonary collateral arteries (MAPCAs) **(Fig. 8.22)**.

All children are cyanosed at birth. The second heart sound will be single but there may be no murmurs unless MAPCAs are present in which case continuous murmurs are often heard throughout the chest.

Where no VSD is present, the absence of flow through the right ventricle in utero results in a hypoplastic right ventricle. Most children with this condition require a modified Blalock-Taussig shunt in the neonatal period followed by a Fontan-type repair when older (discussed later). Some children with Pat/IVS have a reasonably well-developed right ventricular cavity and tricuspid valve. This subgroup may benefit from re-establishing anterograde flow from the right ventricle to the pulmonary artery to encourage further growth of the right ventricle and potentially a biventricular repair.

Where a VSD is present and the pulmonary arteries are confluent, the child will still need initial palliation with a modified Blalock-Taussig shunt; however, at a later stage,

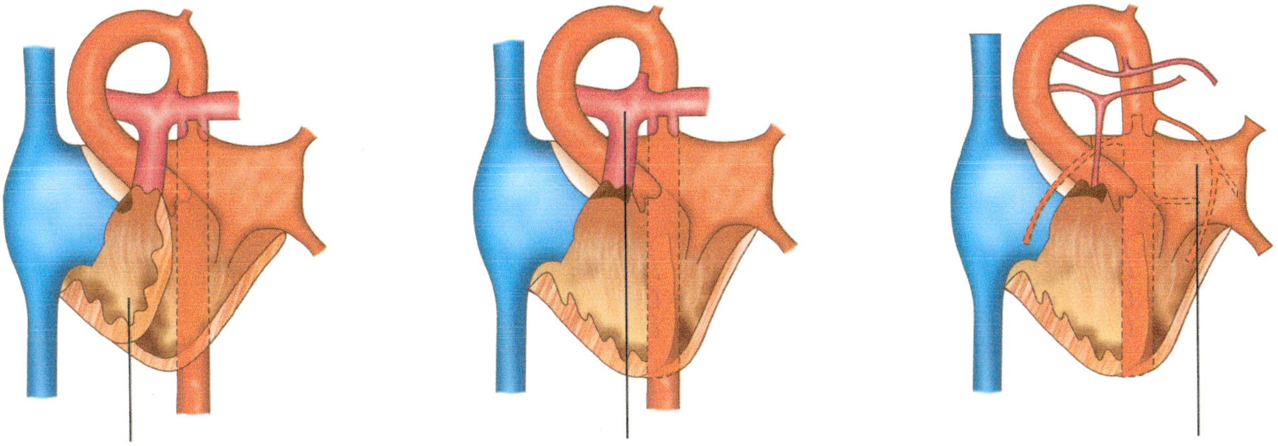

Figure 8.22 Pulmonary atresia variants diagram.

the VSD can usually be closed and a tube interposed between the right ventricle and the pulmonary arteries. Both of these types of PAt are duct-dependent requiring prostaglandin E infusion to maintain ductal patency without which infants will die upon duct closure.

Prognostically, the worst anatomy is PAt with MAPCAs. In these children, MAPCAs arise directly from the aorta and supply individual segments of lung sometimes with little communication between them and any rudimentary main pulmonary artery. Extensive reconstructive surgery is often required to create a pulmonary artery confluence large enough to permit later insertion of a right ventricle to pulmonary artery conduit and VSD closure.

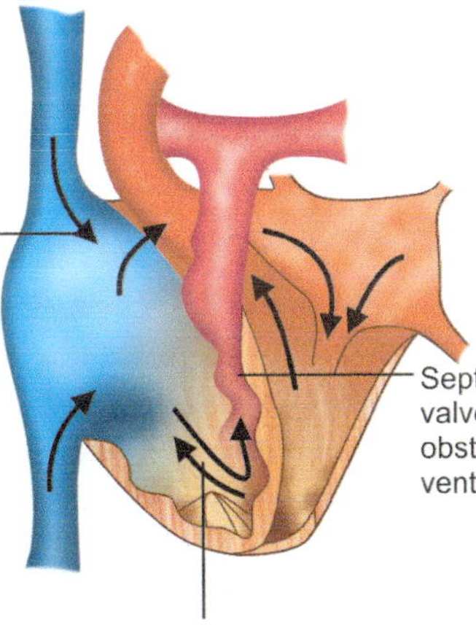

Figure 8.23 Ebstein anomaly diagram.

Ebstein Anomaly

In this rare abnormality, the tricuspid valve annulus has developed within the right ventricle itself. In effect part of the right ventricle functions as part of the right atrium, the right ventricular cavity volume is significantly reduced; the tricuspid valve is abnormal often with significant regurgitation and the right ventricular outflow tract may be obstructed (Fig. 8.23). In severe cases, the abnormality causes huge enlargement of the right atrium in utero such that the sheer size of the heart impedes lung development and the child dies in the newborn period. In less severe cases, the pulmonary artery flow is obstructed and deoxygenated blood tends to shunt right to left across the atrial septum causing cyanosis and poor exercise ability. Mild cases are virtually asymptomatic and present late in life with either right heart failure or arrhythmias.

Clinically there is variable cyanosis and the neck veins may be distended demonstrating prominent V waves due to the tricuspid regurgitation. A systolic murmur and sometimes a late diastolic murmur are heard at the lower left sternal edge often with a gallop rhythm. The ECG shows notched P waves signifying right atrial enlargement, right bundle branch block (Fig. 8.24), and may reveal the short PR interval and delta wave of associated pre-excitation (Wolff-Parkinson-White syndrome). Chest X-ray often shows an increased cardiothoracic ratio, primarily due to right atrial enlargement and oligaemic lung fields. Echo will again confirm the diagnosis and help assess the degree of tricuspid regurgitation and atrial shunting.

Management

Medical treatment is useful only for arrhythmia management. Surgical intervention is difficult and controversial with a significant risk. The exact procedure must be tailored to the individual case and will be determined mainly by the adequacy of the right ventricle.

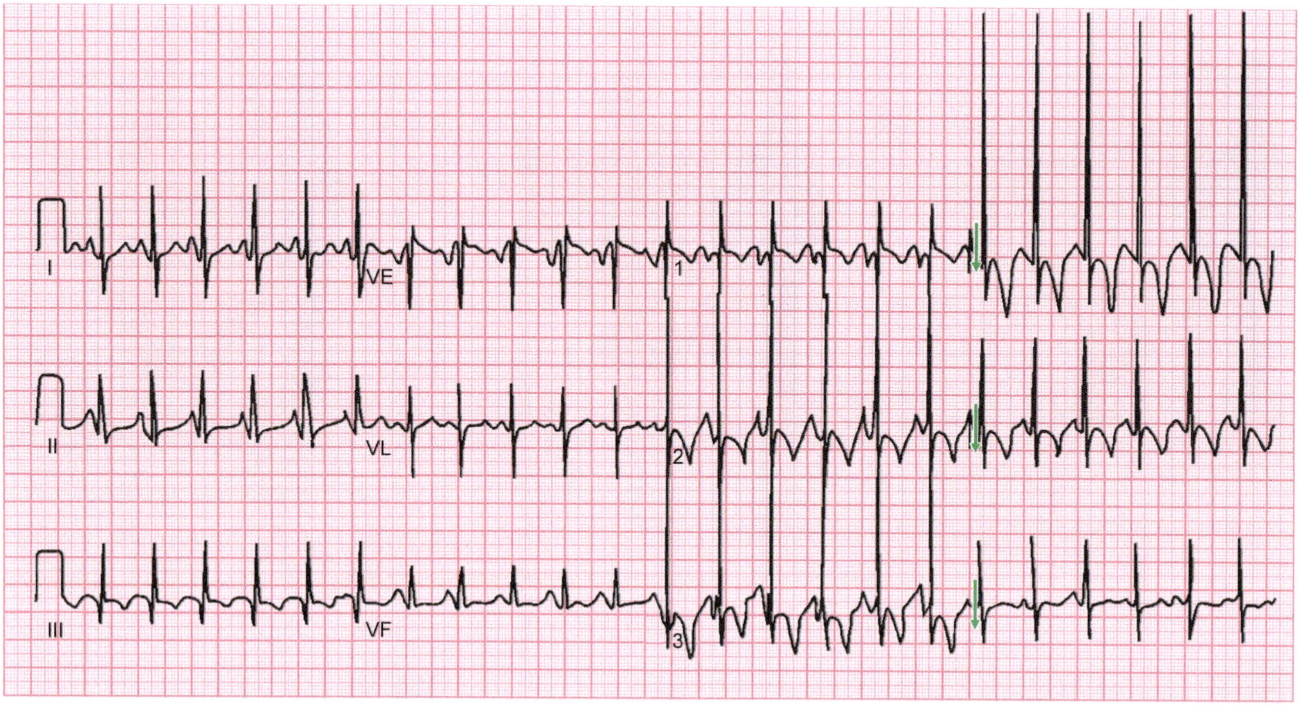

Figure 8.24 Electrocardiography Ebstein anomaly.

Hypoplastic Left Heart Syndrome and Other Forms of Univentricular Heart

Hypoplastic left heart syndrome is the broad term given to describe inadequacy of the left ventricular size in combination with stenosis or atresia of the mitral and aortic valves and hypoplasia of the aortic arch. Coarctation is a common association. As with aortic stenosis, the systemic circulation is dependent on flow through the arterial duct, so duct constriction causes a low cardiac state with severe acidosis and hypoxia. Such children require resuscitation and prompt administration of prostaglandin E as described previously. Despite these measures, infants with HLHS cannot survive without radical surgical palliation in the form of a Norwood procedure. Briefly, this operation bypasses the left heart by removing the atrial septum, transecting the main pulmonary artery above the valve and connecting it to the systemic arterial circulation using a Blalock-Taussig shunt. The proximal pulmonary artery stump is then connected to the side of the ascending aorta to direct the right ventricular cardiac output into the aorta and the aortic arch enlarged using a patch to relieve any further obstruction **(Fig. 8.25)**.

This operation, undertaken in the newborn period, carries a significant risk even in the best centres and is only the first of three operations that will be required for long-term palliation. It is, therefore, unsurprising that after appropriate counselling many families elect not to proceed down a surgical route and opt for medical palliation understanding that the infant will not survive more than a few days.

Other forms of heart disease where only a single functioning ventricle exists do not require such radical early palliation. The key to presentation and early management is pulmonary blood flow. If flow to the pulmonary circulation is obstructed, the child will usually be duct dependent, present early with cyanosis and require a modified Blalock-Taussig shunt to establish effective blood flow to the lungs. Alternatively if there is no obstruction to pulmonary blood flow, the child will present with tachypnoea and failure to thrive as the PVR drops and flow increases. Such children often benefit from having a restrictive band placed around the pulmonary artery to limit flow, protect the pulmonary circulation and prevent volume loading the heart.

Successful long-term palliation of any single ventricle circulation is critically dependent on ventricular function. Therefore, the surgical strategy employed must ensure that the volume load placed on the ventricle is kept to a minimum. Ultimately the palliation diverts the systemic venous drainage around the heart, allowing it to drain directly to the pulmonary artery and this is usually achieved in two stages given as follows: (1) during the first procedure, the superior vena cava is disconnected from the right atrium and reconnected directly to the pulmonary artery, reducing the volume load on the heart but leaving the child still cyanosed. (2) A second and final procedure then redirects the inferior vena caval flow to the lungs, usually by means of an extracardiac conduit. In this way, almost all deoxygenated blood now drains directly to the pulmonary circulation where it is oxygenated before returning to the heart **(Fig. 8.25)**.

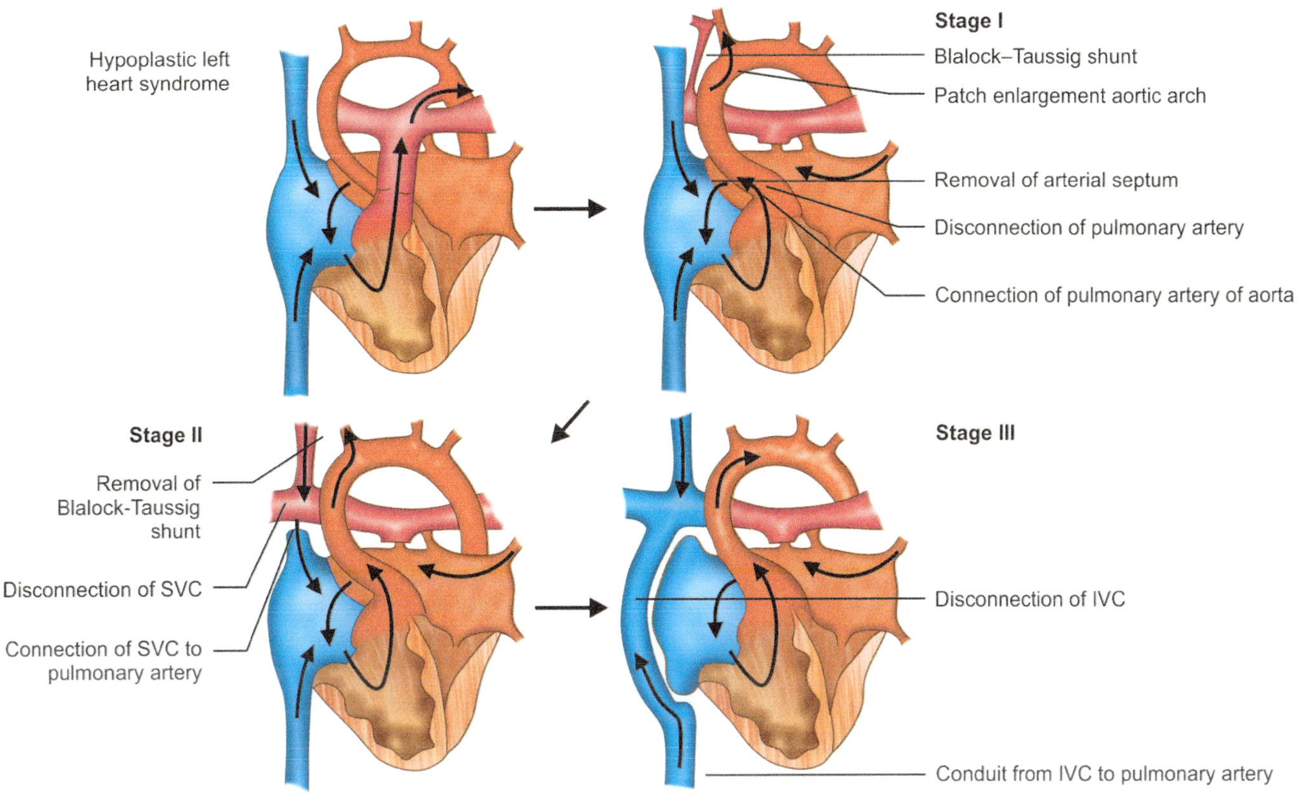

Figure 8.25 Fontan repair.

The long-term prognosis of children with univentricular forms of heart disease is constantly improving as the techniques for repair continue to develop. Currently life-expectancy without a cardiac transplant is in the third decade, and quality of life is reasonable accepting reduced physical capacity. Clearly, given the resources required to palliate children with univentricular circulations for what appears to be a relatively short period of time, harsh decisions must be made regarding appropriateness of treatment where healthcare funding is limited.

Vascular Ring

Numerous abnormalities of great artery development can occur, most of which are rare and many insignificant. A vascular ring exists where there is a continuous ring of structures surrounding the trachea and oesophagus. As the child grows, this ring can result in constriction of the airway and/or oesophagus producing stridor or swallowing difficulties. The most common substrate for this is a right-sided aortic arch with a retro-oesophageal left subclavian artery. The ring is completed by a ductal ligament passing from the left subclavian artery to the pulmonary artery **(Fig. 8.26)**. Alternatively a double aortic arch can also form a ring around the trachea and oesophagus. It should be noted that only one of the aortic arches might have flow throughout its course. Other variations in the anatomy of the head and neck vessels rarely cause symptoms.

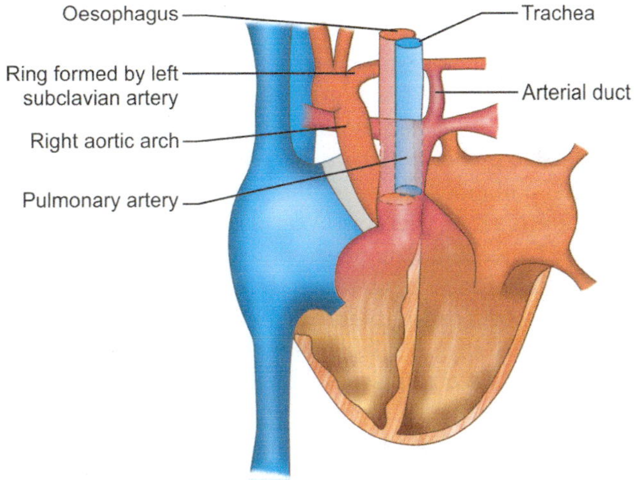

Figure 8.26 Vascular ring.

Vascular rings are best diagnosed by barium swallow where the pattern of indentation seen on the posterior aspect of the oesophagus indicates the type of ring **(Fig. 8.27)**. Further evidence can be obtained from bronchoscopy, CT or MRI scans. Echo is less reliable in these

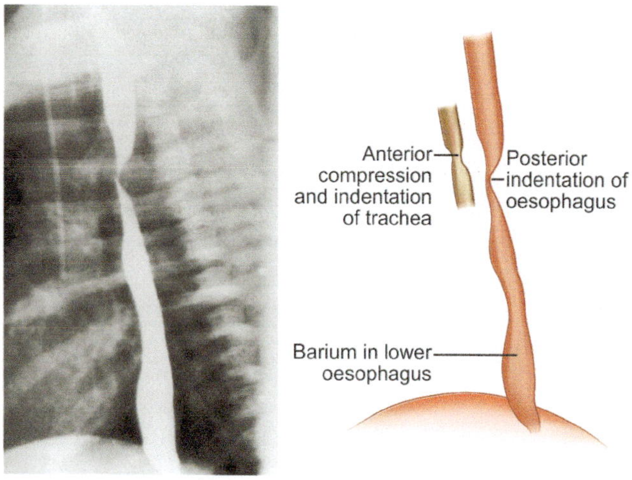

Figure 8.27 Vascular ring due to double aorta (lateral view barium swallow).

situations as at least part of the anatomical substrate often has no lumen or flow.

Treatment is surgical and usually requires simple division of the ligamentous portion of the ring.

ACQUIRED HEART DISEASE

Rheumatic Heart Disease

Outside of the North America and the Europe, rheumatic fever is the most common cause of acquired heart disease in childhood. In the acute phase, rheumatic fever is a systemic disorder that causes cardiac morbidity and mortality from acute valve dysfunction and myocardial involvement. Evolution of the valve abnormality to its more chronic form can lead to problems both in late childhood and adult life.

The pathology seen in the heart results from an immune reaction triggered in certain individuals by exposure to Lancefield group A streptococci, usually acquired through an upper respiratory tract infection. Not all group A streptococci cause rheumatic fever and some conflicting evidence suggests that only those belonging to certain M serotypes are responsible for the disease. There also seems to be a familial tendency to develop the disease and the expression of certain human leukocyte antigen (HLA) groups on a hosts B cells may make them more susceptible to rheumatic fever.

Antibodies produced in response to a streptococcal throat infection in a susceptible host react to both the streptococcal M protein and the myosin and laminin filaments within the hosts' heart. Although antibodies to host myosin cause the myocarditis seen in acute rheumatic fever, it is the reaction to laminin that cause the endocarditis and valve dysfunction so characteristic of acute rheumatic heart disease.

Peak incidence occurs between 10 years and 14 years, but rheumatic fever can be seen in children as young as 3 years and adults as old as 30 years. Carditis is most marked in those affected under 5 years of age.

Acutely the carditis always involves the endocardium, usually the myocardium and occasionally the pericardium. Late sequelae are most commonly related to mitral or aortic valve damage.

Typically the first signs of carditis are a tachycardia and a new murmur. Although the most common murmur seen in acute rheumatic fever is the apical systolic murmur of mitral regurgitation, systolic murmurs are very common in all children particularly when a tachycardia is present so the appearance of a soft diastolic murmur at the apex is much more suggestive of early carditis. These findings in a child with other manifestations of rheumatic fever should prompt urgent further investigation as unrecognised or untreated carditis can result in arrhythmias and heart failure.

Electrocardiography confirms a sinus tachycardia and often shows lengthening of the PR interval, a characteristic finding in acute rheumatic fever. Echo may show early valve dysfunction, usually regurgitation of the left heart valves, reduced ventricular function or a pericardial effusion. Serology will show evidence of streptococcal infection with a raised antistreptolysin O (ASO) titre greater than 200 IU/mL and often much higher. DNase B is a more sensitive indicator of streptococcal infection but will not start to rise for 1–2 weeks. Other non-specific indicators of a systemic inflammatory process will also be raised including C-reactive protein (CRP) and erythrocyte sedimentation rate (ESR).

Management

Management has four distinct aims:

1. The infection that triggered the inflammatory response must be eradicated to remove the immune stimulus. High-dose intravenous or intramuscular benzyl penicillin should be given for 3 days followed by high-dose oral treatment for a further 10 days. Dose will be dependent on weight.
2. The acute inflammatory response must be suppressed. Bed rest and high-dose aspirin are the mainstays of treatment. Some centres advocate the use of corticosteroids, although there is limited evidence for their use. Acute inflammation can be monitored by measuring the ESR on a daily basis. When this has normalised, bed rest can be stopped and moderate exercise positively encouraged. Similarly high-dose aspirin (100 mg/kg per day in four doses) is usually given until at least 2 weeks after the ESR has returned to normal to prevent any rebound inflammation. Whilst using high-dose aspirin, it is sensible to measure serum levels to avoid overdose, maintaining a level of 2 mmol/L (24–30 mg/100 mL).
3. Further streptococcal infections must be prevented. This is adequately achieved using moderate dose

oral phenoxymethylpenicillin (250 mg BD) and encouraging compliance. Where compliance is questionable, an alternative would be intramuscular benzathine penicillin. Currently, it is recommended that prophylaxis be continued throughout childhood and adolescence up to 21 years of age.

4. Treatment of coexisting cardiac dysfunction is largely supportive with diuretics, digoxin and ACE inhibitor. It is best to avoid surgical intervention in the acute phase, although occasionally this is required. Ultimately, chronic valve dysfunction will often require repair or replacement.

Infective Endocarditis

Whenever bacteria enter the bloodstream of a patient with a structural heart abnormality, there is a possibility of seeding and infection at the site of the lesion. Structural heart lesions cause areas of turbulence and stagnant flow where bacteria can dwell and attach/infect the endocardium. This may be at the site of the lesion such as in the case of a regurgitant mitral valve or where the resultant jet hits the myocardium such as where a VSD jet strikes the opposing right ventricular wall. Bacteria can enter the circulation from a variety of sources, although poor dental hygiene and dental procedures causing *Streptococcus viridans* to enter the bloodstream are perhaps the commonest cause. *Staphylococcus aureus* is another common causative organism that enters through infected skin lesions (e.g. eczema) or during tattoos and piercings. When bacteria infect the endocardium, they can form vegetations (small lumps attached to the endocardium by flexible stalks) or they can invade the myocardium causing abscess formation.

Infective endocarditis (IE) should be suspected in any child with a known structural heart abnormality and an unexplained febrile illness. Classically IE has been described as sub-acute bacterial endocarditis (SBE). This name derives from the pre-antibiotic era where the disease often went undiagnosed for many weeks and the child demonstrated signs of chronic infection such as finger-clubbing, painful embolic nodes in the finger tips (Osler nodes), microemboli in the nail beds (splinter haemorrhages), embolic infarctions in the retina (Roth spots) and anaemia of chronic disease. These findings are now rarely seen, and more commonly the child will present with a fever, tachycardia, changing or new murmur, splenomegaly, splinter haemorrhages and haematuria.

Investigation

The most important management step in any child with suspected IE is avoidance of antibiotics before blood cultures are taken. At least three and preferably six sets should be obtained from different venipuncture sites. The microbiologist must be made aware of the suspected diagnosis, as occasionally causative organisms can be very difficult or slow to grow in culture. Blood should also be taken for white cell count, haemoglobin, ESR and CRP. An ECG should be recorded as occasionally IE around the aortic valve can result in heart block and a transthoracic and/or transoesophageal echo should be obtained. It must be emphasised that the absence of vegetations on echo does not exclude endocarditis; however, when seen they confirm the diagnosis.

Management

Appropriate intravenous broad-spectrum antibiotics can be given after blood cultures have been taken. The agents used can be modified once the target organism and its sensitivities have been identified. Usually parenteral therapy is continued for 6 weeks to ensure eradication of deep-seated infection as judged clinically and by inflammatory markers (CRP and ESR). Surgical excision of vegetations may be required where they pose a serious risk in case of embolism or they are affecting cardiac function. Severe valve dysfunction may also require surgical treatment acutely; however, it is best to "sterilise" the area first using prolonged antibiotic therapy prior to attempting to repair or replace a damaged valve.

Prophylaxis

Antibiotic prophylaxis is no longer recommended in the United Kingdom. This decision was based on the lack of evidence that the widespread use of antibiotic prophylaxis influenced the development of endocarditis. Different countries vary widely in their recommendations and for many antibiotic prophylaxis remains recommended for any child with an "at risk" cardiac lesion undergoing an invasive dental or surgical procedure likely to cause a significant bacteraemia. All cardiac lesions producing a high velocity jet or turbulent flow are considered at risk of endocarditis. These include aortic stenosis, mitral regurgitation, VSD and PDA. Antibiotic prophylaxis is not required for low velocity lesions such as ASD, mild pulmonary stenosis or 6 months following complete repair of lesions such as VSD or PDA.

Mucocutaneous Lymph Node Syndrome (Kawasaki Syndrome)

Kawasaki syndrome is an idiopathic vasculitis that is often unrecognised but is important due to potential coronary artery involvement. Key features of presentation are persistent fever, a miserable and irritable child, conjunctivitis, lymphadenopathy, swelling of the lips, tongue, hands and feet followed later by desquamation. Coronary artery inflammation results in aneurysm formation with intraluminal thrombus that may occlude the artery causing myocardial infarction. Early recognition of the disease together with prompt administration of immunoglobulin has reduced the incidence and severity of coronary artery involvement and its potentially fatal sequelae.

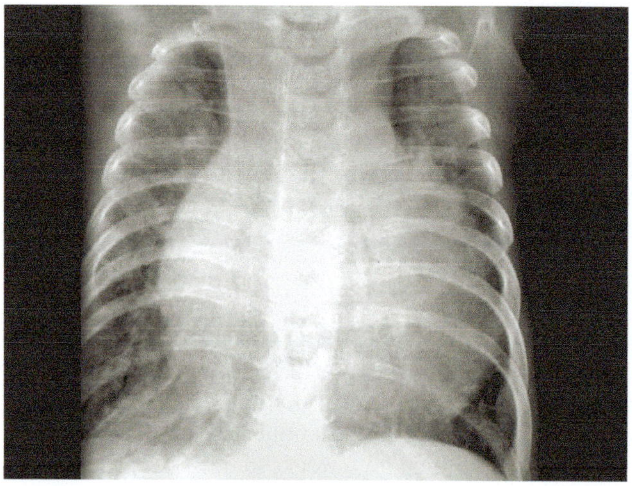

Figure 8.28 Chest X-ray showing pericardial effusion.

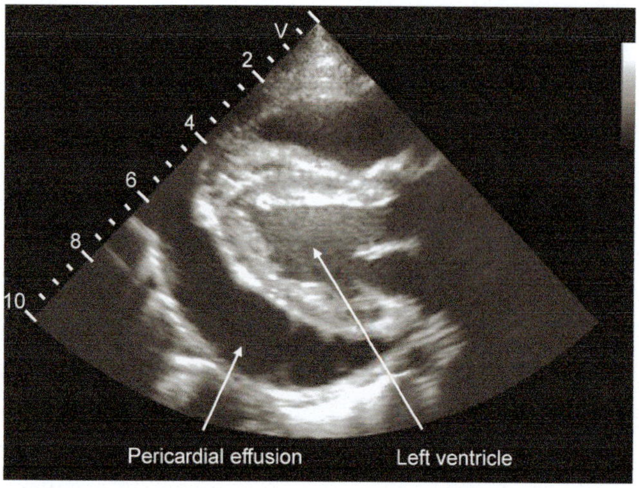

Figure 8.29 Echocardiogram showing pericardial effusion.

If aneurysms are present, long-term treatment with aspirin should be offered, as the risk of future coronary artery disease is raised.

Pericarditis

Inflammation of the pericardium with the accumulation of fluid around the heart may occur for a variety of reasons. Pericarditis resulting from viral infections, rheumatic fever, end stage renal failure, malignancy or systemic inflammatory disorders such as juvenile chronic arthritis now constitutes the bulk of cases. Tuberculosis remains an important if less common cause than previously. Similarly, with the widespread use of antibiotics, bacterial pericarditis usually secondary to pneumonia is also now rare.

Clues to the cause of the pericarditis will often be gained from the history. Most children will have some degree of chest pain that will vary in intensity with cause and degree of fluid accumulation (pain often eases as the volume of pericardial fluid increase or when the child leans forward). A fever is often present as is general malaise and lethargy. Symptoms attributable to pericardial fluid accumulation depend on both volume and rate of accumulation. A small amount of fluid entering the pericardium suddenly (e.g. an intravascular cannula perforating the right atrium) will be more disabling than a considerable volume accumulating over time (e.g. tuberculosis). In general, as more fluid accumulates, the child will become increasingly breathless with worsening exercise tolerance. The child will often be more comfortable sitting forward. The cardinal signs are a pericardial friction rub (a scratching sound varying as much with respiration as it does with the cardiac cycle) and muffled heart sounds. With significant pericardial fluid accumulation, signs of tamponade will be present including raised jugular venous pulsation, pulsus paradoxus, tachycardia and hepatomegaly.

ECG will usually show sinus tachycardia, reduced voltage complexes and "saddle-shaped" ST segment elevation. If the effusion is significant, the heart may "swing" with respiration causing a variation in complex morphology with the respiratory cycle. Chest X-ray may demonstrate a globular, enlarged cardiac silhouette **(Fig. 8.28)**, and the diagnosis is confirmed by echocardiogram **(Fig. 8.29)**, which will also allow estimation of the size of the collection and show signs of impaired systemic venous return (tamponade). Further investigation centres on establishing the cause, ASO titre, viral titres, CRP and ESR should routinely be sent and a Mantoux test performed. Where pericardiocentesis is indicated examination of the fluid aspirated will usually confirm the diagnosis.

Management

In the absence of tamponade, most cases of pericarditis will settle with appropriate treatment of the underlying cause and supportive therapy such as bed rest, oxygen and analgesia. Where tamponade is present, the pericardial fluid should be aspirated and if necessary a drain left in situ. Where bacterial or tuberculous pericarditis is present, surgical exploration and lavage may be required to prevent the later development of pericardial constriction.

Myocarditis

Myocarditis can be caused by viral infection or rarely as part of autoimmune systemic inflammatory disorder. Viral myocarditis results from infection by a wide variety of agents including enteroviruses (particularly Coxsackie B), adenovirus, hepatitis C and HIV. It is unclear why in the majority of children myocarditis is a mild, transient illness, whereas in others it can be rapidly fatal. The degree to which an individual is affected ranges considerably from asymptomatic ECG evidence of myocarditis during viral epidemics to fulminant cardiogenic shock a few days following a usually unremarkable viral illness.

Just as viral myocarditis varies widely in its severity so do signs at presentation. Some children demonstrate only a minor tachycardia and summation gallop; whilst others are peripherally shut down (cold, grey and clammy), have low volume pulses, a marked parasternal heave and hepatomegaly.

Patients with myocarditis have a variable outcome. Those with only minor symptoms will usually fully recover, as surprisingly will those with fulminant myocarditis, if they can be supported through the acute illness. Those children who present with moderate to severe impairment of ventricular function have the worst prognosis, with many having long-term ventricular dysfunction.

The ECG usually shows low voltage complexes and may demonstrate ST changes, QT prolongation and possibly ectopic beats or sustained arrhythmias. Chest X-ray usually demonstrates pulmonary plethora; however, the cardiac outline may or may not be enlarged (acutely, although ventricular function is poor, the ventricle may not have had time to dilate). Blood serology for commonly responsible viral agents should be sent and a metabolic screen should be considered in younger children to exclude rare but treatable causes. The gold standard investigation to confirm the myocarditis is myocardial biopsy; however, many centres rely on a clinical diagnosis with or without serological confirmation of viral infection.

Management

All children with this disease need appropriate treatment for ventricular dysfunction. This will range from diuretics and ACE inhibitors for those with moderate symptoms, up to full intensive care with inotrope support and even mechanical assist devices (if available) for children with fulminant heart failure. Many specific treatments to address the myocarditic process itself have been tried including steroids, pooled immunoglobulin and other more aggressive forms of immunosuppression. Currently, there is no convincing evidence that any are of benefit.

A minority of children may require cardiac transplantation where the heart fails to recover.

Dilated Cardiomyopathy

Dilated cardiomyopathy is usually idiopathic, although approximately 10% are the end result of viral myocarditis. Other causes are familial inheritance, previous anthracycline chemotherapy, a metabolic derangement such as acylcarnitine deficiency and others are part of a systemic myopathic process such as Duchenne muscular dystrophy or a mitochondrial cytopathy. Whatever the underlying process, the left ventricular function is impaired resulting in enlargement which in turn reduces the function further. With increasing enlargement, the mitral valve annulus dilates causing regurgitation, which further strains the failing left ventricle.

Infants typically present with failure to thrive, poor feeding and tachypnoea. Older children generally complain of a gradual decline in exercise tolerance, often culminating in orthopnoea and resting tachypnoea. Examination will demonstrate the classical triad of tachypnoea, tachycardia and hepatomegaly. In addition, there may be a marked heave, gallop rhythm and the apical systolic murmur of mitral regurgitation.

Diagnosis is confirmed on echo and further investigation revolves around finding a treatable cause. In most cases, none is found and treatment is supportive and symptomatic. Children are usually started on diuretics and digoxin, with the addition of ACE inhibitors and beta blockers such as carvedilol now being commonplace. Some form of anticoagulation is often required to prevent thrombus formation in the ventricular chamber.

It is unusual for there to be a significant improvement in function and most will deteriorate with time. Where possible a cardiac transplant may be the only long-term solution.

Hypertrophic Cardiomyopathy

Hypertrophic cardiomyopathy is often inherited in an autosomal dominant manner, although sporadic cases do occur. It is also seen in children with Noonan syndrome. Thickening of the left ventricular wall may be concentric or predominantly within the septum (asymmetrical septal hypertrophy). These changes result in impaired filling of the left ventricle and where asymmetrical hypertrophy is present sub-aortic obstruction develops. Unfortunately, all forms are at risk of ventricular arrhythmias and sudden death particularly on exercise.

Many children are asymptomatic at presentation and discovered during screening where another family member is affected or where a murmur has been detected and referred for investigation. Other children may present with exertional dyspnoea, chest pain, dizziness or syncope.

Diagnosis is by echocardiogram. Whilst the ECG may show changes of hypertrophy and strain, a normal test does not exclude the diagnosis. When a diagnosis has been made, screening should be offered to first-degree relatives.

If significant hypertrophy is present intense, exercise should be avoided and beta blockers may be used for symptom control. Although many treatments including surgical resection of the muscle have been tried, the only measure shown to be of benefit in these patients is an implantable defibrillator.

HEART RHYTHM ABNORMALITIES

Normal

Normal heart rate, like blood pressure, varies with age. A neonate should have a rate of 110–150 beats per minute (bpm), infants 85–125 bpm, 3–5 years 75–115 bpm and over 6 years 60–100 bpm. The heart rate in infants may rise as high as 220 bpm when febrile. Sinus arrhythmia is common in children and can produce a marked drop in heart rate during expiration. Extra beats are also common in childhood. Atrial or junctional ectopic beats can be recognised as narrow complex and may have a preceding abnormal P wave. They are benign and require no further investigation. Ventricular ectopics are broad complex and also occur in healthy children; however, occasionally, they can indicate underlying myocardial disease, electrolyte derangement or drug ingestion. When they can be shown to disappear on exercise they require no further investigation. Three types of rhythm abnormality deserve further attention; (1) supraventricular tachycardia (SVT), (2) ventricular tachycardia (VT) including torsades de pointes and (3) complete heart block (CHB).

Supraventricular Tachycardia

Supraventricular tachycardia in childhood is a narrow complex tachycardia, with rates usually of between 200 and 300. There are many different underlying mechanisms but most fall into two groups.

1. *Reentry arrhythmias*: These arrhythmias are by far the commonest and are caused by an electrical circuit developing either through the atrioventricular (AV) node (e.g., Wolff-Parkinson-White) or within the atria (e.g. atrial flutter) **(Fig. 8.30)**. The electrical impulse passes around the loop repeatedly sending off an action potential to atria and ventricles with each circuit. In most childhood, SVT including Wolff-Parkinson-White syndrome the re-entry circuit involves the AV node and an accessory pathway (extra piece of conduction tissue connecting the atria to ventricles). These arrhythmias tend to be paroxysmal in nature and usually have rate of 200–250 bpm. In atrial flutter, the circuit occurs within the atria often around the foramen ovale and the atrial rate is faster ranging from 500 bpm in the newborn to 300 bpm in adolescents (usually only alternate beats are conducted to the ventricles).
2. *Automatic tachycardias:* These arrhythmias are also known as ectopic tachycardias. They arise from increased automaticity of a group of cells within the myocardium **(Fig. 8.30)**. Essentially the abnormal focus depolarises at a faster rate than the sinus node, thus taking over the role of pacemaker. If the rate of depolarisation exceeds normal for the child concerned, it is designated a tachycardia. These forms of tachycardia tend to be incessant and have lower rates of 160–220 bpm.

Presentation

Infants are unable to communicate symptoms of palpitation. Due to this, SVT lasting less than 24 hours may remain undiagnosed. When prolonged, however, symptoms of heart failure (poor feeding, sweating and

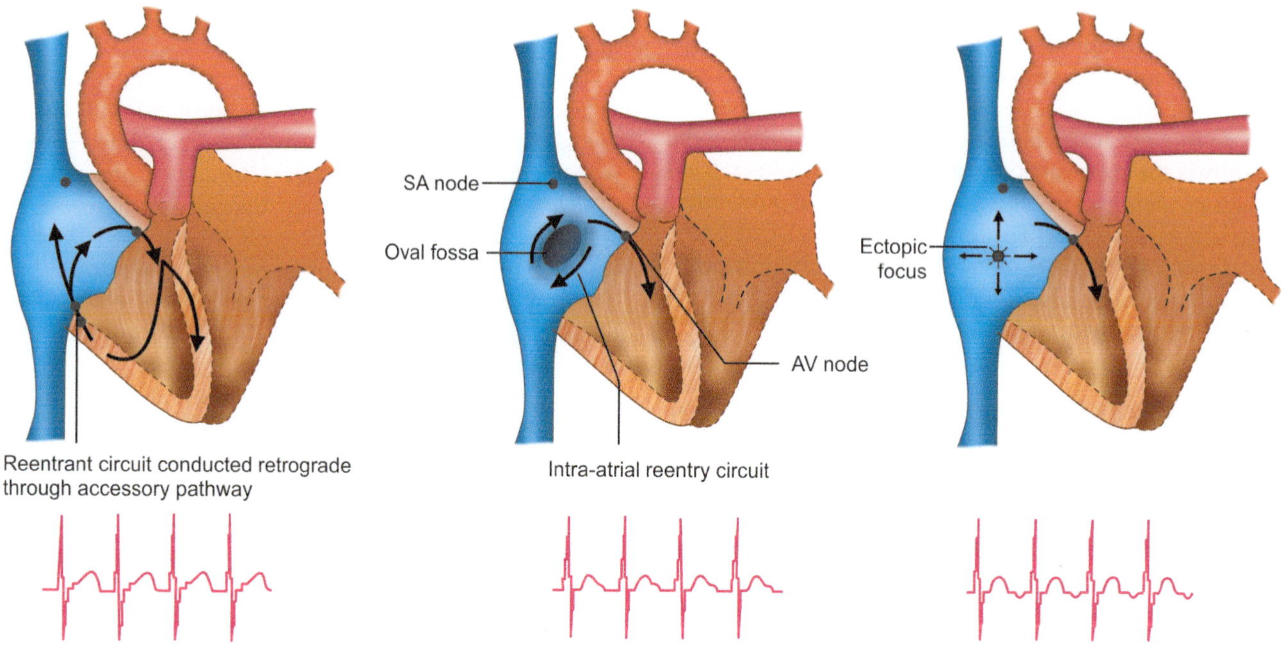

Atrioventricular reentry tachycardia. Atria are depolarised through accessory pathway after ventricles, therefore, P wave is buried in the ST segment

Intra-atrial reentry tachycardia. Rapid narrow QRS complex tachycardia with P wave visible in preceding T wave

Ectopic atrial tachycardia. Area of atrium depolarises at a rapid rate. P wave has unusual morphology and short PR interval

Figure 8.30 Supraventricular tachycardia mechanism.

poor colour) develop, raising awareness of the problem. Incessant, automatic tachycardias tend to have slower rates and cause less haemodynamic compromise. They usually take longer to present and often do so with a form of dilated cardiomyopathy. In contrast to infants, older children will complain of odd feelings, thumping or fluttering within the chest after relatively short episodes. More rapid forms can be associated with chest pain, breathlessness and dizziness, particularly when prolonged.

Investigation

The paroxysmal nature of many tachycardias makes accurate diagnosis difficult. A baseline ECG may reveal the short PR interval and delta wave of Wolff-Parkinson-White **(Fig. 8.31)**, or may show a prolonged QT interval suggesting a VT is responsible for the symptoms (below). Ideally, a 12-lead ECG should be recorded during the tachycardia that will provide the optimum information for an accurate diagnosis. Where episodes are infrequent obtaining a 12-lead ECG may prove impossible in which case ambulatory recordings can be obtained using one of the many systems now available. An echocardiogram is also performed to exclude associated structural heart disease.

Management

Acutely, re-entry forms of tachycardia may respond to vagal manoeuvres. In infants, immersing the face in ice cold water for 5 seconds may be tried. Older children can be taught to perform a Valsalva manoeuvre. If these measures fail, intravenous adenosine is a very effective alternative. Because it has a very short half-life in the circulation it should be injected through a large cannula in a proximal vein with a rapid bolus and flush. By convention a small dose is used initially (0.05 mg/kg) which is increased in steps to 0.25 mg/kg (max 12 mg). If this fails, it is likely the arrhythmia is automatic in nature. Acutely automatic tachycardias are harder to control and often require preloading with an antiarrhythmic agent such as amiodarone prior to synchronised electrical cardioversion (0.5–1 J/kg).

Chronically many children with infrequent short episodes of SVT require no treatment and adequate explanation is sufficient to reassure them and their parents. Where episodes are infrequent but of long duration, patients can be offered a "pill in pocket" form of treatment. This involves the child carrying a supply of verapamil or a beta blocker to take only when an attack starts. The medication is designed to terminate the attack rather than prevent it. Where episodes are frequent many families prefer preventative treatment, usually with digoxin, beta blockers or verapamil. If the baseline ECG demonstrates Wolff-Parkinson-White syndrome, digoxin is considered contraindicated at most ages and should be avoided (it can theoretically accelerate conduction through the accessory pathway allowing rapid ventricular depolarisation and raising the chance of VT or fibrillation). By convention the presence of SVT in an older patient with documented Wolff-Parkinson-White syndrome is considered to be an indication for transcatheter radiofrequency ablation. If other forms of SVT persist despite medical treatment, radiofrequency ablation of the accessory pathway can be offered to abolish the arrhythmia.

Ventricular Tachycardia/Fibrillation

Ventricular arrhythmias are very rare in childhood even after congenital heart surgery. There are, however, an expanding group of inherited conditions known to predispose individual patient to ventricular tachycardiac and sudden death. These comprise the long QT syndromes, Brugada syndrome and arrhythmogenic right ventricular dysplasia. The inheritance of these conditions is complex and sporadic cases occur. Most affected individuals have an abnormal resting 12-lead ECG and many have a prolonged QT interval.

Once an individual patient has been diagnosed with one of these disorders close family members should be offered screening either by 12-lead ECG or where available genetic analysis for the culprit gene.

Where an effected individual is identified treatment with a beta blocker or an implantable defibrillator is usually indicated.

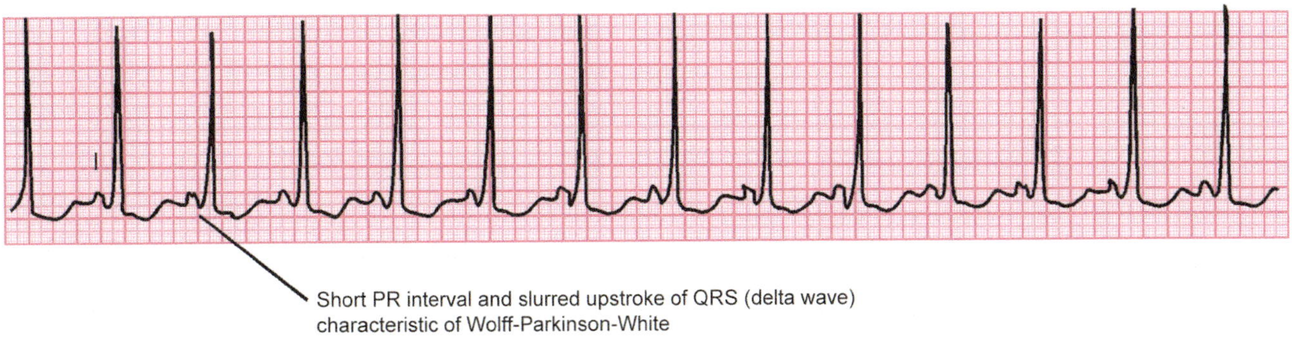

Figure 8.31 ECG showing Wolff–Parkinson–White syndrome.

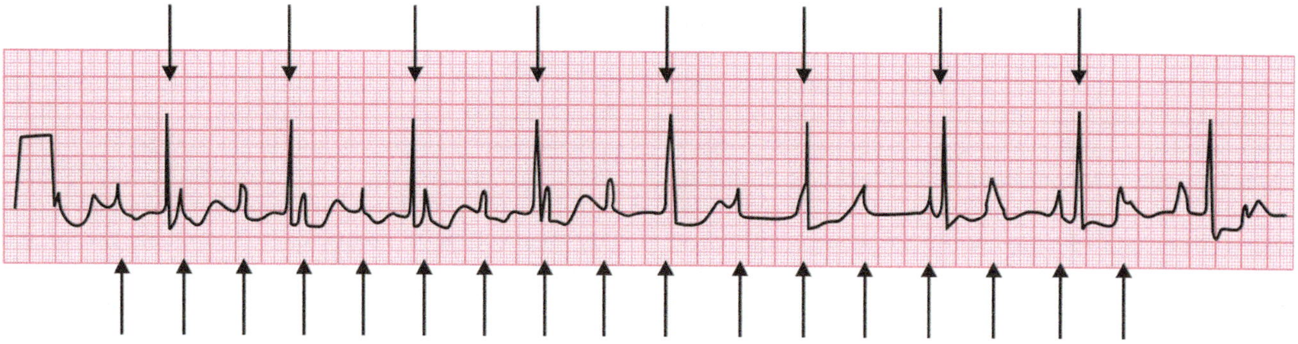

Figure 8.32 ECG showing complete heart block.

Complete Heart Block

In CHB, the electrical activity of the atria is isolated from that of the ventricles. The atria beat at one rate whilst the ventricular rate (effective heart rate) is slower **(Fig. 8.32)**. This is a rare condition. The congenital form is usually seen in newborns where the mother has circulating anti-La and anti-Ro antibodies and may have systemic lupus erythematosus or a related connective tissue disorder. These antibodies cross the placenta and damage the heart particularly targeting the conduction system. Occasionally congenital heart block can also be seen rare forms of congenital heart disease such as congenitally corrected TGA and in atrial isomerism. The most common cause of acquired heart block is iatrogenic and is a complication of open heart surgery when the conduction system is damaged. Often this is a transient problem lasting no more than a few weeks; however, in some children it can persist requiring a pacemaker. Bacterial endocarditis, particularly around the aortic valve, can destroy the junctional tissue and also cause heart block.

In the congenital form, if an infant's heart rate is greater than 55 bpm and there is no heart failure, no treatment is indicated and the outlook is reasonable. Where the heart rate is slower or heart failure coexists then a pacemaker may be required. In acquired forms, where the block is permanent a pacemaker is always indicated.

CHAPTER 9

Paediatric Surgery

Mairi Steven, Robert Carachi

GENERAL PRINCIPLES

Surgical paediatrics is one of the most dynamic, rewarding and exciting fields in hospital medicine. The principles of paediatric surgery are common to all surgical specialties; however, it is important to remember that children are not simply "little adults" and the pathologies dealt with on a daily basis by paediatric surgeons are quite unique to the specialty, and the management of the child very much varies depending on their age. Paediatric surgery is also ever evolving, most notably with improvements in neonatal care and in the era of minimally invasive surgery. In this chapter, we aim to take a "head-to-toe" approach and cover common surgical conditions seen in children as well as rarer congenital conditions, trauma, burns and malignancies.

GENERAL SURGERY OF CHILDHOOD

Head and Neck Swellings

As with any swelling or lump, the size, site, surface, colour, consistency and colour should be described—in addition to whether it is pulsatile, fluctuant, fixed, expansile or reducible. In the neck, it is common to describe whether it is sited in the anterior or posterior triangle. Common lumps include lymphadenopathy (from cat-scratch disease, atypical mycobacterium, tuberculosis or lymphoma). Swellings may also be benign or malignant. Common benign lumps are described in this section. Surgical oncology is dealt with in Chapter 38.

Encephalocele

An encephalocele is a protrusion or outpouching at the cranial end of the neural tube resulting from failure of the neural tube to close (Figs. 9.1A and B). They have an incidence of 1 in 5,000 live births. They can vary dramatically in their appearance and can be classified according to site as nasofrontal, nasoethmoidal, naso-orbital or occipital. Occipital are more common in Europe and frontal are more common in Africa. The cause is unknown but teratogens such as trypan blue and arsenic have been implicated. The encephalocele often contains cerebrospinal fluid (CSF) only, but it may involve brain tissue, referred

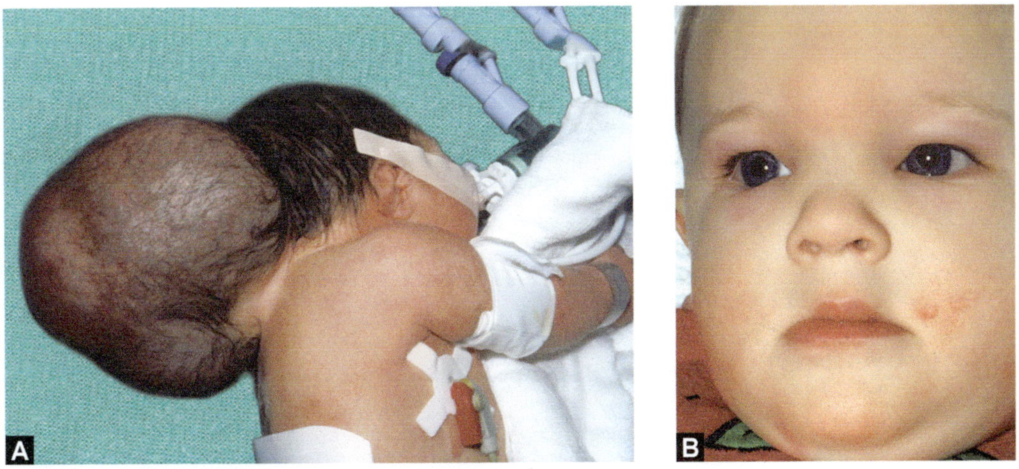

Figures 9.1A and B Encephalocele resulting from failure of closure of neural tube.

to as a meningocele. Magnetic resonance imaging (MRI) and computed tomography (CT) are useful in illustrating what tissues are involved prior to surgery.

Angular Dermoid

Dermoid cysts are extremely common and are often noted around the eye or at the lateral angle of the eyebrow **(Fig. 9.2)**. They are benign and rarely have any intracranial extension. If the mass is midline or its extent cannot be palpated, then further imaging is indicated. These cysts are congenital and result from separation of tissue during development of skin. Rupture can result from trauma and lead to an inflammatory reaction. Treatment is, therefore, by complete surgical excision.

Accessory Auricle

An accessory auricle or pre-auricular skin tags are common and may be bilateral **(Fig. 9.3)**. The incidence is thought to be 3–6 per 1,000 live births and is a congenital developmental abnormality of the first or second branchial arch. They may have a cartilaginous core. Treatment is complete surgical excision and is often requested for cosmetic reasons. Pre-auricular pits or sinuses may also occur and present with infective complications, and once treated they also require excision.

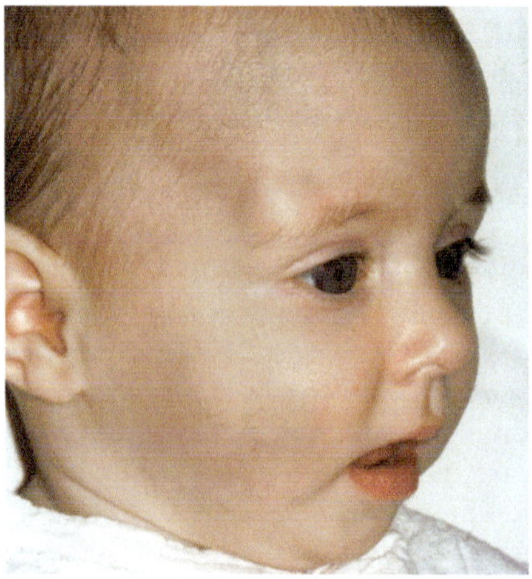

Figure 9.2 Dermoid cysts.

Haemangiomas

Haemangiomas are very common benign tumours seen in childhood presenting at or just after birth **(Fig. 9.4)**. They characteristically display rapid growth over 3–10 months and then have a phase of involution over 5–7 years. They consist of proliferated endothelial cells, in contrast to vascular malformations, which consist of dysplastic vessels with no cellular proliferation. Vascular malformations, however, are biologically inactive. They present at birth and their growth parallels that of the patient. Haemangiomas can occur anywhere on the body and symptoms reflect their site. They are commonly found on the head and neck. They are often referred to as a strawberry naevus. Treatment is often expected as the majority involute. However, if visual fields are involved, then surgery may be considered. Treatment with beta blockers has also more recently been employed with good results. Rarely, haemangiomas can be associated with syndromes such as Kasabach-Merritt syndrome, which can present with bleeding and consumptive coagulopathy.

Thyroglossal Cyst

A thyroglossal cyst is one of the main differential diagnoses of a midline neck lump in a child, in addition to lymphadenopathy, a lipoma, dermoid cyst, goitre or parathyroid swelling **(Fig. 9.5)**. A thyroglossal cyst is a congenital abnormality, although it usually does not present until pre-school age or young adulthood.

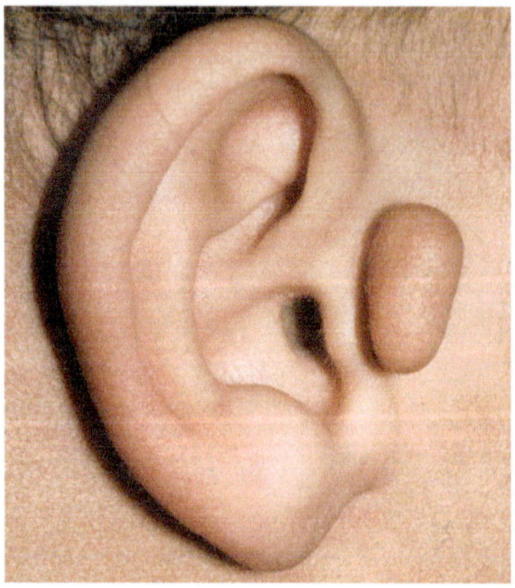

Figure 9.3 Accessory auricle.

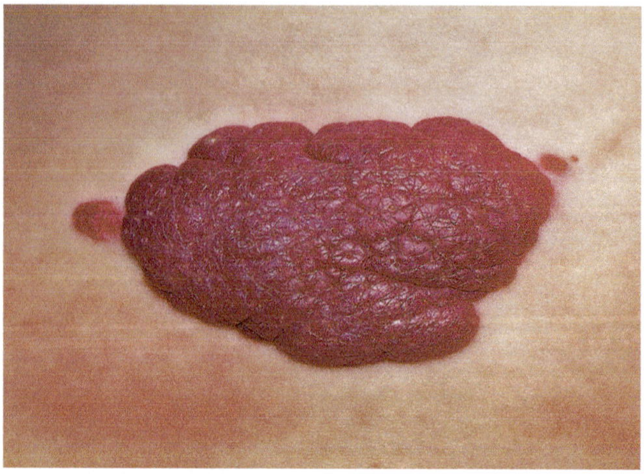

Figure 9.4 Haemangioma.

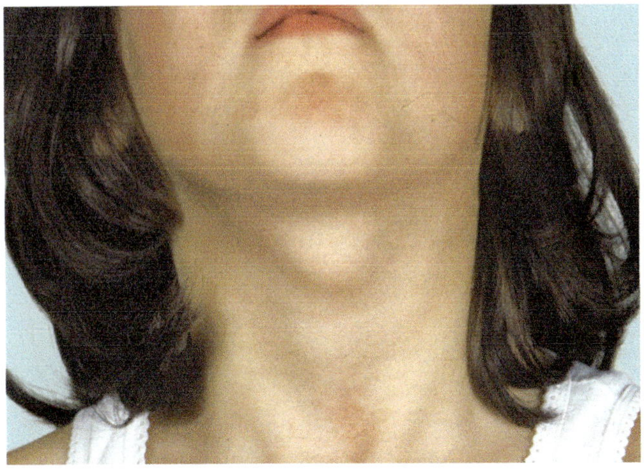

Figure 9.5 Thyroglossal cyst.

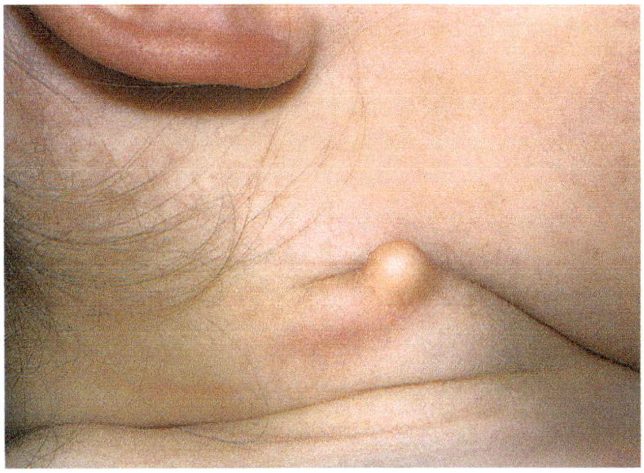

Figure 9.6 Branchial cyst.

It results from failure of involution of the thyroglossal duct following descent of the thyroid gland from its origin at the foramen caecum at the base of the tongue down to its position in the neck below the hyoid bone. A thyroglossal duct cyst may form anywhere down this path. It is vital as always to take a good history from the patient of any thyroid upset and to examine the patient for any mass or palpable thyroid tissue. An ultrasound is often performed to ensure a thyroid is indeed present, prior to excision of the cyst to ensure there is no median ectopic thyroid. Management is complete surgical excision of the cyst and upward tract to prevent any infective complication or malignant transformation, although this is reported to be less than 1%.

Branchial Cyst and Remnants

The embryology of the branchial arches and pharyngeal pouches can be confusing, but is fundamental to understanding the development of important structures in the head and neck. Each arch gives rise to a cartilaginous structure, a muscle, a nerve and an artery (Table 9.1).

Failure of this complicated process can lead to a number of abnormalities. Branchial cysts or remnants account for up to one-third of head and neck swellings (Fig. 9.6). Anomalies of the second cleft are the most common, accounting for more than 90%, and 10% are bilateral. Infective complications can occur, and complete excision to the site of origin often as far as the peritonsillar is recommended.

TABLE 9.1 Branchial acid derivatives.

Arch	*Cartilaginous structure*	*Muscle*	*Nerve*	*Artery*
1	Meckel: mandible, malleus, incus sphenomandibular ligament	Muscles of mastication: temporalis, masseter, lateral and medial pterygoids Mylohyoid Anterior belly of digastric Tensor tympani Tensor veli palatini Anterior two-thirds of tongue	Trigeminal	Maxillary
2	Reichert cartilage: stapes Styloid process Lesser horn of hyoid Stylohyoid ligament	Muscles of facial expression Stapedius Stylohyoid Posterior belly of digastric	Facial	Stapedial
3	Greater horn of hyoid	Stylopharyngeus	Glossopharyngeal	Common carotid/ internal carotid
4–6	Thyroid Cricoid Arytenoids Corniculate Cuneiform	Most pharyngeal constrictors Cricothyroid Levator veli palatini	Vagus	Aortic arch/right subclavian Pulmonary Ductus arteriosus

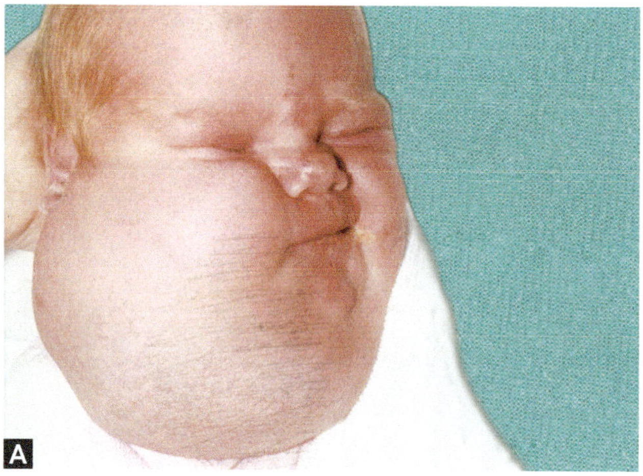

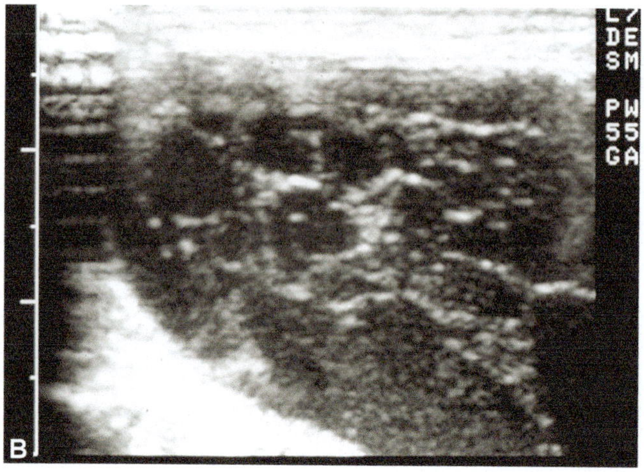

Figures 9.7A and B (A) Cystic hygroma; (B) Ultrasound imaging.

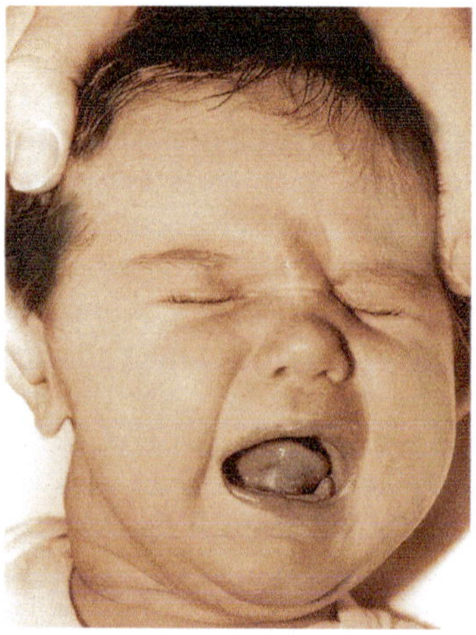

Figure 9.8 sternocleidomastoid tumour.

Parotid Swellings

Parotid swellings are mostly benign in a child, the most common being a haemangioma (discussed earlier). Other causes can include infections such as mumps, staphylococci, atypical mycobacteria and tuberculosis.

Cystic Hygroma

A cystic hygroma is a form of lymphangioma caused by benign aberrant development of lymphatics **(Figs. 9.7A and B)**. Traditionally, the de Serres classification attempts to categorise lymphangiomas according to laterality and whether they are supra- or infrahyoid. They may also be classified according to their cystic element as macrocystic, microcystic or mixed. Patients may present at birth with airway obstruction, which may be anticipated antenatally. Clinical features include a soft, doughy lump which may transilluminate. About 10–15% resolve or involute spontaneously probably after an infective episode. Imaging such as ultrasound, CT or MRI can identify the extent of the lesion. Treatment is by surgery, which may need to be at delivery EXIT (Ex, Utero, Intrapartum, Treatment) procedure. Sclerotherapy can be useful with agents such as OK 432 (Picibanil); however, this is now difficult to source and is not suitable for penicillin-allergic patients. Bleomycin is another option; however, pulmonary fibrosis is a potential side effect. Doxycycline and ethanol are alternatives, and more recently, sildenafil has promising results and may be the drug of choice in the future.

Sternocleidomastoid Tumour/Torticollis

A sternocleidomastoid tumour or fibromatosis coli or dysplasia is a common benign condition **(Fig. 9.8)**. It is often seen in an infant after a traumatic birth. The child presents with a lump and torticollis. The treatment is physiotherapy. If treatment is not given then facial asymmetry or plagiocephaly may result.

Chest Wall Abnormalities

The most common chest wall abnormalities are those of the sternum, known as pectus deformities. They are thought to be caused by aberrant excessive growth or dysplasia of the costal cartilages.

There are three types: pectus carinatum, pectus excavatum and the much rarer pectus arcuatum. A severe mixed form is known as Jeune syndrome. Other associated conditions include Poland syndrome, pentalogy of Cantrell, Marfan syndrome and Ehlers-Danlos syndrome. We will consider the two most common congenital chest wall abnormalities.

Pectus Excavatum

Pectus excavatum or "sunken chest" is the most common chest wall deformity accounting for 88% of all chest wall deformities and occurs in 1 in 1,000 children **(Fig. 9.9)**. It is four times more common in boys. The cause is

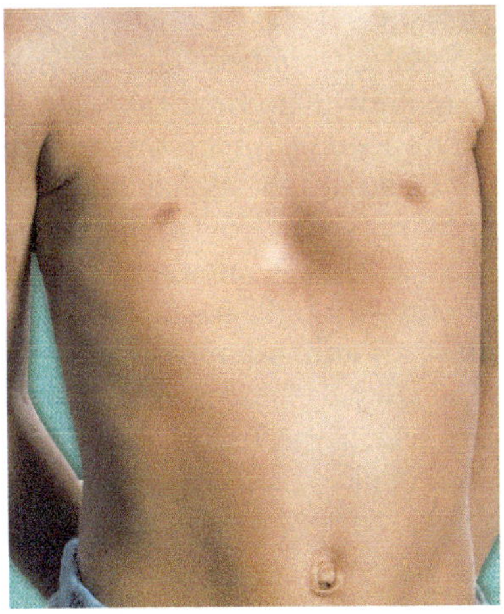

Figure 9.9 Pectus excavatum (sunken chest).

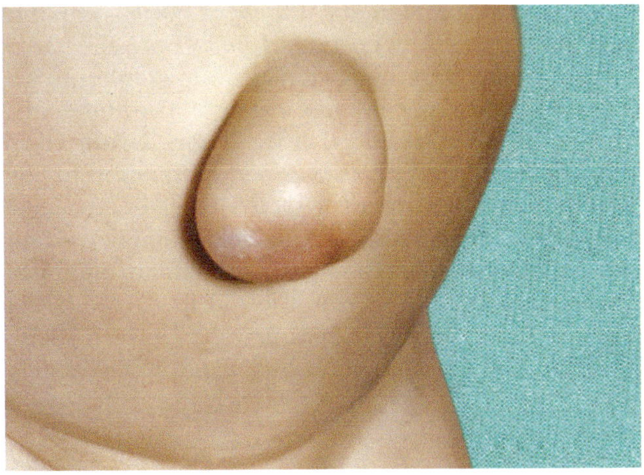

Figure 9.10 umbilical hernia.

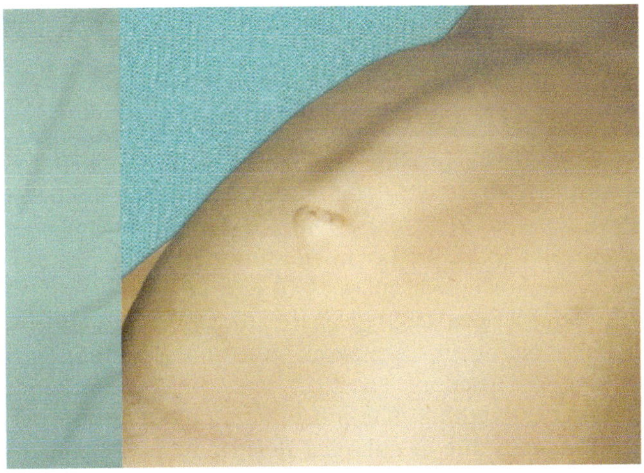

Figure 9.11 Divarication of recti.

unknown, although there is a recognised familial element and many surgeons, including Ravitch, believed in the short diaphragmatic ligament theory pulling excessively on the diaphragm and subsequently the posterior sternum. The degree of depression is variable and may not be symmetrical. Less than a third of patients require surgical correction, usually via the Nuss procedure, which can be performed thoracoscopically. Traditionally, surgery was performed following puberty when the chest is essentially fully grown, but still malleable. There is, however, evidence to support good cosmetic results in both younger children and adults in their 20s and 30s.

Pectus Carinatum

Pectus carinatum or "pigeon chest" is a protrusion deformity of the chest wall and is less common than pectus excavatum, accounting for around 5% of all chest wall deformities. This rarely requires surgical correction and often responds to compression garments and bracing, although in severe cases a modified Ravitch procedure may be considered.

Abdominal Wall Pathologies

Umbilical Hernia

An umbilical hernia results from failure of the umbilical ring or cicatrix to close following birth **(Fig. 9.10)**. It occurs in 3% of the population, and is more common in those of African heritage and is three times more common in females than males. The majority resolve by the age of 3 years and rarely are complicated by incarceration, and thus surgical repair is delayed until after the child's third birthday. Repair is usually performed as a day-case procedure.

Epigastric Hernia and Divarication of Recti Muscle

Epigastric hernia results from defects in or failure of fusion of the linea alba. These require repair because of the risk of incarceration, but must first be distinguished from Divarication of recti muscle **(Fig. 9.11)**, which is a general weakness of the linea alba and is commonly seen in the young and the elderly and does not merit surgical intervention. The hernia should be identified and carefully marked pre-operatively, as the defect can be difficult to feel once the child is under anaesthesia and relaxed. Repair is a day-case procedure through a small transverse incision, identifying the fascial defect and repairing it with an absorbable suture. Recurrence is rarely seen.

A Child with Abdominal Pain

As with any other condition, the acquisition of a full and comprehensive history is paramount. This can be difficult especially in children younger than 5 years. The clinician, however, should ask about the pain [SOCRATES (*s*ite, *o*nset, *c*haracter, *r*adiation, *a*ssociation, *t*ime course, *e*xacerbating/relieving factors, and *s*everity)]. It is also important to ascertain any urinary or bowel symptoms and the last menstrual period in girls. The fasting status of the patient must be documented in addition to any regular medication or drug allergies. The differential diagnosis should be guided by the history and the site of the pain (see diagram below). When examining the child, always remember to check their vital signs, tympanic membranes, and tonsillar beds and examine for lymphadenopathy, in addition to hernial orifices and testes in boys. Investigations can also aid in diagnosis and should start with the simplest first. All children should undergo urinalysis and then, only if deemed necessary, blood tests and possibly imaging such as a plain X-ray or ultrasound.

Appendicitis

Appendicitis is one of the commonest conditions managed by paediatric surgeons with an incidence of 25 per 10,000 before the age of 17 years **(Fig. 9.12)**. Despite its common occurrence, it can be challenging to diagnose, especially in children younger than 5 years. The typical history is that of initial periumbilical pain resulting from distension of the appendix, and this visceral pain presents as a discomfort located at the level of the T10 dermatome. This then commonly shifts to the right iliac fossa, as this is peritoneal pain from the inflamed appendix touching peritoneum. The best way to diagnose appendicitis remains a thorough history and examination and, if possible, repeated examination by the same clinician. A leucocytosis and rise in C-reactive protein can be helpful, but active observation and clinical examination is often the key. A plain abdominal X-ray (AXR) may show features of appendicitis such as scoliosis due to pain, a faecolith, absent right psoas shadow, intraperitoneal gas indicating perforation or abnormal caecal gas or small bowel dilatation. Ultrasound may show free fluid or a non-compressible appendix, but the diagnosis remains clinical. Once the diagnosis has been made, then an appendicectomy is performed often laparoscopically.

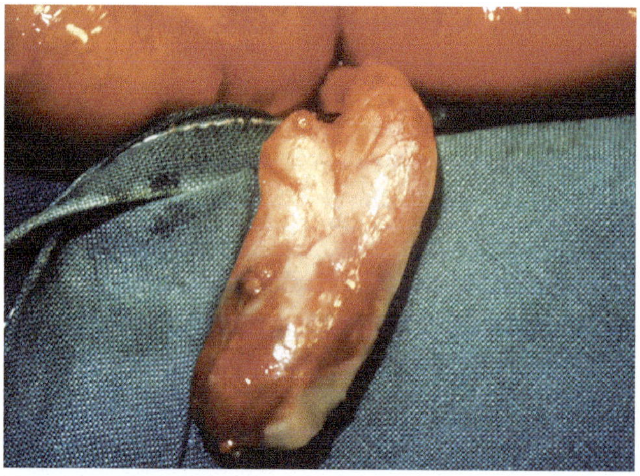

Figure 9.12 Appendicitis.

Intussusception

Intussusception is defined as the full-thickness invagination of the proximal bowel in to distal intestine **(Figs. 9.13A to C)**. About 80–90% occur between 3 months and 3 years. Only 10% have the classic picture of abdominal pain, vomiting and bleeding and a "sausage-shaped" mass. AXR can be helpful but an ultrasound scan (USS) gives the diagnosis. Red currant jelly stools occur because of intestinal oedema, lymphatic obstruction, vascular stasis and subsequent mucosal sloughing. The most common site is ileocolic and is often due to enlarged Peyer patches secondary to a preceding viral illness but may have an anatomical lead point such as a Meckel diverticulum (MD). Treatment is reduction by either air enema or laparotomy. The recurrence rate is between 5% and 10%, depending on the method used.

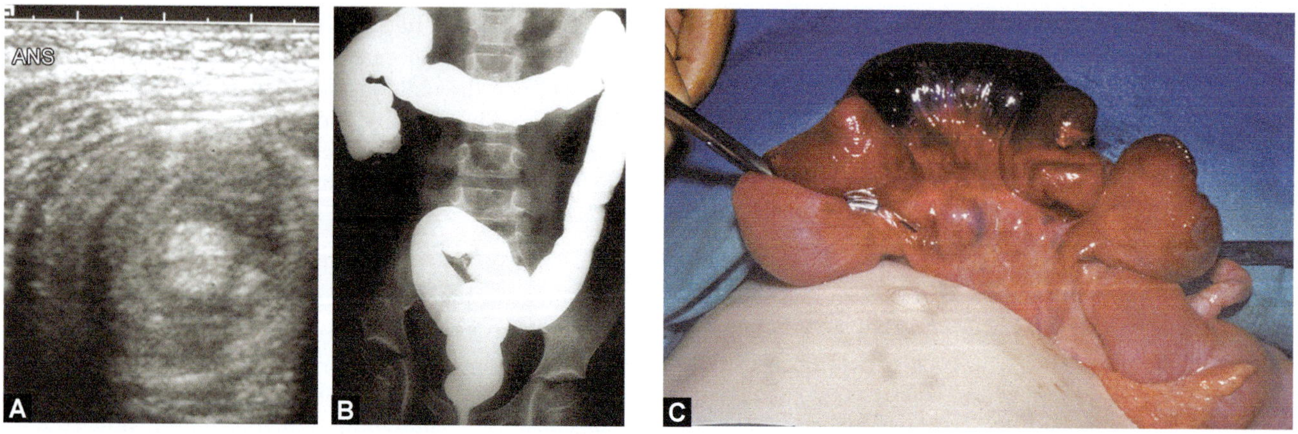

Figures 9.13A to C Intussusception. (A) Ultrasound scan; (B) Abdominal X-ray; (C) Sausage-shaped mass.

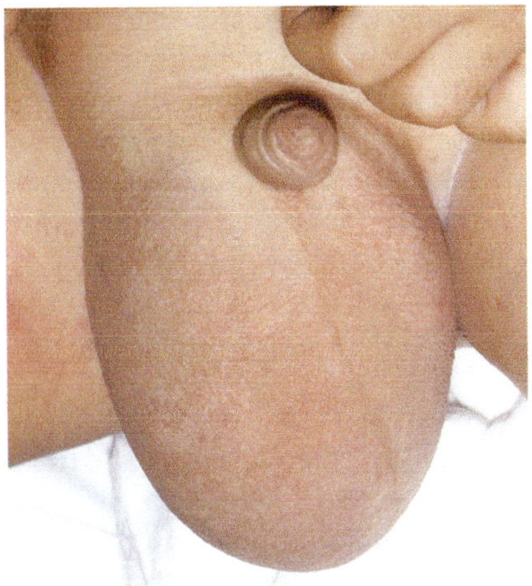

Figure 9.14 Inguinal hernia.

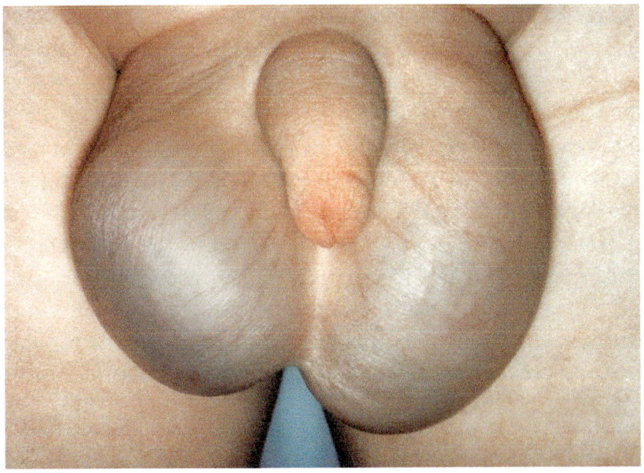

Figure 9.15 hydrocele.

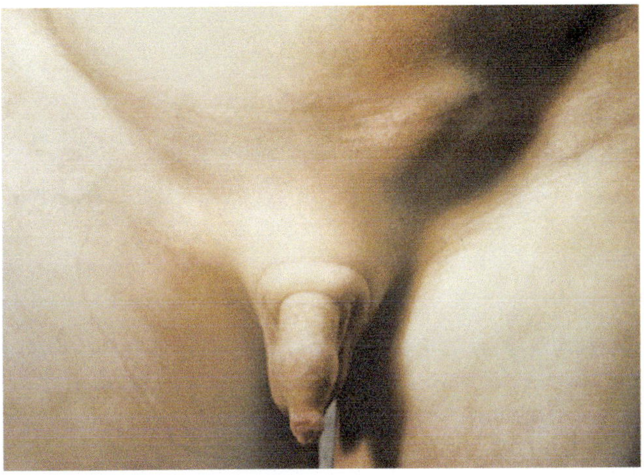

Figure 9.16 Undescended testes.

Groin Conditions

Inguinal Hernia

A hernia can be defined as a protrusion of a viscus or part of a viscus into a cavity where it should not lie. Inguinal hernia is the commonest surgical condition in children (Fig. 9.14). Its incidence is increased in pre-mature and low-birth-weight infants. Inguinal hernia is far more common in boys than girls with a ratio of 10:1. Seventy per cent are right-sided, 25% are left-sided and 5% are bilateral. Ninety-nine per cent are indirect hernias; 30% present within the first year of life. All inguinal hernias need repair because of the risk of strangulation. This is ideally done electively, and in those older than 6 months of age, it is performed as a day-case procedure. If a hernia is incarcerated, the management principle is to "resuscitate, reduce and repair."

Hydrocele

A hydrocele means fluid in the scrotum and is due to a patent processus vaginalis (Fig. 9.15). It is often noticed with or just after a systemic illness. It presents as a swelling with a "blue hue." Typically, on examination, the examining hand can get above it unlike a hernia and it transilluminates. Ninety per cent resolve spontaneously in the first year of life. If it has not resolved by age 3 years, then it is unlikely to and should be repaired by ligation of the patent processus vaginalis.

Undescended Testes

Undescended testes (UDT) or cryptorchidism is another very common condition seen by paediatric surgeons with an incidence of 1–3% of all boys and up to 33% in pre-term infants (Fig. 9.16). They can be classified as impalpable or palpable, unilateral or bilateral. Imaging is seldom of value in identifying impalpable testis, and laparoscopy is required to identify any intra-abdominal gonads. Testes may also be ectopic. Retractile testes are those that are normally descended but, due to the pull of the cremasteric muscle, they retract back up into the inguinal canal. If these testes can be milked down into the scrotum by the examiner and stay down, then they do not require surgery. Much has been written with regard to the optimum age to bring down UDT due to concerns regarding future fertility and malignancy. Boys with unilateral UDT who undergo orchidopexy are thought to have the same paternity rates as the rest of the general population. Boys with bilateral UDT, however, have a 49% paternity rate compared to 81% in the overall population. Cryptorchidism increases the relative risk of testicular malignancy by a factor of between 3 and 7. The recent British Association of Paediatric Urologists consensus 2011 agrees that although there is little prospective evidence, orchidopexy prior to 10 years of age should decrease this risk. The consensus recommends orchidopexy as early as 3–6 months of age, but between 6 and 12 months is acceptable. Hormonal treatment has had variable success in different centres and is not routinely recommended.

Penile Conditions

Phimosis and balanitis/balanoposthitis Phimosis or a non-retractile foreskin is usually physiological before the age of 5 years. Treatment is, therefore, rarely needed before this age. If the boy then becomes symptomatic with ballooning of the foreskin and episodes of infection of the prepuce (balanitis/balanoposthitis), then treatment may be initiated **(Fig. 9.17A)**. This can be with topical steroid cream or surgical options including prepuceplasty or circumcision. Balanitis xerotica obliterans (BXO) is a condition of white scarring of the foreskin and may also affect the glans penis and urethral meatus **(Fig. 9.17B)**. The cause is essentially unknown, although infective and autoimmune causes have been implicated. The treatment is circumcision and meatal dilatation or meatotomy may be needed for more severe cases.

Paraphimosis It is when the foreskin has been pulled back beyond the glans and is unable to be protracted. If left, this can be difficult to reduce. Fifty per cent dextrose topically may help to reduce oedema and facilitate reduction under a penile block, but occasionally theatre is needed to reduce the paraphimosis or to perform a dorsal slit and/or circumcision **(Fig. 9.17C)**.

Acute scrotum

The acute scrotum is a clinical emergency and any testicular pain should be taken seriously and treated as such **(Figs. 9.18A and B)**. The differential diagnosis of testicular pain in boys includes: testicular torsion, torsion of the appendage (hydatid of Morgagni), epididymo-orchitis, hydrocele (rarely painful) and idiopathic scrotal oedema (usually bilateral and rarely painful).

The differences in presentations are shown in **Table 9.2**.

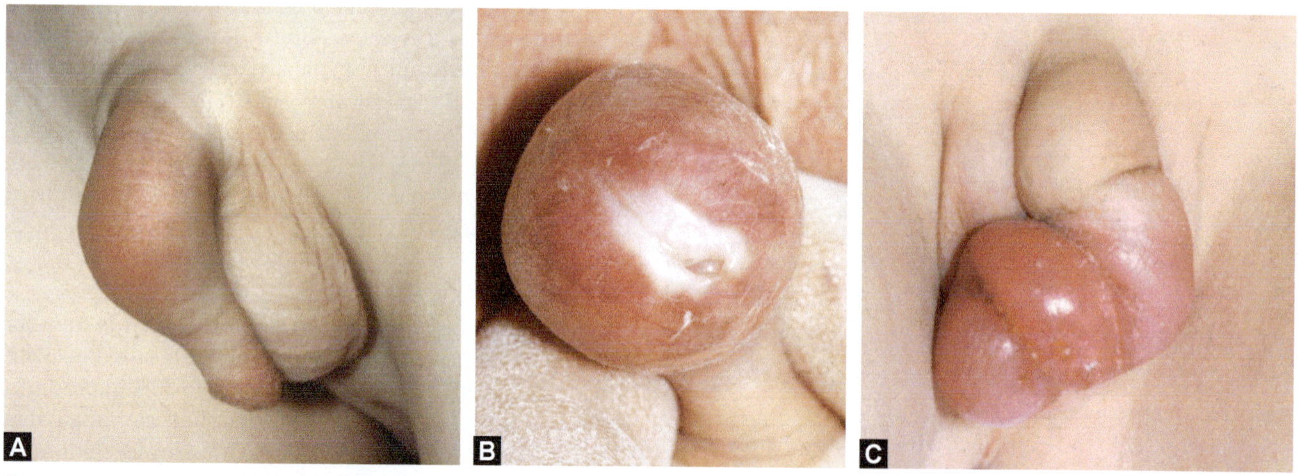

Figures 9.17A to C Different penile conditions.

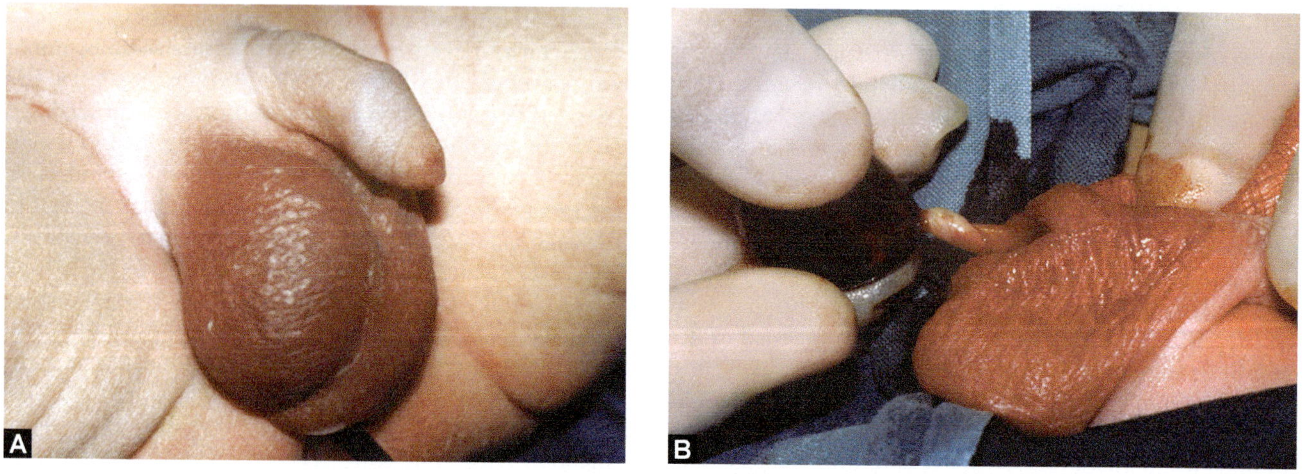

Figures 9.18A and B Acute scrotum.

TABLE 9.2	Difference in presentation of groin conditions.		
	Torted testis	***Torted Hydatid***	***Epididymo-orchitis***
Pain	Sudden Severe	Gradual onset 2–3 days	Gradual Less severe
Associated symptoms	Nausea and vomiting		Dysuria, etc.
On examination	High riding Swollen Red, hard Marked tenderness	Localised to upper scrotum "Blue spot" Reactive hydrocoele	Swelling Erythema Oedema; but less severe

Gastrointestinal Surgery

Pyloric Stenosis

Pyloric stenosis usually presents between 3 and 6 weeks of age. It presents with a history of rapidly progressive projectile vomiting without bile. The baby is hungry, and dehydration and alkalosis are prominent features **(Figs. 9.19A to C)**. It is more common if there is a family history and if the child is a first-born male. The child is examined for signs of dehydration and a test feed is performed, not to see if the child vomits but to establish if there is a palpable "tumour" in right upper quadrant (RUQ). Visible peristalsis may also be seen. If the tumour is not palpable, an ultrasound may be performed. The mainstay of management is then to correct the hypochloraemic hypokalaemic alkalosis with intravenous (IV) fluids prior to pyloromyotomy. This can be performed through an RUQ or supraumbilical incision or laparoscopically.

Intestinal Obstruction

The aetiology of intestinal obstruction in children varies very much in accordance with the child's age **(Fig. 9.20)**. An obstructive picture in a neonate, that is, bilious vomiting, abdominal distension and constipation, is often congenital. Causes include duodenal atresia (DA), small bowel atresias, malrotation and volvulus, necrotising enterocolitis (NEC), meconium disease, Hirschsprung disease (HD), anorectal malformation (ARM) or an incarcerated hernia (see Neonatal Surgery). The clinical picture depends, as in adults, on the level of the obstruction. In infants, intussusception, an MD or appendicitis must be considered. In children, who have had previous surgery, an adhesive obstruction may be the cause. No matter what the age of the child, green or bilious vomiting is obstruction until proven otherwise. If malrotation is suspected, then the child needs an upper gastrointestinal (GI) water-soluble contrast to exclude this. Ultrasound may also be helpful in determining the orientation of the mesenteric vessels and in demonstrating any volvulus. A plain AXR can give a lot of information such as the presence of any dilated loops or air-fluid levels. In a child with a small bowel obstruction thought to be secondary to adhesions, conservative management of "drip and suck" can be employed; however, if not settling after 24 hours or if the child is tender, laparotomy should be considered. Hence, the well-known surgical expression "never let the sun go down on a small bowel obstruction."

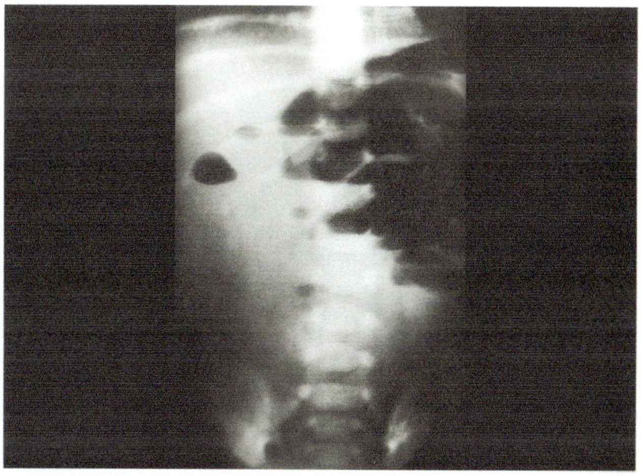

Figure 9.20 intestinal obstruction.

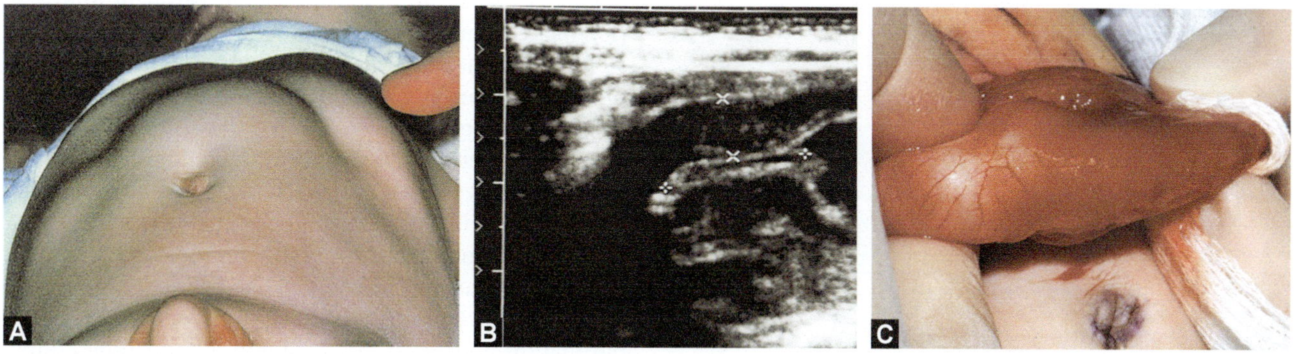

Figures 9.19A to C Pyloric stenosis.

Gastro-oesophageal Reflux Disease

Gastro-oesophageal reflux (GOR) is the involuntary movement of gastric contents back up into the oesophagus and is due to failure of the normal or mature physiological barriers to this such as the angle of His, the lower oesophageal sphincter, the length of the intra-abdominal oesophagus and intra-abdominal pressure. Most babies reflux—however, the term gastro-oesophageal reflux disease (GORD) is used when the condition becomes pathological and the child needs treatment. The majority of GOR resolves spontaneously by the time the child reaches their second birthday. The management is predominantly medical; however, surgical management may be required especially in the neurologically impaired patient. These children can display abnormal posturing and what is referred to as the Sandifer syndrome. Careful history and examination is required followed by a contrast study to ensure no anatomical cause of reflux and to ensure there is normal gastric emptying. Twenty-four-hour pH studies are helpful in the older child, and the pH of the distal oesophagus should be measured. The percentage of time the pH is less than 4 and the number of episodes helps to grade the reflux, and this together with failed medical management such as H2-blockers and proton-pump inhibitors may indicate the requirement for surgical intervention, the most common procedure being a laparoscopic Nissen fundoplication.

Constipation and Rectal Prolapse

Idiopathic childhood constipation can be defined as delay or difficulty in passing stool that causes distress to the patient. The majority of constipation seen in children is idiopathic, but rarer causes such as HD **(Fig. 9.21A)**, ARMs, cystic fibrosis (CF) and hypothyroidism should be borne in mind. Diagnostic clues to pathology include failure to pass meconium in 24 hours, constipation from birth, abdominal distension with vomiting, neurological impairment or asymmetry of the gluteal muscles, any suggestion of spina bifida occulta or sacral agenesis. Surgical causes of constipation are included further on in this chapter. The mainstay of management for idiopathic constipation is dietary modification and laxatives (stimulant, stool softeners or osmotic). It should be explained that the stools need to be of toothpaste consistency with no straining so as to avoid the vicious cycle of painful motions leading to children holding on to stool and resulting in a difficult to treat megarectum. In severe cases of constipation, usually with an underlying pathology, the Irrimatic pump may be of benefit in getting the child empty and keeping them socially clean. An antegrade colonic enema (ACE) is a surgical option for patients with intractable constipation.

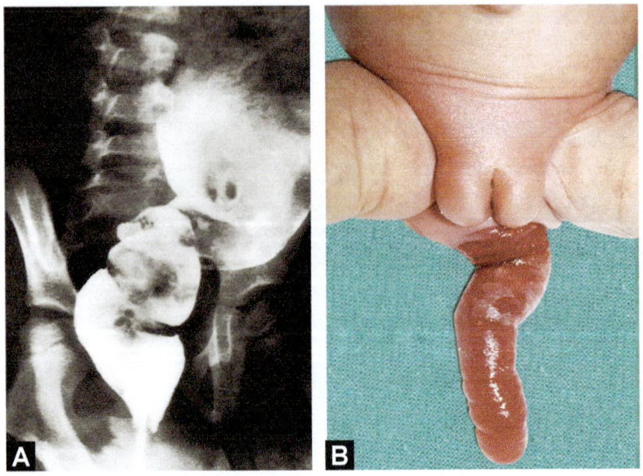

Figures 9.21A and B Rectal prolapse due to constipation.

Gastrointestinal Bleeding

GI bleeding is a common problem encountered in paediatric practice. It can, however, be difficult to reach a diagnosis. It is important to differentiate between upper and lower GI haemorrhage. Haematemesis usually suggests upper haemorrhage, and melaena (passage of dark stool or altered blood) indicates lower GI haemorrhage. Fresh red rectal bleeding usually originates from low down and often within the anal canal. Causes of upper GI bleeding include swallowed maternal blood in the neonate, oesophageal varices, Mallory-Weiss tear, gastric/duodenal ulcer, vascular malformation and non-steroidal anti-inflammatory drugs. Lower GI bleeding may be due to an MD, duplication cyst, intussusception, inflammatory bowel disease (IBD), Henoch-Schönlein purpura, infective diarrhoea and proctitis. In the neonate, especially the pre-mature infant, NEC is an important cause as is malrotation and midgut volvulus (see Neonatal Surgery). Anal fissure as a result of constipation is the most common cause of rectal bleeding. Constipation can also lead to haemorrhoids and rectal prolapse **(Fig. 9.21B)**. Rectal prolapse is more common in children who are malnourished or who are neurologically impaired or have spina bifida. It may also be the presenting symptom of CF and, as such, any child presenting with their first rectal prolapse should have a sweat test performed. Rectal prolapse is usually self-resolving so long as there is aggressive management of constipation so as to avoid any straining during defaecation. It rarely requires surgical intervention in an otherwise normal child. Investigation for lower GI bleeding may include stool for microbiology, routine bloods, enteroscopy, plain AXR, ultrasound, contrast studies and Meckel scan.

Meckel diverticulum: An MD is the remnant of the prenatal yolk stalk **(Figs. 9.22A to C)**. The yolk sac of the developing embryo is connected to the primitive gut by the yolk stalk or vitelline duct. It normally regresses between the fifth and seventh weeks of foetal life. Failure of regression can result in various anomalies. MD occurs in 2% of the population, making it the commonest congenital abnormality of the GI tract. It was first described by the German

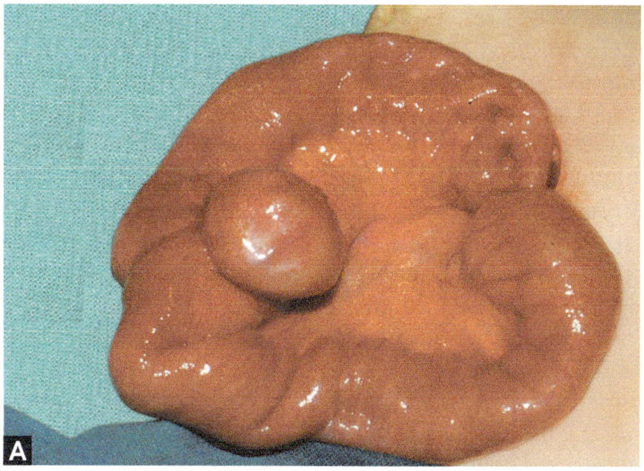

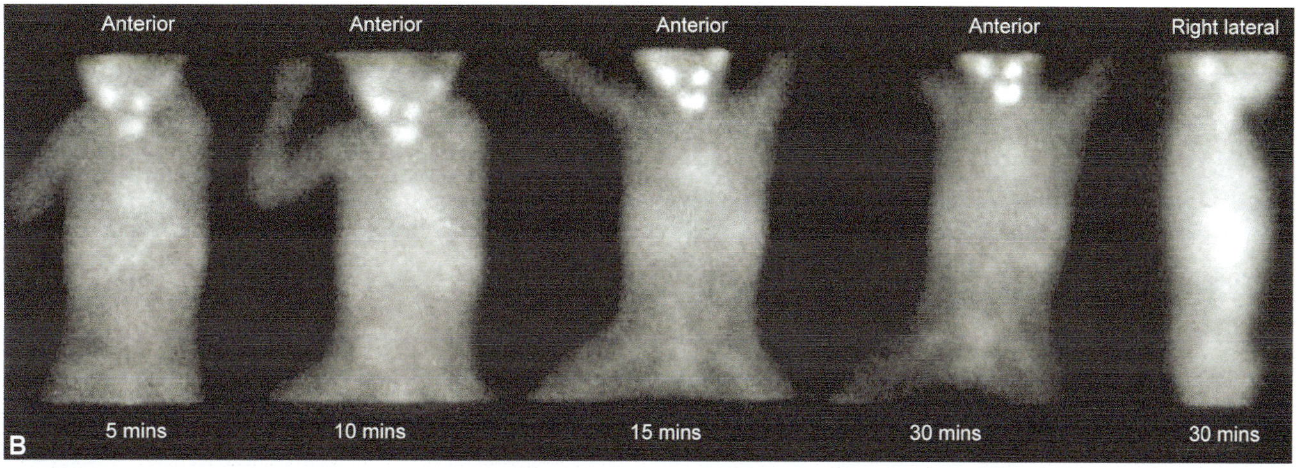

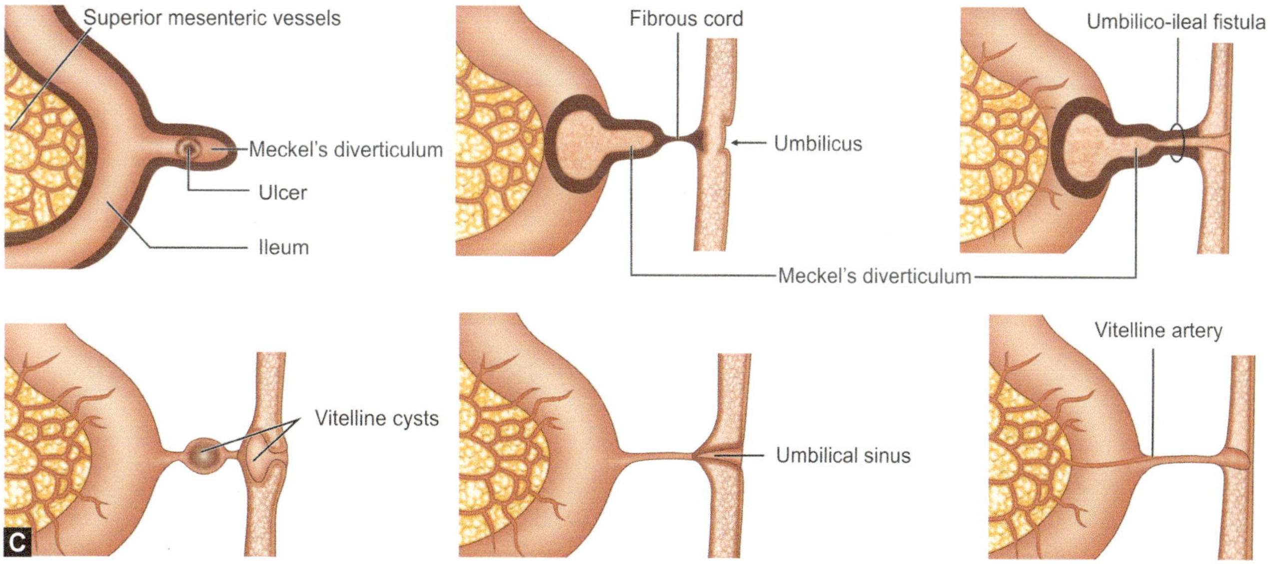

Figures 9.22A to C Meckel diverticulum.

surgeon Wilhelm Fabricius Hildanus; however, it was the German anatomist Johnan Friedrich Meckel who gave the condition his name. The commonly referred to "Rule of 2s" states it is found 2 feet from the ileocaecal valve, is 2 inches long, 2 cm diameter and usually presents within the first 2 years of life. It often contains two types of tissue, typically heterotopic gastric mucosa, and it is this that is responsible for the complication of gastric bleeding. Pancreatic tissue can also be found as can tumours including carcinoid tumours, leiomyomas, GI stromal tumours, angiomas and neurofibromas. An MD may also find its way into an inguinal hernia, so-called Littre hernia, or into a spigelian hernia. In 1933, the American surgeon Charles Mayo was famously quoted as saying that an MD is "frequently suspected, often looked for and seldom found" and poses a diagnostic challenge for paediatricians and surgeons alike. Even with a high index of suspicion and the employment of various radiological modalities, the diagnosis can still be elusive. A radioisotope technetium (Te^{99m}) scan **(Fig. 9.22B)** has for a long time been regarded as the investigation of choice. Te^{99m} is secreted by tubular gland cells in the gastric mucosa and the isotope should only accumulate in the stomach and bladder. The sensitivity of a Meckel scan, however, varies in the literature between 60 and 85% and is less sensitive in patients who are actively bleeding. Pentagastrin increases acid production by parietal cells, and histamine H2-receptor antagonists such as cimetidine decrease the washout of pertechnetate and in the past has been used to improve sensitivity. In the last decade, laparoscopy has been proposed as the diagnostic tool of choice as well as means of definitive treatment, and more recently capsular endoscopy has been proposed as another means of diagnosis.

Inflammatory Bowel Disease

IBD is on the increase in children and has an incidence of 4–6 per 100,000 **(Figs. 9.23 to 9.26)**. Ulcerative colitis (UC) or indeterminate colitis is more common in children

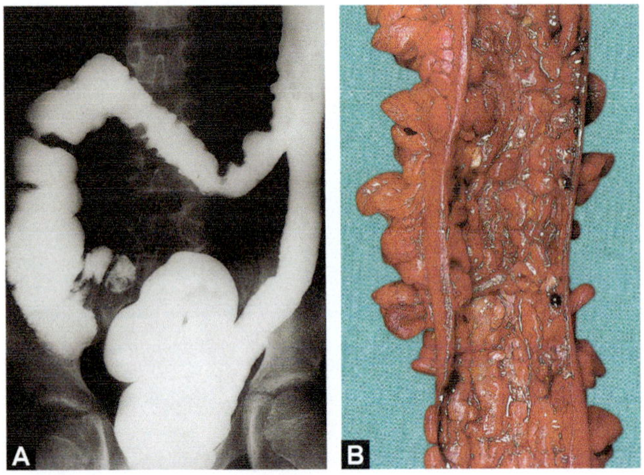

Figures 9.23A and B Ulcerative colitis.

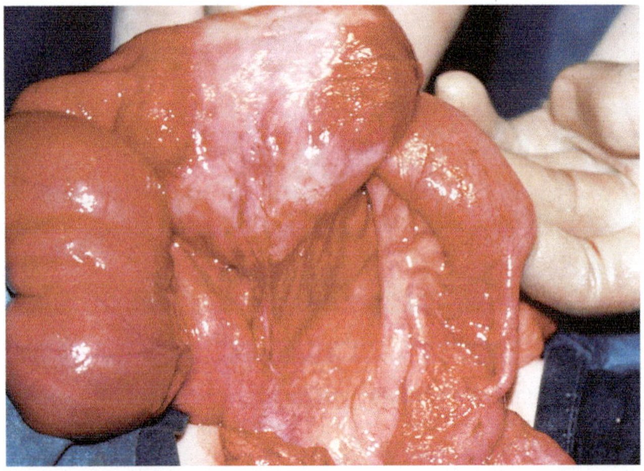

Figure 9.24 Terminal ileal Crohn disease.

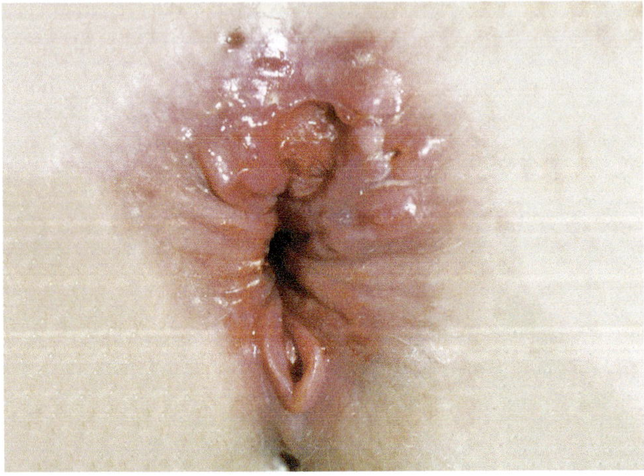

Figure 9.25 Perianal Crohn disease.

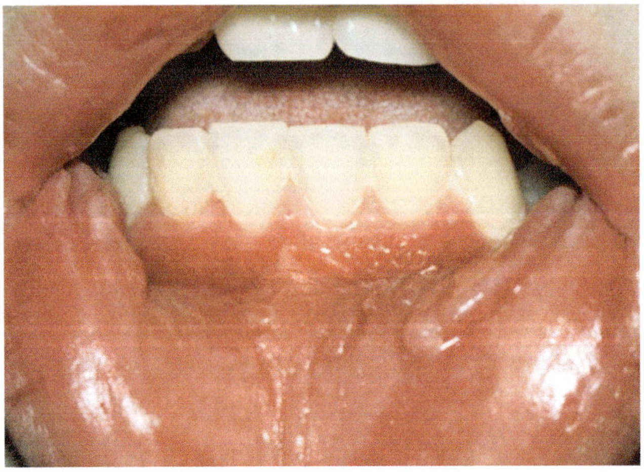

Figure 9.26 Aphthous ulcers.

younger than 5 years and Crohn disease (CD) is more common in children older than 5 years. Unlike in the adult disease, the incidence of CD has doubled in children and is now the most common type of IBD in children and boys are twice as likely to be affected as girls. There is now a known genetic predisposition for IBD, especially in CD and the younger the child is at diagnosis. There are several classical differences between UC and CD, namely that UC affects the rectum and colon for a variable length, whereas CD can be from "mouth to anus." In UC, there is always rectal involvement and it is more common to have severe bloody diarrhoea. Perianal disease with abscesses and fistula is more common in CD, whereas toxic megacolon is more a hallmark of UC. Systemic manifestations such as joint and eye disease are associated with CD rather than UC.

Differences are also seen radiologically, at surgery, and down the microscope. UC classically has a picture of diffuse ulceration, limited to the mucosa, and on X-ray, because of loss of haustrations of the colon, is referred to as a "lead pipe" colon. CD macroscopically shows "cobblestoning" ulceration and typically there are transmural granulomas and the bowel can have skip lesions. Radiologically, narrowed and diseased segments of bowel may give the classic "string sign," cobblestoning may also be apparent and on barium nodular filling defects may be seen.

The management of IBD can be divided in medical and surgical therapies. Medical management comprises anti-inflammatories (5-aminosalicylic acids), antibiotics and steroids, nutritional, immune-suppressors (6-mercaptopurine, azathioprine, cyclosporine, methotrexate) and immunotherapy agents such as infliximab. Surgical management is more common in anti-saccharomyces antibody positive disease and is required when medical treatment fails, when there is refractory illness, growth failure, stricture or abscess formation and perforation or obstruction. Surgical options include resections, commonly terminal ileum or right hemicolectomy in CD, stomas or enteroplasty. Ileal pouch anal anastomosis can be used successfully in UC; however, in CD, proctocolectomy with end ileostomy may be necessary. Fistulotomy may be required for severe fistulas in CD or they be injected with fibrin glue. In refractory cases, advancement flaps are another surgical alternative.

Short Bowel Syndrome

Short bowel syndrome (SBS) is a very challenging condition usually resulting from surgical resection of bowel, which results in an inadequate length of bowel necessary for enteral nutrition and growth of the child. A normal term neonate has 250 cm of small intestine, and by adulthood this has grown to 750 cm. There are many conditions that necessitate extensive small bowel resection. These include atresias, NEC, gastroschisis, malrotation and volvulus in neonates. Congenital SBS is rare. In older children, IBD and intussusception may lead to resection. It has traditionally been taught that at least 40 cm of small intestine is needed for the chance of being successfully enterally fed and not dependent on total parenteral nutrition (TPN). Complete dependence on TPN is referred to as intestinal failure. Less than 100 cm of jejunum usually results in significant malabsorption. It is not, however, simply the length of the bowel that is important but also the type of bowel left and its ability to adapt. It is now known that it is better to lose jejunum as the ileum is better at adapting for absorption of nutrients. The length of ileum preserved is also more important than whether the ileocaecal valve is preserved or not.

Management of SBS is medical or surgical. Medical management includes metabolic and nutritional therapies, and antibiotics for bacterial overgrowth and for complications of TPN, namely liver disease and line sepsis. Medication can also help with associated GOR, malabsorptive diarrhoea and dysmotility.

Surgical interventions fall into three groups: firstly, gaining and maintaining central venous line access for long-term TPN; secondly, bowel-lengthening procedures; and thirdly, intestinal transplantation. Bowel-lengthening procedures include the serial transverse enteroplasty (STEP) and Bianchi procedures. The STEP procedure was first performed in Boston in 2002 and relies on the fact that the bowel's blood supply comes from the mesentery at right angles to the length of the bowel, thus allowing a series of "V" shapes or zigzags to be created, leading to increased length. The Bianchi procedure involves separating a section of bowel into two tubes and then joining them end to end. Neither procedure is without risk or complication, and a recent review compared the two and found that the STEP procedure was less technically demanding and patients were less likely to require transplant. Intestinal transplantation is, of course, a last resort and even when successful involves chronic immunosuppression, long periods in hospital and the risk of infection, graft rejection, graft-versus-host disease and lymphoproliferative disease.

Hepatobiliary

Biliary Atresia

Biliary atresia (BA) is a rare condition that involves a congenital but often progressive obstruction of the biliary tree and is seen in around 1 in 18,000 live births (**Figs. 9.27A and B**). It is the most important surgical cause of a neonate with cholestatic jaundice. It affects slightly more girls than boys and is more commonly seen in Japan and French Polynesia, although no genetic or specific cause has been identified to date. Some potential genes have been identified in so-called syndromic BA, namely *CFC-1*, *IMF*, *jagged-1*, *keratin* 9 and *18*, and increased expression of ICAM 1 is seen with more severe cirrhosis of the liver. Certain infective triggers have been postulated including

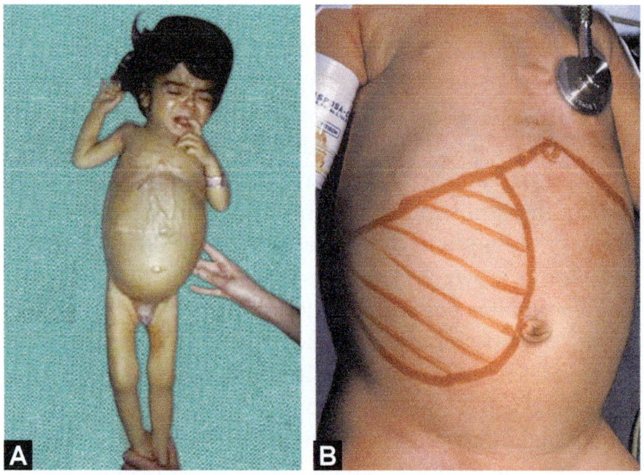

Figures 9.27A and B A child suffering from biliary atresia.

cytomegalovirus, Epstein-Barr virus, human papilloma virus and respiratory syncytial virus, and in mice, reovirus 3 has been shown to induce a BA-type cholangitis, although its link in neonates is still debatable the disease resolves spontaneously. BA, however, may be associated with other congenital malformations such as polysplenia or asplenia, situs inversus, a pre-duodenal portal vein and malrotation. There are three main types of BA. Type I is confined to the common bile duct (CBD); type II involves the common and hepatic ducts; and the commonest type, type III, extends up to the porta hepatis. The classical triad of clinical features which should alert the paediatrician is conjugated jaundice beyond day 14 of life, acholic stool (although some infants may have normal stool) with dark urine and an enlarged liver. An early diagnosis is key to successful treatment. The diagnosis is made by a combination of blood tests [liver function tests (LFTs), coagulation, hepatitis serology, TORCH (Toxoplasmosis, Rubella, Cytomegalovirus, Herpes simplex), α1-antitrypsin deficiency], USS looking for an absent gallbladder and classic "triangular cord sign," scintigraphy [HIDA (hepatobiliary iminodiacetic acid) scan], magnetic resonance cholangiopancreatography (MRCP), cholangiography, liver biopsy and laparoscopy. In the 1950s, Kasai discovered that there may be patent albeit microscopic biliary channels in the region of the porta hepatis and went on to develop the now infamous Kasai procedure or hepatoportoenterostomy. This has been performed laparoscopically, but this is no longer recommended due to poor results. Postoperatively, the patients receive antibiotics; steroids and ursodeoxycholic acid may be given to aid bile flow. By far, the most common complication is cholangitis as a result of biliary stasis. Biliary cysts or "lakes" may be seen on imaging and are often associated with recurrent bouts of cholangitis. Portal hypertension may also lead to oesophageal varices, ascites and hypersplenism; however, this often gets better with time. Rarer later complications include hepatopulmonary syndrome, pulmonary hypertension and hepatic malignancy. Around 20% of patients post-Kasai reach adolescence with a normal functioning liver. The procedure can be repeated in selective cases, but ultimately the patient may well require liver transplantation. Indeed, BA remains the most common indication for paediatric liver transplantation.

Choledochal Cyst

Choledochal cyst is a rare condition seen in around 1 in 15,000 children in the western world, with, again, a much increased incidence in the East—around 1 in 1,000 children affected in Japan. It is four times more common in females. It may present similarly to BA, but presentation depends on the age of the child and the type of cyst. Todani in 1977 classified choledochal cysts into five types: type I, saccular or fusiform dilatation of extrahepatic ducts; type II, a cystic diverticulum of the CBD; type III, a choledochocele; type IV, multiple dilatations of extrahepatic ducts; and type V, intrahepatic bile duct dilatation, also known as Caroli disease. The aetiology is still unclear, but several theories have been proposed including a congenital weakness in the wall of the duct, congenital stenosis and/or reflux of pancreatic enzymes up the CBD causing inflammation and scarring. Increasingly, choledochal cysts are being diagnosed antenatally. In young children, it can present with obstructive jaundice or with a mass with or without jaundice. In older children, it more commonly presents with pain due to pancreatitis (often fusiform cysts) or with an RUQ mass with intermittent jaundice (saccular cysts). The diagnosis is made through blood tests (LFTs, amylase and coagulation), USS, MRCP and cholangiography. The management is by surgical excision. In certain types, simple cyst excision may be possible, or if the cyst is extremely inflamed, mucosectomy may be considered, but the majority require excision with a hepaticojejunostomy and Roux-en-Y loop. Intraoperative endoscopy may be helpful to ensure the cyst is fully resected without damaging the pancreatic duct. Laparoscopy and robotic-assisted excision have been reported. For type V cysts, hepatic lobectomy or even liver transplant may be needed depending on how much of the liver is affected. Complications of cyst resection include cholangitis, pancreatitis, stone formation, anastomotic stricture, portal hypertension and, the most worrying malignancy, cholangiocarcinoma. There is up to a 30% chance of malignancy in a choledochal cyst, which is 20 times that of the average population, and 50% will have developed a malignancy by the age of 50 years; resection, therefore, is always recommended.

Gallstones

Gallstones or cholelithiasis is relatively uncommon in children unless the children have an underlying predisposition such as hereditary spherocytosis. The incidence, however, has been seen to be increasing in children who are obese. In the United States, the primary cause of gallstones now is cholesterol gallstones seen in obese children rather than the traditionally taught haematological causes. Acalculous cholecystitis has also been described in children recovering from other procedures necessitating a long hospital stay such as spinal surgery. As in adults, gallstones are more common in females. Presenting symptoms are the same in adults, that is, colicky RUQ pain which may be associated with jaundice, vomiting, pyrexia which may point to cholangitis or pancreatitis. Investigation and treatment are again similar to those in adults in terms of routine blood tests including LFTs and serum amylase and USS. MRCP may also be needed to make the diagnosis. Depending on the severity of symptoms and the cause, laparoscopic cholecystectomy is the management option of choice.

Urology

Hypospadias

Hypospadias is a congenital abnormality of the position of the urethral meatus **(Fig. 9.28)**. Hypo means low and so the meatus is below where it should be—at the tip of the glans somewhere on the ventral surface. There is a real spectrum of abnormality seen in hypospadias with the site classified as glanular, subcoronal, penile, penoscrotal, scrotal or even perineal. There is often an associated hooded foreskin and ventral bend to the penis, also known as chordee. Glanular, coronal or distal penile hypospadias are the most common types, making up to 70% of all hypospadias. This makes sense embryologically, as the glanular urethra forms last. Hypospadias is a very common abnormality affecting around 1 in 125 boys. The cause is thought to be multifactorial but involves an abnormality in androgen production and the effects this has on the developing penis as well as a possible diminished response to human chorionic gonadotropin (hCG). Environmental factors include winter conception; genetic factors have yet to be identified but are accepted due to the increased incidence in primary relatives. Hypospadias associated with disorders are a different entity and are discussed later in Neonatal Surgery.

Surgery is now being performed earlier around 6–12 months of age. The objectives of surgery are fourfold, that is, to bring the meatus to the tip of the penis, to straighten any chordee, to reconstruct the foreskin where possible and to improve the cosmetic appearance of the phallus. The degree of chordee often dictates the type of repair rather than the site of the meatus alone. There are many procedures described. The most popular are the MAGPI (meatal advancement glanuloplasty procedure), the TIP (tubularised incised urethral plate) and the GAP (glans approximation) procedures. Depending on the severity, surgery may be a single- or two-stage procedure requiring preputial or even buccal grafting. Complications include infection, repair breakdown and fistula formation. Following sound repair, the boys will have a normal functioning penis, that is, they will be able to stand to pass urine and will have normal erections and future fertility will not be compromised.

Epispadias

Epispadias is a rare condition (1 in 100,000 in boys and 1 in 400,000 in girls) and is considered the least severe form of the bladder and cloacal exstrophy spectrum or complex **(Fig. 9.29)**. It is essentially the opposite of hypospadias as the urethral opening opens out onto the dorsal surface of the penis rather than the ventral. The penis often appears flattened and chordee may be present, but again a dorsal bend is seen rather than ventral. The condition can also occur in females with the urethral opening found between a bifid clitoris and the labia minora. In addition to the position of the meatus, epispadias commonly affects the internal sphincter and the pubic symphysis is separated, meaning the child is incontinent of urine.

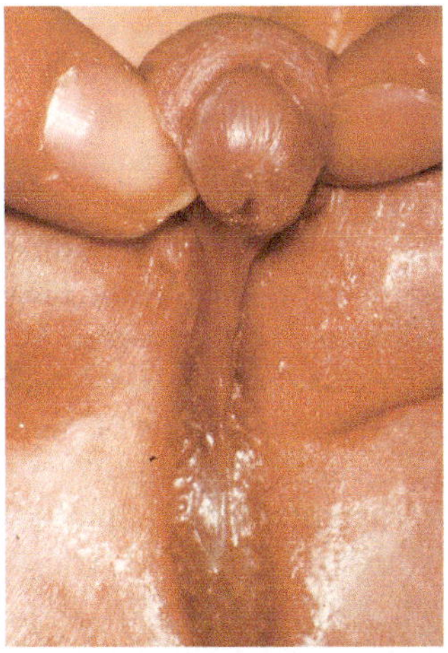

Figure 9.28 Hypospadias.

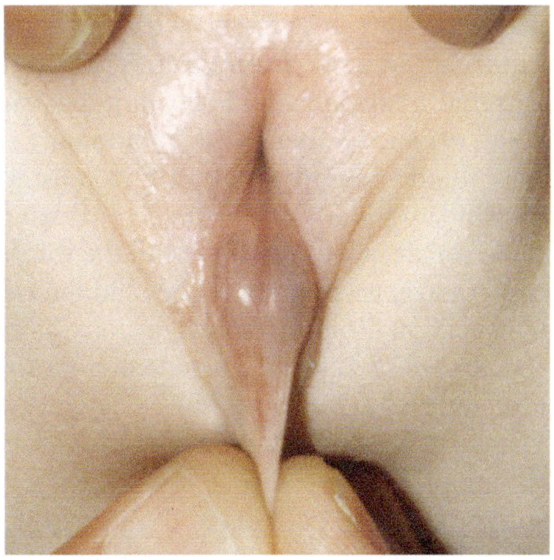

Figure 9.29 Epispadias.

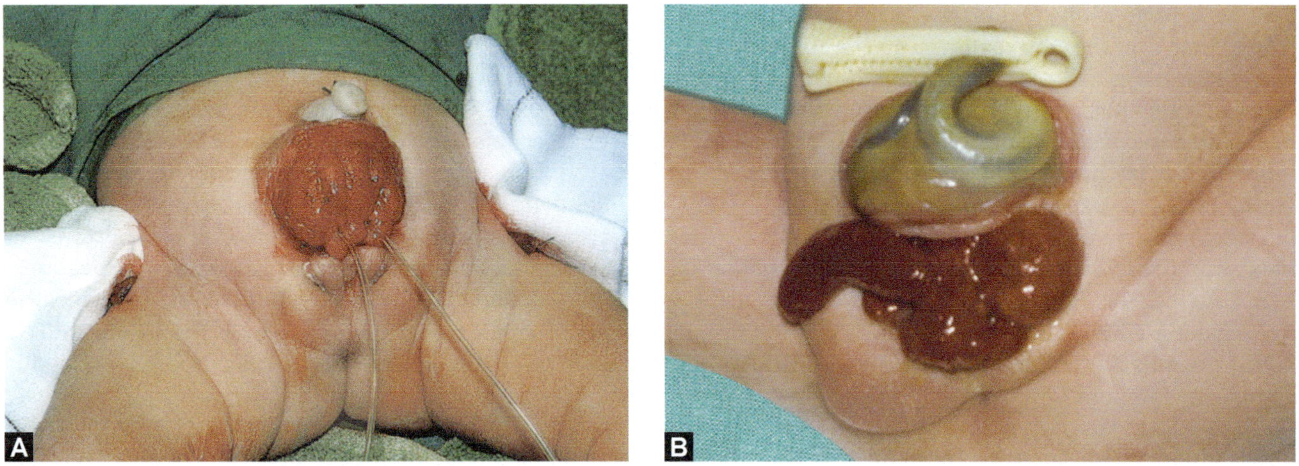

Figures 9.30A and B Bladder exstrophy and cloacal exstrophy.

Bladder Exstrophy and Cloacal Exstrophy

Bladder exstrophy is again part of the bladder and cloacal exstrophy complex and literally means the bladder is turned inside out and is visible below a defect in the umbilicus (Figs. 9.30A and B). In addition to the epispadias abnormalities described earlier, the anus is anteriorly displaced as is the vaginal opening in girls. There is pubic diastasis, as described earlier. Around half of bladder exstrophy patients have this classical type; the rest may have an epispadias or cloacal exstrophy. This is when there are two exstrophic bladders which are separated by a bridge of intestine, which often is in continuity with the terminal ileum. There is always an associated imperforate anus and it may be associated with congenitally short gut or spinal dysraphism. Embryologically, this spectrum of abnormalities is thought to result from abnormal persistence of the cloacal membrane. Most cases are not thought to be inherited; however, there is thought to be a 1 in 100 chance of a further sibling being affected. It is often now diagnosed antenatally and ideally the child should be born near a tertiary referral centre for paediatric surgery. The abnormality is covered with cling film at birth and the child should have chromosomes sent and should have their renal tracts imaged. Following this, surgery is the mainstay of management and traditionally involved three stages: the first shortly after birth to close the bladder, urethra and abdominal wall; the second in the second year of life to repair any epispadias; and the third, undertaken at school age, is to augment the bladder and repair the bladder neck in a bid to achieve urinary continence. More recently, good results have been reported from single-stage total bladder exstrophy (Kelly) repair. Due to the complexity of the surgery involved and the rarity of this condition, two specialist centres now deal with all of exstrophy/epispadias patients in the United Kingdom. Long-term outcomes are that in boys around one in four will be successfully dry and able to void normally. Greater than half will require a catheterisable stoma or have to perform clean intermittent catheterisation (CIC). Renal function is usually normal. There has been a lot of work looking at the psychological outcomes for these patients and the impact this has on their life and future sexual relations. The majority of boys are able to have intercourse; however, due to retrograde ejaculation, fertility may be an issue.

Upper Tract Obstruction

Obstruction of the urinary tract is when flow of urine is impeded so as to have a detrimental effect on the function of the kidney (Figs. 9.31A and B). It commonly encompasses pelvic ureteric junction (PUJ) and vesicoureteric junction (VUJ) obstruction. Obstruction is rarely acute in children and more commonly is intermittent or chronic. Often the child presents before any symptoms occur, as the majority of children are now picked up early with routine antenatal ultrasound screening. The diagnostic challenge is to distinguish through monitoring which of these children are going to spontaneously improve with time and which of them are going to progress and need surgical intervention. Unfortunately, no one test gives a prediction of what children will fall into what category and thus a combination of ultrasound, nuclear medicine and occasionally MRI and pyelography is needed to detect which children need what treatment. Ultrasound can usually identify at what level the obstruction is and can give an indication of the degree of hydronephrosis and parenchymal loss. It is widely accepted that an anteroposterior (AP) renal pelvis of more than 30 mm will lead to significant loss of function and less than 15 mm is unlikely to represent any significant obstruction. Mercapto-acetyltriglycine (MAG3) renograms can diagnose obstruction and can give an idea of differential function, although at the extreme ends of function dimercaptosuccinic acid (DMSA) is better suited for this.

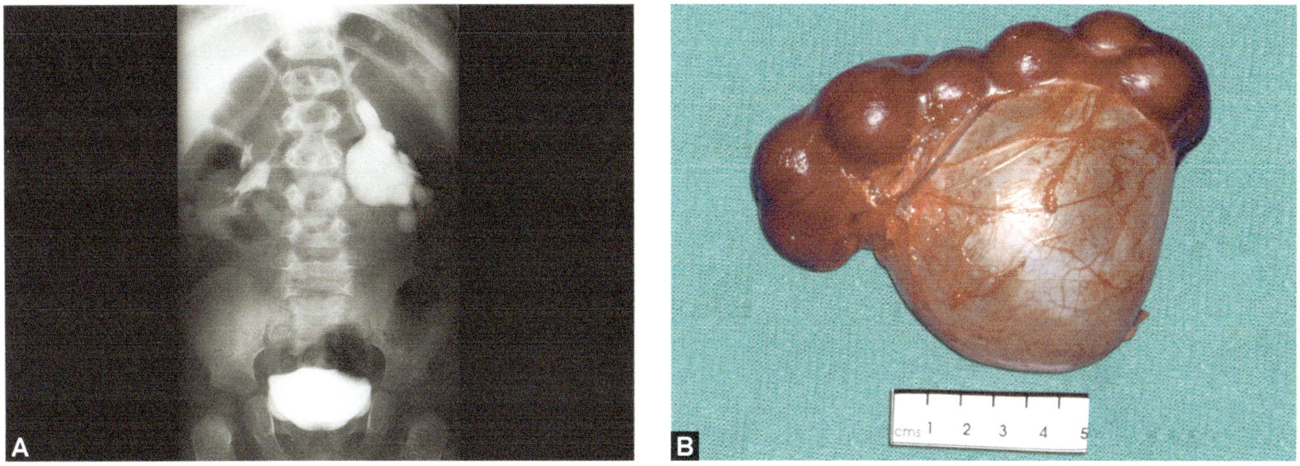

Figures 9.31A and B Urinary tract obstruction at the PUJ.

Pelvic ureteric junction obstruction: It is seen in around 1 in 1,000 children. Boys and girls are equally affected, but the left kidney is twice more likely to be obstructed than the right. It may be associated with other abnormalities of the urinary tract. When considering the aetiology, of which there are many, it is useful to think of intraluminal or extraluminal causes. Intraluminal would include stenosis, ureteric folds or valves within the junction itself. Rarely, epithelial polyps within the ureter may also lead to obstruction. An extrinsic cause is usually what is referred to as a "crossing lower pole vessel." This is an aberrant vessel causing the obstruction which improves following pyeloplasty and is seen more commonly in older patients. Rarely, a retrocaval ureter may be another extrinsic cause, and lastly severe vesicoureteric reflux (VUR) may cause a similar picture. PUJ obstruction does not always progress or need surgery. In a study by Great Ormond Street Hospital, London, 17% needed pyeloplasty because of loss of function, 27% improved and 56% remained stable. Aside from those diagnosed antenatally, children may present with features of urinary tract infection (UTI), abdominal pain, haematuria or even an abdominal mass. Surgery, that is, pyeloplasty, is indicated if the child is symptomatic or if on imaging there is evidence of loss of function, particularly if the AP pelvis is more than 30 mm. If the child is asymptomatic but the MAG3 shows persistent obstruction even in the presence of normal differential function, pyeloplasty is indicated. If function has fallen below 10–15%, then nephrectomy may be considered rather than pyeloplasty. If pyeloplasty is not an immediate option and the child is worsening clinically, then another option is the insertion of a nephrostomy. A dismembered Anderson-Hynes pyeloplasty is still regarded as the operation of choice and may now be performed laparoscopically, and although it is technically very demanding and often has a longer operative time, the cosmetic results are better and the length of stay in hospital is shorter. Robot-assisted pyeloplasty has also been described. A JJ stent or nephrostent is used to bridge the anastomosis for 48 hours prior to being clamped before discharge and removed at 2 weeks postoperatively. Thereafter, the child should be followed up with ultrasound to ensure the system has decompressed and an MAG3 at some point to ensure the obstruction has been relieved. Overall, pyeloplasty is usually a very good operation with success rates of 90% or more.

Vesicoureteric junction obstruction: It affects 1 in 2,000 children and can be grouped according to three principal causes: obstructed megaureter; non-refluxing, non-obstructed megaureter, that is, a burnt-out VUJ obstruction which has since resolved but left a floppy ureter; and lastly a refluxing megaureter. Ten per cent of cases present antenatally, and the remainder may present with loin pain, UTI or calculi. Investigations include ultrasound and always a micturating cystourethrogram (MCUG) so as to separate reflux from obstruction. Nuclear medicine scans should also be performed to assess drainage and function. If the child is symptomatic or there is loss of renal function, then surgery is indicated. If the child is within the first 12 months of life, stent insertion is the preferred option. Following 1 year of age this may be used or open surgery, that is, ureteric re-implantation, may be considered.

Posterior Urethral Valves

The diagnosis of posterior urethral valves is very important, and in order to try to preserve renal function, the diagnosis should not be missed. Valves occur in 1 in 6,000 boys only and often now may be suspected antenatally due to the presence of bilateral hydronephrosis. If diagnosed before 24 weeks of gestation and in the presence of oligohydramnios, the prognosis is worse. Traditionally, three types of valves were described by Young. Type 1 are the most common and, following instrumentation of the urethra, appear as side-by-side leaflets; type 2 are leaflets or folds that project upwards from the verumontanum and are not thought to be clinically significant; type 3 are rare and consist of a membrane in the bulbar urethra with a small perforation, but no attachment to the verumontanum. Valves essentially cause outflow obstruction that leads to abnormal bladder function in addition to renal impairment. In addition to hydronephrosis and dilated upper tract, ultrasound may show a dilated posterior urethra or classic "keyhole sign." The diagnosis is often made, however, on MCUG. Foetal therapy has been used in severe cases by means of a vesicoamniotic shunt. This has been shown to improve lung function of the baby but not renal function. Post-natally, boys should be catheterised and renal function monitored and treated in conjunction with paediatric nephrologists. Depending on the size of the child, endoscopic ablation may be possible. If this is not feasible and the renal function is worsening, a vesicostomy may be needed. In the long term, up to one-third of boys have impaired renal function and 70% have abnormal bladder function despite early diagnosis and treatment.

Calculus Disease

Kidney stones or urolithiasis is much less common in children than in adults with 1 in 10 adults potentially affected compared to 2 per million children in the UK. It is far more common in children from the developing world. The common types of renal calculi in children are those related to infection, most commonly *Proteus* UTI. These stones mostly consist of struvite and most commonly form in the upper urinary tract and maybe "staghorn" in shape. Metabolic stones are another important cause, often as a result from hypercalciuria. Oxalate, cysteine and uric stones may form. Uric acid stones are notably radiolucent; they are more common in developing countries and tend to be found in the lower urinary tract. The child presents with abdominal or loin pain, symptoms or signs of UTI, and more than 90% will have microscopic haematuria. The child may present with a mass and concern may be raised with regard to Wilms' tumour, but the mass may in fact be an enlarged kidney with stones due to xanthogranulomatous pyelonephritis. Children with metabolic conditions such as cystinuria and primary hyperoxaluria are at increased risk of stones as are those on certain medications such as phenytoin because of its metabolites. Other risk factors include children whose mobility is impaired, pre-maturity, CF, those whose urinary tracts are abnormal and those who have undergone bladder augmentation **(Figs. 9.32A and B)**.

Diagnosis is reached by history, examination, urinalysis and renal USS. If a stone is found, then metabolic work-up should be arranged and a urology review may be needed. If the stone has passed, then it should be sent for analysis. Ultrasound-guided extracorporeal shock wave lithotripsy can be used depending on the size and site of the stone, or the stone or its fragments may be removed by percutaneous nephrolithotomy.

Neuropathic Bladder

Neuropathic bladder or more precisely neuropathic bladder–sphincter dysfunction is a condition whereby congenital or acquired conditions damage the nerve supply to the lower urinary tract and as a consequence the bladder and urinary sphincter do not coordinate or function properly. The aetiology may be upper or lower motor-neurone, but in children classification is difficult as lesions may be incomplete and involve different levels, as seen in children with spina bifida. In children, spina bifida remains the commonest cause of neuropathic bladder. Other causes include sacral agenesis, traumatic spinal lesions, iatrogenic damage during pelvic surgery, cerebral palsy, meningitis and encephalitis, transverse myelitis and tumours. A more useful classification of neurogenic bladder is by urodynamics, rather than site of the neurological insult, stratifying those with overactive or underactive bladders and those with coordinated or uncoordinated bladders. Essentially, the bladder is either unable to act as it should as a reservoir or unable to empty adequately. This leads to three main problems; urinary incontinence, UTI and subsequently

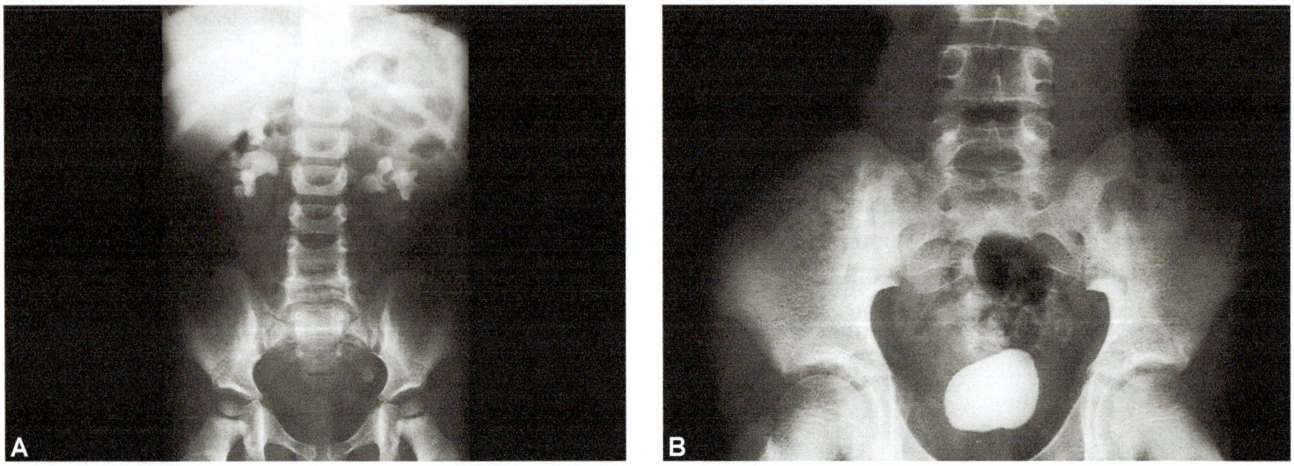

Figures 9.32A and B Intravenous urogram showing bilateral renal calculi.

impaired renal function. Diagnosis is by careful history and neurological examination followed by appropriate investigation, which may include urinalysis, renal and bladder ultrasound, MRI, renograms and video urodynamics. Once thorough work-up is complete, management is broadly medical with early CIC or surgical. The mainstay of medical treatment is prophylactic antibiotics, anticholinergics and in certain situations alpha-blockers and alpha-adrenergics. The main aim is to keep the upper tracts safe. Aside from vesicostomy in babies where decompression of the renal tract is needed to preserve renal function, surgery is not usually offered until the child is of at least school age. Options then include procedures to try and increase the size of the bladder usually with a small bowel augment. A Mitrofanoff procedure may also performed at the same time as continent catheterisable stoma. Many different procedures can be used to try and increase outlet resistance with varying success. These include bladder neck reconfiguration and extension of the posterior urethra and flap-valve mechanisms such as the Young-Dees-Leadbetter, Pippi-Salle or Kropp procedures. Complete bladder neck closure with a catheterisable stomas is another more radical option. Artificial urinary sphincters are more common in adult practice and are rarely used in children.

Duplication of the Urinary Tract

Duplication of the upper urinary tract is common and thought to occur in 1 in 125 children, girls more so than boys (Fig. 9.33). In one in five patients, the duplex system is bilateral. More often nowadays, it is diagnosed antenatally and may indeed lead to recognition of symptoms, requiring no intervention. As with other urinary anomalies, the challenge is to distinguish those that need treatment and those that do not. Following birth, the child should be started on prophylactic antibiotics and should undergo a renal and bladder ultrasound to confirm the diagnosis. An MCUG should be performed to outline any associated ureterocele and VUR. Following this, at around 3 months, a renogram, usually an MAG3, should be performed to elicit any obstruction and split renal function. As discussed in the management of upper tract obstruction, the management is threefold: to prevent UTI, to keep the upper tracts safe and prevent any loss of function and to relieve any obstruction.

VUR is more common in duplex systems especially to the lower moiety and, aside from prophylactic antibiotics and monitoring, it may require subureteric Teflon injection (STING) procedure or re-implantation (discussed later). Ureteroceles or cystic outpouching of the lower ureter into the bladder should be suspected if there is a dilated upper pole of the duplex system on ultrasound. These are usually dealt with by cystoscopic puncture to decompress the ureterocele, but more often in the presence of a duplex system require open resection alongside heminephrectomy. Duplex systems are also associated with ectopic ureters, which should be suspected in girls who are constantly dribbling and have never been dry and in boys who are known to have duplex and have recurrent urinary infections.

Meatal Stenosis

Meatal stenosis is an abnormal narrowing of the distal urethra at the meatus and is more common in boys. Risk factors include circumcision, balanitis, BXO and repeated urinary catheterisation. Symptoms may include spraying of urine, having to push or bear down to pass urine, urinary frequency and urgency. Management is by application of topical steroid in cases associated with BXO and otherwise meatal dilatation which may be repeated or meatotomy. Meatotomy involves surgically widening the meatus and usually has good results.

Vesicoureteric Reflux

The term VUR refers to urine going the wrong way, that is, retrogradely back up the ureter toward the kidney (Fig. 9.34). In the presence of UTI, this carries the risk of renal scarring and loss of function. It is a common

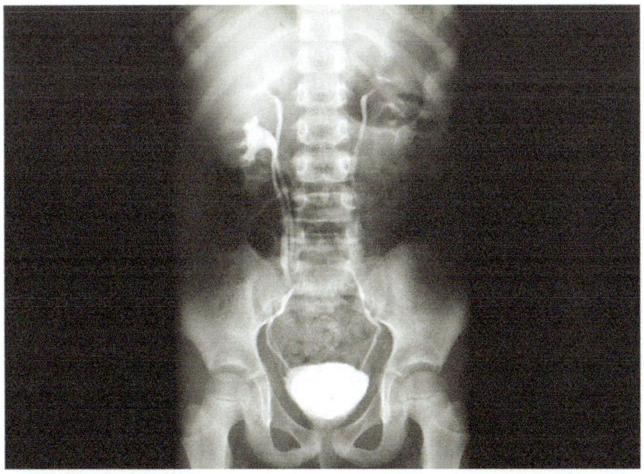

Figure 9.33 Duplex system.

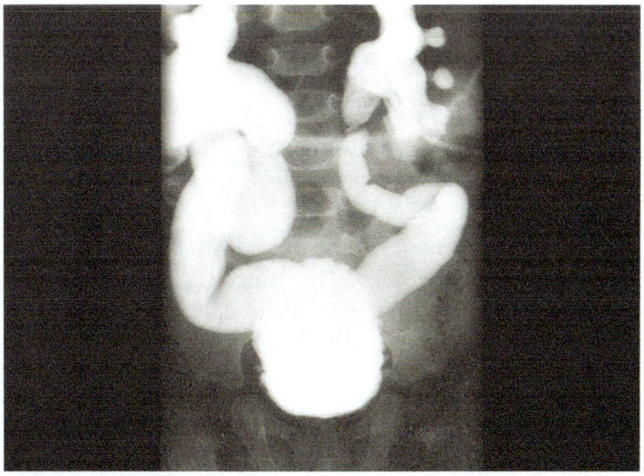

Figure 9.34 Bilateral grade V reflux.

condition occurring in 1 in 100 children and in 1 in 3 children who have a proven UTI. In some children, it causes no symptoms and is self-resolving, but in around a third renal scarring is already evident at the time of diagnosis.

More commonly, however, children are being picked up antenatally because of the presence of hydronephrosis and subsequent investigation. Children with a proven UTI rightly undergo renal ultrasound to identify any predisposing abnormality, but this is not a good modality to identify reflux; MCUG is the investigation of choice. MCUG allows grading of the reflux. There are five grades; grade I involves reflux into the ureter only with no dilatation, grade II is reflux as far as the calyces, but again no dilatation, grade III involves mild dilatation and a tortuous ureter, grade IV progresses to moderate dilatation with blurting of the angle of fornices and grade V is the worse with gross dilatation, tortuous ureter and loss of any clear outline of the calyces. DMSA scans not only can tell split renal function but also can pick up renal scarring.

The natural history of scarring is important and goes by the grades mentioned earlier, that is, 80% of grade I, 60% grade II, 40% grade III and 10% of grades IV and V resolve. The highest risk of scarring is in the neonatal period and in younger patients and, therefore, antibiotic prophylaxis is usually carried on until between the ages of 4 and 7 years depending on grade of reflux seen on repeat MCUG and presence of breakthrough UTI. The vast majority of children with VUR are managed medically; however, some children with recurrent UTIs and worsening renal scarring and renal function may require surgical intervention. Circumcision should be considered in boys; otherwise, the STING procedure is the first option. This term is now out of date as Teflon is no longer used due to previous fear regarding migration to the heart, and usually now another bulking agent such as the polymer Deflux™ is used. It is injected cystoscopically using the hydrodistention-implantation technique and may be repeated before more invasive ureteric re-implantation is considered. In some severe cases, heminephrectomy or complete nephrectomy may be needed in a kidney that has lost more than 90% of its function due to scarring. Nephrectomy is performed to eliminate a nidus for infection and to prevent renal hypertension, which is a complication of VUR seen in later life.

Neonatal Surgery

Spina Bifida

Spina bifida is a neural tube defect which can lead to a spectrum of abnormality. This ranges from spina bifida occulta to meningocele or exposed neural tissue as seen in myelomeningocele (MMC). The incidence of spina bifida and neural tube defects has halved since the recommendation and availability of antenatal folic acid supplementation and now occurs in around 3 per 10,000 live births. MMC is the more severe, but is also the most common neural tube defect. MMC can be diagnosed by antenatal ultrasound but antenatal MRI may be needed. In MMC, the defect extends through the skin, fascial, the posterior elements of the spine and down to neural tissue itself **(Figs. 9.35A and B)**. Parents should be counselled that their baby will require surgery shortly after birth to close the back. This is essential to prevent potentially fatal ventriculitis. The neural placode and dural sac need to be carefully dissected free from its attachment to skin and then the skin needs to be brought together without tension to allow healing and prevent wound breakdown. In larger defect, skin flaps or even grafting may be needed to achieve. The child is often nursed prone following closure so as to avoid pressure on the wound in the immediate post-operative period. Following back closure, head circumference is regularly measured and cranial ultrasound is used to monitor ventricle size and resistive index. Most infants with MMC have a coexisting Arnold-Chiari type 2 malformation leading to hydrocephalus. Around 80% of children with spina bifida will require a ventriculoperitoneal (VP) shunt because of hydrocephalus.

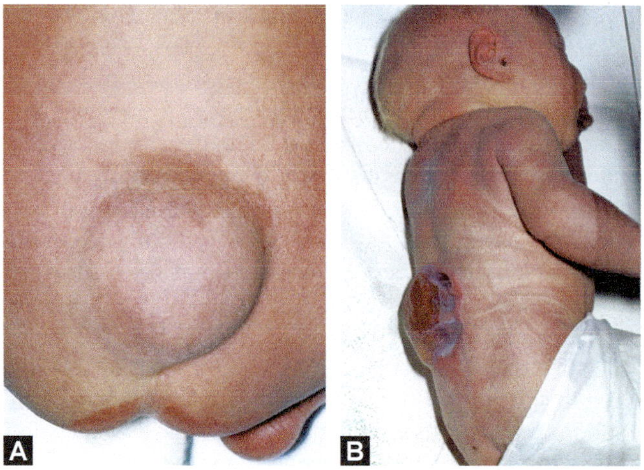

Figures 9.35A and B Meningocele and myelomeningocele.

Meningocele is less common and less severe; essentially the lesion involves fascia, bony elements of the spine and meninges but does not involve neural tissue. It is usually covered with skin and so, unlike in MMC, there is no CSF leak or risk of ventriculitis. These children are therefore usually neurologically normal, although some may have an Arnold-Chiari malformation and subsequent hydrocephalus. In the long term, many children with MMC lead full and active lives and live well into adulthood. The majority are of normal intelligence and the degree of disability very much depends on the level of the lesion and the degree of paralysis and decreased sensation. Many are able to walk with aids, although wheelchair use is common as the child gets older. Other issues that affect day-to-day living are problems with feeding, neuropathic bowel and bladder and a proportion may develop tethered cord syndrome, which may require surgery.

Hydrocephalus

Hydrocephalus literally means "water on the brain." It is commonly divided into congenital and acquired, and communicating and non-communicating hydrocephalus. Congenital hydrocephalus may be syndromic or genetic as in X-linked hydrocephalus or structural as in holoprosencephaly or schizencephaly. In communicating hydrocephalus, there is an obstruction in the subarachnoid space, and this results in dilatation of the entire ventricular system **(Figs. 9.36A and B)**. Causes of this type of hydrocephalus include: meningitis, intraventricular haemorrhage (often a complication of pre-maturity), congenital absence of the arachnoid granulations which should absorb CSF, and the Arnold-Chiari malformation. Non-communicating hydrocephalus, on the other hand, is when the obstruction is within the ventricular system itself and usually results from either congenital or neoplastic lesions. Causes of this type of hydrocephalus include aqueduct stenosis, atresia of the foramina of Magendie and Luschka, ventriculitis, intraventricular tumours and Dandy-Walker syndrome. Management usually consists of surgical placement of a shunt. A shunt is a device that aids permanent CSF drainage by diverting CSF into a body cavity. Options routes include peritoneum, right atrium and the pleural cavity. Most shunts have several common components including a proximal catheter, a one-way valve, a CSF reservoir and a distal catheter. Complications of VP shunts include infection, intracranial haemorrhage, over-drainage, fracture and disconnection and blockage. They should, therefore, be managed in a specialist centre and examined only by experienced clinicians.

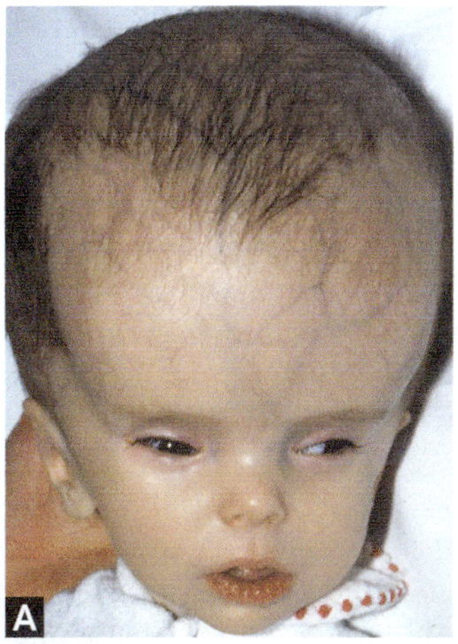

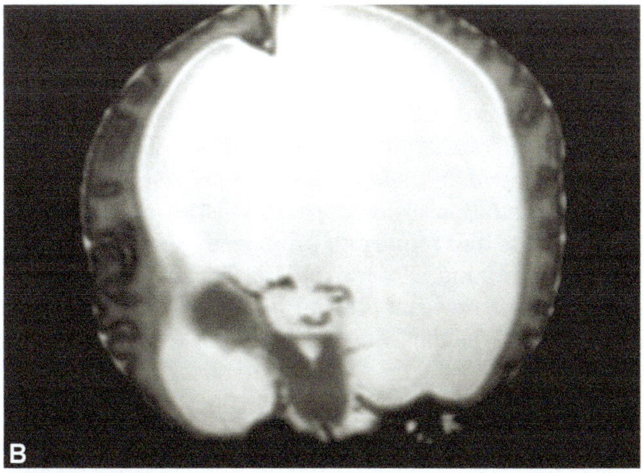

Figures 9.36A and B Hydrocephalus.

Oesophageal Atresia and Tracheoesophageal Fistula

Oesophageal atresia and tracheoesophageal fistula (OA and TOF) occur in 1 in 4,000 live births and result from failure of separation of the mesenchyme of the developing oesophagus and that of the tracheobronchial diverticulum in the first 4–6 months of gestation **(Fig. 9.37)**. There are five main types as classified by Gross (see diagram), the most common being the type C (85%), that is, OA and a distal TOF. Then pure OA with no fistula accounts for 10%, and the other rarer varieties make up the remainder. The condition is commonly associated with cardiac anomalies (33%) and syndromes such as VACTERL (vertebral, anorectal, cardiac, OA and TOF, renal and limb abnormalities) (10%), CHARGE (colobomata, heart defects, choanal atresia, retarded growth, genital and ear anomalies) and trisomies 13 and 18. The diagnosis may be suspected antenatally due to polyhydramnios. A small or absent stomach may also be suggestive of pure OA. Post-natally, the baby presents with frothing at the mouth and increased secretions and inability to pass a nasogastric tube. The initially management is to pass a Replogle tube and to gain IV access and start the child on IV fluids. A chest X-ray is then taken to confirm the diagnosis. Other investigations then need to be carried out to look for any associated anomalies, and include an echocardiogram which may also comment on the side of the aortic arch, and a renal and spinal USS.

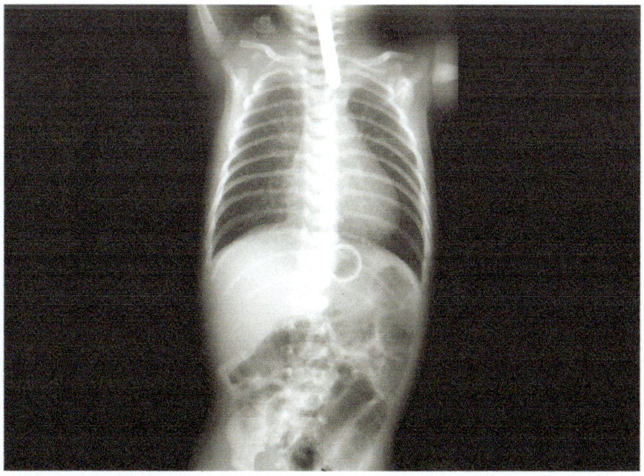

Figure 9.37 Oesophageal atresia (OA) and tracheoesophageal fistula (TOF).

Repair of OA and tracheoesophageal atresia is rarely an emergency except in the case of pre-mature ventilated babies in which the fistula may lead to severe abdominal distension, causing respiratory compromise or gastric perforation. Early ligation of the fistula may also have to be considered in a child with an associated DA or imperforate anus. The operation itself can be open or thoracoscopic and involves going into the right side of the chest, dividing the azygous vein, identifying and ligating the fistula and anastomosing the two ends of the oesophagus over a transanastomotic tube. The child can then be fed by the nasogastric tube until a contrast is performed 1 week post-operatively to confirm the anastomosis is sound and there is no leak before normal feeding can be established and the intercostal drain, if used, is removed. The main early complication is anastomotic leak in 5–50% of patients depending on the approach used. In addition, anastomotic stricture occurs in 10–30% and recurrent fistula in up to 5%. Most small leaks close with conservative management. In terms of long-term outcomes, patients may have problems with dysphagia, feeding issues, reflux, anastomotic stricture, oesophageal dysmotility, recurrent chest infections, scoliosis and chest wall deformities. Long-term outcome is also very much influenced by any associated anomalies such as congenital heart disease.

Congenital Diaphragmatic Hernia

Congenital diaphragmatic hernia (CDH) occurs in 1 in 2,500 live births and is thought to result from failure of closure of the pleuroperitoneal canals. There are two main types: the more common posterolateral Bochdalek defect and less frequent anteromedial Morgagni defect. Left-sided hernias are more common (85%). Often the condition is diagnosed antenatally and there may be a history of polyhydramnios. Early antenatal diagnosis, the liver up in the chest and a lung-to-head ratio of less than 1.0, is associated with a poor outcome **(Fig. 9.38)**. If not picked up antenatally, the neonate classically presents with respiratory distress, a scaphoid abdomen and heart sounds shifted to the right. A plain chest X-ray confirms the diagnosis. The child should be investigated for any associated anomalies seen in up to 40%. These include neurological anomalies, syndromes and cardiac lesions, and often there is evidence of pulmonary hypertension. The baby is quickly ventilated but an effort is made not to use excessive inspiratory pressures so as not to damage the lung. A strategy of permissive hypercapnia or what is referred to as "gentle ventilation" is often employed. Pulmonary hypertension may be treated with pulmonary vasodilators such as prostacyclin and inhaled nitric oxide. In severe cases and for those in respiratory failure, extracorporeal membrane oxygenation may be considered. Once the baby is stable and oxygen requirements have decreased (usually aiming for FiO_2 < 30%), diaphragmatic repair can be undertaken. This is usually performed through an abdominal approach using a left subcostal incision. If the defect is too large for primary closure, a Gore-Tex® patch may be used. If the abdomen is too tight to close, then a silo may be needed. Overall survival is 69%.

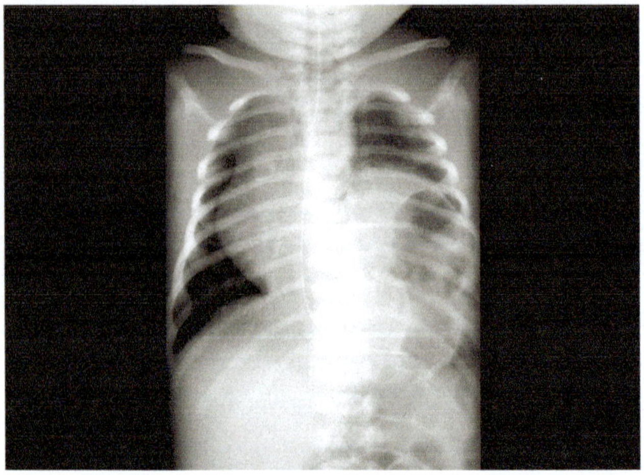

Figure 9.38 Congenital diaphragmatic hernia (CDH).

Abdominal Wall Defects

Gastroschisis: It is often diagnosed antenatally and involves protrusion of a variable amount of bowel out with the abdominal cavity **(Fig. 9.39A)**. There are three main differences between gastroschisis and exomphalos: firstly, there is no covering or sac in gastroschisis; secondly, the defect is usually to the right of the midline in gastroschisis, whereas in exomphalos it tends to be central; and lastly, gastroschisis is not normally associated with any other abnormality unlike exomphalos. The baby should be delivered around 37 weeks of gestation as there is known to be an increased incidence of late miscarriage in gastroschisis and this should be near a tertiary referral centre for gastroschisis. Caesarean section is not recommended routinely unless for other obstetric reasons. The parents should have been counselled antenatally and be aware that the bowel will be wrapped in cling film at birth and will require IV fluids and a nasogastric tube. The bowel is then inspected by the surgical team, and depending on the amount of bowel out and its condition, a primary closure may be possible or a silo may be applied with reduction of the bowel over 3–5 days and subsequent delayed closure. Parents are warned that achieving full enteral feeds in a baby with paediatric surgery is a slow process as the bowel and its motility are not normal. This process can take many weeks and requires a prolonged hospital stay with central access and TPN and the risk of recurrent sepsis and NEC. Overall, however, the mortality from gastroschisis is very low and the majority of babies do extremely well and are able to be discharged on full enteral feeds.

Exomphalos minor and major: Exomphalos is abdominal wall defect and, as mentioned earlier, involves a defect that arises centrally, and the contents may include bowel and, commonly, liver **(Figs. 9.39B and C)**. Again, it

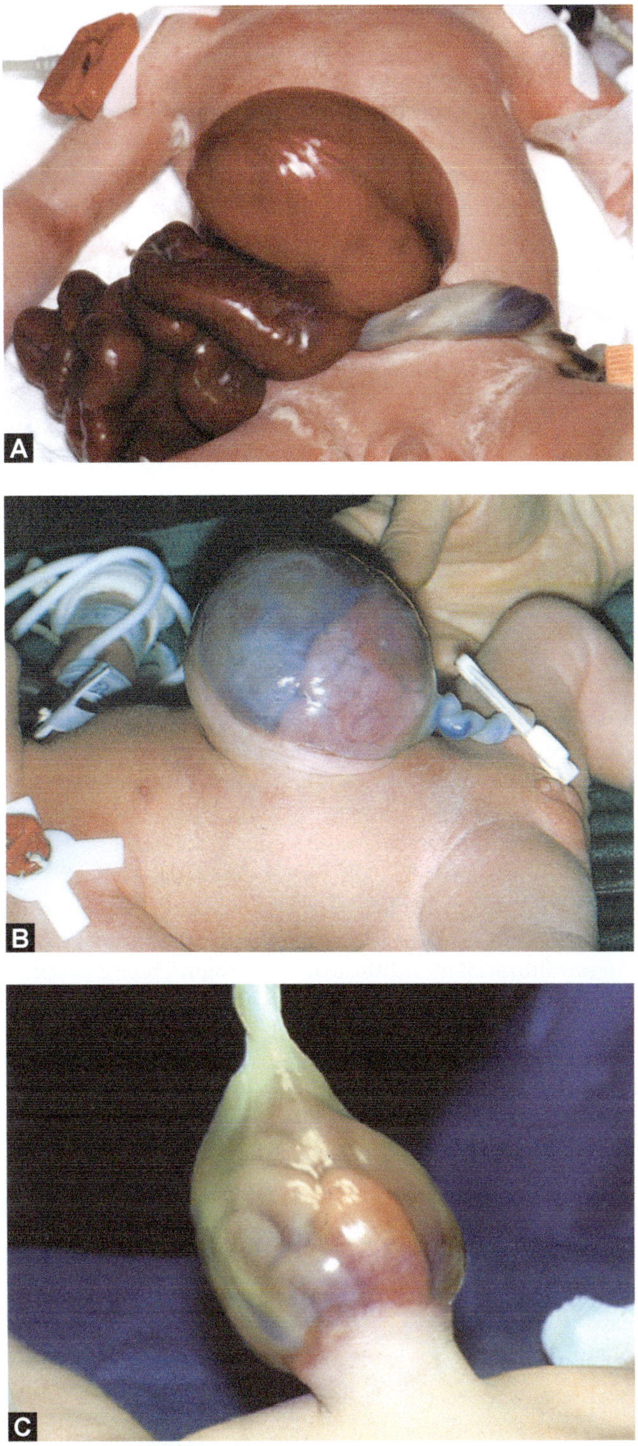

Figures 9.39A to C (A) Gastroschisis; (B and C) Exomphalos and closing gastroschisis.

is often diagnosed antenatally and, depending on size and the presence of the liver being out, may mean that the elective caesarean section is undertaken. Initial management, as for gastroschisis, includes gaining IV access and fluid replacement. A "bowel bag" or cling film is wrapped around the baby to prevent evaporative losses.

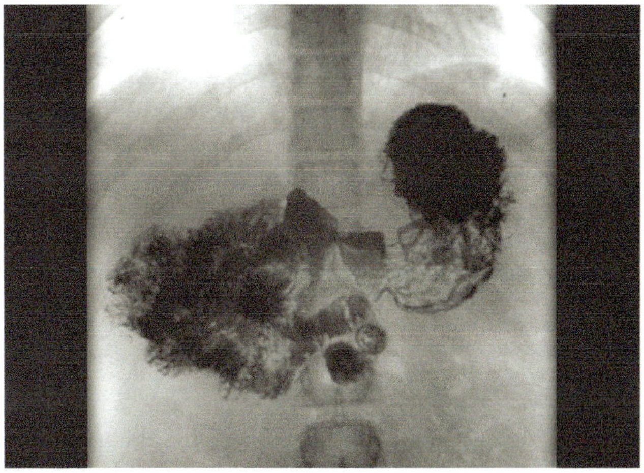

Figure 9.40 Malrotation and volvulus.

Unlike gastroschisis, exomphalos is associated with other abnormalities and syndromes such as Beckwith–Wiedemann and CHARGE syndrome. Investigations should, therefore, be performed to elicit any associated abnormality and should include a plain chest X-ray (often showing a bell-shaped chest with evidence of pulmonary hypoplasia), cardiac, renal and spinal ultrasound. A nasogastric tube should be passed. The operative technique essentially depends on the size of the exomphalos. This is usually graded as small to moderate (<5 cm) and moderate to large (>5 cm). Primary closure should be undertaken where possible to decrease the chance of intra-abdominal sepsis. Most surgeons would excise the sac unless it is adherent to the liver. In moderate to large defects, conservative treatment is appropriate and defects may simply be painted with a disinfectant or Flamazine and observed for development of an eschar. A staged repair is then performed usually at 12–18 months of age and involves excising excess skin and repairing the ventral hernia.

Malrotation and Volvulus

Malrotation of the gut results when the intestinal rotation and fixation that should occur between 4th week and 12th week of gestation does not occur **(Fig. 9.40)**. Normal rotation 270° anti-clockwise around the superior mesenteric artery should result in the duodenojejunal (DJ) flexure lying to the left of the midline, the caecum lying in the right iliac fossa and the transverse colon anterior to the small bowel mesentery. The commonest abnormality with malrotation is that the caecum lies close to DJ flexure, resulting in an abnormally narrow midgut mesentery, which is liable to twist, that is, leading to volvulus. This is a surgical emergency. Any neonate with bilious vomiting has malrotation with volvulus until proven otherwise, that is, the child needs an urgent upper GI contrast. If the child is malrotated, then they should proceed to laparotomy. The bowel is then inspected and any volvulus reduced. A Ladd procedure is then performed. The steps in a Ladd procedure involve straightening or kocherising the duodenum, widening of the small bowel mesentery and then returning the bowel to the peritoneal cavity, and placing all the large bowel on the left and all the small bowel on the right. This is not the anatomically correct position but the best arrangement to prevent any future volvulus. Appendicectomy traditionally is also performed, although some surgeons prefer to leave the appendix in situ and warn the parents that the appendix now resides in the left upper quadrant, should the child develop acute appendicitis in later life.

Necrotising Enterocolitis

Necrotising enterocolitis (NEC) is an acute inflammatory disease occurring in the intestines of 2–5% of pre-mature infants and up to 10% in very-low-birth-weight (VLBW) infants **(Fig. 9.41)**. It can lead to necrosis of the bowel and can be fatal. Clinical features include abdominal distension, blood in the stool, feeding intolerance, vomiting (often bilious) and pyrexia. Bell famously classified NEC in 1978 into three stages: stage 1, suspected NEC; stage 2, definitive NEC; and stage 3, complicated NEC. The aetiology of NEC is essentially unknown, but is most likely multifactorial and a combination of an immature gut mucosal barrier and gut flora. AXR may show fixed, dilated bowel loops, portal gas, pneumatosis intestinalis or perforation. Stage 1 and 2 NECs are often managed conservatively by stopping feeds and giving IV fluids and antibiotics; however, in more complicated NEC, surgical intervention is necessary. The decision to operate is often a very difficult one, especially in VLBW infants who are otherwise unstable. Surgical management includes peritoneal drainage, laparotomy and bowel resection with or without stoma formation. In severe cases, the condition is fatal and operation there may be no salvageable and care is then re-orientated.

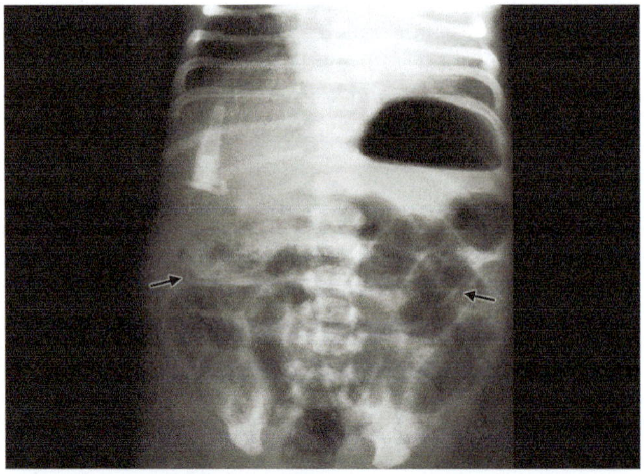

Figure 9.41 Necrotising enterocolitis.

Duodenal Atresia

Duodenal atresia (DA) is often considered a separate entity from the other intestinal atresias **(Fig. 9.42A)**. It is thought to result from a failure of re-canalisation other than a vascular insult as in more distal atresias. DA occurs in 1 in 20,000 to 40,000 births. Approximately, 30% of infants with DA have Down syndrome and over half have an associated anomaly such as a cardiac anomaly. The atresia is usually post-ampullary (80%) and so the child often presents with bilious vomiting. It may be suspected antenatally with the appearance on ultrasound of a classic "double bubble." Further suspicion is raised if the foetus is known or suspected to be trisomy 21. As in other atresias, the different types are classified as type 1 (90%; an intraluminal membrane or diaphragm), type 2 (a cord) and type 3 (a completely disconnected segment of bowel with or without a mesenteric defect). Type 4 atresia is when there are multiple atresias. An annular pancreas is another possible cause of this type of obstruction. Around one in four patients with DA have another anomaly of their GI tract. If not suspected antenatally, the neonate presents with vomiting (often bilious) and distension of

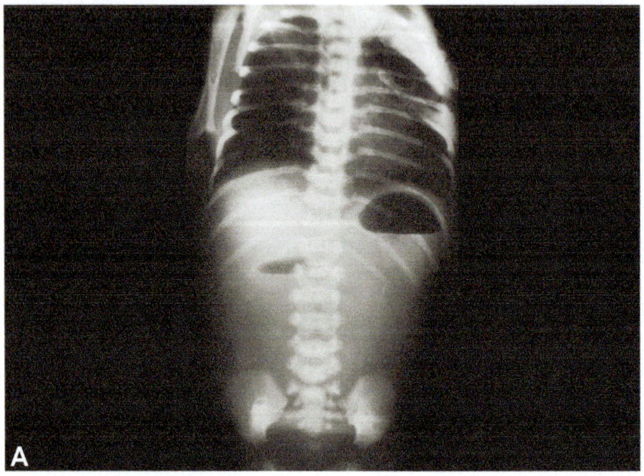

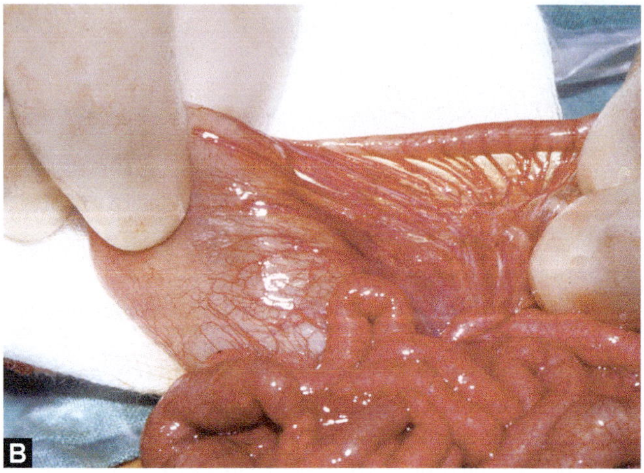

Figures 9.42A and B Intestinal atresia.

the upper abdomen. Plain AXR shows a "double bubble." Management is surgical and is usually in the form of a diamond duodenoduodenostomy. A transanastomotic tube may or may not be passed depending on surgeon's preference. Enteral feeds are gradually increased. Early complications include perforation, wound infection or anastomotic leak. Late complications are often related to the abnormal and dysmotile proximal duodenum and include delayed gastric emptying, GORD, adhesive obstruction and blind-loop syndrome.

Intestinal Atresias

Atresia of the intestine is a malformation where there is a narrowing or absence of a segment of the intestine **(Fig. 9.42B)**. They are classified by the Grosfeld classification into four types as described earlier. Intestinal atresia or stenosis can occur anywhere along the GI tract, and the anatomic location of the obstruction determines the clinical presentation. The most common site of intestinal atresia is the small intestine (jejunum and ileum). The incidence of small bowel atresia is approximately 1 in 5,000 births. It is rarely related to other conditions such as HD, CF, malrotation, Down syndrome, ARMs and congenital heart disease, and other atresias are found in up to one-third of patients. Diagnosis may be suggested antenatally or post-natally; there may be bilious vomiting and features of obstruction. Plain AXR may show dilated loops of bowel with no gas in the pelvis or even meconium calcification. A contrast enema may be performed if meconium disease is suspected or if the diagnosis is not clear. Management is surgical and at laparotomy the bowel is inspected fully and the level of obstruction found. Further atresias should be sought and, depending on presence of these and on the calibre of the bowel, resection and primary anastomosis is performed. Multiple atresias or a significant type 3b or apple peel may lead to extensive resection and SBS (discussed earlier).Colonic atresia is the rarest of all the atresias with an incidence of 1 in 20,000. It presents with more distal obstruction and has a higher chance of perforation than the other atresias. It may be related to HD. Following prompt diagnosis, however, the outcome is generally excellent.

Small Bowel Duplications

Duplications can occur anywhere along the GI tract, for example, thoracic, gastric, pyloric, duodenal, but most cystic duplications in the abdomen are small bowel in origin. They commonly arise on the mesenteric border, and the duplication shares a common blood supply with that of the neighbouring intestine **(Fig. 9.43A)**. They are often suspected antenatally, but may present in the neonate with a mass. The differential diagnosis must include choledochal and ovarian cysts and the presence of a typical bowel signature on ultrasound should confirm the diagnosis. In the older child, they may present with vague abdominal pain and can be wrongly diagnosed as acute appendicitis. Other complications or sequelae of a small bowel duplication include intussusception, perforation or volvulus.

Meconium Disease

Meconium ileus (MI): It is a condition leading to neonatal obstruction due to thickened and inssipated meconium **(Fig. 9.43B)**. It causes one in five neonatal obstructions, and 90% of these infants will have CF, although only 10% of all cases of CF present in this way. MI is classified as simple or complicated, simple being small bowel obstruction alone. Complicated MI means there is something more severe than obstruction, that is, atresia, volvulus or perforation with meconium peritonitis. The neonate presents with bilious vomiting and failure to pass meconium. Diagnosis is made by plain AXR and contrast enema. Contrast enema may show a microcolon and filling defects in the colon and ileum suggestive of MI. The enema itself may be therapeutic in clearing the ileus; however, around a third will not respond to enema and will proceed to theatre. At laparotomy, the bowel is inspected and MI confirmed. An enterotomy is performed in the distal ileum and a Jacques catheter inserted and the bowel flushed with N-acetylcysteine to aid breaking down of the inssipated meconium. Other surgical options are the Bishop-Koop, Santulli or Mikulicz-type stomas.

In complicated MI, ischaemic bowel due to volvulus or perforation may require resection and the formation of a defunctioning stoma is more than likely. The bowel usually starts to move by 5–10 days post-operatively and enteral feeds are slowly increased. The child has genetics sent for CF and, if confirmed, the CF team will initiate management and follow-up of this.

Meconium plug: This syndrome is another cause of neonatal obstruction and is again due to inssipated meconium, but rather than causing ileus, there is concentrated plug of tenacious material, which impedes the motility of the colon **(Fig. 9.43C)**. The cause of meconium plug is essentially unknown; however, it is associated with a number of conditions including maternal diabetes, hypothyroidism, CF, HD and pre-maturity. Passage of the plug often witnessed at contrast enema cures the obstruction; however, all babies with this condition should have a suction rectal biopsy for HD and be investigated for possible CF.

Hirschsprung disease: HD, or congenital aganglionic megacolon, involves an enlargement of the colon, caused by bowel obstruction resulting from an aganglionic section of bowel (the normal enteric nerves are absent) that starts at the anus and progresses upwards **(Fig. 9.43D)**. It occurs in 1 in 5,000 live births, and in 90% of cases, HD presents with delayed passage of meconium; however, it can present later in life with abdominal distension, constipation, failure to thrive and features of obstruction. It may be familial and several genes are now known to be involved in the pathogenesis of HD such as *RET*, *EDNRF* and *PHOX2*. The diagnosis is often suspected following

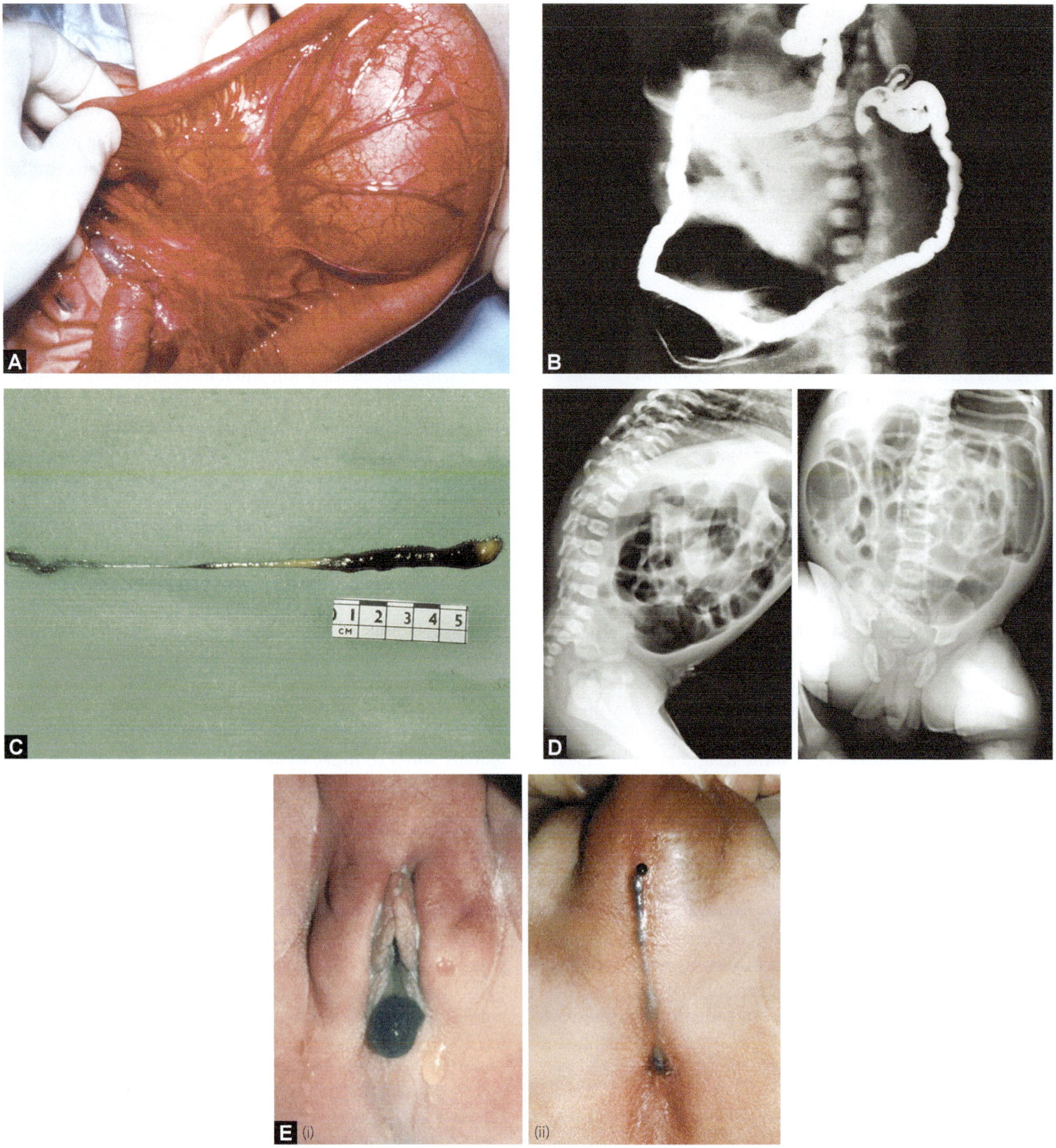

Figures 9.43A to E (A) Duplication cyst; (B) Meconium ileus; (C) Meconium plug; (D) Hirschsprung disease; (E) Anorectal malformations.

decompression, if necessary, by digital rectal examination when there may be a sudden explosion of gas when the examiners finger is withdrawn. Plain AXR and contrast enema may give an indication of the level of the transition, which in around 80% is rectosigmoid. The diagnosis is ultimately confirmed by suction or strip rectal biopsy. The biopsy confirms the presence of thickened nerve fibres and the absence of ganglia in the submucosa. A regimen of rectal washouts is then employed to keep the child decompressed and to prevent enterocolitis. Then when the child is of a good weight, a pull-through procedure is undertaken. There are three common types: the Soave or endorectal pull-through, the Swenson (similar to an anterior resection) and the Duhamel, which involves plugging ganglionic bowel into the back of aganglionic bowel distally. Endorectal pull-throughs are now the most popular procedure and these are usually performed following laparoscopic biopsies at multiple sites to confirm the level of the transition zone. Following surgery, the remainder of the bowel, although ganglionic, is still inherently abnormal and the child still commonly suffers from constipation and is still at risk of developing enterocolitis. The Hirschsprung-associated enterocolitis (HAEC) score may be used to try and predict those who have enterocolitis and treat them early. Overall, the prognosis from HD is good as many of the issues of soiling, incontinence, constipation and psychological issues tend to resolve as the child gets older. HD is, however, a lifelong condition and the risk of enterocolitis should always be considered.

Anorectal Malformations

The term anorectal malformation (ARM) encompasses a real spectrum of congenital abnormalities from a slightly displaced anal opening to an imperforate anus with various types of fistula [**Figs. 9.43E (i) and (ii)**, a female with a vestibular fistula and a male with an anocutaneous fistula, respectively]. The cause is unknown, but it is noted to be more common and often more severe in boys and is associated with various syndromes such as CHARGE and VACTERL. The diagnosis should be made soon after birth or at least at the baby check within the first 24 hours of life. Most neonates can tolerate a lower bowel obstruction for this length of time without becoming dangerously distended. There are several classification systems for ARM by sex as in the Pena classification or by level as in the Wingspread or more widely accepted Krickenbeck classification. The Krickenbeck classification attempts to group those ARM that have common features in terms of both diagnosis, management and outcome.

In females, the most common ARM is a vestibular fistula. This may be difficult to see due to its location within the posterior fourchette of the vagina and all that may be visible at first is meconium staining of the patient's vulva. A vestibular fistula may be a good size or may require dilation. Perineal fistulas occur less commonly in girls or there may be a cloacal anomaly with a common channel or a classic imperforate anus. In boys, there may be an anocutaneous fistula or perineal fistula visible on examination or there may be an imperforate anus with no fistula. The other common scenario in boys with an ARM with no obvious fistula is that there is a fistulous connection but it ends somewhere along the lower urinary tract, that is, rectovesical, rectoprostatic or rectobulbar fistulas. Flattened buttocks suggest a high abnormality. Currarino triad has been mentioned earlier and the most common ARM in this condition is anorectal stenosis. The baby should be kept fasted and a nasogastric tube passed. A pronogram may be performed to try and illustrate the level of the most distal gas. This should not be performed until at least 12 hours of age to allow time for gas to move distally down the gut. Other investigation should be performed to look for any associated abnormality such as seen in VACTERL, that is, a chest X-ray, echocardiogram, renal and spinal ultrasounds. ARM does not usually require surgery urgently if the diagnosis is made promptly after birth. It should, however, be performed in the first 24–48 hours so as to ensure the baby does not become too distended and before the bowel is colonised with pathogens. Unless a very low defect is confidently diagnosed and a cutback procedure performed, the safest management is to perform a divided colostomy. This should be a descending colostomy or at least in proximal sigmoid so as to allow plenty of length for future posterior sagittal anorectoplasty (PSARP) and formation of a neoanus. Transverse colostomies are no longer popular due to the higher risk of prolapse. PSARP is now usually performed around 1 month of age.

Sacrococcygeal Teratoma

Sacrococcygeal teratoma (SCT) is the most common neonatal tumour. As with all teratomas, it is a tumour that is composed of all three germ cells layers, that is, endoderm, ectoderm and mesoderm. Although it is the most common neonatal tumour, it is still incredibly rare with an incidence of 1 in 40,000 live births with four times as many girls affected as boys. It may be diagnosed antenatally and, if particularly large, elective caesarean section may be considered if there is thought to be a risk of dystocia or tumour rupture (**Fig. 9.44A**). SCT was famously classified by Altman in 1974 into four types depending on how much of the tumour is visible externally. In type 1, the most common, the majority is external; in type 2, there is an external component but some pelvic tumour; in type 3, there is less external and more internal pelvic and intra-abdominal tumour; and in type 4, the tumour is not visible externally but is entire presacral or intra-abdominal. It is important to mention that an SCT may also be involved in Currarino triad, that is, a presacral mass which may be an SCT or anterior meningocele or dermoid cyst along with anorectal stenosis and an anterior sacral defect. The majority of SCTs are benign but 1 in 10 can be malignant. Baseline tumour markers (AFP and hCG) are taken at birth and are frequently monitored and an MRI is usually performed to elicit the extent of the tumour prior to surgery in the first few days of life. Complete excision is paramount to prevent recurrence. Surgery is usually performed with the patient prone and using a chevron incision, and classically the patient's coccyx is removed. In larger tumours and those classified as Altman type 3–5, an abdominal approach may be needed. Post-operatively, the patient has serial AFP measured to ensure the level is persistently decreasing and remains at normal levels. It is thought up to a third of patients may be troubled by neuropathic bowel or bladder as a result of either the primary pathology or iatrogenic resulting from the surgery needed to achieve complete resection.

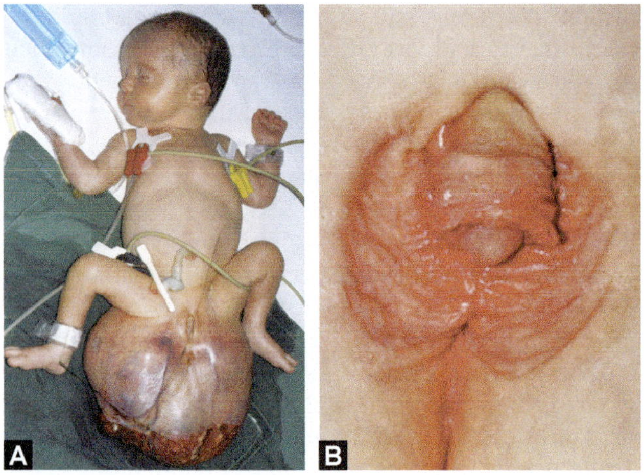

Figures 9.44A and B (A) Sacrococcygeal teratoma (SCT); (B) disorders of sex development (DSD).

Recurrence rates vary in the literature, but are commonly quoted at around 10%. Chemotherapy may be used for recurrence or reoperation may be considered.

Disorders of Sex Development

The previously termed pseudohermaphroditism has been replaced by the term disorders of sex development or DSD and refers to a group of congenital conditions with atypical development of chromosomal, gonadal or anatomic sex **(Fig. 9.44B)**. It is estimated that the incidence of genital anomaly is 2 in 10,000 live births, although some degree of male undervirilization or female virilization may be present in as many as 2% of live births. The new born with suspected DSD should be managed in a tertiary centre by a multidisciplinary team including a paediatric surgeon and a paediatric endocrinologist. The nomenclature of these conditions has also recently changed dividing them into in four categories: 46,XX DSD to replace female pseudohermaphroditism; 46,XY DSD to replace male pseudohermaphroditism; Y dysgenetic DSD to replace the various gonadal dysgenesis syndromes with different karyotypes; and ovotesticular DSD to replace hermaphroditism. In a new born with genital ambiguity, initial investigations often include karyotype with sex-related region Y detection, measurement of 17-hydroxyprogesterone, testosterone, gonadotropins, anti-Müllerian hormone (AMH) and electrolytes. These biochemical investigations together with a pelvic ultrasound should identify the most common form of DSD, 46,XX DSD, mainly due to congenital adrenal hyperplasia. Once 46,XX DSD has been excluded, the diagnostic pathway should consider the rarer forms of DSD. These include XY dysgenetic DSD (mixed gonadal dysgenesis), XY non-dysgenetic DSD (Leydig cell hypoplasia, partial androgen insensitivity syndrome, 5a reductase deficiency, persistence of Müllerian duct syndrome, etc.) and ovotesticular DSD. Examination of the external genitalia, together with biochemical and radiological investigations, is essential in the evaluation of this group of patients. Imaging modalities such as ultrasound and MRI are useful and have in the past been used to identify any persisting Müllerian structures or intra-abdominal gonads; this, however, has been superseded by laparoscopy, which is also often used as a therapeutic modality. The role of the paediatric surgeon in the management of children with DSD is part of a multidisciplinary team and involves not only aiding diagnosis of the underlying condition, but also timely gonadectomy, gonadal biopsies, orchidopexy and, of course, reconstruction of the external genitalia.

Trauma

Trauma is the leading cause of death in young children with road traffic accidents and falls, accounting for 80%. Thoracic and abdominal injuries usually result from blunt trauma. When managing paediatric trauma, it is extremely important to bear in mind that children are not mini-adults and the management needs to take into account the likely injuries in a child of that size and age. Examples of this include the small body size, large surface area-to-body mass ratio, relatively large head, their compliant elastic skeleton and the differences in their airways, that is, small mouth with large tongue, short trachea and the fact that those less than 6 months are obligate nose breathers. As with any trauma case, the first task is the primary survey which involves checking the airway and cervical spine, assessing breathing by looking, listening and feeling, and administering oxygen. Circulation is assessed by monitoring heart rate, blood pressure and capillary refill time. Blood pressure dropping is a late sign in a child and signifies serious injury. Intravenous access should be obtained and bloods taken. GCS is modified for children and practically AVPU is useful. In addition to exposure and temperature of the child, it is important to measure blood glucose. It is also important to know the weight of a child, however, to calculate fluid volumes and drug doses, even before the child arrives, for example, in a "standby" situation, and can be estimated by various formulas depending on the age of the patient. Boluses of normal saline are given in 10 mL/kg aliquots and then the child should be reassessed and the fluids readjusted. If a child requires more than 40 mL/kg of fluid resuscitation, then a member of the surgical team should be consulted. Of intra-abdominal injuries, the spleen, liver and kidney are most commonly involved, but rarely require operation when vital signs and the haematocrit are stable. Much of the focus in terms of research into paediatric trauma is in the setting up of specialist trauma centres and in its prevention.

Burns

A patient with burns has the same priorities as all other trauma patients, that is, to stop the burn and apply first aid.

TABLE 9.3 Syndromes and associations in paediatric surgery.

Syndrome	*Features*	*Associated surgical conditions*
Alagille	Autosomal dominant syndrome associated with abnormalities of the liver, heart, skeleton, eye and kidneys and a characteristic facial appearance	Cholestasis Neonatal jaundice Differential diagnosis of biliary atresia
Beckwith–Wiedemann	Exomphalos, macroglossia, gigantism, increased risk of neoplasm and hypoglycaemia	Exomphalos, umbilical hernia, Wilms tumour and hepatoblastoma
Budd–Chiari	Occlusion of the hepatic veins. Classically presenting with abdominal pain, ascites and hepatomegaly	Abdominal pain, may be associated with tumour, e.g., hepatoblastoma
CHARGE	Coloboma, heart defects, choanal atresia, growth retardation, genital and ear anomalies	OA and TOF Exomphalos ARM
CAIS	Complete androgen insensitivity syndrome (CAIS) phenotypically female but genetically male	Bilateral Inguinal Hernia DSD Gonadectomy
Congenital central hypoventilation syndrome	Congenital or acquired syndrome resulting in respiratory arrest during sleep. Associated with other anomalies of the autonomic nervous system	Hirschsprung disease (HD) Neuroblastoma
Conn	Hyperaldosteronism	Benign tumour of adenoma
Cornelia de Lange	Developmental disorder with slow growth, profound developmental delay, skeletal abnormalities and distinctive facial features (arched eyebrows with synophrys, low set ears and widely spaced teeth)	Feed intolerance, GORD
Crigle–Najjar	Lack or deficiency of the enzyme uridine diphosphate glucuronosyltransferase, autosomal recessive, presents with jaundice	Cause of neonatal jaundice
Denys–Drash	Rare disorder presents in infancy with congenital nephropathy, Wilms tumour and intersex disorders resulting from mutations in the Wilms tumour suppressor (WT1) gene	DSD and Wilms tumour
Di George	Chromosome 22q11.2 deletion syndrome leading to cardiac anomalies, abnormal facies, thymic hypoplasia, cleft palate and hypocalcemia	Increased risk of infectious disease and cardiac anomalies
Down	Trisomy 21. Typical features: mental retardation, epicanthic folds, Brushfield spots, single palmar crease, typical facies, hypotonia, brachycephaly and macroglossia	Down syndrome increases the risk of umbilical hernia, HD, duodenal atresia, annular pancreas, imperforate anus, GORD and coeliac disease
Edwards	Trisomy 18: characterised by severe psychomotor and growth retardation, microcephaly, microphthalmia, malformed ears, micrognathia or retrognathia, microstomia, distinctively clenched fingers and "rocker-bottom feet"	Increased incidence of exomphalos, malrotation, ileal atresia, oesophageal atresia with or without tracheoesophageal fistula, diaphragmatic eventration, prune belly anomaly, absent gallbladder, absent appendix, accessory spleens, pyloric stenosis, imperforate or malpositioned anus, cloacal exstrophy and CDH. In addition to multicystic kidneys, duplex systems, renal agenesis, cryptorchidism and hypospadias
Ehlers–Danlos	11 different types of connective tissue disorder leading to joint mobility, skin extendibility, scarring tendency	Poor wound healing; increased risk of visceral rupture, e.g., spleen
Familial adenomatous polyposis (FAP)	Autosomal dominant condition leading to hundreds/thousands of epithelial polyps within the colon. If left untreated, all patients with FAP will develop colon cancer by the age of 40 years	Bowel surveillance due to increased risk of colon cancer and ultimately colectomy

(Contd...)

(Contd...)

Syndrome	***Features***	***Associated surgical conditions***
Fanconi	Disease of the renal tubules leading to substances excreted in urine that should be absorbed	Can be caused by chemotherapy, e.g., cisplatin
Gardner	Subtype of FAP with colonic polyps, sebaceous cysts, desmoid tumours and osteomas	Bowel surveillance of polyps and possible colectomy
Hunter	Mucopolysaccharidosis type 2—X-linked. Life-limiting, progressive mental retardation and typical facies	As for Hurler (see below)
Hurler	Mucopolysaccharidosis type 1—a lysosomal storage disease which is autosomal recessive. Progressive mental retardation and typical facies	Hepatosplenomegaly, increased incidence of herniae and may need to provide central access if considered for bone marrow transplant
Kartagener	Dextrocardia, bronchiectasis, sinusitis and primary ciliary dyskinesia	Situs inversus, differential of CF
Kasabach–Merritt	Haemangiomas with thrombocytopenia	Haemangiomas
Klienfelter	47,XXY or XXY syndrome, hypogonadism, gynaecomastia, reduced fertility	Hypogonadism, gynaecomastia
Klippel–Trenaunay	KMS or angio-osteohypertrophy syndrome. Features include haemangiomas, varicose veins, hypertrophy of limbs and an abnormal lymphatic system	Haemangiomas
Li-Fraumeni	Autosomal dominant cancer predisposition syndrome (especially sarcoma, breast, leukaemia, and adrenal gland tumours) linked to *TP53* and *CHEK 2* genes	Increased incidence of sarcoma, breast and adrenal gland tumours
Lynch (HNPCC)	Autosomal dominant genetic condition predisposing to colon cancer as well as endometrial ovarian, gastric, skin and brain tumours	Increased risk of tumours
Mayer–Rokitansky	Absence or abnormally developed uterus and vagina, may have associated skeletal, cardiac or renal abnormalities	DSD
Marfan	Autosomal dominant connective tissue disorder (*FBN1* gene), tall, high arched palate, mitral valve prolapse, aortic dissection	Increased risk of hernias and recurrence and pneumothorax
McCune–Albright	Mutations in *GNAS* gene leading to at least 2 out 3 of precocious puberty, polyostotic fibrous dysplasia and unilateral Café-au-lait spots or abnormal pigmentation	Cause of precocious puberty
Multiple endocrine neoplasia	MEN-autosomal dominant cancer syndromes caused by mutations in RET proto-oncogene	MEN 1: Parathyroid tumours, pancreatic tumours and pituitary tumours MEN 2a: Medullary thyroid cancers (MTC), pheochromocytoma and parathyroid tumours MEN 2b: MTC, pheochromocytoma and neuromas
Opitz–Frias	Characteristic facies, hypertelorism, hypospadias and dysphagia and oesophageal defect with swallowing difficulty	Hypospadias and dysphagia
Pallister–Hall	Mutations in the *GLI3* gene leading to a spectrum of hypothalamic hamartoma, central and post-axial polydactyly, bifid epiglottis, imperforate anus and renal abnormalities	ARM and renal abnormalities
Peutz–Jeghers	Autosomal dominant polyposis syndrome associated with hyperpigmented lesions of mouth, hands and feet	Bowel surveillance
Poland	Ipsilateral breast and nipple hypoplasia and/or aplasia, absence of the sternal head of the pectoralis major muscle, hypoplasia of the rib cage and hypoplasia of the upper extremity/hand deformities	Chest wall deformities

(Contd...)

(Contd...)

Syndrome	Features	Associated surgical conditions
Potter	Oligohydramnios and bilateral renal agenesis leading to typical facies, clubbed feet, pulmonary hypoplasia and cranial anomalies	Renal anomalies
Prune belly	Complete absence or lack of abdominal wall muscles, undescended testes (UDT) and renal tract abnormalities	UDT and renal anomalies
Sturge–Weber	Encephalotrigeminal angiomatosis includes facial port wine stain, seizures, mental retardation and brain angiomas	Facial haemangiomas
Triple A	Achalasia, Addison disease, and alacrima caused by mutations in the *AAAS* gene. Autosomal recessive inheritance	Achalasia
Turners	45,X or gonadal dysgenesis, short stature, webbed-neck, primary amenorrhoea, infertility	DSD
Waardenburg	Mutations in different genes including *SOX 10* and *PAX 3*, leading to hearing loss, dystopia canthorum and pigmentary abnormalities of the hair, skin and eyes	Type IV associated with HD
WAGR	Wilms tumour, aniridia, genitourinary abnormalities and mental retardation	Wilms tumour
VACTERL	Vertebral anorectal cardiac tracheoesophageal renal and limb abnormalities	ARMs and OA and TOF

Abbreviations: CF, cystic fibrosis; DSD, disorders of sex development; GORD, gastro-oesophageal reflux disease; KMS, Kasabach–Merritt syndrome; OA and TOF, oesophageal atresia and tracheoesophageal fistula.

In a burn patient, the airway should be checked for signs of smoke or singeing of hair. If there is a history of smoke inhalation, then airway compromise may occur suddenly. Fluid resuscitation and replacement is paramount in burns; compartment syndrome should always be borne in mind; and in terms of exposure, the percentage of the burn as well as its depth should be assessed. To determine the percentage area of a burn in a child, the rule of 9's does not apply in children. However, it is important to calculate percentage accurately as this guides not only management but also appropriate fluid resuscitation. Intravenous access should be obtained and analgesia given. It is very important to find out what first aid has been administered to the patient, what time the injury was and for how long the first aid was given. It is always important to consider continuing first aid measures as this can be done up to 2 hours from the time of the injury and prevent the progression of the depth of the burn. If the patient is on fire, "stop, drop and pat;" rolling is no longer recommended for fear of causing injury. For scalds, remove the hot liquid including clothing, and chemicals should be brushed or washed off. The area should be cooled with tepid water continually for 20 minutes. It is also important to take a detailed history to document who was present at the time of injury, the mechanism of the injury and whether or not this explanation is plausible and consistent with the child's injuries, as non-accidental injury must always be thought of. Percentage area of the burn or percentage of total body surface area (TBSA) is what decides whether the child needs to be admitted and/or whether they need IV fluids. A chart can be used to estimate percentage or the size of the child's palm of their hand is roughly 1%. The depth of the burn is classified as follows—superficial: essentially like sunburn, with no blistering; superficial dermal: again with good blood supply and appears pink and blistered; deep dermal: altered sensation, but not painless and blisters may be present and often well demarcated with a speckled appearance; full-thickness burns: painless and have a white/brown and dry appearance. They are increasingly seen because of the recent popularity of ceramic hair straighteners. Any child with greater than 10% surface area affected will need IV fluids. Greater than 30% merits paediatric intensive care units admission. The amount of fluid to be given is determined by various formulas that are calculated using the percentage of TBSA, for example, the Muir and Barclay or modified Parkland formulas, or a combination of both. Protocols vary from centre to centre. Children with burns in "special" areas such as hands, feet, genitals and around joints should also be assessed by a surgeon and admitted. The child is usually admitted to a warmed room, swabs are taken for microbiology, and dressings are applied. They are then usually taken to theatre the next day for closer inspection. Serial dressings then follow and, if necessary, grafting **(Table 9.3)**.

CHAPTER 10

Dermatology

Ram Gulati, Catherine Jury, Mary Mealyea

INTRODUCTION

The skin is the largest organ of the human body. Its primary function is to act as a barrier between the environment and our internal organs, providing physical, mechanical, chemical and immunological protection. It also has important sensory, endocrine, thermoregulatory and cosmetic functions.

The skin is a complex organ consisting of three layers: (1) epidermis, (2) dermis and (3) subcutaneous fat. Within the three layers, there are many types of cells and structures **(Fig. 10.1A)**.

The epidermis is the outermost layer of skin that is continually regenerating **(Fig. 10.1B)**. More than 90% of its cells are keratinocytes. The keratinocytes are produced in the basal layer, progressively maturing as they move up through the stratum spinosum and stratum granulosum to form an outer layer of dead cells, the stratum corneum. Melanocytes are found in the basal layer of the epidermis. These cells produce melanin, which is taken up by the surrounding keratinocytes. Melanin forms a cap on top of cellular nucleus, protecting the vital nuclear material from photodamage. Melanin absorbs and scatters ultraviolet light, visible light and near-infrared radiation, primarily providing protection against damage from sunlight. Without this protection, skin cancer may develop more readily. Langerhans cells are found suprabasally, and are responsible for immunological surveillance. They act as antigen-presenting cells. Diseases affecting the epidermis usually result in abnormal scale, change in pigmentation or loss of surface integrity.

Dermoepidermal junction is a complex structure responsible for secure attachment of epidermis to dermis. Disorders affecting the junction usually result in blistering conditions.

The dermis contains collagen and elastic fibres, which provide an elastic but tough supportive layer under the epidermis. Specialised structures within this layer include hair follicles with associated pilosebaceous unit and sweat glands. It also contains blood vessels, nerves, and various cells including mast cells, macrophages and lymphocytes. Various inflammatory conditions involve dermis.

The subcutaneous layer provides additional mechanical protection, acting as shock absorber. It is also an important energy store and helps to maintain body heat. This layer is made up of adipocytes that form lobules and are separated by fibrous septae. The neurovascular supply is carried in the septae.

Common Terms Used

Erythema	A patch of redness caused by capillary dilatation or hyperaemia
Macule	A small (<5 mm) circumscribed flat area of altered skin colour
Patch	A large (>5 mm) flat area of altered skin colour
Papule	A small (<5 mm) solid elevated skin lesion
Plaque	A large (>5 mm) solid elevated skin lesion
Nodule	A palpable solid skin lesion, extending deep into dermis or subcutaneous tissue
Vesicle	A small (<5 mm) fluid-filled elevated skin lesion
Bulla	A large (>5 mm) fluid-filled elevated skin lesion
Pustule	A small (<5 mm) pus-containing elevated skin lesion
Abscess	A large pus-containing lesion
Wheal	A transient skin lesion consisting of an elevated pale centre with a surrounding flare of erythema. It is characteristic of urticaria and is produced by the release of histamine in the dermis
Scale	A sheet of adherent corneocytes in the process of being shed

(Contd...)

(Contd...)

Crust	Dried exudate consisting of a mixture of serum and scale, sometimes with erythrocytes and leucocytes
Ulcer	A discontinuity in the skin surface involving the complete loss of epidermis
Erosion	A superficial breach in the skin surface
Excoriation	A scratch mark
Lichenification	An area of skin in which the epidermis is thickened, making the skin darker and the normal skin creases more prominent
Scar	An area of skin in which the skin surface has lost the normal surface markings and skin appendages. This is usually secondary to trauma, but can be seen after severe inflammation
Naevus	Skin lesion, usually hamartomatous, appearing at birth or early in life
Umbilication	Central indentation on a lesion characteristically seen on molluscum lesions

HISTORY

Some conditions in the field of dermatology lend themselves to spot diagnosis; however, as in any other branch of medicine, a careful history is of utmost importance. The history, not only about the skin condition, but also about current general health, past medical and surgical history, details of medications, allergies, family, pets and travel are vital. In children, additional information pertaining to birth, development and immunisation should be obtained. The information will mostly be obtained from a parent or carer, but it should be from the person who is most involved with the care of the child and who can give an accurate history. The child, if at an age when he or she can communicate, should always be involved.

Important Questions about the Rash or Lesion

- When, where and how did it begin?
- Has it changed and if so how?
- Is it intermittent?
- Is it itchy, painful or tender?
- Does anything make it better or worse?
- Does anyone else in the family or child's contact have a similar rash or lesion?
- If the family has a pet, does the pet suffer from a skin condition?

EXAMINATION

Examining the entire skin under a good light is essential. Just looking at the presented lesion or rash can on occasions lead to misdiagnosis. Attention needs to be paid first to the overall appearance of the skin eruption and then on individual lesion(s), as explained in the following paragraph.

Observe the distribution of the rash or lesions. Is it localised or widespread? If localised, is it annular, grouped, segmental, dermatomal or linear? If widespread, is it symmetrical? Are the lesions discrete or confluent?

Note the morphology of the primary lesion. In other words, what does a lesion look like when it first appears? Note the shape, size, colour, contour, surface, edge, consistency and presence of any fluctuation. Secondary changes such as presence of scales, crusts, scabs, excoriations, erosions and lichenification can be important diagnostic pointers too.

INVESTIGATIONS

The history and examination will at times need to be complemented by appropriate investigations. Common outpatient investigations include skin swabs for bacteriology or virology, and skin scrapings, hair or nail clippings for

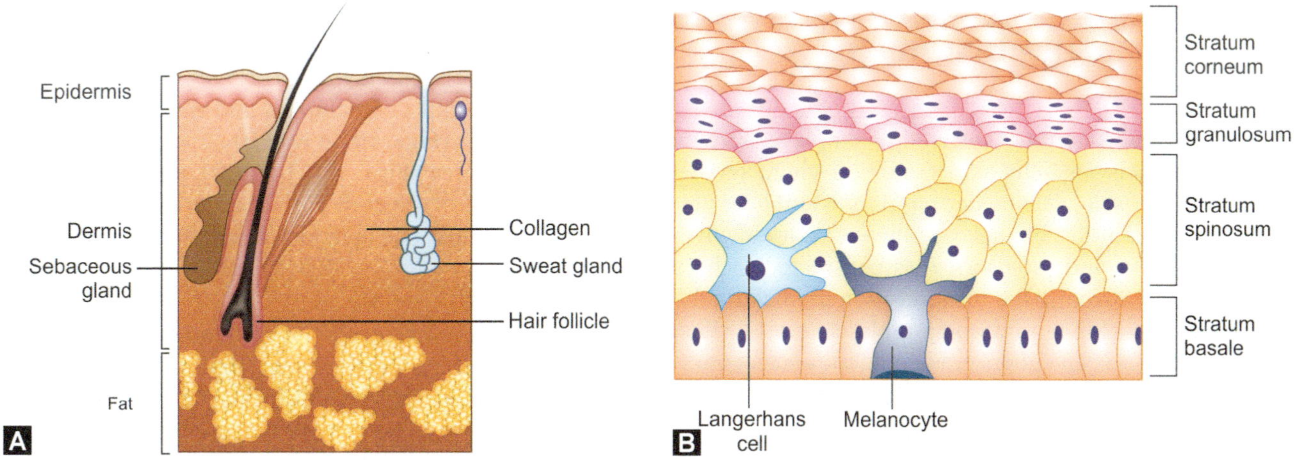

Figures 10.1A and B Structure of (A) skin; (B) Epidermis (not to scale).
(*Courtesy*: (A) M. Mealyea; (B) R. Gulati.)

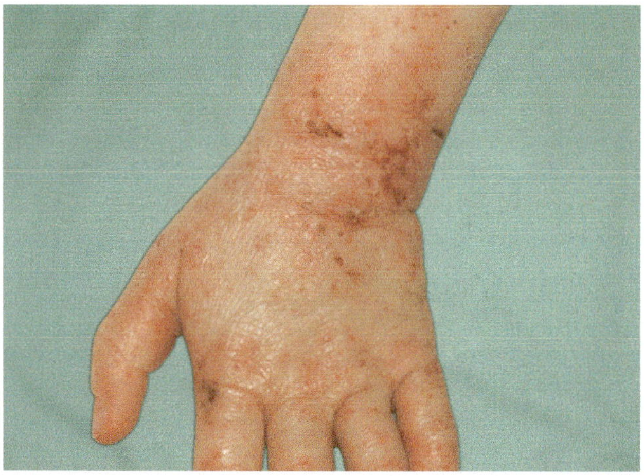

Figure 10.2 Acute excoriated eczema wrist.
(*Courtesy*: M. Mealyea.)

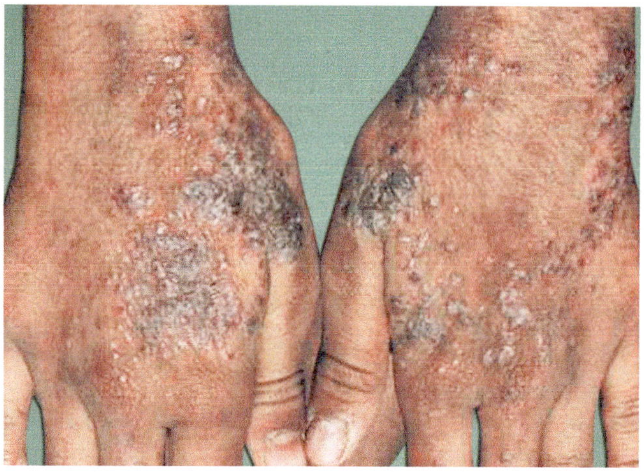

Figure 10.3 Chronic lichenified eczema.
(*Courtesy*: R. Gulati.)

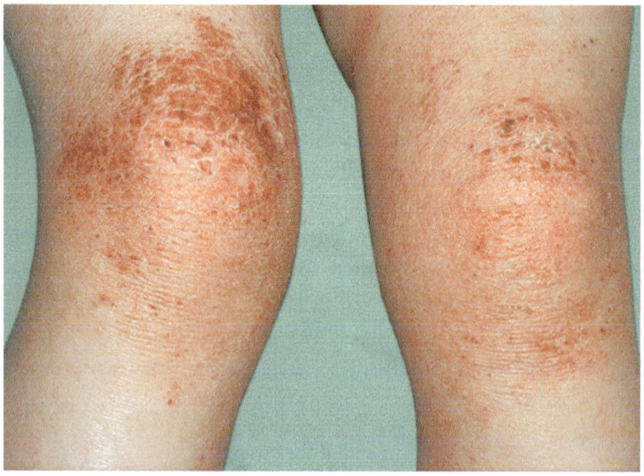

Figure 10.4 Chronic lichenified eczema of the knees.
(*Courtesy*: M. Mealyea.)

mycology. Blood tests may be needed and occasionally a skin biopsy would be helpful in reaching a diagnosis.

INFLAMMATORY DISORDERS

Atopic Eczema

Atopic eczema, sometimes referred to simply as eczema or dermatitis, is an itchy skin condition characterised variably by dry skin, flexural dermatitis and family or personal history of atopy. Infants can, however, have involvement of cheeks and extensors. It is considered to be a barrier defect affecting the filaggrin protein, making the skin more susceptible to dryness and deleterious effect of irritants. This is one of the most frequently seen conditions in paediatric dermatology clinics.

Presentation

It commonly presents within the first few weeks of life as a dry erythematous rash on the face and scalp. It then

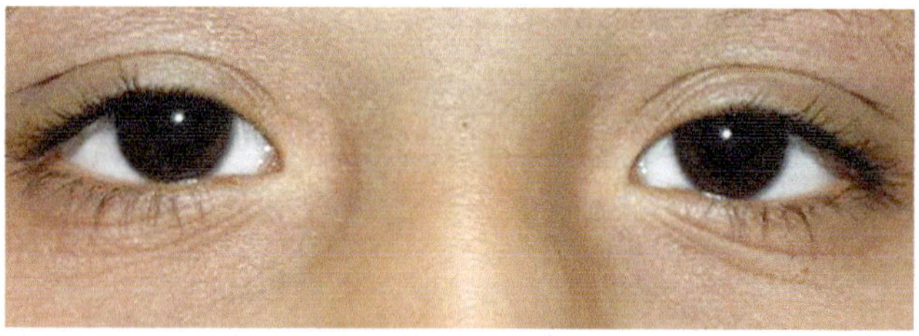

Figure 10.5 Dennie-Morgan lines.
(*Courtesy*: C. Jury, R. Gulati.)

becomes more widespread especially on the extensor aspects of the limbs but usually spares the nappy area. As the child becomes older, the flexures of the limbs become the main site of involvement. Excoriations point towards the itchy nature of the condition, but may be absent in neonates and children with physical weakness, for lack of dexterity.

Acute eczema may present with microvesiculation and weeping **(Fig. 10.2)**, whereas chronic eczema leads to thickened dark skin, a process called lichenification **(Figs. 10.3 and 10.4)**. Children with eczema may also show extra folds or creases below the eyes, termed as Dennie-Morgan lines **(Fig. 10.5)**. Discoid eczema implies discrete well-defined thick areas of eczema, which usually are more resistant to treatment, and necessitate potent topical steroids **(Figs. 10.6A and B)**. Eczema can involve large surface area **(Figs. 10.7A and B)**, and if it involves more than 90% of the body surface area, it is called erythrodermic eczema. The diagnosis is mostly clinical.

Management

Being a barrier defect, emollients remain the mainstay of treatment. Ointments are preferred as they are more occlusive. Creams are helpful for larger areas; however, they have more preservatives, increasing the chances of irritant reactions. Lotions and gels are easy to use on hairy areas. Emollients should be used liberally and regularly as they largely act as preventers. Bath emollients and

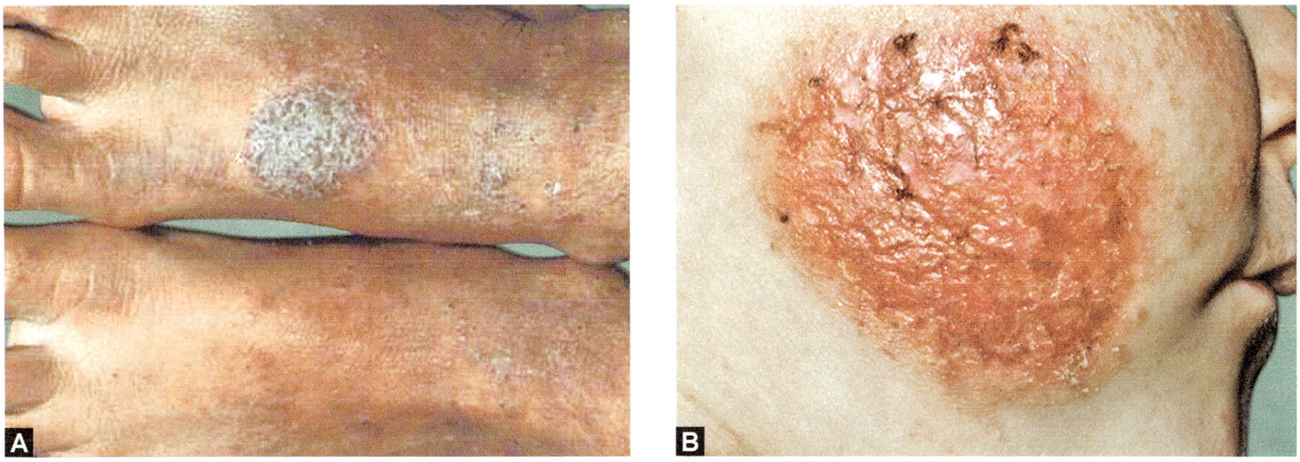

Figures 10.6A and B (A) Discoid eczema of the right foot dorsum. *Note* atopic eczema affecting both feet; (B) Discoid eczema of the cheek.
(*Courtesy*: (A) R. Gulati; (B) M. Mealyea.)

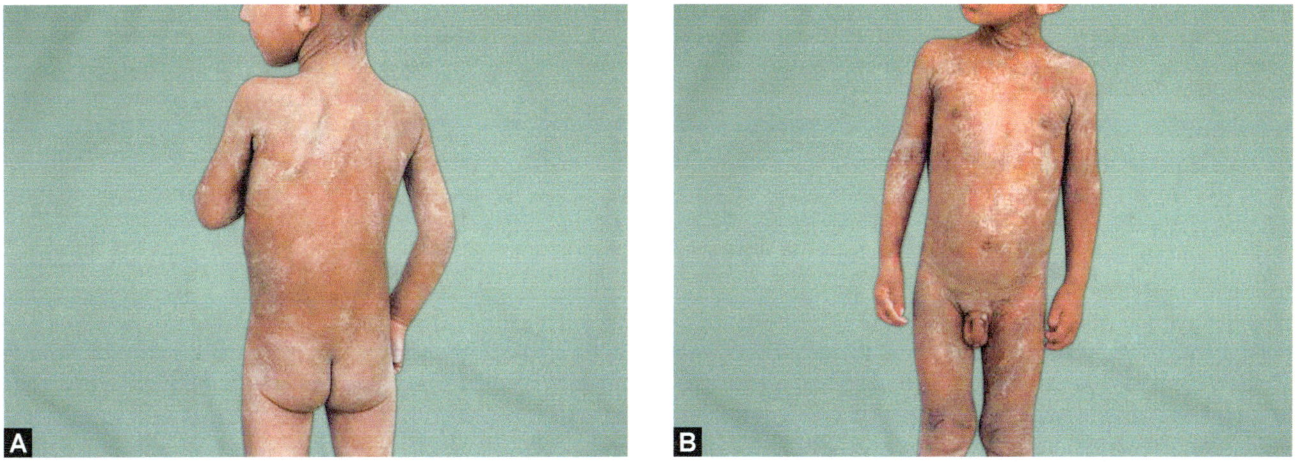

Figures 10.7A and B (A and B) Generalised eczema.
(*Courtesy*: R. Gulati.)

soap substitutes reinforce the moisture retention. Regular soaps, which are alkaline, have a desiccating effect and tend to weaken the skin barrier. Irritants such as woollen or nylon clothing and perfumes, and hot environments can cause a flare of the eczema, and should be avoided.

Flares of eczema need short periods of topical steroids, which act by virtue of their anti-inflammatory effect. Weak steroids such as hydrocortisone 1% are used for the face, folds and napkin area, whereas moderately potent steroids such as clobetasone butyrate 0.05% or potent steroids such as mometasone furoate 0.01% may be required for limbs and trunk. Use of steroids should be restricted to few days at a time, and potent steroids should be used only under specialist supervision.

Topical calcineurin inhibitors such as pimecrolimus and tacrolimus are useful alternatives to topical steroids, particularly on the face, especially around the eyes where prolonged use of steroids are usually contraindicated. These are now approved to be used for up to 1 year for maintenance. Sun protection is advised during their use. A small risk of secondary lymphoma cannot be ruled out, though recent studies consider this less likely.

Complications

Weepy crusty eczema, refractory to adequate topical treatment, may indicate superficial infection **(Fig. 10.8)**. *Staphylococcus aureus* and, less commonly, group A streptococci are implicated. Swabs should be taken and appropriate antibiotics instituted. Recurrent infections may be helped by antiseptic bath emollients and bleach baths.

Acute exacerbation with presence of multiple discrete vesicles or clustered erosions may be due to superinfection with herpes simplex virus (HSV), called eczema herpeticum. Herpes virus can spread quite dramatically in children with atopic eczema and can lead to systemic upset. Oral acyclovir may suffice for localised infection; however, parenteral administration is needed for children with systemic upset. Swabs should be taken for

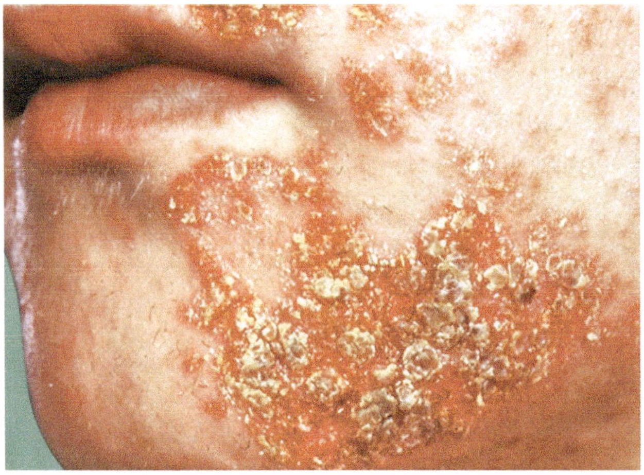

Figure 10.8 Infected atopic eczema.
(*Courtesy*: M. Mealyea.)

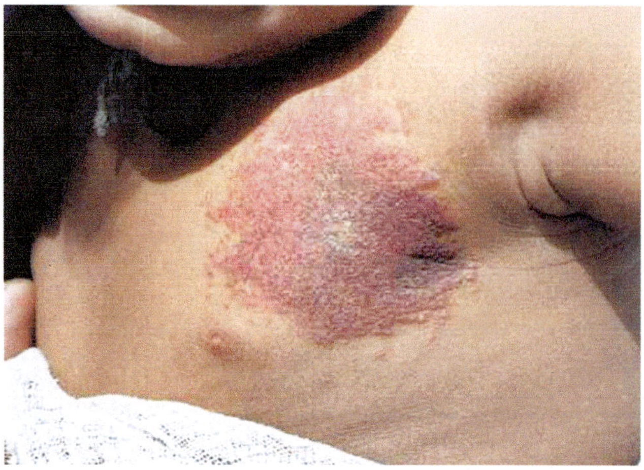

Figure 10.9 Contact irritant dermatitis following application of herbal remedy.
(*Courtesy*: R. Gulati.)

confirmation of the diagnosis. Children with eczema herpeticum are at increased risk for having further similar episodes. It is therefore mandatory to educate parents, so they can look out for the specific signs, leading to early recognition and treatment when the infection is still localised. Children with eczema should avoid close contact with people who have cold sores (herpes simplex).

A small number of non-responders, especially patients with recalcitrant facial eczema, may have associated food allergies, which should be investigated using skin prick testing and/or immunoglobulin E radioallergosorbent test. Patch testing may be useful for resistant eczema affecting certain sites such as eyelids, hands and feet, especially in adolescents, as contact allergens may be implicated. Patch testing has no role in the investigation of food allergy.

Education plays an important part in management of eczema. The first appointment should therefore be seen as an opportunity to make the family understand the nature of the condition and the role of treatment. A written plan and information leaflets are quite helpful. There can be an unintentional information overload, and therefore reinforcement at periodic intervals is helpful. Some children, especially ones with widespread resistant eczema, may need psychological intervention as they may find coping difficult. Widespread resistant eczema may need oral immunosuppressive treatment.

Most children respond well to topical treatment and eventually grow out of their eczema. Children with widespread disease, associated food allergies and/or significant atopic background may continue to be affected in adulthood.

Contact Dermatitis

This implies inflammation of skin secondary to contact with an extraneous trigger. This is broadly divided into two types—contact irritant dermatitis and contact allergic dermatitis.

Contact irritant dermatitis follows contact with an irritant, which is usually acidic or alkaline, leading to inflammation **(Fig. 10.9)**. On the contrary, contact allergic dermatitis is induction of inflammation secondary to contact with a stimulus, which triggers specific type IV immunological reaction. Common contact allergens include nickel, cobalt and chromium. Contact reactions can be diagnosed using patch testing, which includes putting a battery of standard allergens on the back and observing the area in 48 and 96 hours for any inflammation.

Topical steroids are the mainstay of treatment. Avoidance of contact triggers is advocated for avoiding further reaction.

Seborrhoeic Eczema (Cradle Cap)

Seborrhoeic eczema is an inflammatory condition of infancy characterised primarily by thick, greasy yellowish scales on the scalp **(Fig. 10.10)**. It can affect other hairy areas such as the eyebrows, nasolabial folds and ears, and intertriginous areas such as axilla and groin **(Figs. 10.11 and 10.12)**.

Clinical picture can simulate atopic eczema; however, classic rash of seborrhoeic eczema is not itchy and, unlike atopic eczema, quite commonly affects the diaper area. Nonetheless, some authors consider that infants with seborrhoeic eczema may be at higher risk of developing atopic eczema.

Emollients are the mainstay of treatment, although short period of mild to moderate potency topical steroids may be helpful. The condition usually settles within the first year of life.

Psoriasis

Psoriasis is a disorder of rapid epidermal cell turnover causing accumulation of thick silvery white scales on an erythematous inflamed base. It is uncommon

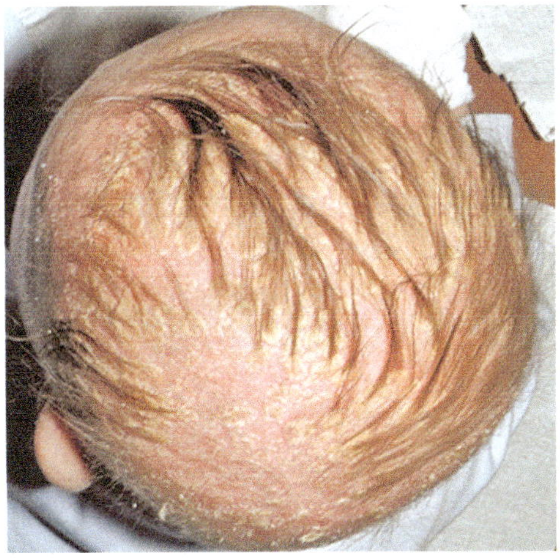

Figure 10.10 Seborrheic dermatitis scalp—cradle cap.
(*Courtesy*: M. Mealyea.)

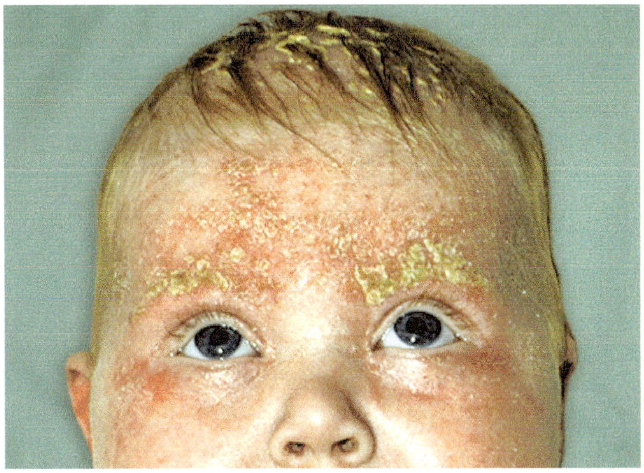

Figure 10.11 Seborrhoeic dermatitis showing yellow scaling of eyebrows, forehead and scalp.
(*Courtesy*: M. Mealyea.)

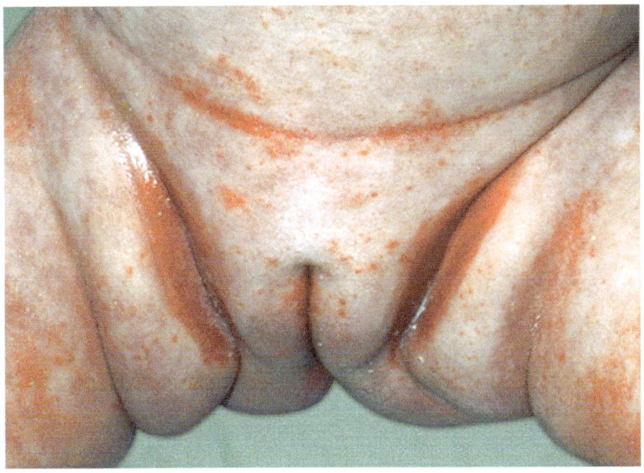

Figure 10.12 Seborrhoeic dermatitis showing involvement of the folds in napkin area.
(*Courtesy*: M. Mealyea.)

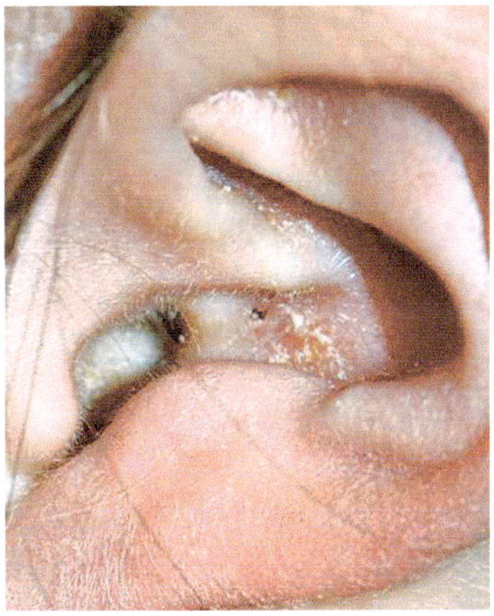

Figure 10.13 Psoriasis affecting the ear concha.
(*Courtesy*: C. Jury, R. Gulati.)

in children younger than 10 years, in whom it tends to affect the seborrhoeic areas such as the scalp, face and ears **(Fig. 10.13)**. Periocular area involvement affecting upper and lower eyelids is a typical presentation **(Figs. 10.14A and B)**. In infants, it may present as persistent napkin dermatitis **(Figs. 10.15A and B)**. The napkin area appears glistening red with involvement of folds. The rash tends to follow a prolonged course. Simultaneous affection of skin or nails may give a clue in some infants. In older children, it follows the adult distribution pattern with involvement of the scalp, ears, periumbilical area and extensors such as elbows, knees and lumbosacral area **(Figs. 10.16 to 10.18)**. This pattern is commonly referred to as chronic plaque psoriasis.

Some children may develop multiple lesions affecting the trunk with subsequent spread to the extremities, termed as guttate psoriasis. This may be secondary to streptococcal sore throat. Guttate psoriasis may clear completely in 8–12 weeks or may evolve into typical psoriasis.

Nail changes in psoriasis include pitting **(Fig. 10.19)**, onycholysis (separation of nail from the nail bed appearing as yellow discoloration) and subungual hyperkeratosis (thickened nail bed).

Psoriasis is a chronic relapsing condition, and treatment largely focuses on keeping it under control. Emollients help in improving the scaling, whereas topical steroids and tar help by anti-inflammatory effect. Topical vitamin D analogues such as calcipotriol are licensed for older children. Dithranol can be used for thick lesions on extremities. Widespread psoriasis resistant to topical treatment may be considered for phototherapy or systemic treatment with immunosuppressives such as ciclosporin or methotrexate.

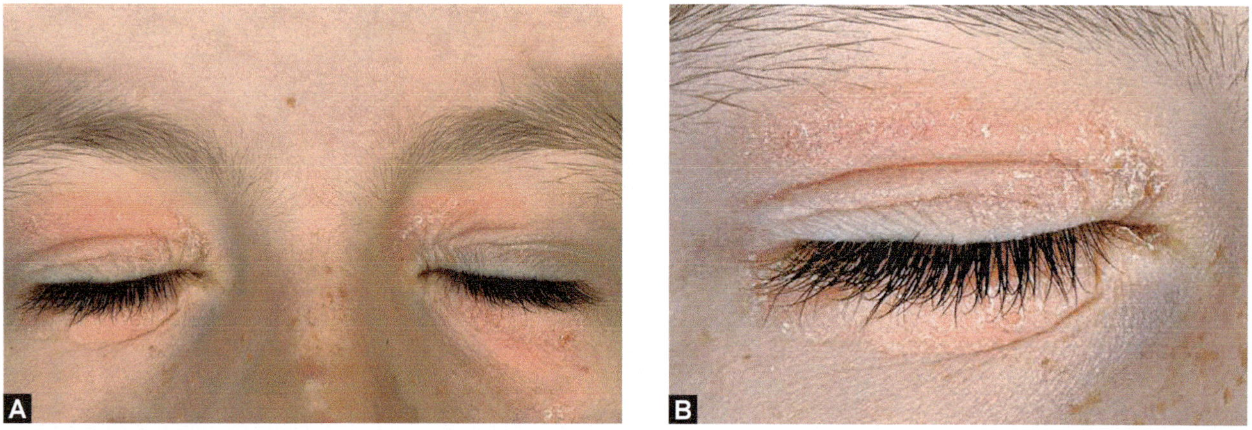

Figures 10.14A and B (A) Psoriasis affecting the periocular areas; (B) Close-up of left periocular area from Figure A.
(*Courtesy*: C. Jury, R. Gulati.)

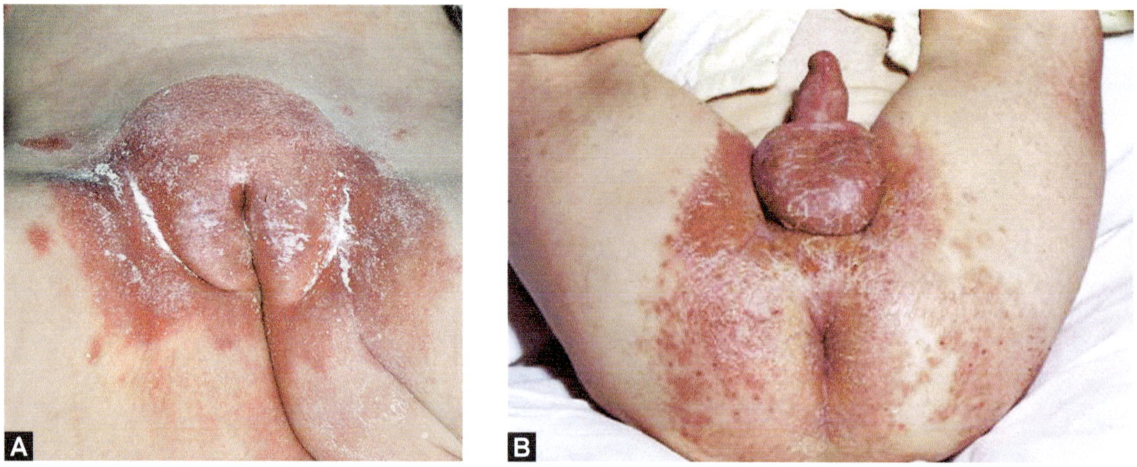

Figures 10.15A and B Napkin psoriasis. *Note*: (A) White deposits represent barrier cream.
(*Courtesy*: (A) C. Jury, R. Gulati; (B) K. Goel.)

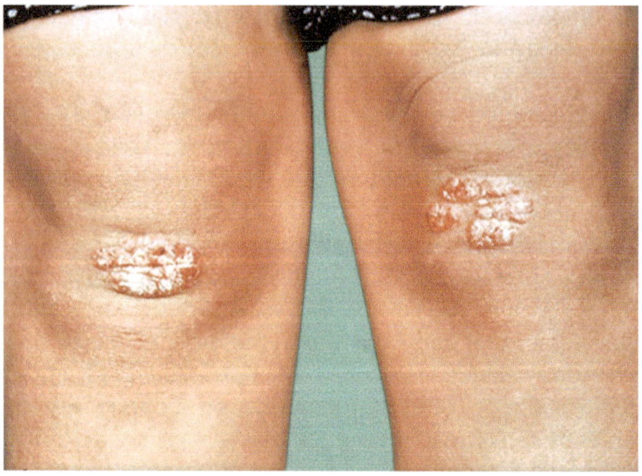

Figure 10.16 Psoriasis—plaque located over the pressure points of the knees.
(*Courtesy*: M. Mealyea.)

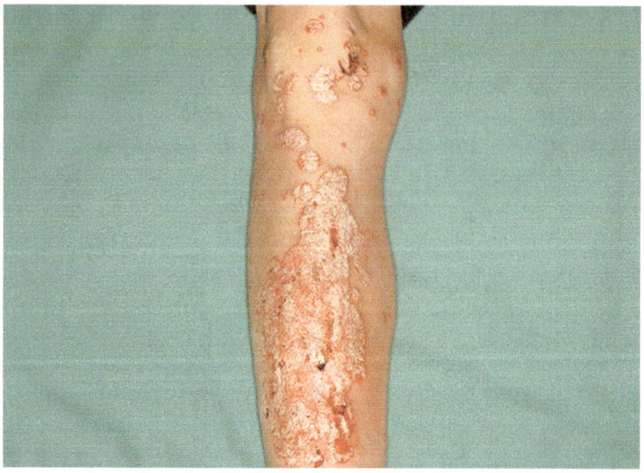

Figure 10.17 Psoriasis—typical plaques with silvery scales.
(*Courtesy*: M. Mealyea.)

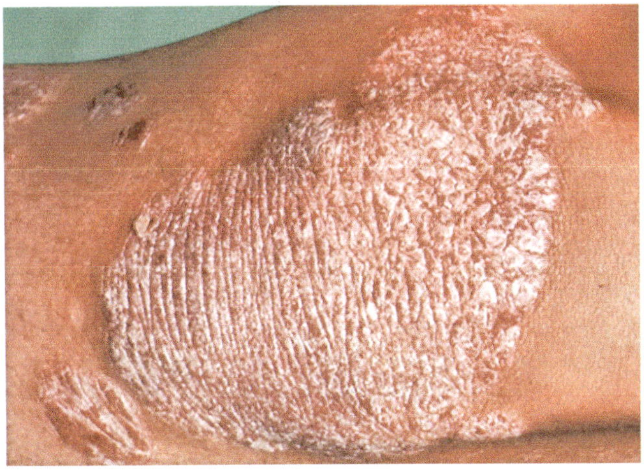

Figure 10.18 Psoriasis—close-up of the plaque.
(*Courtesy*: M. Mealyea.)

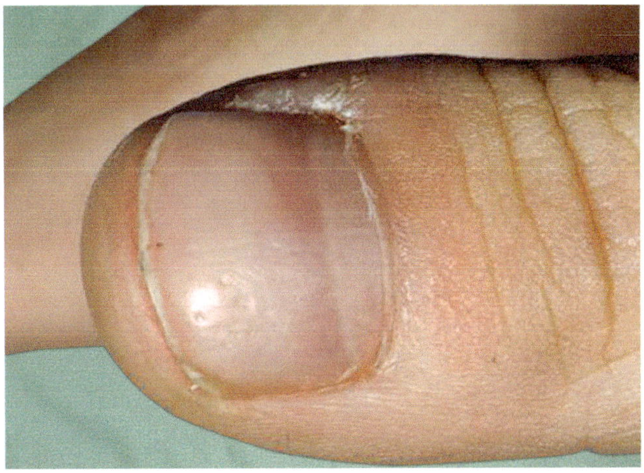

Figure 10.19 Nail pitting in psoriasis.
(*Courtesy*: C. Jury, R. Gulati.)

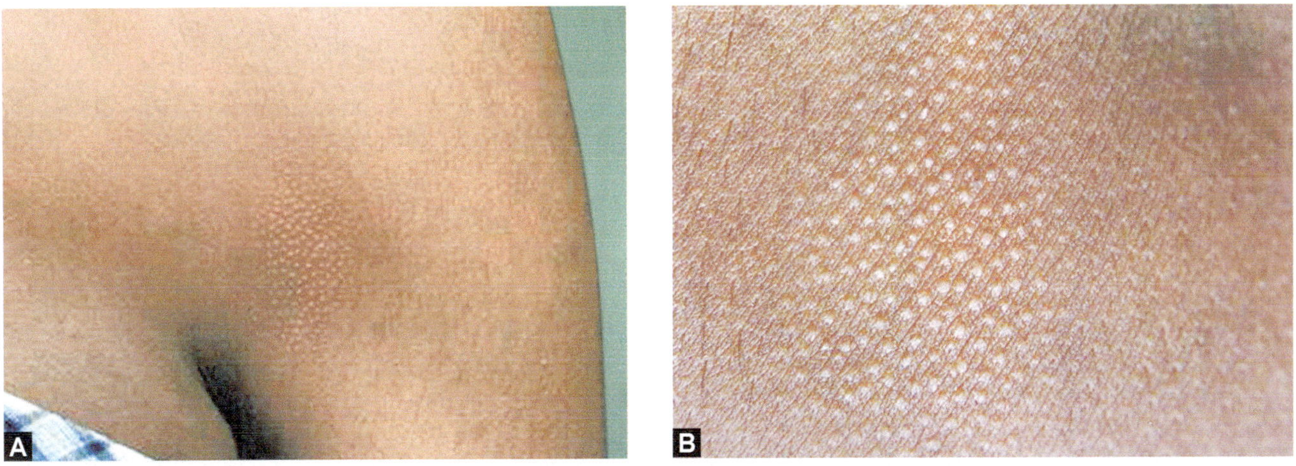

Figures 10.20A and B Lichen nitidus. *Note*: (B) close-up showing clustered monomorphic shiny papules.
(*Courtesy*: R. Gulati.)

Lichen Nitidus

This is an inflammatory disorder characterised by skin coloured flat-topped lesions usually 1–3 mm in diameter, and may be present in clusters **(Figs. 10.20A and B)**. It is usually asymptomatic, although some children complain of itching. In most children, it tends to settle spontaneously over a period of 1–2 years.

Napkin Dermatitis

This is an umbrella term comprising a variety of conditions affecting the napkin area. The most common type of napkin rash is irritant contact dermatitis considered to be caused by the caustic effect of ammonia derived from urine, although role of faeces is also contributory. It tends to affect the convex surfaces, sparing the folds. It can be painful, especially during nappy change. If left untreated, punched-out ulcers and erosions may develop, referred to as Jacquet dermatitis. Treatment aims at frequent nappy change, some time off nappy if possible and regular barrier preparation (such as zinc and ichthammol ointment). Five days of mild topical steroid may help in settling the inflammation.

Candidal diaper dermatitis presents with erythematous perianal rash with small satellite papules and pustules **(Fig. 10.21)**. Groin folds may be affected as well. This may occur in isolation or may be a superinfection over an existing nappy rash. Topical antifungals such as nystatin or imidazole creams for 2–3 weeks are effective. Oral cavity should be checked for thrush, especially in neonates.

As previously mentioned, psoriasis and seborrhoeic dermatitis can present as napkin dermatitis. If napkin dermatitis proves difficult to treat, some uncommon conditions should be considered. Persistent nappy rash having a purpuric element may point to a diagnosis of Langerhans cell histiocytosis and should be biopsied

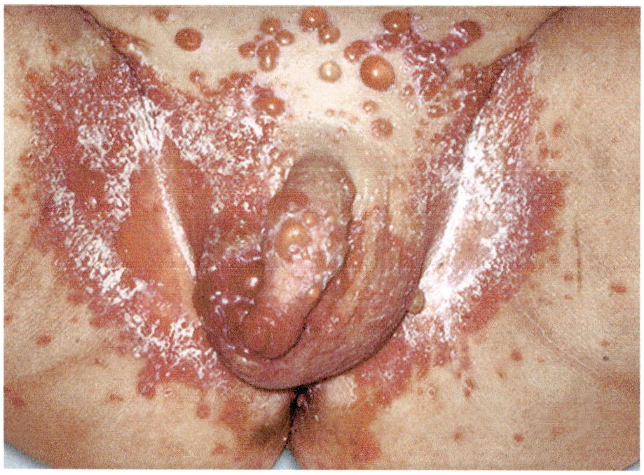

Figure 10.21 Napkin candidiasis with satellite pustules. Bullous lesions represent linear immunoglobulin A disease of childhood.

(*Courtesy*: M. Mealyea.)

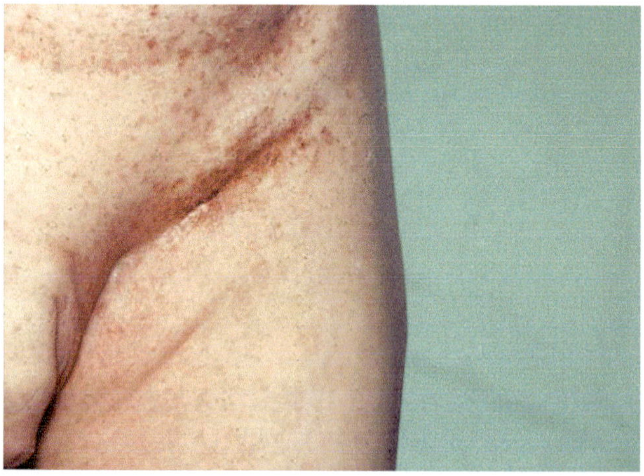

Figure 10.22 Langerhans cell histiocytosis—haemorrhagic rash involving the groins.

(*Courtesy*: K. Goel.)

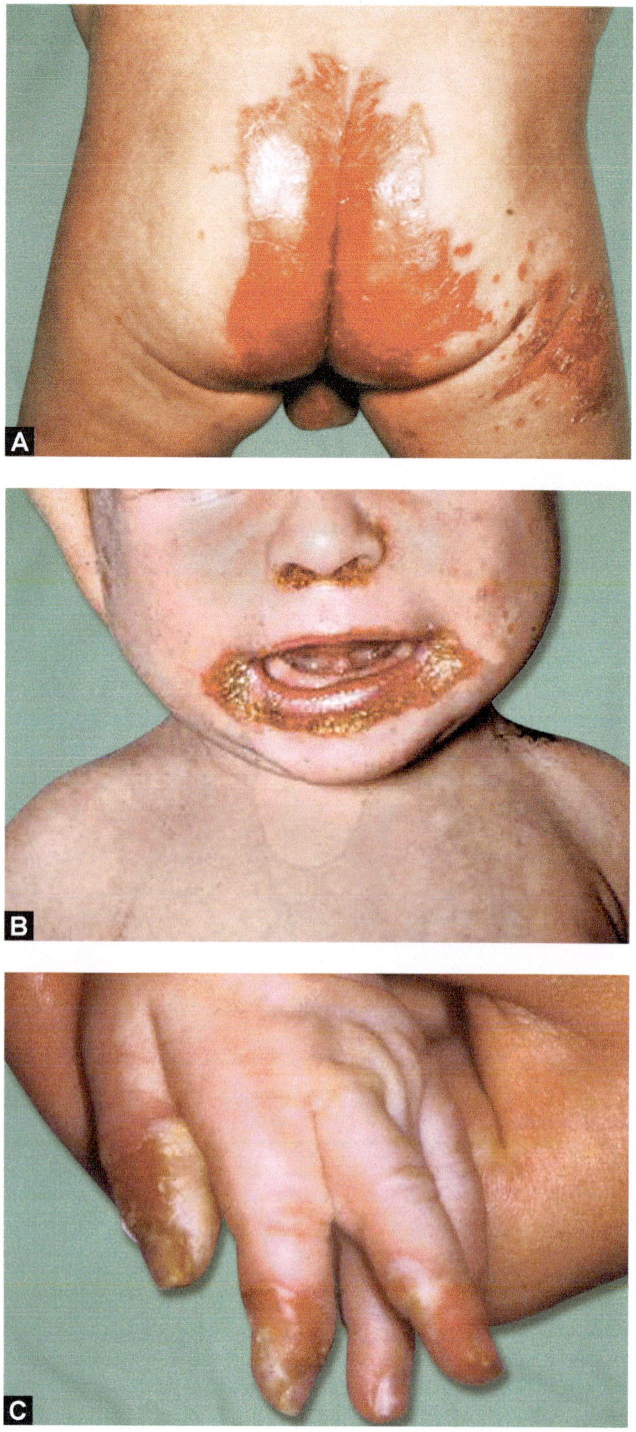

Figures 10.23A to C Acrodermatitis enteropathica. (A) Persistent scaly rash on buttocks; (B) Scaly erythematous perioral rash; (C) Eczematous involvement of acral area.

(*Courtesy*: (A) M. Mealyea; (B and C) K. Goel.)

(Fig. 10.22). A dry scaly erythematous nappy rash with a clear distinct margin **(Figs. 10.23A to C)** associated with similar perioral and acral involvement, diarrhoea, hair loss, irritability and failure to thrive may point to acrodermatitis enteropathica, an autosomal recessive disorder, which causes zinc malabsorption and deficiency. Measuring the zinc level points to the right diagnosis. Secondary causes of zinc deficiency should be considered as well. Oral zinc improves the rash within days. Oral zinc supplementation is needed for life in children with acrodermatitis enteropathica.

Acne

Some infants tend to develop acne in the first few months of life. Like sebaceous hyperplasia, maternal androgens are considered to play a role. Closed comedones are commonly seen, although open comedones, papules, pustules and even cysts can occur. It may settle spontaneously, although topical antibiotics, benzoyl peroxide and tretinoin can be used, the latter two causing irritation in some. Some infants require oral macrolides.

Most infants would be clear by 2 years of age, although a few would have residual scarring. Childhood acne appearing beyond 2 years of age should prompt ruling out hyperandrogenism.

REACTIVE ERUPTIONS

Urticaria

This is a common condition affecting all age groups. It starts acutely with transient, red, raised itchy lesions, with each individual lesion clearing completely within 24 hours, leaving normal skin behind **(Fig. 10.24)**. These lesions are termed as wheals and consist of a central raised white lesion with surrounding flare. The appearance of the lesions can be quite dramatic, sometimes forming giant urticarial plaques with irregular borders. The patient or parent often describes them as blisters in view of their appearance. Urticaria may be associated with angioedema, which presents as swelling of certain sites which have loose tissue such as periocular, lips and sometimes dorsa of hands and feet. Angioedema can occur in isolation as well.

Diagnosis largely rests on clinical history as the examination in clinic is usually normal. The most common cause of urticaria in children is response to a viral infection, termed reactive or viral urticaria. This initially causes the rash to appear daily, but gradually spaces out to settle in few weeks. If the rash lasts more than 6 weeks, it is referred to as chronic urticaria. Drugs and food reactions can cause urticarial reactions as well; however, these tend to be episodic. These should usually be excluded through a thorough history.

Treatment is with non-sedating antihistamines, which should be given on a regular basis for a few weeks.

Angioedema of a more serious nature does occur with anaphylaxis and hereditary angioedema. Anaphylaxis is a medical emergency which presents with associated breathing difficulty and/or hypotension. Laryngeal oedema may result in choking. Intramuscular adrenaline is the treatment of choice.

Hereditary angioedema is due to either deficiency of or loss of function of C1-esterase inhibitor. The diagnosis is suspected on the basis of the symptoms of abdominal pain, vomiting and angioedema, and a family history, but is confirmed by quantitative and functional assay of C1-esterase inhibitor.

Erythema Multiforme

Erythema multiforme (EM) is a reactive rash secondary to infections in children. Herpes simplex and mycoplasma are the most commonly implicated infections. Rash presents with typical target lesions mainly affecting the distal extremities, although it can become widespread **(Fig. 10.25)**. It usually settles in a couple of weeks. Recurrent EM is sometimes secondary to recurrent subtle herpes simplex exacerbations, and a trial of prophylactic oral acyclovir may be helpful.

Erythema Nodosum

This is another reactive process usually caused by infections such as streptococcal and tuberculosis, although other infections such as yersinia and deep fungal infections can be implicated as well. Other causes include sarcoidosis, inflammatory bowel disease and drugs such as sulphonamides and oral contraceptive pills. The condition presents as tender, red nodules often on the anterior lower legs but can sometimes involve other areas **(Fig. 10.26)**. It is due to inflammation of the subcutaneous fat (panniculitis). It usually resolves spontaneously in around 6–8 weeks.

Pityriasis Rosea

This usually represents a hypersensitive rash secondary to a viral infection, although, in minority of the cases, drugs have been implicated. The rash primarily involves

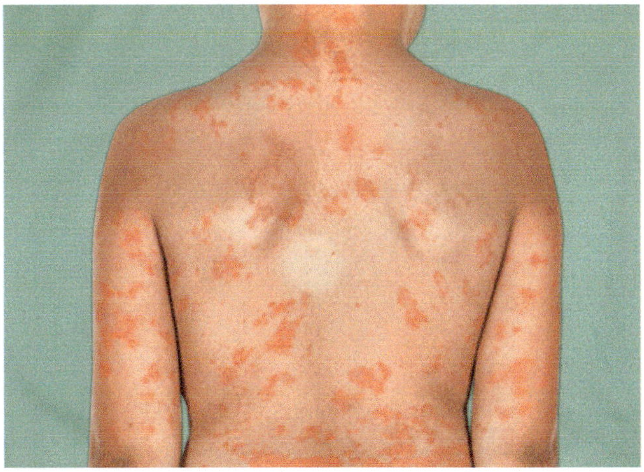

Figure 10.24 Widespread urticaria.

(*Courtesy*: M. Mealyea.)

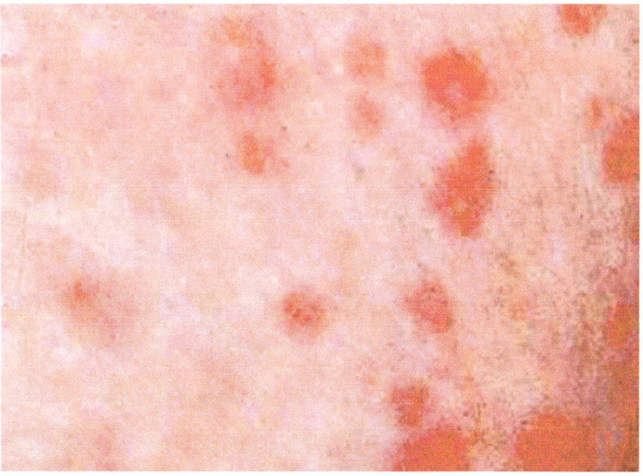

Figure 10.25 Erythema multiforme—target-shaped lesions resembling bull's-eye.

(*Courtesy*: K. Goel.)

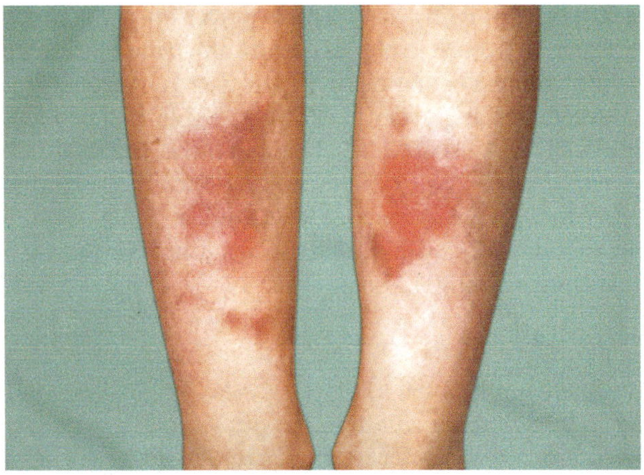

Figure 10.26 Erythema nodosum—tender nodular lesions on shins tending to coalesce.

(*Courtesy*: M. Mealyea.)

the trunk and proximal extremities, and has a characteristic 'fir tree' appearance on the back **(Fig. 10.27A)**. This is secondary to lesions lying along the Langer lines. The individual lesions are oval-shaped patches with a typical collarette of scale at the margins **(Fig. 10.27B)**. In around one-fifth of the cases, the rash is preceded by a larger lesion, termed the herald patch, which is usually seen on the trunk. The condition is asymptomatic, although some feel itchy. The eruption is self-limiting and generally settles in 6–8 weeks.

Gianotti–Crosti Syndrome

This is a reactive papular rash seen in children secondary to a variety of viral infections. The rash generally involves extremities, buttocks and face, and is generally asymptomatic **(Figs. 10.28A and B)**. The papules are firm on

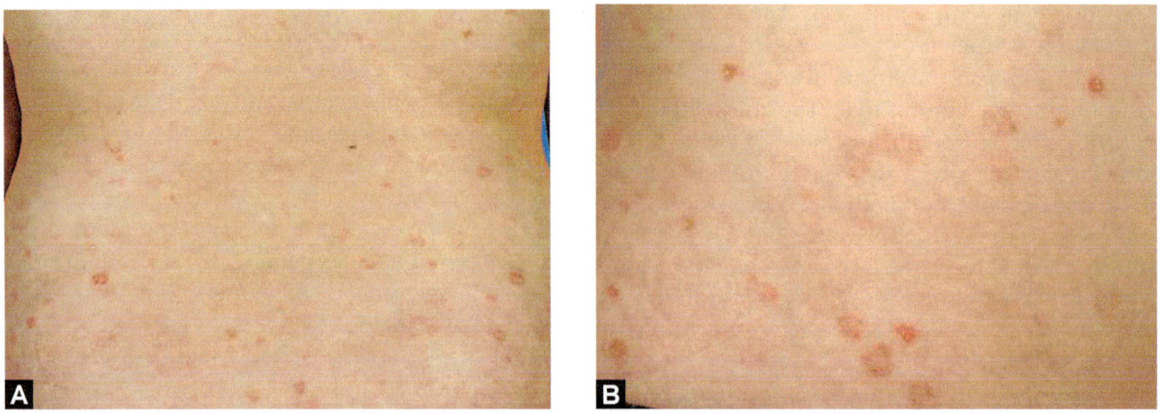

Figures 10.27A and B Pityriasis rosea. (A) Bilateral oval patches with longitudinal axis along the Langer lines; (B) Few lesions showing collarette of scales.

(*Courtesy*: R. Gulati.)

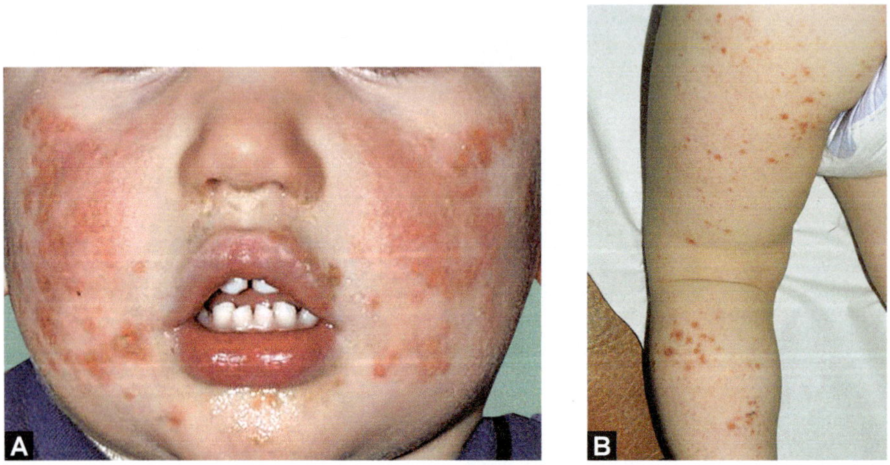

Figures 10.28A and B Gianotti-Crosti syndrome. *Note:* (A) Papular lesions on cheeks.

(*Courtesy*: C. Jury, R. Gulati.)

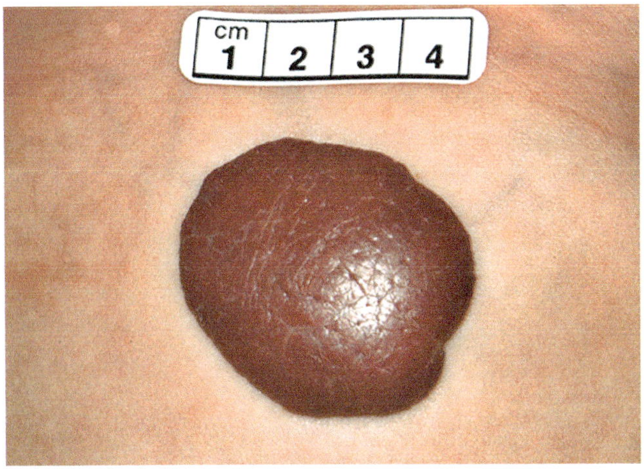

Figure 10.29 Growing superficial infantile haemangioma—bright red, firm.

(*Courtesy*: M. Mealyea.)

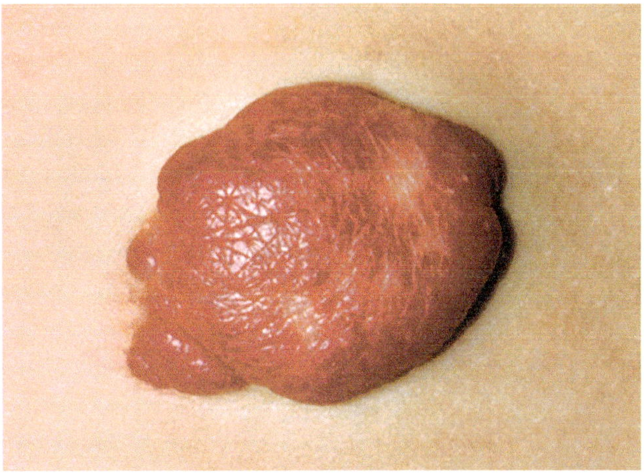

Figure 10.30 Resolving superficial infantile haemangioma—dull red colour, softer.

(*Courtesy*: M. Mealyea.)

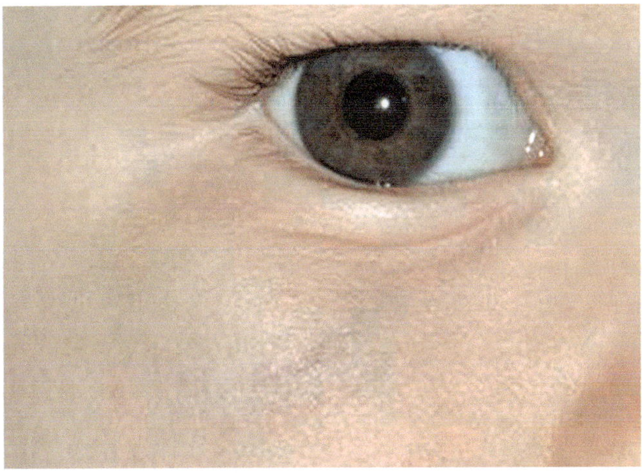

Figure 10.31 Deep haemangioma—notice bluish swelling on the cheek.

(*Courtesy*: C. Jury, R. Gulati.)

palpation. Children are systemically well. The lesions settle over 6–8 weeks.

VASCULAR ANOMALIES

Classification of vascular birthmarks was initially suggested by Mulliken and Glowacki in 1982, which, after slight modification, was accepted by the International Society for the Study of Vascular Anomalies in 1996. The vascular birthmarks were grouped into two large categories: vascular tumours and vascular malformations. The main difference lies in the way these behave clinically. Vascular tumours show endothelial proliferation, thereby showing initial increase in size, whereas vascular malformations are composed of dilated vessels showing no proliferative phase.

Vascular Tumours

Infantile Haemangioma (Strawberry Naevus)

This is the most common vascular tumour, characterised by benign proliferation of endothelial cells. It affects about 10% of infants. It is more common in girls and premature infants. Chorionic villous sampling during pregnancy and multiple gestations also increase the risk.

Haemangiomas are usually not evident at birth; however, some parents do recognise presence of a faint bruise or pale area. They typically become obvious within the first 2 weeks of life, although deeper lesions may become visible only when they have grown a reasonable size. They usually undergo rapid proliferation, mostly within the first 6 months, although they can continue to grow for up to 12 months **(Fig. 10.29)**. This is then followed by a period of slow involution over a number of years **(Fig. 10.30)**.

Infantile haemangiomas can be superficial where the involved blood vessels lie in the superficial dermis and appear red **(Fig. 10.29)** or deep where they lie in deep dermis or subcutaneous tissue giving a blue hue **(Fig. 10.31)**. Most haemangiomas, however, have a mix of both **(Figs. 10.32 and 10.33)**. The diagnosis is made clinically, but can be verified with a Doppler ultrasound, which demonstrates presence of both arterial and venous waveforms.

Most haemangiomas do not require any treatment. After the growing phase, they begin to pale or whiten on the surface, soften and gradually shrink down. Larger lesions leave a residual fibrofatty tissue and may need cosmetic surgery. Residual superficial telangiectasia can be treated using pulsed dye laser.

Lesions at some sites can cause or be associated with significant and serious complications, apart from the potential cosmetic issues. These are listed below **(Table 10.1)**.

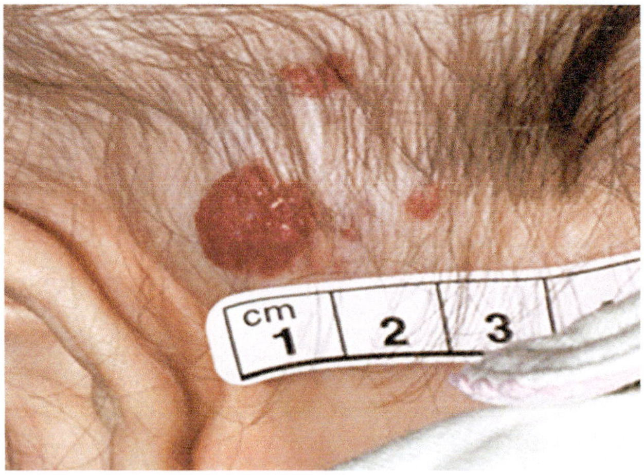

Figure 10.32 Mixed infantile haemangioma—deep component evident as blue hue over which the red superficial component is visible.

(*Courtesy*: M. Mealyea.)

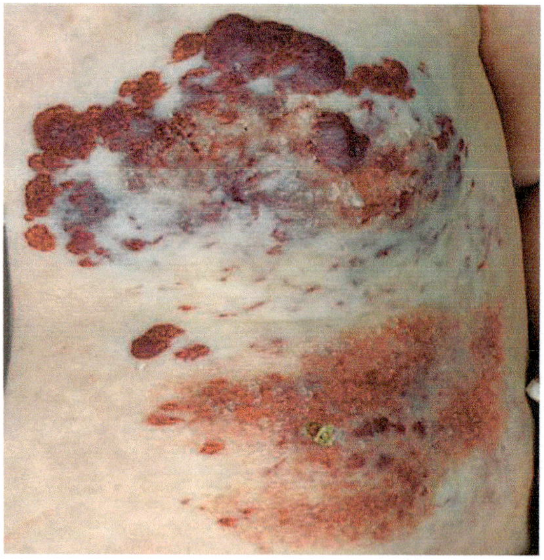

Figure 10.33 Mixed haemangioma—the bluish hue represents deeper component.

(*Courtesy*: C. Jury, R. Gulati.)

TABLE 10.1 Potential complications from haemangiomas present at different body sites.

Site	*Complications*
Around the eye **(Figs. 10.34 and 10.35)**	Obstruction to vision, amblyopia, astigmatism
Lip	Ulceration, feeding difficulty
Perineum	Ulceration, constipation secondary to pain
Beard area	Pressure on larynx and trachea, associated vocal cord lesions
Nose	Cartilage damage, blocked nostril, feeding difficulty
Ear canal	Hearing problems
Segmental facial	PHACES syndrome[a]
Midline lumbosacral	Spinal dysraphism

[a]This is a rare syndrome comprising variably of posterior fossa brain malformation, haemangioma, arterial anomalies, cardiac defects, eye and sternal abnormalities.

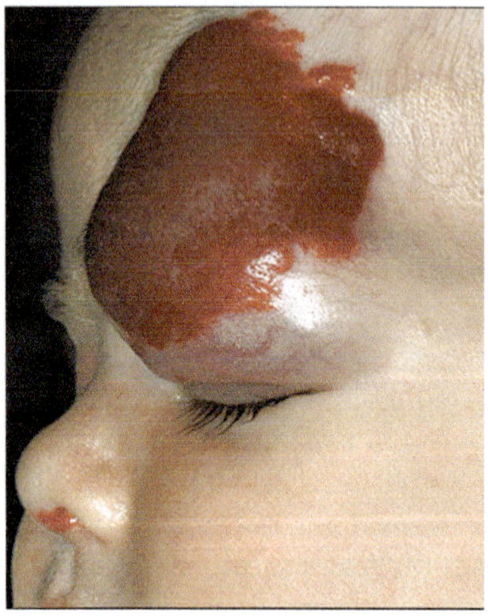

Figure 10.34 Mixed infantile haemangioma involving forehead and upper eyelid.

(*Courtesy*: M. Mealyea.)

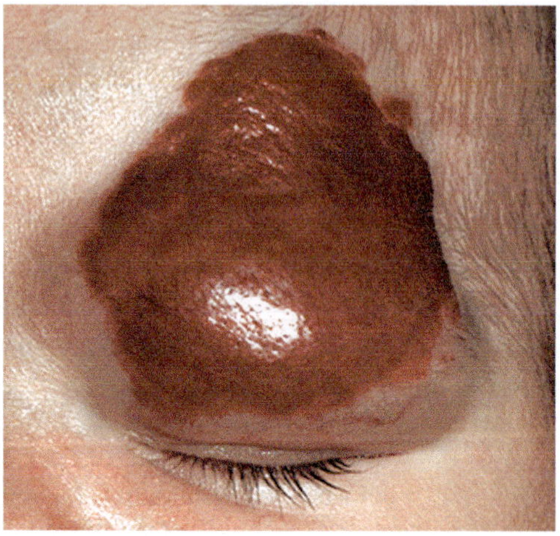

Figure 10.35 Infantile haemangioma on eyelid obstructing vision. Required treatment with oral steroids.

(*Courtesy*: M. Mealyea.)

Multiple cutaneous haemangiomas, usually five or more, can be associated with visceral haemangiomas, most commonly involving liver. Affected children should therefore have an ultrasound of the abdomen. Hepatic haemangiomas can be associated with high-output cardiac failure and hypothyroidism. Some authors refer to this condition as benign neonatal haemangiomatosis if only cutaneous lesions are present, and diffuse neonatal haemangiomatosis if visceral involvement is present as well.

Ulcerated haemangiomas can be quite painful **(Fig. 10.36)** and can lead to scarring. These should be treated quite early on with non-adherent dressings and adequate analgesia.

Rapidly enlarging lesions, if causing functional and/or cosmetic concerns, require early intervention. Oral propranolol in doses of 2–3 mg/kg/d has been used since 2008, and has become the drug of choice in most departments. It is relatively safe, with major side effects being hypoglycaemia, hypotension, bradycardia and exacerbation of wheeze. Previously, high-dose systemic steroids in doses of 2–5 mg/kg/d have been used, although at the expense of significant side effects. Propranolol has been found effective for ulcerated haemangiomas as well.

Other Vascular Tumours

Two other types of vascular tumours can sometimes be confused with infantile haemangiomas. These are: (1) the tufted angioma and (2) the kaposiform haemangioendothelioma. The history and behaviour of these two vascular tumours give a clue to the diagnosis, but usually a biopsy is required for confirmation. They may be present at birth or appear later on. Both these tumours may be associated with Kasabach-Merritt phenomenon, which clinically presents as rapid swelling of the lesion with bruising and purpura. Trapping of platelets can lead to profound thrombocytopaenia, whereas consumption of fibrinogen and coagulation factors can cause consumption coagulopathy. This needs urgent treatment and would necessitate involvement of general paediatrician and paediatric haematologist. High-dose steroids and vincristine have been used along with supportive measures.

Congenital haemangioma: These haemangiomas are fully formed at birth, and mostly show a rim of pallor. They may involute spontaneously over next 12–18 months and are referred to as rapidly involuting congenital haemangiomas. However, if they fail to do so, they are called non-involuting congenital haemangiomas.

Vascular Malformations

Vascular malformations are composed of dilated vessels and can be made up of capillary, venous, arterial, lymphatic or a combination of the above vessels. These lesions are present at birth, although they may become evident later on. Unlike vascular tumours, the lesions do not show any active growth.

CAPILLARY MALFORMATION

Salmon patch is the most common capillary malformation. This presents as a red patch usually on the central forehead and/or nape of neck, sometimes also involving the upper eyelids and upper lip **(Fig. 10.37)**. These patches are present in about 50% of infants and usually disappear by the age of 2 years, although the ones on the nape of the neck often persist. They are of no consequence.

Another variant is a port-wine stain **(Figs. 10.38A and B)**, seen as a flat red patch seen at birth. It can darken with age, and in adulthood it may show palpable purple lesions. Laser treatment may help in fading the lesions. If the capillary malformation involves the ophthalmic division of the trigeminal nerve segment on the face, there is a risk of Sturge-Weber syndrome. This is a triad of capillary malformation in ophthalmic division of the trigeminal nerve, eye involvement (usually glaucoma) and brain

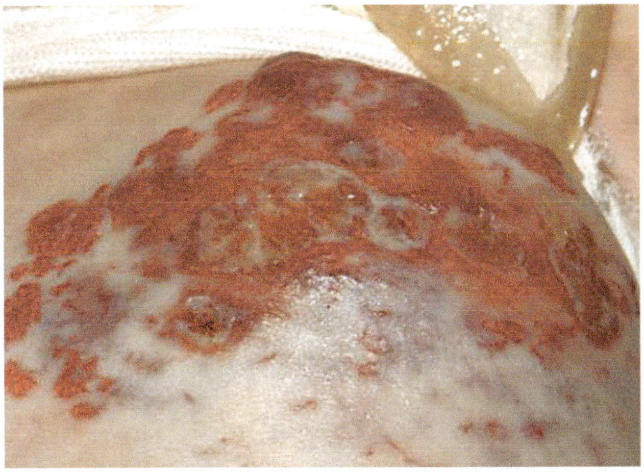

Figure 10.36 Ulcerated haemangioma.
(*Courtesy*: C. Jury, R. Gulati.)

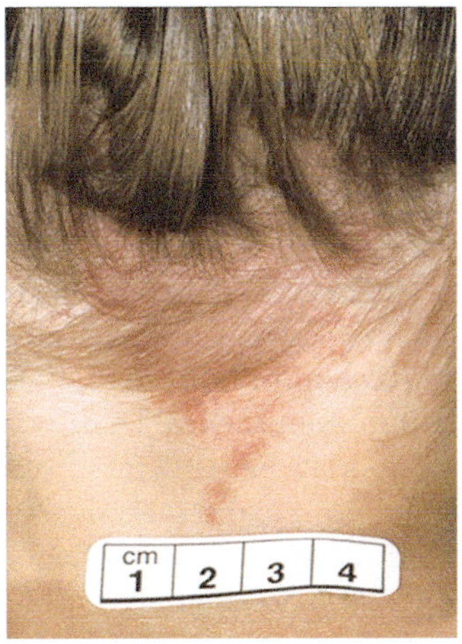

Figure 10.37 Salmon patch on the nape of the neck.
(*Courtesy*: M. Mealyea.)

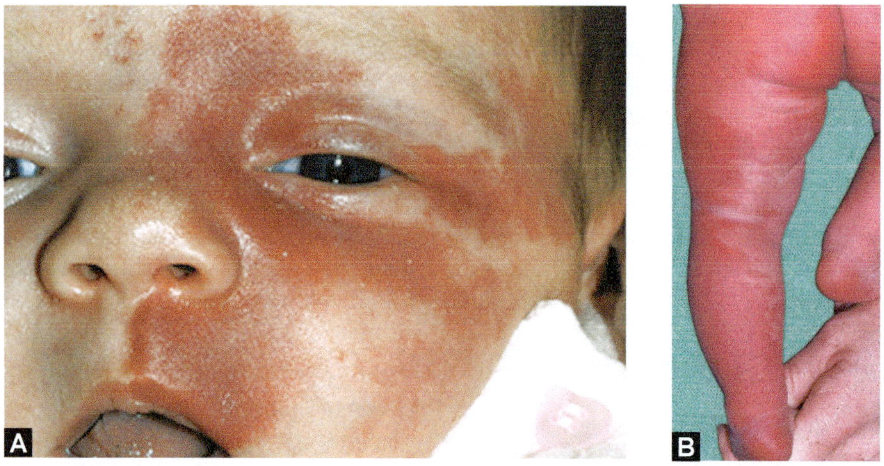

Figures 10.38A and B (A) Capillary malformation (port-wine stain) affecting V1 and V2 area on face; (B) Capillary malformation affecting left lower limb. Limb lengths need to be monitored as they can be associated with limb overgrowth.

(*Courtesy*: (A) M. Mealyea; (B) K. Goel.)

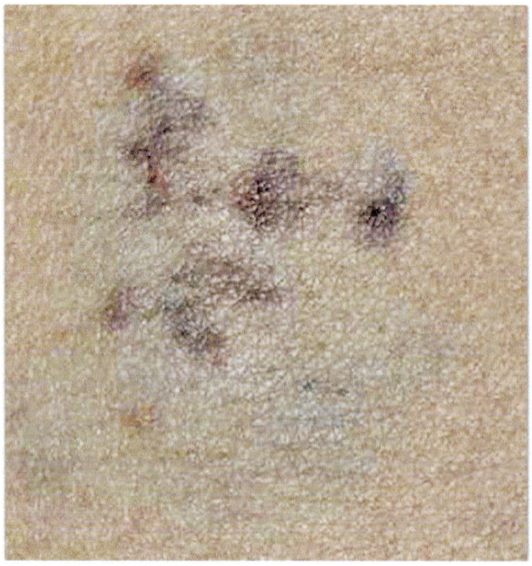

Figure 10.39 Venous malformation.

(*Courtesy*: C. Jury, R. Gulati.)

abnormalities; epilepsy may be a significant problem for these children.

VENOUS MALFORMATIONS

Venous malformations often appear as bluish compressible birthmarks **(Fig. 10.39)**. They can be quite extensive, and radiological imaging may be necessary to determine the extent. Being slow-flow lesions, they are predisposed to formation of intralesional clots. There is some evidence that larger lesions may be associated with pulmonary microembolisation and subsequently secondary right heart dysfunction. Lower extremity malformations may be painful secondary to pooling of blood and stretching of vessel walls. Pressure garments may be helpful. Definitive treatment is challenging, but percutaneous sclerotherapy and, in selected cases, surgical excision may be helpful.

Klippel-Trenaunay syndrome is a rare condition characterised by presence of venous and capillary malformations associated with hypertrophy involving an extremity. Magnetic resonance imaging and Doppler ultrasound help in diagnosis. The condition needs to be monitored to ensure optimal functioning of limbs and avoid complications.

Arteriovenous Malformations

These lesions are high flow and therefore can be life-threatening. Significant bleeding is a risk, especially following trauma and surgery. They may present at any age and diagnosis may be confirmed using Doppler ultrasound.

Lymphatic Malformations

Microcystic lesions are usually superficial, e.g. lymphangioma circumscriptum, which presents as a group of small vesicles, some of which may be haemorrhagic. Macrocystic lesions are usually deeper, e.g. cystic hygroma. Being infiltrative, surgical excision is difficult. Sclerotherapy can be helpful if large lymphatic cysts are present.

DISORDERS OF PIGMENTATION

Pigmentary disturbances are more commonly observed in darker skinned individuals. Either too little or too much pigmentation not only can have medical significance, but also can be cosmetically challenging.

Disorders of Hypopigmentation

Post-inflammatory

Any inflammation involving the skin can be followed by hypopigmentation or hyperpigmentation. When the

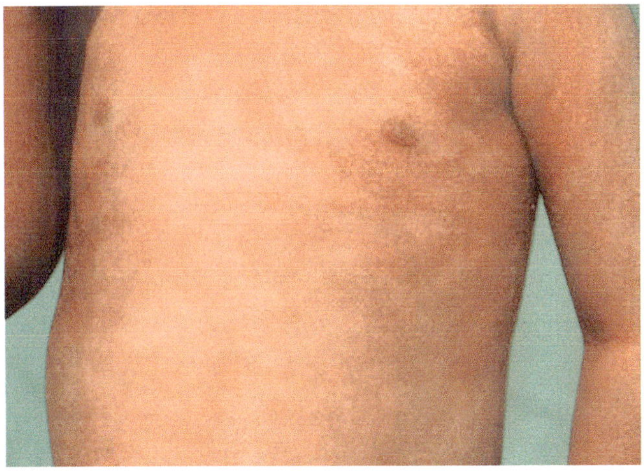

Figure 10.40 Post-inflammatory hypopigmentation following resolved eczema.
(*Courtesy*: R. Gulati.)

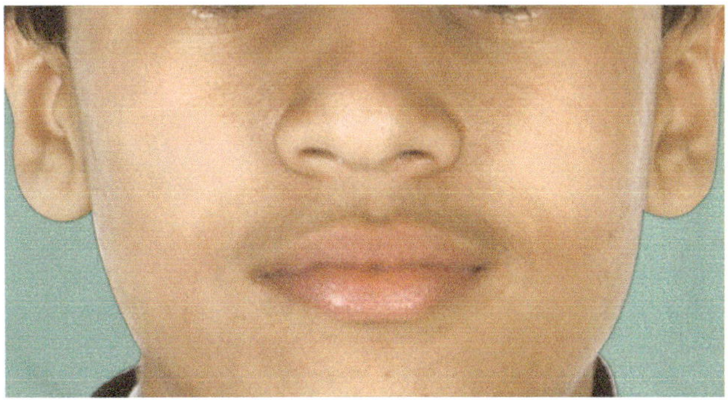

Figure 10.41 Pityriasis alba—ill-defined hypopigmented patches on cheeks.
(*Courtesy*: M. Mealyea.)

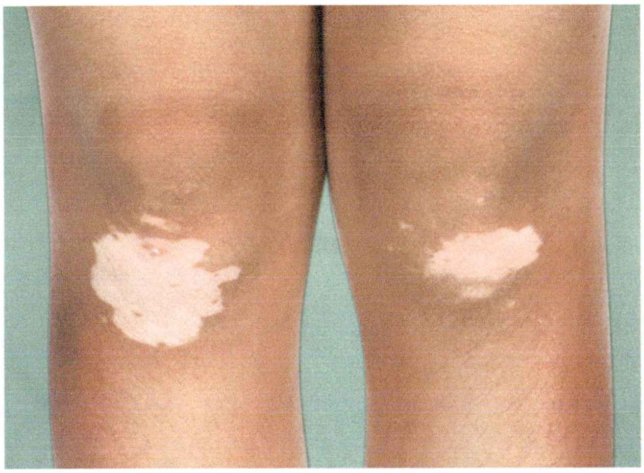

Figure 10.42 Vitiligo—well-defined depigmented patches on knees.
(*Courtesy*: M. Mealyea.)

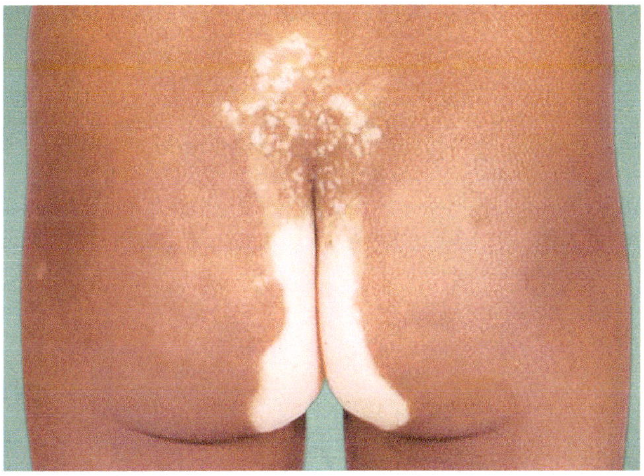

Figure 10.43 Vitiligo—some repigmentation evident on lower back.
(*Courtesy*: K. Goel.)

inflammation subsides, the pigmentary disturbance can take few weeks to months to resolve **(Fig. 10.40)**. This is commonly evident following trauma or inflammatory conditions such as atopic eczema.

Pityriasis Alba

This is a form of post-inflammatory hypopigmentation where pale patches appear mostly on the face **(Fig. 10.41)**. These are more visible in the summer time when the rest of the skin tans secondary to sun exposure. They usually fade over the winter but may become visible again the following summer. The condition is more common in children with eczema. This needs to be differentiated from vitiligo in which the pigment is lost rather than decreased and the skin presents with milk white patches. Pityriasis alba may clear spontaneously. Emollients are the mainstay of treatment, although short period of mild topical steroid may be helpful in improving the appearance more quickly.

Vitiligo

Vitiligo is considered to be an acquired autoimmune condition targeting melanocytes. It presents with localised or widespread white depigmented patches. Twenty-five per cent of cases are seen before 10 years of age. Patches are usually symmetrical involving knees, ankles, elbows, hands and trunk variably **(Figs. 10.42 and 10.43)**. In some children, perioral and periocular areas are involved. Hair in the affected areas can lose pigment as well **(Fig. 10.44)**. There is often a family history of other autoimmune conditions, notably affecting thyroid gland. The condition can raise significant cosmetic concerns, especially for dark-skinned individuals.

Treatment options are limited, more so in children. Potent topical steroids may stimulate repigmentation, usually from the hair follicles where some melanocytes usually survive the autoimmune destruction. Topical

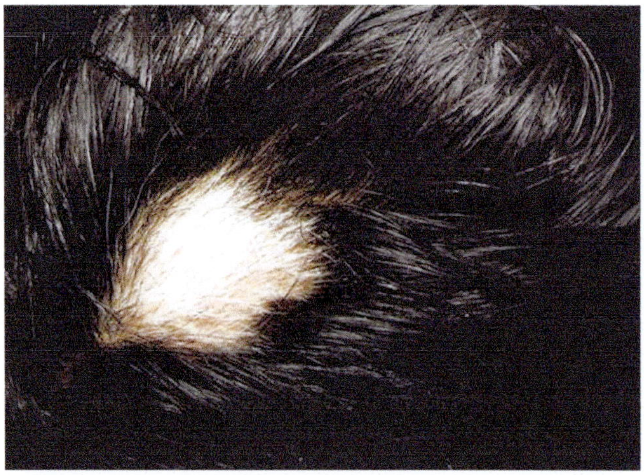

Figure 10.44 Patch of vitiligo in scalp showing loss of hair pigment.
(*Courtesy*: R. Gulati.)

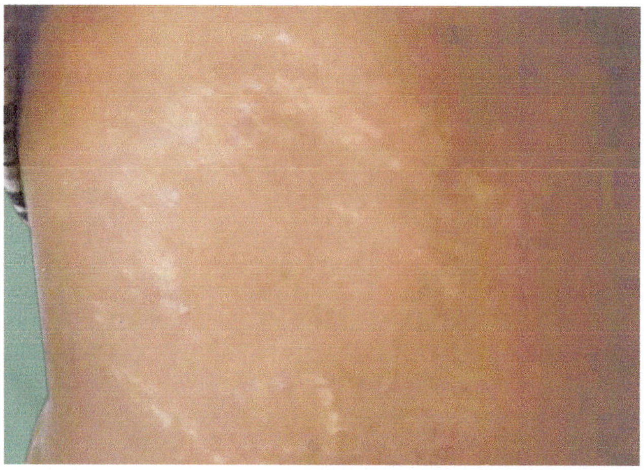

Figure 10.45 Hypopigmented streaks following the lines of Blaschko.
(*Courtesy*: R. Gulati.)

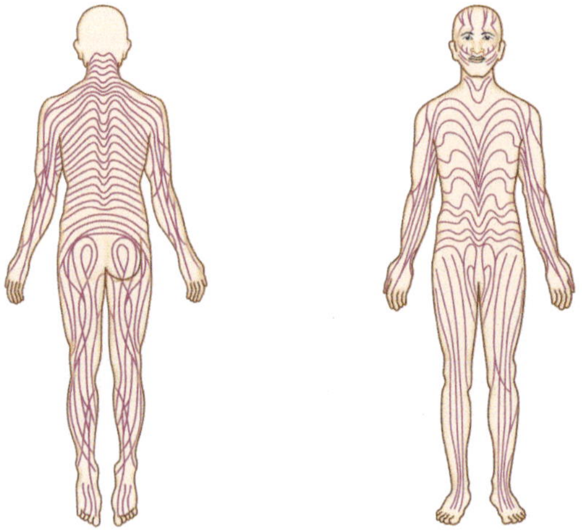

Figure 10.46 Blaschko lines—represent lines of embryological neuroectodermal migration.
(*Courtesy*: M. Mealyea.)

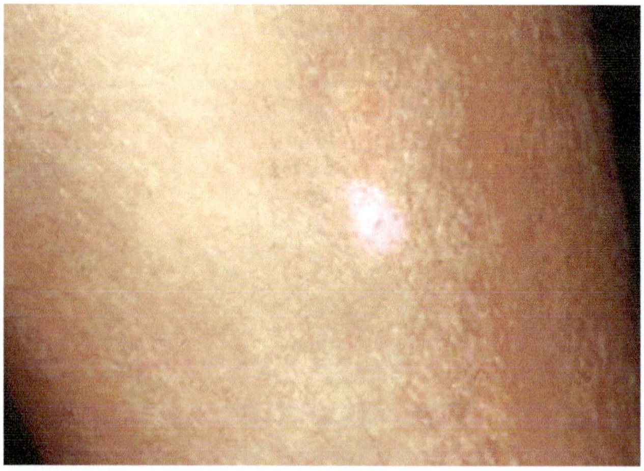

Figure 10.47 Ash-leaf macule—tuberous sclerosis.
(*Courtesy*: K. Goel.)

tacrolimus has recently been used with good effect, especially on face where topical potent steroids can cause significant side effects. As the patches are more susceptible to sun damage, owing to loss of melanocyte protection, sunscreens, preferably with sun protection factor 50 plus, should be used.

Piebaldism

This is an autosomal dominant condition characterised by white forelock and circumscribed depigmented patches affecting the body. It is caused by a defect in the proliferation and migration of melanocytes during embryogenesis. Unlike vitiligo, it is congenital and non-progressive.

Nevoid Hypomelanosis (Hypomelanosis of Ito)

This condition is characterised by hypopigmented patches or streaks **(Fig. 10.45)**, which follow the lines of Blaschko **(Fig. 10.46)**. They are usually present at birth, but may develop in the first 2 years of life. Thereafter, they usually remain stable. In small number of children, there may be associated abnormalities, usually affecting eye, skeleton, teeth and nervous system. The latter associations necessitate careful examination and follow-up.

Tuberous Sclerosis

This autosomal dominant condition variably affects the skin, central nervous system, the eye and viscera. The first sign is usually a small white patch mostly on the trunk, traditionally termed the ash-leaf macule, although the shape can be variably oval **(Fig. 10.47)**, lanceolate or confetti. Other cutaneous features include angiofibromas of the face (adenoma sebaceum) **(Fig. 10.48)**, connective tissue naevi (forehead plaques and shagreen patches) and periungual fibromas. Any child who presents with

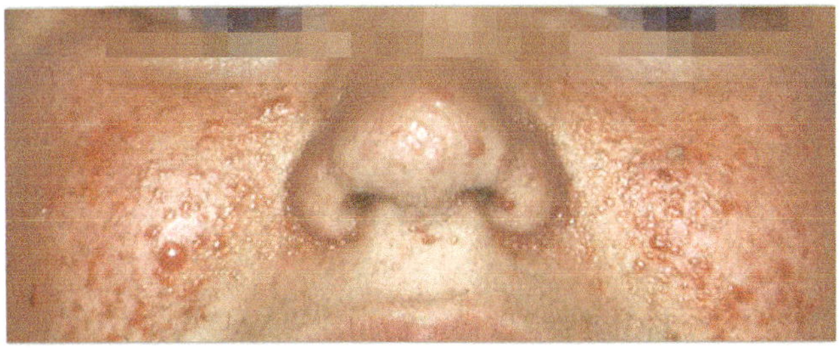

Figure 10.48 Angiofibromas (adenoma sebaceum).
(*Courtesy*: M. Mealyea.)

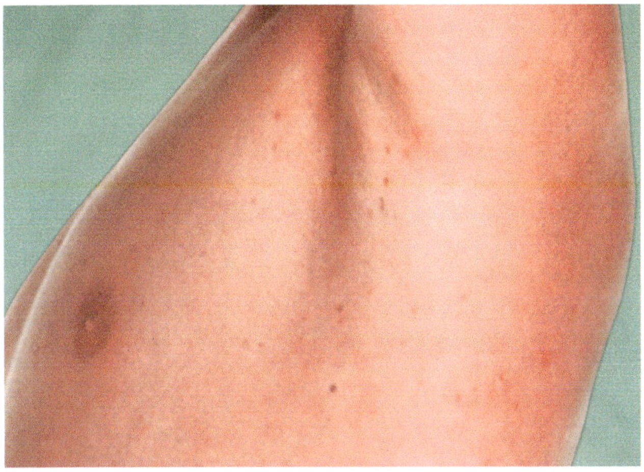

Figure 10.50 Axillary freckling—neurofibromatosis type I.
(*Courtesy*: M. Mealyea.)

a hypopigmented patch should be carefully assessed for other markers of the condition.

Disorders of Hyperpigmentation

Café Au Lait Macules

These are light brown macules which may have an irregular border. These are referred to as macules; however, the size ranges from less than a centimetre to many centimetres. They are present at birth or develop during childhood. They can occur anywhere on the body. Small single lesions are unremarkable; however, the presence of multiple café au lait macules (CALMs) may be a marker for neurofibromatosis type I. Neurofibromatosis type I is an autosomal dominant condition with manifestations in the skin, eye, bone, soft tissues and central nervous system. The diagnostic criteria need at least five CALMs greater than 5 mm in diameter and other signs such as axillary and inguinal freckling, neurofibromas, and Lisch nodules in the eyes, and a family history should be sought **(Figs. 10.49 and 10.50)**. These children should be followed-up and carefully monitored for any changes in their skin. Regular checks on blood pressure, height, and weight and examination of the spine should be carried out. They should be referred to ophthalmology for regular eye examinations.

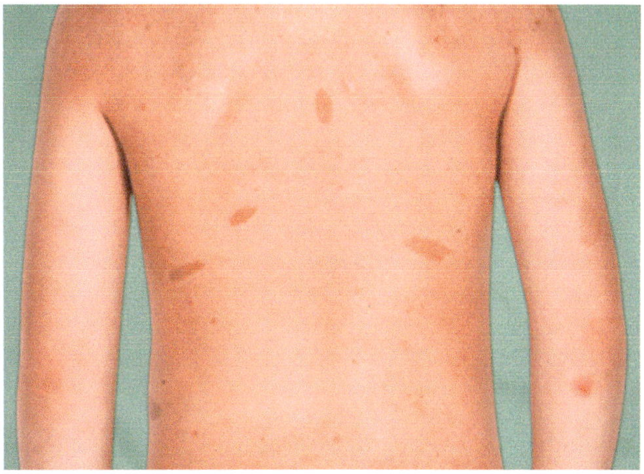

Figure 10.49 Café au lait patches—neurofibromatosis type I.
(*Courtesy*: M. Mealyea.)

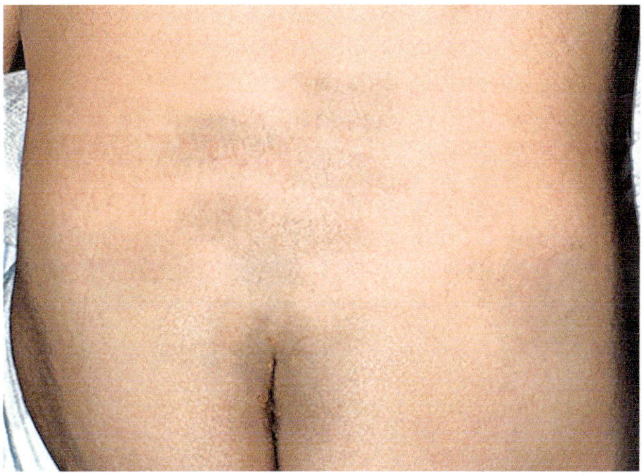

Figure 10.51 Mongolian spots.
(*Courtesy*: M. Mealyea.)

One very large CALM, particularly if segmental with a jagged margin, may be a marker for McCune-Albright syndrome. This syndrome is a triad of CALM, polyostotic fibrous dysplasia and endocrine disorders.

Dermal Melanocytosis

Mongolian spots: These are bluish-grey patches seen most commonly on the lumbosacral area in approximately 80% of Asian and African American and up to 5% of Caucasian babies **(Fig. 10.51)**. More extensive involvement can be seen. They are completely benign and can fade before adulthood. They should be differentiated from a bruise, especially in emergency departments where they are found incidentally. Clinical photography can be helpful here.

Naevus of Ota and naevus of Ito: Blue-grey pigmentation in the periorbital region in ophthalmic and maxillary divisions of the trigeminal nerve is referred to as a naevus

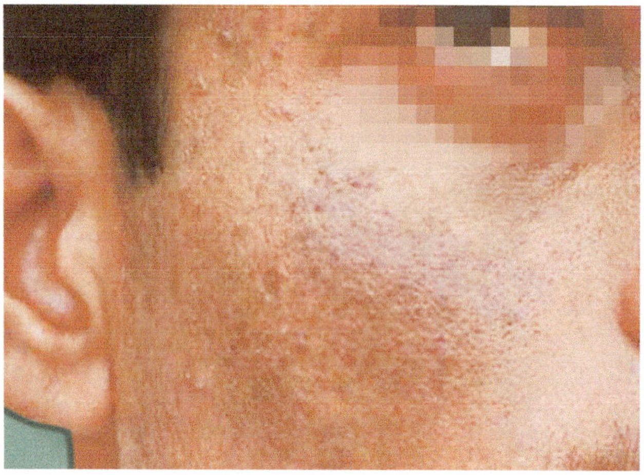

Figure 10.52 Naevus of Ota.
(*Courtesy*: R. Gulati.)

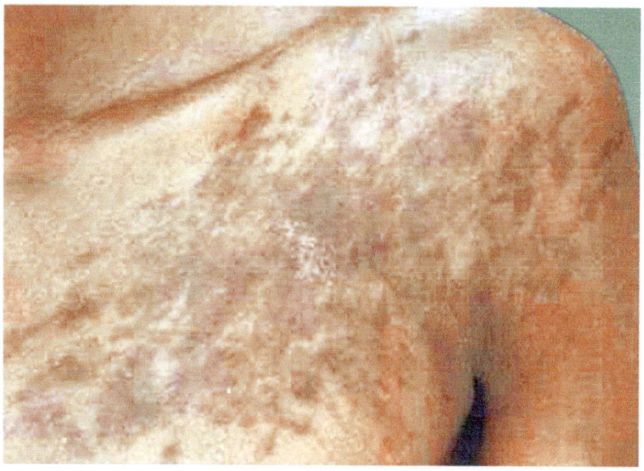

Figure 10.53 Becker naevus.
(*Courtesy*: R. Gulati.)

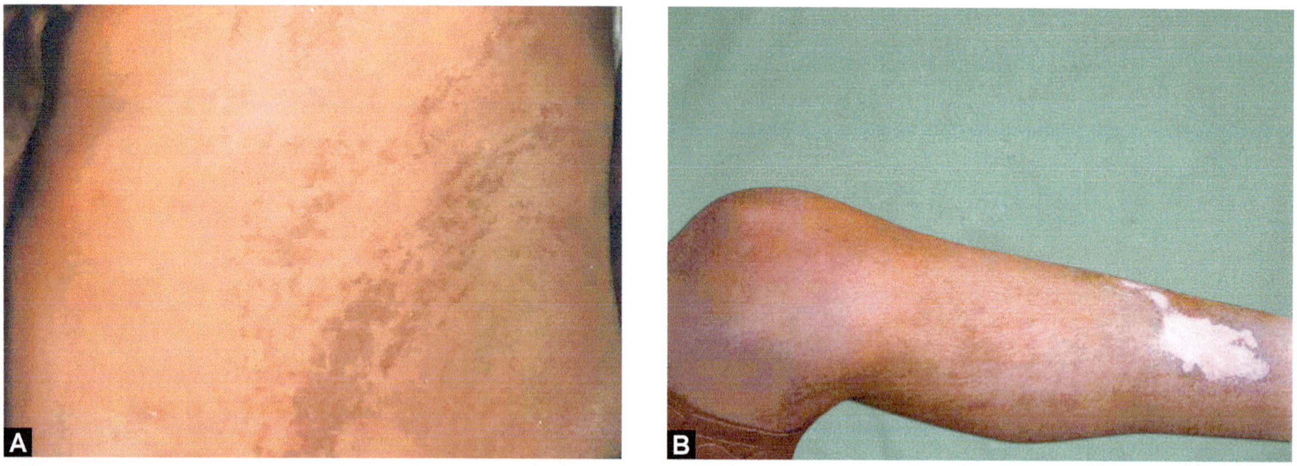

Figures 10.54A and B Linear and whorled nevoid hypermelanosis affecting: (A) The trunk; (B) The leg—also note vitiligo following trauma denoting Koebner phenomenon.
(*Courtesy*: R. Gulati.)

of Ota **(Fig. 10.52)**. Pigmentation can affect the eye in around half the cases. It is more common in Asians and in girls. It is usually present at birth but may not become evident until later in life. It should again be differentiated from a bruise. Ophthalmology review should be done to exclude glaucoma.

Naevus of Ito is similar to the naevus of Ota but the pigment affects the shoulder, neck, upper arms and upper trunk variably. Both naevus of Ota and Ito are generally benign conditions, although rare cases of melanoma have been reported. Laser treatment can lighten the lesions.

Becker Naevus

Becker naevus is a benign acquired pigmented area, often showing increased hair growth, developing after puberty. It is mostly seen in males, and has a predilection for shoulders, chest or upper back **(Fig. 10.53)**. It has increased density of androgen receptors. No definitive treatment is available.

Linear and Whorled Nevoid Hypermelanosis

As the name suggests, this presents as linear or whorled streaks of pigmentation following the Blaschko lines, usually involving the trunk and extremities **(Figs. 10.54A and B)**. The pigmentation is seen quite early in life. Unlike hypomelanosis of Ito, systemic associations are rare.

Melanocytic Naevi

These are localised proliferation of naevus cells, and are seen to develop in early childhood as small dark brown lesions. Histopathologically, these are classified according to anatomic location of the naevus cells. Early lesions tend to be flat (junctional naevi) with naevus cells lying

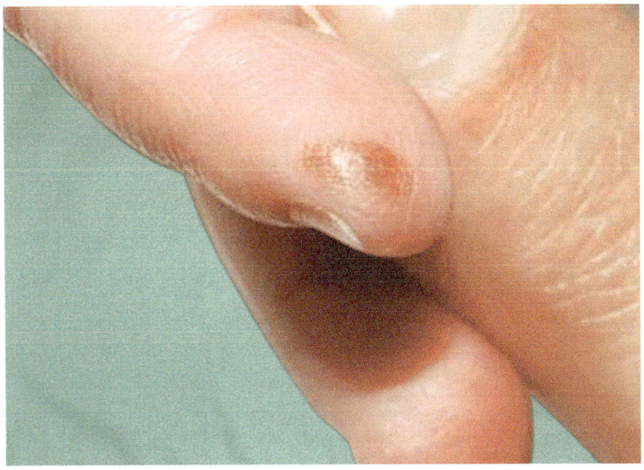

Figure 10.55 Small congenital melanocytic naevus.
(*Courtesy*: C. Jury, R. Gulati.)

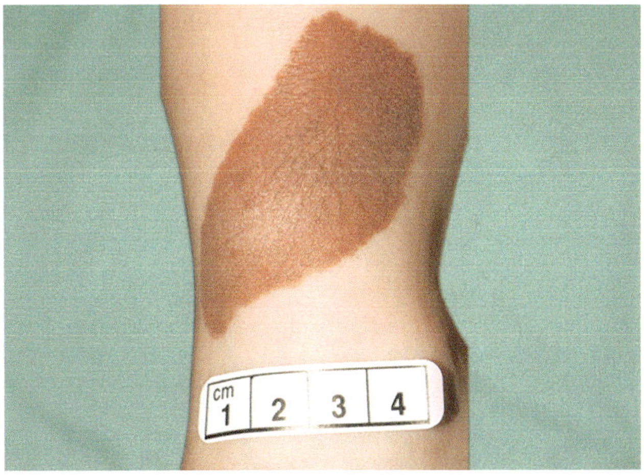

Figure 10.56 Intermediate congenital melanocytic naevus.
(*Courtesy*: M. Mealyea.)

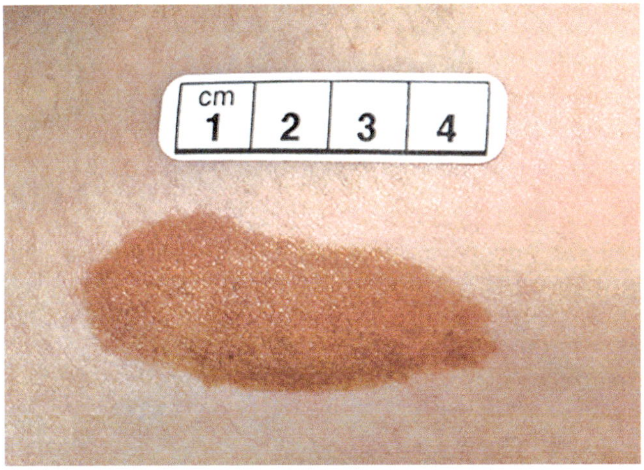

Figure 10.57 Intermediate congenital melanocytic naevus.
(*Courtesy*: M. Mealyea.)

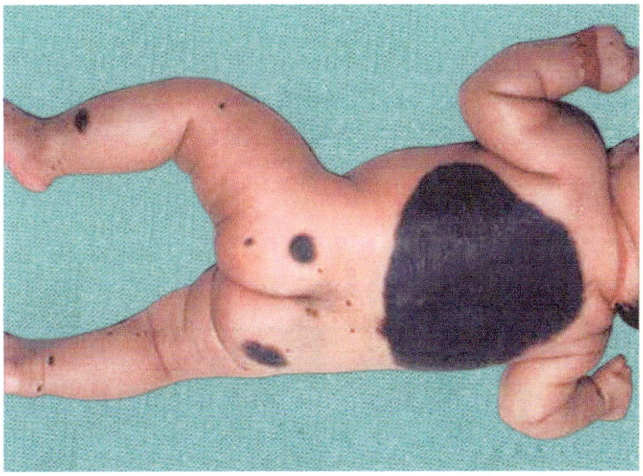

Figure 10.58 Congenital bathing trunk naevus with satellite lesions.
(*Courtesy*: R. Gulati.)

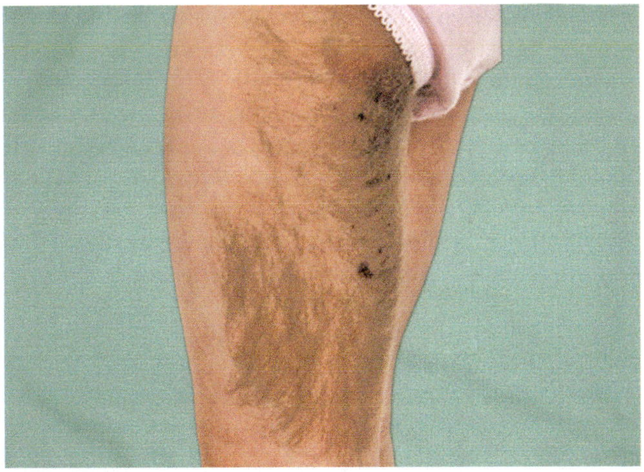

Figure 10.59 Large congenital hairy pigmented naevus.
(*Courtesy*: M. Mealyea.)

at the dermoepidermal junction. As naevi mature, they become elevated (compound naevi) and the cells occupy deeper positions. Naevi may also be classified as congenital and acquired.

Congenital melanocytic naevi (CMNs) present at birth or within the first few months of life **(Figs. 10.55 to 10.57)**. They are usually classified by their size into small (1–1.5 cm), intermediate (1.5–20 cm) and large (>20 cm). Giant naevi can affect large surface areas, and a variant affecting the trunk is called a bathing trunk naevus **(Fig. 10.58)**. Larger naevi are usually associated with smaller satellite naevi. Congenital naevi tend to grow in proportion to child's growth and can become hairy **(Fig. 10.59)**. Often, naevi lighten in colour in the first few years. Large CMNs have up to 10% lifetime risk of developing malignant melanoma, whereas small and intermediate naevi only have a smaller risk. The highest risk of

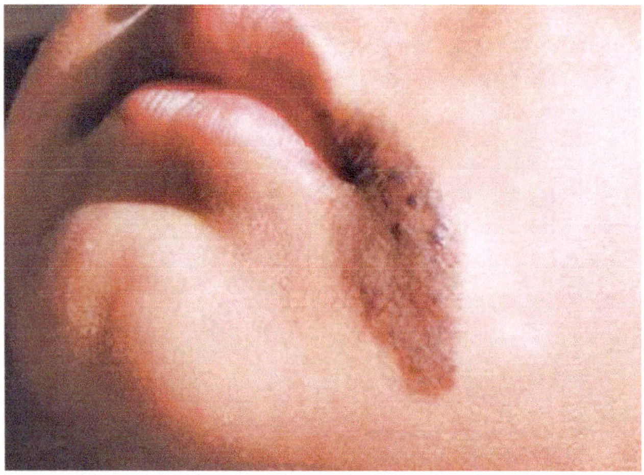

Figure 10.60 Naevus spilus (speckled lentiginous naevus)—sprinkling of small darker lesions on a homogeneous lighter background lesion.
(*Courtesy*: R. Gulati.)

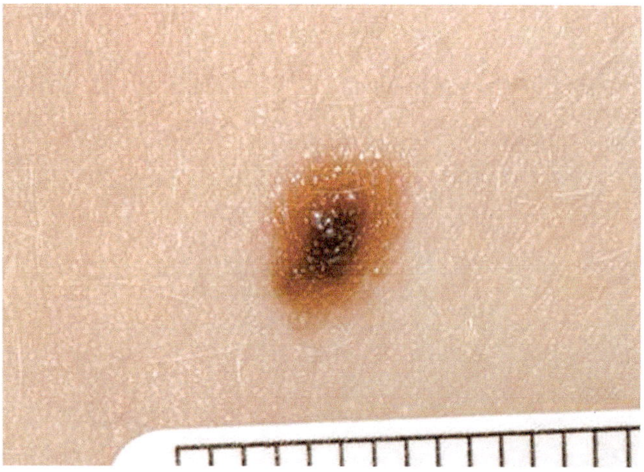

Figure 10.61 Naevus en cocarde.
(*Courtesy*: C. Jury, R. Gulati.)

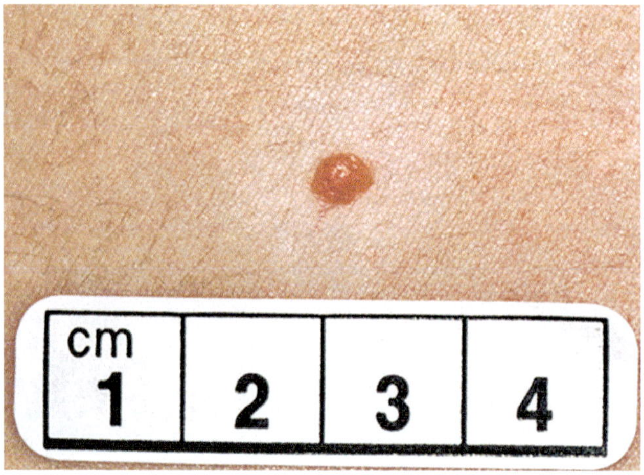

Figure 10.62 Halo naevus.
(*Courtesy*: M. Mealyea.)

melanoma is seen in CMN greater than 60 cm and those with multiple satellite naevi.

Acquired naevi are generally small, brown, evenly pigmented lesions with a regular shape and border. They are mostly less than 5 mm in size. Atypical naevi have irregular border and are usually larger. Malignant melanoma is rare in childhood, but presents with similar features as in adults. Naevi should be monitored using the mnemonic ABCDE (changes in Appearance, Border, Colour, Diameter and Elevation), and any change should be carefully assessed. Children with a family history of malignant melanoma or inherited conditions such as FAMMM (familial atypical mole malignant melanoma syndrome) are at higher risk.

Naevus spilus or speckled lentiginous naevus occurs as a light tan patch, which gradually develops small dark spots within it (**Fig. 10.60**), and usually follows a benign course. Children can have naevi with darker centre and a lighter periphery called naevi en cocarde (**Fig. 10.61**). These lesions can have further outer darker rings of pigmentation. These are more common on scalp and are benign.

Occasionally, naevi can develop a white depigmented halo around them (**Fig. 10.62**). This is considered to be an autoimmune reaction against the naevus cells. The process can lead to disappearance of the naevus, replaced by a patch of vitiligo, which overtime may repigment. This reaction is mostly seen in children and is benign. The development of halo naevus can sometimes herald development of vitiligo.

Pityriasis Versicolor

This is a fungal infection caused by yeast *Malassezia furfur*, which is a common skin coloniser. Pityriasis versicolor is more commonly seen in warm and moist climates. It may present as hypopigmented or hyperpigmented lesions, usually localised on the trunk and proximal upper extremities, although, in children, face can be involved as well (**Fig. 10.63**). The lesions are small and scaly and are usually asymptomatic, although mild itching may be present. Microscopy of scales shows pseudohyphae and spores, an appearance termed as 'spaghetti and meatballs.' Topical antifungal treatment usually suffices, although some recalcitrant cases may need oral treatment usually fluconazole or itraconazole.

Epidermal Naevi

Epidermal Naevus (Keratinocytic Naevus)

Epidermal naevi are developmental lesions typified by proliferation of keratinocytic cells. These naevi usually present at birth or shortly afterward. They are initially light brown in colour and may be slightly raised or

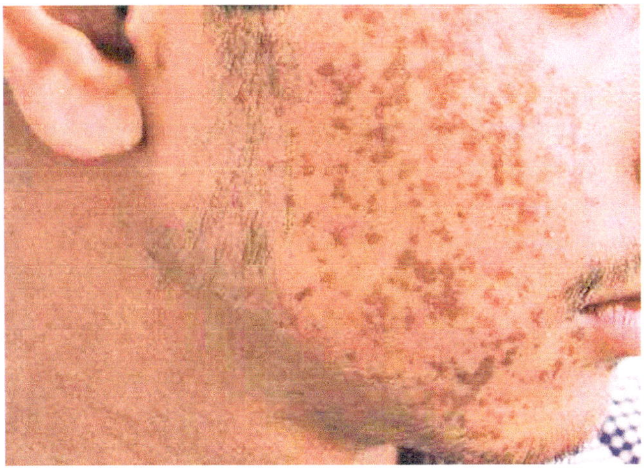

Figure 10.63 Pityriasis versicolor—brown scaly lesions affecting the cheek.

(*Courtesy*: R. Gulati.)

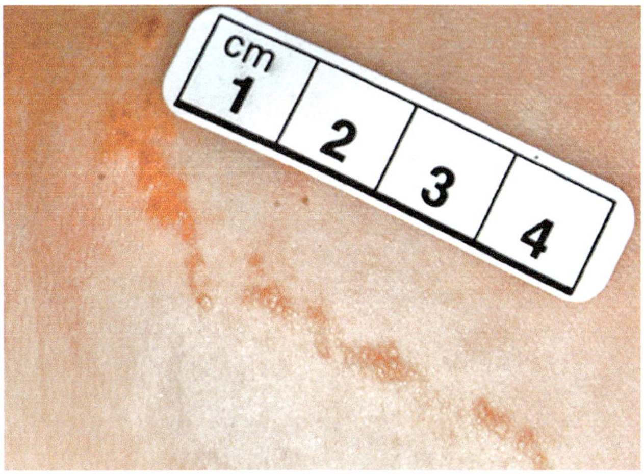

Figure 10.64 Linear epidermal naevus—following the lines of Blaschko.

(*Courtesy*: M. Mealyea.)

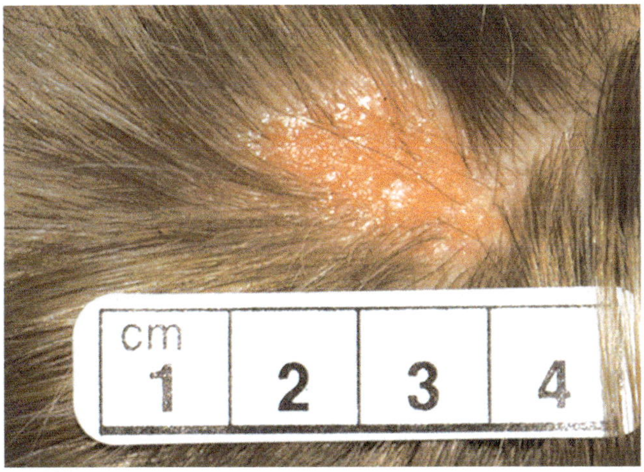

Figure 10.65 Sebaceous naevus on the scalp.

(*Courtesy*: M. Mealyea.)

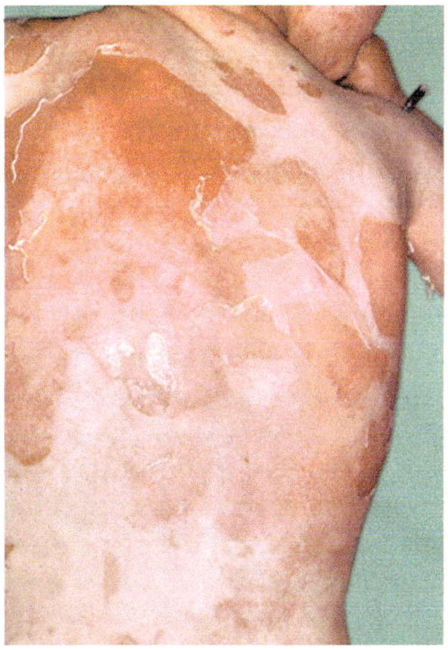

Figure 10.66 Staphylococcal scalded skin syndrome. *Note* the extensive superficial peeling.

(*Courtesy*: M. Mealyea.)

papillomatous. Later, they often become darker and warty and may need differentiating from viral warts. They are mostly linear involving lines of Blaschko **(Fig. 10.64)**. Extensive lesions can be associated with involvement of other ectodermally derived structures, when it is referred to as epidermal naevus syndrome. Surgery or carbon dioxide laser ablation may help some patients but scarring and recurrence are often a problem.

Sebaceous Naevus

Sebaceous naevi are derived from sebaceous glands. They are typically found on the scalp but may also be found on the face or neck **(Fig. 10.65)**. The most common presentation is a yellow orange patch of alopecia on scalp. The patch tends to become raised and papillomatous at puberty as sebaceous glands are activated under hormonal influence. This can make monitoring of lesion challenging, and many parents and children may demand excision. Up to 10% of lesions may show growths, most of which are benign, e.g. trichoblastoma or syringocystadenoma papilliferum. In approximately 1%, basal cell carcinoma can develop. It is uncommon to see growths before puberty.

BLISTERING DISORDERS

Staphylococcal Scalded Skin Syndrome

This is a toxin-mediated condition caused by *Staphylococcus aureus*, resulting in superficial blistering and skin peeling **(Figs. 10.66 and 10.67)**. Young children are mostly affected as their kidneys are unable to clear the bacterial toxin effectively. The affected children look

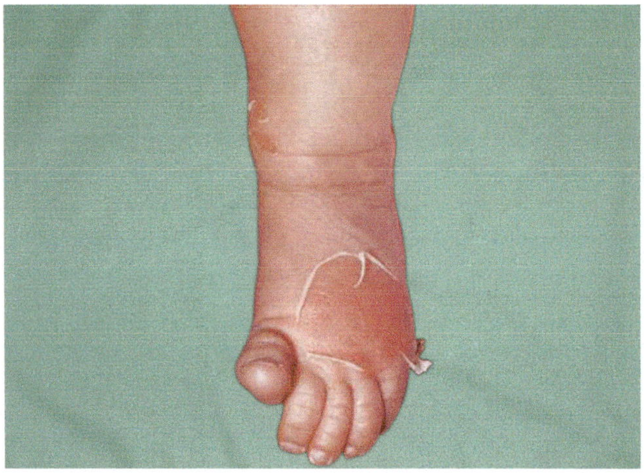

Figure 10.67 Staphylococcal scalded skin syndrome—peeling affecting the extremities.

(*Courtesy*: K. Goel.)

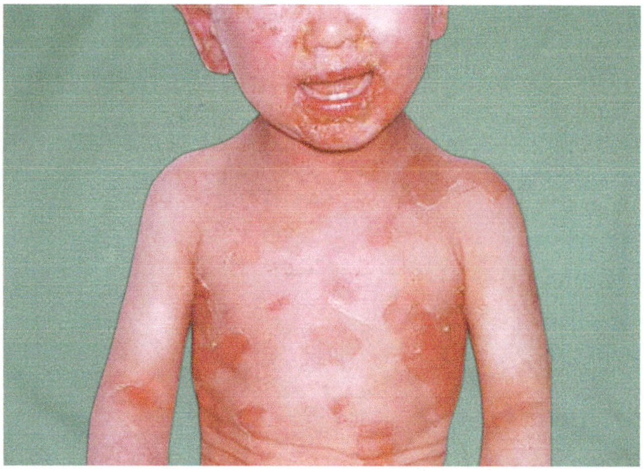

Figure 10.68 Staphylococcal scalded skin syndrome—peeling affecting the trunk and perioral area. *Note* the distress on child's face.

(*Courtesy*: K. Goel.)

toxic with fever, irritability and tender erythema of the skin, often worse in the flexural and periorificial areas **(Fig. 10.68)**. This is followed quickly by the development of large flaccid bullae, which are fragile with a thin roof comprised only of the stratum corneum. These quickly burst, leaving large moist, glistening denuded areas, which are extremely painful. The skin lesions are usually sterile with the source of toxin being remote such as nasopharynx, bone or umbilicus in a neonate. The mucous membranes are not generally involved. The diagnosis is usually made based on the typical clinical picture, but, if there is any doubt, biopsy will confirm the split in the skin to be in the upper epidermis. This differentiates it from toxic epidermal necrolysis (TEN), where the split is basal. TEN is an uncommon condition, usually precipitated by a drug, and tends to affect mucosae as well.

Staphylococcal scalded skin syndrome is potentially life-threatening and prompts immediate treatment with appropriate intravenous antibiotics. Flucloxacillin is most commonly used, although macrolides can be used in penicillin-allergic children. Semi-occlusive non-adherent dressings and analgesics may be required to ease pain. Recovery is usually rapid and healing occurs without scarring.

Chronic Bullous Disease of Childhood (Linear IgA Disease of Childhood)

This is an immunobullous condition affecting children usually between 3 and 10 years of age. It presents with tense bullae usually affecting the genital area, face and extremities **(Fig. 10.21)**. New lesions tend to develop around the previous healed lesions, giving the characteristic 'cluster of jewels' appearance. Direct immunofluorescence shows linear deposition of IgA along the basement membrane. Dapsone is considered the drug of choice, although erythromycin and sulphapyridine have been successfully used as well. The condition tends to resolve in 3–5 years.

Bullous Pemphigoid

Bullous pemphigoid (BP) is an immunobullous disorder that arises due to production of antibodies, most commonly IgG, against target antigens within the basement membrane. Although common amongst the elderly, BP can rarely present in childhood. Clinically, patients develop tense blisters arising on normal or inflamed skin **(Figs. 10.69A and B)**. Urticarial plaques may also be a feature. In young children, activity on acral surfaces and across the oral mucosa may be severe. Diagnosis is made by skin biopsy; microscopic examination shows a sub-epidermal blister with an eosinophil-rich infiltrate. Direct immunofluorescence shows a linear band of IgG and C3 (occasionally IgM or IgA) along the basement membrane. Traditional treatment is usually with systemic steroids (1–2 mg/kg/day); however, steroid-free alternatives such as dapsone, sulphapyridine and erythromycin may also be helpful. Limited disease may be successfully controlled with potent topical steroids. Prognosis is good, with the disease usually resolving in 12–18 months.

INFECTIONS

Bacterial Infections

Impetigo

Impetigo is a superficial skin infection mostly caused by *S. aureus* but occasionally by *Streptococcus pyogenes*. It usually develops secondarily over a primary skin disease such as atopic eczema or an area of skin that has been traumatised by an insect bite, laceration, burn or other

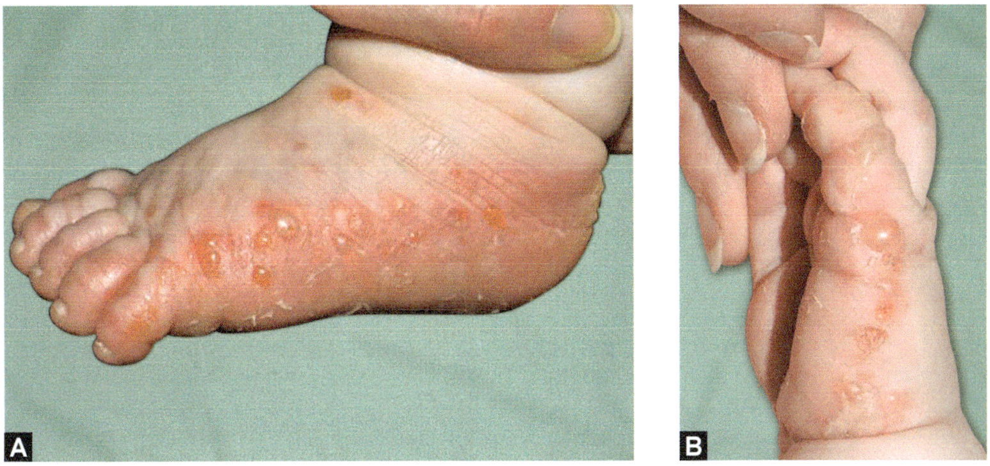

Figures 10.69A and B Bullous pemphigoid. *Note:* (A) Tense bullae.

(*Courtesy*: C. Jury.)

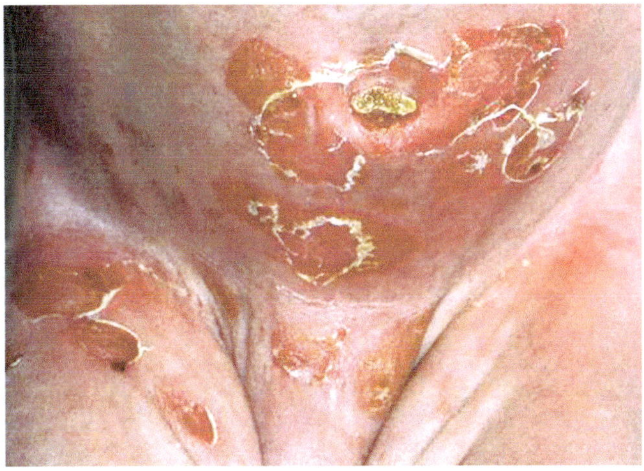

Figure 10.70 Bullous impetigo—the bullae have burst, leaving superficial erosions. *Note* characteristic honey-coloured crusting.

(*Courtesy*: K. Goel.)

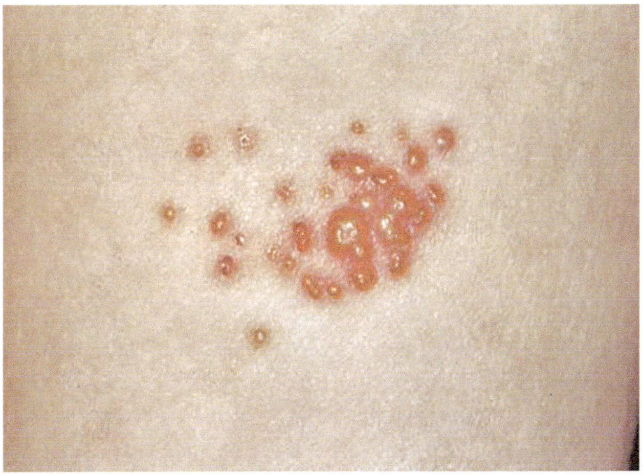

Figure 10.71 Grouped vesicles characteristic of herpes simplex. *Note* umbilication of few lesions.

(*Courtesy*: K. Goel.)

condition resulting in a break in the normal skin barrier. It tends to occur more frequently in hot humid climates.

Impetigo is generally recognised by its honey colour crusts **(Fig. 10.70)**. It can be localised to a small area of skin or become more generalised especially when it is secondarily infecting previously diseased skin. Most children with impetigo remain well. In children with eczema, the infection may be quite subtle and appear only as a flare of the eczema with some yellow crusting. A variant called bullous impetigo presents with flaccid bullae and erosions **(Fig. 10.70)**.

If only a small area is affected, a topical antibiotic such as fusidic acid or mupirocin may be sufficient. Generalised or multiple sites of infection warrant oral antibiotics. Flucloxacillin is usually the antibiotic of choice. Swabs should be taken as some varieties of streptococci may not be sensitive to the above. Good hygiene measures within the family are recommended as impetigo is highly contagious.

Viral Infections

Herpes Simplex

Herpes simplex labialis affecting the oral and perioral areas is the most common presentation. The infection is usually caused by herpes simplex virus type 1. The lesions characteristically present as cluster of vesicles, with few lesions showing umbilication **(Fig. 10.71)**. Primary herpes gingivostomatitis can be quite distressing, presenting with fever, constitutional symptoms and small eroded painful vesicles on the lips and oral mucosa **(Fig. 10.72)**. Recurrent episodes are usually milder and tend to settle within 7–10 days. The lesions can become secondarily infected **(Fig. 10.73)**. Herpetic infections of the hands, including

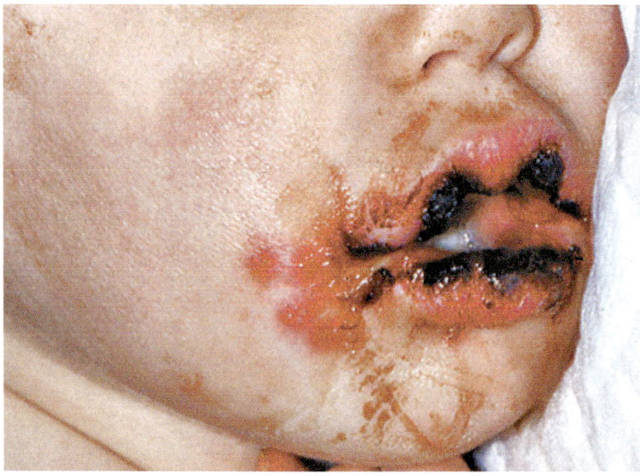

Figure 10.72 Herpes simplex infection—primary gingivostomatitis. *Note* clustered vesicles on the right angle of mouth.

(*Courtesy*: M. Mealyea.)

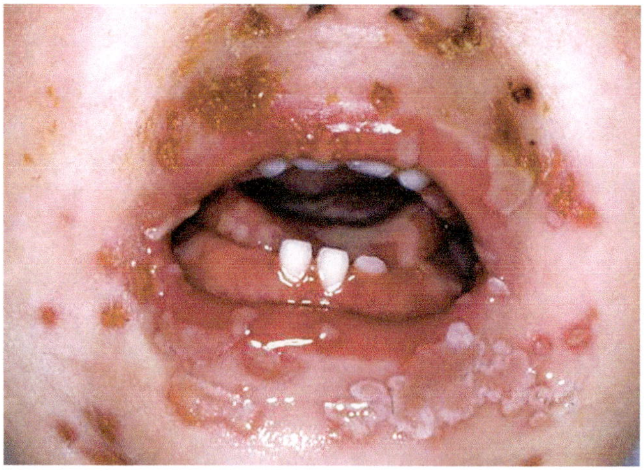

Figure 10.73 Herpes simplex—discrete vesicles with erosions. Lesions below nose show honey coloured crusts typical of secondary impetigo.

(*Courtesy*: K. Goel.)

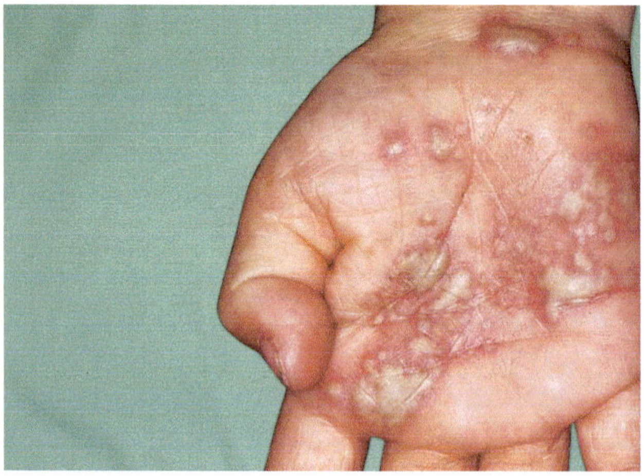

Figure 10.74 Herpes simplex affecting the palm. Thicker roof causes coalescing of vesicles, as they do not rupture readily.

(*Courtesy*: K. Goel.)

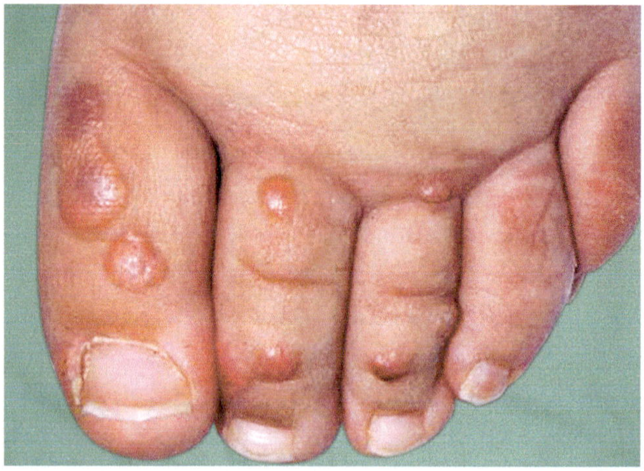

Figure 10.75 Warts affecting dorsa of toes.

(*Courtesy*: K. Goel.)

fingers and thumb, may occur secondary to autoinoculation and are referred to as herpetic whitlow **(Fig. 10.74)**. Herpetic genital infections are much less common in children, and sexual abuse should be considered a possibility. Aciclovir is the drug of choice, and topical, oral and parenteral preparations are available. Recurrent episodes may need regular prophylactic treatment.

Herpes simplex infection in neonatal period can be life-threatening and should be managed aggressively.

Viral Warts

Warts are epidermal growths caused by human papilloma virus. They are quite common in children. They most commonly affect hands and feet, although other areas including face can be involved as well. They initially appear as smooth skin-coloured papules but slowly enlarge and develop an irregular hyperkeratotic surface **(Fig. 10.75)**. They may appear as a slender stalk, in which case they are called filiform warts, which are more common on the face, especially around the nostrils and the lips. Viral warts usually spontaneously resolve once the immune system recognises and overcomes the virus but it may take many months to more than a year.

Treatment consists of physical destruction of the affected keratinocytes. This can be achieved by topical wart paints, which usually have keratolytics such as salicylic acid or lactic acid. These need to be applied daily for a few months, filing the wart once a week to remove the top weakened layer of keratinocytes. Cryotherapy with liquid nitrogen is also usually effective and can be done over a few sittings 4 weeks apart. Other agents such as cantharidin can be used if the above fail.

Genital warts are less common, and should raise suspicion of sexual abuse. However, they can be caused by autoinoculation from warts elsewhere on the child's body or, in case of younger babies and children, from a carer who has hand warts. In infants, they may be caused by vertical spread from the mother *in utero* or during delivery. The virus may lie dormant and not manifest itself for some months or sometimes even years. Warts tend to resolve spontaneously. Topical podophyllotoxin can be used for quicker resolution.

Molluscum Contagiosum

This is a pox viral infection commonly affecting children. It can spread through fomites such as shared baths, towels or swimming pools. It produces crops of pearly dome-shaped papules with an umbilicated centre **(Fig. 10.76)**. The condition is asymptomatic and self-limiting and clears once the individual's immune response kicks in, which can take several months. The lesions tend to become itchy and red when this happens, and scratching can break the skin barrier, making them susceptible to secondary bacterial infection. Topical application of antiseptics can be helpful in preventing this.

Scratching, or any other form of trauma, can lead to further spread of lesions, termed as Koebner or isomorphic phenomenon. This phenomenon can be seen in other conditions such as psoriasis and warts.

Being self-limiting, treatment of molluscum lesions is usually not necessary. Treatment involves physical destruction of lesions and hence is painful and distressing as the lesions are usually multiple. Fewer lesions can be treated with cryotherapy or by piercing the lesions with an orange stick to induce inflammation.

Fungal Infections

Dermatophytes are the commonest group affecting skin. These are keratinophilic fungi and affect stratum corneum. They do not cause systemic infection. As they tend to produce annular lesions on the body, they are also referred to as the ringworm (tinea). Three genera affecting humans are *Microsporum*, *Trichophyton* and *Epidermophyton*. Infection can be acquired from humans, but some are picked up from animals or soil.

Tinea capitis is dermatophyte infection of the scalp. It can have varied presentation, most common being a scaly patch or patches of alopecia, caused most commonly in the western world by *Trichophyton tonsurans*, although *Microsporum canis* and sometimes *Trichophyton violaceum* are found **(Fig. 10.77)**. Dermatophytes from animals can induce marked inflammation, sometimes causing a boggy swelling to develop, which may have pustules. Such swelling is called a kerion. It may mimic a bacterial abscess but a prior history of a scaly patch and concomitant alopecia should point towards the diagnosis. A variant called black dot tinea is more commonly seen in the Asian countries. As the fungal spores largely involve the interior of the hair shaft making it weaker, the hair tend to break near the scalp, producing the characteristic clinical picture **(Fig. 10.78)**. The treatment consists of oral antifungals (griseofulvin or terbinafine). Topical treatments will not clear tinea capitis.

Tinea corporis (fungal infection of the body) appears as annular expanding lesion with scaly edge and central clearing **(Fig. 10.79)**. The appearance may change with use of topical steroids when it is referred to as tinea incognito **(Figs. 10.80A and B)**. The condition needs to be differentiated from other discoid or annular lesions such as eczema and psoriasis. Treatment consists of topical antifungals such as imidazoles for 4 weeks or terbinafine for 2 weeks.

Tinea pedis (fungal infection of the foot) is more common in adults but can be seen in children as well. It usually presents as unilateral scaly lesion involving either the plantar aspect or the interdigital spaces **(Fig. 10.81)**. Topical antifungals are helpful.

Tinea unguium (fungal nail infection) presents as thickened, yellowish and crumbly nails **(Fig. 10.82)**. Systemic

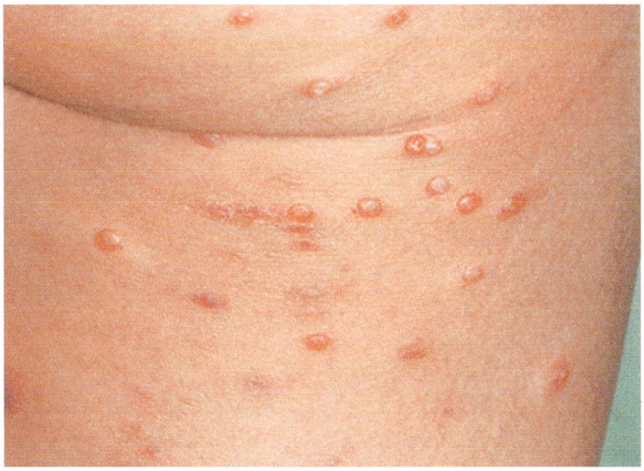

Figure 10.76 Molluscum contagiosum—umbilicated papules.
(*Courtesy*: M. Mealyea.)

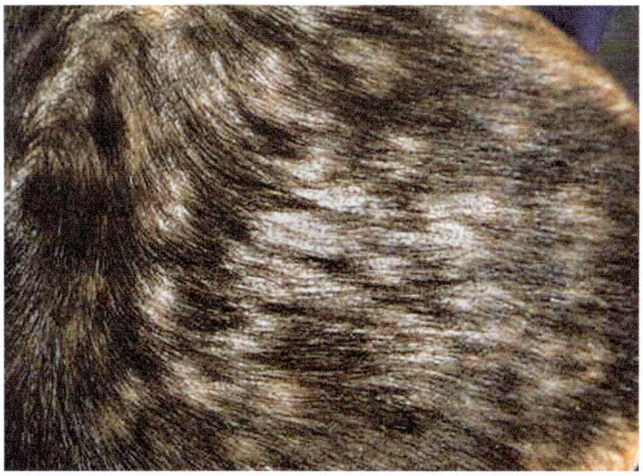

Figure 10.77 Tinea capitis. *Note* scaly areas of alopecia.
(*Courtesy*: R. Gulati.)

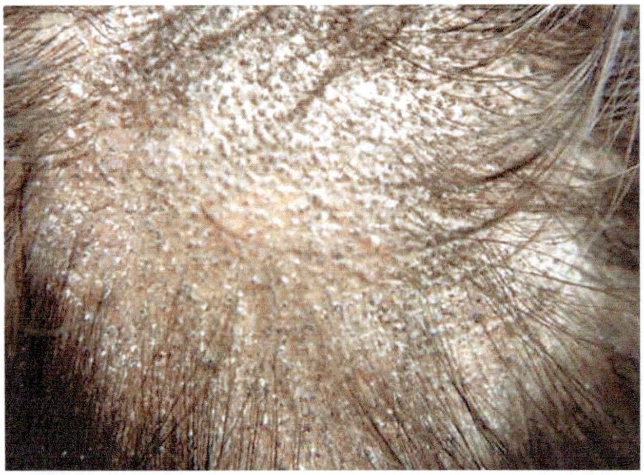

Figure 10.78 Black dot tinea.

(*Courtesy*: R. Gulati.)

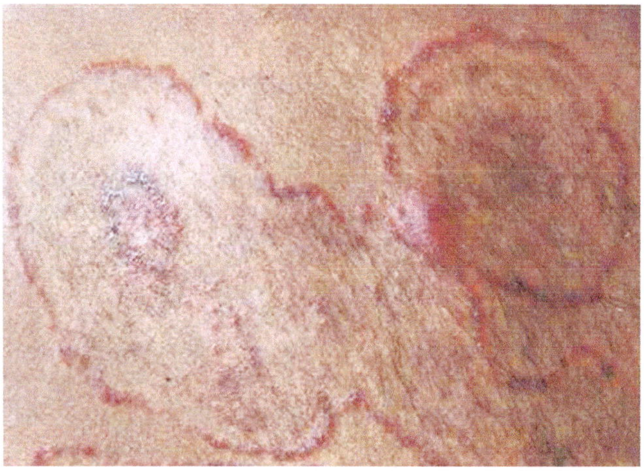

Figure 10.79 Tinea corporis.

(*Courtesy*: R. Gulati.)

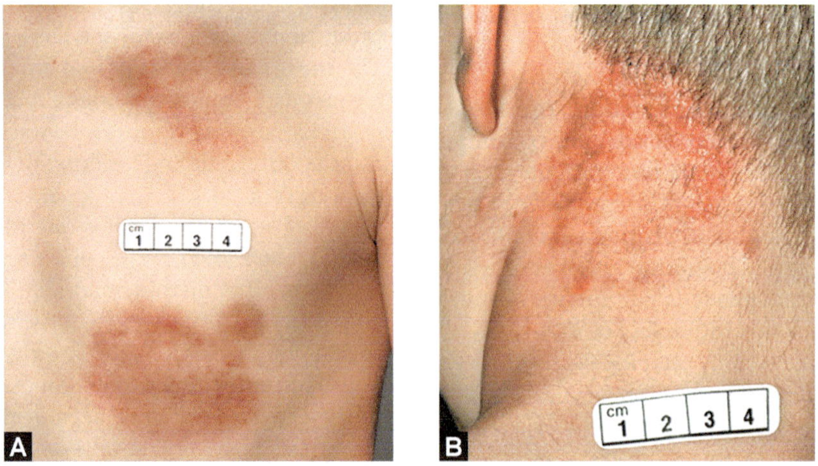

Figures 10.80A and B Tinea corporis incognito. *Note* post-inflammatory hyperpigmentation in Figure A.

(*Courtesy*: M. Mealyea.)

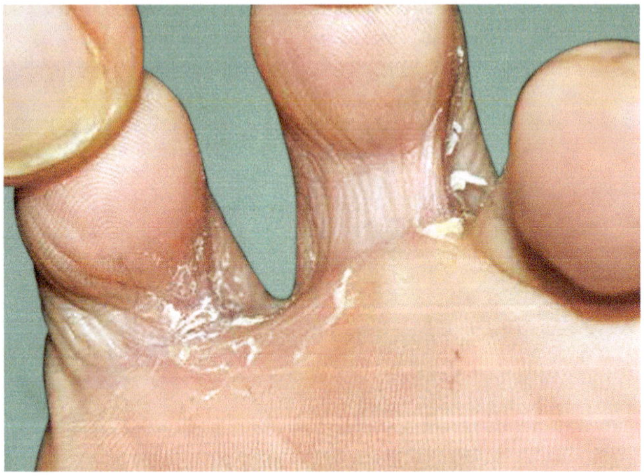

Figure 10.81 Tinea pedis involving the lateral two interdigital spaces.

(*Courtesy*: C. Jury, R. Gulati.)

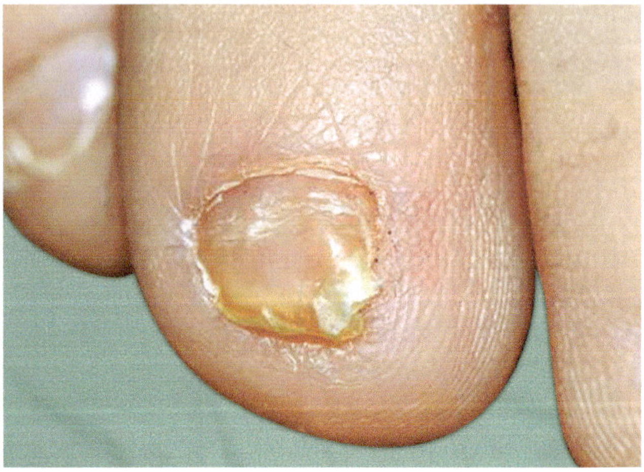

Figure 10.82 Tinea unguium—distal nail shows thickening and yellow discolouration. *Note* associated scaling visible in the interdigital space consistent with interdigital tinea.

(*Courtesy*: C. Jury, R. Gulati.)

treatment with oral griseofulvin for 6–12 months or oral terbinafine for 6–12 weeks is the treatment of choice in older children. Younger children can be tried on topical amorolfine as their nail plates are thinner.

Diagnosis of fungal infection is made by plucking hair samples, taking skin scrapings or nail clippings for microscopic examination and culture, as this may help in identifying the source of the infection. It is important to treat the other sibling(s) or family pet(s) if indicated.

Mycobacterial Infections

Cutaneous Tuberculosis

This is primarily caused by *Mycobacterium tuberculosis,* and other mycobacteria are rarely implicated **(Figs. 10.83 to 10.86)**. Determined by prior sensitisation and immunity of the host, three major clinical presentations are described, namely lupus vulgaris, tuberculosis verrucosa cutis and scrofuloderma. These are summarised in **Table 10.2**.

Diagnosis rests on clinical suspicion, followed by histopathology and mycobacterial culture. Treatment involves 2 months of four drugs, usually rifampicin, isoniazid, ethambutol and pyrazinamide, followed by 4 months of further continuation of rifampicin and isoniazid.

Leprosy (Hansen Disease)

This is a chronic granulomatous disease caused by *Mycobacterium leprae* primarily affecting the skin and peripheral nerves. It can involve other organs such as eyes and respiratory mucosa as well. Clinical presentation is determined by the ability of the host to mount an

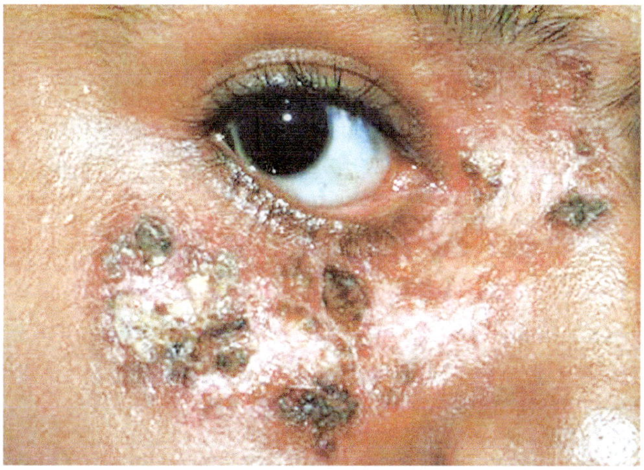

Figure 10.83 Lupus vulgaris—crusted plaque showing some atrophy.
(*Courtesy*: R. Gulati.)

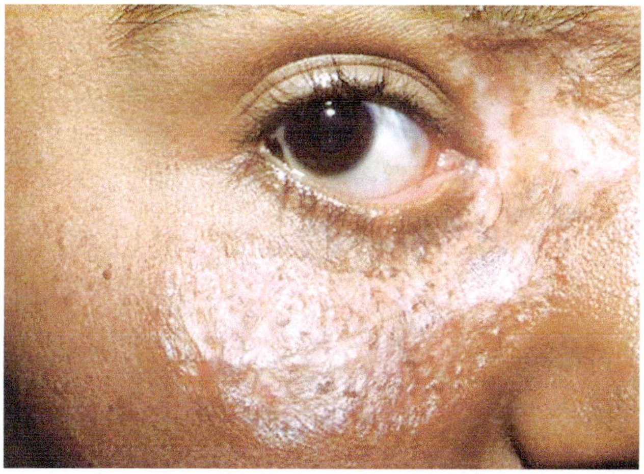

Figure 10.84 Lupus vulgaris (same patient as Figure 10.83)—residual atrophy following 6 months of treatment.
(*Courtesy*: R. Gulati.)

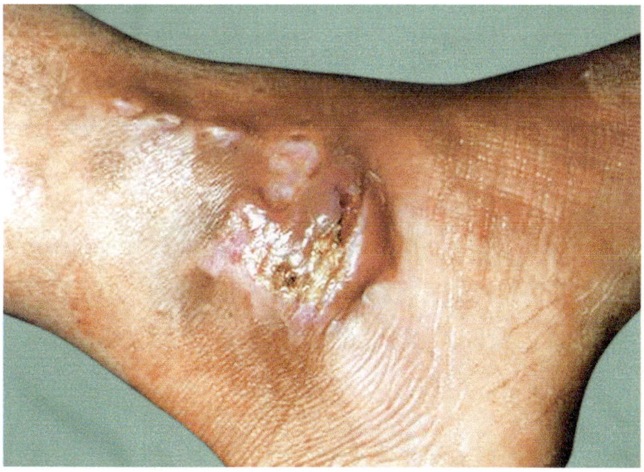

Figure 10.85 Scrofuloderma—ulcer with discharging sinuses and surrounding keloidal reaction. Culture of discharge grew *Mycobacterium tuberculosis*.
(*Courtesy*: R. Gulati.)

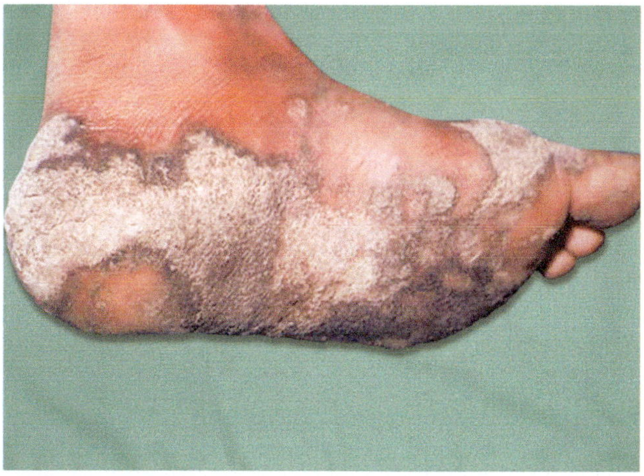

Figure 10.86 Tuberculosis verrucosa cutis (adult patient)—warty plaque covering the plantar and part of dorsal foot.
(*Courtesy*: R. Gulati.)

TABLE 10.2 Clinical presentations of cutaneous tuberculosis.

	Lupus vulgaris	*Tuberculosis verrucosa cutis*	*Scrofuloderma*
Main body site involved	Head and neck	Trunk and limbs	Over lymph nodes or bones (neck, axilla, ankle)
Clinical presentation	Brownish red plaque	Hyperkeratotic warty plaque	Ulcer with draining sinuses
Immunity of host	High	High	Low
Mycobacteria in skin biopsy	Few	Few	Multiple
Pathology	Well-formed non-caseating epithelioid granulomas	Well-formed non-caseating epithelioid granulomas	Granulomas with caseous necrosis

TABLE 10.3 Clinical presentations of leprosy.

	Tuberculoid leprosy (Fig. 10.87)	*Borderline leprosy* (Fig. 10.88)*	*Lepromatous leprosy (Fig. 10.89)*
Immune response of host	Good	Moderate	Poor
Number of lesions	One or few	Few to multiple	Many
Nature of lesions	Well-defined	Well to ill-defined	Nodules, diffuse infiltration of skin
Colour of lesions	Hypopigmented	Hypopigmented to erythematous	Erythematous
Sensation over the lesions	Anaesthetic	Anaesthetic to normal sensation	Hypoesthetic to normal sensation
Number of bacilli in lesions	Few	Few to many	Many
Pathology	Well-defined epithelioid granulomas	Well-defined to loose granulomas	Loose granulomas

*Borderline leprosy is further subdivided into borderline tuberculoid, borderline borderline and borderline lepromatous.

immune response to the bacilli. The major clinical types as described by Ridley and Jopling are summarised in Table 10.3 (Figs. 10.87 to 10.89).

For treatment purpose, classifying leprosy as single-lesion paucibacillary, paucibacillary (two to five lesions) and multibacillary more than five lesions) (WHO classification) is more useful. Single-lesion paucibacillary leprosy is treated by a single dose of rifampicin, ofloxacin and minocycline, not indicated for children below 5 years. Paucibacillary cases are treated with rifampicin and dapsone for 6 months. Multibacillary patients are given rifampicin, dapsone and clofazimine for 12 months.

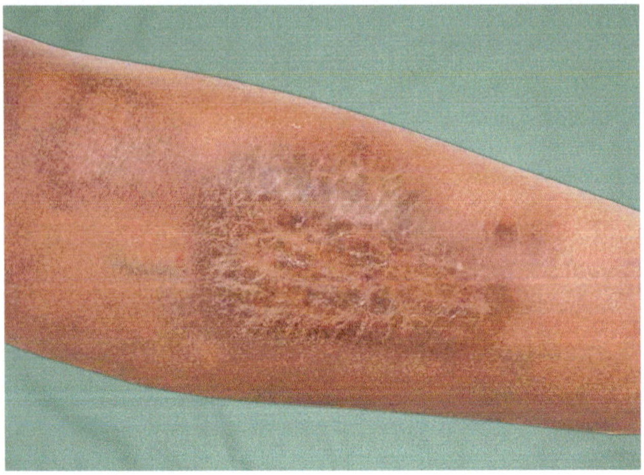

Figure 10.87 Tuberculoid leprosy—dry anaesthetic plaque with central hypopigmentation.

(*Courtesy*: R. Gulati.)

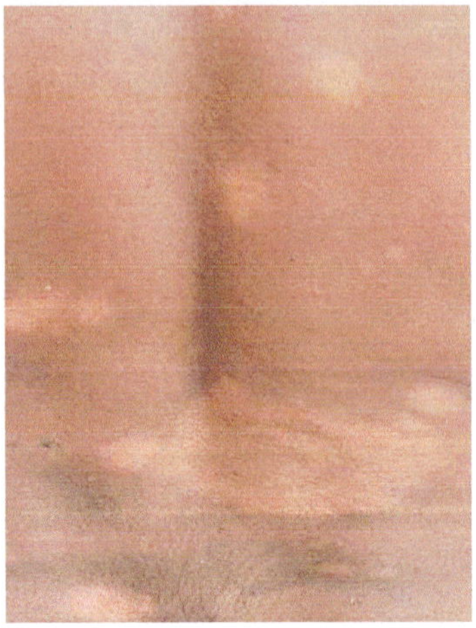

Figure 10.88 Leprosy—borderline leprosy: well-defined to ill-defined lesions.

(*Courtesy*: R. Gulati.)

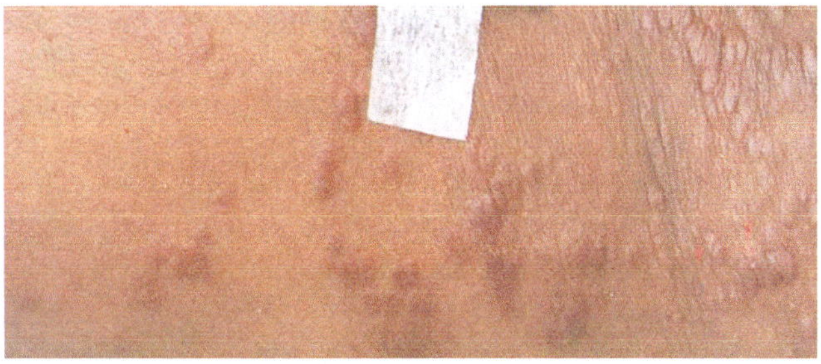

Figure 10.89 Lepromatous leprosy. *Note* papules and nodules.
(*Courtesy*: R. Gulati.)

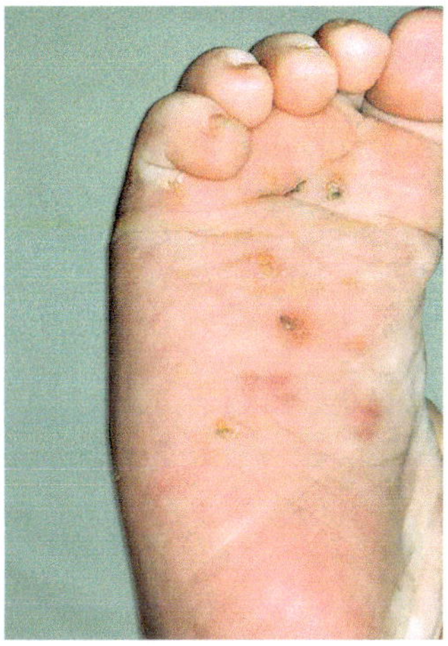

Figure 10.91 Scabies—plantar involvement in an infant.
(*Courtesy*: C. Jury, R. Gulati.)

Other Infections

Scabies

Human scabies is caused by an ectoparasite *Sarcoptes scabiei hominis*. It is a small eight-legged mite affecting all age ranges. Infants present with a generalised rash consisting variably of papules, pustules and excoriations **(Fig. 10.90)**. Burrows constitute typical lesions but are found only in a small number of children. These are linear palpable lesions mostly found on palms, soles, wrists and finger webs. Involvement of head and neck, palms and soles is commonly seen in infants, but is uncommon in adults **(Fig. 10.91)**. Babies are unable to scratch, so the symptoms are often irritability, poor feeding and disturbed sleep. In older children, itch is the predominant feature, especially at night. Scabies should be considered part of the differential diagnosis in any slightly atypical itchy rash especially if other family members are itchy. In children with eczema, it can be the cause of a sudden flare of their eczema. The diagnosis is clinical, although mite, eggs or its faecal matter can be visualised under a microscope if material can be gathered by scraping a burrow.

Treatment is usually with topical permethrin 5% cream, and all family members and regular contacts should be

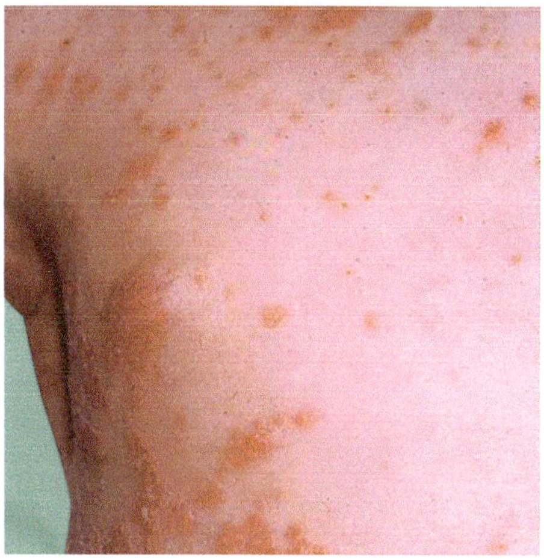

Figure 10.90 Scabies—non-specific rash in an infant. Thorough history and examination is important.
(*Courtesy*: M. Mealyea.)

treated at the same time. Although older children are treated below neck, infants should have the treatment put on the head and neck as well. Treatment involves overnight application, which should be repeated after 7 days.

Pediculosis capitis (Head Lice)

This is an ectoparasite infestation caused by head louse *Pediculus humanus capitis*. The lice are 1–2 mm long. They infest the scalp, laying eggs at the base of the hair, close to the scalp. Eggs hatch in a week, leaving the empty egg shells clinging to the hair shaft. The infestation is spread through close contact. Permethrin lotion applied overnight is safe to use in children. Nit combs help in removing the residual eggs and egg shells. All contacts should be assessed and treated simultaneously to avoid reinfestation.

Genodermatoses

Epidermolysis Bullosa

Epidermolysis bullosa (EB) is group of conditions characterised by skin fragility. Fragility develops secondary to absent or damaged structures within the skin required for its integrity. In the past, classification of these conditions was based on clinical presentation; however, better understanding of their molecular basis has led to refinement of classification, dividing EB into four main groups, namely EB simplex, junctional EB, dystrophic EB and Kindler syndrome (Report of the 3rd International Consensus meeting on diagnosis and classification of EB. J Am Acad Dermatol. 2008;58:931-50).

Epidermolysis bullosa simplex This is the commonest form of EB, usually inherited in an autosomal dominant pattern. It is caused by mutations in keratins 5 and 14, which are found in the epidermis. This gives rise to intraepidermal blisters, usually after mild trauma. Lesions heal without

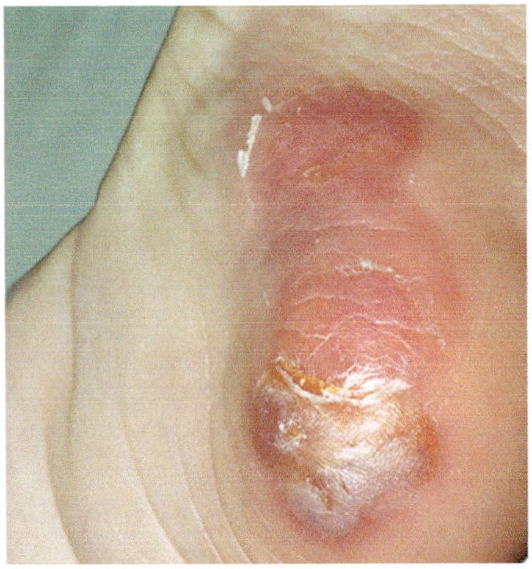

Figure 10.92 Epidermolysis bullosa simplex. *Note* healing blister on heel. (*Courtesy*: C. Jury, R. Gulati.)

scarring. Common sites affected are the hands and feet, although in infants nappy area is frequently involved as well **(Fig. 10.92)**.

Junctional epidermolysis bullosa This is the rarest form of EB and arises due to mutations within the basement membrane (the area that holds the epidermis and dermis together). In the most severe form (Herlitz variant), blistering is usually extensive and severe, often associated with large non-healing areas of over-granulation, involving mainly the perioral area. Involvement of the teeth, oral mucosa and larynx occurs. Nails are shed early. Prognosis is poor with death in early childhood often secondary to infection.

Other forms of junctional EB include non-Herlitz variant, which, although similar to Herlitz, is characterised by absence of granulation tissue formation and associated with a normal life span. Junctional EB with pyloric atresia is usually fatal in early life.

Dystrophic epidermolysis bullosa Dystrophic EB arises due to mutations in collagen VII, which is an important constituent of the anchoring fibrils that loop up from the dermis to connect with the basement membrane. This leads to a deeper plane of cleavage in the skin, thereby causing blisters to heal with scarring. Dystrophic EB can be inherited in an autosomal recessive or dominant fashion.

Recessive dystrophic EB arises due to absent or defective collagen VII and presents with severe skin fragility from birth. Erosions heal with scarring and milia formation. All mucosal surfaces are affected, leading to oral ulceration and microstomia, oesophageal erosions and strictures, pain on defaecation and constipation, ocular erosions and genitourinary scarring. Over time, digits on hands and feet become fused within areas of scarring, leading to "mitten deformity." Multifactorial anaemia develops over time, and growth and development are severely affected. Death usually ensues in the third or fourth decade, mostly from metastatic cutaneous squamous cell carcinoma.

Dominant dystrophic EB has a much less severe clinical presentation, with fragility and scarring limited to areas of friction such as elbows and knees. Nail dystrophy and loss is common, whereas lifespan is normal.

Kindler syndrome This rare genodermatosis is characterised by acral fragility, photosensitivity, poikiloderma and cutaneous atrophy. It is recessively inherited, arising due to mutation in *KIND1* gene, which plays an important role in basement membrane function. It has only recently been included under the EB umbrella.

There is no cure for EB group of conditions, and the child is subject to daily dressings and care of skin. Great care needs to be exercised when handling these babies and children to prevent further blistering. Nutrition may be severely affected. The teeth and eyes may need special care, and mobility is often a problem. The main job of the dermatologist is to make the diagnosis and then coordinate care for these children. They will need special nursing care and may need referral to numerous other specialities.

Ichthyosis

This is a group of inherited disorders where the process of keratinisation is abnormal, resulting in marked scaling and dryness of the skin, ranging from mild to severe and incapacitating.

The most common type is ichthyosis vulgaris, an autosomal dominant condition, which may appear no more than a very dry skin. It affects 1:250 children, and can accompany atopic eczema. It is caused by filaggrin gene mutation. It presents with light-coloured fine scales, usually affecting the limbs and sparing the flexures **(Figs. 10.93 and 10.94)**. Palms and soles show increased creases, termed hyperlinear palms and soles **(Figs. 10.95 and 10.96)**.

X-linked recessive ichthyosis generally affects boys and is much rarer than ichthyosis vulgaris, affecting 1:2,000. It is due to deficiency of the enzyme steroid sulphatase. Both the gene and the enzyme level can be assessed for confirmation of diagnosis. It is characterised by large brown scales, especially seen on the legs and trunk, and affects the flexures **(Fig. 10.97)**. The condition can be associated with cryptorchidism, and therefore, presence of testes in the scrotum should be confirmed on examination. History of difficult labour may be present.

Unlike the above-mentioned conditions, where excessive scale is present, in lamellar ichthyosis, retention of scales leads to dark scales affecting large areas **(Figs. 10.98A to D)**. These children are usually born with a shiny membrane covering the body, called collodion membrane, which clears in the first few weeks, leaving dry

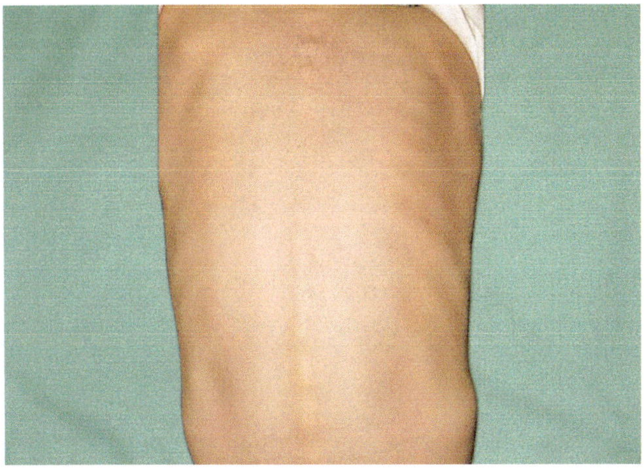

Figure 10.93 Ichthosis vulgaris—generalized fine scales.
(*Courtesy*: C. Jury, R. Gulati.)

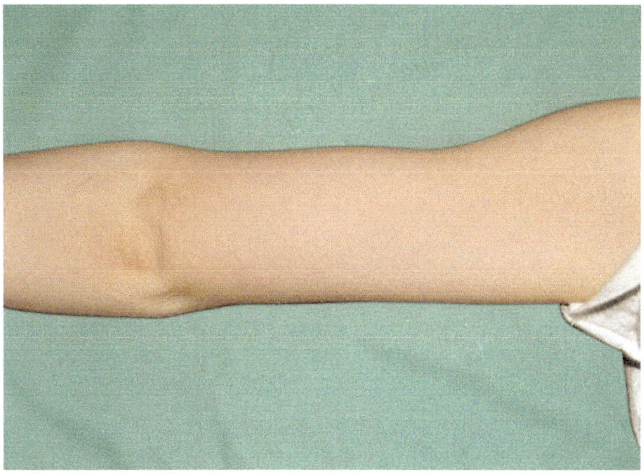

Figure 10.94 Ichthyosis vulgaris. *Note* fine dry scales on upper arm.
(*Courtesy*: C. Jury, R. Gulati.)

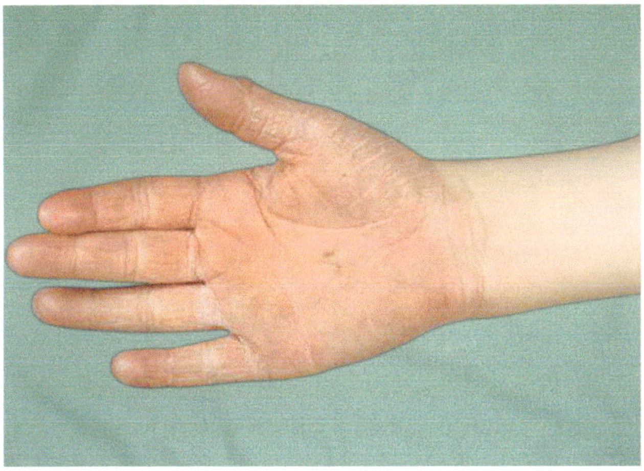

Figure 10.95 Ichthyosis vulgaris—hyperlinear palm.
(*Courtesy*: C. Jury, R. Gulati.)

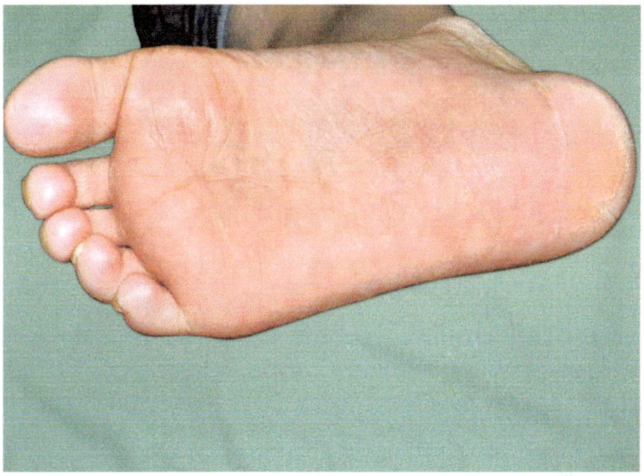

Figure 10.96 Ichthyosis vulgaris—hyperlinearity of sole.
(*Courtesy*: C. Jury, R. Gulati.)

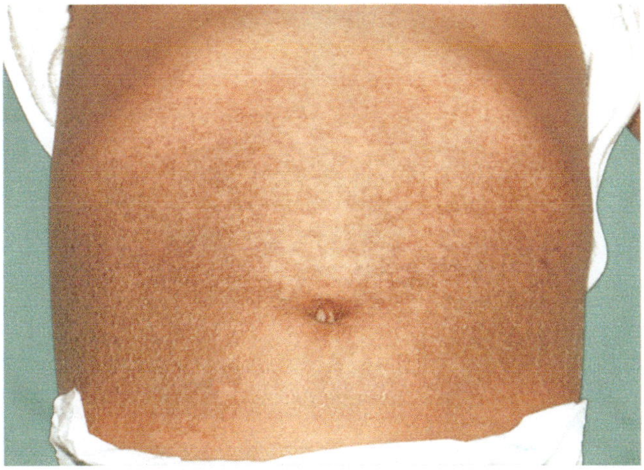

Figure 10.97 X-linked ichthyosis with large dark scales.
(*Courtesy*: M. Mealyea.)

scaly skin. Build-up of thick scales can lead to disfigurement of ears and ectropion. The difference in scale types can be better appreciated in **Figures 10.99A to C**.

Emollients form the mainstay of management, helping to soften the scales. Topical keratolytics and retinoids may help in reducing scales in localised areas but these should be avoided in the neonatal period because of problems with absorption. Severe ichthyosis may be helped by oral retinoids, which tend to improve the process of keratinisation. There is no definitive treatment.

Miscellaneous Conditions and Case Studies

Granuloma Annulare

This presents as an annular ring of firm papules usually on the acral areas such as back of hands or dorsa of

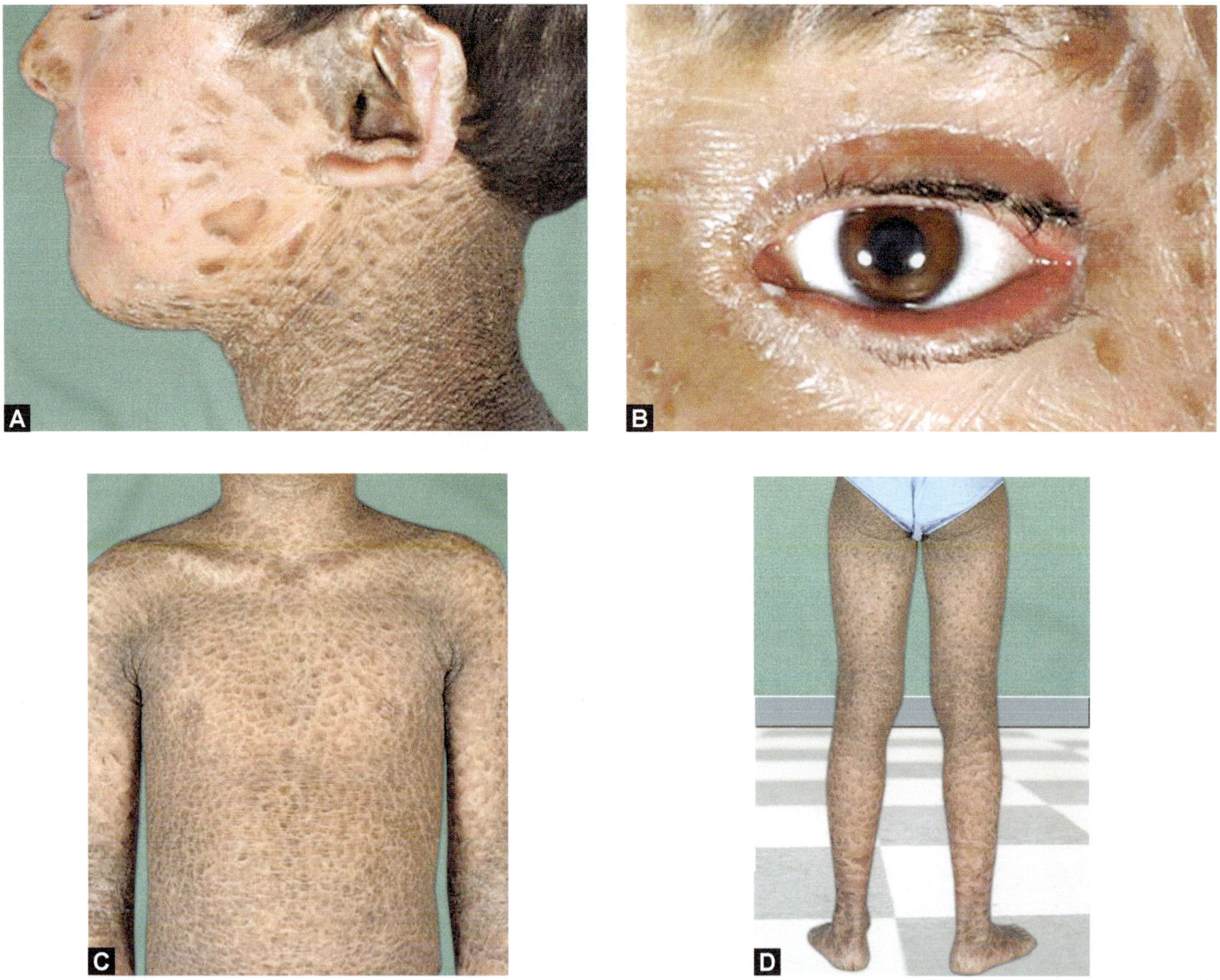

Figures 10.98A to D Lamellar ichthyosis. *Note:* (A) Thick scales disfiguring the ear; (B) Ectropion.
(*Courtesy*: C. Jury.)

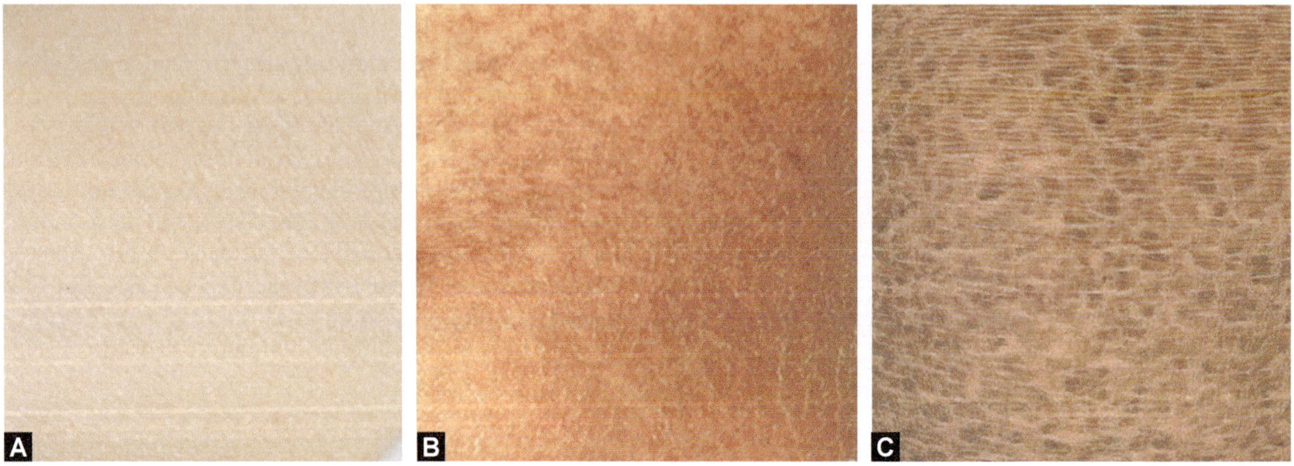

Figures 10.99A to C Scale types in ichthyoses. (A) Ichthyosis vulgaris (fine scales); (B) X-linked ichthyosis (thin dirty scales); (C) Lamellar ichthyosis (thick dirty scales).

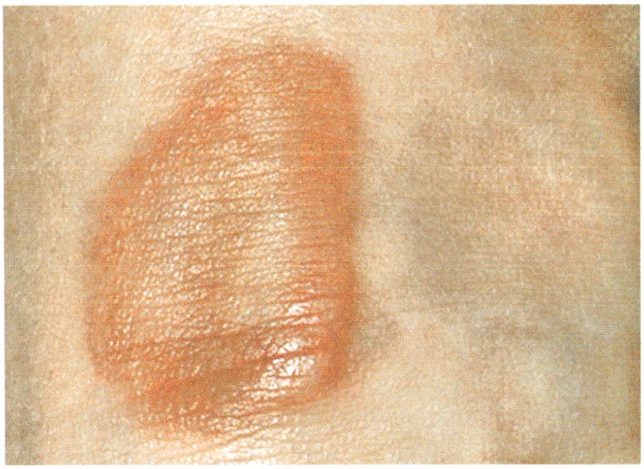

Figure 10.100 Granuloma annulare.
(*Courtesy*: M. Mealyea.)

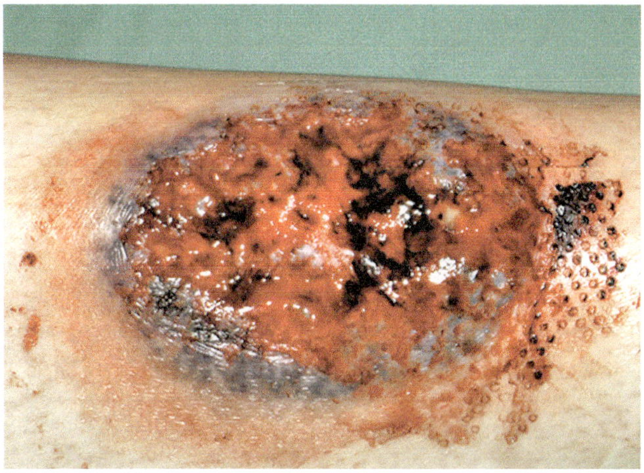

Figure 10.101 Pyoderma gangrenosum.
(*Courtesy*: M. Mealyea.)

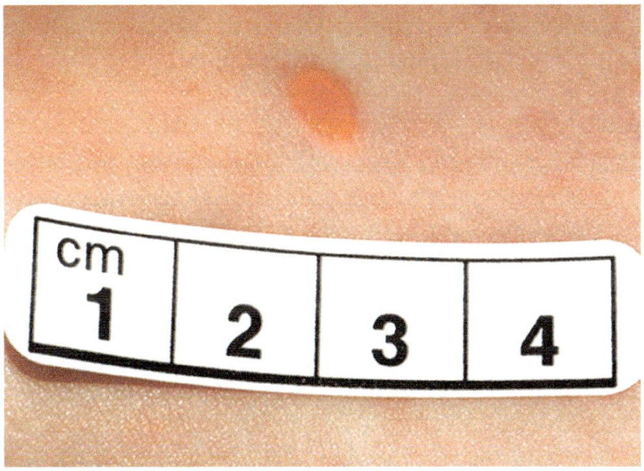

Figure 10.102 Juvenile xanthogranuloma.
(*Courtesy*: M. Mealyea.)

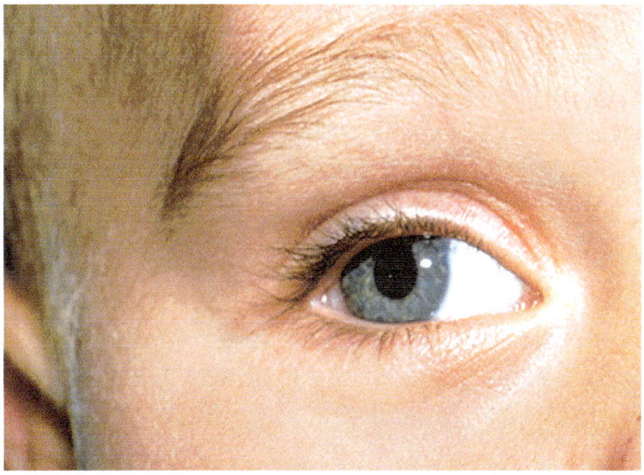

Figure 10.103 Dermoid cyst at the lateral eyebrow area.
(*Courtesy*: M. Mealyea.)

feet **(Fig. 10.100)**; however, it can become widespread. Lesions are asymptomatic. Extensive lesions can be associated with diabetes mellitus, although this is more commonly seen in adults. The diagnosis is clinical but can be confirmed with a biopsy. They need to be differentiated from other annular lesions, most of which are scaly, a feature absent in granuloma annulare. The lesions are self-limiting. Topical and intralesional steroids and cryotherapy may hasten resolution in some.

Pyoderma Gangrenosum

Pyoderma gangrenosum (PG) is a neutrophilic dermatosis that presents as a nodule or a pustule, which evolves into a characteristic ulcer with violaceous undermined edges **(Fig. 10.101)**. It is uncommon in children. PG can be associated with underlying disease such as inflammatory bowel disease, connective tissue disease and haematological malignancy; however, 50% of cases are idiopathic. Treatment involves addressing any underlying disease. For the PG itself, topical and/or oral steroids are the treatment of choice, although recently topical tacrolimus has been found helpful.

Juvenile Xanthogranuloma

Juvenile xanthogranuloma is a non-Langerhans cell histiocytosis presenting early in life as a characteristic yellow/orange-coloured nodule, usually on the head and neck area. It usually presents as a single or few lesions **(Fig. 10.102)**. The condition is self-limiting and tends to resolve spontaneously in few years. Multiple lesions can be associated with neurofibromatosis and myeloid leukaemia.

Dermoid Cysts

These are developmental cysts usually presenting as asymptomatic skin-coloured nodules along the lines of embryonic fusion. They commonly arise in the lateral eyebrow **(Fig. 10.103)**. Midline lesions can have an

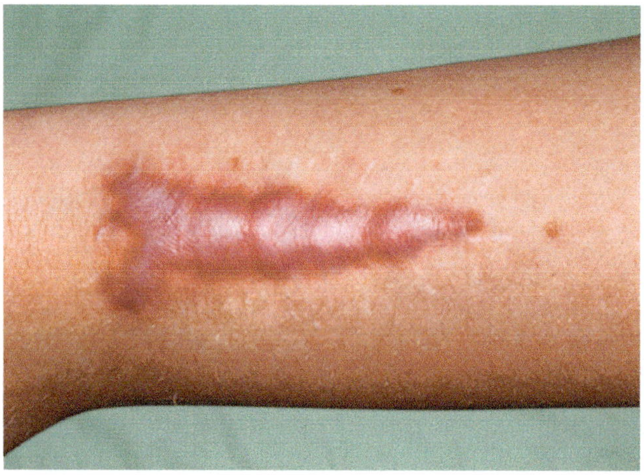

Figure 10.104 Keloid.
(*Courtesy*: M. Mealyea.)

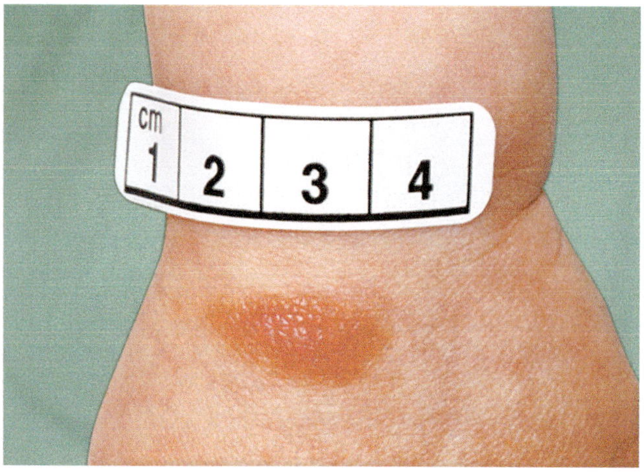

Figure 10.105 Mastocytoma.
(*Courtesy*: M. Mealyea.)

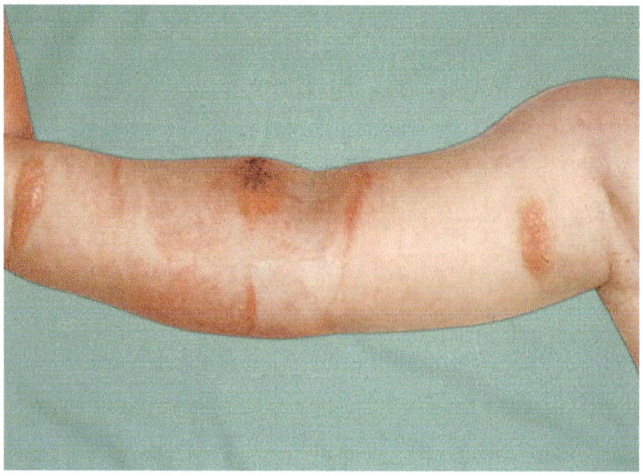

Figure 10.106 Urticaria pigmentosa.
(*Courtesy*: K. Goel.)

intracranial connection, which should be ruled out by radiological imaging. This needs to be done before any surgery is contemplated, as the connection can act as a portal of entry for organisms to cause infection.

Keloid and Hypertrophic Scars

Keloid and hypertrophic scars are caused by an exaggerated fibroblast response to skin injury. They present as firm red nodules or plaques, which can be sore or itchy **(Fig. 10.104)**. Chest and shoulder are the most common locations. Dark-skinned individuals seem to be more at risk and there is sometimes a familial tendency. Hypertrophic scars form at the site of injury, whereas keloids grow beyond the original site of injury.

Topical potent and superpotent steroids and silicone gel may help to flatten the lesion, but may need few months before any effect is noticed. Intralesional steroids can be used if the above fail. If the affected area is excised, steroids may need to be injected in the new scar early on to prevent redevelopment of hypertrophy.

Mastocytosis

This term refers to conditions characterised by collection of mast cells in the skin. Solitary lesions termed mastocytomas present as brown, reddish brown or yellow brown lesions either at birth or early within the first year **(Fig. 10.105)**. Multiple lesions are termed as urticaria pigmentosa **(Fig. 10.106)**. The lesions urticate and may blister with any kind of friction, which results in release of histamine from the cells. This is called Darier sign, and can be a useful diagnostic sign in clinic.

The prognosis is generally good. The blistering usually stops by about the age of 2 years and the lesions themselves often eventually spontaneously clear, although some may leave pigmented areas. Affected children should avoid histamine-releasing agents such as aspirin, opiates and certain anaesthetic agents.

A small number of children, especially those with numerous lesions, may develop systemic symptoms such as flushing, headache, diarrhoea and tachycardia. H_1 antihistamine with or without the addition of H_2 blockers can help. Cromolyn sodium is usually effective for patients with gastrointestinal symptoms.

Neonatal Lupus

This presents in neonates secondary to transplacental passage of anti-Ro and anti-La antibodies. The rash is usually present at birth as annular erythematous lesions with central scale and atrophy. The lesions usually affect the upper body and may be exacerbated by sunlight **(Figs. 10.107A and B)**. Sunlight protection is advised. The lesions tend to settle over the first few months of life as the antibody titre wanes. Topical steroids may help in settling the inflammation quicker. The condition can be associated with varying degrees of heart block, which tends to persist, and may need a pacemaker.

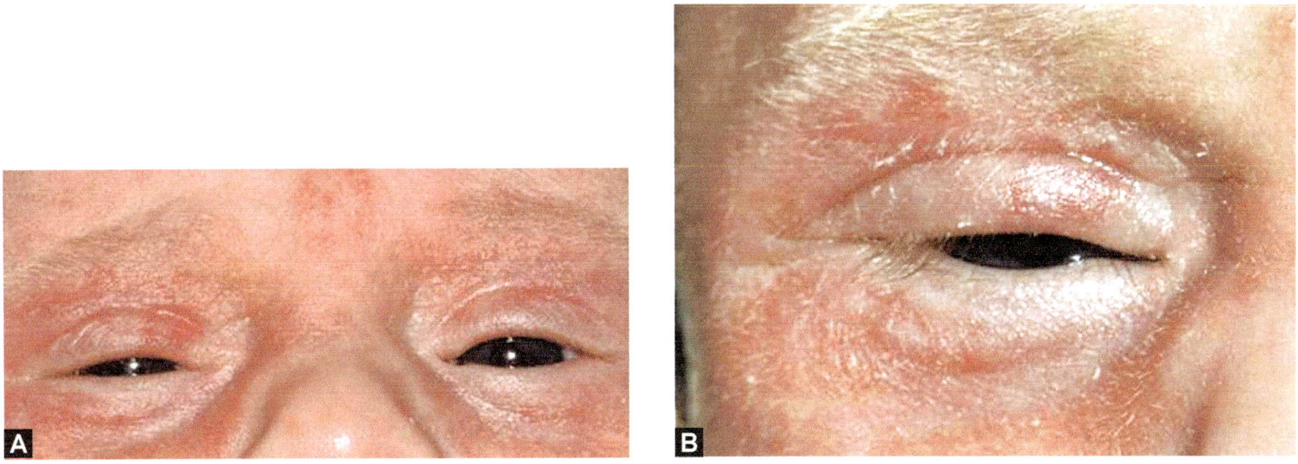

Figures 10.107A and B Neonatal lupus. (A) Note the periocular erythema with some scaling. Infraocular area shows mild post-inflammatory pigmentation; (B) Close-up of right eye of Figure A.

(*Courtesy*: C. Jury, R. Gulati.)

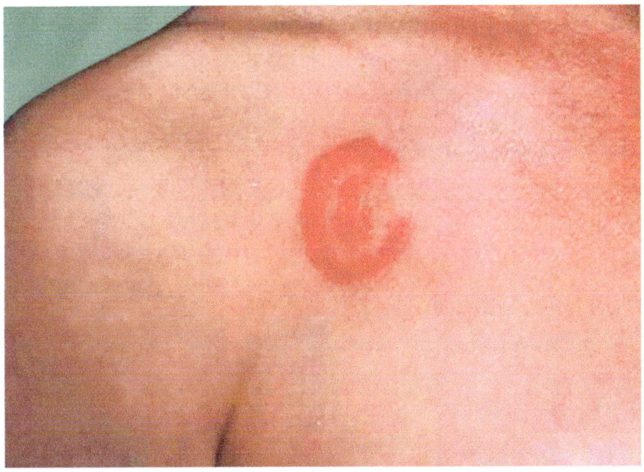

Figure 10.108 Tinea corporis—marked inflammation points towards an animal source.

(*Courtesy*: R. Gulati.)

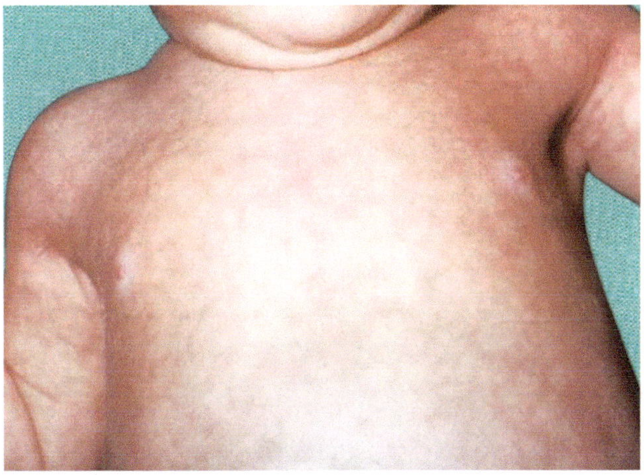

Figure 10.109 Physiological cutis marmorata.

(*Courtesy*: K. Goel.)

CASE STUDIES

Case Study 1

A 5-year-old boy presents with 4-week history of an expanding erythematous itchy lesion on the right chest. He is otherwise well and had attended a cattle farm few weeks before **(Fig. 10.108)**. The lesion appears annular with central clearing. Microscopic examination of scales from the edge of the lesion shows fungal hyphae. Culture shows *Trichophyton verrucosum*. The lesion clears with 2-week application of topical terbinafine.

Diagnosis: Tinea corporis.

KEY LEARNING POINT

Dermatophyte infections derived from animals (zoophilic) cause marked inflammatory response.

Case Study 2

A 3-week-old baby is incidentally noticed to have generalised mottled skin on a doctor's visit **(Fig. 10.109)**. The mottling tends to disappear when the skin becomes warmer. The mottling is likely to disappear beyond neonatal period.

Diagnosis: Physiological cutis marmorata.

KEY LEARNING POINT

Cutis marmorata that fails to respond beyond the neonatal period may be associated with hypothyroidism, trisomy 21 and Cornelia de Lange syndrome.

Case Study 3

A well term baby develops generalised blotchy maculopapular rash with some pustules on third day of life

(Fig. 10.110). The pustules are sterile and contain mainly eosinophils. The rash settles by the 10th day of life.
Diagnosis: Erythema toxicum neonatorum (ETN).

> **KEY LEARNING POINT**
>
> If ETN-like rash is present in an unwell child, generalised staphylococcal infection or candidiasis should be considered. Presence of vesicles should point to possibility of herpes simplex.

Case Study 4

A 7-year-old boy presents with a palpable non-blanching rash. The rash started 3 days back from the ankles and now involves lower limbs and buttocks. He also has painful swollen ankles. He had a viral upper respiratory tract infection 3 weeks back. Biopsy of the rash shows leukocytoclastic vasculitis with deposition of IgA in dermal blood vessels **(Figs. 10.111A and B)**. His urine dipstick is unremarkable and blood pressure is within normal limits. Analgesia is recommended for joint pains. Rash and joints settle in the ensuing 6 weeks.
Diagnosis: Henoch-Schönlein purpura (HSP).

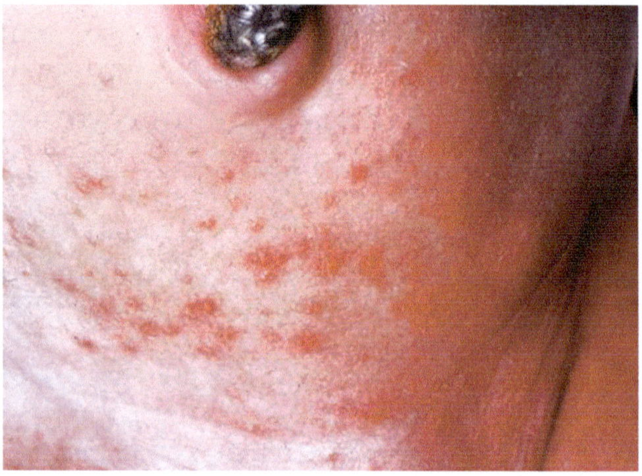

Figure 10.110 Erythema toxicum neonatorum.
(*Courtesy*: K. Goel.)

> **KEY LEARNING POINT**
>
> Small percentage of children with HSP may develop renal damage. It is therefore recommended to monitor blood pressure and urinalysis for 6 months. Presence of abdominal pain or scrotal swelling may warrant oral steroids.

Case Study 5

A 14-year-old girl gives a 2-day history of developing clusters of small vesicles on the right side of neck **(Fig. 10.112)**. The lesion is painful. On examination, the clusters on the right side appear dermatomal. Viral swab from the vesicle fluid grows varicella zoster virus. Analgesia is prescribed. Lesions settle over the next 2 weeks.
Diagnosis: Herpes zoster.

> **KEY LEARNING POINT**
>
> Contact with herpes zoster lesions may cause chicken pox in non-immune individuals.

Case Study 6

A 4-year-old girl was incidentally noticed to have peeling of palms and soles, when seen in the clinic for unrelated condition **(Fig. 10.113)**. History revealed she had a sore throat 8 days back. She was diagnosed with streptococcal

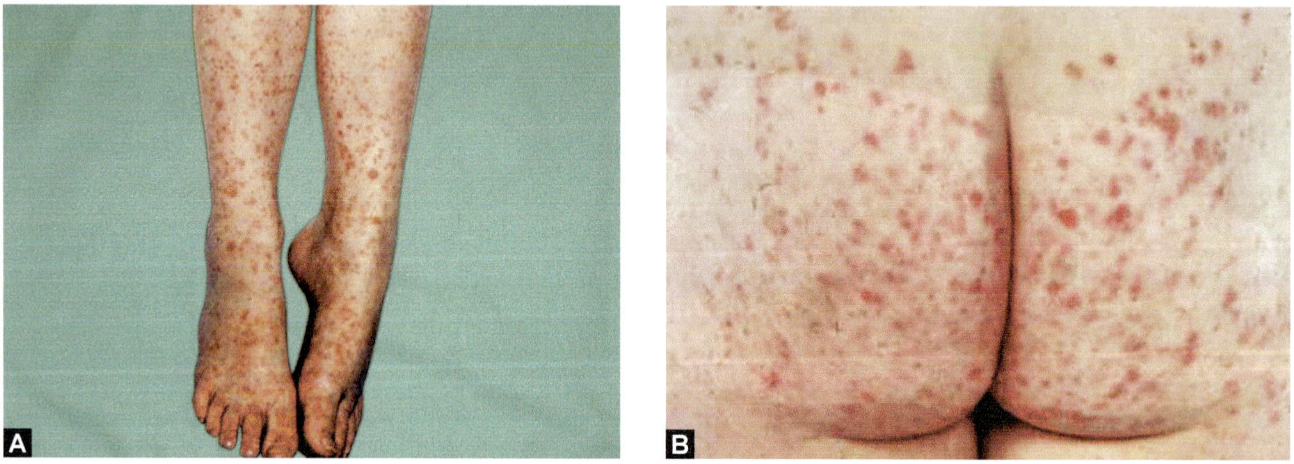

Figures 10.111A and B Henoch-Schönlein purpura. (A) Palpable purpura on lower legs; (B) Involvement of buttocks.
(*Courtesy*: K. Goel.)

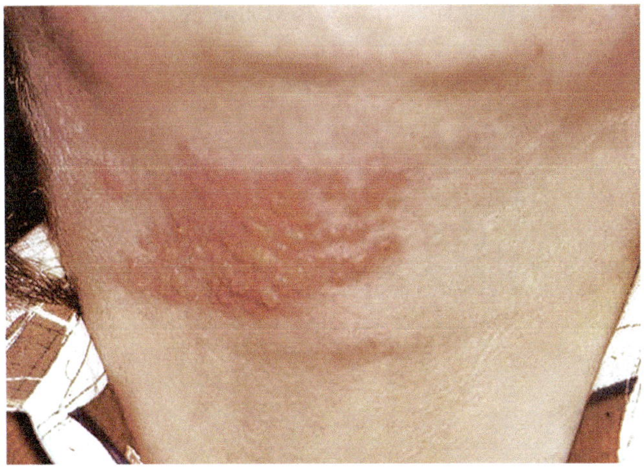

Figure 10.112 Herpes zoster.
(*Courtesy*: K. Goel.)

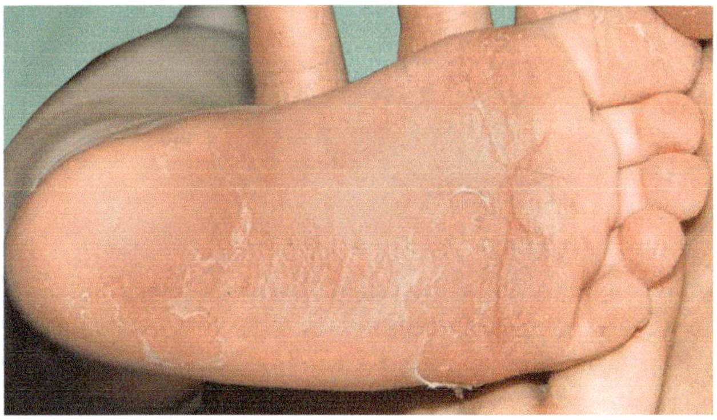

Figure 10.113 Plantar peeling.
(*Courtesy*: K. Goel.)

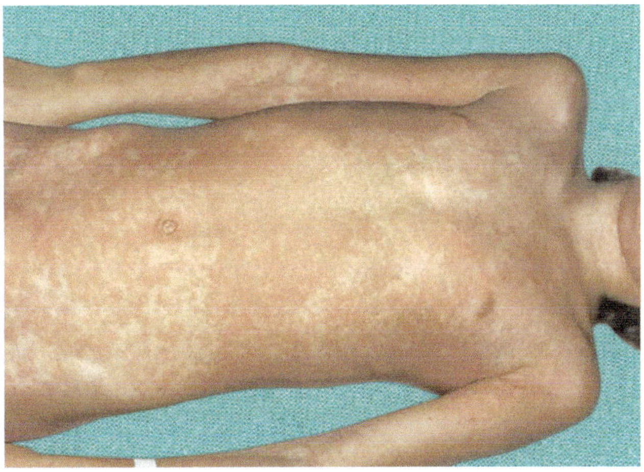

Figure 10.114 Maculopapular drug rash.
(*Courtesy*: K. Goel.)

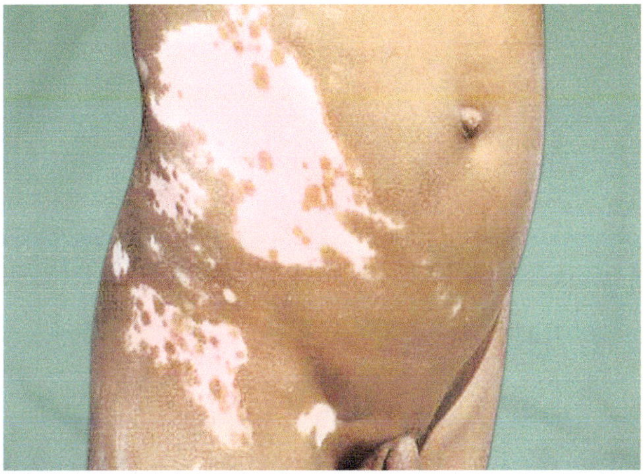

Figure 10.115 Segmental vitiligo.
(*Courtesy*: R. Gulati.)

pharyngitis, which settled with 7-day course of oral penicillin. The palms and soles had shown peeling over the last 3 days. She was advised to use a moisturiser and the peeling settled over the next 10 days.
Diagnosis: Palmoplantar peeling associated with streptococcal infection.

KEY LEARNING POINT

Palmoplantar peeling may also be associated with many viral infections and Kawasaki syndrome. Benign acral peeling syndrome should be considered in a well child with recurrent peeling.

Case Study 7

An 11-year-old girl is seen in accident and emergency with a generalised maculopapular blanching itchy rash **(Fig. 10.114)**. The rash has developed over the last 3 days and is spreading. She was started on amoxicillin for a chest infection 4 days back, which she continues to take. She is switched to a macrolide antibiotic, while an antihistamine is prescribed to control the itch. She is advised to avoid penicillin group of drugs in the future. The rash settles over the next 7 days.
Diagnosis: Maculopapular drug rash.

KEY LEARNING POINT

Drug rash may need to be differentiated from viral exanthems, as they may look similar.

Case Study 8

A 3-year-old boy presents with patchy depigmented skin on the right flank and upper thigh in a segmental distribution **(Fig. 10.115)**. The depigmentation started 1 year back but has been static for about 4 months. The boy is otherwise in good health. Topical steroids were not helpful.
Diagnosis: Segmental vitiligo.

KEY LEARNING POINT

Segmental vitiligo is usually less responsive to treatment. Surgical measures should be considered, if cosmetically concerning.

Case Study 9

A very active 6-month-old baby boy presents with blisters on the feet (Fig. 10.92). Mum tells that he tends to rub his feet quite vigorously. Dad and elder sibling also suffer from acral blistering more commonly affecting the feet, and problematic in summers.
Diagnosis: Epidermolysis bullosa simplex.

KEY LEARNING POINT

Presentation with recurrent blisters on frictional areas with a positive family history should point towards the possible diagnosis of a genetic mechanobullous disorder.

CHAPTER 11

Haematological Disorders

Krishna M. Goel

HAEMATOPOIESIS

Within a few days of embryonic implantation "blood islands" develop in the human yolk sac. Cells from these islands develop into vascular endothelium and primitive blood cells. These pluripotent stem cells known as progenitor or CFU-GEMM (colony forming unit-granulocyte-erythroid/megakaryocyte-macrophage) cells produce red cells, white cells except lymphocytes and platelets (Fig. 11.1). Most haematopoiesis in the foetus takes place from progenitor cells seeded to the liver. Bone marrow haematopoiesis is present from about 10 weeks of gestation and by term has taken over almost all of the foetal haemopoietic function. Control of erythropoiesis in the foetus is through hepatic erythropoietin mediated by foetal tissue oxygen concentration. There is a switch to renal erythropoietin a few weeks after birth.

All of the white cell series and platelets are identifiable in foetal blood by about 14 weeks of gestation, and the granulocyte series is controlled by the hormone gonad stimulating factor and platelets by thrombopoietin.

Modern haematology embraces many complicated techniques that have added greatly to our understanding of the nature of some of the less common disorders, e.g. haemolytic anaemias, haemoglobinopathies, megaloblastic anaemias, etc. Nonetheless, the blood disorders commonly encountered in paediatric practice can most often be dealt with by use of relatively simple standard techniques.

NORMAL BLOOD PICTURE IN INFANCY

Considerable variations in normal values during the early days of life have been recorded by different workers. There are several reasons for this. Blood samples obtained by venipuncture in early infancy have lower values for haemoglobin (Hb) and red cell counts than those obtained by heel prick and individual infants show a wide variation in values. In routine clinical practice, only fairly large departures from normal ranges are likely to prove significant.

Haemoglobin

The Hb concentration in blood from the umbilical cord is high with a mean of 17 g/dL (17 g/100 mL). Values up to 20 g/dL may be recorded. A venous sample of the infant's blood some hours after birth may reveal an even higher Hb level with a mean of 19 g/dL, and a skin-prick sample is likely to be still higher with a mean of 21 g/dL. This rise in Hb values just after birth is probably due to haemoconcentration due to diminution in the plasma volume, in addition to the infusion of red cells which may occur when late clamping of the umbilical cord is practised.

The oxygen-carrying capacity of the blood is related to the total circulating red cell mass (RCM), which can vary in normal infants between 30 and 50 mL/kg depending on whether the cord is clamped early or late. Hb concentration and haematocrit can correlate poorly with the RCM especially in preterm infants. The RCM can vary between 12 and 24 mL/kg in infants with a haematocrit of 0.3 (30%) due to compensatory reductions of plasma volume.

The Hb value falls to 10–11 g/dL by the age of 8–12 weeks but rises again to between 11 and 13 g/dL between the ages of 6 months and a year. Thereafter, the Hb level increases to 11.5–15 g/dL by the age of 10–12 years and reaches normal adult values (men = 13.5–18 g/dL; women = 11.5–16.5 g/dL) by the age of 15 years. The explanation for the fall in Hb level during the early weeks of life is that, although erythropoiesis continues at a high level found in the foetus for about 3 days after birth, an abrupt decline in erythropoiesis then occurs and the marrow erythroid count falls from 40,000 to 6,000/mm^3. This is reflected in a fall in the reticulocyte count from 3% or 4% just after birth to under 1%, 1 week later.

At birth 50–65% of the Hb is of the foetal type (HbF) that resists denaturation with alkalis. It has a slightly different electrophoretic mobility and a quite different oxygen dissociation curve from adult type Hb (HbA). After birth HbF is slowly replaced by HbA so that after a year of age only small amounts of HbF are still present. In certain diseases, such as thalassaemia and sickle-cell anaemia, HbF is

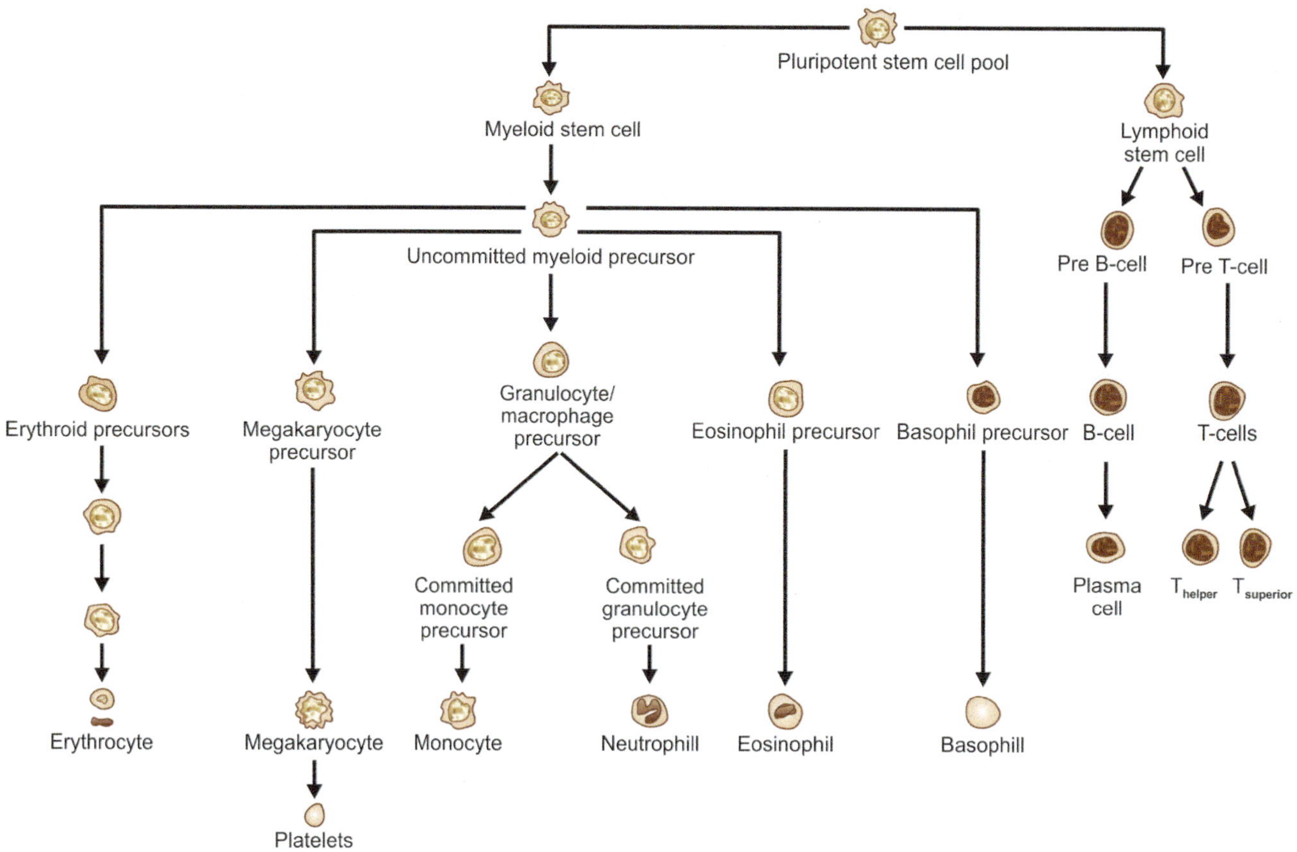

Figure 11.1 Haematopoiesis in the embryo and foetus.

produced in excessive quantity. The value to the foetus of HbF appears to be that of a greater affinity for oxygen at low tensions than HbA and an ability to release CO_2 more readily.

Since the discovery in 1949 of the first abnormal Hb molecule (HbS), a great deal of information has accumulated about the molecular structure of Hb. Over 100 variant forms of human Hb have now been recognised. Some of these are associated with serious disease in various parts of the world.

Red Cells

The red cell count at birth varies between 5.5 and 7.5 million/mm^3. The count falls to about 5–5.5 million after 2 weeks and thereafter runs parallel to the Hb level. Scanty eosinophilic normoblasts are found in the peripheral blood at birth. Erythrocytes at birth have a larger diameter (about 8.4 µm) than in the adult. The mean adult value of 7.2 µm is reached after 1 year.

White Cells

The total white cell count at birth is about 18,000/mm^3. The adult value of 6,000–7,000/mm^3 is not reached for 7–10 years. At birth about 60% of the white cells are polymorphonuclear (11,000/mm^3) and 30% are lymphocytes (5,400/mm^3). During the ensuing 2 weeks, the polymorphonuclear count falls to within the normal adult range (3,500–4,500/mm^3) where they remain during the rest of childhood. On the other hand, the lymphocytes, predominantly of the large type in infancy, rise rapidly to about 9,500/mm^3 at 2 weeks and only slowly fall during the next 12 years to the adult level of about 1,500–2,000/mm^3. It is important to remember the comparatively high lymphocyte count in normal children if mistaken diagnoses such as glandular fever or leukaemia are to be avoided. The monocyte ratio in children tends to be somewhat higher than in adults. Eosinophils and basophils show no special characteristics.

The normal blood volume in infancy is 85 mL/kg.

> **KEY LEARNING POINT**
>
> **Normal values:** It is essential to remember age-related haematology reference ranges for diagnostic purposes.

Iron Deficiency or Nutritional Anaemia in Infancy

This is the only deficiency disease seen commonly among infants and children in the United Kingdom at the present time. The highest incidence of anaemia is found in the lower socio-economic groups.

Aetiology

Several factors, singly or in combination, can result in this deficiency state. Breast milk and cow's milk are low in iron. Therefore, unduly prolonged milk feeding (human or cow's milk) or feeding whole cow's milk in early infancy results in iron deficiency. This is perhaps the most commonly found factor. Another important factor is the influence of birth weight. It is well-known that preterm infants and others of low birth weight (such as twins or triplets) are particularly likely to develop iron-deficiency anaemia. Infants, whatever their maturity, have a body iron content of about 75 mg/kg fat free body weight. The bulk of the infant's iron endowment (66–75%) is represented by Hb iron. One gram of Hb contains 3.4 mg of iron. Complications of pregnancy or the perinatal period that result in blood loss will compromise the infants' iron endowment. The smaller infant grows more rapidly in proportion to his birth weight than the larger with a corresponding need for a larger increase in his red cells and Hb. As the amount of iron absorbed is very low during the first 4 months of life the small infant more rapidly exhausts his storage iron (in liver and spleen) and develops overt signs of iron deficiency. Unless extreme, the presence of maternal iron deficiency does not appear to compromise the iron endowment of the foetus. Infections, to which the iron deficient infant is prone, further aggravate the anaemia. Finally, the possibility of chronic blood loss from, e.g. oesophagitis, a Meckel's diverticulum or hook worm infestation or of iron malabsorption must always be considered in cases of iron deficiency anaemia. Occult gastrointestinal (GI) bleeding can occur in infants who have been started on whole cow's milk early in life. Convenience foods are often low in iron. Red meat, eggs and green vegetables are sources of iron.

KEY LEARNING POINTS

Nutritional iron deficiency anaemia is seen commonly among infants and children during their first year.

Breast milk and cow's milk are low in iron.

Also convenience foods are often low in iron.

Clinical Features

A mild degree of nutritional anaemia probably affects over 25% of infants during their first year. The onset is rarely before the 5th month of life. When the anaemia is severe, there is obvious pallor of skin and mucous membranes. Splenomegaly may be present and there may be cardiomegaly and a haemic systolic murmur. The anaemia is microcytic and hypochromic **(Fig. 11.2)**. Serum iron is markedly reduced (normal mean = 18 μmol/L; 100 mg/100 mL), and the saturation of the iron binding protein of the serum is reduced from 33 to 10% or less. The serum ferritin concentration is reduced (<10 mg/mL). Bone marrow shows normoblastic hyperplasia and an absence of stainable iron. Ferritin is an acute phase protein, and it is increased in inflammatory disease. Thus serum ferritin could be normal even in the absence of iron stores.

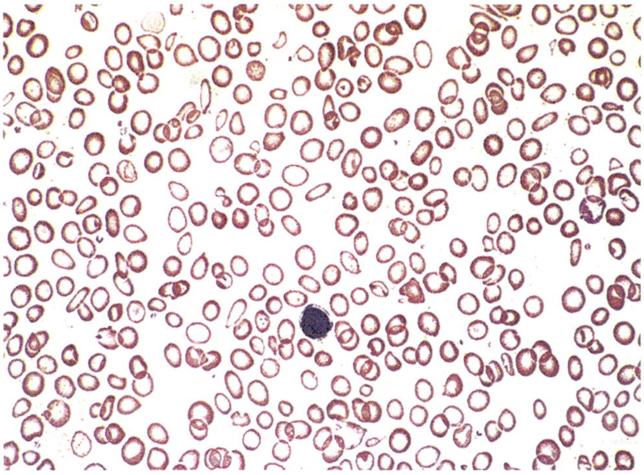

Figure 11.2 Peripheral blood smear of a child with iron deficiency anaemia.

KEY LEARNING POINTS

Ferritin is an acute phase protein and it is increased in inflammatory disease. Thus serum ferritin could be normal even in the absence of iron stores.

Treatment of iron deficiency anaemia:

Treatment with an iron preparation is indicated only in the presence of a clearly demonstrable iron-deficiency state.

It is suggested that the possibility of thalassaemia should always be considered in children of Mediterranean or Indian subcontinent origin, prior to commencing an iron supplement.

Case Study

A 2-year-old Asian girl presented with poor appetite and pallor. Mother's main concern was that her daughter looked pale as compared to her siblings. There was no history of bleeding from any orifice of her body. On examination, she was anaemic and had haemic murmur. Otherwise there was no positive finding. Hb was 6 g/dL.

Hypochromic, microcytic red cells and no target cells were seen. Serum ferritin less than 5 mg/mL. Stools negative for intestinal parasites.

Diagnosis: Nutritional iron deficiency anaemia.

KEY LEARNING POINT

Iron supplements are properly absorbed when taken on an empty stomach, however, they should be taken after food to minimise gastrointestinal side-effects; they may also discolour stools.

MEGALOBLASTIC ANAEMIAS (FOLATE DEFICIENCY AND VITAMIN B_{12} DEFICIENCY)

Folate Deficiency

True megaloblastic erythropoiesis is rare in paediatric practice. Folate is absorbed unchanged in the duodenum and jejunum. It is provided by most foods including meat and vegetables. The most common cause is malabsorption of folic acid in the older child with inadequately treated coeliac disease. However, folate deficiency may also be caused by inadequate intake, increased requirements (haemolytic anaemia), disorders of folate metabolism (congenital and acquired) drugs and increased excretion in children on special diets. The long-term use of anticonvulsants (especially phenytoin) has been associated with megaloblastic anaemia, probably as a result of inhibition of conversion of dietary folate to absorbable monoglutamates. The symptoms of folate deficiency anaemia are similar to vitamin B_{12} deficiency except that neuropathy is not a feature of folate deficiency. Also the peripheral blood and bone marrow changes in folate deficiency are identical to those found in vitamin B_{12} deficiency **(Box 11.1)**.

Hypersegmentation of the neutrophils in the peripheral blood is the single most useful laboratory aid to early diagnosis **(Fig. 11.3)**. The red cell or serum folate assay is a sensitive, reliable guide to the presence of folate deficiency and remains the best way of confirming early folate deficiency. Successful treatment of patients with folate deficiency involves correction of the folate deficiency as well as amelioration of the underlying disorder and improvement of the diet to increase folate intake. It is usual to treat folate deficient patients with 1–5 mg folic acid orally daily. Folinic acid is also effective in the treatment of folate-deficient megaloblastic anaemia, but it is normally only used in association with cytotoxic drugs.

KEY LEARNING POINTS

Megaloblastic anaemia is rare in children.

There is no justification for prescribing multiple-ingredient vitamin preparations containing vitamin B_{12} or folic acid.

Folic acid should never be given alone for vitamin B_{12} deficiency states (because it may precipitate subacute combined degeneration of the spinal cord).

Case Study

An Asian 6-year-old girl had been on phenytoin for 2 years for recurrent seizures. Her seizures were reasonably under control. Over a period of 8 weeks, she developed pallor, weight loss and became anorexic. On her clinical examination, spleen was enlarged 4 cm below the left costal margin. She had no jaundice or oedema.

BOX 11.1 Prevention of neural tube defects.

Folic acid supplements taken before and during pregnancy can reduce the occurrence of neural tube defects.

Couples who are at a high risk of conceiving a child with neural tube defects are:

- If either partner has a neural tube defect
- If either partner has a family history of neural tube defects
- If previous pregnancy affected by a neural tube defect
- If mother taking antiepileptic drugs.

Hb was 4 g/dL, white blood cells (WBCs) 1,500/mm^3 with 700 neutrophils/mm^3 and platelets were within the normal range. Blood film showed marked hypersegmentation of the polymorphs and some late megaloblasts. Reticulocytes were 3%. Serum folate was less than 2 ng/mL and B_{12} 400 pg/mL. She was treated with folic acid 5 mg three times daily orally. A rapid reticulocyte response occurred (12%) and Hb rose to10 g/dL, 3 weeks from the start of folic acid therapy.

Diagnosis: Phenytoin associated megaloblastic anaemia due to folate deficiency.

Vitamin B_{12} Deficiency

Vitamin B_{12} deficiency in children is exceedingly rare. If it occurs it is caused either by a specific malabsorption of vitamin B_{12} or as part of a generalised malabsorption syndrome. Vitamin B_{12} is provided by foods of animal origin, fish, meat, eggs and milk. After resection of the terminal ileum, there is a risk of a megaloblastic anaemia developing 2–3 years later once the liver stores are depleted. Those most vulnerable are children who lose terminal ileum as a result of tumour (lymphoma), necrotising enterocolitis (NEC), Crohn disease or trauma. Most cases of vitamin B_{12} deficiency occur during the

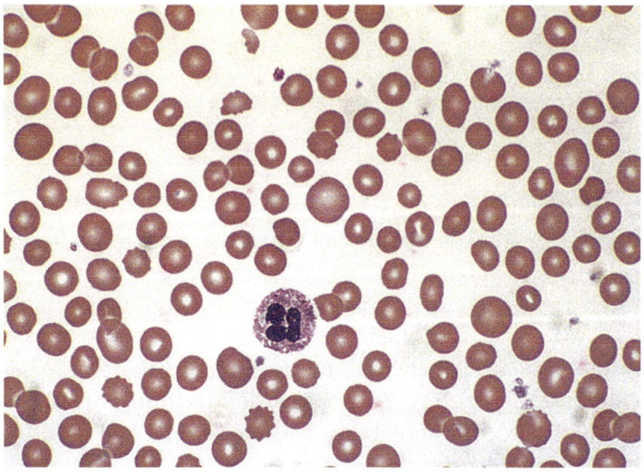

Figure 11.3 Megaloblastic blood picture with oval macrocytic red cells.

first 2 years of life and others manifest later in childhood until puberty.

The clinical signs and symptoms of vitamin B_{12} deficiency are related primarily to the anaemia but can also be complicated by subacute combined degeneration of the spinal cord. Glossitis with papillary atrophy may also be seen.

The haematological findings are indistinguishable from those of folic acid deficiency. The peripheral blood and bone marrow findings can be identical, but the serum vitamin B_{12} level is low. A Schilling test may be necessary to diagnose vitamin B_{12} malabsorption.

HAEMOLYTIC ANAEMIAS

The causes of haemolytic anaemia which may be defined as one in which the life span of the red cells is shortened. The red cell life span in children is 120 days, 60–80 days in neonates and even shorter in premature babies. The classification of haemolytic disorders is as shown in **Table 11.1**.

Hereditary Spherocytosis (Congenital Haemolytic Jaundice)

Aetiology

Hereditary spherocytosis is one of the most common inherited haemolytic anaemias encountered in paediatrics. This disease is inherited in an autosomal dominant fashion but in 25% of the cases neither parent appears to be affected. This is most likely the result of spontaneous mutation. At present, it seems likely that the physiologically important abnormality is an inherent instability of the red cell membrane. It is certain that the major part of the haemolysis of the abnormal red cells takes place in the spleen.

TABLE 11.1 Classification of haemolytic disorders.

(i) Inherited haemolytic disorders
Defects in the structure of the red cell membrane
Hereditary spherocytosis
Hereditary elliptocytosis
Quantitative haemoglobin disorder
Thalassaemias
Qualitative haemoglobin disorder
Sickle cell disease
Defects of red blood cell metabolism
G6PD deficiency
Pyruvate-kinase deficiency
Other enzyme disorders
(ii) Acquired haemolytic disorders
Immune
Autoimmune haemolytic anaemia
Alloimmune haemolytic disease of the newborn

KEY LEARNING POINT

Hereditary spherocytosis is one of the most common inherited haemolytic anaemias encountered in paediatrics.

Clinical Features

The disease is quite variable in its severity. However, most affected children will, at sometimes, manifest one or more of the cardinal features of the disease: anaemia, jaundice (unconjugated bilirubin) and splenomegaly. It can cause haemolytic icterus in the neonatal period and kernicterus has been described. It is, however, rare for the disease to appear in infancy. More commonly, it presents during later childhood with pallor and lassitude; less often with jaundice and highly coloured urine. Children may present with an acute abdomen from splenic infarcts. It may remain symptomless until adult life when biliary colic due to gall-stones is not uncommon. Acute haemolytic crisis with severe anaemia and icterus require emergency treatment but they are, in fact, uncommon. Splenomegaly is usually present whatever the degree of haemolysis in hereditary spherocytosis. The red cells are unable to sustain a normal biconcave shape because of their metabolic defect. They are spheroidal with a smaller diameter than normal. It is usually easy to differentiate microspherocytes in well-stained blood films **(Figs. 11.4A and B)**. They appear unduly dark in colour and small in diameter than normal biconcave erythrocytes. A significant reticulocytosis is usually found. High figures may be reached during a crisis but the absence of a reticulocytosis does not exclude the diagnosis. Increased osmotic fragility of the red cells is an important diagnostic feature. The test is much more reliable when performed on a quantitative basis but is not pathognomonic of hereditary spherocytosis, being sometimes abnormal in acquired haemolytic anaemia, and infrequently it may be normal in the neonatal period. In hereditary spherocytosis, Coombs' test is negative. Routine ultrasound of the gallbladder should be done to determine whether biliary pigment stones have developed. These should be removed at the time of splenectomy **(Box 11.2)**.

Case Study 1

A 4-year-old Caucasian boy presented with pallor and lassitude. On examination, he was anaemic and had slight scleral icterus. He had no lymphadenopathy or hepatomegaly but had 7 cm splenomegaly. His mother had splenectomy at 8 years of age. Hb was 6.2 g/dL, WBC 6.6×10^9/L, platelet count 300×10^9/L, reticulocyte count 40×10^9/L. Blood film revealed numerous microspherocytes. Total bilirubin was elevated at 160 µg/L with an unconjugated bilirubin of 150 µg/L. Aspartate aminotransferase (AST)/alanine aminotransferase (ALT) was normal. Ultrasound examination of gallbladder was negative for gallstones.
Diagnosis: Hereditary spherocytosis.

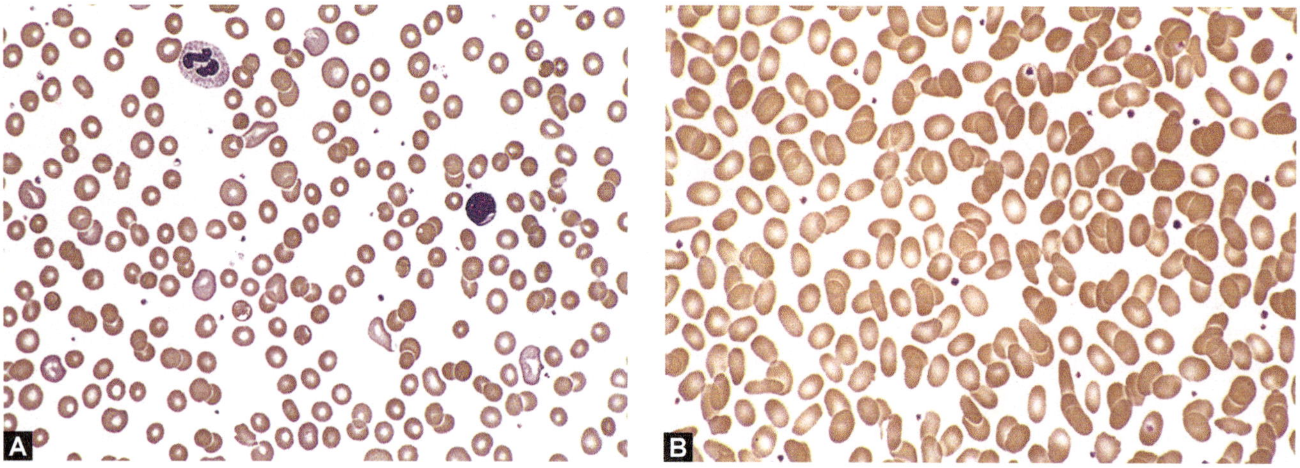

Figures 11.4A and B (A) Peripheral blood film of hereditary spherocytosis showing microspherocytes and polychromasia; (B) Blood film of a child with elliptocytosis.

BOX 11.2 Indications for splenectomy.

Medical
- Hereditary spherocytosis
- Hereditary elliptocytosis
- Severe pyruvate kinase deficiency
- Autoimmune haemolytic anaemia—warm immunoglobulin G antibody type
- Chronic immune thrombocytopenic purpura
- Hypersplenism—who develops significant anaemia or thrombocytopenia
- Sickle cell anaemia—acute splenic sequestration crisis
- Thalassaemia major—increasing transfusion requirements caused by hypersplenism

Surgical
- Splenic trauma, splenic cysts, tumours and Gaucher disease
- Thalassaemia major—massive splenomegaly—for relief from mechanical stress

Case Study 2

A 12-year-old Caucasian boy was admitted with a 48-hour history of jaundice, pain in the right hypochondrium, fever and sweating. He was in severe pain with tenderness in the right upper quadrant and his spleen was palpable 4 cm below the left costal margin. He had previously been seen on several occasions with moderate jaundice and splenomegaly 4–6 cm below the left costal margin. His mother and maternal grandfather had a history of jaundice. His elder brother was well.

Investigations: Blood Hb 13.1 g/dL, mean corpuscular volume 89 fL, mean corpuscular haemoglobin 33 pg, mean cell haemoglobin concentration 37 g/dL, white cell count 7.4 × 10^9/L, neutrophils 5.8 × 10^9/L, lymphocytes 1.6 × 10^9/L, reticulocytes 4%, platelets 500 × 10^9/L, C-reactive protein 4.0 mg/L, urea 6.5 mmol/L, electrolytes normal, total bilirubin 768 umol/L, conjugated bilirubin 430 µmol/L, AST 148 U/L, ALT 329 U/L, total protein 67 g/L and albumin 48 g/L. Urine microscopy negative, culture and blood culture all sterile.

Diagnosis: The most likely diagnosis is congenital spherocytosis.

Thalassaemias

The thalassaemia syndromes are characterised by deficiencies in the rate of production of specific globin chains. A microcytic hypochromic anaemia results.

Developmental Changes in Haemoglobin Synthesis

Normal adult and foetal Hb contains four globin chains **(Table 11.2)**. The thalassaemia syndromes are a heterogeneous group of disorders of Hb synthesis resulting from a genetically determined reduced rate of production of one or more of the four globin chains of Hb—α (alpha), β (beta), δ (delta) and γ (gamma). This results in an excess of the partner chains which continue to be synthesised at a normal rate. The alpha chain types are carried on chromosome 16 and the beta, delta and gamma on chromosome 11. Each type of thalassaemia can exist in a heterozygous or a homozygous state. The most common is beta thalassaemia (Cooley anaemia), which involves suppression of beta-chain formation. In

TABLE 11.2 Globin chains of normal haemoglobins.

Adult	–	Hb A	$\alpha_2 + \beta_2$
	–	Hb A_2	$\alpha_2 + \delta_2$
Foetal	–	Hb F	$\alpha_2 + \gamma_2$
		Hb-Bart's	γ_4
		Hb H	β_4

homozygotes, there is a severe anaemia with a high level of HbF (alpha 2, gamma 2), some HbA2 (alpha 2, delta 2) and a complete absence of, or greatly reduced (normal) HbA (alpha 2, beta 2). Heterozygotes on the other hand suffer from only mild anaemia with reasonable levels of HbA, somewhat raised HbA2, but HbF levels rarely in excess of 3%. Children of the mating of two such heterozygotes have 1 in 4 chance of suffering from the homozygous state for beta thalassaemia. They will not present clinically; however, until later infancy when the effects of beta-chain suppression develop because HbA formation fails to take over from the production of HbF in the normal way. The other main type of thalassaemia involves suppression of alpha-chain production and as alpha-chains are shared by HbA, HbA2 and HbF. It is to be expected that alpha thalassaemia would become clinically manifest in foetal life.

Tetramers of gamma chains may be produced (Hb-Bart's) which result in a clinical picture very similar to that in hydrops foetalis with massive hepatosplenomegaly and generalised oedema, with stillbirth or early neonatal death. In HbH disease, on the other hand, tetramers of gamma chains (HbH) are present in excess and there is considerable clinical variability: From a picture indistinguishable from Cooley anaemia to an absence of specific signs. Heterozygotes for alpha thalassaemia cannot be detected with certainty. Thalassaemias are uncommon in persons of British stock but they are commonly seen in children of Mediterranean, Middle Eastern, Indian, Pakistani origin as well as in South-East Asia where they constitute a major and distressing public-health problem. The distribution parallels with that of falciparum malaria for which the trait appears to have a selective advantage. The clinical account that follows refers only to the most common variety of beta thalassaemia in the homozygous state (beta thalassaemia major—Cooley anaemia).

KEY LEARNING POINT

The clinical severity of beta thalassaemia ranges from thalassaemia minor (usually symptomless), thalassaemia intermedia (with anaemia plus splenomegaly but not transfusion dependent) to thalassaemia major (transfusion dependent).

Clinical Features

This condition is characterised by a chronic haemolytic anaemia which becomes manifest later in infancy, but not in the newborn. Pallor is constant and icterus not uncommon **(Figs. 11.5A and B)**. Splenomegaly increases throughout childhood. Hepatomegaly is also present, largely due to extramedullary erythropoiesis. Pathognomonic skeletal changes can be demonstrated radiographically. Membranous bones of the skull are thickened and lateral views of the skull show the "hair

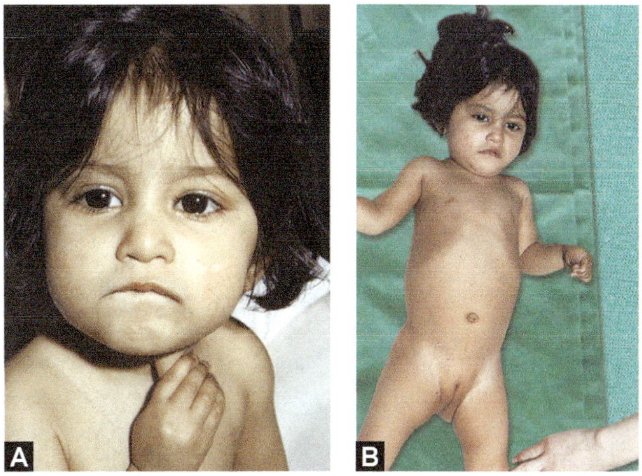

Figures 11.5A and B Clinical photograph of an Asian girl with homozygous beta-thalassaemia. *Note* characteristic facies of thalassaemia major, pallor and jaundice.

on end" appearance **(Figs. 11.6A and B)**. The facies has a Mongoloid appearance due to thickening of the facial bones. The hands may become broadened and thickened due to changes in the metacarpals and phalanges. These bone changes are due to the hyperplasia of the bone marrow **(Fig. 11.7)**. Blood examination shows severe hypochromic anaemia with marked anisocytosis and poikilocytosis. Many microcytic red cells lie side-by-side with large (12–18 mm), bizarre-shaped cells. In some of the latter cells an abnormal central mass of Hb gives them the appearance of "target cells" **(Fig. 11.8)**. Reticulocytosis is marked and Howell-Jolly bodies may be numerous. Serum unconjugated bilirubin concentration is increased. There is increased serum iron while the iron-binding capacity is fully saturated and lower than in normal children. The Hb pattern in beta thalassaemia major consists mainly of HbF, which may amount to 90% of the total and of HbA2; HbA is totally absent or greatly reduced. Most children affected by beta thalassaemia major can be kept in reasonable health, if they are maintained on a high blood transfusion regimen which prevents the Hb level from falling to 11 g/dL. Other laboratory abnormalities commonly found in homozygous beta thalassaemia are mostly due to complications of transfusional haemosiderosis. However, even with the best available treatment, growth failure becomes apparent before puberty. In boys, there is usually a complete or partial failure of pubertal growth and sexual maturation. In girls, the failure tends to be less severe with irregular or scanty menstrual periods. However, secondary amenorrhoea may develop from iron overload. Other effects may include endocrine, hepatic or renal failure and overt diabetes mellitus.

Case Study

A 1-year-old Asian boy presented with pallor, poor feeding, failure to thrive and recurrent upper respiratory

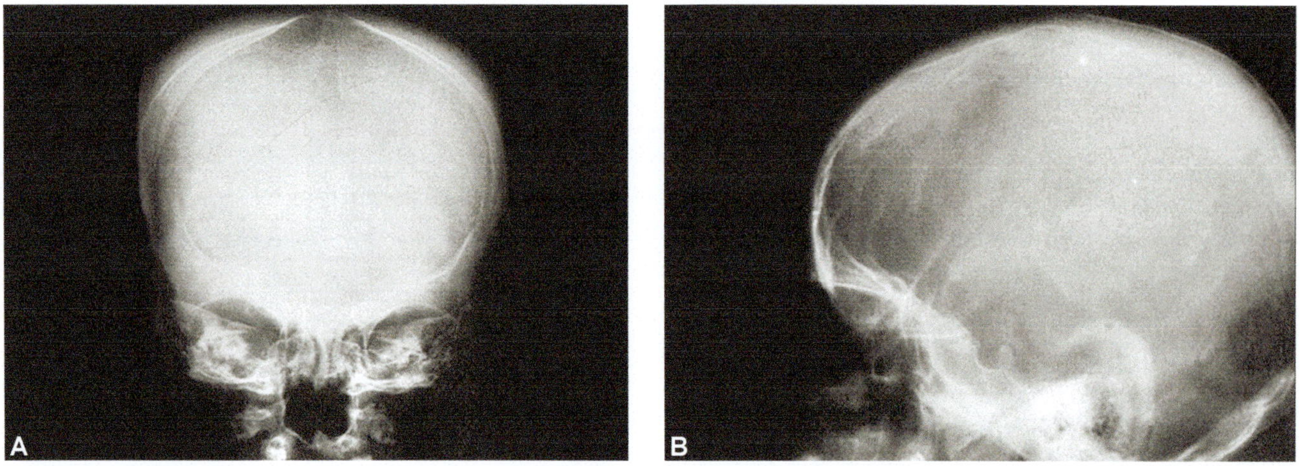

Figures 11.6A and B (A) Lateral view of the skull showing expansion of the diploic space; (B) A hair on end appearance of the skull vault.

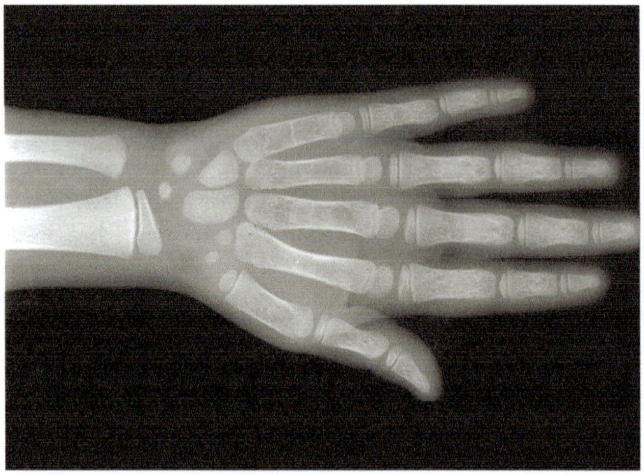

Figure 11.7 Anteroposterior view of the hand showing mild generalised osteopenia; coarsening of the trabecular pattern, medullary widening and cortical thinning.

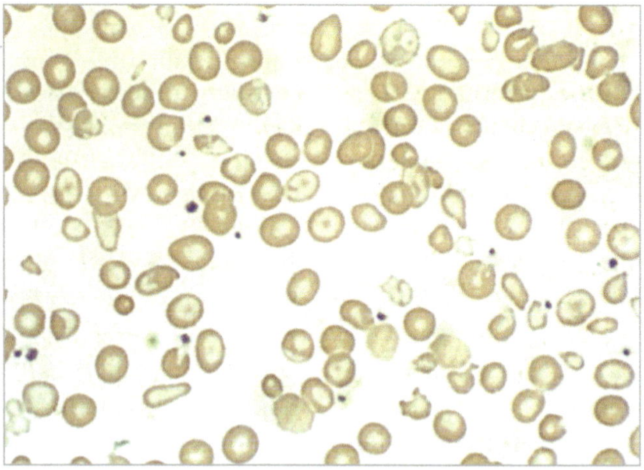

Figure 11.8 Peripheral blood smear of a child with homozygous beta-thalassaemia showing a target cell.

infection. On examination he was anaemic and had a massive hepatosplenomegaly.

Haemoglobin was 5.2 g/dL, WBC and platelet counts were normal. Peripheral blood film showed markedly hypochromic, microcytic red cells, anisocytosis and target cells and some basophilic stippling. Reticulocyte count 10%. He had mildly raised unconjugated bilirubin; otherwise, ALT and AST were normal.

The most likely diagnosis was beta thalassaemia major.

Beta Thalassaemia Minor and Thalassaemia Intermedia

The beta thalassaemia heterozygotes are asymptomatic. The Hb is slightly reduced to 9–12 g/dL and the red cell count is high. On the contrary, patients with thalassaemia intermedia are symptomatic. They have a milder clinical course than those with thalassaemia major and are not blood transfusion dependent and should not be subjected to transfusion inappropriately.

Sickle Cell Disease

Aetiology

This disease is almost confined to the black African races. It is one of the most prevalent autosomal recessive haemoglobinopathies. Homozygotes suffer from sickle cell anaemia (SS) in which all of their Hb is of the HbS variety (homozygous SS disease). The other sickling syndromes are the double heterozygous states such as Hb SC disease and sickle beta thalassaemia (HbS Beta thal). The abnormality in HbS lies in the beta peptide chains, the alpha chains being normal. The aberration in the beta chains is due to the substitution of valine for glutamic acid in the No. 6 position. Heterozygotes reveal the sickle cell trait (AS) and their Hb is composed of about 60% HbA and 40% HbS.

The trait is found in about 7–9% of American black people but it is much more prevalent in some African tribes. It provides increased resistance to malignant tertian malaria. HbS has a distinctive electrophoretic pattern which is due to its abnormal molecular structure. This type of Hb forms crescent-shaped crystals under reduced oxygen tension and it is this property which is responsible for the sickled shape of the erythrocytes in people who possess the gene. Haemolysis in sickle-cell anaemia appears to be due mainly to impaction of the sickled cells in the capillaries, especially in organs where the oxygen tension is low. Capillary obstruction leads to infarcts in various organs, e.g. spleen, intestine, bones, kidneys, heart, lungs and brain.

KEY LEARNING POINT

Most infants with sickle cell disease (SS) are functionally asplenic by 1 year of age because of repeated splenic infarction.

Clinical Features

The sickle cell trait (AS) is symptomless unless it is associated with another haemoglobinopathy or with thalassaemia. SS often presents during the first year with pallor, listlessness and mild jaundice, but not before 6 months of age **(Fig. 11.9)**. The onset of symptoms is, however, delayed for 6 months or longer until the HbF of the infant has been replaced by HbS. In some cases, there are recurrent haemolytic crises with acute symptoms such as severe abdominal pain and rigidity, pain in the loins, limb pains, localised paralyses, convulsions or meningism. Cerebrovascular occlusion can lead to hemiplegia and cranial nerve palsies.

The lung is also one of the major organs involved in sickle cell disease. Clinical lung involvement commonly takes two major forms: (1) the acute chest syndrome and (2) sickle cell chronic lung disease. Acute chest problem is manifested by fever and chest pain and infiltrates in the chest radiograph. Chronic lung disease is due to repeated episodes of infection and infarction.

Symmetrical painful swellings of the fingers and feet (hand foot syndrome—dactylitis) may develop due to infarction of the metacarpals and metatarsals. X-rays show severe bone destruction and periosteal reaction. They may also reveal radial striations in the skull. Chronic haemolytic anaemia interferes with growth and nutrition so that the child is often stunted in later years. Splenomegaly may be marked but sometimes disappears in later childhood. Cholelithiasis may develop as in other haemolytic anaemias. In adults, the large joints may become swollen and painful with serious crippling. The peripheral blood shows a normochromic anaemia, reticulocytosis and polymorphonuclear leucocytosis. In addition, there is an increase in the serum unconjugated bilirubin and a decrease in red cell osmotic fragility. In a crisis, excess urobilinogenuria is marked. Sickled cells may be seen in ordinary blood films **(Fig. 11.10)**. The diagnosis can be confirmed by demonstration of the characteristic mobility of HbS on starch gel electrophoresis. Children affected with SS also have some HbF in their circulation.

Case Study

A 3-year-old Nigerian boy presented with pallor and a painful swollen right index finger. On abdominal examination, he had splenomegaly 4 cm below the left costal margin. Most likely diagnosis is sickle cell disease with dactylitis.

Other Haemoglobinopathies

It has already been noted that there are three normal Hbs each of two identical pairs of globin polypeptide chains with an iron-containing haem group inserted into each chain. In the healthy adult, 98% of the HbA is composed of two alpha and two beta chains ($\alpha_2\beta_2$). About 2% of adult Hb is HbA composed of two alpha and two delta chains

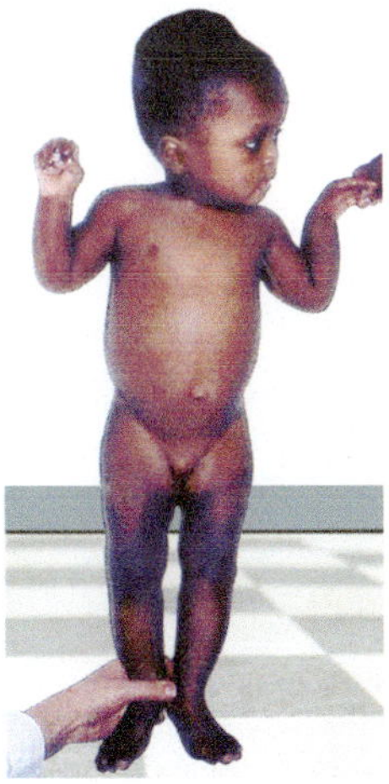

Figure 11.9 Clinical photograph of a Kenyan child with haemoglobin sickle cell anaemia disease showing pallor and jaundice.

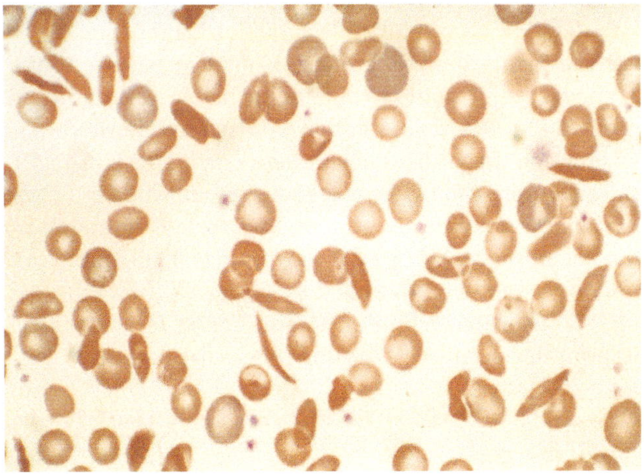

Figure 11.10 Peripheral blood smear of a child with sickle cell disease showing sickled red cells.

($\alpha_2\delta_2$). Foetal Hb or HbF is composed of two alpha and two gamma chains ($\alpha_2\gamma_2$). However, over 100 abnormal Hbs have now been recognised in which the aberration generally consists of a single amino acid substitution in one pair of the peptide chains due to gene mutation. That is to say, they are determined by alleles of the genes for normal HbA, HbA2 or HbF. The different Hbs carry different electrical charges so causing them to move at different speeds in an electrical field and they can usually best be identified by electrophoresis. The different haemoglobinopathies vary widely in their effects, from no apparent effect on health to a fatal disease (e.g. HbS). The homozygote for the gene will, of course always be much more severely affected than the heterozygote, as in sickle cell disease.

The homozygote for HbC presents with manifestations similar to those in SS but sickling and bone changes do not occur. The heterozygote is usually symptomless but blood films show target cells and there is increased osmotic resistance. The homozygote for HbE on the other hand, suffers only from a mild normochromic anaemia with numerous target cells and increase in osmotic resistance, while the heterozygote is asymptomatic. HbM disease is very different in that it causes methaemoglobinaemia.

Having now considered thalassaemia and a few of the haemoglobinopathies in both the homozygous and heterozygous forms, it remains to point out that some anaemic children are found to have inherited the genes for two abnormal Hbs, one from each heterozygous parent, or more commonly for beta thalassaemia and one abnormal Hb. They are, in fact, mixed or double heterozygotes. Thus, there has been described beta thalassaemia with HbS (or C, D or E) as well as S/C, S/D combinations, etc. The effects produced by these states depend upon the peptide chains involved. Thus, if both abnormal genes affect the same type of chain the effects are much more severe than if they affect different chains, i.e. the mixed heterozygous state is more crippling than the double heterozygous state. For example, in both S/C disease and HbS/beta thalassaemia, the beta chains are involved. This means that no HbA can be formed because no normal beta chains can be produced, a state called "interaction" and the resulting clinical manifestations are very similar in severity to the homozygous SS state. On the other hand, when both an alpha and a beta chain abnormalities are inherited (e.g. as in alpha thalassaemia with beta chain Hbs S, C or E), the effects are usually no more severe than when only one of the abnormalities is present because no "interaction" has taken place. Some of these abnormal Hb states can only be accurately identified by family studies, employing sophisticated techniques. The matter is of practical importance because of the differences in prognosis.

Glucose-6-Phosphate Dehydrogenase Deficiency

Glucose-6-phosphate dehydrogenase (G6PD) deficiency is the most common red blood cell (RBC) enzyme abnormality associated with haemolysis. More than 300 types of G6PD have been described. Most of these variants are enzymatically normal and are not a cause of clinical problems. It affects people throughout the world with the highest incidence in individuals originating from most parts of Africa, from most parts of Asia, from Oceania and from Southern Europe. G6PD deficiency is more common in males than it is in females.

Glucose-6-phosphate dehydrogenase A is the commonest variant associated with haemolysis and is found in 10–15% of African-Americans. G6PD B is the normal enzyme found in Caucasians and many Negroes. G6PD Mediterranean is the commonest variant in white people of Mediterranean origin and G6PD Canton is the commonest cause of G6PD deficiency in Asians. It is X-linked and haemolysis is mainly confined to males. The magnitude of haemolysis is variable and is dependent on the degree of oxidant stress. Most variants of G6PD deficiency cause acute haemolysis and not chronic haemolysis on taking a number of common drugs. They are also susceptible to developing acute haemolytic anaemia upon ingestion of fava beans (broad beans, Vicia faba); this is termed favism and can be more severe in children or when the fresh fava beans are eaten raw.

The diagnosis of G6PD deficiency is suggested by Coomb's negative haemolytic anaemia associated with drugs or infection. The specific diagnosis of G6PD deficiency can be made by spectrophotometric enzyme measurements. Special stains of the peripheral blood may reveal Heinz bodies during haemolytic episodes (Fig. 11.11).

Patients should be educated about which drugs to avoid. The risk and severity of haemolysis is almost always dose related. The most common drugs implicated are the sulphonamide antibiotics and antimalarial drugs and other potential sources of oxidant stress (Box 11.3). G6PD deficiency may protect against malaria.

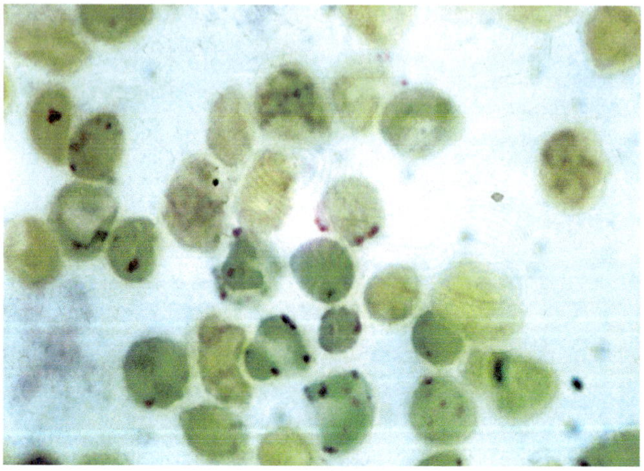

Figure 11.11 Blood film-Heinz bodies: Deep bodies are seen, some lying close to the periphery of the red cells and others attached to the outer surface. Several bodies may be present in the same cell, but when large they are usually found singly. Heinz bodies are the result of polymerisation and precipitation of denatured haemoglobin molecules. Methyl violet × 1200.

BOX 11.3 Drugs commonly associated with acute haemolysis in most G6PD deficiency individuals.

Primaquine
Pamaquine
Sulphanilamide
Sulphapyridine
Sulphamethoxazole
Salazopyrin
Septrin
Dapsone
Thiazolesulphone
Nitrofurantoin
Nalidixic acid
Naphthalene in mothballs, menadione, methylene blue, quinidine, quinine, rasburicase

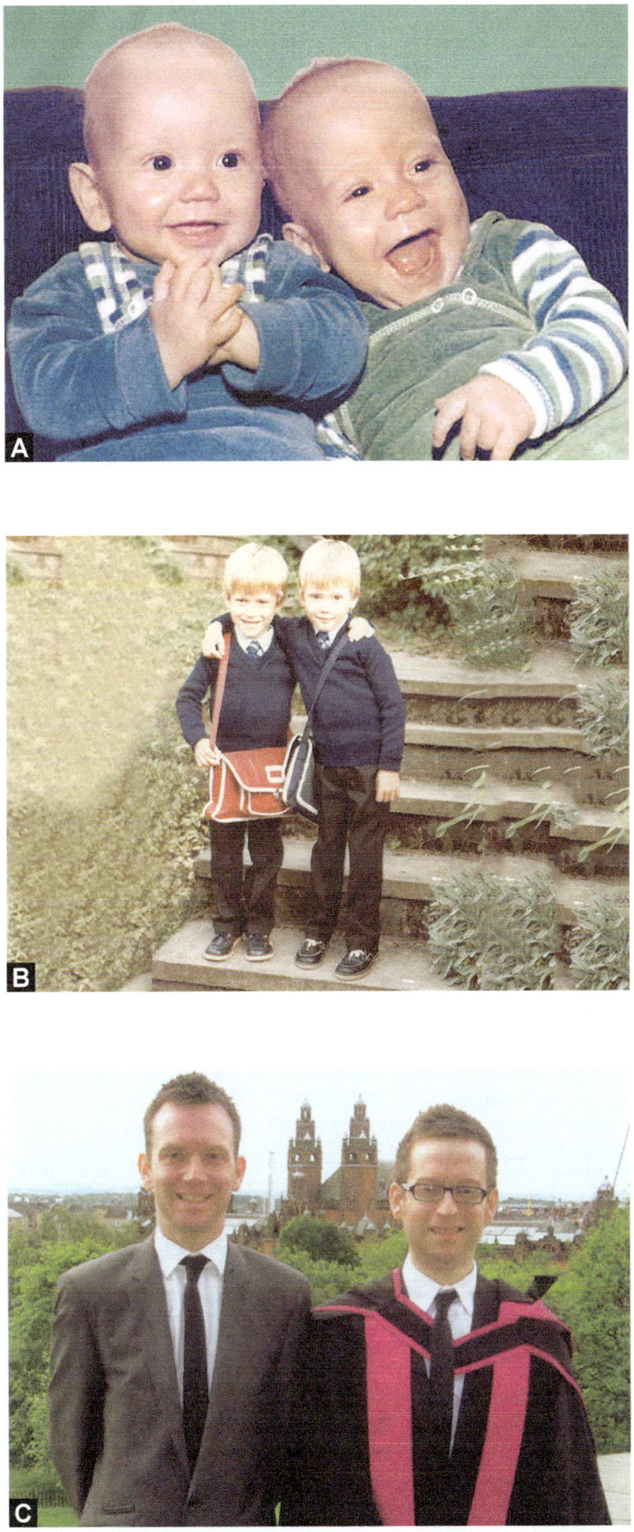

Figures 11.12A to C Pyruvate kinase (PK) deficiency: Photographs of a set of non-identical twins born at 32 weeks of gestation. Developed jaundice on the first day, required two exchange transfusions, thereafter required a few blood transfusions. Diagnosed with PK deficiency at 4 months of age (congenital non-spherocytic haemolytic anaemia). They had splenectomy at 6 years of age to reduce transfusion requirements. They are on prophylactic antibacterial therapy and pneumococcal vaccine against pneumococcal infection. (A) Twins aged 4 months; (B) Aged 5 years, first day at school; (C) As adults and keeping well.

Pyruvate Kinase Deficiency

Pyruvate kinase (PK) deficiency is the commonest red cell enzyme deficiency in north Europeans. It presents in the neonatal period with anaemia and jaundice. Diagnosis requires measurement of PK in the RBCs. The degree of haemolysis varies greatly and is sometimes severe enough to require frequent RBC transfusions. There is a beneficial response to splenectomy **(Figs. 11.12A to C) (Box 11.2)**.

Autoimmune Haemolytic Anaemia

Aetiology

This is not a common problem in paediatric practice but it may present as an acute emergency. There are two major classes of antibodies against red cells that produce haemolysis in man: (1) IgG and (2) IgM. Autoimmune haemolytic anaemia (AIHA) can be warm or cold antibody type. The IgM antibody is generally restricted to the clinical entity of cold haemagglutinin disease because it has a particular affinity for its red cell antigen in the cold (0°–10°C). IgM-induced immune haemolytic anaemia is most commonly associated with an underlying mycoplasma infection or cytomegalovirus (CMV), mumps and infectious mononucleosis infections.

The IgG antibody usually has its maximal activity at 37°C and, thus, this entity has been termed warm antibody induced haemolytic anaemia. IgG-induced immune haemolytic anaemia may occur without an apparent underlying disease (idiopathic disease); however, it may also occur with systemic lupus erythematosus (SLE), rheumatoid arthritis and certain drugs **(Fig. 11.13)**. Warm type AIHA can be severe and life-threatening.

Clinical Features

In some children, the disease has an alarmingly acute onset with fever, backache, limb pains, abdominal pain,

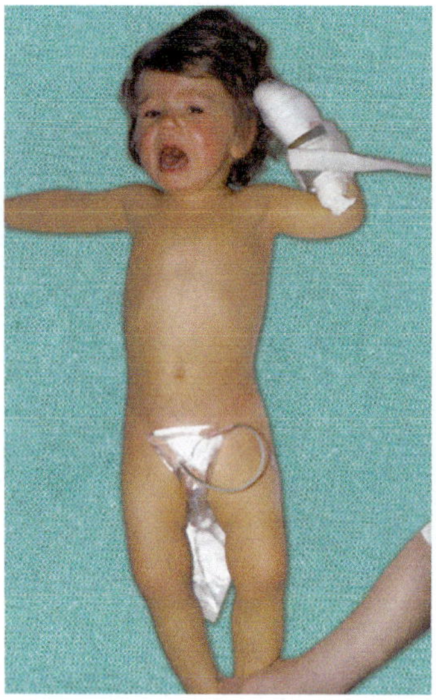

Figure 11.13 Clinical photograph of a child who ingested chemical inorganic copper sulphate. Developed haemolysis resulting in pallor and turmeric yellow jaundice.

vomiting and diarrhoea. Haemoglobinuria and oliguria may be present. Pallor develops rapidly and icterus is common. Frequently, the pallor, listlessness and mild icterus develop more insidiously. Splenomegaly is common. The urine may be dark in colour due to the presence of excess urobilinogen. Reticulocytosis is often marked and there may be many erythroblasts in the peripheral blood. Spherocytosis with an increased fragility of the red cells may simulate congenital spherocytosis. However, in acquired haemolytic anaemia, Coombs' test is positive and serum unconjugated bilirubin concentration is increased.

Case Study

A girl of 14 years was admitted with swollen feet and lower legs for 1 week. She has been unwell with a poor appetite and tired easily. Ten months previously she had been admitted with haemolytic anaemia, from which she recovered after blood transfusion. This had not recurred. On examination, there was pitting oedema of both feet and lower legs. A confluent rash was present on both cheeks and across the base of the nose, with slight scaliness and nodulation. No other abnormalities were present. The blood pressure was 120/80 mmHg. The investigations showed: Blood—Hb 10.6 g/dL, white cell count 13.6×10^9/L, platelets 290×10^9/L, ESR 115 mm per hour, urea 5 mmol/L, albumin 24 g/L, urine contained protein 5.7 g/24 hours, white cell 20 per high power field, epithelial cells present, red cells nil, casts nil, antinuclear antibodies positive, double stranded DNA antibodies positive, direct Coombs' test positive, low C3 and C4 assay and rheumatoid factor negative.
Diagnosis: Paediatric SLE.

Paroxysmal Nocturnal Haemoglobinuria

Paroxysmal nocturnal haemoglobinuria tends to occur in young adult men and is extremely rare in children. As the name suggests, there is a haemolytic anaemia and the urine often contains haemosiderin and may also contain Hb. Patients develop iron deficiency due to haemosiderinuria. Bone marrow transplantation may be curative.

Microangiopathic Haemolytic Anaemia

This condition refers to red cell fragmentation and damage in the microcirculation and appears to be the result of small-vessel disease in part due to endothelial damage and the presence of fibrin strands. In children, the most common cause is haemolytic uraemic syndrome (HUS), although, it is sometimes seen in children with burns and following the insertion of some types of heart valve prostheses.

Aplastic and Hypoplastic Anaemia

This group of anaemias is poorly understood and clearly contains a considerable number of quite separate diseases which present clinically in somewhat similar ways. The defect in erythropoiesis may affect all elements of the marrow or only one, such as the erythropoietic tissue. There may be virtually no formation at all of the precursors or red cells, leucocytes or platelets. Fortunately, these conditions are not common, but those to be considered here occur sufficiently frequent in paediatric practice to merit the attention of all who have to handle sick children.

Congenital Hypoplastic Anaemia (Blackfan Diamond Anaemia)

Aetiology

This disease presents in early infancy as an apparent aplasia of the red cells. Granulocytes and platelets are unaffected. In most cases, the bone marrow shows a gross deficiency or erythroblasts but shows normal maturation of myeloid and megakaryocyte cells. The incidence is the same in boys as in girls but the disease tends to be milder in its effects on boys. Its occurrence in siblings has been reported in several families and family studies have suggested an autosomal recessive mode of inheritance.

Clinical Features

The presenting feature is pallor, which becomes apparent in the early weeks or months of life. Irritability becomes obvious only when the anaemia is severe in degree. Short stature is common and characteristic facial features are described by a snub nose, wide-set eyes and a thick upper lip. There are no haemorrhagic manifestations. Hepatic or splenic enlargement is unusual but may develop as a consequence of cardiac failure. Haemic systolic murmurs are common. The anaemia, often severe, is normocytic and normochromic. Reticulocytes are absent or scanty. WBCs and platelets show no abnormalities **(Fig. 11.14)**.

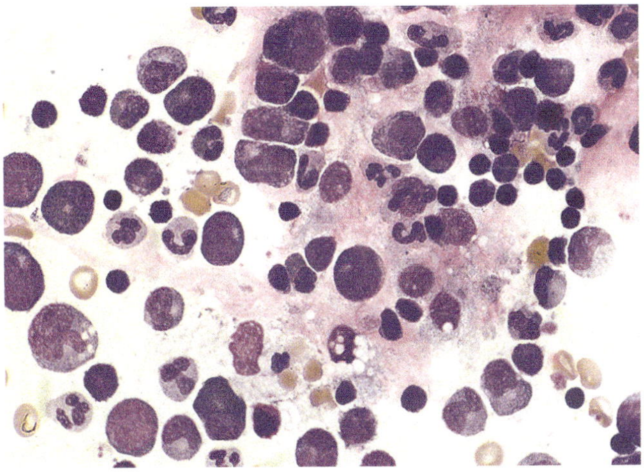

Figure 11.14 Marrow film of a child with Blackfan Diamond anaemia—virtually no red cell precursors on the film.

Fanconi-type Familial Aplastic Anaemia

Aetiology

This autosomal recessive disorder affects all three elements of the bone marrow (pancytopenia). Chromosomal studies in some cases have revealed an abnormally high number of chromatid breaks, endoreduplications and other minor abnormalities.

Clinical Features

Pallor may become obvious in early infancy, but more often the onset is delayed until between the ages of 3 and 10 years. Purpura and ecchymoses are not uncommon and there may be bleeding from mucous membranes. Defects in the radius and/or thumb or accessory thumbs are common. Mild hyperpigmentation, hypogonadism and short stature have frequently been reported and endocrine studies have revealed GH deficiency, isolated or combined with deficiencies of gonadotropins and adrenocorticotropic hormone (ACTH). Other congenital abnormalities are seen less frequently include microcephaly, squints and anomalies of the heart or renal tract. The blood shows a normocytic, normochromic anaemic, leucopenia, granulocytopenia and thrombocytopenia. Reticulocytes are scanty or absent. Leukaemia not infrequently appears in relatives and occasionally in the patient. The diagnosis is readily overlooked in patients who lack the characteristic congenital abnormalities, but useful diagnostic pointers are the presence of HbF, 1-2 g/dL in the blood and of chromosomal abnormalities in the lymphocytes.

Acquired Hypoplastic Anaemia

This is a rare disease in childhood and most cases are "idiopathic." The bone marrow is rarely completely aplastic in such patients. Some cases are secondary to the toxic effects of drugs such as chloramphenicol, phenylethyl acetylurea, carbimazole, thiouracil, phenylbutazone and gold salts.

Clinical Features

The onset may be acute or insidious with increasing pallor, listlessness, malaise, bruises, purpura and sometimes bleeding from mucous membranes. Death is due to haemorrhage into internal organs or to intercurrent infection. The blood shows a normocytic, normochromic anaemia, thrombocytopenia, leucopenia and granulocytopenia. Bone marrow must always be examined by needle biopsy or trephine. Marrow examination is, furthermore, the only way in which hypoplastic anaemia can be distinguished from aleukaemia to leukaemia. The prognosis is grave when the marrow examination reveals gross hypoplasia of all the blood forming elements, but in less severe cases there is always hope of a spontaneous or induced remission.

Albers–Schönberg Disease (Osteopetrosis, Marble Bones)

Aetiology

This is a genetic disorder of bone, usually autosomal recessive. The cortex and trabeculae of the bones are thickened, and the marrow is crowded out. Extramedullary erythropoiesis in the liver and spleen may prevent anaemia for a variable period. It is now recognised that the cause of osteopetrosis is a defect or deficiency of osteoclasts or their precursors which are derived from the pluripotent haemopoietic stem cells. Bone resorption is inhibited.

Clinical Features

The disease may present in infancy with progressive loss of vision due to optic atrophy, with cranial nerve palsies or with deafness. In later childhood, the mode of presentation is a pathological fracture or increasing pallor (**Fig. 11.15**). The anaemia is leucoerythroblastic in type. There is progressive hepatosplenomegaly. The most characteristic diagnostic signs are to be found in radiographs of the skeleton (**Figs. 11.16A to C**). The bones including the base of the skull, ribs, vertebrae, scapulae and pelvis show increased density. Typical zones of decreased density can be seen at the metaphyses and running parallel to the borders of scapulae and ilia; these still contain marrow. This disease should be differentiated from pycnodysostosis.

Pycnodysostosis

Pycnodysostosis is an autosomal recessive disorder of the skeleton characterised by dense but fragile bones, delayed closure of the fontanelle, defective dentition, hypoplastic terminal phalanges, short stature and not associated with haematologic or neurologic abnormalities. The main differential diagnosis of pycnodysostosis is osteopetrosis. Distinction of pycnodysostosis from other conditions is

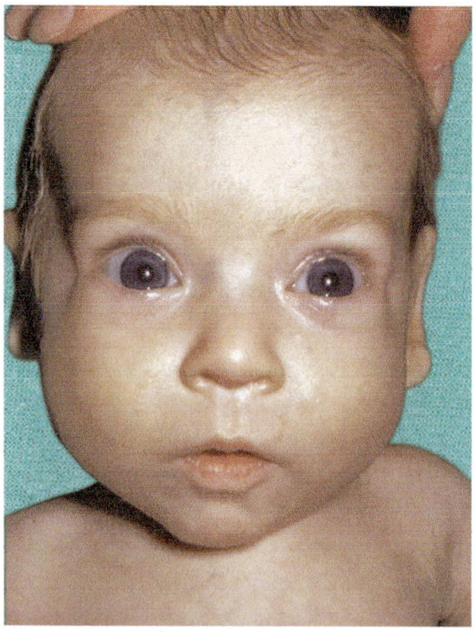

Figure 11.15 Osteopetrosis. *Note* the pallor in this child with osteopetrosis (Marble bones disease, Albers-Schönberg disease).

less likely to give difficulty. Neither craniocleidodysostosis nor acro-osteolysis is associated with generalised osteosclerosis **(Figs. 11.17A to C)**.

Thrombocytopenic Purpuras

Purpura is an extremely common clinical phenomenon in childhood and has many causes. The principal pathogenic factors are capillary defects and thrombocytopenia, sometimes both being present. In most cases, the purpura is symptomatic of another disease. It occurs due to decreased capillary resistance or bacterial micro-emboli in acute infections such as meningococcal (and other) septicaemia, bacterial endocarditis, typhus and typhoid fever, scarlet fever, etc. It may arise in scurvy, uraemia and snake-bite. Severe intrapartum hypoxia sometimes causes petechiae, especially over the head, neck and shoulders of the newborn. A similar mechanical effect is sometimes seen in the child who has had a severe and prolonged convulsion and in whooping cough. Symptomatic thrombocytopenic purpura occurs in leukaemia, hypoplastic anaemia and in states of hypersplenism. Fragmentation of platelets as well as red cells, with thrombocytopenia and haemolytic anaemia may occur in cases of giant haemangioma and after cardiac surgery. Congenital defects in the capillaries are seen in such rare conditions as hereditary haemorrhagic telangiectasia (Osler disease) and cutis hyperelastica (Ehlers-Danlos syndrome). It will be clear, therefore, that purpura reflects a blood disorder in only a minority of cases. Nonetheless, the more important primary diseases in which purpura is a prominent feature are conveniently discussed in this chapter.

Idiopathic Thrombocytopenic Purpura

Idiopathic thrombocytopenic purpura (ITP) accounts for the majority of cases of childhood thrombocytopenia and has been classified into acute and chronic forms. It is a clinical diagnosis reached by exclusion of other causes of thrombocytopenia **(Table 11.3)**.

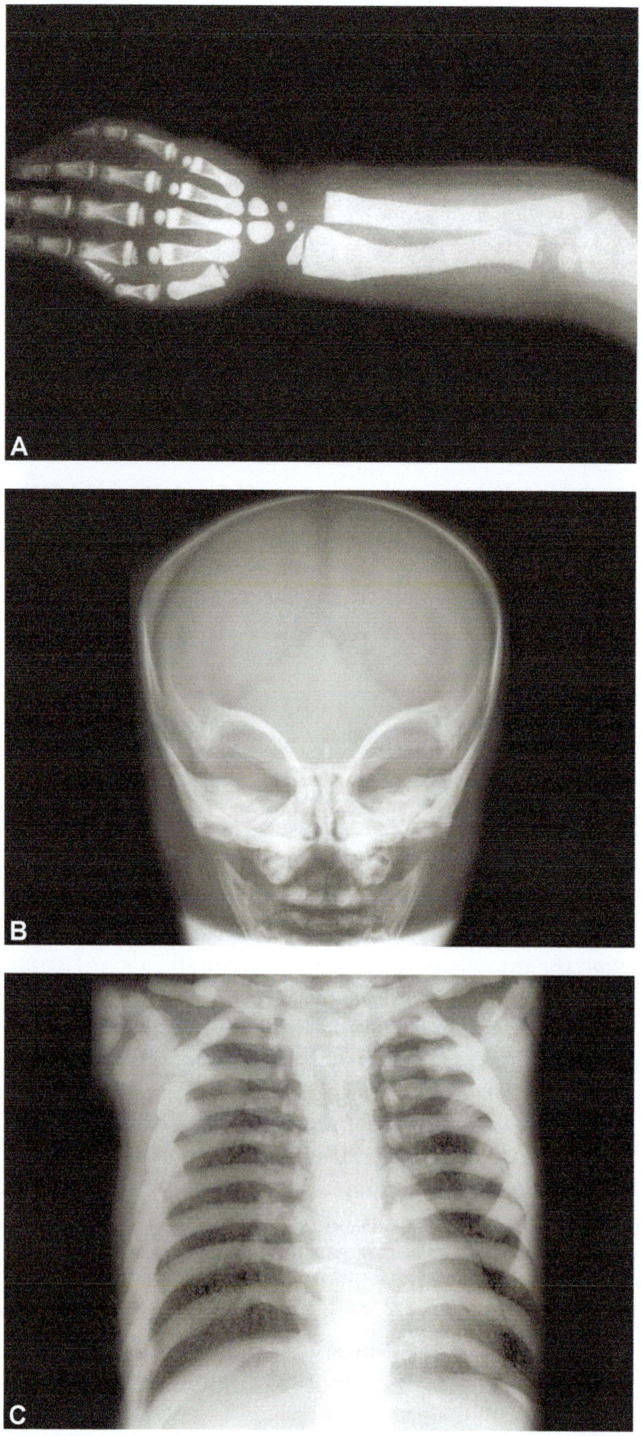

Figures 11.16A to C (A) Osteopetrosis showing zones of increased density of metaphyseal ends of long bones; (B) Face spectacles or showing White spectacle sign; (C) Increased density in ribs.

Clinical Features

Most cases in childhood have an acute onset. The peak age is 2–4 years with a male:female ratio of 1:1. There has

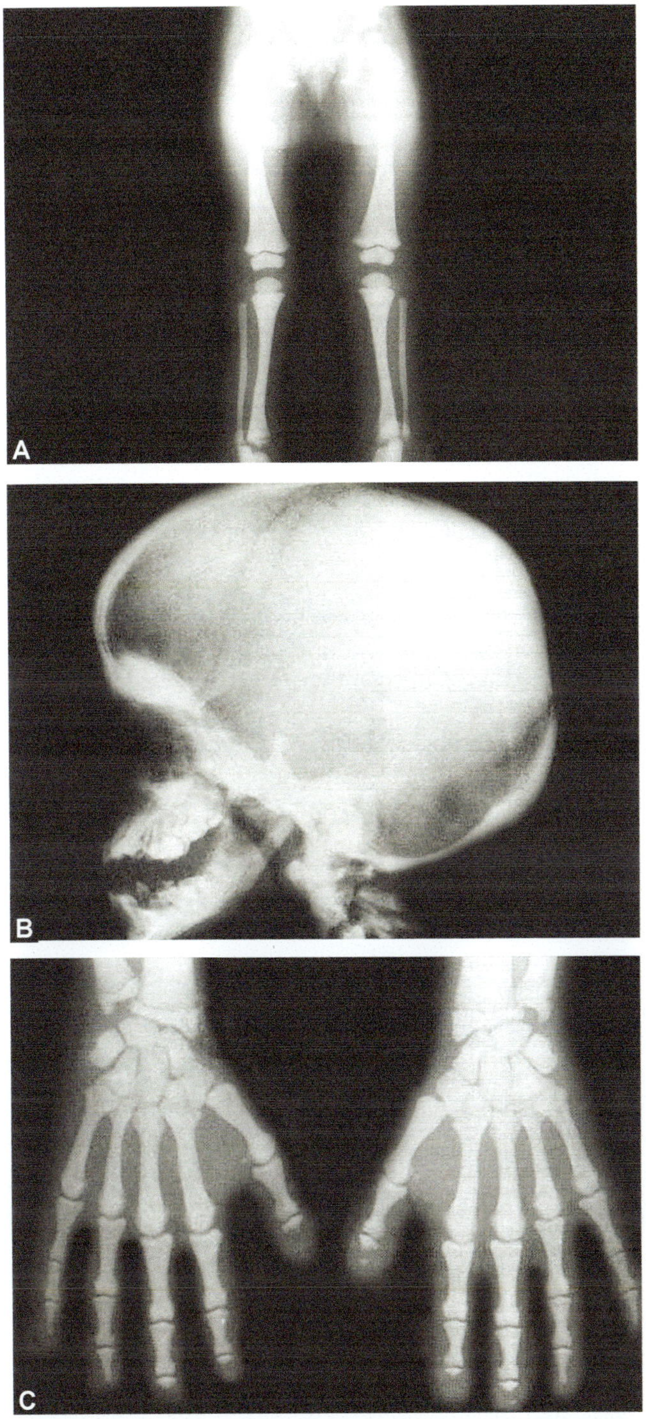

Figures 11.17A to C Pycnodysostosis (A) Lower limbs generalised osteosclerosis; (B) Open fontanelle and loss of mandibular angle; (C) Hypoplastic terminal phalanges.

frequently been a recently preceding, non-specific upper respiratory infection or other common childhood illness and immunisations have been associated. The first manifestation may be bleeding from mucous membranes such as epistaxis, bleeding gums or haematuria. Generalised purpura and/or ecchymoses are characteristic and often profuse (Fig. 11.18). The spleen may be palpable

TABLE 11.3 Thrombocytopenia in childhood.

Disorders of production	*Disorders of destruction*	*Abnormal distribution*
Leukaemia	DIC	Giant haemangioma
Solid tumour	HUS	
Aplastic anaemia	Acute ITP	
TARS	Chronic ITP	
Drug induced, e.g. cytotoxic therapy, sodium valproate, phenytoin carbamazepine	Autoimmune diseases (SLE) TTP, intravascular prosthetic devices, INTP	

Abbreviations: DIC, disseminated intravascular coagulation; HUS, haemolytic uraemic syndrome; ITP, Idiopathic thrombocytopenic purpura; SLE, systemic lupus erythematosus; TTP, thrombotic thrombocytopenic purpura; TARS, thrombocytopenic with absent radius syndrome (giant haemangioma, Kasabach-Merritt syndrome); INTP, isoimmune neonatal thrombocytopenic purpura

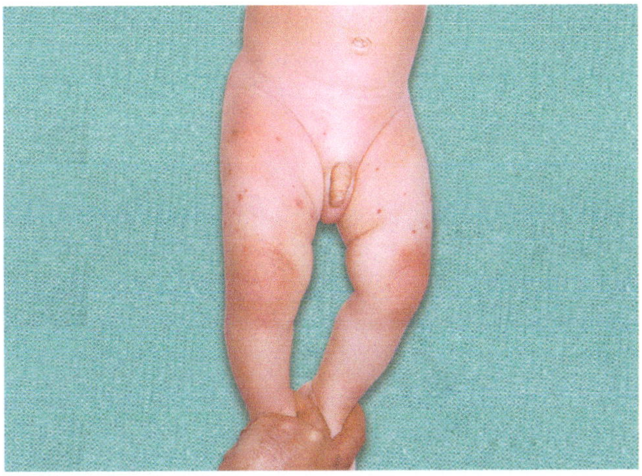

Figure 11.18 A child with Idiopathic thrombocytopenic purpura.

but never becomes very large. Life may be endangered in severe cases by blood loss or by subarachnoid haemorrhage (Fig. 11.19). The differentiating characteristic of this acute form is the spontaneous and permanent recovery within 6 months of onset.

KEY LEARNING POINTS

Meningococcal septicaemia comes into differential diagnosis of a widespread petechial rash but is unlikely in a well-child.

Non-accidental injury with bruises is unlikely because of the abnormal platelet count.

Chronic cases are also seen in which crops of purpura and ecchymosis persist beyond 6 months and occur more

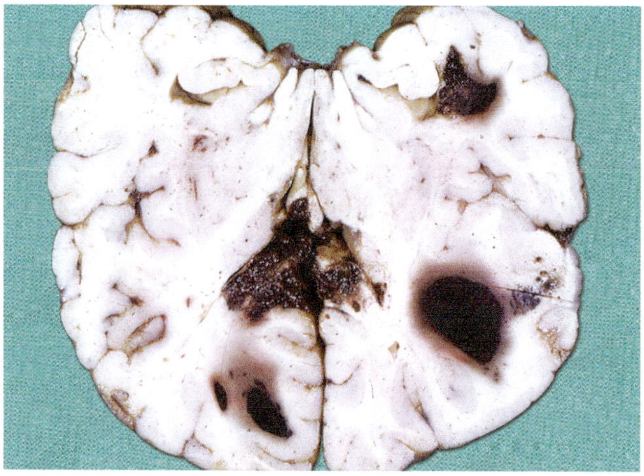

Figure 11.19 Clinical photograph of a child with idiopathic thrombocytopenic purpura developed intraventricular and intracerebral haemorrhage. He required emergency splenectomy but did not survive.

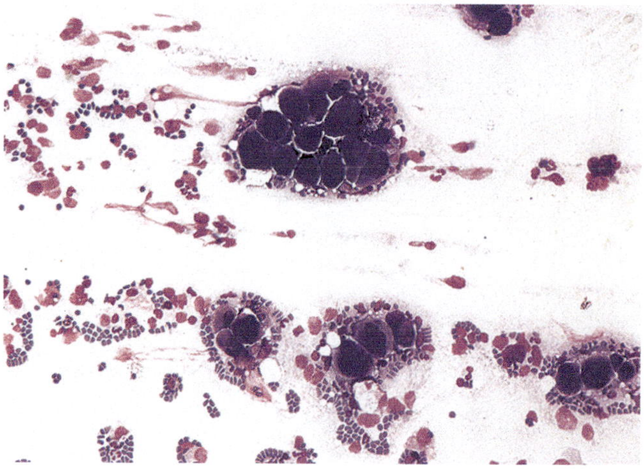

Figure 11.20 Bone marrow of a child with idiopathic thrombocytopenic purpura-showing excess megakaryocytes.

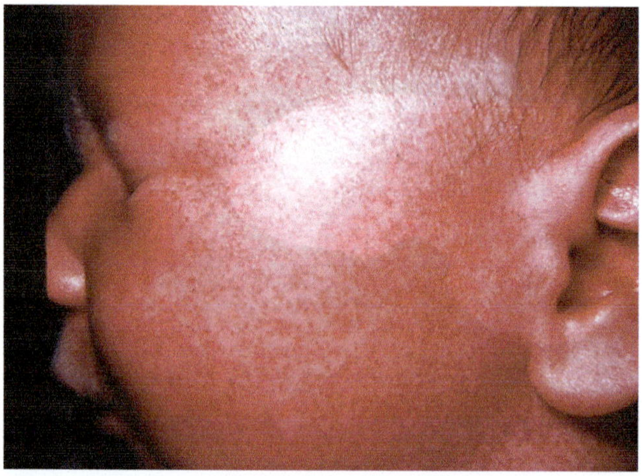

Figure 11.21 Isoimmune neonatal thrombocytopenic purpura; infant with facial petechiae.

frequently in girls. Children who have the chronic form of ITP may present at any age, although children over 10 years of age are at a greater risk than those in the younger age group. The blood shows a diminished platelet count. Spontaneous bleeding can occur when the count will be low and often is less than 10 × 10^9/L. The WBC and Hb are normal. Blood film shows no abnormality other than the absence of platelets.

A bone marrow examination is needed only when there is an atypical presentation or abnormalities other than absent platelets on the blood film or if steroids are going to be used as treatment **(Fig. 11.20)**.

Case Study

A 6-year-old girl presented with a 48 hours history of bruises on her legs and numerous petechiae over face and chest. She had epistaxis a few hours prior to hospitalisation. She had no previous history of easy bruising or being on any medication. In fact, she had been previously healthy. On examination she had widespread petechiae. She had no other positive finding and in particular had no lymphadenopathy or hepatosplenomegaly. Hb was 12.5 g/dL, WBC 10.6 × 10^9/L, neutrophil count 5.6 × 10^9/L and platelet count 1.5 × 10^9/L. The blood film except for the absence of platelets was normal. Immunoglobulin was normal. Blood urea, creatinine and urea and electrolytes were normal.

Diagnosis: The most likely diagnosis in this girl with isolated thrombocytopenia is ITP.

Neonatal Thrombocytopenic Purpura

It is well-recognised that the infant of a mother who is suffering from ITP or thrombocytopenia secondary to SLE may be born with severe thrombocytopenia. The infant usually exhibits generalised purpura and during the first few days of life there is a risk of severe haemorrhage into organs such as the brain, adrenals or pericardium **(Fig. 11.21)**. The pathogenesis has been shown to be the transplacental passage of antibodies which are directed against antigens common to all platelets. If the infant's platelet count falls below 10 × 10^9/L, prednisolone 2 mg/kg per day should be prescribed for 2–3 weeks with later reduction of the dosage. This type of neonatal thrombocytopenia has to be differentiated from neonatal, isoimmune thrombocytopenia in which there is foeto-maternal incompatibility for a platelet antigen absent in the mother and expressed on the foetal platelet membranes [isoimmune neonatal thrombocytopenic purpura (INTP)]. The mother is platelet antigen (PLA-1) negative and anti-platelet antibodies pass to the foetus and destroys the foetal platelets. The situation is analogous to Rh or ABO incompatibility, but there are as yet no reliable tests to predict the birth of an affected baby during pregnancy. In contrast to Rh sensitisation, first born infants may be affected and the risk of recurrence in future pregnancies is high. The diagnosis can be confirmed by the demonstration of antiplatelet antibodies in the maternal serum. These tests, together with a normal maternal platelet count and the exclusion of other known causes of neonatal thrombocytopenia [e.g. neonatal infection—including TORCH infections (toxoplasmosis, rubella, CMV, herpes simplex), syphilis, disseminated intravascular coagulation (DIC), drug induced or autoimmune thrombocytopenia] often establish the diagnosis of neonatal isoimmune thrombocytopenia. The best form of treatment is probably transfusion of platelets lacking the offending antigen, i.e. only the mother's platelets, which can be obtained by plateletpheresis. Exchange transfusion, steroids and intravenous immunoglobulins have also been used but the more effective treatment remains the transfusion of compatible platelets.

Twin–Twin Transfusion Syndrome

Vascular anastomosis is usually present in 85–100% of all monochorial placentae, and may allow the unbalanced transfer of blood from one twin to another. Such vascular communications may be obvious on inspection or on injection of dye into the placental vessels. The most common anastomosis is of direct arterio-arterial type, but some are veno-venous. Perhaps of greater pathological significance is arteriovenous anastomosis between the two circulatory systems. The twin-twin transfusion syndrome is one of the contributory factors to the increased morbidity and mortality in monozygotic twin pregnancies. It has been suggested that two types of twin-twin transfusion syndromes exist—a chronic form existing during pregnancy, and an acute form occurring only during parturition.

In chronic twin-twin transfusion syndrome, the donor twin, owing to an unbalanced transfer of blood, is generally hypovolaemic and anaemic and shows varying degrees of growth retardation. In severe cases, this twin may die in utero resolving in foetus papyraceous at birth. The recipient twin, however, is hypervolaemic and polycythaemic and is often the larger of the two. In severe cases, this twin may develop cardiac hypertrophy and congestive cardiac failure. Furthermore increased urine production by this twin may lead to hydramnios and precipitate premature labour (Figs. 11.22A to D).

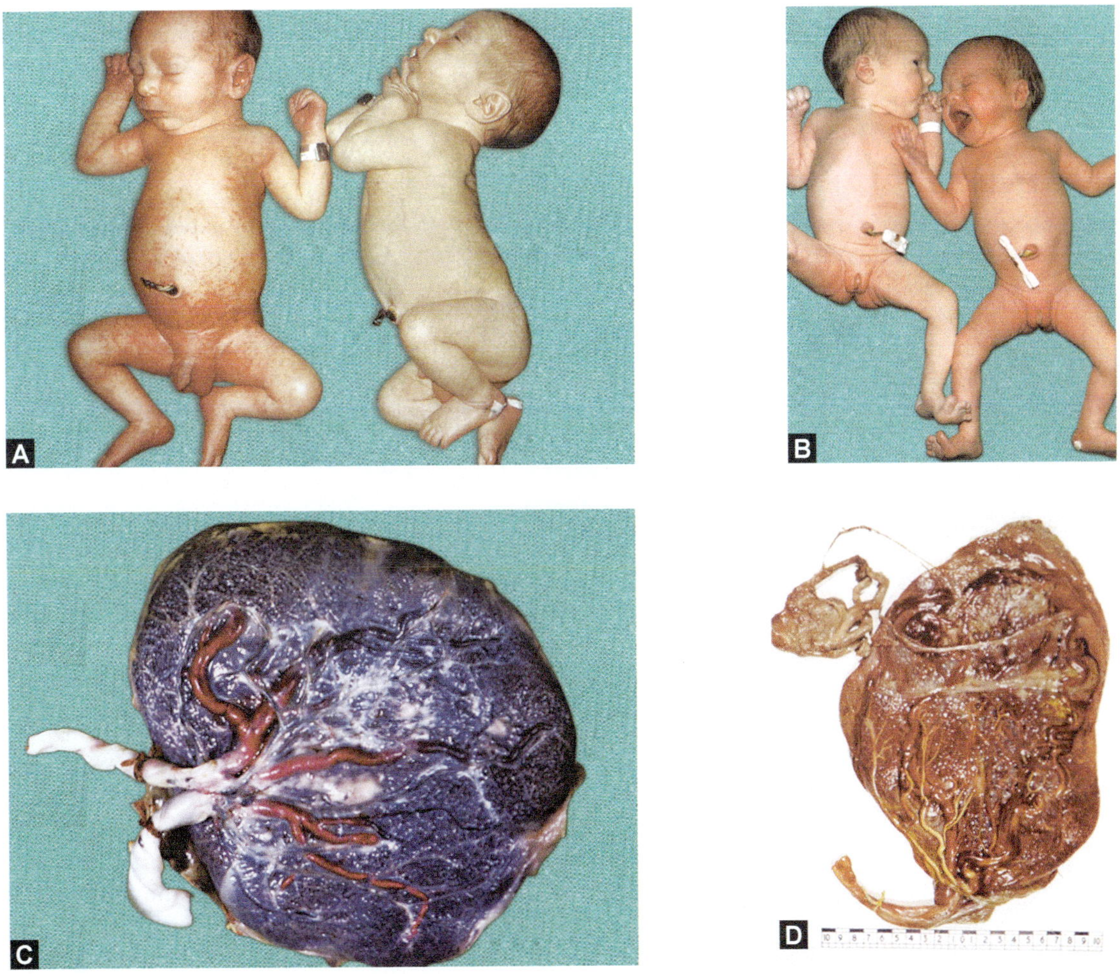

Figures 11.22A to D Twin–twin transfusion syndrome. (A) The infant on the left was born with a haemoglobin (Hb) of 24.4 g/100 mL, that on the right with an Hb of 12.2 g/100 mL; (B) Another set of twins: infant on the left with an Hb of 14.2 g/dL, that on the right with an Hb of 23.4 g/dL; (C and D) Placental vascular anastomoses.

In acute twin-twin transfusion syndrome, the twins are generally similar in weight and length but one is polycythaemic and hypervolaemic and the other anaemic and hypovolaemic.

Wiskott–Aldrich Syndrome

This is a rare X-linked recessive disorder affecting only males. It is characterised by the triad of severe thrombocytopenia, eczema and immunodeficiency. The majority of children die from overwhelming infection at an early age. Those who survive may develop reticuloendothelial malignancies such as lymphoma and myeloid leukaemia. The usual mode of presentation is during infancy with typical atopic eczema which may later be superseded by asthma. The bleeding tendency results in purpura or oozing from mucous membranes. Infections such as otitis media, pneumonia, septicaemia, meningitis and virus diseases constitute the major threat to life. Recent studies have revealed an immunological deficiency in this disease involving both humoral and cellular immunity. There is absence or reduction in isoagglutinins, progressive lymphopenia and failure to produce antibodies to some antigens after an appropriate challenge.

Henoch–Schönlein Purpura

See Chapter 12 on Paediatric Rheumatology.

Blood Clotting Defects

The mechanism of blood clotting is extremely complex and modern tests used to define the various congenital and acquired defects in this mechanism are only for the expert haematologist. The paediatrician must, however, have sufficient knowledge of the clinical types of clotting deficiency to use rationally the help which the haematologist has to offer.

Blood Coagulation Cascade and Screening Tests of Homoeostasis

The classical blood coagulation cascade involves the intrinsic pathway and the extrinsic pathway. Although, the mechanism of blood clotting is extremely complex, it is easier to understand it under these two headings. Intrinsic blood coagulation is initiated by contact of the flowing blood with a foreign surface while the extrinsic pathway is thought to be primarily responsible for initiating haemostasis as shown in Figure 11.23.

Screening Tests

Screening tests of haemostasis include platelet count, the bleeding time-measures platelet function and interaction with vessel wall and clotting factors such as fibrinogen and factor VIII. The precise diagnosis of each coagulation disorder may require very sophisticated coagulation tests.

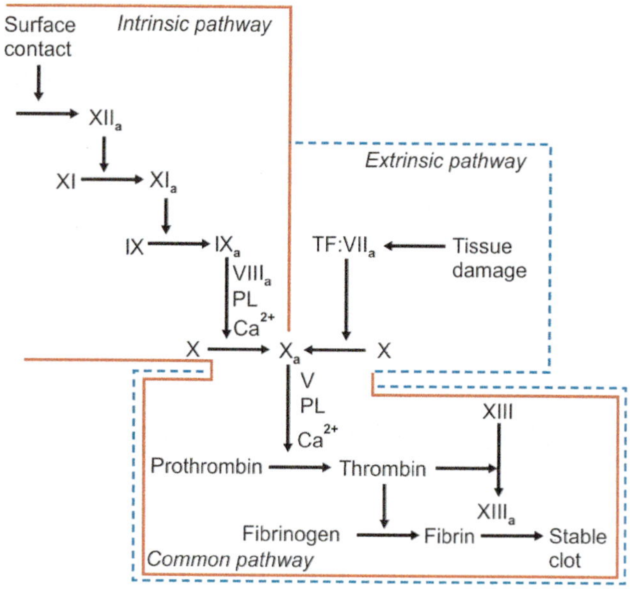

Figure 11.23 Coagulation cascade.

The prothrombin time (PT) measures the extrinsic pathway (factors VII, X, V, II and fibrinogen) and the activated partial thromboplastin time (APTT) measures the intrinsic pathway [measures the coagulation activity of factors XII, HMWK (high molecular weight kininogen), prekallikrein, XI, IX, VIII, X, V, II and fibrinogen]. The thrombin clotting time (TCT) measures the conversion of fibrinogen to fibrin. It is prolonged when fibrinogen is low from consumption, in hypo/dysfibrinogenaemia, in the presence of heparin and fibrin degradation products (FDPs)/D-dimers. Direct estimation of fibrinogen is included since PT, APTT and TCT are insensitive to levels of fibrinogen over 100 mg/dL.

Haemophilia A

Aetiology

Haemophilia A is the second most common inherited haemorrhagic disorder occurring in all ethnic groups. Deficiency of functionally active factor VIII is inherited as an X-linked recessive trait affecting males. Affected females are extremely rare.

Clinical Features

It is rare for haemophilia to become manifest during the first year of life. The outstanding feature is bleeding. The clinical severity of the condition is highly variable. It is classified according to the plasma concentration of factor VIII; severe less than 1 IU/dL, moderate 1–5 IU/dL and mild more than 5 IU/dL. This may take the form of prolonged oozing from a minor injury such as a cut lip or finger, from an erupting tooth, after the loss of a deciduous tooth or from the nose. There may

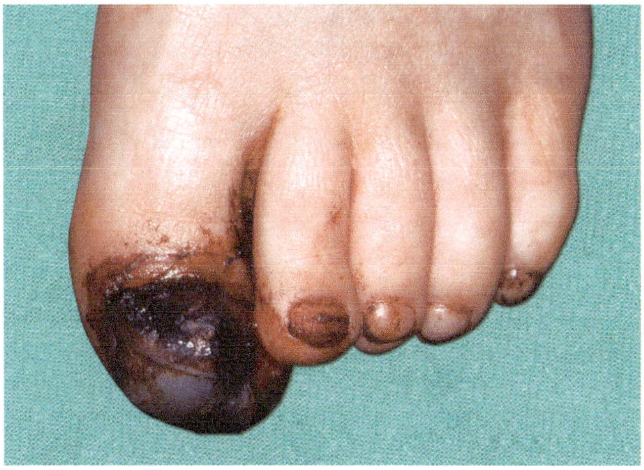

Figure 11.24 Clinical photograph of a boy with haemophilia A. The lesion from an injury to his big toe resulted in subungual haematoma.

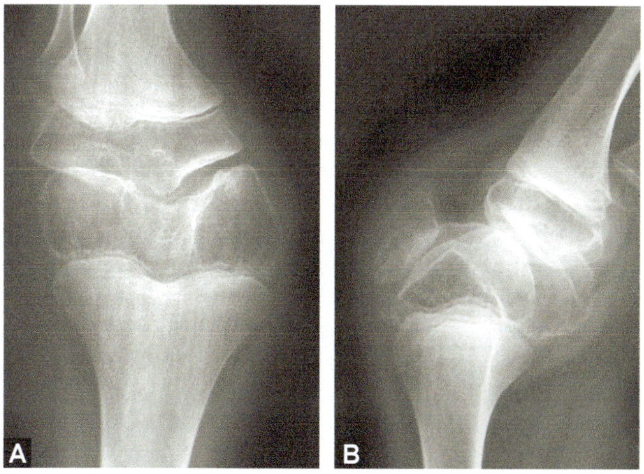

Figures 11.25A and B (A) Anteroposterior view; (B) Lateral view of the knee showing marked enlargement of the epiphyses around the knee, narrowing of the joint space, mild periarticular osteopenia, widening of the intercondylar notch and mild increase in the soft tissue density within the joint itself, corresponding to haemosiderin deposition.

be dangerous and persistent bleeding from circumcision or tonsillectomy if haemophilia has not been discovered. A common event is severe haemarthrosis, especially in a knee-joint after quite minor strain. A blow may result in a massive haematoma on any part of the body (Fig. 11.24). A deeply situated haematoma may threaten life by pressure on vital structures such as the trachea or a large artery. In some children who are severely affected, repeated haemarthroses may lead to fibrous ankylosis and crippling (Figs. 11.25A and B). Bleeding from GI or renal tracts is not rare. Cases vary considerably in severity but run true to type within each individual family. There is a fairly high mutation rate, and the absence of a family history of "bleeders" does not exclude the diagnosis.

Haemophilia B (Christmas Disease)

Aetiology

Deficiency of factor IX is inherited as an X-linked recessive trait. It accounts for about 15% of all "bleeders," being much less common than true haemophilia A.

Clinical Features

The disease cannot be distinguished from haemophilia A on clinical grounds.

Diagnosis of Haemophilia A and B

Both in haemophilia A and B APTT are prolonged because of the low levels of either factor VIII or factor IX. But estimating factor VIII or factor IX levels will help in confirming the diagnosis and classifying the severity. In haemophilia A, the von Willebrand factor antigen (vWF:Ag) and ristocetin cofactor activity (measurement of vWF activity) are normal. In both haemophilia A and B, the bleeding time and PT are normal.

von Willebrand Disease

Aetiology

Von Willebrand disease is caused by a deficiency or defect of vWF, which is responsible for the adherence of platelets to damaged endothelium. This bleeding disorder has been recognised with increasing frequency in children in recent years. It is inherited as an autosomal dominant characteristic and thus affects both sexes equally. The gene is situated on chromosome 12.

Clinical Features

The haemorrhage is of the "capillary" type rather than the "clotting deficiency" type as seen in haemophilia. Common presenting features include epistaxis, prolonged bleeding from cuts or dental extractions and excessive bruising. GI bleeding can occasionally be alarming and menorrhagia may be a problem in the adult.

Diagnosis

The bleeding time is prolonged because of abnormal platelet adhesion. The APTT is prolonged relative to the reduction in factor VIII. The vWF:Ag and ristocetin cofactor activities (measurement of vWF activity) are reduced. The PT is normal.

Case Study

A 4-year-old boy bled on four occasions from the tonsillar bed within 24 hours following tonsillectomy. The investigations showed: Blood—Hb 10.2 g/dL, reticulocytes 2%, white cell count 12.6 × 10^6/L, bleeding time 7 minutes 10 second (normal up to 6 minutes), PT 12.5 seconds (control 13 seconds) and APTT 42 seconds (control 32 seconds). *Diagnosis:* The most likely diagnosis is von Willebrand disease.

Disseminated Intravascular Coagulation Consumption Coagulopathy

Disseminated intravascular coagulation is the commonest acquired haemostatic defect that occurs when there is in vivo activation of the coagulation mechanism resulting in an accelerated rate of conversion of fibrinogen to fibrin. Fibrin may or may not be deposited within blood vessels but resulting in disseminated microthrombi. It is always caused by some underlying disease process. Infection is the most common cause of DIC. Within this category bacterial septicaemia (gram-negative bacterial infections) with associated septic shock is the most frequent infectious cause of DIC. HUS, meningococcal septicaemia, falciparum malaria, haemolytic transfusion reactions and some snake venoms can induce a consumption coagulopathy. Virus-induced DIC occurs predominantly in immunocompromised patients. In children, one of the most fulminant of DICs follows meningococcal septicaemia. Fungal infections are rarely a cause of DIC. Regardless of the underlying primary disease in the majority of patients the main clinical finding is bleeding and only a small number of patients will show thrombosis or thromboembolic episodes. Microthrombi formation can lead to the syndrome of purpura fulminans, which is characterised by peripheral gangrene of fingers and toes **(Fig. 11.26)**.

Diagnosis

The laboratory findings consist of thrombocytopenia, anaemia with red cell fragmentation on the blood film, prolonged PT, APTT and TCT, low fibrinogen and elevated FDPs or D-dimers.

Case Study

A 6-month-old comatosed infant presented with fever, convulsions and numerous petechiae and purpura covering nearly all his skin. The ecchymotic patches on his feet became necrotic and gangrenous. He had meningococcaemia and DIC. He had purpura fulminans.

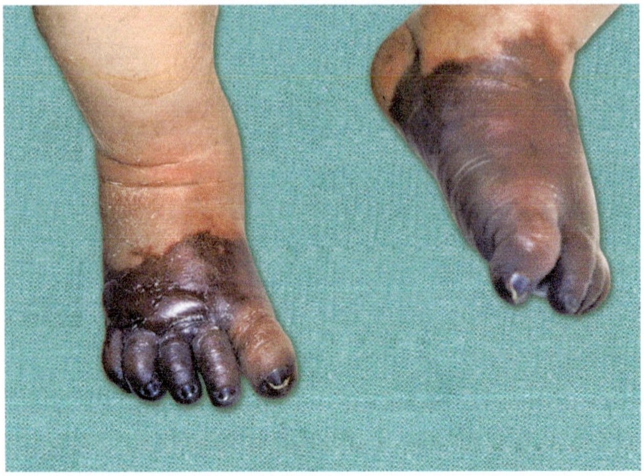

Figure 11.26 A child with purpura fulminans who developed gangrene of both feet.

Acute Leukaemias

In childhood, leukaemia is nearly always of the acute variety. On the basis of morphologic classifications, they are divided into acute lymphoblastic leukaemia (ALL) and acute non-lymphocytic leukaemia or acute myeloid leukaemia (AML) types.

Approximately 80–85% of acute leukaemias in children are ALL, and 15–20% are due to AML. Chronic myeloid leukaemia and myelodysplasia are rare. The exact cause of leukaemia remains unknown although the list of risk factors associated with childhood ALL is substantial.

Clinical Features

The most common symptoms and clinical findings reflect the underlying anaemia, thrombocytopenia and neutropenia that result from the failure of normal haematopoiesis. Therefore, the most common presenting features are rapidly progressive pallor and spontaneous haemorrhagic manifestations such as purpura, epistaxis and bleeding from the gums. These are associated with increasing weakness, breathlessness on exertion, malaise, anorexia and fever. In some cases, the onset takes the form of a severe oropharyngeal inflammation and enlargement of the cervical lymph nodes which does not respond to antibiotics. In two-thirds of children with ALL, the onset is with bone pains and half of these will have radiological bone changes. Arthralgia, secondary to leukaemic infiltration of joints may be difficult to differentiate from other non-malignant disorders such as juvenile idiopathic arthritis or osteomyelitis. Extramedullary leukaemic spread causes lymphadenopathy, hepatomegaly and splenomegaly. In some patients, however, the signs are confined to pallor and haemorrhage of variable severity and distribution. Infrequently, jaundice may develop or there may be early evidence of involvement of the CNS. Ophthalmoscopy frequently reveals retinal haemorrhages.

However, clinicians should be aware of the fact that ALL may mimic a number of non-malignant conditions.

Case Study

A 4-year-old boy presented being pale, toxic and ill looking with generalised bruising for 2 weeks. On examination, he had no lymphadenitis. Liver and spleen were 3 cm and 6 cm respectively. He had no fundal haemorrhages and no soft neurologic signs. Hb was 4.6 g/dL, platelets 4.2 × 10^9/L and WBC 600 × 10^9/L. Blood film showed numerous lymphoblasts. Cerebrospinal fluid (CSF) cytospin, no leukaemic blasts and chest X-ray normal.
Diagnosis: Acute lymphoblastic leukaemia.

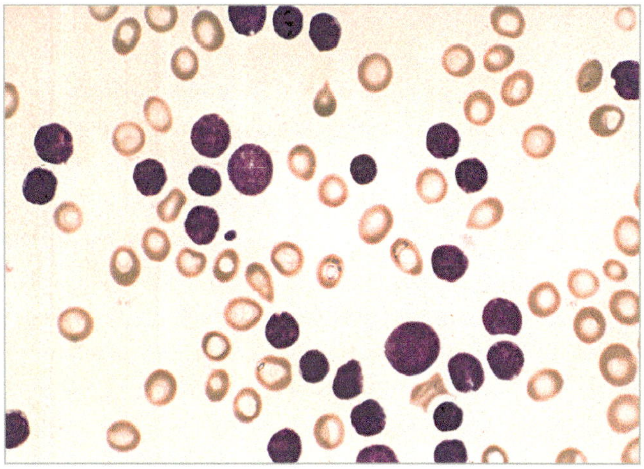

Figure 11.27 Photomicrograph of bone marrow of a child with acute lymphoblastic leukaemia.

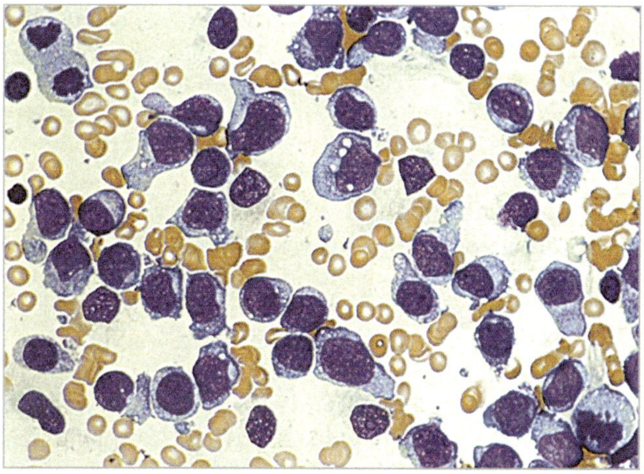

Figure 11.28 Photomicrograph of bone marrow of a child with acute myeloid leukaemia showing myeloblasts.

Blood Pictures and Bone Marrow Findings

In addition to severe anaemia, the peripheral blood films will show immature cells. These are most often lymphoblasts, less commonly myeloblasts and other granulocytic precursors, rarely monoblasts or neoplastic megaloblastic erythroid cells. The total WBC is often raised between 20,000 and 30,000/mm^3; only rarely to a very high figure. Thrombocytopenia is almost invariably found. Reticulocytes are usually scanty. It is, however, rarely justifiable to base the diagnosis of leukaemia on the peripheral blood picture alone. Bone-marrow biopsy will nearly always confirm the diagnosis beyond doubt, the films and sections showing gross leukaemic infiltration by immature or abnormal white cell precursors, diminution in erythropoietic activity and disappearance of megakaryocytes.

The majority of children presenting with ALL will have more than 80% of their marrow cells consisting of lymphoblasts, whereas it is not uncommon to see the presence of only 30–50% blasts in the bone marrow in ALL. The majority of childhood acute leukaemias (85–90%) can be readily separated into lymphoid or myeloid **(Figs. 11.27 and 11.28)** subtypes on the basis of morphology alone. Thus, although in most cases the diagnosis is apparent from the morphology, the final diagnosis of ALL rests on confirmatory cytochemical staining patterns, immunophenotype and cytogenetic studies. These studies are of therapeutic significance in lymphatic leukaemias.

Meningeal and Testicular Leukaemia

Meningeal and testicular leukaemia became a major problem when the duration of life for children with acute leukaemia progressively increased as the result of treatment with modern anti-leukaemic drugs. This manifestation commonly develops in patients who are in complete haematological remission and the incidence has exceeded 50% in some series. Not infrequently the meningeal relapse coincides with a systemic relapse. It is probable that a few nests of leukaemic cells are already present when the patient first presents and as the cytotoxic drugs do not readily cross the blood-brain-barrier these neoplastic cells are able to multiply in the largely protected environment of the brain and meninges. The child, who has been in systemic remission for months or even some years, develops headache, vomiting and meningism. A rapid increase in weight due to the increased appetite because of hypothalamic damage is not uncommon. There may be neurological signs such as squint, ataxia, or visual disturbance, but more often the only signs are of increased intracranial pressure, including papilloedema. CSF will show a pleocytosis due to leukaemic blast cells with increased protein and reduced glucose. The recent introduction of cranial or craniospinal radiation combined with intrathecal methotrexate has drastically reduced the incidence of meningeal relapses.

Testicular Leukaemia

The testes are a major site of extramedullary relapse in boys with ALL. Clinically, overt testicular relapse presents as painless testicular enlargement that is usually unilateral.

Acute Myeloid Leukaemia

The presenting signs and symptoms in this type of leukaemia are similar to those seen in children with ALL. French-American-British M4–M5 subtype manifest with extramedullary disease, including infiltration of gum and skin, lymphadenitis and CNS involvement. Sometimes, there are rare features such as chloromas, which are solid masses of myeloblasts which can develop around the orbits, spinal cord or cranium.

Investigations are similar to those for ALL. The myeloblasts usually contain Auer rods and these are seen only in AML.

Stem Cell Transplantation

Stem cells are primal undifferentiated cells which retain the ability to differentiate into other cell types. This unique ability allows the stem cells to act as a repair system for the body and replenishing other cells as long as the organism is alive, thus change the face of human disease.

The sources of stem cells are bone marrow, blood from placenta and umbilical cord. Stem cell transplantation may be defined as autologous (recipients own stem cells), syngeneic (twins stem cells) or allogenic (stem cells from sibling, non-sibling related or unrelated donor).

Allogenic treatment stem cell transplantation is generally employed in leukaemia and primary bone marrow disorders. Stem cell transplantation has also been used in Hunter syndrome, Hurler syndrome, thalassaemia major, sickle cell disease, immunodeficiency/inborn errors of metabolism, etc.

Langerhans Cell Histiocytosis

The term Langerhans cell histiocytosis is used to include the conditions previously called eosinophilic granuloma (single or multiple), Hand-Schüeller-Christian triad (diabetes insipidus, exophthalmos and large defects in the membranous bones of the skull) and Letterer-Siwe disease. These are not malignancies. They present in a wide variety of ways from non-specific aches and pains to specific lytic bone lesions, to wide spread lymphadenopathy, hepatosplenomegaly and skin rash. Chronic otitis media, diabetes insipidus and weight loss are common in some types.

The old term "histiocytosis X" has been modified into a form of staging system:

- Stage 1: Single lytic bone lesion
- Stage 2: Multiple lytic bone lesions [both previously called eosinophilic granulomata (Fig. 11.29)]
- Stage 3A: Bone plus soft tissue lesions, often associated with diabetes insipidus or exophthalmos (previously termed Hand–Schüller–Christian triad)
- Stage 3B: Soft tissue only, disseminated form (previously termed Letterer–Siwe disease).

The groups are not exclusive and overlap may occur. Stage 3B disease (Letterer-Siwe disease) mostly seen in young infants. They often have wasting, adenopathy, hepatosplenomegaly, anaemia and pancytopenia with red to purple skin rashes, seborrhoeic dermatitis and multiple organ involvement (Figs. 11.30A to D). In most cases of Langerhans cell histiocytosis the disease appears to be self-limiting so that minimal intervention is required except where the disease is clearly progressing.

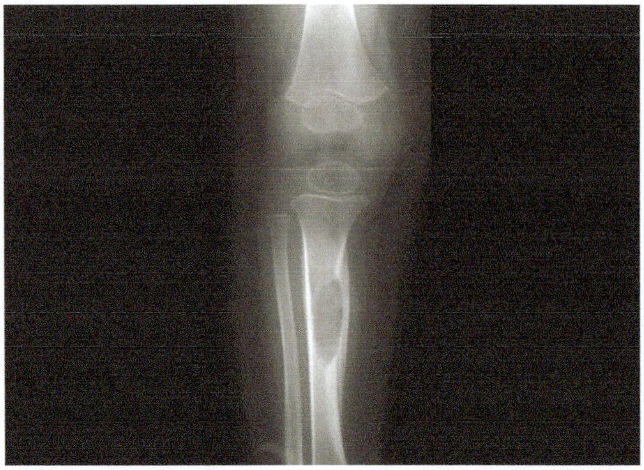

Figure 11.29 Eosinophilic granuloma: The lesions are mostly restricted to the skeleton and almost always are solitary, punched out, subperiosteal new bone formation can simulate neoplastic bone destruction. However, the bone lesions are similar to those that occur in disseminated Hand–Schüller–Christian disease and Letterer–Siwe disease.

Hodgkin Disease (Hodgkin Lymphoma)

Hodgkin disease can affect children at any age but is common in teenagers and young adults. Children with Hodgkin disease present with asymptomatic lymph node enlargement, most commonly in the neck. The lymph nodes appear to be firm and rubbery on palpation. In some cases, respiratory symptoms manifest due to tracheal or bronchial compression or facial oedema and congestion due to pressure on the superior mediastinal great veins, or dyspnoea and wheeze. Involvement of pleura or pericardium may worsen the chest symptoms. In other cases hepatosplenomegaly, jaundice and ascites appear. As the disease progresses increasing anaemia, leucopenia and thrombocytopenia may occur. Eosinophilia in the peripheral blood is rare. Also, fever, weight loss and night sweats are associated with advanced disease. The presence of constitutional symptoms, including unexplained fever more than 38°C, night sweats or weight loss of more than 10% of body weight, these three symptoms are classified as B symptoms and they are used in staging to indicate adverse prognosis. If the child has none of these symptoms, the lymphoma will be classified as A. Biopsy of enlarged lymph nodes is diagnostic (Figs. 11.31A and B).

The recording of disease extent using the staging criteria is essential and is based on the assumption that spread from contiguous node to node. The disease extent is defined as "stage of disease." Patients with different disease stage at presentation have different prognosis, regardless of the ensuing course of disease. Therefore, CT or MRI scanning of the chest and abdomen should be carried out to ascertain the degree of mediastinal involvement and for the assessment of hepatic, splenic and abdominal nodal disease.

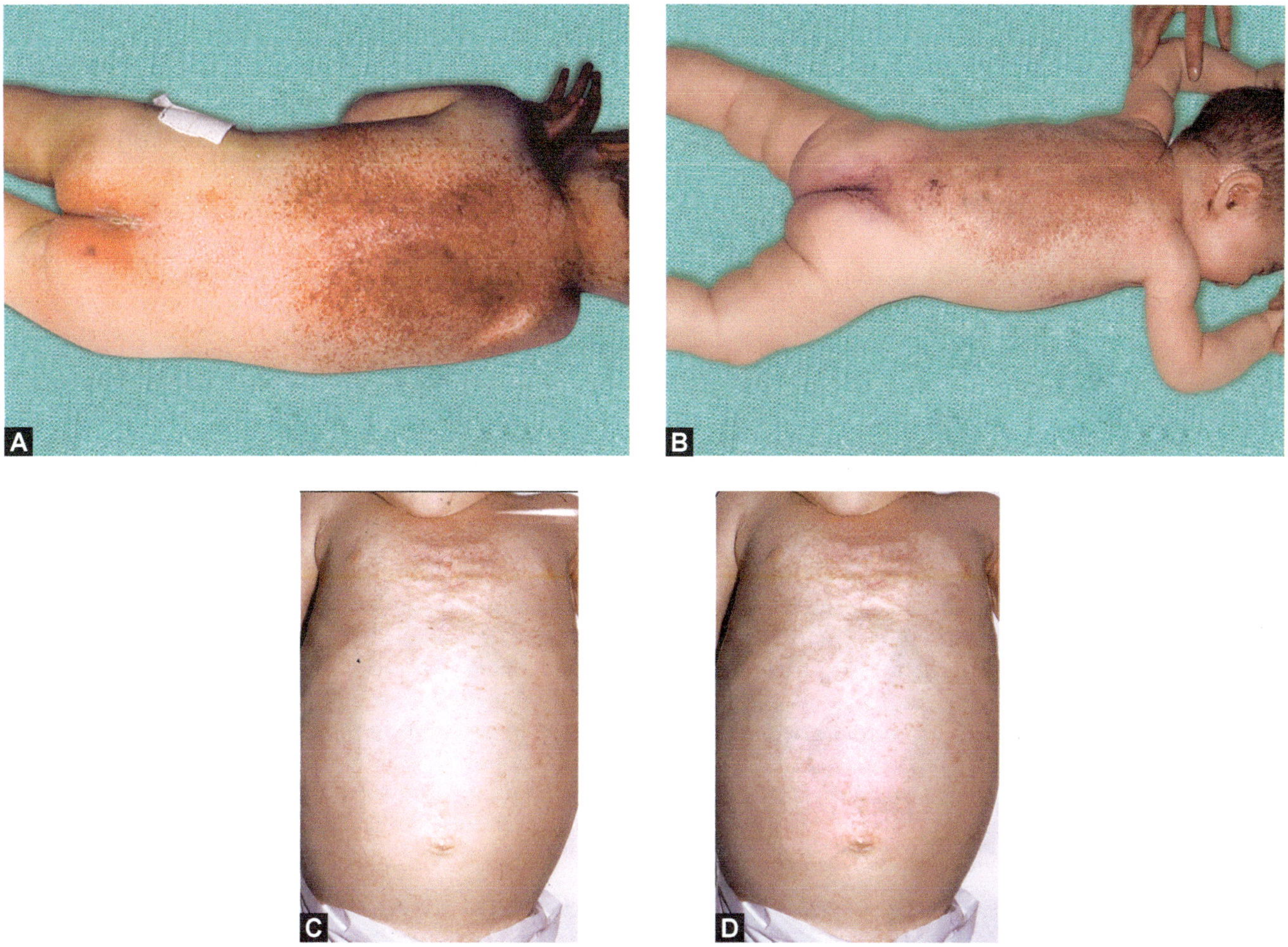

Figures 11.30A to D Clinical photographs of children with Langerhan cell histiocytosis (LCH). These children suffered from the subdivision of Letterer-Siwe disease showing skin involvement. The lesions ranging from seborrhoeic eruptions, erythematous lesions in axillae, groin and scalp. Infants with generalised cutaneous LCH lesions frequently have multisystem disease, with evidence of marrow, lung, and liver failure and systemic upset.

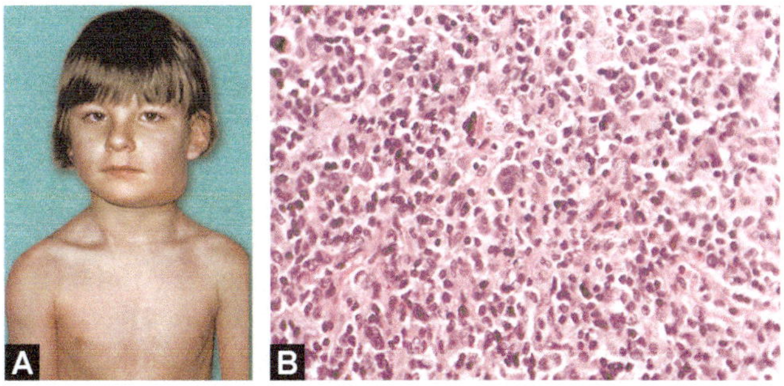

Figures 11.31A and B (A) A 6-year-old boy with Hodgkin disease presented with left cervical lymphadenopathy (stage 1 A disease); (B) Photomicrograph of lymph node biopsy showing Reed–Sternberg cells with two nuclei.

The staging classification for Hodgkin disease is as follows:

- Stage I: Involvement of a single lymph node region of lymphoid structure or involvement of a single extra-lymphatic site
- Stage II: Involvement of two or more lymph node regions on the same side of the diaphragm
- Stage III: Involves lymph node regions on both sides of the diaphragm. Also accompanied by involvement of spleen or localised contiguous involvement of only one extranodal organ site or both
- Stage IV: The lymphoma has spread beyond the lymph nodes, e.g. liver, lungs or bone marrow

CHAPTER 12

Paediatric Rheumatology

Paul Galea, Krishna M. Goel

INTRODUCTION

As most causes of recent onset arthritis are usually the result of trauma or infection, these children fall into the care of the orthopaedic surgeon. Whilst there is considerable overlap, the paediatrician tends to be involved in managing those children with chronic joint pains and arthritis, in whom there is history duration of at least 6 weeks. The aim of this chapter is to discuss the clinical manifestations of the more common conditions dealt with by the paediatrician.

CAUSES OF ARTHRALGIA AND ARTHRITIS IN CHILDREN

The causes of arthritis in children are multiple, and it is important to remember that many children presenting with joint pains do not have arthritis. The initial assessment of the child should include the following questions:

Onset Before or After 6 Weeks

Whilst most cases of trauma and reactive arthritis improve within 1 month of onset, most auto-inflammatory conditions such as juvenile idiopathic arthritis (JIA) persist for much longer.

Single or Multiple Joint Involvements

Single joint involvement is much more likely to signify local conditions such as trauma, sepsis or avascular necrosis as in Perthes disease and osteochondritis dissecans.

Episodic, Continuous, Flitting or Recruiting

Trauma and hypermobility are mostly associated with episodic pain, whilst autoinflammatory conditions such as JIA cause continuing symptoms and recruit new joints. Flitting joint pains are characteristic of rheumatic fever.

Associated Manifestations

The typical rashes in Henoch-Schönlein purpura (HSP), systemic lupus erythematosus (SLE) and dermatomyositis are usually diagnostic. Fever frequently accompanies viral infections but the persistent daily spike of fever in systemic-onset JIA helps to distinguish this condition from viral infections. In nonorganic joint pains, there are usually no associated findings.

Differential diagnosis of arthralgia and arthritis in children is given in **Table 12.1**.

JUVENILE IDIOPATHIC ARTHRITIS

Subtypes of Juvenile Idiopathic Arthritis

The term JIA was first proposed by the International League Against Rheumatism in 1997 to describe the different subtypes of arthritis and to distinguish chronic inflammatory arthritis in children from adult rheumatoid arthritis (RA). Although the condition is known to have an autoimmune and auto-inflammatory origin, its exact aetiology remains unknown. No triggering agent has ever been identified but an autoimmune family background is frequently present, in particular diabetes, RA and thyroid disease. However, sibling pairs with JIA are unusual. The autoimmune dysfunction results in a markedly increased production of intra-articular inflammatory cytokines leading to inflammation and hypertrophy of the synovial lining with production of excess intra-articular fluid and erosion of the cartilage, and ultimately bone, by the hypertrophied synovium. The following JIA subtypes are included in the latest classification:

Oligoarthritis—Involvement of up to four joints (usually large ones).

Extended oligoarthritis—Extension to five or more joints after 6 months from presentation.

Polyarthritis, rheumatoid factor (RF) negative—Five or more joints (large or small) involved at presentation.

Polyarthritis, RF positive—Paediatric equivalent of adult RA.

Psoriatic arthritis—Other features of psoriasis or first degree-relative with psoriasis.

Systemic-onset arthritis—Fever and rash at presentation, arthritis starting later.

Enthesitis-related arthritis (ERA)—Human leukocyte antigen (HLA) B27 positive paediatric equivalent of adult ankylosing spondylitis.

Other chronic arthritides including arthritis in Down syndrome and other chromosomal abnormalities and inflammatory bowel disease.

Oligoarticular Juvenile Idiopathic Arthritis

Oligoarticular JIA is the most frequent type of arthritis in children in North America and Europe. On the contrary, systemic JIA and polyarticular JIA predominate in most parts of Asia including Japan, China and India. Oligoarticular JIA occurs predominantly in young children less than 4 years old. It is defined as persistent oligoarthritis affecting four or fewer joints during and after the first 6 months of disease. It carries a 30% risk of uveitis, especially in antinuclear factor (ANF) positive children **(Fig. 12.1)**. Extended oligoarticular JIA is diagnosed when a child presenting with oligoarthritis continues to recruit new joints 6 months or more after disease onset. The arthritis extends to both large and small joints, becoming more aggressive and resistant to therapy. It carries a bigger risk of uveitis (40%) than oligoarthritis. The knee and then the ankle are the two most commonly involved joints **(Fig. 12.2)**. Oligoarthritis carries the best prognosis for remission though its course is often prolonged. The prognosis is worse for extended oligoarthritis.

Polyarticular Juvenile Idiopathic Arthritis (Rheumatoid Factor Negative, Rheumatoid Factor Positive)

Children with polyarticular JIA have five or more affected joints from outset. Both small and large joints are involved

TABLE 12.1 Differential diagnosis of arthralgia and arthritis in children.

Recent onset		
Arthralgia/arthritis less than 6 weeks duration		
Single joint:		
	Trauma	Accidental and nonaccidental Slipped upper femoral epiphysis
	Infection	Septic arthritis/osteomyelitis Transient synovitis/reactive arthritis
Multiple joints:		
	Reactive arthritis	Streptococcal, mycoplasma, enterovirus and EBV
	Vasculitis	Henoch–Schönlein purpura Kawasaki disease
	Malignancy	Leukaemia, neuroblastoma
Onset of chronic arthritis		
Chronic arthralgia/arthritis more than 6 weeks duration		
	Joint hypermobility	Benign joint hypermobility syndrome (BJHS) Ehlers–Danlos syndrome
	Auto-inflammatory	Juvenile idiopathic arthritis
	Connective tissue disease	SLE, scleroderma, mixed connective tissue disease (MCTD) Juvenile dermatomyositis (JDM)
	Infection	Reactive arthritis Lyme disease Tuberculous arthritis
	Apophysitis	Osgood–Schlatters disease, sever disease, etc.
	Avascular necrosis	Perthes disease, osteochondritis dissecans
	Vasculitis Malignancy Nonorganic	Polyarteritis nodosa, Wegener's granulomatosis Leukaemia, metastatic and primary bone tumours Stress, anxiety related

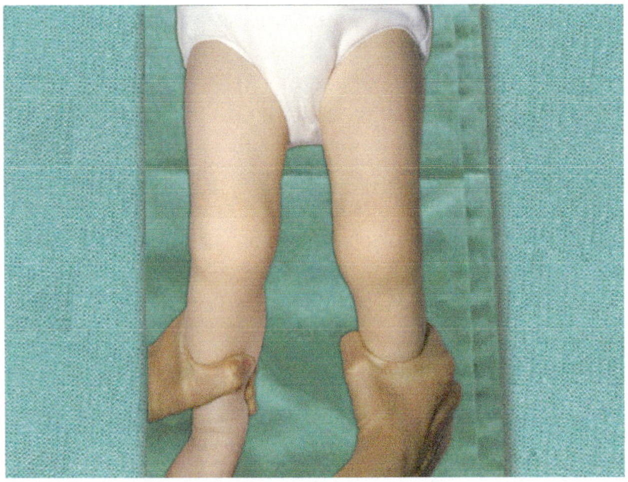

Figure 12.1 Bilateral knee effusions in a young child with oligoarthritis. The knee is the most frequent joint involved at presentation.

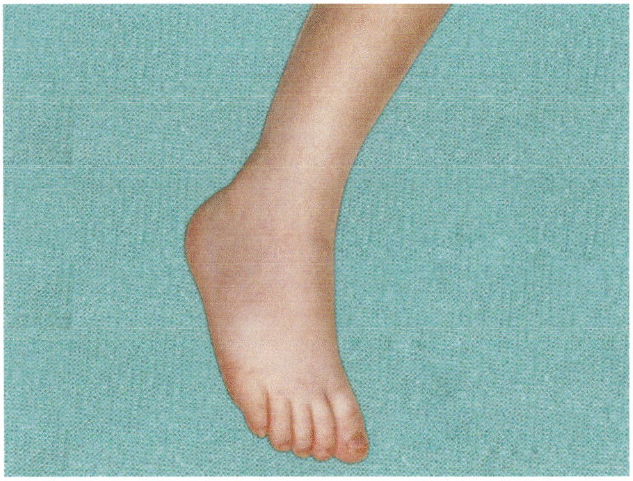

Figure 12.2 Warm swollen ankle in a child with extended oligoarthritis.

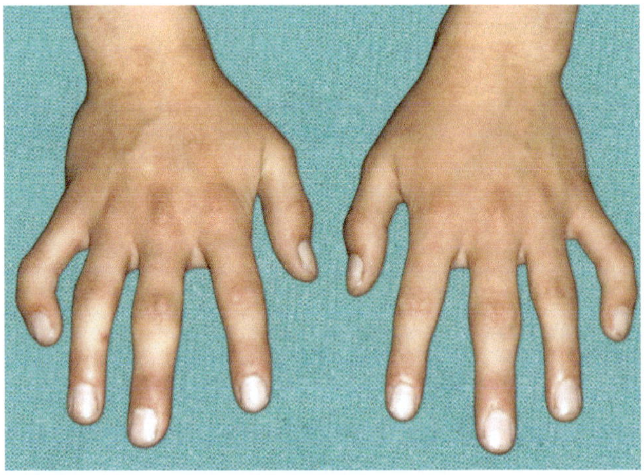

Figure 12.3 Polyarticular juvenile idiopathic arthritis: Swelling of the proximal interphalangeal joints in an adolescent.

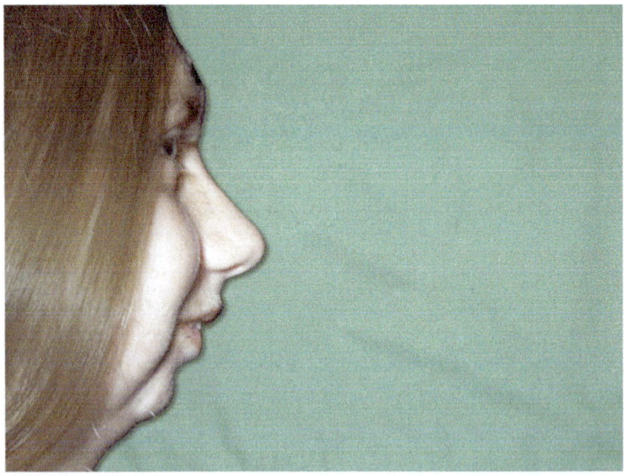

Figure 12.4 Long-standing temporomandibular joints involvement causing severe micrognathia in an adolescent girl with polyarthritis since 18 months of age.

with typically the proximal interphalangeal (PIP) joints of the fingers being affected **(Fig. 12.3)**. There are no systemic manifestations. Whilst most cases are RF negative, about 5% are RF positive. These tend to be girls of about 10 years of age or more and have a more aggressive course of arthritis than RF negative cases. They are the paediatric equivalent of adult RA. The risk of uveitis in RF negative cases is about 10%. Uveitis is very unlikely in RF positive cases. The chance of remission decreases as the number of involved joints increases. Longstanding involvement of the temporomandibular joints can be associated with micrognathia **(Fig. 12.4)**. RF positive cases are lifelong.

Systemic-onset Juvenile Idiopathic Arthritis (Still Disease)

The major signs and symptoms of this subtype of JIA are systemic. The most common age of onset of the disease is under 5 years, but it can occur throughout childhood. Boys are affected as frequently as girls. Characteristic features are high remittent fever and a rash, generalised lymphadenopathy, splenomegaly and polymorphonuclear leucocytosis. The rash has an irregular outline and is coppery red in colour, sometimes pruritic and never purpuric **(Fig. 12.5)**. The best time to look for the rash is just after the child has had a hot bath or at the height of the temperature elevation. The fever shows diurnal swings as large as 2°C or 3°C, which are rarely seen in acute rheumatic fever (ARF). Acute pericarditis is an uncommon manifestation. Endocardial involvement is extremely rare. Joint manifestations are frequently present at an early stage although they may initially amount to arthralgia without visible swelling. Arthritis may present later. Large joints are more commonly involved than small joints. Uveitis is unusual. Some children run a monophasic course with the disease remitting after 2–3 years, but frequently the course is chronic and relapsing,

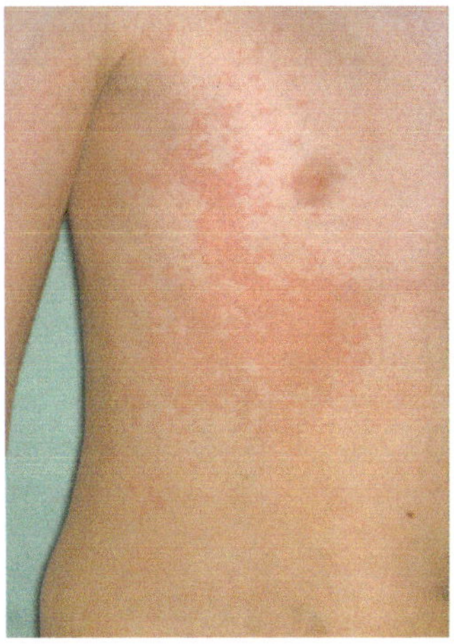

Figure 12.5 Systemic-onset juvenile idiopathic arthritis: Maculopapular confluent rash can appear on any part of the body but more commonly on warmer parts such as axillae and groins. Rash becomes accentuated during febrile periods and may disappear completely when fever settles.

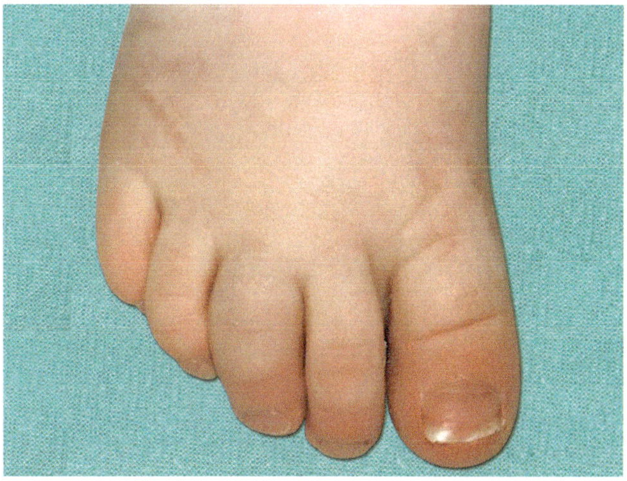

Figure 12.6 Dactylitis of middle toe in a child with psoriatic juvenile idiopathic arthritis.

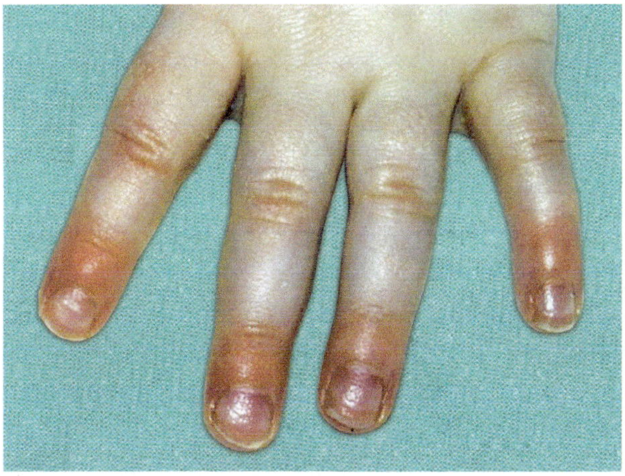

Figure 12.7 Typical pitting of the nails in a child with psoriatic arthritis.

with widespread joint involvement and persistent rash. Laboratory findings include anaemia, leucocytosis, an elevated erythrocyte sedimentation rate (ESR) and C-reactive protein (CRP). Gross elevation of the ferritin level can be a marker for the condition. The anti-nuclear antibody (ANA) is rarely positive. Macrophage activation syndrome is a rare but life-threatening complication of systemic JIA. The major clinical manifestations of macrophage activation syndrome are non-remitting fever, hepatosplenomegaly, lymphadenopathy, bleeding diathesis, altered mental status and rash and may mimic a flare-up of systemic-onset JIA. The typical laboratory findings are leucopenia and thrombocytopenia. A high index of suspicion is required. Early diagnosis and prompt treatment can be life-saving.

Juvenile Psoriatic Arthritis

Arthritis is frequently the initial manifestation of psoriasis in children and should be suspected when there is a family history of psoriasis, especially affecting one of the parents. It is similar to polyarthritis frequently affecting several small and large joints and typically involving both PIP and distal interphalangeal (DIP) joints resulting in a sausage-like swelling of the whole affected digit called dactylitis (Fig. 12.6). In over 50% of cases, skin manifestations appear after the onset of arthritis but close inspection of the fingernails sometimes shows the typical nail changes associated with psoriasis including pitting (Fig. 12.7), horizontal ridging or onycholysis. The risk of uveitis in psoriatic arthritis is minimal. Psoriatic arthritis is an inherited disorder and therefore lifelong.

Enthesitis-related Arthritis

Enthesitis-related arthritis (ERA) is the paediatric equivalent of adult ankylosing spondylitis. It frequently presents with inflammation of the enthesis at the site of insertion of tendons and fasciae into bone (Fig. 12.8). These sites become inflamed, painful and tender, which makes ERA the most painful arthritis of all the JIA subgroups. The arthritis tends to affect mainly the lower limb joints frequently presenting with painful feet due to a combination of arthritis and plantar fasciitis. Hips and knees are commonly affected. Back pain in children tends to be due to sacroiliitis. Axial involvement does not usually manifest itself in the paediatric age group. Ocular involvement is caused by acute uveitis and patients present with a painful red eye. Most children with ERA are HLA-B27 positive and ANA and RF negative.

Other Inflammatory Arthritides

Inflammatory arthritis is associated with several other conditions such as Down syndrome and other chromosomal abnormalities. Inflammatory bowel disease is frequently associated with arthritis of both peripheral

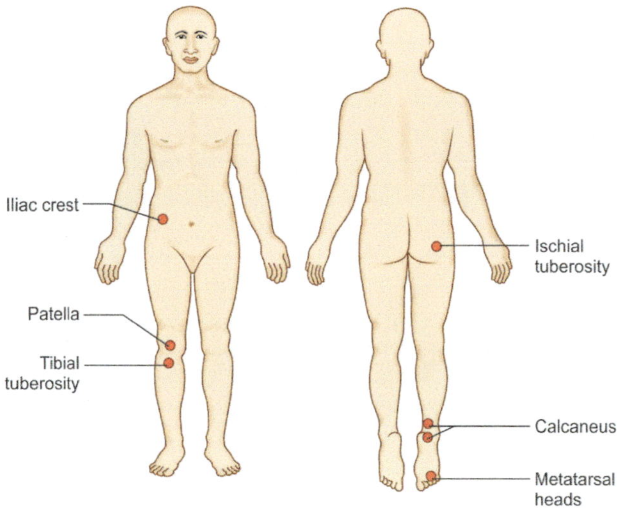

Figure 12.8 Enthesopathic sites in children with enthesitis-related arthritis.

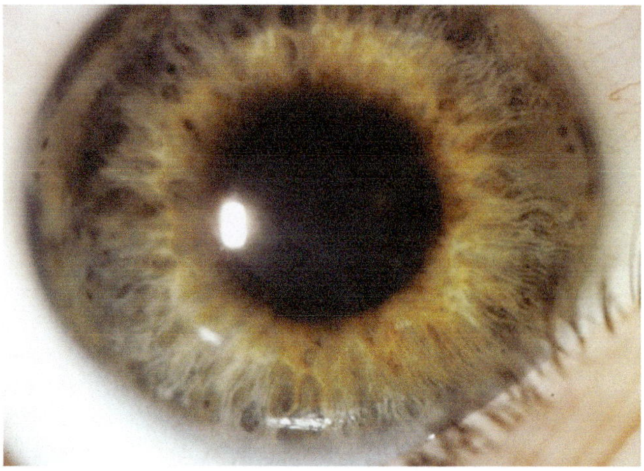

Figure 12.9 Juvenile idiopathic arthritis-associated uveitis causing irregularity of the pupil due to synechiae.

and axial skeleton, the severity of the arthritis tending to reflect the degree of bowel inflammation and improving when the bowel disease is brought under control.

KEY LEARNING POINTS

- Juvenile idiopathic arthritis is different from adult RA.
- Children with JIA often have joint stiffness but little pain.
- Enthesitis-related arthritis is the most painful type of JIA.
- The prognosis for remission in JIA becomes worse with increasing joint involvement.
- The risk of uveitis diminishes with increasing joint involvement.
- All cases of JIA should be screened for uveitis at presentation.
- Uveitis screening should continue for at least 7 years after disease onset.
- Systemic manifestations in systemic-onset JIA frequently precede arthritis.

Juvenile Idiopathic Arthritis-associated Uveitis

Uveitis is the inflammation of the internal lining of the eye. It frequently starts at the same time as the onset of arthritis, but sometimes follows arthritis onset by months and years. Occasionally, it presents before the onset of JIA. It is more common in girls, especially if they are ANA positive, and the risk of developing uveitis is inversely proportional to the number of joints involved. Every child presenting with JIA should have uveitis screening at presentation and this should be continued subsequently at 3–6 monthly intervals until the child reaches 12 years of age. Any delay in detection of uveitis allows complications such as synechiae **(Fig. 12.9)** and band keratopathy **(Fig. 12.10)** cataract **(Fig. 12.11)**, to develop in addition to raised intraocular pressure.

KEY LEARNING POINT

Screening for JIA associated uveitis should start at first consultation and continue 4–6 monthly for up to 7 years after JIA onset or until 12 years of age.

PHYSIOTHERAPY AND OCCUPATIONAL THERAPY

Physiotherapy and occupational therapy are important adjuncts to medication because they help to maintain and improve the range of motion of joints, muscle strength and skills for daily living activities. Exercises may be performed in the warm water of the hydrotherapy pool **(Fig. 12.12)**.

A physiotherapist should plan an exercise programme tailored to the child's needs. The role of an occupational therapist is to keep the child as independent as possible. The occupational therapist assesses any difficulties caused by the arthritis and advises the child, parents, schoolteachers and other carers on ways of helping with these difficulties, e.g. using specially adapted cutlery and pencil grips **(Figs. 12.13A and B)**.

JUVENILE REACTIVE ARTHRITIS

Reactive arthritis occurs when inflammation of the synovium is triggered in response to infection outside the joint. The exact mechanism is not understood but is thought to be an auto-immune response, frequently associated with certain viral infections (such as enterovirus, parvovirus B19, EB virus and rubella) and bacterial infections, typically streptococcal and *Mycoplasma*. Several enteropathic infections may be followed by reactive arthritis including *Salmonella* species, *Shigella flexneri*

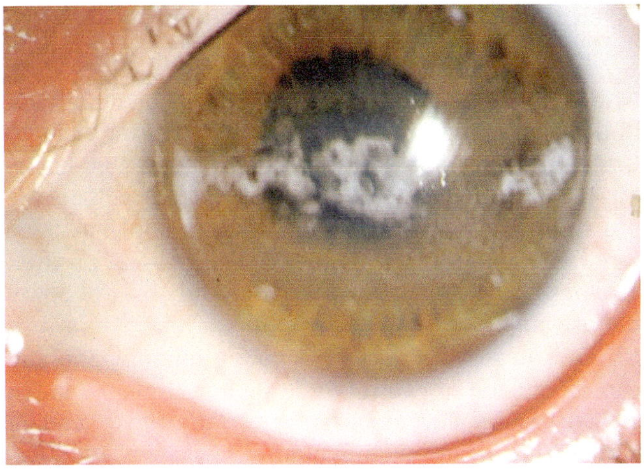

Figure 12.10 Band keratopathy, due to deposition of calcium in Bowman layer in the cornea, complicating poorly controlled, juvenile idiopathic arthritis-associated uveitis.

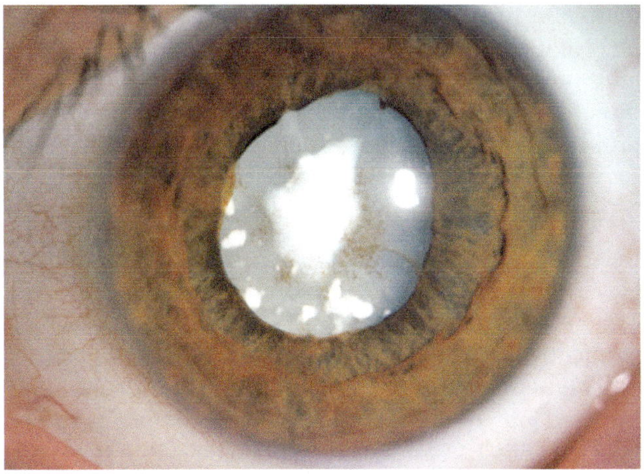

Figure 12.11 Dense cataract and marked pupillary irregularity due to synechiae in a child with severe juvenile idiopathic arthritis-associated uveitis.

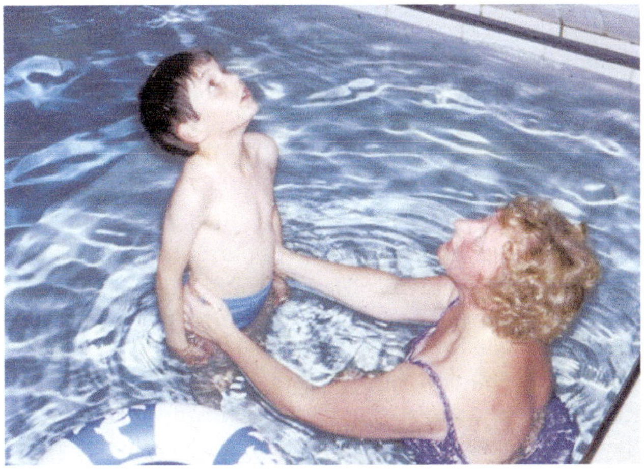

Figure 12.12 Exercises in a warm hydrotherapy pool help to loosen stiff joints and build muscle strength.

and *Campylobacter*. In many cases of reactive arthritis, no etiological agent is identified. The child frequently presents with acute painful swelling of one or both knees having been well the previous day. Other joints may be involved. The condition settles within a few weeks and does not usually persist longer than 1 month, hence the importance of the initial 6-week monitoring period before diagnosing JIA which persists longer and frequently continues to recruit new joints.

Post-streptococcal Reactive Arthritis

Children with sustained fever, arthritis, raised CRP/ESR and a preceding group A, C or G streptococcal infection who do not fulfil the 1992 Jones criteria for acute rheumatic fever (ARF) may be diagnosed as having post-streptococcal reactive arthritis. The arthritis is symmetrical and prolonged in character; knee and ankle

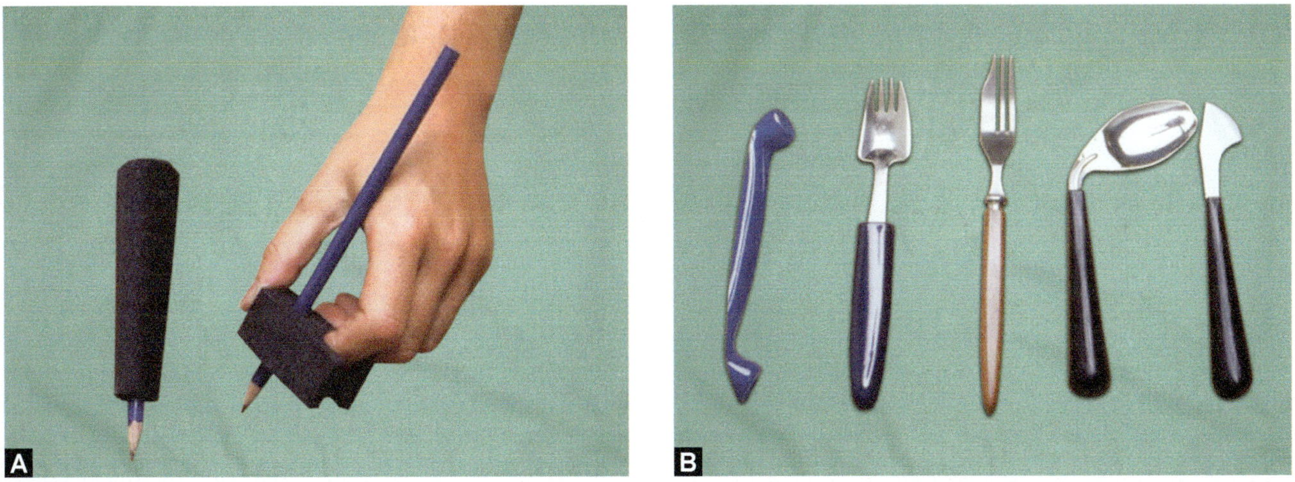

Figures 12.13A and B The occupational therapist assesses hand function and recommends the appropriate utensil to improve the child's grasp and handling ability.

joints are regularly involved but small joints and axial involvement also occurs. It has been suggested that ARF and post-streptococcal reactive arthritis are separate disease entities. Therefore, routine long-term antibiotic prophylaxis is not recommended.

Juvenile Reiter Syndrome

Reiter syndrome includes the typical triad of urethritis, arthritis and conjunctivitis, and is rare in children. The most common cause of this syndrome in childhood is infective diarrhoea, due to *Shigella* or *Salmonella* or other enteric pathogens. The knee is the most commonly involved joint but ankles and single toes or fingers can be affected **(Fig. 12.14)**. Diagnosis of Reiter syndrome is primarily clinical. The prognosis is usually good with gradual amelioration of signs and symptoms.

Lyme Disease

In 1977, Steer and his colleagues announced the discovery of a new disease called Lyme disease which they proved to be transmitted by the deer tick *Ixodes dammini*. The ticks may be carried on the bodies of birds, pets, wild animals or people. In 1982, it was discovered that the infectious agent is a spirochaete (*Borrelia burgdorferi*). The clinical syndrome consists of an initial febrile illness associated with a characteristic rash, erythema chronicummigrans, headache, aseptic meningitis, Bell palsy and vague joint and muscle pains. Left untreated, recurrent episodes of arthritis involving mainly large joints occur, lasting a few weeks at a time, with symptom free intervals in between. The initial phase of the disease may be mild and forgotten so that arthritis may be the initial manifestation of Lyme disease. The diagnosis should be confirmed with Lyme serology [enzyme linked immunosorbent assays (ELISA) and immunoblot assays].

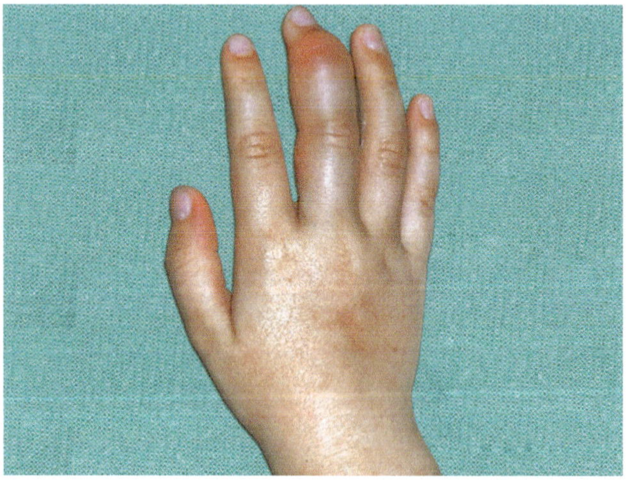

Figure 12.14 Dactylitis of right middle finger with involvement of both proximal interphalangeal and distal interphalangeal joints causing sausage-like swelling of the whole finger.

Arthropathy in Inflammatory Bowel Disease

Arthritis is the most common extra intestinal manifestation of inflammatory bowel disease occurring in both Crohn disease and ulcerative colitis. It predominantly affects large joints, especially the knees and ankles, but axial involvement (spondyloarthropathy) has been reported especially in patients who are HLA-B27 positive. The onset of arthritis usually follows the onset of bowel disease but may precede it by months or years. The arthritis tends to reflect the state of bowel inflammation and can be difficult to control until the bowel inflammation settles. Axial involvement tends to run an independent course from bowel inflammation.

BENIGN JOINT HYPERMOBILITY SYNDROME

Generalised joint laxity is a feature of the hereditary connective tissue disorders such as Marfan syndrome, Ehlers-Danlos syndrome and osteogenesis imperfecta. However, hypermobility without other associations is common in the general population. Hypermobility denotes the ability to move joints through a bigger range than normal. Whist in many children this is asymptomatic, in some it is associated with joint pains, particularly in the lower limbs. This condition is called benign joint hypermobility syndrome (BJHS). The pains typically come on during or immediately after exercise, causing the child to stop and ask to be lifted. They occur mostly in the evenings sometimes waking the child up during the night. They frequently are related to the amount of activity the child performs during daytime. Hypermobile children are frequently described as being clumsy, frequently tripping and falling and being accident prone and have been shown to have poor proprioception. Assessment of the degree of hypermobility includes assessment of the Beighton score. One point is awarded for each of the following:

Ability to hyperabduct the thumbs to touch the forearm	right 1 point	left 1 point
Ability to extend the small finger beyond 90°	right 1 point	left 1 point
Hyperextension of both knees	right 1 point	left 1 point
Hyperextension of elbows beyond 190°	right 1 point	left 1 point
Ability to touch floor with palms while keeping knees straight		1 point

A score of six or more indicates generalised hypermobility **(Figs. 12.15A to E)**. In some children, hypermobility may be localised to only a few joints with symptoms occurring only in affected joints.

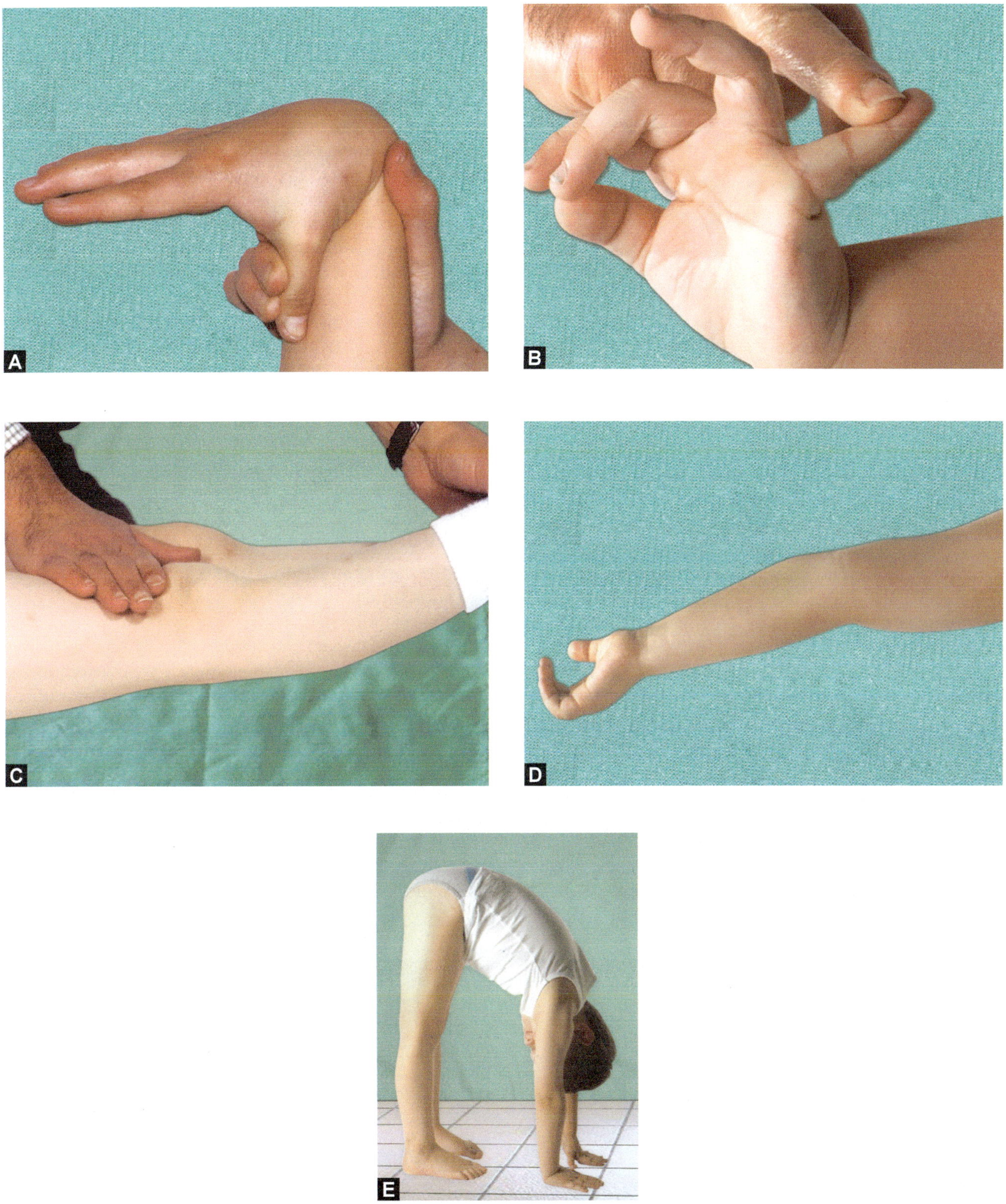

Figures 12.15A to E Assessing degree of hypermobility in a child as described in the Beighton scoring system.

KEY LEARNING POINTS

- Benign joint hypermobility syndrome is a common cause of joint pain in children.
- Pain occurs during exercise and later on in the day.
- Nocturnal pain in the legs frequently occurs.
- About 50% of children continue to have joint pains in adult life.

LIMB PAINS OF CHILDHOOD WITH NO ORGANIC DISEASE (IDIOPATHIC LIMB PAINS)

Growing pains in children occur during the period of rapid growth between 3 and 10 years of age. The child typically wakes up during the night complaining of severe pain in the lower limbs, especially in the legs and knees, without any obvious visible abnormality. Rubbing of the affected area together with simple analgesia helps. The child goes back to sleep after 30–60 minutes, waking up in the morning perfectly well. In most cases, no cause for these pains can be identified. The parents need to be reassured that these pains are common and harmless. In some cases, similar night pain occurs in association with BJHS. Other causes of night pain to be included in the differential diagnosis include bone pain secondary to leukaemia, bony metastasis from a neuroblastoma and more rarely, a bone tumour. In these cases, however, some pain occurs during the daytime and/or may be felt in parts of the body other than the lower limbs.

In older children, particularly in adolescents, pain may be a manifestation of anxiety and stress and not necessarily associated with organic pathology. Pain is usually far in excess of clinical manifestations and when careful examination and investigation fail to identify any abnormality, psychogenic causes for arthralgia should be considered and the opinion of a child psychologist should be sought.

Case Study

A 10-year-old girl presented with nocturnal lower limb pains for 6 months. At no time did she have swelling or tenderness of any of her joints. She had no other symptoms but she had been worried about her exams. Her maternal grandmother had osteoarthritis and maternal aunt was crippled with RA. On clinical examination, no positive finding was detected. In particular, she had no evidence of active synovitis.

Full blood count, urea and electrolytes, liver function test, RF, ANA, ESR and CRP were normal. She was diagnosed as having nonorganic nocturnal lower limb pains. Parents and the child were reassured that she did not have RA. With firm reassurance within a few weeks her symptoms settled and she was discharged from follow-up.

Diagnosis: Idiopathic nocturnal lower limb pains.

JUVENILE DERMATOMYOSITIS

Juvenile dermatomyositis (JDM) is an autoimmune disorder consisting of a vasculopathy affecting primarily skin and muscle and frequently other systems. It occurs in children aged 2 years and over, frequently starting insidiously with increasing proximal muscle weakness and the appearance of a purple red diffuse rash most prominent on bony prominences such as knees, elbows and ankles. On the face, it involves the heliotrope area around the eyes, in particular the upper eyelid **(Figs. 12.16A and B)**. On the hands and fingers, it appears over the metacarpophalangeal, PIP and DIP joints and at the fingertips. This characteristic appearance is described as Gottron rash **(Figs. 12.17 and 12.18)**. Close inspection of the nail folds, eyelid edges and gums shows erythema and

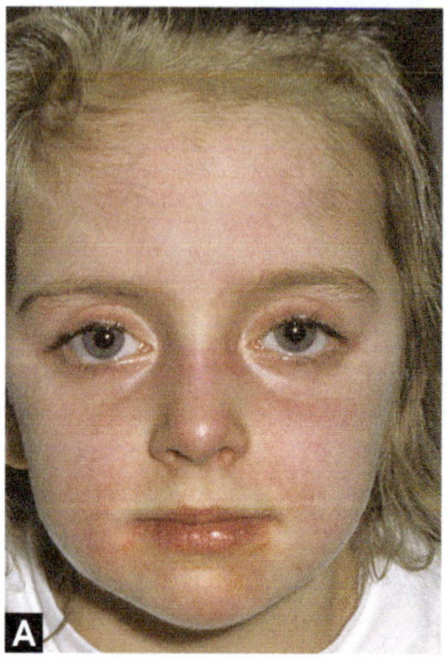

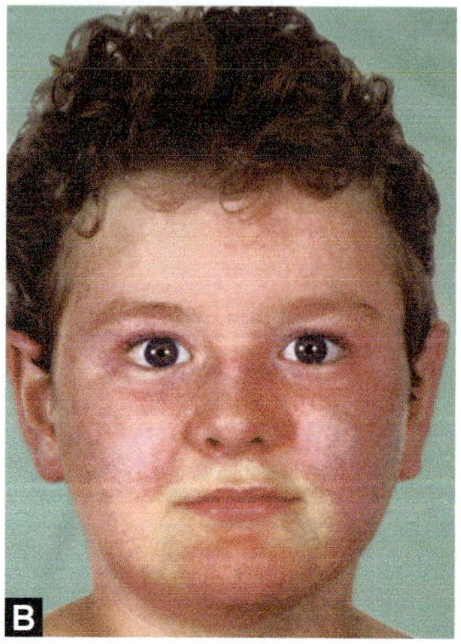

Figures 12.16A and B Juvenile dermatomyositis rash causing red facies in two children with clear involvement of the heliotrope area and sparing of the perioral region.

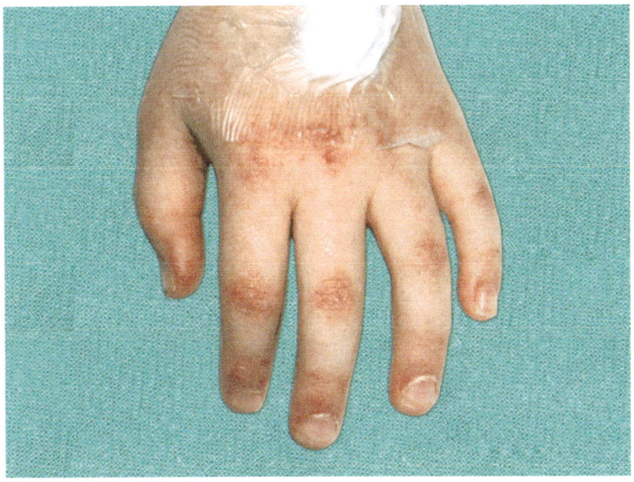

Figure 12.17 Juvenile dermatomyositis: Gottron rash.

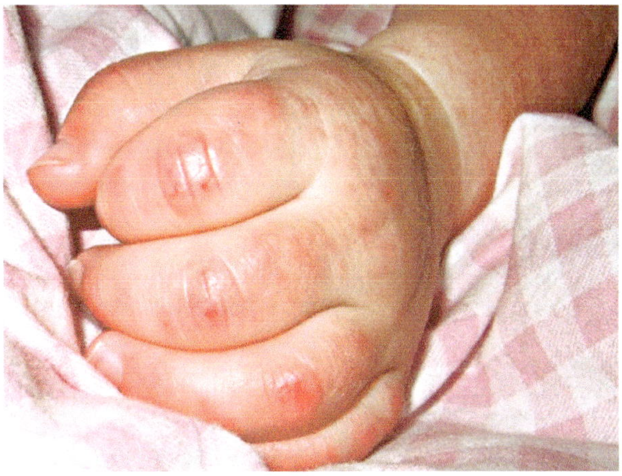

Figure 12.18 Juvenile dermatomyositis: Gottron rash in a young child associated with oedema of the fingers and hand. Generalised oedema can be a presenting manifestation in young children and prior to the appearance of the rash, the picture may resemble that of nephrotic syndrome.

dilated blood vessels suggestive of vasculitis. The myopathy manifests itself with increasing weakness, the child complaining of feeling tired, unable to run, finding difficulty with climbing stairs and having to find support to get off the floor (Gower sign). Occasionally, generalised oedema of subcutaneous tissues occurs causing the facial appearance to resemble nephrotic syndrome. Twenty-five per cent of cases have associated polyarthritis. The younger the child, the more acute tends to be the onset with children becoming very tired and having widespread rash within a few weeks of onset. Rapidly deteriorating cases may have dysphonia, dysphagia, choking due to aspiration and breathing difficulty because of respiratory muscle weakness. In older children, onset may be more insidious. When the child is investigated for lethargy, raised blood transaminases may be mistakenly attributed to liver disease prompting referral to gastroenterology.

The diagnosis of JDM is based on a combination of the clinical findings and biochemical abnormalities. Inflamed muscles frequently cause a rise in the level of aspartate aminotransferase (AST), aldolase, lactic dehydrogenase and creatine kinase in the blood whilst gamma glutamyltransferase remains normal. ESR and CRP may be raised. ANF is usually negative. In some cases, no biochemical abnormalities are present. Confirmation of the diagnosis used to be made by muscle biopsy and/or electromyography, but these invasive procedures have been superseded by muscle magnetic resonance imaging (MRI). Inflamed muscle is oedematous and gives a hyper intense signal on MRI T2 weighted scans. MRI is used to compare the appearance of inflamed muscle with that of subcutaneous fat that appears very hyper intense on T2 weighted scans. The higher the muscle to fat ratio, the stronger is the diagnosis.

Juvenile dermatomyositis runs a variable course in different patients. An acute presentation with rapid deterioration tends to happen in younger children less than 5 years of age. Frequently, this runs a monophasic course lasting 1–2 years and burns itself out. In older children, a more insidious onset tends to occur with low-grade disease activity continuing for several years once it has been controlled with therapy. Occasionally, patients run a multiphasic course, with the disease responding to treatment only to flare up again after a few months.

Calcinosis is a long-term complication in many patients, especially in those with a florid rash. This takes the form of calcific lumps in the skin and subcutaneous tissues particularly on bony prominences although it can occur everywhere. Subcutaneous tissues and fascial planes can become calcified giving a hard feel to the skin and in some cases even interfering with mobility **(Figs. 12.19 and 12.20)**.

In some cases, lipoatrophy may complicate JDM causing localised areas of subcutaneous fat atrophy, leaving the skin thin, wrinkled and lumpy. This is very cosmetically unacceptable to the patient, especially the adolescent.

KEY LEARNING POINTS

- Elevation of plasma AST and alanine aminotransferase (ALT) may be caused by both liver and muscle disorders.
- Some cases of JDM may not be associated with any biochemical abnormalities.

PAEDIATRIC SYSTEMIC LUPUS ERYTHEMATOSUS

Systemic lupus erythematosus is a multisystem autoimmune disease and the literature continually expands our knowledge of the varied and seemingly infinite manifestations and course of this complex disorder. Only a few children develop SLE in the early school years. Most cases

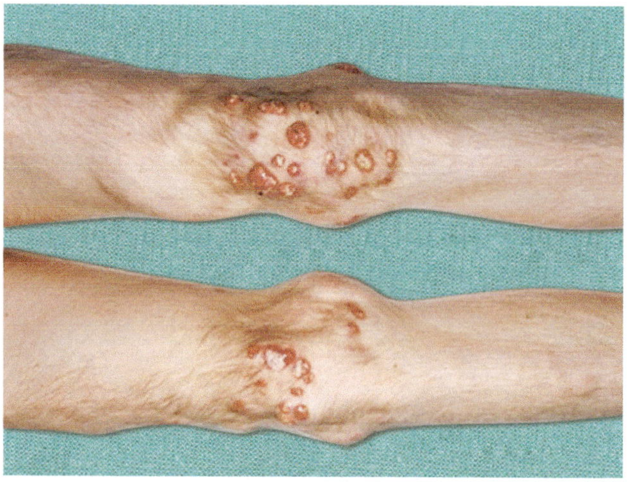

Figure 12.19 Extensive cutaneous calcinosis around the knee in a patient with juvenile dermatomyositis.

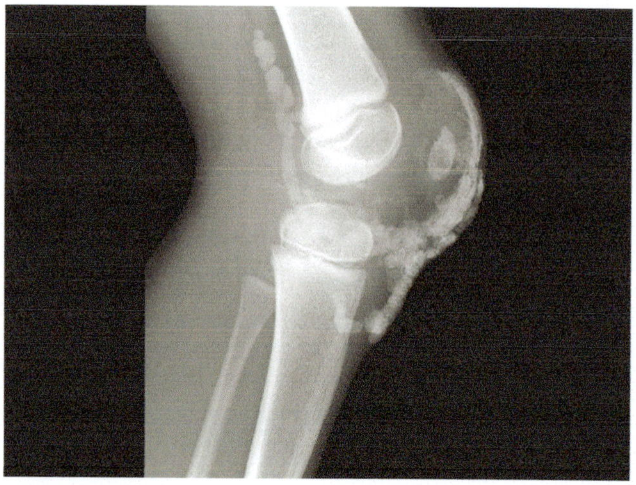

Figure 12.20 Radiograph of the same patient showing extensive cutaneous calcinosis.

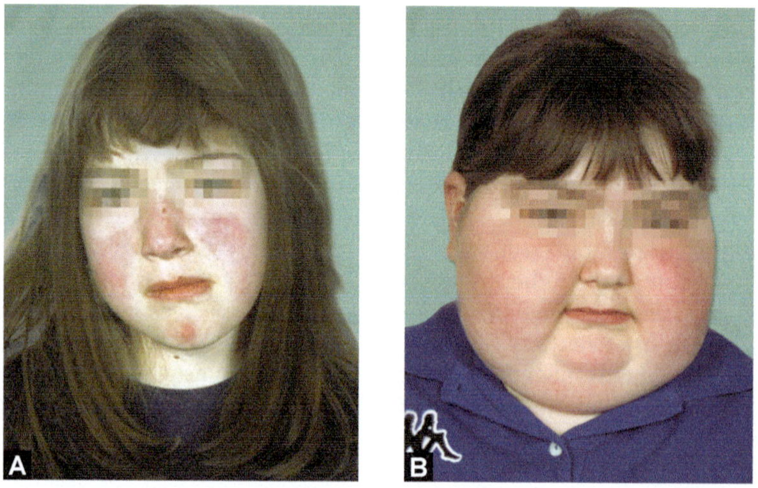

Figures 12.21A and B (A) Butterfly rash in a girl with systemic lupus erythematosus and (B) same patient exhibiting Cushingoid facies following prolonged high-dose steroid therapy.

occur between 11 and 15 years of age and it is more common in girls.

Drug-related lupus is clinically identical with paediatric SLE. In children, the most common cause of drug-related lupus is the administration of anticonvulsants.

Clinical Manifestations

In the childhood form of SLE, as in the adult, the clinical symptomatology may be variable and unpredictable with any number of organ systems eventually becoming involved. The children frequently present with constitutional symptoms and the characteristic erythematous "butterfly" rash on cheeks and bridge of nose, although frequently, the rash consists of erythema of the cheeks with involvement of the lower eyelid **(Figs. 12.21A and B)**. In one-third of patients, the rash is photosensitive. In addition, various skin manifestations may occur such as nonspecific erythemata, purpura, telangiectasia, urticaria, alopecia and abnormal pigmentation. Recurrent mouth ulceration may occur. Raynaud phenomenon is less common in paediatric SLE. Autoimmune haemolytic anaemia, thrombocytopenia and leucopenia may occur.

Lupus nephritis is a grave manifestation, being the most commonly identifiable cause of death in SLE. It is relatively more common and severe in children from China and East Asian countries. Early detection and treatment are essential to prevent progressive and irreversible renal damage and deteriorating renal function.

Joint involvement is common and varies from arthralgia to arthritis closely resembling that of JIA. Cardiac involvement may occur in the form of myocarditis, endocarditis and pericarditis. Manifestations of central nervous system (CNS) involvement include convulsions and mental confusion. Chorea may be a presenting manifestation. Enlargement of the liver and spleen may be found.

Lymphadenopathy with generalised lymph gland enlargement is yet another clinical manifestation. There may be a rapidly progressive retinopathy and extensive retinal haemorrhages, exudates and papilloedema. Antiphospholipid syndrome (APS) has been reported in patients with SLE. The clinical manifestations depend upon the site of the thrombotic process, which may involve arterial and venous vessels of any size in any organ. The diagnosis of APS requires a high degree of clinical awareness. APS is a potentially life-threatening condition.

Laboratory Findings

The diagnosis of SLE is associated with the detection of a large assortment of autoantibodies. One characteristic finding is that of a high ESR in the presence of a normal CRP. The presence or absence of particular autoantibodies influences the confidence with which this diagnosis is made. Antinuclear autoantibodies are present in up to 100% of patients. Anti-double stranded DNA (dsDNA) has 100% specificity for SLE, but only 50% sensitivity. Anti-single stranded DNA (ssDNA) is relatively nonspecific and commonly found in other connective tissue disorders. A detailed autoantibody profile in connective tissue disorders in children is given in **Table 12.2**.

TABLE 12.2 Autoantibodies in connective tissue disorders in children.

Autoantibody	*Disease*
Antinuclear antibody	SLE, JIA, JDM, scleroderma
Antibodies to extractable nuclear antigen	SLE, MCTD
C1q antibody	SLE (particularly lupus nephritis)
Anticardiolipin antibodies	SLE, APS
Double-stranded DNA antibodies	SLE
Histone antibodies	Drug-induced lupus
Lupus anticoagulant	SLE, APS
Rheumatoid factor	JIA
Ro/SS-A	SLE, neonatal lupus
Scl-70	Scleroderma
Anti-Sm antibodies	SLE
U1-RNP	Lupus nephritis, MCTD
Centromere antibodies	CREST syndrome

Abbreviations: SLE, systemic lupus erythematosus; JIA, juvenile idiopathic arthritis; JDM, juvenile dermatomyositis; MCTD, mixed connective tissue disease; APS, anti-phospholipid syndrome; RNP, ribonucleoprotein; CREST, calcinosis, Raynaud, oesophageal dysmotility, sclerodactyly, telangiectasia

NEONATAL LUPUS ERYTHEMATOSUS

Infants born to mothers with active SLE may present with manifestations of SLE such as skin rash **(Figs. 12.22A and B)**, thrombocytopenia, leucopenia and haemolytic anaemia. Most manifestations of neonatal lupus resolve with the clearance of transplacentally transferred maternal antibodies and rarely require treatment. All signs usually clear by 6 months of age. However, in babies of mothers who are anti-SSA/Ro (anti-Ro) positive, there is a risk of complete heart block, which is present form birth, is permanent and usually needs pacing.

Case Study

An 8-year-old girl presented with a 3-month history of feeling very tired, unable to walk, ulcers in her mouth, painful knees, wrists, elbows and fingers and a facial rash. She had been off school for 2 months. On examination, she had a typical butterfly facial rash and active synovitis of knees, wrists and elbows. Blood pressure 100/60 mmHg. No other positive finding was detected. The following investigations were carried out; haemoglobin

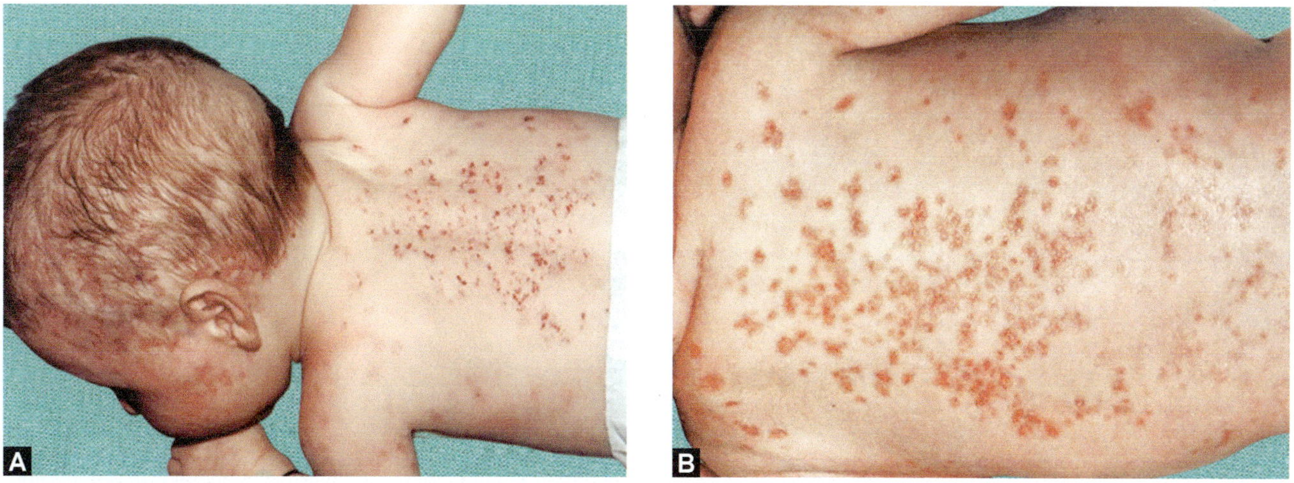

Figures 12.22A and B Rash of neonatal lupus. It gets resolved by 6 months of age.

(Hb) 8.5 g/dL, WBC 3.3 × 10^9/L, neutrophils 2.4 × 10^9/L, platelet count 391 × 10^9/L, ESR 75 mm in first hour, CRP less than 7 clotting profile normal, AST 40 IU/L, ALT 30 IU/L, albumin 31 g/L and protein 80 g/L. Creatinine 36 umol/L, urea 5.2 mmol/L, creatine kinase 42 IU/L, complement C3 0.26 g/L (↓), complement C4 0.06 g/L (↓) urine clear (Dipstix) Direct Coomb test positive, ANA titre 1:2,560, dsDNA more than 1,000 IU/mL, Crithidia test positive, anti-Ro positive, anti-Sm negative, anti-ribonucleoprotein negative, anti-Scl-70 positive, anti-Jo-1 positive, immunoglobulin (Ig) G cardiolipin antibody less than 10 IU/mL(N) and IgM cardiolipin antibody less than 10 IU/mL(N).

She was initially treated with pulse methylprednisolone and a course of oral prednisolone. She responded to this treatment and did not develop lupus nephritis or any other complication.

Diagnosis: Active paediatric SLE.

JUVENILE SCLERODERMA

Scleroderma is a poorly understood autoimmune connective tissue disease. It is rare in children, most cases presenting with localised disease. Systemic disease (systemic sclerosis) is even rarer in children.

Juvenile Localised Scleroderma (Morphea and Linear Scleroderma)

Morphea

Morphea is a rare type of scleroderma. Onset is insidious anytime during childhood and frequently several years pass before a diagnosis is made. Lesions can appear over any part of the body, more frequently on the trunk, starting as erythematous areas which gradually expand in size with a peripheral pink edge and a central slightly pigmented area of atrophic skin through which dilated blood vessels are visible due to atrophy of the subcutaneous fat **(Figs. 12.23A and B)**. Lesions may be slightly pruritic but are not usually painful. They are cosmetically unacceptable, especially on visible parts of the body. Without treatment, new ones continue to appear for several years. Once established lesions tend to persist. They are not usually associated with systemic disease.

Linear Scleroderma

Localised scleroderma is a rare disease. The children present with slowly progressive lesions on their upper and lower limbs, sometimes on the trunk, which consist of localised patches of oedematous, thickened, shiny skin, sometimes tethered to underlying bone. In long-standing cases, the affected limb may be shortened or deformed **(Figs. 12.24A and B)**.

Scleroderma En Coup De Sabre

In this type of scleroderma, lesions appear on the face and scalp consisting of linear depressed areas of atrophied skin and underlying subcutaneous tissue and bone, resembling a sabre cut. They are very disfiguring causing the patient considerable distress. They are not usually associated with systemic disease.

JUVENILE SYSTEMIC SCLEROSIS

Systemic sclerosis is exceptionally rare in childhood, and its course, unpredictable. The patches of skin with scleroderma become oedematous, atrophic and inelastic and adherent to the underlying tissues. The consequent atrophy and tightening of the skin give a characteristic frozen facial appearance of pinched nose and pursed lips. The hands become shiny with tapered finger ends due to loss of pulp **(Figs. 12.25A and B)**. Restricted movement produce claw-like deformities of the hands **(Fig. 12.25C)**, which may also affect the feet. Abnormally dilated nail fold

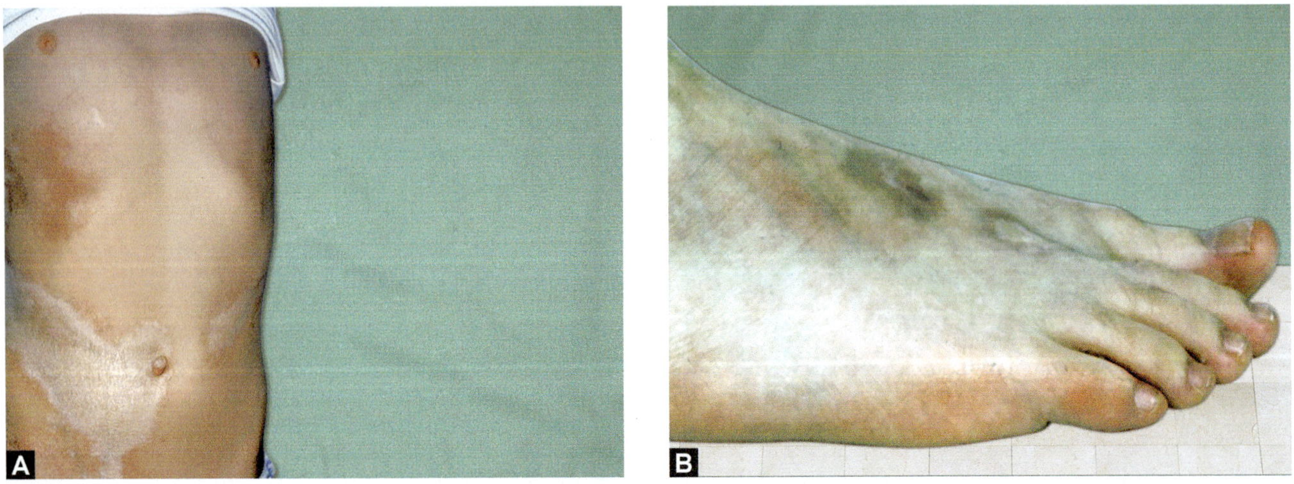

Figures 12.23A and B Extensive patches of morphea, at different stages of progression. At onset areas of depigmentation appear with erythematous edge indicating activity. Older areas become pigmented and thin, have diffuse edge and stop growing.

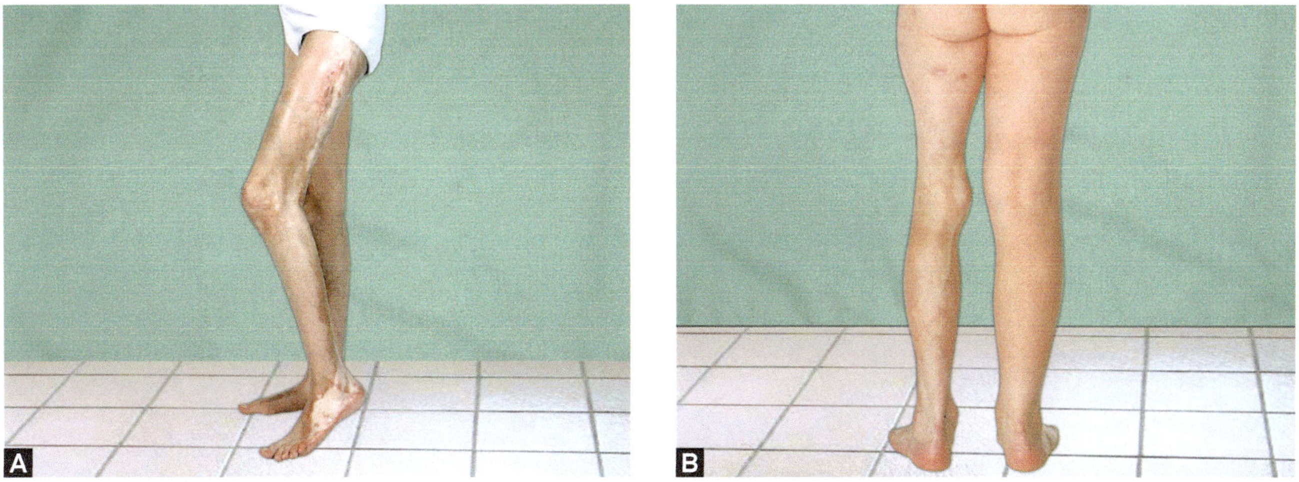

Figures 12.24A and B Extensive linear scleroderma involving left lower limb causing extensive areas of skin depigmentation, thickening and tightening, atrophy of the limb and fixed flexion deformity of left knee.

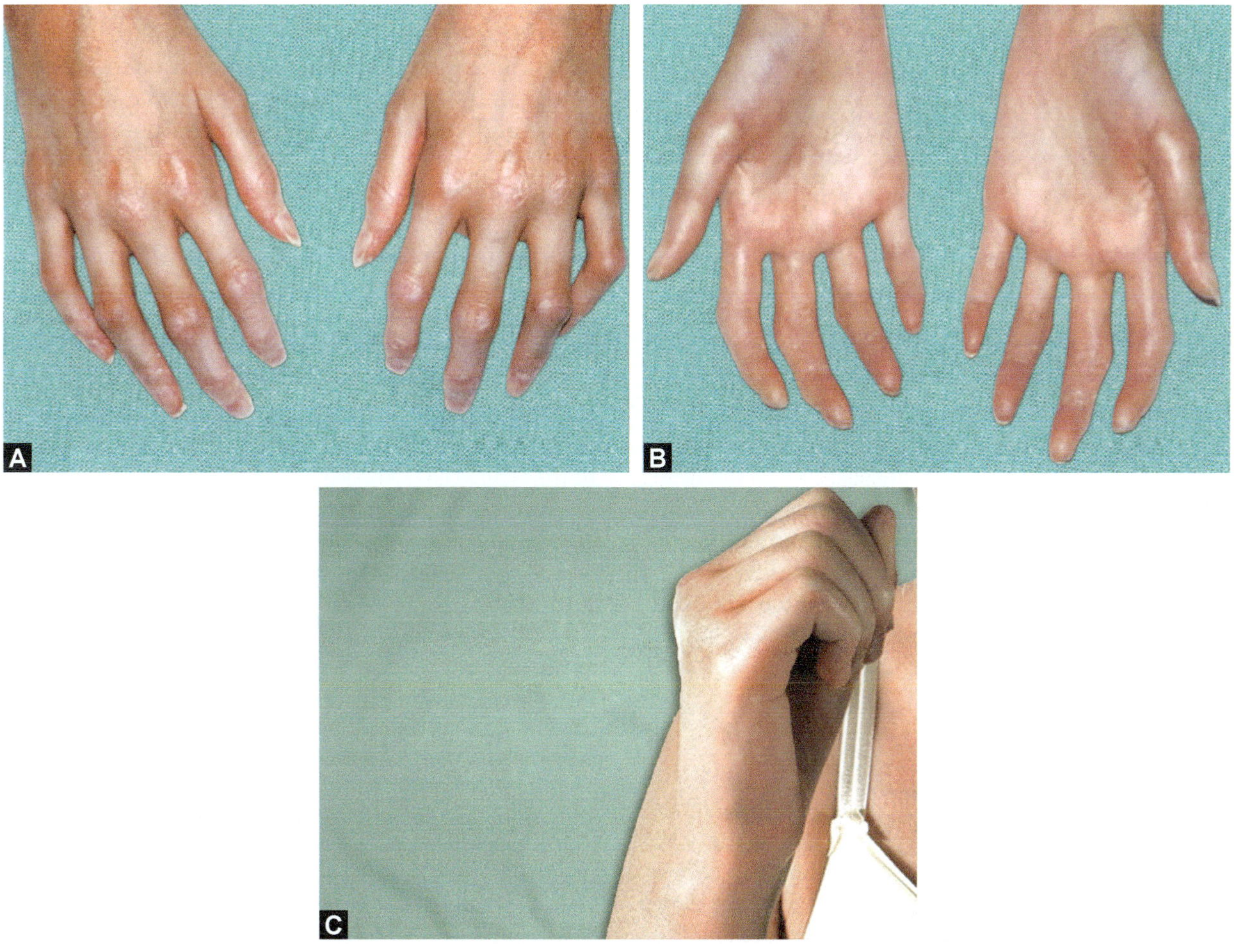

Figures 12.25A to C Systemic sclerosis with extensive cutaneous involvement. The tight skin over the hands and fingers causes marked stiffening of joints, inability to form a fist and loss of pulp at the fingertips.

capillaries may be visible on close inspection (Fig. 12.26). Raynaud phenomenon is common. Gastrointestinal (GI) system involvement with oesophageal dysmotility and dysphagia and long-term fibrosis is much less common in the childhood form of the disease. Pulmonary fibrosis and hypertension and renal involvement may occur. Sjögren syndrome (Sicca syndrome of dry mouth and eyes) is not uncommon in this condition. An apparently

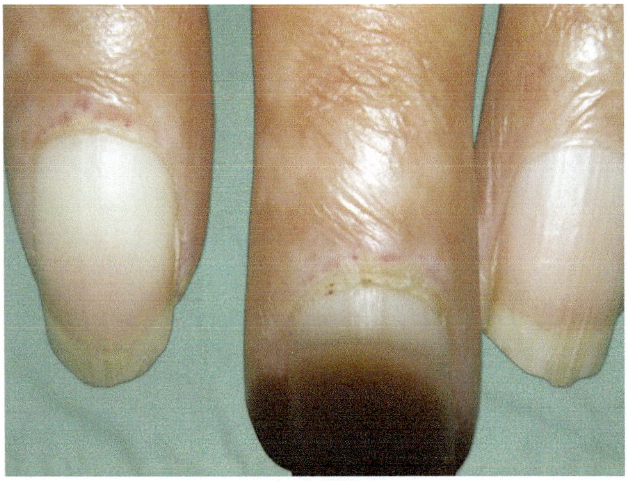

Figure 12.26 abnormally dilated nail fold capillaries as seen in systemic sclerosis and other connective tissue diseases.

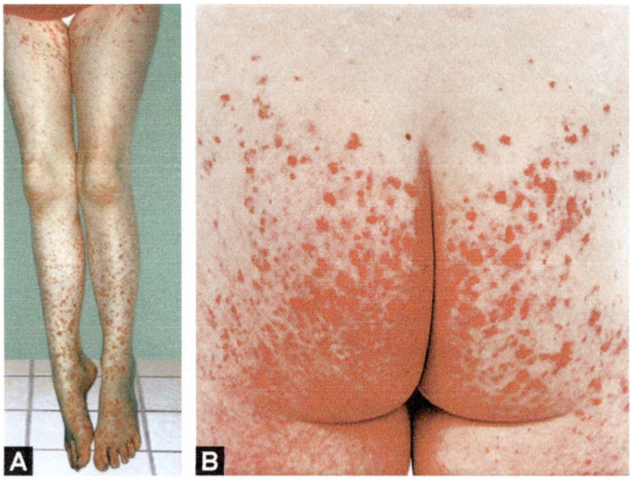

Figures 12.27A and B Henoch–Schönlein purpura: Typical vasculitic rash involving lower limbs and buttocks. The rash is also sometimes present on upper limbs and occasionally on the trunk.

slow developing form of scleroderma, described largely in adults and called CREST syndrome, may be found in children. CREST is an acronym for calcinosis, Raynaud phenomenon, oesophageal dysfunction, sclerodactyly and telangiectasia.

There are no specific laboratory tests diagnostic of scleroderma. ANA are frequently present in sera of children with juvenile systemic sclerosis. The auto-antibody Scl-70 can be identified in some cases.

VASCULITIC SYNDROMES

There are four main groups of vasculitic syndromes of children. The two most common ones are of acute onset and include HSP and Kawasaki disease. More insidious and long-lasting types of vasculitis include polyarteritis nodosa, Takayasu disease and Wegener granulomatosis. Behçet syndrome is more common in Middle Eastern countries than in Western Europe. This section will deliberately concentrate on the vasculitic diseases of significance to the general paediatrician.

Henoch–Schönlein Purpura

Henoch-Schönlein purpura is a systemic small vessel vasculitis, involving skin, joints, abdomen and the kidney. Other organs less frequently affected include the CNS, gonads and the lungs, although less common clinical features may arise from the involvement of virtually every organ system. Certain vaccines, various microbial pathogens, environmental agents and various drugs have been implicated in the aetiology of HSP, but definite supporting evidence for any of them is lacking. IgA1 plays a pivotal role in the pathogenesis of HSP.

The disease has a wide variety of manifestations but the diagnosis is usually obvious when the characteristic purpuric rash on lower and upper limbs is present **(Figs. 12.27A and B)**. The most prominent symptoms arise from swollen painful joints, or from areas of angioedema elsewhere. In some children, the onset is with severe abdominal pain with or without melaena. Intussusception occurs in a small number of cases and when suspected the diagnosis can be confirmed with ultrasound of the abdomen. Another mode of presentation in boys is with an acute scrotal swelling which can be mistaken for torsion of the testis. In the majority of cases, the rash is the most striking feature and causes the parents to seek medical advice but sometimes it may appear after the abdominal pain. Characteristically, the rash appears first as small separate urticarial lesions, both visible and palpable. These soon become dusky red or frankly purpuric. In the typical case, the rash is most profuse over the extensor surfaces of the knees, ankles, dorsum of the feet, arms, elbows and forearms. The face, abdomen and chest are completely spared. This helps to distinguish the HSP rash from the purpuric petechial rash in meningococcal disease which appears on any part of the body. CNS involvement may present as headache, seizure or hemiparesis. Lung involvement presents as pulmonary haemorrhage.

KEY LEARNING POINTS

- Characteristic distribution of HSP rash should help distinguish it from meningococcaemia.
- HSP is the most common vasculitis in children.
- HSP is generally a self-limited condition—lasts an average of 4 weeks.
- Nephritis is one feature of HSP that may have chronic consequences.
- Long-term prognosis is dependent on the severity of nephritis.
- Characteristic distribution of purpuric lesions in HSP should help to distinguish it from meningococcal disease, where the rash may appear on any part of the body.

Renal involvement is more common than is usually recognised and may occur in 20% of children, and presents with microscopic haematuria and/or heavy proteinuria. It is suggested that urinalysis should be carried out for 2 months after resolution of the rash, to ensure that renal involvement is not missed.

There are no specific laboratory tests which would help with the diagnosis of HSP. The platelet count is within the normal range. Coagulation studies are normal.

Kawasaki Disease

Kawasaki disease is the most common cause of multisystem vasculitis in childhood. The vessels most commonly damaged are the coronary arteries, making Kawasaki disease the number one cause of acquired heart disease in children from the developed world. It is characterised by prolonged fever, nonpurulent conjunctivitis, oral mucosal inflammation, skin changes and cervical lymphadenopathy, induration and erythema of the hands and feet. It was described by Dr Tamasaku Kawasaki in the Japanese literature in 1967 and in the English literature in 1974. Since then it has been recognised in children of every ethnic origin although Asian children are affected 5–10 times more frequently than Caucasian children. It is a disease of young children and 80% of cases are younger than 5 years. The peak age of onset is 1 year and the disorder is more common in boys.

A definite diagnosis of Kawasaki disease can be made when at least five of the following six principal signs are present:

1. Fever persisting for 5 or more days.
2. Polymorphous rash.
3. Bilateral conjunctival congestion **(Fig. 12.28)**.
4. Changes of lips and oral cavity including strawberry tongue, red fissured lips, hyperaemia of oral and pharyngeal mucosa **(Fig. 12.29)**.
5. Acute nonpurulent cervical lymphadenopathy.
6. Changes in peripheral extremities including reddening of palms and soles, oedema of hands and feet and membranous desquamation of fingertips **(Figs. 12.30A to C)**.

In the absence of pathognomonic clinical or laboratory signs, it is extremely difficult to diagnose mild or incomplete cases. Therefore, it is essential to keep an open mind and follow a child as a "possible case" with repeated clinical and cardiac evaluations. However, in most cases, the diagnostic criteria are clearly identifiable and a definite diagnosis of Kawasaki disease can be made.

Coronary artery aneurysms develop approximately in 15–20% of untreated children with Kawasaki disease, within 4–6 weeks of disease onset. Two-dimensional (2D) echocardiography will detect nearly all patients with acute coronary artery disease.

Other less frequent features include arthritis, arthralgia, urethritis, diarrhoea, aseptic meningitis, sterile pyuria, myocarditis, pericarditis, alopecia, jaundice, uveitis and hydrops of the gallbladder. Blood tests show leucocytosis, a raised ESR/CRP and during the second week of illness, there may be thrombocytosis.

Case Study

A 2-year-old boy presented with a 5-day history of fever, cough, running nose and a macular rash on his trunk. On examination, he had suffusion of ocular conjunctivae, bilateral cervical lymphadenitis, an inflamed throat, strawberry tongue, induration of palms and soles and a temperature of 40°C. He had no hepatosplenomegaly, no arthritis and no peeling of skin and no neck stiffness. Hb 10 g/dL, WBC 20 × 10^9/L with preponderance of polymorphs, platelet count 600 × 10^9/L, ESR 80 mm in first hour and CRP 60 mg/L. Two-dimensional echocardiography showed dilatation of right coronary artery. Urine was

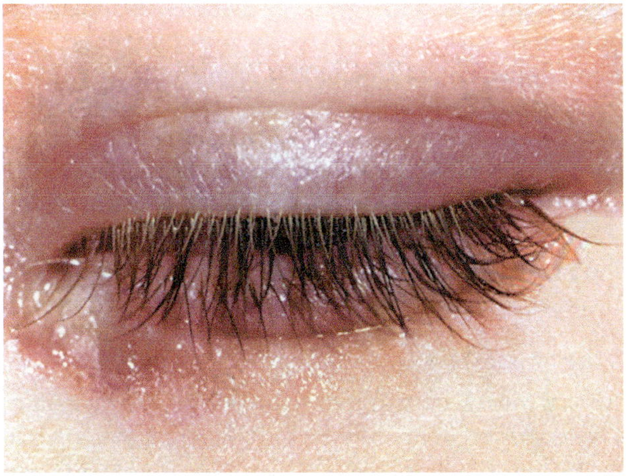

Figure 12.28 Kawasaki disease: Congestion of eyelids associated with conjunctivitis.

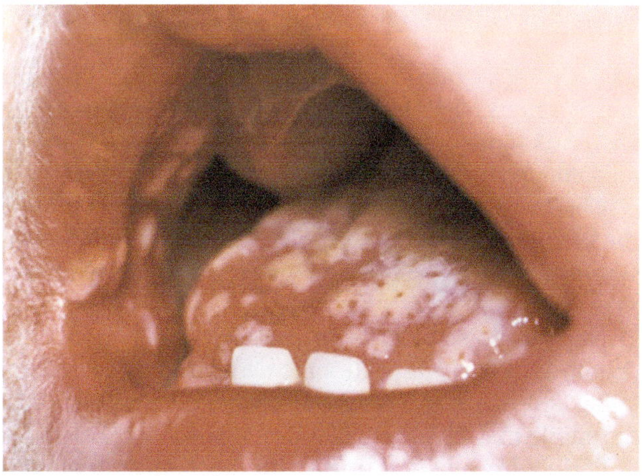

Figure 12.29 Strawberry tongue and dry red and cracked lips as seen in Kawasaki disease.

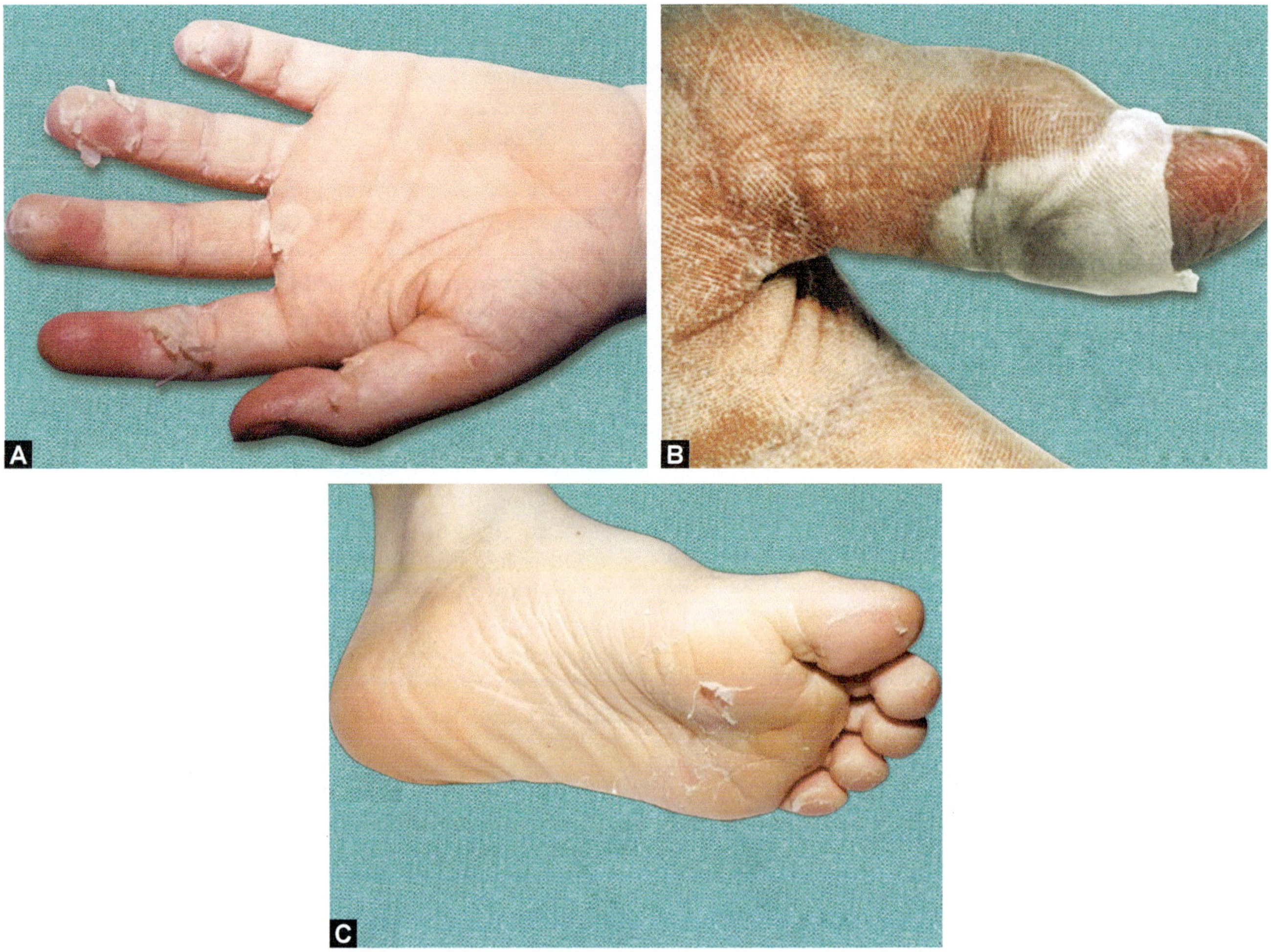

Figures 12.30A to C Kawasaki disease: Typical desquamation of fingertips and toes occurs about 10 days following disease.

clear both biochemically, microscopically and bacteriologically. Viral serology was negative.

The most likely working diagnosis was Kawasaki disease. He was treated with aspirin and intravenous immunoglobulin and made a complete recovery.

Juvenile Polyarteritis Nodosa (PAN)

Juvenile PAN, a rare systemic vasculitis, may present with a wide variety of clinical manifestations. It is a necrotising vasculitis of medium-sized muscular arteries with associated aneurysmal formation.

Clinically, the symptoms are due to involvement of the blood vessels of the kidney, CNS, muscle and viscera. Coronary artery involvement and myocardial infarction may occur.

No specific serological markers are available for the diagnosis of PAN although some patients may have circulating anti-neutrophil cytoplasmic antibody (ANCA). Skin or muscle may be biopsied to detect histological changes of fibrinoid necrosis of small- and medium-sized arterial walls. Renal biopsy may be necessary although it carries a significant risk of bleeding.

Juvenile Takayasu Arteritis

Juvenile Takayasu arteritis (TA) is another vasculitic disorder affecting mainly the aorta and its larger branches causing both stenosis and aneurysms. It is more common in female adolescents, presenting with systemic manifestations of lethargy, fever, myalgia, arthralgia and sometimes arthritis, followed by breathlessness, dyspnoea headaches and palpitations, secondary to severe hypertension. This is a consequence of stenosis of the aorta or its major vessels or renal artery stenosis, which cause severe systemic hypertension and in some cases pulmonary hypertension. Examination of the peripheries reveals absent pulses, and auscultation over the major blood vessels shows the presence of bruits over the stenotic areas. Diagnosis is confirmed with angiography.

Behçets Disease

This is a rare disease in the United Kingdom but is much more common in the Middle East, Japan, especially Turkey, presenting in adolescents between 10 and 16 years of age and continuing into adulthood. It is characterised by the triad of recurrent multiple aphthous stomatitis

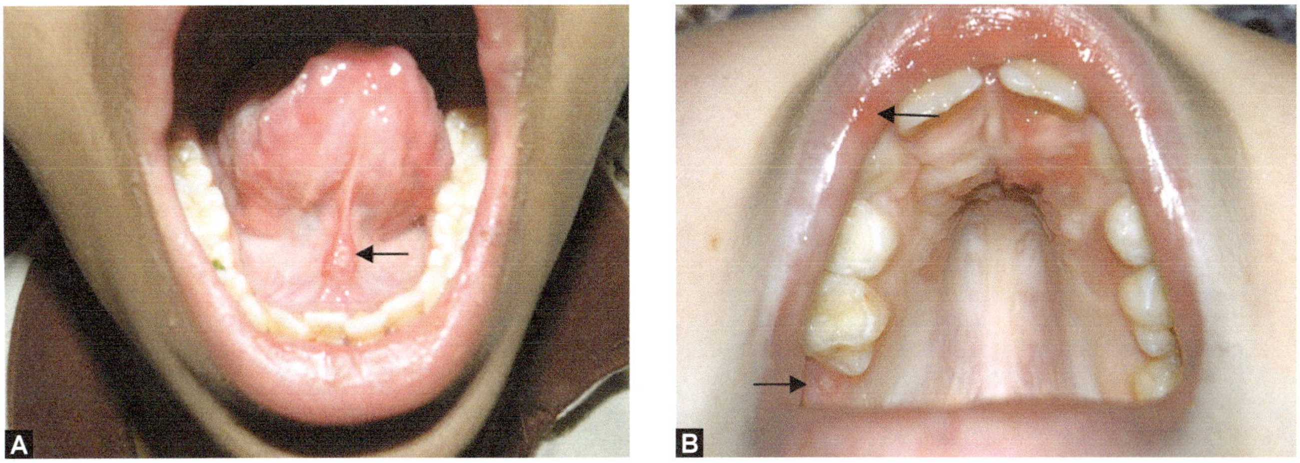

Figures 12.31A and B Behçet disease: Punched out painful recurrent ulcers on lips, gums and frenulum of tongue.

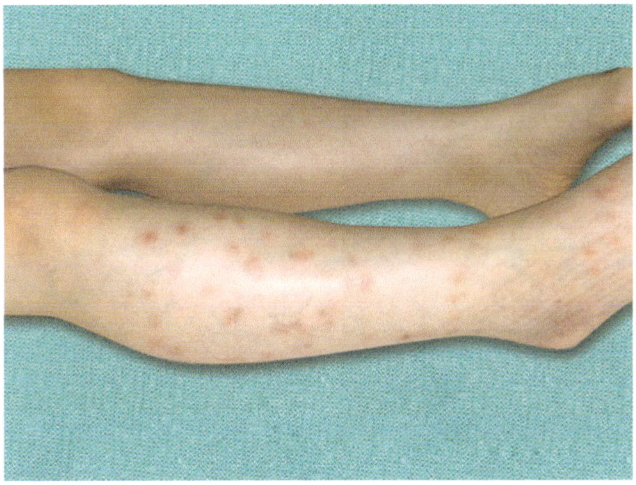

Figure 12.32 Behcet's disease: Rash resembling erythema nodosum over lower limbs complicating deep venous thrombosis.

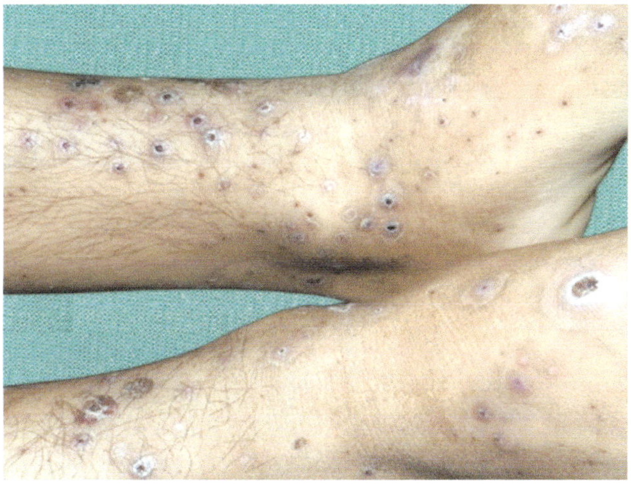

Figure 12.33 Behçets disease: Vasculitic ulcers on lower limbs.

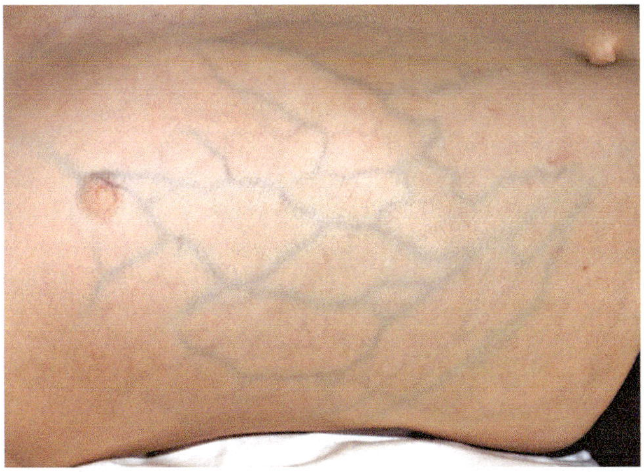

Figure 12.34 Behcet's disease: Marked superficial vein congestion (Caput medusae) due to increased superficial venous return caused by thrombosis of inferior vena cava.

(Figs. 12.31A and B), genital ulceration and severe anterior uveitis. Skin manifestations include erythema nodosum **(Fig. 12.32)** and skin ulcers **(Fig. 12.33)**. Venous thrombosis **(Fig. 12.34)** and aneurysm formation are the result of vasculitis. GI involvement resembles inflammatory bowel disease.

Wegeners Granulomatosis

This granulomatous vasculitis is rare in the paediatric age group. The granulomatous vasculitis has a predilection of the upper and lower respiratory tract, glomerulonephritis and cutaneous vasculitis. Upper respiratory tract involvement includes sinusitis, epistaxis, and nasal mucosal ulceration associated with perforation of the nasal septum and hearing loss. Lower airways disease causes cough, haemoptysis and pleuritis. Glomerulonephritis is encountered in about half the patients and is

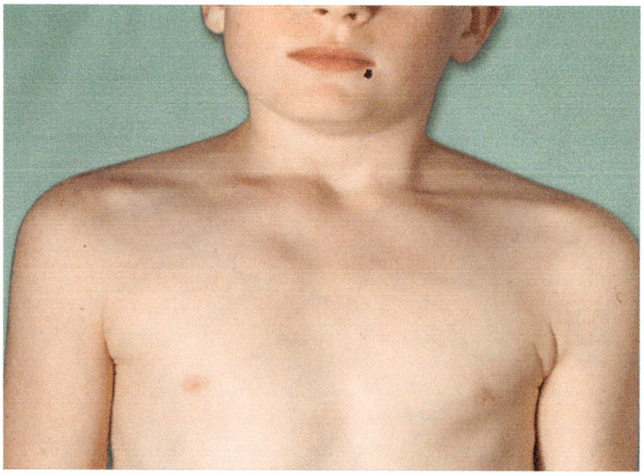

Figure 12.35 CRMO/CNO – Swelling of medial ends of clavicles.

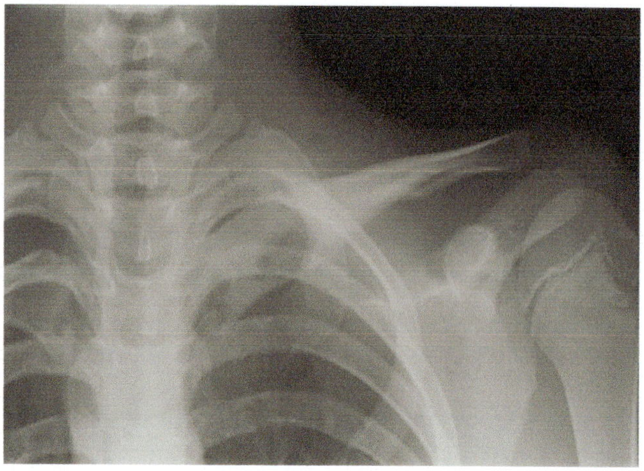

Figure 12.36 X-ray showing osteitis of medial end of left clavicle in CRMO/CNO.

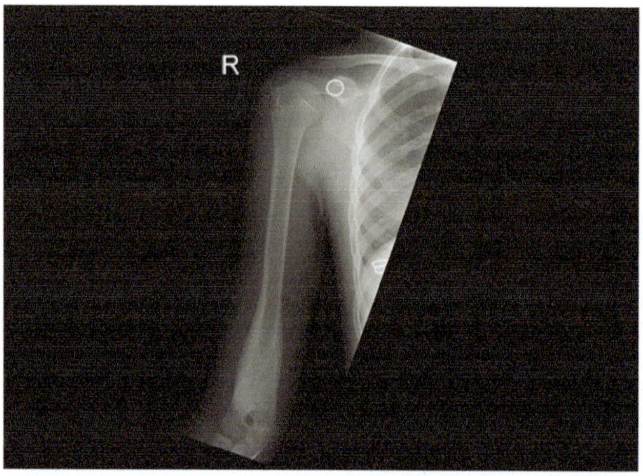

Figure 12.37 X-ray showing hyperostotic osteitis of lower end of right humerus in CRMO/CNO.

rapidly progressive leading to renal failure if not treated. Cutaneous lesions take the form of deep ulcers on face and legs although other sites may also be involved. The ESR is markedly elevated. RF is positive in some patients. Most patients are cytoplasmic ANCA positive.

CHRONIC RECURRENT MULTIFOCAL OSTEOMYELITIS

Chronic Non-infectious Osteitis (CNO)

Chronic recurrent multifocal osteomyelitis (CRMO), more recently renamed as CNO, is a relapsing condition consisting of single or multiple lesions of bone, presenting with constant pain worse at night, local tenderness and swelling, lasting for weeks, months and even years. Histological features resemble osteomyelitis, but repeated cultures are negative. It may run a monophasic course but more frequently it is a relapsing condition affecting all age groups with a peak incidence around 10 years of age and slightly more common in girls. It is diagnosed when other possible etiologies, such as infection and malignancy, have been excluded. In the early stages, there may be no radiographic changes though later on both lytic and hyperostotic **(Fig. 12.35)** areas appear. Lesions are highlighted as "hot areas" on technetium scans and as areas of enhancement on MRI. Sites most commonly affected are the anterior thoracic cage, medial end of the clavicles **(Figs. 12.36 and 12.37)** and long bones **(Fig. 12.35)**, but other sites, such as the mandible, pelvis and axial skeleton, may be affected. Although initially thought to have an autoimmune etiology, it is now considered to be an inherited auto-inflammatory disorder. There is limited or no response to therapy with antibiotics, nonsteroidal anti-inflammatory drugs (NSAIDs) and steroids, but there is usually a rapid and prolonged response to bisphosphonate therapy.

CHAPTER 13

Urinary System

R. Cameron Shepherd, Salvatore Cascio

INTRODUCTION

The kidneys play an important role in metabolic regulation, in fluid and electrolyte balance and in the maintenance of blood pressure (BP). Additional factors in childhood, which are not relevant to adult practice, include the fact that the kidneys do not reach full maturity until the age of 4 years, and disorders of function have an intimate effect on growth and development. The collecting system, the renal pelvis, ureters, bladder and urethra, connects the kidneys to the external environment. The urinary system, the kidneys and the collecting system together, is vulnerable to insults both from a variety of pathological processes within the body and ascending from the external environment. The important presenting complaints of renal disease in childhood are discussed as follows.

Dysuria

Dysuria or painful micturition sometimes accompanied by stranguary, an inability to pass urine due to pain, is an indication of disturbance, usually inflammation, in the lower urinary tract but often pointing to infection throughout the urinary tract [urinary tract infection (UTI)].

Frequency of Micturition and Polyuria

These are symptoms that appear similar but have different origins. Frequency is usually associated with inflammatory processes in the lower urinary tract, possibly a UTI. Polyuria results from a failure to concentrate urine for a variety of reasons.

Incontinence

This is a problem that may be confined to sleep (enuresis) or may be a diurnal problem. It may be either primary (present from birth) or secondary (arising after a period of bladder control). This problem has its own section for discussion.

Abdominal Pain and Loin Pain

Pain is an important symptom indicating renal disease. It most frequently indicates UTI, but other factors such as nephrolithiasis (renal stones) may present with pain in the loin, the abdomen or it may be referred to other parts such as the groin, testes or vulva.

Red Urine

Red urine most commonly indicates blood (haematuria), but other causes may include haemoglobinuria (from the breakdown of blood products) and myoglobinuria (from muscle destruction). Before confirming blood in the urine, even in the context of a positive 'Dipstick' test, urine microscopy must confirm the presence of red blood cells (RBCs). Blood in the urine may only have a 'smoky' appearance. Blood in the urine is the cardinal symptom of glomerulonephritis (GN) but may indicate many other problems including UTI and trauma. Confounding causes of red urine, negative for blood, include the eating of beetroot, the presence of urate crystals and exposure to certain drugs including rifampicin **(Box 13.1)**. The differential diagnosis of paediatric haematuria is outlined in **Table 13.1**.

Proteinuria

Proteinuria is found as the result of investigation, but so ubiquitous it is, as a finding in renal disease that is it a first line test, and even a screening test, for renal disease. It may indicate almost any insult to the renal system, including UTI, but is most important as an indication of glomerular disease. The normal variant of 'orthostatic proteinuria' should be noted where children have proteinuria in the upright position but not while recumbent. The confirmation is to test first morning urine and urine after several hours in the upright position.

Oedema

Oedema is an important sign of renal disease. The oedema may be localized to the lower limbs but is more

BOX 13.1 Causes of dark or discoloured urine in children.

- Rifampicin
- Nitrofurantoin
- Metronidazole
- Desferrioxamine
- Beetroot
- Blackberries
- Urate crystals
- Myoglobinuria
- Haemoglobinuria
- Alkaptonuria, porphyria
- Food colourings (beetroot, berries—anthocyanins and confectionary containing vegetable dyes)

TABLE 13.1 Differential diagnosis of paediatric haematuria.

Glomerular
Acute poststreptococcal glomerulonephritis
Henoch-Schönlein purpura
IgA nephropathy
Systemic lupus erythematosus (lupus nephritis)
Haemolytic–uraemic syndrome
Shunt nephritis
Hereditary nephritis (Alport syndrome)
Urinary tract
Urinary tract infection
Haemorrhagic cystitis
Renal calculi
Urinary schistosomiasis
Vascular
Sickle cell disease
Renal vein thrombosis
Thrombocytopaenia
Interstitial
Renal tuberculosis
Cystic disease
Hydronephrosis
Wilms tumour
Acute tubular necrosis
Drugs, e.g. NSAIDs, chemical cystitis (cyclophosphamide), and so on.
Factitious

Abbreviations: IgA, immunoglobulin A; NSAIDs, non-steroidal anti-inflammatory drugs.

commonly generalized, affecting the face (with periorbital oedema and facial puffiness), the abdomen and, in boys, the genitalia. Isolated periorbital oedema must be distinguished from the (usually) benign condition of angioneurotic oedema.

Abdominal Masses

The finding of an abdominal mass in the renal area may indicate the embryonic tumour nephroblastoma (Wilms tumour). This is dealt with under childhood malignancy. Masses of renal origin may also be the result of renal vein thrombosis or of renal abnormalities such as horseshoe kidney or cystic changes.

INVESTIGATION OF URINARY TRACT COMPLAINTS

A range of investigations is available to explore the nature and severity of renal tract disease.

Urine Examination

Urine examination is the first line of investigation in renal disease and many hold that it is part of the routine examination of all children no matter what their complaints are. Urine examination should include 'Dipstick' testing for albumin, blood, leucocyte esterase and nitrite (indications of pyuria). A positive 'Dipstick' test should, however, be followed-up by urine microscopy with particular attention to the presence and count of white blood cells (WBCs), RBCs and casts, clusters of granular debris sometimes with clumped RBCs, WBCs and hyaline (glassy) material, having a three-dimensional structure and indicating glomerular disease. In certain circumstances, the nature of any crystals present may be of significance **(Fig. 13.1)**. More detailed urine tests will be discussed where appropriate.

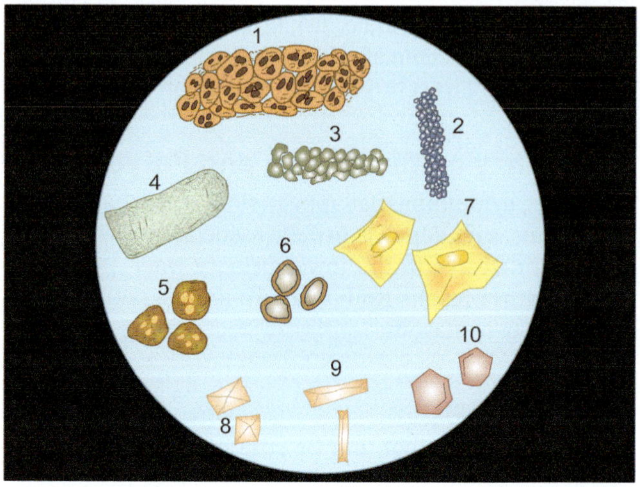

Figure 13.1 Urine microscopy findings: (1) WBC cast, (2) granular cast, (3) RBC cast, (4) hyaline cast, (5) pus cells, (6) RBCs, (7) epithelial cells (not clinically significant), (8) oxalate crystals, (9) phosphate crystals and (10) cystine crystals.

Blood Examination

The primary function of the kidney being the regulation of fluid and electrolytes, and the excretion of metabolites particularly urea, the first line of blood investigation must be the urea and the electrolytes (U&E) such as sodium, potassium and chloride, together with creatinine as a sensitive indicator of function. Phosphate and calcium are important in some renal conditions and should routinely be tested. Where there is likely to be protein loss, the serum protein levels should be checked. Immune mediated mechanisms, often (but not always) endogenous, are important in renal disease and complement C3/4, antinuclear antibody/anti-dsDNA factors and evidence of inflammatory disease such as the erythrocyte sedimentation rate (ESR) or C-reactive protein are appropriate investigations when immune mechanisms are suspected. As the β-haemolytic *Streptococcus* may be responsible for some immune-mediated conditions, the antistreptolysin O titre (ASOT) should be measured in these circumstances.

Renal Function Tests

For all practical purposes in children, especially young children, dynamic scanning using the isotope labelled ^{99m}Tc-diethylentriamene penta-acetate (DTPA) is the most convenient method of measuring renal function. This has the twin advantages of not requiring a timed urine collection and of providing differential function of each kidney

- In older children, the glomerular filtration rate (GFR) may be calculated by a creatinine clearance test requiring timed (preferably 24 hour) urine sampling and a plasma creatinine level. Inulin, given orally, may be used instead of creatinine.

Imaging of the Urinary Tract

A wide range of imaging techniques is available, but the principle should be to use, at each age, the least invasive technique commensurate with the need for appropriate information. Commonly used imaging techniques are:

Ultrasound: Ultrasound (US) provides rapid non-invasive detail of kidney morphology and size, including evidence of scarring and damage, and of the collecting system and bladder, including evidence of distension and bladder wall thickening. It can also indicate the presence of calculi and may define any extrarenal structures of relevance. It has, however, a low sensitivity and specificity, both under and over diagnosing problems. It is the first line imaging investigation on all patients with UTI.

Radionuclide scintigraphy: DTPA has been discussed in relation to renal function testing. ^{99m}Tc-dimercapto-succinic acid (DMSA) is the most sensitive test of parenchymal damage to the kidney. It is the method of choice when investigating UTI and vesicoureteric reflux (VUR), when ectopic elements are suspected and when there is unexplained hypertension. The use of radionuclide labelled ^{99m}Tc-mercaptacetyltriglycine (MAG-3) is a non-invasive test for VUR. Unfortunately, it requires the patient to micturate on demand and is confined to older children who are continent and cooperative.

Micturatingcystourethrogram (MCUG): This remains the best method of defining VUR and other problems with the bladder and urethra. It is less dependent on patient cooperation and is the method of choice in young patients, especially babies. It is, however, invasive, requiring catheterisation and the instillation of radio-opaque dye, and is, therefore, both distressing and potentially dangerous. It is a requirement if surgery to the ureters or bladder is contemplated.

Abdominal X-ray: This is useful for visualising calculi and for detecting abnormalities in the lumbosacral spine (possibly relevant to a neuropathic bladder).

Intravenous pyelogram: With the abundance of other techniques, there are few indications for intravenous pyelogram (IVP). It is generally called for when there is residual doubt about calyceal anatomy or the nature of other abnormalities or when facilities for radionuclide testing are absent.

Others: There are a variety of specialised techniques available in particular circumstances: *arteriography* for suspected renal vascular stenosis, computed tomography (CT) for suspected masses and magnetic resonance imaging (MRI) useful for evaluating the spine and for renal artery stenosis (RAS).

Renal Biopsy

Renal biopsy will be considered when dealing with GN, the main indication in childhood.

URINARY TRACT INFECTION

Urinary tract infection, one of the most common diseases of childhood, occurs in 8% of girls and 1% of boys under 10 years. Only in the neonate is the incidence in boys higher than in girls; it is believed to be because the infection in this age group is bloodborne as opposed to ascending through the renal tract in older children. The organism most commonly involved is *Escherichia coli*, but others including *Enterococcus faecalis*, *Klebsiella*, *Proteus* and *Serratia* species are occasionally found. *Proteus* species is particularly associated with urinary stasis and stone formation. Inadequately treated UTI in childhood may result in chronic renal failure (CRF), hypertension and problems in pregnancy in adult life.

Clinical Features

In the neonate, the features are those of systemic neonatal infection—vomiting diarrhoea, failure to thrive, hyperthermia or (more commonly) hypothermia, jaundice, proceeding to systemic collapse. In older children, symptoms referable to the renal tract predominate—any combination of dysuria, frequency of micturition, urgency, wetting, haematuria and loin pain together with fever, vomiting and malaise. Sometimes, especially in girls, there may be no symptoms and UTI may be found at follow-up examination after a previous infection or on routine screening. So protean are the features of UTI that urine analysis should be part of the routine examination in every infant and child.

Diagnosis

Diagnosis of UTI is based on the following urine findings:

- Any growth on suprapubic aspiration
- A pure growth of more than 10^5 colony forming organisms on mid-stream urine or clean-catch urine (CCU)
- Circumstantial evidence of pyuria on urine microscopy (>10 WBC/mm^3 in boys and >50 WBC/mm^3 in girls) or 'leucocytes' or 'nitrites' on 'dipstick' should ideally await growth on culture.

Management

Early and prompt treatment is important, especially in the neonate where there should be an assumption that there will be a coexisting septicaemia. Older children may have to be treated pending the results of investigation with the 'best guess' antibacterial drug available. Trimethoprim, co-amoxiclav, nitrofurantoin and cephradine are suitable oral preparations and a 2–4 day course seems adequate for first infections. If there is loin pain or other evidence of involvement of the kidney, this should be extended to 7–10 days. Inability to tolerate oral therapy requires admission and intravenous (IV) antibiotics. Prophylactic treatment using a lower dose of the oral antibacterial is usually given (despite minimal evidence) until investigation is complete.

While the majority of children will make a complete recovery with adequate treatment based on urine culture findings, a significant number (up to 50% of girls and 15% of boys) will relapse at some future date, and all children with UTI should be followed up for a minimum of 6 months to 2 years (depending on age and circumstances) with repeat urine examinations and culture. A UTI may indicate an abnormality in the structure or function of the renal tract. All children with UTI must be examined with attention to growth, BP, constipation, and a search made for abdominal masses and congenital abnormalities of their genitalia and lumbar spine.

Investigation depends on the age of the child and aims to determine the functional integrity of the kidneys, ureters, bladder and urethra together with evidence of parenchymal damage to the kidneys and any underlying congenital abnormalities.

A suitable plan for investigation would be as follows:

- Children less than 1 year
    - Renal US
    - Micturating cystourethrogram (delayed for 4–8 weeks postinfection and done under antibiotic cover)
    - DMSA scan
- Children 1–5 years
    - Renal US
    - DMSA scan (if symptoms indicate kidney involvement or recurrence or family history of VUR/renal scarring)
- Micturatingcystourethrogram (if US or DMSA scans show an abnormality or if infection proves recurrent)
- Children more than 5 years
    - Renal US
    - DMSA scan
    - MAG-3 scan and indirect micturating cystogram
    - Micturating cystourethrogram if surgery contemplated

ABNORMALITIES DETECTED ON INVESTIGATION

Scarring

Scarring is an indication of previous infection and occurs in children before the age of 4 years. Its presence in older children suggests they have had past episodes of UTI at a younger age. Scarring can be seen on US but DMSA scan has a greater sensitivity and specificity **(Figs. 13.2A and B)**. Scarring may vary from minor indentation of the capsule to a severely contracted kidney. It indicates a need for functional evaluation, particularly for reflux, and for follow-up urine examination.

Dilatation of the Collecting System

This may vary from mild blunting of the papillae and mild dilation of the calyceal system to gross dilation and tortuosity of the ureters with erosion of the calyces. Dilation usually indicates VUR (see later).

Differential Impairment of Renal Function

The secretory and the excretory functions can be measured selectively in each kidney by the DMSA and DTPA scans and problems in either the secretion of urine or hold up in its passage out of the pelvis of the kidney identified. Evidence of impaired function is an indication for MCUG. Particular attention should be paid to BP when there is a discrepancy of function between the kidneys.

Congenital Abnormalities

Horse-shoe kidney, ectopic kidney, duplex kidneys of various degrees and absence of a kidney may emerge from

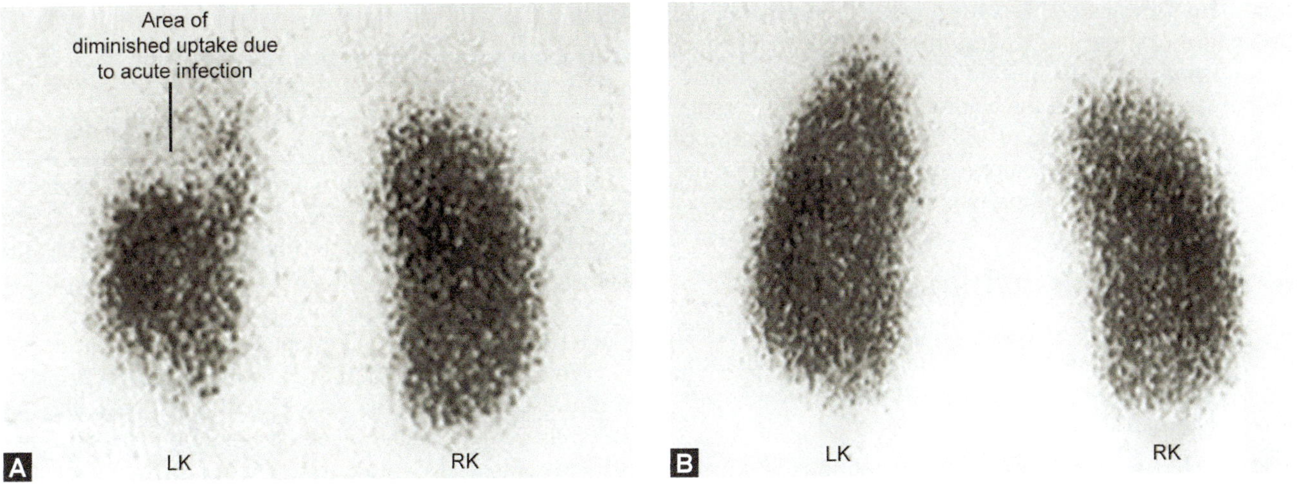

Figures 13.2A and B (A) ^{99m}Tc DMSA (^{99m}Tc-dimercaptosuccinic acid) scan showing an area of reduced uptake of the scanning agent in the upper part of the left kidney at the time of an acute urinary tract infection. The function in the kidney was also reduced; (B) The appearance had returned to normal on a follow-up scan.

investigation of UTI. Minor degrees of spina bifida may also emerge from renal tract investigations.

RECURRENT URINARY TRACT INFECTION

In a variable proportion of children (especially girls), UTI becomes a recurrent problem. There is little convincing evidence that hygiene measures make any significant difference to the recurrence rate but are often advised—cotton underwear, avoidance of bubble baths, double micturition, cleansing the anus from before backwards and a high fluid intake. The only proven effective treatment is long-term prophylaxis with antibiotics sometimes with elective changes in the antibiotic routine. This requires prolonged follow-up and repeat investigation for renal structure and function at 1 or 2 yearly intervals. Recurrent UTI is an indication for MCUG as a proportion of these children will have VUR. The possibility of child sex abuse should be considered, particularly in girls with recurrent UTI with no other predisposing factors.

VESICOURETERIC REFLUX

A functional valve mechanism exists at the vesicoureteric junction to prevent the retrograde flow of urine from the bladder into the ureter. This valve mechanism may be defective either congenitally or as a result of surgery. It has been suggested that the inflammation of a UTI can itself result in dysfunction of the valve leading to reflux. Thus, a UTI may be both a cause and a consequence of VUR. VUR is present in 1% of newborns with UTI and from 30 to 45% of children less than 5 years with UTI. The degree of reflux may be variable from reflux into the ureter only to severe dilatation of the collecting system and damage to the papillae and calyces of the kidney **(Fig. 13.3)**. VUR is an

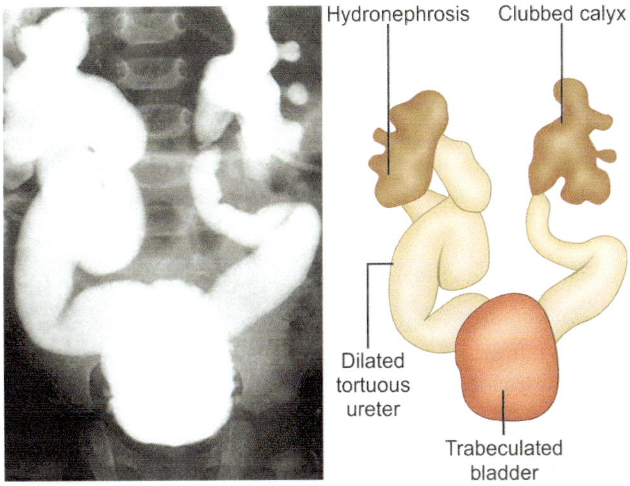

Figure 13.3 Cystogram showing bilateral vesicoureteric reflux.

important cause of renal scarring and end-stage renal failure and there is minimal evidence that treatment either medical or surgical influences the outcome. Investigation of VUR requires an MCUG. This ideally requires the cooperation of the child in passing urine at the appropriate time. This is limited in younger children and babies. A MAG-3 scan is a suitable and less invasive alternative procedure in older children who can micturate on demand.

Management of Vesicoureteric Reflux

Initial management in mild cases with limited evidence of renal damage is conservative—long-term prophylactic antibacterials and follow-up urine cultures at 3-month intervals with repeat US, DMSA and cystography in 1 or 2 years. Where follow-up shows recurrences of UTI or progressive damage on investigation or where there is significant renal tract damage on first examination, surgical treatment is indicated. This may be the relatively benign procedure of subureteric teflon injection ('STING' procedure), when Teflon is injected by cystoscopy at the junction of the ureters and the bladder to restore the patency of the valve mechanism or it may be re-implantation of the ureters by open operation. The success of both procedures is variable and continuing follow-up is necessary.

GLOMERULAR DISORDERS

Diseases of the glomeruli form a large and important body of childhood problems some of which have the potential to progress to acute renal failure (ARF) or CRF. They comprise two broad clinical syndromes:

1. *Glomerulonephritis:* A group of conditions having the common features—haematuria, oliguria, oedema, hypertension and variable proteinuria.
2. *Nephrotic syndrome:* A group of conditions having the common features—proteinuria, hypoproteinaemia and oedema.

The clinical picture is, however, often less neat and cross-over features of both syndromes occur frequently.

Immune mechanisms seem to be a common feature of all glomerular disease, either: immune complex disorders—the deposition of antigen-antibody complexes in the glomeruli or the formation of anti-glomerular basement membrane antibody (anti-GBM disease)

The antigen responsible may be:

- Exogenous, as the result of infection (e.g. β-haemolytic *Streptococcus*)
- Endogenous, as the result of auto-immune processes [e.g. systemic lupus erythematosus (SLE)].

Where renal biopsy is indicated (see later), a variety of pathological changes in the glomeruli may be found using light or electron microscopy and immunofluorescent techniques, but they often correlate imperfectly with the clinical picture. Two main pathological changes may be identified:

Proliferative: These are changes in which there is an increase of inflammatory cells in the glomerulus and mesangium (the matrix holding the glomerular capillaries). This occurs diffusely throughout the glomerulus

Non-proliferative: These are pathological changes in which there may be no changes on light microscopy but changes to the podocytes (see later) on electron microscopy (the so-called minimal change or light-negative variety) or there may be basement membrane thickening or there may be foci of glomerulosclerosis.

Generally, those with the GN pattern tend to show proliferative changes while those with the nephrotic pattern tend to show non-proliferative changes.

The most common glomerular diseases in childhood are as follows.

Acute Post-infective Glomerulonephritis

The most common infectious agent is the Lancefield group A β-haemolytic *Streptococcus* acute poststreptococcal glomerulonephritis (APSGN), but other possible infectious agents include bacteria (*Staphylococcus aureus*, *Streptococcus pneumonia* and *Salmonella* species), viruses (*Herpes* group, *Mycoplasma pneumonia*, *Varicella zoster*), fungi and protozoans (toxoplasmosis, malaria and schistosomiasis). Acute postinfective glomerulonephritis (APIGN) has also occurred in association with subacute bacterial endocarditis and infected ventricular shunts.

Typically a child with APSGN will be over 2 years of age and present with haematuria. The face will be puffy, the BP will be moderately raised (see note on "Blood Pressure Measurement"), and urine microscopy will show the presence of RBCs and granular casts **(Fig. 13.1)**. Chemical testing for blood is insufficient as a positive test may indicate haemoglobinuria (a different set of problems). There is likely to be mild proteinuria but little disturbance of blood proteins and there may be mild elevation of blood urea. Typically, the serum C3 compliment level is markedly lowered, returning to normal as recovery takes place. The C4 level is usually normal. There will usually be a history of tonsillitis or pharyngitis 10 days previously and a throat swab may still grow a β-haemolytic *Streptococcus* on culture, but a small number of cases result from streptococcal skin infections **(Fig. 13.4)**.

Such a typical pattern of APSGN is usually self-limiting and management may be restricted to monitoring the course of recovery, ensuring no complications ensue and treating the causative infection. An appropriate management programme would be:

- Treating any residual pharyngeal or skin infection as indicated by throat swab/skin swab or ASOT.
- Monitoring urine output and fluid intake to ensure they are in balance.

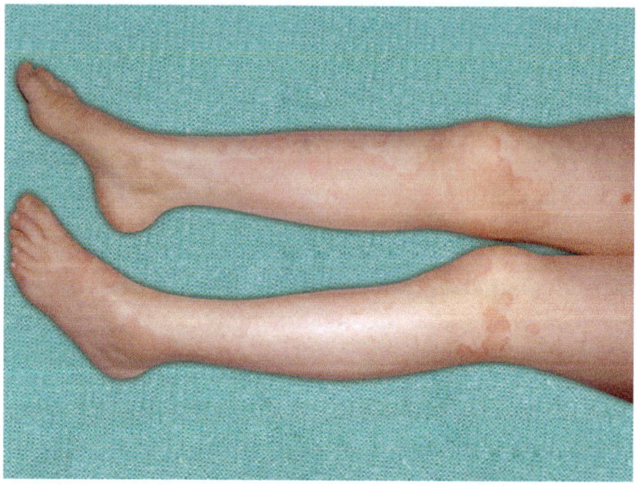

Figure 13.4 A child with cutaneous streptococcal infection developed acute poststreptococcal glomerulonephritis.

- Checking daily urine microscopy and testing for haematuria.
- Monitoring daily weight.
- Monitoring BP.
- Monitoring plasma urea, electrolytes and calcium.

A full blood count (FBC), antinuclear factor (ANF) screen, urine culture, urine protein/creatinine ratio and a renal US would be prudent investigations to exclude other possible causes of haematuria. **Table 13.1** gives the differential diagnosis of haematuria in childhood and **Flow chart 13.1** presents a scheme of management.

Added dietary salt should be avoided, but restricting protein intake and giving a high-carbohydrate intake is unnecessary unless the urea rises. The problem usually resolves itself in 2–3 weeks. Direct intervention is occasionally needed if the BP rises to dangerous levels, in which case, fluid restriction and the use of hypotensive agents may be called for or if potassium levels rise or calcium levels fall significantly. Immunity to nephritogenic streptococci is type specific and long lasting, thus recurrent attacks of APSGN are rare and (unlike acute rheumatic fever) penicillin prophylaxis is unnecessary.

The clinical pattern of other forms of APIGN will vary from that of APSGN and these should be sought where the presentation or course is atypical or where the β-haemolytic *Streptococcus* is not found or where there are other predisposing factors.

Flow chart 13.1 A plan for the investigation of paediatric haematuria.

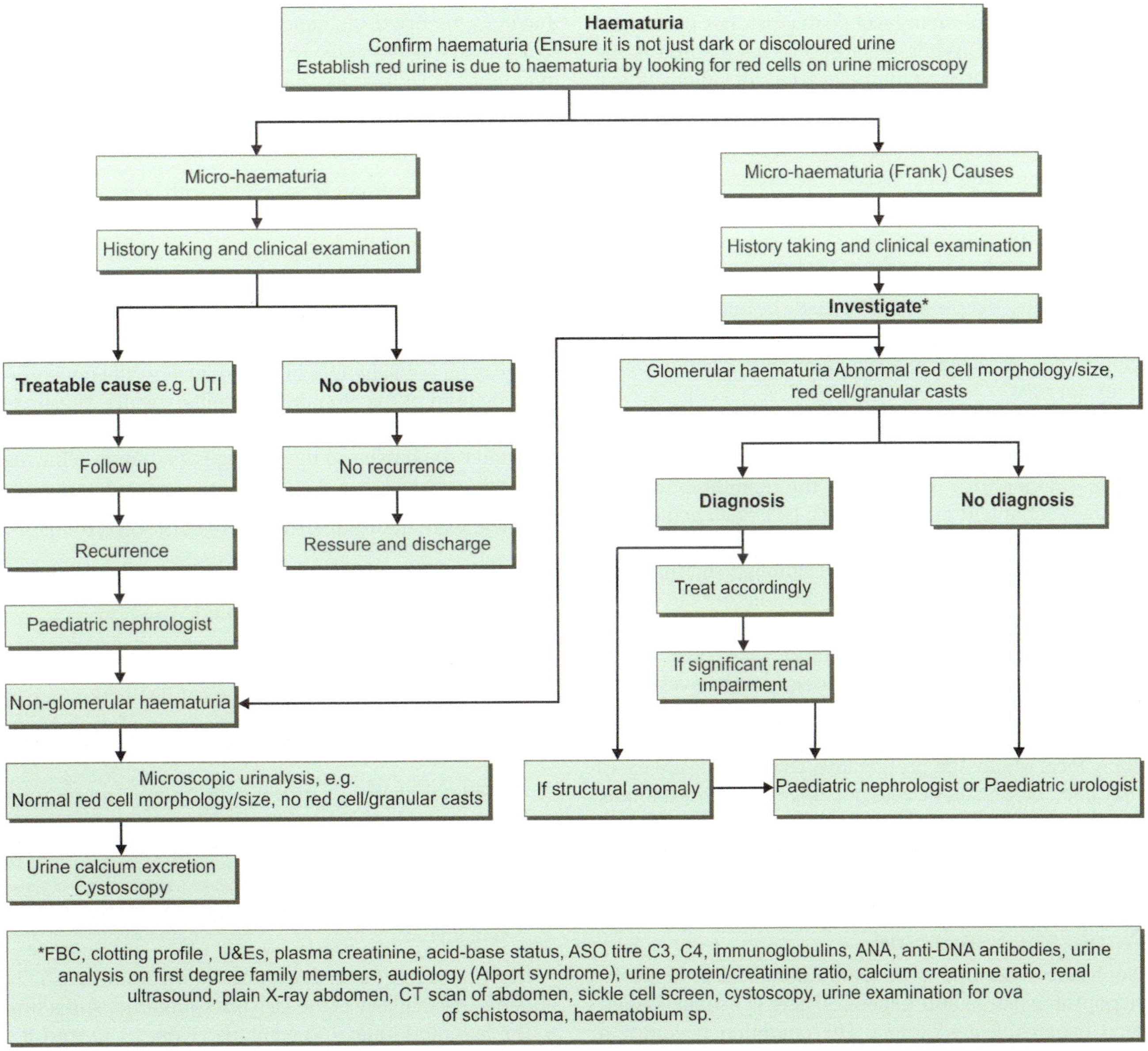

BERGER DISEASE

Immunoglobulin A Nephropathy (Berger Disease)

Immunoglobulin A (IgA) nephropathy results from immune complexes of the IgA type directed against exogenous antigens (viral or bacterial) deposited in the glomeruli. The condition is the most common form of glomerular disease of all ages worldwide but particularly in the second and third decades. Boys are more commonly affected than girls. It has the potential to be a long-term recurrent problem, even to progress to end-stage renal failure.

Typically, recurrent episodes of painless haematuria follow bouts of upper respiratory infection (URI). The interval between the URI and the appearance of haematuria is usually 1–2 days. Plasma IgA levels are typically increased, but compliment levels are normal. The interval between the URI and the appearance of haematuria and the normal compliment level distinguish IgA nephropathy from APSGN. While macroscopic haematuria is the most common presentation, a variety of other clinical patterns may occur including:

- Full-blown acute glomerulonephritis (AGN)
- Asymptomatic microscopic haematuria (which may persist long term)
- Nephrotic syndrome
- Mixed nephrotic/nephritic picture

A definitive diagnosis can be made by immunofluorescent studies of a renal biopsy showing IgA deposits in the glomerulus. A satisfactory treatment of IgA nephropathy does not exist.

Henoch–Schönlein Nephritis

Glomerulonephritis is one of the manifestations of Henoch-Schönlein purpura (HSP). HSP is an acute multisystem disorder resulting from small vessel vasculitis, possibly secondary to infection (although the infection is seldom identified). Renal complications are not invariable, but when they occur, they are potentially the most serious complication of the condition. The spectrum of clinical presentation mimics that of IgA nephropathy with macro- or microscopic haematuria, or a mixed nephrotic/nephritic picture **(Fig. 13.5)**. A renal biopsy in HSP may show focal segmental proliferative changes. Severe cases may need prednisolone with possibly cyclophosphamide, but despite treatment, the end-stage renal failure rate is 1.6–3% with the added hazard that similar changes may occur in a transplanted kidney.

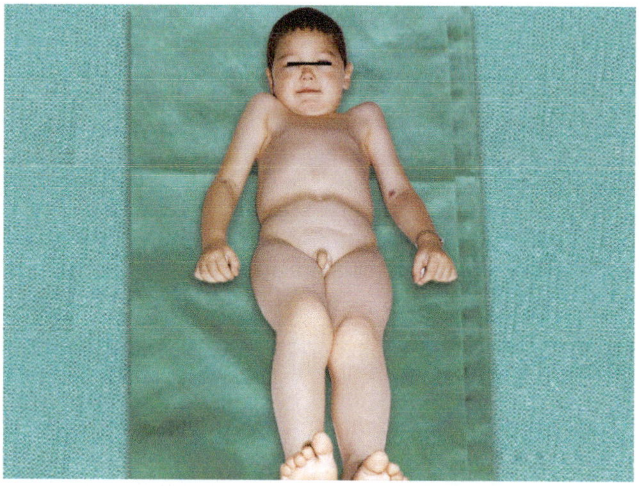

Figure 13.5 A child with Henoch–Schönlein nephritis. *Note* the 'nephrotic' features in this combined 'nephrotic/nephritic picture'.

Nephrotic Syndrome

Nephrotic syndrome is the combination of proteinuria, hypoproteinaemia and oedema. There is usually associated hypercholesterolaemia. The condition is common having a reported incidence in Europe and America of 2–7 cases/100,000 while in the Indian subcontinent the incidence is as high as 16 cases/100,000. The condition may occur at all ages but is most common between the ages of 1½ and 5 years and in boys more commonly than girls.

Nephrotic syndrome is associated with non-proliferative changes in the glomeruli and three histological variants are found:

Minimal-change nephrotic syndrome (MCNS) (85%):

- Here, there is no abnormality on light microscopy (light-negative), but on electron microscopy, there can be seen changes in the podocytes (the outer epithelium of the glomerular capillary wall). These are fused rather than interdigitating and this seems to alter the barrier to the passage of albumin allowing albumin leak.

Focal segmental glomerulosclerosis (FSGS) (10%):

- Here, segments of glomeruli develop sclerosis.

Membranous glomerulonephritis (MGN) (5%):

- Here, there is thickened GBM.

The importance of the pathological distinction lies in the variable response to steroid treatment of each group and thus the ultimate prognosis:

- Minimal-change nephrotic syndrome more than 95% steroid sensitive (SSNS)
- Focal segmental glomerulosclerosis—20% steroid sensitive
- Membranous glomerulonephritis—50% steroid sensitive.

The presenting feature of nephrotic syndrome is usually oedema, particularly of the face but sometimes spreading to the legs, abdomen and genitalia **(Figs. 13.6A and B)**.

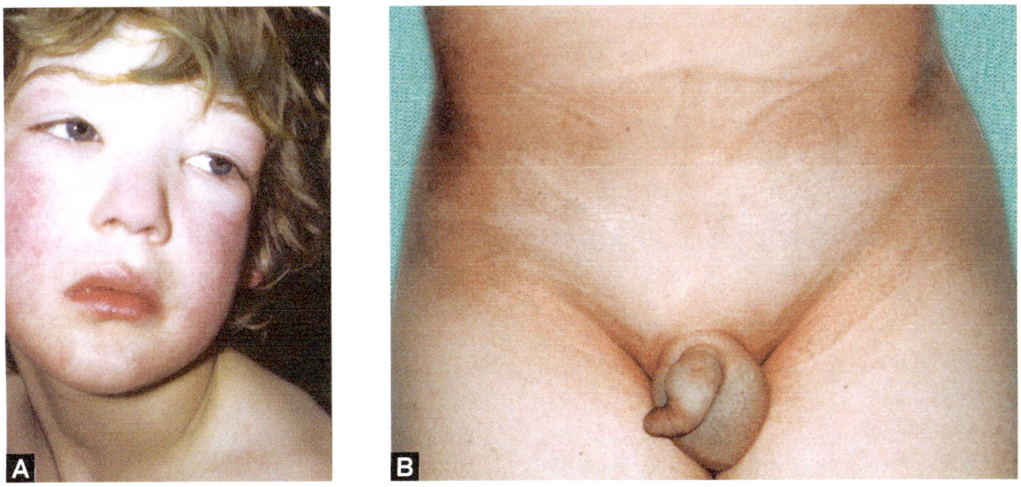

Figures 13.6A and B Nephrotic syndrome. (A) Facial oedema. (B) Scrotal oedema.

Ascites, sometimes gross, may occur. Oedema results from a fall in the serum albumin to 25–30 g/L (normal 36–44 g/L). Urine examination shows gross proteinuria (>50 mg/kg/day or a protein/creatinine ratio of >600 mg/mmol). The proteinuria may be selective (albumin only) or non-selective (including higher molecular weight proteins such as IgG). Haematuria is rare.

Investigation of a suspected case should include:

- Full blood count.
- Urea and electrolytes, and creatinine.
- Throat swab and ASOT (to exclude other glomerular disease).
- Serum proteins and compliment C3/C4 levels.
- Urine culture, chemical testing for protein including protein/creatinine ratio, and microscopy for blood and casts. Protein selectivity tests may be a guide to prognosis.
- Serum total cholesterol, low density lipoproteins and very low density lipoproteins.
- In addition, the following are prudent measures:
- Urinary sodium concentration as a measure of hypovolaemia (a urinary sodium of <10 mmol/L suggests hypovolaemia).
- Varicella zoster status prior to steroid treatment.

Management

There are two possible explanations for the oedema of NS and, as the treatment of each is diametrically opposite and giving the wrong treatment is potentially hazardous, it is important to determine which explanation pertains in each individual patient.

The underfill explanation: The colloid osmotic pressure of the plasma falls as a result of the fall in plasma albumin. In consequence, water transfers to the interstitial fluid space reducing the plasma volume. This is the common explanation in SSNS and the treatment is to raise the blood volume by the cautious infusion of colloids or albumin. A potentially fatal complication of hypovolaemia is thromboembolism.

The overfill explanation: In this explanation, there is impairment of sodium excretion. This leads to water retention, and hence expansion of both the plasma and interstitial fluid volumes. This is the common explanation in steroid resistant nephrotic syndrome. It would clearly be dangerous to increase the fluid volume further by infusion of colloid and it is important to be aware of which problem is present. The treatment in this circumstance is fluid restriction and diuretics.

In the acute phase, therefore, there are three principles of management:

1. The assessment of the height, weight, BP, the state of peripheral perfusion and urinary sodium, followed by a decision on whether the patient needs fluid restriction and diuretics for overfill states or infusion of colloids or albumin for hypovolaemia, recognising the potential hazards of each of the treatment policies.
2. Oral corticosteroids in the form of prednisolone 60 mg/m^2/24 hours (maximum 80 mg) for 4 weeks, reducing by stages over 3 months are recommended for first attacks on the grounds that few will obtain spontaneous remission and most will be of the minimal change—steroid sensitive variety.
3. There should be prevention of infection, which was formerly a major cause of death, due to reduced immunoglobulin levels and to immunosuppression with steroids. *S. pneumonia* is a major potential cause of infection particularly pneumococcal peritonitis. Oral penicillin should be given as a routine to these patients and they should be given pneumococcal immunization. Varicella zoster immunization should be given if indicated by the child's absence of immunity as chickenpox can be devastating to a child

on steroids. In the Indian subcontinent, tuberculosis (TB) is a major infectious complication and should be screened for before steroid therapy commences.

Outcome

One of four measures of outcome may be expected:

1. *Non-relapsing NS* in which recovery takes place and the urine is protein-free at the end of 6 or 9 months.
2. *Infrequently relapsing NS* in which the child seems to make a complete recovery, but recovery is followed by occasional relapses over the next 2–3 years, usually in response to URI.
3. *Frequently relapsing NS* with up to two attacks per 6 months or four attacks per year each attack usually responding to corticosteroid treatment.
4. *Steroid-dependent NS* in which the child, after apparently recovering, has two to four relapses in the next 6 months or relapses while still on treatment or within 4 days of stopping treatment.

Frequently relapsing NS and steroid dependent NS are indications for renal biopsy. As the frequent courses of steroid treatment needed in these circumstances will have an inevitable detrimental effect on the child's growth and development other measures must be sought. A variety of other immunosuppressive drugs have been used including the alkylating agent, cyclophosphamide, cyclosporin A and levamisole. A higher initial dose of corticosteroid, including the use of the powerful IV steroid methylprednisolone, has been tried experimentally. These measures require the supervision of a specialist paediatric nephrology team to whom the child should be referred.

Congenital Nephrotic Syndrome

Congenital nephrosis is a rare disorder of probably autosomal recessive inheritance. It appears to have a particularly high and familial incidence in Finland (Finnish type). The condition is characterised by a large placenta, heavy proteinuria, oedema and ascites. It is unresponsive to steroid therapy and cytotoxic drugs. The affected infants die from intercurrent infections and progressive renal failure.

Another condition causing NS in the first months of life is diffuse mesangial sclerosis. The pattern of inheritance is not clear, but it appears to be genetic.

Indications for Renal Biopsy in Glomerular Disease in Childhood

Features of GN not typical of APSGN
Family history of glomerular disease
Over 15 years of age
Signs of extrarenal disease
Mixed nephritic/nephrotic picture
Persistent macroscopic haematuria at 3 months
Persistent microscopic haematuria at 1 year
Persistent hypocomplementaemia (low C3 at 3 months)
Persistent proteinuria at 6 months (outcomes 3 and 4 above).

ACUTE RENAL FAILURE

The aetiology, mode of presentation and treatment of acute renal failure (ARF) sufficiently differs from those of chronic renal failure (CRF) for them to be considered in different sections. Acute renal failure may be defined as the sudden and often catastrophic reduction in GFR resulting in elevation in plasma creatinine and urea, disturbance in electrolyte balance, most notably with an elevation in potassium (K^+) and with severe metabolic acidosis. Widespread effects of fluid volume overload may result from extreme oliguria or anuria.

Definition of Acute Renal Failure

Oliguria—urine output: less than 300 $mL/m^2/day$ or 0.5 mL/kg/hour
Anuria—urine output: less than 1 mL/kg/day
Hyperkalaemia—potassium more than 6.0 mmol/L
A 50% rise in plasma creatinine over baseline
Clinical fluid overload
Oedema
Hypertension

The causes of ARF may be prerenal (the result of hypoperfusion of the kidneys), renal (the result of intrinsic damage to the kidneys) or postrenal (the result of obstruction to the urinary tract).

Causes of Acute Renal Failure

Prerenal

Hypovolaemia: Gastroenteritis (the most common cause by far in developing countries), blood loss, burns, diabetic ketoacidosis

Peripheral vascular dilatation in severe sepsis

Impaired cardiac output in congestive heart failure (in childhood, this can be a consequence of open heart surgery for congenital heart disease).

Renal

Acute tubular necrosis: dehydration, snake-bite, falciparum malaria, leptospirosis

Acute cortical necrosis

Haemolytic-uraemic-syndrome (HUS) and other forms of IV haemolysis, haemoglobinuria and myoglobinuria and tumour lysis

Drugs: Aminoglycosides, nonsteroidal anti-inflammatory drugs (NSAIDS), IV contrast materials

Renal vein thrombosis

Severe bilateral pyelonephritis

Acute glomerulonephritis.

Postrenal

Calculuses
Posterior urethral valves
Neurogenic bladder
Ureterocoele.

It should be noted that there are causes of ARF prevalent in tropical countries not seen in more temperate regions.

Diagnosis of Acute Renal Failure

When the ARF is prerenal, there will usually be symptoms indicating the underlying aetiology, e.g. diarrhoea, vomiting, fluid or blood loss. Typically there will be a high plasma urea/creatinine ratio, increased urine osmolality (>500 mOsm/kg), urinary sodium concentration less than 20 mEq/L and fractional excretion of sodium less than 1%.

When the cause of ARF is renal there may be manifestations of extrarenal multisystem disease or a history of a precipitating factor (e.g. snake bite, nephrotoxic drugs). The urinary sodium is high (>40 mEq/L), urinary osmolality is low (<300 mOsm/kg) and fractional excretion of sodium is more than 1%.

Ultrasonography is the ideal imaging tool in renal failure because it is not dependent on renal function and is useful in the evaluation of postrenal obstructive causes.

Management of Acute Renal Failure

The management of a child with ARF may conveniently be considered under the following headings:

Fluid Therapy

In the emergency situation before it is clear to what degree the ARF is due to prerenal causes rather than to intrinsic renal damage and where restoring renal perfusion by correcting hypovolaemia might be indicated, a cautious infusion of dextrose saline (appropriate to the age of the infant) can be given. Some would also give a trial of frusemide to stimulate urine output. Fluid and frusemide may be repeated or withheld according to response. Fluid intake thereafter should equal the insensible fluid losses plus output (urine, vomiting, diarrhoea, and so on). Potassium containing fluids should not be given.

Hyponatraemia

Hyponatraemia is the common finding in children with ARF and is most frequently secondary to water excess rather than sodium loss. If doubt exists, it is safer to restrict water intake until the cause becomes clear. Profound hyponatraemia (plasma sodium <120 mmol/L) may cause neurological problems. Therefore, correction of hyponatraemia to a sodium level 125 mmol/L is prudent. Dialysis may be needed for severe intractable hyponatraemia.

Hyperkalaemia

Hyperkalaemia is the most serious problem associated with ARF and causes cardiac dysfunction (peaked T waves, widened QRS complexes, depressed ST segments, dysrhythmias—bradycardia, ventricular tachycardia, ventricular fibrillation and arrest), which may lead to death of the patient. Hyperkalaemia arises from the inability to excrete potassium in the urine and is worse in the presence of acidosis because of the buffering exchange of H^+ for K^+ in the tissues. Potassium intake must be minimised and correction of acidosis undertaken. If electrocardiography (ECG) changes are present or if serum potassium rises above 7 mmol/L, then emergency treatment is indicated—10% calcium gluconate 0.5–1 mL/kg by slow IV infusion over 5–10 minutes will reduce the toxic effect of high potassium on the heart.

A number of emergency measures are available for lowering serum potassium:

- Nebulised salbutamol acts by moving potassium from the extracellular into the intracellular space.
- Cation-exchange resins can be given orally or rectally to expedite the elimination of potassium from the body.
- An IV infusion of insulin 0.1 unit/kg plus dextrose 25% 0.5 g/kg over 30 minutes will reduce the potassium quickly.
- Dialysis is the most effective way of reducing dangerous levels of potassium and hyperkalaemia is the most common indication for emergency dialysis.

Hypocalcaemia

Hypocalcaemia is quite common in ARF, but it rarely causes symptoms. If symptomatic then calcium can be given by slow IV infusion of 10% calcium gluconate 0.5 mL/kg/hour, the infusion rate being titrated according to the blood calcium level. If hypocalcaemia proves resistant, the Mg^{++} should be checked.

Hyperphosphataemia

Phosphate restriction and phosphate binders, e.g. calcium carbonate, should help to deal with this problem.

Metabolic Acidosis

Metabolic acidosis is a constant and early feature of ARF because of the important role of the kidneys in regulating and maintaining acid-base homeostasis. When acidosis is present, it should be treated with sodium bicarbonate. Intravenous 8.4% sodium bicarbonate, 1–2 mL/kg equivalent to 1–2 mmol/kg should be administered where blood pH values are less than 7.25. Adequacy of pH correction should be monitored by regular measurement of blood gases. Rapid correction of acidosis should be avoided as it may cause hypocalcaemia and tetany or seizures.

Anaemia in Acute Renal Failure

Mild to moderate anaemia is often present in ARF and is almost invariable in some causes (e.g. HUS). Anaemia, when present to a significant degree, may potentiate the complications, especially cardiac failure and it may be beneficial to correct this by small transfusions of recently collected packed red cells.

Hypertension

Severe symptomatic hypertension can occur in association with salt and water overload. It is important that hypertension be controlled. Treatment consists of restriction of fluid and sodium intake and antihypertensive therapy.

Infection in Acute Renal Failure

Infection can be both a cause and a serious complication of ARF and every effort must be made to prevent it and to detect it and treat it if it develops.

Nutrition in Acute Renal Failure

Acute renal failure is a hypercatabolic state and requires aggressive nutritional support. The aim of dietary treatment is as follows:

- Control of dietary potassium.
- Control of dietary sodium.
- Control of dietary phosphate.
- To tailor fluid intake to maintain fluid balance.
- Vitamin and micronutrient supplements.

Peritoneal Dialysis or Haemodialysis

While spontaneous recovery from ARF, in whole or in part, may be expected, peritoneal dialysis (PD) may be needed for variable periods of time to support the patient by correcting dangerous degrees of metabolic or other disturbance. The indications for dialysis are as follows:

- A rising serum potassium level is perhaps the most common indication for emergency dialysis.
- Gross fluid overload.
- Severe symptomatic-uraemia with vomiting or encephalopathy.
- Hypertension unresponsive to other therapy.

Peritoneal dialysis is the preferred choice for children in the acute stage. It is available in paediatric units lacking the specialist skills required for haemodialysis and avoids the difficulties of vascular access and anticoagulation. If complications occur with PD or if more long-term dialysis seems needed, then haemodialysis may be necessary. In patients with multiorgan failure, haemofiltration may be required.

Outcomes in Acute Renal Failure

While complete resolution of ARF and return to normal kidney function is possible some degree of long-term or even permanent renal impairment is more likely. The outcome depends to some degree on the underlying cause of the ARF and the speed with which it is dealt.

Prerenal

If the underlying cause, be it hypovolaemia or acute cardiac failure, can be reversed quickly, ARF from this cause has the best prognosis. Any delay, however, leads to intrinsic renal damage and further renal causes of ARF.

Acute Tubular Necrosis

This is usually secondary to prerenal failure. Recovery may be associated with some degree of Fanconi-like syndrome with failure of tubular reabsorption of electrolytes and water and possibly a degree of secondary renal acidosis (*see* Section "Renal Tubular Disorders").

Acute Cortical Necrosis

This is more common in the neonate and is associated with multisystem failure resulting from a severe hypoxic/ischaemic event. The ARF is usually associated with haematuria, oliguria, hypertension and thrombocytopaenia. It has a poor prognosis.

Renal Vein Thrombosis

This is largely a neonatal problem resulting from severe dehydration, especially in the first week of life. The signs of ARF are associated with haematuria, thrombocytopenia and a palpably swollen kidney. When bilateral, it is usually fatal. In addition to other measures, cautious heparinisation can be tried.

Haemolytic–Uraemic Syndrome

See below as discussed in detail.

HAEMOLYTIC–URAEMIC SYNDROME

Haemolytic–uraemic syndrome is the most common cause of ARF in children in developed countries. It is more common in infants and children than in adults. The common pattern is a gastrointestinal (GI) infection, sometimes with scanty and often with bloody diarrhoea, leading to the triad of microangiopathic haemolytic anaemia, thrombocytopenia and ARF. There are two subtypes of HUS. The first is associated with diarrhoeal prodrome (D + HUS) and the second is not associated with antecedent diarrhoea (D-HUS).

The association between HUS (D + HUS) and enteric *E. coli* type 0157:H7 suggests that this is the type responsible for HUS. It produces cytotoxin active on vero-cells (a laboratory cell-culture line derived from kidney cells of African Green Monkeys) called 'verotoxin'. It can be transmitted by ingestion of contaminated food or water, by person to person contact or by contact with animals, especially farm animals. An association of shigellosis with HUS is also well-established; however, the incidence of

HUS in India has declined with the decline in the virulent form of shigella dysentery.

The D-HUS is much rarer in childhood, seen mainly in older children and can be familial, drug induced or recurrent.

Clinical Features

Haemolytic-uraemic syndrome is characterised by abdominal cramps, watery diarrhoea changing to bloody diarrhoea, vomiting, pallor and occasionally accompanied by convulsions. Oliguria is constantly present, but not always appreciated. Hypertension may be severe. The blood shows severe anaemia, thrombocytopaenia and reticulocytosis. Some of the red cells are characteristically misshapen: acanthocytes, burr cells, triangular cells and others with a 'broken egg-shell' shape are common **(Fig. 13.7)**. The blood urea is greatly elevated. The urine shows protein, red cells and granular casts. Proteinuria is in the non-nephrotic range (1–2 g/day). In many cases, sequential studies of the circulating clotting factors will show evidence of a consumptive coagulopathy due to disseminated intravascular coagulation.

Treatment

The mainstay of treatment for children with HUS is the management of ARF as outlined above. In (D + HUS), no specific therapy has proven beneficial. There is no benefit from anticoagulant or thrombolytic therapy or from IV prostacyclin, steroids or gammaglobulins.

Prognosis of Haemolytic–Uraemic Syndrome

In children with HUS, the complete recovery rate is about 70%. A small number die in the acute stage of the illness; some die without recovering renal function after weeks on dialysis while other children are left with hypertension and CRF. In children who develop end-stage renal disease, successful renal transplantation has been reported.

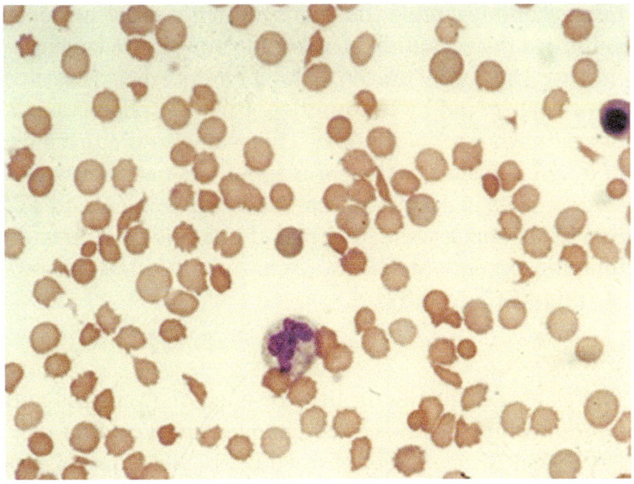

Figure 13.7 Peripheral blood film of a child with haemolytic–uraemic syndrome. (*Note:* Wide variation in shape and size of RBCs including acanthocytes, burr cells, 'broken egg shell' and other fragmented cells and an absence of platelets.)

Prevention

The only way to prevent HUS is to prevent primary infection by developing efficient strategies directed at the known dangers. Control and improvement of food safety procedures, particularly the separation of cooked and uncooked meat in abattoirs, butchers and in the home is paramount, and hygiene procedures should be followed, especially for children in nurseries and when visiting farms and handling animals.

CHRONIC RENAL FAILURE

Chronic renal failure is the end stage of a variety of childhood kidney diseases including congenital abnormalities, hereditary conditions, infection, obstruction, AGN, NS and the various insults leading to ARF. CRF may be asymptomatic in the early stages and may either go undetected until a late stage has been reached or be detected incidentally during the investigation of apparently unrelated complaints (e.g. growth impairment). Reduced renal concentrating capacity may be the first function to be impaired and polydipsia/polyuria, the first symptom. The progress of CRF may be monitored by sequential GFR measurements. Various degrees of CRF may be identified:

- Moderate CRF: GFR = 30–59*
- Severe CRF: GFR = 10–29*
- Kidney failure: GFR = less than 10* (*mL/min/1.73 m^2)

A GFR of less than 10 mL/min/1.73 m^2 indicates end-stage renal failure and suggests the need for long-term dialysis or renal transplant.

Investigation of Chronic Renal Failure

The diagnosis of CRF is based on the GFR and is most conveniently performed by the ^{51}Cr EDTA (chromium ethylenediaminetetraacetic acid) method or inulin clearance. The creatinine is unhelpful as it may remain normal until a late stage. The underlying cause of the CRF may be obvious from the history but if not this should be pursued vigorously. The consequences of CRF on other systems should also be sought, and BP, U&E, acid–base balance, growth and bone changes of renal osteodystrophy are all relevant investigations. US is a quick method of establishing gross abnormalities of kidneys and urinary collecting system.

Management of Chronic Renal Failure

A child with CRF presents a long-term management problem and ideally requires the involvement of a tertiary paediatric nephrology team. The principles of management following the stabilisation of urgent problems are as follows:

- Nutrition: The establishment of estimated average requirements for:
  - Protein (optimising nitrogen intake while reducing catabolism)
  - Energy
  - Vitamins
- Fluid and electrolytes and acid-base balance
  - Free access to water for the child to determine own needs
  - Food low in potassium
  - Sodium supplements if salt losing in polyuria
  - Sodium bicarbonate 2 mmol/kg per day, if in metabolic acidosis
- Control of hypertension
- Management of renal osteodystrophy
  - Hydroxylated derivatives of vitamin D such as 1 alpha hydroxycholecalciferol (alfacalcidol) may be needed as hydroxylation of vitamin D may be one of the failed renal functions
- Management of anaemia
  - Erythropoietin for the normochromic normocytic anaemia which may be present
- Management of growth failure
  - If despite the control of nutrition and management of other aspects of CRF, there is still failure of growth, synthetic human growth hormone may be required
- Renal replacement in the form of regular haemodialysis or renal transplant, if more conservative management fails to stabilise the patient.

RENAL TUBULAR DISORDERS

The renal tubules are responsible for the regulation of fluid, electrolyte and acid-base homeostasis in the body by the selective reabsorption in the proximal or distal tubule of water, sodium, potassium, bicarbonate and phosphate. This function is partly the result of passive ion diffusion and partly under humoral control. Disorders of renal tubular function may result from inborn errors of metabolism or from damage resulting from the causes of ARF discussed earlier. A variety of clinical syndromes result from such renal tubular dysfunction.

Renal Tubular Acidosis

There are two main mechanisms underlying this disorder:

Distal or Type 1 Renal Tubular Acidosis

This appears to be an autosomal dominant disorder in which, in the presence of systemic acidosis, the kidney is unable to secrete sufficient H^+ ion in the proximal part of the distal tubule to lower the urinary pH below 6. An ammonium load test given to stress the system by producing metabolic acidosis fails to reduce urinary pH below 6. There is usually hyperchloraemic acidosis and frequently hypokalaemia. Type 1 renal tubular acidosis (RTA) may be secondary to various renal conditions such as vitamin D intoxication, obstructive uropathies and other insults.

Treatment of type 1 RTA is directed at correcting metabolic acidosis by giving sodium bicarbonate and correcting any associated hypokalaemia with potassium supplements.

Proximal or Type 2 Renal Tubular Acidosis

In type 2 RTA, the proximal tubule is unable to reabsorb filtered bicarbonate leading to bicarbonate wastage. In this form of RTA, the ammonium loading test is normal. As an isolated, sporadic inherited condition, proximal RTA is uncommon, but it may be an association with other renal tubular disorders and will be discussed with them.

Fanconi Syndrome and Cystinosis

Fanconi syndrome comprises a group of renal tubular defects of biochemical origin, either inherited or secondary to a variety of renal insults such as those which cause acute tubular necrosis. Features may include glycosuria, aminoaciduria, RTA, phosphaturia, potassium loss, and occasionally sodium loss and uricosuria. The most common cause is cystinosis in which, as a result of autosomal recessive inheritance, cystine crystals are found throughout the reticuloendothelial system (but with no gross excretion of cystine in the urine as in cystinuria which is a quite separate inborn error of metabolism). Other inborn errors of metabolism causing Fanconi syndrome include galactosaemia, Lowe syndrome and Wilson disease.

Clinical Features

The physical features of cystinosis usually appear in early infancy and resemble those of hyperchloraemic acidosis. Failure to thrive, anorexia, vomiting and severe constipation are constantly present. Thirst and polyuria may also have been noted by the mother. A feature characteristic of cystinosis is photophobia. This is due to the presence of cystine crystals in the cornea, but it is not always present. Rickets makes its appearance after some months of illness. Its appearance in a wasted infant is in contrast to infantile rickets which is more commonly found in growing infants **(Fig. 13.8)**.

Diagnosis

This is based initially on the presence of glycosuria and aminoaciduria. Radiological changes are typical of rickets. Cystinosis can be confirmed by the detection of cystine crystals in the cornea on slit-lamp examination, or by finding them in bone marrow or lymph node biopsy material **(Fig. 13.9)**. White cell cystine levels are raised and this is now used in diagnosis and monitoring treatment.

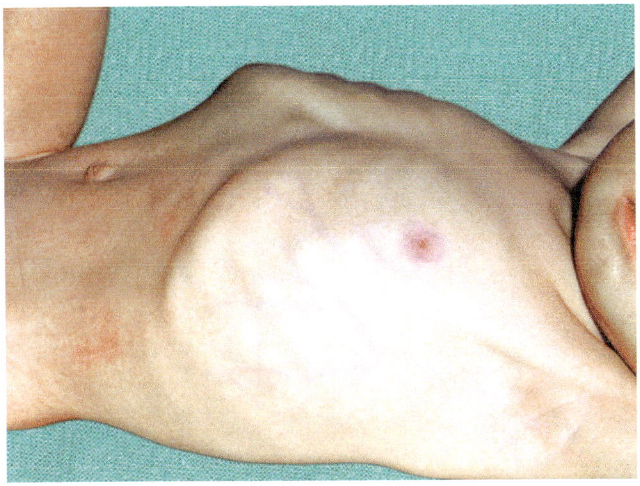

Figure 13.8 Rachitic rosary and generalised wasting.

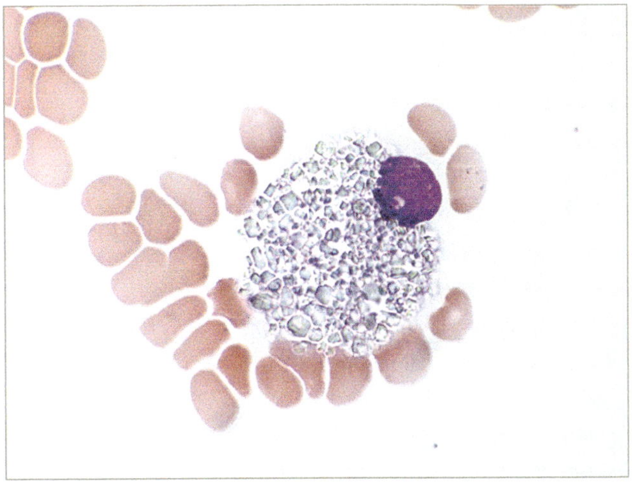

Figure 13.9 Bone marrow showing cystine crystals.

Treatment

Nutritional supplementation with electrolytes, water, bicarbonate, phosphate and calories should be given. Calcium together with 1-α [OH] vitamin D or 1,25 $[OH]_2$ vitamin D are required for treatment of the rickets. Mercaptamine (cysteamine) reduces intracellular cysteine levels and is available for the treatment of nephropathic-cystinosis. Mercaptamine eye drops are available for the management of ocular symptoms arising from the deposition of cystine crystals in the eye. Renal transplantation has been successful in children with cystinosis who develop end-stage renal disease. The other causes of Fanconi syndrome have their own specific treatment requirements.

Bartter Syndrome

This uncommon inborn error of metabolism affects the reabsorption of chloride in the loop of Henlé. It results in the urinary loss of chloride with consequent loss of sodium, potassium and calcium, increased prostaglandin synthesis and stimulation of the renin–angiotensin–aldosterone system. Mutations in up to five genes have been identified in association with this condition and the severity appears to be gene dependent.

Clinical Features

Symptoms are apparent from a young age with failure to thrive, muscular weakness, constipation and sometimes polydipsia/polyuria. Investigation shows hypokalaemia, hypochloraemia, increased renin and angiotensin and normal BP. The urinary potassium, chloride and calcium are raised with osteopenia and sometimes nephrocalcinosis.

Treatment

Treatment aims at keeping the serum potassium level more than 3.5 mmol/L and providing adequate nutrition. It involves oral potassium supplements together with spironolactone (a potassium sparing diuretic) and indomethacin (a prostaglandin antagonist).

Vitamin D Resistant Rickets (Hypophosphataemic Rickets)

Vitamin D resistant rickets, sometimes called hypophosphataemic rickets, is characterised by the typical signs of childhood rickets which fail to respond to treatment doses of vitamin D. It appears to be due to a deficiency in the tubular reabsorption of phosphate and to be transmitted by a dominant gene on the X chromosome, thus affected males have only affected daughters, whereas affected females have equal numbers of affected and healthy children irrespective of sex. The condition, therefore, is more common in girls but, because girls have one normal X chromosome, boys are more severely affected than girls. In a few cases, an autosomal recessive pattern of inheritance has been reported.

Clinical, Biochemical and Radiological Features

On presentation, the typical features of childhood rickets may be present: enlargement of the epiphyses, rachitic rosary and deformities of the limbs including bilateral coxa vara frequently resulting in a waddling 'penguin' gait **(Fig. 13.10)**. Unlike the rickets of vitamin D deficiency, however, where the child is usually quite well grown, in vitamin D resistant rickets, the child is poorly grown with short stature and disproportionate shortening of the lower limbs **(Fig. 13.11)**.

The biochemical findings are the same as those usually found in infantile vitamin D deficiency rickets, namely, normal plasma calcium, reduced plasma phosphate and increased alkaline phosphatase. Despite the low plasma phosphate level [and the low parathyroid hormone (PTH) level], the urinary excretion of phosphate is excessive, the

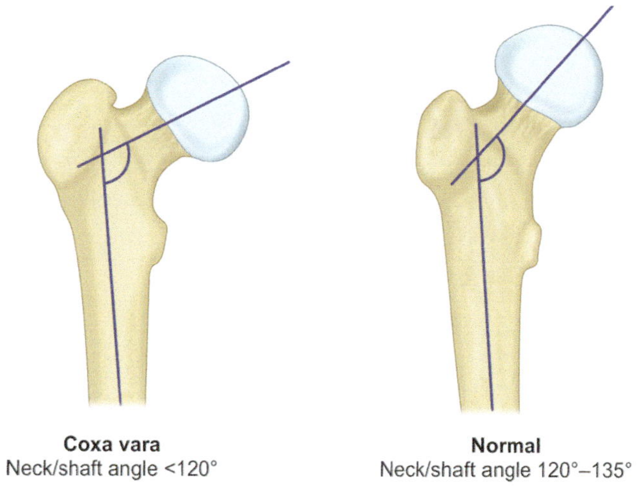

Figure 13.10 Coxa vara.

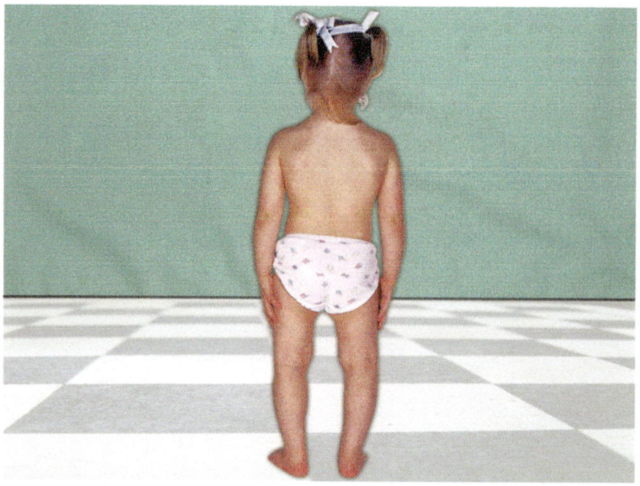

Figure 13.11 A girl with hypophosphataemic rickets showing short stature and bow legs.

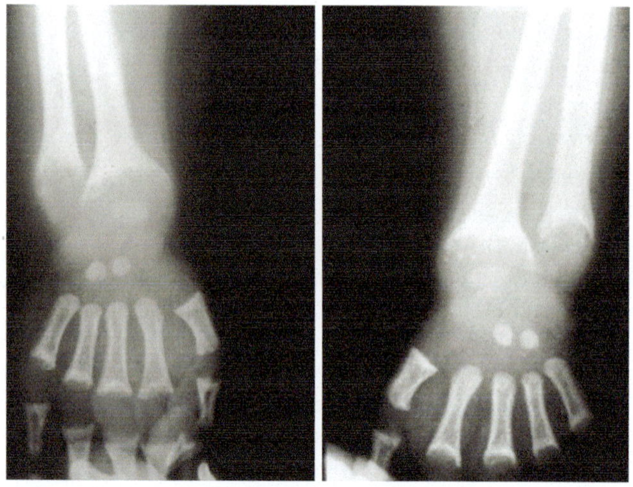

Figure 13.12 X-ray of wrists showing changes of rickets.

phosphate reabsorption percentage being less than 85%. Urinary calcium excretion is usually low. The plasma concentration of 25hydroxyvitamin D_3 25 $[OH]D_3$ is usually normal and that of 1,25 dihydroxyvitamin D_3,1,25 $[OH]_2D_3$ is slightly low or normal. Aminoaciduria that is commonly found in vitamin D deficiency rickets is not a feature of hypophosphataemic rickets. Radiological features are those of rickets, e.g. cupped, frayed and broadened metaphyses, broadened epiphyses, osteoporosis, deformities and pathological fractures **(Fig. 13.12)**.

Treatment

As hypophosphataemic rickets occurs due to abnormal phosphate excretion, treatment with high doses of oral phosphate and hydroxylated (activated) forms of vitamin D allow bone mineralisation and optimise growth. Vitamin D is not a single entity but a group of substances with a specific pattern of activity such as ergocalciferol (vitamin D_2) and cholecalciferol (naturally occurring vitamin D_3 produced by ultraviolet light acting on 7-dehydrocholesterol in the skin). Vitamin D_2 and D_3 are equal in potential potency but are precursors, and two metabolic steps are required to produce active enzymes. The first is in the liver, the second in the kidney. The most effective treatment appears to be a combination of 1-4 g of oral elemental phosphate/day with either oral 1,25 $[OH]_2D_3$ initially 15 nanograms (ng)/kg once daily, increased if necessary in steps of 5 ng/kg daily every 2-4 weeks (maximum 250 ng) or 1,25 $[OH]D_3$ 25-50 ng/kg once daily, adjusted as necessary (maximum 1 μg). Initially phosphate supplementation may cause diarrhoea, but tolerance to the regimen usually develops within 1-2 weeks. Frequent estimations of plasma calcium are necessary to detect hypercalcaemia due to overdosage. Vitamin D therapy alone rarely corrects dwarfism and even if started in early infancy may fail to prevent its development. Patients with residual skeletal deformities may need surgical correction with bilateral tibial and femoral osteotomies, usually after growth has ceased.

Case study: A 5-year-old boy presented to the paediatric clinic with bilateral bowing of the legs. The child was of Scottish origin, had a normal diet and no GI symptoms. On examination, he had short stature, reduced dental enamel and bilateral varus deformity of the knees. He did not have any wrist swelling.

- Investigations performed were as follows:
- Ca 2.31 mmol/L (reference range 2.2–2.7 mmol/L)
- PO_4 0.56 mmol/L (reference range 0.9–1.8 mmol/L)
- PTH 8.5 pmol/L (reference range 0.9–55 pmol/L)
- 25$[OH]D_3$ 74 nmol/L (reference range 15–85 nmol/L)
- Phosphate excretion index high
- Tubular reabsorption rate of phosphate low: less than 85%

Diagnosis: Hypophosphataemic rickets

Cystinuria, Oxaluria and Other Causes of Metabolic Nephrolithiasis

Cystinuria, one of the inborn errors of metabolism, is a rare cause of renal stone formation. In this condition, there is a defect in the tubular reabsorption not only of cysteine but also of lysine, arginine and ornithine. In spite of the passage of the typical hexagonal crystals in the urine (Fig. 13.1), only a minority of affected children develop calculi. This condition must not be confused with the quite separate metabolic disorder called cystinosis in which cystine is deposited in body tissues. Another exceedingly rare cause of renal lithiasis, also an inborn error of metabolism, is primary hyperoxaluria. Other inherited metabolic diseases that increase the excretion of very insoluble substances, and thus formation of renal stones are Lesch-Nyhan syndrome (LNS), 2, 8-dihydroxyadenineuria, xanthinuria and the orotic acidurias.

Nephrogenic Diabetes Insipidus

Nephrogenic diabetes insipidus (NDI) is a rare condition that must be differentiated from central-neurogenic or pituitary diabetes insipidus (CDI) due to failure of production by the posterior pituitary of antidiuretic hormone (ADH) (sometimes known as vasopressin). In NDI, the renal tubules fail to respond to vasopressin and thus fail to reabsorb water normally. The condition is due to a defect in the AVPR2 gene located on the X chromosome and has been transmitted as an X-linked trait in most of the reported families, only males being affected. The concentrating defect can be partial or complete.

Clinical Features

Excessive thirst and polyuria start soon after birth. Failure to thrive, pyrexia, anorexia, constipation and vomiting are common. Deprivation of fluids or a high environmental temperature leads to fever, prostration and hypernatraemic dehydration because these children cannot produce urine of high specific gravity. There is a particular risk during infancy when the patient is unable to determine his own fluid intake and NDI can be a cause of unexplained pyrexia in infants. Usually, the child is non selective in his choice of fluids and will wake from sleep to drink, often drinking from inappropriate sources, e.g. toilet cistern and bath water or any other source of fluid available. Growth may also be retarded.

Diagnosis

Diagnosis can be confirmed by failure to respond to vasopressin (vasopressin test) and by the marked inability to concentrate the urine during water deprivation (urine osmolality after 4 hours water deprivation should be >800 mOsm/kg).

Treatment

In NDI, benefit may be gained from the paradoxical antidiuretic effect of thiazides, e.g. chlorothiazide 10–20 mg/kg twice daily (maximum 500 mg).

- *Note: Vasopressin test*
- In NDI, there is little change in pre- and post-vasopressin urine osmolality
- In CDI, the pre-vasopressin test osmolality is less than 300 mOsm/kg, but post-vasopressin urine osmolality is markedly increased, i.e. more than 800 mOsm/kg.

Case study: 'A 3-month-old boy was born at 38 weeks of gestation with a birth weight of 3 kg. The neonatal period was uneventful. In infancy, he took his bottle feeds satisfactorily but was constantly irritable and the milk offered never seemed to be enough so he was offered flavoured water which he took eagerly. His weight gain was poor. On examination, he was well hydrated and there were no abnormal findings. Urine dipstick and culture were negative, urinary tract US was normal, plasma urea was 12 mmol/L, sodium 164 mmol/L and creatinine 60 μmol/L. He was given DDAVP (desmopressin) 0.5 μg intranasally and urine osmolality 4 hours later was 200 mOs/kg.

Diagnosis: Nephrogenic diabetes insipidus

CONGENITAL RENAL ABNORMALITIES AND INHERITED KIDNEY DISEASES

The frequency of antenatal US screening of pregnancies has led to the early detection of many congenital renal abnormalities. As many as 20% of abnormalities found at the 18–20 weeks scan involve the kidneys. Abnormalities of amniotic fluid volume, either polyhydramnios or oligohydramnios, may indicate a renal abnormality. In addition, many inherited disorders (including metabolic disorders affecting the renal tubules discussed elsewhere) affect the kidneys. Only the commoner will be discussed here.

Dysplastic Kidneys

Dysplastic kidneys are usually associated with oligohydramnios and poor growth of the foetus because the production of amniotic fluid is a function of the foetal kidney. There may be multiple defects in the infant, including facial and limb defects and pulmonary hypoplasia, features sometimes called 'Potter syndrome' a condition almost invariably fatal (Fig. 13.13).

Hydronephrosis

This may be unilateral, the result of pelvi-ureteric junction (PUJ) or vesico-ureteric junction (VUJ) obstruction or to unilateral reflux, or it may be bilateral due to posterior urethral valves, bilateral ureteric reflux or to prune belly syndrome, a condition predominantly of males in

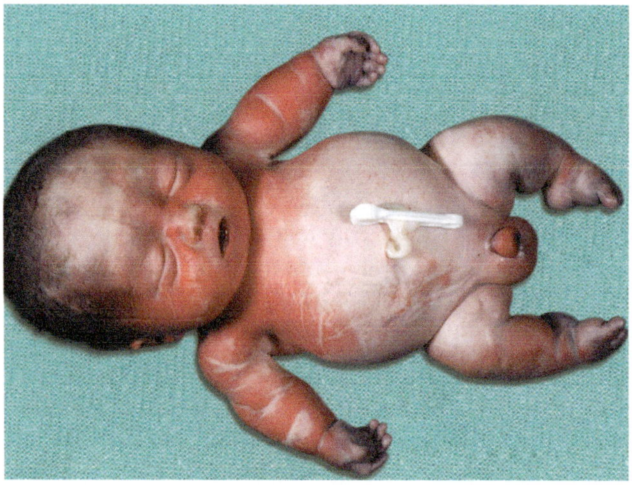

Figure 13.13 Potter syndrome.

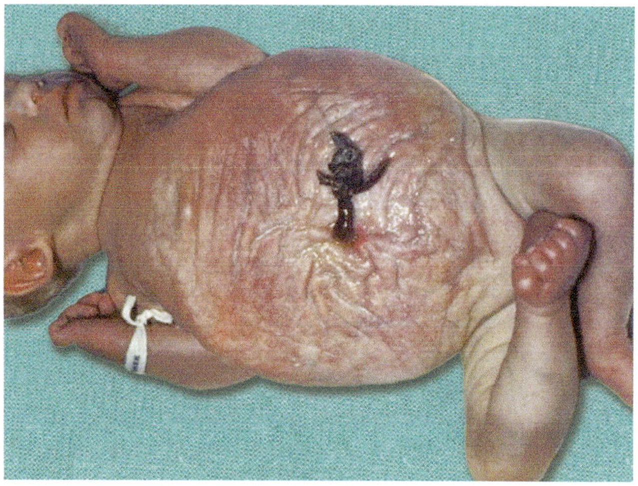

Figure 13.14 Prune belly syndrome.

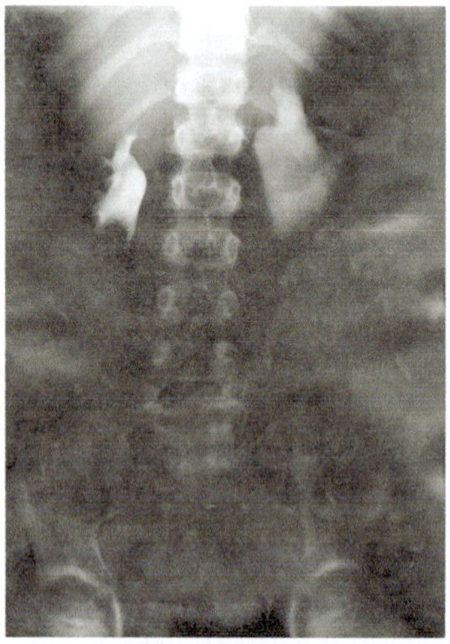

Figure 13.15 Intravenous pyelogram showing hydronephrosis—due to congenital ureteropelvic junction obstruction.

which there is failure of development of the abdominal musculature often with undescended testes and dilatation of the ureters and bladder **(Figs. 13.14 and 13.15)**. The consequences in relation to UTI, kidney growth, hypertension and for renal function are discussed elsewhere. The early discovery of hydronephrosis is an indication for expert renal investigation, renal function testing and possibly surgical intervention.

Polycystic Disease of the Kidney

Inherited as an autosomal dominant, polycystic disease of the kidney (PDK) may not present until the middle adult years, after the next generation of family has been established. Thus, asymptomatic children are often diagnosed as a result of a diagnosis having been made in a parent. A child of any age may, however, present with the complications of PDK, UTI or hypertension. The condition has an inexorable progression to renal failure, severe hypertension and a need for renal replacement therapy (dialysis or transplant). A rarer autosomal recessive form of PDK autosomal recessive polycystic kidney disease (ARPKD) causes severe multicystic kidneys antenatally, oligohydramnios and pulmonary hypoplasia with early death almost constantly. The liver also has cystic changes in ARPKD.

An isolated cyst of the kidney may occasionally be identified when screening for some other reason. This is of no clinical significance.

Duplications and Ectopias

Duplication of the ureters is quite a common finding either incidentally or on the investigation of the renal tract for UTI. They vary from a bifid pelvis to a duplex kidney in which one or both kidneys are doubled, one moiety often in an ectopic position and often subject to reflux and infection. Even without duplication, one or both kidneys may be ectopic usually somewhere in the pelvis. Sometimes the kidneys are fused forming a horseshoe kidney. Horseshoe kidney is sometimes associated with other abnormalities such as Turner syndrome and trisomy 18.

Ureterocoele

This is a cystic dilatation of the end of the ureter as it enters the bladder and is often associated with a duplex kidney. It results in VUR and UTI in a large number of cases and may require excision of the affected part of the kidney and ureter.

Neurofibromatosis and Tuberous Sclerosis

The neurocutaneous syndromes neurofibromatosis (NF) and tuberous sclerosis (TS) may have consequences for the kidney. NF may result in tumours producing vasoactive substances or in RAS from impingement of a neurofibroma on the renal artery. TS may result in cysts in the kidney, angiomyolipomas, either high or low BP and in renal impairment. Therefore, BP and renal function must be monitored in both NF and TS.

RENAL CALCULI (NEPHROLITHIASIS)

There are three main underlying causes of renal calculi in children:

- Infective
- Metabolic
- Endemic.

Infective

By far the most common cause of renal calculi in children is infection of the renal tract, especially by the urea-splitting bacterium *Proteus vulgaris*, which, by maintaining a high urinary pH, favours the deposition of phosphate in combination with calcium, ammonium and magnesium. The typical 'staghorn' calculus fills the renal pelvis and calyces (Fig. 13.16). Calculus formation occurs, especially when there is an obstruction in the renal tract with stasis of urine, e.g. at the PUJ or VUJ.

Metabolic

Cystinuria, oxaluria and other rare metabolic conditions are discussed under renal tubular defects. Very rarely calcium phosphate or oxalate stones are a manifestation of primary hyperparathyroidism or hypervitaminosis D. Calculi may also develop after prolonged immobilisation. Nephrocalcinosis is the deposition of calcium salts within the renal parenchyma, a consequence of a variety of neonatal and metabolic insults.

Endemic

In certain parts of the world, such as India and other developing countries, endemic nephrolithiasis leads to the formation of bladder calculi, which are composed of ammonium acid urate (Fig. 13.17). Dietary factors may be responsible in their pathogenesis where the major source of dietary protein is cereals instead of meat.

Clinical Features

Most children present with UTI and pyuria. Asymptomatic haematuria may be the presentation and requires to be considered together with other causes of this (Table 13.1). Renal colic is relatively uncommon in childhood.

Diagnosis

Calculi have a characteristic US appearance and can be diagnosed by renal US examination. A calculus may, however, be overlooked by US examination and an abdominal X-ray, and IVP may be necessary to establish its presence including the calyceal anatomy prior to lithotripsy. Spiral CT is the most sensitive method for diagnosing renal calculus. In confirmed cases, it is wise to determine the urinary output of calcium, cystine and oxalate and the chemical composition of the stone so that metabolic disorders are not overlooked.

Treatment

This consists of sterilisation of urine by appropriate antibacterial therapy and removal of the calculus either by lithotripsy or by an operation. Percutaneous nephrolithotomy in children before school age is a safe and effective procedure for treating renal stones.

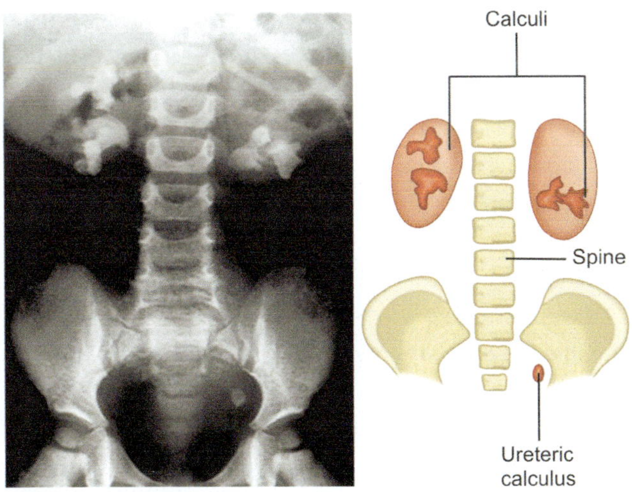

Figure 13.16 Staghorn calculus.

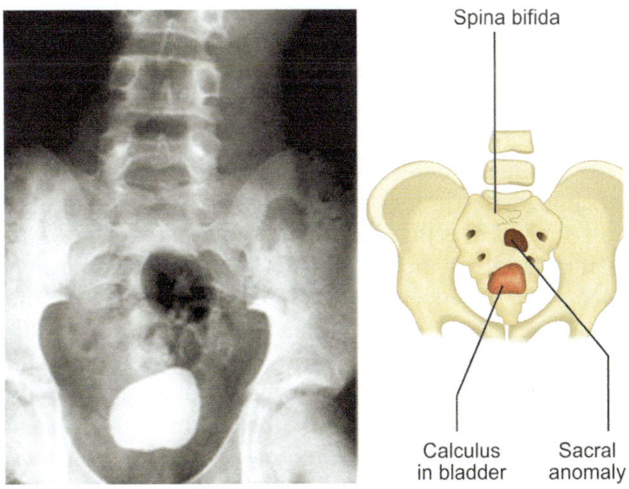

Figure 13.17 Calculus in bladder.

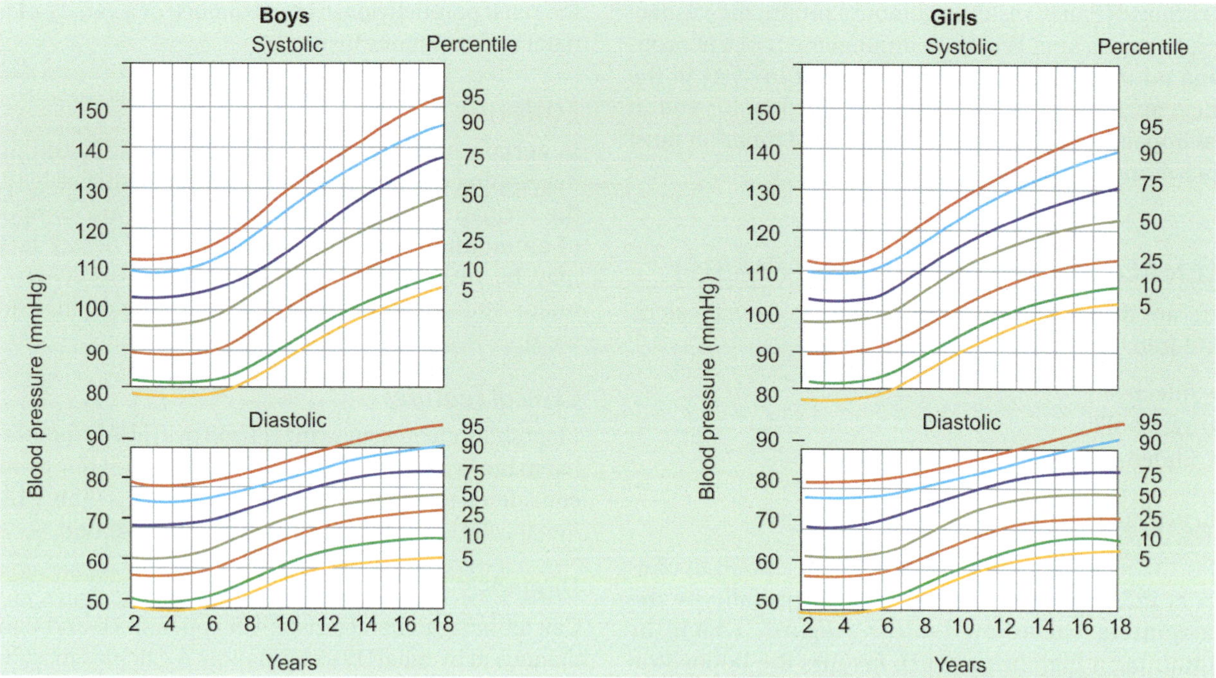

Figure 13.18 Normal blood pressure values in children.

HYPERTENSION

Hypertension may be defined as a systolic or diastolic BP above the 95th percentile for age (**Fig. 13.18**). Thus, the incidence of hypertension in children is 5% by this definition. The top 1% may be said to have 'severe' hypertension. Renal causes account for 80–90% of cases, coarctation of the aorta is another significant cause and all other causes including essential hypertension are uncommon. Only after extensive investigation to exclude secondary causes can a diagnosis of 'essential hypertension' be made. **Table 13.2** lists the causes of hypertension in childhood.

Note on Blood Pressure Measurement

Blood pressure measurement is problematic in children because of the relationship between the width of sphygmomanometer cuff and the length and thickness of child's arm (or leg) and because of confounding factors such as obesity, anxiety and restlessness. The width of the bladder of the cuff should be 70% of the acromion-olecranon distance and should completely encircle the arm. The Doppler US automated device, with auscultatory confirmation using the first and last Korotkoff sounds, is the only practical screening method. The child should be sitting; the infant should be supine. Because of the possibility of coarctation of the aorta, the BP should ideally be taken in all four limbs. This is mandatory if the upper limb BP is raised or if the femoral pulses are difficult to feel.

TABLE 13.2 Causes of hypertension in infants and children.
Renovascular diseases
Renal artery stenosis
Renal artery aneurysm
Renal artery thrombosis
Polyarteritis nodosa
Renal parenchymal disease
Glomerulonephritis, acute and chronic
Polycystic disease of kidneys
Acute renal failure
Haemolytic – uraemic syndrome
Reflux nephropathy
Obstructive uropathy
Chronic renal failure
Renal tumours
Nephroblastoma
Pheochromocytoma
Neuroblastoma
Congenital adrenal hyperplasia
Conn's syndrome and Cushing's syndrome
Neurofibromatosis and tuberous sclerosis
Essential hypertension
Drugs: Corticosteroid therapy (iatrogenic)
Coarctation of aorta

Clinical Features

Only occasionally do symptoms referable to hypertension, headache, nausea and vomiting, cause a child to come to notice. Children with these common symptoms should, however, have BP measurements, as should children with convulsions, epistaxis and facial palsy. More commonly a raised BP is found either incidentally on routine examination or in the investigation of other complaints such as the follow-up of renal disease, or the investigation of features suggestive of Cushing syndrome or NF. Examination of the optic fundi for signs of hypertension, checking for abdominal bruits and checking for cardiomegaly, should be part of the clinical examination of a child with raised BP. Feeling for femoral pulses is part of the routine examination of all children.

Investigation

There are two priorities in the investigation of hypertension:

1. To determine the underlying cause.
2. To assess the severity of hypertensive changes in the cardiovascular system.

If hypertension is found incidentally investigation should include:

- Full blood count, urea electrolytes and creatinine, liver function tests and C-reactive protein
- Urine examination and culture, and an extensive search for RBCs and casts on urine microscopy
- *Renal imaging:* US, DMSA, DTPA and, possibly, Doppler studies and renal angiography if RAS is suspected
- Renal biopsy if unexplained glomerular disease is suspected
- Chest X-ray, ECG and echocardiography
- *If catechol amine excess is proven or suspected:* Abdominal CT or MRI scan, abdominal angiography and selective venous sampling
- *If corticosteroid excess suspected:* Urinary steroid profile, steroid suppression tests, adrenal CT or MRI, and selective adrenal venous sampling.

Treatment

The main indications for antihypertensive therapy in children include symptomatic hypertension, secondary hypertension, hypertensive target-organ damage and persistent hypertension despite life style measures. Most children with hypertension will require general advice regarding diet, exercise and lifestyle, i.e. reduction of dietary salt, reduction of total and saturated fat, increasing exercise, increasing fruit and vegetable intake and not smoking.

Children with retinopathy, encephalopathy, seizure or pulmonary oedema constitute a paediatric emergency and require immediate steps to lower the BP. Controlled reduction in BP over 72–96 hours is essential. Treatment should be commenced with IV drugs; once BP is under control, oral therapy can be commenced. Controlled reduction of BP is obtained by IV administration of labetalol or sodium nitroprusside.

Oral drugs suitable for the first line treatment of children with hypertension belong to five categories:

- Diuretics
- Adrenoreceptor blocking agents
- Angiotensin converting enzyme (ACE) inhibitors
- Calcium antagonists
- Vasodilators.

Other classes of drugs may be used in certain situations. Ideally antihypertensive therapy should be initiated with a single drug at the lowest recommended dose; the dose can be increased until the desired BP is achieved. Once the highest recommended dose is reached, or sooner if the patient begins to experience side-effects, a second drug may be added if BP is not controlled. If more than one drug is required, these should be given as separate products to permit dose adjustment of individual drugs.

ENURESIS (BEDWETTING) AND INCONTINENCE

At the age of 5 years, some 15% of children wet the bed. Each year, without treatment, 12% of the remaining bedwetting population becomes dry, until, at the age of 12 years, only 1% are still wetting. Bedwetting should, therefore, be considered a normal developmental variant, and reassurance and parental support are appropriate managements. Lifting and fluid restriction at bedtime never seem to be effective, perhaps because wetting is said to occur during 'rapid eye movement' (REM)—light or dream—sleep. A minimum investigation should include urine examination with attention to protein, specific gravity and glucose (although diabetes mellitus rarely presents with incontinence. Urine culture would be prudent. There can be no doubt, however, that the complaint is a great nuisance to parents and an increasing embarrassment to the child and there are a number of management strategies available. Opinions vary on what age these should be introduced. Seven or eight years is a reasonable age to try alarm devices, which speed up maturation in a number of children. The ADH like drug desmopressin is effective in a number of patients. BP should be monitored while on the drug and there is a tendency to relapse when treatment stops. The tricyclic antidepressants amitriptyline and imipramine seem to work on some patients perhaps by altering the sleep pattern. The residual 1% of 12-year olds still wetting the bed should be investigated and treated vigorously with all the treatment modalities available.

Daytime incontinence is a different matter. This may be primary incontinence when the child never achieves continence by the usual age of about 2 years or secondary incontinence when the child, having been continent for a period of 6 months, relapses and starts wetting. The possible causes of incontinence are as follows:

Primary

A primary developmental failure as with enuresis

- Chronic pyelonephritis
- Abnormalities of the bladder or urethra (hypospadias in boys or the vulva in girls)
- Some bladders seem hyperactive or have a low bladder capacity
- Ectopic ureter possibly opening in the vagina.

Secondary

Acute or chronic pyelonephritis

- Constipation with faecal impaction
- Emotional problems
- Child sex abuse (this needs to be considered in girls of all ages, especially if resistant to treatment or associated with recurrent UTI).

Examination and investigation must be directed at the possible causes and should include urine examination and culture, examination of the urethra or vulva, palpation for abdominal masses and possibly urinary tract imaging, cystography (preferably noninvasive) and psychiatric and social investigation.

Treatment of diurnal incontinence in the absence of an organic cause is prolonged and intractable and involves bladder training stratagems such as triple voiding, timed micturition and non-tangible rewards such as star charts.

RENAL TUBERCULOSIS

Symptomatic tuberculosis of the kidney and urinary tract is uncommon in children, but endemic in populations where tuberculosis is still prevalent. Renal tuberculosis is evidence of blood-borne spread from a primary lesion, usually pulmonary and frequently inactive. The interval between primary tuberculosis and the development of active renal tuberculosis could be as long as 5–15 years.

Clinical presentation consists of dysuria, frequency of micturition, flank pain and occasionally gross haematuria. Sterile pyuria is typical of renal tuberculosis. The tuberculin test is positive. Positive culture of three morning urine specimens for *Mycobacterium tuberculosis* will establish the diagnosis. Standard anti-tuberculous therapy is recommended. The importance of course completion should be emphasised It would be prudent to search for active tuberculous lesions elsewhere, especially the possibility of open pulmonary TB. Source contact tracing is mandatory.

Antenatal Hydronephrosis

Antenatal hydronephrosis (ANH) is one of the most common abnormalities detected on prenatal ultrasonography (US), reported in approximately 1–5% of all pregnancies. The dilatation of the fetal collecting system is assessed with the measurement of the antero-posterior diameter (APD) of the renal pelvis as visualized in the transverse plane. The APD can be affected by different factors such as gestational age, hydration status of the mother and the degree of bladder distension. The etiology of ANH includes transient dilation of the collecting system, upper/lower urinary tract obstructive uropathy such as pelvi-ureteric junction obstruction (PUJO), ureterovesical junction obstruction (UVJO), duplex kidney with obstructing ureterocele or posterior urethral valves (PUV) and non-obstructive processes such as vesico-ureteric reflux (VUR), multicystic dysplastic kidney (MCDK) and prune belly syndrome.

Pelvi-ureteric Junction Obstruction (PUJO)

Unilateral PUJO is the most common prenatally detected condition leading to hydronephrosis. The obstruction in infants and young children is caused mainly by an intrinsic obstruction caused by a stenotic ureteric segment or by a high insertion of the ureter in the renal pelvis rather than at its most dependent part, while in the older age group may be secondary to an extrinsic obstruction caused by an aberrant lower pole crossing vessels. The diagnostic work up include renal US that shows the dilatation of the renal pelvis and or of the calyceal system with the absence of ureteric dilatation in the flank and behind the bladder. A diuretic renogram (^{99m}Tc MAG3 renal scan) is the most popular study to distinguish between obstructive and non-obstructive hydronephrosis **(Fig. 13.19)**.

The radiopharmaceutical agent is almost exclusively excreted by secretion in the proximal tubules and helps to assess two parameters: (1) the percent extraction of the radioisotope by each kidney following administration of the tracer and (2) the time to half clearance, which is the time taken to drain half of the agent from the renal pelvis following the administration of a standard dose of furosemide (1 mg/kg). Surgery, via the open or laparoscopic approach, is undertaken either in the presence of symptoms, such as pain or urinary tract infections, or when at initial MAG3 delayed drainage is associated with reduced extraction of the tracer (<40%) or when conservative management fails with progression of hydronephrosis on US scan or deteriorating renal function on diuretic renogram. Several retrospective studies have reported a surgical intervention rate of 38–52% with reported successful outcomes in 95% of cases.

Uretero-vesical Junction Obstruction

Congenital anomalies of the vesicoureteral juction (VUJ) are classified into four categories: (1) *obstructed megaureters* (2) *refluxing megaureters* (3) *refluxing with obstruction* and (4) *non refluxing/non obstructing*. Primary

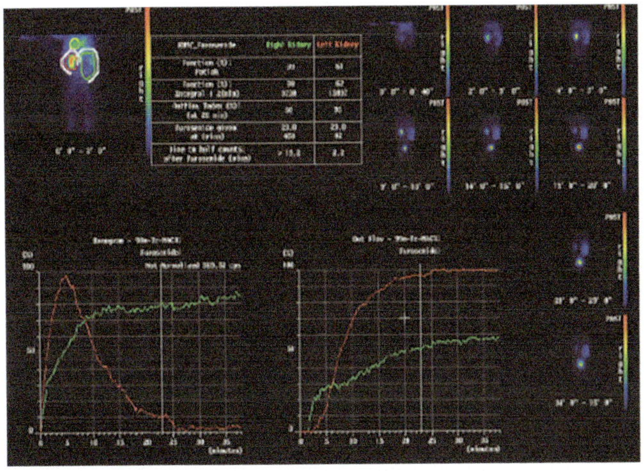

Figure 13.19 Diuretic renogram demonstrating an obstructive curve of the right kidney.

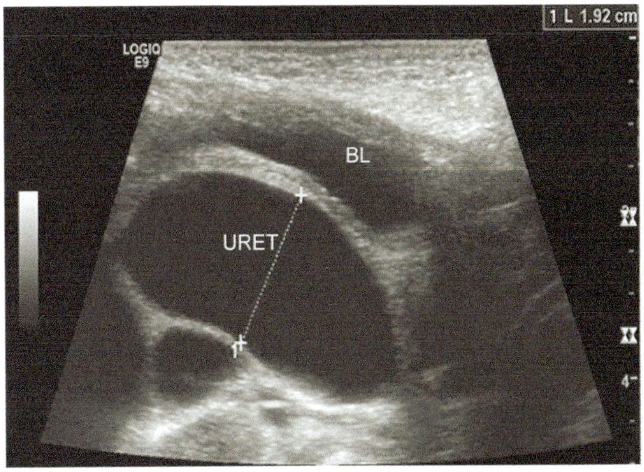

Figure 13.20 Bladder ultrasonography showing an obstructed megaureter behind the bladder.

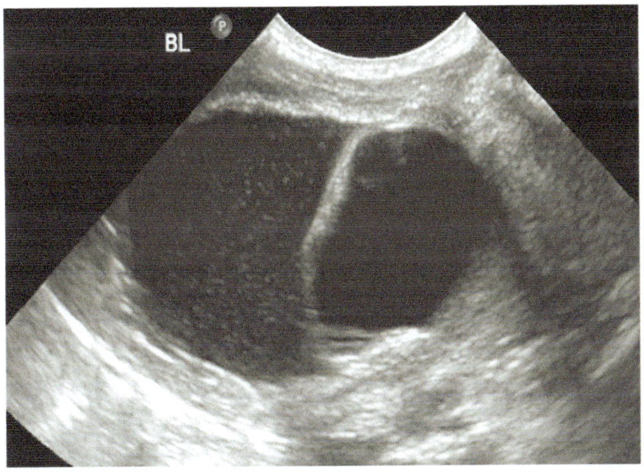

Figure 13.21 Bladder US showing a large ureterocele.

obstructed megaureter also described as VUJ obstruction is due to an intrinsic narrowing of the distal ureter or may be secondary to extrinsic obstruction caused by tumor or iatrogenic scarring. All newborns with a prenatally diagnosed dilatation (>7 mm) of the retrovesical ureter from 30 weeks of gestation should have a postnatal US on days 3–5 **(Fig. 13.20)**.

An early micturatingcystourethrogram (MCUG) is recommended to exclude the presence of bladder outlet obstruction and VUR. Once bladder outlet obstruction and VUR are excluded a diuretic renogram is indicated to look for obstruction at the VUJ. The initial management of megaureters is conservative, based on prophylactic antibiotic, urinary surveillance and regular renal Us scans. Indications for surgical intervention include reduced differential renal function at the initial nuclear scan (<40%) when associated with severe uretero-hydronephrosis or failure of conservative management such as breakthrough febrile urinary tract infections, increasing ureterohydronephrosis on US scans or deteriorating renal function on serial nuclear scans. The surgical options in infants below one year include cystoscopic double J stenting, cutaneous ureterostomy or refluxing ureteric reimplantation. Ureteric reimplantation with or without tapering in the young infant is technically a challenging operation due to the discrepancy in size between the dilated ureter and the small infantile bladder and should be reserved to infants older than 1 year of age.

Duplex Kidney

A duplex collecting system is the most common anomaly of the urinary tract and is defined as a kidney with two pelvicaliceal systems. The incidence in unselected autopsy series is approximately 0.8%. Duplication can be **incomplete** with two ureters joining below the UPJ before entering the bladder (Y or V shaped ureter) or **complete** with two ureters that empty separately. The upper moiety ureter inserts ectopically inferior and medial to the lower pole moiety ureter, often ends in an obstructed ureterocele, which is a cystic dilatation of the intramural ureter, or can insert ectopically into the prostatic urethra in males or vaginal vault in females, while the lower moiety ureter is associated with vesico-ureteric reflux. A renal ultrasound is the first line investigation to assess the dilatation of the upper and or lower moiety, of the ureters and the presence of a ureterocele in the bladder **(Fig. 13.21)**, while a MCUG is recommended to detect VUR in the lower moieties, to look at bladder emptying and at the urethra.

Finally a DMSA scintigraphy, will allow a calculation of the differential renal function of each moiety. The management of duplex kidney is complex and depends on symptoms, degree of obstruction caused by the ureterocele, on the insertion of the ectopic ureter and on the function of the moieties on nuclear scintigraphy. Different management options are available which include endoscopic puncture of ureterocele, partial nephrectomy in cases where the function of upper or lower moiety is severely reduced, excision of ureterocele with ureteric reimplantation in the presence of adequate function of the affected moieties, nephrectomy and pyelopyelostomy.

Vesico-ureteric Reflux

Vesico-ureteric reflux is one of the most controversial topics in paediatric urology. VUR is the retrograde flow of urine from the bladder into the ureter and towards the kidney. It can be primary or secondary. *Primary VUR* is traditionally associated to a shorter intramural and submucosal ureter resulting in deficiency of the antireflux valve mechanism. *Secondary VUR* can be due to bladder outlet obstruction (posterior urethral valves), or by high intravesical pressures caused by neurogenic bladder (neural tube defect) or dysfunctional voiding (detrusor sphincter dyssynergia). It is often diagnosed following investigations for antenatal detected hydronephrosis or a proven urinary tract infection or during screening micturating cysto-urethrogram (MCUG) of asymptomatic siblings or offsprings of patients with known VUR.

An extensive amount of clinical studies in the last 40 years have clearly demonstrated that VUR may resolve spontaneously with time and that in the absence of infection (sterile VUR) at physiologic voiding pressures does not damage the kidneys. In clinical practice, there are five grades of VUR (Fig. 13.22).

MCUG is the gold standard investigation for the diagnosis and evaluation of VUR; it allows the identification of VUR during the filling or voiding phase, the grading of VUR and the assessment of bladder emptying. In toilet trained children MCUG can be replaced by a MAG3 indirect cystogram, which does not require catheterization, radiation exposure is reduced but does not allow visualization of the posterior urethra.

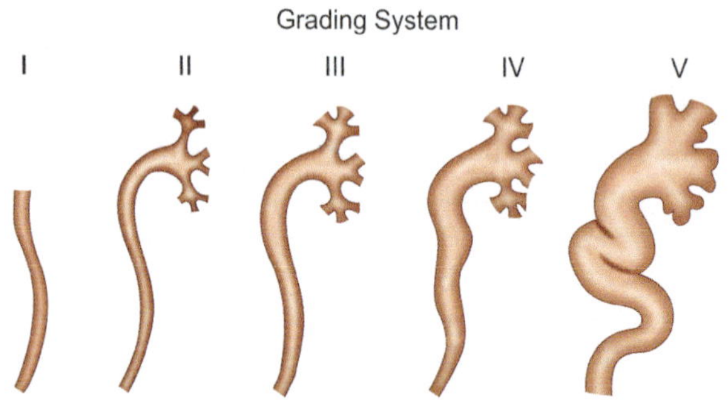

Grade I Into nondilated ureter
Grade II Into pelvis and calyces without dilatation
Grade III Mild to moderate dilation of ureter and renal pelvis
Grade IV Moderate dilatation and/or tortuosity of ureter
Grade V Severe dilatation and tortuosity of ureter, renal pelvis, and calyces

Figure 13.22 Classification of VUR of the International Reflux Study in Children.

The recommended management of VUR is conservative based on continuous antibiotic prophylaxis (CAP) and urinary surveillance. The role of CAP has been recently questioned, especially in low-grade VUR with no significant difference in the incidence of urinary tract infection, acute pyelonephritis and renal scarring in children who take regular CAP compared to placebo. For high-grade VUR (3–5), also described as 'dilating reflux', CAP still remains the most recommended treatment. Indications for surgical intervention are represented by the failure of conservative treatment with breakthrough urinary tract infections or progression of renal scarring on DMSA scan. The endoscopic treatment of VUR, popularized by O'Donnell and Puri as a STING procedure in 1984 and further modified first as HIT (Hydrodistension Injection Technique) and after as double HIT by Kirsch and colleagues has reached a 96% clinical and 92% radiographic success rates at 1-year follow-up. Open ureteric reimplantation is nowadays only reserved for the few selected cases where VUR is associated with anatomical anomalies (VUR associated to large para ureteric diverticulum or ureteral duplication) or where endoscopic treatment has failed.

In boys with high-grade VUR circumcision may be offered, especially in boys younger than 1 year who are at greater risk of febrile UTI and renal scarring. A recent systematic review of the literature has clearly demonstrated a higher risk of UTI's in uncircumcised children which is ninefold higher in the first year of life, 6 times in 1- to 16-year-old children and threefold in children older than 16 years.

The term reflux nephropathy (RN) describes the coarse renal scarring of one or both kidneys associated with VUR. RN can be *congenital*, more common in infants with high grade VUR, which on DMSA scan shows a global reduction of the parenchymal uptake or *acquired*, due to a combination of urinary tract infections and intrarenal reflux, more common in girls with dysfunctional voiding and or constipation. Acquired renal scarring usually demonstrates a patchy uptake, especially at the polar region of the kidneys on DMSA scan.

Posterior Urethral Valves

Posterior urethral valves (PUV) are the most common cause of lower urinary tract obstruction in male infants. PUV in the United Kingdom occur in 1:4000 live born males. The prenatal detection of unilateral or bilateral hydronephrosis associated with a dilated thick-walled bladder and a dilated posterior urethra highly suggests the presence of lower urinary tractobstruction. In newborns with a prenatal diagnosis of bilateral hydronephrosis and a thick walled bladder a period of bladder drainage is recommended with a feeding tube, rehydration, electrolytes correction awaiting stabilization of the creatinine levels. Once the levels of creatinine achieve a plateau a micturatingcystourethrogram is performed to

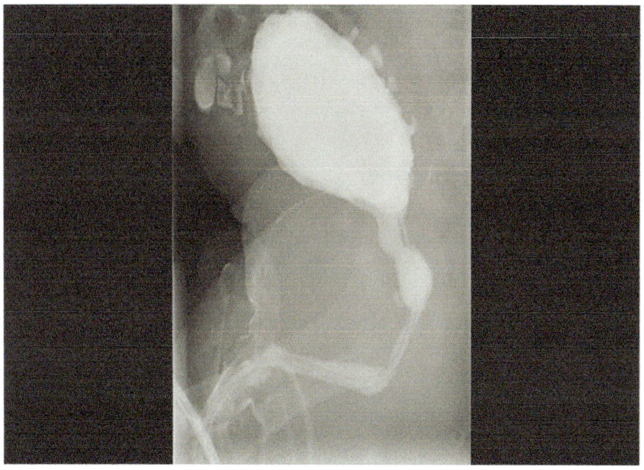

Figure 13.23 Micturatingcystourethrogram showing bladder diverticulae and posterior urethral valves.

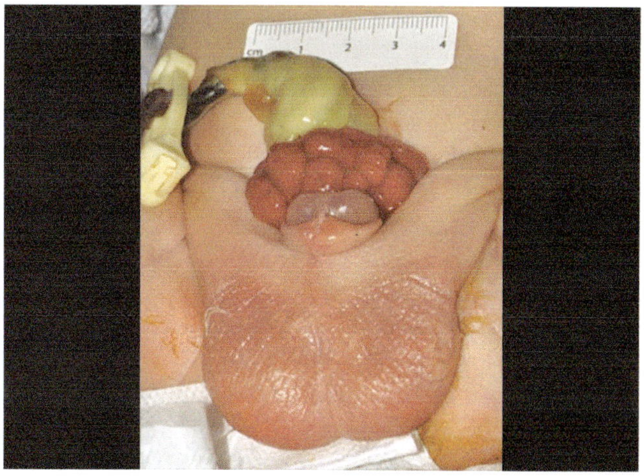

Figure 13.24 Newborn male with bladder exstrophy.

detect the presence of PUV and or vesico ureteric reflux (Fig. 13.23).

Cystoscopy and valve ablation remain the mainstay of treatment with a cold knife at 5, 7 and 12 o'clock position. Nowadays, circumcision is commonly recommended in infants with PUV as it reduces significantly the risk of urinary tract infections and infection-related renal damage. Despite optimal urological management, PUV carries a lifetime risk of end-stage renal disease of 28.5%, with 2/3 progressing before 17 years of age and the remaining third after 17 years.

Multicystic Dysplastic Kidney

Multicystic dysplastic kidney (MCDK) is a congenital condition where the renal parenchyma is replaced by multiple non-communicating cysts whose appearance is similar to that of a cluster of grapes. The presence of a MCDK is detected approximately in 1-1000 to 1-4000 live births and is associated with other genito-urinary anomalies most commonly contralateral or ipsilateral VUR followed by contralateral UPJO, contralateral UVJO, horseshoe kidney and cryptorchidism. Long-term follow-up studies have concluded that the risk of hypertension and of neoplasm are not increased in patients with MCDK. Current management is conservative with limited urological and radiological follow-up. By the age of 10 years, 53% of children with MCDK experience involution of the affected kidney, being children with smaller MCDKs more likely to experience involution and at an earlier age compared to larger MCDKs.

Bladder Exstrophy–Cloacal Exstrophy

Bladder exstrophy-cloacal exstrophy is a spectrum of congenital anomalies that require multiple major surgical reconstructions and lifelong urological follow-up for their implications with continence, renal function, genital appearance and function.

Bladder exstrophy (BE) is a lower midline abdominal defect with an incidence of 1/40,000 live births and is characterized by an exposed bladder plate, low-lying umbilicus, widened pubic symphysis due to malrotation of the pelvic innominate bones, divarication of the recti abdominis and an abnormal pelvic floor musculature, anterior ectopia of anus and vagina and penile epispadias/bifid clitoris (Fig. 13.24).

Cloacal exstrophy (CE) is one of the most severe congenital anomaly compatible with life with a reported incidence of 1/250,000 live births. There are different subtypes of CE; however, the typical presentation include an omphalocele beneath which there are two exstrophied bladders separated by a cecal plate with associated prolapsed terminal ileum and in the lower portion hemi-phalli with a widely spaced pubic diastasis and an underdeveloped blind distal hindgut. Associated anomalies are common in patients with CE and they can affect the gastrointestinal tract (short bowel syndrome), genitourinary tract (renal agenesis, pelvic kidney, hydronephrosis, undescended testis, inguinal hernia), central nervous system (spinal dysraphism, myelomeningocele or lipomyelomeningocele) and the skeletal system (vetebral column, pelvis and limbs).

The management of bladder exstrophy-cloacal exstrophy has changed significantly over the last few decades and is confined to few specialized centers all over the world.

Prune Belly Syndrome

Prune belly syndrome (PBS) is characterized by a classical triad of abnormalities including an absence or deficiency of abdominal wall musculature, cryptorchism and anomalies of the urinary tract. The reported incidence varies between one in 27,000 to one in 40,000 live births. This syndrome occurs almost exclusively in boys. In females, it is extremely rare with less than 50 cases described in the world literature. Over the years numerous studies have

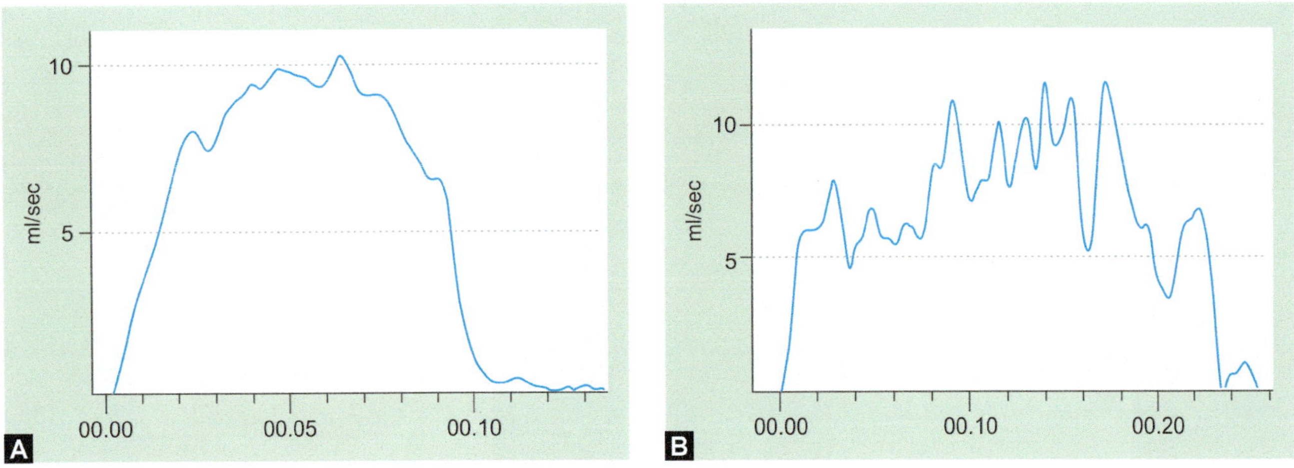

Figures 13.25A and B Normal uroflow curve pattern on the left and staccato-shaped on the right due to dysfunctional voiding.

shown a constant association between PBS and extra-genitourinary anomalies, with the most frequent being orthopedic and gastrointestinal followed by cardiopulmonary and developmental.

Urinary Incontinence

Urinary incontinence is termed by the International Children's Continence Society as the involuntary leakage of urine. The symptom of incontinence requires a minimum age of 5 years and a minimum duration of 3 months. It can be continuous or intermittent. *Continuous* urinary incontinence is associated to congenital causes (ectopic ureter of a duplex collecting system, epispadias, short urethra, urogenital sinus), to neurogenic causes (neural tube defect) or iatrogenic. *Intermittent* urinary incontinence during the day is called *daytime incontinence*, while when intermittent incontinence occurs during sleeping periods it is termed *enuresis. Enuresis* is further termed as primary, since toilet trained, or secondary enuresis reserved for children who had a previous dry period of at last 6 months. Finally enuresis can be isolated, *monosymptomatic enuresis*, or associated to symptoms of bladder dysfunction such as frequency, urgency, post micturition dribbling referred as *non monosymptomatic enuresis*.

The assessment of a child with urinary incontinence include:

- A detailed history and examination: the presence of a meatal stenosis, balanitis xerotica obliterans, epispadias, urogenital sinus, imperforate hymen need to be excluded. The spine should be inspected for the presence of hairy patches, hamangioma, swellings which may suggest an underlying spinal dysraphism.
- Urine examination: to exclude the presence of infection or glycosuria
- Renal and bladder ultrasound
- Bladder and bowel diary: it consists of a 5–7 days recording of incontinence episodes, frequency and volumes of micturition, drinking volumes and a detailed bowel diary using the Bristol Stool Form Scale.
- Uroflowmetry studies: it consists of measuring the flow rate, volume voided, voiding time and the curve pattern of a child who must be toilet trained **(Figs. 13.25A and B)**. Uroflowmetry can be associated to electromyography testing of the perineal muscle to assess the degree of synergy between the bladder and the pelvic floor. In addition, immediately after voiding ultrasound can assess the degree of bladder emptying with measurement of post void residue (PVR). A PVR more than 20% of the expected bladder capacity (EBC) is considered significant, where the EBC is calculated with the formula $30 \times (\text{age} + 1)$ (mL).
- Measurement of nocturnal urinary volumes: nocturnal polyuria is present when nocturnal urinary volumes are >130% of EBC.

The treatment of urinary incontinence is complex and involves addressing the daytime incontinence before achieving success at nighttime. It depends on a careful evaluation and treatment of the underlying condition causing the incontinence. Management options include surgical correction of the underlying anatomical anomaly (ex: ureteric reimplantation for ectopic ureter), treatment of constipation, urotherapy, electric nerve stimulation, biofeedback, alarm and pharmacologic treatment (anticholinergic, desmopressin).

CHAPTER 14(A)

Diseases of the Nervous System

P.D. Moses, M. Thomas, B. Koshy, S. Muthusamy, S. Yoganathan

INTRODUCTION

Diseases of the nervous system contribute to a significant proportion of childhood morbidity and mortality and consequently considerable parental anxiety. Precise and prompt diagnosis helps in cure, limiting disability and proper counselling. This chapter focuses on the common neurological disorders seen in childhood and comprises the following sections:

- Congenital malformations of central nervous system (CNS)
- Infections of the nervous system
- Acute flaccid paralysis
- Convulsions in infancy and childhood
- Childhood stroke
- Movement disorders
- Neurocutaneous syndrome
- Neurodegenerative disorders
- Neuromuscular disorders
- Autonomic nervous system (ANS)
- Brain tumour in children
- Cerebral palsy (CP)
- Learning disorders

CONGENITAL MALFORMATIONS OF CENTRAL NERVOUS SYSTEM

The congenital anomalies of CNS are broadly classified as disorders involving development of the neural tube, forebrain, mid-hindbrain, disorders of brain size, malformations of cortical development, disorders predisposing to hydrocephalus and disorders of skull development. Commonly more than one disorder coexists in a child.

Disorders of Neural Tube Development, Forebrain and Mid-Hindbrain

Neural tube defects include spina bifida occulta (*see* **Figs. 14.83A and B**), meningocoele, myelomeningocoele (*see* **Figs. 14.85A and B**), encephalocoele (*see* **Fig. 14.84**), dermal sinus, dermal tumours, spinal cord lipomas and split cord malformation (**Figs. 14.1A to C**). Myelomeningocoele (**Fig. 14.2B**) is often associated with congenital deformity of the hind brain known as the Arnold-Chiari malformation (**Fig. 14.2A**), in which there is downward displacement of the cerebellar vermis and cerebellar tonsils commonly resulting in symptoms due to progressive hydrocephalus and brainstem dysfunction.

Disorders of forebrain development include holoprosencephaly (*see* **Figs. 14.89 and Fig. 14.3**), agenesis of corpus callosum (**Figs. 14.4A and B**) and septo-optic dysplasia.

Disorders of mid-hindbrain now include a number of disorders with advanced neuroimaging. Common disorders include the Chiari malformations, cerebellar hypoplasia (**Fig. 14.5**), Joubert syndrome and related disorders (**Fig. 14.6**), Dandy-Walker malformation (**Figs. 14.7A and B**), Pontocerebellar hypoplasia (**Figs. 14.8A and B**) and Rhombencephalosynapsis (**Fig. 14.9**).

Disorders of Brain Size

This includes microcephaly and macrocephaly.

Microcephaly is due to failure of normal brain growth and is defined as a head circumference (or occipito-frontal circumference, OFC) that is more than three standard deviations (SDs) below the mean for age and gender.

Microcephaly signifies an underlying neurologic disorder. It is broadly categorised as that of congenital onset and postnatal onset.

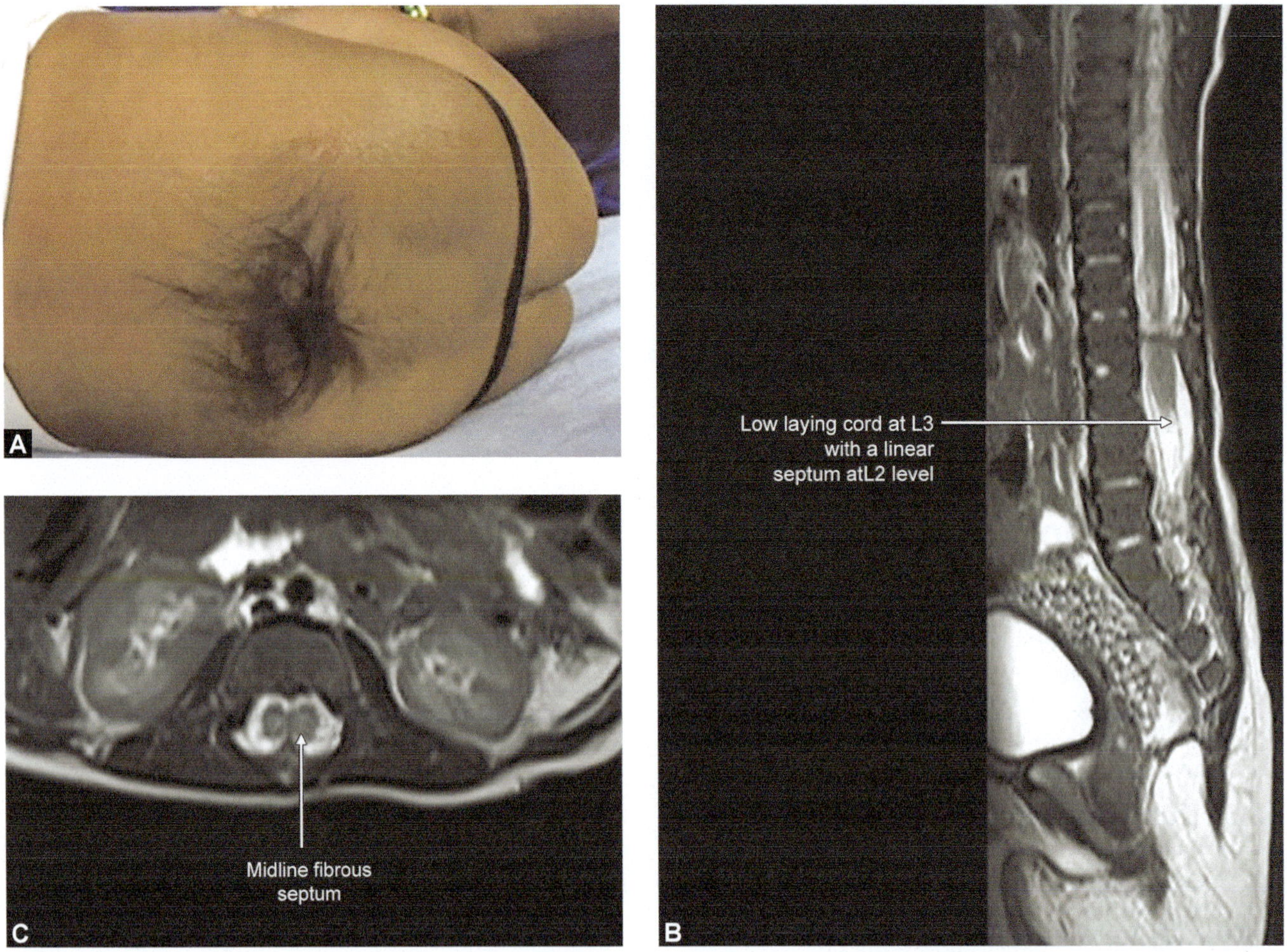

Figures 14.1A to C This infant was noted to have the tuft of hair over low back during antenatal ultrasound (A). Postnatal MRI spine T2 sagittal section (B) of spine showing a low lying cord, with conus ending at lower border of L3 and a fibrous septum splitting the cord into two at the level of L2 seen in the axial image (C). This is a split cord malformation (diastematomyelia) in which a midline septum divides the cord longitudinally into two.

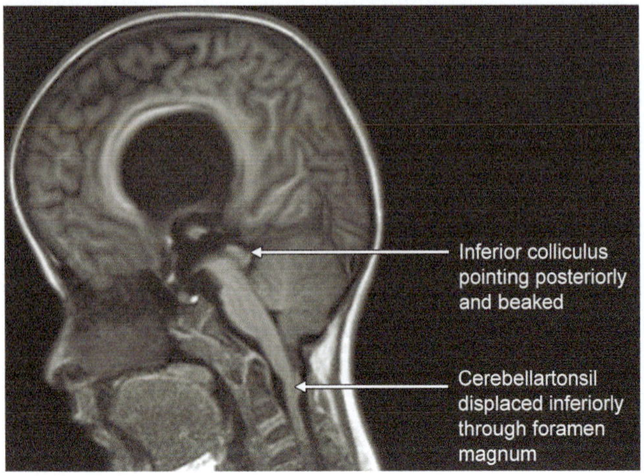

Figure 14.2A T1 sagittal MRI brain of an 8-year old with Chiari II malformation showing small posterior fossa with cerebellar tonsillar herniation. The fourth ventricle is tubular and low lying. There is lateral and third ventriculomegaly and tectal beaking.

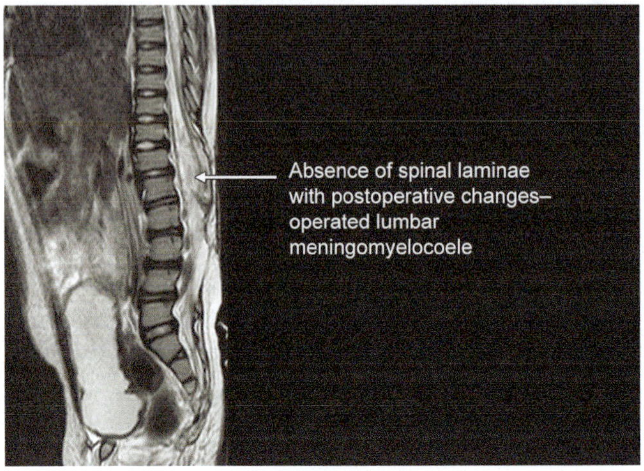

Figure 14.2B The child also had a lumbosacral meningomyelocoele, operated showing postoperative changes seen in the **T11** to sacral levels. The conus is extremely thin and shows syrinx.

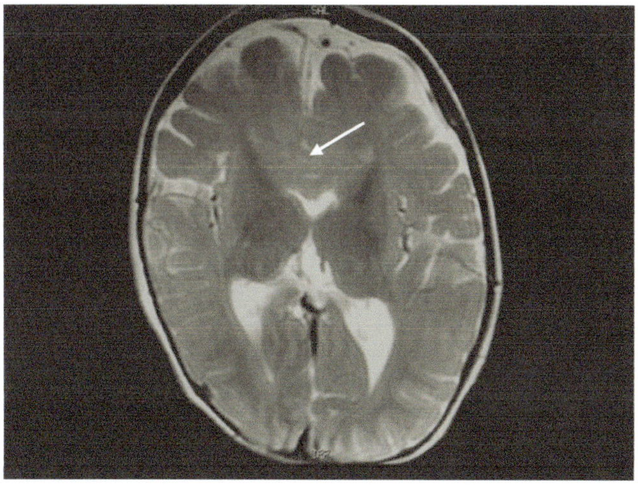

Figure 14.3 Semilobar holoprosencephaly on T2W MRI brain showing lack of separation of the cerebral hemispheres anteriorly and absence of the frontal horns.

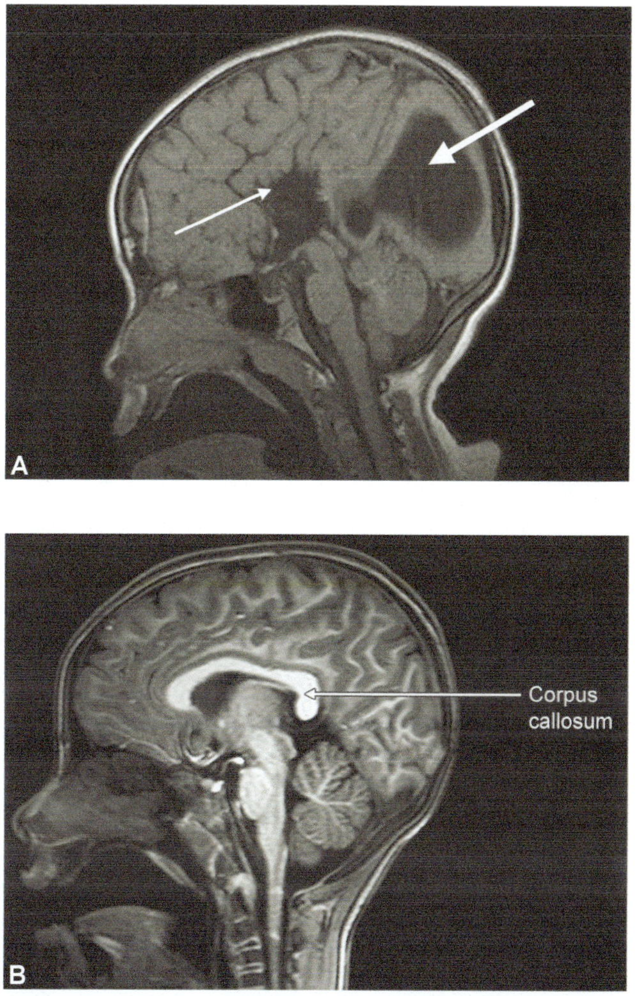

Figures 14.4A and B Corpus callosum agenesis (thin arrow) with colpocephaly (thick arrow) (A). *Note* the normal corpus callosum in MRI. This child had moderate global developmental delay with myoclonic seizures.

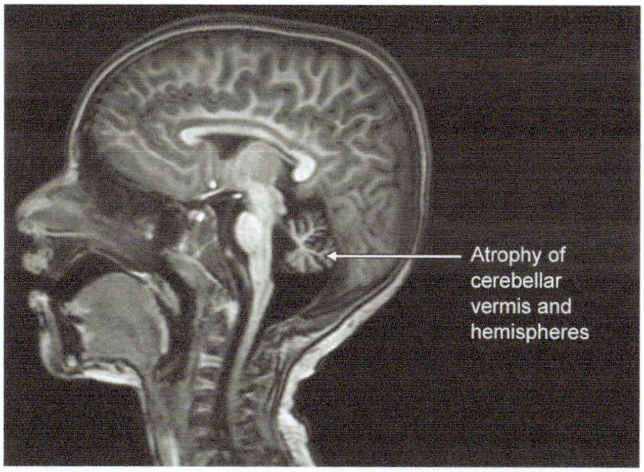

Figure 14.5 Hindbrain malformation showing isolated cerebellar hypoplasia. Clinical picture was that of intellectual disability and static cerebellar ataxia.

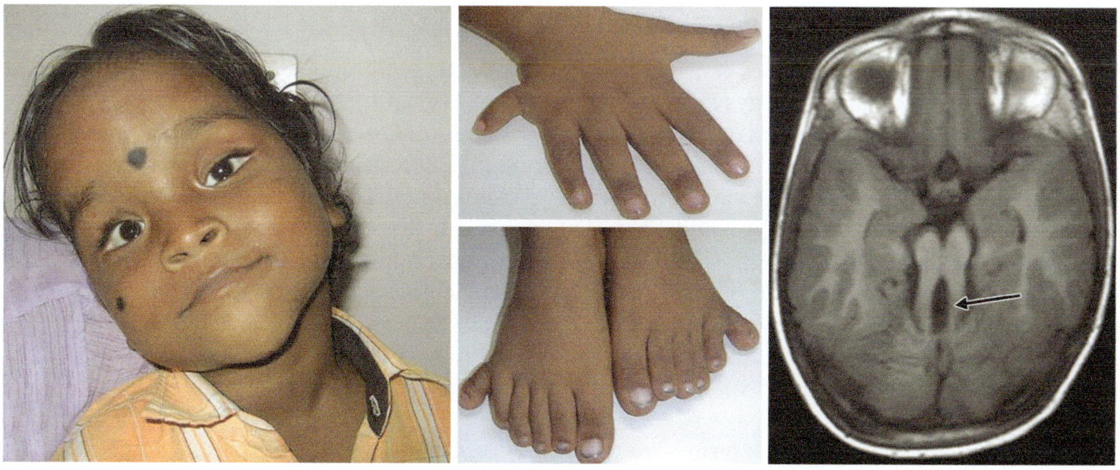

Figure 14.6 A 5-year-old boy with developmental delay, nystagmus, strabismus with bilateral post-axial polydactyly of upper and lower limbs. T1 weighted MRI brain axial image showing molar tooth sign (MTS) suggestive of Joubert syndrome-related disorder (JSRD). Hypertrophy of the superior cerebellar peduncle (arrow) gives this appearance.

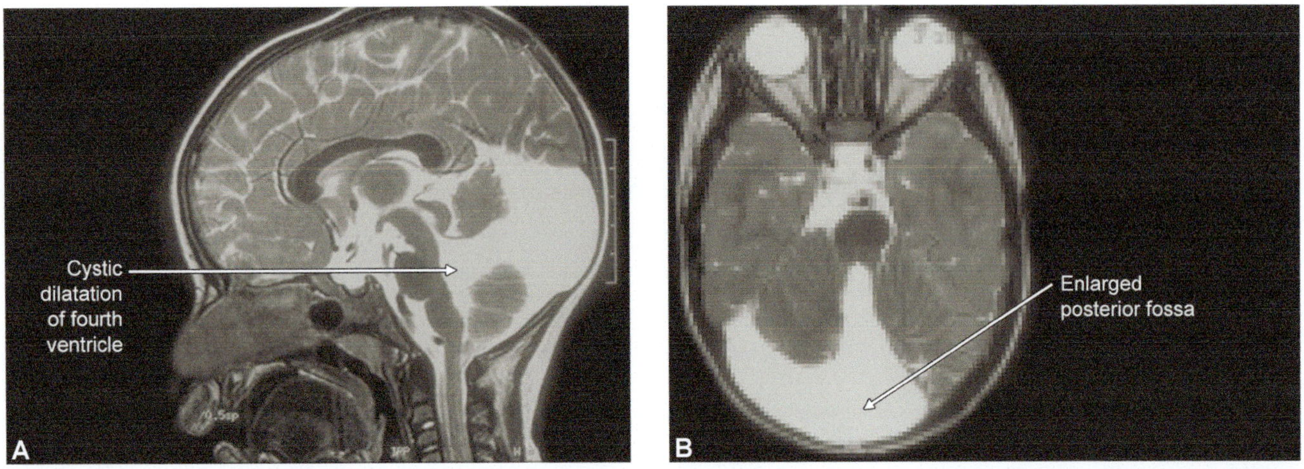

Figures 14.7A and B T2W MRI sagittal (A) and axial (B) sections of brain showing Dandy–Walker malformation. There is complete agenesis of the vermis, cystic dilatation of the fourth ventricle, an enlarged posterior fossa with upward displacement of the tentorium. This 2-year old had moderate global developmental delay and seizures.

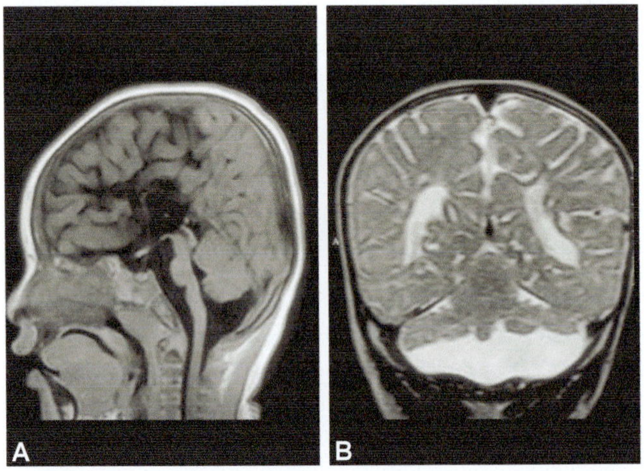

Figures 14.8A and B MRI brain sagittal and coronal T1 images with Pontocerebellar hypoplasia with marked atrophy of the pontine belly (A) and cerebellum on coronal section (B) has a butterfly morphology.

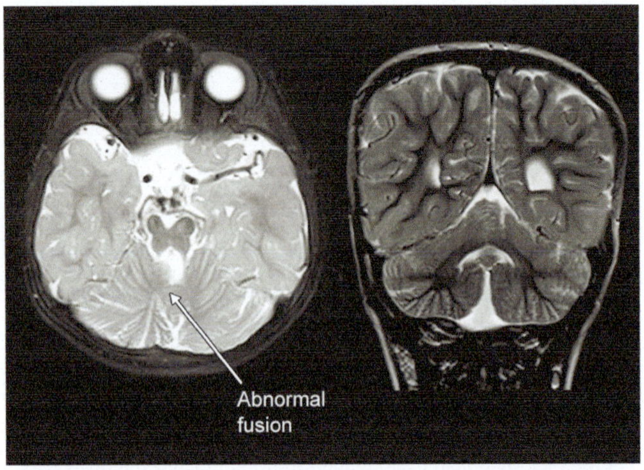

Figure 14.9 Rhombencephalosynapsis. T2W axial and coronal MR images showing fusion of the cerebellar hemispheres in the midline with abnormal orientation of the folia.

Congenital onset microcephaly includes genetic disorders like autosomal-recessive microcephaly **(Figs. 14.10A and B and 14.11)**, autosomal dominant microcephaly and X-linked microcephaly. It is also associated with recognisable malformation syndromes, in particular chromosomal anomalies like trisomy 21, 18 and 13, and in single-gene defects like such as Cornelia de Lange syndrome **(*see* Figs. 14.91A and B)**. Intrauterine insults can also result in congenital onset microcephaly and this includes TORCH infection **(Fig. 14.12)**, toxin exposure or maternal deprivation like maternal hypothyroidism, folate deficiency and malnutrition.

Postnatal onset microcephaly as the term signifies occurs due to insult to the developing brain that may be due to a metabolic disorder like mitochondrial disorder, aminoacidopathies **(Fig. 14.13)**, single-gene disorder like Cockayne syndrome **(Fig. 14.14)**, Aicardi–Goutiere syndrome **(Figs. 14.15A to C)**, traumatic brain injury, hypoxic-ischemic encephalopathy, perinatal stroke **(Fig. 14.16)** and infections like meningitis and encephalitis.

Macrocephaly is defined as OFC of 2 SDs or more above the mean for age, gender and gestation, measured over the greatest frontal circumference. Several different disorders lead to macrocephaly such as hydrocephalus (*see* **Figs. 14.88A and B**), subdural fluid collection **(Fig. 14.17)**, thickening or enlargement of skull **(Fig. 14.18)** and an enlarged brain (megalencephaly) **(Fig. 14.19)**.

Malformations of Cortical Development

Malformations of cortical development (MCD) falls into three major groups—those resulting from abnormalities

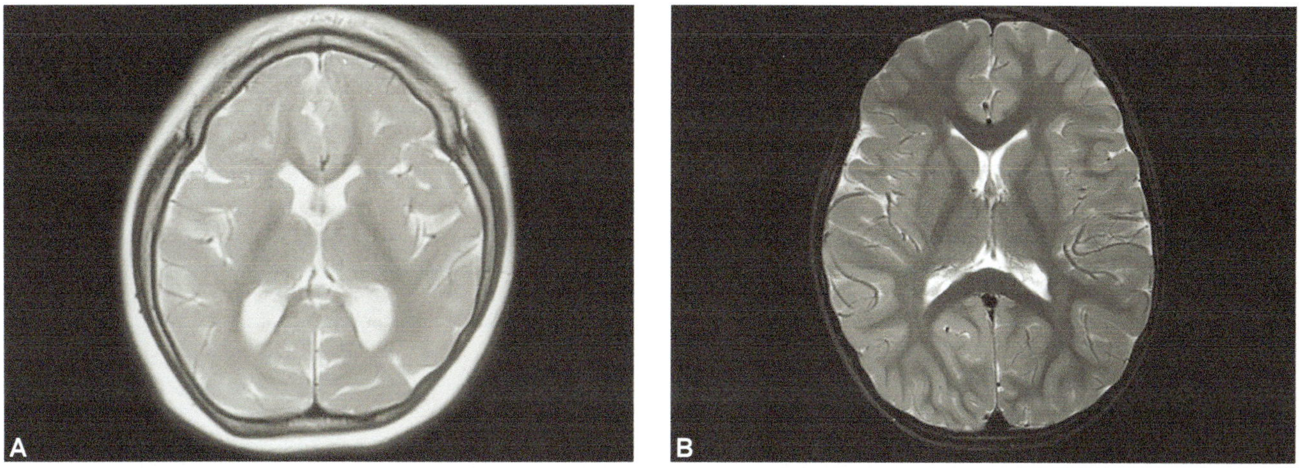

Figures 14.10A and B Simplified gyral pattern in both cerebral hemispheres with thick cortical mantle (A). The child had global developmental delay, microcephaly and generalised seizures. Compare with a normal MRI brain of a 3-year old (B).

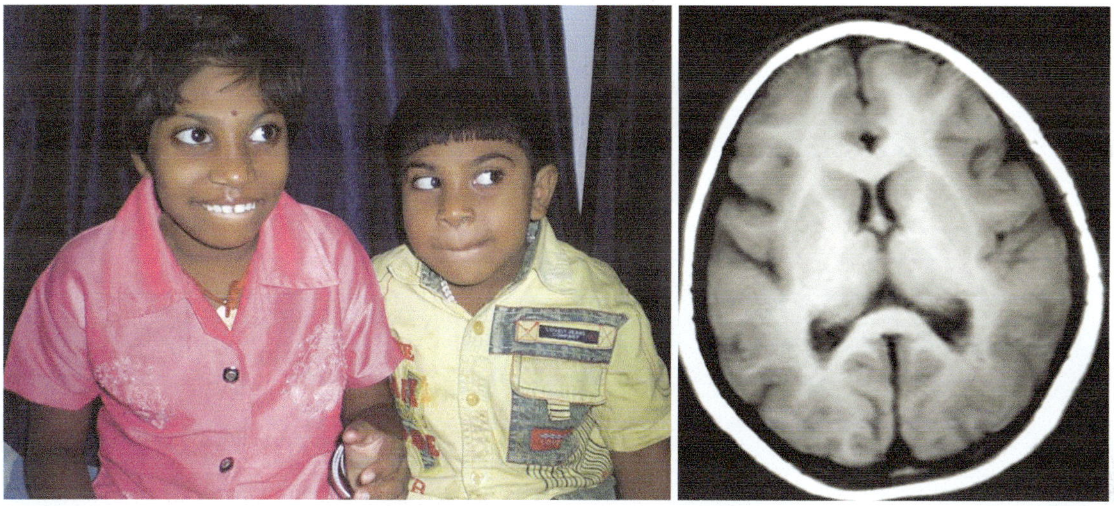

Figure 14.11 Familial microcephaly cerebrum shows less number of gyri with slightly increased cortical thickness mild pachygyria suggestive of simplified gyral pattern. Both siblings had similar looking MRI.

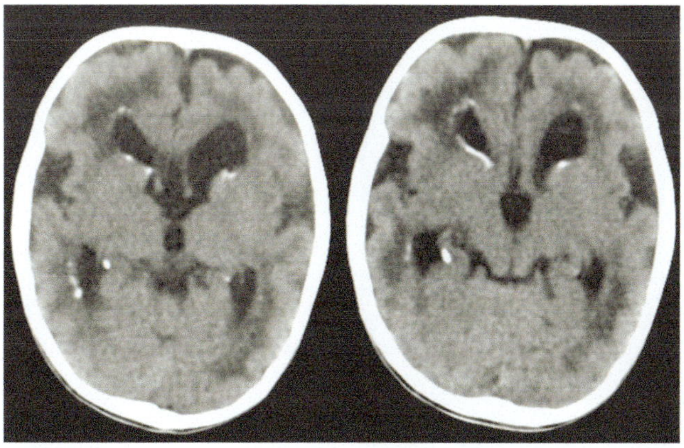

Figure 14.12 Axial CT images of a child with microcephaly and global developmental delay showing circumventricular calcification, mild hydrocephalus and extensive frontal lobe dysplastic thickened cortex suggestive of congenital cytomegalovirus (CMV) infection.

of neural stem cell proliferation, abnormalities of neuronal migration and abnormalities of cortical organisation. These children present with developmental delay and seizures.

Abnormalities of neural stem cell proliferation encompass disorders of brain size.

Abnormalities of neuronal migration result in periventricular heterotopia (abnormal nodules of neurons located along the ventricular wall) **(Fig. 14.20)**, subcortical band heterotopias (a band of subcortical heterotopia neurons, located midway between the ventricles and the cerebral cortex) **(Fig. 14.21)**, lissencephaly (refers to "smooth brain") in which there is loss of the normal gyri and sulci of the brain **(Fig. 14.22)**.

Abnormalities of cortical organisation include polymicrogyria **(Fig. 14.23)**, schizencephaly **(Figs. 14.24 and 14.25)** and focal cortical dysplasia **(Fig. 14.26)**.

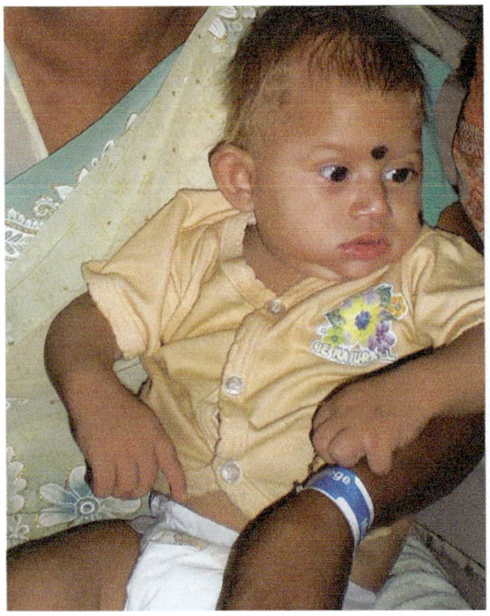

Figure 14.13 Child with untreated phenylketonuria with microcephaly, global developmental delay and light coloured hair. She also had epileptic spasms.

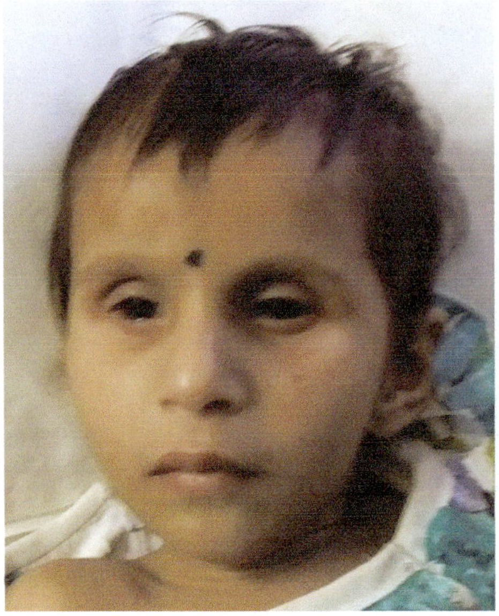

Figure 14.14 Child with Cockayne syndrome. *Note* the microcephaly, deep set eyes and loss of subcutaneous fat.

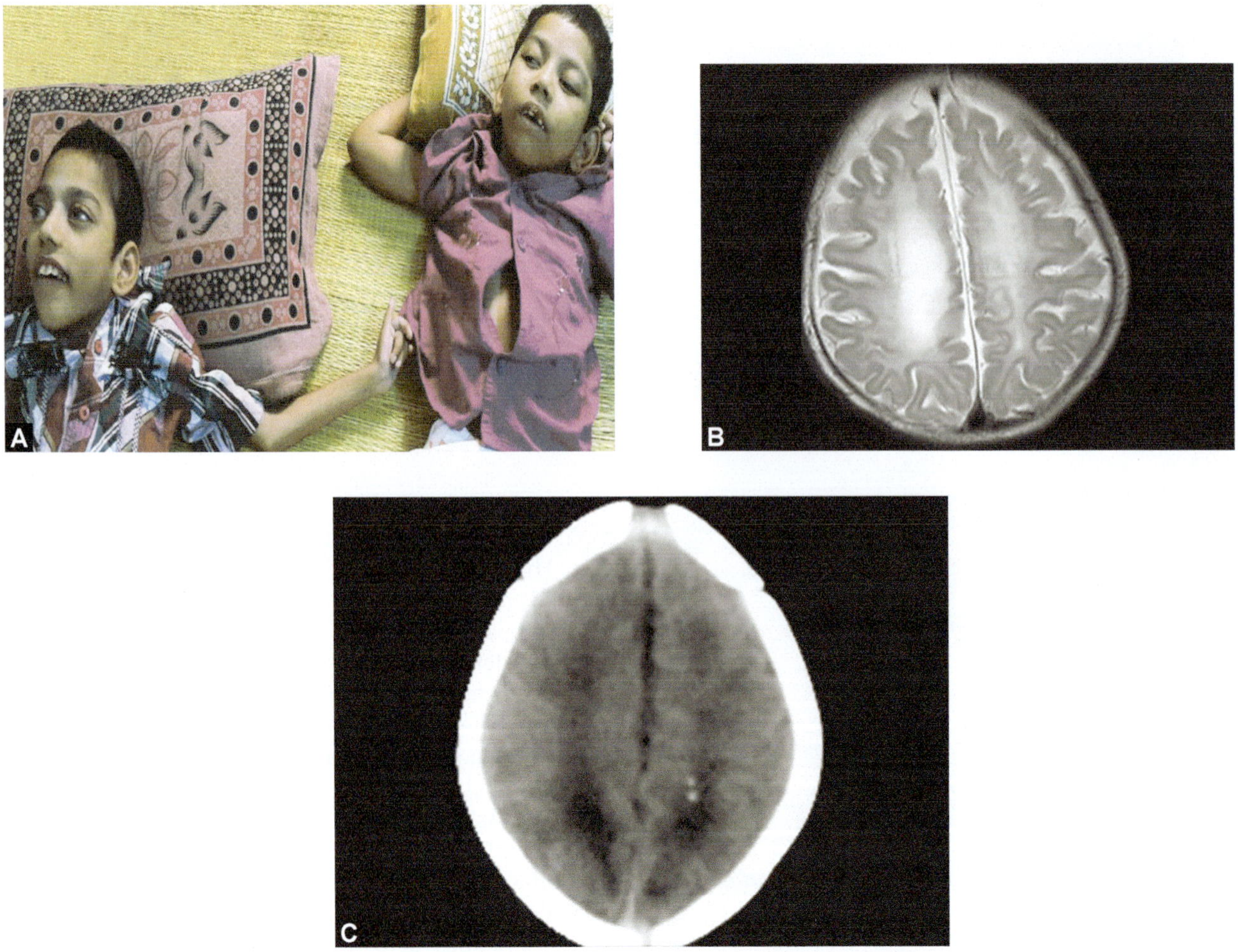

Figures 14.15A to C Siblings with Aicardi–Goutiere syndrome (A). MRI brain (B) with diffuse cerebral atrophy and white matter hyperintensities and CT brain (C) showing the calcifications.

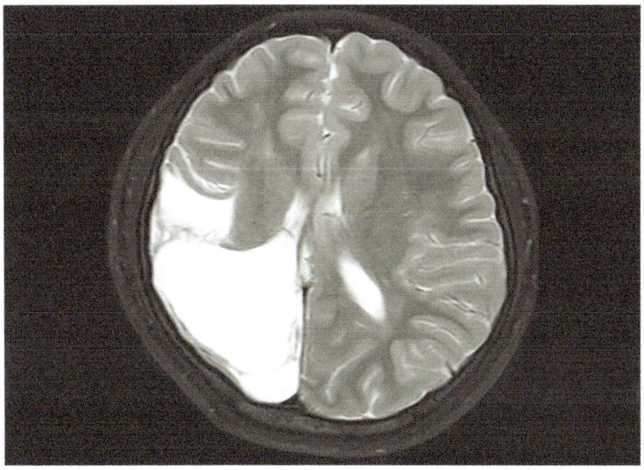

Figure 14.16 Large porencephalic cyst (MRI T2W image) in the right parieto-occipito-temporal region. Here the cyst is communicating with adjacent extra-axial CSF space and the right lateral ventricle. *Note* septations within the porencephalic cyst. Child presented with left hemiparesis and focal seizures and had microcephaly. This probably is the result of a water-shed infarct in the neonatal period as there was history of neonatal sepsis.

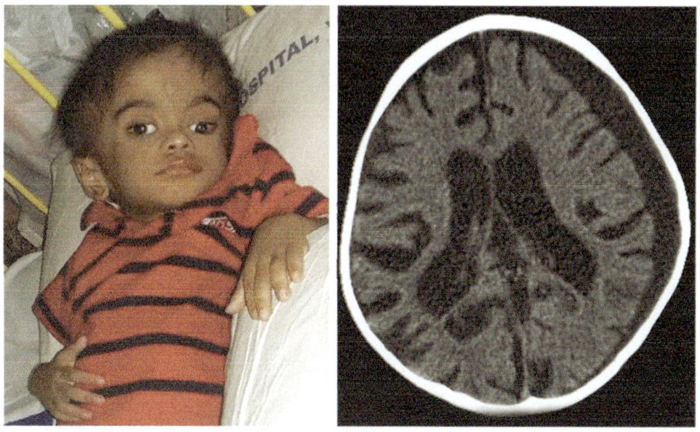

Figure 14.17 Macrocephaly due to chronic subdural effusion in a child with chronic meningitis. Plain CT brain shows diffuse cortical atrophy with prominent ventricles and left subdural effusion.

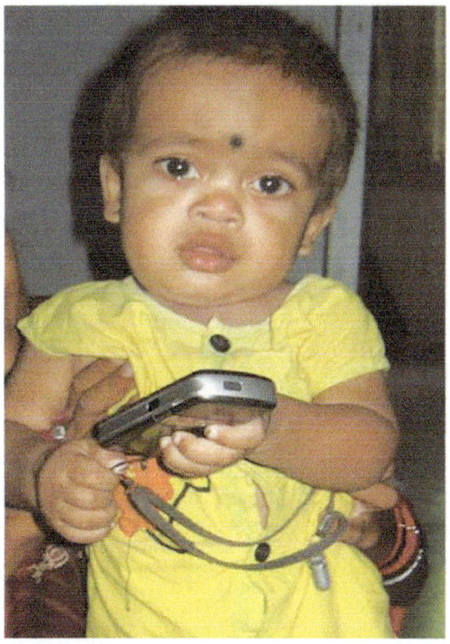

Figure 14.18 Macrocephaly in a child with Hurler syndrome.

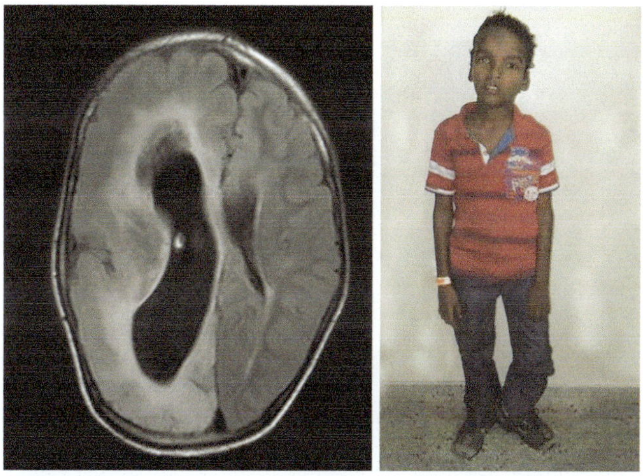

Figure 14.19 Right hemimegalencephaly. Cerebral cortex is thickened and smooth. This child has left hemiparesis and had refractory left focal motor seizures which required right peri-insular hemispherotomy and has since remained seizure-free.

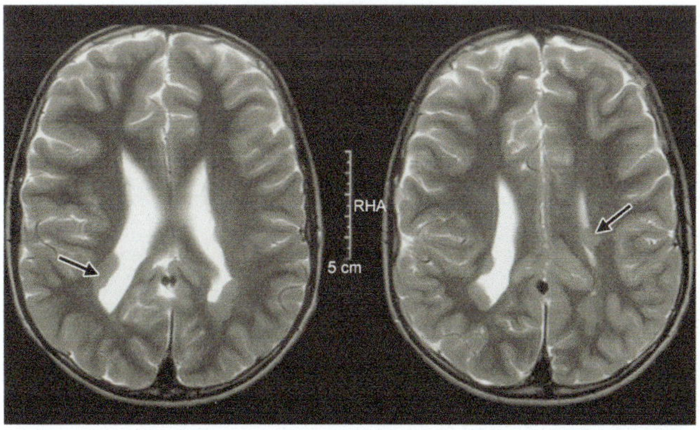

Figure 14.20 Abnormal grey matter (arrow) lining the lateral ventricles suggestive of periventricular nodular heterotopia. This child had intellectual disability and generalised seizures.

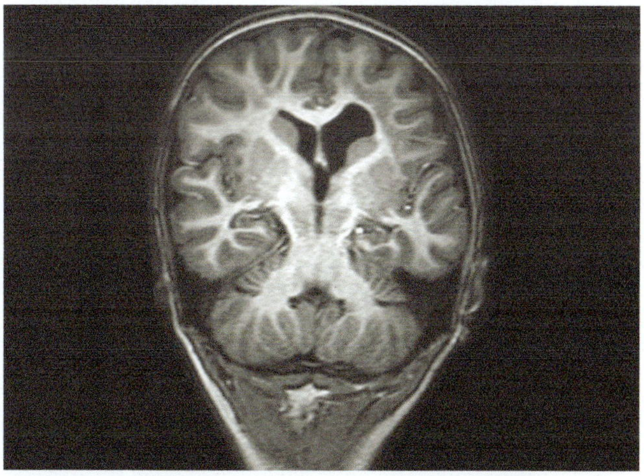

Figure 14.21 Band heterotopia. MRI coronal T1W image showing a band of abnormal grey matter in the left frontal lobe and a smaller band on the right side. There is asymmetric dilatation of the left lateral ventricle.

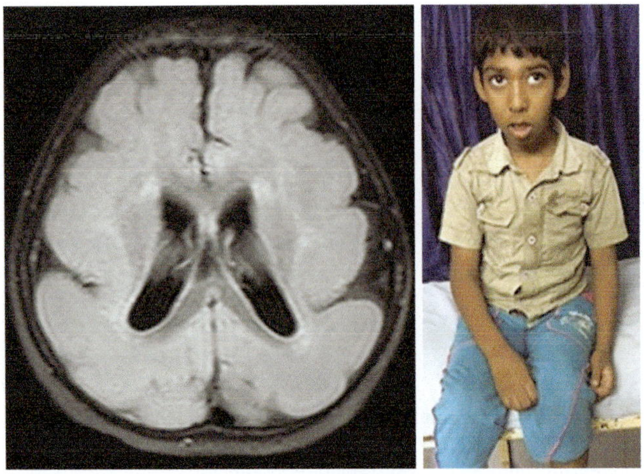

Figure 14.22 MRI brain of a child with epileptic flexor spasms and global developmental delay with microcephaly. MRI brain (T2 FLAIR) showing lissencephaly. *Note* the figure of 8 appearance and smooth thickened gyri.

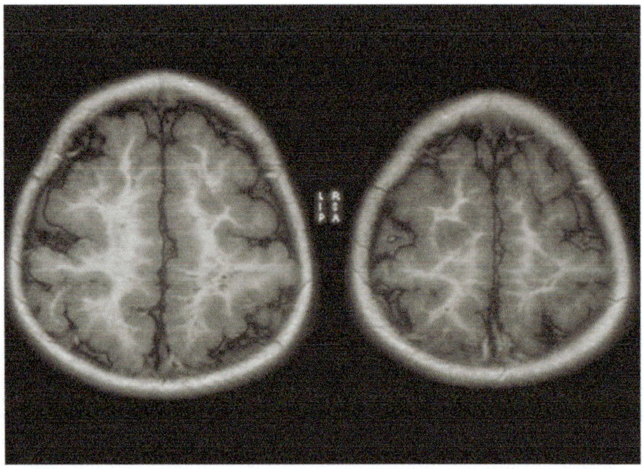

Figure 14.23 MRI brain T1 axial images with bilateral extensive polymicrogyria giving a cobblestone appearance.

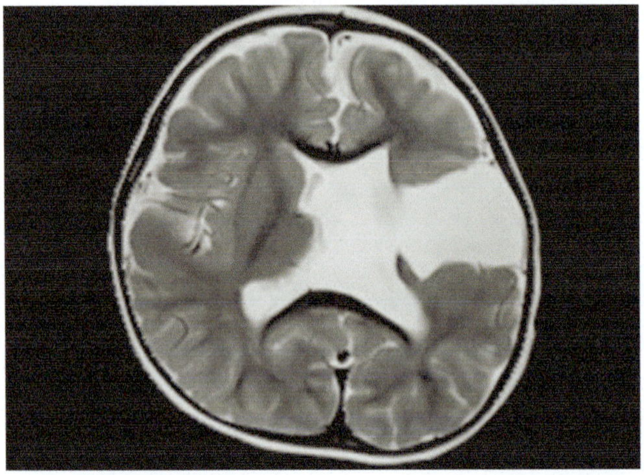

Figure 14.24 Schizencephaly—cleft in the left cerebral hemisphere extending from the lateral ventricle to the subarachnoid space, *note* that the cleft is lined by grey matter (arrows). This child had right hemiparesis.

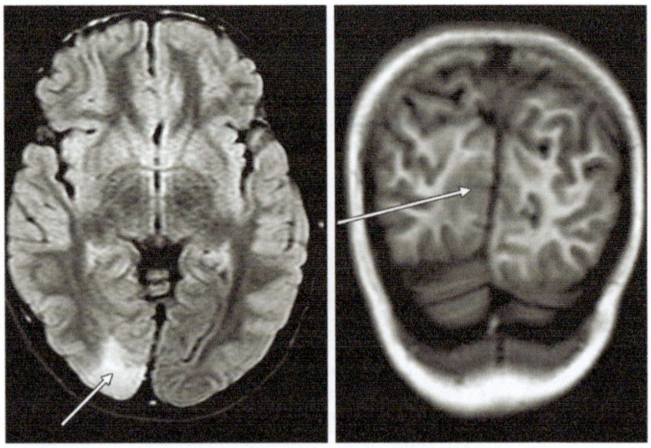

Figure 14.26 Focal cortical dysplasia. T2 FLAIR axial and T1 coronal MR images showing white matter hyperintensity in the right occipital pole which on T1 appears as an area of thickened cortex. This child presented with simple visual hallucination suggestive of occipital epilepsy.

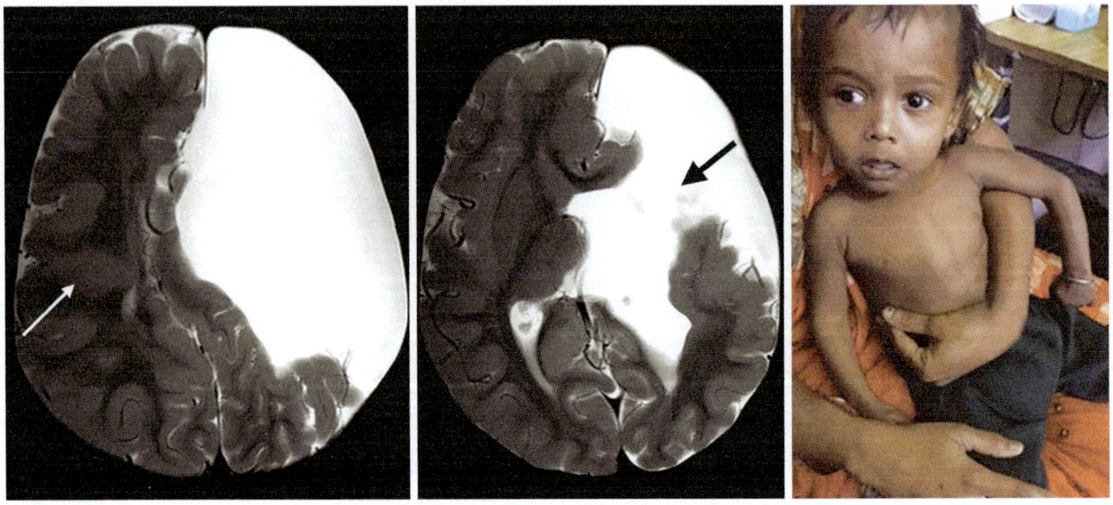

Figure 14.25 This child had right hemiparesis and problems with feeding. He was unable to suck, chew and hold food in mouth. MRI brain shows a large left open schizencephaly (black arrow) and right closed lip schizencephaly (white arrow). In both, the cleft extends from the ventricle to the subarachnoid space.

Hydrocephalus

It is defined as a disturbance of formation, flow or absorption of cerebrospinal fluid (CSF) that leads to an increase in volume occupied by this fluid in the central nervous system. Congenital causes of hydrocephalus include Chiari malformation **(Fig. 14.2)**, Dandy-Walker malformation **(Fig. 14.7)** and aqueductal stenosis **(Fig. 14.27)**.

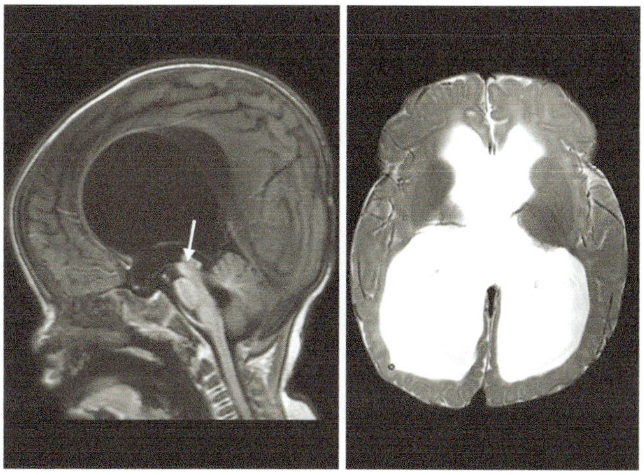

Figure 14.27 MRI brain T1 sagittal and T2 axial sections of the brain showing dilatation of the lateral and third ventricles due to aqueductal stenosis (arrow). The fourth ventricle is normal in size. The cerebral parenchyma is markedly thin with non-visualisation of the white matter.

Craniosynostosis

These are disorders of skull development. Craniosynostosis results from premature fusion of single or multiple cranial sutures leading to deformity of skull and face. The cause of craniosynostosis is unknown but is due to abnormality of skull development. Craniosynostosis can occur isolated or as part of genetic syndromes like Crouzon syndrome **(Fig. 14.28)**, Apert syndrome **(Fig. 14.29)** and Carpenter syndrome. Mutations of the fibroblast growth factor receptor gene family have been shown to be associated with craniosynostosis. Clinical features include abnormal

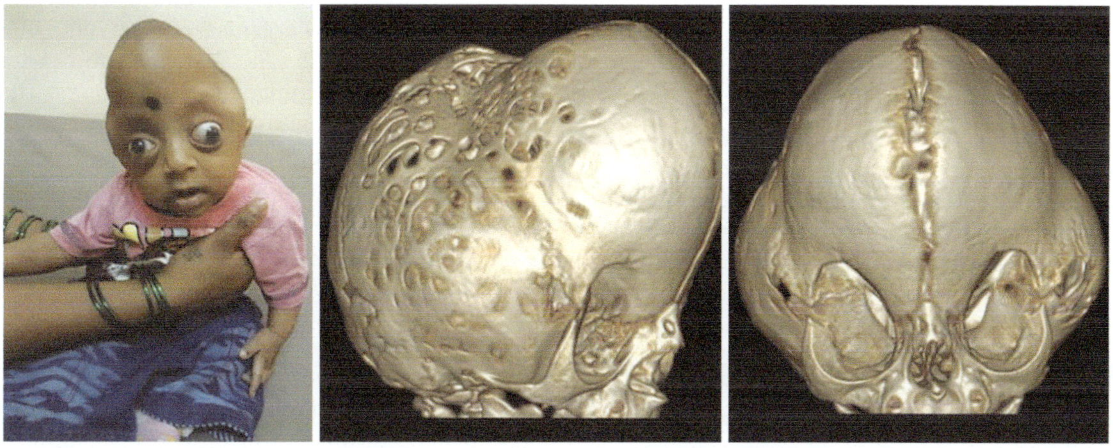

Figure 14.28 Crouzon syndrome. Premature fusion of the coronal and sagittal sutures causing a tower-like skull (turricephaly). This causes raised intracranial pressure and multiple areas of cranial thinning (arrow) giving a 'beaten copper' appearance. This child also had proptosis and optic atrophy.

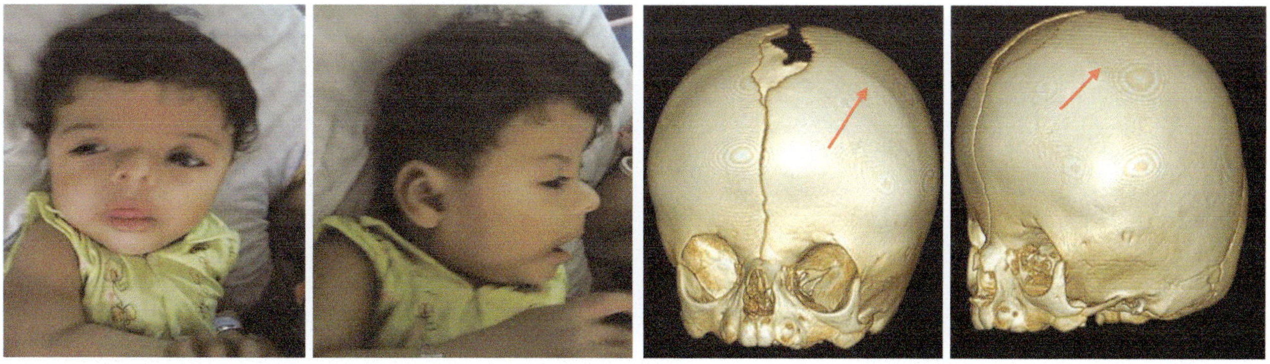

Figure 14.29 Apert syndrome with brachycephaly (anteroposterior shortening). CT reconstruction images of the child showing fusion of the coronal sutures (red arrow).

(*Courtesy:* Dr. Ashish Gupta, Plastic Surgery, Christian Medical College, Vellore, India).

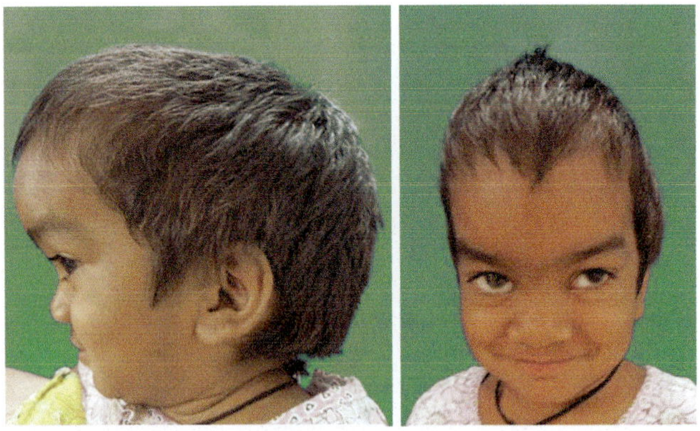

Figure 14.30 Child with dolicocephaly due to premature fusion of the sagittal suture causing increase in the anteroposterior distance.

(*Courtesy:* Dr. Ashish Gupta, Plastic Surgery, Christian Medical College, Vellore, India)

asymmetric craniofacial appearance, suture ridging and premature closure of fontanelles. In sagittal synostosis, lateral growth of skull is restricted, resulting in a long narrow head (scaphocephaly) **(Fig. 14.30)**. In coronal synostosis, expansion occurs in a superior and lateral direction (brachycephaly). This produces shallow orbits and hypertelorism. Involvement of several sutures results in skull expansion towards the vertex (oxycephaly). Frontal plagiocephaly is characterised by unilateral flattering of forehead. Neurological complications include raised intracranial pressure, hydrocephalus, proptosis, optic atrophy and deafness. The diagnosis can be confirmed by plain skull X-ray or computed tomography (CT) scan. Surgical correction to relieve increased intracranial pressure and to improve the appearance of the head with good outcome is possible.

INFECTIONS OF THE NERVOUS SYSTEM

Infections of the nervous system particularly meningitis form a significant proportion of serious infection in childhood.

- Acute bacterial meningitis
- Aseptic meningitis
- Tuberculous meningitis
- Viral encephalitis
- Brain abscess
- Neurocysticercosis

The common types of meningitis are pyogenic, tuberculous and aseptic. Rare forms are mycotic (torulosis, nocardiosis, cryptococcal and histoplasmosis), syphilitic and protozoal (malaria and toxoplasmosis).

Pyogenic Meningitis

Aetiology

Excluding the neonatal period the common bacteria infecting the meninges are pneumococcus *(Streptococcus pneumoniae), Haemophilus influenzae* type B and meningococcus *(Neisseria meningitidis).* Haemophilus infection of the meninges is most common in children 2 months to 3 years of age. The incidence has come down as a result of the conjugated *H. influenzae* vaccine. The next most common meningeal infection is due to pneumococcus; this may be secondary to upper respiratory infection or pneumonia but "primary" meningeal infections are not uncommon. In infants and children meningococcal meningitis is usually sporadic but epidemics can occur. The disease is seen most commonly in the late winter and early spring. In infants both staphylococcal and streptococcal meningitis are occasionally seen, most often secondary to infection elsewhere, e.g. bone, skin, middle ear or lungs. A meningomyelocoele, congenital or acquired CSF leak across cribriform plate, middle and inner ear infections and compound fractures of the skull may also act as portals of entry. In immunosuppressed children and in patients undergoing neurosurgical procedures, including ventriculoperitoneal shunts, meningitis can be caused by a variety of bacteria such as *Staphylococcus, Enterococcus* and *Pseudomonas aeruginosa.*

Clinical Features

Symptomatology is common to all types of bacterial meningitis and the causal organism is most often determined by examination of the CSF. There are a few characteristic signs peculiar to meningococcal infections. The important one from the diagnostic point of view is a generalised purpuric rash although this is seen only in a minority of cases. It is also characteristic of meningococcal meningitis to develop suddenly and unheralded, whereas there is usually a preceding history of respiratory infection in cases due to *Haemophilus* or *Penumococcus.*

The onset of bacterial meningitis is usually sudden with high fever, irritability, refusal of feeds, vomiting, headache in older children and general malaise. Convulsions are common. Young infants show a tense bulging anterior fontanelle, indicative of increased intracranial pressure, and head retraction is common. The older the child the more likely is there to be nuchal rigidity, but its absence in the baby by no means excludes the diagnosis. Kernig sign is useful in older children and may not be observed in infants. Blurring of consciousness of varying degree is the rule and increases in severity as the disease progresses. Hypertonia and decerebrate posturing may be seen in late cases. Focal neurological abnormalities such as paralytic squints, facial palsy sometimes develop. Deafness due to the damage of auditory nerve may be permanent. Papilloedema is infrequently found.

In infants, the disease sometimes has a more insidious onset with diarrhoea and vomiting, irritability and "bogginess" of the anterior fontanelle. The diagnosis is easily missed unless a high index of suspicion is maintained.

Diagnosis

Lumbar puncture is indicated whenever the possibility of meningitis has crossed the physician's mind and ideally treatment should not be started before CSF has been obtained. In pyogenic meningitis, the CSF will be turbid or frankly purulent. The white cell count may be in thousands/mm^3, the majority being polymorphs. The protein content of the fluid is raised (above 0.4 g/L; 40 mg/100 mL), and the glucose is greatly reduced (below 2.5 mmol/L; 45 mg/100 mL). Gram stain films of the centrifuged deposit may reveal Gram-positive diplococci, often very numerous in pneumococcal infection, Gram-negative pleomorphic coccobacilli in *Haemophilus* infection and Gram-negative intra- and extracellular diplococci in meningococcal infection. Rapid identification of bacterial antigen in CSF can be obtained by use of latex agglutination test. The final cause is determined by CSF culture but this may be sterile if prior antibiotic had been administered.

Complication and Sequelae

In the acute stage, raised intracranial pressure due to cerebral oedema, subdural effusion or hydrocephalus may develop. Electrolyte imbalances particularly hyponatraemia may occur as also anaemia. Recurrent convulsions including status epilepticus can further damage the brain. Permanent brain damage with motor and learning deficits is more common in infants, in part due to the greater difficulty and delay in diagnosis. Symptomatic epilepsy is less common. Nerve deafness can develop early in the illness and unpredictably.

The Waterhouse–Friderichsen Syndrome

This is due to acute bilateral adrenal haemorrhage seen most commonly in fulminating cases of meningococcal septicaemia. Death occurs usually before the meningitis has had time to develop, and may, in fact, take place after an illness of only a few hours duration. The characteristic clinical picture is seen in an infant who suddenly becomes ill with irritability, vomiting and diarrhoea, and tachypnoea or Cheyne-Stokes breathing. The heart rate is very rapid. The infant becomes rapidly drowsy and unconscious. Peripheral cyanosis is associated frequently with a patchy purple mottling of the skin, which resembles post-mortem lividity. The child may die at this stage, about 6–8 hours from the onset of the illness. In less fulminating cases, a diffuse purpuric and ecchymotic eruption appears which is the very characteristic of meningococcal septicaemia. The blood pressure may be so low as to be unrecordable. In the toddler, the course of the illness tends on the whole to be less rapid than in the infant. The meningococcus is not always successfully isolated in blood cultures but can sometimes be cultured from the fluid contents of purpuric blebs on the skin. Disseminated intravascular coagulation may also develop in fulminating cases of meningococcal septicaemia and should always be sought by appropriate laboratory tests; blood count with platelet count, blood film for fragmentation of red cells, clotting screen including fibrinogen levels, fibrin degradation products (FDPs) or D dimers.

Aseptic Meningitis

Definition

Aseptic meningitis refers to mostly viral meningitis as well as other forms of meningitis where Gram stain and routine bacterial culture reveal no organisms.

Sporadic cases occur throughout the year, and from time to time sizeable epidemics occur. Hospital based studies looking at the different aetiologies of childhood meningitis have found that aseptic meningitis is two to three times more common than bacterial meningitis; also pyogenic meningitis is more common in younger children whereas aseptic meningitis is seen across all age groups.

Aetiology

Many viruses can cause aseptic meningitis. These include enteroviruses (particularly Coxsackie and Enteric cytopathic human orphan viruses), viruses of mumps, measles, Herpes simplex virus (HSV) and Herpes zoster, the mouse virus of lymphocytic choriomeningitis and Epstein-Barr virus (EBV). Mumps virus can cause aseptic meningitis without any of the other manifestations of this disease. Coxsackie virus can cause meningitis and paralysis, which is indistinguishable clinically from classical poliomyelitis. Non-viral agents, which can cause aseptic meningitis, include *Leptospira* (icterohaemorrhagiae and canicola), *Treponema pallidum, Toxoplasma gondii* and *Trichinella spiralis.*

Clinical Features

The onset is usually sudden with fever, headache, neck pain, vomiting, malaise, diarrhoea or constipation. In some cases, especially of poliomyelitis there is a preceding illness about 1 week earlier with fever, headache, malaise, sore throat and abdominal pain. The temperature chart in such cases shows two "hump," sometimes called "the dromedary chart." The child may be drowsy, apathetic and irritable when disturbed, but marked blurring of consciousness is uncommon. Slight nuchal rigidity is usually found. In the infant, the anterior fontanelle may be tense and full. Compared to bacterial meningitis, meningeal signs and focal seizures are less common in aseptic meningitis. Exanthema may precede or accompany the CNS signs.

Diagnosis

The CSF is clear or only slightly hazy. The cell count varies from 50 to 1,000 mm^3 (may be higher in lymphocytic choriomeningitis) with lymphocytic predominance. The glucose content is normal, but the protein content is moderately elevated (50–200 mg/100 mL). The culture remains sterile. The main differential diagnosis is partially treated pyogenic meningitis. CSF bacterial antigen detection test can be helpful. The causative virus can be identified in the stools. The serum (at least two specimens taken within a 10-day interval) may be tested for neutralising antibody or complement fixation in rising titre. Identification of the viral DNA after polymerase chain reaction (PCR) amplification in CSF is now possible but may give false positive result.

Acute Encephalitis and Encephalopathy

The term encephalitis denotes infection affecting the brain substance. The term encephalopathy is used to describe functional disturbances of the brain without actual infection of the brain.

Aetiology

All of the viruses mentioned in connection with the aseptic meningitis can cause acute encephalitis. Others include arboviruses like Japanese encephalitis virus, Influenza virus, cytomegalic inclusion disease in infancy and the viruses of rabies, human immunodeficiency virus (HIV), encephalitis lethargica and the zymotic diseases such as measles and varicella. Special mention must be made of HSV. In the new born infant HSV type 2 can cause a disseminated infection involving many tissues with a grave prognosis. In the older children, HSV type 1 infection of the brain causes acute necrotising encephalitis affecting particularly the temporal lobe **(Figs. 14.31A and B)**.

In the Indian subcontinent, Japanese encephalitis transmitted by Culex mosquito is common, often in epidemic form, during the monsoon season **(Figs. 14.33A and B)**.

Clinical Features

These are extremely protean. The onset of the illness is usually acute and a prodromal stage with general malaise, fever, headache and vomiting often precedes signs of CNS involvement. The acute encephalitic stage may show varying disturbances of cerebration from the gradual onset of stupor or coma to the sudden onset of violent convulsions. Headache, fever, irritability, mental confusion, abnormal behaviour and seizures may be marked. Focal neurological signs of many kinds are encountered such as cranial nerve palsies, speech disturbances, spastic palsies, cerebellar disturbances and abnormalities in the various reflexes. In cases of acute necrotising encephalitis caused by HSV type 1, in addition to the clinical manifestation described above, some cases have had neurological signs suggestive of an expanding lesion in the brain, particularly in the temporal lobe.

The outcome is always doubtful in every case of encephalitis and especially grave in acute necrotising encephalitis. Death is not uncommon. The case fatality rate in Japanese encephalitis has varied between 25 and 45%. Although complete recovery is possible, many are left with permanent disability such as mental deterioration, hemiplegia or paraplegia, and epilepsy. In some children, an apparently good recovery is followed later by learning difficulties or behaviour problems.

Diagnosis

The diagnosis is usually made on clinical grounds supported by CSF analysis, which shows a mild pleocytosis and increase in protein. Electroencephalography (EEG) typically shows diffuse slow-wave abnormalities. Focal findings and periodic lateralised epileptiform discharges on EEG **(Fig. 14.32)** or CT or magnetic resonance imaging (MRI), especially involving the temporal lobes, suggest HSV encephalitis. Virological studies may be successful in determining the causal agent.

Sclerosing Panencephalitis

There is yet another type of encephalitis produced by measles virus that develops some years after apparent recovery from the measles illness itself. The disease is

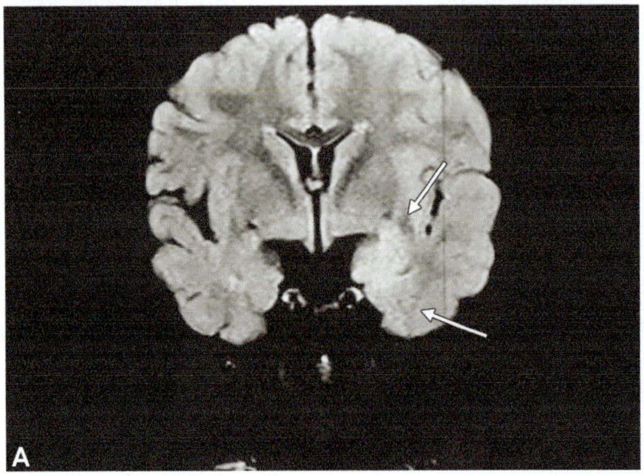

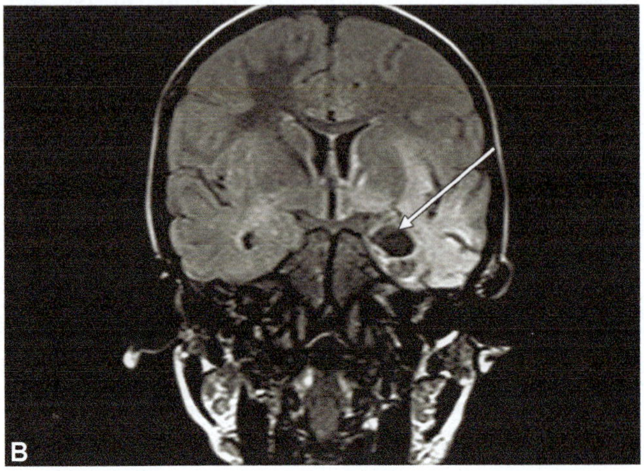

Figures 14.31A and B Herpes simplex encephalitis due to HSV1. MRI brain T2 FLAIR coronal section showing swelling and hyperintensity of the left medial temporal lobe (A) during the first week of illness when the child presented with high-grade fever and seizures. He then went onto develop behaviour symptoms in the form of aggression and spitting and a follow-up MRI showing cavitation of the medial temporal structures and extension of hyperintensity to involve the entire temporal lobe and adjacent insula (B).

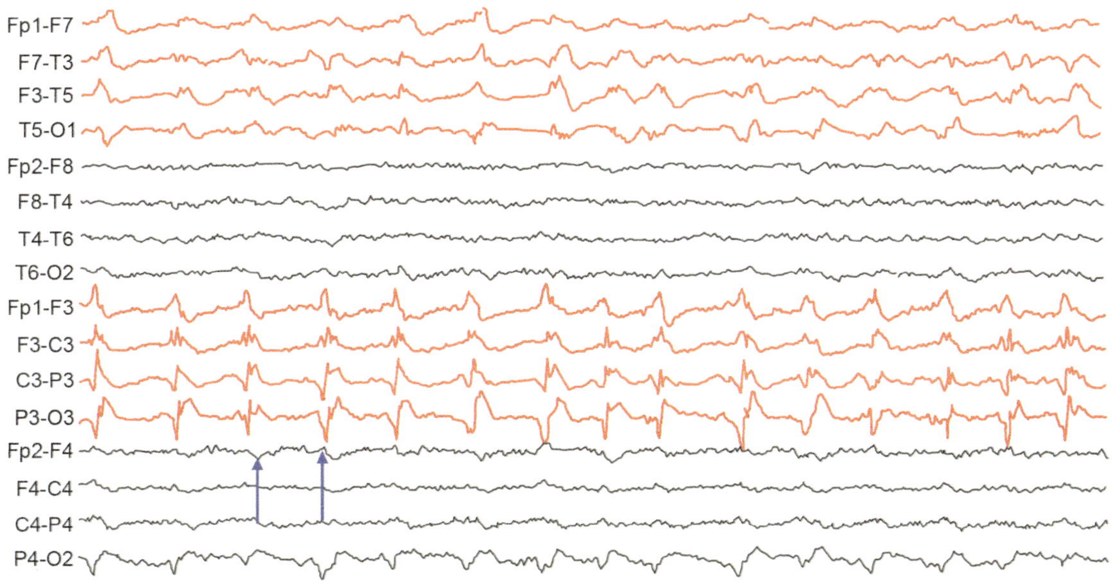

Figure 14.32 Electroencephalogram (EEG) tracing from a child with HSV encephalitis showing periodic lateralised epileptiform discharges (arrow) from the left hemisphere (PLEDS). The discharges are occurring every 1 second.

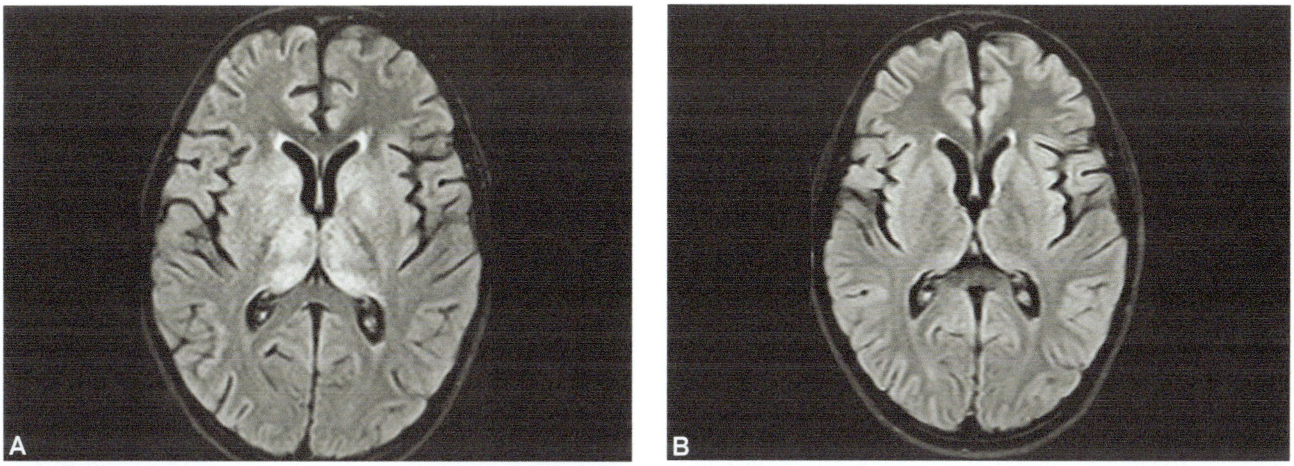

Figures 14.33A and B Japanese B encephalitis—MRI brain T2 FLAIR image (A) showing hyperintensity of bilateral caudate nucleus, lentiform nucleus and thalami. Repeat imaging one year later (B) shows total resolution of the lesions.

called subacute sclerosing panencephalitis (SSPE). Histologically, the disease is characterised by intranuclear inclusions, and under the electron microscopy, these are seen to contain tubular structures typical of the nucleocapsids of Paramyxoviruses. Measles antigen has also been demonstrated in the brain by fluorescent antibody techniques, and measles virus itself has been isolated from brain tissue of patients with SSPE. The initial attack of measles usually antedates the onset of encephalitic manifestation by several years. Infection with measles during infancy seems to increase the risk of SSPE. The disease has also been reported to follow immunisation with live Measles virus vaccine but the risk is very much less than with wild Measles virus infection. Viral mutation, abnormal immune response to Measles virus or subtle predisposing immune deficiency has been proposed to explain the persistent Measles virus infection of the CNS.

Clinical Features

The onset is insidious over a period of months and occurs mostly from 5 to 15 years of age with preponderance among boys. There is insidious deterioration of behaviour and school performance progressing to a state of dementia. Major epileptic seizures may occur. A somewhat characteristic form of myoclonic jerk is commonly seen in which the child makes repetitive stereotyped

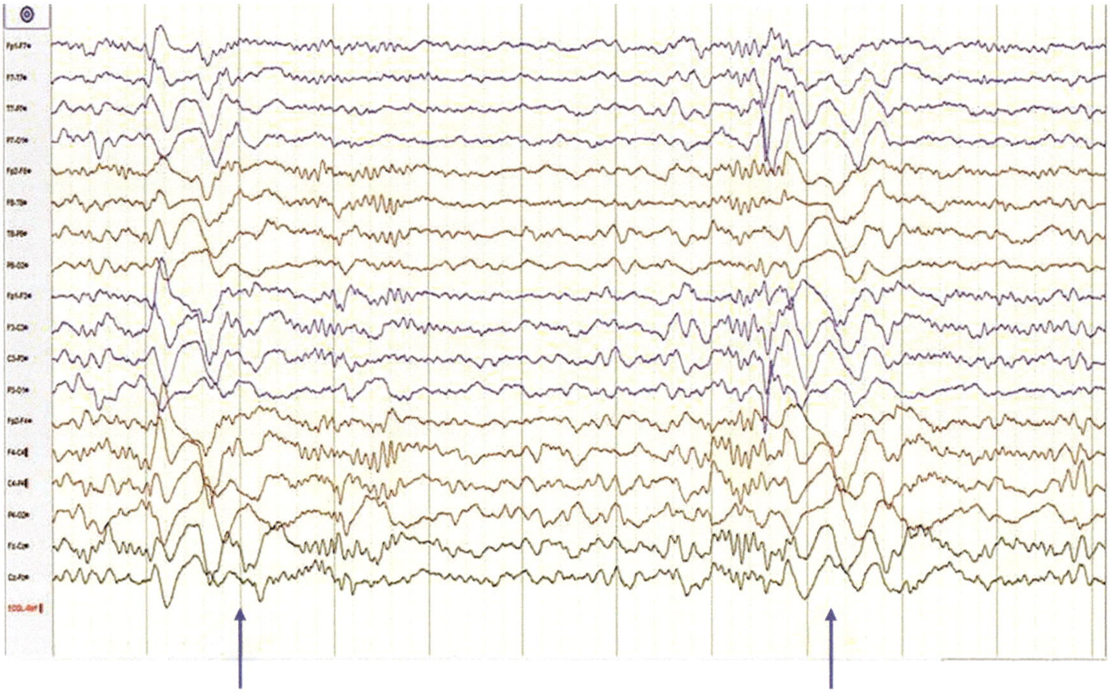

Figure 14.34 EEG of the child with SSPE showing periodic complexes occurring every 4 seconds. These are two to four Hertz high-amplitude delta waves which are usually bisynchronous, symmetrical and repeats once in 5–7 seconds.

movements with rhythmic regularity (2-6 per minute); each begins with shock-like abruptness typical of the myoclonic jerk, but then the elevated limb remains "frozen" for a second or two before, and unlike the usual myoclonic jerk, it gradually melts away. Pyramidal and extra-pyramidal signs are common. The final stage of decerebrate rigidity, severe dementia and coma is reached about 1 year or more from onset and death occurs usually 1-3 years after diagnosis. Rarely, clinical arrest has been reported.

The CSF cell count is usually normal. Although the total protein content of the CSF may be normal or only slightly elevated, the gamma globulin fraction is greatly elevated resulting in a paretic type of colloidal gold curve. On CSF electrophoresis, oligoclonal bands of immunoglobulins (Ig) are often observed. High levels of antibody in CSF in dilutions of 1 equal 8 or more to measles are found. The EEG at the start of the illness may show only some excess slow-wave activity. Later in the illness bilateral periodic complexes typical of the disease appear. The EEG then shows high-amplitude slow-wave complexes, frequently having the same rhythmicality as the myoclonic jerk, sometimes with a frequency of 6-10 seconds (burst-suppression episodes) (Fig. 14.34). Finally, the EEG becomes increasingly disorganised with random dysrhythmic slowing and lower amplitudes. Though it is a disease with predominant cortical involvement in the form of cognitive decline and seizures, initial MRI changes show white matter disease (Fig. 14.35) which then progresses to diffuse involvement (Fig. 14.36).

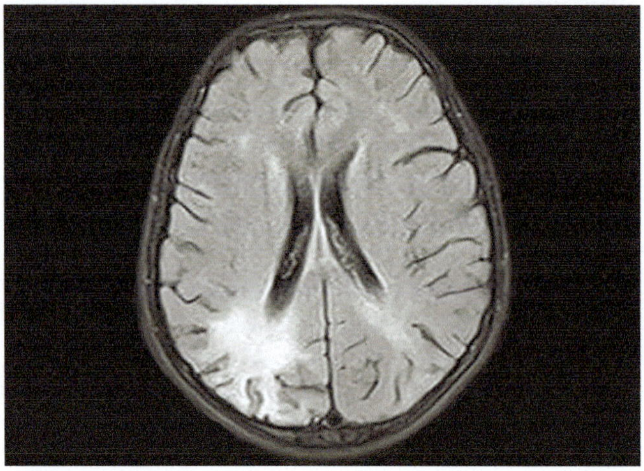

Figure 14.35 MRI brain—T2 FLAIR axial images of a child with subacute sclerosing panencephalitis. This child had subacute cognitive decline and axial myoclonus. MRI shows T2W hyperintensity predominantly involving the right parieto-occipital region.

Acute Encephalopathy

The term acute encephalopathy refers to acute cerebral disorder associated with convulsions, stupor, coma and abnormalities of muscle tone. There is no actual infection of the brain substance. In some cases, there has been a recent preceding virus infection. Rarely, it may be related to the administration of a vaccine. Occasionally, the child may have an underlying inherited metabolic defect such as maple syrup urine disease, organic

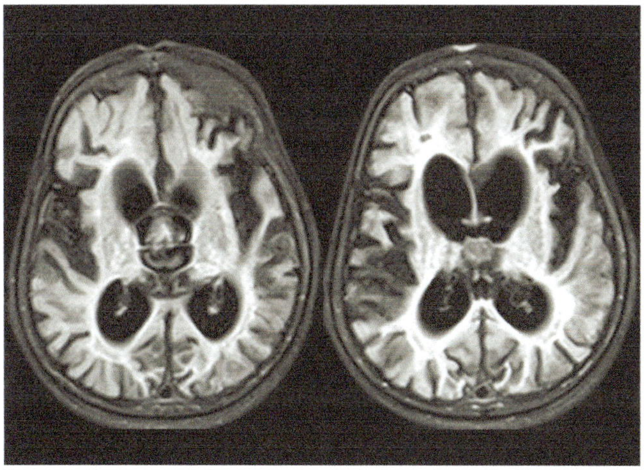

Figure 14.36 End-stage SSPE. T2W MRI brain axial images showing diffuse cortical and subcortical cerebral atrophy with white matter hyperintensities. This child was in a vegetative state with spastic quadriparesis and had no further seizures.

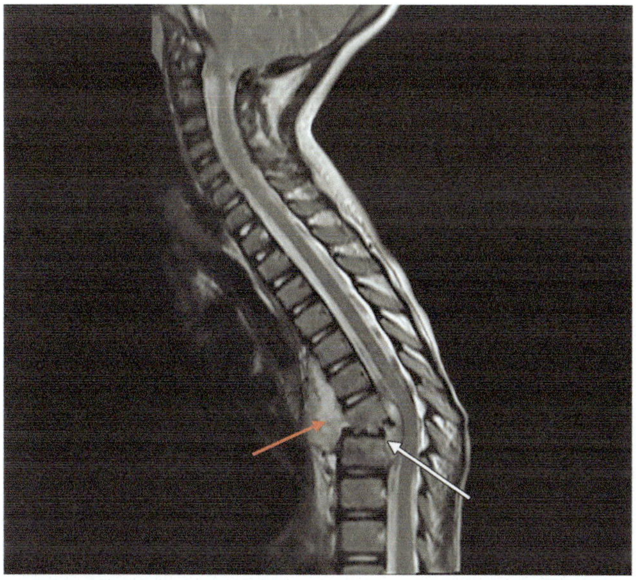

Figure 14.38 Tuberculosis of the spine. MRI T2 sagittal section of spine with gibbus deformity at T7-T8 level due to partial destruction of T7 vertebral body. Intervertebral disc at T7-8 level is destroyed (white arrow) with pre- and para-vertebral collections (red arrow) extending from T5 to T8 level causing compression and posterior displacement of spinal cord.

aciduria or fatty acid, or peroxisomal or mitochondrial metabolic defect. The CSF is usually normal and apart from oedema the findings in the brain are remarkably inconspicuous. One distinct clinicopathological entity is Reye syndrome. Here, an acute encephalopathy with fatty degeneration of the liver in a young child is associated with hypoglycaemia, hyperammonaemia, greatly elevated aminotransferases, metabolic acidosis and respiratory alkalosis with prolongation of the prothrombin time. The CSF generally is clear and acellular

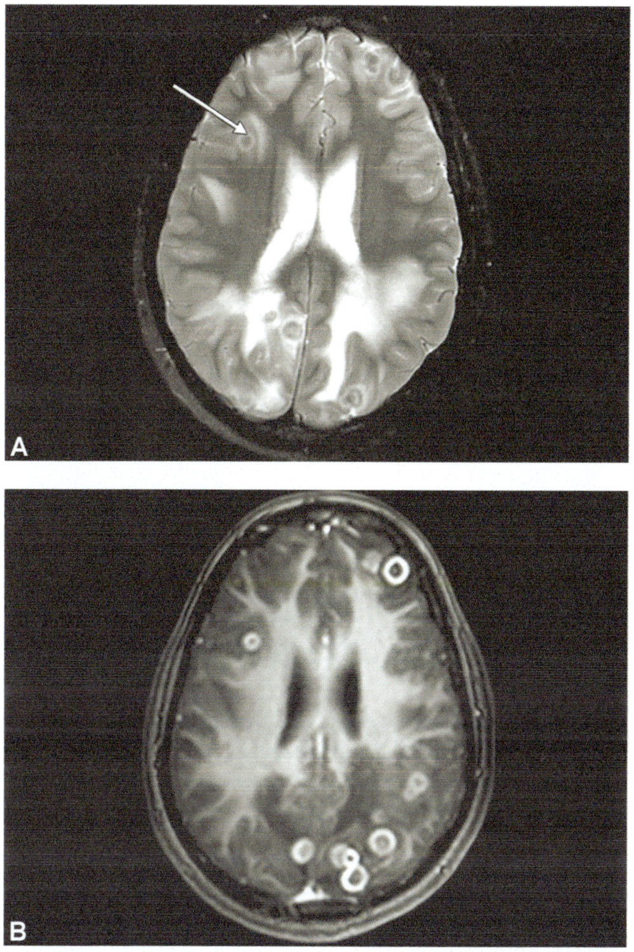

Figures 14.37A and B Tuberculomas. MRI axial T2 (A) and post gadolinium (B) images showing multiple tuberculomas. *Note* the central hypointensity (red arrow) in T2 image due to central caseation. The walls show ring enhancement.

with a normal protein concentration and reduced glucose level. At autopsy, the liver is enlarged and shows gross fatty change, being greasy and pale yellow in colour. The brain shows only oedema. However, electron microscopy reveals distinctive mitochondrial changes in both hepatocytes and neurons. The syndrome follows viral infection with influenza B and varicella. The evidence to support a possible association between Reye syndrome and aspirin ingestion is not absolute but sufficient to discourage the use of aspirin for children.

Tuberculosis of the Central Nervous System

Tuberculosis (TB) of the CNS is the most serious complication of primary TB in children. The clinical presentation commonly takes the form of meningitis. Less commonly, single or multiple tuberculomata enlarge and present as intracranial tumours **(Figs. 14.37A and B)**. TB disease may also be confined to the spinal cord **(Fig. 14.38)**.

Tuberculous Meningitis

This develops following the rupture of a caseous subcortical focus (Rich focus) into the subarachnoid space and is most common in children between 6 months and 5 years of age. Sometimes, it is preceded by a head injury or an intercurrent infection such as measles, mumps or pertussis. HIV infection predisposes children to TB infection including TB meningitis. The onset of symptoms is insidious and progresses gradually over some weeks and may be grouped into stages, which give a guide to prognosis. In infants the disease may run a more rapid course. Initially, the symptoms are non-specific and include lethargy, irritability, anorexia, headache, vomiting, abdominal pain, constipation and low-grade fever. The child's consciousness is unimpaired and neurological signs are absent. Unless there is a high index of suspicion and a positive contact history, the diagnosis is easily missed at this stage. About 2 weeks later the intermediate stage develops with obvious blurring of consciousness, nuchal rigidity, positive Kernig sign and focal neurological signs such as cranial nerve paralysis (ophthalmoplegia and facial paralysis) and hemiplegia. Seizures may develop. Raised intracranial pressure may manifest as full "boggy" fontanelle in an infant and "cracked pot resonance" in the older child. Fundoscopy may reveal choroidal tubercles indicating an associated miliary TB, papilloedema or the development of optic atrophy.

The third and final stage is characterised by coma, decerebrate rigidity, paralytic squints, unequal or dilated pupils, other neurological signs and marked wasting. Convulsions are common. Vasomotor instability and terminal hyperpyrexia may occur. The combination of cerebral vasculitis, cerebral infarction, cerebral oedema and communicating hydrocephalus due to obstruction to CSF flow at the level of basal cisterns leads to severe brain damage with little hope of recovery, and the incidence of permanent brain damage such as hydrocephalus, blindness, deafness, mental retardation and learning impairment is high.

Diagnosis

The diagnosis is based on a positive contact history, clinical examination, positive Mantoux test, chest X-ray and CSF analysis. Mantoux test may be negative in advanced stages and in severe malnutrition. The CSF is often under pressure and may be clear or opalescent depending on the cell count. The CSF cell count varies between 50 and 500/mm^3 with lymphocyte predominance. The protein content is raised above 40 mg/100 mL and may be even in grams/100 mL. The glucose content is low between 20 and 40 mg/dL. The final proof is the detection of tubercle bacilli by acid-fast stain of the CSF sediment or cobweb clot and mycobacterial culture. Identification of specific DNA sequences of *Mycobacterium tuberculosis* after polymerase chain reaction (PCR) amplification in the CSF is possible but there are risks of contamination and false positive results. Cultures of other fluids, such as gastric aspirate or urine, may help confirm the diagnosis. CT or MRI scan of the brain will show basal exudate, communicating hydrocephalus, cerebral oedema and focal ischaemia **(Figs. 14.39A to D)**.

Tuberculous meningitis is most likely to be mistaken for partially treated pyogenic meningitis or aseptic meningitis due to viruses. In these cases, the onset is usually much more acute than in TB cases, with brisk fever and obvious early rigidity of the neck and spine. The CSF may show a lymphocytic pleocytosis but in viral aseptic meningitis there is no fall in sugar content, the protein content is less markedly raised and a spider-web clot rarely, if ever, forms. There will be no other indications of TB in these cases. Detection of bacterial antigen in CSF by latex agglutination test and a positive bacterial CSF and blood culture will help to differentiate pyogenic meningitis. In older children, tuberculous meningitis can simulate brain tumour, but the CSF and CT or MRI scan of the brain will reveal the true state of affairs. Tuberculomas in children are often infratentorial in location and may be single or multiple.

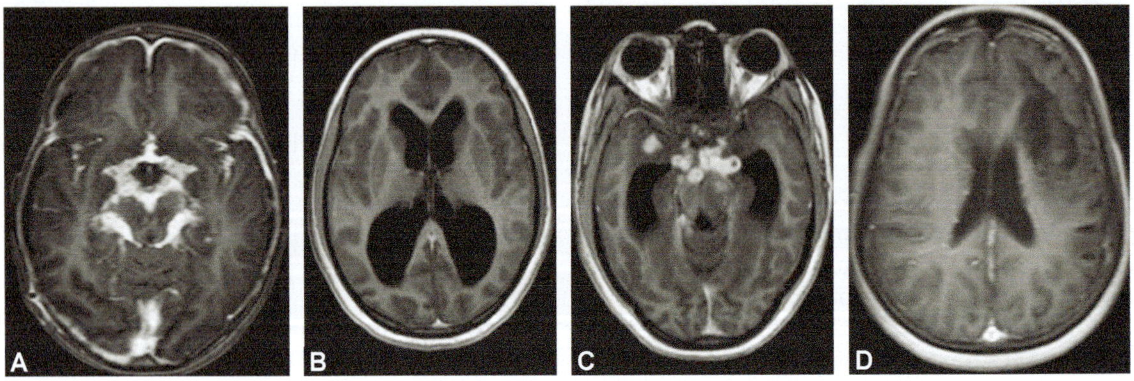

Figures 14.39A to D MRI images showing different complications of CNS tuberculosis. Figure (A) showing thick basal exudates which in turn can cause multiple cranial nerve palsies, Figure (B) showing hydrocephalus which is usually communicating, Figure (C) with multiple tuberculomas in the basal cistern and Figure (D) with an area of infarct in the left middle cerebral artery territory due to tuberculous arteritis.

Complication

During treatment, neurological complications may arise due to obstructive hydrocephalus, thrombosis of cerebral vessels and the involvement of cranial nerves in basal exudate. Serial cranial CT scans should be performed on all patients to detect the presence or development of hydrocephalus. Ventriculoperitoneal shunt surgery may be necessary.

Brain Abscess

Pus accumulation in brain parenchyma may occur as a complication of meningitis, due to haematogenous spread of septic emboli from infective endocarditis and congenital cyanotic heart disease (especially tetralogy of Fallot), extension of infection from chronic otitis media and mastoiditis and penetrating head injuries. The site of abscess depends on the source, e.g. chronic otitis media and mastoiditis leading to abscess formation in temporal lobe and cerebellum. The usual organisms are *streptococcus* (especially *Streptococcus viridans*), anaerobic organisms, *Staphylococcus aureus* and Gram-negative organisms, particularly, *Citrobacter*. In immune compromised children, fungal organisms may be responsible.

The symptoms and signs usually develop over 2–3 weeks and initially are non-specific with low-grade fever and headache. Later signs of raised intracranial pressure, seizures and focal neurological signs develop. Cerebellar signs may be obvious. The diagnosis is confirmed by contrast CT scan which shows a central area of low density with marked "ring" enhancement and surrounding area of low density due to oedema. There may be shift of the midline. Lumbar puncture should not be performed in a child suspected to have brain abscess (*see* Chapter 29: Paediatric Radiology, Fig. 29.126).

Neurocysticercosis

Neurocysticercosis is the most common parasitic infestation of the CNS and is caused by pork tapeworm *Taenia solium* in its larval stage. Human cysticercosis usually results when humans ingest vegetables contaminated with the eggs of *T. solium*. The cysticerci develop almost anywhere but particularly in the skin, muscle, brain and eye. Neurocysticercosis develops with single **(Figs. 14.40A to C)** and multiple cysts **(Figs. 14.41A to C)** and has been reported even in young children. It manifests commonly with seizures but can also cause signs of increased intracranial pressure, meningitis, behavioural disorders, paresis and hydrocephalus. The seizures are mostly focal in nature. A phenomenon peculiar to patients in the Indian subcontinent is the solitary cysticercus granuloma that shows up as a single, small, ring enhancing lesion on the contrast enhanced CT scan, with significant surrounding oedema located superficially near the cortex. The usual presentation is a focal seizure often with post-ictal deficit in the form of monoparesis or hemiparesis. The deficit is usually temporary and the CT lesion resolves spontaneously over a period of time. Serologic tests like enzyme-linked immunosorbent assay and enzyme-linked immunoelectrotransfer blots can be useful to confirm the diagnosis.

ACUTE FLACCID PARALYSIS

Acute flaccid paralysis is defined as onset of weakness and floppiness within 2 weeks in any part of the body in a child less than 15 years of age. The common causes of acute flaccid paralysis are acute paralytic poliomyelitis, Guillain-Barre syndrome (GBS), traumatic neuritis and transverse myelitis. Other causes include non-polio enterovirus infections, encephalitis, meningitis, toxins, etc.

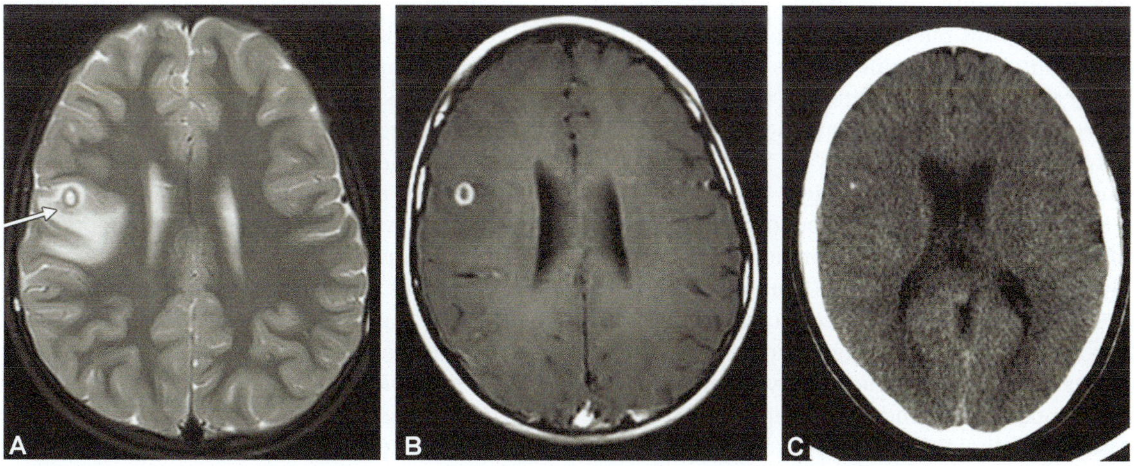

Figures 14.40A to C Solitary cysticercus granuloma (SCG). MRI T2 axial image (A) showing a ring lesion in the right frontal lobe which has central hyperintensity indicating vesicular stage of the *Taenia solium* larvae. Ring enhancement is seen post gadolinium (B). This child presented with left focal motor seizures and was treated with only antiepileptic medication and repeat CT brain (C) after a year shows resolution of the oedema and healing by calcification.

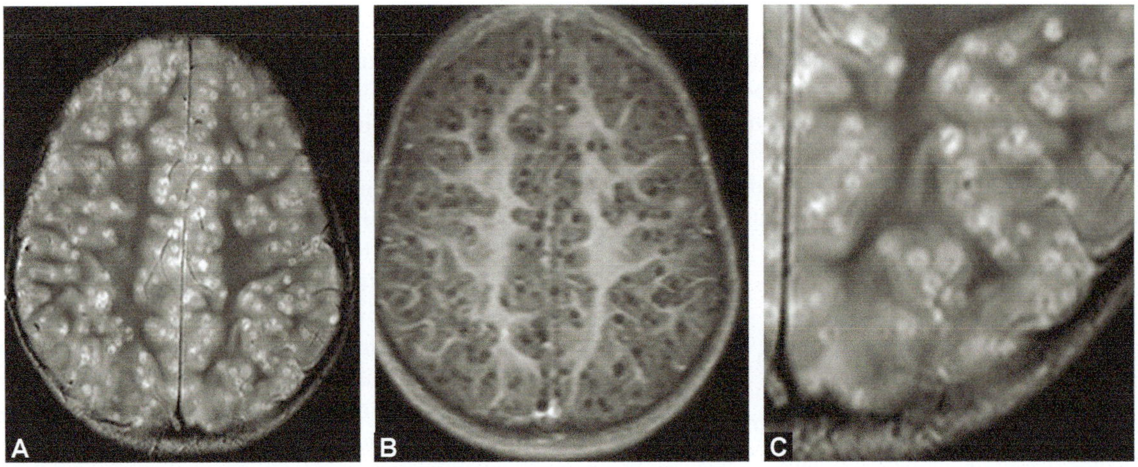

Figures 14.41A to C Multiple neurocysticercosis. MRI T2W axial (A) and post gadolinium (B) images with multiple cysts which are in different stages. There is not much enhancement appreciable. Enlarged image (C) shows the central hyperintensity with an eccentric hypointense dot representing the larval scolex. The cysts have a predilection to remain at the grey white interface.

Acute Poliomyelitis

This is caused by poliovirus, which comprises three serotypes: Types 1, 2 and 3 of which type 1 is the most common cause for poliomyelitis. Transmission is primarily person-to-person via the faecal-oral route. Unimmunised children, 6 months to 3 years of age, are most susceptible. In 90–95% of infected individuals, poliovirus infection is inapparent. In the remaining infected individuals, one of the three syndromes may occur.

Abortive polio is characterised by a minor illness with low-grade fever, sore throat, vomiting, abdominal pain and malaise. Recovery is rapid and there is no paralysis.

Non-paralytic aseptic meningitis is characterised by headache, neck, back and leg stiffness preceded about a week earlier by a prodrome similar to abortive polio. The child may be drowsy and irritable; spinal stiffness is manifested by the tripod sign. There is no paralysis.

Paralytic poliomyelitis occurs in about 1% of infected individuals. Symptoms often occur in two phases with a symptom-free interval. The minor illness consisting of the symptoms of abortive poliomyelitis and the major illness is characterised by high grade fever, muscle pain and stiffness followed by rapid onset of flaccid paralyses that is usually complete within 72 hours **(Fig. 14.42)**.

There are three types of paralytic poliomyelitis:

Spinal poliomyelitis: This accounts for newly 80% of the paralytic poliomyelitis. It results from a lower motor neuron lesion of the anterior horn cells of the spinal cord and affects the muscles of the legs, arms and/or trunk. Paralysis is asymmetrical and the sensory system is intact. The affected muscles are tender and floppy, and tendon reflexes are lost or diminished

Bulbar poliomyelitis results from involvement of lower cranial nerves and can cause facial paralysis, difficulty in swallowing, eating or speech and respiratory insufficiency

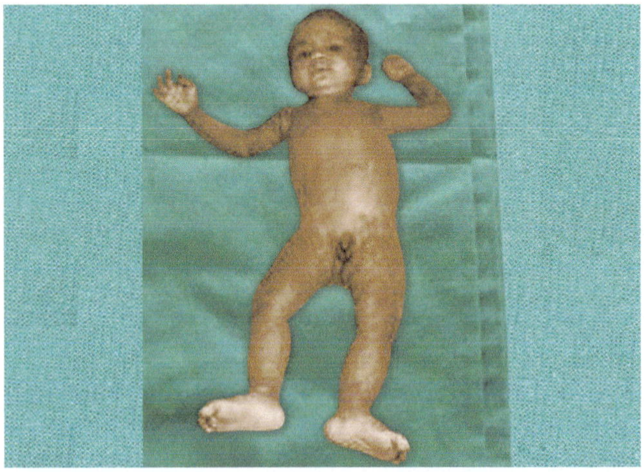

Figure 14.42 Acute flaccid paralysis due to poliomyelitis.

Bulbospinal poliomyelitis involves both bulbar cranial nerves and spinal cord.

Life is endangered in case of bulbar involvement with inability to swallow and obstruction of the airway and when the muscles of respiration are involved.

As the acute phase of paralytic poliomyelitis subsides over 4 weeks, recovery begins in paralysed muscles. The extent of recovery is variable depending upon the extent of damage caused to the neurones by the virus. Maximum recovery takes place in the first 6 months after the illness, but slow recovery can continue up to 2 years. After 2 years, no more recovery is expected and the child is said to have post-polio residual paralysis. Affected muscles atrophy and deformities such as pes cavus, talipes or scoliosis and ultimate shortening of the affected limb may develop.

Poliovirus can be isolated from the stool specimen. Paired serum may be tested for neutralising antibody in rising titre. The CSF is clear or only slightly hazy. The cell count varies from 50 to a few hundreds per cubic millimetre with lymphocytic predominance. The sugar level is normal, but the protein content is elevated leading at times to "cyto-albumino dissociation."

Acute Postinfectious Polyneuropathy (Guillain–Barré Syndrome)

It is an acute inflammatory demyelinating polyradiculoneuropathy affecting the spinal nerve roots, peripheral nerves and cranial nerves. It involves primarily the motor but sometimes also sensory and autonomic nerves. It typically occurs after recovery from a viral infection or in rare cases, following immunisation. The commonly identified triggering agents are *Helicobacter jejuni*, CMV, EBV and *Mycoplasma pneumoniae*. It is believed to be due to a "cross-reactive" immune attack by host antibodies and T-lymphocytes on nerve components. GBS is now appreciated as a heterogeneous spectrum of disorders with distinct subtypes. Some patients have mainly loss of myelin which is the most common type termed acute inflammatory demyelinating polyradiculoneuropathy, while others have predominantly axonal damage involving both sensory and motor nerves termed acute motor-sensory axonal neuropathy. A pure motor axonal form is called acute motor axonal neuropathy, which tend to be more severe. Another subtype, the Miller-Fisher syndrome, consists of acute onset of ataxia, areflexia and ophthalmoplegia. Other variants of GBS include acute pandysautonomia and polyneuritis cranialis.

Clinical Features

After an upper respiratory febrile illness or acute gastroenteritis, the child develops increasing muscle weakness and tenderness with loss of deep tendon reflexes. The lower limbs are the first to be affected followed by involvement of the trunk, upper limbs and finally the bulbar muscles (Landry ascending paralysis). The disease can progress over days to 4 weeks. Proximal and distal muscles are involved relatively symmetrically. Sensory changes tend to be minimal. Intercostal and diaphragmatic paralysis may endanger life. Bilateral facial paralysis is common. ANS involvement may manifest with tachycardia and hypertension. In the typical Guillain-Barre syndrome, the CSF shows a high protein content with little or no pleocytosis, but these changes are inconstant and may be late in appearing. Motor nerve conduction velocities are greatly reduced. Electromyogram shows evidence of acute denervation of muscle.

CONVULSIONS IN INFANCY AND CHILDHOOD

Convulsion is a common acute and potentially life threatening event encountered in infants and children. About 5% of children would have had one or more convulsion by the time they reach maturity. A convulsion (epileptic seizure) is defined as a transient occurrence of signs and/or symptoms due to abnormal excessive or synchronous neuronal activity in the brain. The clinical manifestation consists of sudden and transitory abnormal phenomena which may include alterations of consciousness, motor, sensory, autonomic or psychic events perceived by the patient or an observer.

Classification

Epileptic seizures are generally classified based on the clinical features of the attack and the accompanying EEG. The recent classification of seizures proposed by the International League Against Epilepsy (ILAE) 2017 is shown in **Table 14.1**. Seizures are primarily divided into focal or generalized based on the features at onset and as of unknown onset when information is inadequate. Focal seizures are further classified as those with preserved awareness and those with impaired awareness. Awareness means the person is aware of self and environment during the seizures. A focal aware seizure corresponds to the prior term simple partial seizure. A focal impaired awareness seizure corresponds to the prior term complex partial seizure. Each of this is further classified as those with predominant motor or non-motor symptoms. Since it is difficult to determine the degree of awareness in children, epileptic spasms and atonic seizures are classified as focal aware seizures. Generalized seizures are divided into motor and non-motor (absence) seizures.

Once the seizure type is determined, the epilepsy is then categorized as being a focal, generalized or combined focal and generalized and again unknown when information is inadequate **(Table 14.2)**. Further investigative work up towards aetiology will help to determine if

TABLE 14.1 Classification of Seizures by the International League Against Epilepsy (ILAE 2017).

ILAE 2017 classification of Seizure Types Expanded Version[1]

Focal onset	Generalized onset	Unknown onset
Aware / Impaired awareness	**Motor**	**Motor**
Motor onset	tonic–clonic	tonic–clonic
automatisms	clonic	epileptic spasms
atonic[2]	myoclonic	**Nonmotor**
clonic	myoclonic–tonic-clonic	behavior arrest
epileptic spasms[2]	myoclonic–atonic	
hyperkinetic	atonic	Unclassified[3]
myoclonic	epileptic spasms	
tonic	**Nonmotor (absence)**	
Nonmotor onset	typical	
autonomic	atypical	
behavior arrest	myoclonic	
cognitive	eyelid myoclonia	
emotional		
sensory		
Focal onset		

[1]Definitions, other seizure types and descriptors are listed in the accompanying paper and glossary of terms.
[2]Degree of awareness usually is not specified.
[3]Due to inadequate information or inability to place in other categories.

TABLE 14.2 Categorization of Seizures.

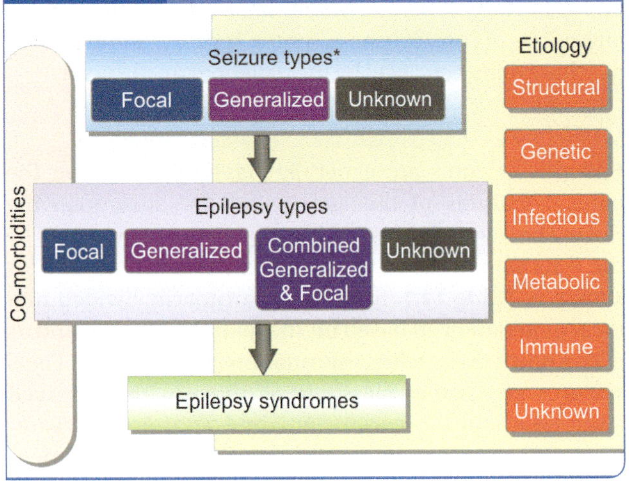

it is of structural, genetic, metabolic, infectious, immune mediated or unknown aetiology.

Some epilepsies have a cluster of features enabling it to be classified as a specific epilepsy syndrome such as childhood absence epilepsy, Dravet syndrome, etc.

The electroencephalographic changes are frequently characteristic in the different clinical types, but this correlation is by no means firm and a good deal of overlap and mixing of types occur **(Figs. 14.43 and 14.44)**. A normal EEG does not preclude the diagnosis of epilepsy especially the interictal recording.

A patient is said to be in **status epilepticus** when seizure lasts or occurs in succession for more than 30 minutes without intervening periods of recovery. All seizures lasting more than 5 minutes have the risk of progressing to status epilepticus and hence are now termed "threatened" or "impending" status epilepticus. The time duration has been modified so that aggressive treatment can start after 5–10 minutes of active seizures to reduce morbidity and mortality. Refractory status epilepticus includes seizures that last beyond 30 minutes despite adequate initial doses of 2 or 3 anticonvulsant medications. It is a true medical emergency and can end fatally or with permanent sequelae of hypoxic brain damage. Secondary metabolic complications appear when convulsive status is prolonged. Initial hyperglycaemia is followed by hypoglycaemia and autonomic dysfunctions appear consisting of hyperthermia, excessive sweating, dehydration, hypotension and eventually shock. Cardiovascular, respiratory and renal failure may result.

CHILDHOOD STROKE

Childhood stroke is defined as a cerebrovascular event occurring between 28 days and 18 years of age. This encompasses ischaemic stroke and haemorrhagic stroke. Ischaemic stroke includes arterial ischaemic stroke and cerebral venous sinus thrombosis while haemorrhagic stroke includes spontaneous intracerebral haemorrhage and non-traumatic subarachnoid haemorrhage. The annual incidence of stroke ranges from 1.5 to 2.5

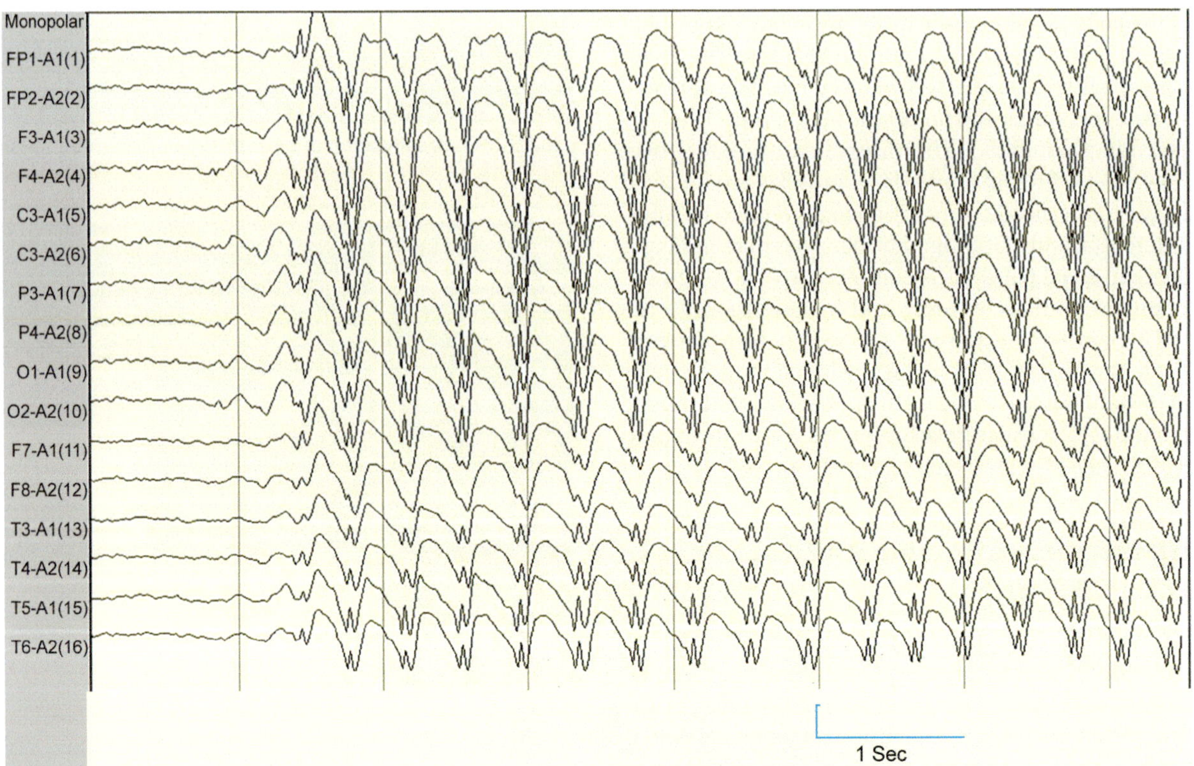

Figure 14.43 Typical EEG pattern in childhood absence epilepsy showing the 3/sec spike wave generalised discharges which are frontally predominant.

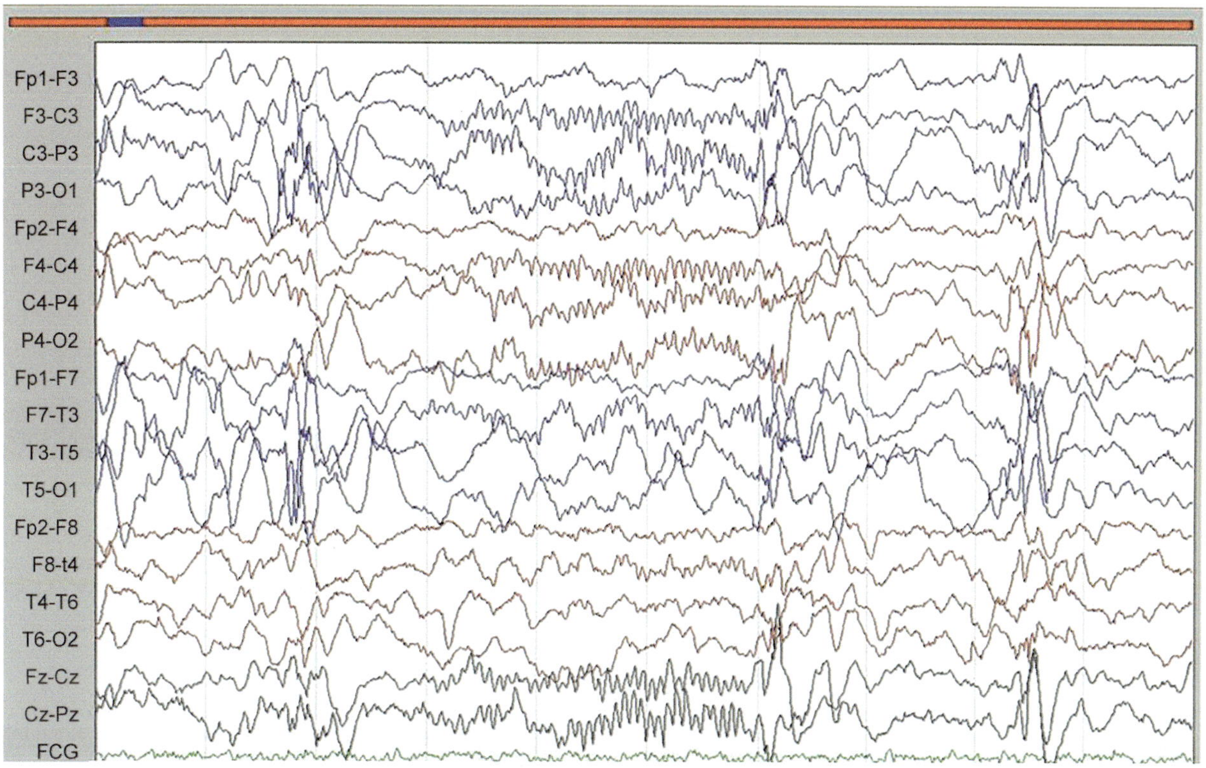

Figure 14.44 Hypsarrhythmia—EEG hallmark of epileptic spasms with high amplitude slow waves and multifocal spikes.

per 100,000 children and of this 50% are arterial ischaemic stroke, 40% haemorrhagic stroke and the rest venous sinus thrombosis. The causes for childhood stroke are many **(Table 14.3)**. One-third of them have an underlying disease, one-third have vascular malformations and in the rest the aetiology remains unclear. Often more than one risk factor is identified. Perinatal stroke includes vascular events which occur between 28 weeks of gestational age and the 7th post-natal day. They are seen later as porencephalic cysts in vascular territory **(Fig. 14.45)**.

Clinical Features

The clinical presentation depends on the territory of ischaemia or bleed. As a rule children with arterial ischaemic stroke present with sudden onset focal neurological deficits without major alteration of consciousness unlike more common paediatric illnesses like encephalitis, complex partial and generalised seizures that often have alteration of awareness. Focal neurological deficits could include hemiparesis, visual field defects, aphasia, cranial nerve palsies, dysphagia and unilateral ataxia. Anterior circulation infarcts are more common. Larger strokes tend to have multiple deficits and alteration of consciousness.

Haemorrhagic strokes have a much more dramatic presentation with alteration of consciousness, nausea, vertigo, vomiting, headache and seizures **(Fig. 14.46)**.

Children with venous sinus thrombosis have protracted severe headache with vomiting as their starting symptoms followed by focal neurological deficits and seizures when they go onto develop venous infarction **(Figs. 14.47A and B)**.

The underlying disease, if already known, will give a clue to the type of stroke. For example, arterial ischaemic stroke is seen in children with cardiac diseases **(Fig. 14.48)**, chronic meningitis like TB **(Figs. 14.49A to C)**, varicella infection **(Fig. 14.50)** and haemoglobinopathies. Thrombosis of the internal carotid artery **(Figs. 14.51A and B)** may result from trauma caused by falls on objects, e.g. a pencil in the mouth, which penetrates the tonsillar fossa. Children with bleeding disorders are more likely to have haemorrhagic strokes and children with dehydration, nephrotic syndrome and older girls on oral contraceptive pills are likely to develop venous sinus thrombosis. Children with moyamoya disease and syndrome present with recurrent transient ischemic attacks (TIA) and seizures **(Figs. 14.52A and B)**.

Stroke Mimics

Acute onset of focal neurological deficit in a child need not be due to a cerebrovascular event and can have multiple other aetiologies. These are called stroke mimics and the differential diagnosis for this includes infectious or inflammatory causes like encephalitis, *H. influenzae*, meningitis, tuberculous meningitis, brain abscess from middle ear infection or congenital heart disease and demyelination like acute disseminated encephalomyelitis. Prolonged focal seizures can cause a temporary paralysis

TABLE 14.3 Causes of childhood stroke.

Types of stroke	*Diseases*
1. ARTERIAL ISCHAEMIC STROKE	
a) Cerebral arteriopathy	Moyamoya disease
	Moyamoya syndrome
	Focal cerebral arteriopathy of childhood
	Post-varicella arteriopathy
	Vasculitis
	Isolated central nervous system vasculitis
	Post-infectious
	Arterial dissection
b) Cardioembolic	Congenital heart disease
	Acquired heart disease
c) Haematological	Sickle cell disease
	Iron deficiency anaemia
	Thrombocytosis
	Protein C/S deficiency
	Factor V Leiden mutation
	Methylenetetrahydrofolate reductase mutation
d) Undetermined aetiology	
2. HAEMORRHAGIC STROKE	
a) Arteriovenous malformation	
b) Cerebral aneurysm	
c) Bleeding disorders	
3. CEREBRAL VENOUS SINUS THROMBOSIS	
a) Dehydration	
b) Hypercoagulable disorders	
c) Iron deficiency anaemia	

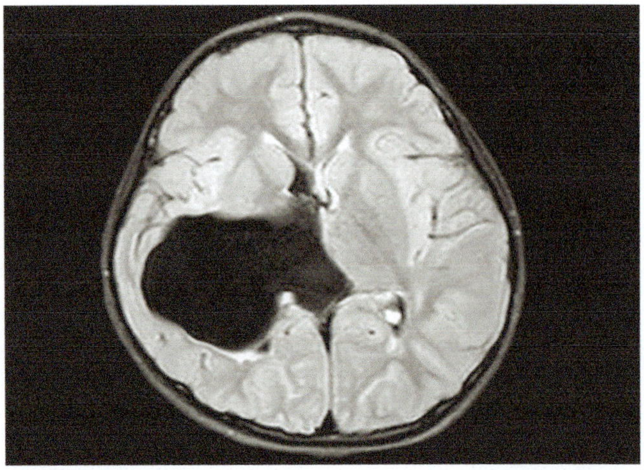

Figure 14.45 Porencephalic cyst (MRI brain T2 FLAIR image) involving the right middle cerebral artery territory in a 4-year-old child who presented with left hemiparesis and left focal motor seizures. Porencephalic cyst is a focal area of cystic encephalomalacia that communicates with the ventricular system and/or the subarachnoid space. This child was noted to have right hand preference from early life and probably had a perinatal stroke.

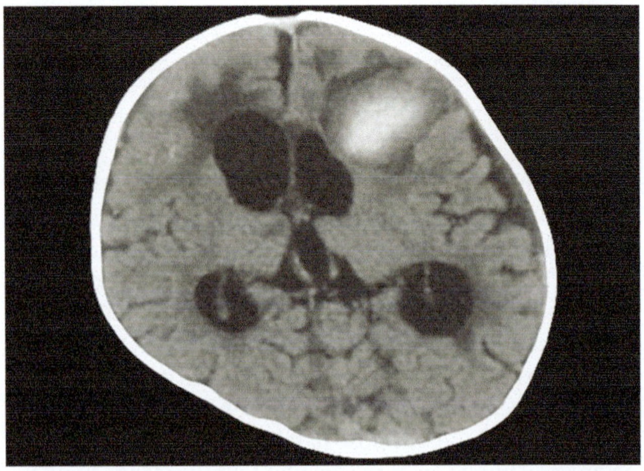

Figure 14.46 Plain CT brain with hyperdensity in the left frontal lobe suggestive of a bleed. This infant had haemorrhagic disease of the newborn and was brought with acute onset lethargy and seizures. CT also shows dilated ventricles with periventricular CSF seepage suggestive of hydrocephalus which is a common complication with large haemorrhagic stroke.

called Todd paresis that can persist for up to 48–72 hours. Metabolic disorders associated with focal neurological deficits include hypoglycaemia, MELAS (mitochondrial myopathy, encephalopathy, lactic acidosis, and stroke syndrome), homocystinuria and Fabry disease.

Diagnosis

Diagnostic evaluation needs to be extensive first to differentiate strokes from stroke mimics and second to determine the cause of the cerebrovascular event. In the acute stage, a plain CT brain will help to identify haemorrhage, abscess and tumours. This has to be followed by an MRI of the brain with diffusion-weighted images to assess acute ischaemic zones. Vascular imaging also needs to be performed along with this like magnetic resonance angiography (MRA) and magnetic resonance venography (MRV). MRA will demonstrate arteriopathy, dissection, stenosis, irregular contour or intra-arterial thrombosis of the head and neck, and MRV will demonstrate cerebral venous sinus thrombosis. Further vascular imaging in the form of CT angiography or conventional angiography is warranted if further neurovascular intervention is planned.

For arterial ischaemic stroke, transthoracic echocardiography is another important diagnostic imaging to detect congenital or acquired cardiac anomalies including patent foramen ovale.

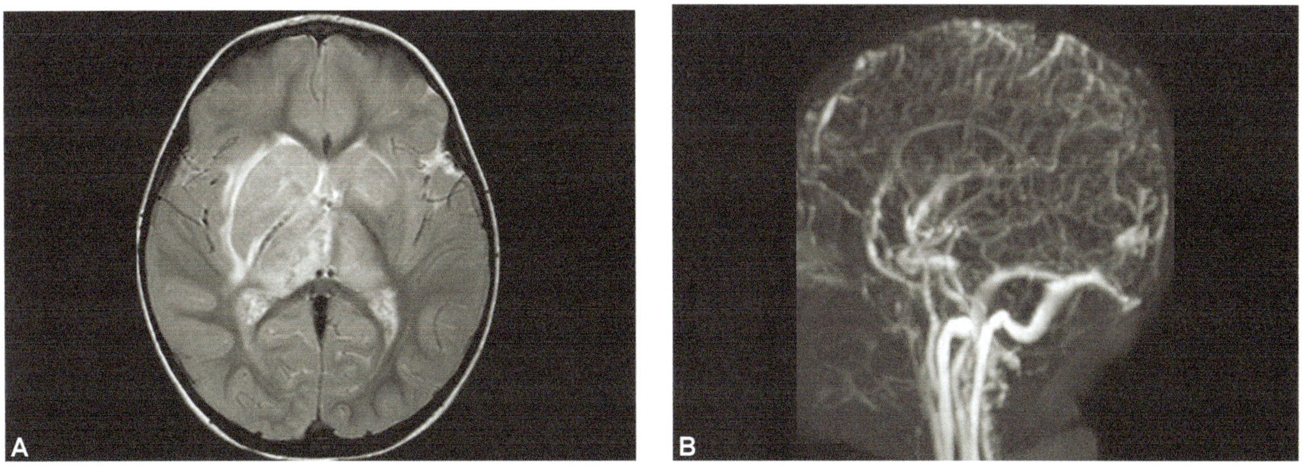

Figures 14.47A and B Cerebral venous sinus thromboses with venous infarcts involving the deep structures namely bilateral thalami, lentiform and caudate nuclei. MRI T2W images (A) showing hyperintensity and swelling of the involved structures and MR venogram (B) showing complete occlusion of the superficial and deep venous sinuses.

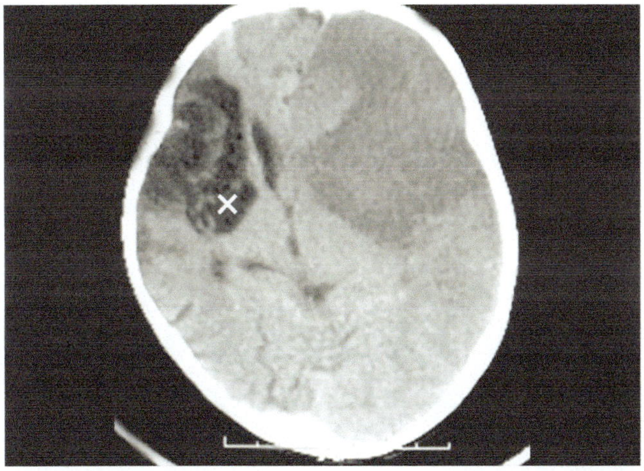

Figure 14.48 Recurrent thrombotic stroke in a child with untreated Tetralogy of Fallot. Imaging will show strokes in different ages. This plain CT brain shows a chronic infarct in the right middle cerebral artery (MCA) territory and an acute infarct in the left MCA territory with oedema and midline shift.

Diagnostic laboratory evaluation has to include complete blood count, complete metabolic panel and erythrocyte sedimentation rate (ESR), C-reactive protein to assess biochemical evidence of systemic inflammation that could suggest vasculitis or infection, and complete thrombotic profile. If vasculitis is suspected, rheumatological evaluation like testing of antinuclear antibody, rheumatoid factor should be considered. A lumbar puncture is indicated if infectious or inflammatory states are considered and in this it would be advisable to perform routinely test for HSV, varicella zoster virus and other enteroviruses.

MOVEMENT DISORDERS

The control of voluntary movement is affected by the interaction of the pyramidal, extra-pyramidal and cerebellar systems. The effects of disease of the extra-pyramidal

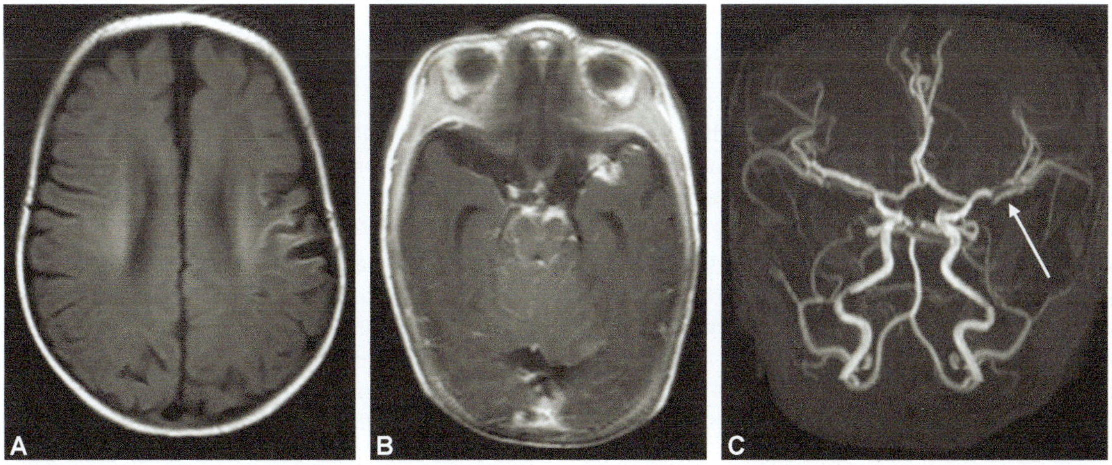

Figures 14.49A to C Tuberculous arteritis with stroke in a child with tuberculous meningitis. MR T2 FLAIR image (A) showing chronic infarct in the left posterior frontal and parietal lobe with the gado image (B) showing exudates in the basal cistern and around the left middle cerebral artery in the left sylvian fissure. MR angiogram (C) shows narrowing at the same site (arrow).

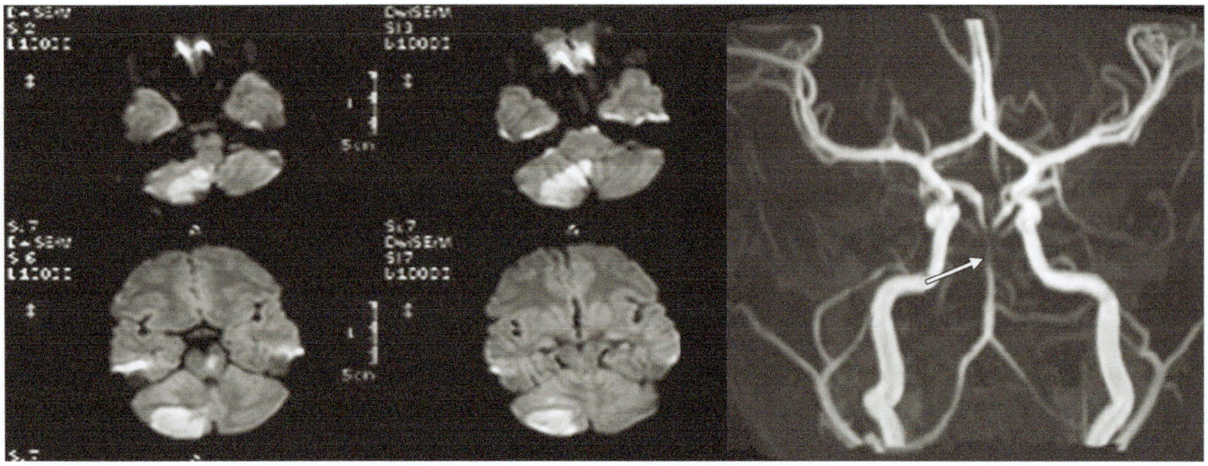

Figure 14.50 Varicella associated vasculopathy. This child after a week of varicella infection presented with acute onset severe neck pain and imbalance while walking. Diffusion weighted MRI shows diffusion restriction in the right superior cerebellar artery territory and MRA with distal narrowing (arrow) of the basilar artery.

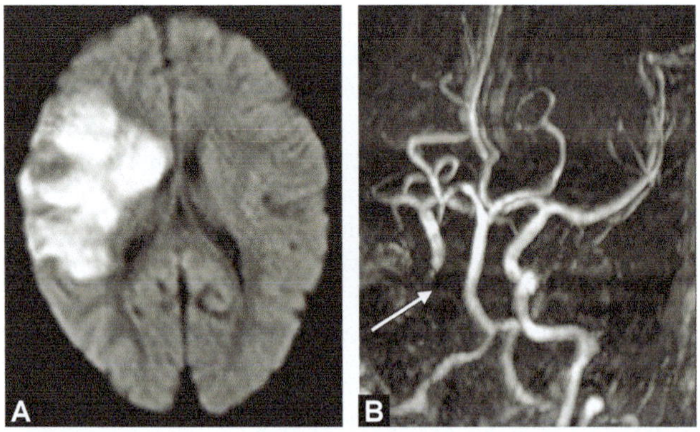

Figures 14.51A and B MR Diffusion weight imaging (DWI) (A) and MR angiogram (B) showing wedge-shaped gyral swelling and hyperintensity with restricted diffusion in the right middle cerebral artery territory distribution. MRA shows non visualisation of the right internal carotid artery which had a subacute thrombus on carotid Doppler. This occurred a day after the 2-year-old child had a fall and rolled over a short distance resulting in dissection of the internal carotid artery and presented with left hemiparesis.

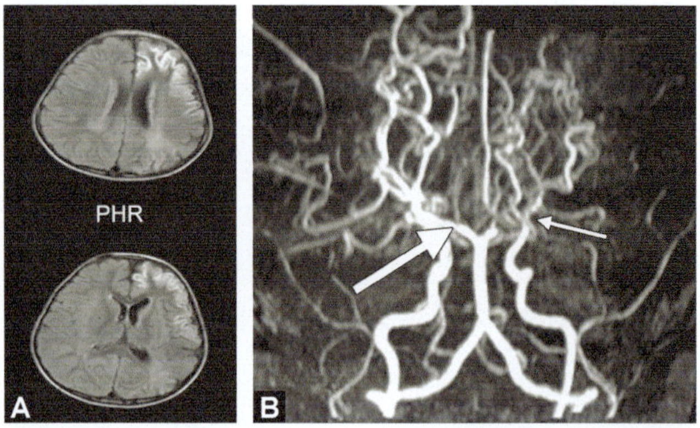

Figures 14.52A and B Moyamoya disease. T2 FLAIR MRI (A) showing hyperintensities in the left anterior and posterior water-shed territories and left middle cerebral artery territory suggestive of chronic infarcts. MR angiogram (B) showing the typical supraclinoid narrowing of the left internal carotid artery (thin arrow) with multiple distal collaterals giving the typical puff of smoke appearance. This child also had involvement of the posterior circulation as well with proximal narrowing of bilateral posterior cerebral arteries (thick arrow).

system on movement are bradykinesia, rigidity, postural disturbance and involuntary movements, namely chorea, athetosis, tremor and dystonia. Chorea is a jerky, semi-purposive, non-repetitive involuntary movement affecting the limbs, face and trunk. Causes of chorea in childhood include rheumatic chorea, extra-pyramidal cerebral palsy, Wilson disease and post-encephalitic sequelae.

Wilson disease

This disease, inherited as an autosomal recessive trait, is an inborn error of copper metabolism resulting in an excessive accumulation of copper in the liver, brain, cornea and other tissues. Wilson disease occurs due to mutation in ATP7B, on chromosome 13 which codes for a copper-transporting adenosine triphosphatase.

Clinical Features

Hepatic presentation in the form of jaundice, hepatomegaly, cirrhosis or portal hypertension is predominant in children younger than 10 years of age. Neurological presentation is predominantly in older children with basal ganglia lesion, e.g. coarse tremors of the extremities (wing-beating tremor), dystonia, dysarthria, dysphasia, drooling, emotional instability, deterioration in school performance and dementia **(Figs. 14.53A and B)**. A characteristic finding is the Kayser-Fleischer (K-F) ring, a golden brown discoloration due to deposition of copper at the corneal limbus **(Fig. 14.53C)**.

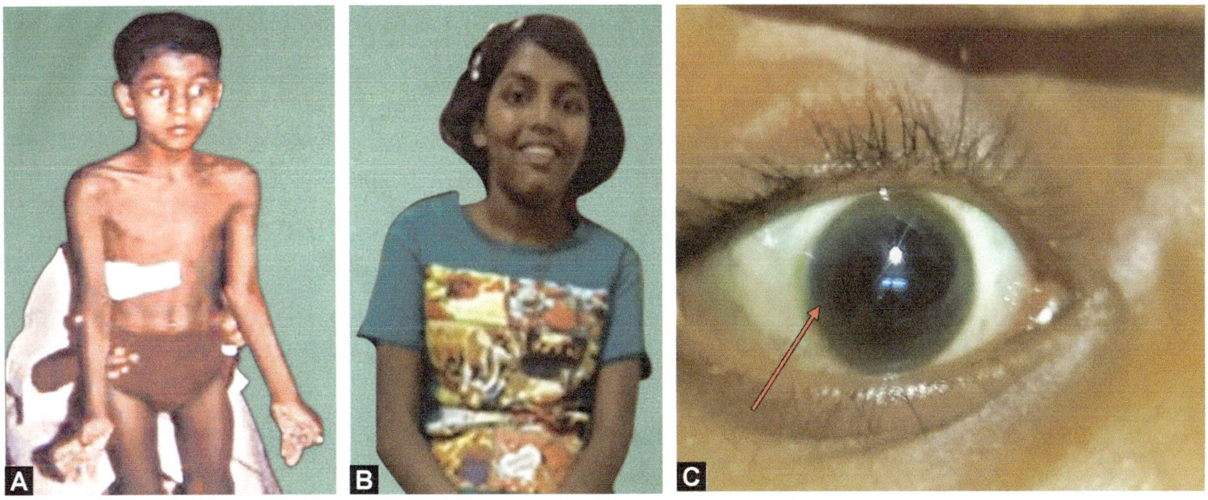

Figures 14.53A to C Wilson disease. Figure (A) showing dystonic posturing of the hands. This child also had hepatic disease and had a liver biopsy. Figure (B) showing the classic vacuous smile due to dystonia of the facial and jaw muscles. She also had mild axial dystonia. All children with Neuro Wilson disease will have the typical Kayser-Fleischer ring at the corneal limbus [arrow in Figure (C)].

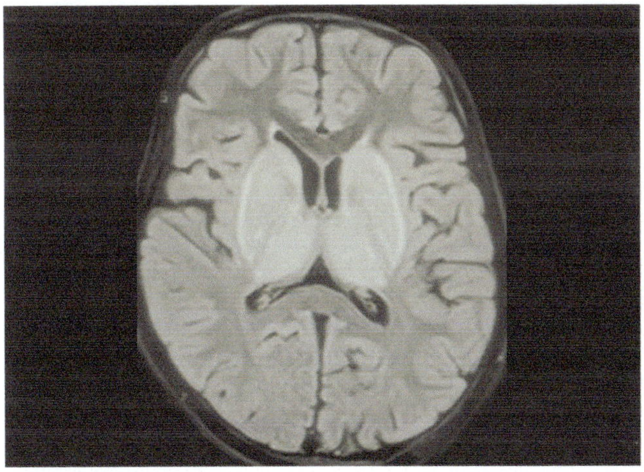

Figure 14.54 MRI brain T2W image showing symmetric hyperintensity of the caudate, lentiform and thalami in Wilson disease.

Diagnosis

The serum ceruloplasmin level is decreased and urine copper excretion is increased particularly after a 1 g D-penicillamine challenge test. Liver function is usually deranged and slit-lamp examination of the eyes reveals K-F ring. Liver biopsy may reveal cirrhosis and excessive copper content. MRI brain has typical findings **(Fig. 14.54)**.

Rheumatic Chorea (Sydenham chorea, Saint Vitus Dance)

This major manifestation of rheumatic fever may occur in association with other manifestations such as polyarthritis and carditis but it frequently appears as a solitary and rather odd phenomenon. It is, in fact, the only major rheumatic manifestation that can affect the same child more than once, and sometimes several times, without the development of any of the other manifestations of acute rheumatic fever. For these reasons and also because the ESR and anti-streptolysin O titre remain normal in uncomplicated chorea, the precise relationship of this disease to rheumatic fever has been the subject of an unresolved controversy. It is more common in girls. The clinical features fall into four main groups.

Involuntary purposeless, non-repetitive movements of the limbs, face and trunk, e.g. grimacing, wriggling and writhing. The movements can be brought under voluntary control temporarily. They are aggravated by excitement and they disappear during sleep. The first indication may be that the child begins to drop things or her handwriting suddenly deteriorates or she gets into trouble with her elders for making faces. Sometimes the movements are confined to one side of the body (hemichorea).

Hypotonia may result in muscular weakness. It also causes the characteristic posture of the outstretched hands in which the wrist is slightly flexed, whereas there is hyperextension of the metacarpophalangeal joints. Occasionally, the child is unable to stand or even to sit up (chorea paralytica).

Incoordination may be marked or only obvious when the child is asked to pick a coin off the floor.

Mental upset is often an early sign. Emotional lability is almost constant. School work usually deteriorates. Infrequently the child becomes confused or even maniacal (chorea insaniens).

Heredodegenerative ataxias

These are inherited progressive ataxias. The most common type is Friedrich ataxia, which is an autosomal recessive

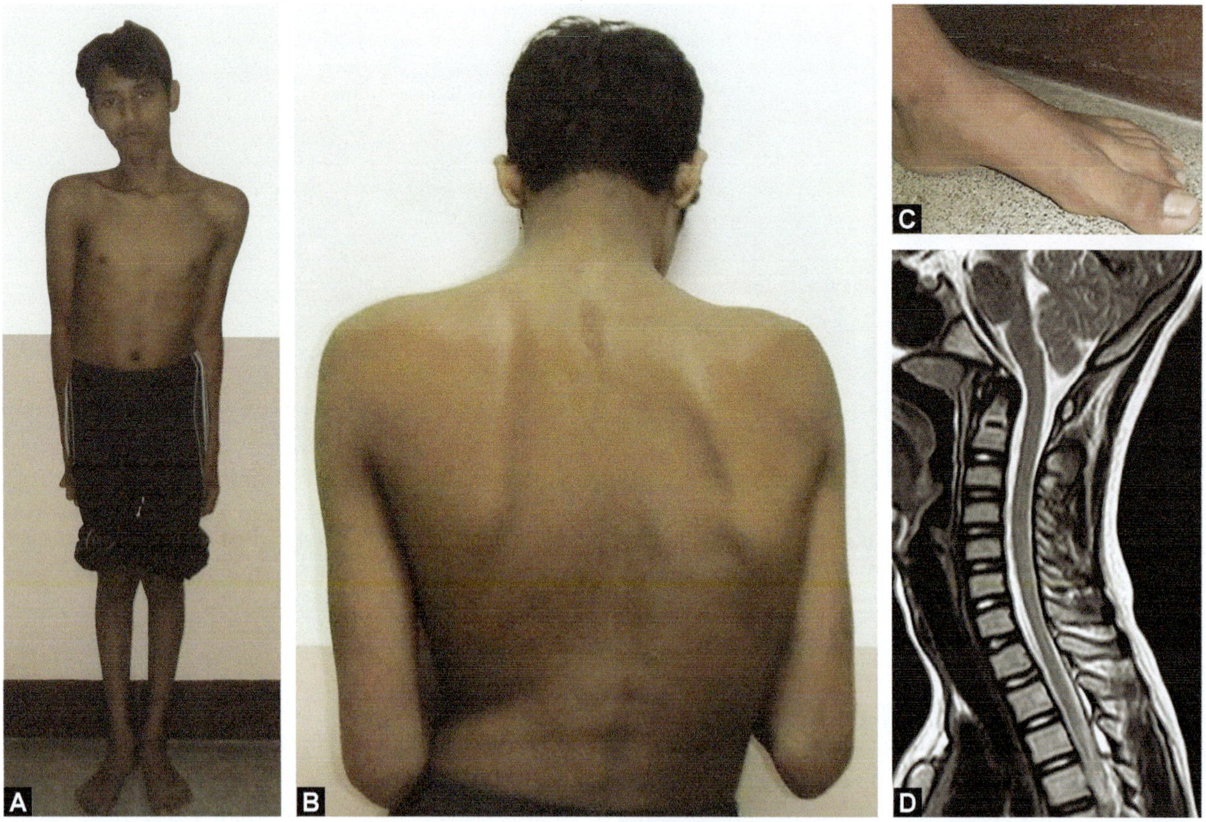

Figures 14.55A to D Friedreich ataxia in an adolescent boy who presented with gait ataxia. *Note* the skeletal deformities—Kyphoscoliosis (B) and pes cavus (C). MRI spine shows cervical cord thinning (D). Brain MRI may show cerebellar atrophy.

disorder caused by decreased expression of the mitochondrial protein, frataxin, encoded in chromosome 9. The onset of symptoms is in childhood and before puberty with pes cavus, kyphoscoliosis and ataxia **(Figs. 14.55A to D)**. There is nystagmus and intention tremor. Involvement of the dorsal columns leads to the loss of vibration and position sense. The deep tendon reflexes are absent, particularly ankle jerk and the plantar response is extensor. Optic atrophy and dysarthria may appear late in the course of the disease. Cardiac involvement can lead to intractable congestive cardiac failure. Death may be delayed for 10–15 years, but it may occur earlier from cardiac failure.

NEUROCUTANEOUS SYNDROMES

Neurocutaneous syndromes (the phakomatoses) are disorders with manifestation in skin and CNS. Most are autosomally inherited and have a high rate of tumour formation. The common phakomatoses are neurofibromatosis (NF), tuberous sclerosis, Sturge-Weber syndrome, von Hippel-Lindau disease and ataxia telangiectasia.

Neurofibromatosis (von Recklinghausen Disease)

This is the most common neurocutaneous syndrome and is transmitted as an autosomal dominant characteristic. There is abnormality of neural crest migration. Two gene defects have been identified; one on chromosome 17q11.2 that causes NF1 with mainly cutaneous features and peripheral nerve abnormalities, and the other on chromosome 22q11 causing NF2 with mainly CNS involvement and vestibular schwannoma formation after the age of 20.

The earliest and pathognomonic signs of NF are the café-au-lait spots or patches **(Fig. 14.56)** that are irregularly shaped hyperpigmented brownish macules often present at or shortly after birth and may vary in size and number with age. Presence of six or more café-au-lait spots greater than 0.5 cm in diameter in prepubertal children is considered diagnostic of NF. Other cutaneous manifestations are axillary or inguinal freckling and presence of pedunculated neurofibromas. Palpable neurofibromata are to be detected along the course of subcutaneous nerves. The brain may be the site of formation of hamartomatous nodules **(Fig. 14.56)**, and various types of tumours (glioma, ependymoma and meningioma) may occur in the brain, optic nerve, spinal cord or spinal nerve roots. Approximately, 10–20% of the patients manifest with seizures, intellectual deficit and speech and motor delay. Lisch nodules are seen in the iris with increasing age. Osseous lesions include progressive kyphoscoliosis in childhood, sphenoidal dysplasia and cortical thickening of long bones with or without pseudoarthrosis.

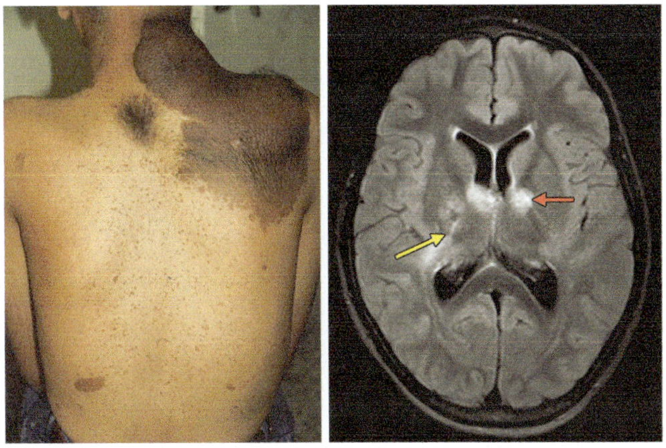

Figure 14.56 Adolescent boy with neurofibromatosis type 1 with multiple café au lait lesions and a plexiform neurofibroma over the right shoulder. The plexiform neuromas are tumours that Involve multiple branches of a major nerve. There is associated thickening and hypertrophy of the overlying skin. MRI brain can show T2 hyperintense lesions in the basal ganglia (red arrow), internal capsule (yellow arrow) and cerebellum.

Tuberous Sclerosis (Epiloia)

Tuberous sclerosis is one of the phakomatoses with manifestations in the skin, CNS and eye as well as hamartomata of internal organs such as kidney, heart, lung and bone. The disease is transmitted as an autosomal dominant trait with gene defects identified on chromosomes 9 and 16. Seizures are the most common presenting symptom and may present in infancy with infantile spasms or partial seizures. Hypopigmented areas of skin, sometimes assuming an ash-leaf shape, are the earliest skin manifestation (Fig. 14.57A). The characteristic rash of butterfly distribution and papular character on the face and nose known as adenoma sebaceum appears later (Fig. 14.57B). Other skin lesions include shagreen patch—a leathery plaque—usually in the lumbosacral area and café-au-lait spots.

The characteristic brain lesion consists of tubers typically present in the subependymal region made of abnormal giant cells and sclerosis due to overgrowth of astrocytic fibrils. These tubers undergo calcification and also at times malignant transformation. Mental retardation is a common feature. Ophthalmoscopy may show characteristic yellowish-white phakomata on the retina. The heart may be the seat of a rhabdomyoma or tubers. In some cases, there are teratomata or hamartomata of the kidneys, liver, bone and lung.

The diagnosis of tuberous sclerosis is based on the combination of characteristic cutaneous lesions, seizures, intellectual deficit and visceral tumours. Neuroimaging studies demonstrate subependymal-calcified nodules adjacent to lateral ventricles and cortical tubers (Fig. 14.58).

Sturge–Weber Syndrome (Encephalofacial Angiomatosis)

This disease consists of cutaneous port-wine haemangioma of the upper face and scalp (Fig. 14.59), which is predominantly limited by the midline, and a similar vascular anomaly of the underlying leptomeninges on the same side. The brain beneath becomes atrophic and calcified particularly in the occipital and parietal regions (Fig. 14.59). The mode of inheritance of this disease is not clear.

The port-wine stain is present at birth. Convulsions confined to the contralateral side of the body develop in infancy. In time a spastic hemiparesis and hemiatrophy may develop on the contralateral side. Mental deterioration ultimately appears and progresses. Glaucoma may also develop in the ipsilateral eye and require surgical intervention. Radiographs of the skull in later childhood show a characteristic double contour or "tramline" type of calcification.

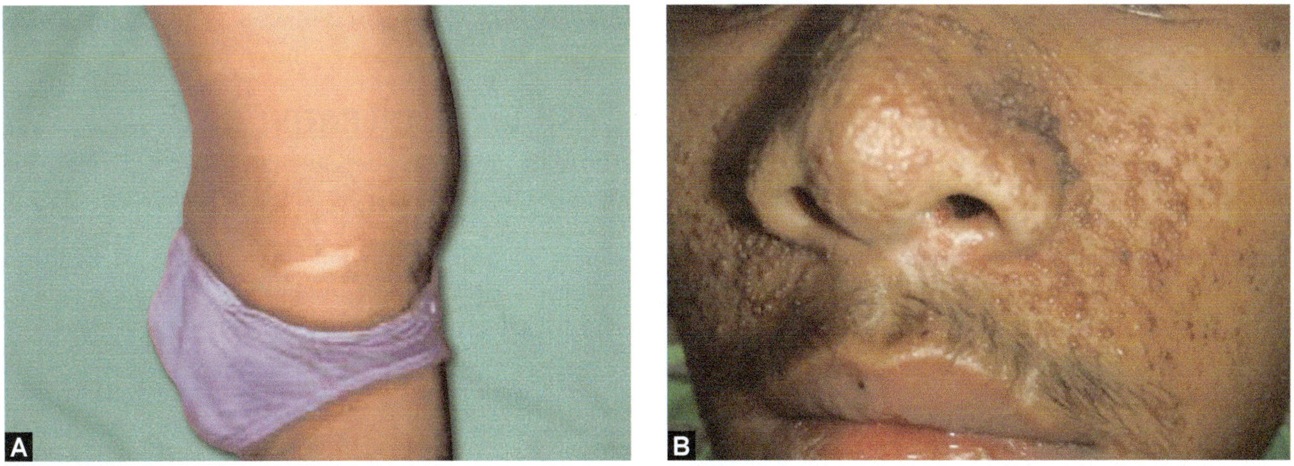

Figures 14.57A and B Tuberous sclerosis with the typical hypopigmented leaf-shaped macule (A) and adenoma sebaceum in a butterfly distribution over the nose and cheeks (B).

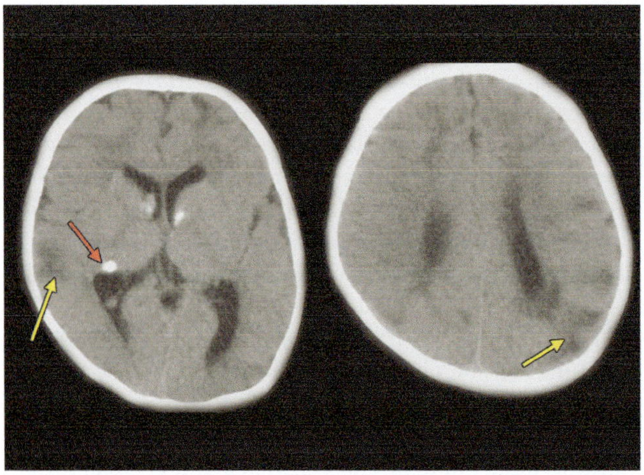

Figure 14.58 Plain CT brain showing the calcified subependymal tubers (red arrow) and hypodensities representing cortical tubers (yellow arrows).

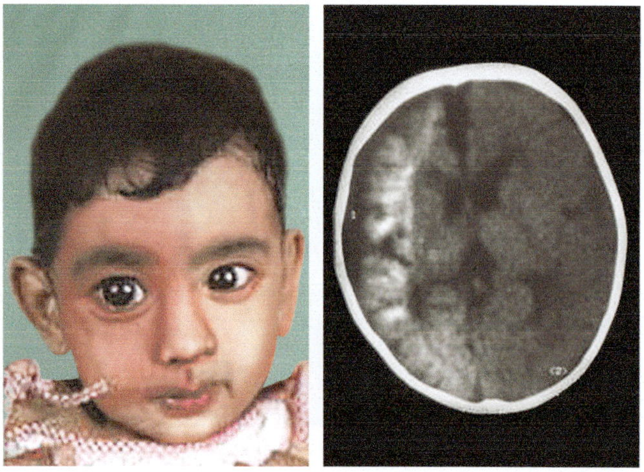

Figure 14.59 Sturge–Weber syndrome. Port-wine non-elevated cutaneous haemangioma in a trigeminal distribution, including the ophthalmic division on the right face. Plain CT brain showing right intracranial calcification and right cerebral hemiatrophy. The child had left hemiparesis and seizures.

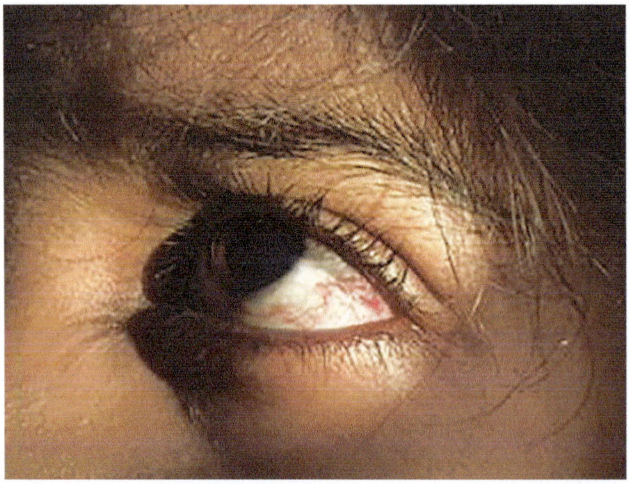

Figure 14.60 Ataxia telangiectasia showing telangiectasia over the bulbar conjunctiva.

Ataxia-Telangiectasia (Louis–Bar Syndrome)

Ataxia telangiectasia is characterised by progressive cerebellar ataxia, oculocutaneous telangiectasia **(Fig. 14.60)**, choreoathetosis, recurrent sinopulmonary infections and immunological dysfunction. It is an autosomal recessive condition with the abnormal gene located to chromosome 11. The first symptom to appear is a progressive cerebellar ataxia beginning in the second or third year of life. There may be, in addition, choreoathetotic movements and a tendency to turn the eyes upwards when focusing. Telangiectasia appear between the ages of 3 and 7 years. They are found on the bulbar conjunctiva, malar-eminences, ears and antecubital fossa. These children suffer severely from infections of the sinuses and lungs; indeed, bronchiectasis is a frequent cause of death. They have a much higher risk of developing lymphoreticular malignancy. These are explained by abnormalities of immunologic function resulting in reduction of serum and secretory IgA, IgE, IgG2 and IgG4. There is hypoplasia of the thymus and cellular immunity is also impaired. Alpha-fetoprotein level is elevated.

Von Hippel-Lindau Disease

This is a rare autosomal dominant inherited disorder characterised by haemangiomatous cystic lesions in the retina and cerebellum, sometime also in spinal cord, kidney, liver and pancreas. It may present with the signs of a cerebellar tumour (progressive ataxia and raised intracranial pressure) or with loss of vision due to retinal detachment. Renal carcinoma and phaeochromocytoma are frequently associated. Surgical treatment is indicated for the cerebellar and visceral tumours, and photocoagulation and cryocoagulation for the retinal angiomas.

NEURODEGENERATIVE DISORDERS

These are progressive degenerative disorders that usually result from specific genetic and biochemical defects. The characteristic features are loss of developmental milestones, intellect, speech and vision often associated with seizures. They may affect primarily the grey matter, i.e. cortical neurons resulting in early symptoms of seizures and intellectual deterioration, or the white matter with early pyramidal tract involvement resulting in spasticity. Degenerative disorders primarily of grey matter include neuronal ceroid lipofuscinosis, Rett syndrome, Menke disease to mention a few. The common ones that primarily involve the white matter include metachromatic leukodystrophy, Krabbe disease and adrenoleukodystrophy.

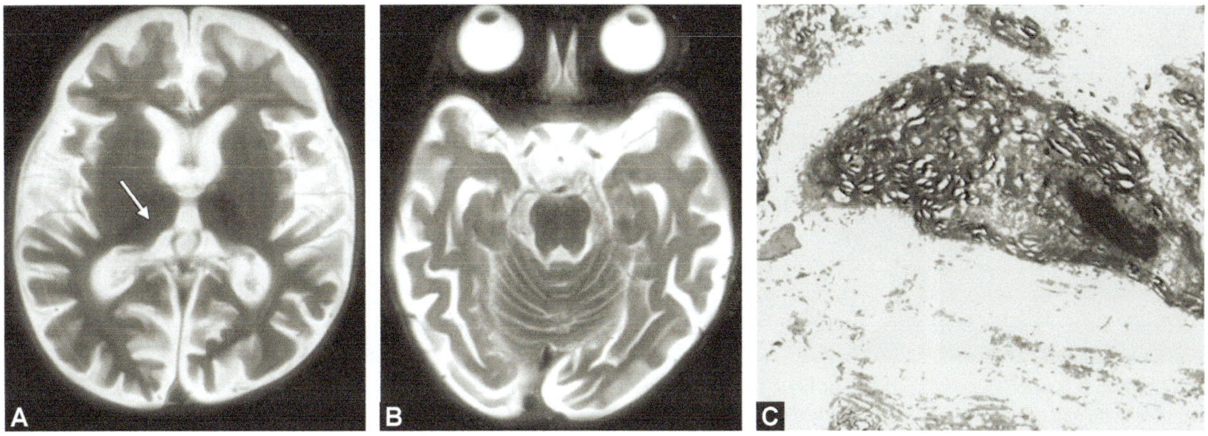

Figures 14.61A to C MRI brain of a child with infantile neuronal ceroid lipofuscinosis (NCL) showing diffuse cerebral (A) and cerebellar (B) atrophy. The cerebral white matter is also abnormal appearing mildly hyperintense with the thalami being hypointense (arrow). This child had low levels of protein palmitoyl thioesterase (PPT1) and EM of skin biopsy (C) showing fibroblasts with lamellated inclusions.

(*EM photograph courtesy:* Dr. Anna Pulimood, Department of Pathology, Christian Medical College, Vellore, India.)

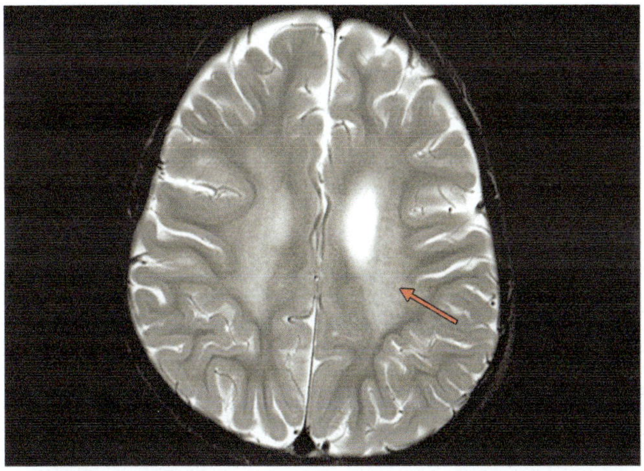

Figure 14.62 Metachromatic leukodystrophy. MRI brain T2W axial section showing hyperintensity of the deep white matter and sparing of the subcortical U fibres. *Note* the faint 'tigroid pattern' (linear dark stripes—arrow) of the white matter which represents normal myelin along the vessels.

Neuronal Ceroid Lipofuscinoses (NCL)

These are autosomal recessive disorders characterised by accumulation of autofluorescent intracellular lipopigment. There are three clinical types namely infantile type, late infantile type and juvenile type. In the types with onset in infancy, myoclonic seizures are a prominent feature with progressive loss of vision and developmental milestones. Diagnosis is based on clinical picture, electron microscopy of axillary skin biopsy. MRI brain demonstrates cerebral and cerebellar atrophy with faint hyperintensities of the white matter **(Figs. 14.61A to C)**.

Metachromatic Leukodystrophy

This autosomal recessive disorder is characterised by accumulation of cerebroside sulphate in the white matter of the brain **(Fig. 14.62)**, the peripheral nerves, the dentate nucleus, basal ganglia and in other organs such as the kidneys due to the deficiency of the enzyme arylsulphatase A. There is a widespread demyelination with neuronal and axonal loss. The sulphatide stains metachromatically with basic polychrome dyes. Three clinical forms of the disease have been described.

Late infantile form: This the most common type with its onset between 6 and 24 months. Deterioration in walking due to progressive and mixed pyramidal and cerebellar damage is soon followed by deterioration in speech and social development, loss of the ability to sit or feed without help, seizures and loss of vision and hearing and finally a decorticate posture leading to death, the time course of which is variable.

Juvenile type: This has an onset between 6 and 10 years. The first signs are educational and behavioural deterioration, followed after some months or years by disorders of gait mostly extrapyramidal with some pyramidal signs. Progression towards dementia and death has a slower course.

Adult type: Onset 16 years to adulthood. Psychiatric changes predominate.

Krabbe Disease or globoid Cell leukodystrophy

Krabbe globoid cell leukodystrophy is characterised by accumulation of globular bodies in white matter due to deficiency of the enzyme galactocerebroside betagalactosidase. The onset is in early infancy with incessant crying followed by apathy. Generalised rigidity, seizures, head retraction, blindness, inability to swallow and death may ensue in a year or so. Peripheral nerve involvement may cause absent deep tendon reflexes. MRI brain provides clue to the diagnosis **(Figs. 14.63A to D)**.

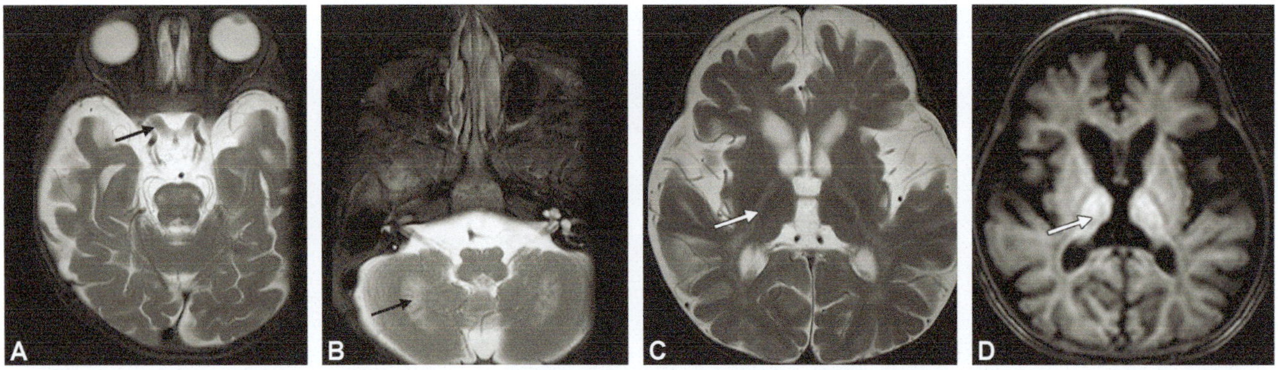

Figures 14.63A to D Krabbe leukodystrophy—MRI brain T2W images of infantile Krabbe disease with enlargement of the optic nerves (A), hyperintensity of the cerebellar (B) and cerebral white matter, marked cerebral atrophy (C), and hyperintensity of the thalami on T1W image (D).

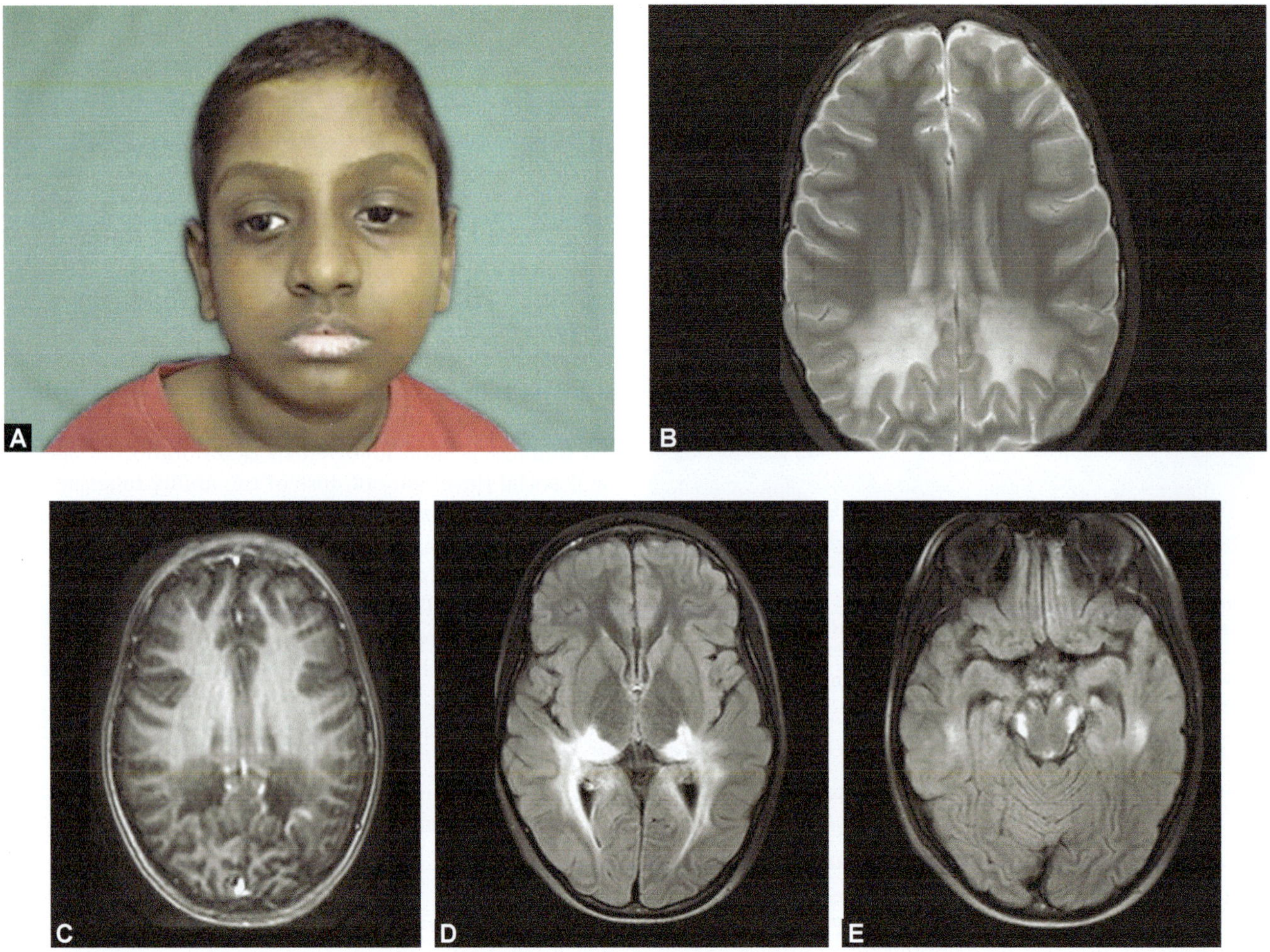

Figures 14.64A to E Child with X-linked adrenoleukodystrophy. He presented initially with features of Addison disease. *Note* the generalized hyperpigmentation (A); MRI brain shows posterior predominant white matter changes (B) with peripheral enhancement post gadolinium (C); The same child had involvement of the optic pathway—optic radiation and lateral geniculate body (D) and acoustic pathway—lateral lemniscus and acoustic radiation (E).

Adrenoleukodystrophy

This is an X-linked recessive disorder with onset usually between 5 and 15 years of age with progressive psychomotor deterioration, ataxia, dementia, loss of vision and hearing. More than two-thirds of them also have associated adrenocortical insufficiency with skin pigmentation. The blood level of very long chain fatty acid is increased. MRI brain in ALD shows typical features **(Figs. 14.64A to E)**. Death occurs within 10 years of the onset. Bone marrow transplant at an early stage is helpful.

NEUROMUSCULAR DISORDERS

Hereditary neuropathies

This group of progressive degenerative disorders of the peripheral nerves can predominantly affect the motor nerves categorised as hereditary motor neuropathy (HMN), sensory and autonomic neurons called as hereditary sensory and autonomic neuropathy (HSAN) or involve both sensory and motor nerves categorised as hereditary motor and sensory neuropathy (HMSN). HMSN also known as Charcot-Marie-Tooth disease includes a wide spectrum of disorders, the classification of which is still evolving.

Charcot-Marie-tooth Disease

This disease starts in late childhood with progressive weakness, and lower motor neurone type of flaccid atrophy of the peroneal and tibial muscles and of the small muscles of the feet resulting in paralaytic talipes equinovarus. Later, wasting of the calf muscles gives the legs an inverted wine-bottle appearance. At a late stage, weakness and wasting affect the hands and forearms. The ankle jerks are lost but the knee jerks remain brisk. Sensory involvement is manifest by some loss of vibration and positional sensation. Most cases are transmitted as autosomal dominant.

Spinal Muscular Atrophy

The principal feature of spinal muscular atrophy (SMA) is progressive degeneration and loss of motor neurons in the anterior horns of the spinal cord. It is caused by homozygous disruption of the survival motor neuron 1 (SMN1) gene by deletion, conversion or mutation located on chromosome 5q13. It is a relatively common disease of infancy inherited as a recessive trait. There are four clinical types differentiated by age of onset and severity of weakness.

Spinal Muscular Atrophy Type 1 (Werdnig-Hoffman Disease)

This is the most severe form and may be present at birth or appear within a few weeks. Its onset in utero may be recognised by the mother because of decreased foetal movements. There is severe flaccidity and weakness of the muscles of the trunk and limbs. The proximal muscles tend to be more severely paralysed than the distal. The deep tendon reflexes are absent. Fasciculation in the muscles of the tongue may be seen. The infant has an alert expression. When the intercostal and other accessory muscles of respiration become affected dyspnoea, intercostal recession and paradoxical respiration develop. Eventually, the diaphragm is involved rendering the infant prone for chest infection and respiratory failure. The loss of power to suck further aggravates the terminal stages of the illness. Death usually occurs before 2 years of age.

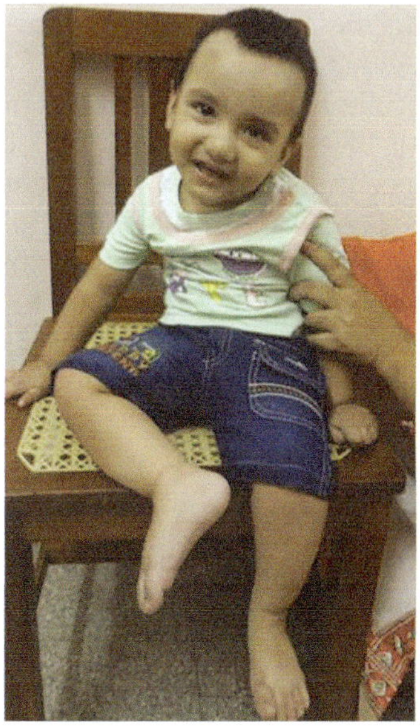

Figure 14.65 Child with spinal muscular atrophy type 2. *Note* the axial and limb hypotonia and requiring assistance to sit.

Spinal Muscular Atrophy Type 2 (Intermediate Type)

This type has a later onset between 7 and 18 months of age (**Fig. 14.65**). There is progressive weakness with severe wasting leading to deformities particularly scoliosis. They are able to sit but rarely learn to walk and are confined to wheelchair. Deaths occur before 10 years of age.

Spinal Muscular Atrophy Type 3 (Kugelberg–Welander Syndrome)

This is a milder type of paralysis with onset after the age of 2 years and is compatible with a prolonged course. There is proximal muscle weakness involving the pelvic and shoulder girdle muscles. Skeletal deformities readily develop. In some cases, the bulbar muscles become involved. These children may learn to walk, but ultimately become confined to a wheel chair. They may live up to middle age.

Spinal Muscular Atrophy Type 4 (Adult Type)

Adults have this disease onset usually in the second or third decade. Motor impairment is mild and they continue to walk with no respiratory complications.

Electromyography (EMG) shows features of denervation with positive sharp waves, fibrillation and occasional fasciculations. Motor unit action potentials show high potentials with decreased recruitment. Muscle biopsy shows atrophic fibres with islands of group hypertrophy.

Treatment is currently aimed at good rehabilitation, prevention of scoliosis and respiratory infections. Trials are on to improve functioning of the SMN protein through non-toxic molecules. Motor neurons derived from stem cells are also being tried in animal trials.

Spinal muscular atrophy has to be differentiated from other causes of "floppy infant syndrome," the causes for which include central hypotonia like cerebral malformations, muscle disorders like congenital myopathy and disorders of neuromuscular junction like congenital myasthenic syndrome (CMS).

In benign congenital hypotonia, hypotonia dates from or soon after birth. The deep tendon reflexes although sluggish can usually be elicited and muscle fibrillation is not seen. The true diagnosis of benign congenital hypotonia becomes clear with the passage of time (5–9 years), when slow but not always complete recovery takes place. Muscle biopsy is normal in benign congenital hypotonia.

Muscular Dystrophy

Muscular dystrophies are a group of inherited disorders characterised by progressive degeneration of muscle fibres.

Duchenne Muscular Dystrophy

This is the most common type of muscular dystrophy. It is inherited as X-linked recessive trait with a high new mutation rate. The abnormal gene is located at Xp21 locus on the X-chromosome, which leads to deficiency of dystrophin protein in the muscle fibre. The onset is usually before the third or fourth years of life. There may be a history of delay in walking. The child may fall unduly often, or has great difficulty in climbing stairs. Weakness begins in the pelvic girdle and the gait assumes a characteristic waddle so that the feet are placed too widely apart and there is an exaggerated lumbar lordosis **(Fig. 14.66)**. A quite characteristic phenomenon Gower sign—is seen when the child, lying on his back on the floor, is asked to stand up. He will roll to one side, flex his knees and hips so that he is "on all fours" with both knees and both hands on the ground; he then extends his knees and reaches the erect posture by "climbing up his own legs," using his hands to get higher up each leg in alternate steps. Weakness of the shoulder muscles may render the child unable to raise his hands above his head. Pseudohypertrophy of the calf muscles with wasting of thigh muscle is characteristic. Tendon reflexes become progressively diminished and finally cannot be elicited. By the age of 10 years the child is usually confined to a wheel chair. Skeletal and postural deformities particularly scoliosis may later become severe. Heart may fail from involvement of the myocardium. Intellectual disability is seen in about 30% of the cases. Death is usual during adolescence from intercurrent respiratory infection, respiratory or cardiac failure.

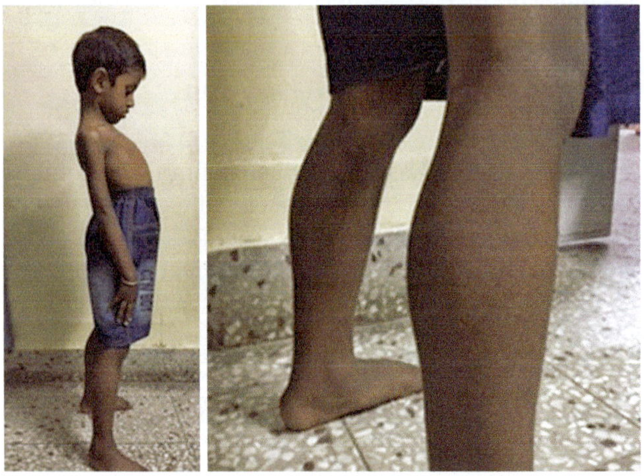

Figure 14.66 Child with Duchenne muscular dystrophy. *Note* the exaggerated lumbar lordosis, wide stance and calf muscle hypertrophy.

The serum creatine kinase is greatly elevated and is often above 10,000 IU/L (normal up to 150 IU/L). EMG shows myopathic changes and muscle biopsy with immunohistochemical staining for dystrophin is confirmatory. Periodic cardiac assessment is necessary. Healthy female carriers often have elevated serum levels of creatine kinase. Antenatal diagnosis is possible using DNA analysis.

Becker Muscular Dystrophy

This sex-linked recessive disorder is similar but milder than Duchenne muscular dystrophy. The progress is slower and affected boys remain ambulatory until late adolescence or early adult life.

The other less common muscular dystrophies include facioscapulohumeral muscular dystrophy, limb-girdle muscular dystrophy and dystrophia myotonica.

Facioscapulohumeral Muscular Dystrophy

This form of dystrophy is transmitted as an autosomal dominant trait and can affect both sexes. The onset may be in early childhood or early adult life, most often with weakness and lack of expression in the facial muscles. In time the child cannot close his eyes, wrinkle his forehead or purse his mouth. The lips project forwards due to weakness of the orbicularis oris to give the appearance of "tapir mouth." Weakness of the shoulder girdle muscles, especially the pectoralis major, serratus magnus, trapezius, spinati, deltoid, triceps and biceps results in winging of the scapulae, inability to raise the arms above the head and looseness of the shoulders. Then the pelvic girdle becomes affected, glutei, quadriceps, hamstrings and iliopsoas, so that there is lumbar lordosis and a broad-based gait. This form of muscular dystrophy usually runs a prolonged and relatively benign course well into adult life. Indeed, the face only may be affected during most of the childhood and severe crippling may be long delayed. The diagnosis can be confirmed by muscle biopsy. Elevated levels of serum creatine kinase are found only in some cases.

Limb-Girdle Muscular Dystrophy

This form of dystrophy affects mainly the muscles of hip and shoulder girdles. It is usually inherited as an autosomal recessive characteristic. Males and females are equally affected.

This rarely appears during the first decade. Weakness first becomes obvious in the muscles of the shoulder girdle with winging of the scapulae and difficulty in raising the arms. Later the muscles of the pelvis girdle become affected. The facial muscles are never affected. The disease runs a slow course but usually leads to death before the normal age. Serum creatine kinase levels may be normal or moderately raised. Muscle biopsy reveals myopathic changes.

Dystrophia Myotonica (Myotonic Dystrophy)

This disorder is inherited as an autosomal dominant with the locus being on the long arm of chromosome 19. Affected children nearly always have affected mothers (rather than fathers). It has been regarded as a disease of adult life, characterised by delayed muscle relaxation and atrophy (especially of the hands, masseters and sternomastoids), baldness, cataract and testicular atrophy. Clinical manifestations in childhood differ from the adult picture.

The clinical features in the neonate or older infant include hypotonia, facial diplegia and jaw weakness, delayed motor development and speech, talipes and respiratory problems **(Fig. 14.67)**. Mental retardation is relatively common. Clinical evidence of myotonia is absent although it may be demonstrated by EMG. Cataracts do not occur. EMG is the most helpful investigation. DNA analysis will demonstrate the abnormal DM gene on chromosome 19.

Congenital Muscular Dystrophy

This disorder involves a heterogeneous group of disorders characterised by hypotonia and weakness from infancy. They also have intellectual disability with some of them having typical MRI features **(Figs. 14.68 and 14.69)**. Serum creatine kinase is elevated and muscle biopsy is required along with genetic studies to determine the specific type.

Myasthenia Gravis

This is an immune-mediated disorder of neuromuscular function caused by a reduction of available acetylcholine (ACh) receptors at the neuromuscular junction due to circulating ACh receptor-binding antibodies. It is an autoimmune disorder and patients with myasthenia gravis have higher incidence of other autoimmune diseases particularly thyroiditis.

Clinical Features Most cases are in girls and the ocular muscles are usually first affected; the child presents with ptosis or complaints of diplopia; the muscle weakness tends to be more severe as the day goes on. The pupillary reflexes are normal. The bulbar muscles are often next affected. The voice is then weak, swallowing and chewing become difficult, and there may be asphyxial episodes due to the aspiration of upper respiratory secretions and saliva. When the facial muscles are affected a lack of expression is a striking feature. Easy fatiguability of muscles is a characteristic feature, but muscle atrophy and fibrillary twitchings do not occur. The deep tendon

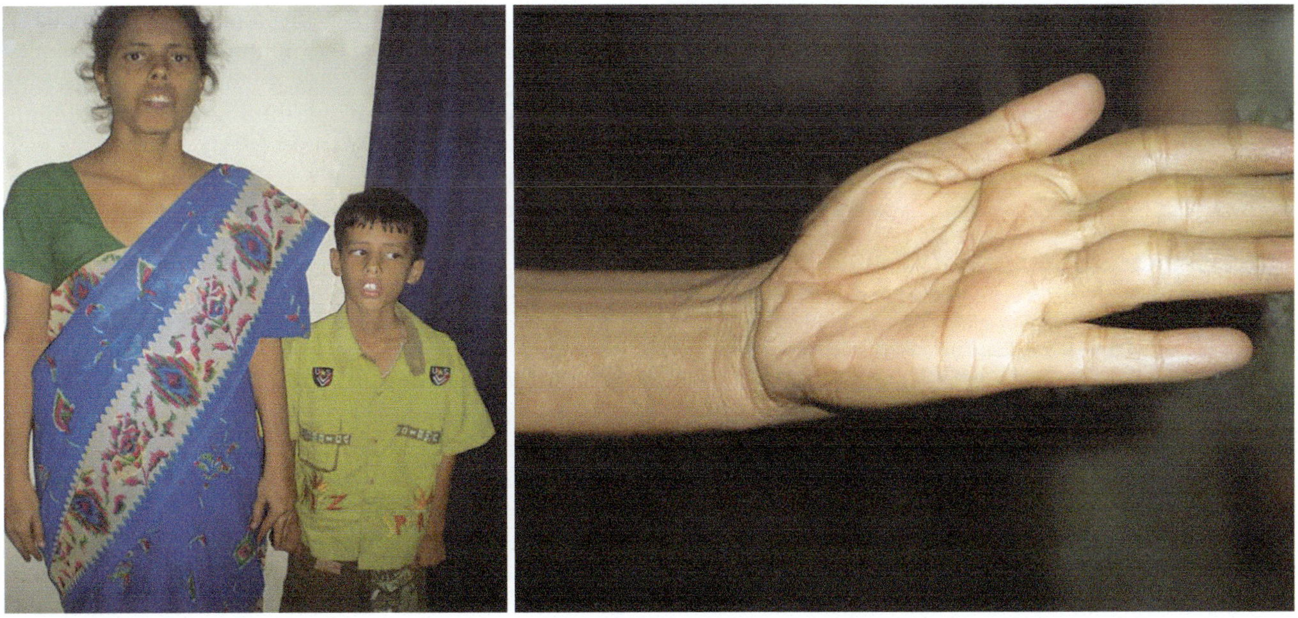

Figure 14.67 Myotonic dystrophy in mother and son. *Note* the elongated facies and distal muscle wasting with percussion myotonia. Son with more severe weakness due to genetic anticipation.

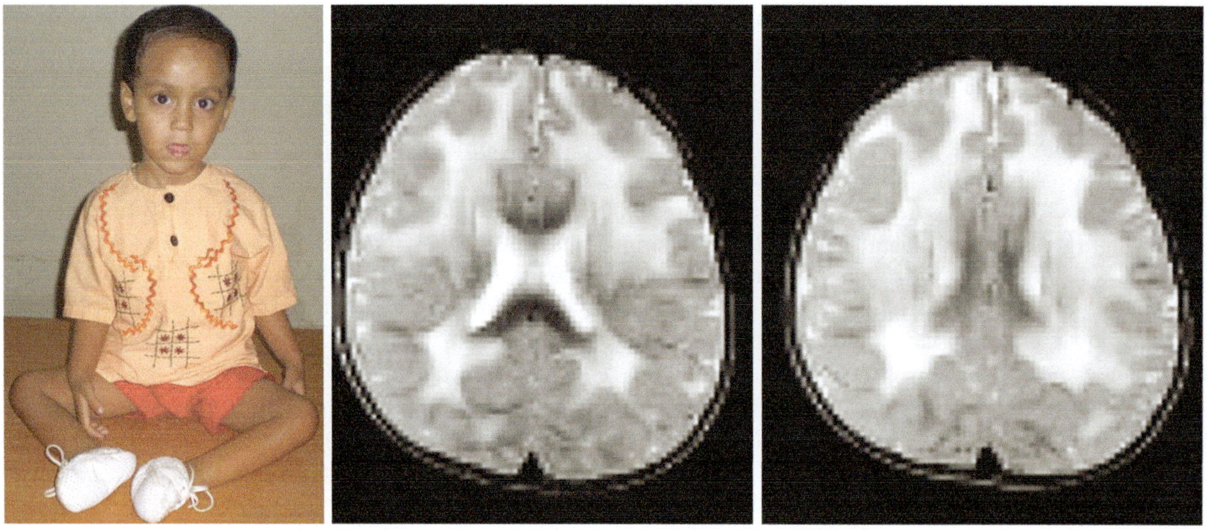

Figure 14.68 Child with merosin negative congenital muscular dystrophy. *Note* the long myopathic facies. Child was hypotonic and unable to stand. They also have MRI brain changes in the form of diffuse hyperintensity of the deep and subcortical white matter.

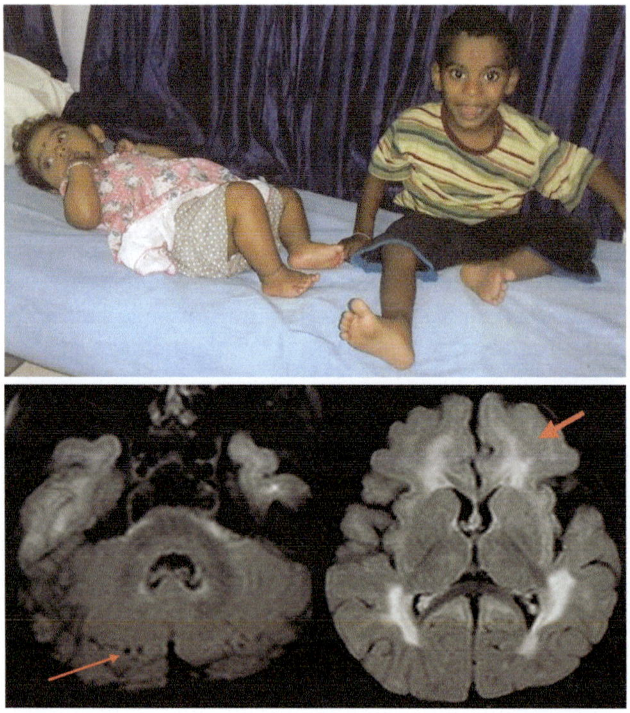

Figure 14.69 Siblings with Fukuyama congenital muscular dystrophy. In addition to presentation as floppy infants, both also had intellectual disability. MRI brain in both showed similar findings of cerebellar cysts (thin arrow), frontal pachygyria (thick arrow) and increased signal in the cerebral white matter.

reflexes are usually present. In the worst cases, the muscles of the limbs and those responsible for respiration are affected. As in the adult, the myasthenic child may run a prolonged course of remissions and relapses, but there is a tendency for the disease to reach a static phase some 5 years from the onset. There is always a risk of death from aspiration of food into the respiratory passages, from respiratory failure due to the involvement of respiratory muscles or from intercurrent respiratory infection.

Neonatal myasthenia gravis occurs in newborn infants born to myasthenic mothers and is due to the placental transfer of antibodies to ACh receptors from mother to baby. The manifestations include a weak cry, generalised severe hypotonia, feeble sucking reflex and attacks of choking and cyanosis. They are temporary and disappear within a few weeks.

Diagnosis Myasthenia gravis should be suspected in the presence of ptosis, strabismus, bulbar palsy or severe muscular hypotonia during infancy or childhood. The diagnosis is confirmed by the immediate response to intravenous injection of edrophonium—a short-acting cholinesterase inhibitor **(Figs. 14.70A and B)**. Atropine sulphate should be available during the edrophonium test to block acute muscarinic effects. Electromyogram demonstrates decremental response to repetitive nerve stimulation. Anti-ACh receptor antibodies may be measured in the plasma. Although the thymus gland is hyperplastic this is not radiologically obvious unless there is an actual thymoma, which is extremely rare in childhood.

Congenital Myasthenic Syndromes

Congenital myasthenic syndromes represent a heterogeneous group of disorders caused due to abnormalities at the neuromuscular junction. The defect may occur at the presynapse, synaptic space or postsynapse. Postsynaptic defects are the most common and include primary acetyl choline deficiency, rapsyn deficiency and sodium channel myasthenia. All these disorders are autosomal recessive except for the slow channel syndrome that has autosomal dominant inheritance.

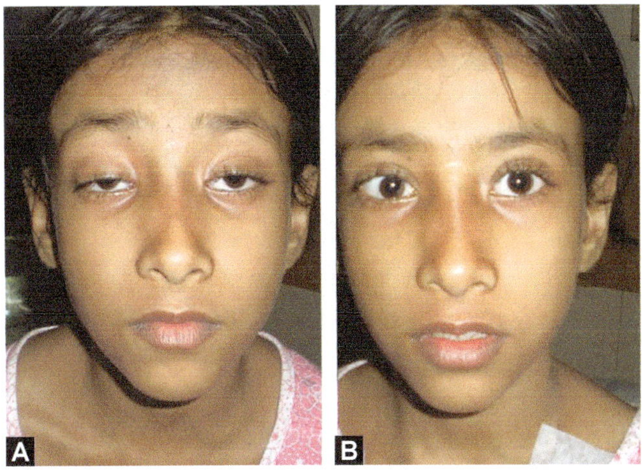

Figures 14.70A and B Child with autoimmune myasthenia gravis—pre (A) and post neostigmine (B), note improvement in ptosis.

Symptoms are present from birth in most forms. All myasthenia, except transient neonatal myasthenia gravis, that begins at birth is genetic. During infancy, most have ophthalmoparesis and ptosis. Limb weakness is mild and respiratory crisis is rare.

AUTONOMIC NERVOUS SYSTEM

Familial Dysautonomia (Riley–Day Syndrome)

This is a rare familial, autosomal recessive disorder, characterised by autonomic neuropathy and peripheral sensory neuropathy. The striking features are severe hypotonia, muscle weakness with areflexia, relative indifference to pain, excessive salivation and sweating, absent tears and recurrent pneumonia. The corneal reflex is usually absent. Difficulty in swallowing is common. There may be delayed psychomotor development and generalised seizures. Recurrent pyrexial episodes are common. In older children, attacks of cyclical vomiting with associated hypertension, excessive sweating and blotching of skin are not infrequent. Urinary frequency has also been noted in some patients.

BRAIN TUMOUR IN CHILDREN

Brain tumours are the second most common tumour in children. Although the aetiology of most brain tumours are unknown, certain neurocutaneous syndromes like neurofibroma and tuberous sclerosis predispose to the development of brain tumours. Infants and young children have higher risk of developing brain tumours. The common histological tumour types are—medulloblastoma/primitive neuroectodermal tumour, astrocytoma, ependymoma and craniopharyngioma.

Most brain tumours in children are malignant and are situated usually in the posterior cranial fossa. The children usually present with signs of raised intracranial pressure which can be mistaken for meningitis. Gait disturbances and ataxia are common with cerebellar tumours. Supratentorial tumours may present with focal seizures and deficits. Craniopharyngiomas occurring in the suprasellar region is minimally invasive and may present with visual disturbances and neuroendocrine deficiencies.

Diagnosis of brain tumour is confirmed by neuroimaging studies (MRI/CT scan) (*see* Chapter 29: Pediatric Radiology, Figs. 29.130 to 29.137). When brain tumour is suspected, lumbar puncture should not be done as it might produce coning and sudden death. Surgery is the preferred mode of treatment. Radiation and chemotherapy have also contributed to improved prognosis.

CEREBRAL PALSY

Cerebral palsy is an umbrella term used for static or non-progressive disorders of the brain affecting the development of movement, posture and co-ordination resulting from a lesion of an immature brain. It is one of the common chronic neurological disorders in children. The International Workshop on Definition and Classification of Cerebral Palsy, held in Bethesda, in 2004 defines CP as follows: "Cerebral palsy describes a group of developmental disorders of movement and posture, causing activity restriction or disability, that are attributed to disturbances occurring in the foetal or infant brain. The motor impairment may be accompanied by a seizure disorder and by impairment of sensation, cognition, communication and/or behaviour."

The incidence of CP is in the region of 2.5 per 1,000 live births and has always varied from one country to another. In the developing world, the incidence may be underrated due to under-reporting and the lack of awareness. However, a significant number of children world over suffer from CP and the issues of healthcare, educational and vocational prospects for these children are mostly overlooked. In spite of improved perinatal and neonatal care, the incidence of CP over the decades has remained the same, as more preterm babies survive with neurodevelopmental morbidities.

Aetiology

The causes of CP can be generally classified as prenatal, perinatal and postnatal causes. However, sometimes, it is impossible to determine the precise cause of CP in the individual patient and in 15% of the children, the aetiology is unknown. The prenatal causes include genetic factors, intrauterine infection during pregnancy, radiation, cerebral infarction, metabolic and toxic factors and hypoxia. Approximately half of all the cases of CP are associated with preterm delivery and low birth weight. The precise nature of this relationship is not clear although hypoxia and hypotension are important factors. Although the perinatal risk factor of birth asphyxia is a well-recognised cause of CP particularly in the

TABLE 14.4 Classification of cerebral palsy: cerebral palsy may be classified in terms of physiologic, topographic, functional and GMFCS categories.

Physiologic	*Topographic*	*Functional*	*GMFCS (Gross Motor Function Classification System)*
Spastic	Diplegia	Class I: No limitation of activity	Level I—Walks without limitation
Dyskinetic	Hemiplegia		
Ataxic	Quadriplegia	Class II: Slight to moderate limitation	Level II—Walks with limitation
Hypotonic	Double hemiplegia		Level III—Walks using a hand-held mobility device
Mixed	Triplegia	Class III: Moderate to severe limitation	Level IV—Self-mobility with limitations; may use powered mobility
	Monoplegia	Class IV: No useful physical activity	Level V—Transported in a manual wheelchair

Source: Adapted from Minear WL. A classification of cerebral palsy. Pediatrics. 1956;18:841 and GMFCS—E and R (Reference: Dev Med Child Neurol 1997;39:214-223)

term baby, the incidence of birth asphyxia among cases of CP is declining. The main pathological lesions found in preterm infants who later develop CP are periventricular leucomalacia and intracerebral haemorrhage. Lesions in the full term infants who develop CP are mainly due to hypoxic ischaemic encephalopathy and are seen in thalami and basal ganglia, or in the cortex and sub-cortical white matter. Postnatal causes of CP include hypoglycaemia, hyperbilirubinaemia, meningitis, subdural haematoma, acute infantile hemiplaegia and trauma.

Classification

It may be classified in terms of physiological, topographical, aetiological and functional categories **(Table 14.4)**. Gross motor functional classification system classifies the motoric ability of child with CP based on the mobility pattern (Reference: Dev Med Child Neurol 1997;39:214-223).

Clinical Features

Spastic cerebral palsy This group shows the features of upper motor neuron type of pyramidal tract lesion such as spastic hypertonicity, exaggerated deep tendon reflexes, ankle clonus and extensor plantar response. It may be symmetric or asymmetric and may involve one or more extremities. In spastic diplegia, the lower limbs are affected more than the upper limbs. In spastic quadriplegia, there is a marked involvement of all four limbs. Involvement of one side of the body is termed spastic hemiplegia.

Spastic diplegia This type of CP, also called Little disease, affects particularly the preterm babies **(Fig. 14.71)**. Term babies with perinatal asphyxia are also prone. Some children go through an initial hypotonic or dystonic phase and then a spastic phase. In the first stage of hypotonia, though the child is floppy, there may be an early scissoring specially in vertical suspension. Dystonia of prematurity is a type of extensor hypertonia seen in preterm babies that emerges around 40 weeks of gestation, peaks by 4 months and may last till 7 or 8 months of age. These babies often have dystonia, opisthotonus and asymmetrical neck reflex, but when turned over into prone, with neck flexed, assume a flexed posture. Dystonia of prematurity resolves spontaneously in some children, while in others, it merges into spasticity.

The spastic phase of diplegia can manifest in two types. The flexor muscles are mainly affected in tonic spasticity and extensor muscles such as triceps and quadriceps in phasic spasticity. The phasically spastic muscles show brisk tendon reflexes and often the clasp-knife phenomenon. Tonically spastic muscles show decreased lengthening reaction and rapidly develop contractures. The hip flexors, hamstrings and calf muscles together with adductors of hip form the main tonic groups in the lower limbs, causing the child to be flexed at hip, knee and in equinus at the ankle with the legs usually internally rotated and the characteristic scissoring posture **(Fig. 14.72)**. The upper limbs are flexed at elbow and wrist, and the fingers are flexed across the adducted thumb with marked spasticity of the pronators. Atrophy below the waist occurs in many

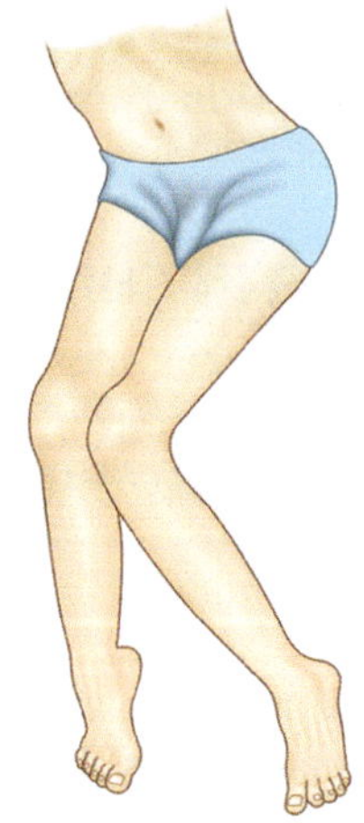

Figure 14.71 Drawing from Little monograph illustrating one of his cases of spastic diplegia (Little deformities of the human frame, 1953).

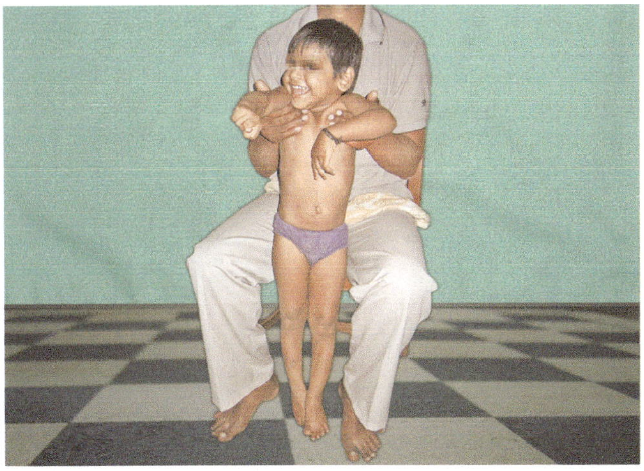

Figure 14.72 Characteristic scissoring posture in a child with spastic diplegic cerebral palsy.

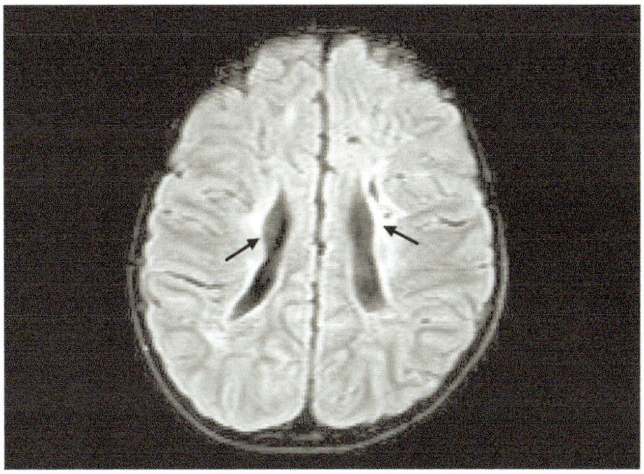

Figure 14.73 Axial T2 FLAIR MRI image of brain showing periventricular leucomalacia and periventricular hyperintensities (arrows) in spastic diplegic cerebral palsy.

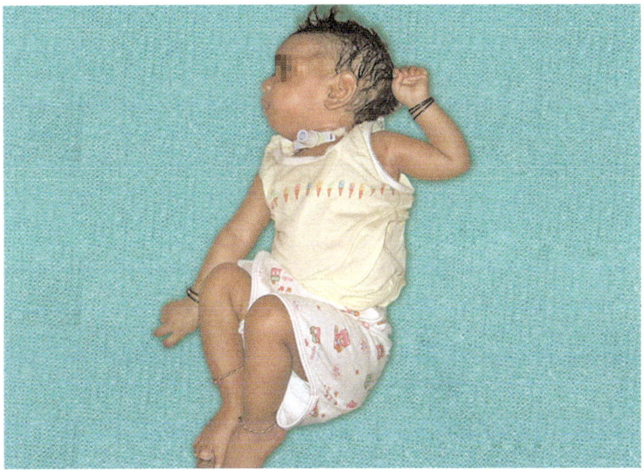

Figure 14.74 Child with spastic quadriplegic cerebral palsy. *Note* the tracheostomy tube and the persistence of asymmetric tonic neck reflex (ATNR).

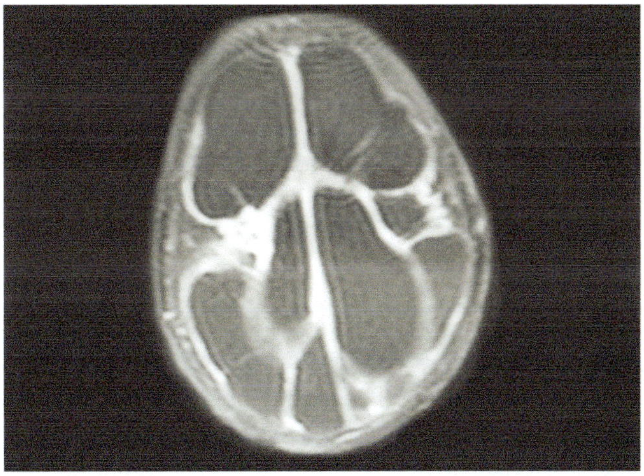

Figure 14.75 Axial MRI image of brain showing multicystic encephalomalacia in spastic quadriplegic cerebral palsy.

patients. In spastic diplegia of preterm babies, epilepsy is uncommon and intelligence is only moderately reduced; whereas in diplegia of term asphyxiated babies, epilepsy, mental retardation, microcephaly, speech and behaviour disorders are more common. The most common neuropathologic finding in spastic diplegic CP is periventricular leucomalacia (PVL) **(Fig. 14.73)**, which occurs when the periventricular structures are vulnerable between 26 and 36 weeks of gestation, usually *in utero*.

Spastic quadriplegia: This is the most severe form of CP, often as a result of intrauterine disease or malformation and in some cases due to hypoxic ischaemic encephalopathy (especially in term new borns). There is a marked motor impairment of all four extremities. Feeding is difficult because of pseudobulbar palsy with increased incidence of gastro-oesophageal reflux and aspiration syndrome **(Fig. 14.74)**. There is a high association with mental retardation and seizures. Speech and visual abnormalities are common. Neuropathologic findings include severe PVL, multicystic encephalomalacia **(Fig. 14.75)** and cerebral dysgenesis. Positional deformities are common resulting in windswept posture of lower limbs, dislocation of hip, pelvic tilt, scoliosis and chest deformities.

Spastic hemiplegia This type of CP affects one side of the body. The majority are congenital and the result of maldevelopment, prenatal circulatory disturbances or perinatal stroke in the distribution of middle cerebral artery. Postnatal causes include acute CNS infection, acute infantile hemiplegia, cerebral thrombosis particularly in congenital cyanotic heart disease and subdural haematoma. The right side is more often affected than the left and the arm more severely than the leg.

Children usually present in the second half of first year with asymmetric crawling, tip toeing on the affected side

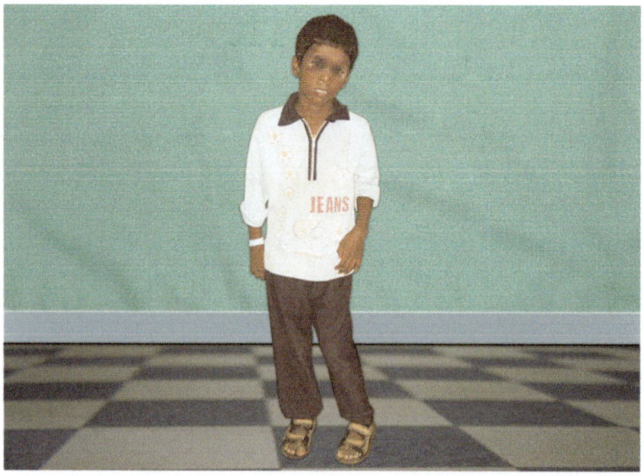

Figure 14.76 Child with left hemiplegic cerebral palsy with flexed and pronated upper limb, and flexed and adducted lower limb.

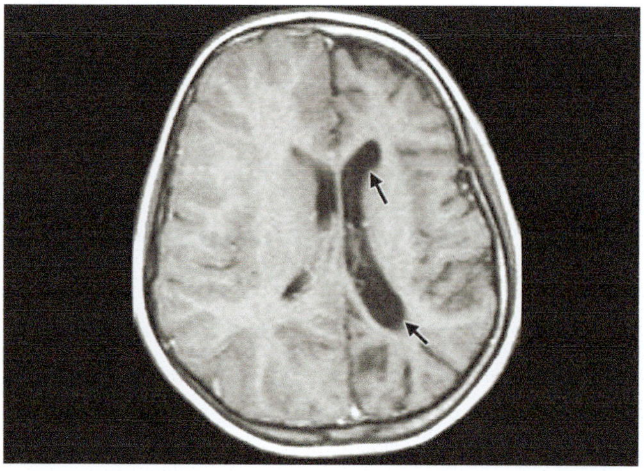

Figure 14.77 Axial T1W MRI image of brain showing atrophy of the cerebral hemisphere with prominent ventricles (arrows) in hemiplegic cerebral palsy.

while walking, asymmetric hand skills, persistence of fisting of the affected side or unusual dominance of the unaffected side. The child walks with a circumduction gait with the affected upper limb adducted at shoulder, flexed at elbow and wrist, with forearm pronated and the lower limb partially flexed and adducted at hip, the knee flexed and the foot in equinus position **(Fig. 14.76)**. There is growth arrest of the affected extremities, particularly the hands and the feet. Cortical sensory loss and haemianopia are not infrequent. Convulsions and mental retardation are seen in about one-fourth of these children. Children with right hemiplegia also have a delay in acquiring language skills and speech. Neuropathologic findings show an atrophic cerebral hemisphere **(Fig. 14.77)** or a porencephalic cyst.

Dyskinetic cerebral palsy This type of CP results from damage to the extrapyramidal system usually the result of neonatal jaundice or acute severe perinatal asphyxia. There is defect of posture and involuntary movement in the form of athetosis, choreoathetosis, rigidity or dystonia **(Figs. 14.78A to C)**. Pathologic findings include lesions in the globus pallidus, subthalamic nucleus and status marmoratus (lesions in the basal ganglia and thalamus with a marbled appearance).

Athetosis The affected infants go through an early hypotonic phase characterised by lethargy, poor head control and feeding difficulty. This is followed after 4 months of age by the dystonic phase associated with extensor hypertonia, arching attacks, mass body movements and abnormal persistence of primitive reflexes. The stage of involuntary movement is obvious after 2 years consisting of slow writhing distal movements. When athetosis is caused by kernicterus there is often an associated high-tone deafness. Some children who had neonatal jaundice also have associated G6PD deficiency. The child with athetosis is usually dysarthric and drooling may be prominent. Seizures are uncommon and intelligence may be well preserved but difficult to be quantified by the routine intelligence tests.

Choreoathetosis In this type the writhing athetotic movements have in addition jerky, irregular, rapid movements involving the face and proximal extremities. Stress and excitement may exacerbate the chorea.

Dystonia This type affects the trunk and proximal muscles of the limbs and consists of abnormal twisting and sustained movements, which may be either slow or rapid. These children tend to be more severely affected.

Ataxic cerebral palsy In a small proportion of children with CP, the clinical manifestations indicate a cerebellar defect, e.g. ataxic reeling gait, intention tremor and past pointing, dysdiadochokinesia and muscular hypotonia. Most of these cases are congenital in origin and due to malformations of the cerebellum and may have an autosomal inheritance. A few cases are due to perinatal asphyxia and hydrocephalus. Most patients have congenital hypotonia. Motor milestones and language skills are typically delayed. Truncal ataxia predominates over appendicular signs.

Hypotonic cerebral palsy In a few children CP takes the form of a hypotonic quadriplegia without any spasticity. Many infants destined to develop typical spastic diplegic or choreoathetoid CP pass through a hypotonic phase and require continued observation for a definitive diagnosis. In benign congenital hypotonia, there has usually been a normal birth and later normal development, whereas in hypotonic CP there has often been perinatal asphyxia and is associated with learning difficulties.

Mixed Cerebral Palsy Mixed CP includes manifestations of two or more types usually of both spastic and extrapyramidal types. Often an ataxic component is present.

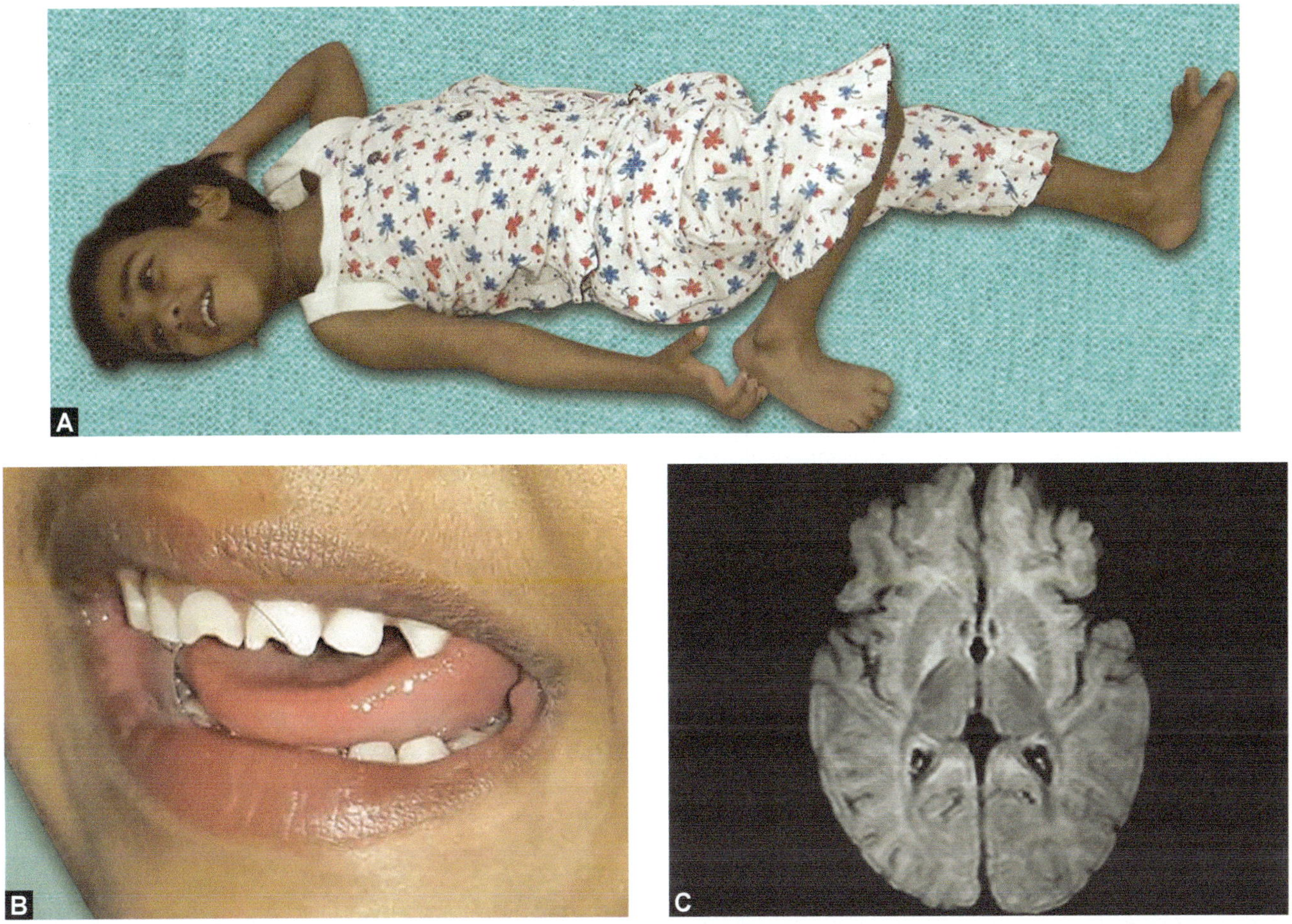

Figures 14.78A to C Child with dystonic cerebral palsy due to bilirubin encephalopathy in the newborn period which occurred as a result of G6PD deficiency (A). Enamel hypoplasia is an associated finding with bilirubin encephalopathy (B). T FLAIR axial MRI brain with hyperintensity and atrophy of bilateral basal ganglia (C).

These patterns of motor impairment are the result of involvement of large areas of brain affecting the cortex, subcortical areas and basal ganglia.

Associated Disabilities

Children who suffer from CP frequently have other disabilities, which are most significant when it comes to everyday life. The associated co-morbid conditions result mostly from damage to other parts of the brain by the same damaging event. Approximately 50% of the cerebral palsied children have an intelligence quotient (IQ) below 70, as compared with 3% of the general population. Epileptic seizures are common in cerebral palsied children and speech defects occur in about 50%. Deafness, frequently unexpected, is common in choreoathetoid CP particularly high-tone deafness. Squints occur in almost one-half of all affected children. Refractive errors are common. Dental problems are also common, such as gingivitis and caries due to defective chewing, tooth grinding and malocclusion. Gastro-oesophageal reflux disease and pseudobulbar palsy affect feeding and nutrition in these children and often results in malnutrition. Many children have emotional and behavioural problems during growing up years, particularly during adolescence.

A holistic and complete diagnosis of CP should include in addition to the physiologic and topographic type, the functional class, all co-morbidities, neuroradiological features or a possible neuroanatomical level and probable aetiology. The type, severity and timing of the insult and the present developmental level will also aid in planning for management.

Early Diagnosis of Cerebral Palsy

The diagnosis of CP depends upon a combination of motor delay, neurologic signs, persistence of primitive reflexes and abnormal postural reactions. An early diagnosis helps in early intervention preventing the secondary deformities. Infants with an abnormal obstetric or perinatal history are at increased risk to develop CP and should be monitored closely. Clues to an early diagnosis include abnormal behaviour, psychomotor delay and abnormal oromotor or oculomotor patterns.

Neurobehavioural signs suspicious of CP are excessive docility or irritability. A typical history includes poor feeding in the neonatal period. The baby often is irritable, sleeps poorly, vomits frequently, is difficult to handle and cuddle and has poor visual attention.

Motor tone in the extremities may be normal or increased. Persistent or asymmetric fisting may be present. Poor head control and excessive head lag may be early motor signs. However, increased neck extensor and axial tone may make head control appear early in CP. In many cases, spasticity may not be identified until 6 or 7 months of age. Dyskinetic patterns are not typically apparent until approximately 18 months. Ataxia may not become obvious until even later.

Primitive reflexes in CP may be asymmetric or persistent. In normal infants, most primitive reflexes related to posture (tonic labyrinthine, tonic neck and neck-righting and body righting reflexes) disappear when the infants are between 3 and 6 months of age. These reflexes often are not appropriately integrated or inhibited in children with CP. Thus, delay in the disappearance or exaggeration of a primitive reflex may be an early indicator of CP. Other abnormal signs can be elicited when the infant is held in vertical suspension. During the first few months, the appropriate response is for the baby to assume a sitting position (sit in the air). An abnormal response is persistent extension of the legs and crossing (scissoring), which is due to adductor spasm.

LEARNING DISORDERS

Words used to describe individuals with learning disorders such as the terms mental deficiency, mental retardation or mental handicap are taken to mean a failure of development of the mind. This is in contrast to dementia, which means a disintegration of the fully developed mind. As a group these children have in common learning difficulty. The severely affected have difficulty learning to walk, feed, dress and communicate. The more mildly affected have difficulty in acquiring social and physical skills to enable them to earn a living and cope with the demands of the society. Words used to describe the severity of the learning difficulty, e.g. idiot, imbecile, feeble-minded, moron have become terms of abuse and even the terms mental retardation and handicap are being abandoned. The term learning disability is preferred now and can be either global or specific.

Learning Disability (Developmental Retardation)

When the abilities of a child fall below the –2 SD as compared with the normal population, which translates into an IQ of less than 70, learning disability or more specific global learning disability is considered. However, caution needs to be exercised in blindly following IQ, without looking at the abilities and needs of child, as most intelligence tests assess only a few components of the multiple intelligences.

The World Health Organisation classifies this mental handicap into profound (IQ 0–20), severe (IQ 20–34), moderate (IQ 35–49) and mild (IQ 50–70). The child with an IQ between 50 and 70 is educable and may require additional educational concessions and inputs. The child with an IQ between 35 and 49 is trainable and requires special curriculum and school settings and may become functionally independent. The child with an IQ less than 35 requires regular care and is sometimes even dependent for his self-care skills. Such children may require an institutionalised care later on.

Aetiology

The vast majority of cases of learning disorder can be placed in one of two broad aetiological groups, primary amentia which is due to inheritance or defects in the child's genetic material and secondary in which the brain, derived from a normal germ plasma, has been damaged by environmental influences which may be operative prenatally, perinatally or postnatally. In some cases, both genetic and environmental factors combine to result in brain damage. It must be stressed, however, that in individual patient, it is quite often impossible to determine the precise cause of the mental retardation. For example, in the case of a severely retarded child, apnoeic and cyanotic attacks in the first week of life could indicate brain damage resulting from anoxia or respiratory difficulties due to malfunctioning of an abnormally formed brain.

Genetic causes A large number of single gene defects have been uncovered as causes of learning disorder. Many of these fall into the category of inborn errors of metabolism. They are now numerous and include phenylketonuria, maple syrup urine disease, the organic acidurias, homocystinuria, argininosuccinic aciduria, Hartnup disease, galactosaemia, pyridoxine dependency, Niemann-Pick disease, Gaucher disease, Tay-Sach disease, mucopolysaccharidoses and others such as Sturge-Weber syndrome, tuberous sclerosis and Neurofibromatosis. Some cases of sporadic cretinism and all cases of non-endemic familial goitrous cretinism are also due to single gene defects. Another rare example is familial dysautonomia (Riley-Day syndrome). While the single gene defects cited above are each relatively rare, it has been recognised that X-linked genes are quite frequently responsible for non-specific mental retardation. In many of the affected males a marker X-chromosome has been identified. The marker in this "fragile X syndrome" is a "fragile site" occurring at band q27 or q28 (i.e. towards the end of the long arm) of the X-chromosome. However, not all males with X-linked non-specific mental retardation have this fragile site on the X-chromosome. At least three distinct forms of X-linked mental retardation have been described which seem to breed true within families. The most clearly definable is found in males with the marker X-chromosome and macro-orchidism. The enlarged testes become obvious after puberty and are only occasionally noticeable at birth. The degree of learning difficulty is usually severe but may be mild **(Fig. 14.79)**. Specific speech delay is common

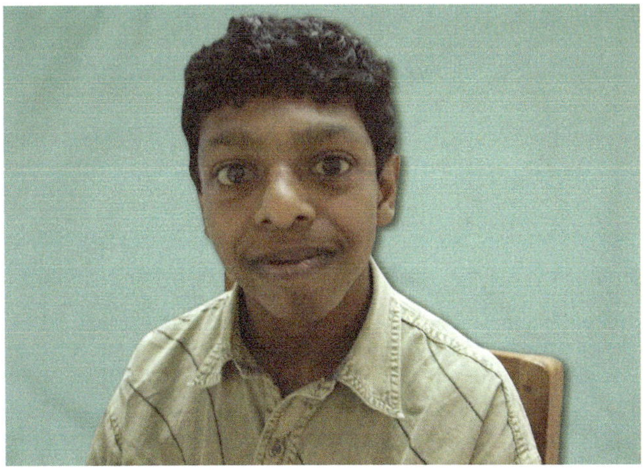

Figure 14.79 Child with Fragile X syndrome. He had intellectual disability, prominent jaw and macro-orchidism.

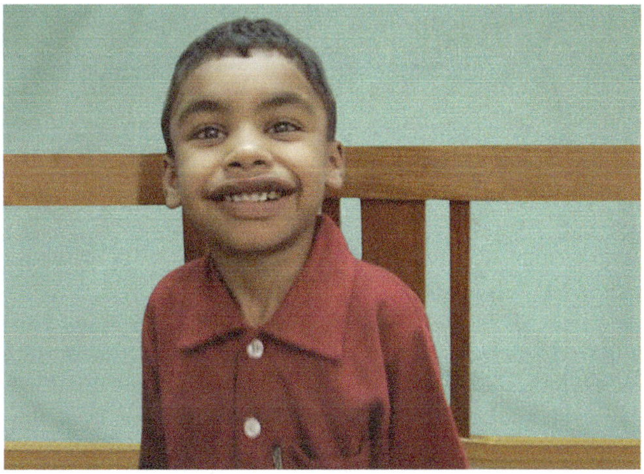

Figure 14.80 Child with Angelman syndrome. This child had predominant speech delay, seizures and autistic behaviour. *Note* the happy facial profile with prominent lips and large mouth.

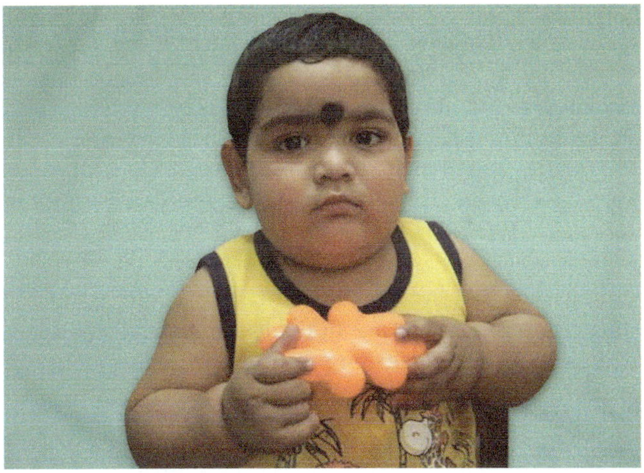

Figure 14.81 Child with Prader Willi syndrome. *Note* obesity and small hands.

and is associated with a characteristic rhythmic quality of "litany speech." Epilepsy may be a feature in some severely affected boys. In another group of families both the marker X-chromosome and macro-orchidism are absent but the other clinical features are indistinguishable from those described above. In the third type of X-linked mental retardation there is no marker chromosome, but the affected boys show microcephaly, severe retardation and small testes. The female carriers of the marker X-chromosome are generally of normal intelligence although some have mild disability, possibly related to non-random X-inactivation in the CNS. Chromosome analysis of boys with non-specific learning disorder is essential for genetic counselling. When the characteristic clinical features described above are present in a boy with no family history the recurrence risk seems to be about 10%.

Some types of mental retardation have been clearly related to gross chromosomal abnormalities. The most severe degrees are usually produced by non-dysjunction during gametogenesis in the mother, leading to trisomy for one of the small acrocentric autosomes. In these conditions the long-recognised correlation with advancing maternal age has been explained on the assumption that the aging ovum is more prone to favour non-dysjunction. Down syndrome (*see* **Fig. 14.96**) is the most common of the trisomies (about 1.8 per 1,000 live births) and has a wide range of disabilities including learning disability.

The next most common autosomal trisomies in live-born children are trisomy 13 (Patau syndrome) (*see* **Fig. 14.94**) and trisomy 18 (Edward syndrome) (*see* **Fig. 14.95**) with frequencies of about 0.5 and 0.1 per 1,000 live births respectively. Each causes such severe and multiple abnormalities including profound learning disorders that those affected rarely survive infancy.

A variety of structural chromosome anomalies have also been found associated with severe learning disability. The best defined of these is the Cri-du-Chat syndrome, which is due to partial deletion of the short arm of chromosome 5. About two-thirds of the patients have been females and its frequency at birth is 1/50,000–1/100,000 or less. The name of this syndrome derives from the characteristic mewing-like cry, which is present from the neonatal period. The birth weight is low. Both physical and mental developments are markedly retarded. In Wolf-Hirschhorn syndrome many features similar to the Cri-du-Chat syndrome occur, although the cat-like cry is often absent. It is due to partial deletion of the short arm of chromosome 4.

Some children can have defects of genomic imprinting such as uniparental disomy where both copies of the gene are inherited from one parent. Angelmann syndrome has both 15q12 copies from the father while Prader-Willi syndrome has from the mother. Children with Angelman syndrome have short stature, severe intellectual disability, seizures and characteristic facial and gait pattern known as "happy puppet" **(Fig. 14.80)**. Children with Prader-Willi syndrome have short stature, obesity, intellectual disability, small hands and feet and hyperphagia **(Fig. 14.81)**.

Rett Syndrome

In 1966, Rett described 22 mentally handicapped children, all of them were girls, who had a history of regression in development and displayed striking repetitive hand movements. It is now evident that this clinical disorder affects between 1 in 10,000 to 1 in 30,000 female infants, with signs of developmental regression appearing during the first year of life and accelerating during the second year of life.

These girls, who have normal antenatal, perinatal and postnatal periods have normal development till 6 months of age. Slowing head growth beginning 6 months of age usually precedes the stagnation stage which moves into regression by the second year of life. The regression stage is characterised by rapid developmental deterioration, autistic features and stereotyped hand movements with loss of purposeful hand use. Rhythmic hand movements with fingers usually adducted and partly extended are characteristic with patting or lightly clapping them, banging the mouth or wringing and squeezing intertwined fingers **(Fig. 14.82)**. In some girls there are choreiform trunk and limb movements and dystonia. As they grow older the girls become more placid, their lower limbs progressively stiff with wasting, scoliosis and respiratory dysrhythmias, hyperventilation and apnoeic episodes. A defect in the methyl CpG binding protein 2 (MECP2) gene on X-chromosome has been linked with most Rett syndromes.

Most of the genetically determined types of disordered mental function discussed so far have been of severe to moderate degree. On the other hand, rather more than 75% of all learning disorders fall into the mild learning disability category (IQ 50–70) and cannot be attributed to single gene or gross chromosomal abnormalities. Although, it is accepted that genetic influences play a major part in determining the child's intelligence, there is a good evidence that environmental influences also affect intelligence.

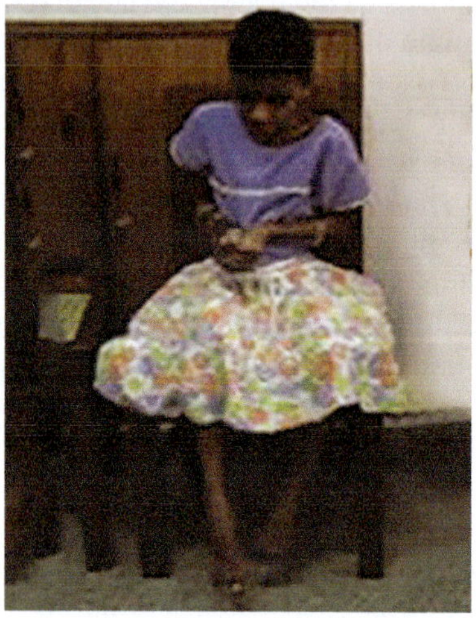

Figure 14.82 Girl with Rett syndrome. Note the midline hand wringing movements.

Environmental Causes

In some cases, learning disability has resulted from damage to a normally developing brain by some noxious environmental influence. They may operate at various periods in the stage of development. Microbial causes of brain damage account for about 10% of all the cases of learning disorder associated with microcephaly.

Prenatal Rubella during the first 12 weeks of pregnancy can certainly damage the foetal brain. Toxoplasmosis may also be associated with mental retardation. CMV is the most common known viral cause of mental retardation. About 40% of the women enter pregnancy without antibodies, about twice the number who are susceptible to rubella. It has been estimated that about 1% of the pregnant women in London undergo primary infection and that half of their infants are infected in utero. While most of these congenital infections are asymptomatic and only a few exhibit the severe illness, proportions are subsequently found to have learning disorders or to suffer other neurological deficits. HIV infection is a well-known cause of mental retardation. Maternal irradiation has been shown to result in mental retardation with microcephaly, and sometimes microphthalmia as in the survivors of the Hiroshima and Nagasaki atomic attacks. Antenatal exposure to alcohol can result in Foetal alcohol syndrome **(*see* Fig. 14.92)**. The effect upon a child's intelligence of adverse environmental factors during the mother's pregnancy, such as poverty, malnutrition, excessive smoking and emotional stress are difficult to assess. They might increase the risk of learning disorder by their association with intrauterine foetal malnutrition.

Perinatal There is a well-documented association between some of the complications of pregnancy and abnormalities of the brain including mental retardation. These complications such as antepartum haemorrhage, pre-eclampsia, breech presentation and complicated or instrumental delivery are frequently associated with intrapartum foetal anoxia. It is, however, extremely difficult to assess the importance of intrapartum or neonatal anoxia as a cause of later neurological disability.

Postnatal Postnatal causes of mental retardation include meningitis, encephalitis, hypoglycaemia, bilirubin encephalopathy, subdural haematoma, hypernatraemia and head injury. Lead encephalopathy is a rare but undoubted cause of permanent brain damage. Even low-level lead exposures especially in the critical 1,000 day period of brain development can cause some cognitive impairment and possibly behavioural abnormalities.

Diagnosis

In most cases, the diagnosis of disordered learning ability can be made in the first year of life, provided the physician is familiar with the stages of development in the normal baby and that he realises the variations, which may occur in perfectly normal babies. It is essential that a thoughtful history be obtained from the parents, to be followed by a detailed physical examination of the child. Frequently the child must be seen on several occasions before a final conclusion is possible. There may be factors which indicate that the child is "at risk" and more likely to be retarded than others. These include prematurity, complications of pregnancy or labour, a history of asphyxia neonatorum, intra or periventricular haemorrhage, jaundice in the newborn period, convulsions or cyanotic attacks, maternal rubella or a family history of learning disorder. The basis of the diagnosis of learning disorder may be conveniently discussed under four headings.

Physical abnormalities Certain physical features are undoubted evidence of associated mental defect. These include the characteristic signs of Down syndrome (*see* **Fig. 14.96**), microcephaly, cretinism and gargoylism. Other physical abnormalities are often, although not invariably, associated with learning disorder. In this group are CP, the bilateral macular chorioretinitis of toxoplasmosis, Turner syndrome (*see* **Fig. 14.99**) and hydrocephalus. Certain other physical "stigmata" are seen more commonly in learning disordered than in normal people, but in themselves they can do no more than direct the physician's attention towards a more careful assessment of the child's intellectual development. Such peculiarities are a high narrow (saddle-shaped) palate, abnormally simple ears, hypertelorism, marked epicanthic folds and short, curved fifth finger (clinodactyly). A distinctive pattern of altered growth and morphogenesis can be recognised in the children of mothers who consume alcohol during pregnancy known as Foetal alcohol syndrome (*see* **Fig. 14.92**). They exhibit both pre- and post-natal growth failure involving weight, length and head circumference. Neurological abnormalities include hypotonia, irritability and jitteriness, poor co-ordination, hyperkinesis, and learning difficulties, which may vary from severe to mild. Dysmorphic features include short palpebral fissures (canthus to canthus), epicanthic folds, and hypoplastic or absent philtrum, thin upper lip, broad nasal bridge with upturned nose and mid-facial hypoplasia. Other congenital anomalies may involve the heart, genitourinary system, eyes, ears, mouth or skeleton. Haemangiomata and herniae are not uncommon. Abnormal palmar creases and hirsutism have also been recorded.

Delayed psychomotor development It is characteristic of the learning disordered child that his development is delayed in all its parameters. He is slow in showing an interest in his surroundings, slow in attempting to handle or play with objects, slow to sit or stand unsupported or to walk on his own, late in speaking, and late in acquiring bladder or bowel control. A lack of concentration or sustained interest is also obvious. Thus, after handling a new toy or object for a minute or two he loses interest and throws it down. His lack of interest in things around him may raise the suspicion of defective vision, just as his lack of response to sounds is apt to lead to a mistaken impression of deafness. Infantile practices tend to persist beyond the normal period, e.g. putting objects into his mouth, excessive and prolonged posturing of his hands and fingers before his eyes, drooling and slobbering. The physician must obviously be familiar with the various developmental stages of normal infants and children before he is in a position to make a judicious assessment of an individual patient. A brief outline of the more positive developmental steps is shown in **Table 14.5**. The best assessment is to be expected from the doctor who has had long and intimate contact with normal children in the child health clinic or in their family practice, provided that during their undergraduate period they have developed the capacity to observe, and to appreciate the significance of their observations.

Abnormal behaviour and gestures Learning disordered children frequently engage in types of behaviour and mannerisms, which are obviously abnormal for their age. Thus, in early infancy the child with delay may be excessively "good" in that he will lie in his bed for long periods without crying or showing restlessness, interest in surroundings, or boredom. In other cases, there is constant or prolonged and apparently purposeless crying. Teeth grinding when awake is a common and distressing habit of many with profound learning disorders. The older child may exhaust his mother by his aimless over-activity, which may at times endanger his life. Certain repetitive and rhythmic movements, although by no means confined to learning disordered children, are more commonly present in them and for more prolonged time periods. These include head banging, body-rocking to-and-fro, and head rolling. Profoundly disordered children frequently lack the normal capacity for affection, they may be prone to sudden rages, and they may assault other younger children.

Convulsions Most epileptics are of normal intelligence. None the less, epileptic seizures occur more frequently among mentally retarded children than those who are normal. Frequently repeated generalised seizures lead to slowly progressive intellectual deterioration. The association of infantile spasms (hypsarrhythmia) with severe learning difficulties has been described previously.

DIFFERENTIAL DIAGNOSIS

The diagnosis of learning disorder is obviously one in which the physician must not be wrong or he will cause the parents unjustifiable and unnecessary grief and anxiety. Some infants have a "slow start" but catch up later, and in the absence of manifested physical signs, such as microcephaly or Down syndrome, a firm diagnosis of learning disorder should only be made after a period of observation

TABLE 14.5 Developmental steps in the normal child.

Age	***Development***
4 weeks	Head flops back when lifted from supine to sitting position
	Sits with rounded back while supported
	Primitive grasp reflex elicited by placing object in palm
	Responds to sudden noise
8 weeks	Minimal head lag when pulled into sitting position
	Primitive grasp reflex slight or absent
	Smiles readily: vocalises when talked to
12 weeks	Horizontally tracks objects with head and eyes
	No head lag when pulled into sitting position
	Sits supported with straight back: head almost steady
	No grasp reflex: holds objects in hand for short time
	Watches own hand movements
	Turns head towards sounds
6 months	Lifts head from pillow
	Sits unsupported when placed in position
	Rolls from supine to prone position
	Grasps objects when offered
	Transfers objects from one hand to the other
	Responds to name
	Held standing, can bear weight on legs and bounces up and down
	No more hand regard: finds feet interesting
12 months	Understands simple sentences and commands
	Can rise to sitting from supine position
	Pulls to standing position by holding onto cot side
	Walks holding hand or furniture
	Speaks a few recognisable words
	Points to objects which are desired
	Throws objects out of pram in play
15 months	Walks unsteadily with feet wide apart; falls at corners
	Can get into standing position alone
	Tries untidily to feed himself with spoon
	Plays with cubes: places one on top of another
	Indicates wet pants
	Now seldom puts toys in mouth
	Shows curiosity and requires protection from dangers
18 months	Can walk upstairs holding onto hand or rail
	Can carry or pull toy when walking
	Can throw ball without falling
	Points to three or four parts of body on request
	Indicates need for toilet
	Lifts and controls drinking cup
	Points to three to five objects or animals in picture book
	Runs safely on whole foot: can avoid obstacles, can kick a ball without losing balance
	Can walk upstairs: holding rail coming downstairs
	Turns door handles
	Demands constant adult attention

(Contd...)

(Contd...)

TABLE 14.5 Developmental steps in the normal child.

Age	Development
3 years	Walks upstairs with alternating feet
	Washes and dries hands with supervision
	Rides tricycle
	Draws a man on request—head, trunk and one or two other parts
	Can count up to ten
	Discusses a picture
	Listens to and demands stories
	Likes to help mother in house, father in garden
	Eats with fork and spoon
	Can dress and undress
	Asks incessant questions
	Climbs ladders and trees
4 years	Engages in role play, e.g. doctor or nurse
	Uses proper sentences to describe recent experiences
	Can give name, age and address
	Draws man with features and extremities
	Matches four primary colours correctly
	Plays with other children
	Alternately cooperative and aggressive with adults or other children
5 years	Runs quickly on toes: Skips on alternate feet
	Can tie shoelaces
	Can name common coins
	Draws recognisable complete man
	Names four primary colours; matches 10–12 colours
	Cooperates more with friends: accepts rules in games
	Protective towards younger children and pets
	May know letters of alphabet and read simple words

during which the rate of development is assessed. There are now available developmental screening protocols in which a child's development can be charted in a longitudinal fashion, making it easier for the less experienced doctor to detect early departures from the normal. It is easy to confuse learning disorder with cerebral palsy. Indeed the two frequently coexist. Careful neurological examination, repeated on several occasions, will reveal the motor handicaps of CP. The deaf child has frequently been diagnosed as mentally retarded, sometimes with tragic results. This mistake should not occur when the physician takes a detailed history and follows it with a careful physical examination. The deaf child will, of course, show a lively visual interest and his motor skills will develop normally. A difficult if not very common problem is the child who fails to develop speech (developmental dysphasia). He is readily confused with the learning disordered child although here too a careful history and period of observation will reveal that in other respects his psychomotor development is proceeding normally. Particular caution is required in the intellectual assessment of the child who has been emotionally deprived by the break-up of his home, death of his mother or who has been otherwise bereft of normal security. The child may require a long period outside an institution in a comforting and reassuring environment, before he can be assessed.

Until recently many autistic children were wrongly labelled mentally defective. Autistic children have a varied profile ranging from superior intelligence to severe learning disability. The most characteristic features of infantile autism are a complete lack of interest in personal relationships which contrasts with an interest in inanimate objects; frequently a preoccupation with parts of the body or a toy; a tendency to react violently and unhappily to changes in environment; loss of speech or failure to acquire it, or the meaningless use of words or phrases and grossly abnormal mannerisms such as rocking, spinning or immobility (catatonia). Some children with autism spectrum disorder may reject or ignore social contacts. Some of their repetitive movements and stereotypy are shown to correlate with abnormal sensory perception and integration as well as to anxiety. There is an odd high incidence of professional and educated people among the parents of autistic children. Such children, of course, are wrongly placed in institutions for profound and severe learning disorders. Some have responded considerably to behavioural and developmental therapy.

Intelligence Tests

Psychological testing and evaluations are of considerable although limited value in providing an estimate of a child's probable potential ability. They cannot, naturally, take into account the influence of such variables as zeal, ambition, interest, encouragement or the lack of it, good or bad teaching so forth. There are many aspects of intelligence and personality, and the various tests assess these in different degrees. It is not proposed here to describe these tests in detail; they are reliable only in the hands of the expert. The most commonly used are Bayley Scales of Infant Development (BSID) and Griffith Mental Developmental Scale (GMDS); for older children, the Stanford-Binet scale and the revised test of Terman and Merrill, also the Wechsler Intelligence Scale for Children; for adolescents and adults, the Wechsler Adult Intelligence Scale and Raven Progressive Matrices. There are also several useful personality tests of which the best for the mentally retarded are the Rorschach test and the Goodenough "Draw-a-Man" test. In the case of the school child it is also important to enquire about educational progress. An evaluation of the results of various tests competently performed is of great value in planning suitable education or training for the mentally handicapped child.

Investigations: Depending on the history and physical examination the following investigations may be done: thyroid function test, metabolic screening for inborn error of metabolism, cranial CT or MRI scan, EEG, karyotyping including examination for fragile-X syndrome, TORCH infection screen, etc.

Specific Learning Disability

Specific learning disability (SLD) is a disorder in one or more of the basic psychological processes involved in understanding or using language, spoken or written is affected and is not the result of visual, hearing or motor handicaps or global learning disability. There is a discrepancy between aptitude, measured by intelligence tests and achievement, as reflected in academic performance. The SLD can be of reading (dyslexia), writing (dysgraphia) or mathematics (dyscalculia). Some children may have associated behavioural problems like attention deficit hyperactivity disorder. The children with SLD require bypass strategies and concessions based on the primary deficit. They learn to adapt well and most have a remarkable ability to learn, when provided proper strategies.

Prevention of Learning Disorders

The prevention of neurological disorder has become increasingly possible in recent years. Indeed, the more efficient application of knowledge, which has been available to us for some years, would considerably reduce the present incidence of brain damage from such disturbances as perinatal hypoxia, hypoglycaemia, kernicterus and hypernatraemia and the prevalence of maternal rubella by the institution of anti-rubella vaccination. Screening programmes during the neonatal period for several of the treatable inborn errors of metabolism such as phenylketonuria, homocystinuria, maple syrup urine disease, galactosaemia as well as congenital hypothyroidism are making some impact upon the number of learning impaired children.

A most common development in the field of prevention is to be found in prenatal diagnosis. This is most often based upon examination of the amniotic fluid obtained by transabdominal amniocentesis between the 14th week and 16th week of pregnancy and supported by ultrasonography. Sampling of chorionic villi or foetal blood or tissue may also be employed in selected cases. Chromosome analysis of amniotic cell cultures may reveal abnormalities such as trisomies 21, 13 and 18, or trisomy affecting the sex chromosomes (XXX and XXY). It may, on the other hand, lead to a diagnosis of 21/14 translocation in the foetus when one of the parents is known to be a translocation carrier and other more complex translocations have also been demonstrated. The sex of the foetus can also be determined when there is a known sex-linked inherited disease in a family, and where the risk to male progeny is 50:50. While most of the X-linked disorders are not associated with learning disorder (e.g. haemophilia) a few, such as Hunter syndrome do lead to progressive mental deficiency.

Recent years have seen a rapid increase in the number of inborn errors of metabolism, which are capable of prenatal diagnosis. A considerable number of these are associated with progressive neurological deterioration. Most are autosomal recessives although a few are X-linked. The laboratory techniques involved include enzyme assays on cultured amniotic fluid cells, measurement of metabolites and biochemical analysis of the liquor.

Analysis of foetal blood obtained by umbilical cordocentesis has also been applied in the prenatal diagnosis of the haemoglobinopathies. Molecular genetic techniques allow earlier diagnosis and intervention.

When severe and irreversible disorders of the foetus are recognised prenatally, therapeutic abortion may be considered. This is a complex problem with ethical, legal and religious implications. Occasionally, prenatal testing will reveal a treatable disease, as when congenital adrenal hyperplasia due to 21-hydroxylase deficiency is confirmed by a high level of 17-hydroxyprogesterone in the amniotic fluid, when no delay should arise in instituting appropriate treatment from the time of the infant's birth. In practice, it has been found that in the majority of cases involving prenatal diagnosis the extreme parental anxiety, which is common in this situation, is relieved because in most instances the foetus is found not to be carrying the chromosomal or enzyme abnormality.

Prenatal diagnosis demands careful selection of patients as the techniques are not entirely devoid of risk and there can be no absolute guarantee of success. Not only must there be full discussion and investigation of the family problems, but there must also be close liaison between the clinicians, geneticists and the laboratories. This should preferably be undertaken before and not after the female partner has become pregnant. Suitable indications for prenatal diagnosis include:

- Advancing maternal age, where the risk of chromosome abnormalities, particularly trisomy, is increased
- When either parent is a translocation carrier or has chromosomal mosaicism with a high risk of an abnormal foetus
- When there has previously been a child with a chromosomal abnormality such as Down syndrome

In families with X-linked and certain autosomal recessive diseases.

Illustrations of a few conditions (Figs. 14.83 to 14.114) are shown below. They consist of congenital anomalies and paediatric syndromes as follows:

- Spina-bifida occulta (Fig. 14.83)
- Occipital encephalocele (Fig. 14.84)
- Myelomeningocele (Fig. 14.85)
- Anencephaly (Fig. 14.86)
- Congenital hydrocephalus (Fig. 14.87)
- Hydranencephaly (Fig. 14.88A)
- Transillumination of skull (Fig. 14.88B)
- Holoprosencephaly (Fig. 14.89)
- Achondroplasia (Fig. 14.90)
- Cornelia de Lange syndrome (Fig. 14.91)
- Foetal alcohol syndrome (Fig. 14.92)
- Williams syndrome (Fig. 14.93)
- Trisomy 13 (Patau) syndrome (Fig. 14.94)
- Trisomy 18 (Edward) syndrome (Fig. 14.95)
- Down syndrome (Fig. 14.96)
- Prader-Willi syndrome (Fig. 14.97)
- Klippel-Feil syndrome (Fig. 14.98)
- Turner syndrome (Fig. 14.99)
- Lowe syndrome (Fig. 14.100)
- Beckwith-Wiedmann syndrome (Fig. 14.101)
- Crouzon syndrome (Fig. 14.102)
- Treacher Collins syndrome (Fig. 14.103)
- Noonan syndrome (Fig. 14.104)
- Klinefelter syndrome (Fig. 14.105)
- Dystrophia myotonica (Fig. 14.106)
- Myasthenia gravis (Fig. 14.107)
- Infant with meningococcal meningitis (Fig. 14.108)
- Mumps meningitis (Fig. 14.109)
- Duchenne muscular dystrophy (Fig. 14.110)
- Ocular torticollis (Fig. 14.111)
- Tuberous sclerosis (Figs. 14.112 and 14.113)
- Neurofibromatosis (Fig. 14.114)

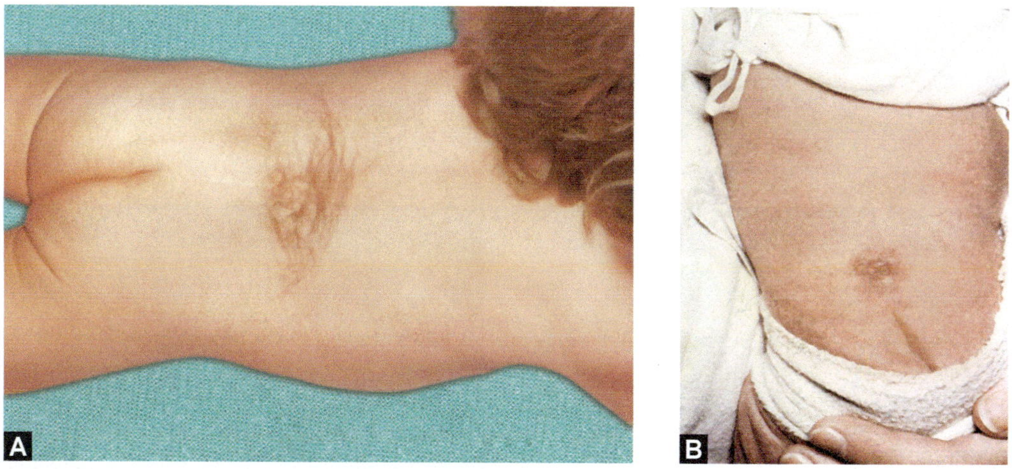

Figures 14.83A and B Spina bifida occulta: (A) Lumbosacral hypertrichosis. (B) Lumbar haemangioma—are indicative of spinal defect but are seldom associated with neurological disability.

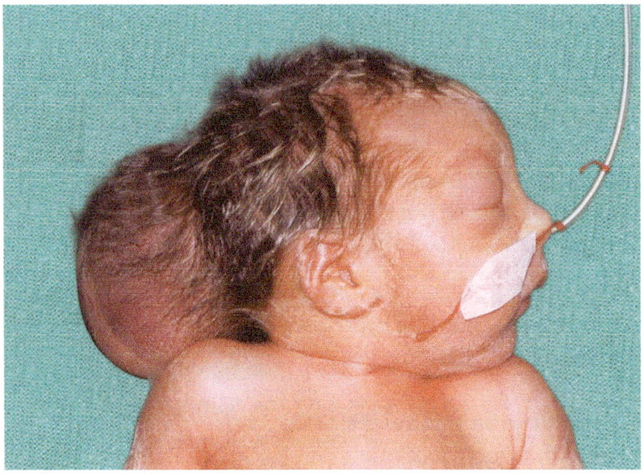

Figure 14.84 Occipital encephalocele: newborn infant with massive occipital encephalocele. It is a neural tube defect that involves extrusion of cranial contents through a bony defect.

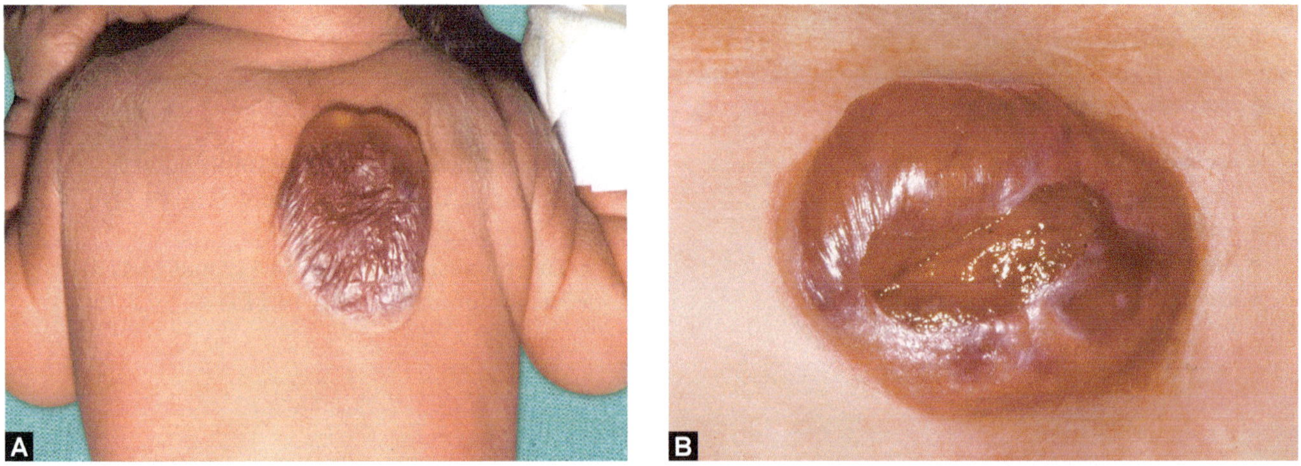

Figures 14.85A and B Myelomeningocele: symptoms vary depending on the level of the lesion. (A) Thoracic myelomeningocele; (B) Lumbar myelomeningocele.

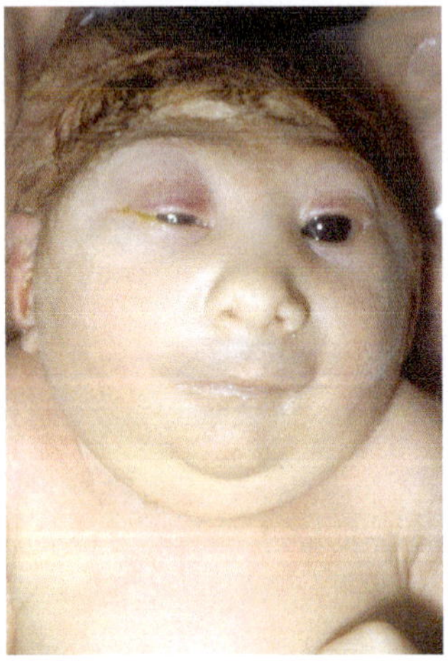

Figure 14.86 Anencephaly: The lack of normal development of the brain, skull and scalp. Diagnosed prenatally by maternal AFP screening and foetal ultrasonography.

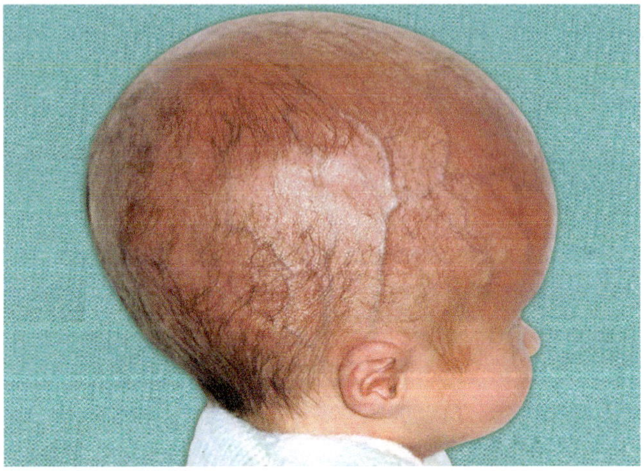

Figure 14.87 Congenital hydrocephalus: showing large head with dilated scalp veins.

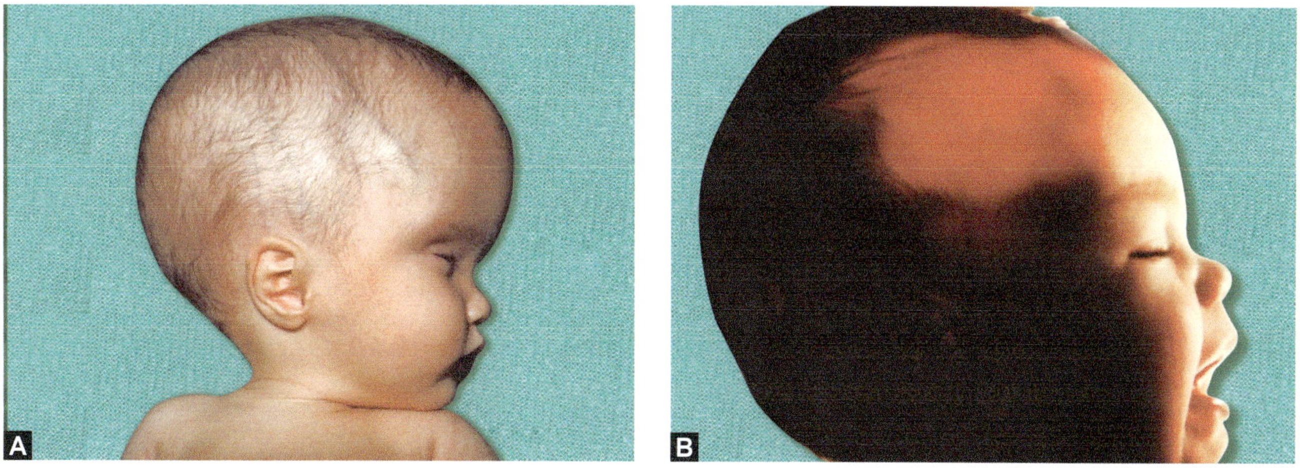

Figures 14.88A and B (A) Hydranencephaly: Hydranencephaly may be confused with hydrocephalus. In hydranencephaly, the cortical hemispheres are absent or represented by membranous sacs with remnants of frontal, temporal or occipital cortex dispersed over the membrane; (B) Positive transillumination of skull.

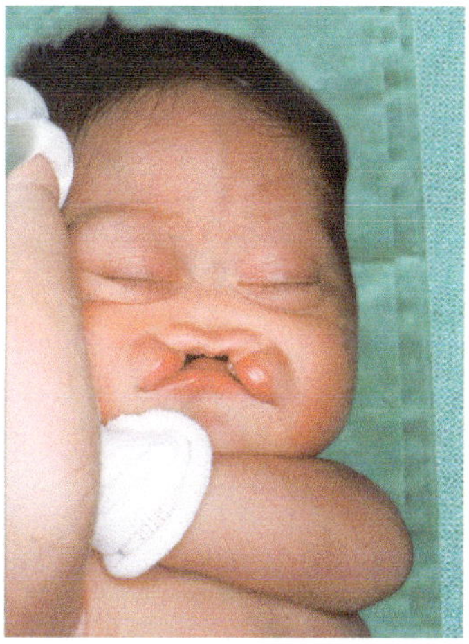

Figure 14.89 A child with holoprosencephaly: In this condition, there is a single spherical cerebral structure with a single ventricular cavity, often associated with midline facial defects and single nostril.

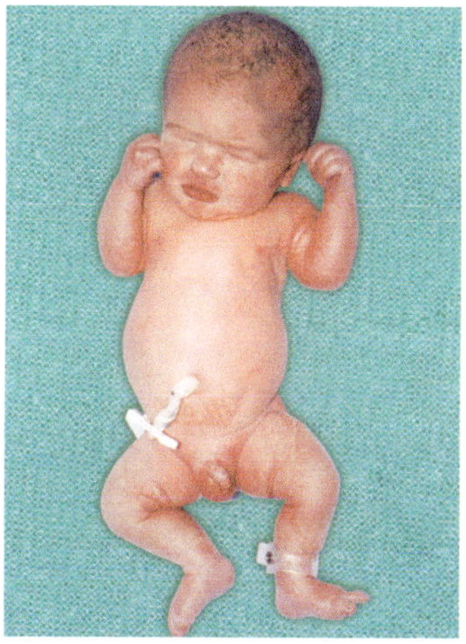

Figure 14.90 Achondroplasia: Frontal view of a child with typical features of achondroplasia. It is characterised by significant macrocephaly, short stature and normal trunk size.

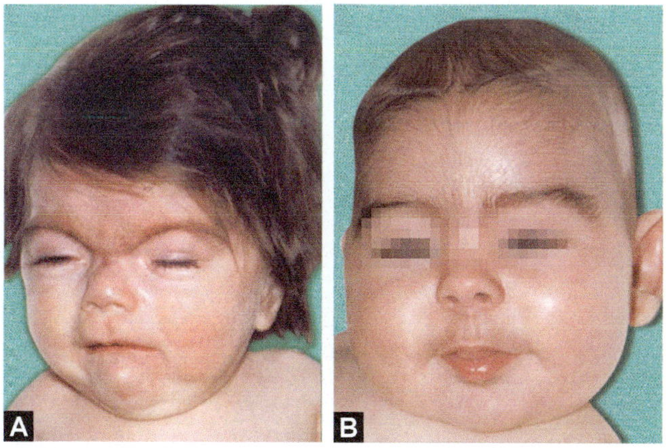

Figures 14.91A and B Cornelia de Lange syndrome: *Note* small round head, bushy eyebrows and synophrys (eyebrows run together), long curly eyelashes, small nose, anteverted nostrils, long philtrum and generalised hirsutism.

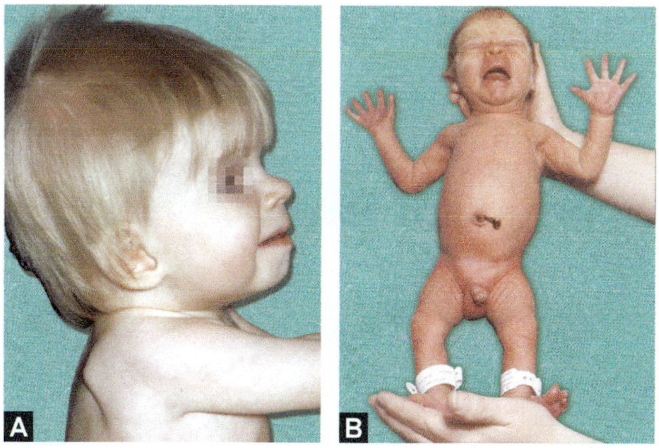

Figures 14.92A and B Foetal alcohol syndrome (FAS): Infants with abnormal facial features consistent with FAS. *Note* the short palpebral fissures, hypoplastic philtrum with thinning of upper lip, flattening of the maxillary area.

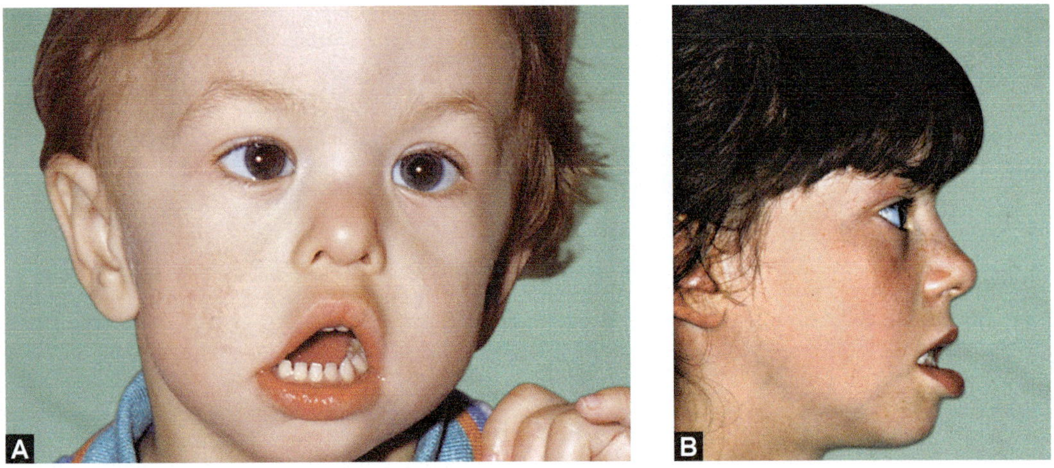

Figures 14.93A and B Williams syndrome: It is a relatively common disorder and is easily diagnosed because of characteristic facial appearance. *Note* the epicanthic folds, flattened bridge of the nose, short nose and upturned nares, long philtrum and prominent lips being typical of the "elfin" facial features.

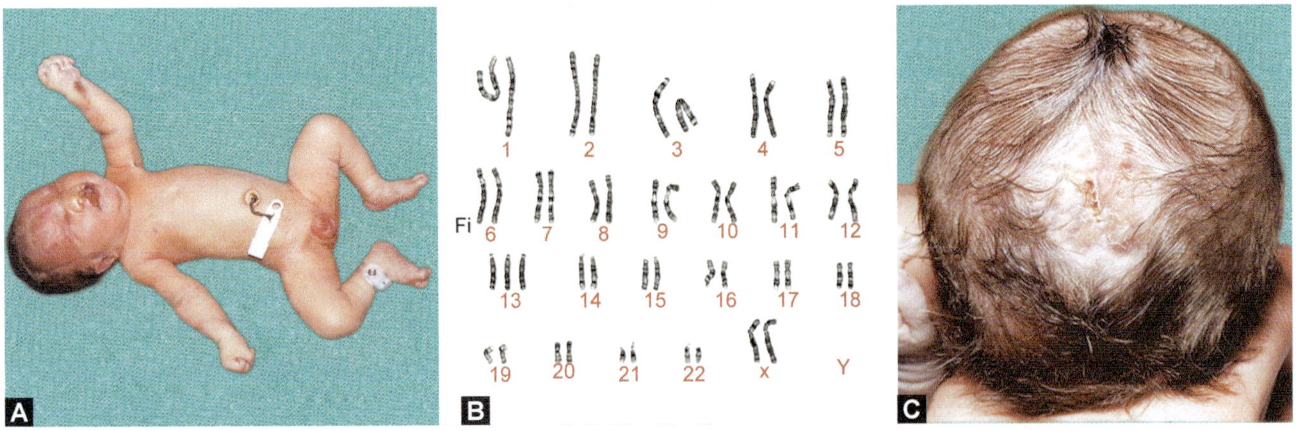

Figures 14.94A to C (A) An infant with Trisomy 13 (Patau syndrome); (B) Karyotype of trisomy 13; (C) Scalp defect in trisomy 13 is helpful diagnostically as it rarely appears in other chromosome abnormalities.

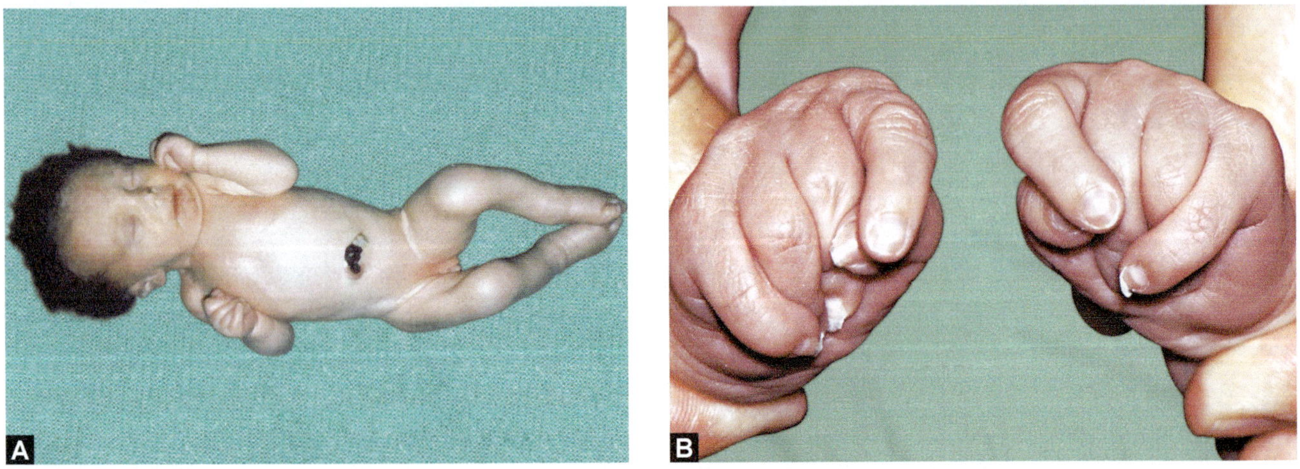

Figures 14.95A and B Trisomy 18 syndrome (Edwards syndrome). (A) An infant with trisomy 18: prominent occiput, low set ears, long cranium; (B) Overlapping fingers.

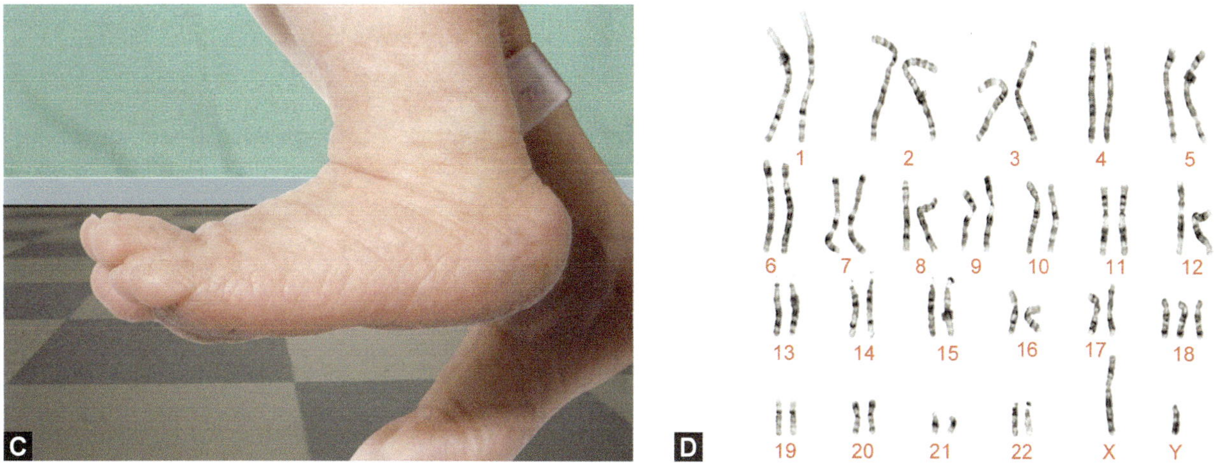

Figures 14.95C and D Trisomy 18 syndrome (Edwards syndrome). (C) Rocker-bottom feet; (D) Karyotype of trisomy 18.

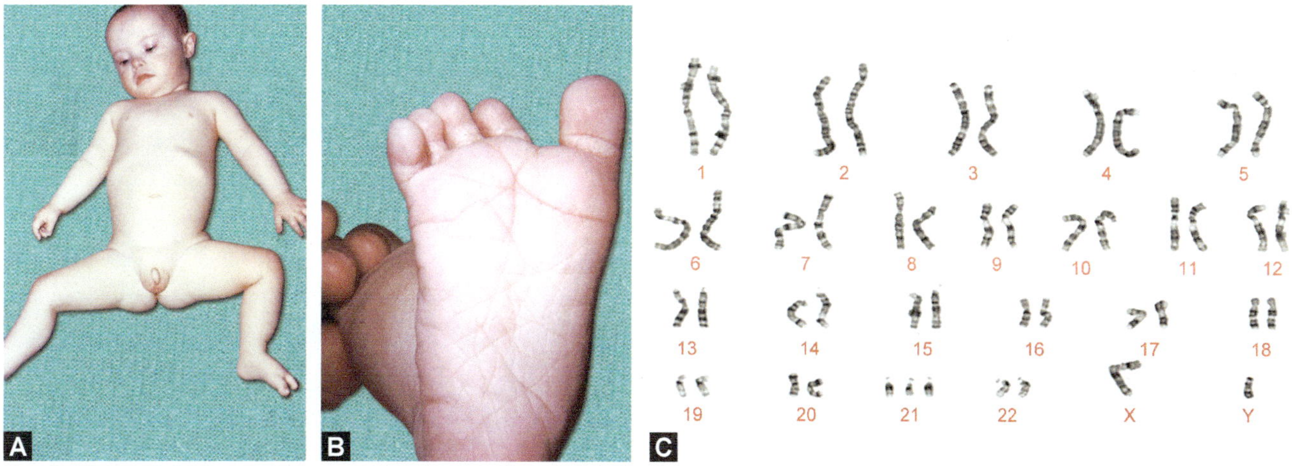

Figures 14.96A to C Down syndrome: (A) A child with many typical physical features of Down syndrome; (B) Foot-saddle sign; (C) Chromosomal karyotype showing typical trisomy 21.

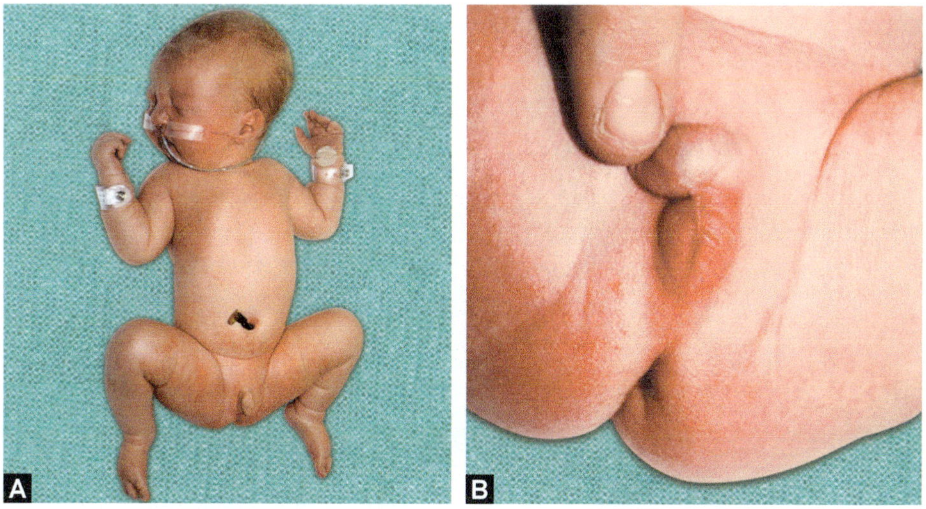

Figures 14.97A and B Prader–Willi syndrome (PWS): (A) It is characterised by decreased foetal movement, infantile hypotonia and feeding difficulties; (B) Genitalia—small penis and cryptorchidism.

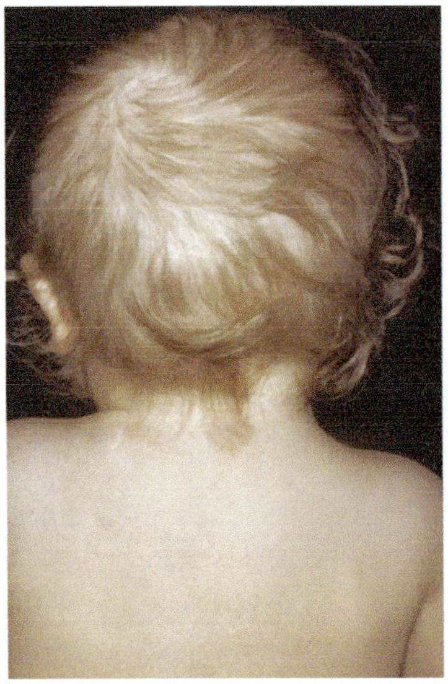

Figure 14.98 Klippel–Feil syndrome: It consists of a congenital fusion of cervical vertebrae. *Note* a short neck, low hair line posteriorly.

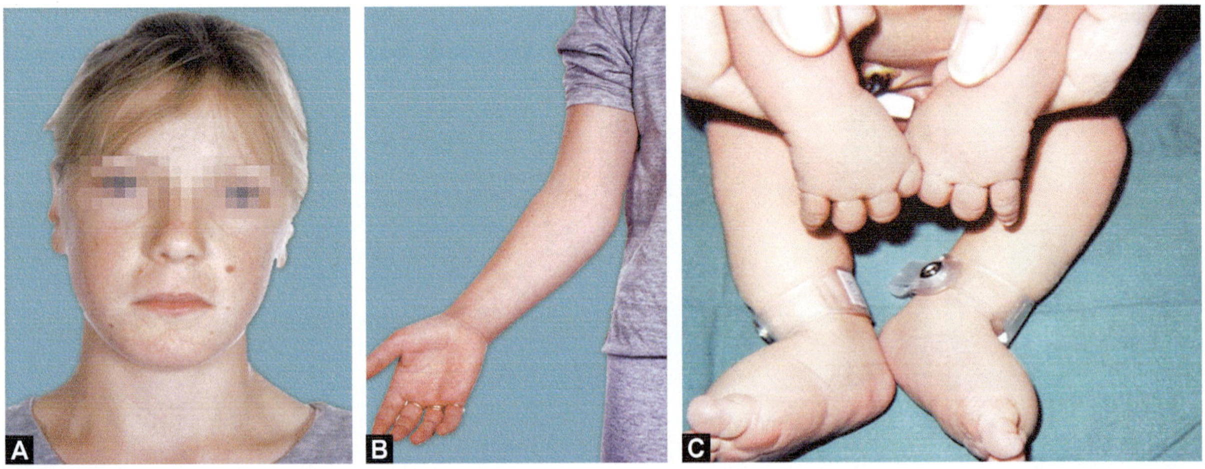

Figures 14.99A to C Turner syndrome, 45X: (A) Somatic features in Turner syndrome; (B) Increased carrying angle; (C) Neonatal Turner syndrome: Lymphoedema of feet and hands.

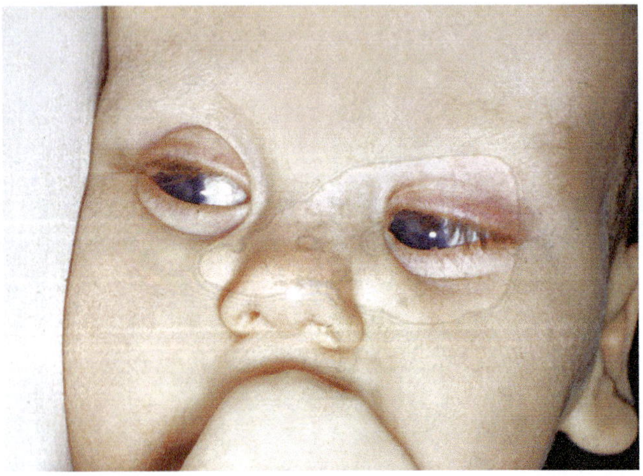

Figure 14.100 Lowe syndrome (oculocerebrorenal dystrophy). A child with Lowe syndrome. *Note* cataracts and megalocornea.

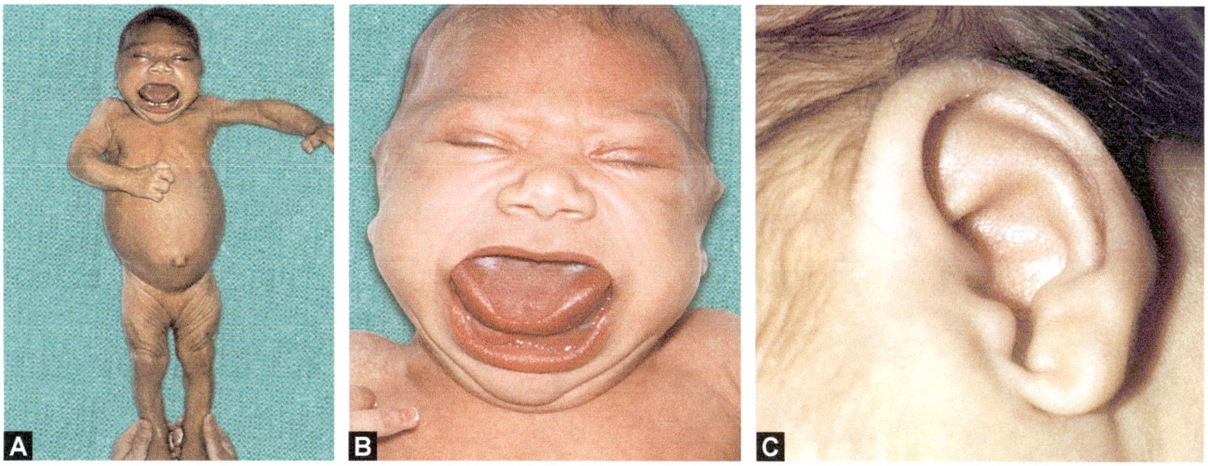

Figures 14.101A to C Beckwith–Wiedemann syndrome: (A) A child with typical features of Beckwith–Wiedemann syndrome; (B) Tongue-macroglossia; (C) Ear-lobe-indentations in the ear lobe.

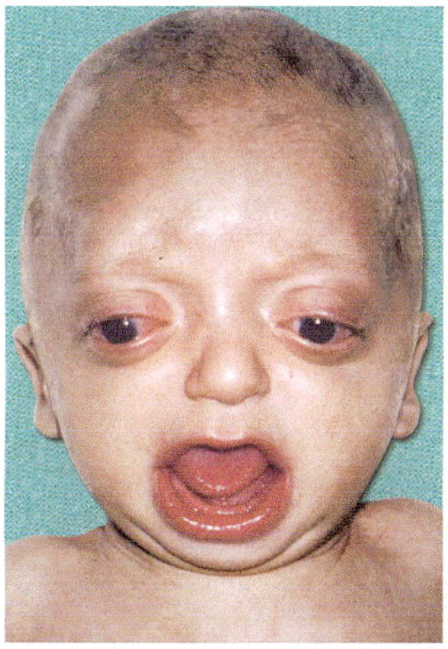

Figure 14.102 Craniofacial dysostosis (Crouzon syndrome): A child with typical facial features, consisting of hypertelorism, exophthalmos with shallow orbits, a beaked parrot nose, rather low-set ears, short upper lip and relative prognathism.

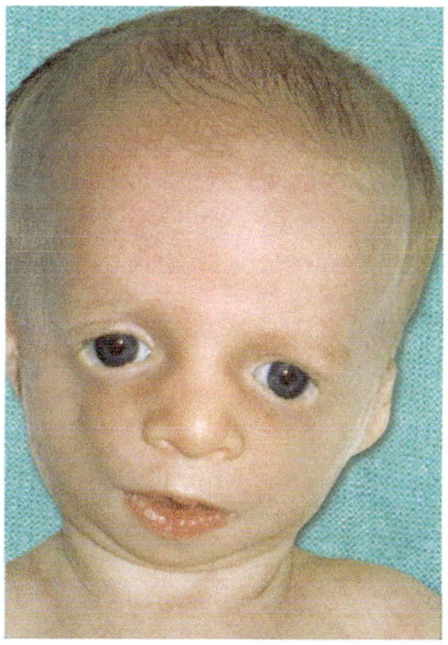

Figure 14.103 Treacher Collins syndrome: A child with Treacher Collins syndrome showing downwards sloping palpebral fissures, sunken cheek bones, receding chin, large mouth and deformed pinnae.

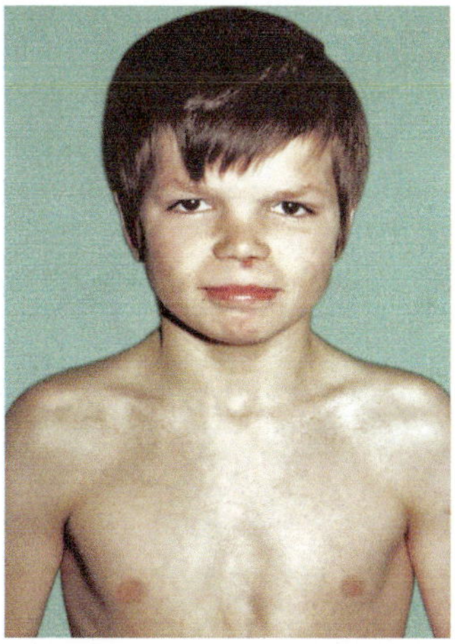

Figure 14.104 Noonan syndrome: *Note* broad forehead with hypertelorism, epicanthic folds, ptosis, downwards slanting palpebral fissure, neck webbing.

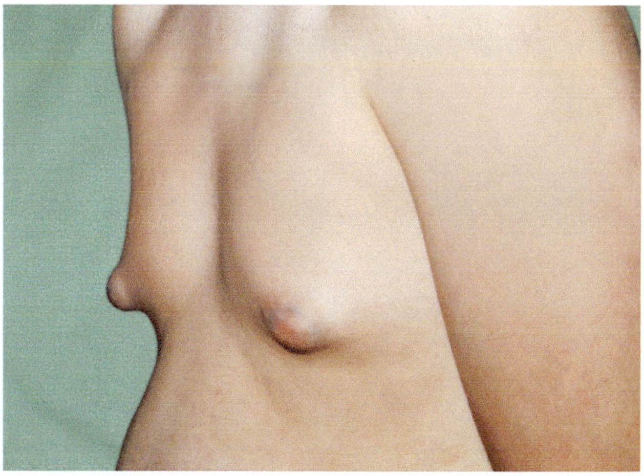

Figure 14.105 Klinefelter syndrome (47,XXY): *Note* gynaecomastia in a boy with Klinefelter syndrome.

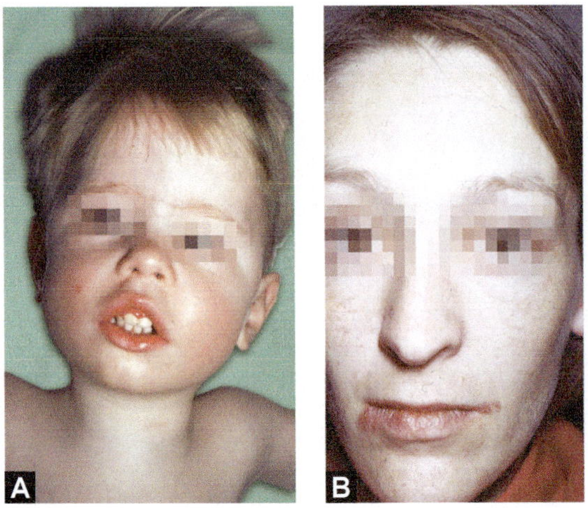

Figures 14.106A and B Dystrophia myotonica: (A) *Note* the characteristic droopy myopathic, rather shiny face, and tenting of upper lip; (B) Affected mother.

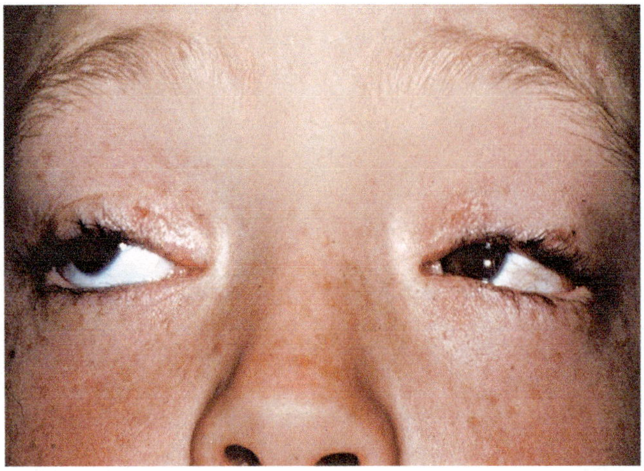

Figure 14.107 Myasthenia gravis: *Note* bilateral ptosis and facial weakness.

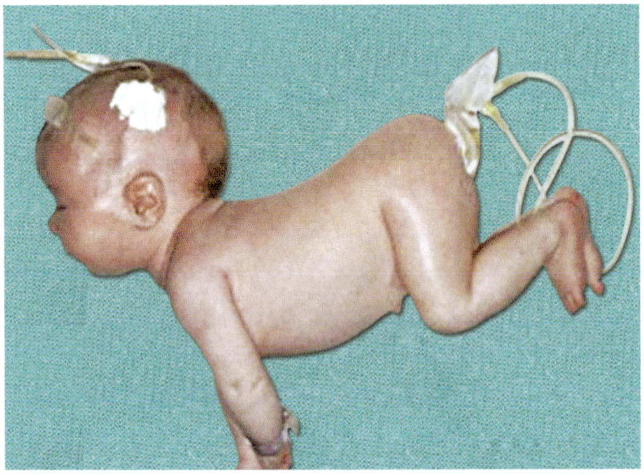

Figure 14.108 Infant with meningococcal meningitis: *Note* marked head retraction.

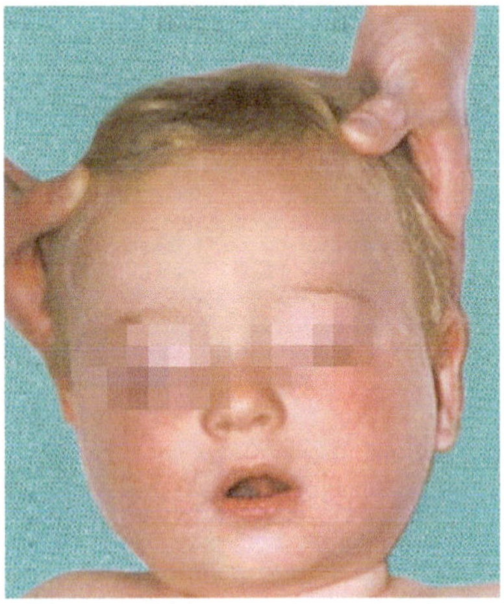

Figure 14.109 Mumps meningitis: *Note* parotid swelling mainly on the left side with left ear protruding.

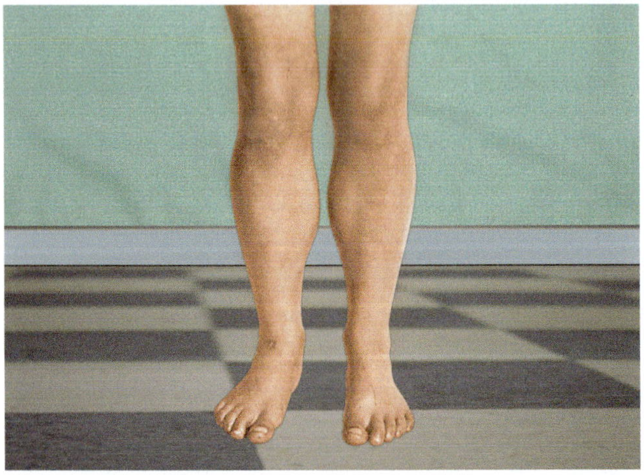

Figure 14.110 Duchenne type of pseudohypertrophic muscular dystrophy: *Note* hypertrophy of calf muscles.

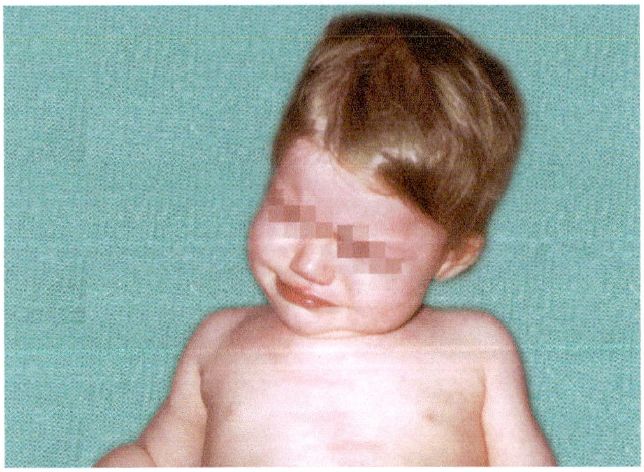

Figure 14.111 Ocular torticollis (head tilt): Due to posterior fossa tumour.

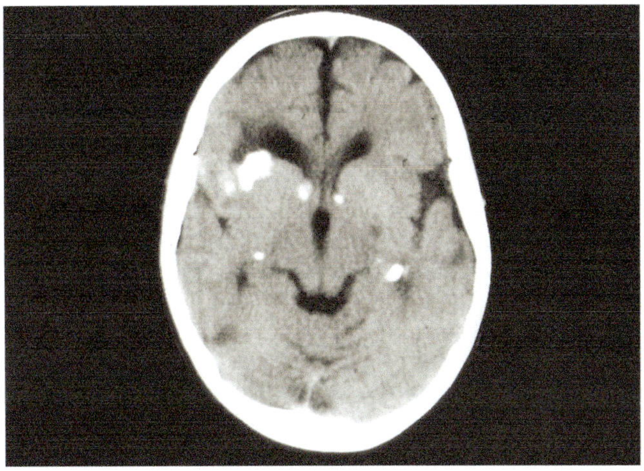

Figure 14.112 Tuberous sclerosis: MRI scan head showing nodular intracranial opacities representing adenoma formation.

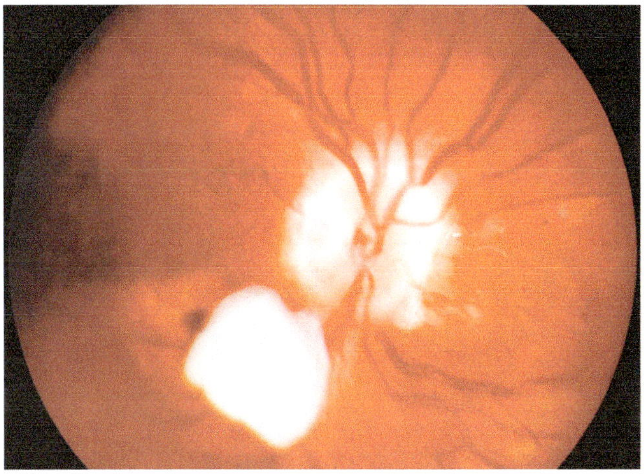

Figure 14.113 Tuberous sclerosis: ocular fundus: this shows an early hamartomatous lesion near the disc in the retina of a child with TS.

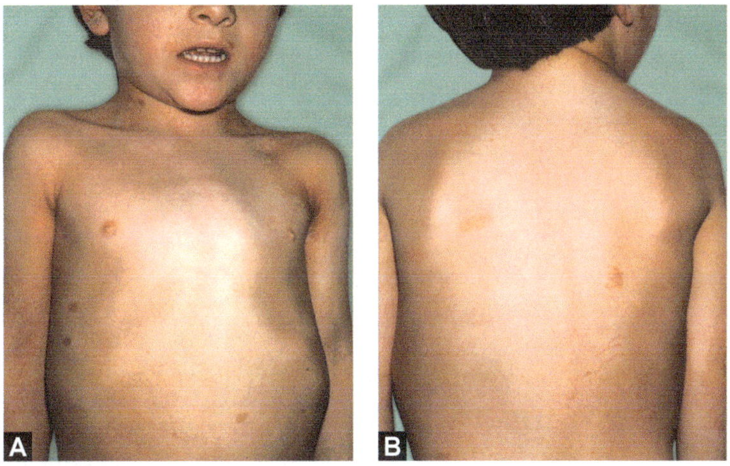

Figures 14.114A and B Neurofibromatosis Café-au-lait spots. They typically increase in pigmentation, number and size throughout early childhood.

CHAPTER 14(B)

Neurosurgical Diseases of the Nervous System

Roddy O'Kane, Maya Kommer

INTRODUCTION

Paediatric surgical neurology is a rapidly evolving field dealing with neurological conditions in children with potential operative treatment strategies. The specialty involves close working with many disciplines including paediatric neurologists, intensivists, neonatologists, neuroradiologist and pathologists.

The specialty covers a diverse spectrum of pathologies including congenital malformations, neuro-oncology, CSF disturbance/hydrocephalus, trauma, craniofacial, vascular and functional neurosurgery

We will give an overview of the more common pathologies; congenital malformations, neuro-oncology and hydrocephalus.

CONGENITAL MALFORMATIONS OF THE CNS

Dysraphism

Dysraphism refers to the variety of cranial and spinal abnormalities that result from erroneous closure of the neural tube during embryological development. There is a wide geographical variation in the incidence of dysraphism. Genetic and environmental factors play a key role in their formation. There is good evidence that maternal folate ingestion during conception and pregnancy reduces the incidence of neural tube defects. The majority of dysraphic defects can be detected on foetal anomaly ultrasound.

Dysraphic abnormalities of the neural axis include:

- Anencephaly
- Encephalocoele
- Craniorachischisis
- Neurenteric cyst
- Myelomeningocoele
- Lipomyelomenigocoele
- Diastematomyelia
- Myelocystocoele
- Spinal dysraphism
- Failure of the caudal neuropore to close properly can result in a spectrum of spinal abnormalities

The least severe of these abnormalities is known as spina bifida occulta—in these patients a bony deficit of the posterior elements of the spine occurs but often does not result in any clinical findings and may be discovered incidentally on imaging. It is thought to affect up to 5% of the population.

Sometimes there is an overlying cutaneous abnormality such as a dimple, sinus, skin discolouration or a tuft of hair. In these patients an underlying defect such as tethered cord, cord lipoma, dermoid cyst or diastomatomyelia (split or duplicated cord) is more likely.

If a cystic herniation of the meninges without any neural tissue through the bony defect occurs this is known as a meningocoele. Much more commonly the spinal cord, cauda equina or spinal roots herniate in addition to the meninges; this is known as a myelomeningocoele **(Figs. 14.115A to E)**. The degree of neurological impairment of the neonate with myelomenigocoele should be assessed; bladder and bowel dysfunction is common. Surgery to return the neural tissue into the spinal canal should occur as soon as possible after birth; this does not improve neurological function but aims to reduce the risk of CNS infection. These children will require long-term multidisciplinary follow up. Myelomeningocoeles are associated with a range of other CNS abnormalities such as hydrocephalus (80% requiring CSF diversion surgery) and type II Chiari malformation.

Cranial Dysraphism

Cranial dysraphism is much less common than spinal dysraphism and is a result of erroneous closure the anterior neuropore. The most severe of this is anencephaly in which all or a large part of the cranium is absent.

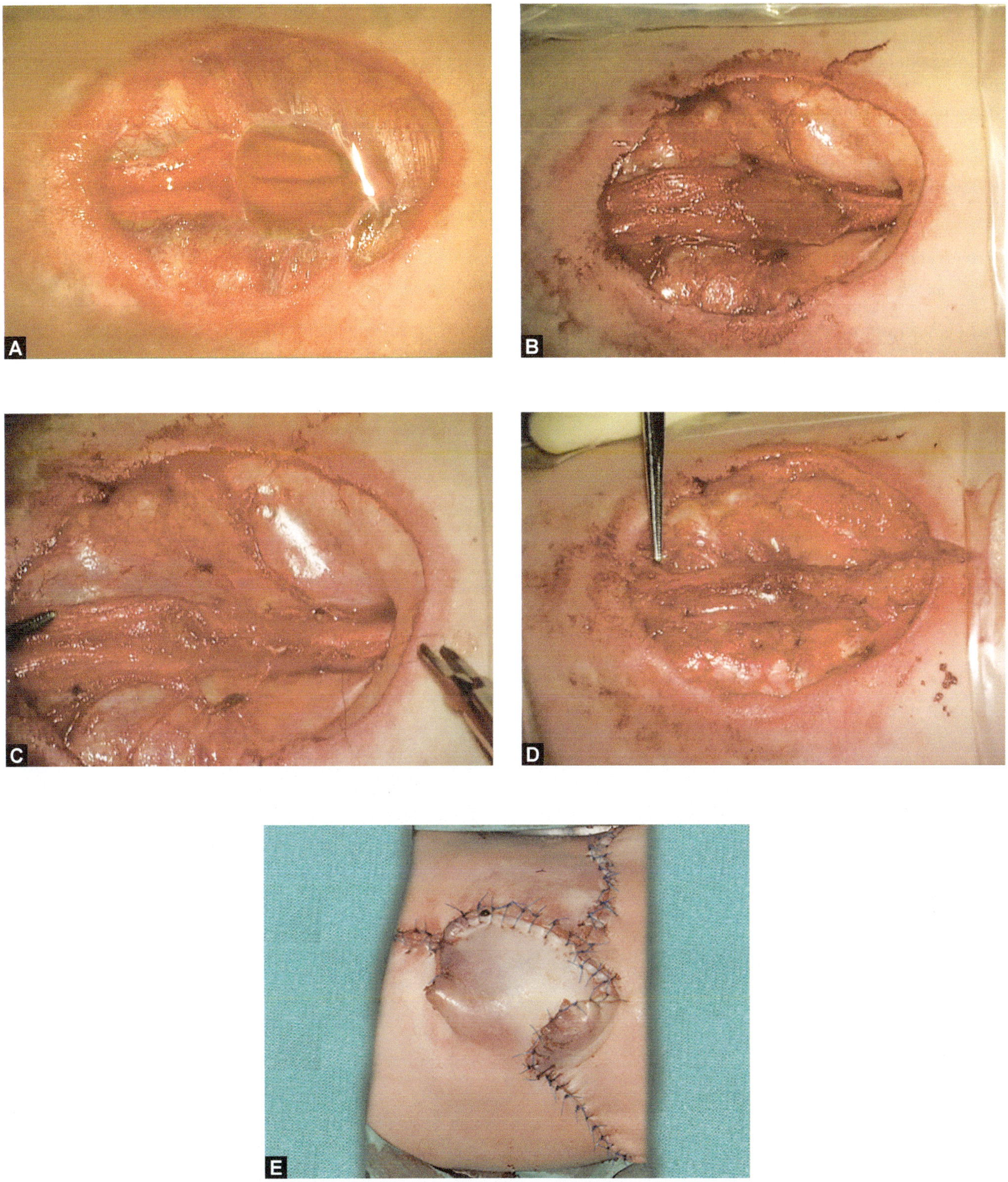

Figures 14.115A to E (A) A large thoraco-lumbar myelomeningocoele is shown. The neural placode is seen in the centre and the rootlets of the cauda equina can be visualised under the junctional tissue which represents arachnoidal tissue; (B) The junctional tissue has been removed from the neural placode and the skin margin. The dura is represented by the "white" tissue lying to either side; (C) The distal cord has been neuralated restoring it to an anatomical cylindrical structure; (D) The dura mater has been dissected free and closed over forming a water tight CSF closure; (E) Rotational skin flaps were utilised for closure due to the large defect.

Anencephalic fetuses have an absent cranial vault, most are stillborn, and the remainder die shortly after birth.

Congenital encephalocoeles are extensions of the cranial contents through a defect in the skull. As with spinal dysraphism, meningocoeles may occur which do not contain neural tissue. Encephalocoeles contain brain tissue and occur most commonly in the midline with the herniation point located between the occipital region through to the basifrontal region. The most common location is the occipital region of the skull, with the second most common location being through the skull base at the anterior cranial fossa.

They are generally skin covered abnormalities. They may be asymptomatic or present with neurological deficits, seizures or hydrocephalus.

Several associated genetic syndromes have an association with encephalocoeles including Meckel Gruber syndrome and Walker-Warburg syndrome.

The tissue within the encephalocoele is often not functional and the treatment is surgical excision of dysplastic cerebral tissue and removal of the sac **(Figs. 14.116A to D)**.

CNS TUMOURS IN CHILDHOOD

Brain tumours are the second most common type of childhood cancer; every week 10 children and young people are diagnosed with a brain tumour in the United Kingdom.

A large variety of pathologically diverse tumours can occur in the CNS. The classic consideration of tumour biology; benign versus malignant is not an appropriate dichotomisation when considering CNS tumours. Slow growing, histologically "benign" tumours can infiltrate extensively into neural and surrounding vascular structures making excision impossible. Furthermore, transformation of slow growing tumours to more aggressive histological tumour types can occur over time.

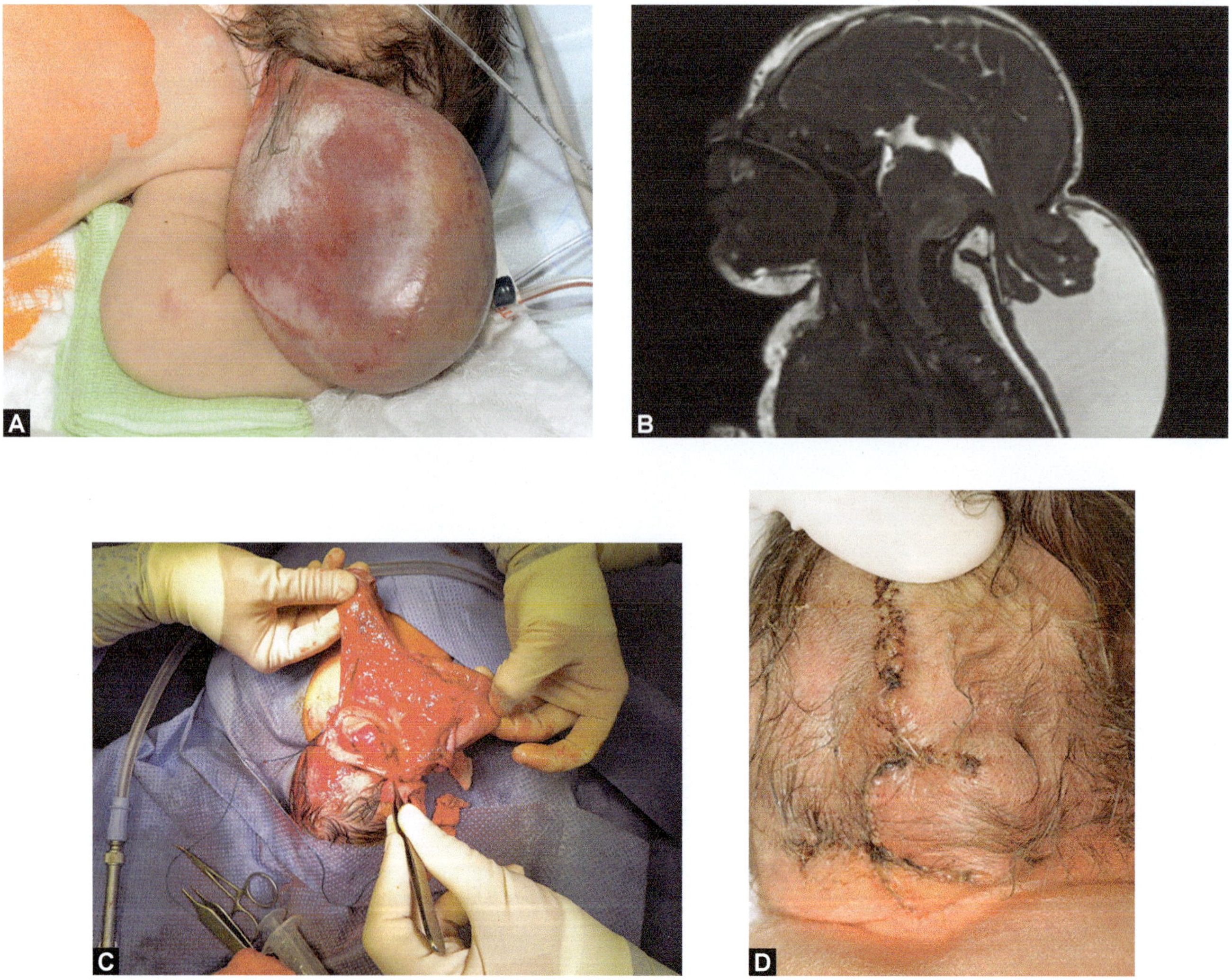

Figures 14.116A to D (A) A large occipital encephalocoele is noted; (B) MRI reveals a large CSF filled sac with herniation of occipital cortex into the sac; (C) At operation dysplastic occipital cortex was excised; (D) The sac was excised and skin closure completed.

As such tumours are generally considered on a grading scale by the World Health Organisation (WHO) ranging from grade 1 to 4. Grade 1 and 2 tumours are often considered low grade and grades 3 and 4 high grade.

There is increasingly a shift within neuro-oncology to define tumour types not only by the histopathology but also by genetic/molecular makeup. The most recent update of the WHO classification of CNS takes this into account.

Tumours have differing presentations based on location within the CNS and the age of the child. The following text provides a brief overview of the more common diagnoses of paediatric central nervous system tumours. We have described them in relation to anatomical location within the neuroaxis.

The management of CNS tumours is multidisciplinary and includes neurosurgeons, oncologists, radiation oncologists, neuropathologists and neuroradiologists.

Posterior Fossa Tumours

Tumours of the posterior fossa can present in a number of ways. Obstruction of CSF flow pathways causes hydrocephalus resulting in features of raised intracranial pressure. Disturbed function due to local effects of the tumour may result in cranial nerve palsies, long tract signs, impaired eye movements, pupillary abnormalities, tremor and vomiting. Cerebellar dysfunction results in ataxia, nystagmus, intention tremor, dysmetria and dysarthria.

Medulloblastomas **(Figs. 14.117A and B)** are the most common type of high grade (Grade 4) posterior fossa brain tumour. It is now recognized that there are 4 genetically characterized sub types of medulloblastoma. Treatment includes maximal safe resection followed by post-operative chemo- and radiotherapy tailored to patients' circumstances.

Pilocytic astrocytomas **(Figs. 14.118A and B)** are one of the most common neoplasms of childhood. They are

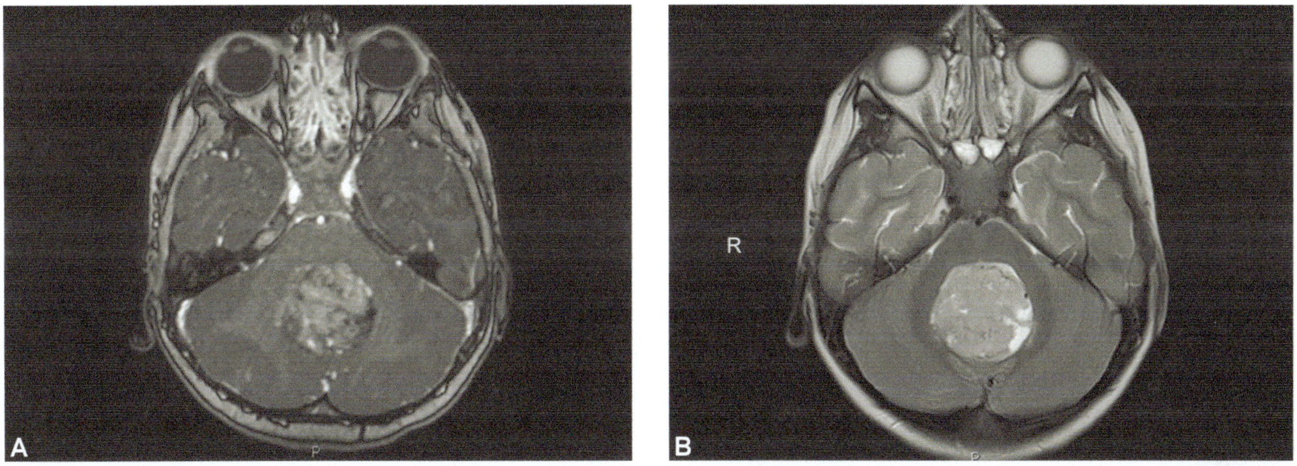

Figures 14.117A and B (A) T1 post Gad axial MRI reveals a heterogeneous mass within the fourth ventricle; (B) T2 MRI delineates the abnormality clearly from the neural tissue of brainstem and cerebellum.

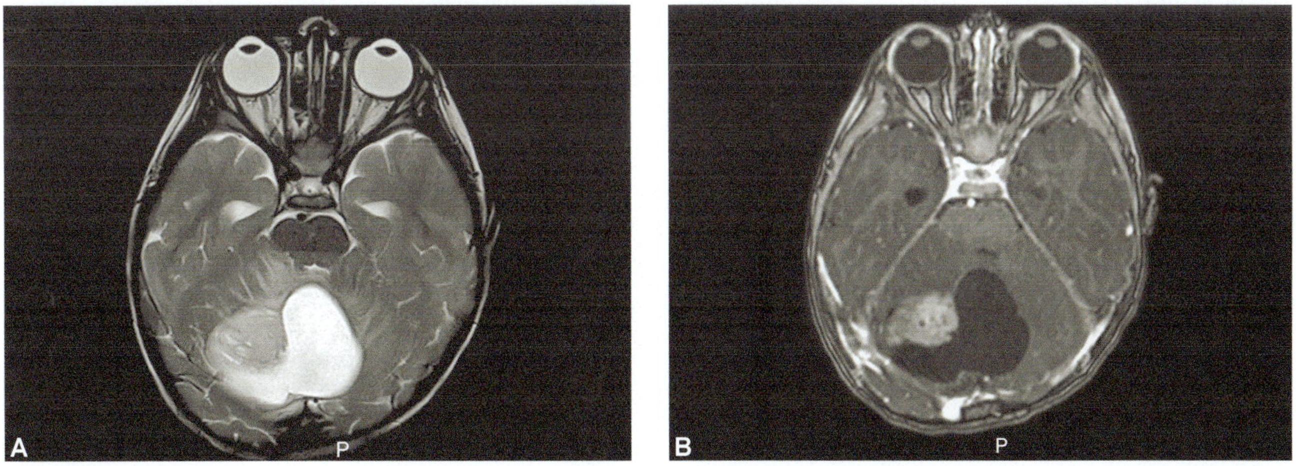

Figures 14.118A and B (A) Pilocytic astrocytoma demonstrated on T2 MRI, note solid nodule with associated cyst with same intensity as CSF. Note effacement of the fourth ventricle; (B) T1 post Gad MRI of same lesion. Note uniform enhancement of solid tumor nodule.

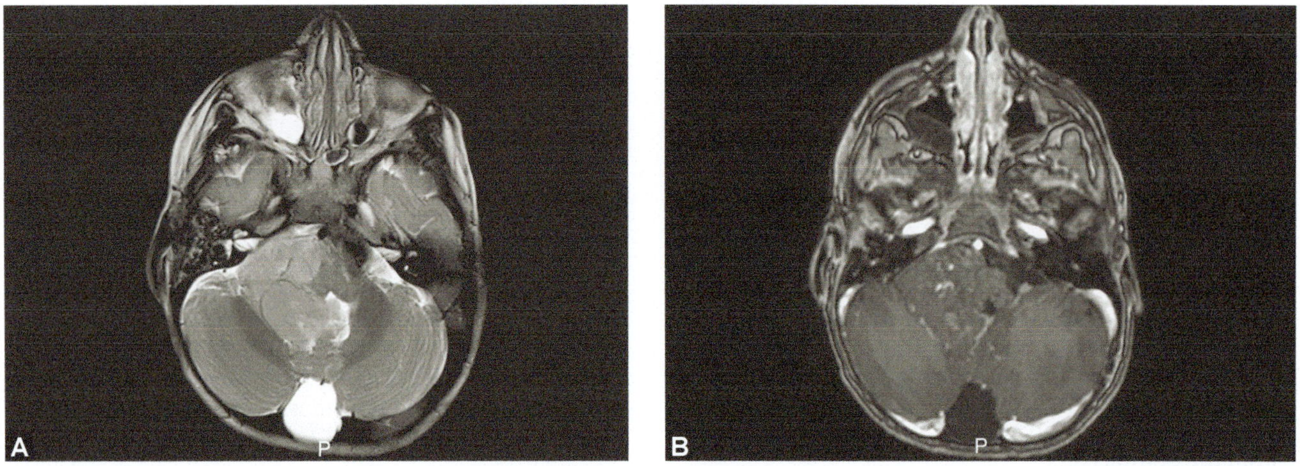

Figures 14.119A and B (A) T2 MRI reveals lesion within the fourth ventricle extending out of the foramen of Luschka and displacing the medulla oblongata to the left (B) T1 post Gad reveals patchy enhancement and tissue density similar to surrounding neural structures.

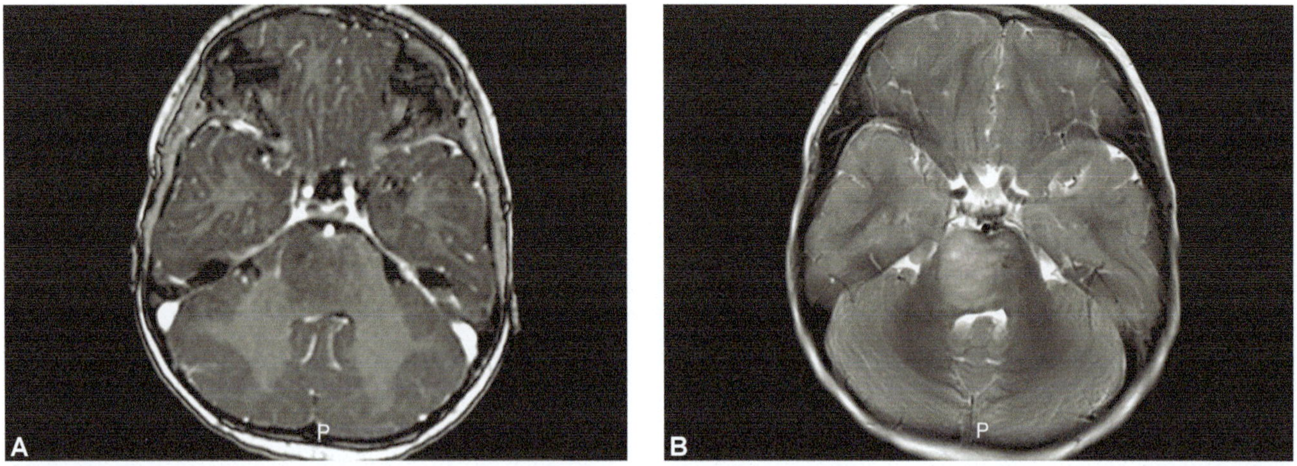

Figures 14.120A and B (A) T1 post Gad MRI reveals a lesion in the pons, this is difficult to delineate from normal brain tissue. This is diffuse intrinsic pontine glioma (B) T2 MRI reveals hyperintensity of the diffuse lesion.

WHO grade 1 tumours that can grow very slowly and cure can be achieved with surgery alone.

Ependymomas **(Figs. 14.119A and B)** occur most commonly in the posterior fossa but can also occur supratentorially. The extent of surgical resection is the single most important determinant of outcome. The use of post-operative chemotherapy is not clear. Radiotherapy is often utilised after surgical resection.

Other paediatric tumours of the posterior fossa include atypical teratoid/rhabdoid tumour (ATRT) and diffuse intrinsic pontine glioma (DIPG) **(Figs. 14.120A and B)**, both of which carry a grave prognosis.

Supratentorial

In addition to features of raised intracranial pressure, supratentorial tumours present with seizures and disturbed function related to the cortical area affected. Frontal lobe tumours cause contralateral face, leg or arm weakness and expressive dysphasia if the dominant hemisphere is affected. Parietal tumours can result in sensory disturbance, visual field defects, neglect and apraxias as well as problems with recognition, reading and counting.

Common supratentorial tumours in children are astrocytic tumours, embryonal tumours and choroid plexus tumours **(Figs. 14.121A and B)**.

Sellar Region Tumours

The sellar region contains the pituitary stalk and gland, the optic apparatus, arterial vessels of the circle of Willis, midbrain and diencephalon and upper cranial nerves, base of the frontal and medial temporal lobes.

Tumour in this location can cause a wide variety of symptoms when considering the potential disruption to these structures.

Endocrine dysfunction due to pituitary compression can manifest as short stature, failure to thrive, precocious puberty, diabetes insipidus as well as non-specific symptoms such as lethargy.

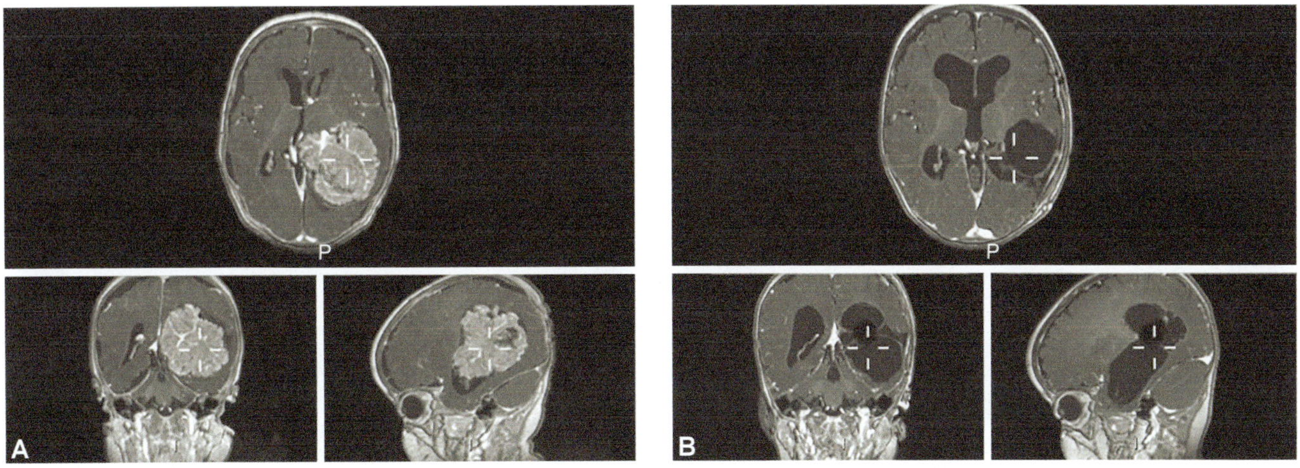

Figures 14.121A and B (A) Choroid plexus papilloma evident on preoperative T1 post Gad. The tumour has a frondular appearance and occupies the trigone of the left lateral ventricle; (B) Postoperative T1 post Gad reveals complete excision of the tumour.

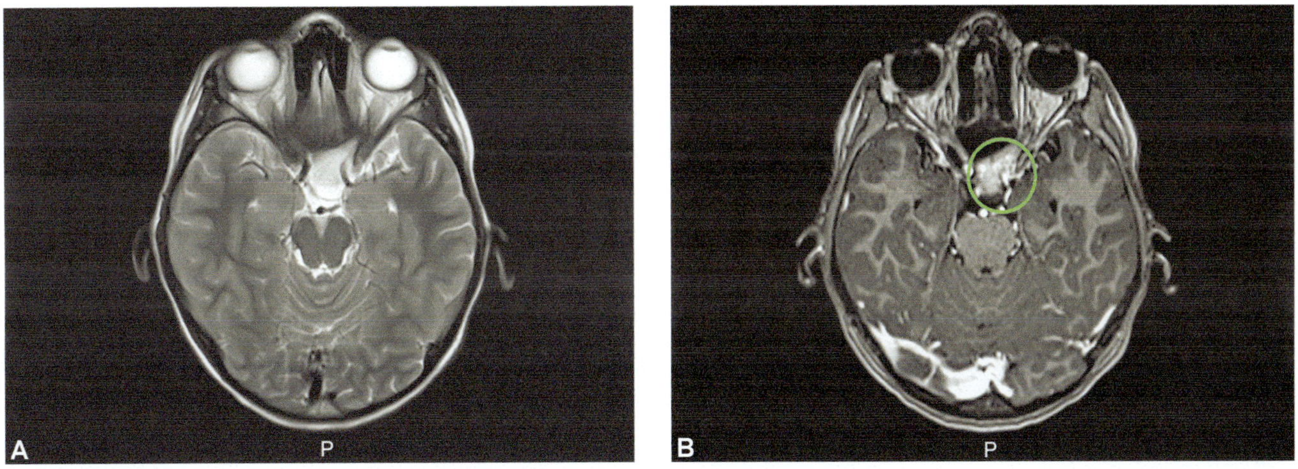

Figures 14.122A and B (A) T2 MRI reveals poorly visualized lesion along optic apparatus; (B) T1 post Gad reveals a uniform enhancing lesion along the left optic nerve extending back to the chiasm (green circle).

Visual field defects occur due to compression or disruption of the optic apparatus pre-, post- infra- and supra-chiasmatically.

Hydrocephalus can result from obstruction of CSF by tumour extending into the third ventricle.

Psychobehavioural impairments occur due to diencephalic/limbic system disruption.

Optic Pathway Gliomas

These tumours can involve any part of optic pathway and surrounding diencephalon. Histologically they are usually pilocytic astrocytomas. These tumours are often associated with NF1 when they portend a more indolent course (Figs. 14.122A and B).

Tumours that do exhibit clinical or radiological progression may require intervention. Given the location with surrounding eloquent cerebrum surgery carries significant risk of incurring neurological damage and as such chemotherapy has become the first line of treatment for these lesions.

Craniopharyngioma

These are histologically benign epithelial tumours. They are thought to arise from epithelial cell remnants along the embryological migration path of the anterior pituitary lobe pouch and the hypophyseal pharyngeal duct/craniopharyngeal duct (Figs. 14.123A and B).

Complete surgical resection is difficult to achieve without inflicting damage to structures in this region resulting in long-term impairments. The benign, slow growing pathology makes them less susceptible to chemotherapeutic and radiation modalities. Treatment of these tumours poses great challenges.

Intracranial Germ Cell Tumours

Germ cell tumours (Figs. 14.124A and B) arise from primordial germ cell rests resulting in a diverse group of histological tumours. They tend to occur in deep midline areas, notably the pineal region and the sellar region. Six subtypes are recognized but they are generally classified

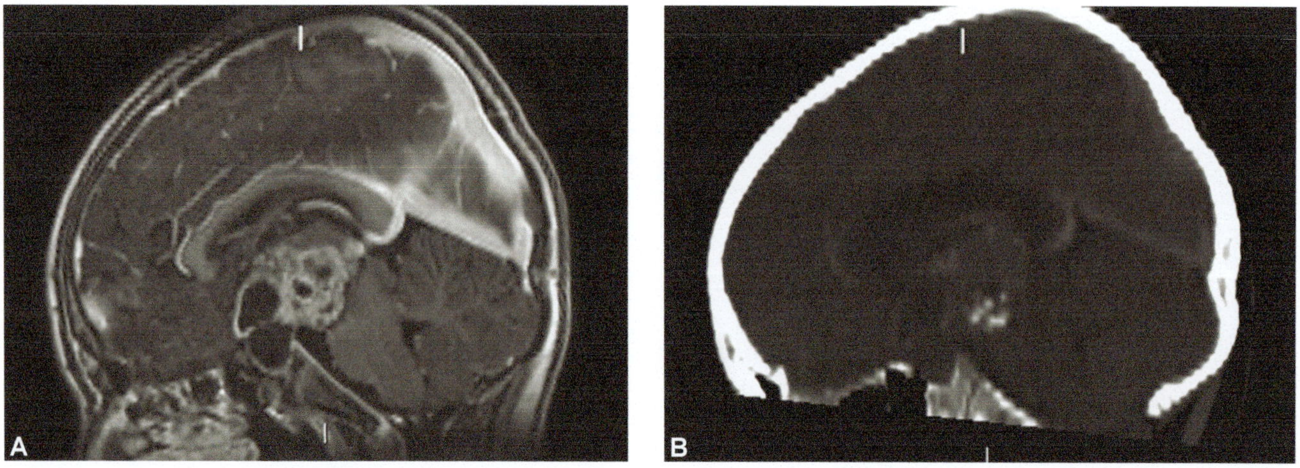

Figures 14.123A and B (A) T1 post Gad sagittal MRI showing cystic lesion with enhancement of the cyst walls in the suprasellar lesion. This is craniopharyngioma (B) Mid sagittal CT of same patient reveals calcification within the lesion a feature characteristic of craniopharyngioma.

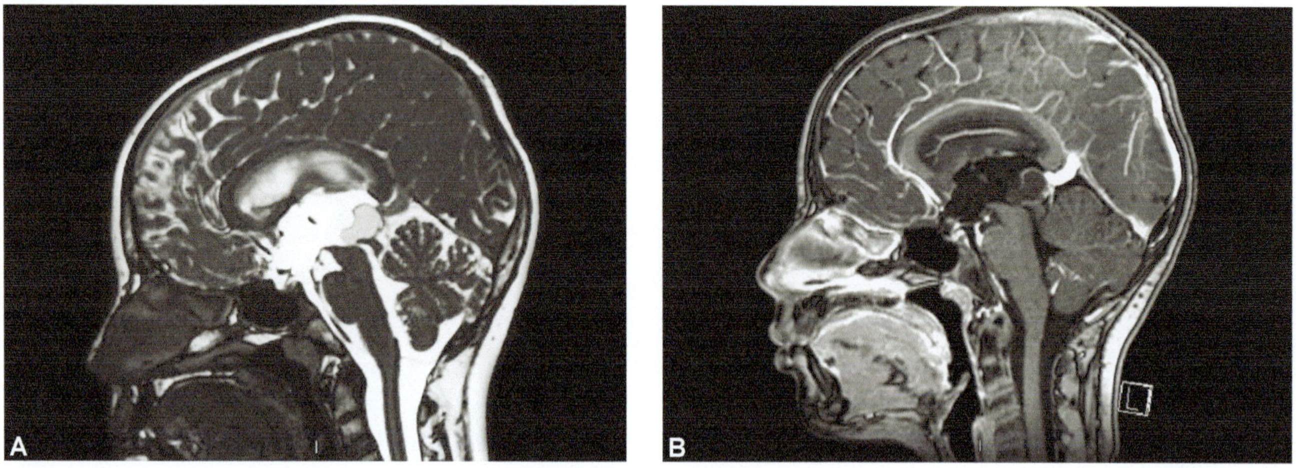

Figures 14.124A and B (A) T2 sagittal MRI demonstrating pineal region germinoma; (B) T1 post Gad reveals peripheral enhancement of the lesion.

into germinomas, non-germinomatous germ cell tumours and teratomas. Tumours with mixed types occur.

Pineal region tumours may lead to hydrocephalus with obstruction at the cerebral aqueduct. Parinaud syndrome may arise.

These tumours may secrete alpha-fetoprotein or beta-human chorionic gonadotrophin. These can be detected in the serum and CSF and not only provide diagnosis but allow evaluation of treatment

CSF DISORDERS IN CHILDHOOD

Cerebrospinal fluid disorders are amongst the most commonly treated paediatric neurosurgical disorders. The classic model states that CSF is produced predominantly by the choroid plexus. The normal pathway of flow proceeds from the lateral ventricles, though the foramen of Munro into the third ventricle then through the cerebral aqueduct into the fourth ventricle. CSF exits the fourth ventricle via the foramen of Magendie and Luschka into the cerebral sub-arachnoid space and spine. CSF is finally absorbed back into the blood stream via the arachnoid villi situated along the superior sagittal sinus.

A universally accepted definition of hydrocephalus has not been agreed however an inadequate passage of CSF from the point of production to the point of absorption in the systemic circulation broadly covers most conditions considered under the umbrella of hydrocephalus.

Whilst the classic model is an over simplification of a much more complex system it provides a good scaffold to consider treatment options for disturbances in CSF disorders.

Hydrocephalus can result from many underlying pathological processes. Examples of some of these processes are illustrated in **Figure 14.125**.

Before fusion of the cranial sutures hydrocephalus presents with enlarging head circumference crossing centiles **(Graph 14.1)** tense fontanelle, dilated scalp veins, lid retraction and failure of upgaze. Irritability, impaired

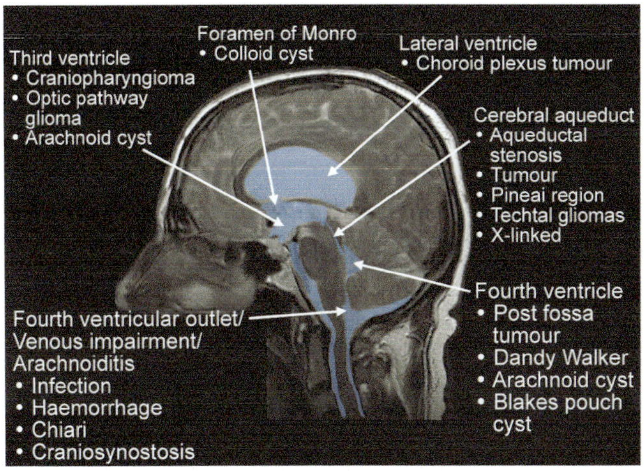

Figure 14.125 MRI investigation of hydrocephalus.

conscious level, vomiting and cardiorespiratory abnormalities may occur. If the onset is more gradual regression of developmental milestones and failure to thrive may become evident.

Older children with closed sutures will present with signs and symptoms raised intracranial pressure including headache, vomiting, papilloedema, deterioration of conscious level, 6th nerve palsies and gait disturbance.

The mainstay of investigation of hydrocephalus is imaging with either CT or MRI. Ultrasound is a useful investigation in the infant with an open fontanelle.

Treatment of hydrocephalus requires consideration of underlying aetiology and the clinical status. Temporary cannulation of the ventricular system with an external ventricular drain will provide an immediate relief of elevated ICP and is used in emergent situations.

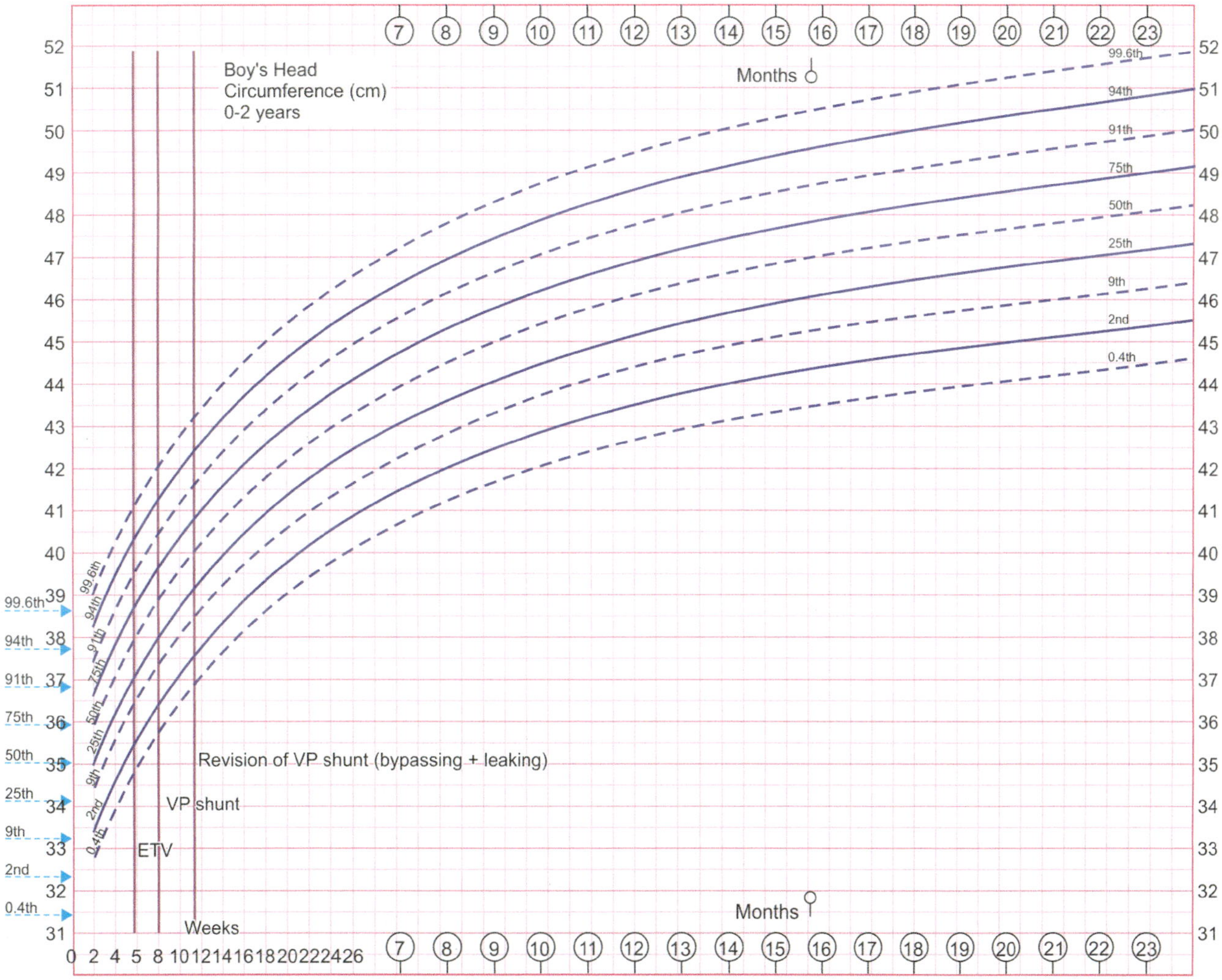

Graph 14.1 A boy's head circumference chart. In this patient a rapid increase in OFC is noted in the first 6 weeks of life. A diagnosis of hydrocephalus was established. He was initially treated with an ETV at 6 weeks of age. This was not successful as evidenced by progressing macrocrania. As such a VP shunt was sited at 8 weeks of age. OFC started to fall. However 3 weeks post op the child became irritable and OFC was noted to increase. VP shunt revision revealed a blocked proximal catheter, this was revised. The child has remained well since that time and OFC have stopped jumping centiles

TABLE 14.6 Adapted from Kulkarni et al. Predicting who will benefit from endoscopic third ventriculostomy compared with shunt insertion in childhood hydrocephalus using the ETV Success Score.

Score	*Age*	*Aetiology*	*Previous shunt*
0	< 1 month	Post-infectious	Yes
10	1–6 months		No
20	6 months – 1 year	myelomeningocoele, intraventricular haemorrhage, non-tectal brain tumour	
30	1 year – < 10 years	aqueductal stenosis, tectal tumour, other	
40	>10 years		
50			

(*Source:* J Neurosurg Pediatr. 2010 Oct; 6(4):310-5)

Permanent CSF diversion using a shunting system is the mainstay of long term treatment. This consists of a ventricular catheter, a valve and a distal catheter which may be placed into the peritoneum (most common) **(Figs. 14.126A to F)**, pleura or atrium of the heart. CSF shunts are mechanical devices that have a failure rate necessitating surgical revision; failure rates of 40% at 1 year, 50% at 2 years and 60% at 4 years are generally reported figures.

The presence of foreign material provides a potential nidus for infection, shunt infection rates are in the order of 10% necessitating shunt removal and antibiotic treatment.

The use of endoscopic third ventriculostomy **(Figs. 14.127A to F)** is becoming increasingly popular in appropriate cases. In this procedure, an endoscope is inserted into the third ventricle and a stoma is created in the floor of the third ventricle to allow an alternative CSF flow pathway. The success of an endoscopic third ventriculostomy is determined by a number of factors; these have been studied extensively by Kulkarni et al. and a predictive score has been devised. The age of the child, aetiology of the hydrocephalus and presence of previous shunt are assigned a score and the total is expressed as a percentage reflecting the likelihood of ETV success. These factors are shown in **Table 14.6**.

Success of ETV may be improved with choroid plexus coagulation **(Figs. 14.128A to C)** as reported by the Uganda series.

As described above a number of different causes of hydrocephalus exist. Certain cause merit further discussion

Post-haemorrhagic Hydrocephalus

One of the most common causes of hydrocephalus in preterm child is intraventricular haemorrhage. Haemorrhage arises from the germinal matrix which is a highly vascular region from which developing cells of the CNS migrate, it usually involutes before the 36th gestational week. The severity of the haemorrhage is classified by the Papile grading system from being confined to within the germinal matrix (grade 1) to intraventricular haemorrhage with intraparenchymal extension (grade 4). The higher the grade of haemorrhage, the worse the prognosis and the more likely that hydrocephalus requiring permanent treatment will be required. Intraventricular haemorrhage should be suspected in any preterm infant with a rapidly increasing head circumference. Haemoglobin should be monitored as substantial blood loss into the ventricular system may occur.

Treatment of these premature children poses a very difficult challenge due to their size; VP shunt generally cannot be sited in a child weighing under 1.5 kg. They also have an immature immune system rendering the use of foreign materials a considerably higher infection risk.

Temporising surgical interventions in the form of a subgaleal shunt **(Figs. 14.129A to H)** have proven useful to allow a time period for growth prior to permanent treatment with a VP shunt. In this procedure the lateral ventricle is cannulated with a catheter that drains into the subgaleal space. CSF drains into this space for a period of several weeks. Ultimately the subgaleal space shuts down and the subgaleal shunt fails. At this juncture the child has developed and can now proceed to a VP shunt.

Arachnoid Cysts

These are congenital, non-neoplastic abnormalities that may occur throughout the central nervous system; the lining may actively secrete CSF. They are often an incidental finding on imaging performed for other reasons and do not require treatment. They may, however, present with features of raised intracranial pressure, hydrocephalus, seizures or with an acute deterioration due to haemorrhage associated with the cyst.

Anatomical locations vary, sylvian fissure arachnoid cysts are the most common (40%), followed by post fossa (25%), suprasellar (10%), quadragemminal cistern (10%) and interhemispheric (10%) and cerebral convexity (5%) **(Figs. 14.130A to O)**.

Treatment may involve cyst aspiration, endoscopic fenestration, open surgical excision excision/fenestration or cystoperitoneal shunting.

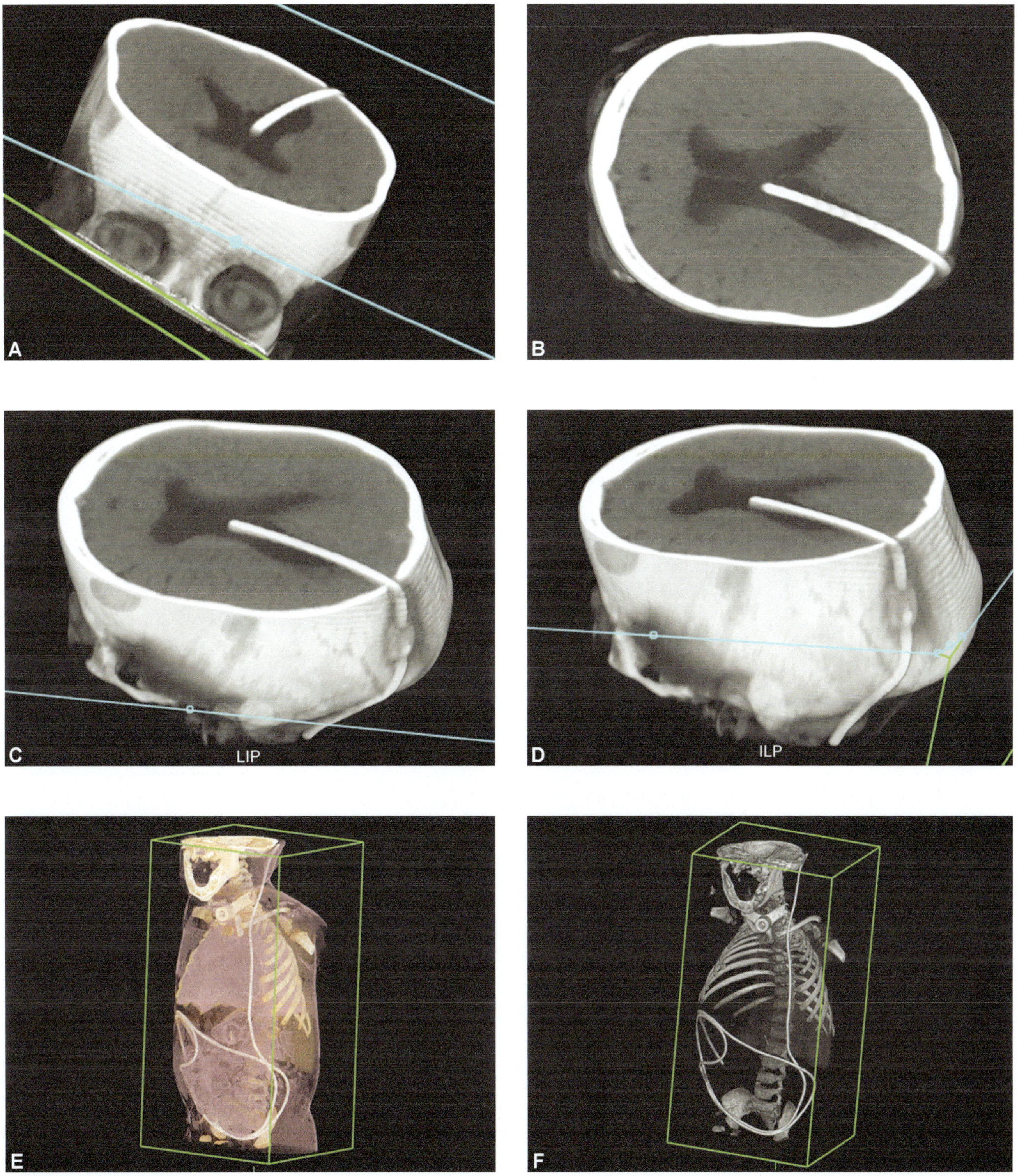

Figures 14.126A to F Ventriculo-peritoneal shunt in situ. The shunt is made up of 3 components: (A) The ventricular catheter sited in the lateral ventricle; (B) The ventricular catheter sited in the lateral ventricle; (C) The valve that regulates the flow of CSF from the ventricle to the peritoneum; (D) The distal catheter that connects the valve to the peritoneal cavity; (E) The distal catheter that connects the valve to the peritoneal cavity; (F) The distal catheter that connects the valve to the peritoneal cavity.

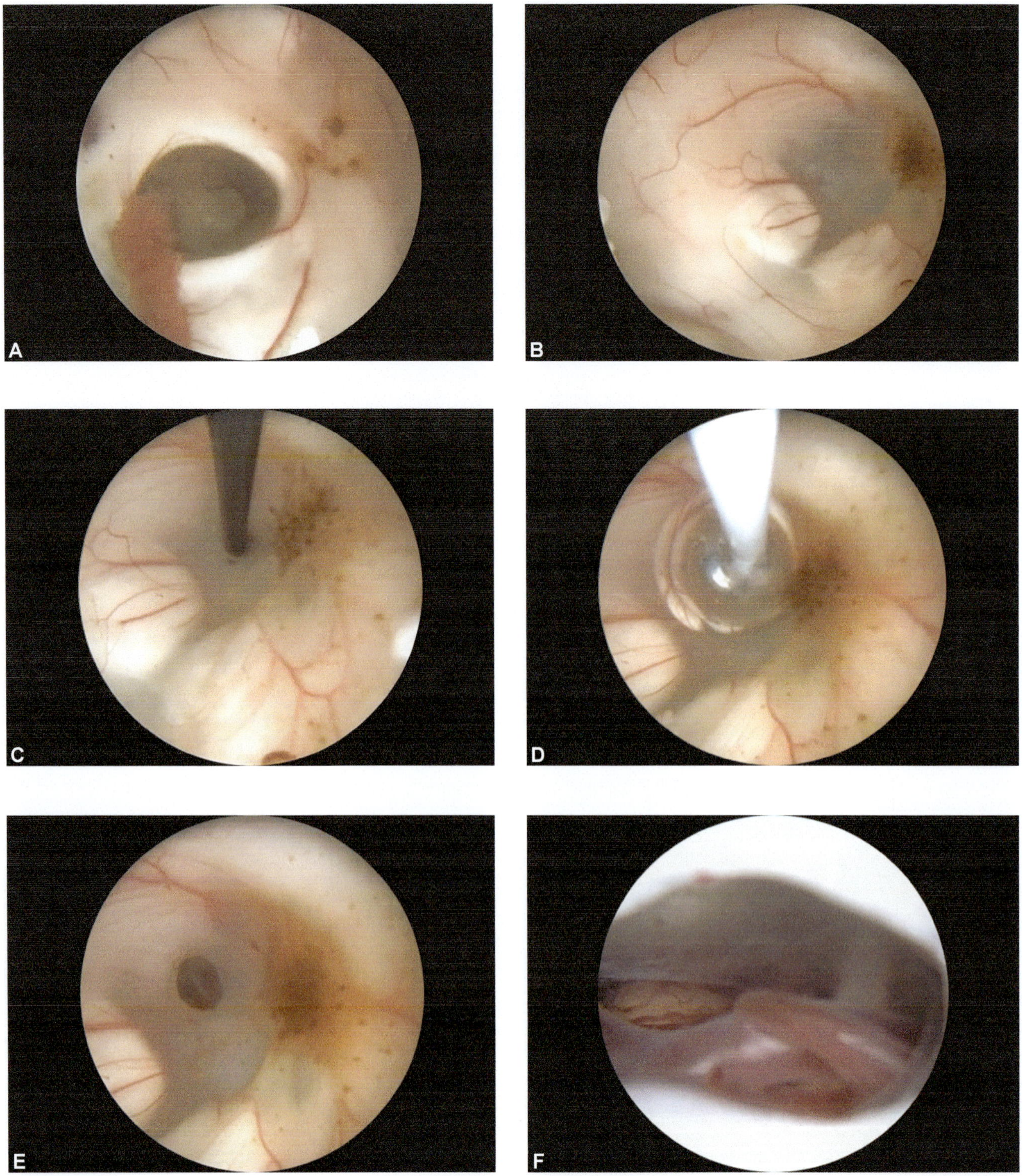

Figures 14.127A to F (A) Endoscope is in the right lateral ventricle. The foramen of Munro is visualised with choroid plexus entering the foramen; (B) The endoscope has been advanced through the foramen of Munro into the third ventricle. The floor of the third ventricle is visualized with the two mammillary bodies evident; (C) The stoma/ventriculostomy is created by perforating the floor anterior to the mammillary bodies; (D) The stoma is widened using a balloon; (E) Stoma is now evident; (F) The endoscope is advanced through the stoma to visualize the prepontine space. The anterior pontine surface is visualized with the basilar bifurcation and right posterior cerebral artery. The third nerve is visualized just below the posterior cerebral artery.

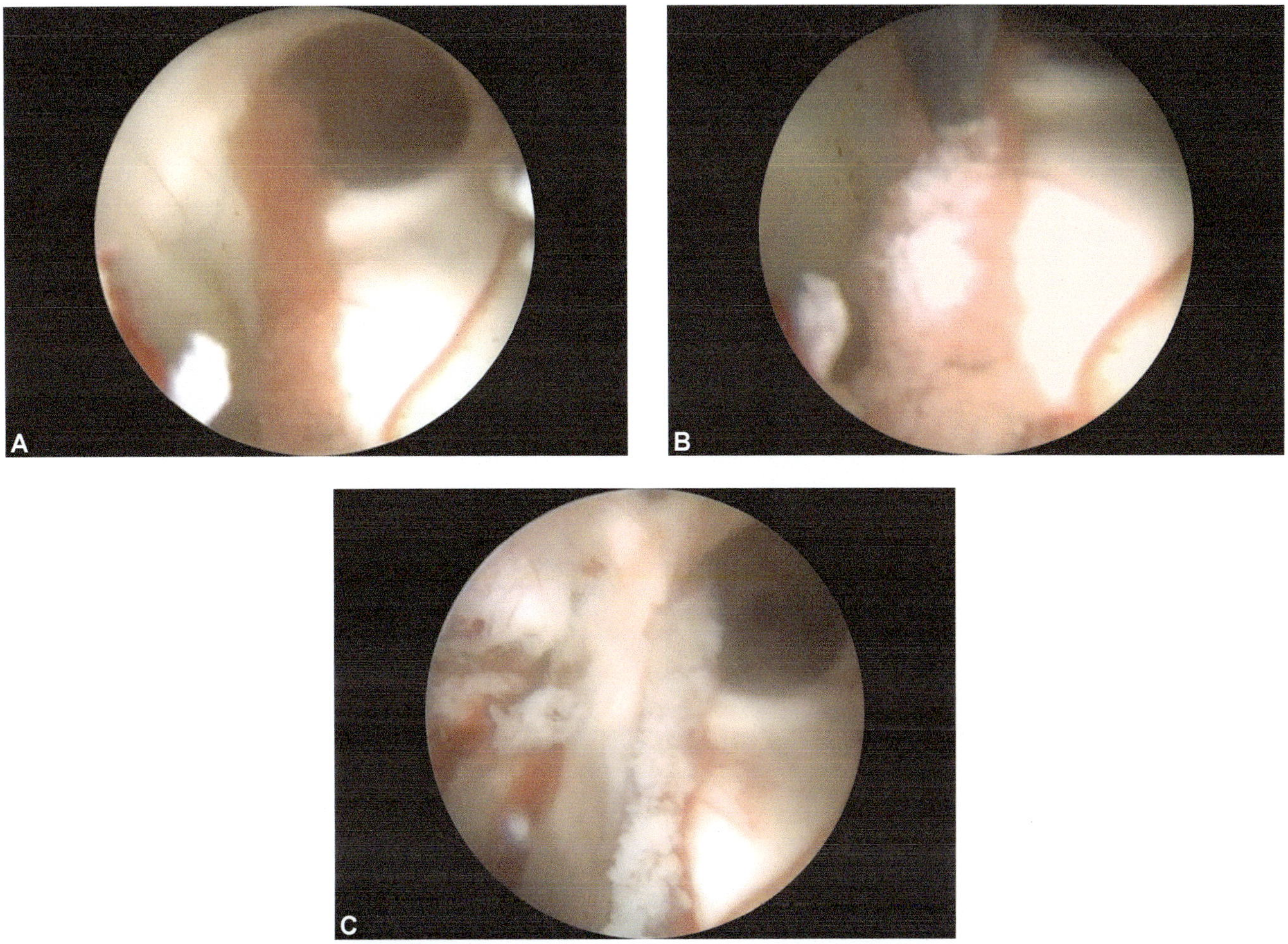

Figures 14.128A to C (A) The choroid plexus in the right lateral ventricle is visualized leading to the foramen of Munro; (B) Monopolar coagulation is utilised to coagulate the choroid plexus. *Note* thechange in colour from red to white as the choroid plexus is coagulation; (C) The choroid plexus has been completely coagulated in the right lateral ventricle.

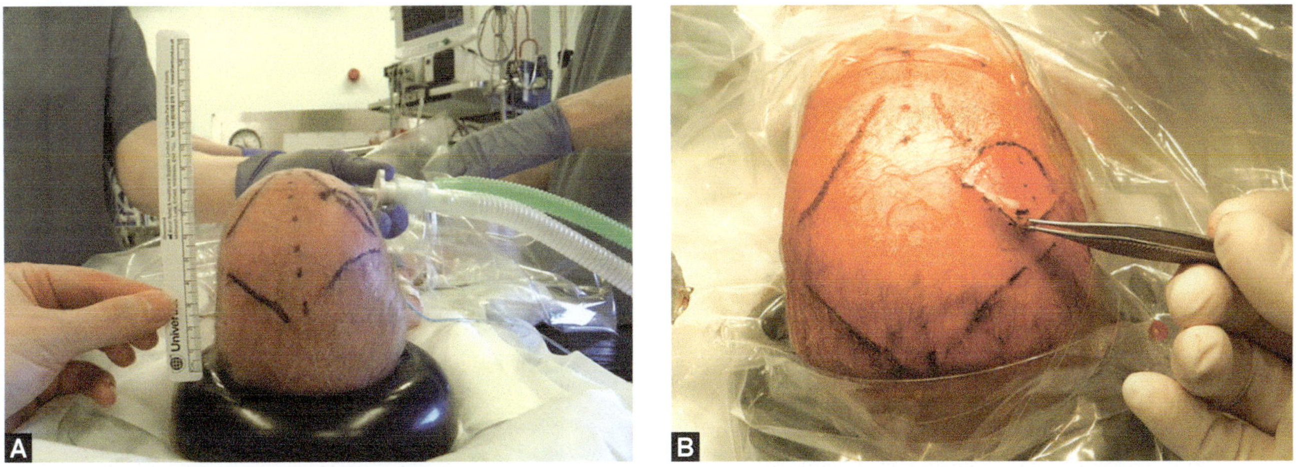

Figures 14.129A and B (A) Insertion of subgaleal shunt in premature child. Midline and fontanelle have been marked out; (B) Curvilinear incision over the anterior border of the anterior fontanelle.

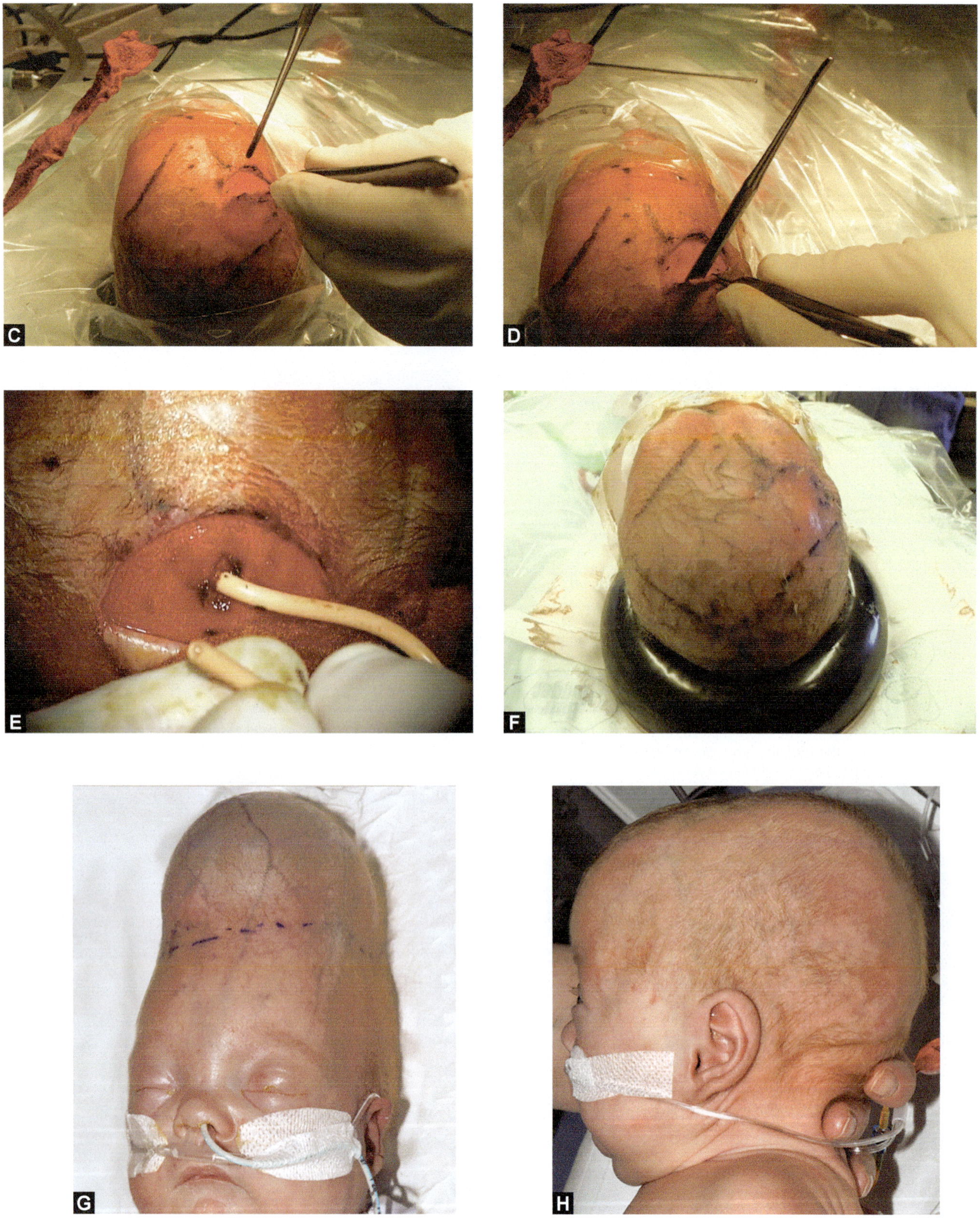

Figures 14.129C to H (C) the subgaleal pocket is created by blunt dissection (D) the subgaleal pocket is created by blunt dissection (E) the lateral ventricle is cannulated with a catheter (F) after closure the fontanelle is sunken after drainage of CSF (G) 4 weeks post procedure; the expansion of the subgaleal space with CSF (H) 8 weeks post procedure the subgaleal space has c with resolution of the cystic space. The child went onto have a VP shunt sited.

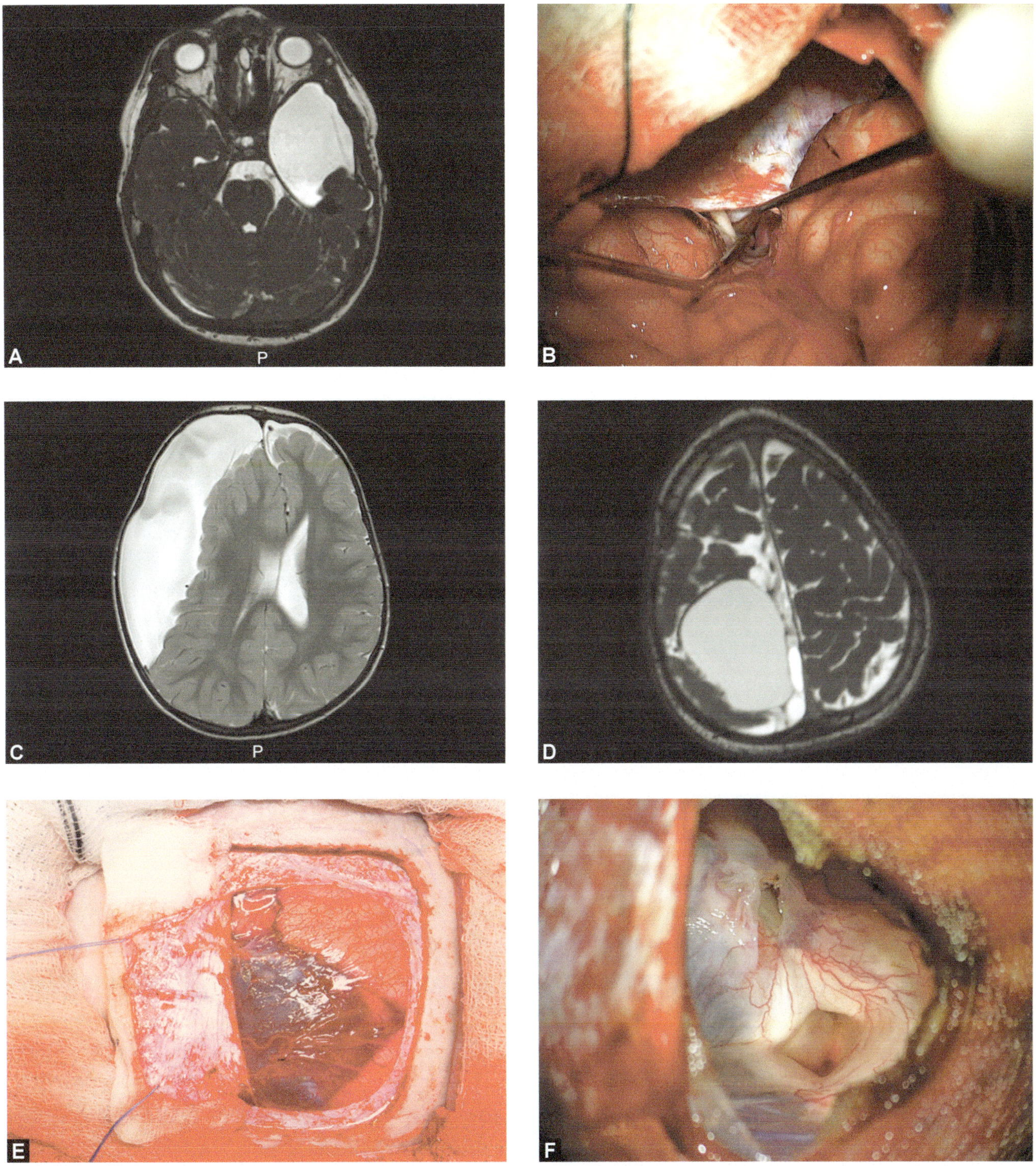

Figures 14.130A to F (A) Left sylvian arachnoid cyst (B) Fenestration of cyst in medial aspect. Atrophic temporal lobe is to the right and frontal lobe to the left. The right optic nerve and internal carotid artery are visualised at the sucker and the dissector (C) Right hemispheric arachnoid cyst (D) Right interhemispheric arachnoid cyst (E) Operative photo of (D) showing surface of cyst with cortex laterally (F) The superior cyst wall of (D) has been excised and the inferior wall has been fenestrated.

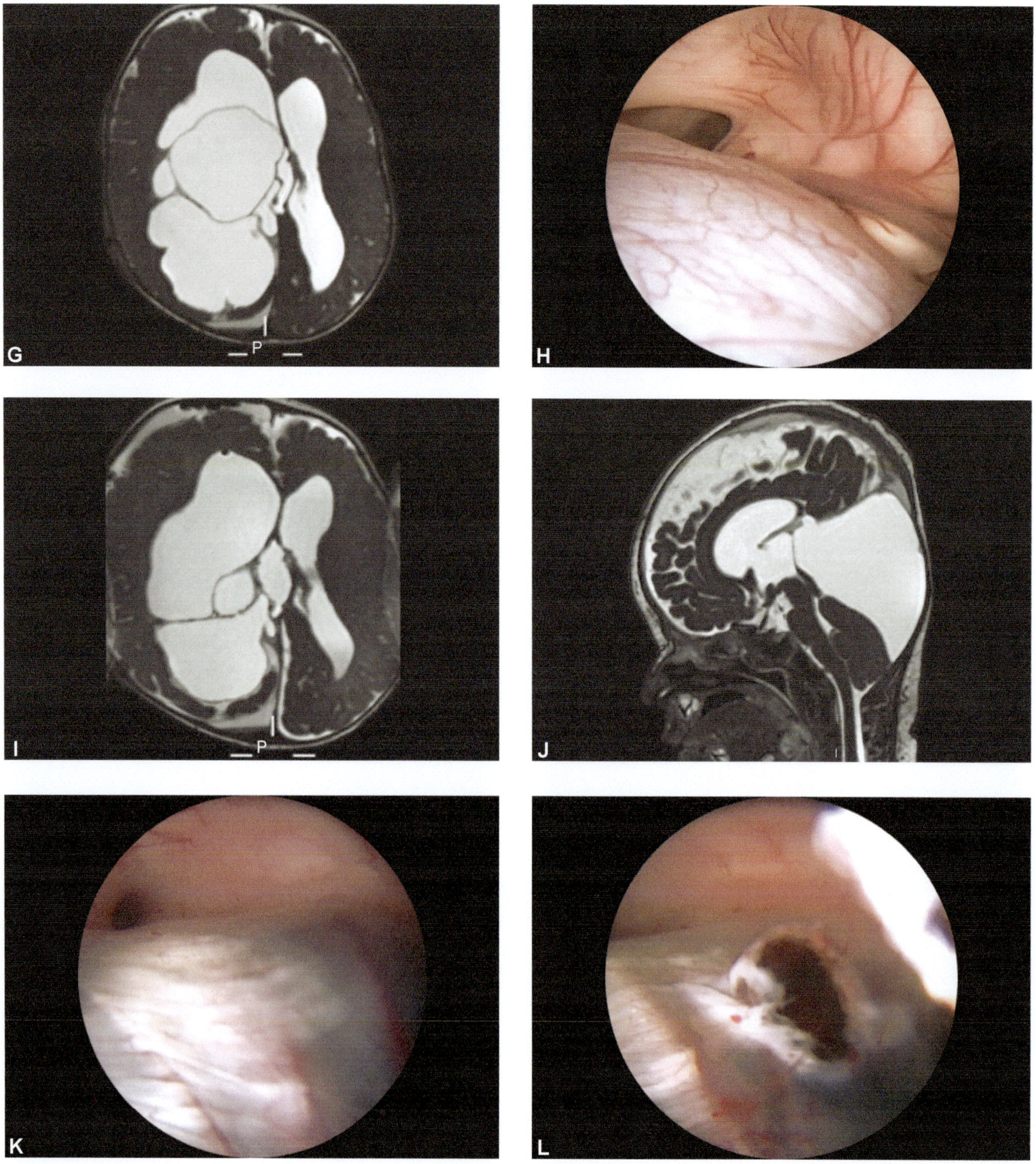

Figures 14.130G to L (G) Intraventricular arachnoid cyst in the right lateral ventricle; (H) Endoscopic view of the cyst in (G) with the foramen of Munro visualized at 10 o'clock position; (I) Post operative MRI revealing reduction of cyst post endoscopic cyst fenestration; (J) Large quadrigeminal arachnoid cyst causing aqueduct compression with resultant hydrocephalus. *Note* the downward displacement of the cerebellum; (K) Endoscopic view of the posterior wall of the third ventricle revealing the arachnoid cyst. The cerebral aqueduct is visualized; (L) Fenestration of the arachnoid cyst allows cyst decompression and resolution of hydrocephalaus.

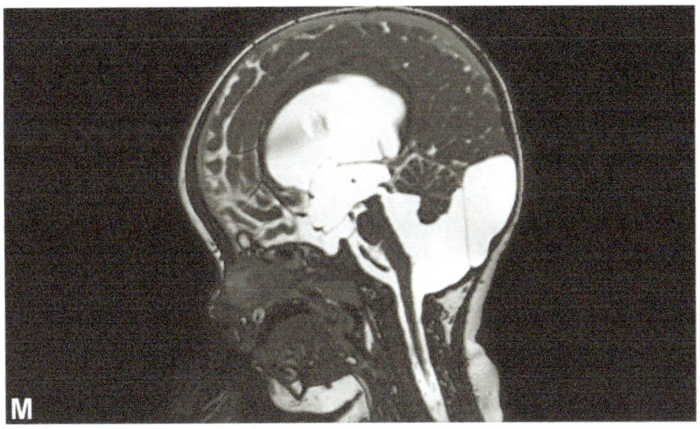

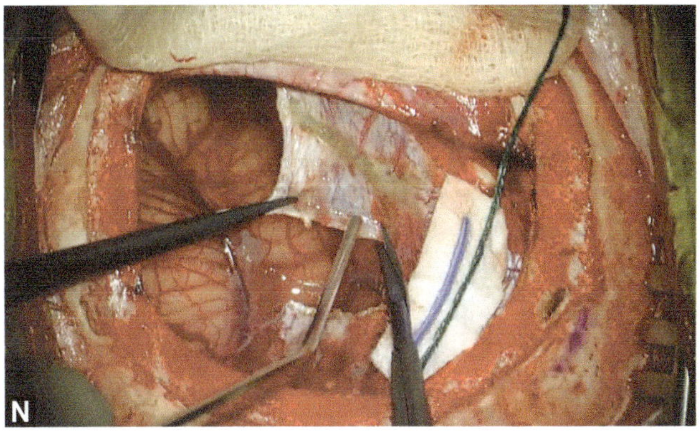

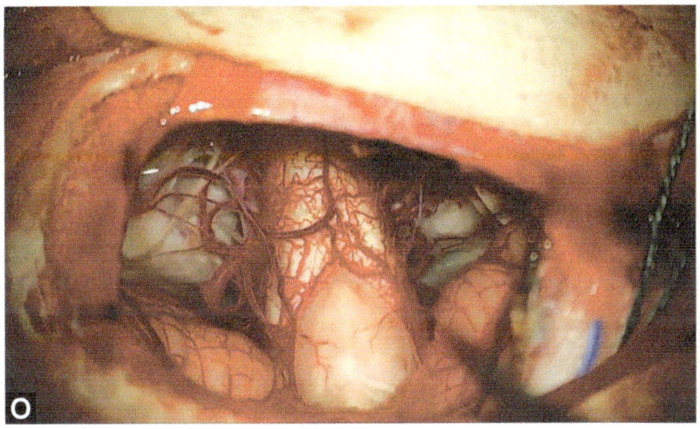

Figures 14.130M to O (M) Posterior fossa arachnoid cyst. The cyst wall can be seen running vertically dorsal to the cerebellum; (N) Open craniotomy and cyst excision of (M). The cyst wall is being excised (O) after complete cyst (M) excision the upper cervical cord, medulla oblongata and 4th ventricle are visualized. Cerebellar tissue is noted laterally. The ascending rootlets of the spinal accessory nerve are also visualized on the left side of the picture.

CHAPTER 15

Accidental Poisoning in Childhood

Krishna M. Goel

INTRODUCTION

In spite of the many educational programmes aimed at prevention and exposure to a poison, it remains the most common childhood accident. Paediatric poisonings involve three distinct groups. Poisoning in children is quite different from that in adults. Children have their special physiology and react differently to medicament as well as to poisoning. Most childhood poisoning is accidental. Other causes include intentional overdose, drug abuse, iatrogenic and deliberate poisoning. The drugs most commonly involved in childhood poisoning are paracetamol, ibuprofen, orally ingested creams, aspirin, iron preparations, cough medicines and the contraceptive pill.

The first group involves children between the ages of 1 and 4 years. Certain children with strong oral tendencies can be identified as especially likely to poison themselves by ingesting tablets or liquids, particularly if these have a pleasing colour or are held in an attractively labelled bottle or container. Poisoning can also occur by absorption through the skin and infiltration of the eyes, that is, ocular instillation. Patterns of accidental poisoning have been changing in recent years, and while the number of children poisoned remains high, the incidence has shown a fall. There has also been a steady decline in the number of childhood deaths from poisonings. This is related to a number of factors including changes in prescribing practices, educational programmes directed towards prevention, safer packaging of dangerous drugs and safe storage of household products. Child-resistant containers have been particularly effective in reducing the incidence of death from the ingestion of prescription drugs by children. In a recent survey, the rank order of poisons, drugs and chemicals, which have most often led to hospital admission, were petroleum distillates, antihistamines, benzodiazepines, bleach and detergents, and aspirin. However, when the ratios of fatalities to ingestion were analysed to give an index of the practical danger of the substances to which children are exposed, the rank order became cardiotoxic drugs, tricyclic antidepressants, sympathomimetic drugs, caustic soda and aspirin. While noxious plants such as laburnum, foxglove and deadly nightshade continue to be ingested, a fatal outcome is exceedingly rare. Ingestions of petroleum distillates, insecticides such as chlorinated hydrocarbons and organic phosphates and weed killers, particularly paraquat, are commoner in rural areas. Lead poisoning is in a different category as it usually involves ingestion over a fairly prolonged period.

The second distinct population involved in paediatric poisoning is the young 12–17-year-old adolescents who ingests medications in a suicide attempt or gesture. They may require full psychiatric and social assessment. Also on the increase is 'glue sniffing', that is, inhalation of various solvent vapours and ingestion of 'ecstasy' and alcohol used by teenagers as recreational drugs.

The third group is the result of parents deliberately giving drugs to their children as a manifestation of Munchausen syndrome by proxy. The most common poison given by parents is table salt, anticonvulsants and opiates. In certain situations, identifying poisoning can be difficult even when the doctor is alert to the possibility.

The possibility of poisoning should always be entertained in acute illness of sudden onset if no cause is immediately discoverable, particularly if it is associated with vomiting and diarrhoea or if there are marked disturbances of consciousness or behaviour.

ASSESSMENT OF THE CHILD AND MANAGEMENT

The primary assessment of the child with acute poisoning is essential for management. This should be done under the following acronym: *'ABCDE'*.

Assessment of Airway

If at first, it is found that the child can speak or cry, this means that the airway is patent and breathing is taking place and the circulation is satisfactory. Otherwise, due to the effects of poisoning, there could be loss of consciousness and this would lead to a complete or partial closure of airway. However, if the airway is not patent, it should be made patent and intubation may be needed.

Assessment of Breathing

The child's respiratory rate should be checked. Tissue oxygen saturation must also be measured by pulse oximeter, and arterial blood gas estimation should be done. There are a number of ingested substances, such as opiates, which can induce respiratory depression. In such cases, oxygen should be given if there is respiratory depression, cyanosis or shock. However, if the child is breathing inadequately, support should be given by bag-valve mask with oxygen or by intermittent positive pressure ventilation in an intubated patient.

Ventilatory Support

Ventilatory support is indicated if:

- Respiratory rate is less than 10/min
- There is poor air entry despite airway being fully open
- There is arterial blood gas measurement showing falling PO_2 and rising partial pressure of carbon dioxide (PCO_2).

BOX 15.1 AVPU assessment.

A = Awake or alert

V = Responds to verbal stimuli (voice)

P = Responds only to pain

U = Unresponsive to all stimuli—sternal pressure, supraorbital ridge pressure or pulling hair

Children in categories P and U will require careful assessment of their airways and ventilation. Intubation should be considered before carrying out gastric lavage or instilling activated charcoal in categories P and U.

Assessment of Conscious Level

A rapid assessment of conscious level should be made by assigning AVPU method (alert, responds to voice, responds to pain, unresponsive) (**Box 15.1**). A detailed assessment can be made by using the Glasgow Coma Scale and Children's Coma Scale (**Table 15.1**).

Assessment of Circulation

It is important to assess the adequacy of the child's circulation by the following:

- Heart rate, rhythm and pulse volume
- Blood pressure

TABLE 15.1 Glasgow coma scale and children's coma scale.

Glasgow coma scale (4–15 years)		***Children's glasgow coma scale (<4 years)***	
Response	***Score***	***Response***	***Score***
Eye opening		**Eye opening**	
Spontaneously	4	Spontaneously	4
To verbal stimuli	3	To verbal stimuli	3
To pain	2	To pain	2
No response to pain	1	No response to pain	1
Best motor response		**Best motor response**	
Obeys verbal command	6	Spontaneous, obeys verbal command	6
Localises to pain	5	Localises to pain or withdraws to touch	5
Withdraws from pain	4	Withdraws from pain	4
Abnormal flexion to pain (decorticate)	3	Abnormal flexion to pain (decorticate)	3
Abnormal extension to pain (decerebrate)	2	Abnormal extension to pain	2
No response to pain	1	No response to pain	1
Best verbal response		**Best verbal response**	
Oriented and converses	5	Alert, babbles, coos words to usual ability	5
Disoriented and converses	4	Less than usual words, spontaneous irritable cry	4
Inappropriate words	3	Cries only to pain	3
Incomprehensible sounds	2	Moans to pain	2
No response to pain	1	No response to pain	1
Normal aggregate score = 15			

Peripheral perfusion: Signs of poor end-organ perfusion (shock) are as follows:

- Poor peripheral pulses
- Capillary refill more than 2 seconds
- Blood pressure may be normal in compensated shock
- Low blood pressure indicates decompensated shock.

Disability: Assessment of neurological function.

It is assessed by assessing the level of consciousness, posture, pupillary size and reaction to light.

Exposure

Exposure is essential for external evidence of drug abuse and drug-induced rashes (e.g. purpura, swelling of lips or tongue, urticaria, angio-oedema). Record child's core and toe temperatures, because a number of drugs can cause hypothermia or hyperthermia.

POISON IDENTIFICATION AND ASSESSMENT OF THE SEVERITY OF OVERDOSE

Subsequent to the primary assessment of the child, it is important to evaluate the severity of the overdose. To assess this properly, obtain the identity of the substance ingested, the amount taken and the length of time the child has been in contact with poison. Sometimes, it may not be easy to gather this vital information.

However, some clues about the substance taken may be obvious from the clinical signs noted during full clinical examination. An essential part of substance identification is to match the collection of signs and associated toxic effects and the offending substance as shown in Table 15.2.

KEY LEARNING POINT

Base line monitoring in a child with poisoning

- ECG
- Pulse oximetry
- Core temperature
- Blood glucose level
- Urea and electrolytes and liver function tests
- Blood gases

KEY LEARNING POINT

Amount of poison ingested

- Some idea of the maximum amount of substance that could have been ingested can be obtained from counting the number of remaining tablets or volume of liquid left in the bottle and details on packaging.
- Poison identification: Routine toxicology screen on urine sample.
- Substances identifiable: Benzodiazepines; cocaine metabolites; methadone; opiates and amphetamines.

SALICYLATE POISONING

Accidental poisoning in children due to salicylate has recently declined in incidence following the packaging of salicylates in child-resistant containers and also because aspirin is being superseded by paracetamol and ibuprofen as the standard domestic analgesic. Salicylate is usually ingested in the form of aspirin (acetylsalicylate). This is often accidental but sometimes it has been given with therapeutic intent by the parents and even by the doctor. On occasion, oil of wintergreen (methyl salicylate), a source of the salicylate, has been swallowed, one teaspoonful of which contains

TABLE 15.2 Drugs and associated toxic effects.

Associated signs	*Possible toxin*
Tachypnoea	Salicylates, CO, theophylline
Bradypnoea	Opiates, barbiturates, sedatives
Convulsions	Phenothiazines, aminophylline, salicylates, tricyclic antidepressants, insecticides, organophosphate
Hyperpyrexia	Salicylates, aminophylline, amphetamine, cocaine
Hypothermia	Aminophylline, barbiturates, phenothiazines
Hypertension	Aminophylline, amphetamines, cocaine
Hypotension	Tricyclic antidepressants, aminophylline, barbiturates, benzodiazepines, opiates, iron, phenytoin
Large pupils	Atropine, cannabis, carbamazepine, tricyclic antidepressants
Small pupils	Opiates, phenothiazines, organophosphate, insecticide
Tachycardia	Aminophylline, antidepressants, amphetamine, cocaine
Bradycardia	Tricyclic antidepressants, digoxin
Metabolic acidosis	Salicylates, ethanol, CO

the equivalent of 4 g aspirin. Salicylate poisoning can also occur due to local application of ointments containing salicylic acid.

Prognosis in the individual case is determined much more by the interval of time, which has elapsed between the ingestion of the poison and the start of treatment than by the level of the serum salicylate. Indeed, the toddler can show signs of severe poisoning with a salicylate level as low as 2.9 mol/L (40 mg/100 mL). With the exception of rheumatic fever, juvenile idiopathic arthritis and Kawasaki disease, aspirin should not be prescribed for infants or children.

Clinical Features

Rapid, deep, regular, acyanotic breathing or air hunger is almost diagnostic of salicylate poisoning. Cases may be misdiagnosed as 'pneumonia', but the hyperpnoea of salicylate poisoning is quite different from the short, grunting respirations of pneumonia. Other early manifestations of salicylate poisoning such as nausea and vomiting are difficult to evaluate in infants and toddlers and they cannot often describe tinnitus.

The hyperpnoea has a double aetiology. It is initially due to direct stimulation by salicylate of the respiratory centre of the brain. The resultant overbreathing washes out CO_2 from the lungs and causes a respiratory alkalosis with a blood pH (>7.42) and lowered PCO_2 (<33 mmHg). This alkalotic phase is commonly seen in adults with salicylate poisoning, but in young children, an accelerated fatty-acid catabolism with excess production of ketones results in the early establishment of a metabolic acidosis. By the time, the poisoned toddler reaches hospital; the blood pH is usually reduced (<7.35). The compensatory hyperventilation of metabolic acidosis adds to the stimulant effect of salicylate on the respiratory centre so that the overbreathing of the poisoned child is often extreme. A side effect of salicylate overdosage is fever. There is also a disturbance of carbohydrate metabolism and the blood glucose may rise above 11.1 mmol/L (200 mg/100 mL) although not above 16.7 mmol/L (300 mg/100 mL). Hypoglycaemia has been recorded but it is uncommon.

The child with salicylate poisoning shows peripheral vasodilatation until near to death. Death is preceded by cyanosis, twitching, rigidity and coma.

Case Study

A 12-year-old boy presented with severe ichthyosis. He was treated with topical 2% salicylic acid in simple cream applied to the whole body twice daily. The salicylate concentration was increased to 5% on day 3 of treatment and 10% on day 5. On day 8, he developed symptoms of salicylate toxicity. His blood salicylate level was 3.3 mmol/L. Topical salicylate treatment was stopped. Intravenous fluids and bicarbonate were given and complete clinical and biochemical recovery was achieved after 2 days.

This case illustrates that significant percutaneous salicylate absorption can occur especially when salicylate preparations of increasing strength are used.

Diagnosis: Salicylate poisoning in dermatological treatment

PARACETAMOL POISONING

While paracetamol accounts for a large number of attempted suicides in adults (either alone or in combination with dextropropoxyphene as 'Co-proxamol'), cases of serious poisoning are rare in children. Paediatric paracetamol elixir preparations ingested by the toddler very rarely cause toxicity. Nonetheless, as it can lead to irreversible liver and renal failure, any child who may have ingested in excess of 150 mg/kg should be admitted to hospital without delay. However, children are more resistant to paracetamol-induced hepatotoxicity than adults. Doses of less than 150 mg/kg will not cause toxicity except in a child with hepatic or renal disease.

Clinical Features

The first symptoms are nausea, vomiting and abdominal pain. Evidence of severe liver damage may be revealed by elevated levels of aspartate aminotransferase and alanine aminotransferase over 1,000 IU/L and of renal impairment by a plasma creatinine concentration over 300 μmol/L (3.4 mg/100 mL). Liver damage is maximal 3–4 days after ingestion and may lead to encephalopathy, haemorrhage, hypoglycaemia, cerebral oedema and death.

IBUPROFEN POISONING

Ibuprofen is a nonsteroidal anti-inflammatory drug (NSAID). It is available over the counter and is commonly ingested by children and adolescents.

Clinical Features

Most children after oral overdose remain asymptomatic but a few may require hospitalisation. They may manifest with bradycardia, apnoea, hypotension, severe metabolic acidosis, polyuria with renal failure, coma and seizures.

ACUTE IRON POISONING

Iron poisoning is most common in childhood and is usually accidental. The most common source of acute iron poisoning is ferrous sulphate tablets, which the young child mistakes for sweets. Other ferrous salts such as gluconate or succinate are less dangerous. If over 20 mg/kg of elemental iron has been taken, toxicity is likely. Over 150 mg/kg may be fatal.

Clinical Features

The symptoms are vomiting, diarrhoea, haematemesis, melaena, pallor and metabolic acidosis. Hypotension, coma and hepatocellular necrosis occur later. Coma and shock indicate severe poisoning.

Case Study

A 2½-year-old Asian boy was found with an empty bottle of ferrous sulphate tablets (ferrous sulphate 200 mg containing 65 mg of ferrous iron). His mouth was full of crushed pieces of tablets. His mother took him to a nearby paediatric accident and emergency unit. On examination, he had a temperature of 98.4°C, pulse 120/min, respiratory rate 40/min and blood pressure 90/55 mmHg. He was drowsy; otherwise clinical examination was unremarkable. Hb 12.6 g/dL, WBC and platelet count normal, urea and electrolytes and lever function tests normal, HCO_3 16 mmol/L and serum iron 60 µmol/L.

He was gastric lavaged with normal saline. He was treated with desferrioxamine 15 mg/kg per hour intravenously for 24 hours. He did not develop any complications and recovered unscathed. He was discharged home, well, 2 days later.

BARBITURATE POISONING

Barbiturates are now much more commonly prescribed and are rarely encountered as a cause of poisoning in children.

Clinical Features

In most cases, the child is only extremely drowsy. Infrequently, the child may be flushed, excited, restless and may vomit. In severe cases, the child is comatose, unresponsive to stimuli and may show respiratory depression with cyanosis, absence of deep reflexes and circulatory failure with hypotension. Skin blisters mainly over bony prominences, peripheral nerve pressure lesions may develop.

POISONING BY ANTIHISTAMINES

The common prescribing of antihistamines of many kinds has, unfortunately, increased the opportunity for young children to ingest them accidentally. There is sometimes a fairly long period between ingestion and the appearance of symptoms. These include anorexia, progressive drowsiness, stupor and signs such as incoordinated movements, rigidity and tremor. Poisoning by two of the newer nonsedating antihistamines, terfenadine and astemizole may predispose to the development of ventricular tachyarrhythmias.

Poisoning by Tricyclic and Related Antidepressants

The frequent use of antidepressants for adults has resulted in a rapidly increasing incidence of their accidental ingestion by children. Moreover, these drugs are prescribed for enuresis in children and the fact that overdosage can produce dangerous toxic effects in a young child is not sufficiently stressed to the parents.

Clinical Features

Mildly affected children develop drowsiness, ataxia, abnormal postures, agitation when stimulated, dilated pupils and tachycardia. Thirst and nystagmus have been present in some cases. In severely affected children, convulsions may be followed by coma and severe respiratory depression. Cardiac arrhythmias such as ventricular tachycardia and various degrees of heart block with profound hypotension in children are prominent and dangerous.

ATROPINE POISONING

This type of poisoning may arise from ingestion of the plant 'deadly nightshade'. It may also occur when drugs such as tincture of belladonna, atropine or hyoscine are taken accidentally or prescribed in excessive doses. Antidiarrhoeal agent Lomotil that contains diphenoxylate and atropine is toxic to some children at therapeutic dosage.

Clinical Features

The onset of symptoms is soon after ingestion, with thirst, dryness of mouth, blurring of vision and photophobia. The child is markedly flushed with widely dilated pupils. Tachycardia is severe and there may be high fever. Extreme restlessness, confusion, delirium and incoordination are characteristic. In babies, there may be gross gaseous abdominal distension. In fatal cases, circulatory collapse and respiratory failure precede death.

POISONING BY ANTIMALARIALS

The toxicities of antimalarial drugs vary according to the differences in the chemical structure of antimalarial compounds. Of the currently used antimalarials most are quinolone derivatives. The quinolone derivatives, especially quinine and chloroquine, are very toxic in overdose.

Clinical Features

The toxic manifestations are mainly due to antimalarials quinidine like actions on the heart and thus include circulatory arrest, cardiogenic shock, conduction disturbances and ventricular arrhythmias. Other clinical features are coma, convulsions, respiratory depression. Hypokalaemia is consistently present in severe chloroquine poisoning. Amodiaquine may induce side effects such as gastrointestinal symptoms, agranulocytosis and hepatitis. The main clinical manifestation of primaquine overdose is methaemoglobinaemia.

Poisoning with quinacrine may result in nausea, vomiting, confusion, convulsion and acute psychosis. The other drugs used in malaria treatment are sulfadoxine, dapsone, proguanil, trimethoprim and pyrimethamine. Most of these drugs are used in combination. Convulsion, coma and blindness have been reported in pyrimethamine overdose. Sulfadoxine can induce Stevens-Johnson syndrome. The main clinical feature of dapsone poisoning is severe methaemoglobinaemia.

POISONING BY DIGOXIN

The increasing number of older adults taking digitalis preparations in the community is resulting in accidental ingestion by children of cardiac glycosides. The most commonly involved preparation is digoxin. Children require treatment if they have ingested more than 100 μg/kg body weight. The toxic effects may not become marked for some hours and it is important to treat every case as potentially dangerous.

Clinical Features

The most striking presenting feature is severe and intractable vomiting, which is largely due to the action of digoxin on the central nervous system. Other neurological manifestations include visual disturbances, drowsiness and convulsions, which are usually delayed for several hours in their appearance. The cardiac manifestations of digoxin intoxication in a previously healthy child are exaggeration of normal sinus arrhythmia, which is a common early finding, and sinus pauses with nodal escape beats may occur. Other findings include sinus bradycardia, nodal rhythm, coupled idioventricular rhythm and complete heart block.

POISONING BY PETROLEUM DISTILLATES, INSECTICIDES AND WEED-KILLERS

Ingestion of petroleum distillates is a common childhood problem because they are readily available in most households, including developing countries where kerosene, in particular, is used for heating, cooking and lighting. Petroleum distillates (petrol, paraffin, turpentine, turps substitute, white spirit and kerosene) cause irritation of mucous membranes, vomiting and diarrhoea, when ingested, and respiratory distress, cyanosis, tachycardia and pyrexia, when inhaled. Ingestion of more than 1 mg/kg body weight will cause drowsiness and depression of the central nervous system. Children can develop symptoms up to 24 hours following ingestion. Chlorinated hydrocarbon insecticides such as DDT, dieldrin, aldrin and lindane can be absorbed through the skin and respiratory tract as well as from the gastrointestinal tract and can cause salivation, abdominal pain with vomiting and diarrhoea and central nervous system depression with convulsions. Contaminated clothing should be removed, the child washed with soap and water and convulsions treated with diazepam.

Organophosphorus insecticides such as malathion, chlorthion, parathion, phosdrin and tetraethyl pyrophosphate are cholinesterase inhibitors, which can also be absorbed from skin, lungs and intestines. The accumulation of acetylcholine in tissues causes nausea, vomiting, diarrhoea, blurred vision, miosis, headache, muscle weakness and twitching, loss of reflexes and sphincter control, and finally, loss of consciousness. Weed-killers of the paraquat type may also be absorbed through skin, respiratory tract and intestinal tract particularly when concentrated solutions of paraquat have been swallowed; children can experience a burning sensation in the mouth, nausea, vomiting, abdominal pain and diarrhoea, which may be bloody. Hours later, ulceration of the mouth, throat and gastrointestinal tract may occur. The absence of initial symptoms does not exclude a diagnosis of paraquat poisoning.

When low to moderate doses of paraquat have been ingested, the signs of kidney and liver damage may occur after 2–3 days. Both types of damage are irreversible. After 5–10 days, or very occasionally up to 14 days after poisoning, the child may develop signs of lung damage, which is almost always irreversible. When relatively large doses of paraquat are ingested, multiorgan damage and failure occurs quickly and death usually occurs within a few hours or days. Tissue damage is probably caused by local hydrogen peroxide and this might be aggravated by giving oxygen to breathe. Paraquat absorption can be confirmed by a simple qualitative urine test.

ACUTE ALCOHOL POISONING

Episodes of acute alcohol (ethanol) poisoning occur predominantly in infancy and preadolescence with peaks at ages 3 and 12 years and are commoner in boys. In the younger age group, ease of access to spirits and fortified wines allied with poor parental surveillance in the home are important factors. Household ethanol sources include perfumes, colognes, aftershaves, mouthwashes and antiseptics. In the older children, the episodes are more likely to occur outside the home, thus increasing the risks of physical danger from accidents and hypothermia. The younger infants are at risk of significant hypoglycaemia especially if they drink alcohol in the early morning after an obligate overnight fasting. The lethal dose of ethanol in children is only 3 g/kg, compared with the adult lethal dose of 5–8 g/kg.

Clinical Features

Nausea, accompanied by vomiting, ataxia and progressive loss of consciousness are the usual features. Aspiration pneumonia, hypoxic and alcoholic brain damage with cerebral oedema, hypothermia, hypoglycaemia and convulsions are not uncommon complications.

Diagnosis

This is based predominantly on history and on the finding of an elevated blood alcohol concentration. The blood glucose concentrations must be measured.

LEAD POISONING

Lead is usually ingested in small quantities over a long period and the manifestations of poisoning develop insidiously. There are various possible sources of lead such as lead-containing paint that may be used on a child's cot, flakes or paint from plasterwork or woodwork in old Victorian houses, burnt out lead batteries or swallowed pieces of yellow crayon and lead water pipes. Pica is common in children suffering from lead poisoning and is a valuable clue to the diagnosis. It is more common in children from the poorest homes. Asian mothers, mainly for cosmetic reasons, apply Surma, which contains lead sulphide, to the eyelids and conjunctivae of infants and children **(Fig. 15.1)**. It seems that an appreciable absorption of lead in these children occurs from drainage down the tear duct or from rubbing the eyes and then licking the fingers. Other sources of environmental lead contamination are the gasoline exhaust fumes of motorcars and lead in soil. An early diagnosis is extremely important in lead poisoning because, if it is left untreated, lead encephalopathy may result in death or permanent brain damage. Lead poisoning is now defined as a blood lead level equal to or greater than 10 μg/dL (0.50 μmol/L).

Clinical Features

The earliest signs such as lethargy, anorexia, vomiting and abdominal pain are too common to arouse suspicion in them, but their persistence without other discoverable cause should do so. The pallor of anaemia is a frequent and characteristic sign. Insomnia and headache frequently precede the onset of lead encephalopathy with convulsions, papilloedema and a cracked-pot sound on percussion of the skull. Radiographs of the skull may then reveal separation of the sutures **(Fig. 15.2)**. Peripheral neuropathy is uncommon in the young child but may develop with paralysis of the dorsiflexors of either the wrist or foot. Radiographs of the bones may show characteristic bands of increased density at the metaphyses **(Fig. 15.3)** but this is a relatively late sign and, therefore, of limited diagnostic value. Excess aminoaciduria is a common manifestation of renal tubular damage and glycosuria may also occur. Renal hypertension has also been reported. Elevated blood lead levels are also associated with neurodevelopmental abnormalities, behavioural disturbances, learning disabilities, and defects in fine and gross motor development.

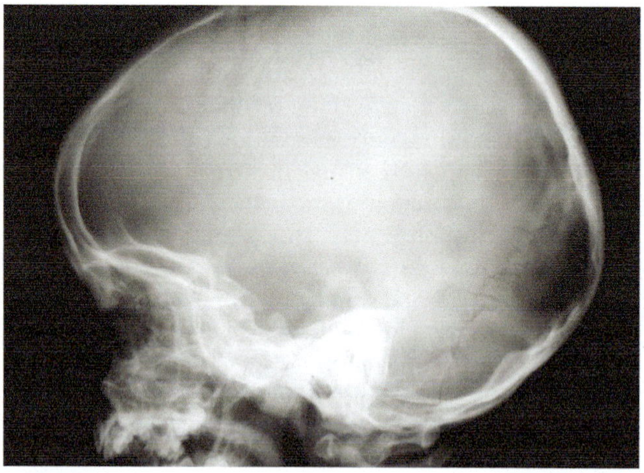

Figure 15.2 X-ray of skull showing splitting of cranial sutures due to raised intracranial pressure. This child had lead encephalopathy due to inhalation of lead fumes from burning of lead-containing batteries.

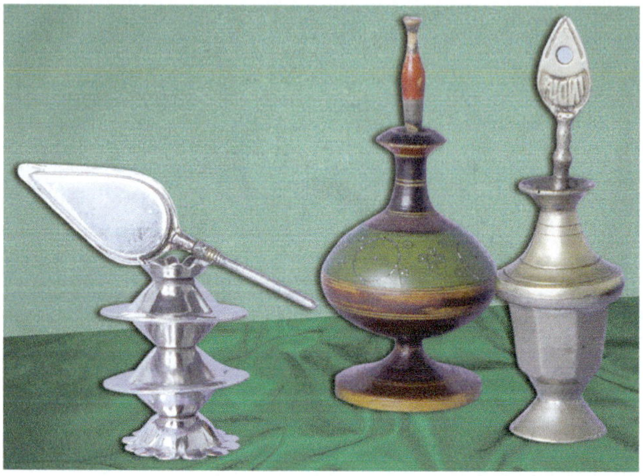

Figure 15.1 Lead poisoning: Surma containers: Surma contains lead and is used as a cosmetic. It could be a source of exposure to lead among some countries.

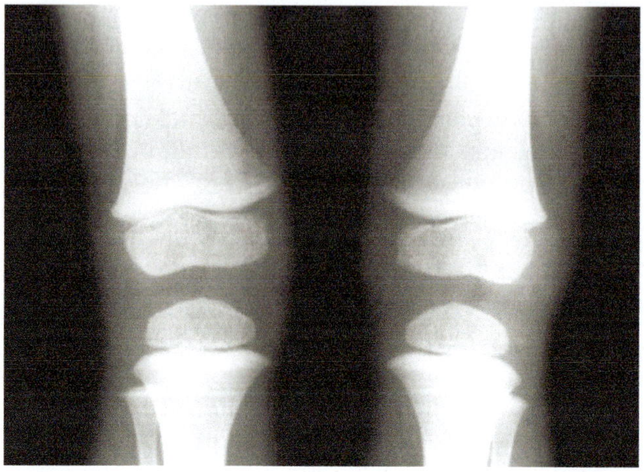

Figure 15.3 Radiograph of lower limbs in chronic lead poisoning. *Note* bands of increased density 'lead lines' at metaphyseal ends of the long bones.

The most dangerous development, both with regard to life and future mental health, is lead encephalopathy. Depending upon the amount of lead ingested, this dreaded complication may develop quite quickly or only following a long period of relatively mild ill health.

Diagnosis

The diagnosis of lead poisoning can be justified in the presence of two or more of the following findings:

- Microcytic hypochromic anaemia with punctate basophilia
- Radio-opaque foreign bodies in the bowel lumen and lines of increased density at the growing ends of the long bones
- Coproporphyrinuria
- Renal glycosuria and aminoaciduria
- Raised intracranial pressure and protein in the cerebrospinal fluid

Interpretation of the blood lead concentration is, unfortunately, much more difficult. While levels below 1.9 mmol/L (40 mg/100 mL) exclude lead poisoning and levels in the region of 2.9 mmol/L (60 mg/100 mL) are associated with clinical signs, it is possible that behaviour and learning difficulties occur at values between these levels.

CAUSTIC INGESTION

Accidental ingestion of caustic substances by inquisitive toddlers may result in serious injury to the mouth, oropharynx, oesophagus or stomach **(Fig. 15.4)**. The most corrosive and commonly ingested caustics are the liquid form of sodium or potassium hydroxides used as drain cleaners. Other less caustic alkalis, which may be ingested, are bleach (sodium hypochlorite), laundry and dishwasher detergents, and disinfectants usually kept in the kitchen.

Ingestion of these substances is most likely to result in injury to the oesophagus, but if ingested in large amounts, they can produce extensive damage to the upper gastrointestinal tract **(Figs. 15.5A and B)**. If the hydroxide concentration is high, it may lead to perforation of the oesophagus and thus penetration into the perioesophageal tissues, which may cause mediastinitis. The presence of oral burns confirms that ingestion of a caustic substance has taken place but it does not suggest the degree of oesophageal damage. Dyspnoea, stridor or hoarseness suggests laryngeal injury. Products that become trapped in the oesophagus cause the most damage, e.g. batteries or dishwasher tablets.

SWALLOWED FOREIGN BODIES

Foreign body ingestion is common in children because they have a tendency to explore and to taste new objects and, thus, they swallow bizarre and multiple objects. Most foreign bodies swallowed pass through the alimentary tract without symptoms. However, if the foreign body is lodged in the oesophagus, it should be removed immediately through an endoscope to avoid serious complications of oesophageal obstruction, asphyxia or mediastinitis. In the absence of symptoms, the management simply consists of an X-ray of the abdomen to confirm the presence of a radio-opaque object and a careful watch kept on the stools until the foreign body is recovered.

Disc batteries (button batteries) are often ingested in young children these days due to their widespread use in electrical products in the home. These batteries contain alkalis in sufficient concentration to cause caustic injuries and mercury in sufficient quantities to create problems. However, the highly toxic mercuric oxide is converted to essentially nontoxic elemental mercury on leakage or complete disintegration of the battery **(Figs. 15.6A and B)**.

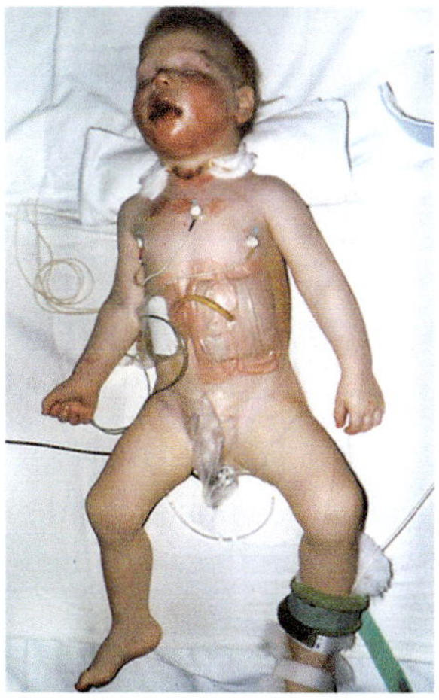

Figure 15.4 Ingestion of caustic materials—caustic soda can produce injury to the oral mucosa, oesophagus, and stomach. Children can have significant oesophageal injury even in the absence of visible oral burns.

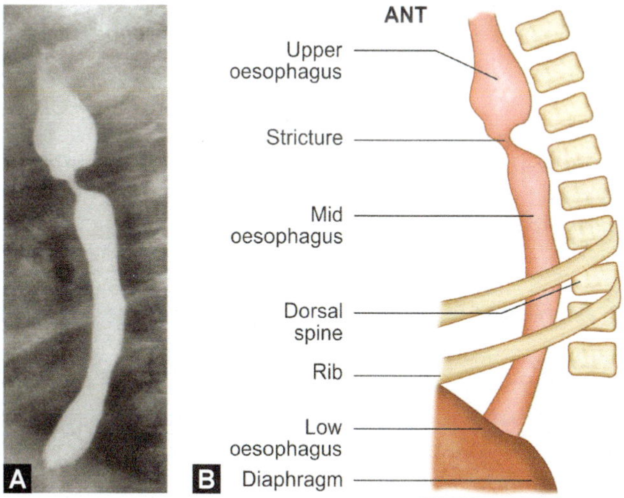

Figures 15.5A and B Oesophageal stricture: barium swallow showing short smooth stricture secondary to caustic soda.

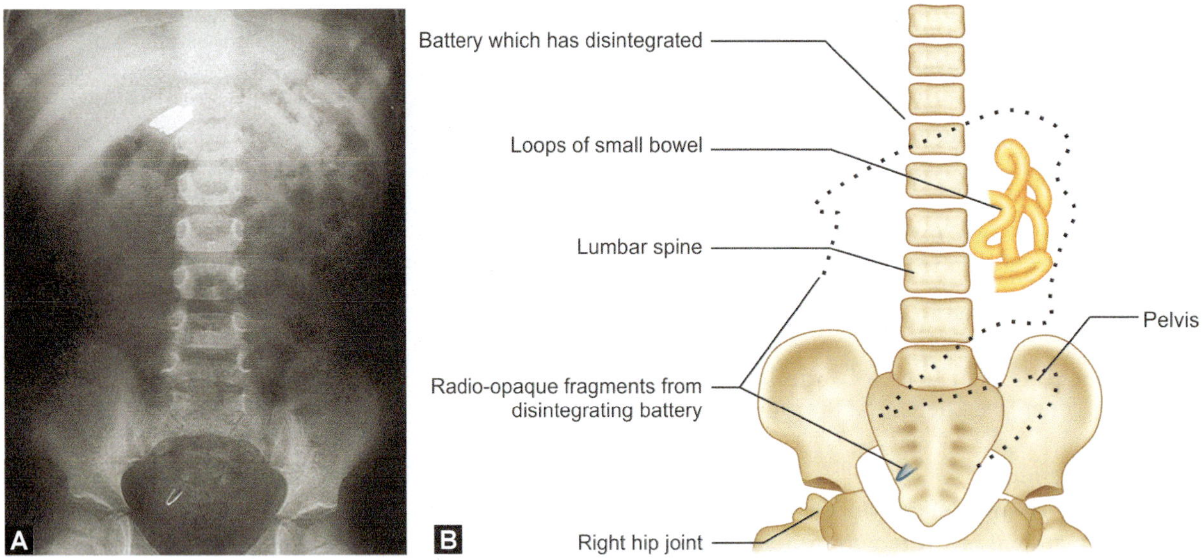

Figures 15.6A and B (A) X-ray of abdomen showing disintegrating battery; (B) Schematic diagram of Figure A.

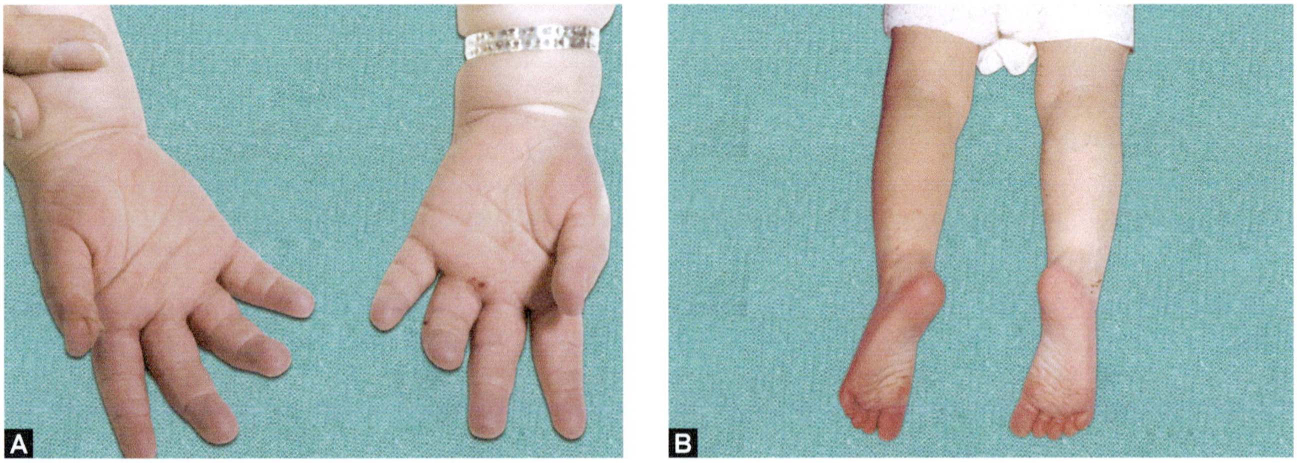

Figures 15.7A and B Clinical photographs of a child with acrodynia or pink disease. *Note* diffuse painful swelling and redness of hands and feet.

In addition, mercuric oxide is poorly soluble and not well-absorbed and this may account for the very low incidence of mercury poisoning and, therefore, children may not need chelation therapy.

ACRODYNIA (PINK DISEASE)

Chronic exposure to elemental mercury can give rise to the syndrome of acrodynia. It is also called pink disease. Pink disease is a form of childhood mercury poisoning. It occurs due to a prolonged exposure to mercury. Agents containing mercury can raise the blood pressure even when used as topical preparations (teething powders) or nose drops. Diffuse painful swelling, redness of hands and feet and peripheral neuropathy are characteristic of pink disease. These days application of mercury salts is rarely seen and mainly of historical interest **(Figs. 15.7A and B)**.

ACUTE CARBON MONOXIDE POISONING

Carbon monoxide (CO) is an odourless, colourless gas and its poisoning causes hypoxia, cell damage and death.

Carbon monoxide is produced by the incomplete combustion of carbon containing fuel, such as gas (domestic or bottled), charcoal, coke, oil and wood. Gas stoves, fires, car exhaust fumes, paraffin heaters are all potential sources.

The symptoms of CO poisoning are nonspecific and include headache, fatigue, confusion, nausea, dizziness, visual disturbances, chest pain, shortness of breath, loss

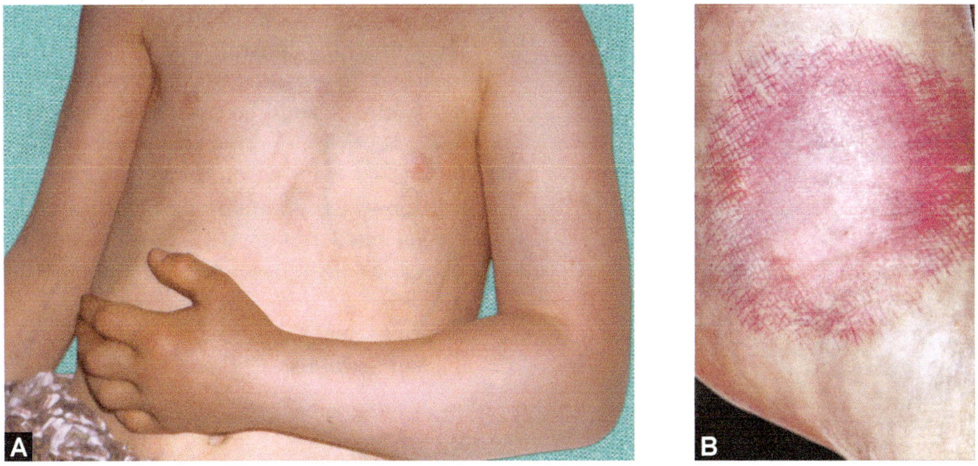

Figures 15.8A and B The site of a snakebite by an adder. *Note* the minimal swelling and erythema.

of consciousness and seizures. The classical signs of CO poisoning, such as cherry-red lips, peripheral cyanosis and retinal haemorrhages, are uncommon. A carboxy-haemoglobin level of 10% or more or the presence of clinical signs and symptoms after known exposure to CO are indicative of acute CO poisoning.

SNAKEBITE

Snakebite is a major medical problem in many parts of the world. The snakes of medical importance are the vipers (e.g. carpet viper, Russell viper, adder, etc.) and the elapids (cobra, mamba, krait, etc.). In the Indian subcontinent, the most important species are cobra, common krait, Russell's viper, but in South East Asia the Malayan pit viper, green pit viper and the monocellate cobra cause most bites and deaths. In Britain, the adder or viper is the only venomous species.

Clinical Manifestations

The earliest symptoms related to the bite are local pain, bleeding from the fang puncture, followed by swelling and bruising extending up to the limb, and tender enlargement of regional lymph nodes **(Figs. 15.8A and B)**. Clinical effects of systemic envenomingusually involve haemorrhage and coagulation defects resulting in incoagulable blood. Systemic elapid poisoning usually causes neurotoxic effects, which, in untreated cases, results in ptosis and life-threatening paralysis of the respiratory muscles. In victims of envenoming by sea snakes and Russell's vipers in Sri Lanka and South India, muscles become tender and painful and develop myoglobinuria. In rural and coastal regions of India and Thailand, snake-bite is a frequent cause of acute renal failure.

Insect Stings

Stings from ants, wasps, hornets and bees cause local pain and swelling but seldom cause severe toxicity unless

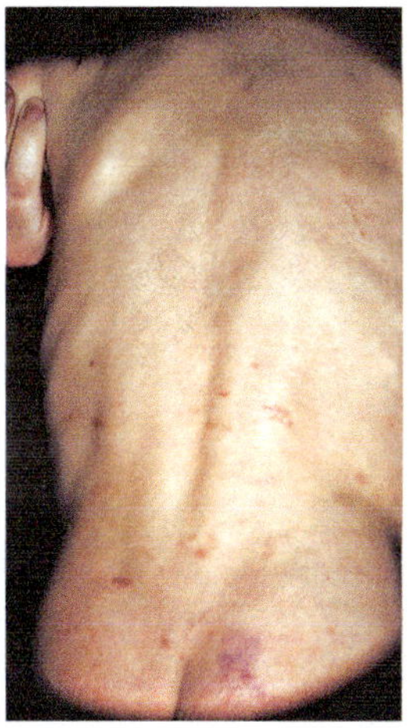

Figure 15.9 Insect bites. Group 1 reactions consist of a local response at the site of the bite or sting.

many stings are inflicted at the same time **(Fig. 15.9)**. If the sting is in the mouth or on the tongue, local swelling may threaten the upper airway. The stings from these insects are usually treated by cleaning the area. Bee stings should be removed as quickly as possible. Anaphylactic reactions require immediate treatment.

MARINE STINGS

Children stung by jellyfish should be removed from the sea as soon as possible. Adherent tentacles should be lifted off or washed off with sea water. Ice packs will reduce pain and a slurry of baking soda (sodium bicarbonate), but not vinegar, may be useful for treating stings.

PLANT AND MUSHROOM POISONING

Plants found in the home, garden and field now constitute the most common source of ingested poison in children. The fruits, seeds or roots of many common plants are

BOX 15.2 **Symptoms of mushroom poisoning. Symptoms typically appear 6–8 hours after eating but the symptoms can develop as soon as 2 hours and as late as 12 hours after ingestion.**

Symptoms

- Bloated feeling
- Nausea and vomiting
- Watery or (bloody) diarrhoea
- Muscle cramps
- Abdominal pain

Severe cases can include

- Liver damage, high fever, convulsions and coma
- Death (usually 2–4 days after ingestion)

poisonous. Fortunately, poisonous plants are rarely ingested in quantities sufficient to cause serious illness. However, the symptoms of poisoning from plants can include:

- Vomiting
- Stomach cramps
- Irregular heart beat
- Burning to the mouth
- Convulsions.

The type and severity of symptoms will vary according to the type of plant eaten. Any amount of any wild mushroom is considered to be very dangerous (**Box 15.2**). Deliberate ingestion of magic mushroom is also a potential source of poisoning. Identification of the plant must be attempted early and a computerised database can be accessed through the poisons centres.

Caution should be used in accepting common names of plants or in identifying a plant from a verbal description of its fruit or foliage. If substantial doubt exists, a portion of the plant should be brought for identification. However, each plant ingestion in a child must be viewed as potentially toxic until the plant has been positively identified or sufficient time has passed for a conclusion on nontoxicity. There is no way to tell by looking at a plant if it is poisonous.

DROWNING AND NEAR DROWNING

Drowning is defined as death, if the child dies within 24 hours as a result of a submersion accident and a near drowning accident if the child survives at least 24 hours after an episode of submersion. Drowning is now the most common cause of accidental death in children for a water-oriented society. Most drownings and near-drownings occur in the age group of 1–2 years.

The complications of drowning are directly related to anoxia and to the volume and composition of water that is aspirated. Both fresh and salt water damage alveoli and result in pulmonary oedema. The most important complication of near-drowning accidents in addition to pulmonary injury is the anoxic-ischaemic cerebral damage. As soon as water has entered the mouth, it causes the epiglottis to close over the airway. Without oxygen, the child will lose consciousness. Thereafter, bradycardia, cardiac arrhythmias, cardiac arrest and death occur.

CHAPTER 16

Metabolic Diseases

Peter Galloway, Rajeev Srivastava

INTRODUCTION

Inborn errors of metabolism (IEM) are often viewed with concern and suspicion due to their complexity and diverse clinical presentations. While there are over 550 disorders, some are incredibly rare being reported in one or a few families. The more common ones usually have clinically similar presentations, though like in all specialities of medicine unusual presentations do occur. Improved diagnostics and clinical awareness has resulted in recognition in adults often with milder clinical manifestations. Similarly, female carriers (heterozygotes) of X-linked disorders, e.g. ornithine transcarbamylase deficiency and Fabry disease, presenting in later life with milder manifestations defy classical genetic teaching.

This chapter outlines the basic pathophysiology and clinical-diagnostic features of selected IEMs. Specific therapies are beyond the scope, but by considering the pathophysiology, logical therapeutic approaches can be deduced.

BASIC PATHOPHYSIOLOGY

Difficulties in metabolising compound A to B resulting in problems either from accumulation of A [e.g. leucine in maple syrup urine disease (MSUD) or from inability to break down complex material, e.g. lysosomal disorders]; problems because B becomes deficient [e.g. in glycogen storage disorder (GSD) 1a inability to release glucose from liver from glucose-6-phosphate results in hypoglycaemia once no further absorption from gut]; or an enhanced production of C (e.g. sulphocysteine in molybdenum cofactor deficiency) which itself is toxic **(Fig. 16.1)**.

A few disorders are due to compartmentalisation of metabolites or substrates, e.g. in cystinosis there is an inability to export cysteine due to transport defect in lysosomes; in hyperammonaemia-hyperornithiniaemia-homocitrullinaemia syndrome, ornithine does not gain access to the mitochondria preventing the urea cycle from functioning normally; or in familial hypercholesterolaemia (FH), there is a failure to endocytose low density lipoprotein (LDL) particles by the liver results in progressive endothelial accumulation and accelerated atherosclerosis.

Therapeutic Options

Depending on the pathophysiology, a number of potential therapeutic options are available **(Fig. 16.2)**.

Exclude the substrate (A) which is unable to be metabolised, e.g. in phenylketonuria (PKU) low phenylalanine diet with amino acid supplement with extra tyrosine and minimal natural protein.

Supply sufficient end product (B), e.g. in GSD type 1a it is important to feed regularly during the day and overnight either with nasogastric feeding or by taking complex starch at bed time that is broken down overnight.

Replace enzyme AB, e.g. Gaucher disease has been treated with enzyme replacement therapy for 20 years and bone marrow transplant for some lysosomal storage disorders.

Cofactor to stimulate AB—half the cases of homocystinuria are pyridoxine response with pyridoxine enhancing activity of the enzyme cystathionine beta synthase.

Blocking conversion of substrate to new toxic metabolite C, e.g. in tyrosinaemia type 1, the failure to metabolise fumarylacetoacetate leads to its accumulation and conversion to succinylacetone, which inhibits the final steps in the porphyrin pathway giving rise to its neurological features. This induces a type II/III scenario with painful red eyes and planter/palmer hyperkeratosis from tyrosine accumulation. To treat this, a diet low in tyrosine is used, i.e. amino acid supplement without phenylalanine and tyrosine.

Further therapies: (1) more recently gene therapy has been proposed but is in its infancy, (2) liver transplantation has been used in a number of disorders, e.g. combined renal and hepatic transplantation in methylmalonic aciduria and (3) encouraging breakdown of substrate A to harmless product D, e.g. proposed in PKU with phenylalanine

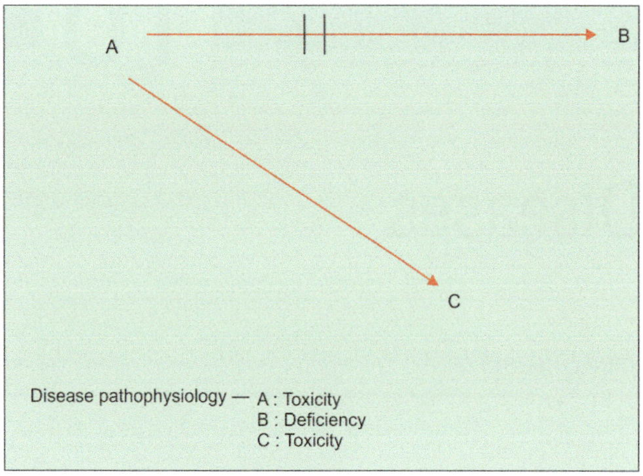

Figure 16.1 Basic pathophysiology.

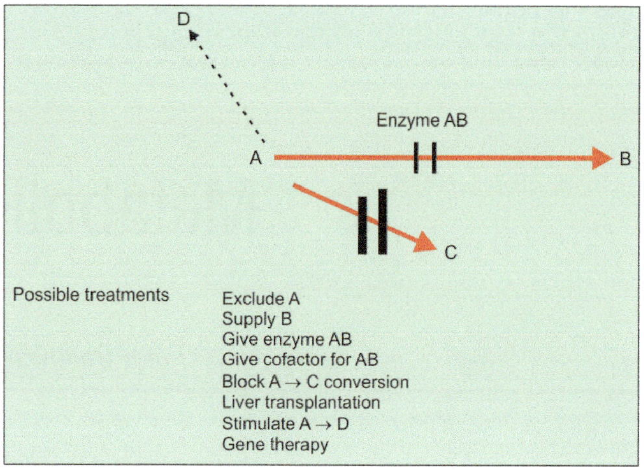

Figure 16.2 Therapeutic options.

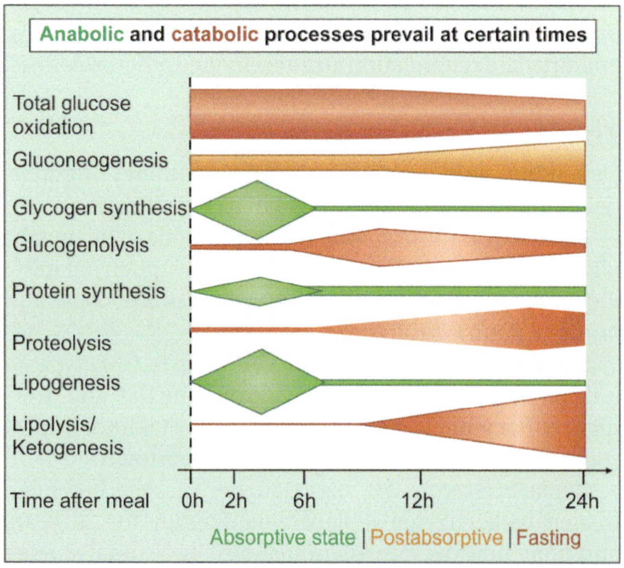

Figure 16.3 Normal physiological changes during fasting.

ammonia lyase converting phenylalanine to harmless trans-cinnamic acid.

Transport Defects

These have been approached in different ways:

Cystinosis: Cysteamine converts cysteine in lysosomes to cysteine and cysteamine-cysteine which are exported by two different transporters from the lysosomes.

Hyperammonaemia-hyperornithnaemia-homocitrullinaemia syndrome: Since problem relates to urea cycle failure, limiting protein intake and alternative pathways for nitrogen excretion with sodium benzoate and phenylbutyrate.

Familial hypercholesterolaemia: Prevention of accumulation of LDL particles by inhibiting cholesterol synthesis with HMG CoA reductase inhibitor or in homozygous state by plasma apheresis to remove the LDL particles.

PHYSIOLOGICAL CONSEQUENCES OF FASTING

It is useful to appreciate what happens during fasting particularly when assessing hypoglycaemia or catabolic responsive to inadequate feeding. Maintenance of blood glucose concentration is primarily due to insulin, with cortisol and growth hormone only being released if glucose falls below 2.5 mmol/L. After a meal, absorption of food and glucose usually lasts for 3-4 hours. (Complex starch can take approximately 8 hours, hence used overnight in GSD1a). The initial high insulin released in response to high portal glucose concentrations stimulates glycogen synthesis. As the gut stops absorbing glucose, the portal glucose concentration falls resulting in reduced insulin release from pancreatic beta cells. This removes the inhibition of glycogenolysis. The liver glycogen stores are broken down over a further 6–8 hours.

After 12 hours following the last meal, the liver glycogen stores are exhausted and plasma glucose falls further with insulin being suppressed further. As a result, there is no inhibition of the action of adipose tissue hormone-sensitive lipase causing breakdown of triglycerides to fatty acids and glycerol.

The glycerol is taken up into the liver and via gluconeogenesis produces glucose. The fatty acids are also taken up by liver and metabolised generating ketones. The brain which requires glucose progressively adapts to ketones over approximately 36 hours but all other tissues will preferentially use ketones or free fatty acids (FFAs). Thus, the glucose requirement to maintain normoglycaemia is reduced by the presence of ketones.

A child with hypoglycaemia thus needs endocrine and metabolic testing to identify the underlying disorder. However, in those over 6 months of age, hypoglycaemia occurring within 4-6 hours of food suggests a GSD and that after 12 hours suggests a fatty acid oxidation defect (FAOD) **(Fig. 16.3)**.

CLINICAL APPROACH TO DIAGNOSIS

Many classifications of IEM were based around a specific metabolite or cellular organelle. An example of the former is disorders of fructose metabolism: (1) Essential fructosuria—a benign problem where the proximal convoluted tubule fails to reabsorb fructose resulting in urine testing positive for reducing substances, but glucostix negative (which uses a specific glucose oxidase method), (2) Fructose 1, 6-bisphosphatase—rapid onset of hypoglycaemia from failure of gluconeogenesis, 2–3 hours after feeding associated with gross lactic acidaemia and (3) Hereditary fructose intolerance—severe liver failure may result following ingestion of fructose. An example of organelle disorders is lysosomal disorders: (1) I-cell disease—presenting with hydrops foetalis or early onset dysostosis multiplex, (2) Glycogen storage disease type II (Pompe disease)—presenting with cardiac failure or (3) Mucopolysaccharidosis (MPS) type IV (Morquio disease)—presenting with coarse features and short stature. Clinically, this approach offers limited utility.

A more useful clinical approach has been developed, in which disorders are classified according to common clinical presentation or specific signs, e.g. cherry-red spot on the macula. There are four groups of clinical scenarios where a metabolic disorder should be considered:

1. Acute neonatal presentation, e.g. MSUD
2. Late onset acute and recurrent attacks of symptoms such as ataxia, vomiting or acidosis, e.g. female with ornithine transcarbamylase deficiency
3. Chronic and progressive generalised symptoms—usually gastrointestinal (chronic vomiting, failure to thrive); muscular or neurological deterioration, e.g. Refsum disease with ataxia and progressive night blindness
4. Specific and permanent organ presentations suggestive of an IEM, e.g. cataract in galactokinase deficiency

Approximately, 2% of all newborns have an IEM. Within this group, the autosomal dominant conditions usually present in adulthood and are the most common, e.g. FH (~1 in 500). In X-linked conditions, where there is no male-to-male transmission within a family, females were considered only carriers; increasingly they are noted to have variable features dependent upon lyonisation and the specific organs which have the defective X-chromosome active. However, the vast majority of conditions are autosomal recessive and present before puberty.

NEONATAL PRESENTATIONS AND EARLY INFANCY (<1 YEAR)

Inborn errors of metabolism most commonly present in the neonate. Suspicion of an IEM is raised in families with first cousin marriages; where a previous sibling has unexplained failure to thrive or death—particular care is required when a term neonatal death is attributed to sepsis, intraventricular haemorrhage (premature babies) or lactic acidosis—this is a common feature of multiple IEM. Clues can include abnormal odour in cot (e.g. MSUD); marked acidosis with neutropenia (e.g. organic aciduria), maternal ill health in pregnancy (e.g. HELLP and LCHAD) or rarely intrauterine hiccups and pyridoxine responsive seizures.

Pathophysiology of Neonatal Presentations

There are three common pathophysiological processes involved:

- *Group 1 (Disorders giving rise to intoxication):* These neonates are usually healthy term babies who after a delay, develop symptoms as a toxic metabolite accumulates. Neonates have limited repertoire of responses, therefore, the signs are nonspecific—poor sucking, drowsiness, floppiness, abnormal tone/posture, breathing changes (tachypnoea and apnoea), bradycardia and temperature instability. Biochemical abnormalities include acid-base disturbance (pH increase hyperammonaemia, pH reduced organic acidurias) and liver/dysfunction especially abnormal clotting. Diagnosis is usually based on plasma amino acid and urine organic acid analysis.
- *Group 2 (Disorders involving energy deficiency):* Symptoms arise in part to deficiency in energy production or utilization with liver, heart, muscle and brain signs and symptoms, e.g. hypoglycaemia—GSD, FAOD or lactic aciduria, e.g. pyruvate metabolism defects and mitochondrial disorders. Signs include severe generalised hypotonia, cardiomyopathy/cardiac failure, conduction defects and abnormal creatine kinase/liver function tests (CK/LFTs) in biochemical testing.
- *Group 3 (Disorders involving complex molecules):* The signs are permanent, progressive and independent of intercurrent events or food intake.

Clinical Patterns

In neonates, IEM either present with a specific organ affected, e.g. cataract, or as a generalised disorder. The latter group may be classified into predominant neurological, hepatological or dysmorphological presentations.

Neurological Presentations

Two patterns of metabolic intoxication exist:

1. Generalised hypotonic episodes with opisthotonus with or without boxing/pedalling movements or slow limb elevation

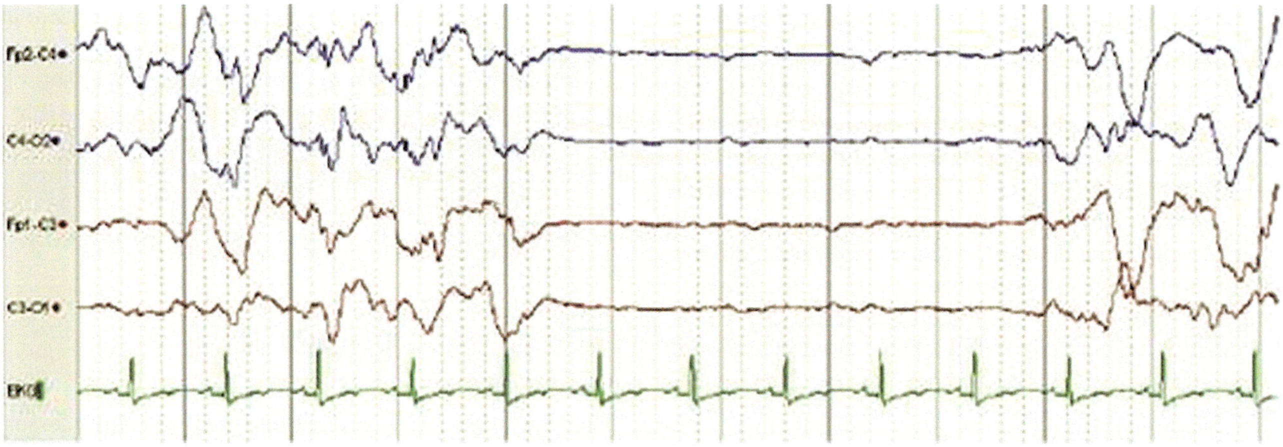

Figure 16.4 Electroencephalogram (EEG); Burst suppression EEG; Pattern of high amplitude EEG activity interrupted by relatively low amplitude activity, typically under 20 V peak-to-peak, classified as an EEG abnormality due to its relation to severe encephalopathy: Clinical conditions causing BS pattern:- Head trauma, stroke, coma, anaesthesia, hypothermia, prematurity.

2. Axial hypotonia and limb hypertonia with large amplitude tremors and myoclonic jerks. Seizures are a late aspect of progressive encephalopathy except in a small group where EEG may show burst suppression patterns **(Fig. 16.4)**. Other neurological presentations can be split conveniently into those with and those without acidosis

Seizures

Seizures associated with IEM are intractable and respond poorly to conventional antiepileptic therapy. If occurring in the first 4 days of life, they point towards a small group of specific but unrelated disorders, the four commonest being: (1) pyridoxine responsive seizures, (2) nonketotic hyperglycinaemia, (3) molybdenum cofactor deficiency and (4) peroxisomal disorders. A trial of treatment with pyridoxine is, therefore, appropriate along with consideration of other much rarer treatable disorders—congenital magnesium deficiency, folinic acid responsive seizure and biotin responsive seizures **(Fig. 16.4)**.

Encephalopathy without Acidosis

Maple syrup urine disease and urea cycle disorders are the important disorders included in this group. The clue to the latter is early development of respiratory alkalosis though this may disappear with the onset of severe illness. Aggressive intervention to lower leucine and ammonia concentrations, respectively, may be sufficient to prevent death, but varying degrees of permanent neurological deficit is often unavoidable. Definitive diagnosis, however, allows close monitoring of future siblings in early postnatal life where prospective support can lead to a very good clinical outcome.

Encephalopathy with Acidosis

Three major disorders can present within the first 2 weeks with very negative base excess. The three enzyme deficiencies—(1) holocarboxylase, (2) propionyl CoA carboxylase and (3) methylmalonyl CoA mutase—are differentiated by urine organic acid analysis. Treatment with N-carbamyl glutamate (to reduce hyperammonaemia), biotin, bicarbonate and dietary protein restriction is associated with clinical improvement. The other group of acidotic encephalopathies such as mitochondrial and pyruvate disorders are associated with lactic acidosis but have limited effective therapies.

Hepatological Presentation

This group can also be subdivided into three: (1) jaundice, (2) hypoglycaemia and (3) gross liver dysfunction.

Jaundice

Unconjugated hyperbilirubinaemia can occur early in galactosaemia though classically these patients often develop *Escherichia coli* septicaemia and conjugated hyperbilirubinaemia. Other causes of unconjugated jaundice include hypothyroidism, breast milk jaundice and rarely Crigler-Najjar syndrome.

With conjugated hyperbilirubinaemia and failure to thrive, two common diagnoses to consider are alpha 1-antitrypsin deficiency and cystic fibrosis.

Hypoglycaemia

While significant hypoglycaemia is usually secondary to hyperinsulinism, progressive liver enlargement and hyperlactic acidaemia merit consideration of GSD type I (von Gierke) and fructose 1,6-bisphosphatase deficiency in the differential diagnosis. With milder hepatomegaly associated with features of encephalopathy, acylcarnitine profiling to exclude FAODs is appropriate.

Gross Liver Dysfunction

While viral infections remain a very common and important cause, metabolic disorders such as mitochondrial mutation defects, neonatal haemochromatosis (an

TABLE 16.1	Liver disorders.
In utero	Hepatic enlargement—sterol metabolism defect lysosomal storage disorder
1st week	Mitochondrial especially mitochondrial DNA depletion
2nd week	Galactosaemia
Neonatal jaundice	Alpha 1-antitrypsin deficiency Peroxisomal disorders Niemann Pick C Bile salt disorder
Later in first year	
Coagulopathy ± ascites	Tyrosinaemia Congenital disorder of glycosylation type 1a

alloimmune disease offering therapeutic options in future pregnancies) and tyrosinaemia type 1 should be considered in those with gross liver dysfunction presenting with a coagulopathy.

The following **Table 16.1** incorporates age during first year of life and timing of likely liver disorder presentations.

Storage Presentations Dysmorphology

The clinical pattern gives the clue to diagnosis: A floppy child with a large anterior fontanelle would suggest Zellweger syndrome (peroxisomal disorder), while infection, haemolytic anaemia and cardiac disease are common aetiologies for hydrops foetalis. Hydrops is also associated with a vast array of metabolic disorders, particularly lysosomal disorders.

While rarely seen since the introduction of neonatal screening in early 1970s and treatment during pregnancy, an infant of a mother with untreated hyperphenylalaninaemia may have microcephaly (90%), mid-facial abnormalities including cleft palate and congenital heart disease (10%) including ventricular septal defect (VSD) and coarctation of aorta. Some organic acidaemias and X-linked pyruvate dehydrogenase deficiency cause facial features similar to those in foetal alcohol syndrome suggesting a common mechanism.

Table 16.2 gives a list of initial investigations, which can help categorise the metabolic disorders. More specialised investigations such as amino acid and organic acid analyses can then be arranged.

COMMON METABOLIC SCENARIOS AFTER 6/12 OF AGE

Hypoglycaemia

Beyond the neonatal period, children can present often during intercurrent illness with hypoglycaemia. Careful examination looking for liver enlargement (e.g. in severe liver disease and GSD) and buccal hand pigmentation (e.g. in adrenal insufficiency). A range of investigations should be undertaken **(Box 16.1)**.

The child needs to be given glucose rapidly. Where the parents report concerns that the child remains encephalopathic, particular attention is required to exclude FAOD, MSUD or an organic aciduria.

While many children under the age of 6, ultimately have idiopathic ketotic hypoglycaemia, this is a diagnosis of exclusion only. FAOD (relative hypoketotic with very high FFA (BOH butyrate/FFA ratio <0.7), adrenal insufficiency, late onset MSUD and multiple carboxylase deficiencies need to be excluded.

TABLE 16.2	Initial investigations to help categorise metabolic disorders.
Urine	Smell Ketones Reducing substances Ketoacids (dinitrophenylhydrazine test) Sulphites (Sulfitest, Merck) pH
Blood	Blood cell count Electrolytes (look for anion gap) Calcium Glucose Blood gases (pH, PCO_2, HCO_3, PO_2) Ammonia Lactic acid 3-hydroxy butyrate Uric acid
Store at-20°C	Urine (as much as possible) Heparinized plasma (2–5 mL), do not freeze whole blood! Cerebrospinal fluid (0.5–1.0 mL)
Miscellaneous	Electroencephalogram, bacteriological samples, chest X-ray, lumbar puncture, cardiac echography, cerebral ultrasound

BOX 16.1	Hypoglycaemia investigations.
Require	UE LFT Ammonia Lactate BOH butyrate NEFA Cortisol Insulin GH Acylcarnitine Organic acids

Reye Syndrome/Reye-like Illnesses

Reye syndrome is defined as an acute noninflammatory encephalopathy [<8 wc/mm^3 cerebrospinal fluid (CSF)] with elevated ammonia and aspartate transaminase (both 3 × upper limit of normal) and no more reasonable explanation for the condition. It often has a biphasic course with a prodromal virus type illness, followed by period of apparent recovery then onset of intractable vomiting and subsequent rapid neurological deterioration demonstrated by early irritability, confusion and aggressiveness.

Since the withdrawal of aspirin in under 16 years, except under medical guidance, the incidence has fallen. Aspirin uncouples oxidative phosphorylation within the cells. However, a number of IEM may mimic Reye syndrome.

- Fatty acid oxidation defects
- Primary carnitine deficiency
- Organic aciduria
- Urea cycle defects
- Respiratory chain defects
- Maple syrup urine disease
- Hereditary fructose intolerance
- Fructose-1, 6 bisphosphatase deficiency.

Developmental Delay

Biochemical metabolic investigations are not indicated in isolated delay in speech and language development, autistic or motor development. However, those with more severe signs and symptoms should be further investigated (Table 16.3). The history is important but care is required in assuming whether loss of acquired skills or slow acquisition of new skills is progressive. Coarse facial features, bone abnormalities, skin feature, eye signs, deafness, cataract, parental consanguinity and recurrent and unexplained illnesses may be useful clues.

Mucopolysaccharidosis III (Sanfilippo) is easily overlooked in a child with hyperactive features as physical signs may be mild. Demonstrating loss of skills with motor dysfunction (usually 9 months to 3 years) after encephalopathic episode is suggestive of GA1. Sphingolipidoses, e.g. Tay-Sachs, Gaucher type III, may have severe early onset developmental failure or with regression in older child, e.g. metachromatic leukodystrophy/Niemann Pick C. From 5 years onwards any boy with adrenal insufficiency (excess pigmentation often present) or neurological signs, e.g. hyper-reflexia/leg spasticity must have very long-chain fatty acids (VLCFAs) performed to exclude X-linked adrenoleukodystrophy (ALD).

Hyperammonaemia

Any child with encephalopathy, altered consciousness, acute disorientation/combative or altered consciousness without history of epilepsy or head injury should get plasma ammonia measured. Presence of focal signs does not rule out hyperammonaemia.

TABLE 16.3 Generalised investigations in a child with developmental delay without specific features.

First line
Chromosomes including fragile X
Calcium (hypoparathyroidism)
Thyroid function test
Creatine kinase (exclude Duchenne muscular dystrophy)
Blood lead
Biotinidase (treatable disorder)
Urate (very high in Lesch-Nyhan Syndrome)
Second line
Lactate
Amino acids especially if not screened at birth for phenylketonuria
Total homocysteine
NH_3
Free carnitine
Very long-chain fatty acid
Organic acids
GAGs

Causes in children include urea cycle disorders, organic acidurias, advanced liver disease, Reye syndrome and two unusual but well described associations—idiosyncratic response to sodium valproate and urinary tract infection in obstructed kidney with a urea splitting organism usually Proteus species.

Early diagnosis and aggressive therapy prevents devastating and irreversible brain damage.

Hyperlactic Acidaemia

In neonates, high lactate often reflects underlying cardiac disease including hypoplastic left heart disease or major VSDs. In older children, lactate tends to reflect inadequate oxygenation of the tissues. However, a large number of secondary metabolic causes exist. These include hepatomegaly in GSD and organic acidurias. Rarely primary lactate acidaemia is present with disorders of pyruvate metabolism often with dysmorphic and brain abnormalities or mitochondrial disorders. This latter group has a vast array of presentations particularly multisystem effects with no apparent connection, which may manifest at different times, e.g. brain abnormalities with abnormal CK and LFTs.

Dysmorphological

Lysosomal Storage

While some MPS disorders present at birth with hydrops foetalis or early coarse features (e.g. mucolipidosis II), many present from 1 year onwards. Early signs are corneal clouding, claw hands and lumbar abnormalities. Recurrent upper airway infections, glue ear, deafness and hernias may be present. Oligosaccharidoses may have similar dysmorphic features and often angiokeratoma. Sphingolipidoses present with neurological abnormalities especially regression of skills. Other rarer presentations include Pompé disease presenting with enlarged heart in first year, hepatosplenomegaly in Wolman disease and Cystinosis—commonest cause of Fanconi syndrome with rickets, salt loss and failure to thrive under the age of 3 years.

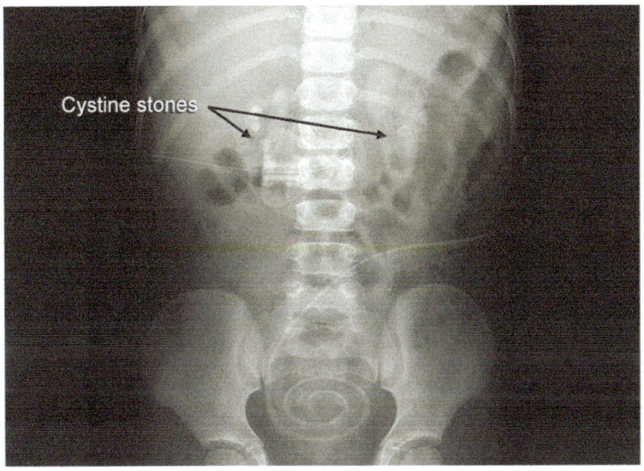

Figure 16.5 X-ray showing renal stones.

Peroxisomal Disorders

These disorders encompass the child with Zellweger at birth (floppy, large anterior fontanelle, hepatomegaly, stippled epiphyses); Rhizomelic chondrodysplasia punctata (RCDP) with short humeri and femora and cataracts at birth; Refsum disease (night blindness around teenage years—leading to progressive blindness, cerebellar ataxia, cardiomyopathy and neuropathy); hyperoxaluria (renal stone from early life with haematuria—see below); neurological regressive disease, e.g. Infantile Refsum Disease (IRD). Diagnosis is through measurement of VLCFAs, phytanic and pristanic acid and plasmalogens.

Renal Haematuria/Stones

Children presenting with renal stones or unexplained persistent haematuria should be investigated for cystinuria **(Fig. 16.5)**. This is an autosomal recessive disorder resulting in transporter defects (both in the kidney and intestine) of the dibasic amino acids—cysteine, ornithine, arginine and lysine **(Fig. 16.6)**. Cysteine precipitates out in neutral or acidic urine resulting in calculi and nephrolithiasis. Diagnosis is by urinary amino acid analysis and urine cysteine concentrations are monitored while

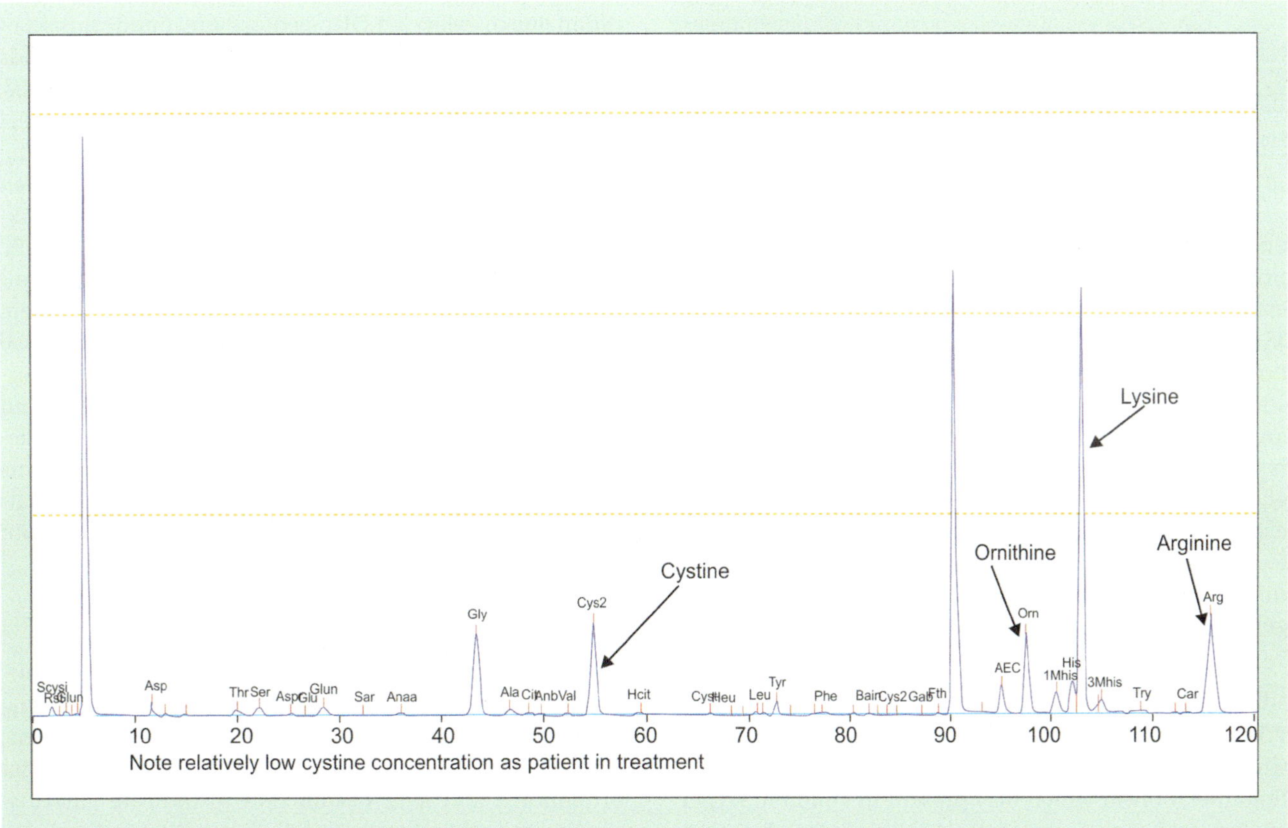

Figure 16.6 Amino acid chromatogram showing cystinuria.

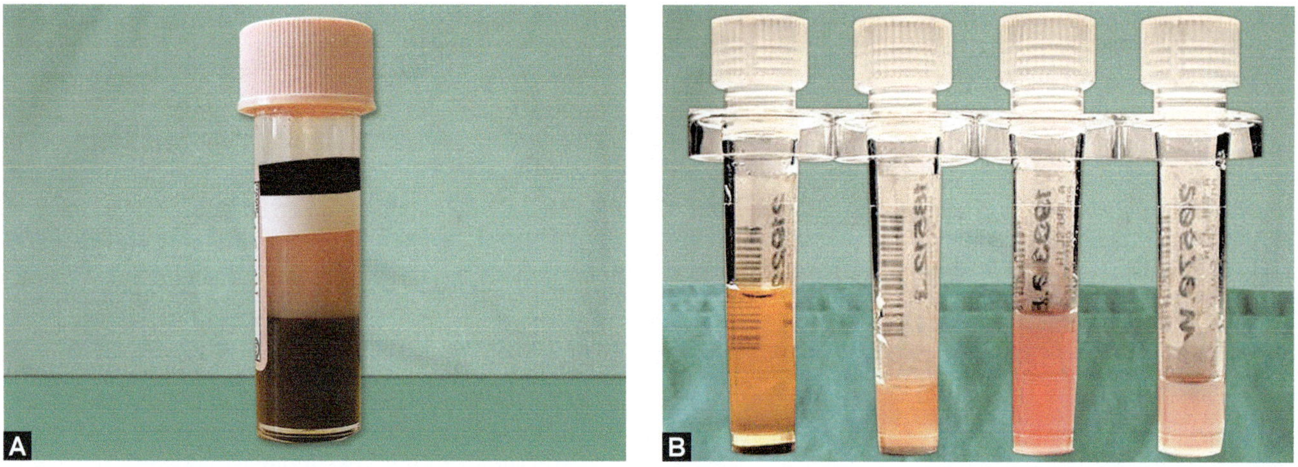

Figures 16.7A and B Presence of chylomicronaemia in spun sample.

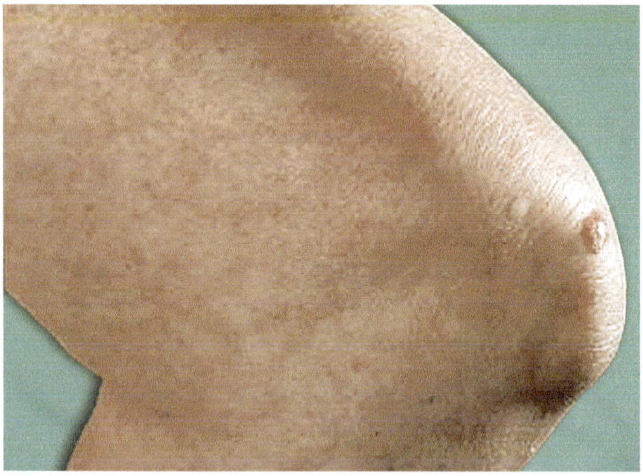

Figure 16.8 Xanthomata at elbow.

on treatment. Another rare, but important condition is primary hyperoxaluria which results in increased urinary excretion of oxalate resulting in calcium oxalate stones. Type 1 is due to deficiency of alanine-glyoxylate aminotransferase and is normally found only in liver peroxisomes. This leads to increased excretion of glycolic acid and oxalic acid, which quickly converts to oxalate. Type 2 is the rarer form and is due to deficiency of the enzyme glyoxylate reductase, which results in increased urinary excretion of oxalate and glycerate. Untreated, they lead to renal failure. Diagnosis is by demonstrating increased urine excretion of oxalate and confirmation of molecular genetics.

Lipid Disorders

While lipid disorders are almost always seen in adults, it is worth mentioning some important inherited disorders of lipid metabolism which may present in children. Hyperchylomicronaemia syndrome is due to excessive accumulation of chylomicrons in the plasma, resulting from (1) lipoprotein lipase deficiency or (2) apo-CII deficiency. Clinical presentation is of xanthomatous deposits, hepatosplenomegaly, lipaemia retinalis and recurrent abdominal pains often due to acute pancreatitis. Biochemically, serum triglycerides (the likely cause of acute pancreatitis) and total cholesterol are very high. The high triglycerides impart a tell-tale sign—the presence of a "milky" layer on top of the serum after centrifugation of the blood sample **(Figs. 16.7A and B)**, which exaggerates if the sample is refrigerated overnight. Genetic testing though feasible is not always performed. FH is an autosomal dominant condition due to defect in LDL receptors, preventing uptake of LDL from the circulation into the hepatocytes. This leads to very high total and LDL cholesterol and increased risk of premature cardiovascular disease. Heterozygous FH has a prevalence of 1 in 500 and usually manifests in the form of myocardial infarction before the age of 60 (often earlier). Tendon xanthomatas—around the tendo Achilles, over the knuckles and elbows—are pathognomonic **(Fig. 16.8)**. Homozygous FH is very rare (1 in a million) and can present with cardiovascular disease in children. Even in heterozygous FH, the vascular pathological changes start as early as the first decade of life. It is estimated that there are 120,000 people with FH in the UK but only 15% of these are diagnosed. This has resulted in cascade screening of family members of known FH patients in an effort to make an early diagnosis and initiate treatment. Population screening has also been considered but in most countries is not thought to be cost-effective.

Metabolic Investigations

A wide variety of metabolic tests are now available. Useful clues in ill children are obtained by measuring ammonia and lactate. Simple spot tests still have a use, e.g. urine reducing substances in child with early onset of jaundice and liver dysfunction to indicate galactosaemia [though more specific diagnostic confirmatory tests galactose-1-phosphate uridyl transferase enzyme activity (GAL1PUT) is required] and 2,4-dinitrophenylhydrazine (DNPH) to rapidly exclude MSUD in a neonate with encephalopathy while awaiting amino acids analysis (Figs. 16.9A to D).

It is interesting to appreciate the historical line of diagnostic developments. Prior to the early 1980s, gas chromatography with flame ionisation was available. While useful in identifying major peaks (in g/g creatinine), e.g. methylmalonate and glutarate, it was not good with minor peaks. The advent of benchtop gas chromatography-mass spectrometry (GC-MS) compared to earlier massive machines with magnetic separation of ions, allowed development of small volume analysis leading to ability to detect minor peaks (10–50 mg/g creatinine) such as suberylglycine and phenyl propionyl glycine in MCAD. This technology became available in most specialist metabolic laboratories during the late 1980s.

Tandem mass spectrometry (TMS) followed and its increased sensitivity (around 100–1,000 fold more sensitive) allowed assessment of plasma carnitines. While initially described in 1968, suitable benchtop rapid analysers required powerful pcs and it was not until the millennium that most specialist metabolic laboratories obtained a TMS. Thus we can now screen for MCAD and use this technology to identify many disorders (Fig. 16.10).

The polymerase chain reaction technique was developed in the 1980s to look for specific mutations. Subsequently, we have been able to sequence the genome.

The human genome was sequenced costing $13 billion and was first reported in 2000. It is expected by 2015 to be able to perform this for $1,000. However, interpreting abnormalities will be complex. Targeted approaches to clinical scenarios are likely to be implemented with biomarkers to confirm or refute potential diagnoses.

Future techniques including time of flight (TOF)—TMS are increasingly being used to identify complex molecules such as Lysosomal storage disorders or defects in proteins. Proton nuclear magnetic resonance spectroscopy is being used to identify new disorders. The field of metabolomics (a systematic study of unique chemical fingerprints that specific cellular processes leave behind) will also soon have an impact like gene sequencing. This will generate a lot of data requiring complex statistical packages to accurately analyse and interpret the data.

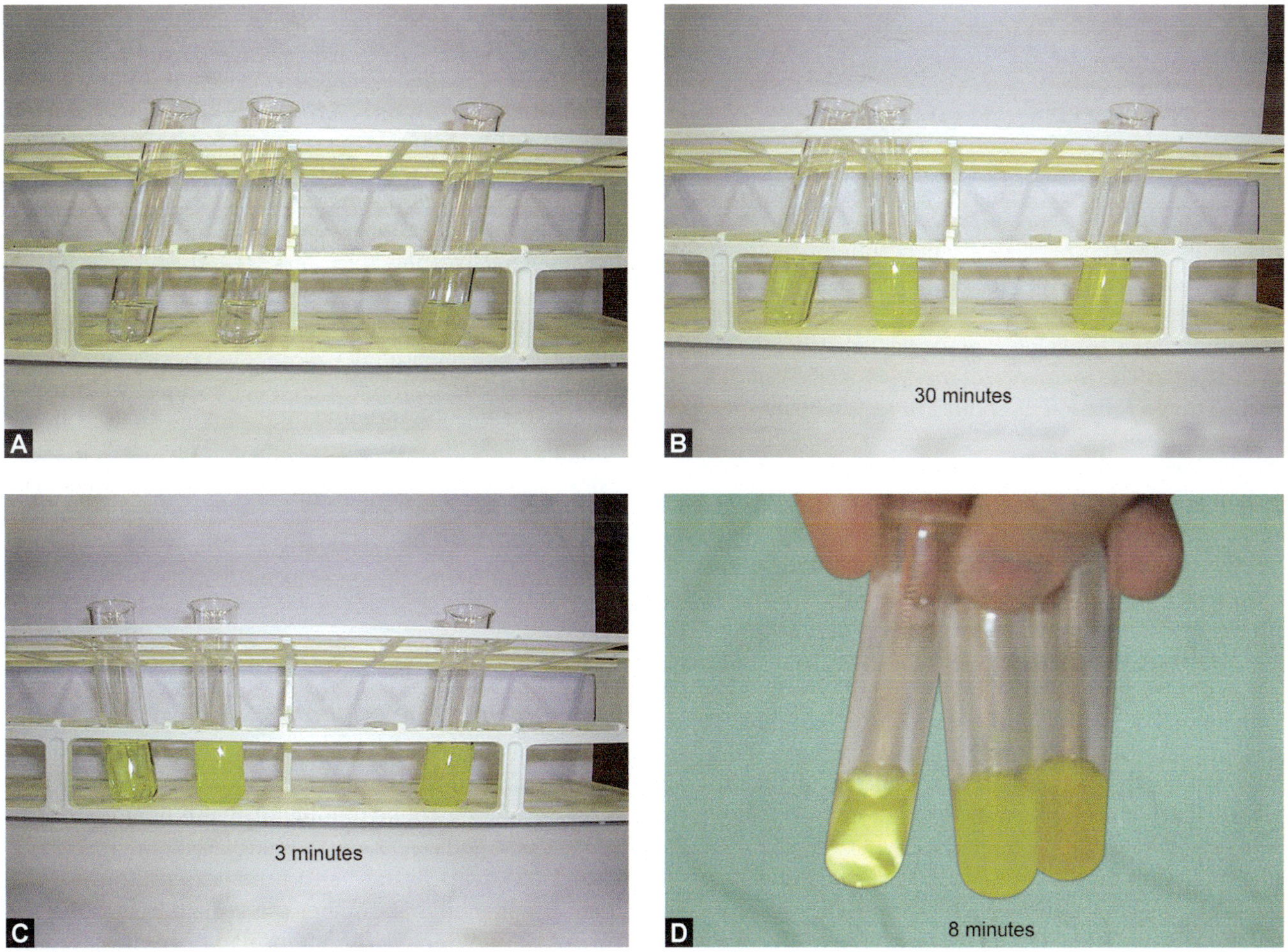

Figures 16.9A to D Positive dinitrophenylhydrazine (DNPH) reaction; negative and two positive responses to DNPH reaction with increasing yellow precipitate.

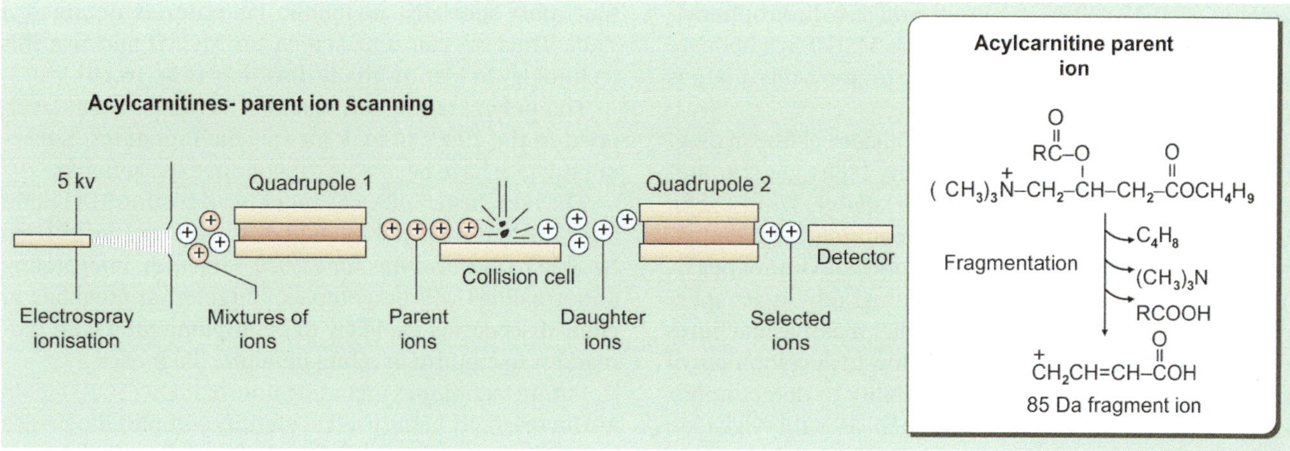

Figure 16.10 Schematic representation tandem mass spectrometer.

Why Investigate Further?

Even where a disease is untreatable, confirming the specific diagnosis often to DNA mutation level, allows prenatal testing of future pregnancies. In certain cultures, this may not be acceptable, but the more specific the diagnosis, the better the risk of future pregnancies can be explained to the parents of an affected child.

SPECIFIC COMMON DISORDERS

Amino Acid Disorders

Phenylketonuria

Classical PKU (persistent hyperphenylalaninaemia >360 μmol/L, relative tyrosine deficiency and excretion of an excess of phenyl-ketones) is an autosomal recessive condition due to deficiency of the enzyme phenylalanine hydroxylase. The incidence of the "classical" form of PKU in the United Kingdom is about 1 in 12,000 births.

Pathogenesis Deficiency of phenylalanine hydroxylase results in accumulation of blood phenylalanine, which is converted by phenylalanine transaminase to phenylpyruvic acid and other degradation products such as phenyllactic acid, phenylacetic acid and ortho-hydroxyphenylacetic acid. The precise chemical cause for the inevitable mental retardation in "classical" PKU is not known but is probably related to the high phenylalanine concentration and to deficiencies of the neurotransmitters noradrenaline, adrenaline and dopamine. The fair hair and blue eyes are due to the deficient availability of melanin, which is synthesised like the neurotransmitters from tyrosine. Mild to moderate hyperphenylalaninaemia (with normal enzyme activity) may be due to defects in the biopterin pathway. As tetrahydrobiopterin is the cofactor for phenylalanine hydroxylase, its deficiency prevents the conversion of phenylalanine to tyrosine even though the phenylalanine hydroxylase enzyme is normal. Deficiencies of tetrahydrobiopterin will also interfere with the conversion of tyrosine to dihydroxyphenylalanine (DOPA) and noradrenaline and the conversion of tryptophan to serotonin, as tetrahydrobiopterin is also a cofactor for the enzymes involved. These tetrahydrobiopterin defects are found in about 1% of hyperphenylalaninaemic children and treatment is with tetrahydrobiopterin, L-DOPA (dihydroxyphenylalanine) and L-5 hydroxytryptophan and a peripheral decarboxylase inhibitor. There is a blood spot-screening test available for total blood biopterin and this should be performed in all hyperphenylalaninaemic children **(Fig. 16.11)**.

Clinical features Patients with untreated "classical" PKU have severe learning disorders (IQ 30 or lower). They are frequently blue-eyed, fair-haired and with fair skins. Eczema is often troublesome. Some have convulsions, athetosis and electroencephalographic changes. Many show psychotic features such as abnormal posturing of hands and fingers, repetitive movements such as head-banging or rocking to-and-fro and complete lack of interest in people as distinct from inanimate objects. The tendon reflexes are often accentuated. It should be noted that infants born homozygous for the phenylketonuric trait are not brain-damaged at birth. They only become so after they start to ingest phenylalanine in their milk **(Fig. 16.12)**.

Maternal Phenylketonuria

As a consequence of defects of phenylalanine and tyrosine metabolism in the mother, abnormalities have been reported among a large number of infants of mothers with PKU. These include mental retardation, microcephaly, congenital heart disease and intrauterine growth retardation. Congenital anomalies are uncommon in the offspring of mothers with phenylalanine concentrations less than 600 μmol/L at the time of conception. However, head size, birth weight and intelligence have been shown

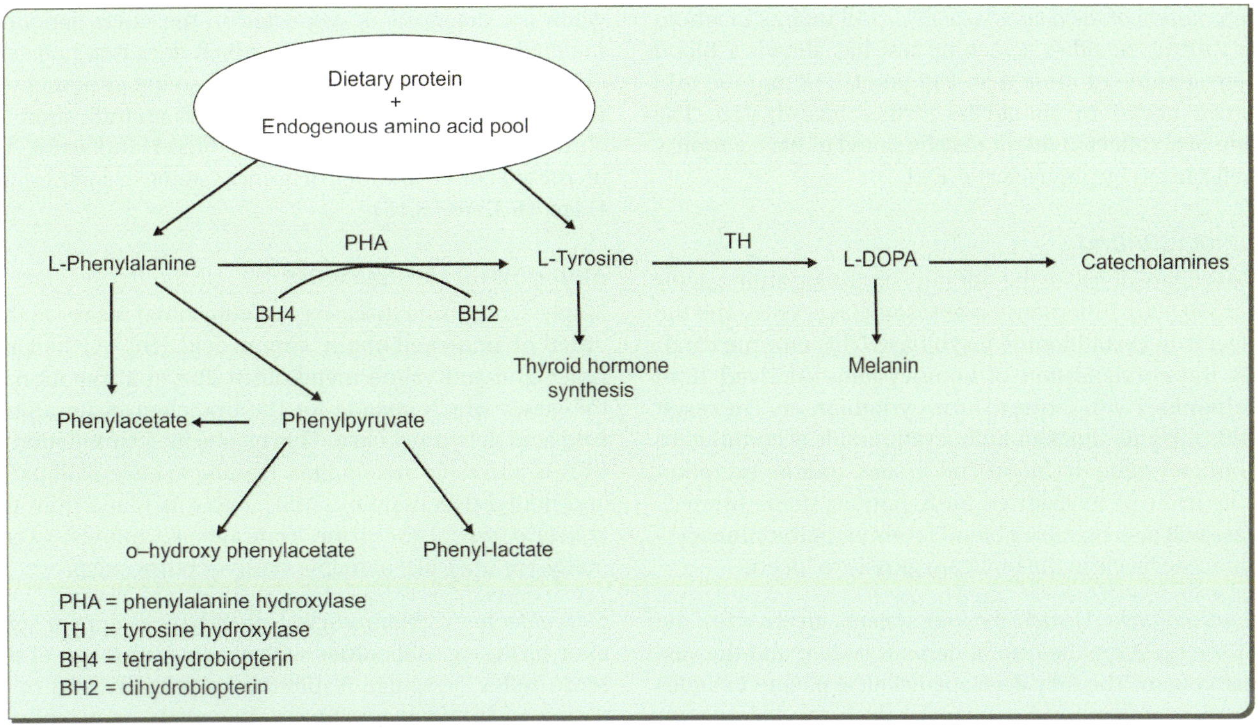

Figure 16.11 Phenylalanine metabolism showing role of biopterin.

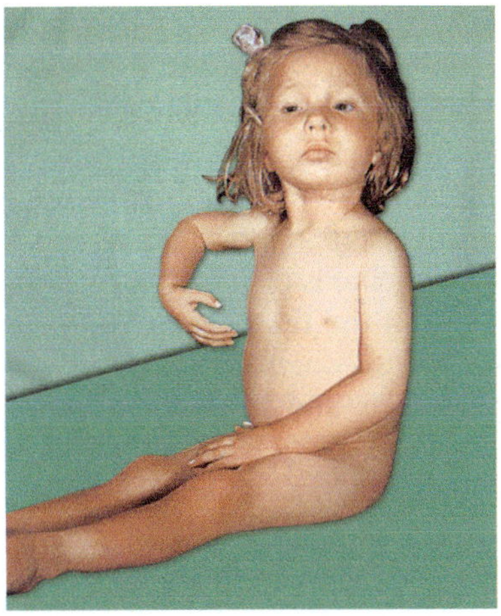

Figure 16.12 Child with untreated phenylketonuria.

to be inversely and linearly associated with maternal phenylalanine concentrations. Phenylalanine concentrations during pregnancy and in the period prior to conception should be maintained between 60 and 250 μmol/L. Effective contraception should be continued until control has been achieved. Biochemical monitoring should be at least twice weekly and careful foetal ultrasound examinations to assess foetal growth and anatomy should be performed. Restriction of maternal dietary phenylalanine with tyrosine supplementation when necessary begun prior to conception controls the blood phenylalanine level and metabolite accumulation in the pregnant mother with PKU just as it does in the child with PKU. Dietary treatment begun after 8th week of conception is much less effective. It is essential, therefore, those women with PKU should be appropriately counselled and supported so that their children are conceived under the best possible phenylalanine control.

Diagnosis When it became clear that a low-phenylalanine diet improved the intelligence of patients with PKU, the need for early diagnosis, before intellectual impairment had occurred, was recognised. This requirement demands the "screening" of all newborn infants in a community. Those infants found to give a positive result with the screening test require to be submitted to more detailed confirmatory tests.

The neonatal screening programmes, which are now used, permit the accurate detection of infants who have raised blood phenylalanine levels from the 5th day of life. The most commonly used screening test for raised blood phenylalanine in the United Kingdom was initially the Guthrie bacterial inhibition test, which has been proved to be extremely reliable. Both the Guthrie test and chromatography can be modified to "screen" for several other inborn errors such as galactosaemia, tyrosinaemia, homocystinuria and maple-syrup urine disease. Techniques have evolved from Guthrie bacterial inhibition tests to TMS which can potentially identify a vast array of conditions. The objective is to identify as soon after birth as possible and before the onset of recognizable clinical symptoms, specific metabolic disorders that can then be treated to ameliorate the consequences of untreated disease.

Confirmation of the diagnosis of PKU All infants in whom the Guthrie or other screening test has shown a blood phenylalanine of more than 240 μmol/L (4 mg/100 mL) on two occasions should be further investigated. The urine of an affected infant may be noted to have a mousy smell caused by phenylacetic acid.

Homocystinuria

This is a rare defect of the sulphur containing amino acids (1 in 350,000). Inheritance is autosomal recessive, and the defect is in cystathionine β-synthase. This enzyme catalyses the condensation of homocysteine (derived from methionine) with serine to form cystathionine. The result of this enzyme block in homocystinuria is accumulation of homocysteine in blood and tissues, and its excretion in the urine in its oxidized form, homocysteine (dimer). There will also be raised blood levels of methionine; cystathionine levels in the brain are grossly reduced.

Clinical features Usually the four systems involved are the eye, the skeleton, the central nervous system and the vascular system. The fully developed clinical picture includes mental retardation, seizures, malar flush, fair hair, downward dislocation of the lens, livedo reticularis and thromboembolic episodes in both arteries and veins. Skeletal changes have been common, e.g. genu valgum, pes cavus, arachnodactyly, irregular epiphyses, vertebral changes, osteoporosis and pectus carinatum or excavatum. The fully developed picture resembles that of Marfan syndrome (Marfanoid habitus of the body) but in the latter there is no mental retardation, no osteoporosis, no thrombotic tendency, the dislocation of the lens is upwards and inheritance is dominant. Epileptic seizures may also occur. A considerable number of patients have a normal level of intelligence.

Diagnosis The diagnosis can be made early in infancy during screening programmes, and before clinical abnormalities have become manifest. A simple screening test when the diagnosis is suspected in the older patient is the nitroprusside/cyanide test, which does not, however, discriminate between an excess of cysteine or homocysteine in the urine. A positive reaction is an indication for chromatographic examination of blood and urine for increased concentrations of homocysteine or methionine **(Figs. 16.13 to 16.15)**.

Maple Syrup Urine Disease

Maple syrup urine disease is an autosomal recessive disorder of branched-chain amino acid (BCAA) leucine, isoleucine and valine metabolism due to a mutation in the genes which encode for the branched-chain alpha-keto acid dehydrogenase. This results in accumulation of BCAAs and their metabolites, leading to encephalopathy and neural degeneration. MSUD gets its name from the typical odour of the urine from affected infants: sweet, malty, caramel-like of maple syrup or burnt sugar.

Clinical features Neurological disturbances appear soon after birth, e.g. difficulties with feeding, absence of the Moro reflex, irregular respirations, spasticity and opisthotonus. Intercurrent illness, starvation or injury can precipitate symptoms by increasing the catabolism of endogenous symptoms. Pronounced dehydration and metabolic acidosis are usually not features of acute MSUD in contrast to disorders of organic acid metabolism.

Diagnosis Early diagnosis and management are essential to prevent permanent brain damage or death. Plasma and urine amino acids chromatography shows significantly elevated branched leucine, isoleucine and valine. Presence of allo-isoleucine is diagnostic (though may appear towards the end of the first week of life). Urine organic acid analysis reveals increased excretion of branched chain hydroxyl acids and keto acids. Demonstration of decreased enzyme activity in lymphocytes or fibroblasts is not essential for diagnosis **(Fig. 16.16)**.

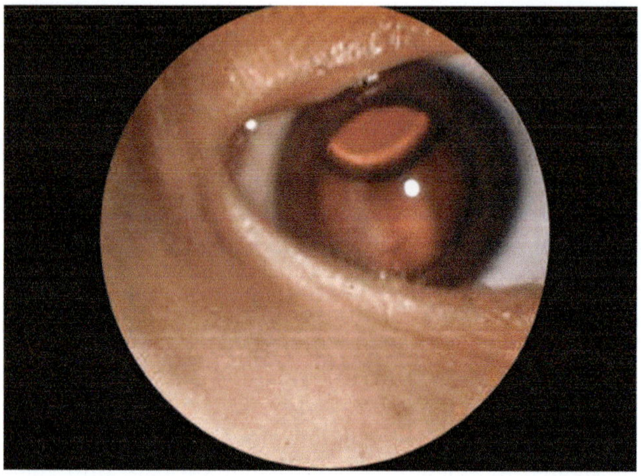

Figure 16.13 Lens dislocation in homocystinuria.

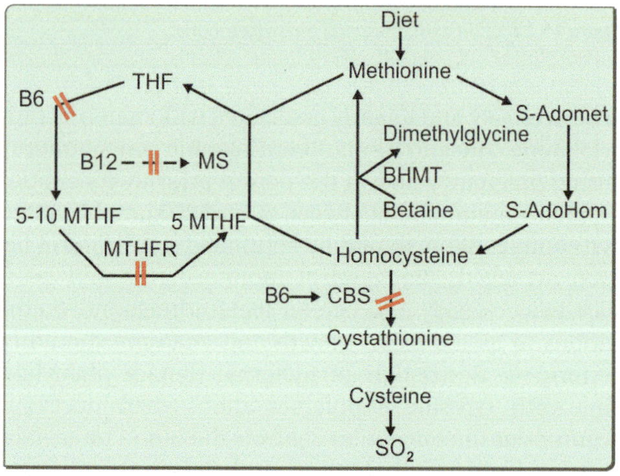

Figure 16.14 Pathways in homocysteine metabolism.

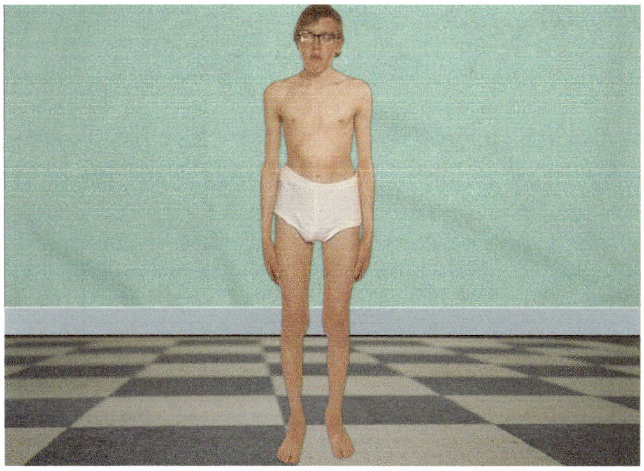

Figure 16.15 Marfanoid habitus present in two-thirds of cases of homocystinuria.

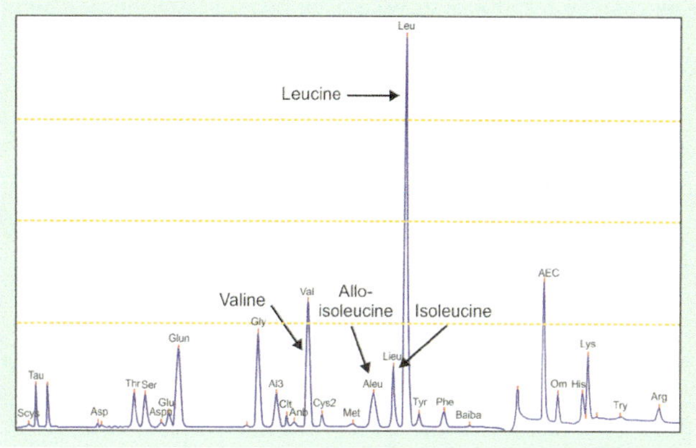

Figure 16.16 Amino acid chromatogram showing maple syrup urine disease.

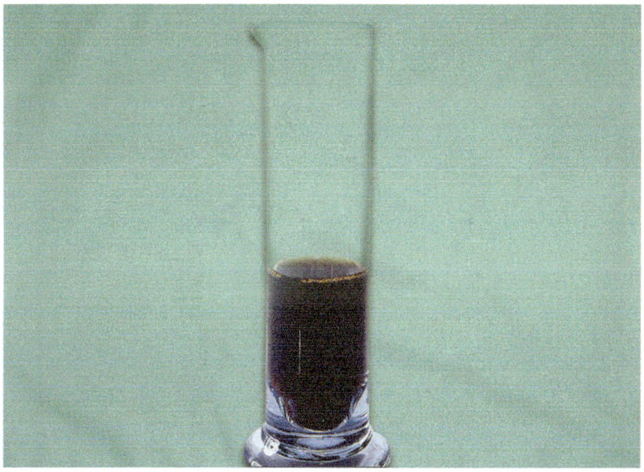

Figure 16.17 Homogentisic acid—darkening urine as left in sunlight.

Alkaptonuria

Alkaptonuria is due to deficiency of the enzyme homogentisic acid oxidase so that homogentisic acid, instead of being converted to maleylacetoacetate, accumulates in the tissues and is excreted in the urine. The urine is noted to turn dark on standing as the homogentisic acid is oxidized to a melanin like product or it can be made to do so immediately by the addition of ammonia or sodium hydroxide. The alkaptonuric is symptomless in childhood but in adult life develops ochronosis and arthritis. This causes an ochre-like pigmentation of sclerae, ears, nasal cartilages and tendon sheaths, also kyphosis and osteoarthritis of the large joints. The disease is usually inherited as an autosomal recessive. A few families have shown dominant inheritance **(Fig. 16.17)**.

Organic Acidaemias

There are now described more than 30 inherited conditions characterised by an excessive urinary excretion of acidic metabolites of amino acids, carbohydrates and fats. Infants with otherwise unexplained metabolic acidosis, who become acutely ill, should have urine levels of organic acid and its by-products analysed by GC-MS in order to detect conditions such as isovaleric acidaemia, glutaric aciduria, propionic acidaemia and methylmalonic aciduria. Of these, propionic and methylmalonic aciduria constitute the most commonly encountered abnormal organic acidurias in children.

Infants with isovaleric, propionic and methylmalonic acidurias have many symptoms in common. After an initial symptom-free period, babies may present with feeding difficulties, vomiting, lethargy, respiratory distress, hypotonia and generalised hypertonic episodes. Metabolic acidosis, ketonuria, hyperammonaemia, hypocarnitinaemia, neutropaenia and thrombocytopaenia are almost constant findings. The acute presentation is frequently precipitated by infection or some other form of stress. Treatment includes stopping all protein intake and maintenance with dextrose and bicarbonate to control acidosis. The emergency treatment of organic acidurias consists of removal of toxic metabolites by haemo- or peritoneal dialysis and/or exchange transfusions. The use of N-carbamyl glutamate 100 mg 6 hourly acutely has revolutionised the correction of hyperammonaemia by replacing the absent promoter of carbamoyl phosphate synthetase. The long-term treatment involves reducing accumulated toxic products, maintaining normal nutritional status and preventing catabolism. Therefore, in these children protein intake is largely restricted **(Flow chart 16.1 and Fig. 16.18)**.

Urea Cycle Disorders

Six well-documented diseases have been described, each representing a defect in the biosynthesis of one of the normally expressed enzymes of the urea cycle, which converts nitrogen in amino acids into urea and CO_2 **(Fig. 16.19)**. Carbamyl phosphate synthetase converts

Flow chart 16.1 Pathways showing major organic acid metabolic defects.

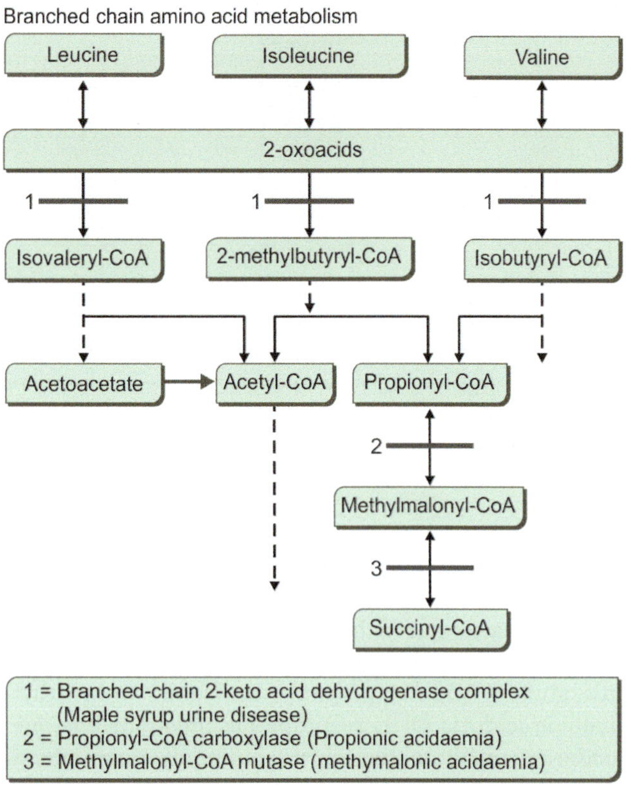

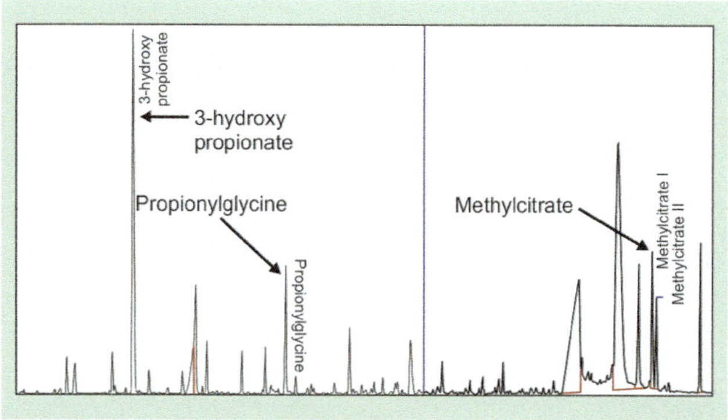

Figure 16.18 Organic acid chromatogram confirming propionic acidaemia with no increase in methylmalonate.

ammonia and bicarbonate to carbamyl phosphate, which then condenses with ornithine under the action of ornithine transcarbamylase to form citrulline. The conversion of citrulline to argininosuccinic acid is catalysed by argininosuccinate synthetase, and argininosuccinic acid is cleaved to form arginine and fumaric acid by argininosuccinate cleavage enzyme (argininosuccinase). The enzyme arginase finally converts arginine into urea and ornithine. The synthetic process takes place in the liver. The mechanisms leading to the toxicity of ammonia are not fully understood. The clinical manifestations of urea cycle disorders are mainly abnormalities secondary to hyperammonaemia and protein intolerance. A rapid diagnosis and institution of dietary treatment is essential for a good prognosis.

All enzyme defects have autosomal recessive inheritance, except for ornithine transcarbamylase, which is inherited as an X-linked trait with variable expression in the female. The increased amounts of orotic acid indicate carbamoyl phosphate was synthesised and along with the plasma amino acid pattern indicates the specific disorder.

Arginase Deficiency/Argininaemia

Arginase deficiency presents in childhood with hyperammonaemia, vomiting and retarded development with spastic quadriplegia, convulsions and hepatomegaly. Plasma and CSF arginine concentrations are grossly

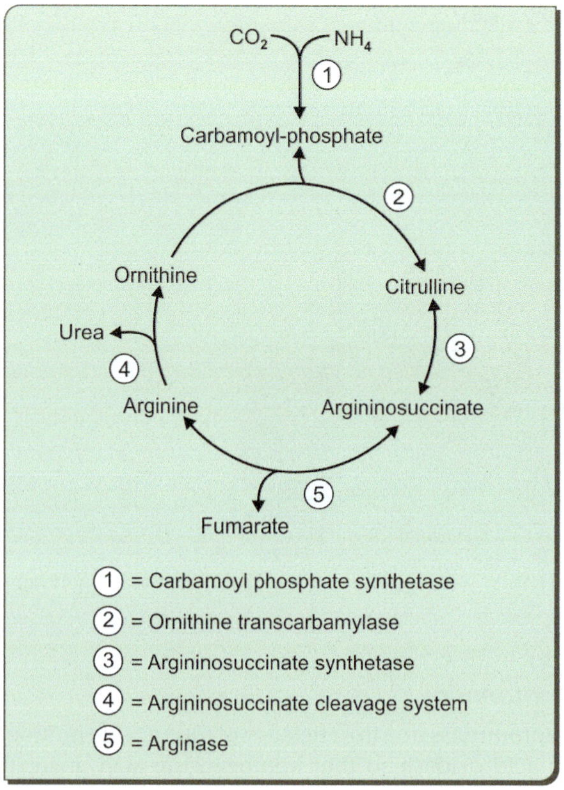

Figure 16.19 Ornithine urea cycle.

elevated. Arginase deficiency can be demonstrated in erythrocytes and is rare (1 in 500,000).

Disorders of Specific Sugars

Galactosaemia

Galactose is ingested as lactose in milk, which undergoes splitting in the intestine into its component monosaccharides glucose and galactose. Milk and its products are virtually the sole source of dietary galactose in man. Galactose is then converted to glucose or energy in a series of enzyme steps **(Fig. 16.20)**. Although, the liver is the main site of this conversion, the demonstration of

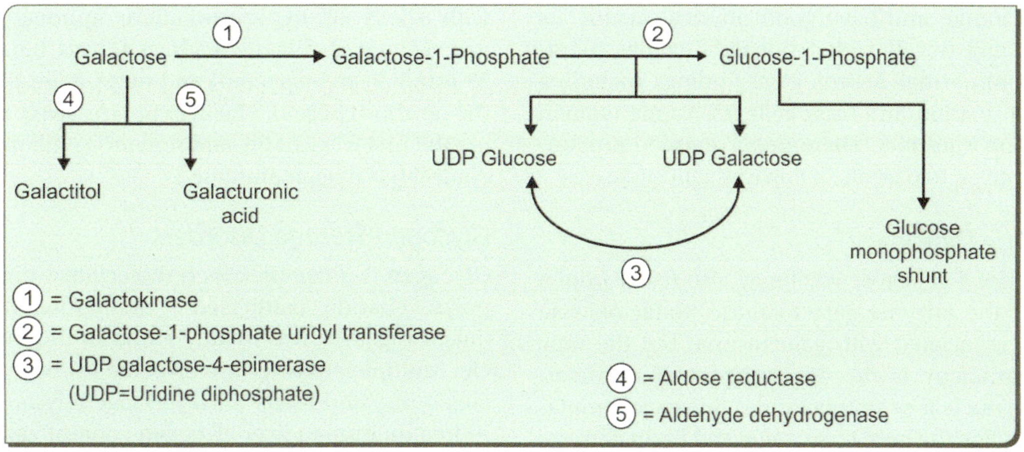

Figure 16.20 Enzyme steps in galactose metabolism in erythrocytes.

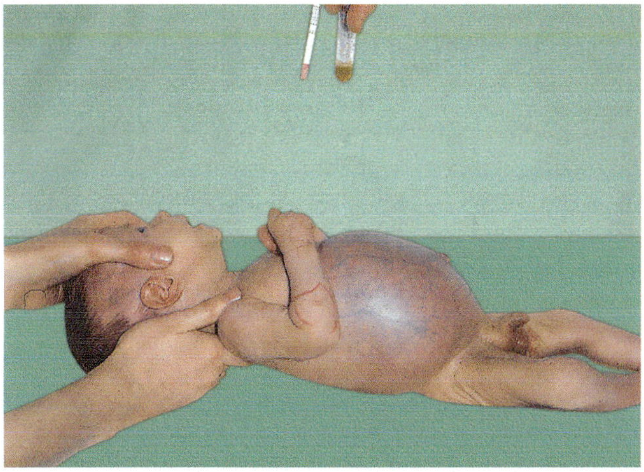

Figure 16.21 Severely ill neonate with galactosaemia, with positive Benedict's test and liver enlargement.

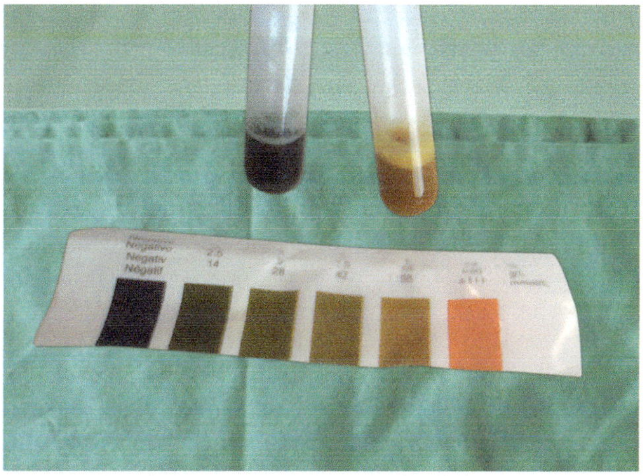

Figure 16.22 Urine—Positive Benedict's test.

a similar series of enzyme reactions in red cells and the excess accumulation of galactose-l-phosphate (Gal-1-P) in the erythrocytes makes red cells, the diagnostic material of choice.

Clinical features Two main clinical types occur. The more severely affected children develop clinical features within 2 weeks of birth, after milk-feeding has been started, with vomiting, disinclination to feed, diarrhoea, loss of weight, dehydration, hypoglycaemia, hepatocellular damage and renal tubular damage. The liver is enlarged with a firm, smooth edge and there may be jaundice. Splenomegaly is common. Cataracts may be seen with a slit-lamp. Finally, the infant becomes severely marasmic with hepatic cirrhosis, ascites and hypoprothrombinaemia. Obvious signs and symptoms are later to appear in the less severe type, although a history suggesting some early intolerance to milk may be obtained. The child may present with mental retardation, bilateral cataracts and cirrhosis of the liver. All the abnormalities, except for mental retardation, may regress rapidly on a galactose-free diet. It is, therefore, of prime importance that the diagnosis is made before irreversible brain damage has occurred. Undiagnosed cases may succumb to gram-negative sepsis **(Fig. 16.21)**.

Diagnosis The first clue to the disease may be a positive Benedict's test for the presence of a reducing substance in the urine. However, care must be taken as due to developing tubulopathy, specific test for urine glucose (Clinistix, which uses the enzyme glucose oxidase) may be positive; proteinuria may also be present. Chromatography is required to confirm the reducing substance as galactose. There may be significant aminoaciduria and proteinuria due to renal tubular damage. Galactitol can be detected in blood and urine. The demonstration of the absence of Gal-1-P uridyl transferase activity in the red cells confirms the diagnosis **(Fig. 16.22)**.

Outlook Unfortunately, galactosaemic children (despite treatment, avoiding milk and its products from the diet) tend to fall below the average in mental development in spite of dietary treatment, although they remain within the educable range and have good physical health. As adolescents, some develop educational difficulties, memory loss and abnormal neurological findings including ataxia, incoordination and brisk reflexes. Young women usually develop infertility. Therefore, a guarded prognosis should be given to parents of newly diagnosed cases.

Galactokinase Deficiency

An elevated blood galactose level may also result from a deficiency of the enzyme galactokinase. Galactokinase deficiency is associated with galactosuria, but the only significant pathology is the development of cataracts, which may be nuclear or zonular and is due to accumulation of galactitol in the lens. Liver, renal and brain damage do not occur. The dietary treatment as for galactosaemia prevents the development of cataracts and should be started as early in infancy as possible.

Hereditary Fructose Intolerance

Aetiology This disease causes severe metabolic disturbances. It must be clearly distinguished from benign fructosuria which is due to a deficiency of fructokinase and is of no clinical consequence.

Pathogenesis The metabolic pathways of fructose are complicated. The primary enzymatic defect is in fructose-1-phosphate aldolase, which in the liver and intestine splits fructose-l-phosphate into two trioses, glyceraldehyde and dihydroxyacetone phosphate. This defect results in the accumulation of fructose-1-phosphate, which inhibits fructokinase and leads to high blood levels of fructose after its ingestion in the diet. The intracellular accumulation of fructose-1-phosphate prevents the conversion of liver glycogen to glucose.

Clinical features Symptoms only appear when fructose is introduced into the diet as sucrose (glucose + fructose) in milk feeds, as sorbitol or as fruit juices. The condition varies in severity, partly according to the amounts of fructose ingested, and the wholly breast-fed infants remain symptomless. Common features are failure to thrive, anorexia, vomiting, diarrhoea and hepatomegaly; these may lead to marasmus. Hypoglycaemia may cause convulsions or loss of consciousness. Liver damage may result in jaundice, and LFTs are abnormal. Albuminuria, fructosuria and excess aminoaciduria may be present. Hyperfructosaemia and hypoglycaemia develop following upon the ingestion of fructose or sucrose. Death ensues in undiagnosed infants. In milder cases, i.e. in older children gastrointestinal symptoms predominate, and in some, a profound distaste of anything sweet develops spontaneously as a protective mechanism.

Hereditary Fructose-1,6-Bisphosphatase Deficiency

Hepatic fructose-1,6-bisphosphatase deficiency is usually classified as an error of fructose metabolism. It manifests with spells of hyperventilation, apnoea, hypoglycaemia, ketosis and lactic acidosis (levels between 10 and 25 mmol/L are expected) and may be life-threatening in the newborn period. The liver progressively enlarges during the first week of life and remains so till period of good control has been maintained.

Glycogen Storage Disorders

Glycogen is a complex high molecular weight branched polysaccharide, composed of numerous glucosyl units linked together. It is mainly found in the liver and muscle. Multiple enzymes are involved in the synthesis (glycogenesis) and breakdown (glycogenolysis) of glycogen. In health, human liver glycogen content varies from 0 to 5%, while muscle glycogen is rarely as high as 1%. Hepatic glycogen functions as a reserve of glucose and is utilised during fasting to maintain normoglycaemia.

Glycogen storage disorders comprise a group of disorders, some of which have hepatic presentations with liver enlargement and hypoglycaemia. In addition, there are a number of subtypes with exercise-induced myalgia and cramps often leading to rhabdomyolysis. Two of these (myopathic GSD III and GSD V) give rise to a chronic myopathy affecting trunk, limb and respiratory muscles. GSD II (Pompe disease) is a specific defect affecting lysosomal breakdown of glycogen presenting with cardiomyopathy in infancy.

Type I Glycogenosis (von Gierke Disease; Glucose-6-Phosphatase Deficiency)

Pathogenesis The enzyme glucose-6-phosphatase normally liberates free glucose from glucose-6-phosphate in the liver. Its absent activity results in GSD type Ia, seriously limiting the ability to release glucose from glycogen or gluconeogenesis.

Clinical features Gross enlargement of the liver is the most constant feature and it is often recognised in early infancy. In the severe form, it may present in the neonatal period with profound hypoglycaemia and acidosis. Growth is stunted and the protuberant abdomen is often associated with an exaggerated lumbar lordosis. Genu valgum (knock knees) is common. There may be an excess deposition of subcutaneous fat, leading to affected infants developing a characteristically round (doll-like) face **(Fig. 16.23)**. Xanthomatous deposits are commonly found on the knees, elbows and buttocks. There is no splenomegaly and there are no signs of cirrhosis. Gout and uric acid nephropathy may develop and there are reports of hepatic adenomata formation. The presence of fever may lead to an erroneous diagnosis of sepsis.

Type Ib has a similar clinical course with the additional findings of neutropenia and impaired neutrophil function resulting in recurrent bacterial infections. Oral and intestinal mucosa ulceration commonly occurs.

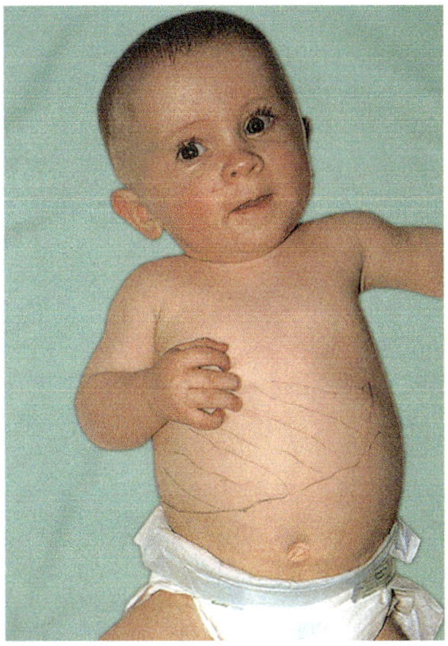

Figure 16.23 4-month-old infant with GSD 1a. Note rounded facies and gross hepatomegaly.

Biochemical findings Hypoglycaemia may be so severe as to precipitate convulsions and even lead to mental impairment. Hyperlipaemia and hypercholesterolaemia are marked and may even interfere with accurate measurement of plasma electrolytes. Episodes of severe metabolic acidosis develop in some cases. Plasma pyruvate and lactate concentrations are increased and phosphate may be reduced. Renal damage from glycogenosis can cause glycosuria and aminoaciduria.

Diagnosis Hepatomegaly with the combination of hypoglycaemia, hyperlactic acidaemia and hyperuricaemia is virtually diagnostic of type I glycogenosis. Further evidence of von Gierke disease may be obtained from a variety of tests:

The glucose tolerance test (after 1.5 g glucose/kg) shows paradoxical fall in plasma lactate.

Another indirect measurement of glucose-6-phosphatase activity can be obtained after an intravenous dose of galactose 1 g/kg, or fructose 0.5 g/kg. Blood glucose concentrations at 10-minute intervals are compared with the preinjection value. In healthy persons, galactose and fructose are converted via glucose-6-phosphate to free glucose, but this metabolic pathway is blocked in von Gierke disease.

Conclusive proof of the diagnosis, however, can only be obtained from a liver biopsy for low glucose-6-phosphatase activity or DNA mutation analysis in blood.

Glycogenosis of the Heart (Pompe Disease; GSD Type II)

Pathogenesis The disease may involve the CNS and skeletal muscles as well as the myocardium. The primary defect is of the lysosomal enzyme acid alpha-1,4-glucosidase (acid maltase).

Clinical features Clinically, the enzyme deficiency results in two major presentations. The first was originally described by Pompe. The infant becomes ill in the early weeks of life with anorexia, vomiting, dyspnoea and failure to thrive. The heart is enlarged, tachycardia is present and a systolic murmur is commonly heard. Oedema may also develop. The electrocardiography shows a shortened P-R interval, inverted T waves and depression of the ST segments. When skeletal muscles are severely involved the degree of hypotonia may simulate Werdnig-Hoffmann disease. In some infants, macroglossia has been so marked as to arouse the suspicion of cretinism. On the other hand, hepatomegaly is not prominent until cardiac failure is advanced. The diagnosis may be established by muscle biopsy and the demonstration of increased glycogen content. There will also be low acid maltase activity in the leucocytes.

The second presentation is of a more slowly progressive muscle disorder, with symptoms beginning in childhood or in adult life and manifestations limited to skeletal muscle. The muscle involvement is mainly proximal muscle weakness including impairment of respiratory function. Death results from respiratory failure **(Figs. 16.24 and 16.25)**.

Type III Glycogenosis (Debrancher Enzyme Deficiency)

Pathogenesis The debrancher enzyme (amylo-1,6-glucosidase) is absent from liver, skeletal and cardiac muscle, resulting in glycogen deposition in these organs (unlike von Gierke disease, where glycogen deposition does not occur in heart and skeletal muscles).

Clinical features Hepatomegaly is marked but hypoglycaemic problems are less troublesome and there is less interference with growth. It is common to find the same plump appearance and round face as in von Gierke disease. In some cases, the involvement of skeletal muscles gives rise to weakness and hypotonia.

Diagnosis De-esterification of glucose-6-phosphate to glucose can proceed normally and there is, therefore, a normal hyperglycaemic response to intravenous galactose or fructose. The serum lactate level is not often raised but rises during an oral glucose tolerance test; there is dyslipidaemia. The liver glycogen content is increased and it is abnormal in structure with short external chains and an increased number of 1,6 branch points. Activity of liver amylo-1,6-glucosidase is not detectable. It is also possible to demonstrate an elevated erythrocyte glycogen of the limit dextrin type. Direct assay of the enzyme in liver and muscle tissue is confirmatory.

Type IV Glycogenosis (Familial Cirrhosis of the Liver with Abnormal Glycogen; Brancher Enzyme Deficiency)

This appears to be an extremely rare disease in which amylo-(1,4-1,6)-transglucosidase deficiency results in deposition of an abnormal glycogen with a molecular

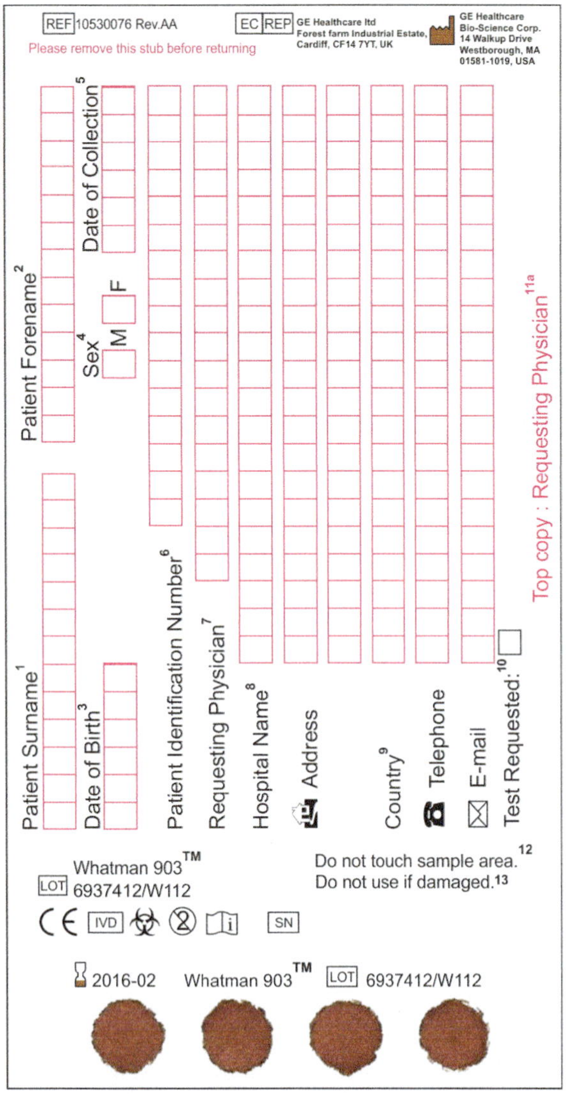

Figure 16.24 Blood spot card (previously known as Guthrie test) increasingly being used to measure lysosomal enzymes and basis for screening analysis by fluorometric assays on plate readers or tandem mass spectrometer analysis for complexes failing to be metabolised.

structure resembling the amylopectins of plants. This substance is toxic so that the patient presents with cirrhosis of the liver, splenomegaly and jaundice. LFTs yield grossly abnormal results and death is preceded by the development of ascites and deep jaundice. This diagnosis should be considered in all cases of familial hepatic cirrhosis. Deficiency of the branching enzyme can be demonstrated in liver and leucocytes. There is no specific treatment for GSD type IV.

Type V Glycogenosis (Myophosphorylase Deficiency; McArdle Disease)

Children with myophosphorylase deficiency are asymptomatic at rest but muscle cramps occur with moderate exercise. These symptoms are usually absent or minimal during the first decade. A diagnosis is made on the basis of history and the absence of elevation of lactate after exercise

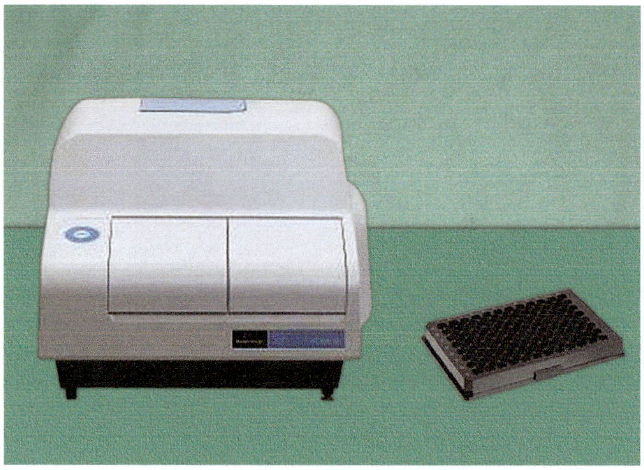

Figure 16.25 Fluorometer plate reader with 96 well plates which after controls allows 40 samples in duplicate with minimal reagent use.

Forearm exercise test

Time (mins)	0	1	2	3	5	10
	Plasma Ammonia (umol/L) Plasma lactate (mmol/L)					
Normal response	45 0.8	85 1.5	155 2.8	202 5.1	125 3.6	85 2.9
McArdle disease	45 0.8	85 1.1	155 1.2	202 0.9	125 1.4	85 1.0

Figure 16.26 McArdle's ischaemic forearm exercise test in normal and affected cases.

(forearm exercise test). It may remain undiagnosed during childhood and presents in adult life with muscle weakness, cramps and a characteristic "second-wind" phenomenon (marked improvement in tolerance to aerobic exercise, like walking or cycling, after about 10–20 minutes, especially after a brief rest). Severe exercise risks rhabdomyolysis; at rest, the patients remain asymptomatic.

No specific treatment is available, but the patient should continue regular exercise such as walking to keep fit and develop physiological adaptation **(Fig. 16.26)**.

Purine Disorders

Lesch-Nyhan syndrome This is an X-linked recessive disorder caused by deficiencies of the enzyme hypoxanthine-guanine phosphoribosyltransferase, resulting in excessive quantities of uric acid in blood, tissue and urine.

Clinical features It is characterised by central nervous system disorders of various types and excessive urate. Male infants are generally normal at birth but soon develop mental retardation and have choreoathetosis, spasticity and distressing compulsive self-mutilation, or they may present with gouty arthritis and pain from ureteric colic caused by urates.

Diagnosis High blood and/or urine urate concentrations should raise suspicion. A definite diagnosis can be made

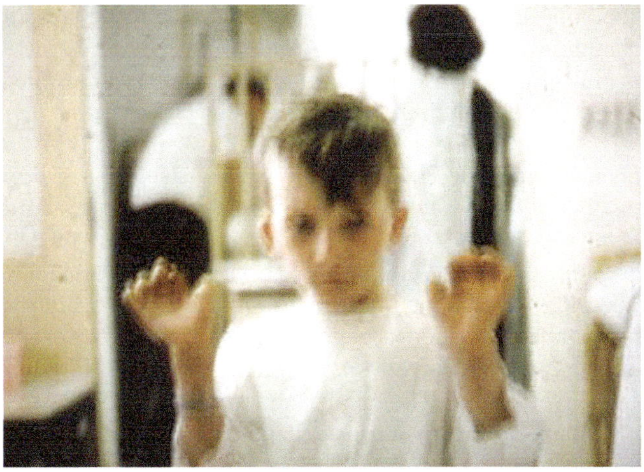

Figure 16.27 Child with Lesch–Nyhan syndrome.

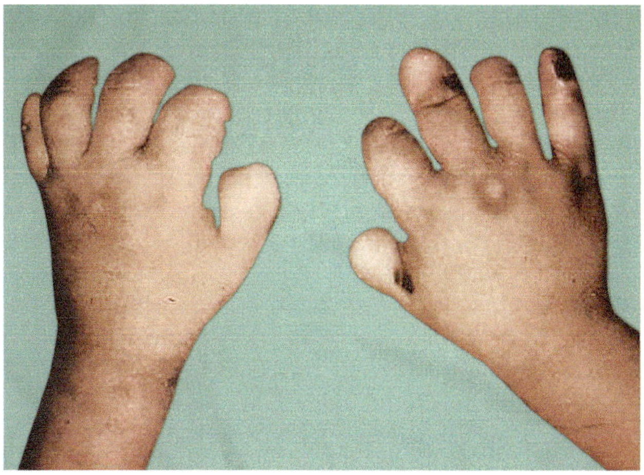

Figure 16.28 Hands of child demonstrating self-mutilation.

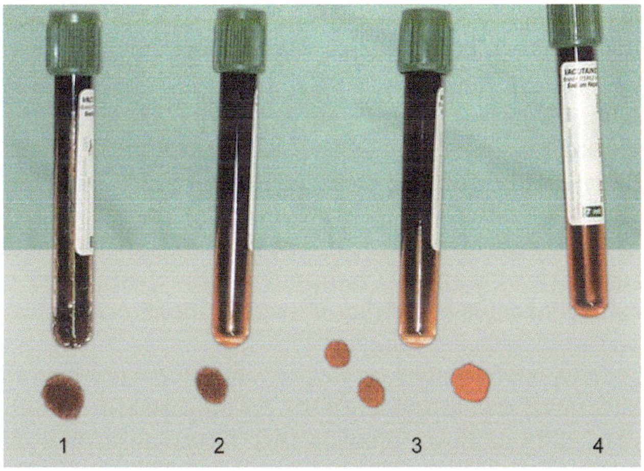

Figure 16.29 Methaemoglobinaemic samples; 1 and 2 ~ 70% methaemoglobin; 3 ~ 20% and 4, normal asymptomatic till >20% deficiency.

by the absence of hypoxanthine-guanine phosphoribosyltransferase enzyme activity in peripheral circulating erythrocytes **(Figs. 16.27 and 16.28)**.

CONGENITAL METHAEMOGLOBINAEMIA

Aetiology

The most common form of congenital methaemoglobinaemia is inherited as an autosomal recessive trait and it is due to the absence of a normal intraerythrocytic enzyme activity. A rare type, inherited as an autosomal dominant, has a quite different aetiology in that it is due to the formation of haemoglobin M with a defective globulin component.

Pathogenesis

In normal haemoglobin, the iron of the four-haem groups is in the reduced or ferrous state. In methaemoglobin, the iron is in the oxidised or ferric state and it is incapable of combining with oxygen. In normal erythrocytes, methaemoglobin is constantly being formed and detectable in small amounts but is being continuously reduced back to haemoglobin by a complex series of enzymatic steps. Congenital methaemoglobinaemia is caused by an intraerythrocytic defect in one of these enzymes. Alternatively, congenital methaemoglobinaemia is caused by haemoglobin M.

Clinical Features

The primary sign is a dusky slate-grey type of cyanosis, which is present from birth. The child is free from respiratory or cardiac symptoms and clubbing of the fingers and toes does not develop. Some patients develop compensatory polycythaemia and some may go onto become severely mentally retarded.

Diagnosis

The presence of excess methaemoglobin in the blood should be demonstrated by spectrophotometry.

It is important to distinguish the congenital and permanent form of methaemoglobinaemia from the temporary but dangerous acquired form, due to toxins such as aniline dyes, nitrites, acetanilide and potassium chlorate. It is important to remember that cyanotic children without heart murmurs may have methaemoglobinaemia **(Fig. 16.29)**.

Inborn Errors of Lipid Metabolism (Lipidoses)

This group includes Gaucher disease, Niemann-Pick disease, Tay-Sachs disease, metachromatic leukodystrophy and Krabbe's leukodystrophy. In the lipidoses, there is an abnormal intracellular deposition of sphingolipids, often widely spread throughout many organs and tissues as in Gaucher and Niemann-Pick diseases.

Gaucher Disease

Aetiology In Gaucher disease, a glucocerebroside (glucosylceramide) is deposited in the tissues. The glycolipids from which glucocerebroside is generated are derived from senescent leucocytes and erythrocytes. They are normally broken down by a series of enzymes, one of which is glucocerebrosidase. In the type 1 form of the disease, the spleen has only about 15% of normal enzyme activity whereas in the type 2 acute form glucocerebrosidase is completely absent from the spleen and other organs (including the brain).

Clinical features This disease appears to occur in three forms: (1) type 1 adult, chronic, non-neuropathic form, (2) type 2 infantile, acute, neuropathic form and (3) type 3 juvenile sub-acute neuropathic form.

Type 1 Gaucher disease: The type 1 chronic form is the most common. It presents at any age from a few months to late adulthood with gross splenomegaly. Hepatic enlargement may also be marked. There is also a progressive anaemia, and leucopenia and thrombocytopenia due to hypersplenism developing early in its course. Bone involvement may give rise to limb pains. Radiographs reveal a characteristic flaring outwards of the metaphyseal ends of the long bones with thinning of the cortex. This is most marked at the lower ends of the femora, which have an Erlenmeyer flask appearance. These features develop in childhood or early adult life. In older patients especially, the face, neck, hands and legs may show a characteristic brownish pigmentation, and the conjunctiva may show a wedge-shaped area of thickening with its base to the cornea (pinguecula). The diagnosis can be confirmed by finding the lipid-filled cells, which have a typical fibrillary appearance of the cytoplasm. These should be sought in material obtained by needle puncture of the bone marrow, spleen or lymph nodes. The disease runs a slow course but death is inevitable.

Type 2 Gaucher disease: The type 2 infantile acute form is a rare presentation confined to infancy. In addition to hepatosplenomegaly, there is evidence of severe cerebral involvement, which is rarely seen, in the chronic form. There may be hypertonia, catatonia, trismus, opisthotonus, dysphagia, strabismus and respiratory difficulties. Death occurs by the age of 3 years.

Type 3 Gaucher disease: The type 3 juvenile sub-acute form shares some characteristics of types 1 and 2. Neurological features may appear early in addition to hepatosplenomegaly but the time course of progression is slower. Spasticity, ataxia, ocular palsies, mental retardation and seizures are later features. Ultimate proof of diagnosis requires tissue or white blood cell beta glucosidase (glucocerebrosidase) assay, or liver or spleen glucocerebroside determination. Prenatal diagnosis is routinely available for all types of Gaucher disease.

Niemann–Pick Disease

Aetiology Sphingomyelin, a component of myelin and other cell membranes, accumulates within cells throughout the CNS and other tissues. Sphingomyelin is normally catabolised by the action of sphingomyelinase but in Niemann-Pick disease type A or B, this enzyme activity is only about 7% of normal. In type C, there is a complex defect in cellular cholesterol trafficking.

Clinical features This disease also consists of a group of disorders characterised by hepatosplenomegaly and accumulation of sphingomyelin (ceramide phosphorylcholine) in organs and tissues. Three clinical forms have been identified. In type A (acute neuropathic), which is the commonest, there is hepatosplenomegaly by 6 months of age and there are severe feeding difficulties related to CNS involvement. The infant's abdomen becomes greatly protuberant due to massive hepatosplenomegaly. Skin pigmentation is common and severe wasting is invariable. Deterioration in cerebral functions appears early and progresses to a state of severe incapacity with generalised muscular weakness and wasting. Pulmonary involvement is commonly found. Anaemia of severe degree is an early sign but thrombocytopenia develops late, in contrast to its early appearance in Gaucher disease. In some affected infants, ophthalmoscopy reveals a cherry-red spot at the macula resembling the retinal appearance in Tay-Sachs disease and corneal opacities may be found.

Confirmation of diagnosis depends on demonstration of increased sphingomyelin levels in tissue specimens (usually liver or spleen) and/or identification of a specific sphingomyelinase deficiency in white blood cells, fibroblasts or visceral specimens.

In type B (chronic non-neuropathic), there is a slightly later onset and no evidence of CNS impairment. Pulmonary infiltration can predispose to recurrent respiratory infections. In type C (chronic neuropathic), there is gradual onset, usually after the age of 18 months, of neurological impairment manifest as ataxia, loss of speech with dysarthria and convulsions. Most die before the age of 15 years **(Fig. 16.30)**.

GM2 Gangliosidosis (Tay–Sachs Disease; Sandhoff Disease)

Aetiology An abnormal accumulation of GM2 ganglioside is confined to the brain resulting in progressive cortical failure and death by 2.5–5 years of age. These are complex lipids and their catabolism involves a succession of enzymes of which hexosaminidase is lacking in Tay-Sachs disease. There are two hexosaminidases in the body, hexosaminidases A and B. In classical Tay-Sachs disease (type 1)—commonly seen in Ashkenazi Jews—only hexosaminidase A is lacking; in the non-Jewish form (type 2: Sandhoff disease), which is clinically indistinguishable, both A and B are absent. There are also extremely rare adult and juvenile forms that have their onset after the age of 1 year and in which hexosaminidase A activity is from 10 to 12% of normal. All types are inherited as autosomal recessive.

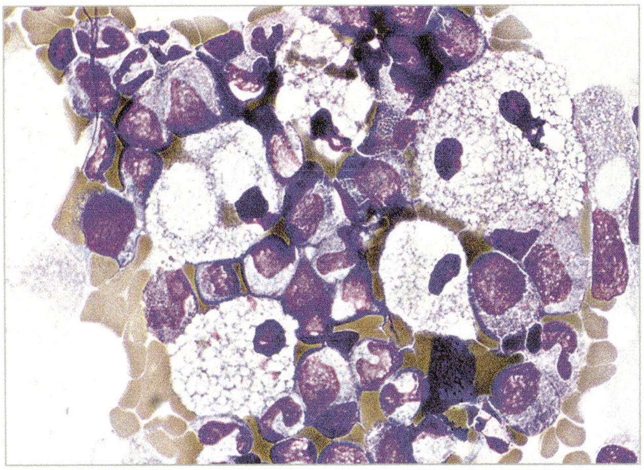

Figure 16.30 Niemann–Pick disease—foamy or mulberry-like cells in the bone marrow.

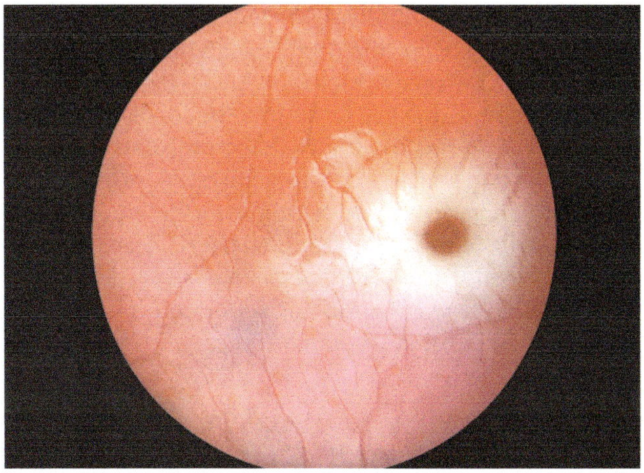

Figure 16.31 Cherry red spot in the fundus of child with Tay–Sachs disease.

Clinical features In this disease because the deposition of lipid is confined to the CNS the features are neurological in character. They appear between the ages of 4 and 6 months as delay in psychomotor development, irritability, hyperacusis for sudden noises, spasticity, generalised weakness and muscle wasting. An outstanding feature is progressive loss of vision leading to complete blindness. The deep reflexes are exaggerated, at least to begin with, and the plantar responses are extensor. Ophthalmoscopy reveals primary optic atrophy and the diagnostic macular cherry-red spot on each side, surrounded by a greyish-white halo appearance **(Fig. 16.31)**. Convulsions may occur. Ultimately there are dysphagia, dementia, blindness and a tendency to repeated respiratory infections due to accumulation of mucus. Diagnosis can be confirmed by enzyme estimations on leucocytes or in skin fibroblasts grown in tissue culture. Death usually occurs before the age of 3 years.

GM1 Gangliosidosis

Aetiology There is accumulation of GM1 gangliosides due to defect in beta-galactosidase activity. There are two distinct forms: (1) juvenile GM1 gangliosidosis (type II) and (2) generalised gangliosidosis (type I). In type I, gangliosides accumulate in the brain, viscera and bones; in type II, the accumulation is only in the neurones.

Clinical features In generalised GM1 gangliosidosis (type I) neurological manifestations—hyperacusis, muscle weakness, incoordination, convulsions, loss of speech, mental retardation—develop during infancy and progress inexorably. Splenomegaly and hepatomegaly develop, and in due course facial and skeletal changes resembling those of gargoylism become more obvious. Eye changes include macular degeneration, cherry-red spot, nystagmus and blindness. The full clinical picture is rarely present before the age of 18 months. Diagnosis can be based upon enzyme assays in leucocytes, and rectal biopsy will also reveal characteristic changes. Death occurs before the age of 5 years.

In the juvenile form (type II), the viscera are not involved and the bones only to a slight degree. Slowly progressive neurological deterioration is the principal feature. Diagnosis is suggested by MPS type dysmorphism (with normal urinary mucopolysaccharides), eye changes, multi-vacuolated foam cells in the bone marrow and vacuolisation of lymphocytes in peripheral blood smear.

MUCOPOLYSACCHARIDOSES

This group of disorders, classified into six types, is characterised by the widespread intracellular deposition of complex substances called mucopolysaccharides or sulphated glycosaminoglycans. They present primarily as disorders of the reticuloendothelial system or as progressive disorders with visceral and skeletal manifestations. The mucopolysaccharides, which appear in the urine, show variations between the different clinical types and this is of help in differential diagnosis. All types are inherited as autosomal recessive, except Hunter syndrome (MPS type 2) in which transmission is sex-linked recessive. The aetiology appears to be a defect in the degradation of the mucopolysaccharides to their constituent sugars, this being related to a deficiency of one of the several lysosomal enzymes, each of which normally breaks a specific bond in the mucopolysaccharide molecule. Specific enzyme deficiencies have now been identified. In Hurler syndrome (MPS type 1-H), the missing enzyme activity is α-L-iduronidase and in Scheie syndrome (MPS type 1-S), the same enzyme is absent in spite of marked clinical differences. In Hunter syndrome, the missing enzyme is iduronate-2-sulphatase. Sanfilippo syndrome (MPS type 3), however, appears in biochemical terms to be four diseases: (1) Sanfilippo A—due to deficiency of heparan sulphatase, (2) Sanfilippo B—related to

N-acetyl-α-glucosaminidase, (3) Sanfilippo C—related to acetyl CoA: α-glucosaminidase N-acetyl-transferase and (4) Sanfilippo D—related to N-acetyl-α-D-glucosamine-6-sulphatase. There are two forms of Morquio disease (MPS type 4), types A and B, due to defect in galactosamine-6-sulphate sulphatase and β-galactosidase, respectively. In the Maroteaux-Lamy syndrome (MPS type 6), the enzyme deficiency is of arylsulphatase B. A few cases of "atypical" Hurler syndrome has been described in which β-glucuronidase was the missing factor and is referred to as MPS type 7 or Sly syndrome.

Mucopolysaccharidosis Type 1 (Hurler Syndrome)

This type of MPS is associated with excessive amounts of dermatan sulphate and heparan sulphate in the urine in a ratio of about 2:1. There is deficiency of α-L-iduronidase. The superficial appearances in a typical case of "gargoylism" allow immediate diagnosis **(Figs. 16.32A to C)**. The head is large and scaphocephalic. The eyes are set wide apart and there are heavy supraorbital ridges and eyebrows. The nose is broad with a flattened bridge and the lips are thick. The skin is dry and coarse. The cornea usually shows a marked spotty type of opacity or cloudiness. The neck is short, there is a lumbodorsal kyphosis and the protuberant abdomen often has an umbilical hernia. The spleen and liver are considerably enlarged. The hands tend to be broader than they are long. There is characteristic limitation of extension (but not of flexion) in many joints, most marked in the fingers. The fourth and fifth fingers may be short and curved towards the thumb. Genu valgum and coxa valga are common. There are also very characteristic radiological changes in the bones. The skull shows an elongated sella turcica, widened suture lines and an unduly large fontanelle. The long bones and phalanges are broader and shorter than normal and they are often bizarre in shape. The ribs too are excessively thick. The pelvis is distorted with abnormal acetabula. The vertebral bodies have an abnormal shape with concave anterior and posterior margins and there is often a hook-like projection from the anterior border of the first or second lumber vertebra, which tends to be displaced backwards. Bone age is usually delayed. Affected children are severely mentally retarded. They show diminished physical activity. This is partly due to excessive breathlessness on exertion when the heart is involved. Cardiomegaly, precordial systolic and diastolic murmurs and electrocardiographic evidence of left ventricular hypertrophy are commonly found. Death takes place before adult life from congestive cardiac failure or intercurrent respiratory infection.

While the child with this disorder somewhat resembles a cretin, there are very obvious clinical differences, e.g. corneal opacity, hepatosplenomegaly, limitation of extension of the interphalangeal joints and characteristic radiological findings in the skeleton. The precise diagnosis should be based on demonstration of the specific enzyme deficiency in leucocytes or cultured fibroblasts.

Mucopolysaccharidosis Type 2 (Hunter Syndrome)

This form of MPS is X-linked. It differs from Hurler syndrome in usually being less severe, but there is a severe form which results in death by the age of 15 years and a milder variety with survival to middle age. Clouding of the cornea does not occur but deafness is common. The urine contains large amounts of dermatan sulphate and heparan sulphate in approximately equal quantities. By 12 months of age radiographs show a mild but complete pattern of dysostosis multiplex.

Mucopolysaccharidosis Type 3 (Sanfilippo Syndrome)

In this variety, heparan sulphate is excreted in the urine almost exclusively. Mental deficiency is severe and there

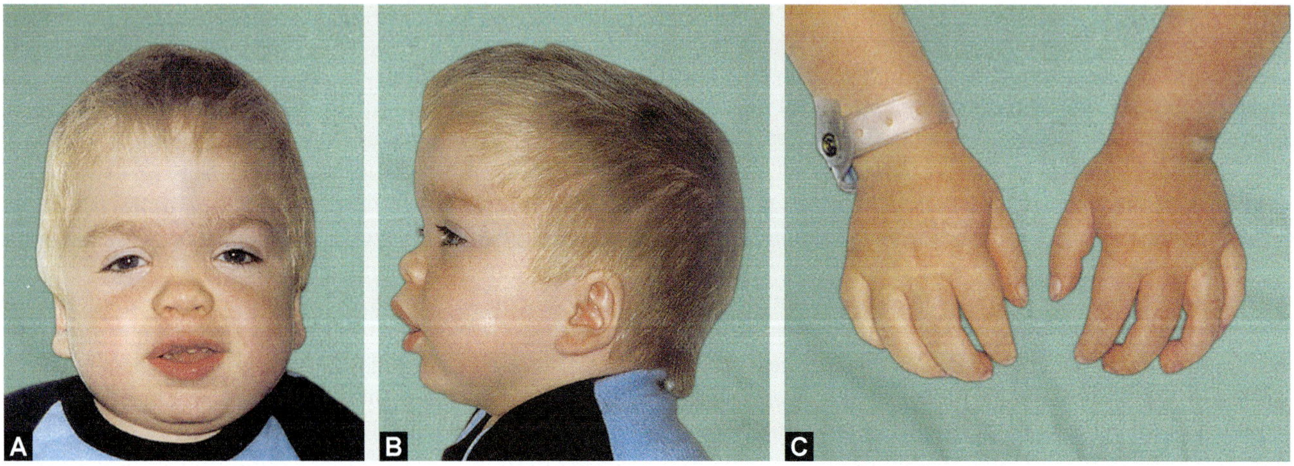

Figures 16.32A to C Mucopolysaccharidosis type 1-H, Hurler syndrome.

may be hyperactivity and destructive behaviour. Visceral and corneal involvement is relatively mild and the only skeletal signs may be biconvexity of the vertebral bodies and some degree of claw hand. There may also be a very thick calvarium.

Mucopolysaccharidosis Type 4 (Morquio Syndrome)

This is probably the disease first described by Morquio in Montevideo in 1929. The urine contains large amounts of keratan sulphate, a mucopolysaccharide that is unrelated to dermatan or heparan sulphate. Mental deficiency is not a usual finding and the face and skull are only slightly affected. The neck is short, there is marked dorsal kyphosis and the sternum protrudes. The arms are relatively long for the degree of dwarfism and may extend to the knees. There is, however, no limitation of flexion of the fingers. Genu valgum with enlarged knee joints and flat feet are present. There is a waddling gait. Radiographs may reveal platybasia, fusion of cervical vertebrae and flattening of the vertebral bodies; odontoid dysplasia predisposes to atlantoaxial subluxation with the risk of acute or chronic cervical cord compression. The metaphyses of the long bones may be irregular and the epiphyses are misshapen and fragmented. Mild degrees of corneal opacity may appear at a late stage of the disorder.

Mucopolysaccharidosis Type I-S (Previously Type 5): Scheie Syndrome

The outstanding features are stiff joints, aortic regurgitation and clouding of the cornea (most dense peripherally). The facies shows the characteristics of gargoylism to a lesser extent than in Hurler syndrome, intellect is but mildly impaired and survival to adulthood is common. The urine shows the same distribution of mucopolysaccharides as in Hurler syndrome.

Mucopolysaccharidosis Type 6 (Maroteaux–Lamy Syndrome)

The principal features are severe corneal and skeletal changes as in Hurler syndrome and valvular heart disease, but mental deficiency does not occur. Hepatosplenomegaly is usually of mild degree. The somatic features in the severe form of Maroteaux–Lamy syndrome are similar to that in Hurler syndrome (Fig. 16.33). The urine contains dermatan sulphate almost exclusively.

Mucopolysaccharidosis Type 7 (Sly Syndrome)

The principal features are unusual facies, protruding sternum, hepatomegaly, umbilical hernia, thoracolumbar gibbus, marked vertebral deformities and moderate mental deficiency.

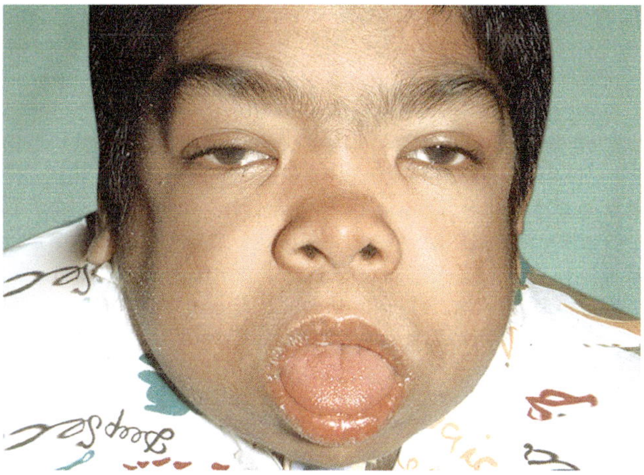

Figure 16.33 MPS V1 Maroteux–Lamy syndrome.

MITOCHONDRIAL DEFECTS

Energy, in the form of adenosine triphosphate (ATP), is generated by oxidative phosphorylation of breakdown products of metabolic fuels such as glucose, fatty acids, ketone bodies and organic and amino acids in the mitochondria. Mitochondria can be reviewed as the cell's batteries. This breakdown of nutrient fuels (oxidation) generates reduced factors such as NADH and reduced flavoproteins. These must be reoxidised for reutilisation in this process by the respiratory chain. The mitochondrial respiratory chain is a series of five complexes situated within the inner mitochondrial membrane. There are also two small mobile electron carriers (ubiquinone and cytochrome c) involved in the process. Energy substrates cross the double phospholipid mitochondrial membrane usually with a specific carrier (L-carnitine). The proton pumps of the respiratory chain components produce an electrochemical or proton gradient across the inner membrane and this charge is subsequently discharged by complex V and the energy thus released is used to drive ATP synthesis.

Clinical Presentation

The first of the mitochondrial respiratory chain diseases were described in relation to disorders of muscle and this resulted in the term mitochondrial myopathies. It is now known that other tissues particularly the brain may be involved. Respiratory chain defects may produce isolated myopathy, eye movement disorder (ophthalmoplegia) with or without myopathy and occasionally with CNS dysfunction such as ataxia, multisystem disease, fatal lactic acidosis of infancy and single organ dysfunction such as cardiomyopathy. The encephalopathies contain a number of recognisable syndromes such as the Kearns–Sayer syndrome characterised by progressive external ophthalmoplegia, pigmentary retinopathy and heart block, myoclonus epilepsy with ragged-red fibres where in addition to myoclonic seizures there is weakness, ataxia, deafness and dementia. Myopathy, encephalopathy, lactic acidosis and stroke-like episodes is characterised by the recurrence of stroke-like episodes with onset usually before the age of 15 years. Cortical blindness and hemianopia usually accompany the stroke-like episodes which may be preceded by a migraine-like headache, nausea and vomiting. Dementia frequently ensues. Another syndrome known as NARP is comprised of neurogenic weakness, ataxia and retinitis pigmentosa. Unlike the other syndromes described, there are no morphological changes in skeletal muscle and the mitochondrial DNA (mtDNA) defect affects ATP synthesis.

Leigh syndrome of sub-acute necrotising encephalomyopathy presents with vomiting, failure to thrive, developmental delay, muscular hypotonia and respiratory problems. There may also be ophthalmoplegia, optic atrophy, nystagmus and dystonia. The disorder usually presents at around the age of 6 months but may be present from birth or may not appear until late teenage. In Leigh encephalopathy like many of the mitochondrial syndromes, it is difficult to pinpoint a single biochemical abnormality. There are defects of the respiratory chain, pyruvate dehydrogenase complex and biotinidase, which variably present with this syndrome. Lactate and pyruvate concentrations are frequently elevated in blood and CSF and MRI scans show characteristic low density areas within the basal ganglia or less commonly the cerebellum. There is occasionally an autosomal recessive pattern of inheritance in Leigh syndrome, which suggests that it may be caused by a nuclear gene rather than a mitochondrial defect. However, in some patients mutations have been found in mtDNA. There are some patients who do not fit into these clinical patterns of disease and many have been shown to have multiple defects of respiratory chain complexes due to mtDNA disorder.

Leber hereditary optic neuropathy is one of the commonest inherited causes of blindness in young men due to a disorder of mtDNA. Some men with the disorder have an encephalopathy with deafness and dystonia and a few develop cardiac conduction defects. There is some evidence that a gene on the X-chromosome may be linked with this disorder.

There are a variety of syndromes with non-neuromuscular presentation, which involve the gastrointestinal tract with anorexia and vomiting and occasionally hepatic failure; yet others have cardiomyopathy with different degrees of heart block, renal disease with generalised aminoaciduria and haematological disorders affecting bone marrow function. In Pearson syndrome, which presents at birth or early infancy there is refractory sideroblastic anaemia, thrombocytopenia, neutropenia, metabolic acidosis, pancreatic insufficiency and hepatic dysfunction. Renal tubular disorder, diarrhoea, steatorrhoea and skin lesions with eventual liver failure have been described. Deletions of mtDNA have been identified.

Many of the respiratory chain disorders may present in the very young but there are three specific syndromes affecting the infant. The first is fatal infantile lactic acidosis. Infants present with hypotonia, vomiting and ventilatory failure and die often before the age of 6 months. A generalised aminoaciduria (de Toni-Fanconi-Debré syndrome), grossly increased plasma lactate concentrations, hypoglycaemia, liver dysfunction, convulsions and increased plasma calcium have been reported. The second clinical presentation is benign infantile lactic acidosis, which may present with failure to thrive, respiratory failure and hypotonia with increased plasma lactate concentrations but the condition gradually remits and by 12–18 months these infants are often normal. There is a cytochrome oxidase defect, which appears to improve with age and may be related to a switch from a foetal to an adult form of complex IV. The third syndrome is the mtDNA depletion syndrome in which the infant is weak, hypotonic and has respiratory difficulties together with renal tubular disorder and convulsions. The condition is usually fatal before the age of 1 year.

PEROXISOMAL DISORDERS

Peroxisomes are present in every body cell except the mature erythrocyte and are particularly abundant in tissues active in lipid metabolism. They do not contain DNA and are, therefore, under the control of nuclear genes. Peroxisomes have a number of metabolic functions—particularly:

- Fatty acid β-oxidation of very VLCFAs, pristanic acid and cholestanoate compounds which are intermediates in biosynthesis of bile acids
- Plasmalogen synthesis
- Phytanic acid oxidation—a branch-chain fatty acid formed from chlorophyll metabolism.
- Glycolate detoxification preventing formation of oxalate.

Over 16 clinical and biochemical disorders have now been ascribed to disorders of peroxisomal metabolic functions.

Table 16.4 gives a tentative classification of the peroxisomal disorders. In the group l disorders, there is a reduction or absence of functional peroxisomes. Zellweger syndrome is a lethal disease presenting with severe hypotonia, typical craniofacial abnormality with a high domed forehead, severe developmental delay with neurosensory defects and progressive oculomotor dysfunction. These neurological abnormalities may be related to the neuronal migration disorders found in the brain at post-mortem. There is also progressive liver dysfunction with chondrodysplasia calcificans of the patellae and the acetabulum. In neonatal ALD, there is progressive demyelination of the cerebral hemispheres, cerebellum and brainstem with neuronal migration disturbances and perivascular

TABLE 16.4	Classification of peroxisomal disorders.
Peroxisome deficiency disorders	
Neonatal adrenoleucodystrophy	
Infantile Refsum disease	
Hyperpipecolic acidaemia	
Disorders with loss of multiple peroxisomal functions and peroxisome structure in fibroblasts	
Rhizomelic chondrodysplasia punctate	
Zellweger-like syndrome	
Disorders with an impairment of only one peroxisomal function and normal peroxisomal structure	
Disorders of peroxisomal β-oxidation:	
Adrenoleucodystrophy (X-linked) and variants	
Acyl-CoA oxidase deficiency	
Bi (multi) functional protein deficiency	
Peroxisomal thiolase deficiency	
Other disorders:	
Acyl-CoA: Dihydroxyacetone phosphate acyltransferase (DHAPAT) deficiency	
Primary hyperoxaluria type I	
Acatalasemia	
Glutaryl oxidase deficiency	

lymphocytic infiltration. There is also adrenal atrophy. In IRD, there is developmental delay, retinitis pigmentosa, failure to thrive and hypocholesterolaemia. In the group 2 disorders, RCDP is an autosomal recessive disorder characterised by short stature, a typical facial appearance, joint contractures and X-ray changes showing stippling of the epiphyses in infancy and severe symmetrical epiphyseal and extra-epiphyseal calcifications in later life. Only few patients have been described as having the Zellweger-like syndrome which is clinically indistinguishable from the classical Zellweger but shows abundant peroxisomes in the liver. In the group 3 disorders with impairment of a single peroxisome function and with a normal peroxisome structure ALD, an X-linked recessively inherited disorder, usually affects males between the ages of 4 and 10 years.

Initially, there may be attention deficit noticed in school followed by convulsions, visual disturbance with the later manifestations of paralysis and death. This phenotype known as childhood ALD has been treated with long-chain polyunsaturated fatty acids but there is some doubt as to the overall benefit of this form of therapy. About 25% of ALD cases present in adulthood with paraparesis whilst a few may exhibit adrenocortical insufficiency without

Flow chart 16.2 Metabolic pathways (peroxisomal β-oxidation) in peroxisomes.

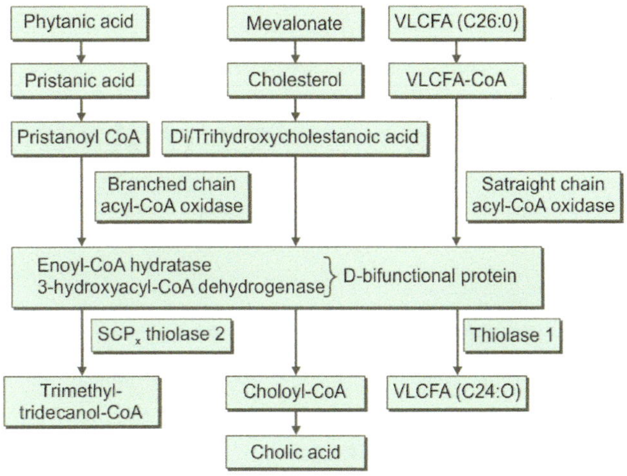

TABLE 16.5	Results from a child with Zellweger syndrome elevated long chain fatty acids in a patient with Zellweger spectrum disorder.	
Fatty acid	***Result***	***Reference interval***
C26	+ 12.91	(0.33-1.39)
C26/C22	+ 0.421	(<0.030)
C24/C22	+ 1.88	(0.32-1.07)
Pristanic acid	0.6	(<3.0)
Phytanic acid	2.9	(<16.0)

(Note: Pristanic and phytanic acid concentrations are diet dependent and often not found to be elevated especially in young infants.)

neurological involvement. About 20% of female heterozygotes develop mild or moderate progressive paraparesis after the age of 40 years.

The other disorders are also rare apart from primary hyperoxaluria type I, an autosomal recessive disorder of glyoxylate metabolism, in which there is recurrent calcium oxalate nephrolithiasis and nephrocalcinosis presenting during the first decade. There are a few, however, who present with an acute neonatal form of the disorder and early death **(Flow chart 16.2 and Table 16.5)**.

SUGGESTED READING

1. Saudubray, Baumgartner, Walter (Eds). Inborn Metabolic Diseases: Diagnosis and treatment, 6th edition. Heidelberg: Springer; 2016.

CHAPTER 17

Endocrine Disorders

Louis C.K. Low

HYPOPITUITARISM

Embryologically the pituitary gland is formed from the Rathke's pouch, a diverticulum of the stomodeal ectoderm and the neuroectoderm of the floor of the forebrain. A number of signalling molecules and transcription factors are involved in pituitary organogenesis and the differentiation of the different cell lineages somatotropes [growth hormone (GH)], lactotropes (prolactin), corticotropes [adrenocorticotropic hormone (ACTH)], thyrotropes [thyroid-stimulating hormone (TSH)] and gonadotropes luteinising hormone (LH), [follicle-stimulating hormone (FSH)]. Multiple pituitary hormone deficiencies can result from malformations of the hypothalamus and pituitary gland or mutations of these transcription factors. Patients with mutations in the pituitary transcription factors have other anomalies associated with hypopituitarism. POU1F1 is the first pituitary transcription factor to be cloned and mutations result in defects in somatotrope, lactotrope and thyrotrope development. Mutations in prophet of PIT1 (PROP1) lead to combined pituitary hormone deficiency including GH, TSH, prolacti and ACTH in later life. Mutations in PROP1 accounts for 50% of the cases of genetically determined combined pituitary hormone deficiency. Secretion of hormones from different lineages of pituitary cells is dependent on hypothalamic-releasing factors [gonadotrophin-releasing hormone (GnRH), thyrotrophin-releasing hormone (TRH), corticotrophin-releasing hormone (CRH), growth hormone-releasing hormone (GHRH)] or suppressive hormone-like somatostatin. Two hormones are secreted by the posterior pituitary gland: vasopressin and oxytocin. Vasopressin is important for the reabsorption of water by the distal renal tubules and collecting ducts. Vasopressin release is stimulated by rising plasma osmolality; fall in blood volume or blood pressure; or by stress. Oxytocin release is stimulated by suckling and its role is limited to the puerperal period. Causes of hypopituitarism are shown in Box 17.1. Extent of the anterior and posterior pituitary dysfunction depends on the extent of the damage.

Clinical Features

The usual presenting features include symptoms and signs relating to the hormonal deficiencies or the underlying cause of hypopituitarism. Patients with mutations in the LIM homeobox genes (LHX3, LHX4) have hypopituitarism and malformation of the skull base and cervical spine. Other pituitary transcription factors mutations can be associated with abnormalities of the development of the eye and forebrain structures. Intracranial tumours in the suprasellar region can lead to visual field defects, neurological symptoms and symptoms and signs of raised intracranial pressure such as headache and vomiting and papilloedema. Polyuria, polydipsia and dehydration may or may not be present depending on whether there is posterior pituitary involvement. Short stature and infantile body proportions are common due to GH and thyroid hormone deficiencies. Adrenal insufficiency can lead to lethargy, hypoglycaemia, nausea, vomiting or even shock when the patient is under stress. In infants with hypopituitarism, the presenting features include recurrent hypoglycaemic attacks, micropenis in males (stretched penile length <2.5 cm), and persistent neonatal jaundice resembling the neonatal hepatitis syndrome. Microphthalmia, pendular nystagmus, optic nerve hypoplasia and signs of hypopituitarism suggest septo-optic dysplasia. Early onset of symptoms indicates a congenital or genetic cause of hypopituitarism. A proper history can usually shed light on the aetiology of postnatal damage to the hypothalamus and pituitary gland.

Investigations

Assessment begins with the documentation of anthropometric data using standard techniques and the state of the development of the genitalia and pubertal staging.

BOX 17.1 Causes of hypopituitarism.

Cerebral malformations—holoprosencephaly, midline facial defects, septo-optic dysplasia, congenital hypopituitarism (transection of pituitary stalk, adenohypophysis hypoplasia, ectopic position of posterior pituitary signal on MRI scan)

Mutations of pituitary transcription factors genes (multiple pituitary hormone deficiency) or of pituitary hormone or pituitary hormone-releasing hormone genes (isolated pituitary hormone deficiency)

Postnatal damage of hypothalamus or pituitary gland—

- Traumatic or breech delivery
- Head Injury
- Suprasellar or pituitary tumours, e.g. craniopharyngioma, germ cell tumour, astrocytoma, glioma, prolactinoma
- Infiltrative lesions, e.g. Langerhans cell histiocytosis, sarcoidosis, lymphocytic hypophysitis
- Pituitary apoplexy
- Infection, e.g. meningitis, encephalitis
- Autoimmune
- Cranial irradiation
- Pituitary haemosiderosis, e.g. transfusion dependent thalassaemia major

An X-ray for bone age as assessed by the Greulich and Pyle and Tanner-Whitehouse Atlas will usually show retardation of skeletal maturity (Fig. 17.1) relative to the chronological age. Baseline fasting, morning cortisol, thyroid hormone, TSH, prolactin, gonadotrophins and sex steroids (in pubertal age group) should be taken and one should proceed to combined pituitary hormone assessment (tests for stimulating GH and cortisol secretion) together with TRH and luteinising hormone-releasing hormone (LHRH) test if there is a strong clinical suspicion of hypopituitarism.

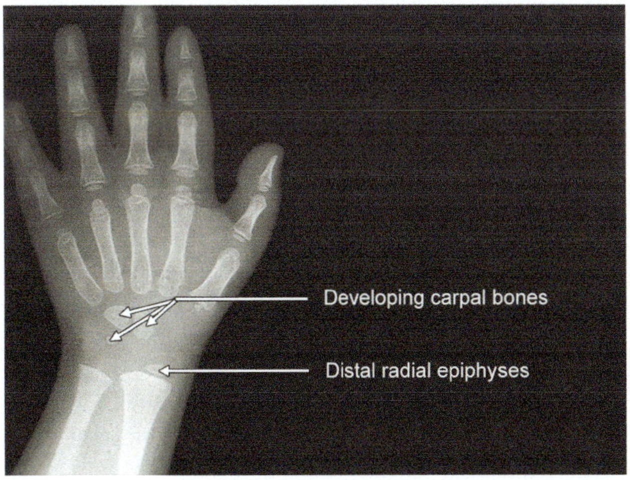

Figure 17.1 Bone age: X-ray of the left hand and wrist of a boy aged 4 years and 3 months. The bone age using the TW II 20-bone score (Tanner–Whitehouse) is 3.8 years, which is just below the 50th percentile for his age.

Imaging of the hypothalamus and pituitary preferably with magnetic resonance imaging (MRI) is required after establishing a hormonal diagnosis of hypopituitarism.

DISORDERS OF THE POSTERIOR PITUITARY

Diabetes Insipidus

The prohormone of vasopressin is synthesised in the cells of the supraoptic and paraventricular nuclei, and granules of propressophysin are rapidly transported through the axons by axoplasmic streaming and stored in the axon terminals in the posterior pituitary gland. Central diabetes insipidus (CDI) is due to vasopressin deficiency and the causes are shown in Box 17.2. The patients present with polyuria, polydipsia, nocturi or secondary enuresis, passing inappropriate large volumes of dilute urine (>2 L/m^2 per day). Affected children could be admitted in a severe dehydrated state. Patients with craniopharyngioma or other suprasellar tumours can present with signs of raised intracranial pressure, visual field defects, growth failure or symptoms of pituitary hormone deficiencies. Central DI must be distinguished from other causes of polyuria such as diabetes mellitus (DM), nephrogenic diabetes insipidus (NDI), renal tubular disorders, hypokalaemia, hypercalcaemia and obstructive uropathy. More than 90% of NDI results from mutations in the vasopressin receptor (V2R) on chromosome Xq28-qter. Autosomal recessive form of (NDI) is due to mutations in the aquaporin 2 gene (AQP2) on chromosome 12q12-q13. Patients usually present in infancy with polyuria, polydipsia, failure to thrive, unexplained fever and constipation. The baby often prefers water to milk. Developmental delay can occur due to severe hypernatraemic dehydration in infancy.

BOX 17.2 Causes of vasopressin deficiency.

Tumour (38%)
- Craniopharyngioma, optic glioma, germinoma

Vascular
- Sickle-cell disease, haemorrhage, shock infection

Hereditary
- Familial central diabetes insipidus, X-linked diabetes insipidus, Wolfram syndrome

Cerebral malformation (3.2%)
- Septo-optic dysplasia, empty sella, Bardet–Biedl syndrome

Trauma (1.6%)

Infiltrative
- Histiocytosis (8%), leukaemia

Miscellaneous
- Idiopathic (20–30%), autoimmune

In a patient suspected of suffering from DI, an accurate documentation of the daily fluid intake and urine output is required. If the patient is admitted in dehydration with serum sodium of greater than 150 mmol/L and a plasma osmolality greater than 300 mOsmol/kg, a simultaneous urine osmolality less than 750 mOsmol/kg is suggestive of DI. A water deprivation test is required for diagnosis in a patient who can compensate for the defect in urine concentration by excessive water drinking.

The water deprivation test must be done under medical supervision. The patient must be allowed to drink ad libitum overnight and the patient must be well-hydrated in the morning before the test. (1) Fluid is then withheld with hourly monitor of: urine volume and osmolality; (2) body weight; (3) plasma sodium and osmolality and (4) clinical status, pulse, blood pressure and perfusion. The end-point of the test is (1) loss of 3–5% body weight and (2) serum sodium more than 150 mmol/L and osmolality more than 300 mOsmol/kg, and the diagnosis of DI is reached if the urine osmolality fails to reach more than 750 mOsmol/kg at the end-point of the test. Vasopressin responsiveness is established by giving desmopressin (1 month to 2 years—5–10 µg as a single dose and 2–12 years, 10–20 µg as a single dose intranasally) or arginine vasopressin (1 unit/m^2 subcutaneously) at the end of water deprivation and urine volume and osmolality should be assessed hourly for a further 3 hours after desmopressin. In CDI, urine volume will fall and there should be a rise of the urine osmolality at least by 120 mOsmol/kg above the peak value achieved during the water deprivation test.

After reaching a diagnosis of CDI, one should look for an underlying cause. Investigations should include a full blood count (FBC), skeletal survey (for osteolytic lesions), alpha-fetoprotein and human chorionic gonadotrophin (hCG) (germinoma) and MRI of the brain. MRI of the brain is preferred to look for suprasellar lesions (craniopharyngioma, optic glioma, germinoma), thickening of the pituitary stalk (histiocytosis, germinoma, lymphocytic hypophysitis) and loss of posterior pituitary "bright spot" on T1-weighted images.

Syndrome of Inappropriate Antidiuretic Hormone Secretion

Syndrome of inappropriate antidiuretic hormone (SIADH) comprises aetiologically heterogeneous conditions leading to retention of water with plasma hypo-osmolality (<270 mOsmol/kg), normal or slightly increased effective blood volume with less than maximally dilute urine (>100 mOsmol/kg) and absence of adrenal, thyroid or renal insufficiency. Causes of SIADH are shown in **Box 17.3**. The symptoms consist of apathy, confusion, anorexia, headaches, muscle cramps and in several cases convulsion and coma.

Severe symptomatic hyponatraemia can be corrected by slow infusion of 3% sodium chloride 4–6 mL/kg over 1 hour and this will raise the serum sodium by about 5 mmol/L and the correction of hyponatraemia should not be faster than a rise of serum sodium concentration of 10–12 mmol/L per day due to the risk of central pontine myelinolysis. Milder cases should be managed by fluid restriction. Ideally one should anticipate and prevent the development of SIADH by monitoring the fluid balance, body weight and electrolytes in at-risk patients.

BOX 17.3 Causes of syndrome of inappropriate antidiuretic hormone (SIADH).

- Central nervous system disorders
  - Meningitis, encephalitis, intracranial tumours or haemorrhage
- Respiratory tract disease and infection
- Decreased left atrial filing
  - Positive pressure ventilation, pneumothorax, cystic fibrosis
- Drugs
  - Carbamazepine, vinca alkaloids
- Malignancies
  - Thymoma, bronchogenic carcinoma, lymphoma, Ewing sarcoma
- About 35% of HIV patients have SIADH due to Pneumocystis infection or malignancy

SHORT STATURE

The factors governing human growth have already been described in the Chapter 2: Growth and Development. Short stature is common, but short stature due to an endocrine cause is less common. Children with a height below the 0.4th percentile (below-2.67 SD) with correction for the mean parental height (1.6 SD below the corrected mean parental height) or growing with a subnormal growth velocity should be referred for specialist care. A genetic cause of GH deficiency can be suspected if there is an early onset of growth failure, a positive family history or consanguinity, extreme short stature and an extremely low GH response to GHRH, low serum insulin-like growth factor 1 (IGF-1) and insulin-like growth factor binding protein 3 (IGFBP-3) levels (see later). The causes of growth failure are shown in **Box 17.4**. Idiopathic short stature accounts for 60–80% of children with a height below -2 SD and includes constitutional delay in growth and puberty (CDGP) and familial short stature.

Assessment of Short Stature

The height, span, upper to lower (U/L) segment ratio and previous growth record are important axiological data. Disproportionate short stature is indicative of skeletal dysplasia. Initial investigations should include FBC, sedimentation rate, serum calcium, phosphate, alkaline phosphatase, IGF-1, renal and liver function tests, acid-base status, thyroid hormone, TSH and X-ray for bone age.

BOX 17.4 Causes of short stature.

- Genetic short stature
- Constitutional delay in growth and puberty
- Undernutrition
- Chronic illness of all major systems, e.g. chronic renal failure, inflammatory bowel disease, congenital heart disease, inherited metabolic diseases, thalassaemia major
- Psychosocial deprivation
- Syndrome and chromosomal disorders, e.g. Turner syndrome, Noonan syndrome, Silver–Russell syndrome, Prader–Willi syndrome
- William syndrome, Down syndrome
- Skeletal dysplasia, e.g. hypochondroplasia, achondroplasia, spondyloepiphyseal dysplasia

A short child with normal growth velocity and no bone age delay and a plasma IGF-1 level above the mean for age does not require GH testing. If the serum IGF-1 and IGFBP-3 are lower than -1 SD for age in a child with significant short stature and subnormal growth velocity, then the GH/IGF-1 axis should be investigated. GH deficiency is diagnosed by an inadequate GH response of less than 20 mIU/L measured by a polyclonal radioimmunoassay (RIA) or an equivalent lower value using a two-site GH immunoassay, to two pharmacological stimuli like clonidine, L-dopa, arginine, glucagon, GHRH or insulin induced hypoglycaemia. The latter test is not favoured by some paediatric endocrinologists and should not be used in children under 5 years of age. Assessment of the hypothalamic-pituitary adrenal axis and the gonadotropins and TSH responses to their respective hypothalamic-releasing hormone should be performed when pituitary dysfunction is suspected (glucagon and LHRH and TRH test). It is important that hypothyroidism be diagnosed and adequately treated before any investigation of the GH/IGF-1 axis. Adrenal insufficiency is diagnosed when the plasma cortisol fails to reach 500 nmol/L in response to glucagon or insulin induced hypoglycaemia. Neuroimaging with MRI is indicated in patients diagnosed with GH deficiency or multiple pituitary hormone deficiency. Children with(CDGP) have slow physical and pubertal maturation and a delay in bone age. The diagnosis can only be made after the other causes of short stature have been excluded.

TALL STATURE

The referral of children with tall stature to the endocrine service is not common and the patients are usually very tall girls who are worried about their heights. The causes of tall stature are shown in **Box 17.5**.

Beckwith-Wiedemann syndrome is characterised by prenatal and postnatal overgrowth, visceromegaly, omphalocoele, hemihypertrophy and neonatal hypoglycaemia. This condition is due to epigenetic errors of the imprinted gene cluster on chromosome 11p15 or mutations of cyclin-dependent kinase inhibitor gene (CDKN1C) on chromosome 11p15. Patients with Sotos syndrome have macrodolichocephaly with prominent forehead and jaw and a characteristic growth pattern of rapid growth in early life followed by slowing of the growth velocity to normal by mid-childhood. Sotos syndrome is due to microdeletion of paternal chromosome 5 in the region of the nuclear receptor binding SET-domain containing gene 1 (NSD1) or intragenic mutation of NSD1. Epigenetic mutations in the imprinted gene cluster on chromosome 11p15 have been found in patients with the Sotos phenotype without NSD1 mutations. This suggests that an overlap of the molecular basis of overgrowth syndrome exists.

BOX 17.5 Causes of tall stature.

- Prenatal overgrowth—Beckwith-Wiedemann syndrome, Sotos syndrome, Weaver syndrome
- Postnatal overgrowth—familial tall stature, Marfan syndrome, homocystinuria, Klinefelter syndrome
- Secondary causes—obesity, precocious puberty, growth hormone-secreting tumour, hyperthyroidism

Skeletal features of Marfan syndrome include pectus excavatum or carinatum, scoliosis, reduced U/L segment ratio and a span to height ratio more than 1.05. Other features include ectopia lentis, dilatation of the ascending aorta or pulmonary artery, mitral valve prolapse, spontaneous pneumothorax and lumbosacral dural ectasia. A positive family history (autosomal dominant inheritance) is helpful in the diagnosis. Marfan syndrome is due to mutation in the fibrillin gene (FBN1) on chromosome 15q21.1 or rarely mutation in transforming growth factor beta receptor 2 (TGFB2) on chromosome 3p22.

Assessment of children with tall stature includes identification of syndromal disorders. The pubertal status, parental stature, thyroid status and body mass index should be noted. GH excess usually resulting from a GH-secreting pituitary tumour, leads to growth acceleration, coarse facial features, prognathism and enlarging hands and feet. Glucose intolerance or hypertension may occur. A large pituitary tumour can cause visual field defects and headache. GH excess is occasionally associated with the McCune Albright syndrome. Further investigations include measurement of thyroid hormone, testosterone, oestradiol, LH, FSH, prolactin, IGF-1 and 17α-hydroxyprogesterone (17α-OHP). The failure of suppression of the serum GH level below 10 mIU/L during an oral glucose tolerance test (1.75 g/kg to a maximum of 75 g) remains the gold standard for the diagnosis of GH hypersecretion. Karyotyping, X-ray for skeletal maturation and

MRI scan of the brain and pituitary should be performed where indicated.

Girls may seek treatment and those with a predicted final adult height more than +3 SD could be considered for hormonal therapy (100–300 μg ethinyl oestradiol or 7.5 mg premarin combined with medroxyprogesterone acetate 5–10 mg from day 15 to day 25 of each calendar month). Testosterone enanthate 250–1,000 mg intramuscularly every month can be used to accelerate skeletal maturation and reduce final height in tall boys. However, the use of sex hormone therapy for limiting adult height should be reserved for selected patients because knowledge in potential long-term effects and fertility is still scanty. Calf cramps and weight gain are the common side effects of high-dose oestrogen in girls. In boys, acne, aggressive behaviour and hypertrichosis are the common complaints. For the other secondary causes of tall stature, treatment should be directed at the underlying condition. A pituitary GH-secreting tumour is managed by trans-sphenoidal surgery.

OBESITY

In 1997, the World Health Organisation (WHO) press release declared that "Obesity's impact is so diverse and extreme that it should now be regarded as one of the greatest neglected health problems of our time with an impact on health, which may well prove to be as great as that of smoking". The prevalence of obesity is on the rise in both developed and developing countries. There is currently no consistent evidence that the current epidemic of obesity is due to increased fat or caloric intake. There is an enormous range of energy intakes by children of the same age and there is little correlation between intake for age and weight for height for age. Technological advances have caused a marked reduction in the average daily energy expenditure and it appears to be the key determinant of the current obesity epidemic. Television viewing and use of the computer for leisure have now been viewed as surrogate measures of physical inactivity. As much as 28% and 46% of all children and non-Hispanic black children in the United States National Health and Nutrition Examination Survey III (NHANES III) survey reported watching television more than 4 hours per day. The best estimate of genetic contribution to obesity is about 25% whereas cultural transmission of lifestyle accounting for obesity is estimated to be about 30%. As of October 2005, 176 cases of obesity due to mutations in 11 different genes have been reported, and the molecular basis of at least 25 obesity syndromes is now known. There are 253 quantitative trait loci (QTLs) for obesity-related phenotypes from 61 genome-wide scans and of these 52 genomic regions harbour QTLs replicated among two to four studies (The Human Obesity Gene Map—the 2005 update). The complications of childhood obesity are shown in **Box 17.6**.

BOX 17.6 Complications of childhood obesity.

- Insulin resistance and type 2 diabetes mellitus
- Hyperlipidaemia
- Hypertension
- Steatohepatitis
- Respiratory inadequacy including obstructive sleep apnoea syndrome
- Musculoskeletal problems including slipped capital femoral epiphysis, genu valgum
- Tall stature and early puberty
- Gynaecomastia or adipomastia
- Oligomenorrhoea and hyperandrogenism
- Psychological sequence like poor self-image, disordered eating and nonspecific behaviour disturbances

The increase in the prevalence of obesity has been associated with a similar increase in the prevalence of type 2 diabetes in many countries. It is recommended that screening for type 2 diabetes mellitus (T2DM) be performed every 2 years in obese children and adolescents who have acanthosis nigricans, a family history of type 2 diabetes and evidence of insulin resistance (acanthosis nigricans, hypertension, dyslipidaemia and polycystic ovary syndrome).

Obese infants and children under the age of 3 years without obese parents are at low risk of becoming obese as an adult, whereas obese adolescents are at increased risk of developing adult obesity. The doctor should be able to identify obesity-related syndromes and to monitor for and treat any obesity-related complications developing in these obese children. Investigations to exclude a pathological cause should be undertaken if there is severe early onset of obesity or when obesity is associated with short stature or features suggestive of a syndromal disorder, e.g. Prader-Willi syndrome, pseudohypoparathyroidism, glucocorticoid excess, hypothalamic syndrome and Bardet-Biedl syndrome.

A preventive programme needs to have commitment from all stakeholders and be directed at the whole population. The preventive messages must be free from harm to those in the community who are not obese. Prevention should be directed towards developing a healthier lifestyle in the family and the community like increased physical activity, decreased dependence on television and computer games for entertainment and healthy eating. As children spend a significant part of the day at school, much can be done by schools to combat this epidemic by health education, providing healthy snacks, drinks and meals at school and encouraging increased physical activity and fitness.

Once a child has developed significant obesity, measures to encourage weight loss and weight maintenance have proved disappointing in achieving these aims. Education on the nature and complications of obesity, healthy eating and lifestyle and psychological support on a regular basis by a team of professionals consisting of paediatricians, dietician, exercise physiologist and psychologist have frequently been suggested, but the cost-effectiveness and sustainability of such programmes have been called into question. Pharmacotherapy should be restricted to treat the most severe cases of obesity associated with complications. Bariatric surgery employing roux-en-y gastric bypass or adjustable gastric banding has been increasingly used to treat patients with morbid obesity and severe medical complications.

THYROID GLAND

Disorders of the thyroid gland are, with the exception of DM, the most common endocrine problems of childhood. The advent of immunoassay techniques has been followed by a vast increase in our knowledge of the physiology and disturbances of thyroid function and molecular mechanism of disease.

Hypothyroidism

A classification of the causes of hypothyroidism is shown in Box 17.7. It is designed upon an aetiological basis which will permit the clinician to systematically approach diagnosis and treatment. Of the various causes of hypothyroidism in childhood only endemic iodine deficiency, congenital hypothyroidism and autoimmune thyroiditis will be described in this chapter.

Endemic Iodine Deficiency

Iodine deficiency is now recognised as the most common preventable cause of mental retardation in the world today. If the foetus and developing children in a community are not provided with sufficient quantities of iodine, the entire population will have decreased intelligence quotient (IQ), impaired motor function and hearing defect. The WHO estimates that there are still over 100 countries in our world with a significant problem with iodine deficiency. In areas of the world where iodine deficiency is found, up to 8% of the population may have deficient thyroid hormone production, TSH hypersecretion and increased iodine trapping with goitre and raised plasma T_3:T_4 ratio. Iodine deficiency in utero results in increased perinatal mortality, risk of abortion and congenital anomalies, neurological cretinism (development delay, deafness, spastic diplegia, squint) or myxoedematous cretinism (developmental delay and dwarfism). Iodine deficiency in the neonate leads to neonatal goitre, congenital hypothyroidism and hyperthyrotropinaemia. Iodine deficiency in childhood can manifest as retarded growth and development and goitrous hypothyroidism. In a recent meta-analysis of studies in China on the effects of iodine on intelligence, it was found that there was an IQ difference of 12.45 points in children living in iodine deficient areas as compared to those living in iodine sufficient areas. Neonatal serum TSH is included by WHO, The United Nations Children's Fund (UNICEF) and International Council for the Control of Iodine Deficiency Disorders (ICCIDD) in 1994 as one of the indicators for iodine deficiency disorders. If 3–19.9% of the neonatal TSH values exceed 10 mIU/L, mild iodine deficiency exists in that community. Regional differences in the incidence of congenital hypothyroidism could be due to differences in population iodine intake. The prevalence of goitre in

BOX 17.7 A classification of hypothyroidism in childhood.

- Dysgenesis of the thyroid gland (may present as congenital hypothyroidism or juvenile myxoedema in childhood in milder cases)
  - Congenital athyreosis
  - Maldescent
  - Maldevelopment
- Deficiency of iodine (endemic cretinism)
- Genetic basis of congenital hypothyroidism
  - Mutations in transcription factors resulting in thyroid dysgenesis (FOXE1, PAX8, NKX2.1)
  - Mutations in the monocarboxylate transporter 8 gene (MCT8 or SLC16A2)
- Dyshormonogenesis
  - Hyporesponsiveness to thyroid-stimulating hormone (TSH or GNAS1 mutations)
  - Iodide transport defects (mutations in natrium-iodide symporter gene SLC5A5)
  - Thyroglobulin synthesis defects (defective TG gene)
  - Iodide organification defects (mutations in thyroperoxidase gene (TPO) or genes of dual oxidase proteins (DUOX1 and DUOX2)
  - Pendred syndrome (SLC26A4 gene and FOXI1 gene mutations)
  - Dehalogenase defects (mutations in iodothyrosine deiodinase gene IYD)
- Thyroid hormone resistance (thyroid hormone receptor gene TRβ mutations)
- Ingestion of goitrogens (accidental or therapeutic)
  - Antenatal (iodine, thionamides in pregnancy)
  - Postnatal (iodine-containing radiographic contrast medium, amiodarone)
- Primary thyroid disease, e.g. autoimmune thyroiditis, carcinoma, and so on
- Pituitary hypothyroidism
  - Malformation of the brain, e.g. holoprosencephaly
  - Mutations of pituitary transcription factors
  - Secondary to disruption of the hypothalamus–pituitary–thyroid axis, e.g. tumour, infection, irradiation, haemosiderosis

the childhood community is also an indicator of iodine nutrition status. Iodination of salt supplies can effectively reduce the prevalence of this condition.

Congenital Hypothyroidism

Apart from the rare genetic causes of thyroid dysgenesis, the causes of thyroid dysgenesis in which thyroid tissue may be absent (aplastic), deficient (hypoplastic) or abnormally sited (ectopic) are unknown but affect about 1 in 3,600 of all newborns and more commonly affect female infants. Dyshormonogenesis (inborn errors of thyroid hormone biosynthesis) accounts for about 10% of all cases of congenital hypothyroidism, that is, 1 in 40,000. These autosomal recessively inherited disorders may present with goitre.

Clinical features The diagnosis of severe congenital hypothyroidism should not be difficult. Indeed, the manifestations are present within a few days of birth. The presenting symptoms that are usually mild consist of feeding difficulties, skin mottling, noisy respiration and constipation. The undue prolongation of 'physiological jaundice' should always arouse the suspicion of hypothyroidism. The appearance of the infants is typical if they remain undiagnosed after 3–4 months of age. The facial features are coarse with often a wrinkled forehead and low hairline. The posterior fontanelle remains patent in early infancy. The hair may be dry and scanty. The large myxoedematous tongue protrudes from the mouth and interferes with feeding and breathing **(Fig. 17.2)**. The cry has a characteristic hoarseness. The neck appears short due to the presence of myxoedematous pads of fat above the clavicles. The skin, especially over the face and extremities, feels dry, thick and cold. An umbilical hernia is common. The hands and fingers are broad and stumpy. The hypothyroid infant is frequently apathetic and uninterested in his surroundings. As times goes by, psychomotor retardation becomes obvious and partially irreversible. Patients with Pendred syndrome have sensorineural hearing deficit in addition to hypothyroidism.

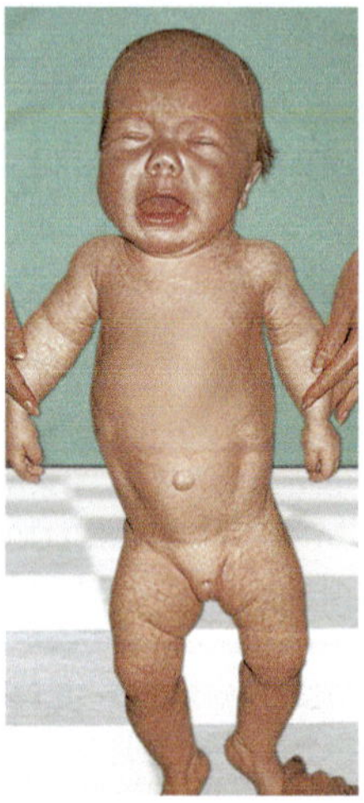

Figure 17.2 Sporadic cretin aged 4 months. *Note* coarse features, large myxoedematous tongue and umbilical hernia.

However, most infants with congenital hypothyroidism are born with few symptoms or signs. Nonetheless, the marked delay in diagnosis so commonly encountered is unnecessary and it results often in avoidable intellectual impairment. The possibility of hypothyroidism should be considered in every infant or child in whom growth is retarded. Most cases of congenital hypothyroidism are diagnosed by neonatal screening by the detection of increased TSH concentrations in Guthrie card blood spots, but cases with delayed rise in TSH will be missed.

In the undetected or untreated child, the body proportions remain infantile with long trunk and short legs. A tendency to stand with exaggerated lumbar lordosis and slightly flexed hips and knees is common. The anterior fontanelle is late in closing and the posterior fontanelle remains patent. The deciduous teeth are slow in erupting and radiographs may show defects in the enamel. The face and hands are frequently mildly myxoedematous, and the cerebral activities are slow and sluggish. The mandible is often underdeveloped and the nasolabial configuration may be obviously that of a much younger child. The deep tendon reflexes are sometimes exaggerated with slow relaxation and there may be mild ataxia.

Juvenile Hypothyroidism

Short stature is one of the only two invariable findings in hypothyroidism. The ratio of the U/L skeletal segment is also abnormal (infantile) in hypothyroid children. The lower segment is the distance from the top of the symphysis pubis to the ground; the upper segment is obtained by subtracting the lower segment from the total height. The mean body U/L ratio is about 1.7 at birth, 1.3 at 3 years and 1.1 after 7 years of age. Hypothyroid children have an unduly long upper segment due to their short legs. Patients are lethargic and have waxy complexion, dry skin and coarse hair. Constipation and cold intolerance are common. Sexual development is often delayed. Rarely in some children with severe hypothyroidism, precocious sexual development can occur, but the underlying mechanism is unknown. The sella turcica is enlarged, and serum prolactin and FSH levels are elevated. Early sexual development will regress when the hypothyroid state is alleviated by treatment.

Delayed ossification to a more severe degree than that retardation in linear growth is the other constant finding in hypothyroidism. The assessment of bone age is based on radiographs of various epiphyseal areas, chosen according to the child's age, and their comparison with an ossification chart showing the normal ages at which the different centres should ossify **(Fig. 17.1)**. Dysgenesis of the epiphyses is pathognomonic of hypothyroidism. It may be florid at one area and absent at another, so that radiographs should always be taken of several areas

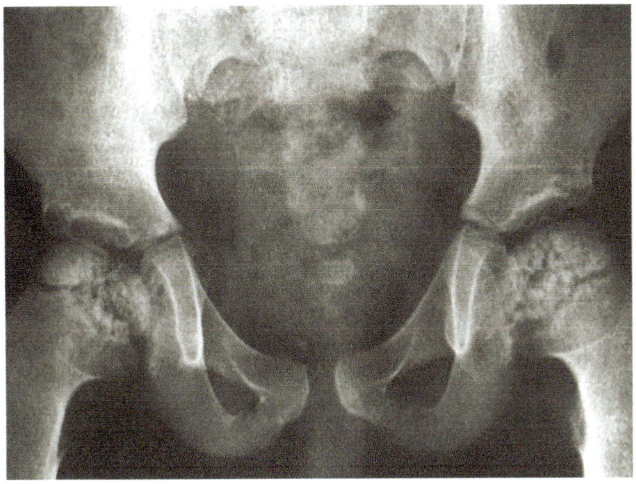

Figure 17.3 Epiphyseal dysgenesis in femoral heads. *Note* stippling and fragmented appearance.

of the skeleton. In some cases, dysgenesis only appears after thyroid treatment has been started, but then only in those ossification centres which should have appeared in the normal child before that age. The presence of dysgenesis indicates that hypothyroid state existed before the affected centre would be normally due to ossify and it permits an assessment of the age, foetal or postnatal, at which the hypothyroidism developed. The characteristic X-ray appearance is of a misshapen epiphysis with irregular or fluffy margins and a fragmented or stippled appearance (Fig. 17.3). In older children, skeletal maturations are assessed with an X-ray of the non-dominant hand and wrist using the Greulich and Pyle or Tanner-Whitehouse skeletal atlas. In the great majority of cases of hypothyroidism, measurements of the linear height, the upper and lower segments and a few well-chosen radiographs will establish or exclude the diagnosis of hypothyroidism beyond doubt. They will also determine the age of onset of the hypothyroid state.

Investigations

The circulating free thyroxine (fT_4) and free triiodothyronine levels (fT_3) are low. A particularly sensitive biochemical test for hypothyroidism lies in measurement of the serum TSH using a suprasensitive assay. The TSH level (normal range <0.5–5.5 mIU/L) is markedly raised (above 50 mIU/L) in primary hypothyroidism, whereas it will be low in pituitary hypothyroidism. In countries where screening for congenital hypothyroidism is carried out, neonates with a serum TSH more than 40 mIU/L or between 20 and 40 mIU/L on two occasions in the confirmatory samples will be regarded as suffering from primary hypothyroidism. A test of the TSH response to TRH given intravenously in a dose of 10 µg/kg is rarely necessary except in neonates with persistent mild elevation of serum TSH levels. Serum thyroglobulin level is low in thyroglobulin gene defect or thyroid agenesis but is elevated in patients with organification disorders and TSH receptor defects. In babies with congenital hypothyroidism, X-ray of the knee and ankles should be done to assess skeletal maturity. Thus, foetal hypothyroidism can be presumed in the full-term baby if the upper tibial or lower femoral epiphyses (which normally ossify at 36 weeks of gestation) are absent or if they show epiphyseal dysgenesis.

Radioactive iodine (RAI) test is never necessary to establish the diagnosis of hypothyroidism, but it can be used to provide information about the pathogenesis. With the exception of iodide transport defects, patients with dyshormonogenesis have increased RAI uptake with the thyroid gland in the normal position. Patients with thyroid peroxidase (TPO) defect, Pendred syndrome and mutations in dual oxidase gene 2 (DUOX2) have excessive discharge of RAI to perchlorate after its uptake into the thyroid gland. For the detection and location of thyroid activity in congenital hypothyroidism, ^{123}I or ^{99m}Tc can be safely given followed by scanning of the neck for radioactivity. Absent or decreased uptake in the neck is suggestive of thyroid dysgenesis and activity in the lingual location suggests an ectopic gland. Ultrasound examination of the thyroid gland is often helpful. Absence of radionuclide uptake in the presence of ectopic thyroid gland on ultrasound is suggestive of an iodine trapping defect.

Neonatal Screening for Congenital Hypothyroidism

Irreversible brain damage is a common sequel to a delayed clinical diagnosis and treatment of congenital hypothyroidism. Newborn screening for congenital hypothyroidism has been highly successful in improving the prognosis for mental development in hypothyroid neonates. The incidence of congenital hypothyroidism has been reported to be in the region of 1 in 3,600. Thyroid agenesis, hypoplasia or ectopic thyroid gland accounts for 80% of the cases of congenital hypothyroidism. Ten percent of the cases are due to inborn errors of thyroid hormone biosynthesis. Congenital hypothyroidism due to pituitary or hypothalamic dysfunction has an incidence of 1:25,000 births. Screening is usually carried out between the third day and seventh day of life. In Europe and Britain, the favoured technique is by RIA or more commonly enzyme-linked immunosorbent assay (ELISA) of TSH levels on dried filter paper blood spots obtained by heel stab. It involves an extremely low recall rate for repeat tests but is unable to detect the rare cases of secondary (pituitary) hypothyroidism. This disadvantage does not apply to measurement of T_4 levels followed by TSH assay, which is confined to specimens with low T_4 values. This latter method is favoured by some American centres. While both methods are highly reliable, it is essential that infants with results in the hypothyroid range have confirmatory tests, which should include clinical assessment, TSH assays, quantitative measurements of T_4 and T_3 and assessment of bone maturation by X-ray of the knee.

Infants are missed despite newborn thyroid screening programmes due to human error or problems in the infrastructure of the screening programmes. Treatment should be started as early as possible. The incidence rate of congenital hypothyroidism has been noticed to be rising in the United States, and thyroid-blocking antibodies, maternal ingestion of antithyroid drugs (ATDs), iodine deficiency or excess have not been found to be contributing factors. It is possible that transient hypothyroidism and hyperthyrotropinaemia are being misclassified as cases of true congenital hypothyroidism.

Physiological hypothyroxinaemia is common in premature infants and significant hypothyroxinaemia occurs in 15–20% of extreme low birth weight (ELBW) babies and 5–10% of very low birth weight (VLBW) neonates. Also transient primary hypothyroidism occurs in 0.41% of VLBW infants and transient secondary hypothyroidism can occur in up to 10% of VLBW newborns. Nonthyroidal illness syndrome is common in VLBW neonates due to their stormy postnatal course. All these factors need to be taken into account to plan for screening for congenital hypothyroidism in premature infants. The Clinical and Laboratory Standards Institute recommends collection of blood spot specimen from premature neonates on admission to the neonatal intensive care unit or special care baby unit, a repeat specimen at 48–72 hours and a final sample at 28 days of life or on discharge whichever comes first.

Autoimmune Thyroiditis (Hashimoto Thyroiditis)

Autoimmune thyroiditis is the most common cause of hypothyroidism in childhood. It is one of the best examples of an organ-specific autoimmunity and the immunological phenomena are usually confined to the thyroid gland. It is caused by an interaction of multiple genetic and environmental factors like infection and dietary iodine intake. The outstanding feature is infiltration of the thyroid by lymphocytes, plasma cells and reticular cells. Hyperplasia of the epithelial cells is commonly seen. In more advanced cases, the epithelial cells show degenerative changes and there may be extensive fibrosis with final destruction of the gland. Occasionally autoimmune thyroid disease may be associated with other autoimmune endocrine gland dysfunction as part of the autoimmune polyendocrine syndrome, including DM, adrenal insufficiency, candidiasis, hypoparathyroidism and pernicious anaemia.

Clinical features In most children, the only sign is goitre and the onset of the disorder is usually insidious. It rarely has the firm, rubbery consistency so typical of the adult form of the disease. Presentation is usually with euthyroid goitre but in up to 10% of the cases, particularly in adolescence, there may be signs of thyrotoxicosis. Only a minority of affected children go on to develop hypothyroidism, but it is important to monitor for signs of this state in every case as the onset of hypothyroidism is insidious and may be missed. The patient may have weight gain, slowing of growth, cold intolerance, constipation and deteriorating school performance. In adolescent patients, there may be delayed puberty or rarely precocious puberty. Hypothyroidism is diagnosed by a low or normal total or free thyroxine level together with elevated TSH concentrating (>10mU/L). The classical antithyroglobulin and thyroid antimicrosomal antibodies titres are markedly elevated.

Hyperthyroidism

In contrast to hypothyroidism, thyrotoxicosis is a less common disorder in childhood. It usually takes the form of Graves' disease with diffuse thyroid enlargement and thyrotoxic ophthalmopathy. The incidence varies from 0.1 per 100,000 in young children to 14 per 100,000 among adolescents in some countries. About 35% of monozygotic twins as compared to 3% of dizygotic twins have been found to be concordant for Graves' disease suggesting the importance of genetic relative to the environmental factors (stress and smoking) in disease susceptibility. The HLA-DRB1 locus and A-G polymorphism of exon 1 of the cytotoxic T-lymphocyte-associated antigen-4 (CTLA-4) have been found to be associated with Graves' disease. Association between autoimmune thyroid disease and polymorphisms of the genes of tumour necrosis factor receptor superfamily member 5 (TNFRSF5), vitamin D receptor (VDR), (TPO) and Pendred syndrome [solute carrier family 26 (anion exchanger) member 4 (SLC26A4)] have been reported but not always replicated by others. Chromosomal regions (5q31, 14q31, 20q11) linked to autoimmune thyroid disease have been identified by linkage analysis using the genome scan approach.

About 85–95% of cases of hyperthyroidism are due to Graves' disease and other causes include thyroiditis, hyper-functioning thyroid adenoma, germ-line activating TSH receptor mutation, McCune Albright syndrome, pituitary resistance to thyroid hormone and iodine induced hyperthyroidism.

Clinical Features

The disease is more common in girls and rare before the age of 7 years. The parents may bring their child for medical advice with a variety of symptoms, such as irritability, fidgetiness, deterioration in school performance, loss of weight in spite of good appetite, excessive sweating, palpitations or nervousness. The child looks thin, and often startled due to her stare and wide palpebral fissures. There may be obvious exophthalmos **(Fig. 17.4)**. Other eye signs include lid retraction, lid lag and ophthalmoplegia. There may be conjunctival injection because of exposure due to the proptosis. The skin will be flushed, warm and moist. A fine tremor of the outstretched fingers is common. The abnormal cardiovascular signs in the child include sinus

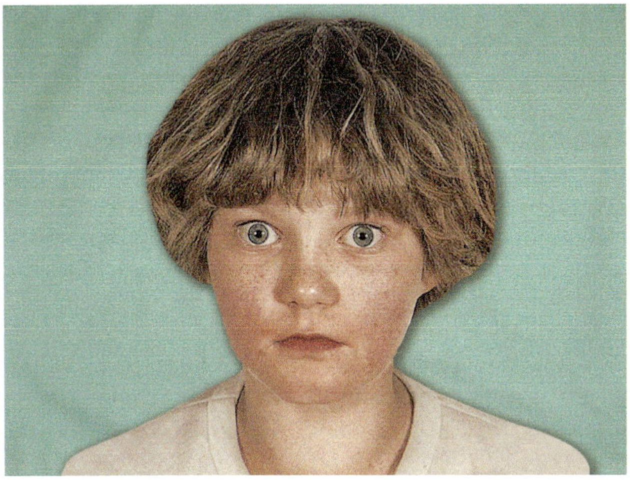

Figure 17.4 Thyrotoxicosis showing exophthalmos, lid retraction and goitre.

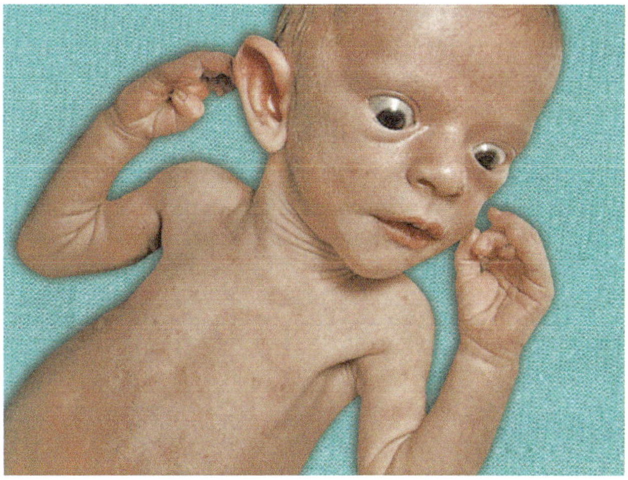

Figure 17.5 Neonatal thyrotoxicosis.

tachycardia, raised systolic blood pressure and a large pulse pressure. The thyroid gland is visibly enlarged and feels soft. A bruit may be audible over the gland. Emotional liability is frequently very obvious. Menstruation may be delayed or irregular in untreated adolescent girls and growth acceleration is commonly seen at diagnosis. Neuropsychiatric complications include attention deficit, emotional liability, delusion and thyrotoxic autoimmune encephalopathy presenting with profound personality change, bizarre motor automatism and seizures. Thyrotoxic periodic paralysis is rare in Caucasians but occurs in 2% of Chinese and Japanese thyrotoxic patients with a strong male predominance.

Diagnosis

This is usually obvious on simple clinical observation. The most reliable biochemical feature is an elevated total and free serum T_3 and T_4 levels with suppressed TSH documented with a suprasensitive TSH assay. Both thyroid-stimulating antibody (TSAb) and thyroid-blocking antibody (TBAb) epitopes are close together and are both detected in the commercially available thyroid-binding inhibiting immunoglobulin (TBII) assays. TSAb bioassays are limited to specialised centres. TBIIs are disease-specific and are never present in normal euthyroid individuals. TBIIs are present in 80–90% of children with Graves' disease. ELISA assays for human autoantibodies against thyroid-stimulating hormone receptor (TRAb) are also available as commercial assay kits. The antithyroglobulin and thyroid antimicrosomal antibodies are present in 68% of paediatric patients.

Transient Neonatal Thyrotoxicosis

There have been a considerable number of instances in which women who have or have had thyrotoxicosis, given birth to infants with the unmistakable signs of hyperthyroidism in the neonatal period. The infants are restless, agitated, excessively hungry and they exhibit warm, moist flushed skin, tachycardia (190–220 per minute), tachypnoea, exophthalmos and goitre (Fig. 17.5). The diagnosis has been made antenatally due to foetal tachycardia. Some mothers have been previously treated by partial thyroidectomy; others have received thyroid-blocking drugs during pregnancy. When the mother is thyrotoxic and not on ATDs up to the time of delivery, the hyperthyroid state is present in the infant from birth. If the mother has been rendered euthyroid by drugs and ATD therapy is continued until the time of delivery, neonatal thyrotoxicosis does not develop for some days because the thyroid gland is suppressed in utero and during the infant's first day of life.

There is good evidence that neonatal Graves' disease is caused by the transfer of maternal TSAbs/thyroid-stimulating immunoglobulins (TSIs) across the placenta from mother to foetus. The presence of such immunoglobulins in the mother and infant at the same time has been demonstrated both by bioassay techniques and the radioreceptor assay method. The TSIs disappear from the infant's blood after about 3 months, so that the disorder is a temporary one. Diagnosis in the neonate is confirmed by demonstrating increased levels of total and free T_4 and T_3 and suppressed levels of TSH.

The degree of thyrotoxicosis can be alarmingly severe and prompt treatment of the newborn infant is essential.

PARATHYROID GLANDS

Primary disorders of the parathyroid glands are exceedingly rare in paediatric practice. Much has been learned about the molecular structure and physiological activities of parathyroid hormone (PTH) in recent years and circulating PTH can be measured by RIA. PTH increases renal tubular calcium absorption and phosphate excretion and intestinal calcium absorption. PTH also maintains serum calcium levels by stimulating osteoclastic bone resorption. It is hardly possible to consider the actions of PTH without consideration of calcitonin. Calcitonin is also a polypeptide and is secreted from the parafollicular "C" cells of the thyroid gland. It inhibits the resorption of bone and acts as a physiological antagonist to PTH, causing hypocalcaemia. The only disorder associated with excessive calcitonin production is medullary thyroid carcinoma which may occur as part of multiple endocrine neoplasia type 2b (MEN 2b) caused by mutations in the RET proto-oncogene.

Hypoparathyroidism

Hypoparathyroidism may occur after thyroid or parathyroid surgery or rarely radiation damage. In Asia and the Mediterranean basin, hypoparathyroidism can result from haemosiderosis in transfusion-dependent thalassaemia major patients. A rare autoimmune polyendocrine syndrome due to mutations in the autoimmune regulator gene (AIRE) can result in hypoadrenalism, which develops in childhood and is associated later with hypoadrenocorticism, and sometimes with steatorrhoea, pernicious anaemia, DM or elevated sweat electrolytes; moniliasis frequently precedes the endocrine manifestations. Rarely hypoparathyroidism can result from mitochondrial cytopathy. Apart from transient neonatal hypoparathyroidism due to maternal parathyroid disease, congenital hypoparathyroidism can be due to dysgenesis of the parathyroid gland, familial forms of disease (antosomal recessive, autosomal dominant, X-linked recessive), heterozygous gain-of-function mutations of the calcium-sensing receptor gene (CASR) or the DiGeorge syndrome (thymus hypoplasia, hypoparathyroidism, malformations of the outflow tracts of the heart) due to microdeletion of chromosome 22q11. Familial hypoparathyroidism may be associated with sensorineural deafness and renal anomalies (haploinsufficiency of GATA3).

Clinical Features

The diagnosis of hypoparathyroidism is not difficult when a child presents with recurrent tetany. Other symptoms include paraesthesia ("pins and needle"), muscle cramps and carpopedal spasm. Chvostek and Trousseau signs may be elicited. More often the outstanding feature is the presence of recurrent convulsions when an erroneous diagnosis of epilepsy may easily be made. Newborn infants with hypoparathyroidism presents with jitteriness or convulsions. Some affected children have also been mentally retarded and intracerebral calcification may occur. Useful diagnostic clues are delay in the second dentition and defective enamel, ectodermal dysplasia and deformed nails, loss of hair and moniliasis in the mouth or nails. Cataract develops later in 50% of cases. The characteristic biochemical changes are a low serum calcium (below 2.25 mmol/L) and raised serum phosphate (above 2.25 mmol/L) and normal serum alkaline phosphatase and low PTH levels by RIA in the absence of rickets, renal disease and steatorrhoea. The urine calcium concentration is low but hypercalciuria is present if the patient has a gain of function mutation of CASR.

Pseudohypoparathyroidism gives rise to a very similar clinical presentation, hypocalcaemia and hyperphosphataemia, but in addition, some patients have features of Albright hereditary osteodystrophy, a stocky figure with dwarfism and a rounded face, brachydactyly with shortening of the metacarpals and metatarsals of the first, fourth and fifth fingers and toes, subcutaneous calcification, developmental delay and obesity. Pseudohypoparathyroidism type 1a is due to maternal transmission of GNAS1 mutation. The serum PTH levels are markedly elevated in the presence of hypocalcaemia, hyperphosphataemia and the phosphaturic and cyclic adenosine monophosphate (cAMP) responses to PTH are blunted. The biochemical abnormalities usually present at a mean age of 8 years.

Hyperparathyroidism

Hypercalcaemia due to adenoma or hyperplasia of the parathyroid glands are very rare in childhood. Neonatal primary hyperparathyroidism is caused by homozygous or compounded heterozygous mutations of the CASR and is associated with hypotonia, anorexia, respiratory distress, dehydration and a high mortality. Urgent parathyroidectomy is required. In older children, parathyroid tumour leading to hyperparathyroidism can be associated with multiple endocrine neoplasia syndrome type I (MEN I) (parathyroid, pancreatic, pituitary tumours due to mutation in MEN I gene) or multiple endocrine neoplasia type II (MEN II) (MTC, phaeochromocytoma, parathyroid tumour due to mutations in the RET proto-oncogene).

Clinical Features

In older children with hyperparathyroidism, bone pains and muscular weakness are the first symptoms. Peptic ulceration is unduly frequent in these patients. Anorexia, polyuria, polydipsia, vomiting, and severe constipation are common and attributable to the hypercalcaemia. The bone changes of osteitis fibrosa cystica are found. These include osteoporosis with patches of osteosclerosis. This produces a characteristic granular mottling or discrete rounded translucent areas in radiographs of the skull. Similar appearances are commonly found in the clavicles and iliac bones. Pathognomonic changes are frequently seen in the terminal phalanges of the hands where there is subperiosteal resorption of bone with a crenellated appearance. The lamina dura, a dense line of alveolar bone surrounding the roots of the teeth, disappears. A giant-cell tumour (osteoclastoma) may appear as a multilocular cyst on radiographs of the mandible or long bones. Occasionally, the presenting sign is a pathological fracture at the site of such a tumour. Hypercalcaemia can lead to nephrocalcinosis and renal calculi.

The most common biochemical features are a raised serum calcium level (over 2.74 mmol) and lowered serum phosphate (below 1 mmol). These values fluctuate and several estimations in the fasting patient at intervals may be required before the diagnosis is confirmed. The plasma alkaline phosphatase is frequently but not invariably raised. There is an increased urinary output of calcium (over 10 mmol/24 hours while on an ordinary diet). This observation should be followed by estimating the 24-hour calcium output on a low-calcium diet (120 mg/day); an output in excess of 4.5 mmol/24 hours is abnormal. When the kidneys have been severely damaged by nephrocalcinosis a high serum phosphate level may simulate secondary hyperparathyroidism. In children, however, renal osteodystrophy includes the changes of rickets that are rare in primary hyperparathyroidism. Furthermore, hypocalciuria is the rule in renal failure, but hypercalciuria usually persists in primary hyperparathyroidism even when there is severe renal damage.

RICKETS

Rickets and osteomalacia are the consequences of decreased mineralisation of the bone osteoid caused by deficiencies of calcium, phosphate or vitamin D. Rickets in childhood can be due to nutritional deficiency of vitamin D from low intake or disordered absorption of fat soluble vitamins due to diseases of the hepatobiliary and gastrointestinal systems. The condition could also result from renal tubular disorders, X-linked familial hypophosphatamic rickets or genetic defects like loss of function mutation of the genes for VDR or 25-hydroxyvitamin D3 1α-hydroxylase (CYP27B1).

Nutritional rickets has emerged again as a paediatric health issue in several parts of the world. The vitamin D intake in most adults should be more than 200 international unit (IU) per day and pregnant and lactating women would not meet the recommended daily vitamin D intake without adequate exposure to sunlight. Dark-skinned infants breastfed by vitamin D deficient mother, who remain covered for cultural reasons, are particularly at risk. The American Academy of Paediatrics recommends that infants, children and adolescences should have a minimum daily vitamin D intake of 200 IU per day. Low calcium, high oxalate and phytate intake in Asian diet contribute to nutritional rickets. The clinical features of rickets are shown in **Box 17.8**.

BOX 17.8 Clinical features of rickets.
Expanded wrist, knee and ankle joints
Rachitic rosary (swelling of costochondral junctions of the anterior chest cage)
Bowing deformity of lower limbs in weight-bearing children
Craniotabes
Hypotonia, muscle weakness and delayed motor development
Enamel hypoplasia and delayed tooth eruption

The biochemical abnormalities in nutritional rickets include hypocalcaemia, hypophosphataemia, elevated PTH and alkaline phosphatase levels in the blood. The 25-hydroxyvitamin D level is less than 50 nmol/L. Radiologically, there is cupping and fraying of the metaphyses of the long bones and osteopaenia. Treatment with vitamin D 3,000 IU daily for 3 months and maintenance of a daily vitamin D intake of 400 IU daily should be continued.

In most developed countries, the most common form of rickets is X-linked familial hypophosphataemia rickets, which is caused by loss of function mutation of the phosphate-regulating gene with homologies to endopeptidases on the X-chromosome gene (PHEX). The incidence is reported to be 1 in 25,000. Apart from clinical features of rickets, these patients present with short stature, bone pain, joint stiffness, dental abscess but craniotabes and muscle weakness are not present. The clinical expression is variable and male patients are more severely affected than heterozygous females. Biochemical abnormalities include low normal serum calcium, low serum phosphate and elevated alkaline phosphatase levels. The serum PTH and vitamin D levels are normal, but the $1,25(OH)_2D_3$ (1,25-dihydroxyvitamin D3)concentration is inappropriately low for the degree of hypophosphataemia. The urine calcium concentration is normal and there is no aminoaciduria. The urine hydroxyproline is increased. Nephrocalcinosis is a common complication, and is due to deposition of calcium and phosphate in the kidneys, and it has been shown to have a stronger link with phosphate dosage and urine phosphate excretion. Treatment include phosphate supplement (not more than 70 mg/kg per day) and rocaltrol (20–60 ng/kg per day), and regular monitoring is required to avoid hypercalcaemia, hypercalciuria (calcium/creatinine ratio >0.7 mmol/mmol) and nephrocalcinosis.

Autosomal dominant hypophosphataemic rickets is due to activating mutations of fibroblast growth factor 23 gene (FGF23), which prevents the degradation of FGF23. Hereditary hypophosphataemic rickets with hypercalciuria is due to loss of function in sodium-phosphate cotransporter type 2 gene (SLC34A3) and long-term phosphate supplement alone is adequate to treat these patients. Other causes of phosphaturic rickets include the Fanconi syndrome and other types of renal tubular acidosis, oncogenic osteomalacia and McCune Albright syndrome.

GONADS

The development of the pituitary gland, the control of pubertal development and development of secondary sexual characteristics have already been described. Secretion of GnRH by GnRH neurons is inherently pulsatile. GABAergic receptors mediate inhibitory and NMDs (N-methyl-D-aspartats) receptors mediate facilitatory input. Oestradiol directly stimulates or inhibits GnRH gene expression under different conditions and the

BOX 17.9 Causes of hypogonadism.

hypogonadotrophic hypogonadism
Congenital defects in hypothalamic-hypophyseal formation associated with midline facial defects
Mutations in genes of pituitary transcription factors, gonadotrophin-releasing hormone receptor and gonadotrophin
Genetic hypothalamic defects (Kallmann syndrome, Prader–Willi and Bardet–Biedl syndrome)
Acquired
- Suprasellar tumours
- Infiltrative disease
- Damage from radiation, trauma, haemosiderosis, intracranial Infection

Functional hypothalamic hypogonadism
- Drugs and contraceptive pills
- Systemic illness and eating disorder
- Exercise-induced amenorrhoea in girls
- Stress and cortisol excess

Hypergonadotropic hypogonadism in girls
Gonadal dysgenesis—Turner syndrome (45,X) and trisomy syndrome, Wilms' tumour 1 mutations
Autoimmune ovarian failure
Damage by radiation, cytotoxic drugs and infection
Genetic causes due to mutations of steroidogenic factor 1, gonadotrophin receptor gene, fragile X premutation, Noonan syndrome
hypergonadotrophic hypogonadism in males
Klinefelter syndrome (47,XXY)
Damage from orchitis, radiation and chemotherapeutic agents
Noonan's syndrome, cystic fibrosis and rare genetic causes

stimulation of GnRH and LH surge in mid-cycle by oestrogen seems to involve induction of progesterone receptors in the hypothalamus. Prolactin suppresses both hypothalamic and gonadotrope GnRH receptor expression. Hypothalamic endorphins suppress GnRH secretion and interleukins inhibit gonadotrophin release.

Hypogonadism

Adolescents without signs of puberty by 13 years in girls and 14 years in boys, or failing to progress in the development of secondary sexual characteristics warrant further assessment. Primary amenorrhoea is defined by the absence of menstruation by 14 years of age in a girl with no secondary sexual characteristics or by 16 years in a girl with some development of secondary sexual characteristics. The causes of hypogonadism are shown in **Box 17.9**.

Clinical Features

With the exception of cryptorchidism and micropenis suggestive of congenital hypopituitarism, the features of hypogonadism in the male only become manifest after the time of normal puberty. Growth continues for an abnormally long

BOX 17.10 Investigations of hypogonadism.

Serum LH, FSH, prolactin, oestradiol or testosterone levels
Morning cortisol, fT_4, TSH concentrations
X-ray for bone age
Karyotype
GnRH/GnRH-analogue test to distinguish hypogonadotrophic hypogonadism from CDGP
Combined pituitary stimulation test and MRI scan of the brain, hypothalamus and pituitary gland if indicated

Abbreviations: LH, luteinising hormone; FSH, follicle-stimulating hormone; ft_4 free thyroxine TSH, thyroid-stimulating hormone; GnRH, gonadotrophin-releasing hormone; CDGP, constitutional delay in growth and puberty; MRI, magnetic resonance imaging.

period, but at a slower growth rate due to delay in fusion of the epiphyses. There is a falloff in the growth velocity in hypogonadal adolescents and this pattern of growth is different from that seen in adolescents with CDGP. Children with CDGP grow at a normal rate below the third percentile and the onset of puberty is delayed. The bone age is frequently delayed by more than 2 years when compared to the chronological age. Both males and females with hypogonadism have a low U/L segment ratio. Clinicians should be aware of the clinical features of syndromes associated with hypogonadism like Prader-Willi, Noonan, Bardet-Biedl, Klinefelter and Turner syndromes. Gynaecomastia is usually seen in hypergonadotrohic hypogonadism. hypogonadotrophic hypogonadism associated with anosmia is suggestive of Kallmann syndrome, which can be inherited in the X-linked (KAL1 mutation) or autosomal recessive [fibroblast growth factor receptor 1 (FGFR1 mutation)] fashion. Clinical evaluation should be done to exclude acquired hypogonadism **(Box 17.9)**. Suggested investigations for hypogonadism are shown in **Box 17.10**.

In adolescents with hypogonadism, induction of puberty should be started no later than 14 years in girls and 15 years in boys.

Precocious Puberty

Pubertal development in girls has been reported to occur earlier in recent years in many populations, but there has been a less dramatic change in the age of onset of menarche. The age of onset of puberty in boys has not advanced significantly in recent years. Precocious puberty is defined as breast development before the age of 7 years, menstruation before the age of 10 years in girls and testicular or penile enlargement before the age of 9 years in boys. The causes of precocious puberty are shown in **Box 17.11**.

Clinical Features

In premature thelarche, there is isolated development of the breasts without significant acceleration of growth or skeletal maturation or the development of other secondary sexual characteristics. The condition frequently occurs

BOX 17.11 Causes of precocious puberty.

Gonadotrophin-dependent or central precocious puberty
- Idiopathic
- Intracranial tumours—hypothalamic hamartoma, pineal region tumour, tumour in posterior hypothalamus, germinoma, craniopharyngioma (rare), optic nerve glioma
- Cranial irradiation
- Head trauma
- Neurological disorders—hydrocephaly, intracranial infection, cerebral palsy, epilepsy
- Hypothyroidism
- Neurofibromatosis type 1

Gonadotrophin-independent sexual precocity
- McCune Albright syndrome
- Familial testotoxicosis

Pseudoprecocious puberty
- Congenital adrenal hyperplasia
- Oestrogen or androgen-secreting tumours from the gonads or adrenal glands
- Human chorionic gonadotrophin-secreting tumour (boys)
- Autonomously functioning ovarian cysts in girls

Incomplete precocious puberty
- Premature thelarche
- Premature adrenarche

in the first 18 months of life. There may be fluctuations of the breast size but the condition is not progressive. Occasionally, no-progressive breast development can occur in girls in the peripubertal age group (5–7 years of age) and the condition is sometimes referred to as the larche variant but should be distinguished from the early stage of central precocious puberty. Premature adrenarche refers to early isolated development of sex hair without other signs of puberty. Premature adrenarche is more prevalent in African Americans and East Asian Indians. Care must be taken to exclude the possibility of late-onset congenital adrenal hyperplasia (CAH) or androgen-secreting tumour from the adrenal glands or gonads.

Patients with true precocious puberty have rapid physical growth and advanced skeletal maturation. In addition to the development of secondary sexual characteristics, behavioural change like emotion liability and aggression may occur. The behaviour of children with precocious puberty is more appropriate to their chronological age rather than the degree of sexual development. Other changes include increased sebaceous gland secretion (greasy skin and hair), acne and body odour. Children with precocious puberty who are untreated usually have an increased U/L segment ratio. Most cases of precocious puberty in girls are idiopathic, but about 5–10% of girls and 40% of boys with precocious puberty have an occult or known intracranial pathology.

Patients with the McCune Albright syndrome have the characteristic triad of irregular café-au-lait pigmentation, gonadotrophin independent sexual precocity and polyostotic fibrous dysplasia but sometimes, the complete triad is not present. The condition is due to a somatic activating mutation of the GNAS1 gene. The patients typically have breast development due to oestrogen production from an autonomously functioning ovarian cyst. When the cyst ruptures, menstruation occurs as a result of acute oestrogen withdrawal.

Familial testotoxicosis is inherited in an autosomal dominant male limited fashion. There is autosomal dominant presentation of early sexual development in males of the affected families. The condition manifests itself usually by 2–3 years of age and is due to activating mutations of the LH receptor gene. Females carrying the mutation will not develop precocious puberty. There is some seminiferous tubule development and spermatogenesis due to the high intratesticular concentrations of testosterone present in affected patients even though the gonadotrophin levels are suppressed.

A germ cell tumour producing HCG can lead to pseudoprecocious puberty in boys only. However, germ cell tumours can also cause true precocious puberty due to the location of the tumour in the posterior hypothalamus distorting the hypothalamic "gonadostat". An autonomously functioning ovarian cyst producing oestrogen can cause premature breast development. These cysts should be distinguished from juvenile granulosa tumours of the ovaries by serial ultrasound assessment. Persistence of cystic lesions with a significant solid component and persistent elevation of serum oestradiol concentration for more than 3 months should alert the doctor to the possibility of an ovarian tumour.CAH can cause isosexual pseudoprecocious puberty in boys and heterosexual pseudoprecocious puberty in girls (refer to subsequent section of this chapter). Differentiation of virilisation due to CAH from an adrenal tumour is important in virilised patients.

Investigations

Suggested investigations and interpretation of the hormonal tests are shown in **Box 17.12** and **Table 17.1**, respectively.

BOX 17.12 Investigations and interpretations for precocious puberty.

- Baseline oestradiol or testosterone, LH, FSH levels and the LH and FSH response to GnRH (2.5 mg/kg intravenously)
- X-ray for bone age
- Ultrasound examination of the pelvis in girls for ovarian volume and cysts, uterine size and cervix to uterus ratio
- MRI of the brain
- Investigations for involvement of other pituitary hormones where indicated: fT_4, TSH, prolactin levels, and cortisol and GH reserve

Abbreviations: LH, luteinising hormone; FSH, follicle-stimulating hormone; GnRH, gonadotrophin-releasing hormone; fT_4, free thyroxine; TSH, thyroid-stimulating hormone; GH, growth hormone.

TABLE 17.1 Sex steroids and gonadotropins in precocious puberty.

	E2/testosterone	*LH (basal)*	*LH (peak)*	*FSH (peak)*
Premature thelarche (girls)	Prepuberty	<0.5 IU/L	Prepuberty	↑↑
Early precocious puberty	Prepuberty or ↑	<0.5 IU/L	<7 IU/L	↑↑
Established precocious puberty	↑–↑↑	>0.6 IU/L	>9.6 IU/L in boys	↑
			>7 IU*/Lin girls	
Pseudoprecocious puberty	↑–↑↑	↓↓	↓↓	↓↓
Gonadotrophin-independent sexual precocity	Prepuberty – ↑	↓↓	↓↓	
HCG tumour (boys)	↑	Slight ↑	No change	↓↓

*The levels of LH are for reference only and the cut-off levels for definition of puberty depends on the performance of the immunoassay used in the laboratory.

Abbreviations: LH, luteinising hormone; FSH, follicle-stimulating hormone; HCG, human chorionic gonadotrophin.

ADRENAL GLAND

Adrenal steroidogenesis is controlled by a number of cytochrome P450 and hydroxysteroid dehydrogenase enzymes **(Flow chart 17.1)**. The adrenal cortex produces cortisol, mineralocorticoid (aldosterone) and sex steroids (androgens), whereas the adrenal medulla secretes adrenaline, noradrenaline, catecholamines and dopamine.

Cushing Syndrome

Cushing syndrome in children is commonly iatrogenic in nature due to steroids given by the oral, topical or inhalational routes. Rarely steroid excess state can become manifest due to adrenal tumour, primary pigmented nodular adrenal disease, ectopic ACTH-secreting malignancy or Cushing's disease (ACTH-secreting pituitary adenoma). Apart from iatrogenic Cushing syndrome, adrenal tumours account for 80% of Cushing syndrome in children less than 7 years of age and 40% are malignant. Pseudo-Cushingoid states can be due to stress, depression and alcoholism.

Clinical Features

The clinical features of Cushing syndrome result from the excessive secretion of adrenal hormones and are dominated by the effects of cortisol. Growth retardation, fatigue and emotional liability are common symptoms. Those due to an increased production of glucocorticoids

Flow chart 17.1 Pathways of steroid metabolism.

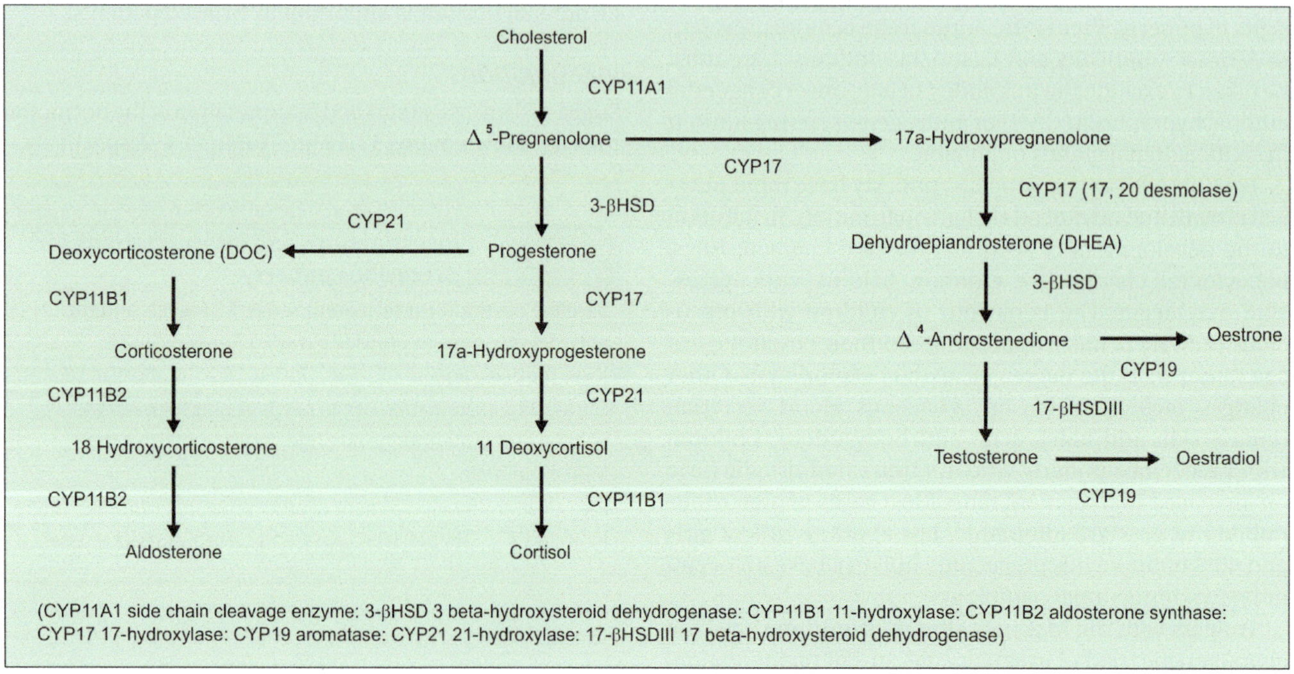

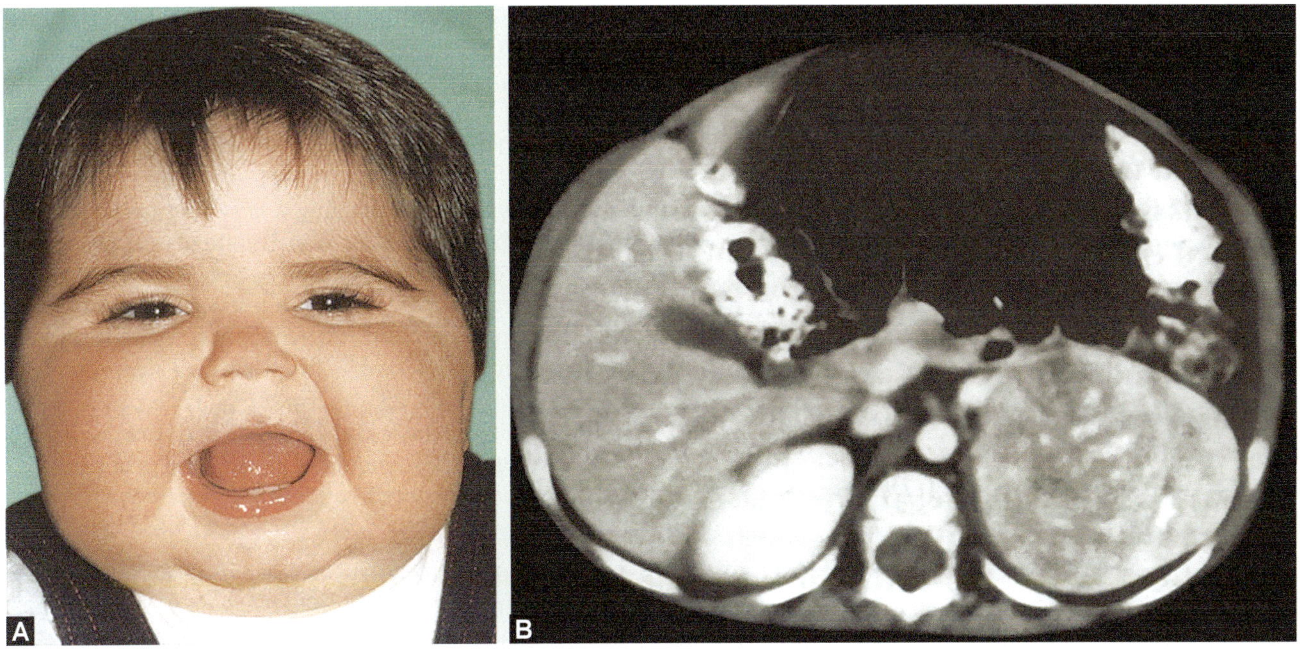

Figures 17.6A and B A child with Cushing syndrome; (B) CT scan showing a large well-encapsulated tumour with calcification of the left adrenal gland.

include buffalo hump fat pad over the back of the neck, obesity, moon face, purple striae over abdomen, flanks and thighs, easy bruising, muscle wasting and weakness, osteoporosis, latent DM and polycythaemia **(Figs. 17.6A and B)**. Increased output of mineralocorticosteroids and aldosterone accounts for the hypertension and hypokalaemic alkalosis. Excessive secretion of androgens may cause hirsutism and clitoral enlargement in females, baldness and acne. These patients are, in addition, highly susceptible to infections.

Diagnosis

In patients with Cushing syndrome due to exogenous steroids given in excess (>6–8 mg/m^2 per day of hydrocortisone equivalent), the endogenous secretion of glucocorticoids will be suppressed. Excessive doses of glucocorticoids such as prednisolone or dexamethasone (1 mg prednisolone equivalent to 4 mg hydrocortisone and 1 mg of dexamethasone is equivalent to 30 mg of hydrocortisone) will result in features of Cushing syndrome but the morning plasma cortisol and 24-hour urine free cortisol and 17-oxogenic steroids will be suppressed. Endogenous excessive secretion of glucocorticoids due to an adrenal tumour or ACTH-secreting pituitary tumour will result in loss of diurnal cortisol rhythm with elevated morning and evening plasma cortisol levels, and a midnight plasma cortisol of greater than 207 nmol/L is highly specific for the diagnosis of Cushing syndrome. The urinary free cortisol will be elevated more than four times the upper limit of normal corrected for the creatinine level. Frequently, the 24-hour urinary oxogenic steroids concentration is also elevated. A plasma ACTH level is useful and measurable or elevated levels is suggestive of ACTH-dependent Cushing's disease or ectopic ACTH production. The change in plasma cortisol and urinary free cortisol levels to low dose (30 mg/kg per day divided in four doses) and high dose (120 μg/kg per day in four divided doses) dexamethasone suppression is a useful test. Failure of adrenocortical suppression by high dose dexamethasone is strongly suggestive of an adrenal tumour. In difficult cases, the CRH test and bilateral inferior petrosal sinus venous sampling may be required to localise a pituitary ACTH-secreting adenoma. Biochemical diagnosis must be complemented by MRI scan with gadolinium enhancement of the pituitary and adrenal glands.

Adrenal Insufficiency

Adrenal insufficiency can be caused by disorders involving the hypothalamus and pituitary gland **(Box 17.1)** or those affecting primarily the adrenal gland. The causes of primary adrenal insufficiency are shown in **Box 17.13**.

Clinical Features

In the most common form of autoimmune polyendocrine syndrome, the children present with cutaneous candidiasis, hypoparathyroidism (tetany and convulsions) and adrenal insufficiency. Allgrove syndrome is characterised by alacrima, achalasia, ACTH-resistance and neurological symptoms. In the older child, the manifestations closely resemble those seen in the adult—extreme asthenia, cachexia, hypotension and microcardia. Pigmentation of skin and mucous membranes tends to be less marked in children. Dangerous adrenal crises may occur, often

BOX 17.13 Causes of adrenal insufficiency.

DAX1 mutation
SF1 mutation
IMAGe syndrome
P450 oxidoreductase deficiency (± Antley–Bixler syndrome phenotype)
Adrenocorticotropic hormone unresponsiveness
Familial glucocorticoid resistances
Autoimmune adrenal insufficiency (APS1 AIRE; APS2 HLADR3 CTLA-4)
X-linked adrenoleucodystrophy
Inherited defects of adrenal steroidogenesis
Mitochondrial cytopathy
Triple A syndrome (ALADIN-WD-repeat protein)
Acquired adrenal insufficiency
Infections—tuberculosis, fungal infection, CMV, HIV *Meningococcus, Pseudomonas, E. coli*
Haemorrhage/thrombosis—SLE, polyarteritis, antiphospholipid syndrome, anticoagulant therapy
Infiltration—tumour, sarcoidosis, amyloidosis, haemosiderosis
Drugs—cyproterone acetate, ketoconazole, aminoglutethimide, mitotane, rifampicin

Abbreviations: CMV, cytomegalovirus; HIV, Human immunodeficiency virus; *E. coli*, *Escherichia coli*; SLE, systemic lupus erythematosus.

precipitated by infections. Hypoglycaemic convulsions may first bring the child to the physicians.

In the congenital form of the disease, acute adrenal failure may develop with alarming rapidly during the neonatal period. Newborn infants with adrenal insufficiency frequently present with hypoglycaemia and prolonged neonatal jaundice. Increased skin pigmentation is also seen. Vomiting, diarrhoea and extreme dehydration can lead easily to an erroneous diagnosis such as pyloric stenosis, high intestinal obstruction or gastroenteritis. The pointer to adrenal insufficiency is the presence of abundant sodium and chloride in the urine and hyponatremia and hyperkalaemia in the serum. Congenital adrenal insufficiency is due to a number of rare genetic disorders and the diagnosis and genetic analysis and management should be performed in a tertiary referral centre. Tuberculous adrenalitis is now a rare cause of primary adrenal insufficiency in childhood. Exogenous corticosteroid therapy can induce adrenal suppression in patients if used in dosages above the cortisol secretion rate for over 3 weeks.

Diagnosis

During a crisis, characteristic blood chemical changes include low serum chloride and sodium, elevated serum potassium (with changes in the electrocardiography (ECG)] and hypoglycaemia. In the absence of a crisis, the blood chemistry may not be grossly abnormal and more refined tests are necessary. In primary adrenal insufficiency, the plasma ACTH concentration will be elevated. The early morning plasma cortisol level will be low and fails to rise in response to low dose synacthen stimulation (1 μg/1.73 m^2 intravenously) or standard dose synacthen test (250 μg intravenously). In neonates and young infants, a synacthen test using a dose of 1 μg/kg intravenously has been recommended. Failure of the plasma cortisol to increase by 200 nmol/L and reach to an absolute level of more than 500 nmol/L in response to synacthen is suggestive of adrenal insufficiency. If secondary adrenal insufficiency is suspected, appropriate investigations of the hypothalamic pituitary axis like the glucagon stimulation test or insulin tolerance test should be performed.

In further assessment of the aetiology of primary adrenal insufficiency, recommended investigations include:

- Plasma very long-chain fatty acids.
- Auto-antibody levels against adrenal, thyroid, gastric parietal cell and islet cell.
- Serum thyroid hormones, calcium, phosphate, vitamin B_{12} and folate concentrations.
- Recombent and erect plasma renin activity, aldosterone, electrolytes and urine sodium concentrations to assess mineralocorticoid activity.
- Plasma lactate.
- Skeletal survey.
- Appropriate molecular genetic diagnosis.

Congenital Adrenal Hyperplasia

Deficiencies of the enzymes involved in adrenal steroidogenesis will lead to different varieties of CAH **(Flow chart 17.1)**. 21α-hydroxylase deficiency accounts for 95% of the cases of CAH seen in childhood and will be discussed in detail. The incidence varies from 1:15,000 to 1:20,000 births and is inherited in an autosomal recessive manner. The incidence of CAH has been reported to be higher in India, Philippines and South America. 21α-hydroxylase deficiency results from mutations of the CYP21B gene which is situated on chromosome 6 in close proximity to the human leukocyte antigen (HLA) genes. There is a reasonable genotype-phenotype correlation with drastic mutations causing salt-wasting 21 hydroxylase deficiency (21-OHD) and severe mutations leading to virilising form of the disease. Nonclassic form of 21α-hydroxylase deficiency occurs if one of two mutations is mild and female patients present with premature adrenarche or hyperandrogenism in adolescence.

Newborn Screening for Congenital Adrenal Hyperplasia

Salt-wasting form of CAH is a life-threatening disorder leading to circulatory collapse and disorder of sex development in girls. In Sweden, the mortality rate of CAH without screening was 2.2% from 1969 to 1986. First-tier screening tests measure 17α-OHP levels in dried blood spots collected

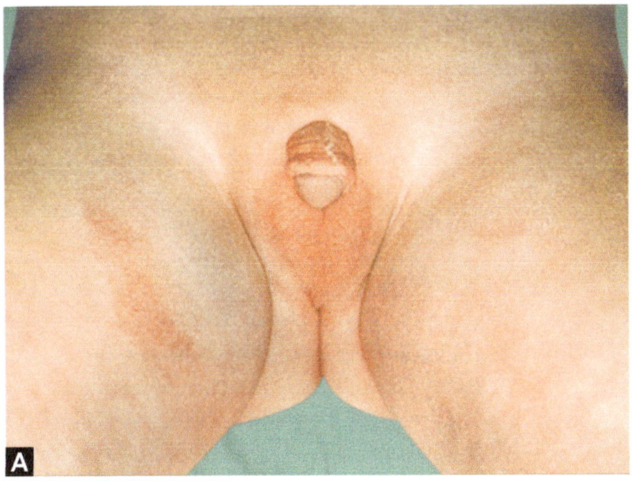

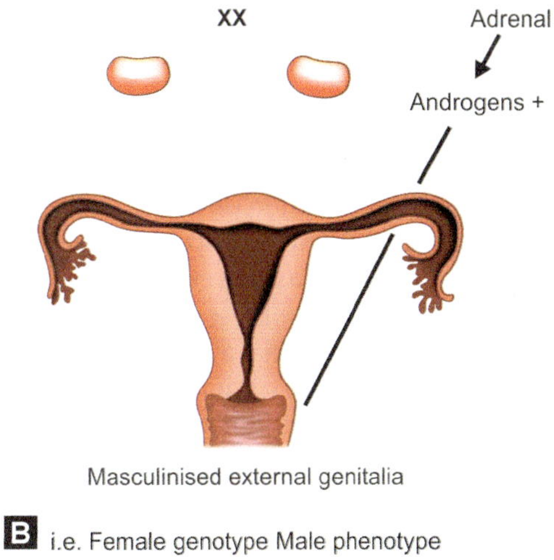

Figures 17.7A and B Masculinisation of female genitalia due to congenital adrenal hyperplasia.

on filter paper cards by enzyme-linked immunoassay or by time-resolved dissociation-enhanced lanthanide fluorescence immunoassay (DELFIA). The serum 17α-OHP levels in the newborn are affected by birth weight, gestational age and timing of the sample. Stratification of recall 17α-OHP cut-off values according to birth weight categories and the use of second-tier screening of measuring 17α-OHP by tandem mass spectrometry or molecular diagnosis have been used to improve the positive predictive value of the screening test. The cost-effectiveness of neonatal screening for CAH remains controversial.

Clinical features Male infants with 21α-hydroxylase deficiency appear normal at birth apart from rather marked pigmentation of the scrotum. After a short time virilisation is revealed in the virilising form of 21-OHD by enlargement of the penis, growth of pubic hair, excessive muscular development and advanced skeletal maturation due to the action of the excess androgens. The testes, however, remain small and undeveloped. The increased stature ultimately gives way to short adult stature due to premature fusion of the epiphyses. In the salt wasting form of the disease, male patients present in a salt-losing crisis at the end of the first week or in the second week of life with vomiting, diarrhoea, severe dehydration and shock. The correct diagnosis is easy enough in the virilised female infant, but in the male an erroneous diagnosis of pyloric stenosis, gastroenteritis or septicaemia is easily made. The serum sodium and chloride levels are reduced, and the serum potassium level is high with corresponding ECG changes. There is also metabolic acidosis, elevated serum urea and increased fractional excretion of sodium. The salt-losing form of 21-OHD accounts for 60–75% of cases. In all types of adrenal hyperplasia excessive skin pigmentation is common.

In female infants, the excessive androgenic effects upon the foetus produce more striking and unwelcome changes. In mild cases, there is marked clitoral enlargement. In an extensively virilised newborn female, there is marked clitoral enlargement, fusion of the labia majora and the vagina, and urethra may enter a single common urogenital sinus **(Figs. 17.7A and B)**. An extensively virilised infant can readily be mistaken for a cryptorchid male. Similarly, females with drastic CYP21B mutations present in salt-losing crisis in the neonatal period. Without treatment, a girl with virilising 21-OHD becomes progressively masculinised with hirsutism, clitoromegaly, muscularity and advanced bone age **(Fig. 17.7)**.

Diagnosis In countries where there is screening for CAH in the neonatal period, patients with the classical form but not necessarily the nonclassical form of 21-OHD will be identified. Biochemical confirmation of a clinically diagnosed case is shown by elevated plasma ACTH, 17α-OHP, high plasma renin activity levels and low plasma cortisol and aldosterone levels in patients with salt-wasting 21-OHD. In simple virilising 21-OHD, the morning 17α-OHP levels are high, but the plasma renin activity and serum electrolytes may be normal. Advanced skeletal maturation is seen in untreated or undertreated patients with classical 21-OHD. In a virilised female, chromosomal analysis and ultrasound examination of the pelvis for the presence of female internal genital organs are necessary.

DISORDERS OF SEX DEVELOPMENT

Sexual development is a complex process that is dependent on a variety of molecular signals working in concert to specify sex-specific differentiation and organogenesis. In humans, the process of sex determination commits the bipotential gonads to become either a testis or an ovary depending on the genetic sex of the foetus. The process of sexual differentiation follows when the gonads release sex-specific signalling molecules and hormones which are responsible for shaping the phenotypic sex of the individual. Genes of several transcription factors including steroidogenic factor 1 (SF1) and Wilms tumour 1 (WT1) are required for the formation of the indifferent genital ridges in humans. The sex determining region of the Y-chromosome gene (SRY gene) expression must reach a threshold level at a critical time in the cascade of early events leading to testis differentiation, before male sex determination can occur. SOX9 encodes a transcription factor downstream of SRY and is a crucial component of the male sex-determining pathway. Loss of function mutation in SOX9 results in gonadal dysgenesis and campomelic dysplasia. Other transcription factors and signalling molecules are important in the differentiation of peritubular myoid cells, endothelial cells, Leydig cells, Sertoli cells and germ cells within the developing testes. Both the Müllerian and Wolffian ducts are present in male and female embryos. Anti-Müllerian hormone (AMH), which is secreted by Sertoli cells of the testes, stimulates the production of matrix metalloproteinase 2 (MMP2) which induces apoptosis in the Müllerian duct epithelial cells. The Wolffian ducts develop into the epididymis, vas deferens and seminal vesicles under the influence of testosterone produced by Leydig cells of the developing testes. A number of enzymes are responsible for testosterone biosynthesis **(Flow chart 17.1)** and mutations in these genes will result in under masculinisation of a genetic male. Testosterone is converted to dihydrotestosterone (DHT) by 5α-reductase encoded by the SRD5A2 gene. DHT signals through the androgen receptor present in the developing external genitalia to bring about the development of the phallus and scrotum which is completed by about 8 weeks of gestation. Further development of the penis in males is stimulated by gonadotrophin secreted from the foetal pituitary from mid-gestation onwards. The transabdominal phase of descent of the testes is controlled by the enlargement of the caudal genitoinguinal ligament and the gubernaculum mediated by the hormone insulin-like 3 produced by the Leydig cells. The inguinoscrotal phase of descent of the testes is controlled by the neurotransmitter calcitonin gene-related peptide produced under the control of androgens.

In the absence of SRY, the Wolffian ducts regress and the Müllerian ductal system develops into the uterus, fallopian tubes and part of the vagina. Although ovarian and female genital development has been regarded as a default pathway, recent evidence suggests that there are genes important in female sexual development.

A recent suggested classification of disorders of sexual development (DSD) is shown in Table 17.2.

A newborn with DSD should be referred for assessment and management by a multidisciplinary team of surgeon, paediatric endocrinologist, geneticist, neonatologist, psychologist and nurse specialist in a tertiary centre. Although not easy, an attempt should be made to decide whether the newborn infant is a virilised female or an under-masculinised male. The degree of masculinisation can be assessed according to the Prader staging. Whenever a gonad is palpable, then the newborn is a genetic male. The nature of the opening below the clitorophallus, position of the anus should be noted, and the urethral and vaginal opening identified if possible. Increased skin pigmentation in a virilised female newborn is suggestive of 21-OHD, and the circulatory and hydration status should be assessed. Any dysmorphic feature should be noted.

TABLE 17.2	Classification of disorders of sex development.
Sex chromosome DSD	Turner syndrome 45,X and variants Klinefelter syndrome 47,XXY; 45,X/46,XY mixed gonadal dysgenesis 46,XX/46,XY ovotesticular DSD
46,XY DSD	Disorders of gonadal development— Complete gonadal dysgenesis Partial gonadal dysgenesis Ovotesticular DSD Disorder of androgen synthesis or action— Defect in androgen action Androgen biosynthetic defects Luteinising hormone receptor gene mutations Mutations of AMH or its receptor gene
46,XX DSD	Disorder of gonadal development Ovotesticular DSD Testicular DSD (SRY+, SOX9 mutation) Gonadal dysgenesis Androgen excess, e.g. 21-OHD

(*Source:* Adapted from Lee PA, Houk CP, Ahmed SF, et al. Consensus statement on management of intersex disorders. International Consensus Conference on Intersex. Pediatrics. 2006;118:e488)
Abbreviations: DSD, disorder of sex development; AMH, anti-müllerian hormone

Diagnosis

Most of the virilised female infants will have 21-OHD, while a definitive molecular diagnosis can only be reached in less than half of the children with 46, XY DSD. Initial investigations should include karyotyping with X and Y specific probe detection, and measurement of plasma 17α-OHP, androstenedione, dehydroepiandrosterone sulphate (DHEAS), testosterone, DHT, gonadotrophins, AMH, ACTH, cortisol and serum electrolytes concentrations. An ultrasound examination of the pelvis should be performed to assess the presence or absence of female internal genital organs. Further assessments of urinary steroid profile or androgen levels after hCG stimulation may be required beyond the first 3 months of life.

DIABETES MELLITUS

Diabetes mellitus is a common chronic childhood disorder in the Western World but is less common among Asians. As of 2009, there are 479,600 children with

BOX 17.14 Classification of diabetes mellitus.

Type 1 diabetes mellitus (absolute insulin deficiency)—
- Autoimmune
- Idiopathic

Type 2 diabetes mellitus (insulin resistance with relative insulin deficiency)

Other specific types—
- Genetic defects of β-cell function
- Genetic defects of insulin action
- Diseases of the endocrine pancreas endocrinopathies
- Drug- or chemical-induced infections
- Uncommon immune-mediated
- Diabetes
- Genetic syndromes associated with diabetes

Gestational diabetes

BOX 17.15 Diagnosis of diabetes mellitus.

Classical symptoms of polyuria, polydipsia and presence of glycosuria and ketonuria, a random sugar greater than 11 mmol/L

In cases of asymptomatic glycosuria
- Fasting blood sugar greater than 7 mmol/L
- Two-hour blood sugar after oral glucose load (1.75 g/kg) greater than 11 mmol/L

Prediabetes
- Impaired fasting glycaemia (IFG) if fasting blood sugar between 5.6 and 6.9 mmol/L
- Impaired glucose tolerance (IGT) if blood sugar 2 hours after oral glucose load of 7.8–11 mmol/L

type 1 diabetes mellitus (T1DM) in the world, of which 23% comes from Southeast Asia and 6.3% comes from the Western Pacific region. The annual increase in incidence is 3% per year worldwide. A classification of DM is shown in Box 17.14 and DM can develop as a result of several pathogenic processes. The diagnostic criteria for DM are shown in Box 17.15.

Type 1 Diabetes Mellitus

The aetiology of T1DM has remained elusive, but genetic and environmental influences are thought to be important. In Caucasians, there is an association between T1DM and the HLA histocompatibility complex on chromosome 6 and the insulin gene variable number of tandem repeats polymorphism on chromosome 11. These associations are less strong in Asian diabetic patients. It is likely that T1DM is a polygenic disorder. Recently, many genome wide association studies of T1DM have identified at least 24 genes and chromosomal loci each conveying a small increase in risk of developing T1DM. Ethnic groups with low incidence of disease take on a higher incidence when they migrate to another country where the incidence of diabetes is higher. This suggests that environmental factors are important. Enterovirus RNA is detected in the blood of 34% of patients with newly diagnosed T1DM. Early exposure and high dietary intake of cow's milk protein past infancy increase the risk of T1DM. Prolonged breastfeeding and vitamin D supplement decrease the risk of T1DM. Consumption of food high in preservatives and nitrosamines is associated with increased risk of T1DM. The 'hygiene hypothesis' suggests that good hygiene, vaccination and decreased childhood infections in early life lead to modulation of the immune system favouring an increased risk of development of autoimmune diseases like T1DM. There is a wide geographic difference in the incidence of childhood and adolescent DM. The lowest incidence is found in Asia (0.23–2.4 per 100,000 children in China) and highest in Sardinia and Finland (over 40 per 100,000 children). A significant increase in the incidence in recent years has been documented in 65% of the populations worldwide and the relative increase is more evident in populations with a low incidence of T1DM.

Clinical Features

Diabetes mellitus is potentially a much more acute disease in the child than in the adult. The onset is marked by polyuria, excessive thirst and rapid loss of weight over a period of 2–6 weeks. Other patients may present with secondary nocturnal enuresis, vomiting, abdominal pain and abdominal distension, which can mimic an acute abdomen. In females, pruritis vulvae may be a presenting complaint, and recurrent skin infections can occur. Frequently children are reported to be irritable and there is deterioration in school work. The presentation of DM can be preceded by an intercurrent infection.

In the untreated state, a child can present with diabetic ketoacidosis (DKA) and be admitted in a state of profound dehydration with sunken eyes, dry tongue and scaphoid abdomen. The child can lapse into a coma. Respiration is rapid, sighing and pauseless (Kussmaul breathing). Nausea, vomiting, abdominal pain and distension may mimic an acute abdomen. The biochemical criteria for the diagnosis of DKA include hyperglycaemia (blood sugar >11 mmol/L), metabolic acidosis (pH <7.3 and bicarbonate <15 mmol/L) and ketonaemia and ketonuria. DKA is the result of absolute insulin deficiency and an excess of circulating counter-regulatory hormones such as glucagon, cortisol, catecholamines and GH. The incidence of DKA at presentation inversely correlates with the incidence of T1DM in that population and ranges from 15 to 70%. DKA at diagnosis is more common in children under 5 years of age. The risk of DKA in established T1DM varies between 1 and 10% per patient per year and at-risk patients include poorly controlled diabetics, adolescents, patients with eating disorder, young children and those who inappropriately manage insulin pump failure. DKA carries a mortality rate of 0.15–0.3% with cerebral oedema accounting for 60–90% of the deaths. Other causes of morbidity and mortality include pulmonary oedema, aspiration pneumonia, venous thrombosis, rhabdomyolysis and acute pancreatitis. Cerebral oedema usually occurs within 4–12 hours after starting treatment but can be present at presentation before treatment. Warning signs are headache, vomiting, slowing of heart rate, rise in blood pressure and change in the sensorium and development of neurological signs (cranial nerve palsy, incontinence). Epidemiological studies have identified factors associated with increased risk of cerebral oedema in patients with DKA and understanding these risk factors can guide our treatment of DKA:

- Young age of new-onset diabetes with long duration of symptoms
- Severe metabolic acidosis and hypocapnoea
- An attenuated rise in serum sodium level during treatment
- Elevated serum urea
- Greater volume of fluid given in the first 4 hours
- Administration of insulin in the first hour of fluid replacement
- Treatment of acidosis with bicarbonate.

Diagnosis

In the presence of classical symptoms of polyuria, polydipsia and the documentation of glycosuria and ketonuria, a random blood sugar more than 11 mmol/L is diagnostic of T1DM. A glucose tolerance test is not usually necessary for diagnosis. DKA is present if the blood pH is less than 7.3, bicarbonate is less than 15 mmol/L in the presence of hyperglycaemia (blood sugar >11 mmol/L), and heavy glycosuria and ketonuria. At diagnosis, the serum electrolytes, acid-base status, haemoglobin A1C, glutamic acid decarboxylase (GAD), anti-islet cell antibody and anti-insulin antibody should be measured. These antibodies are present in 85–90% of newly diagnosed Caucasian diabetic children and adolescents, but the autoimmune form of diabetes is less common in Asians. Tests for thyroid function, thyroid antibodies and anti-gliadin, anti-endomysial and tissue transglutaminase antibodies for coeliac disease should also be performed. Children may have evidence of infection at presentation and appropriate investigations should also be undertaken. AFBC will reveal leucocytosis with left shift and fever is present if there is intercurrent infection. There may be nonspecific elevation of amylase. The serum sodium and phosphate potassium levels may be low.

Type 2 Diabetes Mellitus

Type 2 diabetes mellitus is usually regarded as a disease of people older than 40 years of age. However, with the increase in prevalence of obesity in childhood and adolescence, type 2 diabetes is increasingly reported in adolescents especially of ethnic minority or Polynesian origins. In countries where there is annual screening for type 2 diabetes in childhood and adolescence like Japan and Taiwan, the incidence of type 2 diabetes has surpassed that of type 1 diabetes. It has been recommended that obese children and adolescents with a family history of type 2 diabetes and presence of acanthosis nigricans or other cardiovascular risk factors be screened for type 2 diabetes in every 1–2 years. The percentage of T2DM among newly diagnosed diabetic children has been reported to be increasing worldwide and T2DM seems to be less prevalent in Europe as compared to Asian and North American countries. The rising trend of obesity worldwide is an important risk factor for the development of T2DM. A recent meta-analysis reaffirmed the U-shaped association between birth weight and T2DM risk, and the high prevalence of low birth weight births in Asia puts Asian populations at risk. Asians have more visceral fat and less muscle mass than Caucasians with the same body mass index. Asian diets also have a high glycaemic index and glycaemic load, and in South Asian, consumption of n-6 polyunsaturated fatty acid correlated with fasting hyperinsulinaemia. Southeast Asians and South Indians have higher postprandial blood sugar and lower insulin sensitivity as compared to Caucasians.

Recent genome wide association studies have revealed more than 22 genes and chromosome loci that are associated with T2DM, but all these T2DM risk variants explain at most 5–10% of the genetic basis of T2DM.

Clinical Features

Although most of the children and adolescents with T2DM do not have any symptoms, 5–25% can present with ketoacidosis. Up to 85% of the patients have first- or second-degree relatives with type 2 diabetes. Acanthosis nigricans, polycystic ovary syndrome, hypertension and dyslipidaemia are common associated disorders. The differentiation of T2DM from T1DM has become increasingly difficult especially in Asians. Only 60–85% of adolescent T2DM patients are obese. Approximately 15–40% of phenotypic Caucasian T2DM patients have islet cell and insulin antibodies, GAD and tyrosine phosphatase antibodies. Antibody-positive T2DM patients are reported to have insulin deficiency while antibody negative T2DM patients are more insulin resistant. Only 40–60% of Asian children with T1DM are antibody positive and a slowly progressing form of autoimmune T1DM reported in Japan further complicates this issue. The rarer form of maturity onset diabetes of youth (MODY) is characterised by onset of noninsulin dependent diabetes before 25 years of age with autosomal dominant mode of inheritance involving a minimum of two but preferably three consecutive generations affected by type 2 diabetes in the family. The majority of the individuals with insulin resistance who can compensate by an adequate insulin secretion do not develop T2DM but they are still prone to the complications associated with type 2 diabetes.

HYPOGLYCAEMIA

Blood glucose is the main metabolic fuel of the brain and it is maintained in a relatively narrow normal range of 4.4–6.7 mmol/L by a number of hormones including insulin, glucagon, cortisol, GH and catecholamines. Hypoglycaemia in neonates is defined as a blood sugar below 2.6 mmol/L and would require further investigation, but autonomic and neuroglycopenic symptoms will appear when the blood sugar falls below 3.5 mmol/L in older children. The common causes of hypoglycaemia in infants and children are shown in Box 17.16.

Clinical Features

Mild to moderate hypoglycaemia can result in autonomic nervous system activation including hunger, trembling of extremities, pallor, sweating and palpitations and manifestation of neuroglycopaenic symptoms. Neuroglycopaenia leads to confusion, irritability and abnormal behaviour, jitteriness, headaches, paraesthesia of the extremities and dizziness. Severe hypoglycaemia can result in coma and convulsion. Prolonged and severe hypoglycaemia with coma and convulsion can lead to permanent neurological sequelae.

Investigations

Although hypoglycaemia require prompt treatment once identified (usually by a low glucometer sugar reading at the bedside), it is important to document the true blood sugar and obtaining critical samples (blood for GH, cortisol, insulin, free fatty acids, blood ketones and b-hydroxybutyrate, lactate, ammonia and urine for ketones and toxicology). Nonketotic hypoglycaemia is due to hyperinsulinism or fatty acids oxidation defects. Hyperinsulinaemic hypoglycaemia is diagnosed when in the presence hypoglycaemia, insulin level is inappropriately elevated (>3mU/mL), plasma free fatty acids (<1.5 mmol/L) and β-hydroxybutyrate (<2.0 mmol/L) are low, a high glucose infusion rate is required to maintain euglycaemia (>10–12 mg/kg per min) and the presence of an exaggerated glucose response to glucagon. Hyperinsulinaemic hypoglycaemia with hyperammonaemia is suggestive of a gain of function mutation of the glutamate dehydrogenase gene. Perinatal stress hyperinsulinism is reported in 10% of small for gestational age neonates. Fatty acid oxidation defect can be diagnosed by measurement of plasma acylcarnitine profile and urine organic acids. Ketotic hypoglycaemia commonly occurs in young children following prolonged fasting, decreased intake or repeated vomiting. It is always important to look for sepsis (especially with gram-negative organisms) as a treatable cause of hypoglycaemia. Further assessment for hypopituitarism should be carried out where indicated.

BOX 17.16 Causes of hypoglycaemia in infants and children.

- Intrauterine growth retardation and prematurity
- Perinatal asphyxia
- Infant of diabetic mother
- Intrauterine infection and sepsis
- Rhesus incompatibility
- Inborn errors of metabolism
  - Amino acids and organic
  - Disorders of carbohydrate metabolism, e.g. glaucoma storage disease, fructose intolerance, lactosaemia
  - Fatty acid oxidation defects
  - Urea cycle defects
- Endocrine causes
  - Hypopituitarism
  - Growth hormone or adrenal insufficiency
  - Persistent hyperinsulinaemic hypoglycaemia of infantry
  - Beckwith–Wiedemann syndrome
  - Insulinoma
- Ketotic hypoglycaemia
- Drugs including alcohol, aspirin, β-blockers
- Sepsis especially due to gram-negative organisms

CHAPTER 18

Paediatric Orthopaedics

Benjamin Joseph

INTRODUCTION

Children may present with a variety of symptoms related to the musculoskeletal system (**Box 18.1**). It is important to be aware of symptoms that are likely to be innocuous and those that may herald serious underlying disease that requires early treatment. Several conditions need no active treatment; reassurance to allay parental anxiety is all that is required. Another group of conditions may need to be monitored as spontaneous improvement occurs with growth in most cases but in a few instances deterioration may occur, warranting some intervention. The third group of conditions always needs elective, early or urgent immediate treatment. In other words, the children may be managed in one of three ways:

1. Reassurance (no active intervention)
2. Observation (often no treatment is needed but treat later in selected situations)
3. Active intervention (elective intervention, early intervention or urgent intervention).

It is vitally important that this third group is identified and referred to the paediatric orthopaedic surgeon without any delay. In order to try to work out that in which of these groups the symptom of a particular child would fall into, there are some basic questions that need to be answered. Throughout this chapter the relevant questions to be asked regarding each symptom would be indicated and an attempt will be made to clarify which of these three approaches is appropriate for the particular condition.

DEFORMITIES

By far the most common reason for a child being referred for an orthopaedic opinion is the presence of a deformity. The questions that need to be asked regarding a child with a deformity of the upper or lower limbs are listed in **Table 18.1**.

Some of the common deformities seen in paediatric orthopaedic clinics are shown in **Table 18.2**. It is clear that a quarter of these conditions need no active treatment. However, it needs to be emphasised that these benign conditions form a much larger proportion of the cases seen in the clinic.

GAIT ABNORMALITIES

The common gait abnormalities seen in children are shown in **Box 18.2**. The questions that need to be asked while evaluating a child with a gait abnormality are listed in **Table 18.3**. With the exception of a painful limp, all other gait abnormalities do not require urgent intervention and hence can be evaluated without undue haste.

DELAYED WALKING

Delayed walking is quite alarming for parents and a thorough examination of these children is warranted to determine if there is global developmental delay. The most common cause of delayed walking that is associated with global developmental delay is cerebral palsy (CP). Some children with some forms of severe ligament laxity syndromes tend to walk late without demonstrating any other developmental delay. It had been assumed in the past that developmental dysplasia of the hip (DDH) with an established dislocation delays walking. However, there is little evidence to support this assumption.

TOE-WALKING

Children who walk on their toes again need to be evaluated carefully. Among causes for toe-walking are CP, some forms of myopathies and muscular dystrophies, and a very benign condition known as habitual toe-walking. Habitual toe-walking is a diagnosis of exclusion and it is important that the more serious causes of toe-walking are definitely excluded before this diagnosis is made. Initially, these children can bring their heels down to the ground while standing but go onto their toes when they start walking. In due course, the Achilles tendon may get

BOX 18.1 Common symptoms with which children may be brought to an orthopaedic surgeon.

Deformities

Gait abnormalities

Musculoskeletal pain

Paralysis and pseudoparalysis

Joint stiffness and limitation of movement

Other, e.g. soft tissue swelling/bony swelling/frequent fractures/limb deficiencies

BOX 18.2 Common gait abnormalities seen in children.

Delayed walking

Toe-walking

Intoeing gait

Out-toeing gait

Short-limbed gait

Waddling gait

Painful (antalgic gait)

Paralytic gait pattern—high stepping gait/hand-to-knee/crouch gait/scissor gait, etc.

TABLE 18.1 Questions to be asked regarding a limb deformity in a child.

Question	*Relevance*
Is the deformity unilateral or bilateral?	Unilateral deformity is more likely to be pathological.
Was the deformity present from birth?	Most deformities that are present from birth either resolve or remain static; only a few progress.
Is the deformity remaining static or is it resolving or progressing?	A deformity that is progressing may indicate that the growth mechanism is affected and would probably need early treatment. A deformity that is resolving just needs to be periodically observed.

TABLE 18.2 Common deformities seen in the paediatric orthopaedic clinic.

Region	*Aetiology*	*Condition*	*Management*
Foot	Congenital	Clubfoot	Treat early
		Metatarsus adductus	Observe/Treat electively
		Calcaneovalgus	Observe
		Vertical talus	Treat early
	Developmental	Mobile flatfoot	Observe
		Rigid flatfoot	Treat electively
	Paralytic	Equinus	Treat electively
		Equinovarus or equinovalgus	Treat electively
		Calcaneus or calcaneovalgus	Treat early
		Cavus	Treat electively
Leg	Congenital	Anterolateral bowing	Treat early
		Posteromedial bowing	Observe
		Internal tibial torsion	Observe
Knee	Congenital	Hyperextension	Treat early
		Flexion	Treat electively
	Developmental	Physiological genu varum or valgum	Observe
		Unilateral genu valgum or varum	Treat electively
Hip	Congenital	Acetabular dysplasia with neonatal hip instability	Treat early
		Femoral anteversion	Observe
	Developmental	Coxa vara	Treat electively
Spine	Congenital	Scoliosis	Treat electively
	Developmental	Infantile scoliosis	Observe
		Adolescent scoliosis	Treat early
	Paralytic	Scoliosis	Treat early

TABLE 18.3 Questions to be asked while evaluating a child with a gait abnormality.

Question	*Relevance*
Does the child have pain on walking?	If there is pain on walking, urgent investigations are needed to establish the definitive diagnosis as some conditions that cause a painful limp require immediate treatment.
Is the gait abnormality unilateral or bilateral?	Unilateral gait abnormality is more likely to be pathological.
Has the gait abnormality been present from when the child started to walk?	If present from when the child started to walk, it is likely to be due to a congenital abnormality.
Does the child run, play and do normal activities with peers?	If the child does play normally, it indicates that there is negligible pain and that the underlying problem is probably not serious.
Is there an improvement in the gait pattern with growth?	If the gait improves as the child grows, the underlying problem is likely to be "physiological."
Is there a deterioration of the gait pattern with growth?	If gait deteriorates as the child grows, there is some underlying pathology.

contracted and then they would also stand on tip toe. At this stage, lengthening of the Achilles tendon is indicated.

INTOEING GAIT

This is a very common complaint and parents are often very concerned about this gait abnormality. The child typically sits in the "W" position **(Fig. 18.1)** and examination of the range of passive hip motion would demonstrate excessive internal rotation of the hip with a reduction in the range of external rotation. This is characteristic of excessive femoral anteversion. The anteversion tends to reduce spontaneously as the child grows. There is no functional disability though these children tend to be a bit clumsy and some parents feel that they tend to trip more frequently. The parents need to be reassured that gradual resolution of the torsional deformity will occur. Bracing and shoe modifications that have been tried in the past have been quite clearly shown to be totally ineffective and should not be used. Surgical intervention is not justified in these children except in the very rare instance where the deformity persists till the age of 10 years and is still severe at this age.

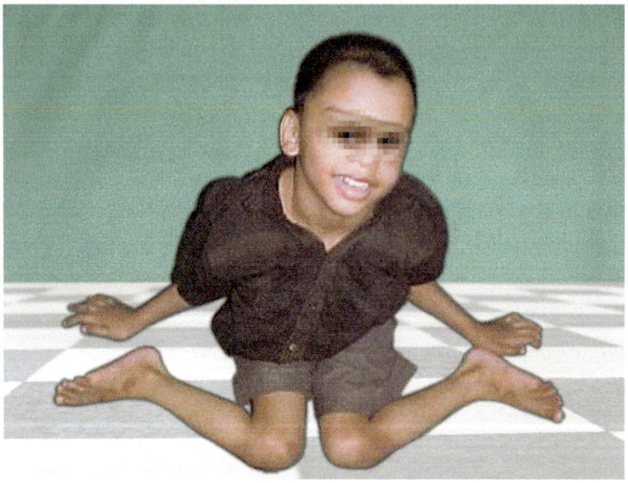

Figure 18.1 This posture while sitting is characteristically seen in children with excessive femoral anteversion. It is referred to as the "W" pattern because the legs and the thighs of both the limbs together are aligned in the form of a "W."

OUT-TOEING GAIT

This is less frequently seen and may be due to retroversion of the femur or external tibial torsion. Again, there is no functional disability in these children and no active treatment is required.

SHORT-LIMBED GAIT

A short-limbed gait indicates that there is a structural abnormality of one limb. While more commonly the shorter limb is at fault due to reduced growth, occasionally the longer limb may be abnormal. Lengthening of one limb is often seen in association with vascular malformations such as haemangioma, lymphangioma and arteriovenous fistula. The decision to correct the limb-length inequality is governed by the magnitude of the discrepancy that is likely to be present at skeletal maturity. If the difference at skeletal maturity is likely to exceed 2–3 cm, intervention may be considered.

WADDLING GAIT

A waddling gait or a Trendelenburg gait is characteristically seen when the hip abductor power is weak. This may be seen in the relatively uncommon situation where there is actual paralysis of the hip abductors. Far more commonly, this gait pattern is seen when the hip abductor mechanism is rendered ineffective either due to dislocation of the hip or due to a reduction of the angle between the neck and shaft of the femur as in coxa vara deformity. This gait pattern signals serious hip pathology and so children with a waddling gait must be evaluated carefully and must have radiographs of the pelvis to exclude these conditions that require surgical intervention.

ANTALGIC GAIT

An antalgic gait or painful gait signifies that bearing weight on the affected limb causes pain. Children who demonstrate this abnormality of gait should undergo a meticulous examination to identify the source of pain and in the vast majority of instances the site of pain can be located by clinical examination alone. Appropriate imaging may then be done to confirm the nature of underlying pathology. Treatment would depend on the nature of the pathological process that is producing pain. Of all conditions that can manifest with a painful limp the one that requires immediate surgical invention is osteoarticular infection. The urgency for establishing a diagnosis and the need for immediate intervention cannot be overemphasised.

PARALYTIC GAIT PATTERNS

Depending on the pattern of paralysis, typical gait aberrations may occur. Paralysis of the ankle dorsiflexors will produce a high-stepping gait. A hand-on-thigh gait is seen when there is paralysis of the quadriceps muscle. Characteristic abnormal gait patterns such as scissor gait, crouch gait, stiff-knee gait and toe-toe gait are seen in CP depending on which muscles are most spastic.

MUSCULOSKELETAL PAIN

When a child complains of pain in the limbs or back, it is imperative that a careful examination is performed and this should be followed by appropriate imaging. It will become clear from the list of painful conditions seen in children (Table 18.4) that most of these conditions can be confirmed by a combination of clinical examination and imaging (Table 18.5).

It will also be evident that several of the conditions listed in Table 18.4 require urgent or early treatment. This is distinctly different from that seen in the conditions listed in Table 18.2.

PARALYSIS AND PSEUDOPARALYSIS

When an infant stops moving a limb, a distinction needs to be made between true paralysis and pseudoparalysis.

TABLE 18.4 Causes of musculoskeletal pain in children.

Region	*Condition*	*Imaging modality to supplement clinical examination*	*Management approach*
Foot	Sever disease	X-ray	Observe
	Kohler disease	X-ray	Observe
	Tarsal coalition	X-ray/CT scan	Treat electively
Calf	Growing pains	No imaging	Reassure
Tibia	Osteoid osteoma	X-ray/CT scan	Treat electively
	Acute osteomyelitis	No imaging/ultrasound scan	Treat urgently
	Osteosarcoma	X-ray/CT/MRI	Treat urgently
	Ewing tumour	X-ray/CT/MRI	Treat urgently
Knee	Osgood-Schlatter	X-ray	Observe
	Septic arthritis	No imaging	Treat urgently
	Tubercular arthritis	X-ray	Treat early
	Referred pain from the hip		
Hip	Transient synovitis	Ultrasound scan	Treat early
	Perthes disease	X-ray	Treat early
	Slipped capital femoral epiphysis	X-ray	Treat urgently
	Septic arthritis	No imaging	Treat urgently
	Tubercular arthritis	X-ray	Treat early
Back	Disc prolapse	MRI	Treat early
	Pyogenic discitis	X-ray/CT/MRI	Treat early
Generalised bone pain	Osteogenesis imperfecta	X-ray	Treat early
	Adolescent osteoporosis	X-ray/CT/Dexa scans	Treat early

Abbreviations: CT, computed tomography; MRI, magnetic resonance imaging.

TABLE 18.5 Questions to be asked while evaluating a child with musculoskeletal pain.

Question	*Relevance*
Can the pain be localised consistently?	Likely to be caused by localised pathology.
Is the pain brought on by movement of a joint?	Likely to be due to pathology in the joint.
Is the pain present at rest and on bearing weight on the limb?	Likely to be due to disease of bone.
Is the child able to run and play normally but has pain at rest after physical activity?	The cause is likely to be innocuous.
Is the child unable to bear weight on the limb?	If the child cannot bear any weight on the limb, it is likely that there is serious underlying pathology.

The later phenomenon is on account of pain and this is typically seen when there is osteoarticular infection. Since the infant cannot indicate the site of pain it is important to do a meticulous examination to try to ascertain the site of pain. In the older child with true paralysis, it is necessary to differentiate between flaccid, lower motor-neuron paralysis and spastic, upper motor-neuron paralysis.

JOINT STIFFNESS

Stiffness of a joint or limitation of joint movement can occur on account of abnormalities within the joint itself (intra-articular pathology) or due to contracture or shortening of soft tissue structures outside the joint (extra-articular). Intra-articular stiffness can be caused by adhesions between the articular surfaces or due to actual bony continuity between the bones that form the joint. Bony continuity can be of congenital origin due to failure of segmentation and formation of a joint space resulting in a synostosis. The common sites of synostosis include the proximal radioulnar joint, the carpus and the tarsus (Fig. 18.2). If the articular cartilage is dissolved in septic arthritis, the raw bony surfaces may fuse together. This is referred to as bony ankylosis. When either a congenital synostosis or an acquired bony ankylosis is present no movement will be present at all in the affected joint.

CONGENITAL ANOMALIES

Congenital Clubfoot

Treatment Approach: Treat Early: Congenital clubfoot (congenital talipes equinovarus) is probably the most common congenital anomaly of the musculoskeletal system that requires treatment (Fig. 18.3). Clubfoot may occur as an isolated anomaly (idiopathic clubfoot) or may occur in association with spina bifida or with multiple congenital contractures (MCC—formerly called arthrogryposis multiplex congenita). Idiopathic clubfoot is far more common than the neurogenic form that occurs with spina bifida or MCC. Idiopathic clubfoot may either be postural or rigid. The postural variety is due to intrauterine moulding; the foot is structurally normal and responds well to nonoperative management. On the other hand, the rigid variety is characterised by contractures of muscles and joint capsules and the bones of the foot are structurally abnormal. Despite this, a proportion of these rigid feet do respond to nonoperative treatment.

The deformity is a complex one with individual deformities at the ankle, subtalar and the midtarsal joints (the calcaneocuboid joint and the talonavicular joints function together in unison and are referred to as the midtarsal joint). These individual deformities are caused

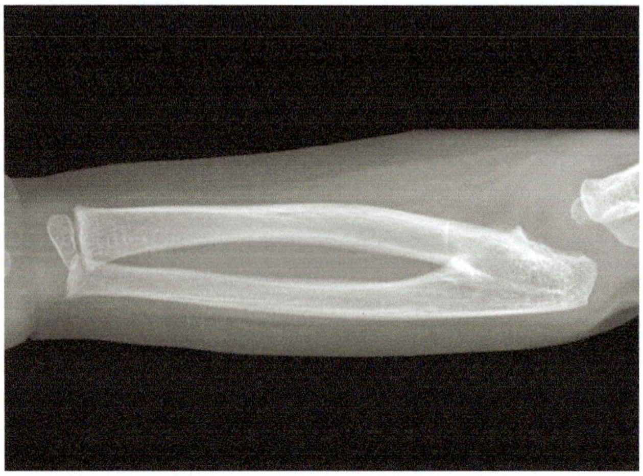

Figure 18.2 Radiograph of a child's elbow showing congenital synostosis of the radius and ulna.

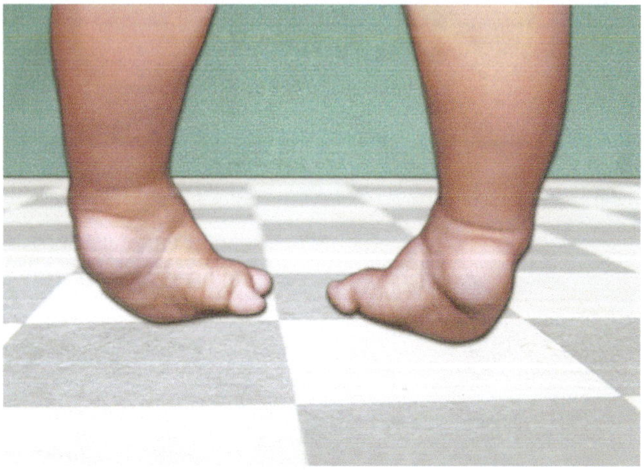

Figure 18.3 Appearance of congenital clubfoot—equinus and varus deformities of the hindfoot and forefoot adduction are clearly seen.

TABLE 18.6	Deformities of clubfoot and the underlying contractures that contribute to these deformities.			
Region of the foot	***Joint***	***Deformity***	***Primary muscle contracture***	***Secondary contracture***
Hindfoot	Ankle subtalar joint	Hindfoot equinus Hindfoot varus (a combination of adduction and inversion)	Gastrocsoleus Tibialis posterior	Posterior capsule of ankle joint Medial capsule of the subtalar joint
Midfoot	Midtarsal joint	Forefoot adduction	Abductor hallucis	Medial capsule of the talonavicular and calcaneocuboid joints
		Forefoot inversion Forefoot equinus	Tibialis posterior Short plantar muscles	Plantar aponeurosis

primarily by contractures of muscles that act on these joints, and secondary contractures of the joint capsules make the deformities more rigid **(Table 18.6)**.

Management of clubfoot should first begin with a careful examination to determine whether the deformity is associated with a swelling in the lumbosacral region (spina bifida) or with symmetrical deformities of the knees, elbows and wrists (MCC). Once these conditions have been excluded, an attempt is made to gently correct the deformity **(Fig. 18.4)**. If the deformities can be completely corrected by passive stretching, the clubfoot is likely to be a postural clubfoot.

SERIAL MANIPULATION

To begin with, all idiopathic clubfeet should be given a trial of serial manipulation. Treatment should be started as soon as possible after birth. The feet are manipulated without sedation or anaesthesia to ensure that excessive force is not used. At the first sitting, partial correction of the deformity is achieved and with each subsequent sitting more and more correction is achieved. After each manipulation a plaster of Paris cast that extends from the tips of the toes to the groin is applied with the foot in the position of correction that has been achieved. The forefoot deformities and the hindfoot varus are corrected first. Only after these deformities are well corrected should any attempt be made to correct the hindfoot equinus. Full correction of the deformity may be achieved after four or five manipulations. If the hindfoot equinus cannot be corrected by manipulation, percutaneous tenotomy of the Achilles tendon would be needed. A small proportion of feet will not respond to this treatment and these feet would need surgical correction. The success with this method of manipulative correction steadily decreases with increasing age and often this method will not be effective in infants over 6–9 months of age.

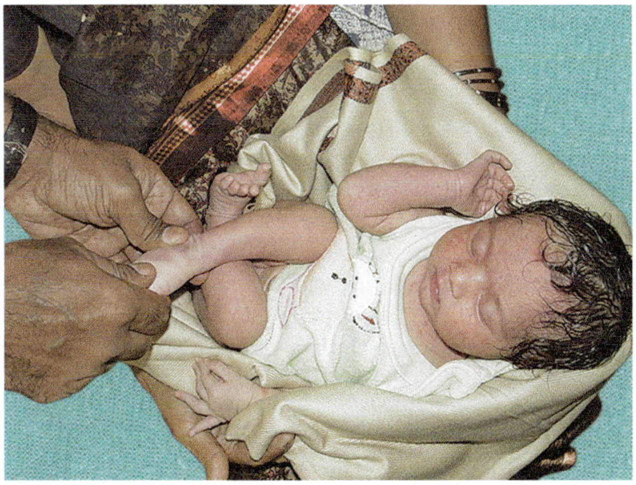

Figure 18.4 Gentle passive correction of clubfoot in a neonate should be done without causing any pain.

SOFT TISSUE RELEASE

Soft tissue release is indicated in children who have not responded well to serial manipulation and in children who are too old for serial manipulation. Soft tissue surgery entails lengthening of the tendons of the contracted muscles and division of the contracted capsules. Since structures on the back and medial aspect of the foot need to be released, the operation is referred to as a posteromedial soft tissue release.

Ideally, soft tissue release should be performed by 9 months of age so that by the time the postoperative plaster immobilisation for 3 months is over the child will be able to start walking.

Satisfactory correction of the deformity should result in a supple, normal looking foot that functions well throughout life.

BONY SURGERY

Children with clubfoot who present after 4 or 5 years of age would need additional surgery on the bones of the foot in order to correct the deformity as the tarsal bones

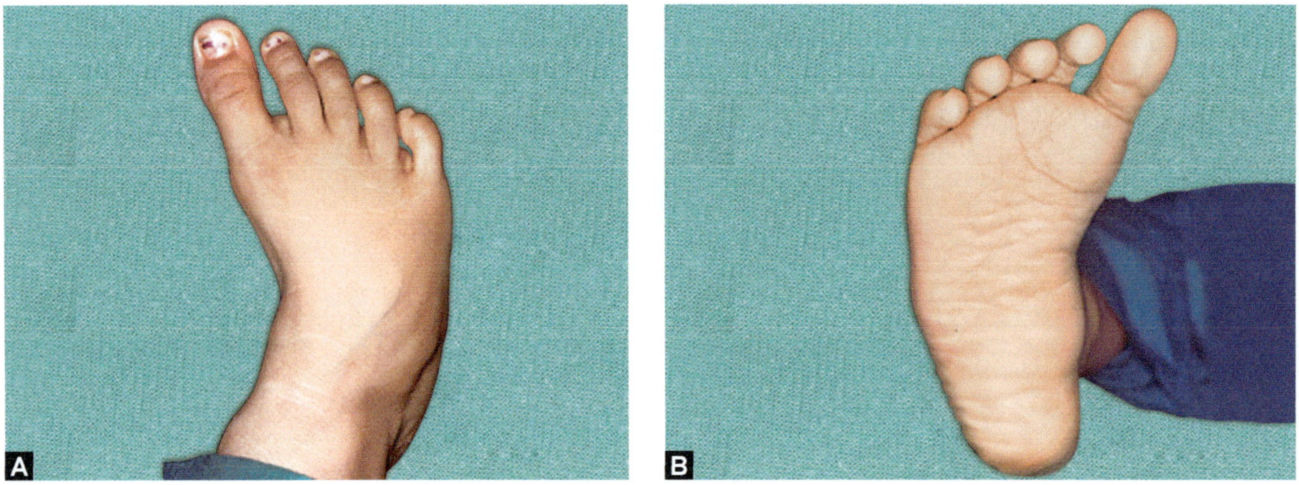

Figures 18.5A and B Clinical appearance of the foot of a child with metatarsus adductus.

would have been deformed by weight-bearing. The common operations include osteotomies of the calcaneum to correct the hindfoot varus, and osteotomies of the cuboid and cuneiform bones aimed at shortening the lateral border of the foot or lengthening the medial border of the foot.

Occasionally, one may encounter an older child or an adolescent with untreated clubfoot. It is possible to correct the deformity even at this age by either resecting wedges of bone from the dorsolateral aspect of the foot or by distracting the contracted soft tissues with the help of an external fixator mounted on the limb through wires that pass through the leg and foot. It needs to be emphasised that any form of surgery to correct clubfoot in the older child will result in a stiff foot even if the deformity can be completely corrected.

CLUBFOOT IN SPINA BIFIDA

Clubfoot in spina bifida is more difficult to treat. Manipulation and plaster casts are better avoided on account of the risk of producing pressure sores on the anaesthetic feet. There may also be muscle imbalance due to paralysis of some muscles acting on the foot and ankle, and this must be addressed or else the deformity will recur.

CLUBFOOT IN MULTIPLE CONGENITAL CONTRACTURES

Clubfoot in MCC is far more rigid than idiopathic clubfoot, and hence nonoperative methods are not likely to succeed. There is also a very high chance of relapse of the deformity following surgical correction. In view of this, surgery should be more radical with excision of segments of the contracted tendons rather than mere lengthening as done in idiopathic clubfoot.

METATARSUS ADDUCTUS

Treatment Approach: Observe/Treat Electively

Metatarsus adductus is a congenital anomaly where the forefoot is adducted. It resembles the forefoot adduction component of clubfoot, but the deformity is at the tarsometatarsal joints rather than at the midtarsal joint as in clubfoot (Figs. 18.5A and B). Metatarsus adductus may be associated with other deformities such as infantile scoliosis, torticollis and plagiocephaly all of which may be part of the moulded baby syndrome.

Milder degrees of metatarsus adductus tend to resolve and hence one can wait for a few years to see if resolution of the deformity occurs. The more severe deformity may need release of the abductor hallucis muscle or osteotomies of the bases of the metatarsal bones.

CALCANEOVALGUS

Treatment Approach: Observe

Congenital calcaneovalgus deformity may occur in isolation or with congenital posteromedial bowing of the tibia. Calcaneovalgus deformity is a postural deformity that develops on account of intrauterine moulding. At birth, the foot is dorsiflexed and everted; the dorsum of the foot may be in contact with the shin (Fig. 18.6). Despite this apparently severe deformity, rapid spontaneous resolution occurs. Spontaneous resolution can be facilitated by gentle stretching of the foot into plantar flexion and eversion by the mother several times a day. Very occasionally, a few casts holding the foot in plantar flexion and inversion may be needed.

If there is an associated posteromedial bowing of the tibia, the parents need to be reassured that the tibial deformity again is likely to resolve spontaneously. However, these children do need to be followed-up as residual

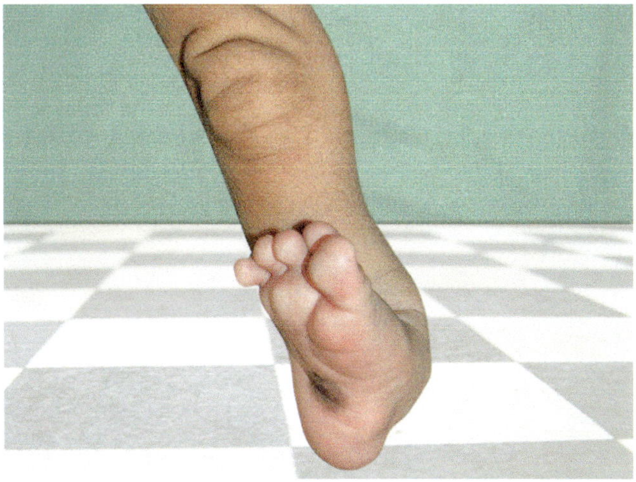

Figure 18.6 Calcaneovalgus deformity of the foot in a newborn infant.

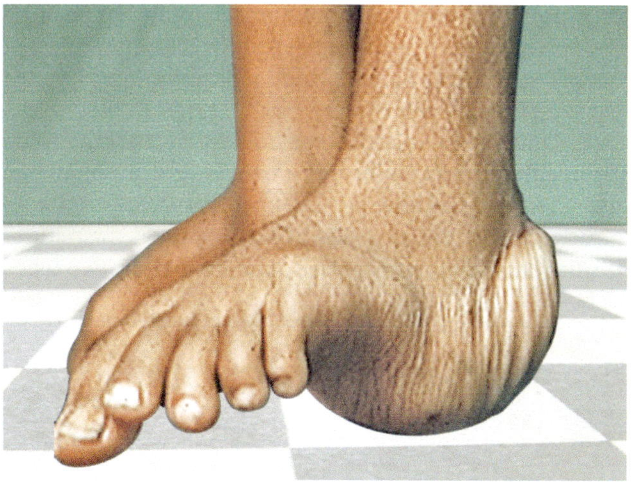

Figure 18.7 In congenital vertical talus, the medial longitudinal arch of the foot is reversed and this is described as a rocker-bottom deformity.

tibial deformity and shortening of the limb that may occur in some children may need to be addressed later in childhood.

CONGENITAL VERTICAL TALUS

Treatment Approach: Treat Early

Congenital vertical talus is a complex, rigid deformity of the foot that is often associated with spina bifida, chromosomal anomalies (Trisomy 13 and 18) and MCC. The ankle is plantar flexed and the forefoot is dorsiflexed; consequently there is a total reversal of the normal longitudinal arch of the foot. This is referred to as a rocker-bottom deformity **(Fig. 18.7)**. The talus is severely plantar flexed (hence the name of the condition) and the talonavicular joint is dislocated. There is also a valgus deformity of the foot **(Table 18.7)**. Nonoperative treatment in the form of serial manipulations should be started early. However, the deformities usually will not correct completely by nonoperative treatment and surgery is needed to release the contracted structures and to restore normal tarsal relationships. The extent of surgery may be minimised by serial manipulation and casting.

ANTEROLATERAL BOWING OF THE TIBIA

Treatment Approach: Treat Early

Bowing of the tibia may be present at birth. The location and the direction of the convexity of the bowing should be identified. When the child is born with anterolateral bow of the tibia, a careful examination must be made to look for pigmented spots (café-au-lait spots) on the trunk or limbs. These spots suggest that the child has neurofibromatosis. If these spots are not present on the baby, examination of the parents may show features of neurofibromatosis in either of them. The radiograph of the limb may show narrowing of the tibia at the junction of the middle- and lower-third of the leg with obliteration of the medullary cavity. If these changes are noted, the limb needs to be protected in a splint to prevent the tibia from fracturing. If the tibia does fracture, union will not occur

TABLE 18.7 Deformities of congenital vertical talus and the underlying contractures that contribute to these deformities.

Region of the foot	*Joint*	*Deformity*	*Primary muscle contracture*	*Secondary contracture*
Hindfoot	Ankle subtalar joint	Hindfoot equinus Hindfoot valgus (a combination of abduction and eversion)	Gastrocsoleus Peroneus longus and brevis	Posterior capsule of ankle joint Lateral capsule of the subtalar joint
Midfoot	Midtarsal joint	Forefoot abduction	Peroneus brevis	Lateral capsule of the calcaneocuboid joint
		Forefoot dorsiflexion	Tibialis anterior, extensor hallucis, extensor digitorum, peroneus tertius	Dorsal capsule of the talonavicular joint

by simple immobilisation (fractures in infants and young children normally heal quite quickly by immobilisation in a cast) and will go on to develop a pseudarthrosis that is exceedingly difficult to treat.

In contrast to anterolateral bowing of the tibia, posteromedial bowing is far more benign and spontaneous resolution of the bowing will occur. It is important to clearly identify the direction of the bowing as the natural history and the prognosis are so different in the two types of bowing.

DEVELOPMENTAL DYSPLASIA OF THE HIP

Treatment Approach: Treat Early

The term "developmental dysplasia of the hip" has replaced the older term "congenital dislocation of the hip" since true dislocation of the hip is not present at birth though the factors that predispose to dislocation are present at birth. DDH covers a spectrum of hip abnormality that includes neonatal hip instability, subluxation and dislocation of the hip, and acetabular dysplasia without hip instability. The cause of DDH is multifactorial and among the causes are two clearly defined heritable predisposing factors, namely, ligament laxity and acetabular dysplasia. DDH occurs six times more commonly in girls than in boys; it occurs far more frequently in breech deliveries and in those with a definite family history of DDH.

Unlike most other musculoskeletal congenital anomalies, DDH is not apparent unless one specifically examines the newborn for signs of neonatal hip instability. If the diagnosis of neonatal hip instability is not made, the hip may dislocate in early infancy and this too may remain undetected till the child begins to walk with a limp. Treatment of neonatal instability is relatively simple both for the baby and the treating surgeon, while treatment becomes increasingly difficult as the child grows older. Furthermore, the results of treatment deteriorate as the age at treatment increases; the best chance of obtaining an excellent outcome is if treatment is instituted in the neonatal period itself. Hence, it is imperative that every newborn child is screened for hip instability.

Screening for Developmental Dysplasia of the Hip

The two main methods of screening are clinical and ultrasonographic. For obvious logistic and economic reasons, it would just not be feasible to screen every newborn in a developing country by ultrasound and hence clinical screening will remain the mainstay of diagnosis of DDH for a long time to come. It is important that every clinician who attends to the newborn is adept at performing the screening tests for neonatal hip instability. This is particularly vital in situations where a paediatric orthopaedic surgeon may not be available.

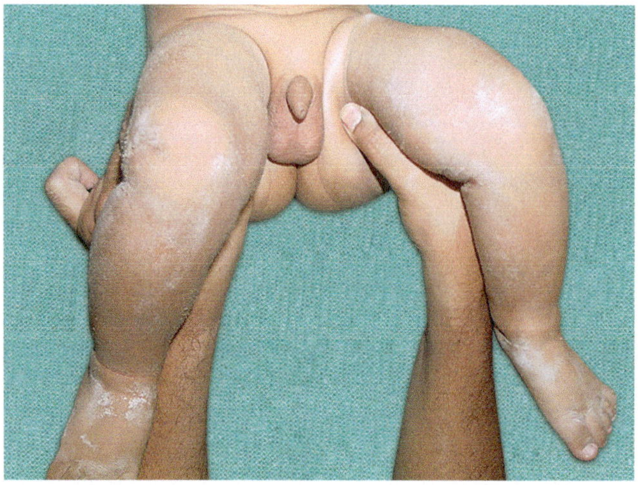

Figure 18.8 The method of holding the infant's thighs while performing the Barlow's and Ortolani's tests for detecting neonatal hip instability.

The two clinical tests for detecting hip instability in the newborn are the Barlow's test and the Ortolani's test. Both these tests should be performed with the baby lying on its back. The thigh is grasped with the thumb of the examiner on the medial side of the thigh, and the index and middle fingers over the greater trochanter **(Fig. 18.8)**. The hip is flexed to 90° and the Barlow's test is first performed.

The hip is adducted and at the same time, pressure is applied by the thumb on the medial aspect of the thigh to attempt to push the femoral head posteriorly and laterally. If the hip is unstable, the femoral head can be clearly felt moving out of the acetabulum. This provocative test, if positive, signifies that the hip is "dislocatable." Then the Ortolani's test is performed. Pressure is applied on the greater trochanter by the index and middle finger attempting to push the femoral head medially and anteriorly while the hip is abducted. The femoral head can be felt reducing into the acetabulum with palpable click. This is the Ortolani's test which when positive implies that the hip is "reducible."

Treatment of Neonatal Hip Instability

If either of these tests is positive, the hips are splinted in flexion and abduction in a Pavlik harness **(Fig. 18.9)**. The harness is maintained for 6 weeks, by which time the hip ought to have become stable. If the hip has not stabilised by this time, closed reduction must be performed under anaesthesia as outlined below. In infants over 6 months of age the Pavlik harness is not likely to be effective.

Treatment of Developmental Dysplasia of the Hip in Infants under 6 Months of Age

If the hip does not become stable in spite of splinting in a Pavlik harness, the child needs to be anaesthetised and

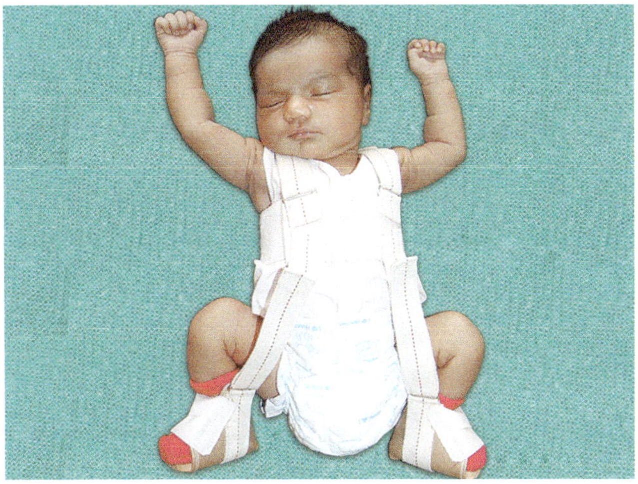

Figure 18.9 The hips of a neonate with neonatal hip instability are splinted in flexion and abduction in a Pavlik harness.

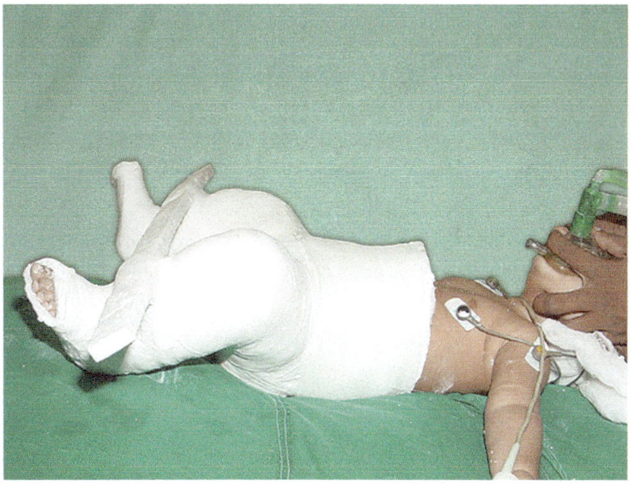

Figure 18.10 Spica cast applied after closed reduction in an infant with developmental dysplasia of the hip.

then the hip is examined, to see if it will reduce. In the vast majority of instances, the hip will reduce. Once it is noted that the hip does reduce, a careful assessment is made to determine the position in which the hip remains reduced. If the hip remains reduced in around 45° of abduction and neutral rotation of the hip, a spica cast extending from well above the costal margin to the tips of the toes is applied with the hips flexed to 90° and abducted to 45° **(Fig. 18.10)**. The spica is changed under anaesthesia at monthly intervals and at each change the stability of the reduction is assessed. Usually, the hip will become quite stable within 3–4 months, at which time the spica cast can be abandoned. If the hip has to be abducted over 60° or if the hip has to be internally rotated a great deal in order to keep the hip reduced, surgical open reduction of the hip should be undertaken as immobilisation in these positions of excessive abduction and internal rotation can jeopardise the blood supply to the femoral head. Open reduction is also indicated in children under 6 months of age if the hip cannot be reduced by closed reduction under anaesthesia.

Treatment of Developmental Dysplasia of the Hip between the Age of 6 and 18 Months

Once the hip dislocates and remains dislocated, soft tissue contractures will develop and they would prevent the hip from being reduced. This is seen in a proportion of children over 6 months of age. These children would have to undergo an open reduction of the hip. During the operation, the soft tissue impediments to reduction need to be identified and removed; these include contracture of the inferomedial capsule, iliopsoas tendon, the ligamentum teres and fibro-fatty tissue in the floor of the acetabulum. The hip is immobilised in a spica cast for 3 months following the open reduction. If on the other hand, the hip does reduce when examined under anaesthesia the treatment can be as for children under 6 months of age.

Treatment of Developmental Dysplasia of the Hip in Children between the Age of 18 Months and 3 Years

Adaptive changes will develop in the femur and the acetabulum in a child who has been walking with a dislocated hip, and these would need to be addressed in order to obtain a stable reduction. The femur may be excessively anteverted and the neck may develop some degree of valgus. The acetabulum may become even more dysplastic and sloping. In addition, the muscles that cross the hip would become excessively contracted. Consequently the femur may need to be shortened in order to reduce the hip. Varus derotation osteotomy may be needed to ensure that the femoral head is directed towards the centre of the acetabular floor. The normal slope of the acetabulum may need to be restored in order to prevent the hip from subluxating again after the reduction has been achieved **(Figs. 18.11A and B)**. All or some of these bony operations may be needed in addition to an open reduction in these older children.

It is important to follow-up all children who have been treated in early childhood for DDH till they are skeletally mature as late subluxation and acetabular dysplasia may occur in a few children. These problems can be promptly addressed if children are reviewed on a regular basis through their childhood.

CONGENITAL SCOLIOSIS

Treatment Approach: Treat Electively

Congenital scoliosis occurs on account of anomalous development of the vertebral column; this may be failure

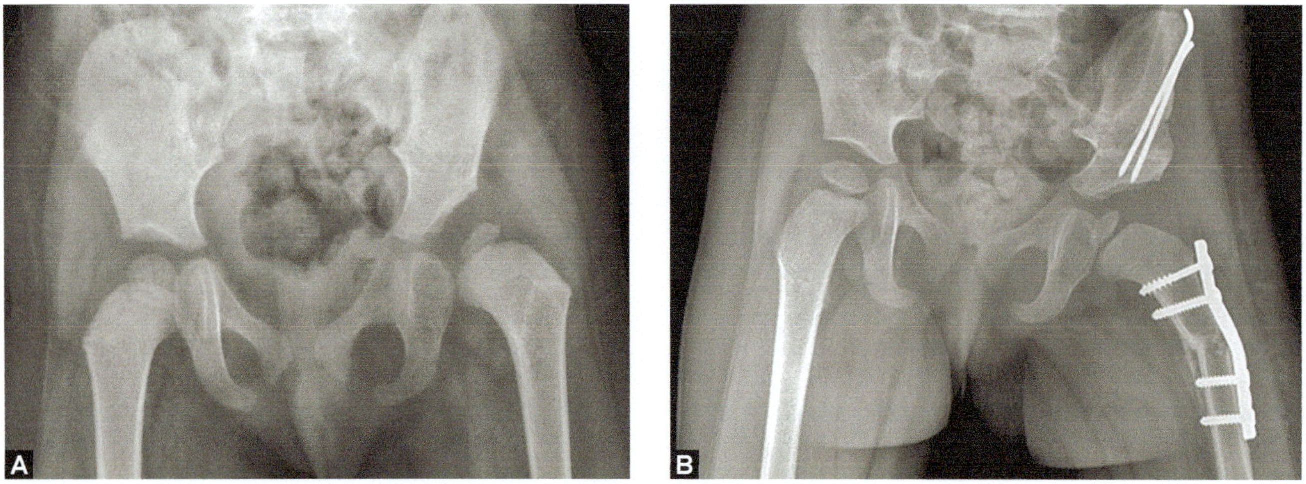

Figures 18.11A and B (A) Acetabular dysplasia in a child; (B) It has been corrected by an osteotomy of the pelvic bone.

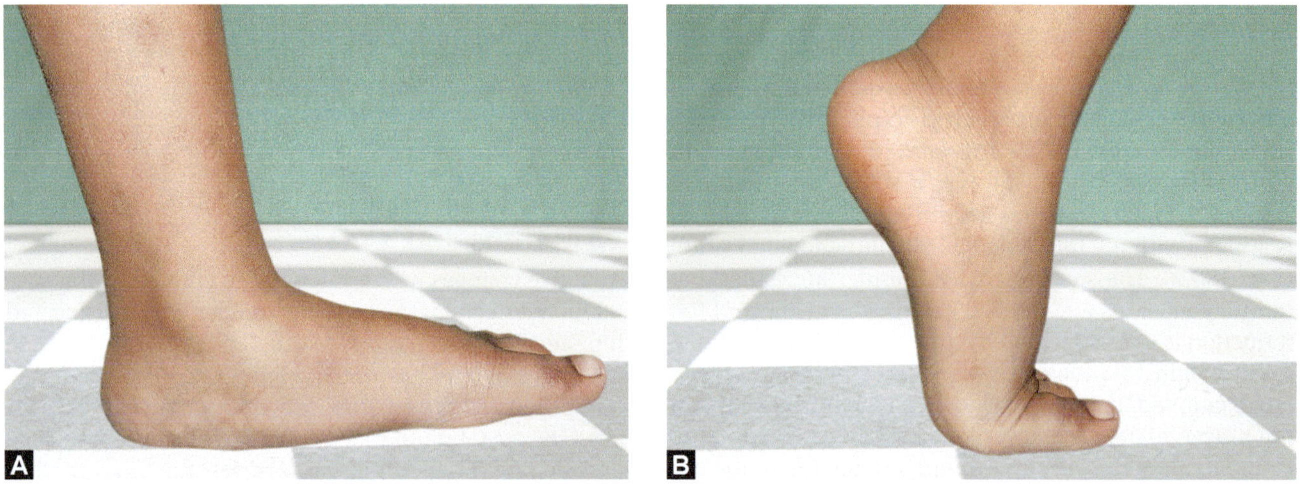

Figures 18.12A and B (A) An arch of the foot of a child with flexible flatfoot; (B) It is restored on standing on tip-toe.

of development of a part of the vertebra or failure of segmentation. Failure of formation of part of the vertebra results in a hemivertebra, while failure of segmentation can result in block vertebrae or unsegmented unilateral bars. The embryonal mesodermal tissue of the sclerotomes from which the vertebrae develop, is very close to the mesoderm that goes to form the urogenital tract. Consequently, very often, children with congenital scoliosis have associated anomalies of the renal tract. This must be borne in mind and children with congenital scoliosis should be screened for renal and other visceral anomalies.

Due to asymmetric growth of the spine, the deformity may progress relentlessly and neurological deficit may develop in the limbs on account of stretching of the spinal cord. Surgical intervention may be needed in early childhood to prevent rapid progression of the scoliosis. This may involve excision of the hemivertebrae and spinal fusion.

DEVELOPMENTAL PROBLEMS

Flatfoot

Flatfoot is a condition where the medial longitudinal arch of the foot is not well formed or has collapsed. At the outset it is imperative that a distinction is made between a mobile, flexible flatfoot and a rigid flatfoot. This distinction can be made very easily by simply asking the child to stand normally and then to stand on tip-toe. While the child is standing normally it would be seen that the medial longitudinal arch is collapsed and the instep of the foot is resting on the ground. However, as the child stands on tip-toe the arch is completely restored **(Figs. 18.12A and B)**. Such a flatfoot is a mobile or flexible flatfoot. In children with rigid flatfeet, no restoration of the arch will be noted on standing on the toes.

It is important to be aware that the foot appears flat in the vast majority of infants on account of fat in the instep region. In addition to this, the joints of young children are more lax and consequently the ligaments that support the arch are not taut and the arch flattens when the child bears weight on the foot. By around 5 or 6 years of age, the ligaments of most children tighten up and the medial longitudinal arch forms. There is evidence to suggest that the arch develops better in children who do not wear footwear. Among children who use footwear from early childhood, those that wear closed-toe shoes appear to have poorer development of the arch than children who wear sandals or slippers.

Flexible Flatfoot

Treatment approach—reassurance: Flexible flatfoot is far more common in children who have hypermobile joints and in children who are obese. Less than 1% of children with flexible flatfeet have any symptoms related to the foot. Yet parents are often very concerned about flatfeet in their children. There is also an unsubstantiated notion that flatfeet function badly and limit the activity of the child. It is important that parents are counselled and informed that there is no need to treat asymptomatic flatfeet. The tendency to prescribe shoe modifications for young children with asymptomatic flexible flatfoot should be strongly discouraged for two very compelling reasons. First, there is no evidence at all to show that the use of any form of shoe inserts or shoe modification corrects flatfoot. Second, in the light of evidence that shoe-wearing may actually be detrimental to development of the arch the wisdom of prescribing a modified shoe would be questionable. In the very rare situation where there is pain in the foot on standing or walking, an arch support may be worn.

Rigid Flatfoot

Treatment approach—treat electively: The common cause for rigid flatfoot is tarsal coalition or an abnormal bony bar between two tarsal bones. The two most common coalitions are talocalcaneal coalition and calcaneonavicular coalition. The coalition may be cartilaginous to begin with and then may ossify. Pain often appears when the child reaches 10–12 years of age. Examination will reveal that the arch cannot be restored by standing on tip-toe and that there is limitation of movement of the subtalar or midtarsal joints. Calcaneonavicular coalitions can be demonstrated clearly on an oblique-view radiograph of the foot **(Fig. 18.13A)**. Computed tomography (CT) scans may be needed to clearly demonstrate a talocalcaneal coalition. If pain has developed, the coalition can be excised and fat or muscle tissue needs to be interposed into the gap to prevent the coalition from reforming **(Fig. 18.13B)**. This form of surgery usually relieves pain but the movements of the subtalar and midtarsal joints are seldom restored to normal. Occasionally, painful arthritis may develop in the adjacent joints; excision of the coalition will be ineffective at this stage and the arthritic joint would need to be arthrodesed.

PHYSIOLOGICAL GENU VARUM AND GENU VALGUM

Treatment Approach: Reassurance

Several children between the ages of 1 and 3 years have genu varum (bow-legs) and children between 3 and 7 years of age often have genu valgum (knock-knees). These deformities spontaneously resolve completely in the vast majority of instances and hence are referred to as physiological genu varum and valgum **(Figs. 18.14A and B)**. However, one needs to be certain that the deformities are not due to any underlying pathology. Among the various causes of genu varum and valgum, rickets is a common cause in developing countries and must be excluded before assuming that one is dealing with physiological

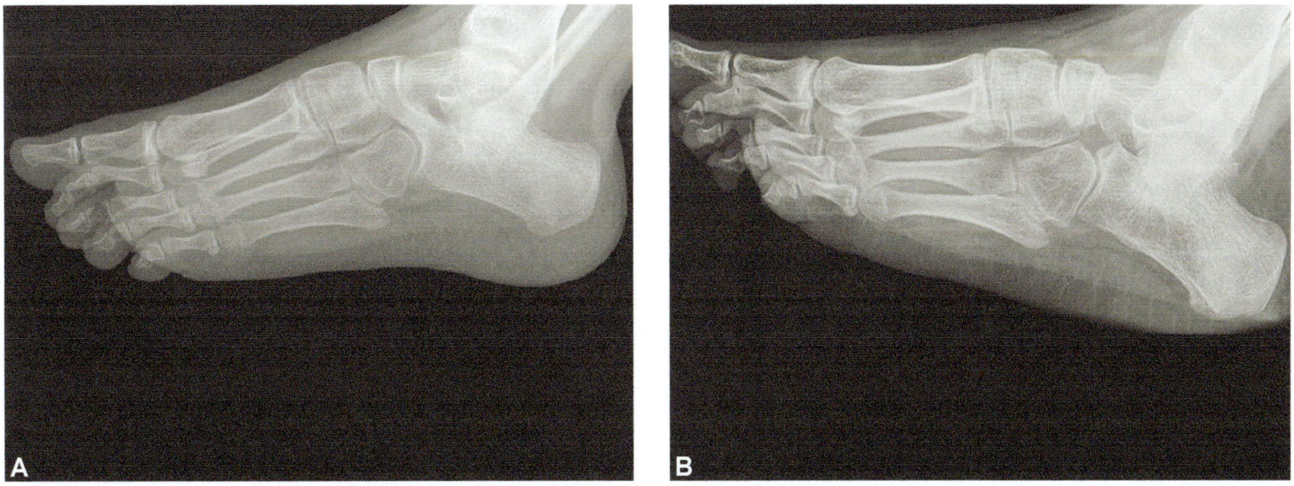

Figures 18.13A and B (A) Oblique radiograph of the foot of a child with calcaneonavicular coalition; (B) The radiographic appearance of the same foot after excision of the coalition was performed.

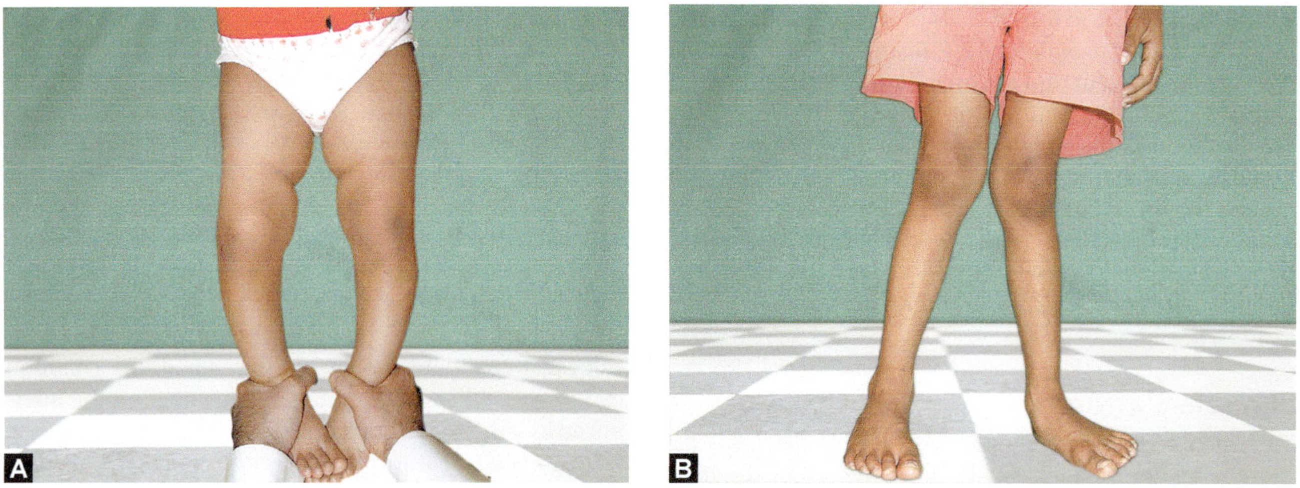

Figures 18.14A and B (A) Physiological genu varum; (B) Physiological genu valgum.

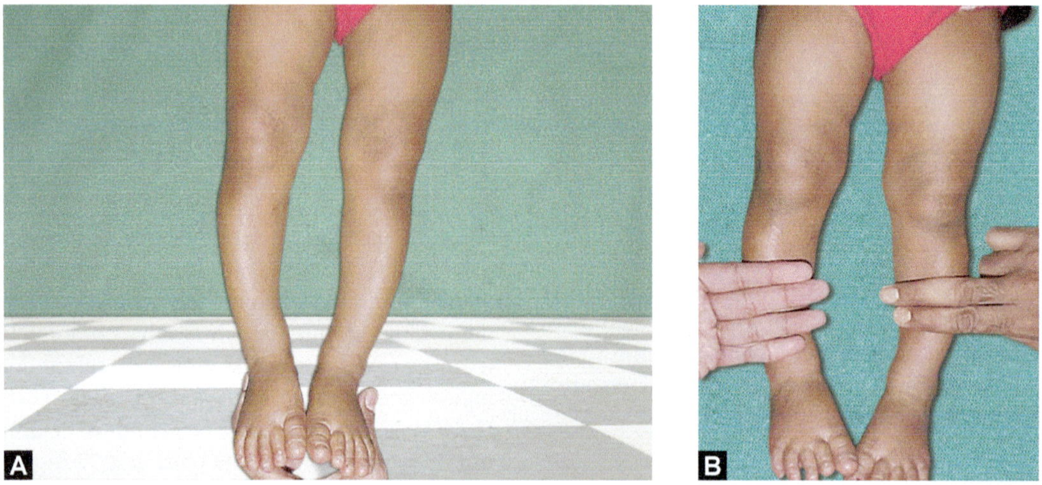

Figures 18.15A and B (A) Cover-up test showing valgus alignment of the proximal tibia in a child with bow-legs; (B) This indicates that the child does not have Blount disease.

genu varum or valgum. Plain radiographs and biochemical investigations can exclude active rickets. Physiological genu varum also needs to be differentiated from infantile Blount disease which requires early treatment. A clinical sign that appears to be quite reliable in making this distinction is the cover-up test **(Figs. 18.15A and B)**. While the examiner covers the middle- and lower-third of the bowed leg with the palm, the alignment of the proximal third of the leg in relation to the thigh is noted. If the proximal third of the leg is in valgus, Blount disease is excluded.

Children with physiological genu varum and valgum need to be periodically reviewed to ensure that resolution of the deformity is occurring. The parents can be reassured that the deformity is likely to correct over time. Bracing, night splints and shoe modification have no effect on the natural history of these deformities and are not warranted.

ADOLESCENT IDIOPATHIC SCOLIOSIS

Treatment Approach: Treat Early

Scoliosis or lateral bending of the vertebral column often develops in adolescent girls. The deformity is not merely lateral curvature of the spine but has rotational and sagittal plane components also. The rotation of the spinal column results in an asymmetry of the rib cage; a prominence or rib hump develops on the side of the convexity of the spinal curvature. It is the rib hump that attracts the attention of the parents. The deformity tends to progress during the pubertal growth spurt. If diagnosed early, spinal instrumentation and fusion can correct the deformity satisfactorily. However, if treatment is delayed, surgery may succeed in reducing the deformity but seldom completely corrects it. For this reason the diagnosis needs to be made early. In conservative societies where it is uncommon for the parents or friends to see the

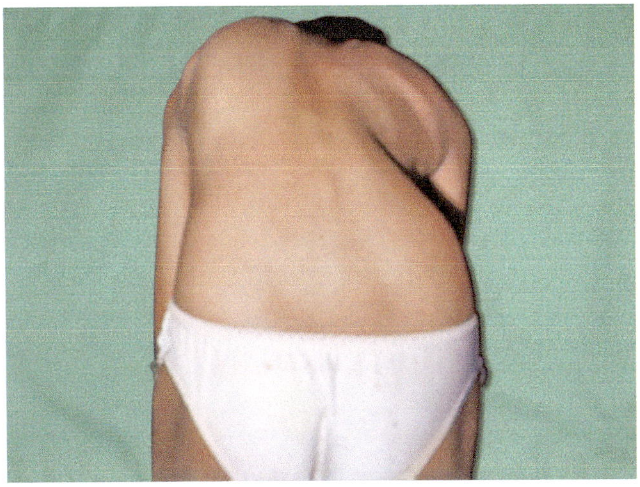

Figure 18.16 Forward bending test used to detect scoliosis. The rib hump that is evident indicates that there is thoracic scoliosis.

adolescent girl's bare back the diagnosis may be delayed till the rib hump is severe enough to attract attention through the girl's loose clothing. For this reason, school-screening for scoliosis is recommended. The screening test is the forward bending test where each student bends forwards and the examiner views the back to identify a rib hump (Fig. 18.16).

PARALYTIC CONDITIONS

Obstetric Brachial Plexus Palsy

Treatment Approach: Treat Early: Injury to the brachial plexus commonly follows shoulder dystocia during labour. Loss of spontaneous movements of the upper limb would be apparent soon after birth. Often what initially appears to be a whole-arm type of paralysis will turn out to be a more localised paralysis; most commonly the upper two roots (C5 and C6) or the upper trunk of the brachial plexus is involved. The severity and the location of the injury determine the extent of recovery. If the injury involves avulsion of the roots of the plexus within the spinal canal (preganglionic injury) no recovery can be anticipated, while if the injury is an extraforaminal (postganglionic) neuropraxia complete recovery can be anticipated. Electrodiagnostic tests are unreliable in accurately differentiating between the different grades of severity of injury in the first few weeks and hence are not recommended. A careful clinical recording of the muscle function of each muscle group is made periodically to map the recovery. If shoulder abduction and elbow flexion of more than Grade III power (antigravity function) is restored within 2 months of birth, the prognosis for full recovery is excellent. If antigravity function of the elbow flexors is restored by 3-6 months, some useful recovery of function would occur. However, if no elbow flexor power is restored within 3 months the prognosis for recovery is poor. In such a child electrodiagnostic tests need to be done at this stage to determine if the injury is preganglionic or postganglionic, and exploration and repair of the brachial plexus needs to be considered.

Fortunately, in the majority of instances elbow flexor power does return by 3 months. Several of these children will have some residual weakness and many develop contractures of the shoulder. The most common contracture that develops is an internal rotation contracture, which can result in posterior dislocation of the shoulder. Since these contractures can develop within a few months, it is imperative that passive stretching exercises to prevent contractures are begun soon after birth and continued regularly for several months. In the past, splints that held the arm abducted and externally rotated were used but currently no form of splintage is recommended. If an internal rotation contracture develops, it needs to be identified early and surgery done in order to correct it and prevent it from going on to produce a dislocation of the shoulder.

POLIOMYELITIS

Treatment Approach: Treat Electively

Although the incidence of polio has reduced in most parts of the developing world, children with postpolio residual paralysis would be encountered for several years to come. The vast majority of children with postpolio residual paralysis have deformities in addition to paralysis. The two causes of deformity in these children are abnormal posture and muscle imbalance. It follows that deformities in polio can be prevented by ensuring proper posture and by recognising muscle imbalance early and restoring muscle balance before the deformity develops. The fact that most children do develop deformities clearly indicates that sufficient attention has not been paid to prevention of deformities.

PREVENTION OF DEFORMITIES

During the acute paralytic phase of polio, the paediatric orthopaedic surgeon should be involved in planning appropriate bracing to prevent postural deformities. During the stage of recovery again bracing of the paralysed extremity can minimise the onset of deformity. Once the stage of recovery is over, careful muscle charting needs to be done in order to identify if muscle imbalance exists. At this stage, if muscle balance is restored by surgery, deformities can be avoided.

CORRECTION OF ESTABLISHED DEFORMITIES

Deformities secondary to poor posture result in contracture of fascia, muscles and joint capsules. Muscle imbalance primarily results in joint deformity due to contracture of the stronger muscle group acting on the joint. Secondarily, the joint capsule may get contracted. If the deformity remains uncorrected, adaptive bony changes take place. This emphasises the need to intervene before bony changes develop.

The milder degrees of deformity will get corrected by releasing the contracted fascia and lengthening the tendons of the contracted muscles. In moderately severe deformities, the contracted capsule would also have to be released; additional osteotomies of the bone adjacent to the joint would be needed to correct severe deformities.

DEALING WITH PARALYSIS

The best option for restoring function of a paralysed muscle is to perform a tendon transfer. However, in order to do so, a muscle that is transferred should have normal (Grade V) muscle power and transferring the muscle should not cause secondary disability. Tendon transfers are most commonly done around the foot and ankle in polio.

TREATING JOINT INSTABILITY

When all the muscles acting on a joint are paralysed, the joint is rendered flail and unstable. Unstable joints need to be stabilised either externally by the use of an orthosis or by fusing the joint. Such an intentional fusion of a joint is referred to as an arthrodesis.

BRACING

If there are no muscles available to consider a tendon transfer, an orthosis may be needed to facilitate ambulation. The extent of bracing would depend on the extent of paralysis. An orthosis that stabilises the paralysed foot and ankle (below-knee brace) is referred to as an ankle-foot orthosis or AFO; an orthosis that stabilises the knee, ankle and foot is called a knee-ankle-foot orthosis or KAFO. In the past, these braces were made of metal uprights and leather belts. Currently they are made of light-weight thermoplastic materials like polypropylene.

SPINA BIFIDA

Treatment Approach: Treat Early (Incipient Neuropathic Ulcer: Treat Urgently)

Spina bifida is primarily a congenital anomaly of development of the neural tube. Secondarily, the neural arches of the vertebrae at the level of the neural tube defect fail to fuse in the midline. Either the meninges alone bulge through the vertebral defect (meningocoele) or neural tissue of the spinal cord and the meninges protrude through the defect (myelomeningocoele) (Fig. 18.17). Varying degrees of neurological deficit will be present in these children depending on the level of the defect. Motor deficit, sensory loss and autonomic dysfunction, that affects bowel and bladder continence, may all be present in children with myelomeningocoele.

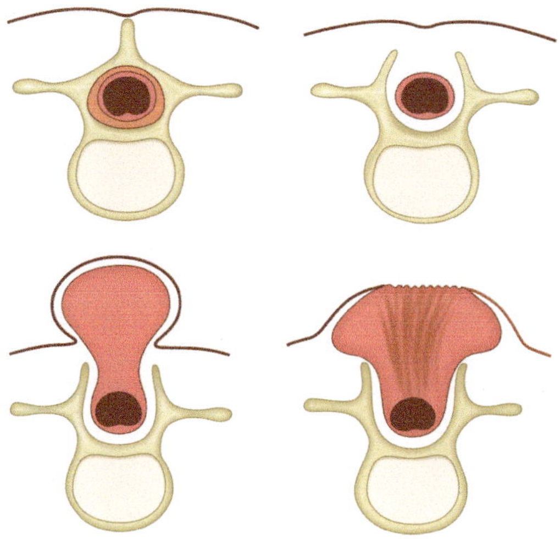

Figure 18.17 Meningocoele in a newborn.

The level of the neurological damage, to a large extent, determines the likelihood of the children retaining their ability to walk outside their homes in adult life (community ambulators). In general, if the child has functioning quadriceps muscles of both lower limbs, the potential for remaining a community ambulator is good. If, however, the level of the damage is higher and the quadriceps muscles are paralysed, the child is likely to end up in a wheel chair by adolescence even if the child does walk with braces in early childhood.

MANAGEMENT OF PARALYSIS

The management of paralysis in children with spina bifida is very similar to that in polio. Wherever tendon transfers are feasible, they should be considered and when there are no tendons available for transfer bracing is needed.

CORRECTION OF DEFORMITIES

In spina bifida, deformities of the spine, hips, knees and feet are all common. Scoliosis and kyphosis occur frequently in these children and their management is particularly difficult. Once the scoliosis becomes severe sitting balance may be lost and the child may only be able to sit with the support of both hands on the cot or chair. The scoliosis must be corrected if this happens or else the child would not be able to use the hands for any other useful activity while seated.

The deformities of the lower limbs in spina bifida again are largely due to muscle imbalance. These deformities can be minimised if muscle balance is restored by appropriate surgery.

In a child who is wheel chair bound, any deformity of the lower limb that precludes sitting should be corrected. In a child who needs to use an orthosis, any deformity that interferes with the fitting of the orthosis must be corrected. Any deformity of the foot that prevents the foot from resting flat on the ground (plantigrade tread) should be corrected in all children with spina bifida who can walk.

PREVENTING NEUROPATHIC ULCERS

One of the most distressing complications of spina bifida is neuropathic ulceration or pressure sores. These occur in regions of sensory loss over bony prominences. The two common regions where these ulcers develop are the ischial region and the soles of the feet. It is important to understand how these ulcers develop and plan strategies to prevent them because getting an ulcer to heal once it develops is often very difficult. If the ulcer does not heal the underlying bone can get infected **(Fig. 18.18)**.

Neuropathic ulcers develop when insensate tissue overlying a bony prominence is either subjected to excessive pressure or to shearing forces. Since pressure is force per unit area any reduction in the area of contact will result in excessive pressure. This is typically seen when the foot is deformed and not plantigrade; the entire sole will not rest on the ground. Since a smaller area of the sole rests on the ground when the foot is deformed, greater pressure is borne on the sole than when the child stands on a normal plantigrade foot. Hence, it is vitally important to correct any deformity that may be present and restore a plantigrade tread. However, it is also important to be aware that operations performed to get the foot plantigrade should not make any joint of the foot stiff. It is important to restore a plantigrade tread while retaining the suppleness of the foot. This is because the frequency of neuropathic ulceration is high if the feet are stiff and rigid even if they are plantigrade.

Similarly, a lumbar scoliosis will cause pelvic obliquity and then more pressure will fall on the ischial tuberosity that is lower when the child is seated and this increases the risk of development of an ischial pressure sore. This underscores the importance of correcting the spinal deformity to overcome the pelvic obliquity.

The second factor that can cause a neuropathic ulcer is shearing forces on tissue overlying a bony prominence. If a child shuffles on its bottom the tissue overlying the ischial tuberosity is subjected to shearing forces and so it is important to educate the parents about the potential risk of ulceration and ensure that the child does not bottom-shuffle. Another example of a situation where shearing forces cause neuropathic ulceration is a calcaneus deformity in an ambulant child. A child with paralysed plantarflexors of the ankle with functioning dorsiflexors will develop a calcaneus deformity. When such a child walks, there is uncontrolled dorsiflexion of the foot during the latter part of the stance phase of gait; quite significant shearing forces develop under the heel when this occurs. Consequently, these children are very prone to develop ulcers on the heel **(Fig. 18.19)**.

Apart from correcting deformities that predispose to neuropathic ulcers and avoiding activity that can cause abnormal stresses on the insensate tissue in susceptible areas, the parents and the child need to be educated about the care of the anaesthetic regions. Children with anaesthetic feet should use soft-lined foot wear and should not walk without this foot wear. Any orthotic that is used should be lined with soft lining material. Parents (and children who are old enough to cooperate) should be taught to inspect the soles of the feet every day. If redness or early blistering is noted, a day's bed rest should be enforced to enable the incipient ulcer to heal. If the redness does not resolve with rest, the orthopaedic surgeon must be consulted immediately.

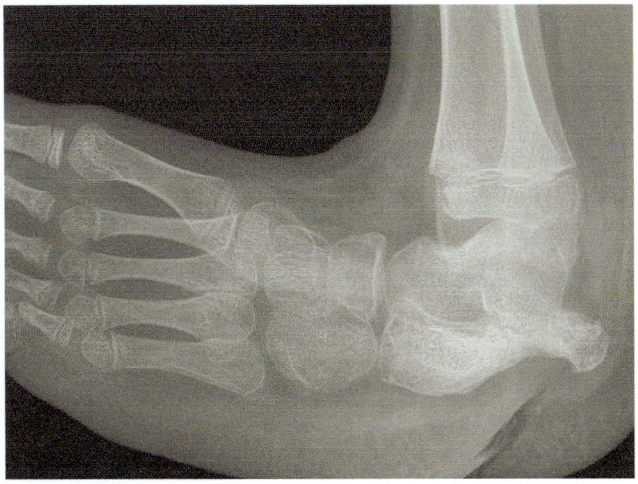

Figure 18.18 Radiograph of a child with spina bifida who developed osteomyelitis of the calcaneum.

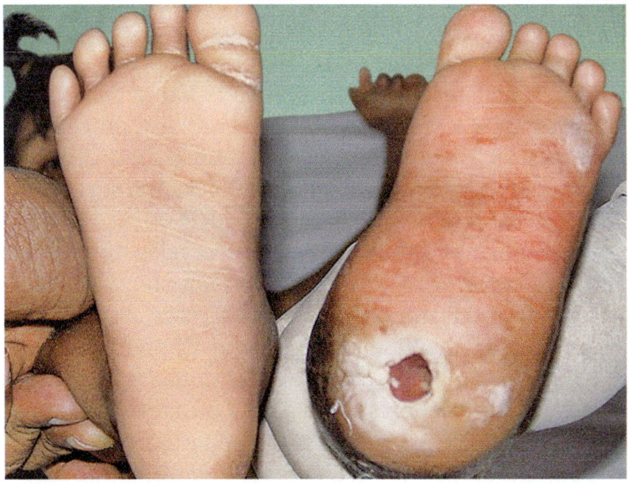

Figure 18.19 Neuropathic ulcer of the heel in a child with spina bifida and paralysis of the gastroc soleus.

CEREBRAL PALSY

Treatment Approach: Treat Early

Though the motor system involvement in CP is the most overt, it is extremely important to note that there are several other impairments in children with CP including speech defects, visual disturbances, hearing defects, behavioural disorders and epilepsy. Several of these associated impairments often need to be addressed before dealing with the motor deficit. (These issues are dealt with in Chapter 14.)

Motor system involvement in CP compromises upper limb function and the activities of daily living. Involvement of the lower limb in CP results in abnormalities of gait. The manifestations of motor system damage include spasticity, in-coordination, paresis, muscle imbalance, lack of selective motor control and involuntary movements. Uncontrolled spasticity will lead to contracture of the spastic muscle and this in turn will lead to deformities. Among these specific problems, spasticity, muscle imbalance and deformities can be modulated by treatment. It needs to be emphasised that treatment can frequently improve these problems but the function can never be made normal.

The ideal aim of treatment of CP is to make the child totally independent. However, in several instances this may not be feasible. It is important to clearly spell out the aims of treatment and communicate these aims to the parents of the child. Every effort must be made to minimise dependence in children who cannot be made totally independent. In children who are severely affected and are likely to remain totally dependent for life, the aim of treatment would be to facilitate care of the child and to make the caregiver's job a bit easier. In addition to these aims of treatment, in all children with CP complications such as hip dislocation should be prevented.

MANAGEMENT OF SPASTICITY

There are several ways to reduce spasticity of muscles. These include physiotherapy, myoneural blocks, oral or intrathecal medication, splinting and casting, surgery on the muscles and tendons, and neurosurgical procedures such as selective dorsal rhizotomy. Among these different options, physiotherapy, myoneural blocks and surgery on muscles and tendons are the most widely used.

Physiotherapy needs to be done every day throughout the period of growth. The need for regular physiotherapy till skeletal maturity needs to be emphasised at the outset. Often parents abandon physiotherapy when they do not see any dramatic improvement. The compliance can be improved if the patients are reviewed on a regular basis in a special clinic. This would give the opportunity to remind the parents about the need for pursuing with physiotherapy and interaction with parents of other children can also have very positive effect in this regard.

Myoneural blocks either into the muscle belly or in the vicinity of the nerve supplying the spastic muscle can appreciably reduce spasticity. Currently injection of botulinum toxin into the muscle at the motor point is widely practised. This reduces spasticity and the effect lasts up to 6 months or more. Unfortunately, the cost of botulinum toxin is prohibitive. Alcohol (40%) has a comparable effect and is a great deal cheaper.

The aim of surgery on the muscles or tendons is to weaken the spastic overactive muscles. The force of muscle contraction can be reduced if the resting length of the muscle fibres can be reduced and this can be achieved by either lengthening the tendon or aponeurotic insertion of the muscle or by erasing the muscle from its origin and permitting the muscle to slide distally.

RESTORING MUSCLE BALANCE

Spastic muscles that are overactive cause reciprocal inhibition of the antagonistic muscles and this results in muscle imbalance. Once the spastic muscle is weakened, the antagonistic muscle can be strengthened by physiotherapy.

INFECTIONS OF BONE AND JOINTS

Acute Septic Arthritis

Treatment Approach: Treat Urgently: Acute septic arthritis is a surgical emergency that develops following haematogenous seeding of bacteria in the synovium. The bacteria and the macrophages secrete very potent proteolytic enzymes which can degrade and destroy hyaline cartilage of the articular surfaces, the epiphysis and the growth plate. Enzymatic degradation of cartilage can begin within 8 hours of colonisation of bacteria in the synovial tissue. If adequate treatment is delayed beyond 3 days after the onset of symptoms, damage to the joint is almost inevitable (Fig. 18.20).

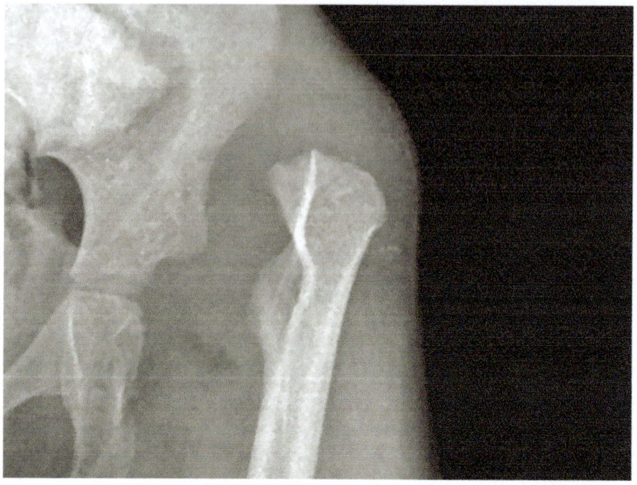

Figure 18.20 Destruction of the head and neck of the femur following acute septic arthritis in infancy.

The most common causative organism is *Staphylococcus aureus*. Neonates and children under the age of 5 years are most susceptible to developing septic arthritis, though septic arthritis can occur at any age. The hip and the knee are the most commonly involved joints. In neonates, it is not uncommon to have more than one joint simultaneously affected.

In neonates, the most common presentation is pseudoparalysis; no spontaneous movement of the affected limb will be seen. True paralysis, fracture of a bone in the limb or septic arthritis may all present with lack of spontaneous movement of the limb. A careful examination can help the clinician to differentiate these conditions. Attempting passive movement of the affected joint causes the baby to cry and there may be some swelling around the joint.

X-rays and other imaging modalities are not helpful in confirming the diagnosis of septic arthritis. Similarly, no laboratory test apart from actual demonstration of bacteria in the synovial fluid is diagnostic of septic arthritis. In a sizeable proportion of cases of true septic arthritis, bacteria may not be demonstrable on a Gram stain of the synovial fluid and on culture. On account of the unreliability of laboratory tests and imaging studies in confirming the diagnosis of septic arthritis, treatment needs to be instituted on the basis of the clinical features. Treatment should not be withheld for want of laboratory confirmation.

Intravenous antibiotics that are effective against Staphylococci should be started immediately. If clear improvement in the swelling of the joint and reduction in pain on passive movement are not noted within 8–12 hours the joint must be explored and drained. Lavage of the joint with copious quantity of saline at the time of surgery will help to reduce the bacterial load. Joints such as the hip that have a propensity to dislocate need to be immobilised in a plaster cast for a few weeks while other infected joints should be immobilised till the inflammation subsides. The intravenous antibiotics may be replaced by oral antibiotics once clinical improvement is noted.

ACUTE OSTEOMYELITIS

Treatment Approach: Treat Urgently

Acute pyogenic osteomyelitis again most commonly is due to haematogenous spread of bacteria from a source elsewhere in the body. The infection starts in the metaphysis due to peculiarities of the blood vessels in this region. If the infection is not controlled, pus will collect in the metaphysis and then track under the periosteum. Gradually, pus will fill the entire medullary cavity and the endosteal blood vessels will get occluded. At the same time the periosteum will get elevated circumferentially over the entire length of the diaphysis by pus, resulting in loss of the periosteal blood supply to the cortex. The diaphysis which now is devoid of both endosteal and periosteal sources of blood supply will undergo necrosis and become a sequestrum. It is of paramount importance to diagnose osteomyelitis early and prevent this catastrophic complication.

The femur and tibia are most commonly affected. If the metaphysis is situated within a joint, as in the proximal femur, arthritis may ensue very soon and then the clinical features would be those of the arthritis.

The initial mode of presentation in neonates is the same as for acute septic arthritis—as pseudoparalysis. Careful examination of a child with acute osteomyelitis may demonstrate tenderness in the region of the metaphysis with no aggravation of pain on gently moving the adjacent joint. As in the case of septic arthritis, imaging modalities and laboratory investigations are not useful in the first few days after the onset of osteomyelitis. Aspiration of the metaphysis with a wide-bore needle may yield pus, if frank suppuration has begun. Ultrasonography and magnetic resonance imaging scans can delineate the extent of a subperiosteal abscess, if it has formed. However, ideally a diagnosis of acute osteomyelitis should be made on clinical grounds even before the subperiosteal abscess forms and appropriate treatment should be instituted without any delay. Intravenous antibiotics that are effective against the most likely pathogens should be started immediately. Staphylococci are the most common group of organisms responsible for acute haematogenous osteomyelitis, while in children with sickle cell disease, *Salmonella* may be the causative organism. If the pain and fever subside and the local warmth and tenderness reduce within 24–48 hours, antibiotics and bed rest may suffice. If, on the other hand, there is no definite clinical improvement within 48 hours, surgery should be undertaken. The involved metaphysis (the diaphysis in *Salmonella* osteomyelitis) is explored. If a subperiosteal abscess is present, it is drained. A couple of drill holes are made in the underlying bone and a small quantity of pus may exude through the drill holes. This serves as effective decompression of the bone, if the infection is localised. If a large quantity of pus is evacuated, a small cortical window is made in the bone to facilitate irrigation of the medullary cavity. The limb is protected in a plaster of Paris cast to prevent a pathological fracture. Once clinical improvement is documented, intravenous antibiotics may be replaced by oral antibiotics which are then continued for 4–6 weeks.

INHERITED DISORDERS OF BONE

Osteogenesis Imperfecta

Treatment Approach: Treat Electively: Osteogenesis imperfecta is an inherited disorder of the skeleton characterised by frequent fractures. The frequency of fractures varies with the severity of the disease. There may be associated ligament laxity, blue sclera and abnormal dentition. In the most severe variety, fractures occur in utero

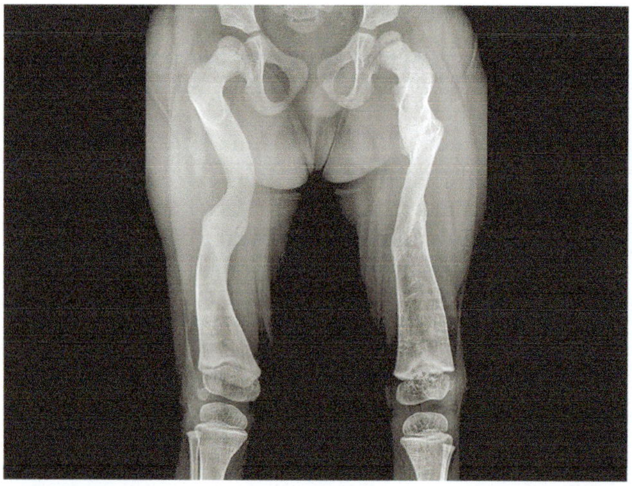

Figure 18.21 Severe deformities of the femur and tibia seen in osteogenesis imperfecta.

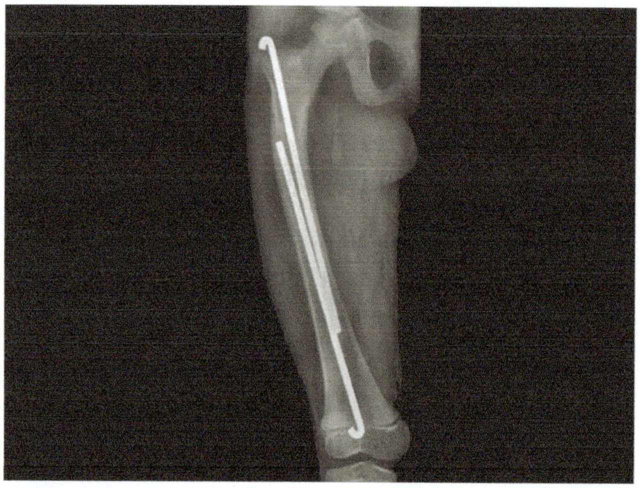

Figure 18.22 Fractures in osteogenesis imperfecta can be minimised by inserting intramedullary rods into the long bones.

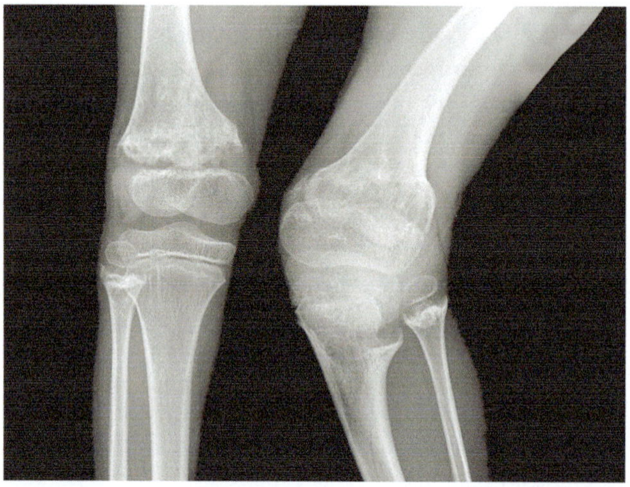

Figure 18.23 Deformity of the knee seen in a form of skeletal dysplasia.

and the baby is often still born. In the less severe varieties, fractures may commence soon after birth and in the mild form may not occur till early childhood. The child may be unable to stand or walk as the femur or tibia may fracture. The fractures often malunite and over a period of time quite horrendous deformities may develop **(Fig. 18.21)**. Generalised bone pains and the pain of repeated fractures make the quality of life very poor.

Bisphosphonates appear to reduce the pain and the frequency of fractures. In addition, correction of the deformities and insertion of rods into the medullary cavity of the bones of the limbs markedly reduce the frequency of fractures **(Fig. 18.22)**. Since the bones outgrow the rods as the child grows, the rods would have to be removed and longer rods need to be inserted or else, fractures will occur in the unsupported part of the bone. The propensity for fractures tends to reduce as the child approaches skeletal maturity.

SKELETAL DYSPLASIAS

Treatment Approach: Treat Electively

Skeletal dysplasias include a large variety of genetically determined abnormalities of the skeleton that manifest as abnormalities in growth of part or the entire skeleton. In some forms, the appendicular skeleton is predominantly involved with little abnormality in the spine, while in other forms both the axial skeleton and the limbs are involved. The pattern of involvement of the skeleton varies with the form of skeletal dysplasia. In some forms, the proximal segments (femur and humerus) are most affected, while in other forms the tibia, fibula, radius and ulna are the most severely affected and in a few types, the hands and feet are most affected. The abnormalities of growth may also result in dwarfism or angular deformities due to asymmetric growth at the growth plates of long bones **(Fig. 18.23)**. These deformities result in abnormal stresses on joints and this contributes to very early onset of secondary degenerative arthritis of the weight-bearing joints. In addition to aberrant growth, joint instability or joint stiffness may be present in some dysplasias.

Whenever there is evidence of dwarfism or abnormal body proportions, radiographs of the skeleton need to be obtained to exclude skeletal dysplasia. Some skeletal dysplasias can be diagnosed at birth (e.g. achondroplasia) while in some dysplasias the growth abnormality may only become evident in early or even late childhood (e.g. spondyloepiphyseal dysplasia tarda). Orthopaedic intervention for skeletal dysplasia in childhood is mainly to correct deformities.

TUMOURS OF BONE

Benign Tumours

Treatment Approach: Treat Electively: One of the common benign tumours of bone is osteochondroma, which

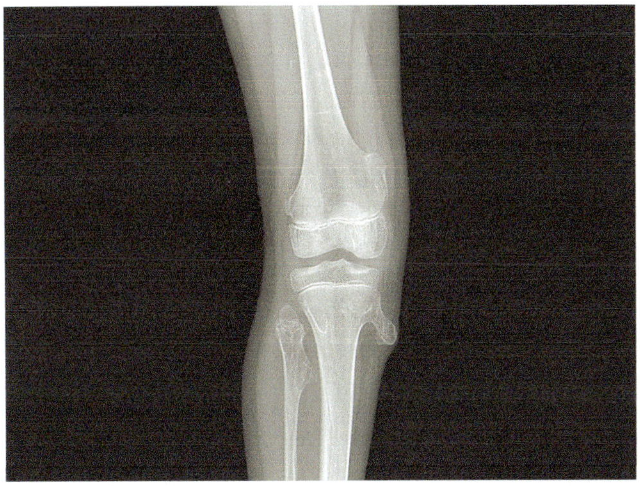

Figure 18.24 Multiple osteochondromata seen in the distal femur and proximal tibia of both limbs.

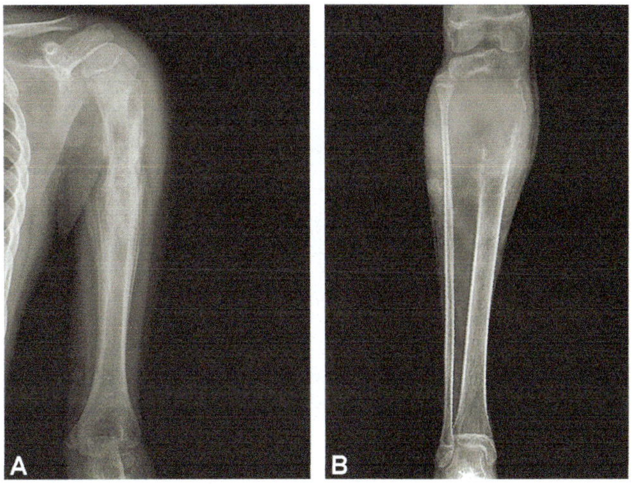

Figures 18.25A and B Radiographic appearance of: (A) Ewing tumour; (B) Osteosarcoma.

as the name implies has a cartilaginous and a bony component. The tumour typically occurs in the metaphyseal region of long bones and may be either solitary or multiple (Fig. 18.24). Multiple osteochondromatosis is an inherited disorder, which is associated with a remodelling defect of the long bones and growth abnormalities. The solitary variety, on the other hand is not associated with growth abnormalities or a remodelling defect. The osteochondromata grow till skeletal maturity and then cease to grow unless they have undergone malignant transformation. Malignant transformation to a chondrosarcoma is very rare in solitary osteochondromas but may occur in about 10% of patients with multiple osteochondromatosis. Unless the osteochondroma causes pressure on an adjacent nerve or impairs movement of a joint it can be left alone. If symptoms warrant it, the osteochondroma may be excised along with the periosteum surrounding the base of the osteochondroma.

Malignant Tumours

Treatment Approach: Treat Urgently: The two important malignant tumours of bone seen in children are osteosarcoma and Ewing tumour. Ewing tumour occurs most commonly in the first decade of life while osteosarcoma occurs in the second decade of life. The presenting features may be pain or swelling in the thigh, leg or arm which are the common sites for these tumour to occur. Unexplained pain or swelling of the limb should be investigated carefully. A radiograph of the limb is mandatory and if either of these tumours is present, characteristic changes may be seen. In the case of Ewing tumour, a lesion would be seen more commonly in the diaphysis with areas of patchy osteolysis, cortical erosion and periosteal reaction that may have a very typical "onion peel" appearance (Fig. 18.25A). Osteosarcoma, on the other and is metaphyseal and the lesion is predominantly sclerotic in appearance; early breach of the cortex with extension of the tumour under the periosteum produces a typical "sun ray" appearance (Fig. 18.25B). Though these radiographic appearances are quite characteristic of these tumours, similar appearances can occur in other less morbid conditions. Radiographic changes in the bone that are similar to those of Ewing tumour may occur in osteomyelitis, while changes akin to those of osteosarcoma may occur with exuberant callus formation after a fracture in spina bifida or osteogenesis imperfecta. Therefore, it is mandatory to perform a biopsy to confirm the diagnosis. Unless a pathologist who is experienced in interpreting needle biopsies is available, it is preferable to perform an open biopsy.

Ewing tumour is treated with cyclical chemotherapy and in some instances with additional radiotherapy and surgery. Osteosarcoma is treated with adjuvant chemotherapy followed by surgery. If strict criteria are fulfilled, limb salvage surgery may be considered or else an amputation is performed. Cyclical chemotherapy is resumed again following surgery. Limb salvage surgery would require some form of reconstruction after resection of the diseased bone segment.

HIP PAIN IN CHILDREN AND ADOLESCENTS

Among all the joints of the body that may be a source of pain in children, the hip joint is most frequently affected. Apart from trauma and bone and joint infection, there are some other causes of hip pain that warrant a brief mention; these include transient synovitis, Perthes disease and slipped capital femoral epiphysis. The age at which each of these conditions occurs varies (Table 18.8) and the knowledge of the typical ages at presentation can alert the clinician to the possible diagnosis. Though the

TABLE 18.8 Typical ages at which painful conditions of the hip occur.

Condition	*Common age at presentation*
Septic arthritis	Under 5 years
Transient synovitis	5–10 years
Perthes disease	5–12 years
Slipped capital femoral epiphysis	12–15 years

pathology in these conditions is in the hip, the child may complain of pain in the knee as pain arising from the hip may be referred to the knee. This emphasises the need to carefully examine the hip in addition to examining the knee when a child complains of knee pain.

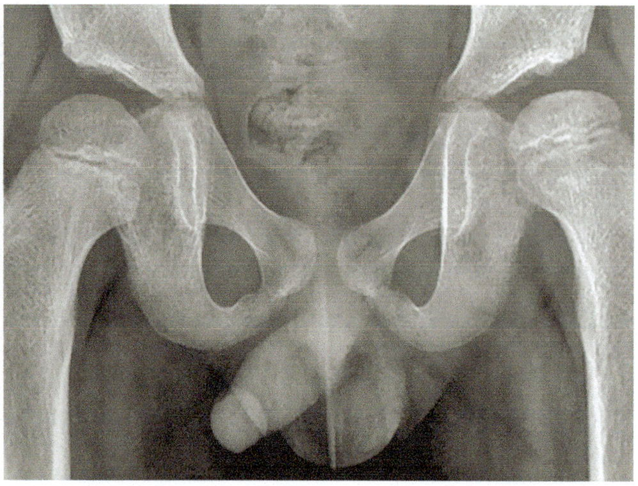

Figure 18.26 Radiographic appearance of a boy with Perthes disease. The epiphysis is sclerotic and flattened.

TRANSIENT SYNOVITIS

Treatment Approach: Treat Early

Transient synovitis affects children between 5 and 10 years of age. The child presents with a limp and pain in the hip or knee. The onset of pain may be preceded by an upper respiratory infection in a proportion of cases. Extremes of hip movement are painful and there may be a mild flexion or abduction deformity. All these signs point to the presence of an effusion in the hip which can be clearly demonstrated by ultrasonography. The clinical features, including the absence of fever, normal blood counts and erythrocyte sedimentation rate help to exclude septic arthritis. A few days of bed rest and traction usually relieves the pain completely and the synovitis settles without any permanent sequelae. However, since Perthes disease may present in the same manner in the very early stages, these children should be followed up with a radiograph of the hips after 6–8 weeks to see if the changes of Perthes disease are visible.

PERTHES DISEASE

Treatment Approach: Treat Early

Perthes disease is a form of osteochondrosis that affects the capital femoral epiphysis **(Fig. 18.26)**. Part or all of the femoral epiphysis becomes avascular, the precise cause of which is unknown; the blood supply gets restored spontaneously over a period of 2–4 years. The prevalence of Perthes disease varies profoundly from region to region. In India, the disease is exceedingly common in the South-West coastal plain but is quite uncommon in other parts of the country. In India, the disease affects children mainly between the ages of 5 and 12 years; the peak age at onset of symptoms is around 9 years. This is distinctly older than the age of onset reported in the Western literature. The classical presentation is with a limp and pain of insidious onset and moderate limitation of passive abduction and internal rotation of the hip. The X-rays will show characteristic changes of flattening and sclerosis of the capital femoral epiphysis. In the younger child, the prognosis is generally good; the blood supply gets restored and healing of the epiphysis occurs without any deformation of the femoral head. In the older child, however, the femoral head tends to get deformed during the process of healing. Consequently, surgery aimed at preventing femoral head deformation is often needed in the older child. It is important that such surgery is performed early in the course of the disease if it is to be effective. If the femoral head does get deformed, secondary degenerative arthritis may develop by the third or fourth decades of life.

SLIPPED CAPITAL FEMORAL EPIPHYSIS

Treatment Approach: Treat Urgently

Slipped capital femoral epiphysis or adolescent coxa vara occurs commonly between 12 and 15 years of age. There may be an underlying endocrine disorder or chronic renal disease in a proportion of these patients and it is important that these are excluded. Majority of the patients are obese though the epiphyseal slip can occur in children with a normal body habitus.

The growth plate of the proximal femur gets disrupted and the epiphysis slips medially and posteriorly off the neck of the femur **(Figs. 18.27A and B)**. The slip is heralded by pain in the hip and in the majority of instances tends to occur gradually. The patient continues to walk albeit with a limp and the slip is referred to as a stable slip. On the other hand, if the slip occurs suddenly the pain is severe and the patient will be unable to bear weight on the limb; this is an unstable slip. Complications are far more common in patients with unstable slips and hence the importance of this classification. Complications of slipped femoral epiphysis include progression of the slip,

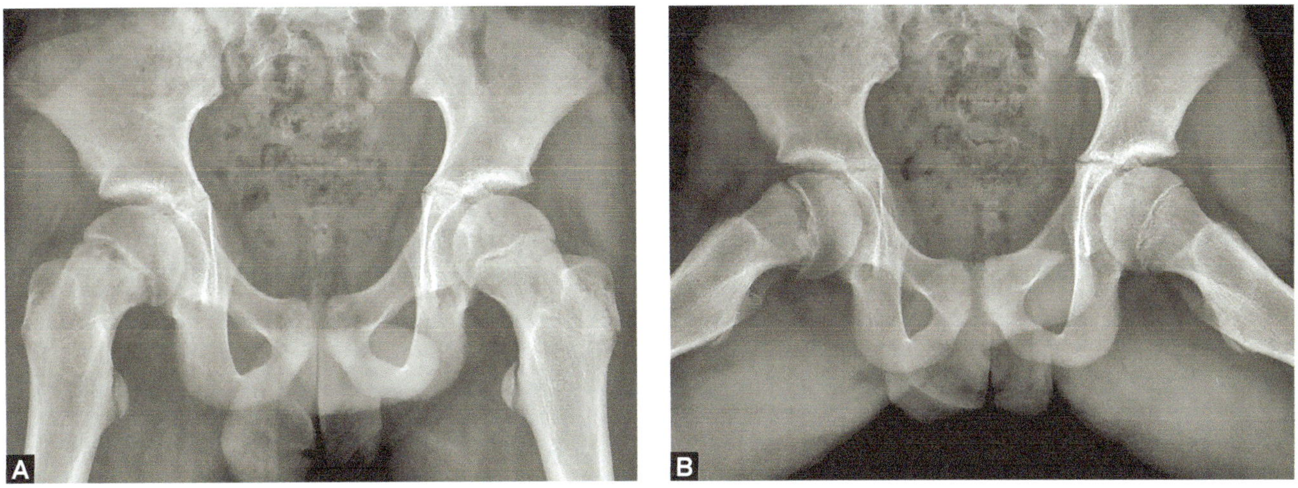

Figures 18.27A and B Radiographic appearance of a slipped capital femoral epiphysis in an adolescent.

avascular necrosis of the femoral epiphysis and chondrolysis which results in extreme hip stiffness. Secondary, degenerative arthritis may occur in early adult life. The aim of treatment is to prevent the slip from progressing and to prevent other complications listed above. Since the risk of complications increase with delay in treatment, it is recommended that the femoral epiphysis is fixed to the femoral neck with a screw as soon as possible. There is a risk that a slip can occur in the opposite hip and because of this some surgeons fix the opposite epiphysis also prophylactically. If prophylactic fixation of the unaffected hip is not done, these patients should be periodically reviewed to ensure that a slip of the epiphysis has not occurred in the second hip.

CHAPTER 19

Paediatric Dentistry

Richard Welbury, Alison M. Cairns

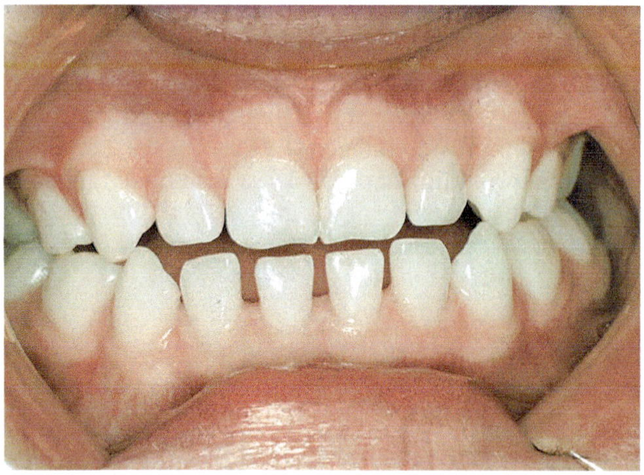

Figure 19.1 Normal primary dentition.

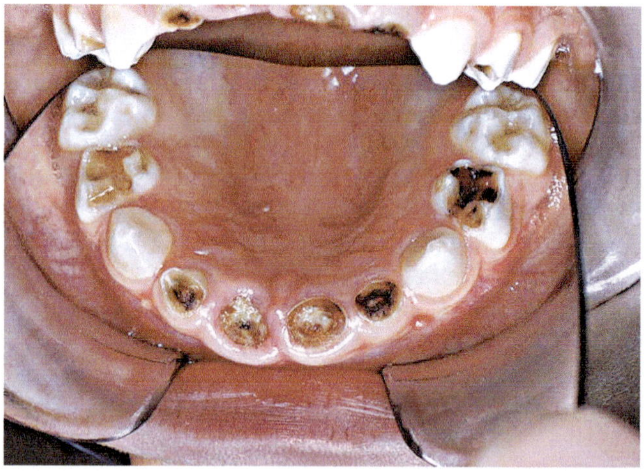

Figure 19.2 Nursing caries in infant 1.

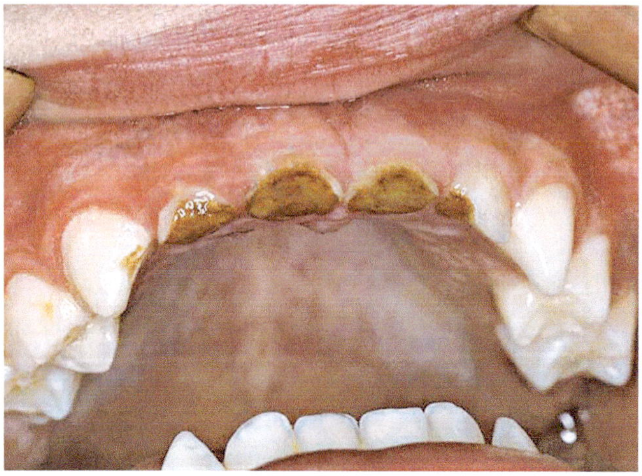

Figure 19.3 Nursing caries in infant 2.

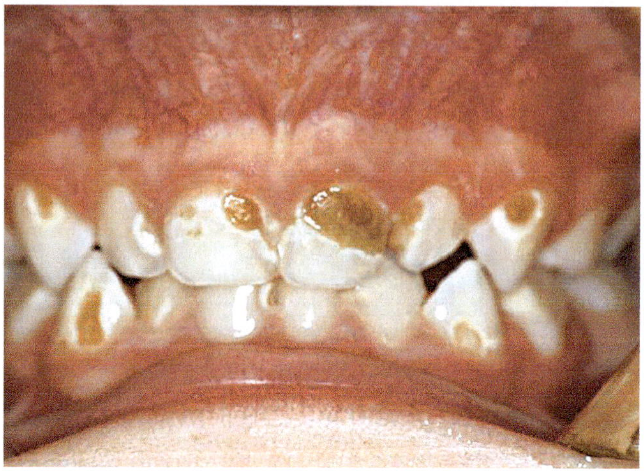

Figure 19.4 Nursing caries in infant 3.

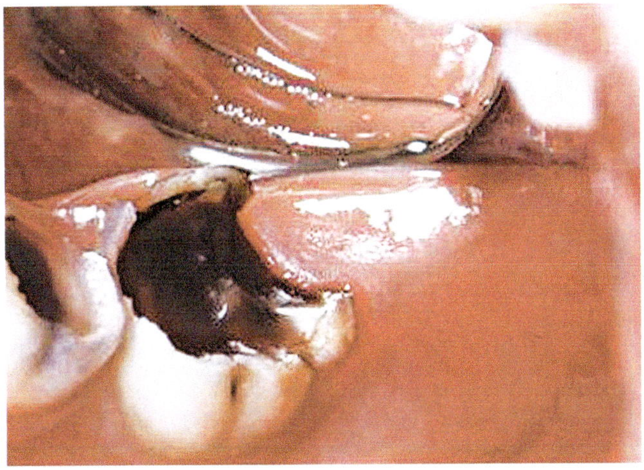

Figure 19.5 Arrested caries in primary teeth.

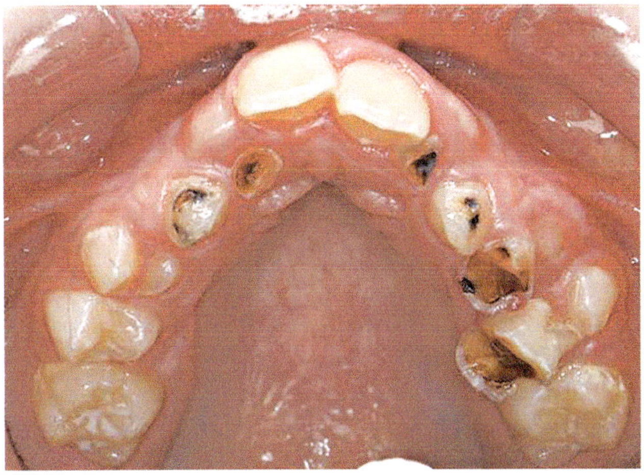

Figure 19.6 Caries in primary teeth close to exfoliation.

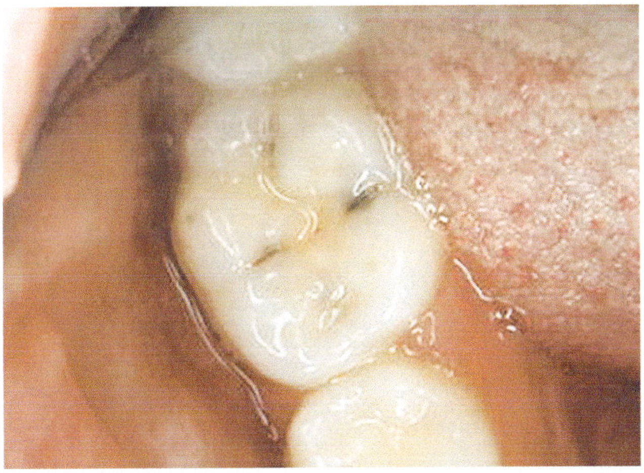

Figure 19.7 Stained fissures of permanent molar.

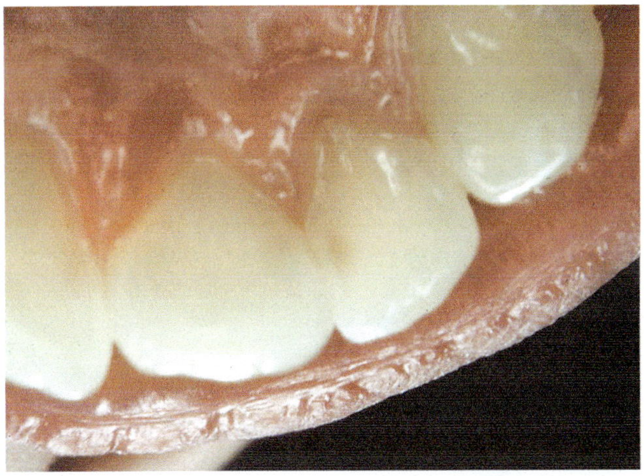

Figure 19.8 Interproximal caries.

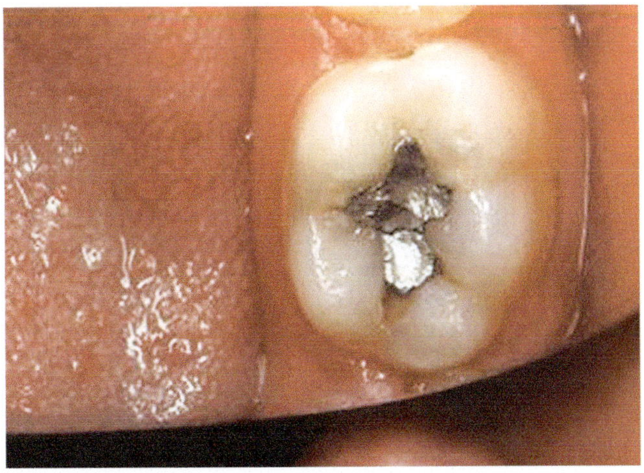

Figure 19.9 Secondary caries around restoration.

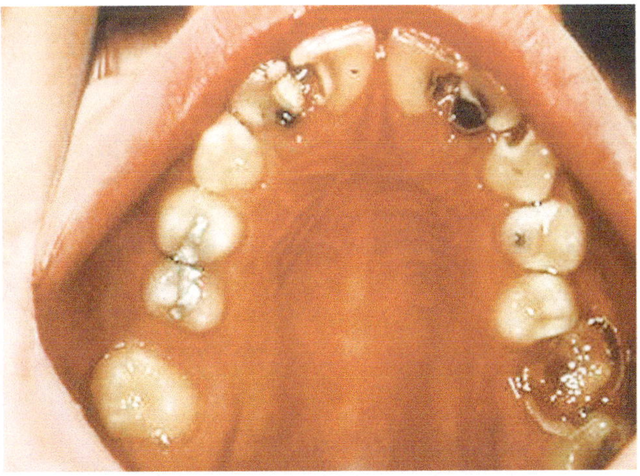

Figure 19.10 Rampant caries in permanent dentition.

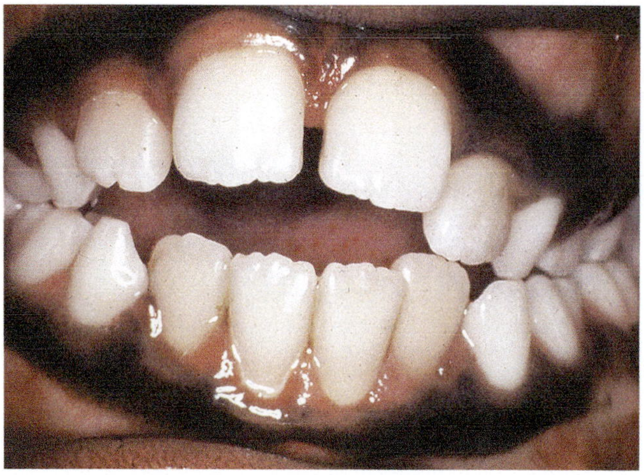

Figure 19.11 Anterior open bite due to digit sucking.

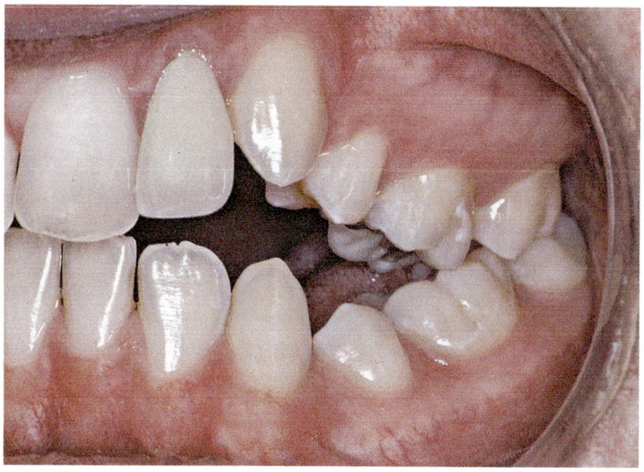

Figure 19.12 Lateral open bite.

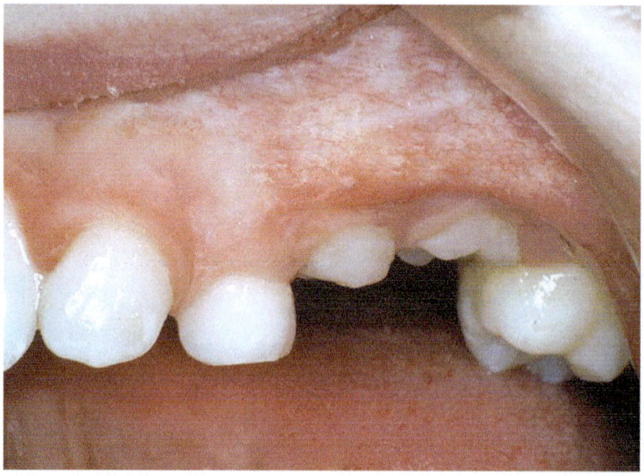

Figure 19.13 Infraocclusion.

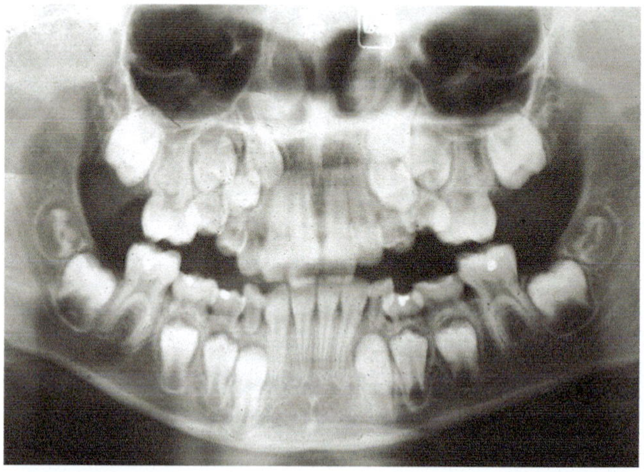

Figure 19.14 Infraocclusion radiograph.

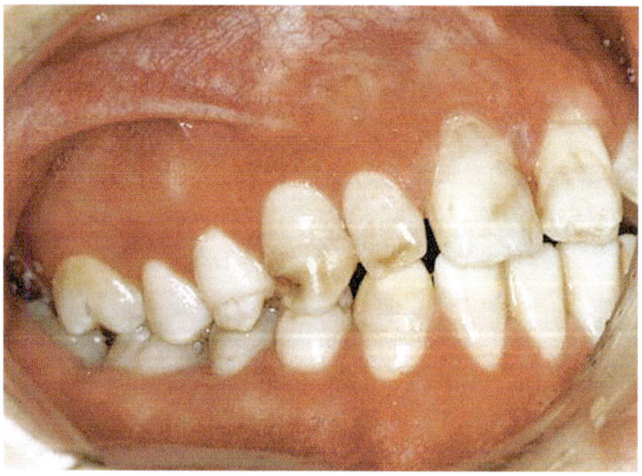

Figure 19.15 Enamel defects: Chronological hypoplasia 1.

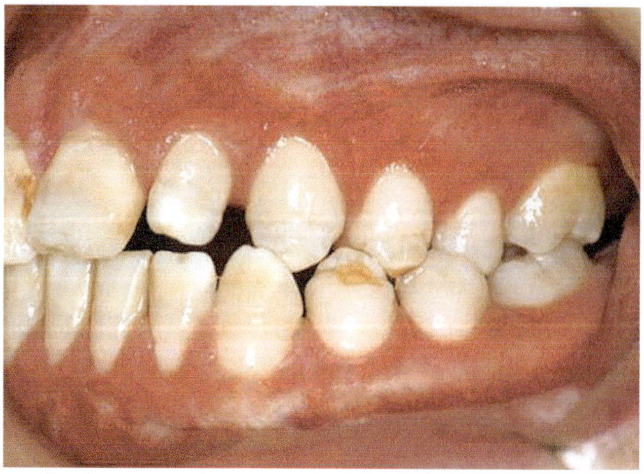

Figure 19.16 Enamel defects: Chronological hypoplasia 2.

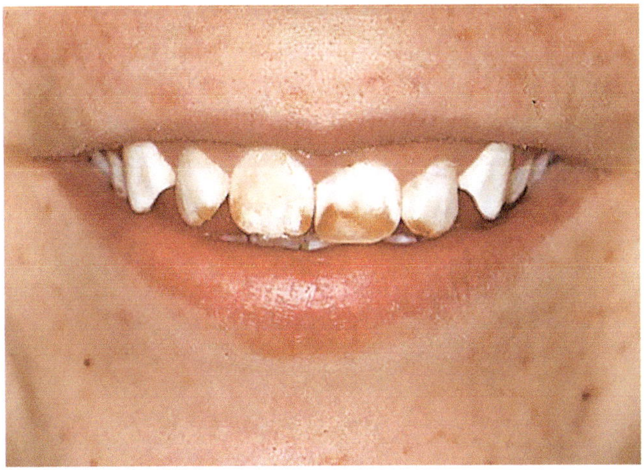

Figure 19.17 Enamel defects: Fluorosis 1.

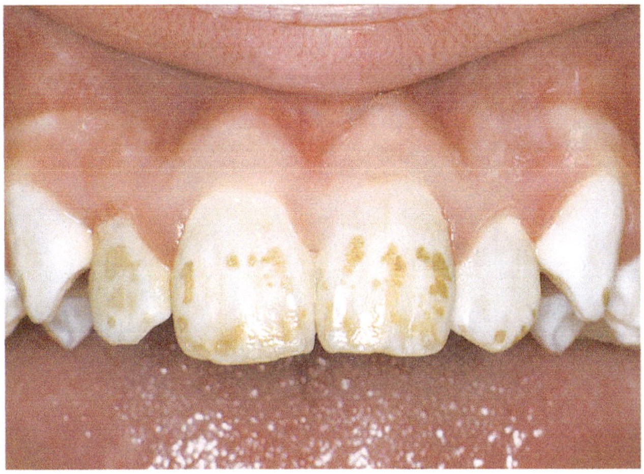

Figure 19.18 Enamel defects: Fluorosis 2.

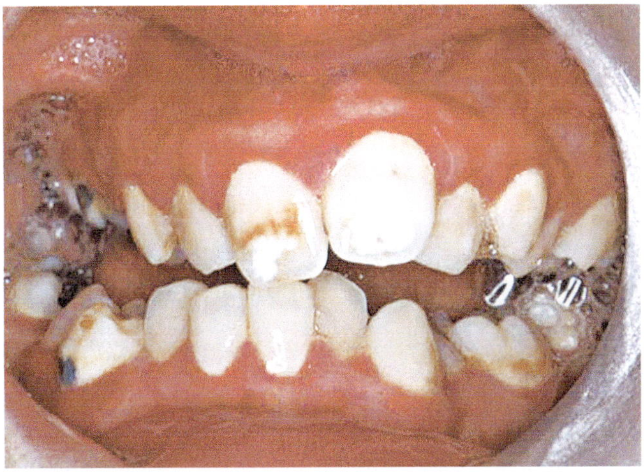

Figure 19.19 Enamel defects: Hypomineralised.

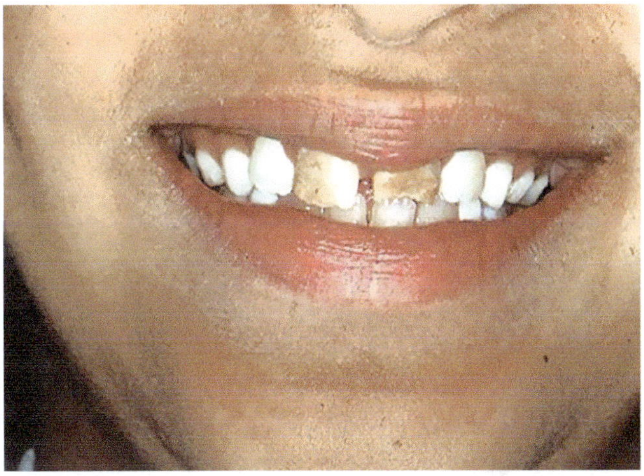

Figure 19.20 Enamel defects of permanent incisors post primary tooth trauma.

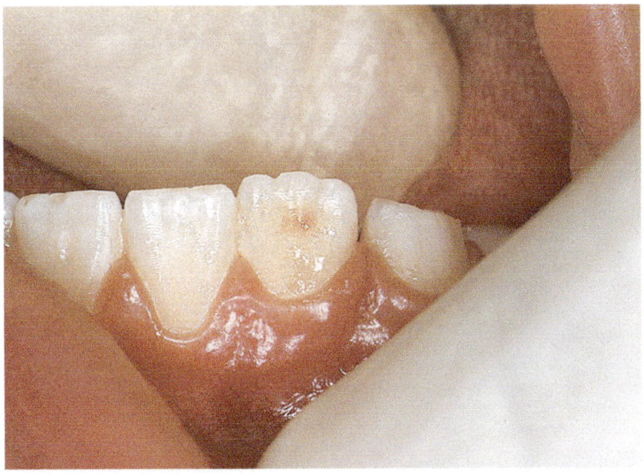

Figure 19.21 Turner's tooth post infection of primary predecessor.

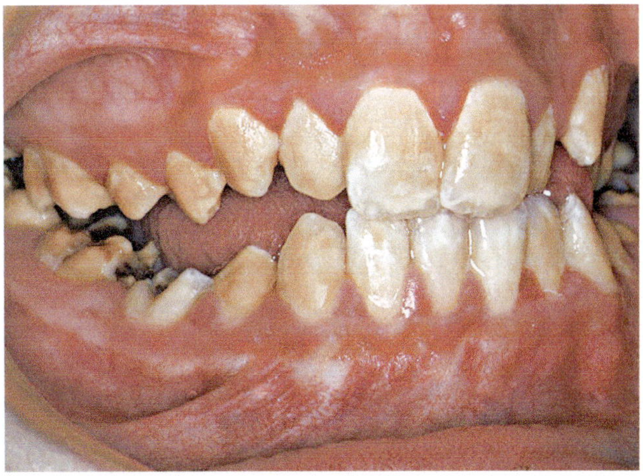

Figure 19.22 Enamel defects of amelogenesis imperfecta.

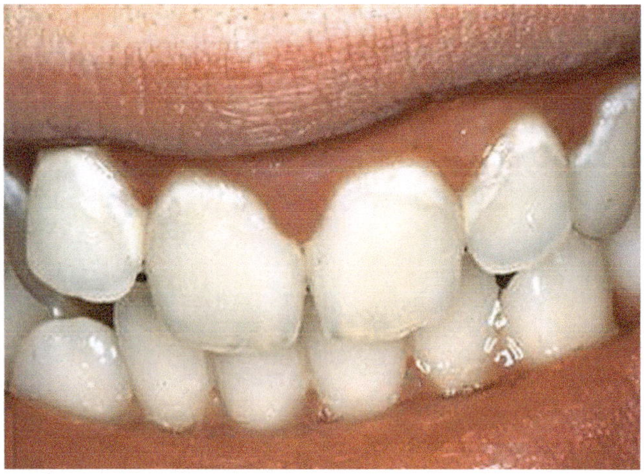

Figure 19.23 White decalcification due to poor oral hygiene.

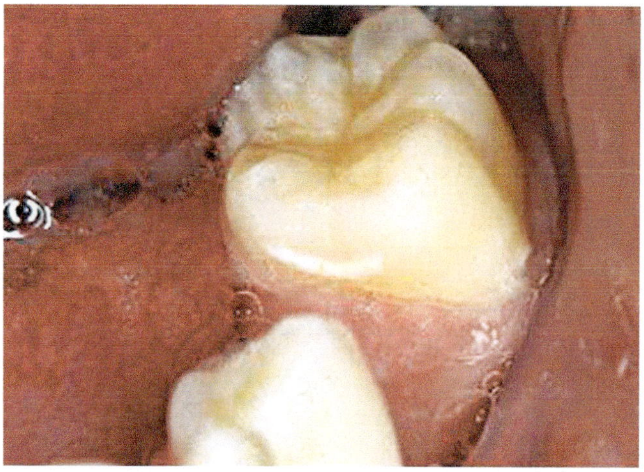

Figure 19.24 White spot lesion on mesial enamel.

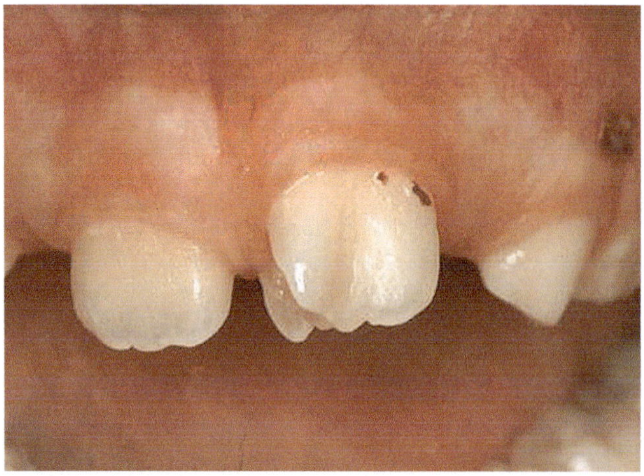

Figure 19.25 Talon cusp.

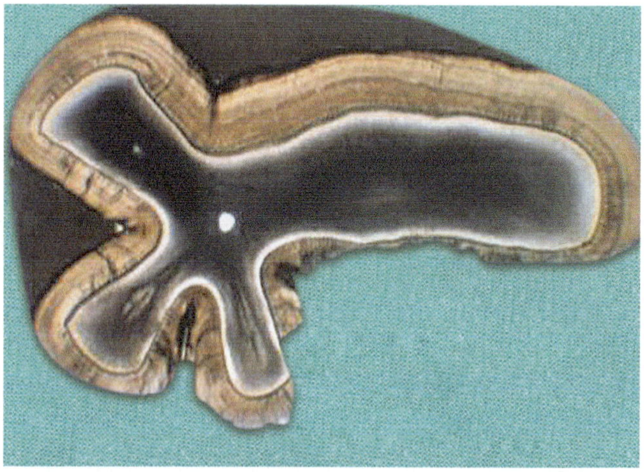

Figure 19.26 Talon cusp histology.

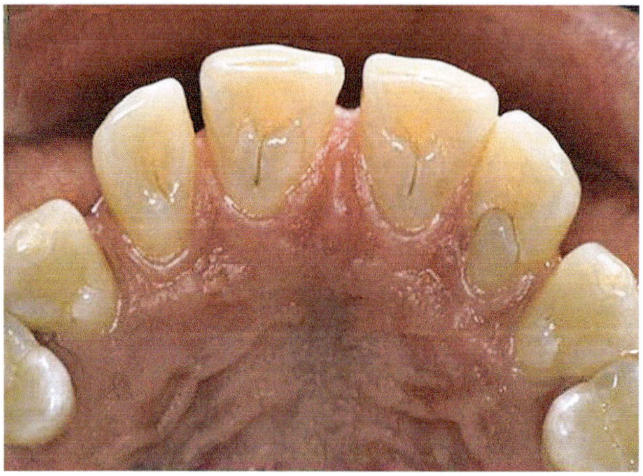

Figure 19.27 Clinical appearance of dens in dente.

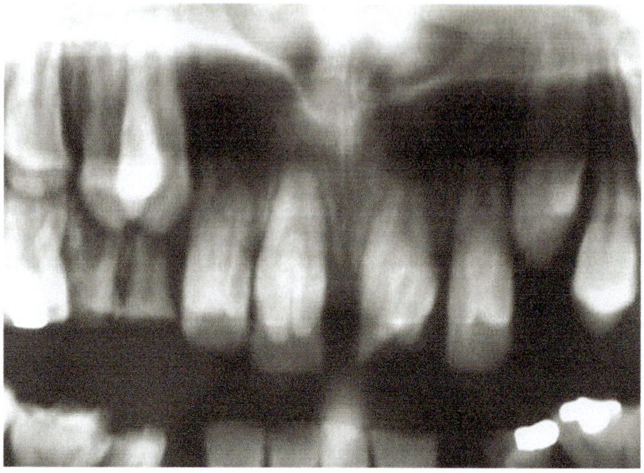

Figure 19.28 Radiographic appearance of dens in dente teeth 2.

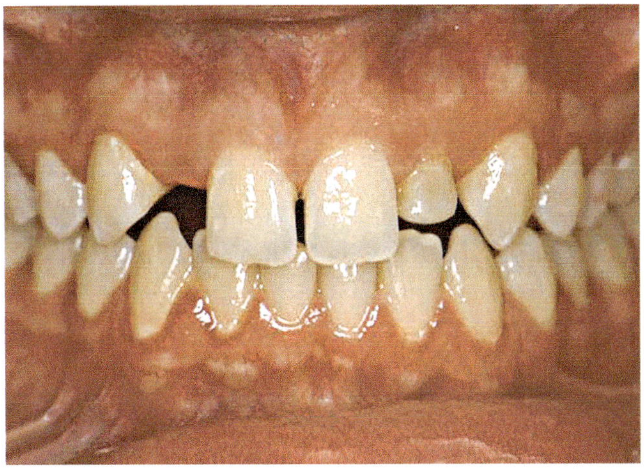

Figure 19.29 Missing laterals pre-restoration.

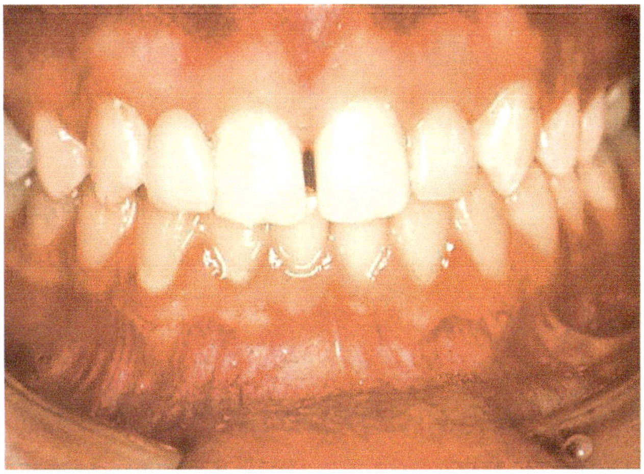

Figure 19.30 Missing laterals restored.

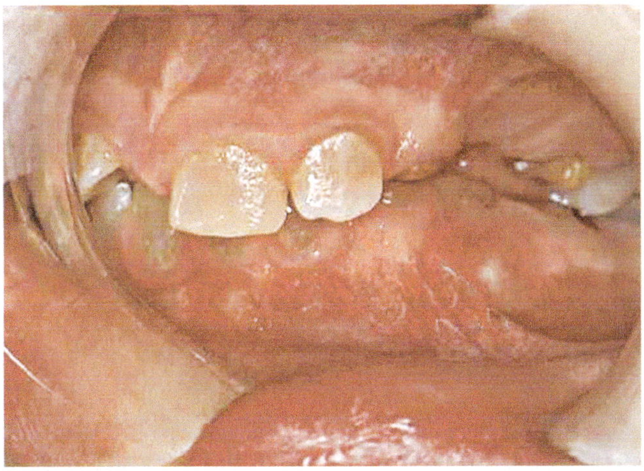

Figure 19.31 Amber opalescent appearance of teeth in dentinogenesis imperfecta.

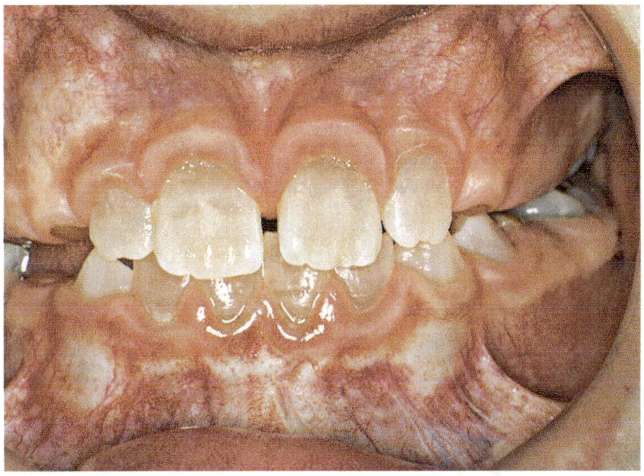

Figure 19.32 Grey opalescent appearance of teeth in dentinogenesis imperfecta.

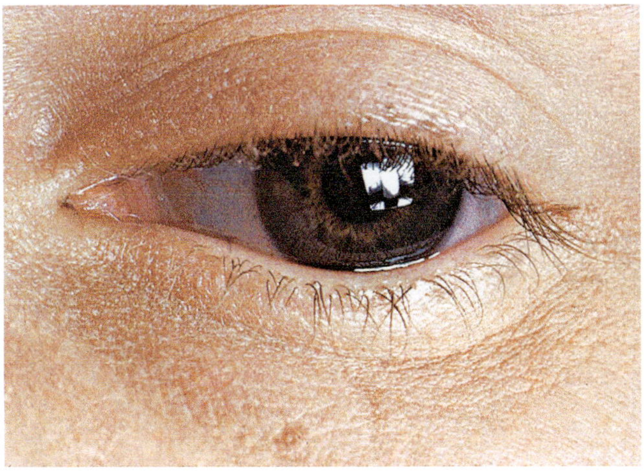

Figure 19.33 Blue sclera of osteogenesis imperfecta often associated with dentinogenesis imperfecta.

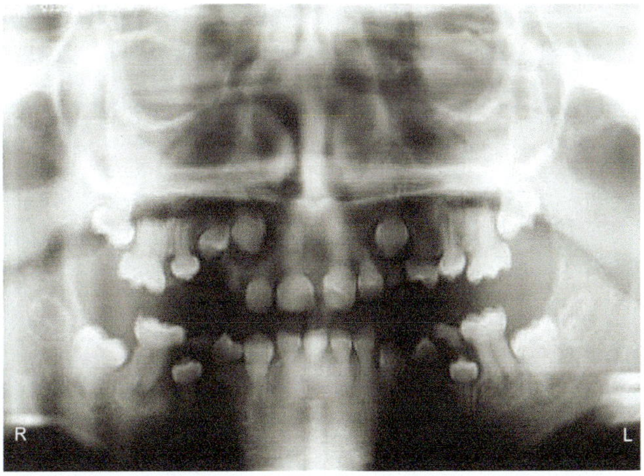

Figure 19.34 Radiographic appearance of teeth in dentinogenesis imperfecta.

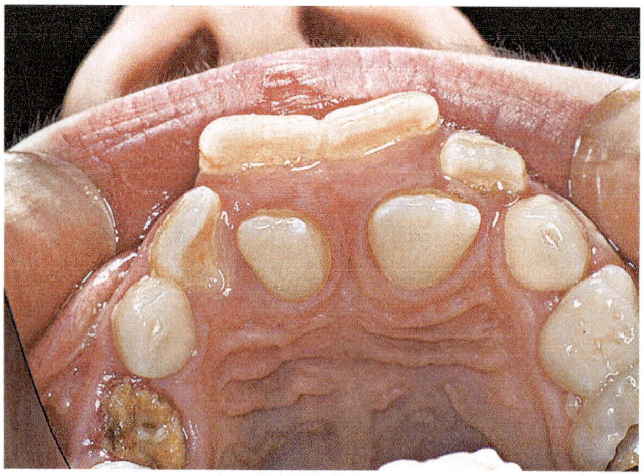

Figure 19.35 Erupted palatal supernumerary teeth.

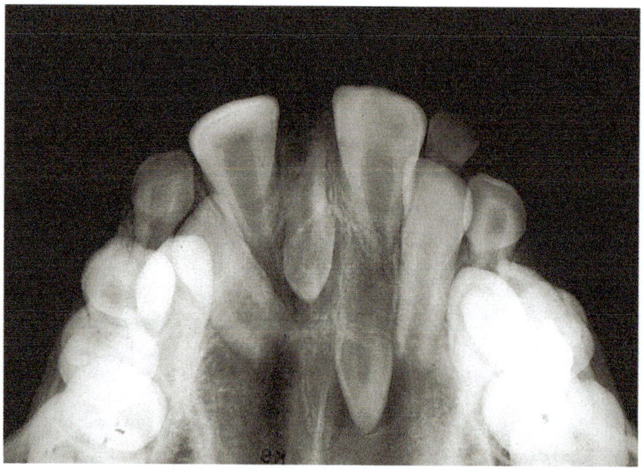

Figure 19.36 Inverted supernumerary teeth.

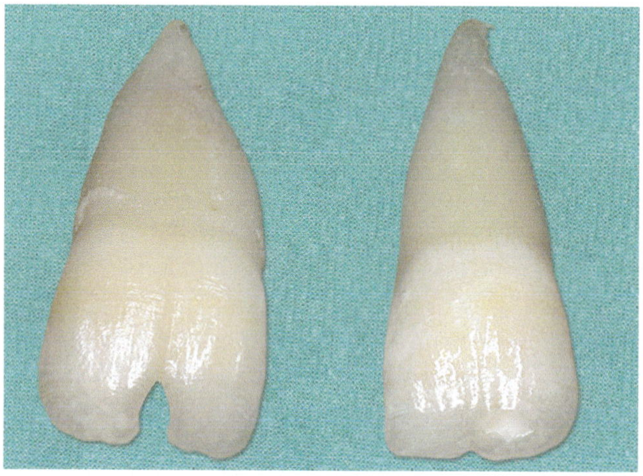

Figure 19.37 Megadont teeth.

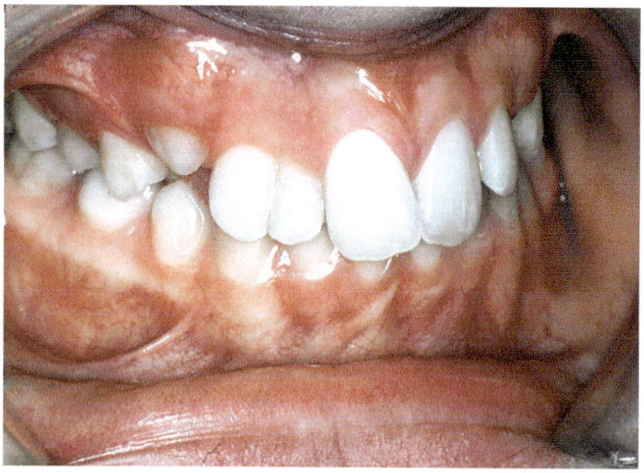

Figure 19.38 Double tooth.

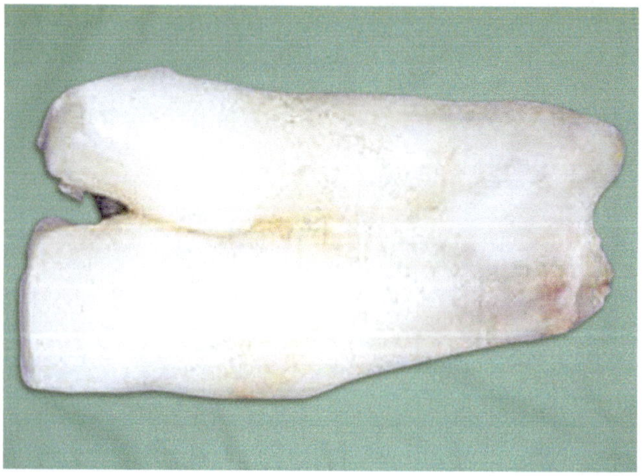

Figure 19.39 Double tooth post extraction.

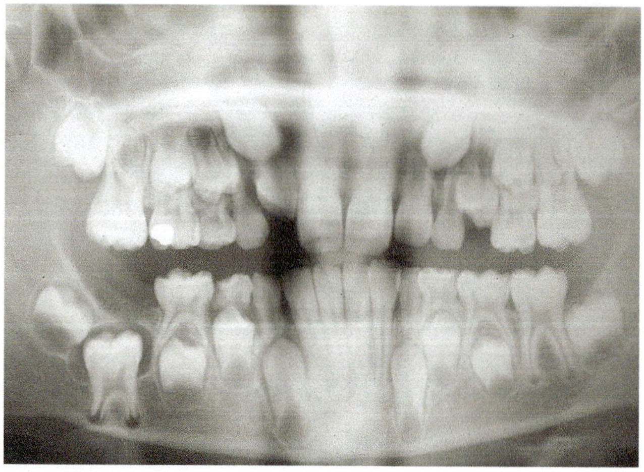

Figure 19.40 Dentigerous cyst and failure of eruption.

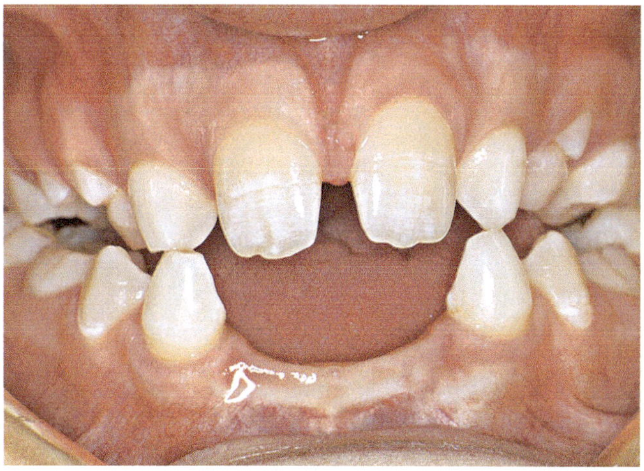
Figure 19.41 Hypodontia.

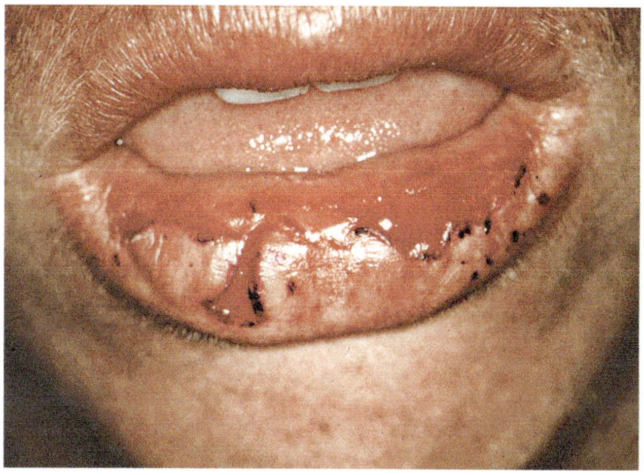
Figure 19.42 Actinic burn due to excessive sun exposure.

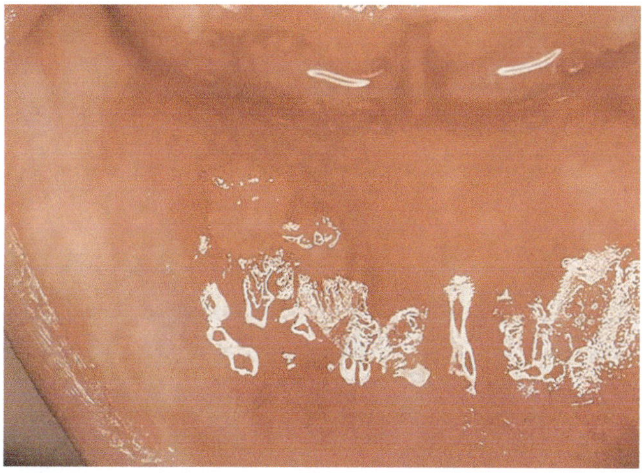
Figure 19.43 Traumatic ulceration.

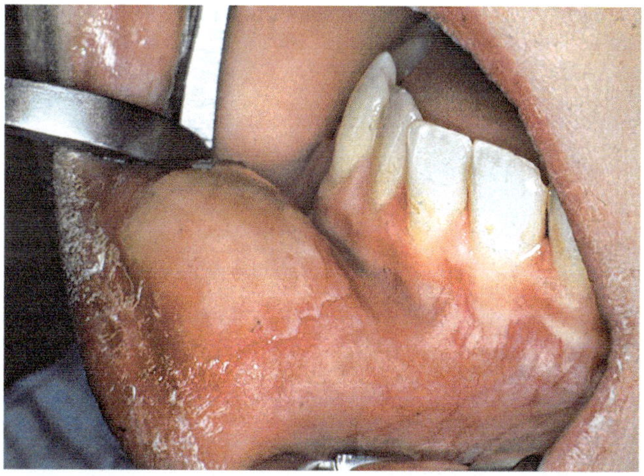
Figure 19.44 Thermal burn 1.

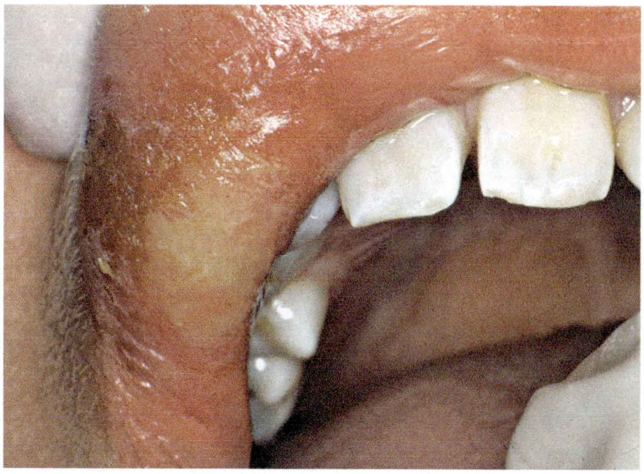
Figure 19.45 Thermal burn 2.

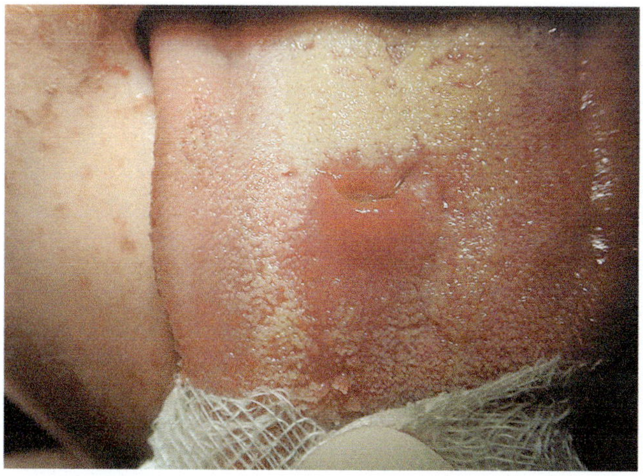
Figure 19.46 Tongue bite.

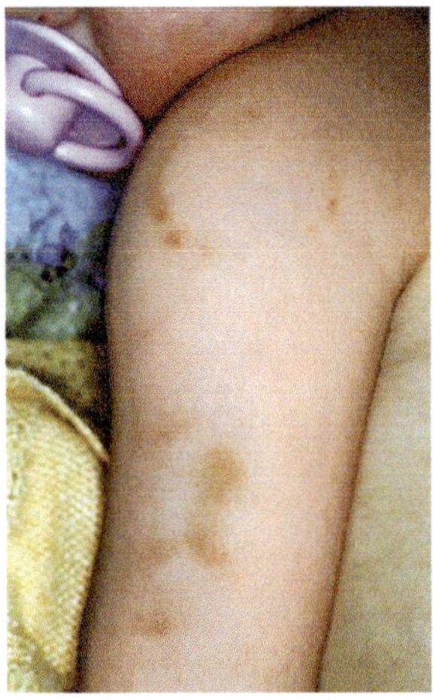

Figure 19.47 Nonaccidental injury bite mark and grip mark.

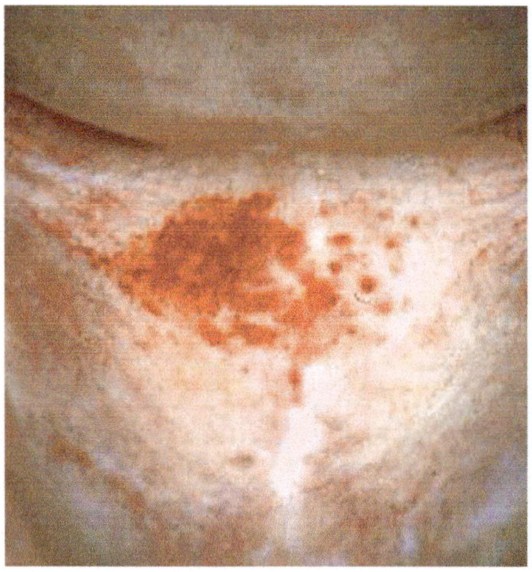

Figure 19.48 Nonaccidental injury palatal petechiae.

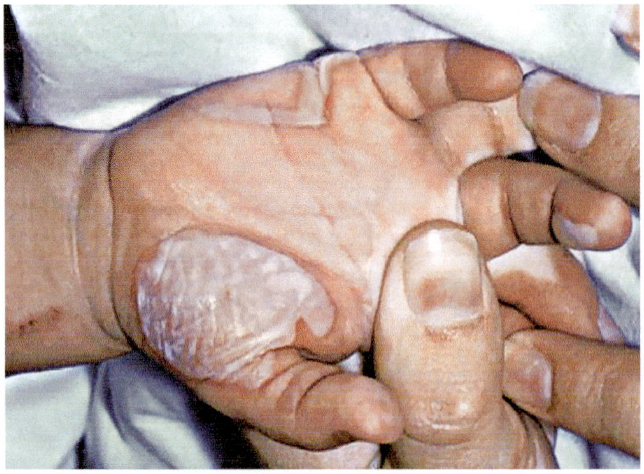

Figure 19.49 Nonaccidental injury tatoo burns.

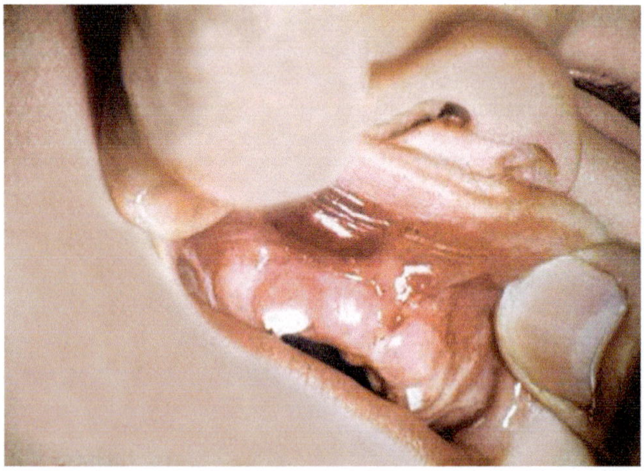

Figure 19.50 Nonaccidental injury torn upper labial fraenum.

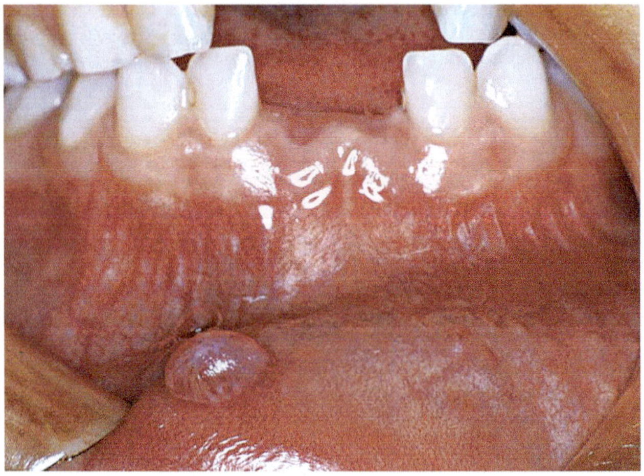

Figure 19.51 Mucocoele.

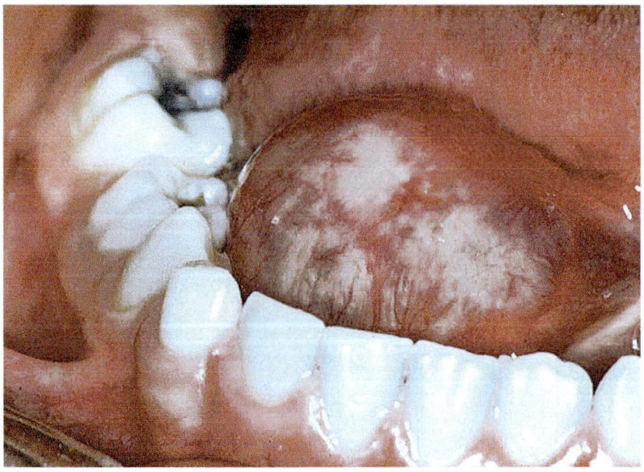

Figure 19.52 Ranula mucocoele from sublingual gland.

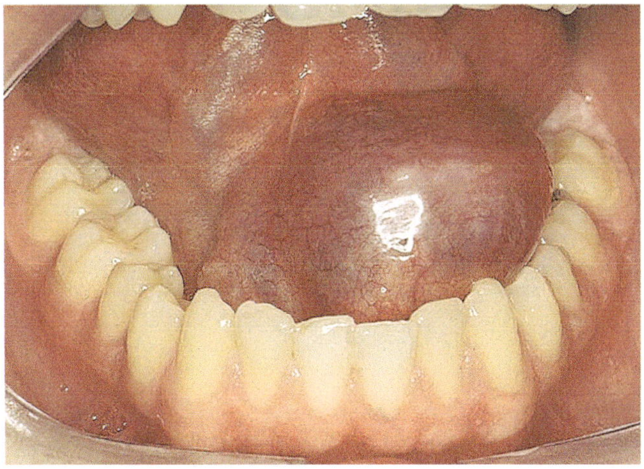

Figure 19.53 Ranula 2.

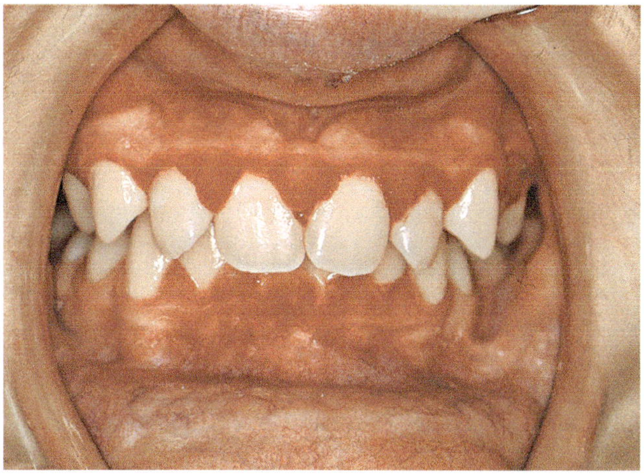

Figure 19.54 Chronic marginal gingivitis.

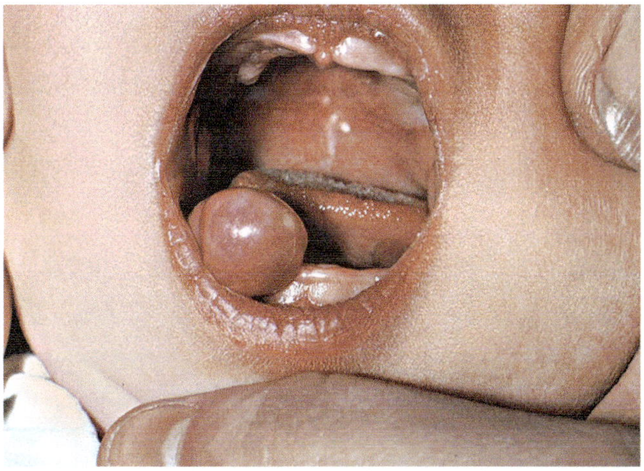

Figure 19.55 Congenital epulis of the newborn.

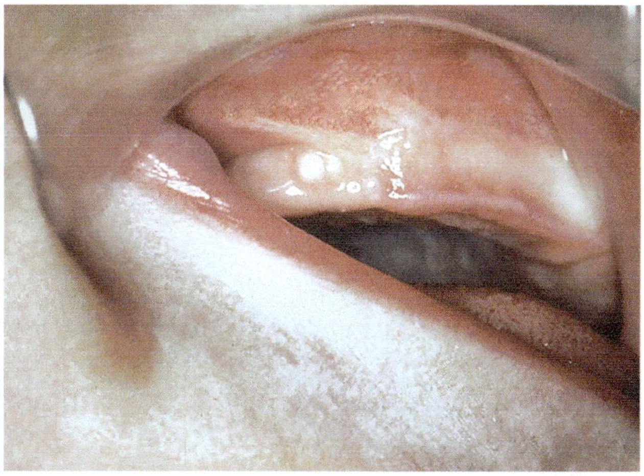

Figure 19.56 Gingival cysts of newborn.

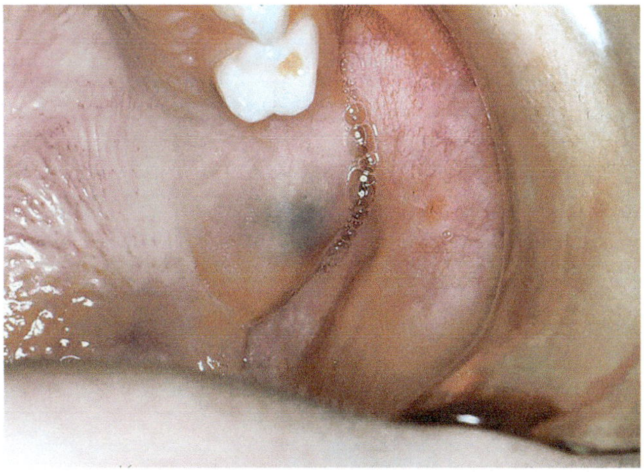

Figure 19.57 Eruption cyst 1.

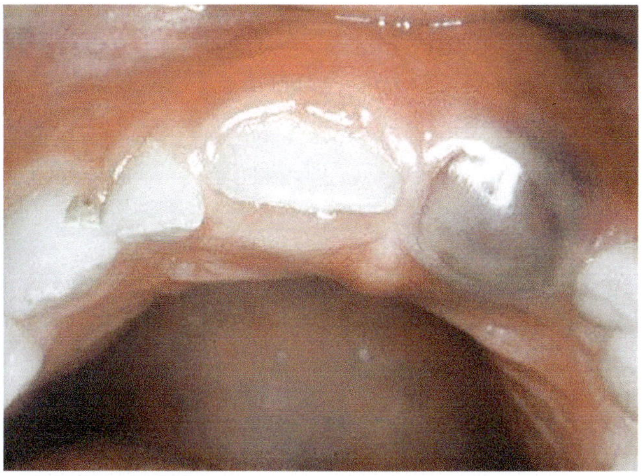

Figure 19.58 Eruption cyst 2.

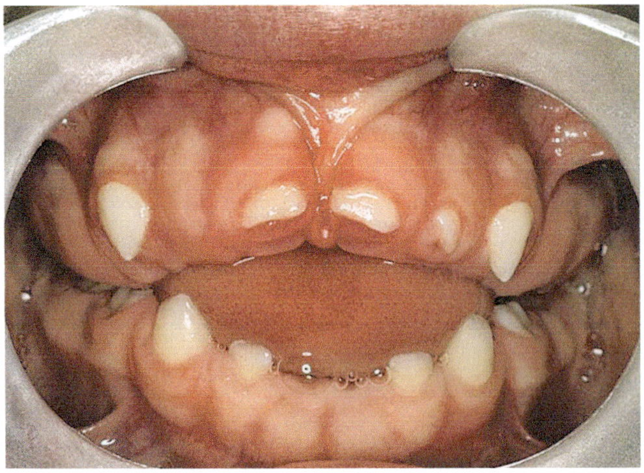
Figure 19.59 Hereditary gingival fibromatosis 1.

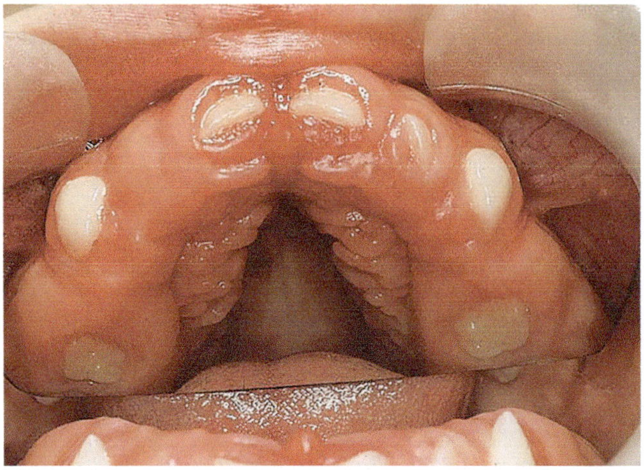
Figure 19.60 Hereditary gingival fibromatosis 2.

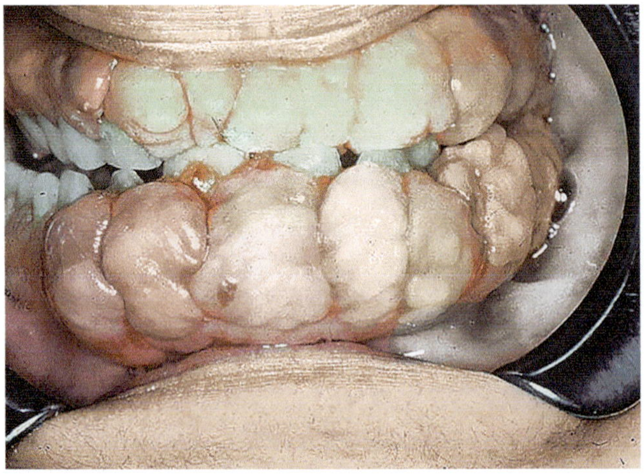
Figure 19.61 Severe cyclosporin-induced gingival hyperplasia.

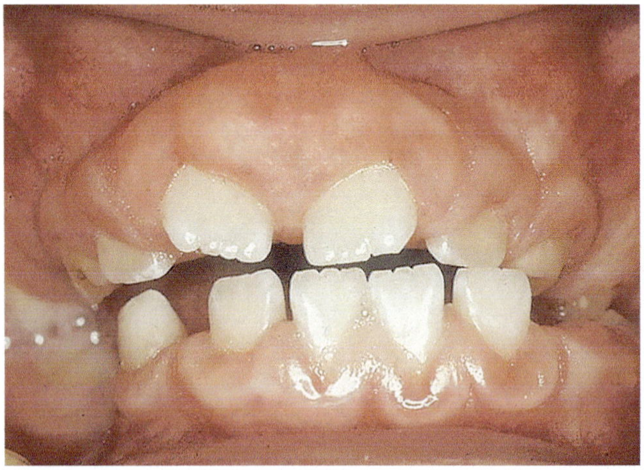
Figure 19.62 Moderate drug-induced gingival hyperplasia.

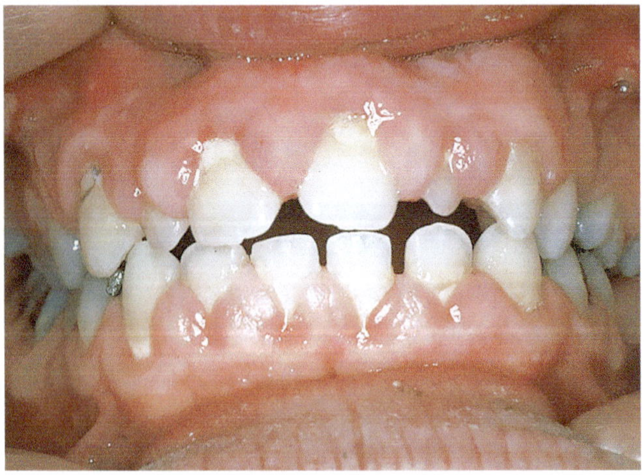
Figure 19.63 Moderate drug-induced gingival hypertrophy 2.

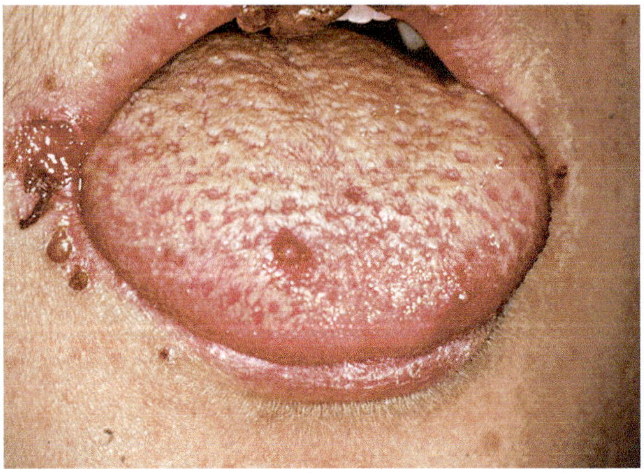
Figure 19.64 Lesions in primary herpetic gingivostomatitis 1.

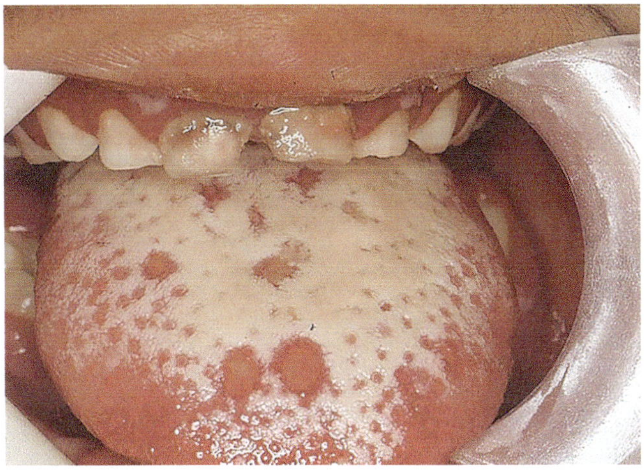

Figure 19.65 Primary herpetic gingivostomatitis.

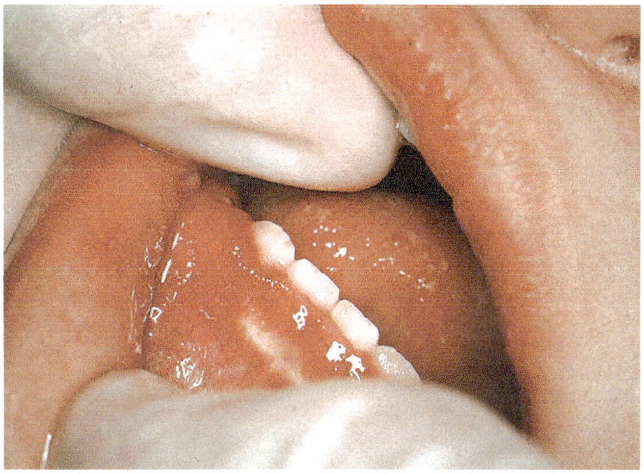

Figure 19.66 Gingivae in primary herpetic gingivostomatitis 2.

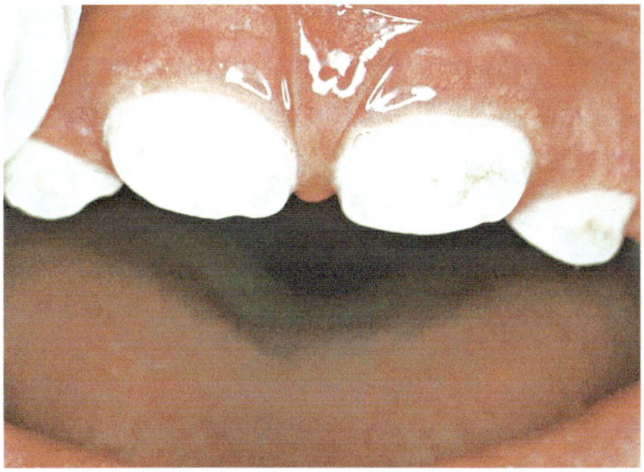

Figure 19.67 Gingivitis associated with primary herpes.

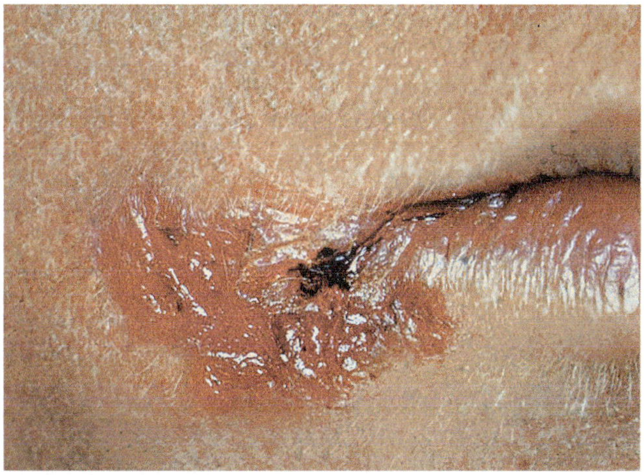

Figure 19.68 Recurrent herpes simplex.

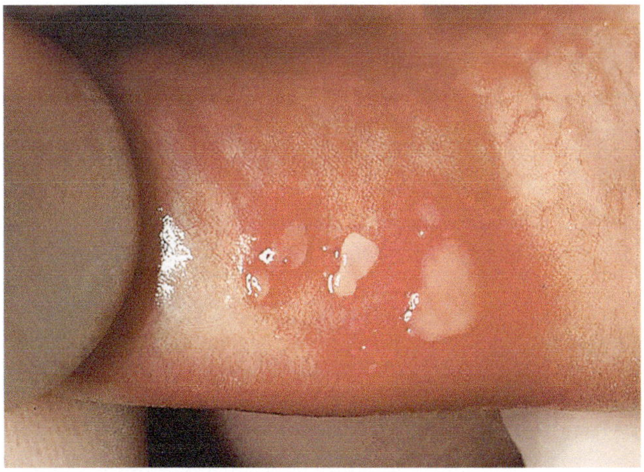

Figure 19.69 Oral lesions of hand, foot and mouth.

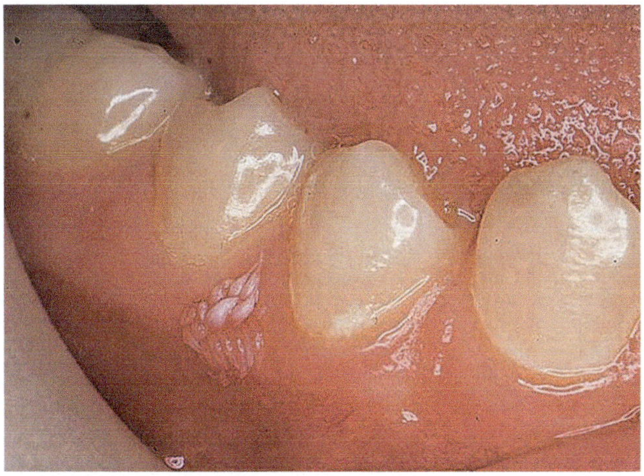

Figure 19.70 Human papillomavirus.

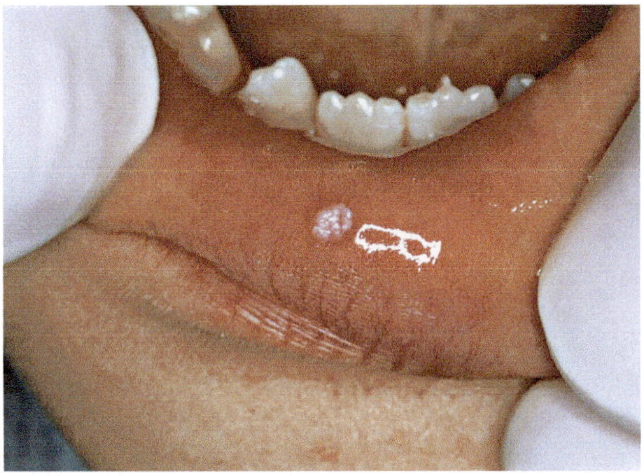

Figure 19.71 Squamous cell papilloma.

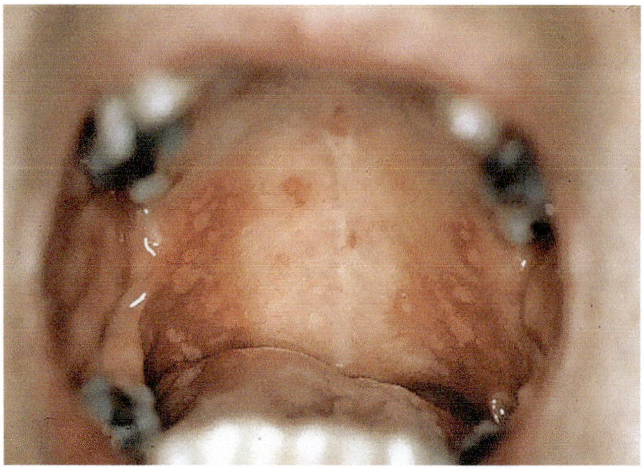

Figure 19.72 Herpangina.

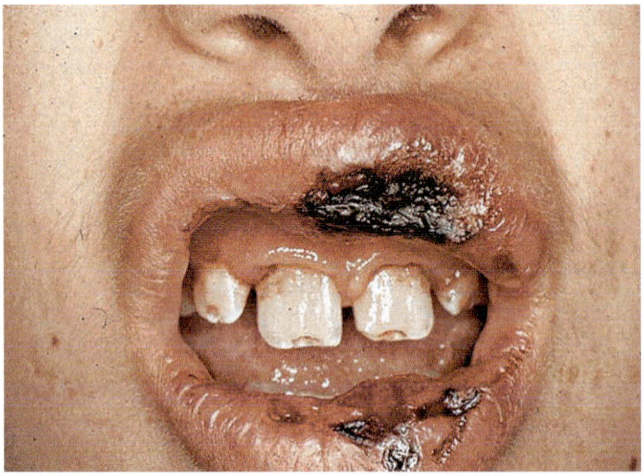

Figure 19.73 Secondary infection of lip lesions in leukaemia.

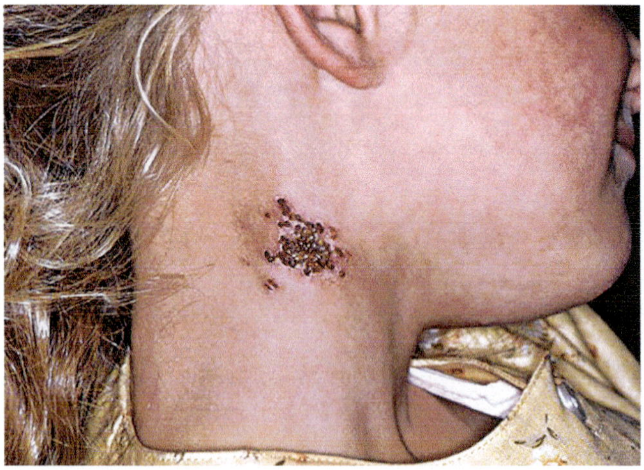

Figure 19.74 Shingles.

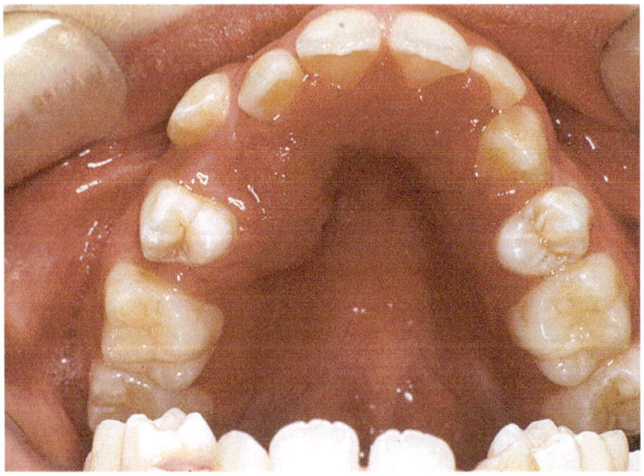

Figure 19.75 Denture-induced stomatitis.

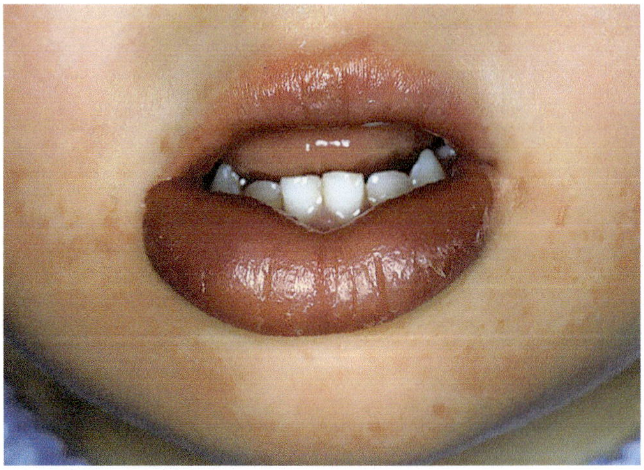

Figure 19.76 Lip swelling in orofacial granulomatosis 1.

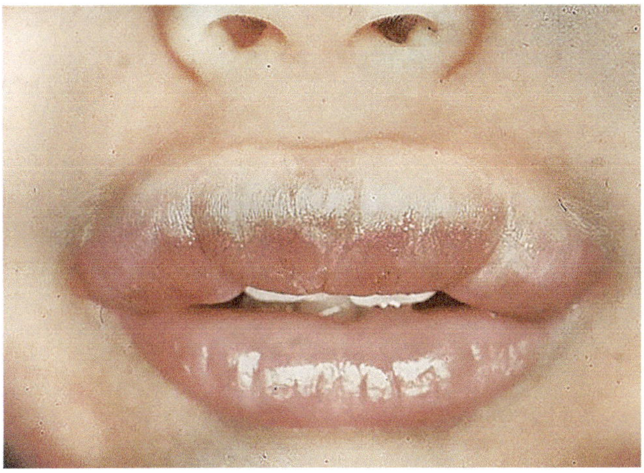

Figure 19.77 Lip swelling in orofacial granulomatosis 2.

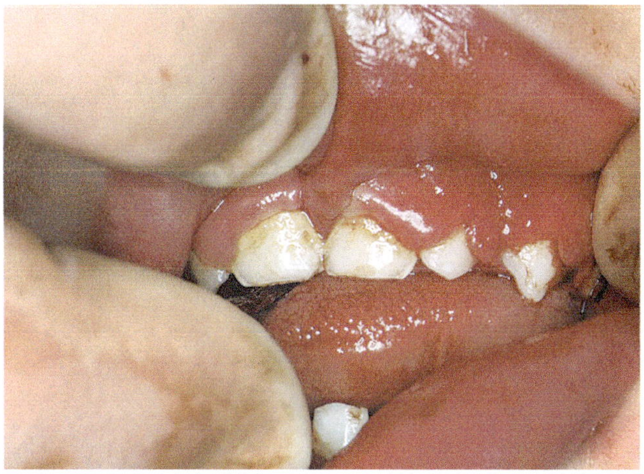

Figure 19.78 Full width gingivitis in orofacial granulomatosis.

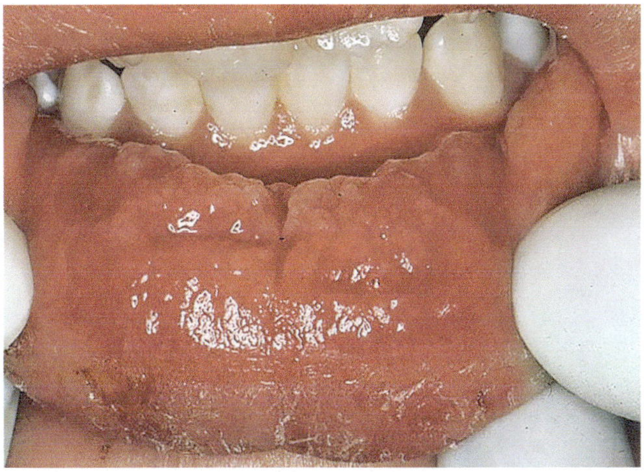

Figure 19.79 Orofacial granulomatosis cobblestone appearance of mucosa.

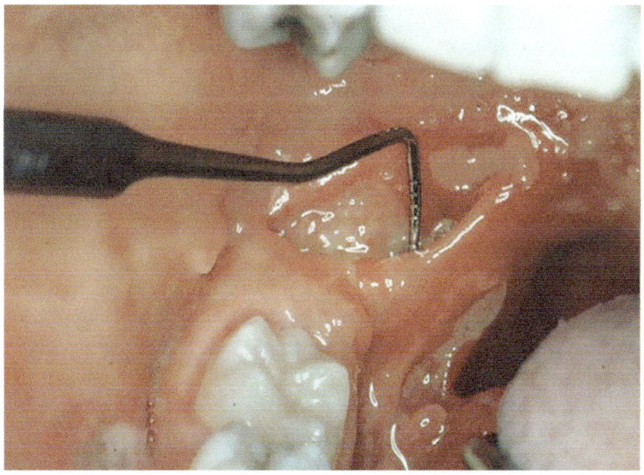

Figure 19.80 Orofacial granulomatosis penetrating ulceration.

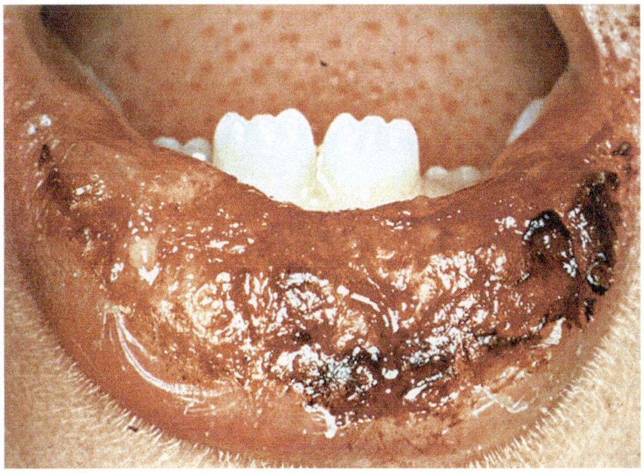

Figure 19.81 Erythema multiforme.

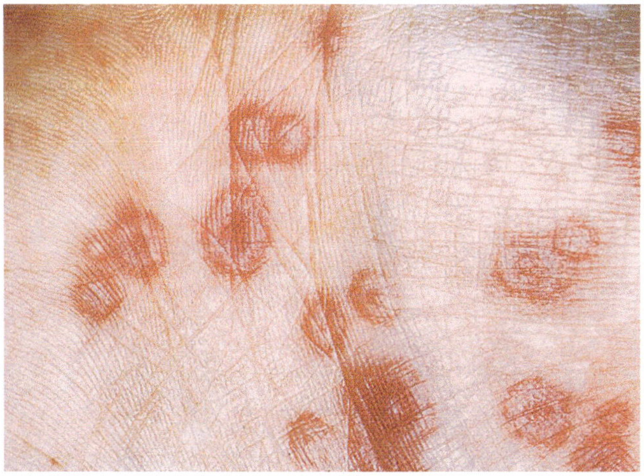

Figure 19.82 Target lesions of Steven–Johnson syndrome.

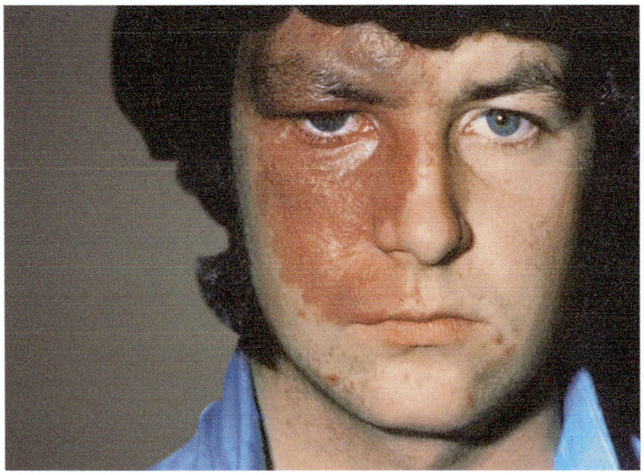

Figure 19.83 Haemangioma of Sturge–Webber syndrome.

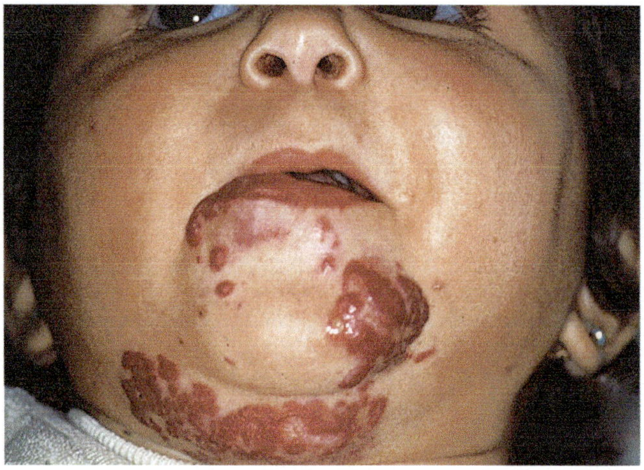

Figure 19.84 Cavernous haemangioma.

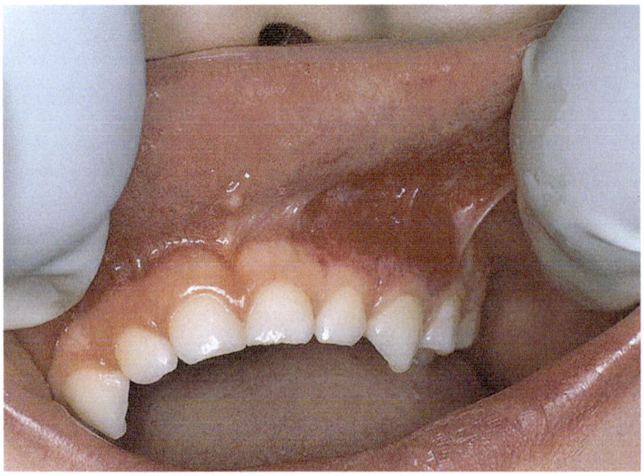

Figure 19.85 Intraoral capillary haemangioma.

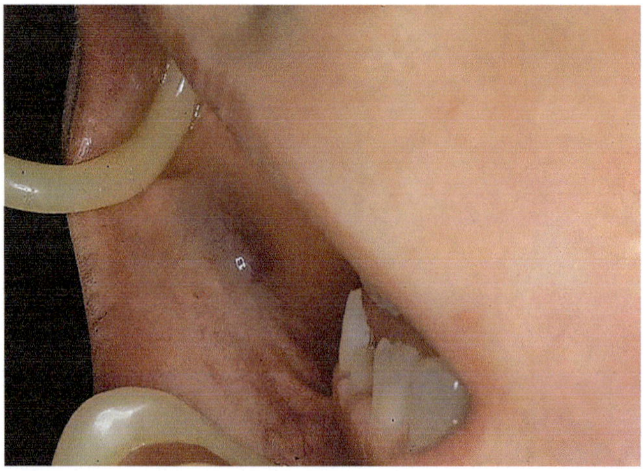

Figure 19.86 Intraoral haemangioma.

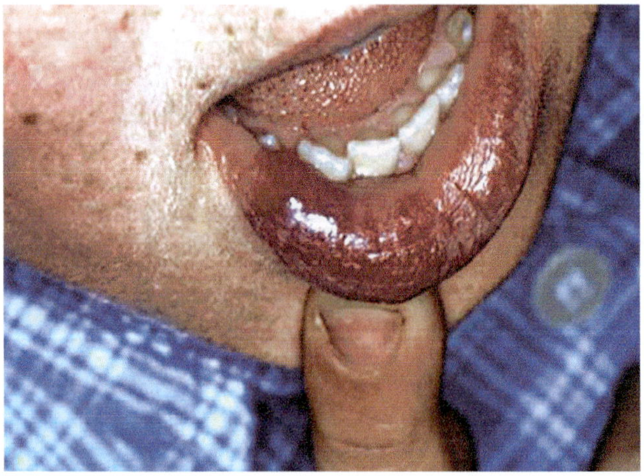

Figure 19.87 Haemangioma birth mark.

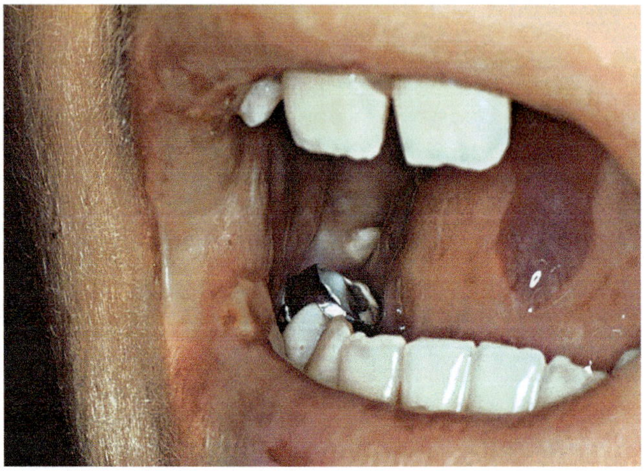

Figure 19.88 Oral bullae in epidermolysis bullosa.

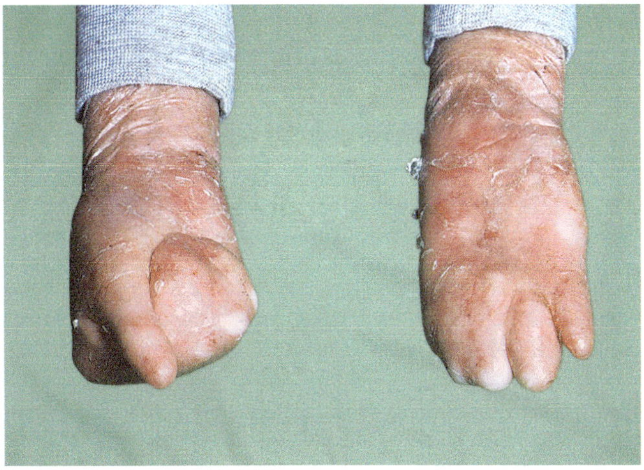

Figure 19.89 Hands in epidermolysis bullosa.

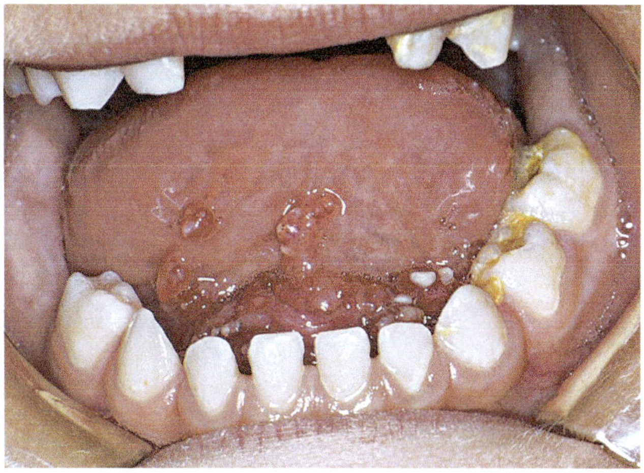

Figure 19.90 Lymphangioma.

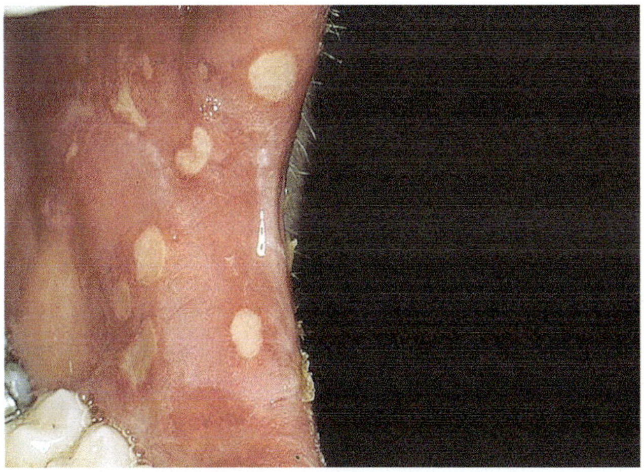

Figure 19.91 Minor aphthous ulceration.

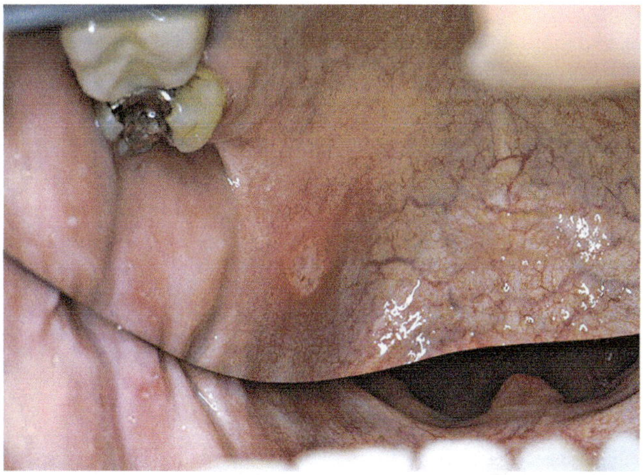

Figure 19.92 Aphthous ulceration.

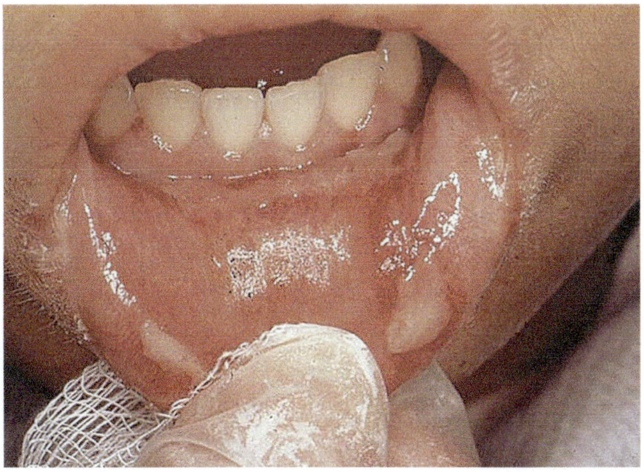

Figure 19.93 Radiation mucositis.

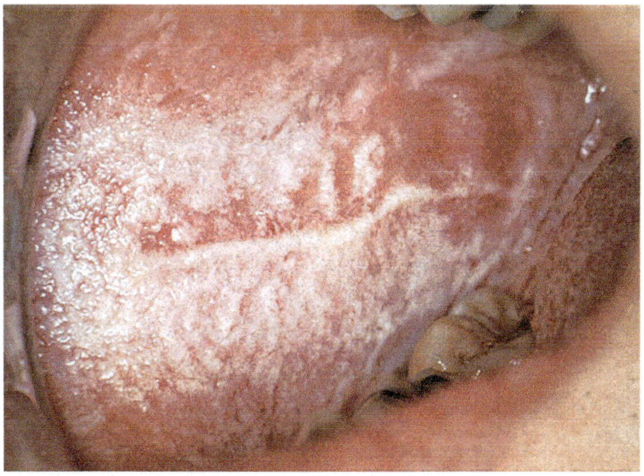

Figure 19.94 Leukoderma.

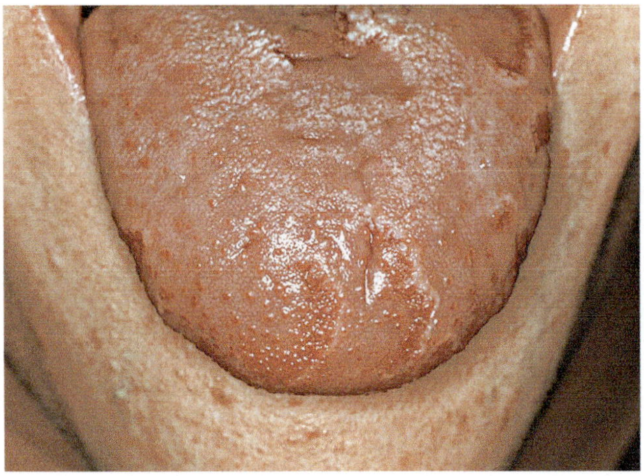

Figure 19.95 Geographic tongue 1.

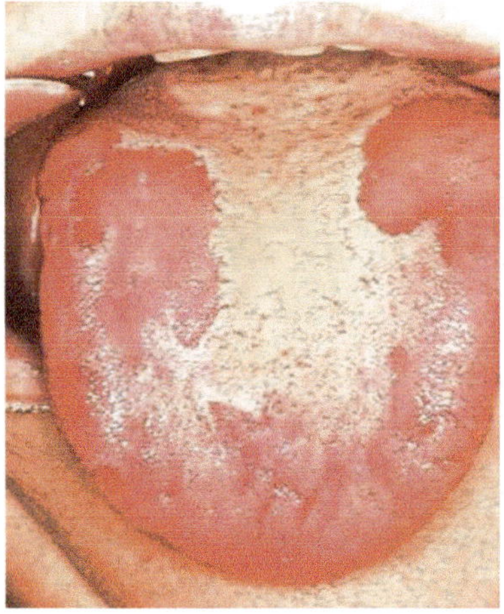

Figure 19.96 Geographic tongue 2.

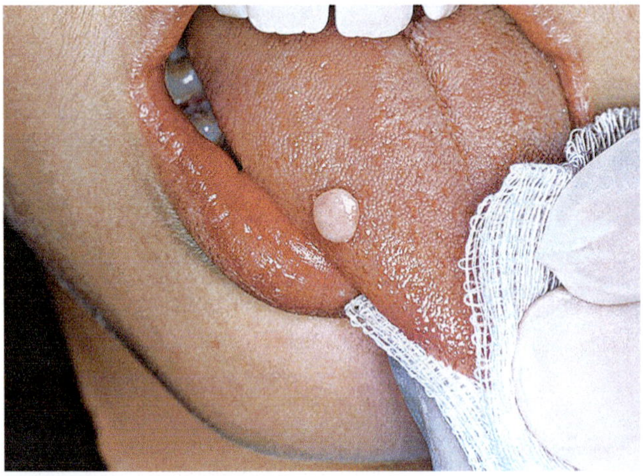

Figure 19.97 Fibroepithelial polyp 1.

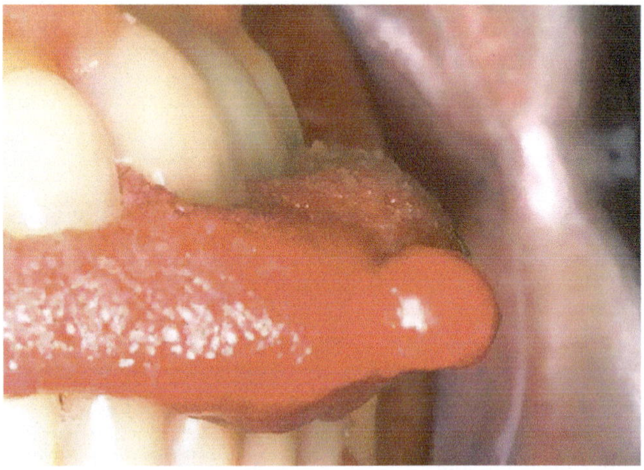

Figure 19.98 Fibroepithelial polyp 2.

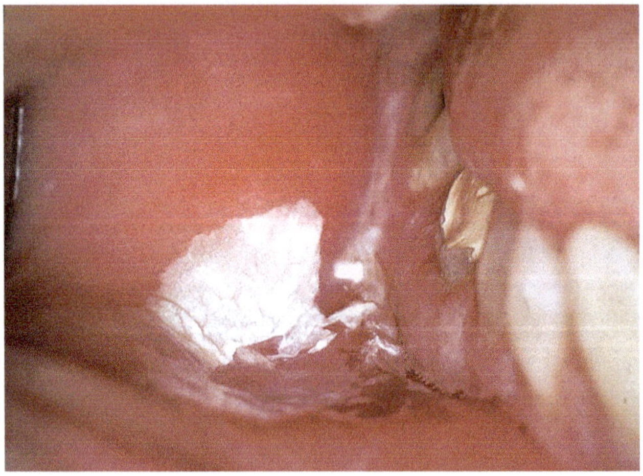

Figure 19.99 Aspirin burn.

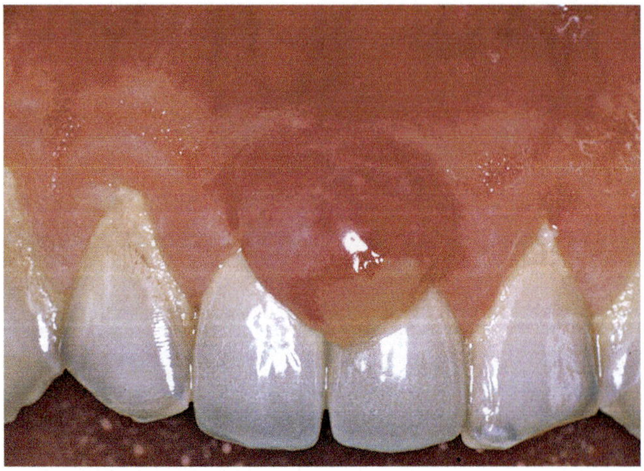

Figure 19.100 Pyogenic granuloma.

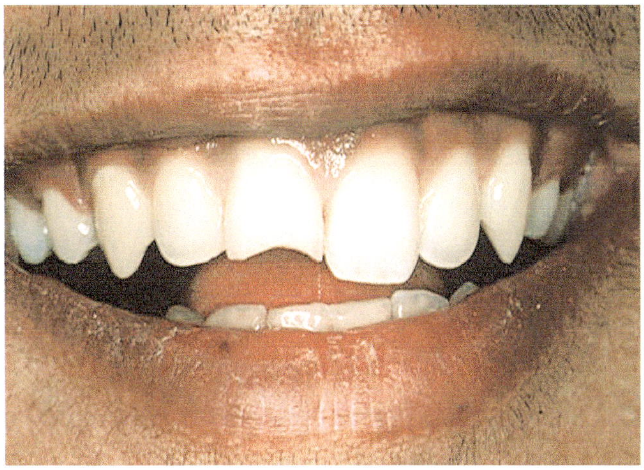

Figure 19.101 Trauma dentine enamel fracture 2.

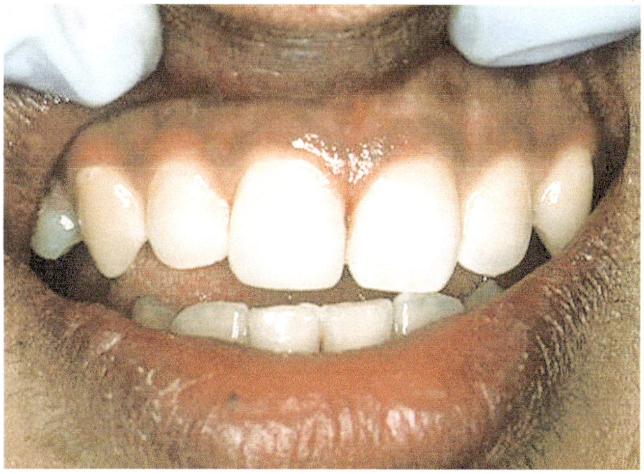

Figure 19.102 Trauma dentine enamel fracture 2 restored.

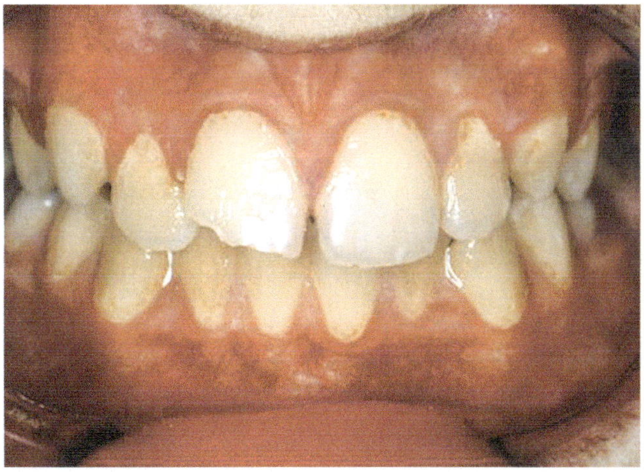

Figure 19.103 Trauma dentine enamel fracture 1.

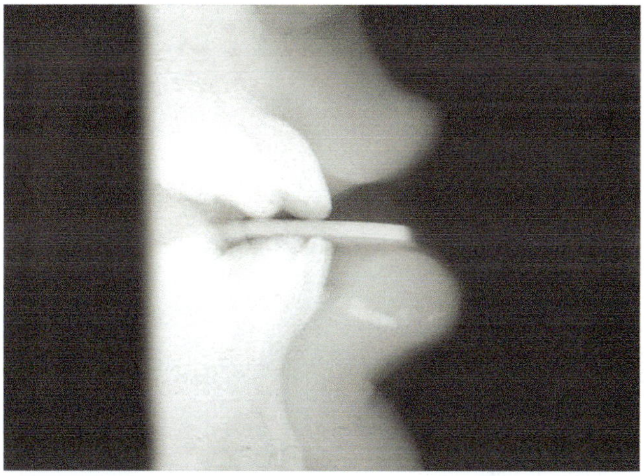

Figure 19.104 Foreign body in lip from dentine enamel fracture in Figure 19.103.

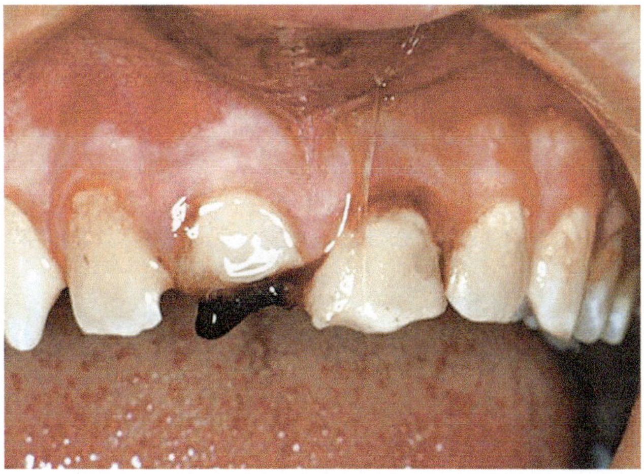

Figure 19.105 Trauma dentine enamel pulp fracture.

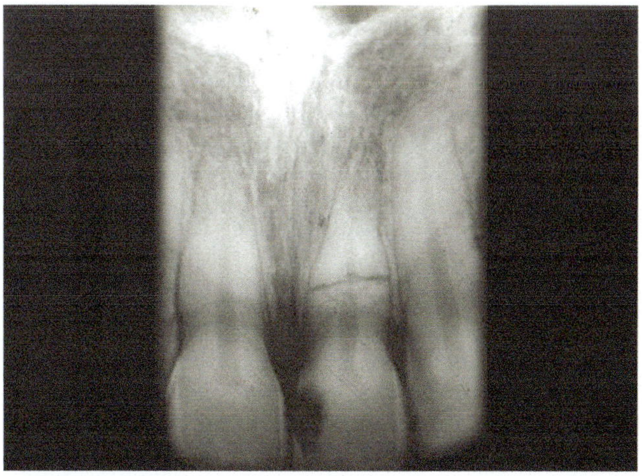

Figure 19.106 Trauma root fracture radiograph.

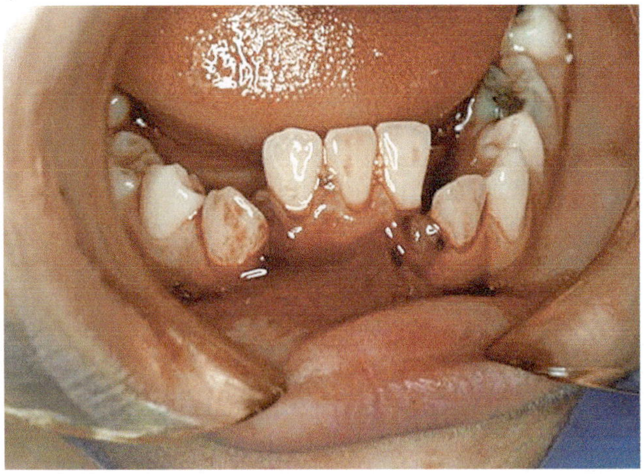

Figure 19.107 Trauma dentoalveolar fracture.

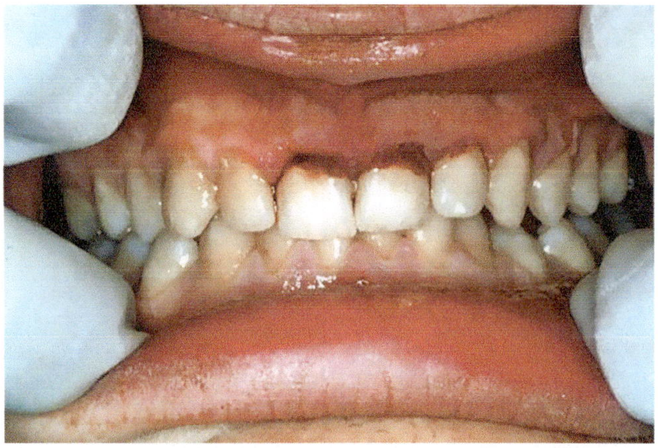

Figure 19.108 Trauma subluxation injury.

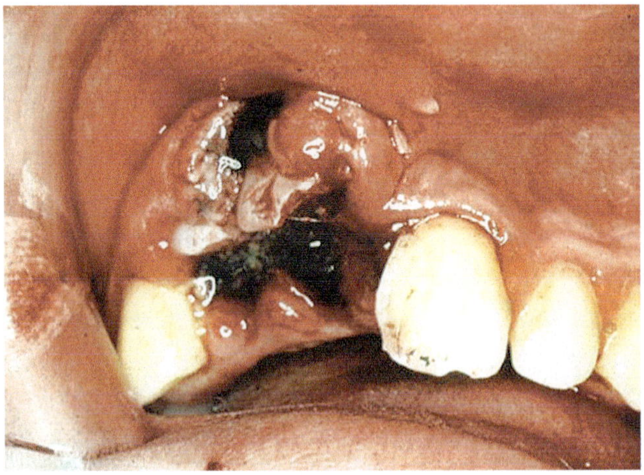

Figure 19.109 Trauma intrusion injury.

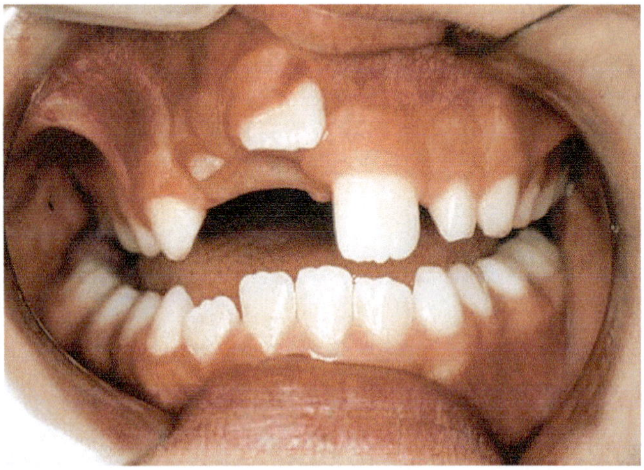

Figure 19.110 Trauma intrusion injury same as Figure 19.109.

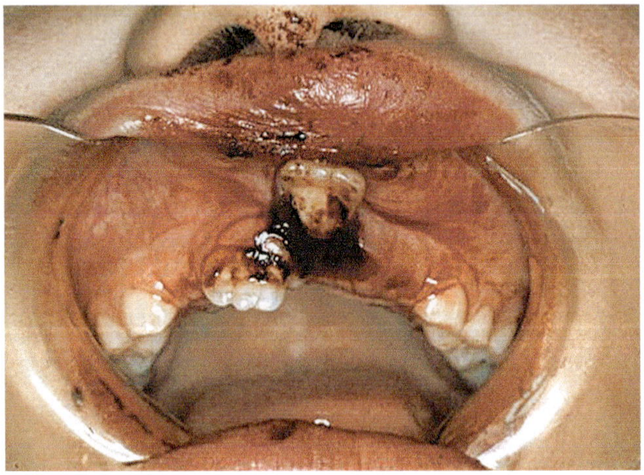

Figure 19.111 Trauma lateral luxation injury.

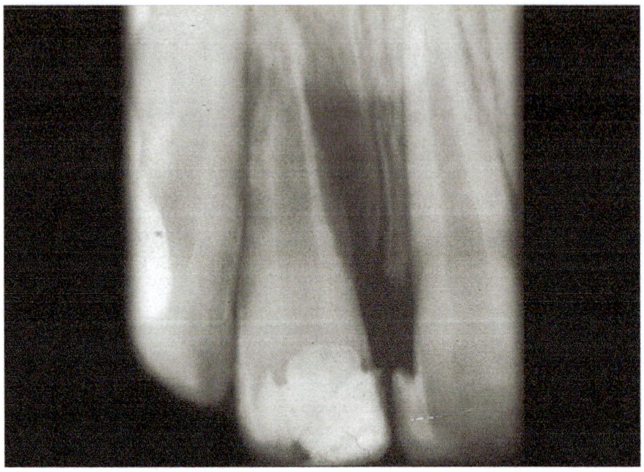

Figure 19.112 Trauma external inflammatory resorption.

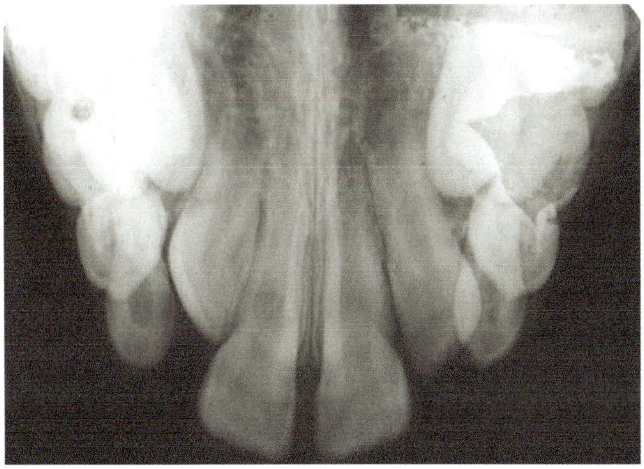

Figure 19.113 Trauma internal inflammatory resorption.

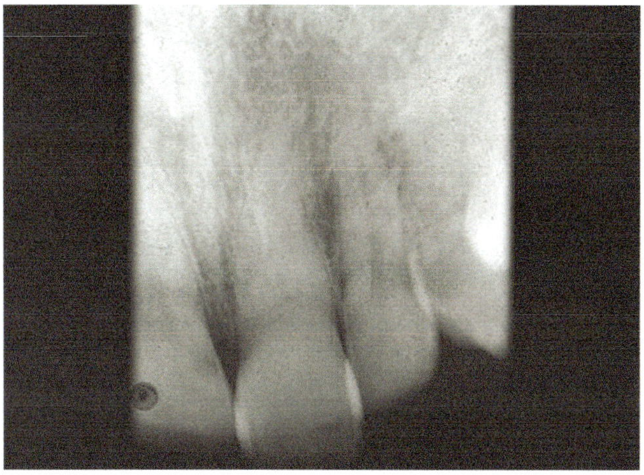

Figure 19.114 Trauma pulp canal obliteration radiographic.

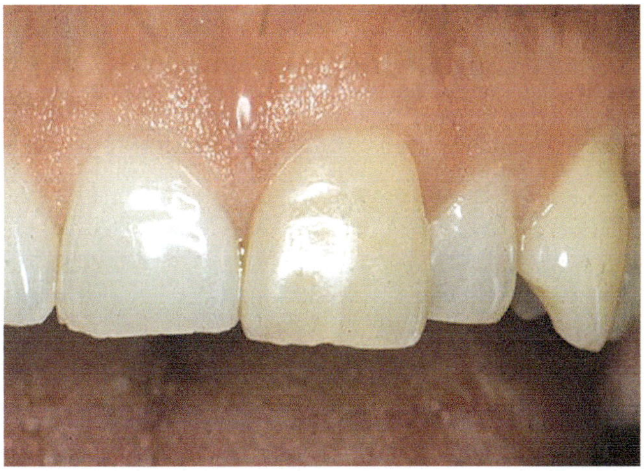

Figure 19.115 Trauma pulp canal obliteration.

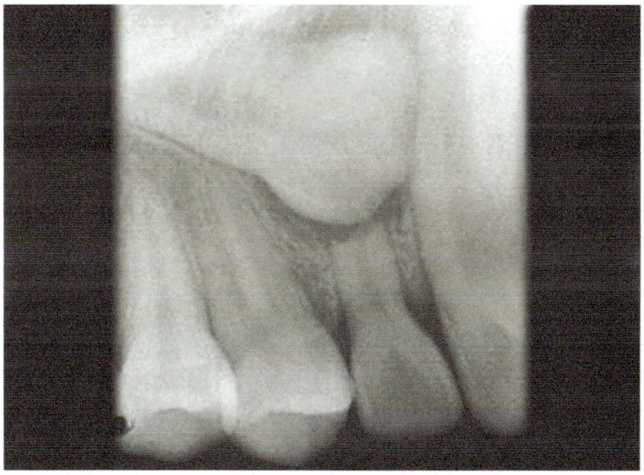

Figure 19.116 External surface resorption 1.

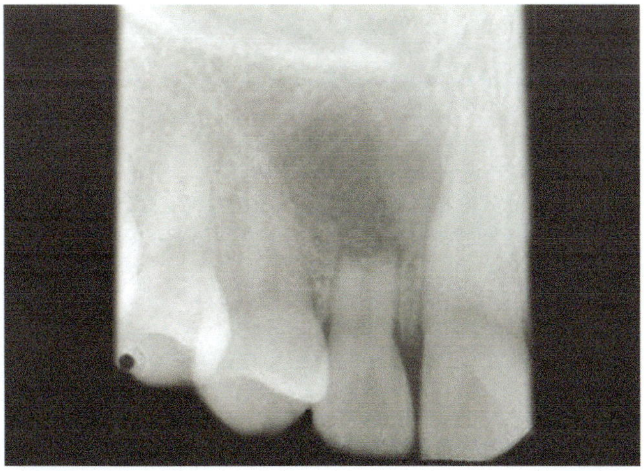

Figure 19.117 External surface resorption 2.

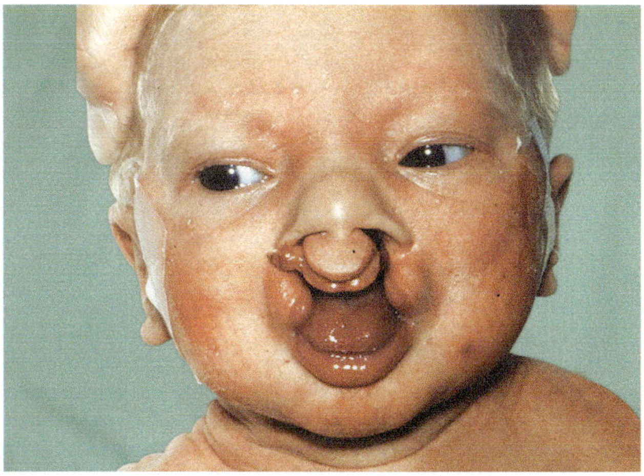

Figure 19.118 Facial view of bilateral cleft lip and palate 1.

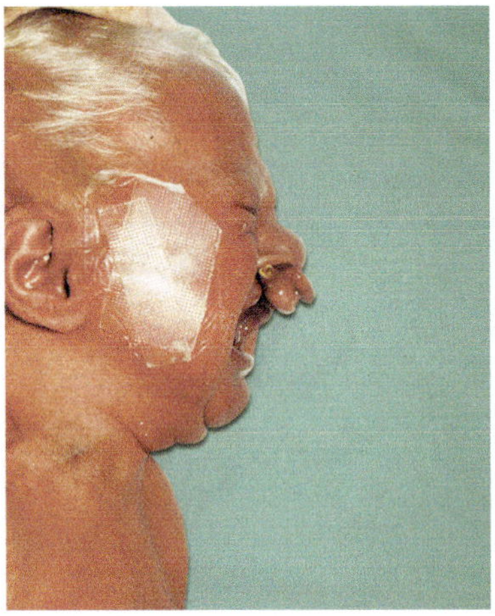

Figure 19.119 Lateral view of bilateral cleft lip and palate.

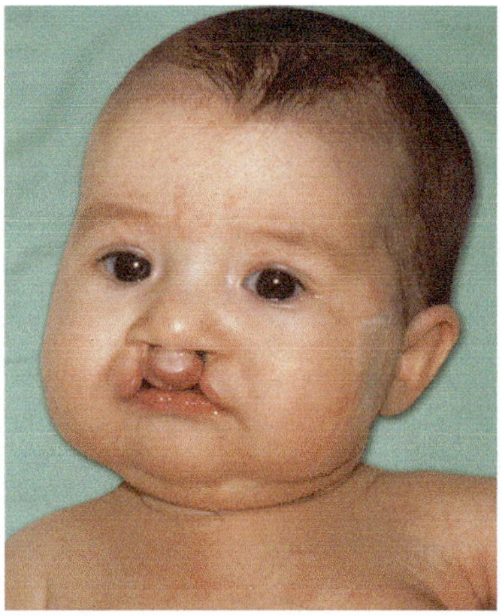

Figure 19.120 Facial view of bilateral cleft lip and palate 2.

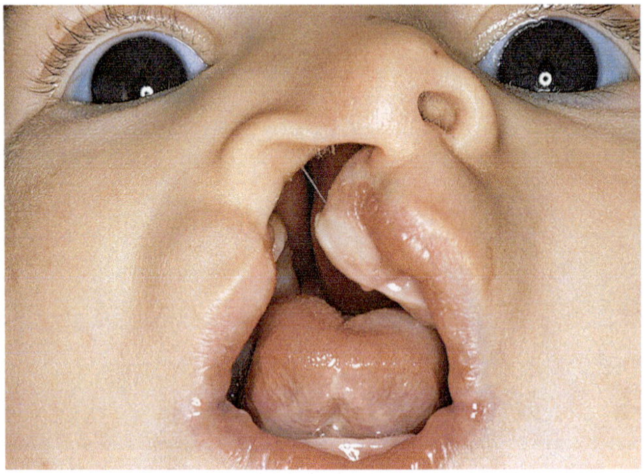

Figure 19.121 Unilateral cleft lip and palate.

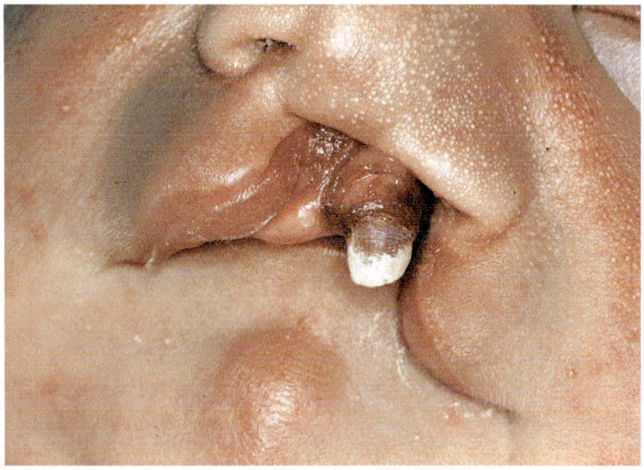

Figure 19.122 Tooth protruding from premaxillary cleft site 2.

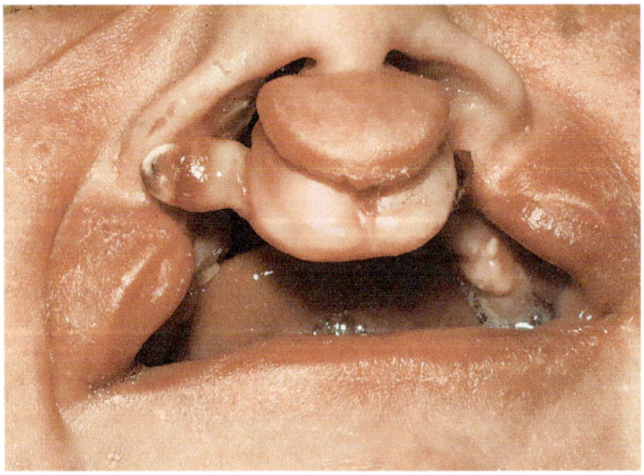

Figure 19.123 Tooth protruding from premaxillary cleft site.

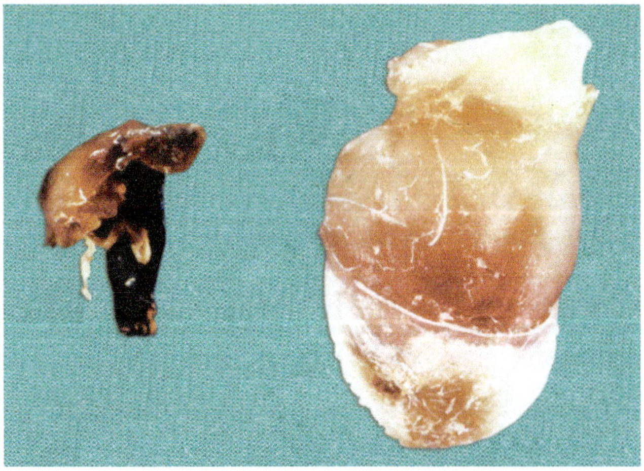

Figure 19.124 Deformed and carious teeth removed from cleft site.

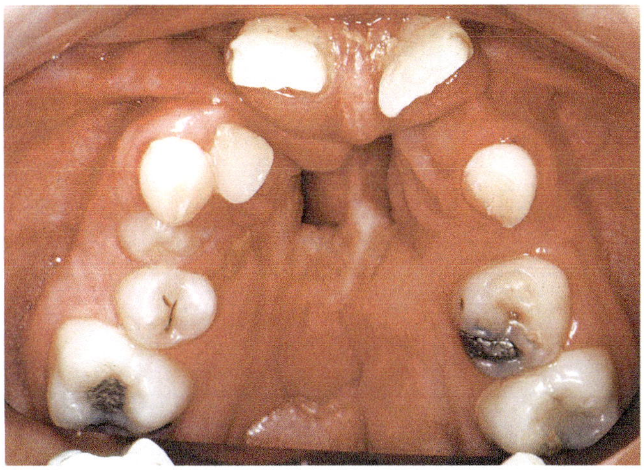

Figure 19.125 Residual fistula following bilateral cleft repair.

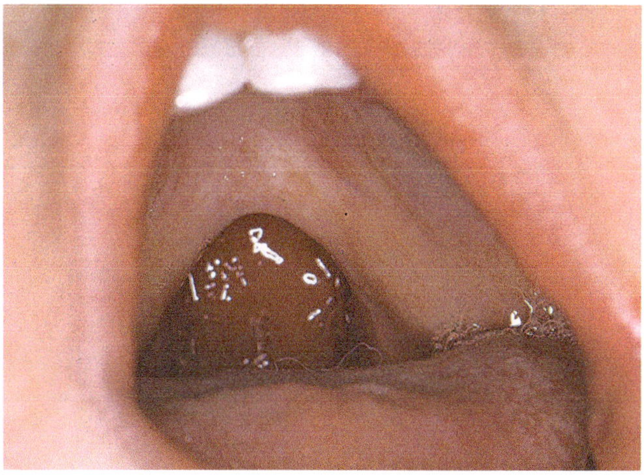

Figure 19.126 Missing uvula.

CHAPTER 20

Immunity and Allergy

Rosemary Anne Hague

IMMUNITY

In order to grow and develop normally, we have to develop methods of protecting ourselves from organisms that have the potential for invasion and to cause damage. Pathogenesis of infectious disease is not only dependent upon characteristics of the pathogen but also upon our immune response to it. As children develop from foetal life through infancy into childhood, so their immune systems are continuing to mature. Hence, susceptibility to different infectious agents varies with age.

COMPONENTS OF THE IMMUNE SYSTEM

The first line of defence against infection is the physical barrier formed by the skin and mucous membranes.

Skin

The epidermis is made up of four layers of densely packed cells, through which bacteria cannot penetrate. The outer layers are shed, taking organisms with them. Its dryness, together with the high salt content due to sweat, and low pH due to sebum and lactobacilli inhibit bacterial growth. Sweat also contains lysozyme, which is an antimicrobial enzyme, particularly for Gram-positive organisms. Sebum from hair follicles contains lipids, salts and proteins, which have antimicrobial properties, but it also provides nutrition for commensal organisms such as *Corynebacteria*. Skin cells can also secrete antimicrobial peptides such as cathelicidins, defensins and dermcidins. These peptides do not only have a direct effect, but they also stimulate components of the innate and adaptive immune system. Organisms that are able to colonise the skin surface inhibit pathogens, and many secrete proteins toxic to other species, known as bacteriocins.

Cells of the innate immune systems (Langerhans cells, mast cells) and adaptive immune system (lymphocytes) are also found in the dermis should the superficial epidermis be penetrated.

Mucous Membranes

These are body surfaces not covered by skin. They are, therefore, protected by viscous mucus, which traps microorganisms, and by washing. E.g., tears wash organisms from the conjunctiva, and saliva and chewing of food has the same function in the mouth.

Respiratory Tract

The nasal turbinates are designed to trap large particles, preventing their travelling down the respiratory tract. Smaller particles get further down, but cough and irritant receptors stimulate cough and bronchoconstriction, enabling them to be cleared. The mucociliary blanket is the chief means of clearing the respiratory tract from the smallest bronchioles to the larynx. In addition, compounds secreted onto the surface of the respiratory epithelium enhance bacterial killing. These include lysozyme, transferrin, alpha 1 antitrypsin, opsonins, interferon as well as immunoglobulins (Ig) and complement.

Gastrointestinal Tract

In contrast to the respiratory tract, where potential pathogens are swept proximally in the gut, peristalsis keeps bacteria moving distally to be eliminated. Gastric acid creates a stomach pH, which is toxic to many bacteria, and those surviving to pass into the small intestine encounter bile and pancreatic secretions. The gut is not a sterile environment, and the normal gut flora is important in keeping pathogenic bacteria at bay. The intestinal wall is protected from invasion by these organisms by intestinal mucins which bind potential pathogens. Molecules such as lysozyme and immunoglobulins are secreted onto the epithelial surface. The epithelial cells themselves are joined by tight junctions, which limit the passage of antigens across the barrier.

Urogenital Tract

The flow of urine washes microorganisms away from the mucosal surface. Vaginal mucus performs the same function. In addition, the vesicoureteric junction acts as a one way valve, preventing urine (and micro-organisms) flowing towards the kidneys.

THE NEXT LINE OF DEFENCE: INNATE (NONSPECIFIC) IMMUNITY

Both humoural (chemical) agents and cells play major roles.

Humoural Agents

These agents are as follows:

Acute-phase Proteins

These are proteins produced by the liver whose plasma levels rise in response to inflammation.

C-reactive protein assists complement in binding to foreign or damaged cells.

Mannose-binding lectin binds to carbohydrate moieties on the surface of bacteria and fungi, thus activating the lectin pathway of the complement system.

Alpha 1 antitrypsin and *alpha 2 macroglobulin* inhibit the activity of harmful proteases produced by bacteria.

Ferritin binds iron, which is necessary for bacterial growth.

Others include coagulation factors (fibrinogen, plasminogen, factor VIII, von Willebrand factor), components of complement, amyloid P and amyloid A.

Antibacterial Agents

These include lysozyme, defensins, lactoferrin and myeloperoxidase.

Complement

This is a series of blood proteins which, when activated, lead to lysis of bacteria and also stimulate chemotaxis and phagocytosis.

The *classical pathway* is activated by bacterial antigen bound to antibody. The *alternative pathway* is activated directly by bacterial or fungal oligosaccharide, endotoxin and immunoglobulin aggregates. The *lectin pathway* is activated by mannose-binding lectin bound to its receptor on the bacterial surface (Fig. 20.1).

Cells of Innate Immune System

Phagocytes

These include monocytes/macrophages and neutrophils. They engulf opsonised bacteria and kill them within the phagosome. The most important mechanism for bacterial killing is the oxidative burst, illustrated in Figure 20.2. The oxygen radicals, hydrogen peroxide and hydroxyl ions, all mediate killing.

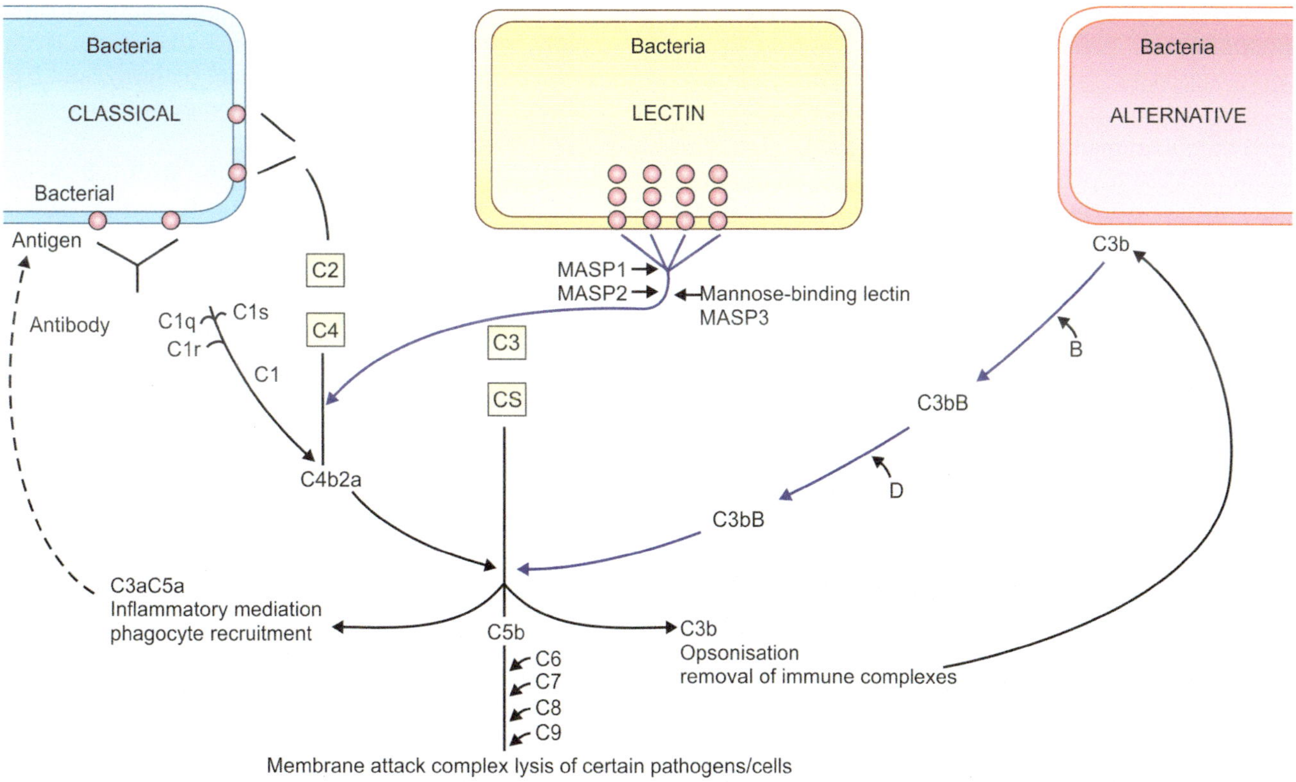

Figure 20.1 Complement cascade—classical, all ± lectin pathways.

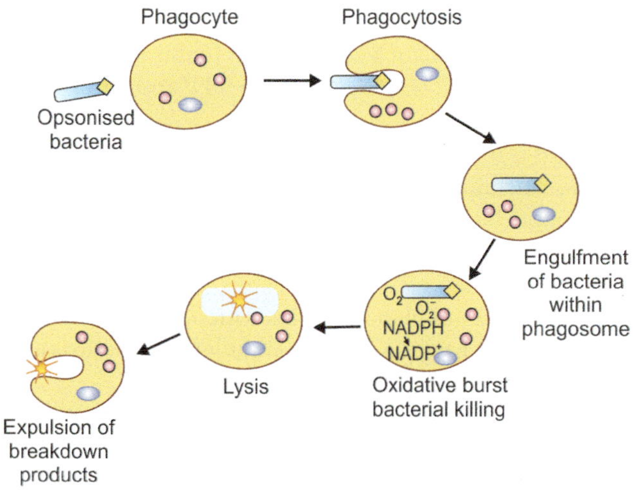

Figure 20.2 Phagocytosis with oxidative burst.

Eosinophils

These comprise 1–3% of circulating white blood cells. They are less efficient at phagocytosis and bacterial killing than neutrophils. They can kill parasites opsonised by antibody or complement. Eosinophil granule protein contains some powerful inflammatory mediators, which can kill helminths directly, and induce basophil histamine release. It has long been assumed that they have a major role in defence against parasites, but their true function is unclear. When activated during an allergic response, these mediators cause tissue damage, particularly to the respiratory epithelium, causing chronic inflammatory change.

Basophils

These cells develop from promyelocytes in the bone marrow. They have granules containing many of the same mediators of immediate hypersensitivity as mast cells, but do not release heparin or arachidonic acid metabolites. They are found in the circulation. Again, it is assumed that they have some role in defence against parasitic disease.

Mast Cells

These cells develop from pluripotential stem cells (CD34+ cells), which migrate into tissues, and mature into mast cells, which are differentiated from each other, depending on their site. They are activated in allergy, but can also be activated by pathogens or their products, peptide mediators such as substance P, endothelin and components of complement. They have high affinity for IgE and release chemicals such as histamine, neutrophil chemotactic factor, inflammatory proteases and heparin, which are preformed inflammatory mediators contained in granules. When stimulated, they also produce arachidonic acid metabolites and platelet-activating factor.

Natural Killer Cells

These are large lymphocytes that recognise and kill cells infected with viruses or intracellular pathogens such as *Listeria* and *Toxoplasma*. They also recognise tumour cells. They recognise these cells either because of reduced expression of class I human leucocyte antigen molecules on their surface, or by binding to CD16 receptor on an antibody-coated target cell (antibody dependent cellular cytotoxicity). They release granules that increase the permeability of the target cell (perforin) and cytokines which promote apoptosis.

THE ADAPTIVE (ACQUIRED) IMMUNE SYSTEM

Humoural Agents: Immunoglobulins

These are proteins, which mediate antibody responses, and are found in blood, tissues and secretions, and also as part of the surface membrane of B cells. They combine with antigen to form immune complexes and can opsonise bacteria, fix complement and neutralise viruses.

Figures 20.3A to E show the basic structure of immunoglobulin. Each molecule consists of two heavy chains and two light chains, joined by disulphide bridges. The characteristics of the five classes are shown as follows:

1. *IgG:* It activates complement via the classical pathway, opsonises organisms and mediates antibody-dependent cytotoxic responses.
2. *IgM:* It is important for clearing bacteria from the blood stream by agglutination and opsonisation. It is the most efficient fixer of complement by the classical pathway.
3. *IgA:* IgA in its secretory form is important for antiviral and antibacterial activity on mucosal surfaces. It can fix complement via the alternate pathway, and has bactericidal activity when combined with lysozyme and complement.
4. *IgD:* The majority of IgDis bound to B cell membranes, where it acts as an antigen receptor, and is important in the development of B cell responses.
5. *IgE:* It triggers immediate hypersensitivity. This may be important in defence against worm infection, by binding to the worm, and stimulating mast cell degranulation, leading to the worm being flushed from the mucosal surface.

Cells of Adaptive Immune System

T Cells

These are the co-ordinators and regulators of specific immunity. They interact with cells of the innate immune system (antigen-presenting cells) and with B cells and produce cytokines which stimulate or suppress the activity of other inflammatory cells.

Antigen Presentation and T Cells

In the process of phagocytosis and elimination of organisms within the phagosome, not all foreign

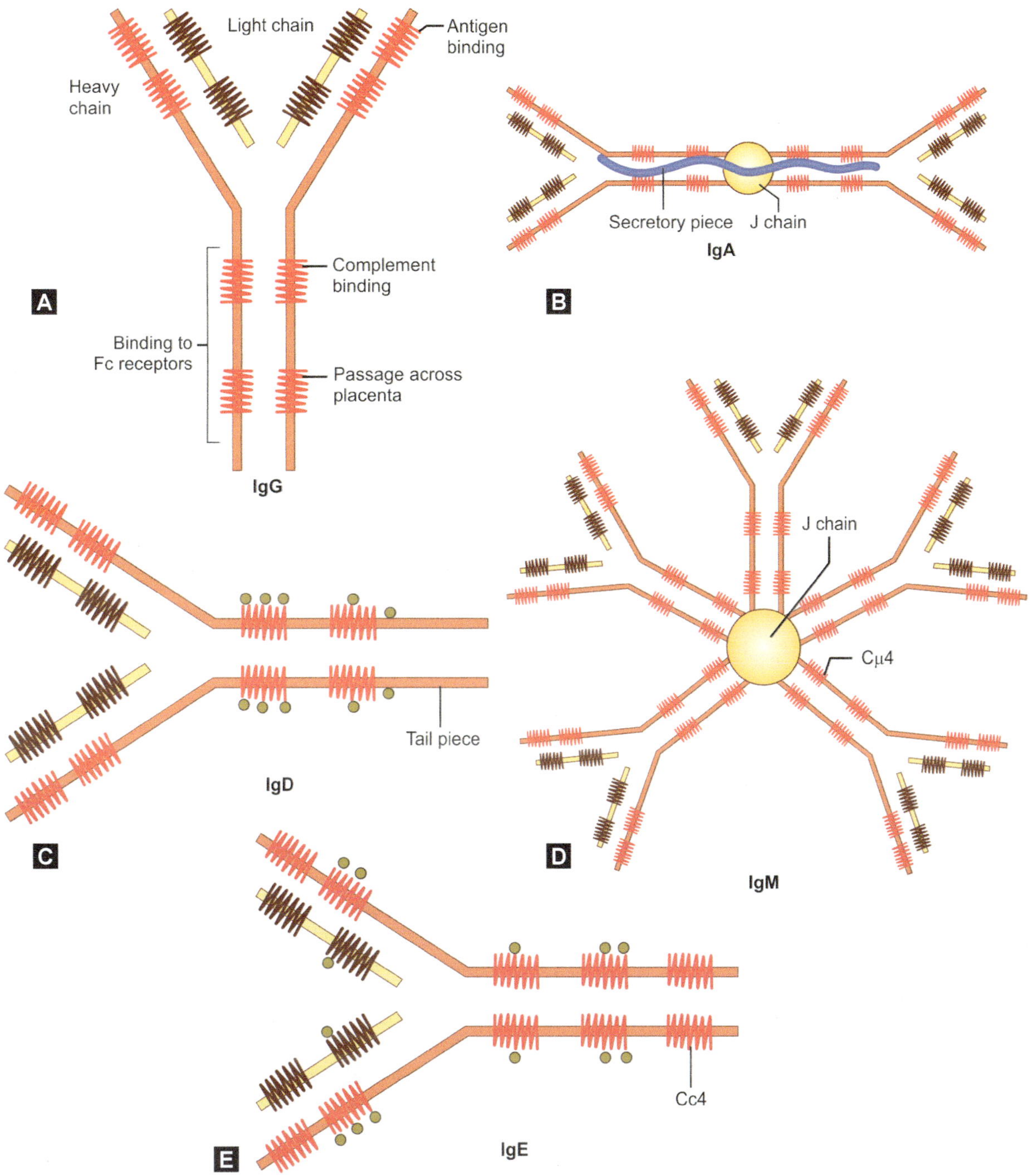

Figures 20.3A to E Basic structures of type of immunoglobulins and classes.

protein is destroyed. A small portion is preserved and then presented on the surface of the cell associated with molecules of the major histocompatibility complex (MHC). The T cell receptor binds to this complex, and is activated, as illustrated in **Figure 20.4**. Macrophages function both as phagocytes and antigen-presenting cells, whereas the major role of dendritic cells is to capture antigen for presentation. Other cells, such as B cells and virus infected cells, can also present antigen + MHC.

T cells are classified according to their surface markers and function.

T Helper Cells

T helper (Th) cells have the CD4 marker. They recognise antigen associated with class II MHC.

Th1 cells They differentiate under the influence of interferon gamma and interleukin 12 (IL12). Activation leads to release of IL2, interferon gamma and tumour necrosis

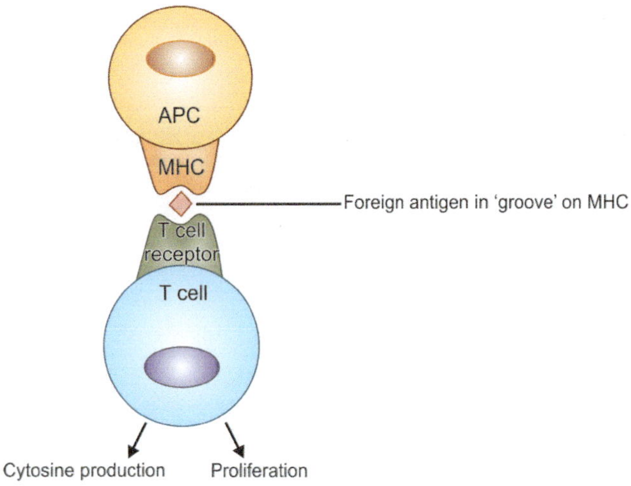

Figure 20.4 Antigen presentation.

factor. These stimulate cytotoxic T cells and cell-mediated immune responses, including delayed hypersensitivity.

Th2 cells These are the main co-ordinators of B cell responses. They possess CD40 ligand which binds to CD40 on the immature B cell surface. This leads to B cell isotype switching and production of B cell memory cells. The main cytokine involved is IL4. Activation of Th2 also leads to stimulation of IgE production, and so mediates immediate hypersensitivity.

Th0 cells They initially produce both Th1 and Th2 cytokines. However, either response may predominate, depending on genetic predisposition, type of antigen exposure and influence of costimulatory molecules.

Cytotoxic T Cells

These are characterised by the CD8 marker, which binds to MHC class I. They are responsible for killing virus-infected cells.

The Thymus and T Cell Immunity

Early in foetal life, immature lymphocytes enter the thymus. Once within, the genes that encode for the variable region of the T cell receptor are sequentially rearranged. This results in thousands of T cells with different receptors, recognising different MHC/antigen combinations. Those which recognise foreign antigen bound to self MHC are preserved, while those recognising non-self MHC or self-antigen are eliminated.

During the maturation process, T cells acquire the surface markers CD3, CD4, CD8 and differentiate into helper and cytotoxic/suppressor cells.

B Cells

These bone marrow-derived cells are the immunoglobulin factory. The immunoglobulin that is bound to the surface binds antigen, and with the help of T cell, the B cells proliferate. Once stimulated with antigen, IgM-producing plasma cells are formed, while other B cells become memory cells. If exposed to the same antigen again, these produce mature plasma cells, and a larger IgG response. B cells respond to polysaccharide antigen (surrounding encapsulated organisms) without T cell help, but the response is limited, resulting mainly in IgM, and no B cell memory.

Why are Neonates and Infants Prone to Infection?

Cells of the immune system develop early in foetal life. However, the main defences at this stage are the physical barriers of the uterus and the placental barrier. Infants born prematurely lack the same degree of physical protection, with thinner skin and less effective mucous membranes, in addition to immature immune responses.

By the time of birth at term, physical barriers have matured. Acute-phase proteins are present, but neonates lack terminal components of complement activation, particularly C9. These are important for lysis of Gram-negative bacteria, such as *Escherichia coli*, to which infection they are particularly susceptible.

Neutrophils comprise only 10% circulating white cells in the second trimester, but 50–60% by term. However, neonates often respond to sepsis with neutropaenia. Their neutrophils do not adhere as well to the endothelium, inhibiting migration. Chemotaxis and phagocytosis are less efficient, but bacterial killing and antigen presentation are as good as in adults.

T cell numbers are more in infancy than in adult life, but the majority of them are naïve, whereas in adults, they are primed to proliferate rapidly following repeated antigen exposure. Cytokine production, cytotoxicity, delayed hypersensitivity and B cell help are all reduced.

During the last trimester, maternal immunoglobulin (IgG) crosses the placenta, conferring passive immunity to the neonate. B cells are present at birth and can differentiate into IgM-producing plasma cells. The ability to produce T cell-dependent responses to protein antigens such as tetanus toxoid and *Haemophilus influenzae* type B (Hib) conjugate is also present at birth. However, the development of IgG-producing plasma cells and T cell-independent responses are delayed until around 2 years of age. As the normal response to polysaccharide antigens, such as those in the cell wall of encapsulated organisms requires B cells to work without T cell help, this may account for the increased susceptibility of infants to infections with organisms such as *Pneumococcus*, *Neisseria meningitidis* and *Haemophilus influenzae*. Normal immunoglobulin levels rise with age **(Fig. 20.5)**. IgA is the latest antibody to be produced, and IgA-producing plasma cells are not found until around the age of 5 years.

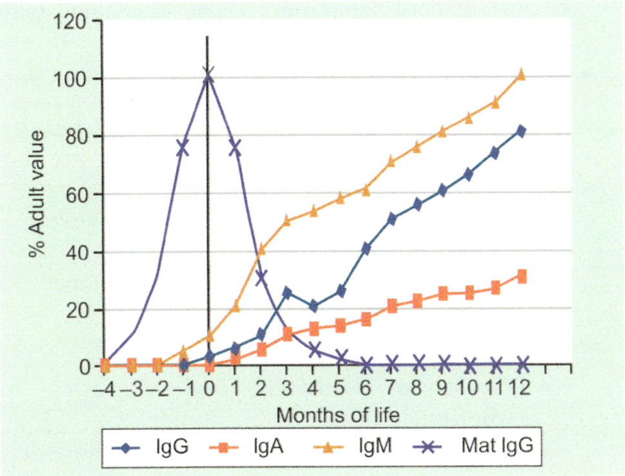

Figure 20.5 Normal level of immunoglobulin with age.

NUTRITION AND IMMUNITY

The association of undernutrition and increased susceptibility to infections, particularly respiratory and gastrointestinal (GI) infection, has long been recognised. The reasons are multifactorial, in that conditions leading to undernutrition are also associated with over-crowding, lack of sanitation and access to clean water, increased risk of prematurity and lack of vaccination. In turn, episodes of infection increase metabolic demand for nutrients and decrease appetite and intake, thus increasing malnutrition in a vicious cycle.

Bacterial infections, such as pneumonia, tuberculosis, and Gram-negative GI infections are particularly common in children sufficiently malnourished to be hospitalised. Mortality from measles due to giant cell pneumonia is high. These children may suffer from severe herpes fungal and parasitic infections.

Undernutrition has adverse effects on all parts of the immune response. Protein-calorie malnutrition (PCM) leads to atrophy of the skin and mucous membranes. Vitamin deficiencies, particularly A (xerosis), C (scurvy), E and B (dermatitis, cheilitis), and deficiencies of trace elements such as iron (cheilitis), zinc (acrodermatitis), selenium and copper can disrupt these physical defences.

Protein calorie malnutrition compromises lysozyme and interferon production, and components of complement, particularly C3, C4, however, tends to be raised. Leptin levels are reduced. This hormone promotes Th1 responses, and has an anti-apoptotic effect, important for normal haemopoiesis. Phagocytic function is decreased, with impaired bacterial killing, despite increased production of reactive oxygen species. Natural killer (NK) cell's function is reduced in PCM, and deficiencies in zinc, selenium and vitamins A and D.

T cell responses are profoundly affected by PCM, and also vitamin A, zinc, selenium and iron deficiency. Thymic atrophy occurs, together with the depletion of lymph node germinal centres. There can be lymphopaenia with decreased CD4/CD8 ratio. Reduced delayed hypersensitivity responses and T cytotoxicity lead to lack of response to BCG (Bacillus Calmette-Guérin) and susceptibility to tuberculosis, reactivation of viral infections and other opportunistic infections.

In contrast, levels of immunoglobulin are usually well maintained. There can be particularly high levels of serum IgE, which is not necessarily related to helminth infestation, but probably represents dysregulation. Antibody responses are usually preserved, although some studies suggest decreased response to vaccines in severe PCM.

PROBLEMS WITH THE IMMUNE SYSTEM

How Many Infections are Too Many?

The normal range for number of infectious episodes/year in an immunocompetent child is extremely wide and dependent on factors including the risk of exposure to environmental pathogens (e.g. water-borne organisms, malaria), over-crowding and exposure to other children either at home or in nurseries or school. Lack of breast feeding and parental smoking influence the infection rates. Children with medical conditions, such as sickle cell syndrome, nephrotic syndrome, cystic fibrosis, are atopic, have injuries breeching physical barriers, such as compound fractures or burns, or who have implanted foreign bodies will have an increased risk. Immune dysfunction may also be secondary to malignant disease, immunosuppressive agents, infections such as human immunodeficiency virus (HIV), Epstein-Barr virus (EBV) or result from splenectomy.

When to Suspect Immune Deficiency?

An underlying problem with immunity should be suspected in children who have more frequent episodes of infection than expected, given the factors above. Children may suffer recurrent infections with a particular type or organism, or the course of an infectious episode with a particular pathogen is unusual in length, severity or character. Children may become infected with organisms, which would not usually be pathogenic (opportunistic organisms).

Immune deficiency should also be considered in children who have other features of a syndrome known to be associated with immune problems, such as DiGeorge syndrome (DGS), ataxia telangiectasia, Wiskott-Aldrich syndrome (WAS) and so on. Early diagnosis (before the onset of severe infections) can sometimes be achieved by taking note of abnormal results of tests performed for other reasons, e.g. neutropaenia or lymphopaenia from a full blood count.

DIAGNOSIS OF IMMUNE DEFICIENCY

History

From this information, a number of patterns may emerge—invasive bacterial infections, problems with opsonisation (complement, immunoglobulin), phagocyte numbers or function (chemotaxis, phagocytosis and killing), recurrent infection with encapsulated organisms and so on.

A careful history is the key to diagnosis throughout medicine, and immune deficiency is no exception. A detailed history should include:

- Documentation of episodes of infection, their frequency, their course, character, duration, treatment given, effect of treatment, necessity for hospitalisation, clinical diagnosis given and whether confirmatory tests performed
  - From this information, a number of patterns may emerge:immunoglobulin, phagocyte numbers or function (chemotaxis, phagocytosis, killing and so on)
  - *Recurrent infections with encapsulated organisms:* Antibody deficiency, complement defects (especially recurrent meningococcal disease), etc.
  - *Recurrent/persistent/severe viral infections:* Cytotoxic T cells, NK cells and so on.
  - *Fungal infections:* Neutrophil number/function, T cell function and so on.
  - *Opportunistic pathogens, e.g. pneumocystis:* T cell function
- Periodicity of infections: Problems occurring at 3-weekly intervals, particularly associated with mouth ulcers is suggestive of cyclical neutropaenia
- Age of onset:
  - From birth suggestive of cellular defect, e.g. congenital neutropaenia, T cell immunodeficiencies
  - 6–9 months: Recurrent sinopulmonary infection suggestive of antibody deficiency
  - After 2 years of age—consider common variable immune deficiency
- Birth history:
  - Gestation
  - Birth weight: Intrauterine growth retardation is associated with nutritional immune dysfunction and specific syndromes
  - Neonatal problems:
    - Jitteriness/seizures due to hypocalcaemia or heart failure/cyanosis due to congenital heart disease may indicate DGS
    - Petechiae/bleeding from cord in WAS
    - Severe erythroderma in congenital graft versus host disease
    - Neonatal sepsis in reticular dysgenesis and severe neutropaenia and severe T cell defects
  - Time of cord separation: Delay associated with lymphocyte adhesion defect
- Other medical problems:
  - Growth problems:
    - Severe failure to thrive in T cell defects
    - Short stature in Bloom syndrome
  - Developmental delay/neurological problems
    - Ataxia telangiectasia
    - Purine nucleoside phosphorylase deficiency
    - HIV
  - Skin problems:
    - Eczematoid dermatitis and abscesses in Hyper-IgE
    - Recurrent abscesses in chronic granulomatous disease (CGD)
    - Eczema and petechiae in WAS
    - Skin sepsis in antibody deficiency, neutrophil disorders, complement defects
- Immunisations given and reactions:
  - Neonatal BCG: Reaction/dissemination—T cell deficiency, interferon gamma/IL12 dysfunction
  - Symptomatic disease following live vaccine, e.g. measles—T cell function
  - Abscess/reaction at site; neutrophil function complement
- Allergies
- Current and past medication, including "over the counter" and alternative/herbal remedies
- Family history:
  - Family members with similar features
  - Deaths early in life
  - Consanguinity
- Social history:
  - Housing
  - Occupants of house
  - Attendance at nursery/school
  - Risk behaviours for blood-borne virus infection
  - Parental occupations
  - Smoking
  - Pets/animals/birds.

Diagnostic Tests

Selection of appropriate tests should depend upon the differential diagnosis obtained as a result of the history and examination, and also on the resources available.

Full Blood Count

Haemoglobin is reduced in chronic infection and inflammatory conditions.

- *Neutrophil count* will identify chronic neutropaenia. Serial tests over a 3 weeks period are needed to diagnose cyclical neutropaenia. A neutrophil leucocytosis is seen in disorders of neutrophil function such as CGD and lymphocyte adhesion defect.

- *Lymphocyte count* is low in T cell immunodeficiencies such as severe combined immunodeficiency. Note that the lymphocyte count is normally higher in infants, so values persistently below 2.8 × 10^9/L should prompt further investigation.
- *Platelet count* and platelet size are reduced in WAS.
- *Blood film* microscopy may identify Howell-Jolly bodies in asplenia.

TESTS FOR CELL-MEDIATED IMMUNITY

Skin Testing

Delayed hypersensitivity is mediated by cell-mediated responses, and so it is possible to test for this in vivo. The problem in infants and children under 2 years is to find a suitable antigen to which they have previously been exposed and sensitised. Children who have had BCG may respond to tuberculin, and those who have had tetanus immunisation may respond to tetanus toxoid. Candidal antigen may also be used. Testing involves an intradermal injection of the antigen and recording of the resulting erythema and induration at 24–48 hours.

Lymphocyte Subset Quantification

If monoclonal antibodies labelled with fluorochrome are generated against lymphocyte surface markers, they can be used to identify lymphocyte subsets using a flow cytometer or fluorescence activated cell scanner machine. The most common monoclonals used are against CD3 (all mature T cells), CD4, CD8, CD19/20 (B cells) and CD16/56 (NK cells). Normal ranges for numbers and proportions vary with age.

Lymphocyte Function

In vitro, this can be assessed by incubating lymphocytes with mitogens such as phytohaemagglutinin and pokeweed mitogen. The degree of proliferation is measured by assessing the uptake of tritiated thymidine, compared to that of a normal control sample.

Cytokine and Receptor Assays

These are not widely available, but they can diagnose rare immunodeficiencies.

TESTS FOR HUMOURAL IMMUNITY

Immunoglobulin Assays

Normal plasma concentration of immunoglobulin classes also vary with age. Low levels of all classes are found in T cell immunodeficiencies, such as severe combined immunodeficiency, and in antibody deficiencies such as X-linked agammaglobulinaemia (XLA). High levels are found in chronic infection, CGD and HIV.

B Cell Function

B cell function can be assessed by measuring the titre of antibody to a specific antigen following exposure to the antigen, e.g. anti-tetanus antibody, pre- and post-vaccination. Antibody to *Pneumococcus* can also be measured, but as this is a polysaccharide antigen, children under 2 years do not normally respond.

Phagocyte Function

There are no reliable tests of chemotaxis. The respiratory burst can be measured using the nitroblue tetrazolium test during which normal cells phagocytose the colourless dye and reduces it to a purple compound. Neutrophils from children with CGD phagocytose normally, but there is no colour change.

Complement Function

It is possible to measure levels of individual complement components—the most straightforward being C3 and C4. CH50 is a dynamic assay of total haemolytic complement and is reduced in defects of the classical pathway.

Genetic Tests

Chromosome analysis can diagnose conditions such as DGS, which is associated with a deletion on q22. The exact genetic defect has been identified for some inherited immune deficiencies, and in these analyses of DNA or assay of the gene product (e.g. B tyrosine kinase in XLA) can be performed.

PRIMARY IMMUNODEFICIENCY DISORDERS

These conditions are individually quite rare, with an estimated prevalence of 1 in 5,000 population. The most common are antibody deficiencies accounting for approximately 65% total, cellular deficiencies comprise 20%, phagocytic disorders 10% and complement disorders 5%. Those with an autosomal recessive mode of inheritance may be more common in societies with a high incidence of marriage within the extended family.

Severe Combined Immune Deficiency

Severe combined immune deficiency (SCID) is a group of conditions characterised by low or absent T cells and hypogammaglobulinaemia. B and NK cell numbers may be normal or absent, depending on the type. It may present with congenital graft versus host disease due to engraftment of maternal T cells, or following neonatal transfusion of non-irradiated blood. More commonly, the infant develops recurrent or chronic mucocutaneous candidiasis, chronic diarrhoea and failure to thrive due to persistent viral gastroenteritis and chronic respiratory viral infection (e.g. Respiratory syncytial virus,

Adenovirus), leading to respiratory failure. Acute sepsis can occur, as can opportunistic infection with agents such as Pneumocystis and Cytomegalovirus. Without treatment (bone marrow transplantation), it is unusual to survive beyond the first year of life. There are X-linked (e.g. common gamma chain deficiency) and autosomal recessive (e.g. adenosine deaminase deficiency) forms of the condition, and for some the underlying defect is unknown.

DiGeorge Syndrome

The main features of this syndrome are conotruncal cardiac anomalies (e.g. interrupted aortic arch, truncus arteriosus), hypocalcaemia and hypoplastic or absence of thymus. Children with this syndrome have characteristic facies, with hypertelorism, antimongoloid slant of the eyes, micrognathia, cleft or high-arched palate and ear malformations. These defects are due to failure of migration of neural crest cells into the third and fourth pharyngeal pouches early in embryological life. This is commonly associated with a microdeletion on chromosome 22 (q2211). Many cases are sporadic, but there is, therefore, an autosomal dominant inheritance.

Most children present with symptoms of their congenital heart disease or with neonatal hypocalcaemia, and although they may have low T cell numbers compared with normal infants, immune function is well preserved. However, those with absent or severely hypoplastic thymus can have features of severe T cell immunodeficiency similar to SCID. They can have normal immunoglobulin levels, but reduced specific antibody production. There is also an increased risk of autoimmune disease.

X-linked Agammaglobulinaemia

This condition is due to a lack of the enzyme Bruton's tyrosine kinase (Btk), which is essential for B cell maturation. Circulating B cell numbers are very low or absent, as are levels of circulating immunoglobulin. Children are normal at birth, protected by passive maternal antibody, but develop recurrent bacterial infections, particularly sinopulmonary infections, usually becoming symptomatic between 6 and 18 months of age. As T cell function is normal, they cope with childhood exanthemata such as varicella normally. Immunoglobulin can be replaced with regular intravenous (IV) or subcutaneous infusions, and in those who are treated adequately, prognosis is good. Ongoing problems with chronic sinusitis, purulent rhinitis and conjunctivitis, can occur despite replacement, and chronic lung disease is particularly likely in those not maintaining adequate trough levels of immunoglobulin.

CD40 Ligand Deficiency

This condition is also X-linked and shares many characteristics with XLA. However, CD40 ligand is a T cell receptor, binding with CD40 on the B cell to enable B cell proliferation and isotype switching. Children with this condition have normal numbers of circulating B cells, and normal or high levels of serum IgM, but absent IgG, IgA and IgE. This T cell ligand has other functions in host defence, in addition to B cell stimulation, so unlike XLA, children can present with pneumocystis carinii pneumonia and fail to clear pathogens such as *Cryptosporidium*. Even with immunoglobulin replacement, the prognosis is much poorer. This is due to the risk of liver failure due to sclerosing cholangitis, which may result from chronic biliary infection with organisms such as *Cryptosporidium*, and of malignancy, particularly abdominal malignancies.

Common Variable Immunodeficiency

This is another form of antibody deficiency, but unlike XLA, symptoms can start at any age, but after 2 years at the earliest. The most common presentation is with recurrent or chronic sinopulmonary infection, which can lead to chronic lung disease. These children have B cells, but low levels of immunoglobulin, and poor or absent specific antibody responses. In addition to infections, they may develop granulomatous disease or autoimmune features and have an increased risk of malignancy. Treatment is with immunoglobulin and antibiotic prophylaxis.

Chronic Granulomatous Disease

This is a disorder of phagocytes in which there is a defect in NADPH (nicotinamide adenine dinucleotide phosphate) oxidase, the enzyme involved in the respiratory burst. There are both X-linked and autosomal recessive forms of the disease. Children with CGD are at particular risk of infection.

With catalase positive bacteria (such as *Staphylococcus* organisms and coliforms) and fungi such as *Aspergillus*, they can present with recurrent lymphadenitis, invasive bacterial infection such as pneumonia, liver abscess, osteomyelitis or life-threatening sepsis. Prophylactic antibiotics and antifungals have improved prognosis, but many succumb to invasive fungal infection in the second and third decades of life.

Complement Deficiencies

These are individually very rare and tend to present with recurrent bacterial infection, due to poor opsonisation, glomerulonephritis or features suggestive of rheumatological disease. Some, such as properdin deficiency, lead to increased susceptibility to infection with encapsulated organisms, particularly *N. meningitidis*, which should be considered if children present with recurrent meningococcal disease. It has X-linked inheritance.

Wiskott–Aldrich Syndrome

This results from a mutation on the X chromosome of a gene encoding for WAS protein. This protein is important for the normal development of the cytoskeleton and plays a role in apoptosis. The main features are thrombocytopaenia, recurrent infections and eczema. Those affected often present in the neonatal period with petechiae and bleeding. Not only are platelet numbers reduced, but they are smaller than normal and function less well, so bleeding may be more severe than would be expected from the platelet count alone. Boys suffer recurrent bacterial infections, such as otitis media, pneumonia and meningitis, particularly with encapsulated organisms. They also suffer from viral infections, such as recurrent herpes simplex and severe varicella. Their eczema has the same characteristics as classic atopic eczema. Other atopic symptoms such as food allergy can develop. Some boys develop autoimmune problems, and the long-term risk is from malignancy, particularly EBV driven B cell lymphoma. Treatments include splenectomy, intravenous immunoglobulin and antibiotic prophylaxis. However, bone marrow transplant can be curative.

Hyperimmunoglobulin E (Job) Syndrome

Children with this condition suffer from recurrent severe staphylococcal infection, particularly skin abscesses and pneumonia. They have a dermatitis, which may be diagnosed as eczema, but the characteristics and distribution of the lesions are different from atopic eczema. Children can have coarse facies and skeletal abnormalities. As the name suggests, levels of serum IgE are extremely high (often many thousand international units per litre). The gene and underlying defect for this condition are unknown, and there is no specific treatment apart from long-term prophylactic antistaphylococcal antibiotics.

Ataxia Telangiectasia

This is caused by a mutated gene on chromosome 11, which encodes for a protein which is important for repair of double stranded DNA. The cells of those affected are, therefore, abnormally sensitive to irradiation. Children are normal at birth, and early development is normal. They tend to drool, and speech is slow. They begin walking at the usual age, but become more wobbly. Unlike many other cerebellar disorders, the ataxia of AT results in a narrow-based gait, and children have difficulty keeping their head and trunk still when standing. From around the age of 7 years, there is progressive neurological deterioration. Conjunctival telangiectasia is often the first to appear, with cutaneous lesions appearing between the ages of 3 and 6 years (Fig. 20.6).

The immunodeficiency associated with condition is variable, both in clinical manifestation and laboratory findings. Children with AT may suffer from severe or recurrent sinopulmonary infection and also chronic or recurrent warts. They commonly have low or absent IgA levels, but can have low specific antibody responses to polysaccharide antigens or T lymphopaenia. They have a very high risk of cancer, chiefly leukaemias and lymphomas, but other solid tumours can occur. Most sufferers die in the second or third decade from chronic lung disease or malignancy.

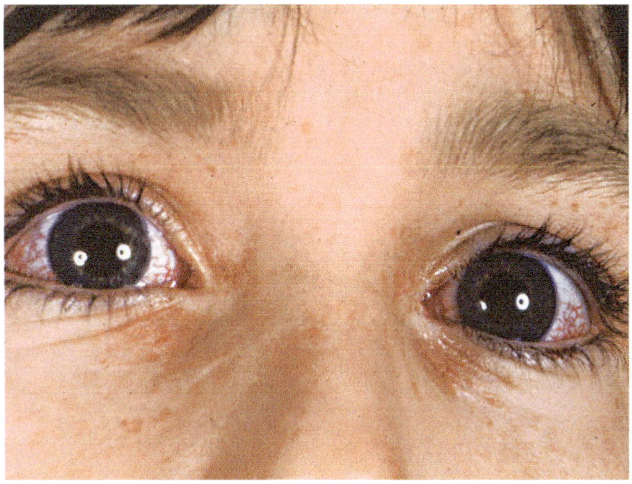

Figure 20.6 Telangiectasia on the bulbar conjunctivae.

ALLERGY

Allergy can be defined as an immunologically mediated response whose effects are detrimental to the host.

These responses are much more common in individuals described as *atopic*. *Atopy* is highly genetic and characterised by an individual or familial tendency to become sensitised to common protein allergens at normal levels of exposure. This response is usually mediated by IgE. Atopic individuals tend to have higher levels of circulating IgE than those who are nonatopic.

Hypersensitivity can be defined as the development of reproducible symptoms and signs following exposure to a particular stimulus at a dose which would normally be tolerated (e.g. peanut allergy). However, it can also be used more widely to describe allergic reactions, some of which are universal (e.g. reaction to mix-matched blood).

IMMUNOLOGY OF ALLERGIC DISEASES

Traditionally, hypersensitivity reactions have been classified into four types. Although we now recognise that many complex interactions occur between different parts of the immune system, it is still a useful way of understanding allergy.

Type I (Immediate/Anaphylactic)

Symptoms occur within minutes/hours of exposure to the allergen, which forms a complex with specific IgE and is bound to the surface of effector cells, such as mast cells (Fig. 20.7A). This leads to the release of chemical mediators which cause the changes associated with observed symptoms and signs, e.g. vasodilatation, capillary leak,

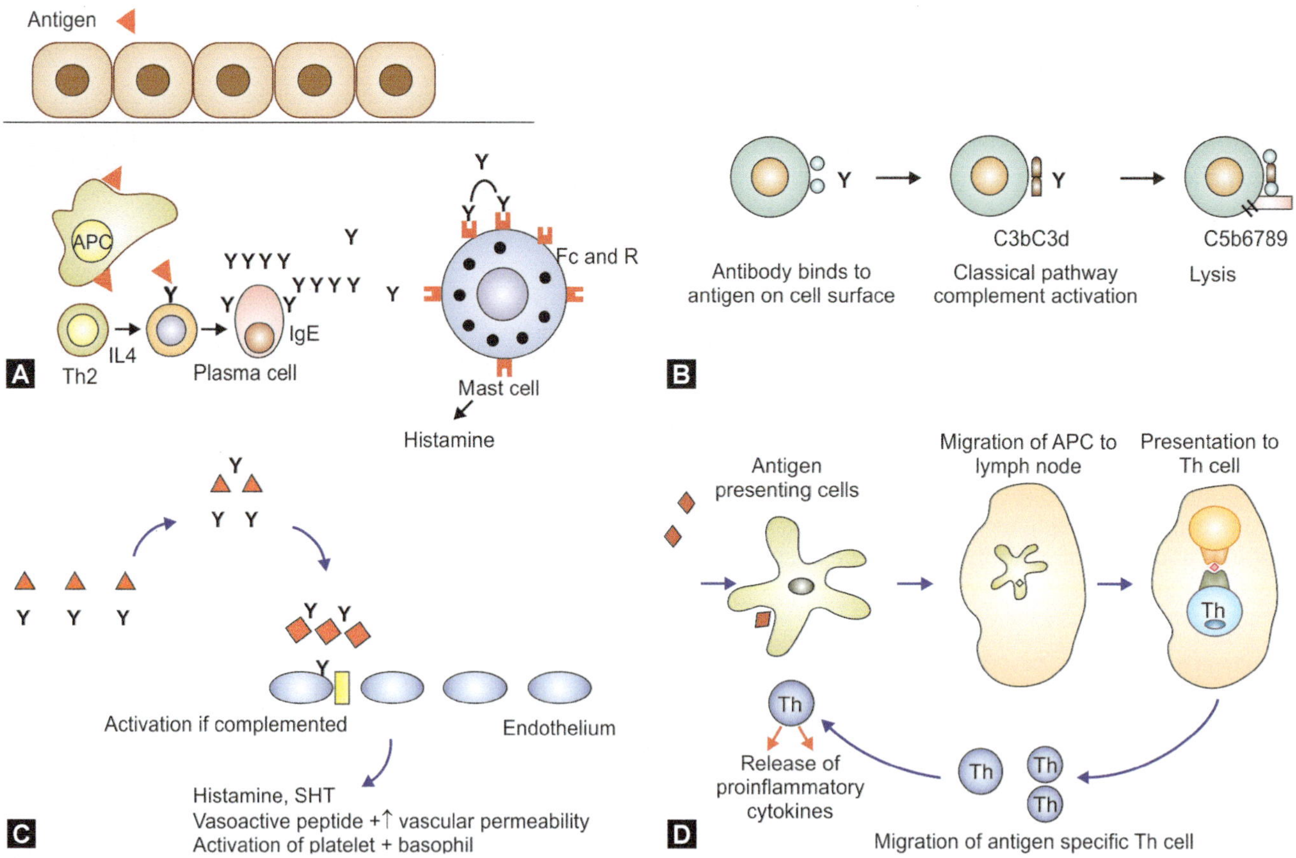

Figures 20.7A to D (A) Type I reaction: pathogenesis of type I hypersensitivity; exposure to antigen immunoglobulin E production, mast cell sensitisation; (B) Type II reaction: pathogenic mechanism in type II hypersensitivity; (C) Type III reaction; (D) Type IV reaction.

bronchoconstriction and increased gut peristalsis. This is the mechanism behind peanut allergy, drug reactions, allergic rhinitis and acute asthma.

Type II (Cytotoxic)

In this reaction, antibody (IgG or IgM) binds directly to tissue bearing the specific antigen, resulting in complement activation and tissue damage **(Fig. 20.7B)**. Examples are transfusion reactions, to which all are susceptible, but they also occur in diseases such as autoimmune haemolytic anaemia, Goodpasture syndrome and some drug-induced cytopaenias.

Type III (Arthus/Immune Complex)

In these reactions, antibody is bound to antigen to form immune complexes, some of which are cleared by the reticuloendothelial system. However, some are deposited in blood vessels or tissues, inducing complement activation and tissue damage **(Fig. 20.7C)**. This is the pathogenesis of serum sickness and glomerulonephritis.

Type IV (Delayed/Cell Mediated)

Unlike the first three types, delayed hypersensitivity is not mediated by antibody, but by T cells. The maximum inflammatory response may not occur until 48–72 hours after exposure. As a result of interaction between local antigen-presenting cells (principally dendritic cells) and T cells, T cells proliferate and produce cytokines which mediate a local inflammatory response. Reactions are universal following exposure to antigen such as poison oak or poison ivy. Induction of this type of reaction is the basis of the tuberculin skin test (Mantoux).

Some allergic conditions involve both immediate and delayed hypersensitivity responses to the same stimulus. E.g., exposure to egg in a young child may cause urticaria and angio-oedema within minutes, due to IgE-mediated hypersensitivity. Forty-eight hours later, a flare of atopic eczema may result from the influx of mononuclear cells associated with a type IV response **(Fig. 20.7D)**.

MEDIATORS OF THE ALLERGIC RESPONSE

T and B Cells

Immunoglobulin E-producing plasma cells develop following T cell stimulation, first of all by cytokines (chiefly IL4) released as a result of interaction between antigen (allergen) presented in association with class II MHC and T helper cells. The interaction between CD40 ligand on the Th2 cell and the CD40 B cell receptor is also necessary. In atopic children, there is an increased number of allergen-specific T cells, which when stimulated, produce IL4, IL5 and IL13. These cytokines induce allergic inflammation by their action on mast cells, basophils and eosinophils.

Mast Cells, Basophils and Eosinophils

These play a large role in the allergic response and resulting inflammation. Their functions have already been outlined.

Histamine

This is the major mediator of type I hypersensitivity. Different tissues have different histamine receptors, determining the response.

- *H1 receptors* are found in blood vessels, and smooth muscle of the respiratory and GI tract. The action of histamine on these receptors results in increased vascular permeability, GI muscle contraction, bronchoconstriction, increased chemotaxis and decreased chemokinesis.
- *H2 receptors* are found in the gastric mucosa, the heart, uterus and central nervous system. Stimulation results in increased gastric acid and pepsin production, increased chemotaxis and chemokinesis, with a negative effect on lymphocytotoxicity, and on further histamine production.
- Both types of receptor contribute to vasodilatation, flushing, headache, tachycardia, hypotension, and the wheal and flare reaction.
- *H3 receptors* modulate cholinergic sensory nerves and inhibit histamine release from mast cells.

Leukotrienes

These are fatty acids whose active inflammatory metabolites cause vasodilatation, swelling of the mucosa, increased mucous production and bronchoconstriction. Metabolism is governed by the 5-lipoxygenase pathway, which can be stimulated by certain antigens. They have an important role in the pathogenesis of asthma and allergic rhinitis.

Other Chemical Mediators

These include kinins, complement, interleukins and cell adhesion molecules.

EPIDEMIOLOGY

The prevalence of atopic disease varies greatly throughout the world, being much more common in the developed world with "Western" lifestyle. There has also been a dramatic increase in prevalence, particularly in the developed world over time. The rise in sensitisation to aeroallergens probably began in the 1920s, but the large increase in symptomatic disease started in the 1960–1970s, with some evidence that the rates have now stabilised, with rates of asthma between 20 and 40%, depending on the criteria used, compared with 2–3% in the developing world. Similarly rates for hay fever, at the age of 16 years are around 20–25% in the UK, and 6% for atopic eczema. Within the developing world, a shift from rural to urban habitat results in increased prevalence, and immigrants from areas of low to high prevalence reach rates similar to the indigenous population in a generation.

Why is Atopic Disease Increasing?

We believe that the immune system is "primed" to generate predominantly Th1 or Th2 responses to a given stimulus early on in life. This process may, therefore, be influenced by the nature of the antigens to which the infant is exposed at this stage. In the West, the burden of infectious disease is much lower than in the developing world now and in Western society in the past. Moreover, even in developing countries where the overall prevalence is still low, there is an increased risk associated with change from rural to urban environment. Some studies have suggested that large family size, attendance at day nursery, and living on a farm particularly with animals are all associated with a lower rate of atopic diseases. The reasons for these differences are complex. A popular theory is the "hygiene hypothesis", which in some ways, is a misleading title, as it could imply that good standards of hygiene are bad for your health, which is far from the case. It is certainly true, however, that one of the most striking differences between rural life in a developing country, and Westernised society, is in the nature of exposure to microbial and parasitic organisms. The degree of exposure early in life to agents such as bacterial endotoxin, environmental mycobacteria, and to helminths, particularly hookworm, may be important for the manner in which mechanisms which regulate the immune response develop.

Clinical Presentation of Allergic Disease

These include acute anaphylaxis, food allergy and atopic diseases such as asthma, eczema, allergic rhinitis and conjunctivitis. Allergic asthma and eczema have been described elsewhere in the sections on respiratory medicine and dermatology, respectively (Chapters 6 and 10).

Acute Immediate Hypersensitivity and Anaphylaxis

In some references, the term anaphylactic is used to describe type I hypersensitivity reactions of any severity. Here anaphylaxis is defined as a sudden life-threatening systemic reaction which is immune mediated. As such it is an acute medical emergency. It usually results from a type

I hypersensitivity reaction, mediated by histamine, and other active chemicals released during IgE-associated mast cell degranulation. Type III reactions can sometimes give a similar clinical picture.

If exposure to the allergen has been cutaneous or mucosal, there may initially be local symptoms at the site of contact, such as tingling lips and tongue with local swelling, sneezing, conjunctival irritation or localised urticaria. Urticaria may progress to become widespread, with intense itch. There may be angio-oedema with facial swelling, hoarse voice and a feeling of a lump in the throat, with coughing and choking, if this affects the upper airways. Bronchospasm may also lead to audible wheeze. Some children vomit profusely or complain of abdominal cramps or diarrhoea.

In the most severe cases, the onset is sudden and heralded by a "sense of impending doom", and a sudden feeling of weakness. The child experiences palpitations, becomes cold and clammy, with poor peripheral perfusion. They may develop severe difficulty in breathing, either secondary to upper airways obstruction or to severe bronchospasm. This is followed by circulatory collapse and unconsciousness. Although uncommon, particularly in childhood, deaths do occur.

Anaphylaxis can result from exposure of the sensitised child to food allergens such as peanut. It can also be triggered by venoms, such as bee and wasp, or plants, such as strawberry and natural rubber latex. A wide variety of drugs can cause it, particularly antibiotics such as penicillin, sulphonamides or anaesthetic agents.

Anaphylactoid Reactions

The term anaphylactoid is used to describe a clinical picture which closely resembles anaphylaxis, i.e. urticaria/ erythema, respiratory difficulty, shock, but in which the pathogenesis is not immune mediated. It may result from direct action of chemicals such as drugs on cells, leading to the release of vasoactive peptides. Vasoactive agents may also be released through stimulation of intermediate pathways such as the complement cascade. It may result from drug interactions, or from infusion of large volumes of plasma products, in which immunoglobulins form aggregates in the circulation. Reactions due to underlying pathology (e.g. tumours) or surgical stimulation causing release of vasoactive peptides is very rare in children. Very occasionally, the cause may be psychosomatic, and the possibility should be considered in teenage patients, when no other explanation can be found.

FOOD ALLERGY

While food is essential for our survival, it can also cause a number of well-recognised adverse events. Moreover, children and their families may attribute all sorts of symptoms which they suffer due to "food allergy". Some beliefs regarding the association of certain foods and ill health are routed deep in the culture of the society to which the family belongs. Many have their base in philosophies other than "conventional" medicine and are not amenable to application of the scientific method to explore.

There are a number of recognised mechanisms for adverse reactions to food, only one of which is IgE-mediated immediate hypersensitivity. Others are immune mediated, but not through IgG. Examples include cow's milk protein intolerance and gluten enteropathy (coeliac disease). Some foods can lead directly to histamine release, or actually contain histamine, such as strawberries and tomatoes. Localised urticaria after ingestion is commonly described in atopic children, particularly those with eczema, who show no evidence of IgE-mediated sensitivity. In some cases, symptoms are due to pharmacological effects of ingredients, such as caffeine in soft drinks, leading to vomiting and diarrhoea, or tartrazine (yellow colouring used in soft drinks) causing bronchospasm, particularly in those with underlying asthma. Reactions can reflect lack of necessary enzymes, such as disaccharidase deficiency in lactose intolerance, or in inborn errors of metabolism, such as galactosaemia. Neurological symptoms following food ingestion can result from build-up of a toxin within the food, such as in scombrotoxic fish poisoning, or in botulism, due to contamination of food with *Clostridium*. To some children, certain food smells act as noxious stimuli leading to retching and vomiting and aversion to that food. However, for the purpose of this discussion, we will concentrate on "true" IgE-mediated allergic reactions.

Like other atopic disorders, the incidence of food allergy has been increasing. This is reflected in the number of children presenting to clinics with symptoms, but also in admissions to hospital with significant reactions or anaphylaxis. Death from such reactions can occur, but is extremely rare in childhood (0.006/100,000 children aged 0–15 years in the UK). The prevalence in the UK is quoted in the region of 2–6%, with peanut allergy at 0.8%. Many children with food allergies have other atopic diseases. A third of children with atopic eczema in infancy and 1 in 10 children with asthma report food-related symptoms.

In many parts of the world, the most common food allergens in infants and young children are eggs and milk. There is, however, a wide geographical variation, not only in the incidence of food allergy but also in the foods causing these reactions. In the UK and Australia, peanuts and tree nuts are the next most common. Fish is the most common allergen in Italy. Sesame allergy is common in the Middle East, seafood in Japan and Singapore and legumes (lentils, peas, beans) in India and Pakistan.

Children who are allergic to one food allergen have an increased likelihood of also being allergic to related foods. For instance, the majority of milk allergic children are also allergic to egg. Allergy to pulses can be associated with peanut allergy. Those with peanut allergy may also be allergic to other nuts and seeds (e.g. sesame seed); although an allergy to one individual nut (e.g. Brazil nut) can occur. There can also be cross-reactivity between sensitivity to inhaled allergens and foods. E.g., allergy to birch pollen is associated with reactions to apples, pears and other fruit, as well as to hazelnuts. Reactions to melon and banana, and ragweed sensitivity are similarly related.

The prognosis for food allergy varies, depending on the allergen. Ninety per cent cow's milk allergic infants will become tolerant by the age of 3 years. Egg allergy commonly resolves before school age. However, allergies to pulses and nuts are usually lifelong, with only around 5% resolving by the age of 7 years.

Oral Allergy Syndrome

Children with this condition develop an itchy mouth and tongue, sometimes with localised urticaria and swelling after eating a variety of fresh fruit or vegetables. The same foods may be eaten if they are peeled and/or cooked, as the sensitivity is to proteins which are destroyed by this process. A common association is that of hay fever symptoms in the spring and early summer due to allergy to birch pollen and symptoms on eating whole apple, while the child can still drink apple juice. Although symptoms can be unpleasant, and their precipitants best avoided, these reactions do not carry a risk of anaphylactic shock.

Exercise-induced Anaphylaxis

This is very unusual before teenage years. It occurs when ingestion of a particular food is followed within a few hours by moderate to intense exercise. Both elements are necessary to produce the reaction, and so the causal relationship with the food allergen may not be made, if a history of tolerating the same food on other occasions (when such exercise has not taken place) is elicited. Changes in metabolism associated with the exercise result in the mast cells becoming more activated, and thus more likely to degranulate after a given IgE/allergen stimulus. This effect can also be seen in children who normally suffer only mild reactions after exposure to a food allergen but who may develop anaphylaxis following the same degree of exposure, following exercise.

Latex Allergy

Allergy to natural rubber latex is strongly associated with exposure to settings where a lot of latex material is used. Thus health care workers and those exposed to industrial latex have a high risk of developing sensitivity. In children, high-risk groups are those with spina bifida or with genitourinary abnormalities, which is likely to be due to repeated exposure of mucous membranes to latex urinary catheters. Children with a history of repeated surgery in the first year of life are also at risk, presumably because of repeated exposure to latex gloves and other latex containing equipment. Because of this problem, other materials, such as nitrile, are being substituted for latex where this is possible.

Around half of the children with latex allergy also experience symptoms on exposure to various foods. These include banana, avocado, chestnut, potato, kiwi and other tropical fruits. In children with allergies to these foods, the possibility of latex allergy should, therefore, be considered.

Latex is used very widely in clothing, for mattresses, bicycle or wheelchair tyres, balls, erasers, computer mouse mats and so on. Total avoidance of all such products is almost impossible, but thankfully seldom necessary. While contact with the skin can lead to urticaria or contact dermatitis, severe reactions usually occur only after significant mucosal or systemic exposure. The main risks, therefore, surround episodes of medical or dental care. If latex allergic children need such care, it is very important that every effort is made to ensure the environment is latex free. Where the risk of exposure cannot absolutely be eliminated, e.g. during major surgery, premedication with hydrocortisone and antihistamines is advised, with careful observation peri- and postoperatively.

Allergic Rhinitis

Allergic rhinitis is very common in industrialised societies, with a prevalence of up to 40% in children. Some suffer symptoms all year round (perennial rhinitis), whereas for others the problem is restricted to times of year when there is exposure to the causal allergen (seasonal rhinitis). The allergens responsible for perennial rhinitis tend to be those encountered in an indoor environment such as house dust mite, animal dander and so on. Those developing seasonal rhinitis in the spring are allergic to tree pollen, whereas symptoms of grass pollen allergy peak in the mid-summer. Those who have their main problems in the autumn may be allergic to leaf mould or weed pollen.

There are two phases of response. After exposure in a sensitised child, there is a type I reaction, in which the nasal passages leads to nasal vasodilatation, capillary leak and increased mucus production. This leads to nasal congestion, and a watery runny nose with itching and sneezing. In around 50% of sufferers, this is followed by a late response, induced by inflammatory cells, causing ongoing nasal congestion, with runny nose and postnasal drip, which may last for days. Nasal symptoms are often accompanied by itching of the eyes (allergic conjunctivitis), ears, throat and palate.

Although the consequences are rarely life threatening, these symptoms are a major cause of morbidity in school-aged children. Those who are severely affected with chronic nasal obstruction suffer recurrent or chronic headache, tiredness and sleep disturbance, sometimes resulting in sleep apnoea. It can lead to day time somnolence, poor concentration and poor school performance. The effect on children's emotional and psychological development can, therefore, be profound.

There is a close association between allergic rhinitis and asthma. Half of children with asthma also have rhinitis, and around a third of children with rhinitis also have asthma. Furthermore, allergic rhinitis is a risk factor for the subsequent development of asthma.

DIAGNOSIS OF ALLERGY

History

Once again, a careful history is the key to diagnosis of allergy. This should include the nature of symptoms experienced, the evolution of symptoms, from the first symptom experienced onwards, time taken to resolution, and whether any treatment was administered. Details of exposure to potential allergens should be obtained, and the length of time between the suspected exposure and onset of symptoms should be known. It is important to take a history of any previous reactions and their suspected precipitants in a similar way. Also, a history of any previous exposure to the same potential allergen, and whether or not any symptoms developed is important. It should be noted whether or not related allergens are tolerated. If the suspected allergen is a food, whether the food was raw or cooked may be relevant, as may the circumstances in which the reaction took place (e.g. following exercise).

A common acute presentation is urticaria. Although urticaria is one of the signs of immediate hypersensitivity, this is not the only mechanism. Many viral and other infectious agents are associated with an immune reaction leading to urticaria which is not IgE mediated. Children developing such rashes are often diagnosed with "allergy". In general, if a child wakes up in the morning in his usual environment with an urticarial rash which lasts for a number of days, and does not resolve with antihistamine, the rash is not due to immediate hypersensitivity, and a "trawl" for possible precipitants is unlikely to be helpful.

In children suspected of allergic rhinitis or asthma, history of nasal and respiratory symptoms should be taken. These include itching, sneezing, rhinorrhoea, nasal congestion, worsening of symptoms is the first thing in the morning after exposure to allergen the night before, cough (including nocturnal cough), sleep disturbance, mouth breathing and snoring. Any seasonal variation should be noted.

A past history of any other atopic conditions, e.g. eczema, asthma, rhinitis should be taken. In particular, if the child has asthma, it is important to assess how well controlled the asthma is, in terms of frequency and severity of symptoms, precipitants of symptoms and what prophylactic and rescue medication the child is using. Any current medication should be noted, together with details of any adverse reactions to medications in the past. A picture should be built up of the child's home environment, or any other place where they regularly spend time, including pets, other animal or bird exposure, dust, mould, vegetation and so on.

Examination

A full general examination may reveal the skin features of eczema. Those with allergic rhinitis may be obvious mouth-breathers with dark rings round the eyes due to suborbital oedema. They can also develop an "allergic crease" across the nose just above the tip, formed after constant rubbing, redness around the eyes, again due to rubbing, and excoriation above the upper lip, caused by nasal drip.

Those with asthma may show signs of chronic chest deformity with increased anteroposterior diameter of the chest, and splaying of the lower ribs (Harrison's sulcus). There may be signs of hyperinflation or wheeze on auscultation.

Investigations

Investigation of Acute Anaphylaxis

For children who present with severe symptoms, it can be difficult to establish clinically whether this is a type I reaction, or whether the reaction is anaphylactoid. True anaphylactic reactions are associated with histamine release, which, therefore, could be measured. However, the rise and fall in histamine levels following an anaphylactic reaction is very steep and short-lived, and therefore, likely to escape detection by the time the child presents.

True anaphylactic reactions are caused by mast cell degranulation. While it is histamine which is the major mediator of the resulting symptoms, other chemicals, such as tryptase are also released. The half-life of mast cell tryptase in the circulation is considerably longer than histamine **(Fig. 20.8)**. Serial measurements can, therefore, be taken over the first 12 hours after the reaction, a rise and subsequent fall to baseline being indicative of true anaphylaxis. If no such change is demonstrated, an alternative mechanism for the symptoms should be sought, and further investigation to identify a particular allergen is likely to be fruitless.

Skin Prick Testing

This is a quick method of diagnosing immediate hypersensitivity. A drop of a standard solution containing the allergen is put on the skin. The most common sites used are the forearm in older children and the back in younger children, avoiding skin affected by eczema. A calibrated

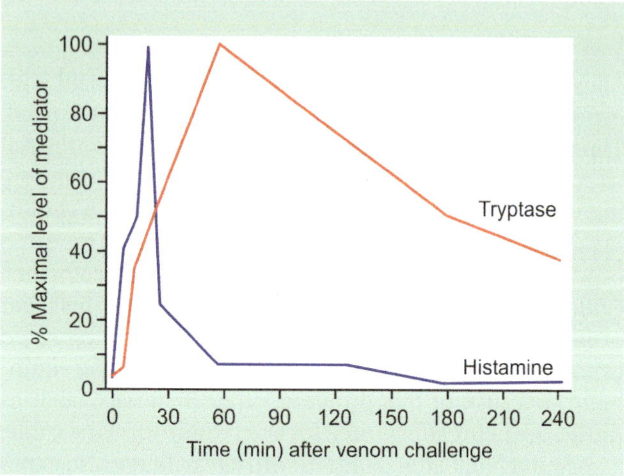

Figure 20.8 Half-life of mast cell tryptase.

lancet is used to prick the epidermis to a depth of a couple of millimetres only. Excess solution is removed, and after 15–20 minutes, any resulting wheal is measured, and compared with a positive and negative control. A positive test should have a wheal at least 3 mm greater than the negative control or equivalent to the positive control. For some foods, such as fruits, the fruit itself can be pricked, and then the skin pricked in a similar way ("prick test"). False-negatives can occur if the child has recently taken an antihistamine. While it is extremely rare for a systemic reaction to occur as a result of this degree of allergen exposure, these test should always be performed where staff are trained in the management of anaphylaxis and appropriate equipment for resuscitation is available.

Serological Testing

Titres of specific IgE directed against a wide variety of allergens can be assayed in the blood using radioallergosorbent test (RAST) or similar techniques. Such tests are more invasive, and often more traumatic for children, but can be performed in settings where no trained staff are available, and the results are not influenced by antihistamine usage. The concentration of specific IgE with a high positive predictive value for clinical hypersensitivity varies between different allergens. E.g., a titre of 14 kU/L has a 95% positive predictive value for peanut allergy. Care should be taken not to over-interpret results reported as positive, but with lower titres, as highly atopic children may have detectable specific IgE to many potential allergens which they tolerate with no obvious adverse effects.

Provocation Test

This is usually performed to investigate food allergy, but can be used for other potential allergens such as latex or drugs. It can be used when the diagnosis remains uncertain following the other tests detailed above. It is also useful to determine whether a child with a history of allergy has become tolerant (e.g. in milk allergy), or to investigate possible non-IgE-mediated or delayed reactions.

In an open challenge, the child is gradually exposed to increasing amount of the allergen until either a reaction occurs, or until they have tolerated an amount as large as a normal exposure would be expected to be. This should only be performed by staff trained in the early recognition and treatment of reactions, and where there are facilities for the management of anaphylaxis. In a food challenge, the food is first applied to the skin, then the lips, before small amounts are ingested.

In a double-blind placebo-controlled challenge, the allergen is "hidden" so that the child, the parents and the administering staff are unaware which of two foods/solutions contains the potential allergen. The procedure for each arm is the same as in the open challenge. A sufficient interval between the two arms is necessary to ensure that any delayed symptoms can be attributed to one arm or the other.

Patch Testing

This is often confused with skin prick testing, but this technique is used for the diagnosis of delayed (type IV) reactions, particularly involving the skin, such as contact dermatitis due to perfumes, metals and other chemicals. Adhesive patches containing the allergen are applied to the skin (usually on the back) and left in place for 24 hours. Positive and negative controls are applied to distinguish between true hypersensitivity and irritant reactions. Erythema and induration at the site of contact at 48–72 hours is indicative of sensitivity.

MANAGEMENT OF ALLERGY

Management of Anaphylaxis

If a child presents with symptoms, which include severe difficulty in breathing or shock, they should be given high-flow oxygen via a face mask and epinephrine by intramuscular injection (preferably midpoint in anterolateral thigh) of 1 in 1,000 (1 mg/mL) solution. A second dose of epinephrine can be given after 5 minutes if there is no improvement after the first. Antihistamine (e.g. chlorpheniramine) should also be given parenterally. Hydrocortisone is useful in helping to prevent recurrence of reaction, particularly if the precipitating cause has not been completely removed. All children with wheeze as part of the reaction, or who have underlying asthma, should also have hydrocortisone to prevent an acute asthma exacerbation. Its effects are not seen for 4–6 hours; however, it has a limited role in immediate resuscitation. Children with severe shock will benefit from a bolus of IV fluid once IV access can be established (the intraosseous route may be used in young children).

It is essential that epinephrine is given by the intramuscular route, the lateral thigh being the most appropriate site. Its mode of action is to stimulate alpha-adrenoreceptors, which cause vasoconstriction, thus reducing the excess peripheral blood flow and preventing capillary leak. However, beta receptor stimulation is also required for the bronchodilator effect, and also to stimulate myocardial contractility, and suppress further release of histamine and other mediators. In addition, beta-2 receptor stimulation leads to vasodilatation. These receptors are found in muscle, allowing increased blood flow to muscles (for "fight or flight"). This means that epinephrine administered via this route enters the circulation rapidly, enabling its systemic effects. In contrast, subcutaneous tissue only has alpha receptors. The resulting local vasoconstriction inhibits the circulation of epinephrine from the point of injection, limiting its action. It is, therefore, important to choose a needle of sufficient length to ensure that the muscle is reached.

In profound shock, IV epinephrine can be given. However, it is potentially very dangerous. A more dilute solution (1:10,000) is used, and it is extremely important that it is given slowly by a doctor experienced in its use.

Allergen Avoidance

The most important measure in all allergic conditions is to avoid the allergen as far as possible. In food allergic children, they and their parents need detailed information regarding which foods may contain the allergen and how to avoid them. If children have multiple food allergies, or are allergic to major sources of essential nutrients, such as milk, it is also important to ensure that their restricted diet is nutritionally replete, and they have access to appropriate substitutes. The input of a paediatric dietician is therefore invaluable.

In children allergic to inhaled allergens, such as animal dander, house dust, etc., total avoidance can be impossible. Measures to reduce exposure can, however, be effective in controlling symptoms. For those allergic to house dust mite, these include using impermeable covers for mattresses and pillows, and washing bed linen frequently in hot water (60°C), removing soft toys, replacing carpet with hard flooring and minimising soft furnishings.

Exposure to pollens can be reduced by shutting windows and doors and limiting outdoor activities on days with high pollen counts. If the child is allergic to animal dander, if possible, the pet should be removed. If this is not feasible, then dogs and cats should be washed frequently (which may not be popular with the animal!), and it should not be allowed in the child's bedroom. The animal should be kept outside as much as possible. Hands should be washed immediately if the pet is handled.

Antihistamines

For conditions where the allergen cannot be completely avoided, such as seasonal rhinitis and conjunctivitis (hay fever), regular long-acting antihistamines such as cetirizine and loratadine can be used. These are less sedative than first-generation antihistamines, and so have less effect on cognition, which is important particularly for school-aged children who need to use these on a long-term basis.

For conditions where the allergen can usually be avoided, but accidental exposure can occur, such as food allergy, it is important to have antihistamine, such as chlorpheniramine immediately available, so that it can be given at the first hint of symptoms of immediate hypersensitivity. This means in practice that children or their carers should carry the medication at all times. It should also be available in schools and other settings where the child spends time, where those responsible for the child's care should be trained to recognise and treat the signs of a reaction.

PROPHYLACTIC MEDICATIONS

Cromoglycate

Cromoglycate is a mast cell stabiliser, which also has other anti-inflammatory properties. It is no longer as widely used for the prophylaxis of asthma, as it has limited efficacy compared with inhaled corticosteroids. For those who can tolerate the irritation on initial application, it is a useful agent in allergic conjunctivitis when used regularly.

Corticosteroids

Steroids have a broad anti-inflammatory action. In addition to reducing inflammation, they decrease vascular permeability, increase the responsiveness of smooth muscle to B agonists and reduce arachidonic acid metabolite production. Their effects can be seen 4–6 hours after administration, so they are mainly useful in modifying late phase or delayed responses and resulting chronic inflammation. Used systemically, they prevent late-phase response following anaphylaxis, particularly where wheeze is part of the presentation. They are also used in the treatment of acute exacerbations of asthma, and occasionally in severe allergic rhinitis or dermatitis. The disadvantages of systemic use are the unwanted side effects such as growth retardation, immunosuppression and adrenal suppression.

Topical steroids are the mainstay of management of chronic allergic conditions such as asthma (inhaled), rhinitis (nasal spray) and eczema (topical creams). Given in sufficiently high doses they can have the same side effects as systemic steroids, but even in lower doses may predispose to local infection, such as candidiasis and herpes simplex, and impair wound healing.

Leukotriene Antagonists

These agents have a more specific anti-inflammatory action than corticosteroids, and also directly inhibit bronchoconstriction. They reduce bronchial responsiveness in both immediate and delayed reactions, including drug and exercise induced symptoms. An example is montelukast, which has been used as a single agent for prophylaxis of asthma, but is recommended as second line treatment for asthma in those not well controlled on moderate doses of inhaled steroids. Montelukast is also effective in the treatment of allergic rhinitis, by causing mucosal vasoconstriction and reducing oedema and mucous production. It has fewer side effects than steroids, but is not as effective in all patients.

Injectable Epinephrine

Epinephrine autoinjectors, such as the Epipen or Anapen, are now available. They can be carried by children (or their carers) who are at significant risk of anaphylaxis following accidental exposure to an allergen to which they are sensitised. These may include bee or wasp venom, latex or food allergens such as peanut. They administer a single dose, which delivers 0.15 mg or 0.3 mg epinephrine; the "pen" used being determined by the weight of the child (15–30 kg, or >30kg, respectively). They are designed for use in the emergency situation, to "buy time" until medical help can be obtained, rather than to be a substitute for it.

Who should Carry Epinephrine?

The answer to this question involves a risk assessment of the individual child. Factors to be taken into account include the following:

- Risk of inadvertent exposure to the allergen, despite reasonable precautions being taken to avoid it
- *Severity of reaction after previous exposure*: The child with a history of previous anaphylaxis after minimal exposure would be considered at high risk compared with a child who developed localised symptoms only
- *Concomitant asthma*: Those with severe or poorly controlled asthma are at greater risk of developing severe breathing difficulties following allergen exposure
- Lifestyle where co-factors may increase the risk, e.g. competitive aerobic sport
- *Adolescence*: Risk-taking behaviour and use of alcohol or other drugs that may impair judgement
- Proximity to back-up medical help. Those in remote areas need to "buy more time"
- Parental anxiety.

Those for whom an autoinjector is prescribed must undertake to carry both antihistamine and epinephrine at all times, and all carers must be trained in the management of reactions, and in the technique for use of the autoinjector. As it will be used only rarely, if ever, regular updates need to be given to maintain proficiency. The training is required not only for parents, but day care, nursery or school staff, and any adult who undertakes the supervision of the allergic child. This may mean that the child's life is restricted as some people may be unwilling to undertake this responsibility, and therefore the child may be excluded from certain activities. For these reasons, it is important that the advantages and disadvantages of such medication should be carefully weighed up before it is prescribed.

Immunotherapy

The aim of specific immunotherapy is to modify the immune response following allergen exposure. The mechanism by which this is achieved is known as immune deviation. Therapy leads to the reduction of activity of the allergen-specific Th2 cells, which mediate allergic inflammation, and producing alternative responses, including the upregulation of Th1 responses, and the production of interferon gamma, and the induction of regulatory T cells, which produce IL10. At one time, it was thought that blocking IgG antibodies had a major role in this process, but it is now thought that the cellular mechanisms are more important.

Traditional specific immunotherapy involves the subcutaneous injection of allergen once or twice weekly, starting with a dose below that is required to cause a reaction, and gradually building up until a maintenance dose is achieved, which is greater than that likely to be encountered by natural exposure. This can take a considerable amount of time, and even when the maintenance dose is achieved, periodic injections need to be continued for 2–3 years. There is a risk of both local and systemic reaction, and rarely anaphylaxis, and so immunotherapy should only be performed in a setting where staff is trained to deal with anaphylaxis, and resuscitation facilities are readily available. It also entails multiple injections, which limits its tolerability, particularly in young children, and so this restricts its use in this age group.

This form of immunotherapy has been shown to be effective in allergy to bee and wasp venom, and also in allergies to inhaled allergens, such as tree and grass pollen, and animal dander, such as cat. The benefits can last for many years after discontinuation of treatment. There is some evidence that early treatment can prevent further sensitisation to other allergens. Therapy in children with allergic rhinitis can also prevent the subsequent development of asthma. It would appear that it is less effective in children who are allergic to multiple allergens at presentation. It has been tried in food allergies, such as peanut allergy, but the problem is finding a small enough starting dose to which the child does not react. There have been attempts made to modify the peanut protein in order to reduce the undesirable IgE-mediated response, while still inducing the immune deviation. So far, there has been limited success with these attempts.

Because of the difficulties inherent in repeated injections, alternative routes have been tried. The most successful of these has been sublingual immunotherapy. The allergen is placed under the tongue, and subsequently swallowed. Although some patients do describe itching of the mouth and tongue, and sometimes abdominal pain after swallowing the allergen, systemic effects are rare. Preparations are available for use via this route for inhaled allergens such as pollens. Studies suggest that the beneficial effect may be long-lasting as is the case for subcutaneous therapy, and that there may be a similar effect on the subsequent development of asthma.

FUTURE DEVELOPMENTS

DNA Vaccines

An alternative approach to injecting allergen is to give the complementary DNA of allergens directly. This approach has been used to develop vaccines against infectious diseases and cancer. It has been shown that if a plasmid-containing sequences encoding for the allergen, a specific immune response involving Th1 and CD8 cells can be induced. Potentially this would mean that a short course of only one or two doses would be needed to produce the desired clinical outcome.

Anti-immunoglobulin E

Humanised monoclonal antibodies have been produced, which bind to the high-affinity binding site on the IgE molecule. Trials have been performed with such products in asthma, and also in peanut allergy. In asthma, a beneficial effect on symptoms and also on the requirement for corticosteroids was seen. The role of this mode of therapy in asthma management is not yet clear.

In peanut allergy, treated patients could tolerate a much larger amount of peanut protein before reacting than they were previously able to do. While this is certainly not a "cure" as the effect only lasts while the passive antibody remains in the circulation, such treatment may allow the administration of allergen and escalation of therapy in conventional immunotherapy in children who would previously not have been able to tolerate sufficient exposure.

At the present time, we have little influence over the underlying disease process and concentrate mainly on avoidance of the precipitating allergen, and treating symptoms which arise. We would hope that in the future, research in this field may lead to developments which enable us to offer our patients a true cure, or preferably better strategies for prevention of atopic disease.

CHAPTER 21

Infectious Diseases

Jugesh Chhatwal, Daniel Reid, Ian W. Pinkerton

DIPHTHERIA

Aetiology

Diphtheria is caused by *Corynebacterium diphtheriae*, also known as Klebs–Löeffler bacillus. *C. diphtheriae* is an aerobic, polymorphic, gram-positive bacillus. The disease-causing potential is in the exotoxin produced by the bacillus. Three biotypes of the bacillus, namely, mitis, intermedius and gravis have been differentiated with varying disease-causing capabilities.

Epidemiology

C. diphtheriae resides mainly on human mucous membranes and skin, although it can be viable in dust or on fomites for about 6 months. The disease is transmitted from person to person, either through carriers or patients. It spreads primarily by airborne droplets or direct contact with respiratory secretions. The most susceptible age group is in unimmunised children below 15 years but can occur in unprotected adults also. Asymptomatic carriers are an important source of infection.

Pathogenesis

After infection, *C. diphtheriae* remains in the respiratory mucosa. They induce a local inflammatory reaction and elaborate an exotoxin, which is responsible for the virulence of the disease. Locally, there is necrosis of the mucous membrane along with collection of fibrin, leucocytes and red blood cells (RBCs). Together they form the characteristic dirty grey-coloured membrane seen in the upper airways of a patient with diphtheria. Attempts to remove this thick adherent membrane lead to bleeding, as superficial epithelium is part of the membrane. The membrane can cause life-threatening obstructive respiratory symptoms by blocking the air passages from the pharynx to larynx and even trachea. The toxin affecting the nervous tissues, cardiac muscles, renal tubules and platelets causes the other serious manifestations.

Clinical Features

The usual incubation period of diphtheria is 2–5 days but is occasionally longer. The major symptoms and signs are related to the respiratory tract but other parts of the body can also be affected, viz. skin (cutaneous diphtheria), ears, eyes or genital tract. The presentation due to the local involvement varies according to the site, whereas the features due to exotoxin occur irrespective of the site. The most common site of involvement is tonsillopharyngeal area followed by nose and larynx.

Nasal

It frequently resembles the common cold. It is seen more often in infants. There is serosanguineous nasal discharge that may be unilateral with mild constitutional symptoms. Often there is a membrane seen on the nasal septum.

Tonsillopharyngeal

The typical membrane is the hallmark of the disease. This can have a variable extent from unilateral to bilateral involving all the pharyngeal structures and can lead to respiratory obstruction. Accompanying symptoms may be mild initially but toxaemia can set in early. The surrounding soft tissue and the draining lymph nodes can enlarge and give the appearance of 'Bull-Neck.'

Laryngeal

The membrane can extend from the pharynx to larynx causing severe respiratory obstruction or difficult, noisy breathing with hoarse voice and stridor. From the larynx, the membrane can further extend to the trachea, and the respiratory symptoms can become more severe.

Differential Diagnosis

- Streptococcal membranous pharyngitis
- Vincent angina
- Viral laryngotracheobronchitis.

TABLE 21.1 Neurological complications of diphtheria.

Site of involvement	*Time of onset*	*Clinical presentation*
Palatal paralysis	2–3 weeks	Weakness of pharyngeal muscles, hoarse voice, nasal twang, swallowing difficulty and aspiration
Ocular paralysis (oculomotor ciliary paralysis)	3–5 weeks	Strabismus, blurred vision and accommodation paralysis
Polyneuropathy (symmetric)	2 weeks to 3 months	Proximal muscle weakness, motor deficits with decreased deep tendon reflexes
Phrenic nerve paralysis	2 weeks to 3 months	Diaphragmatic paralysis
Vasomotor centre	2–3 weeks	Hypotension, cardiac failure

Complications

Most of the complications are caused by the exotoxin.

Toxic Myocarditis

It occurs in 10–25% of patients and is responsible for almost half the deaths due to diphtheria. Typically, it is seen during second to third week but can occur as early as first week and as late as sixth week. Tachycardia with soft heart sounds, heart failure or sudden respiratory distress may indicate the onset. Cardiac dysrhythmias may also occur.

Toxic Neuropathy

Diphtheria toxin can lead to a variety of neurological involvements in a multiphasic manner. The different manifestations are shown in **Table 21.1**. The recovery from most of these is likely although residual weakness may sometimes persist.

Diagnosis

The diagnostic investigation for diphtheria is the demonstration of *C. diphtheriae* either by smear examination or by culture. For this purpose, a swab should be taken from under the edges of the membrane or the membrane itself. The smear is preferably stained by Albert stain. A negative smear is not reliable and culturing the organism is necessary. For culture, selective media, potassium tellurite should be used.

Case Study

A 4-year-old boy from poor socio-economic strata was brought to the emergency paediatric service with a history of cough and a low-grade fever for 4 days. He had developed difficulty in breathing over 4 hours prior to hospitalisation. His father did not know the child's immunisation status. On arrival, he was dysphonic, pale, malnourished and temperature was 38°C. There was a diffuse swelling of his neck. Throat examination revealed a dirty grey membrane over his tonsils, tonsillar pillars and extending to the soft palate. The membrane could not be removed easily and bled from underneath. Pulse 120/min. He had marked suprasternal and subcostal retractions. Otherwise, systemic examination was unremarkable. Throat swab for *C. diphtheriae* was positive. He was given diphtheria antitoxin intravenously 60,000 units after sensitivity testing and benzyl penicillin. He developed sudden onset acute respiratory distress. He underwent tracheotomy to relieve the obstruction caused by the membrane in the upper airways. Thereafter, he made an uneventful recovery.

Diagnosis Tonsillar diphtheria.

PERTUSSIS (WHOOPING COUGH)

Pertussis means intense cough in Latin. Pertussis is an acute infectious disease of the respiratory tract occurring in susceptible hosts of all ages.

Aetiology

The main causative organism for pertussis is *Bordetella pertussis*. Few cases are attributable to other *Bordetella* species such as *B. parapertussis* or *B. bronchiseptica*. These organisms are tiny, gram-negative and coccobacillary in shape.

Epidemiology

Pertussis has been prevalent worldwide for many centuries and has been a leading cause of death in children, especially in the pre-vaccination era. Whooping cough may occur at any age, even in the first few weeks of life. Placental transfer of antibody does not protect young infants passively. With effective coverage of pertussis vaccine, the incidence of disease as well as attributable mortality have markedly decreased. The immunity conferred by vaccine as well as the disease wanes over a period of time. Hence, older children and adults with poor vaccine updates become susceptible to active disease and/or act as reservoir of infection.

Pathogenesis

Bordetella pertussis produces a pertussis toxin as well as few other biologically active substances. All together are responsible for various inflammatory changes with pertussis toxin playing a central role. The mucosal lining of the respiratory tract is inflamed with necrosis and desquamation of epithelial cells leading to obstruction, atelectasis and accumulation of secretions. The resultant hypoxia can affect liver and brain also.

Clinical Features

The incubation period of 3–12 days is followed by three characteristic stages of pertussis. The first stage, the catarrhal stage begins with low-grade fever, nasal symptoms and conjunctival redness with watering of eyes, just like any other upper respiratory infection. Coughing indicates the beginning of paroxysmal stage, which can last 2–6 weeks. Initially, the cough is dry, irritating and hacking and gradually becomes paroxysmal. The paroxysms of cough can soon be accompanied by the characteristic whoop. The whoop is a forceful inspiration through partially closed airways, which follows a bout of coughing. During the paroxysms of cough, the child has incessant coughing which increases in crescendo with flushing of face, bulging of eyes and gasps of respiration. During severe bouts of coughing, there may be cyanosis also. Very often vomiting follows the bouts of coughing. The infant or young child usually appears quite well in between these paroxysms of coughing, although the frequency of such bouts can keep on increasing progressively. Gradually, the patient passes into the convalescent stage where the coughing episodes become less severe and less frequent. The cough can persist for sometime and, hence, the disease has also been called 'Cough of 100 days'. The young infant or a sick child may not have the characteristic whoop, as they cannot generate enough pressures in their respiratory passage.

Complications

Respiratory system is the site for most complications, especially secondary bacterial infections. Otitis media, emphysema, air leaks in the form of pneumothorax or pneumomediastinum and even subcutaneous emphysema can occur. During the paroxysmal stage, serious central nervous system (CNS) complications, such as seizures and encephalopathy, can occur. A number of complications associated with the severe cough or whoop can also occur. The raised pressure in various blood vessels can lead to subconjunctival haemorrhage, facial petechiae, retinal haemorrhage, epistaxis and even intracranial haemorrhage **(Figs. 21.1 and 21.2)**. Increase in intra-abdominal pressure can cause inguinal hernia, rectal prolapse and rarely diaphragmatic rupture. Due to the protracted course, vomiting and poor feeding, malnutrition is a frequent occurrence. Flaring of underlying tuberculosis (TB) can also occur.

Differential Diagnosis

- Viral infections, e.g. adenovirus, influenza, respiratory syncytial virus
- Mycoplasma infection
- Foreign body aspiration
- Endobronchial TB.

Diagnosis

- Diagnosis is mainly based on the history and clinical examination. None of the investigations is very efficient in diagnosing pertussis. The following investigations maybe helpful:
- Leucocytosis especially increased the number of lymphocytes
- Low erythrocyte sedimentation rate
- Isolation of *B. pertussis*
  - Deep nasopharyngeal swab/cough plate cultures
  - Direct fluorescent antibody testing
  - Polymerase chain reaction (PCR) on nasopharyngeal swab

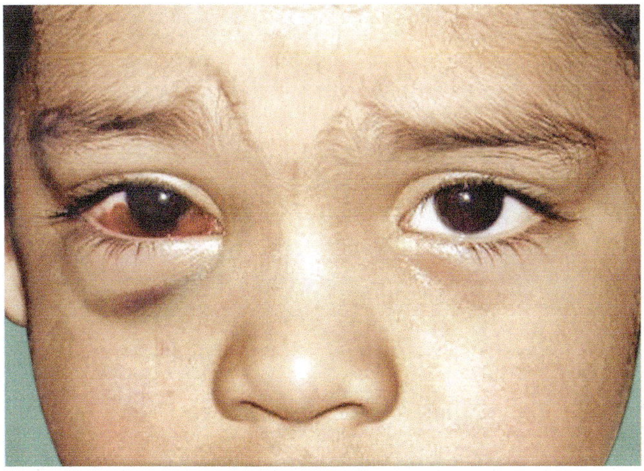

Figure 21.1 Subconjunctival haemorrhage and black eye in a child with pertussis.

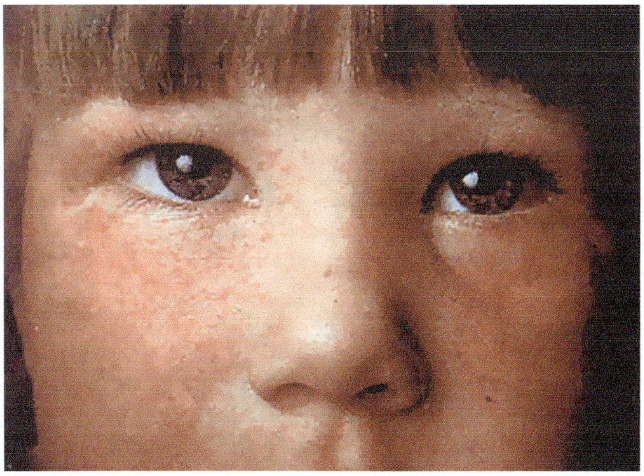

Figure 21.2 Facial petechiae in whooping cough.

- Serological tests during convalescent stage to detect specific antibodies.

TETANUS

Tetanus, also known as lockjaw, is an illness caused by *Clostridium tetani*. Despite the availability of safe and effective immunisation, tetanus is still a serious health problem worldwide especially in many developing countries.

Aetiology

C. tetani is a gram-positive, anaerobic organism. It forms spores, which are resistant to boiling but are destroyed by autoclaving. *C. tetani* is not an invasive organism. On entering the human body, it elaborates two exotoxins, namely, tetanospasmin and tetanolysin. Tetanospasmin is responsible for all the manifestations of tetanus.

Epidemiology

Tetanus occurs all over the world. The resistant spores of *C. tetani* are ubiquitous in nature and can be present in several dirty objects. They also inhabit the human intestines or animal oral cavities and intestines.

Tetanus occurs in unimmunised children and adults exposed through dirty or contaminated injuries and wounds. The other susceptible group is pregnant women undergoing unsterile methods of delivery. Along with them, the newborns are another major susceptible population. Neonatal tetanus is reported from many developing countries where unimmunised women give birth in unclean conditions. The umbilical cord is the portal of entry for the neonate born through such a process. Occasionally, tetanus occurs with no history of trauma. In such cases, chronic supportive otitis media or intestinal colonisation with *C. tetani* leads to an invasive infection.

Pathogenesis

After entering through a portal, the tetanus spores germinate, and the vegetative bacterial cell dies releasing the exotoxin. Tetanospasmin binds the neuromuscular junction and then enters the major nerves and travels to the spinal cord. There it blocks the inhibitor pathways of muscular contraction leading to sustained spasm of muscles. The autonomic nervous system is also affected. *C. tetani* by itself causes little local inflammatory reaction.

Clinical Features

The incubation period of tetanus is usually from 3 to 21 days, although it may range from 1 day to several months. The presentation is most often generalised but sometimes can be localised also. The usual early symptoms may be irritability or headache, which is soon accompanied by the classical presentation of trismus or lockjaw in 50% of cases. These are followed by stiffness of whole body, difficulty in chewing and swallowing and then muscle spasms. The typical risus sardonicus occurs because of spasm of masseter muscles of face. The stiffness and spasms lead to neck retraction and an extreme opisthotonus position, i.e. arching of the back. There can be involvement of laryngeal and respiratory muscles also. With all this, the patient is generally conscious and, hence, has extreme pain. The spasms can be caused by minor stimuli, such as noise, light and touch, but can occur spontaneously. The autonomic involvement can cause tachyarrhythmias, hypertension, urinary and bowel involvement. There is accompanying fever of variable level.

Neonatal Tetanus (Tetanus Neonatorum)

Tetanus in neonates is an important cause of neonatal mortality. As stated earlier, unimmunised mothers undergoing unclean delivery is the cause, the portal of entry being the umbilicus. The first symptom is sudden inability to suck. The infant rapidly develops stiffness of the body, followed by generalised spasms. Persistent risus sardonicus is common. Spasms of the larynx occur early in the course of neonatal disease and the infant is unable to swallow. Aspiration pneumonia and gastroenteritis are common complications. The differential diagnosis includes intracranial injury secondary to birth trauma, meningitis, hypocalcaemic tetany, sepsis and seizures of any other aetiology **(Fig. 21.3)**.

Complications

Respiratory complications occur due to heavy sedation and laryngeal spasms. Cardiac arrhythmias, hypotension are seen in some patients. Severe spasms can cause rhabdomyolysis, myoglobinuria and fractures.

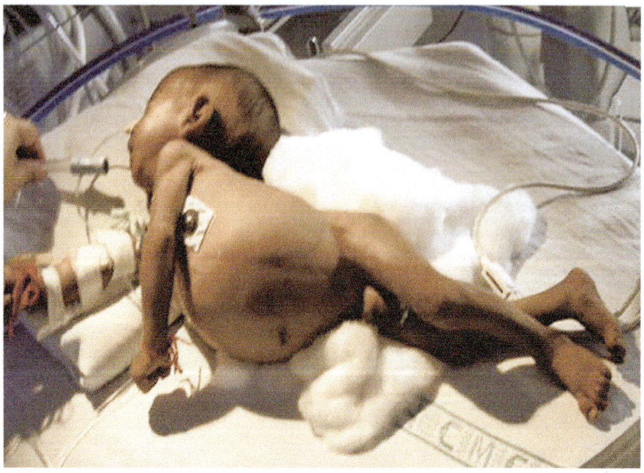

Figure 21.3 Marked opisthotonus seen in tetanus neonatorum due to intense contraction of the paravertebral muscles.

Differential Diagnosis

- Abscess in pharyngeal areas can sometimes produce trismus
- Acute encephalitis
- Rabies
- Strychnine poisoning.

Diagnosis

The diagnosis is based on classical clinical picture. Attempts to isolate *C. tetani* are not successful and not required. The routine laboratory investigations are more helpful for assessing secondary bacterial infections.

KEY LEARNING POINTS

- Exotoxin produced by tetanus bacilli, tetanospasmin is responsible for the clinical features.
- A tetanus patient usually remains conscious even with severe spasms and opisthotonus.

Other Clostridial Infections

Clostridium botulinum

Clostridium botulinum causes botulism, of which three presentations are known:

1. Infantile botulism due to intake of contaminated honey or similar items
2. Food-borne botulism seen in older age groups or adults due to ingestion of food contaminated with *C. botulinum*. This contamination can occur in canned as well as non-canned foods
3. Botulism due to wound infection is less common.

Clostridium difficile

Clostridium difficile has been associated with pseudomembranous colitis or antibiotic associated diarrhoea. It produces two types of toxins, which are responsible for death of intestinal cells, inflammatory response and the formation of a pseudomembrane. The clinical presentation can range from mild diarrhoea to an explosive onset of watery diarrhoea with blood fever and abdominal pain.

ENTERIC FEVER (TYPHOID FEVER)

Enteric fever or typhoid fever is caused by strains of the *Salmonella* group of organisms. *Salmonella* are gram-negative bacilli with flagellar motility. There are 2,463 serovars of *Salmonella*, which are broadly classified as typhoidal or non-typhoidal.

Aetiology

The 'typhoidal' Salmonellae are comprised of *S. typhi*, *S. paratyphi* A, B and C. The classical typhoid fever is caused by *S. typhi*, while *S. paratyphi* causes a less severe febrile illness.

Epidemiology

Typhoid fever occurs worldwide but the incidence differs according to the sanitation and hygiene levels. In developing countries where insanitary conditions are prevalent, it continues to be a significant infectious disease and a public health problem. Man is the only reservoir. Infection occurs through the faeco-oral route due to ingestion of contaminated water and food. As asymptomatic persons can continue to excrete the bacilli for months to years, food handlers can be an important source of infection. Contaminated water cultivation of oysters and shellfish can also cause infections. *Salmonella* can cross the placental barrier in a pregnant mother to infect the foetus.

Pathogenesis

During a variable incubation period ranging from 1 to 3 weeks depending on the size of the infecting dose, the organisms invade the intestines through Peyer patches and then travel via lymphatics to mesenteric nodes to reach bloodstream through the thoracic duct. This leads to primary bacteraemia followed by proliferation of the bacilli in the reticuloendothelial organs. From there the organisms re-enter the bloodstream causing secondary bacteraemia and the clinical illness. The proliferation in Peyer patches causes sloughing, necrosis and ulceration of the intestinal mucosa. These typhoid ulcers can become deep and lead to haemorrhage or perforation. During the second phase of bacteraemia, the gallbladder is seeded and can become a reservoir of bacilli in carriers from where the organism is excreted through bile into the intestines and faeces. The organism has a somatic antigen (O), flagellar antigen (H) and a capsular antigen (Vi). The Vi antigen interferes with phagocytosis. It also produces an antitoxin, which causes the toxic symptoms of typhoid.

Clinical Features

Typhoid fever occurs at all ages including neonates. The clinical presentation may vary a little with age but fever is a universal symptom. Initially, it may be low grade but increases in few days to become high grade and persistent. The fever is soon accompanied by abdominal symptoms such as diarrhoea, abdominal pain, vomiting and loss of appetite. There may also be cough and myalgia. The child by the second week appears sick and toxic with a coated tongue, hepatomegaly and a tender abdomen. Soft splenomegaly may also be present. The rashes of typhoid, rose spots, are frequently transient and faint and, hence, not easily visualised **(Fig. 21.4)**. Some respiratory signs may also appear. A tender mass palpable in right hypochondrium suggests a calculus cholecystitis. Sometimes liver involvement can lead to jaundice and tender hepatomegaly. In severe cases, an encephalopathy-like

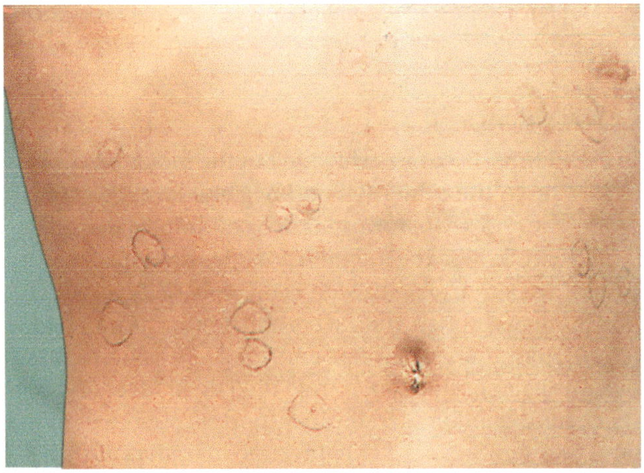

Figure 21.4 Rose spots—one of the clinical features of typhoid.

picture and coma can occur. The patient lies in bed with open eyes but may be oblivious of surroundings.

Complications

Complications are less frequent in children than adults. Two important intestinal complications, which usually occur in second or third week of illness, are haemorrhage and perforation. In both situations, patients can suddenly collapse with shock, tachycardia and drop in temperature. Perforation may be indicated by increase in abdominal pain, distension and features of peritonitis. *S. typhi* can invade any organ of the body to cause inflammation ranging from meningitis, endocarditis, myocarditis to osteomyelitis and arthritis. Certain late neurological complications, such as acute cerebellar ataxia, chorea, and peripheral neuritis, have also been reported.

Diagnosis

Blood culture for *S. typhi* is the confirmatory test. It becomes positive in the first week itself. Bone marrow aspirate culture has a higher sensitivity of 85–90%. PCR has also been used to detect typhoid and has a good specificity and sensitivity. Cultures of urine and stool can be positive for *Salmonella* but are not considered useful in diagnosis.

The Widal test, a serological test, used to measure antibodies against O and H antigens is commonly used for aiding in diagnosis. It has fairly high rates of false positivity and negativity. In addition, the baseline antibody levels of different communities may differ according to the endemicity of the disease in the region. The immunisation may also affect the antibody levels. A careful interpretation of Widal results is required keeping in mind the clinical picture of the patient and the above factors.

Haematological investigations can show anaemia due to infection or blood loss as well as poor intake. Leucopenia is the usual finding in typhoid but in younger children leucocytosis is more common.

KEY LEARNING POINTS

- Fever with abdominal symptoms and signs are a common presentation of typhoid fever.
- The gold standard, confirmatory test for typhoid is blood culture.

Non-typhoidal Salmonellosis

Non-typhoidal salmonellosis is caused by a number of organisms similar to *S. typhi* but have different serotypes (e.g. *S. dublin, S. typhimurium, S. choleraesuis, S. marina*). Unlike *S. typhi*, animals are important source of human infection for non-typhoidal salmonellae. Poultry and related products are responsible for a number of outbreaks. The infection has a short incubation period of 6–72 hours. The common clinical presentation is of acute enterocolitis. In neonates, young infants, malnutrition and other immunocompromised states they can cause a more invasive disease leading to a septicaemia-like picture and meningitis. Seeding of bones can lead to osteomyelitis especially in children with sickle cell anaemia. The diagnosis is by culturing the organism from the stool or other areas of involvement.

CHOLERA

Cholera, caused by *Vibrio cholerae*, is an acute gastrointestinal infection. It is a major public health problem, especially in developing countries.

Aetiology

Vibrio cholerae is a gram-negative, motile, comma-shaped organism with a flagellum. Two pathogenic strains *V. cholerae* 01 and 0139 are known. The 01 strain has two bio groups, i.e. Classic and El Tor and there are further serogroups of O antigens, viz. Ogawa, Inaba and Hikojima.

Epidemiology

Cholera has been known to occur for centuries in various parts of the world. It has not only an endemic or sporadic presence but has caused epidemics as well as pandemics. The route of infection is faecal-oral. Contaminated water serves as a reservoir and frequently the source of the infection. Other sources of infection include contaminated foodstuffs, utensils and houseflies. There are no animal reservoirs of infection.

Pathogenesis

Cholera has one of the shortest incubation periods of 6 hours to 5 days. After ingestion, the organisms have to pass through the acid barrier of stomach. Once they survive that, they colonise the upper small intestines. For colonisation, a relatively large inoculum of *V. cholerae* is required. The organisms produce an enterotoxin, cholera toxin, which causes the symptoms. The toxin enters the intestinal epithelial cells, binds and activates the enzyme adenyl cyclase. As a result, cyclic adenosine monophosphate levels increase. This leads to decreased absorption of sodium and chloride from villous cells and also an active secretion of chloride. As sodium absorption is impaired, water is poured out from intestinal epithelium. The outpouring of fluid and electrolytes produces the watery diarrhoea and the related changes.

Clinical Features

Cholera infection can be a mild self-limiting disorder or even asymptomatic. Severe infection leads to profuse watery diarrhoea accompanied by vomiting. In young children, there can be significant fever. The stools are watery with a fishy odour and the mucus flakes give it the typical rice water appearance. The fluid and electrolyte loss can be massive leading to symptoms and signs of severe dehydration and even circulatory collapse and acute renal failure. The outpouring of watery diarrhoea can continue for 5–7 days.

Diagnosis

Examination of fresh stool sample as a hanging drop preparation under the microscope can show the darting motile *V. cholerae*. There are generally no faecal leucocytes. Stool culture confirms the diagnosis as well as helps in identifying the type. *V. cholerae* is best cultured on thiosulphate citrate bile sucrose media.

The estimation of serum electrolytes and blood sugar levels is useful for appropriate management of sick children.

Case Study

An 8-year-old boy was brought to the emergency service with a history of frequent, profuse watery stools, fever and vomiting for 1 day. The stools were whitish, watery with a peculiar fishy odour. The child was severely dehydrated and was in shock. He was resuscitated with intravenous (IV) fluid therapy. His serum sodium was 265 meq/L, potassium 3.5 meq/L and chloride 85 meq/L. Stool hanging drop preparation showed organisms with *Vibrio* like morphology and motility. He was given oral doxycycline and continued on IV fluids. He made a complete recovery in 4 days.

Diagnosis Cholera.

KEY LEARNING POINTS

- Cholera has a short incubation period of 6 hours to 5 days.
- Typical cholera stools are watery, rice water in appearance with fishy odour.

SHIGELLOSIS

Shigellosis is caused by *Shigella* group of organisms. There are four aetiological species, namely, *Shigella dysenteriae, S. flexneri, S. sonnei* and *S. boydii.*

Epidemiology

Shigella dysenteriae is endemic in Asia and Africa and can cause epidemics. The infection is more common during warm season and source is contaminated water and food. *Shigella* can survive in milk for up to 30 days. Flies also excrete *Shigella*. Unlike cholera, a small inoculum of 10–100 bacteria is adequate to cause disease. Asymptomatic individuals can carry *Shigella* organisms and be a source of infection. Person-to-person transmission due to poor hand washing also occurs.

Pathogenesis

Shigellas are invasive organisms and affect the colon. There is colitis with mucosal oedema, ulceration and bleeding. The deeper layer of colonic wall, i.e. muscularis mucosa and submucosa can also be affected by the inflammatory process. *S. dysenteriae* also produces an exotoxin, shiga toxin, which can cause watery diarrhoea.

Clinical Features

All four types cause similar clinical picture although the severity may vary. After an incubation period of 12 hours to several days, the clinical presentation may start with loose stools, abdominal pain, fever and vomiting. Soon the fever becomes higher; there are severe abdominal cramps and tenesmus with blood in stools. Abdominal examination may reveal distension and tenderness. There can be accompanying features of fluid and electrolyte loss. In some children, neurological manifestations, such as convulsions, headache and lethargy, may occur.

Complications

- Dehydration and electrolyte disturbance
- Sepsis and bacteraemia can occur with *S. dysenteriae* and organisms may be isolated from blood culture
- Haemolytic uremic syndrome is mediated by shiga toxin
- Persistent diarrhoea and malnutrition
- Rectal prolapse in malnourished children tenesmus may cause rectal prolapse.

Diagnosis

Stool examination can show numerous leucocytes. Culture of stool for *Shigella* confirms the diagnosis. There is leucocytosis, and in some children leukemoid reaction can also occur. In sick and toxic looking children, blood culture should also be obtained.

STREPTOCOCCAL INFECTIONS

Streptococcus pyogenes or group A *Streptococcus* is known to cause acute infection of the respiratory system and skin. It is also responsible for certain clinical conditions such as scarlet fever, necrotising fasciitis and toxic shock syndrome and post-infectious entities such as acute rheumatic fever and acute glomerulonephritis.

Aetiology

Streptococci are gram-positive cocci seen in chains. They are categorised into three categories depending on their ability to cause haemolysis, i.e. (1) beta (β)-haemolytic causing complete haemolysis, (2) alpha (α) causing partial haemolysis while (3) gamma (γ) causing no haemolysis. The β-haemolytic streptococci are further classified based upon polysaccharide components in their cell wall. This serological classification ranges from A to T.

Epidemiology

Group A streptococci cause highly contagious disease and all persons not having immunity to it are susceptible. Humans are the source of infection and transmission occurs by droplet infection from respiratory passages. Overcrowding and close contact favour the spread of infection. Skin infections occur only after a break in the normal barrier, as streptococci do not penetrate intact skin.

Pathogenesis

The pathogenesis and virulence of group A *Streptococcus* is related to the presence of M proteins. M protein-rich streptococci resist phagocytosis and also generate a protective antibody response. The streptococci produce a variety of toxins and enzymes. Streptococcal erythrogenic or a pyrogenic toxin is one of these and responsible for causing invasive diseases. Certain other substances also cause antibody production but not immunity. One of these is streptolysin O (antigen) and the antibody is antistreptolysin O (ASO). The ASO levels are measured as an evidence of a recent streptococcal infection. Another similar antibody is anti-deoxyribonuclease (anti-DNase).

TABLE 21.2 Diseases caused by group *A Streptococcus*.

Infective conditions	*Non-infective conditions*
Acute pharyngitis/pneumonia	Acute rheumatic fever
Scarlet fever	Post streptococcal glomerulonephritis
Impetigo	Post streptococcal reactive arthritis
Bullous	Paediatric autoimmune neuropsychiatric disorders associated with *Streptococcuspyogenes* (PANDAS)
Non-bullous (Figs. 21.5A and B)	
Erysipelas	
Perianal dermatitis	
Vaginitis	
Toxic shock syndrome	
Necrotizing fasciitis	

Clinical Features

In addition to the common respiratory and skin infections, *Streptococci A* are also associated with a number of other acute infective as well as non-infective conditions (**Table 21.2 and Figs. 21.5A and B**).

Scarlet Fever

The illness starts as an upper respiratory infection. Soon, within 24–48 hours, a rash appears, first around the neck and then spreads to trunk and extremities. The rash is brightly erythematous, diffuse, and finely papular giving a sand paper feel of the skin (**Figs. 21.6 and 21.7**). The face

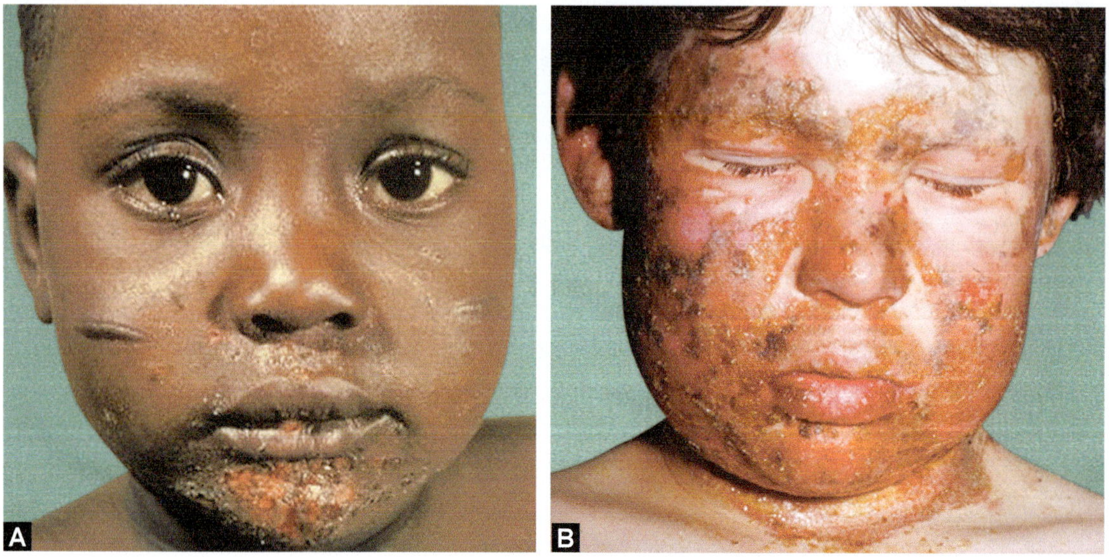

Figures 21.5A and B Impetigo lesions.

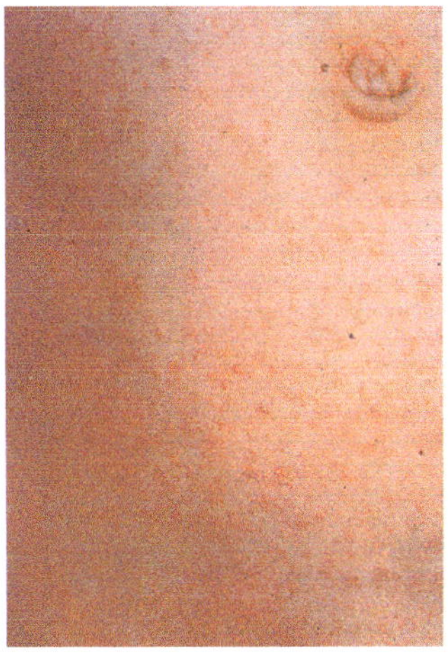

Figure 21.6 Punctate erythematous rash of scarlet fever.

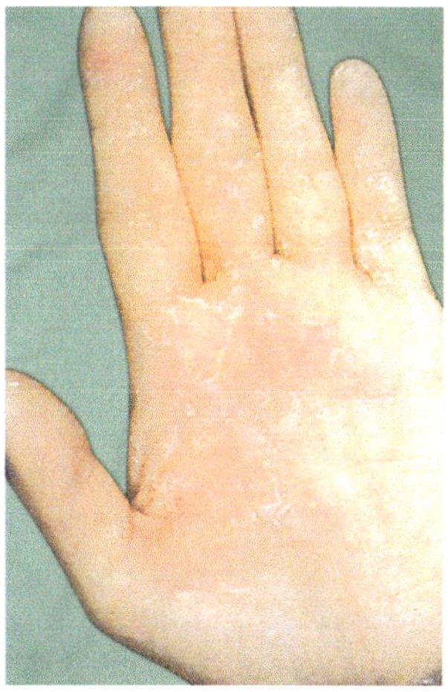

Figure 21.7 Characteristic scaling of the epidermis during convalescence from scarlet fever.

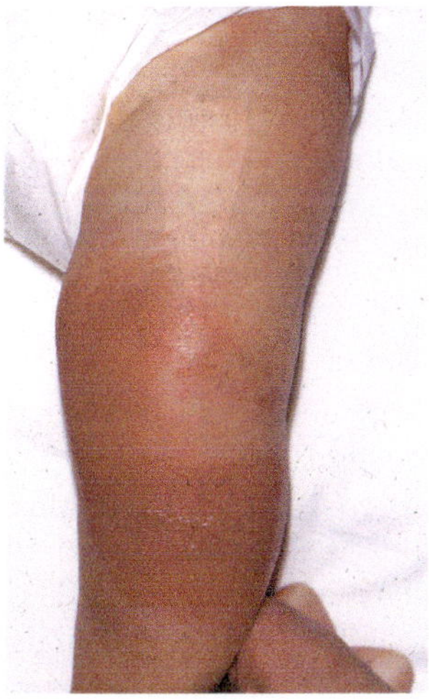

Figure 21.8 Erysipelas: Well-demarcated area of erythema and induration.

is usually not involved with the rash but there is characteristic peri-oral pallor. The rash fades in 3–4 days leading to desquamation. During the acute stage, the pharynx is also inflamed and tongue is coated and inflamed. Later, the papillae appear swollen and red giving rise to the 'strawberry tongue'.

Erysipelas

Streptococcal infection of the subcutaneous deeper layers and connective tissue is known as erysipelas. The child has fever and other constitutional symptoms. The involved area has the signs of inflammation and is very tender. There may be few overlying blebs. There is a sharp demarcation of the involved area (Fig. 21.8).

Invasive Streptococcal Disease

Isolation of streptococci from sterile body sites with serious systemic manifestation is taken as invasive disease. This can be in the form of toxic shock syndrome, necrotising fasciitis or other systems involvement, e.g. meningitis, septicaemia, osteomyelitis, and so on.

Diagnosis

Isolation of *Streptococcus* A from the site of infection is confirmatory. The only exception to this can be asymptomatic chronic carriers with organism in the pharynx. Rapid antigen detection test with high specificity but medium sensitivity are available and are useful for a quick diagnosis although they are expensive. Evidence of a recent streptococcal A infection can be seen from ASO titres, especially increasing titres. ASO titres of 320 Todd units are significant in children while for anti-DNase the value is 240 Todd units or greater. The values in adults are 240 and 120 Todd units, respectively.

PNEUMOCOCCAL INFECTIONS

Pneumococcus or *S. pneumoniae* is a frequent inhabitant of upper respiratory tract. It is a common cause of meningitis and acute respiratory infection. *S. pneumoniae* is gram-positive capsulated diplococci and based on capsular polysaccharide, 90 serotypes have been identified.

Epidemiology

More than 90% of children below 5 years of age have pneumococci in their respiratory tract sometime or other. The route of infection is by droplet infection. Children with asplenia, sickle cell disease and immunecompromised states are more susceptible to pneumococcal infections.

Pathogenesis

Normal defence mechanisms of the respiratory passages, e.g. ciliary movements, epiglottic reflex, and so on inhibit infection of lower passages with organisms, such as pneumococci, which colonise the upper passages. Any conditions altering these mechanisms like a preceding viral infection or allergy can predispose to pneumococcal disease. The commonly involved sites are lungs, ears and CNS. The spread of infection is facilitated by the antiphagocytic properties of the capsular polysaccharide of bacteria.

Clinical Features

Clinical presentation depends on the site of involvement. Upper respiratory tract infection may present predominantly as an otitis media, tonsillopharyngitis or sinusitis. Lower respiratory tract involvement may be seen as pneumonia. An invasive infection can cause bacteraemia and septicaemia. Pneumococcal peritonitis occurs rarely as a spontaneous infection. Serious systemic involvement can also occur as meningitis, osteomyelitis, arthritis or endocarditis.

Diagnosis

Culturing pneumococci from the site of infection, viz. throat, blood or cerebrospinal fluid (CSF) establishes the diagnosis.

MENINGOCOCCAL DISEASE

Meningococcal meningitis was described over two centuries ago, but it still remains a feared public health problem.

Aetiology

The causative organism *Neisseria meningitidis* is a gram-negative kidney-shaped diplococcus. Humans are the only source of infection. Many individuals carry the organism in their nasopharynx. The polysaccharide capsule of the organism has antigen variation and based on that 13 serotypes have been identified. The well-known serotypes are A, B, C, W135 and Y.

Epidemiology

Meningococcal infections are endemic in many parts of the world and are marked by periodic outbreaks in geographical areas. Overcrowding, low socio-economic status and viral infections are risk factors for the infection. The route of infection is through respiratory droplet infection. Serotypes A, B and C are variably responsible for endemic disease as well as outbreaks.

Pathogenesis

The meningococci first attach themselves to non-ciliated epithelial cells and gain entry to the bloodstream. They are protected by their polysaccharide capsule, which resists phagocytosis. After invasion, there is an acute inflammatory response, diffuse vasculitis, disseminated intravascular coagulation (DIC), leading to focal necrosis and haemorrhage. Any of the organs can be affected. In meningococcaemia, myocarditis occurs in more than half the fatal cases. Waterhouse-Friderichsen syndrome due to adrenal haemorrhage can be another fatal complication.

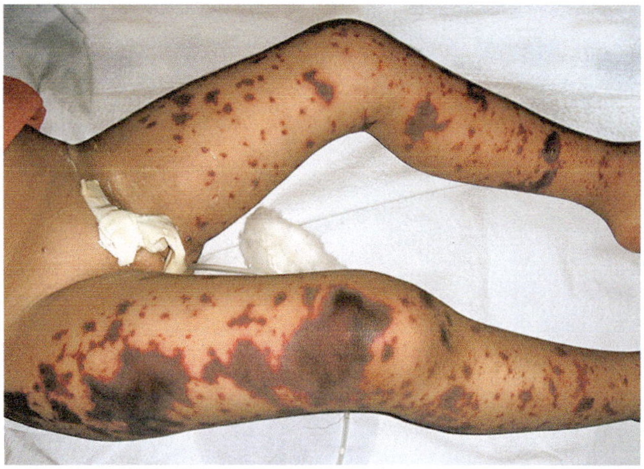

Figure 21.9 Extensive purpuric lesions in a child with overwhelming meningococcaemia.

Clinical Features

Meningococci can cause clinical disease in the form of meningitis, septicaemia or meningococcemia.

Acute meningococcaemia is a fulminant disease. The initial presentation is similar to a viral illness with fever, headache, myalgia and pharyngitis. An erythematous generalised maculopapular rash may also be seen. The disease can rapidly progress to hypotension, DIC, septic shock, adrenal haemorrhage, myocarditis or renal failure. Multiple petechiae, purpuric spots and purpura fulminans may be seen. Meningitis is not a necessary feature (Fig. 21.9).

Meningococcal meningitis can occur with or without meningococcemia. All the features of meningitis are seen. Occasionally, only cerebral involvement is present. Rarely meningococci can cause pneumonia, osteomyelitis, cellulitis, otitis media and empyema.

Diagnosis

Culturing meningococci from CSF or blood is diagnostic. Rapid diagnostic tests like latex agglutination are helpful, especially in seriously ill patients (Fig. 21.10).

HAEMOPHILUS INFLUENZAE

Aetiology

Haemophilus influenzae is a gram-negative, pleomorphic coccobacillus. Serotype B is the most common and most virulent strain.

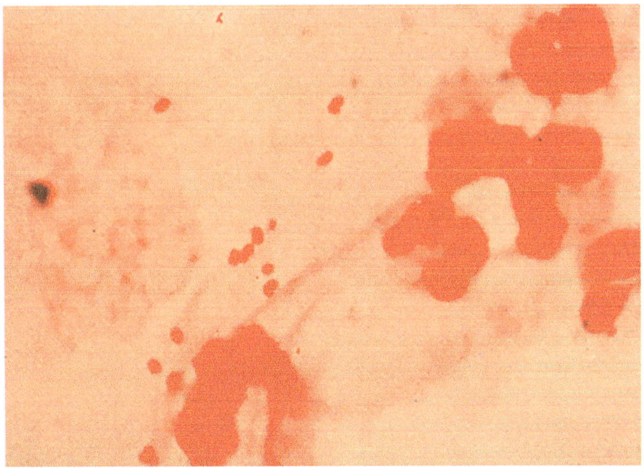

Figure 21.10 Gram-stained film of cerebrospinal fluid from a patient with meningococcal meningitis showing pus cells and meningococci.

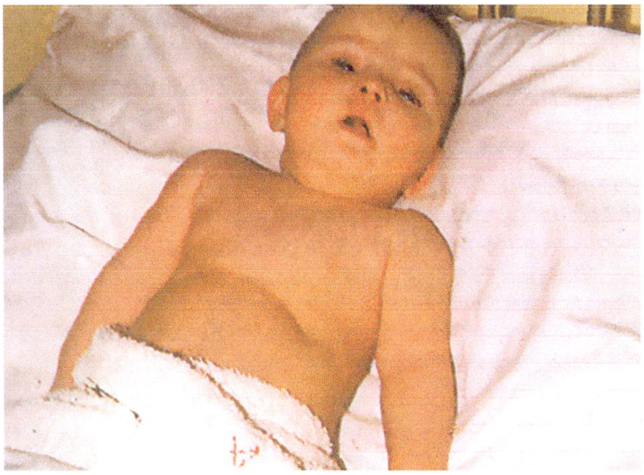

Figure 21.11 A child with croup showing the characteristic indrawing of the chest.

Epidemiology

Haemophilus influenzae is seen in the respiratory flora of normal healthy persons. Humans are the only reservoirs. The mode of transmission is from droplet infection.

Clinical Features

Haemophilus influenzae can cause a wide range of illness primarily affecting the respiratory system and meningitis (**Table 21.3**).

Meningitis

The clinical presentation is like any other form of meningitis. It is often associated with post-meningitic sequelae in the form of sensorineural hearing loss, developmental retardation, seizures, ataxia and hydrocephalus.

Croup

Croup is a heterogeneous condition of varying pathogenesis and prognosis. Laryngeal obstruction by spasm, oedema or secretion is the essential feature, with a characteristic barking cough, stridor, dyspnoea and indrawing of the chest (**Fig. 21.11**).

Diagnosis

Haemophilus influenzae is a fastidious organism to culture. The specimens must be promptly transported without drying or at extreme temperatures. Positive culture or smear from the affected site confirms the diagnosis.

TUBERCULOSIS

Tuberculosis, an ancient disease, occurs in all parts of the world with variable frequency. It has been given many names and has a very diverse spectrum of clinical presentation.

Aetiology

The causative organism, *Mycobacterium tuberculosis* belongs to family mycobacteriaceae. The tubercle bacilli are pleomorphic, weakly gram-positive, non-motile, nonsporing organisms. The characteristic feature of all mycobacteria is their resistance to acid decolouration after staining, a property attributed to the mycolic acid in their cell wall. Most mycobacteria are slow-growing organisms. Their generation time is 12–24 hours and cultures require at least 3–6 weeks.

Epidemiology

World Health Organisation (WHO) estimates that one-third of the world's population has latent TB, which means people have been infected by TB bacteria but not (yet) ill with disease and cannot transmit the disease. The ongoing human immunodeficiency virus (HIV) epidemic, poverty, crowded populations and inadequate TB control programs have all contributed to this.

The most common route of infection is through respiratory secretions containing tubercle bacilli. Patients with sputum positive for acid-fast bacilli (AFB) are the source of infection. Persons with copious sputum or a severe, forceful cough and a closed ill-ventilated environment increase the likelihood of transmission. There is no transmission from fomites or from direct

TABLE 21.3 Clinical disease caused by *Haemophilus influenza* type B.

Respiratory	***Miscellaneous***
Epiglottitis Sinusitis Otitis media Pneumonia	Cellulitis Arthritis Pericarditis Septicaemia
Eye	***Neonatal infection***
Conjunctivitis Orbital cellulitis	

contact with secretions. Young children are usually not infective. Other possible route of infection is through gastrointestinal system if the bovine strain, *M. bovis*, is ingested. Congenital TB occurs if mother has TB during pregnancy, which is transmitted through placenta to the foetus.

Human immunodeficiency virus and TB share a symbiotic relationship. TB is more common, widespread and severe in persons with HIV infection.

Pathogenesis

After infection through the respiratory route, the TB bacilli start multiplying in the lung alveoli. Most are killed but some bacilli survive which are intracellular in the macrophages. The macrophages carry them along the lymphatics to the lymph nodes, usually the hilar nodes or in case of upper lobe the paratracheal nodes. The organisms multiply and lymphatic reaction increases over the next 12 weeks. There is also development of tissue hypersensitivity. The whole complex of parenchymal lesion along with the involved lymphatics and the draining lymph nodes are known as the primary complex. The infection at this stage can become dormant with healing of the primary complex by fibrosis or calcification. The tuberculin skin test is positive at this stage. Or there can be progression of the disease, the risk being greatest in children within 2 years of infection. The risk gradually decreases till adulthood.

Immunity

Immunity in TB is an important determinant of the spread of the disease as well as the presentations. The primary immune response is cell-mediated immunity (CMI), which develops 2–12 weeks after infection. Progression from TB infection to TB disease is affected by CMI. In individuals with decreased CMI due to any reason the disease disseminates whereas in those with good CMI and tissue hypersensitivity there is a granuloma formation restricting the infection to a localised area.

Progress of Primary Infection

The primary infection in the form of primary complex can have variable outcome.

- Progressive primary complex
- The primary complex enlarges with pneumonitis and pleuritis. There can be associated caseation and liquefaction. The radiological appearance shows a segmental lesion with lymph node enlargement
- Partial obstruction of a bronchus due to enlarged lymph nodes can cause emphysematous appearances (Figs. 21.12A and B).
- The caseous nodes can erode through a bronchus and empty into the distal lung giving rise to a bronchopneumonia

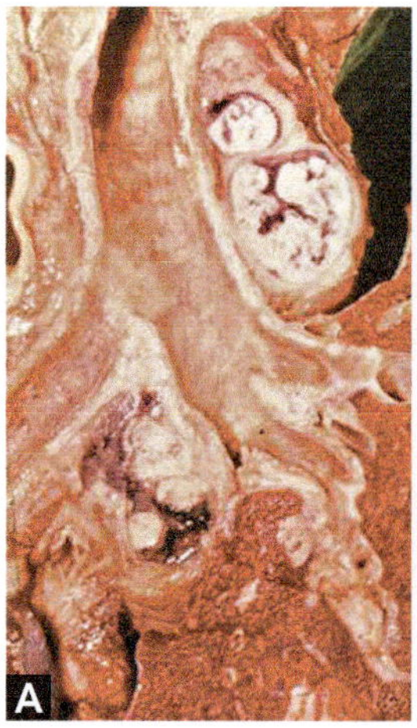

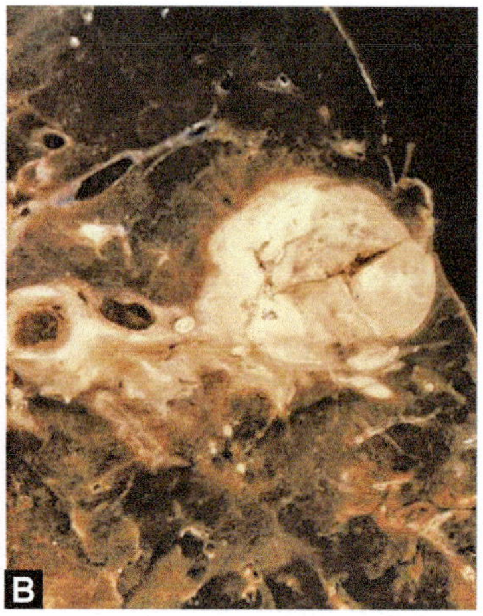

Figures 21.12A and B Tuberculous lymph nodes compressing the trachea.

- The bronchi adjacent to the tuberculous nodes can get thickened and develop endobronchial TB
- The haematogenous spread from a primary infection can cause miliary TB.

During the primary infection, the TB bacilli seed various organs through blood borne or lymphatic spread. If the number of bacilli are more and the host immunity inadequate, disseminated TB occurs. In children with good immunity and less bacilli, the seeding of the organs becomes dormant. This can get reactivated at any time when the balance of immunity changes. The presentation of the involvement of these organs can be variable (Table 21.4).

Clinical Features

The clinical presentation of TB can be either of pulmonary symptoms and signs only or of any other organ system involvement or a mixed picture. In children, approximately 25–30% cases are of extrapulmonary TB.

Pulmonary TB The symptomatology of pulmonary TB is almost uniform across various types of involvement in the lungs. Children tend to have more non-specific symptoms. Cough, low-grade fever, loss of appetite, lethargy and weight loss are usual symptoms. Failure to thrive is one of the most common presentations. The additional clinical signs of the disease depend upon

TABLE 21.4 Time interval from primary infection.

Primary infection	*Time interval*
Disseminated tuberculosis (TB)	2–6 months
TB meningitis	2–6 months
Osteomyelitis/arthritis	Several years
Renal TB	Decades

the type and extent of the involvement. There may be no clinical signs or range from findings of pleural effusion, consolidation and bronchopneumonia. In miliary type of pulmonary TB, there may be high-grade fever, toxic look and splenomegaly.

Extrapulmonary TB Any organ can be involved by tuberculous infection. In children, CNS TB is a frequent occurrence. Depending upon the extent of involvement, CNS TB can have variable clinical picture (*see* Chapter 14).

Tuberculosis lymphadenitis Lymphadenitis due to *M. tuberculosis* is one of the common forms of extra-pulmonary TB seen at all ages. The nodes draining the lungs fields are usually involved. The common groups of nodes involved are cervical and axillary but other groups can also be involved especially secondary to drainage from an infected organ. The node involvement usually occurs 6–9 months after primary infection. The affected nodes are firm, non-tender, fixed and often matted due to periadenitis. There may be an accompanying low-grade fever. When a node breaks down, this may lead to sinus formation.

Disseminated TB Two forms of disseminated spread are seen. In disseminated TB, the organs seeded during the haematogenous spread begin to get active involvement. Usually, there is fever, hepatosplenomegaly and lymphadenopathy. Other organs may also be involved.

In the other more serious disseminated form of TB, there is a large haematogenous spread and in a patient with inadequate immune response there may be miliary TB. It can occur at any age but is more common in young children. It usually occurs 2–6 months after primary infection. Miliary TB may start with an insidious fever, malaise and loss of appetite. Soon fever rises and there is lymphadenopathy with hepatosplenomegaly. There can be an acute presentation of miliary TB also. The child looks toxic with high fever, has dyspnoea along with crepitations in the chest and hepatosplenomegaly. There can be extrapulmonary involvement with meningitis in which there may be characteristically choroid tubercles on fundoscopy. Choroid tubercles indicate end artery embolisation with formation of tubercles **(Fig. 21.13)**.

Tuberculosis of bones/joints Skeletal TB is a late complication. The commonest site of involvement is in the vertebrae leading to the classical Pott spine with a formation of gibbus and kyphosis. TB of any bone can occur. Dactylitis of the metacarpals is seen in children. Tuberculous arthritis of any of the joints can occur.

Abdominal TB In the abdomen, there are two major clinical presentations, viz. tuberculous peritonitis and tuberculous enteritis.

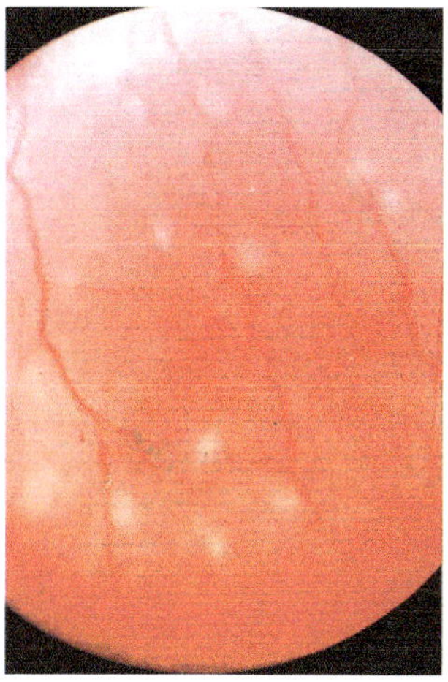

Figure 21.13 Choroidal tubercles.

Tuberculous peritonitis is uncommon in children but can occur due to either haematogenous spread or local extensions from abdominal lymph nodes or intestines. Low-grade fever and pain, ascites, weight loss are the typical features. Tuberculous infection of the intestines occur either secondary to haematogenous spread or from ingestion of TB bacilli from sputum. The small intestine and appendix are the usual sites of the involvement. Tuberculous ulcers or later strictures can cause the clinical features. Low-grade fever, weight loss, diarrhoea or constipation or features of subacute intestinal obstruction can be the presenting features.

Genitourinary TB Renal TB has a long incubation period and, hence, is generally seen in older children or adolescents. Kidneys as well as other parts of the urinary system can be involved. Renal involvement is usually unilateral and initially present as sterile pyuria and microscopic haematuria. Later abdominal pain and mass, dysuria and frank haematuria with progression to hydronephrosis or urethral strictures may be seen.

Congenital TB Perinatal transmission of TB can occur as a haematogenous spread through the placenta in the mother with active disease. Inhalation/ingestion of infected amniotic fluid or exposure after birth to a positive contact can also cause infection in a neonate. The transplacental infection presents with a primary complex-like manifestation in the abdomen. The liver has the focus with the nodes in porta hepatis also involved. If the infection is through inhalation or the haematogenous spread occurs further to lungs then respiratory signs are predominantly present. The neonate can have acute onset respiratory distress, fever, poor weight gain, lymphadenopathy and hepatosplenomegaly. Occasionally, meningitis can also occur. The clinical signs and symptoms can be similar to other infections. A maternal history or contact with an AFB-positive person should raise the suspicion.

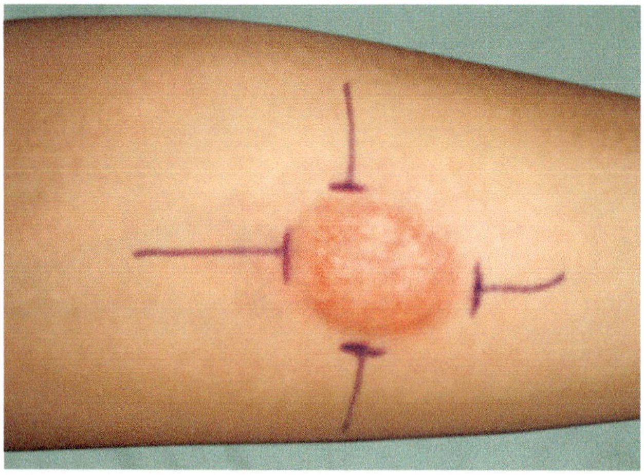

Figure 21.14 A positive Mantoux test.

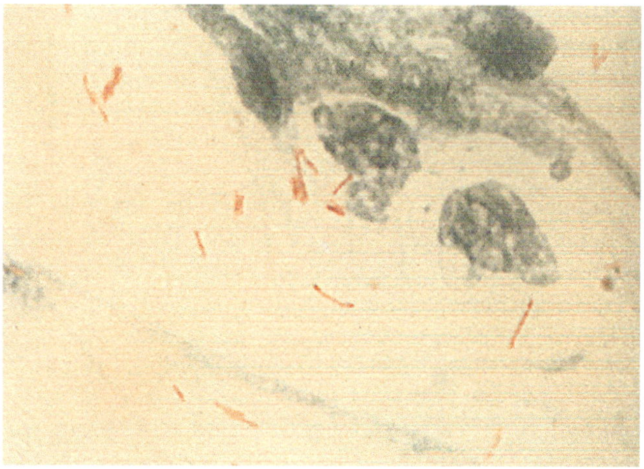

Figure 21.15 Tubercle bacilli.

Diagnosis

Diagnosis of TB in children is not simple. A high index of suspicion in the endemic area is important. The modalities most frequently used for diagnosis are as follows:

- Mantoux test **(Fig. 21.14)**
- Radiological examination
- Gastric aspirate/sputum AFB smear and culture **(Fig. 21.15)**
- Polymerase chain reaction

LEPROSY

Leprosy also known as Hansen disease is an ancient disease. It is a chronic infection of skin, peripheral nerves and respiratory system.

Aetiology

The causative organism is *M. leprae*, an intracellular acid-fast bacillus from the Mycobacteriaceae family, closely related to *M. tuberculosis*. Illness usually results from prolonged exposure to infected persons. The bacterium only affects humans under natural conditions. Transmission of the disease to experimental animals is difficult. This fact hampers research into many aspects of the disease.

Epidemiology

Throughout the world there has been a steady decline in the prevalence of leprosy. Presently, more than 90% of cases of leprosy are in 10 countries of the world, located in Africa, South-east Asia, Central and South America, with 70% in India alone. Transmission occurs from person to person among those in close contact, especially the family members. The infection is transmitted through breast milk but nasal and respiratory secretions are the ones with highest bacterial load and are the usual source. Infection rarely occurs in infants but is common in the 5–14 years age group. In-utero transmission has been considered a possibility. The incubation period is between 2 and 5 years, but may be much longer. Infection spreads only by the lepromatous type of the disease.

Pathogenesis

Most of the persons coming in close contact with *M. leprae* develop immunity without an evident disease. *M. leprae* and host immunity are two major determinants of the extent and severity of the disease in an individual. After entering through the respiratory mucosa, especially the nose, the bacilli spread hematogenously to skin and peripheral nerves. The organisms colonise the perineural and endoneural spaces and the Schwann cells. In hosts with good cell-mediated immune response, the presentation is in form of tuberculoid leprosy (TL). The tissues show granuloma formation with epithelioid cells, lymphocytes and scanty bacilli. There is no caseation or intracellular bacilli in macrophages. The cutaneous nerve fibres are destroyed with extensive cellular infiltration of the dermis.

On the other extreme in the presentation of lepromatous leprosy (LL) where there is almost no immune response to *M. leprae*. A large number of bacilli invade the skin, peripheral nerves, nasal mucosa as well as other organs with the exception of CNS, which is not involved. There are poorly formed granulomas with foamy histiocytes and macrophages with numerous intracellular bacilli. In between the two extremes of the spectrum of presentation of leprosy lie three other forms of borderline (BB), borderline tuberculoid (BT) and borderline lepromatous (BL) pictures with in between features.

Clinical Features

Tuberculoid leprosy The usual presentation is with a large skin lesion (>10 cm). The lesion has a well-demarcated

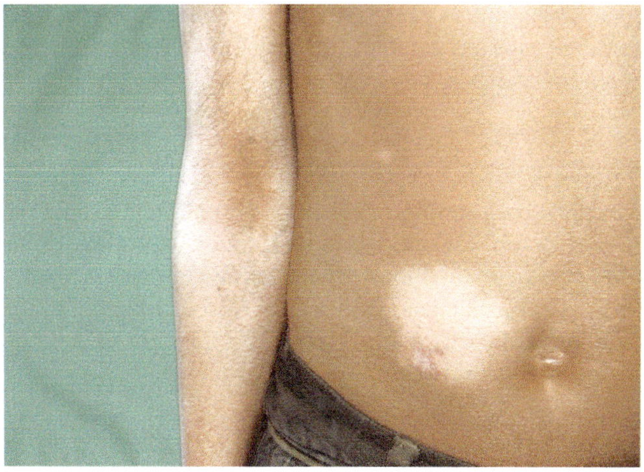

Figure 21.16 Hypopigmented patch in tuberculoid leprosy.

erythematous rim with atrophic, hypopigmented, anaesthetic areas. There can be more than one lesion sometimes. The peripheral nerve closest to the area involved is usually thickened. The lesion can continue to enlarge and there is irreversible loss of skin appendages, i.e. hair follicle, sweat glands as well as cutaneous receptors **(Fig. 21.16)**.

Indeterminate leprosy This is the earliest clinically detectable stage from which most patients will pass. There is a skin lesion, which is a single hypopigmented macule of 2–4 cm size with minimal anaesthesia. A high index of suspicion in close contacts of leprosy patients is required to diagnose this stage. In majority, this lesion may heal without any treatment while in some it progresses to other forms of the disease.

Borderline leprosy Features, which do not clearly belong to either TL or LL and are ill-defined, are taken as borderline leprosy. There can be three further subdivisions BT, BB, or BL. There can be shift from one category to the other depending upon host and bacterial factors, which change the clinical picture.

Lepromatous leprosy The initial skin lesions are macular or diffuse skin infiltration. Later they progress, become papular and nodular, and innumerable and confluent. The characteristic facial features—leonine facies, loss of eyebrows and distorted earlobes develop. There may be accompanying anaesthesia and later peripheral sensory neuropathy which may go on to deformities such as claw hand, dropped foot, inversion of the feet and claw toes. Trophic ulcerations follow with loss of peripheral tissues, such as the nose or digits.

Reactional states Changes in the immunological balance between host and bacteria especially on treatment can cause following acute clinical reactions:

- *Type I (reversal) reactions:* Acute pain and swelling of existing skin and neural lesions occur. The acute neuritis can cause irreversible nerve injuries, e.g. facial paralysis, foot drop and claw hand. The skin lesions ulcerate and can leave severe scars. This results from a sudden increase in CMI and is seen predominantly in BL. Type I reaction is a medical emergency requiring immediate treatment.
- *Type II reactions [erythema nodosum leproticum (ENL)]:* This reaction is seen in LL or BL. The skin nodules become red and tender resembling erythema nodosum. There is accompanying fever, polyarthralgia, tender lymphadenopathy and splenomegaly. This is caused by a systemic inflammatory response to the immune complexes.

Diagnosis

Anaesthetic skin lesions are pathognomonic of leprosy. A skin biopsy from an active lesion provides confirmation. To classify patients for treatment categories, slit and smear preparations are made. The disease is classified as Paucibacillary if there are less than five skin lesions and no bacilli on smear; multibacillary if less than six skin lesions with bacilli on smear. No other investigations are required.

SYPHILIS

Aetiology

The causative organism for syphilis is *Treponema pallidum* from the Spirochaeteae family.

Epidemiology

Syphilis is either an acquired infection or transmitted transplacentally. The acquired infection occurs most commonly through sexual contact with an infected person and very infrequently through blood or blood products.

A pregnant woman, who is in either the primary or secondary stage of syphilis or less often while in latent stage, transmits congenital syphilis.

Clinical Features

Congenital syphilis The transplacental transmission rate of syphilis is almost 100% with foetal loss in little less than half of the pregnancies. If born alive, then the baby goes through early and late signs of congenital syphilis. The infant may be asymptomatic at birth or develop early manifestations. One of the characteristic presentations is a maculopapular rash along with hepato-splenomegaly, lymphadenopathy and bone involvement in the form of osteochondritis and periostitis leading to pseudoparalysis. There can be involvement of any of the systems like the CNS, renal and gastrointestinal systems. Late signs of syphilis appear after the first 2 years of life and are primarily related to the involvement of the bones and CNS **(Table 21.5)**.

TABLE 21.5 Late signs of congenital syphilis.

Signs	*Description*
Olympian brow	Periostitis of frontal bone and bony prominence of forehead
Higoumenaki sign	Unilateral or bilateral thickening of the sternal head of clavicle
Saber shins	Anterior bowing of tibia
Hutchison teeth	Peg-shaped upper central incisors
Mulberry molars	Excessive cusps in lower molar
Saddle nose	Depressed nasal root
Rhagades	Linear scars around mouth
Juvenile tabes	Spinal cord involvement
Clutton joints	Unilateral/bilateral synovitis of lower limb joints, especially knee
Interstitial keratitis	

Diagnosis

Direct examination for *T. pallidum* under dark field microscopy from any lesion is diagnostic

Serological tests:

- Non-treponemal serological tests
  - VDRL (Venereal disease research laboratory test)
  - RPR (Rapid plasma regain test)
- Treponemal serological tests:
  - TPI (Treponema immobilisation test)
  - FTA-ABS (Fluorescent Treponemal antibody absorption test)
  - MHA-TP (Micro haemagglutination assay for antibodies to *T. pallidum*).

The treponemal antibody tests in congenital syphilis have to be interpreted in context of the maternal antibody titres. (If the infant's titre decreases by 3–6 months, it confirms transplacentally transferred maternal antibody titres). If initial titres of non-treponemal serology are 4 times more than the maternal levels, this indicates that the infant has been infected.

LEPTOSPIROSIS

Leptospira are aerobic spirochetes occurring worldwide. There are more than 200 pathogenic sero-varieties of *Leptospira* with clinically overlapping presentations.

Epidemiology

Most of the cases occur in tropical and sub-tropical areas. *Leptospira* infects many species of animals, but the rat has been the principal source of infection for man. Pets, especially dogs, can also cause infection if good hygiene is not maintained. *Leptospira* can cause disease in animals as well. The animals excrete the bacteria in urine and contaminate surface water and soil from which infection travels to humans.

Pathogenesis

The portal of entry for *Leptospira* is usually a break in skin like abrasions or mucous membranes. The *Leptospira* after entry into the bloodstream, spread to various organs and get lodged in liver, kidneys or CNS for a long time. The primary pathology seen is damage to the endothelial lining of small blood vessels.

Clinical Features

Leptospiral infection can present as an asymptomatic or a mild illness or a typical biphasic illness with severe organ dysfunction and death. The incubation period is 7–12 days. The initial phase of bloodstream invasion is called septicaemic phase and lasts 2–7 days. During this time, the child has fever with chills, headache, vomiting and myalgia. Lymphadenopathy and hepatosplenomegaly may also occur. The septicaemic phase may be followed by a brief asymptomatic period and followed the immune phase. The immune phase is characterised by the appearance of antibodies to *Leptospira* while the organism itself disappears from circulation and is present in the organ systems. This phase can last for several weeks. There is a recrudescence of fever and depending on the extent of the organ involvement; the clinical presentation can be variable. Neurological involvement is seen as meningoencephalitis and neuropathies. Liver involvement is generally a severe disease with jaundice and elevation of enzymes (Weil disease). Renal dysfunction can range from abnormal urinalysis, azotaemia to acute renal failure. Haemorrhagic manifestations and circulatory collapse are uncommon manifestations.

Diagnosis

During first week, *Leptospira* can be cultured but requires prolonged period for same. Dark-field microscopy of blood (first week) and fresh urine (second week) may show *Leptospira*. Serological tests: (1) microscopic agglutination test is the specific test but difficult to do as it involves live cultures of *Leptospira*; (2) enzyme-linked immunosorbent assay (ELISA) test—tests immunoglobulin (Ig) M antibodies and is positive early in disease and (3) slide agglutination test.

MEASLES

Measles, also known as rubeola, occurs worldwide and is an important cause of childhood morbidity and mortality.

Aetiology

Measles is caused by a ribonucleic acid (RNA) virus belonging to Paramyxoviridae family, genus *Morbillivirus*. There is only one serotype known.

Epidemiology

Measles has been identified to occur in history from ancient times. Epidemics have occurred in various parts of the world. With the widespread use of measles vaccine, the epidemiology has changed. The unimmunised children of all ages are susceptible. Infants younger than 6–9 months have protective antibodies transferred from their mothers transplacentally and hence are protected. As the measles vaccination coverage is increasing, it has been suggested that the transplacental antibodies of vaccine-immunised mothers may protect the infant for a lesser time.

Measles is a highly contagious disease with secondary attack rate as high as 90% among susceptible close contacts. The infection occurs through droplets and there are no other hosts or vectors. The period of infectivity is 5 days before and 4 days after the appearance of rash.

Pathogenesis

The measles virus enters the body via respiratory epithelium causing a viraemia and then lodges in the reticuloendothelial system. A second phase of viraemia occurs infecting various organs. There is an inflammatory reaction in the mucosa of respiratory tract with exudation and proliferation of mononuclear cells. An interstitial pneumonitis can result—Hecht giant cell pneumonia. The intestinal tract is also involved and there can be hyperplasia of lymphoid tissue especially in appendix where multi-nucleated giant cells (Warthin-Finkeldey cells) are seen. The skin rash (exanthema) of measles is accompanied by a similar reaction (enanthem) in the mucosa characteristically seen as Koplik spots in buccal mucosa. Enanthems occur in the mucosal lining of respiratory and gastrointestinal systems also.

Clinical Features

Three clinical stages have been described in measles including the incubation period, which is of 10–12 days duration. This is followed by the 2nd stage or the prodromal period. During this stage, the child has cough, coryza, conjunctivitis and the pathognomonic Koplik spots. Koplik spots are seen on buccal mucosa opposite lower molar and appear as pale white or greyish tiny dots over reddish mucosa. They are seen for 1–2 days only. The conjunctival inflammation initially has a characteristic erythematous line at the lid margin but later becomes more diffuse. The 3rd stage, the stage of rash, is heralded by a sudden rise of fever to 40°C or even higher and the appearance of rash. The erythematous, maculopapular rash first appears behind ears, along hairline and neck, spreads to face, arms and chest within 24 hours **(Fig. 21.17A)**. The rash spreads further to abdomen, back and lower limbs. As it starts appearing on feet, it begins to fade from the face and downwards in the order of appearance. The whole stage takes 3–4 days. The fever drops to normal as the rash reaches the lower limbs. Persistence of fever indicates a secondary bacterial infection. The measles rash on fading leaves a branny desquamation and a brownish pigmentation, which persists for 2 weeks or more **(Fig. 21.17B)**. The clinical appearance of rash can vary from mild to confluent and completely covering the body. Occasionally, there can be a haemorrhagic rash (Black Measles), and this may be accompanied by bleeding from other sites as well **(Figs. 21.18 to 21.21)**.

Involvement of reticuloendothelial system is apparent clinically as enlargement of lymph-nodes in the neck, splenomegaly and abdominal pain due to mesenteric lymphadenopathy.

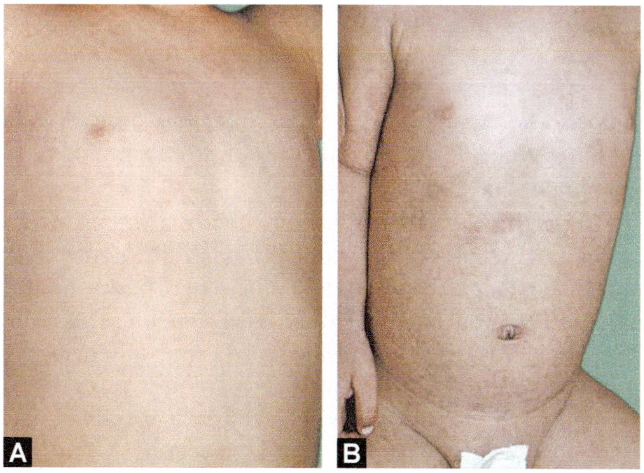

Figures 21.17A and B (A) Erythematous maculopapular rash of measles; (B) Postmeasles brownish pigmentation.

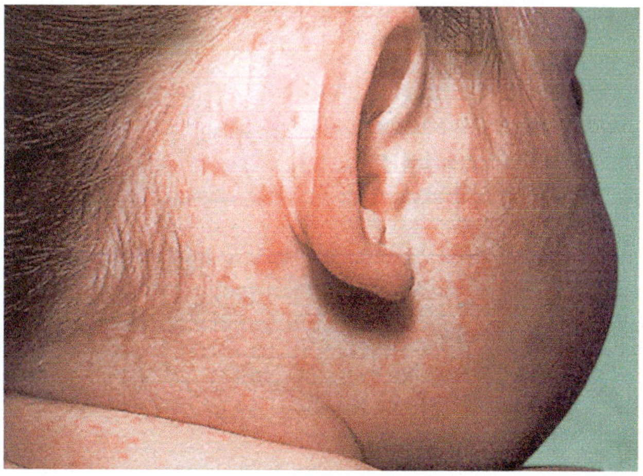

Figure 21.18 Measles rash on the first day. The face is heavily covered but elsewhere the spots are scanty.

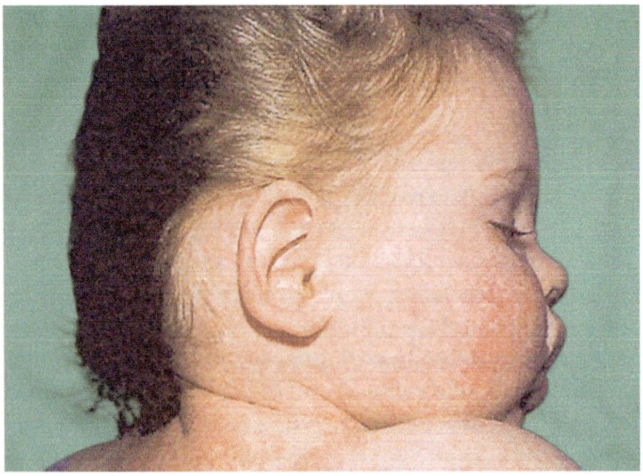

Figure 21.19 Measles rash on the second day. Large blotches appear on the trunk.

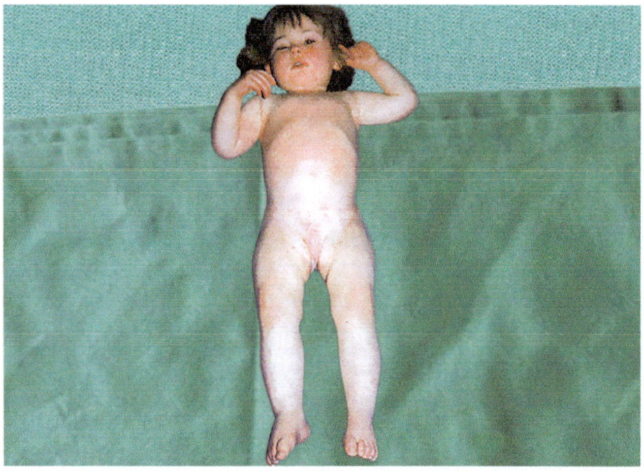

Figure 21.20 Measles rash on the third day. By now, the rash may have become spread over most of the body, but some discreet spots remain.

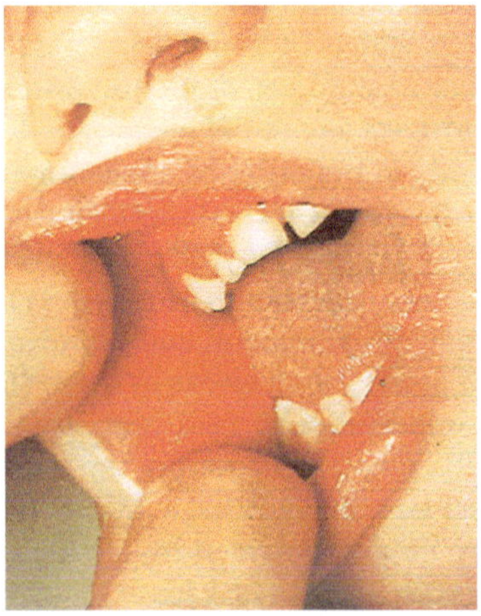

Figure 21.21 Koplik spots found on the mucosa of the cheeks opposite the molar teeth during the prodromal stage of measles.

Diagnosis

No investigations are required to diagnose measles in a typical case. In doubtful cases, measles IgM antibody can be estimated. Paired sera (acute and convalescent phases) estimation will be more reliable.

Complications

Respiratory complications Secondary bacterial infection can cause otitis media and other upper respiratory system involvements. Interstitial pneumonitis can occur due to measles virus itself. Secondary bacterial pneumonia or viral infections are also common.

Myocarditis is an infrequent occurrence.

Gastrointestinal complications Acute diarrhoeal disease is a common complication, especially in developing countries. Due to decreased immunity, dysentery can also occur.

Neurological complications Measles infection has been associated with various types of encephalomyelitis, as listed below:

- Early encephalitis-like picture thought to be due to direct viral invasion of the CNS
  - A later post-measles encephalitis due to demyelination, may be an immunological reaction
  - Chronic encephalitis—subacute sclerosing panencephalitis (SSPE)
  - In addition, other neurological complications, such as Guillain-Barré syndrome or retrobulbar neuritis, can also occur.
- Ocular involvement can cause keratitis and corneal ulceration
- Skin infection can cause gangrene of cheeks known as noma
- Malnutrition
- Flaring of underlying pulmonary TB.

Subacute sclerosing panencephalitis It is also known as Dawson encephalitis and occurs due to persistent measles virus in CNS. It is a rare disorder occurring worldwide. The onset generally occurs at 5–15 years of age. A higher risk has been seen for measles infection occurring at a younger age, for boys and children from rural or poor socio-economic background.

The pathological picture shows necrosis and inclusion body panencephalitis picture. It has an insidious onset with behaviour changes or declining school performance. This is followed by myoclonic jerks and there may be frank seizures also. Cerebellar ataxia and other abnormal movements may also be seen. There is progressive dementia, stupor and coma. The course is variable ranging from few months to few years (1–3 years).

Diagnosis is by demonstrating IgG and IgM measles antibodies in CSF. These are markedly elevated in CSF. There are no diagnostic EEG or MRI pictures of SSPE.

MUMPS

Mumps is an acute viral infection of the salivary glands.

Aetiology

Mumps virus, with only one serotype, is an RNA virus from Paramyxoviridae family.

Epidemiology

Mumps is known to occur worldwide. Unimmunised children are at risk. The mode of transmission is by airborne droplets or contaminated fomites. There is no other reservoir of infection. The infective period extends from 24 hours before the appearance of swelling to 3 days after it has subsided.

Clinical Features

A little less than half of the infections by mumps virus are subclinical. The incubation period is 2–4 weeks. The prodromal features are minimal. The primary manifestations of mumps are related to salivary glands. The parotid salivary glands are the most commonly involved structures. The glands swell and increase in size to obliterate the angle of jaw and reach the ear, which gets displaced upwards and outwards (Fig. 21.22). The glands are tender with pain in the ear and also on salivation. The opening of Stensen duct near the upper molars may show redness and oedema. The involvement of the parotid glands may be unilateral or bilateral. The submandibular salivary glands are affected less frequently. There is swelling and tenderness in the submandibular area and the Wharton duct opening is inflamed. Sublingual salivary glands are still less commonly involved. There can be accompanying low-grade fever. The swelling of the salivary glands subsides in a week's time.

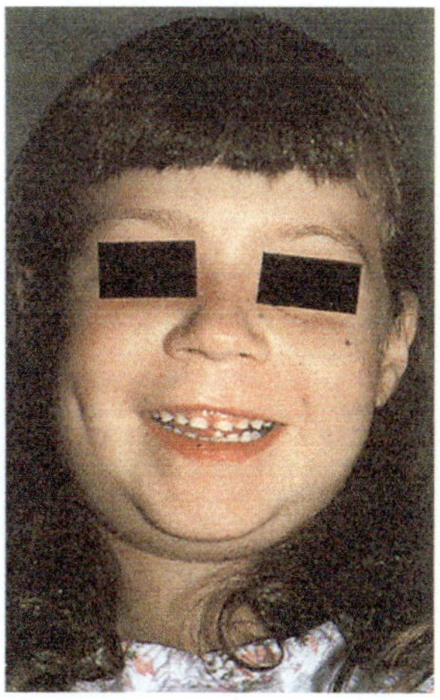

Figure 21.22 Characteristic bilateral parotid gland enlargement in mumps.

Differential Diagnosis

- Other viruses causing parotitis, e.g. influenza, parainfluenza, coxsackie, cytomegalovirus (CMV), HIV
- Bacterial parotitis
- Salivary calculus
- Cervical lymphadenitis.

Diagnosis

Viral confirmation of a diagnosis of mumps depends on isolation of the virus or the demonstration of a significant rise in antibody titre during the illness.

Complications

Central nervous system complications are the most frequent in children:

- Aseptic meningitis
- Mumps encephalitis
- Post-infectious demyelination encephalitis
- Aqueduct stenosis and hydrocephalus.

Orchitis and epididymitis Commonly seen in adolescents or adults. This may follow salivary gland involvement by a week or so. There can be bilateral orchitis. The symptoms of fever, vomiting and lower abdominal pain with testicular swelling and pain last for about 4 days. In one-third of cases affected testis may undergo atrophy. Infertility is rare:

- Oophoritis in post pubertal females is seen
- Pancreatitis
- Myocarditis
- Arthritis
- Sensorineural deafness.

KEY LEARNING POINTS

- Central nervous system involvement in mumps can precede parotitis.
- Mumps rarely causes sterility in males.

Case Study

A 4-year-old partially immunised child was hospitalised with fever for 3 days, seizures and altered sensorium for 1 day. Systemic examination was normal except for positive meningeal signs and altered sensorium. A diagnosis of acute meningoencephalitis was made. CSF examination showed pleocytosis of 400 WBCs/mm^3 with 50% lymphocytes and 50% polymorphs and normal sugar and protein levels. Over the next few days in hospital, the child developed a tender swelling over the left parotid region indicative of parotitis.

Diagnosis Mumps with meningoencephalitis.

RUBELLA

Rubella or German measles is a milder viral infection as compared to measles. The major clinical significance of rubella is in the transplacental transmission to the embryo and foetus from an infected mother leading to congenital rubella syndrome.

Aetiology

Rubella virus, the causative agent, is an RNA virus from the family Togaviridae.

Epidemiology

As with measles, the human is the only host for rubella virus. It has a worldwide presence. The route of usual infection is through droplet spread except for congenital rubella. It is also highly contagious with outbreaks occurring in hostels or institutions with a closed environment. The period of infectivity is from 7 days before the rash to 7 days after the disappearance. Even subclinical cases can be a source of infection.

Clinical Features

The incubation period of 14–21 days is followed by a prodrome of mild catarrhal symptoms, which are of short duration. Before the appearance of rash, the typical tender lymphadenopathy of rubella is seen. The posterior-auricular, posterior-cervical and posterior-occipital groups of lymph nodes are involved. The lymphadenopathy can last up to 1 week. The rash begins on face and spreads fast to the rest of the body, generally within 24 hours and then fades in the next 1–2 days leaving minimal desquamation **(Figs. 21.23 and 21.24)**. The fever may be absent or low grade.

Diagnosis

Confirmation of the diagnosis, if required, is by serology and sometimes by cultures. Haemagglutination inhibition (HI) antibody test, EIA and fluorescent immunoassay have been found to be sensitive tests.

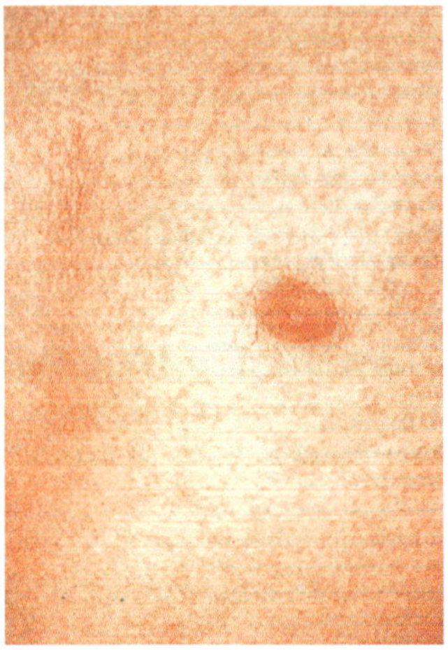

Figure 21.23 The pink macular rash of rubella on the first day.

Complications

Unlike measles, few complications occur. A rare progressive rubella pan encephalitis similar to SSPE has been described.

Congenital Rubella Syndrome

Active infection during pregnancy can lead to transplacental infection of the embryo or foetus depending upon the gestation. The risk is greatest (90%) during first trimester and decreases to 70% in second and lesser in third trimester. The foetus develops intrauterine growth retardation. The virus infects all the organs **(Box 21.1)**. The diagnosis is confirmed by rubella IgM antibodies in the neonate or by isolating the virus, as it is present in the tissues and nasopharynx. It is excreted in urine for 1 year or more. The outcome of congenital rubella is highly unfavourable as disease can progress even after birth.

CHICKENPOX AND ZOSTER

Varicella zoster virus is responsible for two clinical entities, chickenpox and herpes zoster (shingles).

Aetiology

Varicella virus belongs to human herpes virus group.

Epidemiology

Varicella has a worldwide distribution and is almost a universal infection. Prior to vaccination, by 15 years of age, most of the children were infected with less than 5% remaining susceptible, especially in temperate climates.

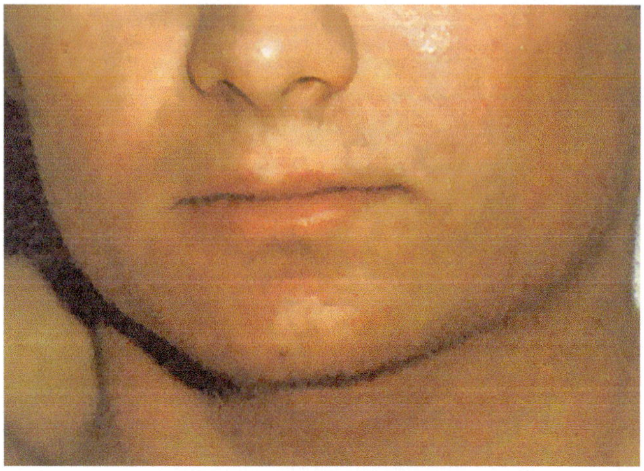

Figure 21.24 Rubella on the second day. The individual lesions have coalesced to provide a pinkish flush, closely resembling the rash of scarlet fever, but lacking the punctuation.

BOX 21.1 Features of congenital rubella.

- General
  - Intrauterine growth retardation
  - Skin rashes—blueberry muffin
- Eyes
  - Cataracts
  - Micro-ophthalmia
- Ears
  - Sensorineural hearing loss
- Others
  - Pneumonia
  - Hepatitis
- Central nervous system
  - Meningoencephalitis
  - Mental retardation
  - Microcephaly
- Cardiovascular system
  - Myocarditis
  - Patent ductus arteriosus, pulmonary artery stenosis
- Haematological
  - Anaemia
  - Thrombocytopaenia

In warmer climates, there may be a shift to older age infection. It is a highly contagious disease with high secondary attack rates. The source of infection is either droplet or contact with the lesion fluid. The period of infectivity is 1–2 days before the rash and till all the lesions have crusted. There is usually no asymptomatic infection, although the disease may be very mild in young children. Herpes zoster is caused by reactivation of the virus, which has become latent after the primary infection. It is uncommon in children and is a milder disease in childhood.

Pathogenesis

The varicella virus enters the respiratory epithelium where it multiplies and causes viraemia. A second viraemic phase occurs during which the cutaneous lesions appear in crops. The virus enters the sensory ganglia and becomes latent there. The subsequent reactivation of this leads to herpes zoster rash and the neurological features.

Clinical Features

Chickenpox is a febrile, exanthematous illness. The incubation period is 10–21 days following which prodromal symptoms of fever, malaise and headache may occur for 1–2 days. The fever can rise to 104–106°F. The rash starts from face or trunk as erythematous papules. It evolves through the stages of clear fluid filled vesicles, which then become pustules and finally there is crusting of the lesions. The evolution can take 1–2 days. Fresh crops of rashes keep erupting and at a time in the illness one can find all stages of the rash **(Figs. 21.25 to 21.28)**. The rash has a centripetal appearance with more lesions in the trunk. The palms and soles are also involved, as are oropharynx and vagina. There is intense itching of the lesions. By the end of 1 week, usually most lesions have become scabs. The scabs fall off leaving faint scars, which usually disappear.

Diagnosis

The classical skin lesions help in making the diagnosis on clinical basis. There may be leucopenia for few days. Liver enzymes also show transient elevation.

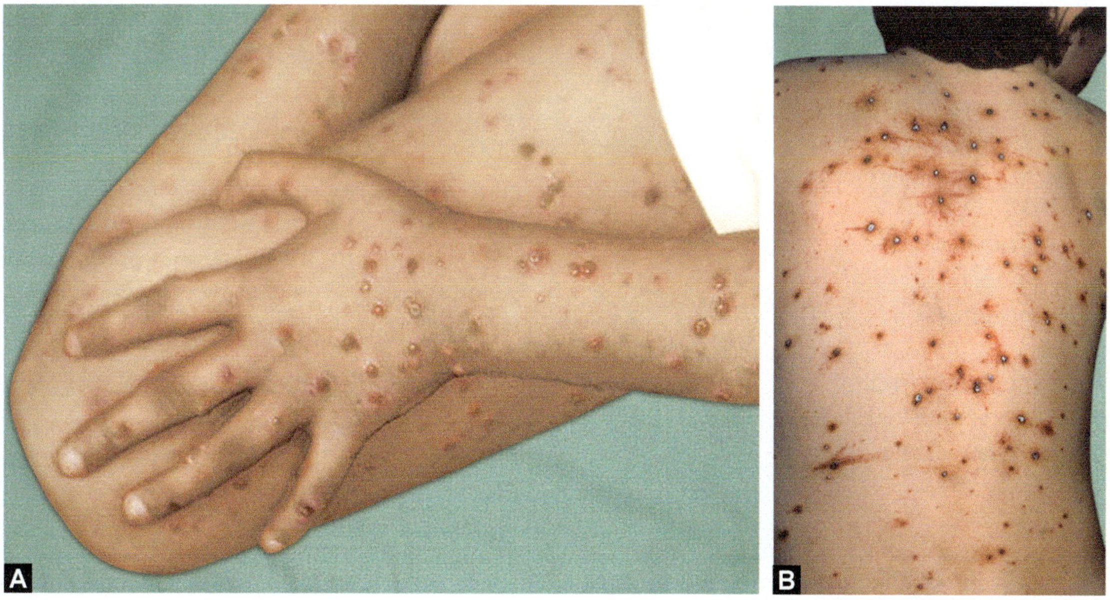

Figures 21.25A and B Polymorphic lesions of chickenpox.

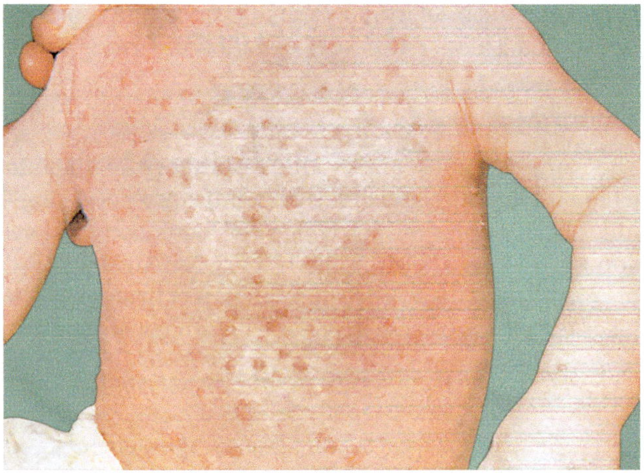

Figure 21.26 A typical chickenpox rash.

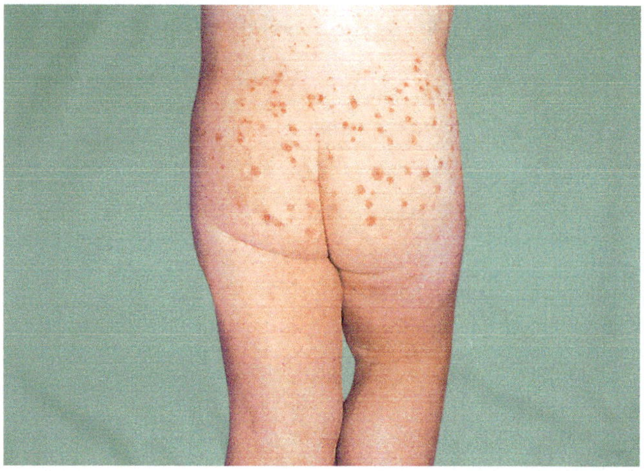

Figure 21.27 Chickenpox rash on the 'nappy area'. Distribution of the rash may be influenced by the condition of the skin; it is concentrated on the nappy area.

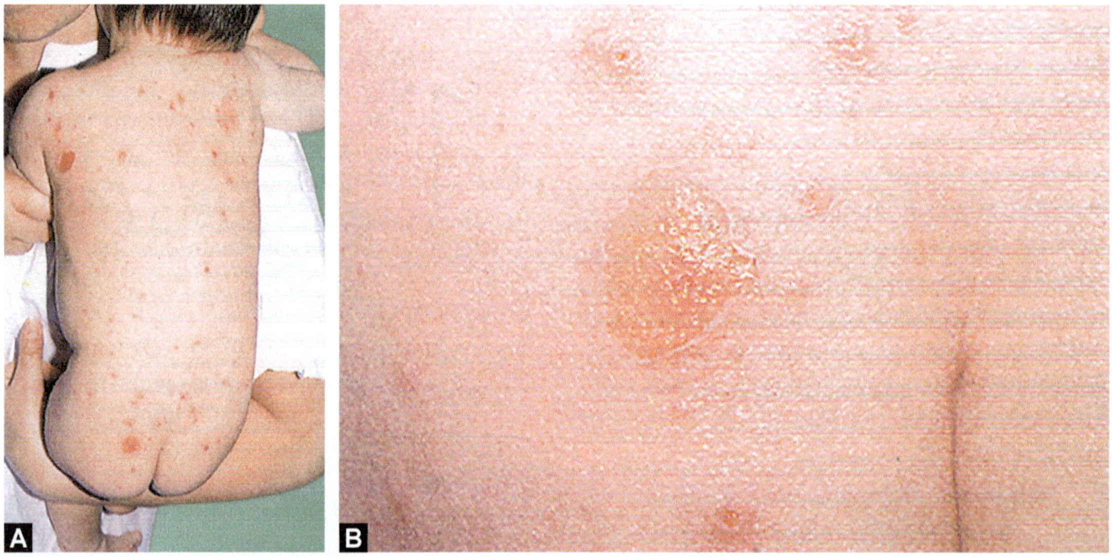

Figures 21.28A and B A dark red areola indicates secondary infection of lesions.

Complications

- Thrombocytopenia
- Cerebellar ataxia
- Varicella encephalitis
- Pneumonia
- Nephritis/nephrotic syndrome
- Haemolytic uraemic syndrome
- Secondary bacterial infections.

Herpes Zoster

In herpes zoster, the skin rash is similar to chickenpox but has the characteristic dermatomal distribution and the vesicles can coalesce to become large bullae. The rash is accompanied by pruritus, pain and hyperaesthesia **(Figs. 21.29A to F)**. Unlike adults, post-herpetic neuralgia is not common in children. Immunocompromised children, e.g. with HIV infection, tend to have severe zoster disease and may even have recurrent episodes. Oral acyclovir is effective in herpes zoster.

Neonatal Chickenpox

Neonatal chickenpox can be a severe disease with high mortality. It occurs if the baby is born within a week of onset of maternal varicella rash, as the virus will pass to the baby. If maternal illness occurs more than 1 week before delivery, the maternal antibodies may form and protect the neonate. Neonatal varicella requires vigorous treatment with IV acyclovir and zoster immune globulin.

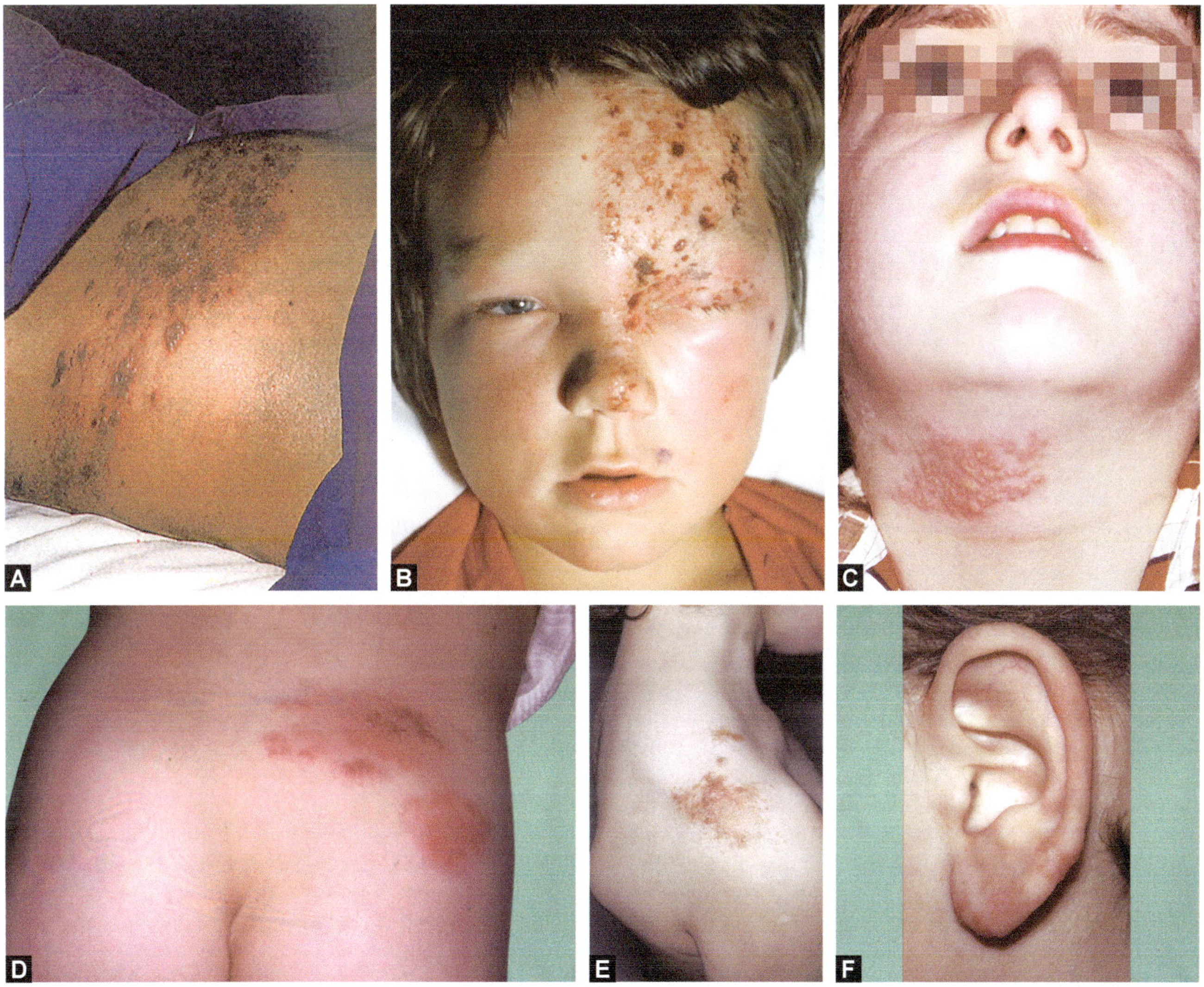

Figures 21.29A to F (A) Abdominal zoster of 1-week duration showing early crusting; (B) Zoster ophthalmicus; (C) Zoster over neck; (D) back; (E) Shoulder; (F) Ear.

Varicella Fetopathy

Varicella fetopathy has been described if maternal infection occurs before 20 weeks of gestation. A number of malformations can occur. There are cicatricial skin lesions with limb defects and damage to eyes and CNS.

KEY LEARNING POINTS

- All types of skin eruptions, i.e. papules, vesicles and pustules, are seen at one time in chickenpox.
- Lesions are infective till completely scabbed.

POLIOMYELITIS

Poliomyelitis is an acute viral illness caused by poliovirus and has a wide spectrum of presentation ranging from a mild disease to acute flaccid paralysis. Because of the success of poliovaccine there has been a marked fall in the number of cases of polio **(Fig. 21.30)**. It is covered in the chapter on Diseases of Nervous System (*see* Chapter 14).

RABIES

Rabies, a viral infection of warm-blooded animals; its occurrence has been known for a very long time and finds mention in ancient texts.

Aetiology

The rabies virus belongs to the Rhabdoviridae family and is an RNA virus.

Epidemiology

Rabies can also affect susceptible animals. Although dogs are the most well-known vectors, there are many other

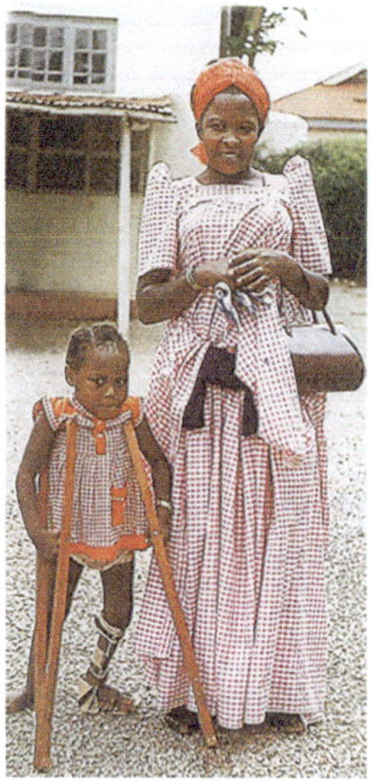

Figure 21.30 Poliomyelitis remains a serious risk in many warm countries.

animals that transmit rabies, including bats, skunks, raccoons, foxes and cats. With the vaccination of pets becoming widespread, other animals are becoming an important source of infection. In areas with substantial population of stray animals, the virus remains in circulation. The main source is the virus shedding in the saliva by the infected animal. The incubation period in the dog ranges from 2 weeks to 6 months. The shedding of virus occurs only 3-6 days before visible symptoms. The viral shedding may be variable and only less than half of bites from proven rabid animals result in rabies. Claw scratches by animals are also considered dangerous as they lick their paws and leave the virus there. Human-to-human transmission has not been reported except for transplants from infected individuals.

Pathogenesis

After the bite, the virus enters the skeletal muscles, multiplies and enters the nerves, ascends along the axons to the spinal cord and eventually brain causing neuronal destruction. The areas involved include medulla, pons, brainstem, floor of the fourth ventricle, hippocampus, thalamus and basal ganglia. Characteristically, the cerebral cortex is spared. The typical Negri bodies are cytoplasmic inclusions of the virus in the neurons. These can be absent in proven cases. The combination of brain stem encephalitis with an intact cerebral cortex is seen in rabies only.

Clinical Features

The incubation period of human rabies is extremely variable. The usual is 20-180 days but the extremes have been 9 days and 7 years. There may be a prodrome of non-specific symptoms for the first week before entering the acute neurological phase. The neurological illness can be of two types, the furious variety seen in 80% of cases or the paralytic variety in 20%.

Furious Rabies

The pathognomonic sign of this is hydrophobia. It is presumed to be occurring due to an inspiratory muscle spasm secondary to destruction of brain stem neurons inhibiting the nucleus ambiguous controlling inspiration. Whenever the patient attempts to swallow liquids, there is possible aspiration into the respiratory passages leading to a respiratory muscle spasm. With this reflex spasm, even the sight of water causes distress to the patient. A similar response is seen to the air currents fanning the patient—aerophobia that is another pathognomonic sign. Along with these two characteristic signs, there are behavioural changes in the form of disorientation, violent behaviour and there may be seizures. The patient may have brief lucid intervals.

Paralytic Rabies

There is an ascending, symmetrical flaccid paralysis.

Differential Diagnosis

The classical signs of rabies help in differentiating from encephalitis due to any other cause. The paralytic rabies may be mistaken for other causes of acute flaccid paralysis like Guillain-Barré syndrome or poliomyelitis.

Diagnosis

Rabies virus can be isolated from saliva, conjunctival epithelial cells or skin cells at the hairline. The method used can be fluorescent antibody stain or reverse transcriptase PCR. These tests can be done on the brain tissue also after the death of a patient.

JAPANESE ENCEPHALITIS

Aetiology

Japanese encephalitis (JE) is caused by an RNA virus from Flaviviridae family and is an arboviral disease.

Epidemiology

Japanese encephalitis, as the name suggests, was reported from Japan in late 19th century and the virus identified in early 20th century. It has also been called Japanese B encephalitis to differentiate from another type of viral encephalitis called type A. The distribution of JE is mainly in the eastern part of the world, i.e. Japan, Korea, China, Philippines, Indonesia and the Indian subcontinent. The vector for this arbovirus is a mosquito, *Culex tritaeniorhynchus* that usually bites large animals and birds or humans at night time. *C. vishnui* is another related species of mosquito, which spreads the disease in India. As mosquito population is closely related to seasonal changes, so JE outbreaks also follow the seasonal pattern.

Clinical Features

The incubation period of 4–14 days is followed by four stages of JE:

Prodromal stage	2–3 days
Acute stage	3–4 days
Subacute stage	7–10 days
Convalescence stage	4–7 weeks

The illness starts with a sudden onset of fever accompanied by respiratory symptoms and headache. This is soon followed by some behavioural changes such as disorientation, delirium or excessive sleepiness. Seizures of generalised variety may occur in a quarter of patients. The neurological signs fluctuate from hyper-reflexia to hyporeflexia, intention tremors and cogwheel rigidity. Patient may progress to coma. A rapid progression of disease is often seen in young children with high fatality.

Diagnosis

The CSF shows pleocytosis (100–1,000/mm^3) with initial polymorph predominance followed by lymphocytosis. Confirmation of the diagnosis can be by checking for specific IgM antibodies in the serum or CSF early in the illness or an increase of IgG antibodies in paired sera. EEG shows diffuse slowing. Cranial MRI/CT may show white matter oedema and hypodense lesions in thalamus, basal ganglia and pons.

DENGUE FEVERS

Dengue fevers comprise a group of febrile illnesses caused by arthropod-borne viruses (Arboviruses) including dengue haemorrhagic fever (DHF) and dengue shock syndrome (DSS).

Aetiology

The dengue viruses belonging to family Flaviviridae have four distinct antigenic types. In addition, there are a few other arboviruses, which cause a similar clinical picture.

Epidemiology

The principal vector for all dengue viruses is a mosquito, *Aedes aegypti*. Other *Aedes* species have also been reported to carry these viruses. At present, the disease is endemic to areas, which have suitable breeding environment for the specific mosquito. Hence, it is the tropical areas, such as Asia, Africa, Caribbeans and South America, which have majority of cases. Explosive outbreaks of dengue occur in urban areas where A. *aegypti* is breeding. This mosquito lives in areas where stored or pooled water is collected and is a day-biting mosquito. The biting rates increase with increase in temperature and humidity. The mosquito does not have a wide flight ranges so the outbreaks and epidemic are usually due to viraemic humans travelling to different areas.

Pathogenesis

The exact pathogenic mechanism for the diverse clinical presentations of dengue fevers is not yet known. No single characteristic pathological change has been noticed in the autopsy of patients dying with dengue. It has been observed that a second exposure or infection by the dengue viruses is more likely to lead to a significant disease. There are infection-enhancing antibodies formed as a result of first infection, which, on second exposure, cause higher degree of viraemia and consequently a more severe disease. The second infections activate the complement system and there are many factors which together interact to produce increased vascular permeability. This allows fluids to move from intra- to extravascular spaces leading to haemoconcentration and hypovolaemia.

The mechanism of bleeding in DHF is not exactly clear. It may be a combination of factors such as thrombocytopaenia, DIC and liver damage. The cause of thrombocytopaenia is also not well established. There is a maturational arrest of megakaryocytes in bone marrow. Other mechanisms, such as antibodies on platelet surface or cross-reacting antibodies, have also been considered.

Clinical Features

The incubation period of dengue fever is 1–7 days. The clinical presentation can be variable.

There may be an initial flu-like illness for few days or a sudden rise of temperature even up to 106°F. There is an accompanying frontal headache and retrobulbar pain with severe myalgia and arthralgia. There may also be severe backache before the fever. A transient erythematous rash may also appear early in the febrile phase. Towards the end of first week of illness, there is a typical cutaneous hyperaesthesia and hyperalgesia with marked loss of appetite and taste. As the fever comes down, there is a second phase of rash, which is generalised, erythematous with a morbilliform or a lacy appearance. There can be accompanying diffuse oedema, especially of palms and soles. The rash lasts 1–5 days followed sometimes by desquamation and intense itching. There may be a slight fever also at this stage. In some patients, there is thrombocytopaenia and neutropaenia with variable bleeding manifestations ranging from epistaxis to menorrhagia. The platelet count can drop to 10,000/mm^3 and WBC count to even 1,000/mm^3. Usually, the patient makes a quick recovery in 2–4 days.

Dengue Haemorrhagic Fever

The initial mild onset of dengue fever may rapidly change its course towards rapid deterioration after 2–5 days. The patient appears ill with flushed and cold extremities, restlessness and has bleeding from venepunctures or spontaneous petechiae and ecchymoses. There is significant hepatomegaly. Few patients may have gastrointestinal bleeding also.

Dengue Shock Syndrome

In few patients, the DHF may be complicated by a shock-like state due to the accompanying hypovolaemia (Leaky capillaries) and also bleeding.

Some patients have significant extravasations into pleural spaces (pleural effusion, unilateral or bilateral) as well as ascites. The liver involvement occasionally can be clinically manifested as mild icterus also. After 1–2 days of critical illness, the patient can make a quick recovery with return to normal temperature, blood pressure and pulse. There is reabsorption of the intravascular fluid. During this phase, careful attention to fluid intake and balance is required as the patient may develop congestive heart failure. There have been few reports of dengue encephalitis also in children similar to other viral encephalitis.

Differential Diagnosis

A clinical suspicion in the setting of dengue fever endemicity is usually used to make a diagnosis. As there are other viruses causing similar diseases, the term 'Dengue-like disease' should be used in the absence of specific diagnosis. WHO has given guidelines for diagnosing DHF/DSS.

WHO Criteria for Dengue Haemorrhagic Fever/Dengue Shock Syndrome

Dengue Haemorrhagic Fever

- Fever
- Minor/major haemorrhagic manifestations
- Thrombocytopenia less than 100,000/mm^3
- Increased capillary permeability (increase in haematocrit of >20%)
- Pleural effusion (X-ray chest)
- Hypoalbuminaemia.

Dengue Shock Syndrome

- DHF criteria Plus
- Hypotension
- Pulse pressure less than 20 mmHg.

Diagnosis

Complete blood counts including haematocrit and platelets will show the already mentioned changes. Liver function test may show elevation of enzymes, hypoproteinaemia and prolonged prothrombin time. Chest radiographs show pleural effusion in many patients.

Specific virological investigations are based on serological tests or virus isolation. In dengue infection, first episode IgM levels rise for 6–12 weeks but in second infection IgG rise is much more. Fourfold rise in paired sera help in diagnosis. A single serum sample for antibodies collected at least 5 days after the onset and up to 6 weeks can also be used.

Case Study

A 13-year-old boy was hospitalised with a history of fever with body ache for 1 week, generalised rash and epistaxis on the day of admission. On examination, he had a low-grade fever, a generalised morbilliform erythematous rash and a few petechiae on limbs. He had tachycardia otherwise examination of respiratory and cardiovascular system was normal. There was hepatomegaly on abdominal examination. Investigations: Haemoglobin (Hb) 14 g/dL, total white cell count 3,000/mm^3, P45%, L42% M5%, E3%, platelets 20,000/mm^3.

Diagnosis Dengue fever.

HUMAN IMMUNODEFICIENCY VIRUS INFECTION/AIDS

Infection with HIV is one of the recently identified diseases. The first case of HIV infection in paediatric age group was reported in 1983. HIV infection eventually leads to acquired immunodeficiency syndrome (AIDS), a disease with a very high mortality.

Aetiology

Human immunodeficiency virus is of two types, viz. HIV-1 and HIV-2. They are both RNA viruses of family Retroviridae. HIV-2 is a rare cause of infection in children.

Epidemiology

According to WHO in 2005, it was estimated that 38,600,000 persons are living with HIV or AIDS. Out of these children comprise about 6%. The sub-Saharan Africa, South East Asian countries such as India, Thailand, Vietnam and China dominate the picture. In children, more than 90% of infection is through vertical transmission, i.e. from mother to child. A small percentage is through blood or blood products and transmission through sexual contact or IV drug use seen in the adolescent age group.

Perinatal Transmission

In HIV-positive women, the perinatal transmission rates can vary from 16 to 40% if no protective measures are undertaken. The risk factors for higher rates of transmission are advanced maternal HIV disease, delivery less than 37 weeks, prolonged rupture of membranes, vaginal delivery, chorioamnionitis, invasive procedures (e.g. amniocentesis) and haemorrhage in labour. The transmission of infection can occur any time during pregnancy or intrapartum period. In utero transmission can occur as a transplacental infection or through inflammation of the membranes or by materno-foetal transfusion. With early infection, foetal loss is more likely. The most frequent timing of transmission of infection is intrapartum (60–75%) and occurs through materno-foetal transfusion. Postpartum transmission can occur through breastfeeding. The risk of HIV transmission to baby from breastmilk ranges from 12 to 14%. The risk is higher in babies on mixed milk feeding as compared to exclusive breastfeeding.

Pathogenesis

The first cells to be infected through mucosal entry of HIV are the dendritic cells. These cells transport the virus to the lymphatic tissues where it selectively invades the HIV helper cell count (CD4) lymphocytes, monocytes and macrophages.

After infecting CD4 cells, there is progressive viral replication followed by a viraemic phase 3–6 weeks after infection. This is associated with influenza-like symptoms sometimes. Subsequently, there is a decline in the viraemia due to the normal immune response of the body. HIV suppressor cell count (CD8 cells) are of help in containing the initial infection. A variable period of clinical latency follows but during this phase viral multiplication continues. The cytokines play an important role in sustaining viral load during this phase.

Following perinatal transmission of infection, there is little evidence clinically or virologically of HIV infection at birth. The viral load increases after first month and viral isolation by laboratory tests is more likely to be positive between 1 and 4 months of age. The immunological abnormalities in HIV-infected children are similar to changes in adults except that, as there is a physiological lymphocytosis, hence, the values for labelling CD4 depletion are different in children. There is also B cell activation leading to an increased antibody production and resultant hypergammaglobulinaemia.

Clinical Features

After perinatal transmission, there are three types of clinical presentations described. The first presentation is of rapid progression where the infant presents with features of AIDS in the first few months of life. There is a rapid deterioration with poor survival beyond the first year of life. Majority of the children have the second type of presentation. The child is asymptomatic during initial 1–2 years and, later, presents with lymphadenopathy, failure to thrive and other features of AIDS. The median survival in this pattern is about 6 years. The third pattern is of a delayed presentation, which is seen infrequently. The child has no significant features till 8–10 years of age followed by full AIDS presentation.

The usual presenting features in developing countries are chronic or recurrent diarrhoea, failure to thrive and wasting. There may be accompanying chronic or recurrent mucocutaneous candidiasis, lymphadenopathy and hepatosplenomegaly. In infants, the initial presentation may be a severe respiratory distress due to *Pneumocystis carinii* infection. CNS involvement is also more common in children. The symptoms have been categorised by Centres for Disease Control and Prevention (CDC) as described here.

Staging of Paediatric AIDS [Centers for Disease Control and Prevention (1994) Criteria]

Category N: Asymptomatic, no signs or symptoms or only one of the conditions listed in Category A.

Category A: Mildly symptomatic or two or more of the following conditions:

- Lymphadenopathy
- Hepatomegaly
- Splenomegaly
- Parotitis
- Dermatitis
- Recurrent or persistent upper respiratory infection.

Category B: Moderately symptomatic conditions attributed to HIV infection:

- Severe bacterial infections
- Lymphoid interstitial pneumonia
- Anaemia
- Neutropaenia
- Thrombocytopenia
- Cardiomyopathy
- Nephropathy
- Hepatitis
- Diarrhoea
- Candidiasis.

Category C: Severely symptomatic, two serious bacterial infections:

- Encephalopathy (acquired microcephaly, cognitive delay and abnormal neurology)
- Opportunistic infections (*P. carinii* pneumonia, CMV, toxoplasmosis, disseminated fungal infections)
- Disseminated mycobacterial diseases
- Cancer (Kaposi sarcoma, lymphomas).

ASSOCIATED INFECTIONS

As HIV causes serious disturbances in immune system, associated infections are almost universal and very often the presenting feature. Any organism bacteria, viruses, protozoa or fungi can cause serious systemic sepsis in HIV-infected children. Opportunistic organisms are also frequent causes of serious disease in such children. Various opportunistic infections are listed as follows.

Opportunistic Infections

- *Pneumocystis carinii* pneumonia
- Candidiasis—oesophageal or pulmonary
- Tuberculosis
- *Mycobacterium avium*
- Cytomegalovirus

- Cryptosporidiosis
- Non-tuberculous mycobacteria
- Herpes zoster
- Toxoplasmosis.

Mycobacteria and HIV share a symbiotic relationship in HIV-infected patients. Both TB as well as non-TB mycobacteria, can cause difficult to treat, disseminated and resistant disease.

Candidal infections also occur in a more widespread fashion often involving oesophagus along with oral cavity. Out of viruses, herpes group, both zoster and simplex are frequent offenders.

Diagnosis

If any one of the parents is known to be having HIV infection, the infant/child must be screened for it. In others, the indications for HIV testing are given below.

In asymptomatic children:

- Parent at high risk for HIV infection, e.g. truck drivers, IV drug users.
- Children receiving transfusion or blood products, etc.

In symptomatic infants and children:

- Recurrent, severe bacterial infections
- Opportunistic infections
- Poor response to antitubercular treatment
- Evidence of congenital toxoplasmosis, rubella, cytomegalovirus and herpes simplex virus (TORCH)
- Unexplained wasting, neuroencephalopathy, myopathy, hepatitis, cardiomyopathy and nephropathy
- Hyperimmunoglobulinaemia.

Viral cultures are the gold standard for diagnosis of HIV and have 100% specificity. The culture requires 2–3 weeks, is labour-intensive and expensive. The alternative, PCR for viral deoxyribonucleic acid or RNA, is also specific and sensitive. The assay for p24 antigen of HIV has also been frequently used with good specificity but less sensitivity.

PERINATAL TRANSMISSION

At birth, all infants born to HIV-positive mothers have placentally transferred antibodies. These declines slowly in 6–12 months time. Only at the age of 18 months or more, if the antibody test is positive, that can be used as an indicator of infection in the child. In a neonate born to an HIV-positive mother, virological assay (PCR/culture/p24 antigen) provide reliable results. If anti-retroviral therapy is to be started, it is recommended that testing should be done within 48 hours of birth, at 4–6 weeks of age and/or 4–6 months of age. Two positive tests from different samples confirm the transmission of HIV infection to the infant. On the other hand, if two different tests, of which one should be at 4–6 months of age are negative, then HIV infection can be excluded. At 18 months of age, in an asymptomatic infant, two negative antibody tests exclude HIV infection.

Older Infants and Children

In older infants and children, two or more HIV antibody tests done by different techniques on different samples are recommended to make a diagnosis. Once HIV infection is diagnosed in a child, further evaluation is done by complete blood count along with CD4 and CD8 lymphocyte counts. Additional tests depend on the extent and type of systemic involvement.

MALARIA

Aetiology

Intracellular protozoa, *Plasmodium*, cause malaria. There are four species of *Plasmodium* that infect humans, viz. *P. vivax*, *P. falciparum*, *P. malariae* and *P. ovale*. Female anopheles mosquitoes transmit it during a blood meal on humans. It can also be a transfusion-transmitted infection or a transplacental infection from mother to the foetus.

Epidemiology

Malaria occurs worldwide but the endemicity depends on the mosquito population. In areas with suitable environment for mosquito breeding, the incidence of malaria is high, e.g. Africa, Asia and South America. *P. falciparum* and *P. vivax* are more commonly seen in sub-Saharan Africa and the Indian subcontinent. *P. ovale* is rare and seen mainly in Africa. *P. malariae* is the rarest.

Pathogenesis

Plasmodia have two parts of their life cycle, sexual and asexual phase, in vector mosquito and human host, respectively. In the humans, there are two stages: first stage in the liver, the exo-erythrocytic phase, and the second one in RBCs, the erythrocytic phase. Mosquito bites the human host and releases sporozoites in the bloodstream, which quickly enter the hepatocytes. In the hepatocytes, the sporozoites multiply, become schizonts and rupture the cell. On rupture of hepatocytes, thousands of merozoites are released into the circulation. *P. vivax* has two types of schizonts, a primary type, which follows the above cycle, and a secondary type, which becomes dormant in the hepatocytes for weeks and months causing frequent relapses. The merozoites released into the circulation enter the RBCs and become the ring form, which later grows to become trophozoite. The trophozoite multiplies again and gives rise to merozoites in RBCs, which rupture releasing them in circulation. The release of merozoites is associated with a sharp rise in fever. Some of the merozoites develop into male and female gametocytes, which are ingested by the female anopheles mosquito during a blood meal. The gametocytes undergo the sexual phase of development in the stomach of the mosquito

BOX 21.2 Incubation period of malaria species.

P. vivax	12–17 days
P. falciparum	8–14 days
P. malariae	18–40 days
P. ovale	16–18 days

where a zygote is formed and develops into sporozoites, which enter the mosquito salivary glands ready to inject the new host.

In the pathogenesis of malaria, fever results from RBC rupture and release of merozoites. The other common feature, anaemia, is a result of breakdown of RBCs, i.e. haemolysis. There are two more mechanisms responsible for other clinical features. An immune-pathological process leading to release of cytokines, which cause many features. In *P. falciparum*, another pathological change is the adherence of infected RBCs to the endothelial lining of blood vessels. This results in damage to various organs such as brain, kidneys, intestines, and so on.

Clinical Features

Incubation period for each species is different (**Box 21.2**).

The onset of the disease is marked by a sudden rise of fever, which may be periodic. Rigors and sweating, headache, body ache, nausea and vomiting accompany the fever. There may be diarrhoea and cough also sometimes. The gastrointestinal and respiratory symptoms are seen more often in young children and infants. After a few days of fever, the patient begins to appear pale and may even have jaundice. In adults, there is a definite periodicity of fever, which is generally not seen in children. The clinical presentation in some children may be different with low-grade fever, hepatosplenomegaly, anaemia and thrombocytopenia.

Congenital malaria is considered in a neonate whose mother was symptomatic during late pregnancy. The neonate may manifest with symptoms between 10 and 30 days of age. The neonate may or may not have any fever along with poor feeding, lethargy and vomiting. Unexplained anaemia and severe jaundice (indirect hyperbilirubinaemia) are additional features.

Black water fever is a severe form of falciparum malaria with haemolysis, haemoglobinuria and severe anaemia. The mortality can be high with this presentation of malaria.

Algid malaria is a severe infection with *P. falciparum*. There is hypotension, shock, shallow respiration, and pallor with a rapid fatality. Gram-negative sepsis is often associated.

Diagnosis

Peripheral blood smear, thin and thick smear should be examined. From the thick smear, the diagnosis can be

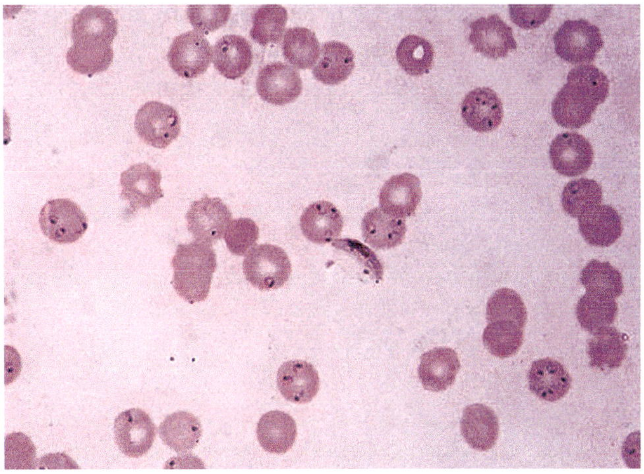

Figure 21.31 Ring forms and gametocytes of *Plasmodium falciparum*.

made more quickly while thin smear helps in identifying the species and the parasitic load. Several smears over different days may be required to confirm the diagnosis (**Fig. 21.31**).

The newer diagnostic tests include an antibody test as well as a PCR. A test based on malarial antigen has also been available for sometime, although sensitivity and specificity are still a problem.

Complications

Cerebral malaria: P. falciparum causes this serious life-threatening complication, especially with a heavy parasitaemia. The child presents with high fever even up to 108°F (hyperpyrexia) accompanied by alteration of sensorium, coma, twitching and seizures. There may be retinal haemorrhages and neurological deficits also. The CSF does not show any significant abnormality except for raised pressure. Cerebral malaria is associated with high mortality and requires intensive treatment at the earliest possible.

- Renal failure may occur due to haemoglobinuria and tubular damage.
- Hypoglycaemia.
- Thrombocytopenia.
- Splenic rupture may occur if spleen is greatly enlarged or there is trauma.

Case Study

An 8-year-old girl was brought to the paediatric service with a history of fever for 4 days, which went up to 104°F, accompanied by a feeling of chills. She also had mild cough and vomiting. Examination showed pallor and no jaundice. Examination of abdomen revealed a mild hepatomegaly of 3 cm while spleen was enlarged to 4 cm and was firm in consistency. Rest of the systemic examination was normal. Investigations: Hb 9 g/dL, total leucocyte count (TLC) 5,400/mm^3, P 60%, L 40%. Peripheral smears showed *Plasmodium vivax* schizonts.

Diagnosis Malaria caused by *P. vivax*

TOXOPLASMOSIS

Toxoplasmosis is a disease with many varied presentations. It occurs in neonates as a transplacental infection and in immunocompromised older individuals. Healthy immunocompetent persons rarely manifest clinical disease.

Aetiology

The causative organism is an intracellular protozoan, *T. gondii*. The infection occurs after ingesting oocysts, which may be present in the contaminated foodstuff, especially infected meat. The oocysts are released in the environment by cats in their faeces. Cats acquire the infection after ingesting mice infected with encysted bradyzoites of *T. gondii*.

Epidemiology

Toxoplasma gondii occurs as a latent infection among humans throughout the world with a higher prevalence in warmer, humid area. The route of infection is by ingestion of contaminated meat containing oocysts or transplacental or transfusion transmitted. There is no direct person-to-person transmission. The oocysts ingested by cats undergo schizogony and gametogenesis in the intestines and form sporocysts, which are excreted in the faeces and remain viable in a suitable environment for 1 year. They can be destroyed by drying, boiling or by some strong chemicals. Other animals, e.g. sheep, pigs and cows become infected by ingesting the cysts and develop viable tissue cysts in muscles and brain. Humans eating partially cooked or uncooked meat of these animals ingest these cysts.

Congenital toxoplasmosis occurs in case the mother acquires the infection during pregnancy. In the first trimester, the likelihood of transmission is low but the resultant foetal infection is severe. In the third trimester, almost 65% of foetuses are infected but the disease is either mild or inapparent.

Pathogenesis

Toxoplasma gondii can multiply in any mammalian tissue. They cause necrosis and an immunological reaction. In healthy persons, the tachyzoites soon disappear from the tissues to become latent. They cause characteristic changes in lymph nodes. In congenital toxoplasmosis, CNS, eyes, heart, lungs, liver, spleen and muscles can be involved with the necrotic lesions.

Clinical Features

The majority of healthy individuals do not have any clinical features. Occasionally, there can be features ranging from fever, myalgia, CNS involvement, rashes, lymphadenopathy, which may be present for a variable period of time. Lymphadenopathy can wax and wane for 1–2 years. One of the frequently caused presentations is of chorioretinitis.

Congenital infection can present as intrauterine growth retardation, prematurity and prolonged jaundice. The classical triad is of chorioretinitis, hydrocephalus and cerebral calcification. Severe manifestations include hydrops foetalis and perinatal death. The infants with inapparent infection often present with ocular involvement later in life.

Diagnosis

Toxoplasma gondii can be isolated from body fluids or from tissues. Cultures are done by inoculating into mice or tissue cultures. The tachyzoites of *T. gondii* can be demonstrated in bone marrow aspirates, CSF, amniotic fluid or in biopsy specimens.

Serological testing: A number of serological tests are available for toxoplasmosis. It is important that these tests have appropriate quality control measures. Some of the tests used are as follows:

- Sabin-Feldman dye exclusion test
- IgG or IgM indirect fluorescent antibody test
- Double sandwich ELISA
- Polymerase chain reaction.

AMOEBIASIS

Aetiology

Amoebiasis is caused by *Entamoeba histolytica*. There are a few non-pathogenic *Entamoeba* also, which are present in the gastrointestinal tract of human beings, e.g. *Entamoeba coli*.

Epidemiology

Amoebiasis is more commonly seen in tropics and in areas of low socio-economic status with poor sanitation. It is estimated that amoebiasis is the third leading parasitic cause of death worldwide. The transmission is through faeco-oral route. The cysts of *E. histolytica* are the infectious form while the trophozoites do not transmit infection. The amoebic cysts are nucleated. They are resistant to low temperature and chlorination of water. On ingestion, they are resistant to gastric acidity and the digestive enzymes. Trophozoites succumb to the environmental factors.

Pathogenesis

After ingestion, the amoebic cysts reach the small intestine and give rise to eight trophozoites, which are actively motile and reach the large intestines. In the colon, they attach to the mucosa and cause tissue destruction by various cellular products. This leads to ulceration of the mucosa, but surprisingly there is little local inflammatory response. The organisms spread laterally from the ulcerated areas causing further destruction and leading to the typical 'flask-shaped' ulcers. The trophozoites invade liver also producing similar lesions but again with no inflammatory reaction.

Clinical Features

The spectrum of amoebic disease varies from asymptomatic carriers to severe intestinal or extraintestinal disease. More severe disease is likely in young or malnourished children and those on corticosteroid therapy.

Symptomatic Intestinal Amoebiasis

The symptoms of intestinal amoebiasis can occur any time after infection and even an asymptomatic carrier can develop invasive disease later on. The presentation starts with abdominal colic, loose stools with or without blood, tenesmus and occasionally there may be fever. In young children, the onset can be of more acute colitis with dehydration and dyselectrolytaemia. Chronic amoebiasis is more commonly seen in adults.

Systemic or Extraintestinal Amoebiasis

Liver can be affected in amoebiasis as a diffuse hepatitis like picture with hepatomegaly. The more severe and less common is the formation of an amoebic liver abscess, which is seen in less than 1% of infected persons. The abscess is usually in the right lobe and single. There may be a history of associated intestinal symptoms. The presentation is with high fever, abdominal pain and tender hepatomegaly. There may be reactionary changes in the adjacent right lung or pleura. The abscess can rupture into the abdominal or thoracic cavity. The contents of the abscess are characteristically described as 'anchovy sauce' and contain lysed RBCs.

Diagnosis

Detection of the amoebic trophozoites in stool sample is diagnostic. A fresh stool sample, i.e. within 30 minutes of passage, can show motile trophozoites with ingested RBCs. Repeated stool examination, at least three, increases the yield. Serological tests are helpful in diagnosis but may be positive in asymptomatic carriers also. Indirect haemagglutination is the most sensitive serological test.

Case Study

A 10-year-old boy was hospitalised with a history of high-grade intermittent fever for 1 week, pain in abdomen for 4 days. He had diarrhoea for about 2–3 weeks previously. On examination, he was mildly icteric, pale, febrile and sick looking. His vital signs were stable. On chest examination, the movements and breath sounds were diminished in the right lower zone but there were no adventitious sounds. Abdomen had an enlarged, tender hepatomegaly of 8 cm in mid-clavicular line. There was no splenomegaly. Hepatic punch was positive. Investigations: Hb 9 g/dL, TLC 20,000/mm^3, P80%, L20%, blood film showed normocytic, normochromic anaemia. Serum liver function tests were abnormal. Ultrasonography of abdomen showed a large 6 × 8 cm abscess in right lobe of liver near the dome of diaphragm with restricted mobility of diaphragm.

Needle aspiration of the abscess revealed chocolate brown thick fluid.

Diagnosis Amoebic liver abscess

GIARDIASIS

Aetiology

Giardia lamblia is a flagellate protozoon, which causes primarily an intestinal infection. *Giardia* cysts are infective in even small numbers.

Epidemiology

Giardiasis is the commonest intestinal parasitic infection the world over. It is more common in areas of poor sanitation and hygiene and in institutionalised children. Drinking contaminated water is a frequent source of infection but other foodstuffs can also transmit infection. The cysts are resistant to chlorination and ultraviolet radiation but boiling inactivates them.

Pathogenesis

After ingestion, the cysts produce trophozoites, which colonise the duodenum and jejunum. They attach to the brush border of the intestinal epithelium and multiply there. The trophozoites pass to intestines and are encysted to form the cysts, which are then excreted in the stools.

Clinical Features

The incubation period is usually 1–2 weeks but can be longer. Most infections may remain asymptomatic. In children with no prior exposure to *Giardia*, the presentation can start as acute diarrhoea. In another manifestation, the child may have intermittent diarrhoea, which is accompanied by abdominal cramps, distension, flatulence and loss of appetite. There may be features of increased gastrocolic reflex. The stools become greasy and foul smelling. There are no blood, mucus or pus cells in stools. Chronic giardiasis can present as malabsorption with significant weight loss.

Diagnosis

Demonstration of *Giardia* cysts or trophozoites in stool sample is diagnostic. A fresh stool sample (within

1 hour of passage) is more likely to be positive and repeated examinations are helpful. In some cases, if necessary, duodenal aspirates or a biopsy can show the trophozoites.

Case Study

A 7-year-old child had history of recurrent diarrhoea for 6 months. The stools were pale yellow, foul smelling, greasy and did not contain blood or mucus. He had abdominal pain off and on and an urge to pass stool after every meal. He had lost weight and looked pale. There were no other findings on examination. A fresh stool examination showed trophozoites of *G. lamblia*.

Diagnosis Giardiasis.

KEY LEARNING POINT

- Giardiasis can cause a clinical presentation similar to malabsorption syndrome. Examination of fresh stool or duodenal aspirate confirms the diagnosis.

KALA AZAR (VISCERAL LEISHMANIASIS)

Leishmania are a group of organisms causing diverse diseases transmitted by sandflies. There are a number of species, which cause cutaneous or mucosal disease and also visceral disease.

Aetiology

Leishmania are protozoa belonging to trypanosomatidae family. They have two morphological forms, a flagellate organism in the insect known as promastigote and the aflagellate form in the humans, amastigote.

Epidemiology

Leishmaniasis occurs in most parts of the world except Australia and Antarctica. The various types of leishmaniasis are specific to the regions of the world. *Leishmania* causing cutaneous disease does not cause visceral involvement. *Leishmania* enters the vector sandfly and changes from promastigote to an infective stage and migrates from the gut to mouth of the sandfly. From the mouth, they are inoculated into the host during a blood meal. In endemic areas, leishmanial cycle is continued as a zoonosis with humans being incidental hosts. The reservoir for the visceral forms is dog.

Pathogenesis

Leishmania after inoculation into the host enters the macrophages. Inside the macrophages, the promastigote form change to amastigote form and start multiplying. They rupture the cell to infect more macrophages.

Clinical Features

The children may have an asymptomatic infection. Some children develop a symptomatic illness with fever, malaise, fatigue accompanied by a mild hepatomegaly. In all but few, this resolves spontaneously. In some, it progresses slowly over weeks and months to kala azar. There is intermittent fever, weakness and splenomegaly. As the disease progresses, fever becomes higher, there are weight loss and hepatosplenomegaly. The patient has severe anaemia and may develop heart failure due to this. Oedema and jaundice are also present. As spleen becomes massive, features of hypersplenism in the form of thrombocytopaenia and pancytopenia develop.

Differential Diagnosis

The conditions causing pyrexia with hepatosplenomegaly, anaemia are to be considered in differential diagnosis of visceral leishmaniasis.

Diagnosis

Amastigote forms, also known as *Leishmania donovani* bodies, are found intracellularly in tissues such as liver, spleen and bone marrow. A positive bone marrow or spleen aspiration for *L. donovani* bodies provides confirmation of diagnosis **(Fig. 21.32)**. An ELISA test using a recombinant antigen also has high sensitivity and specificity.

Case Study

A 9-month-old girl was admitted to a children's hospital, with a 10-day history of lethargy, pallor, fever and poor feeding. On examination, she was found to have a mass in the left hypochondrium. She was febrile and miserable. Her Hb was 65 g/L, white cell count 6.3×10^9/L and platelets 41×10^9/L. Initially, she was thought to be suffering from a malignant condition and was investigated accordingly. Bone marrow examination, blood culture, chest radiography, skeletal survey and urine catecholamines

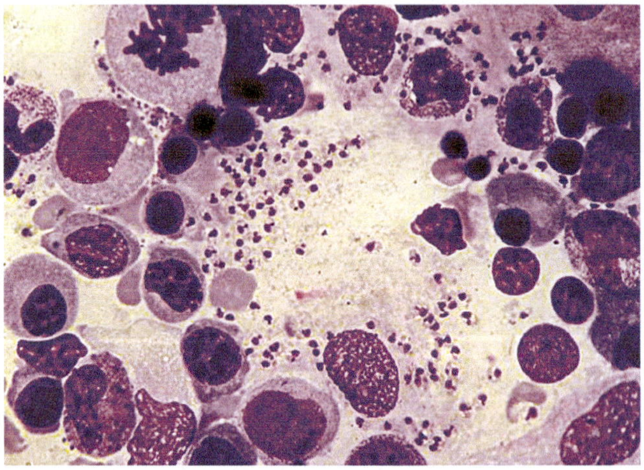

Figure 21.32 *Leishmania donovani* bodies seen in bone marrow.

were all normal. Abdominal ultrasound examination showed the mass to be a massively enlarged spleen.

She was given a blood transfusion and antibiotics after which her general condition improved, although she continued to spike a fever two to three times a day. By the third day after admission, the results of the above investigations were all negative and the possibility of visceral leishmaniasis was raised. The child had been on a holiday to an endemic area where leishmaniasis is known to occur. The bone marrow examination showed the presence of Leishman-Donovan bodies. Also *Leishmania* serology became positive 5 weeks after presentation.

She was treated with sodium stibogluconate 20 mg/kg per day for 10 days followed by 10 mg/kg per day for another 10 days. Her temperature settled within 2 days of starting treatment. Her platelet count returned to normal within 7 days and, by the 10th day of treatment, her white cell count reached normal values. She made an uneventful recovery.

Diagnosis Visceral leishmaniasis

HAND, FOOT AND MOUTH DISEASE

The syndrome of hand, foot and mouth disease (HFMD) should not be confused with foot and mouth disease of cattle, which is caused by a different virus. It is caused by coxsackie viruses A16, A5, A10, B2 and B5. However, coxsackie virus A16 has continued to predominate as the most common cause of HFMD in numerous reports from many parts of the world.

Epidemiology

Although sporadic cases can occur, the disease is usually associated with outbreaks appearing approximately every 2 or 3 years. Cases are usually seen during the summer and early autumn, predominantly in rural and suburban areas. Although older patients can be affected, most are children under 10 years. The illness is highly infectious. Outbreaks also frequently occur in crèches, nursery schools, childcare centres, and so on. Transmission is usually by droplet spread or direct contact with discharges from the nose and throat and from the faeces of the affected people. The disease is communicable during the acute stages of illness, but because the virus can persist in faeces for several weeks, the infectious phase may last longer. Contact in communal swimming pools has also been implicated as a possible method of spread.

Clinical Features

After an incubation period of 3–7 days, malaise and anorexia may occur, particularly in children. If fever is present, this rarely exceeds 38°C and lasts only for 1 or 2 days. A sore mouth can precede the development of the scanty mouth lesions, which are red macules or small vesicles surrounded by a zone of erythema. They can appear on the tongue, mucous membranes of the lips and cheeks and the soft and hard palates. In about 75% of patients, there is an exanthema consisting of a few mixed papules and vesicles with, surrounding erythema usually on the exterior surfaces of the hands and feet or on the palms and soles **(Figs. 21.33A and B)**. Occasionally, the buttocks or genitalia are affected. Resolution of the lesions takes place in 5–10 days. In chickenpox, similar lesions may be evident but usually the skin rash is centripetal, and unlike HFMD, the vesicles usually progress to pustules or form scabs.

Virology and Laboratory Tests

The growth and detection of the group of viruses most commonly associated with HFMD is usually slower, e.g. 7–14 days, than that of most other *Enteroviruses*. As in all suspected enterovirus infections. Diagnosis is best carried out by attempted isolation of virus from the faeces. Paired sera are essential to exclude other non-enteroviral causes, e.g. chickenpox.

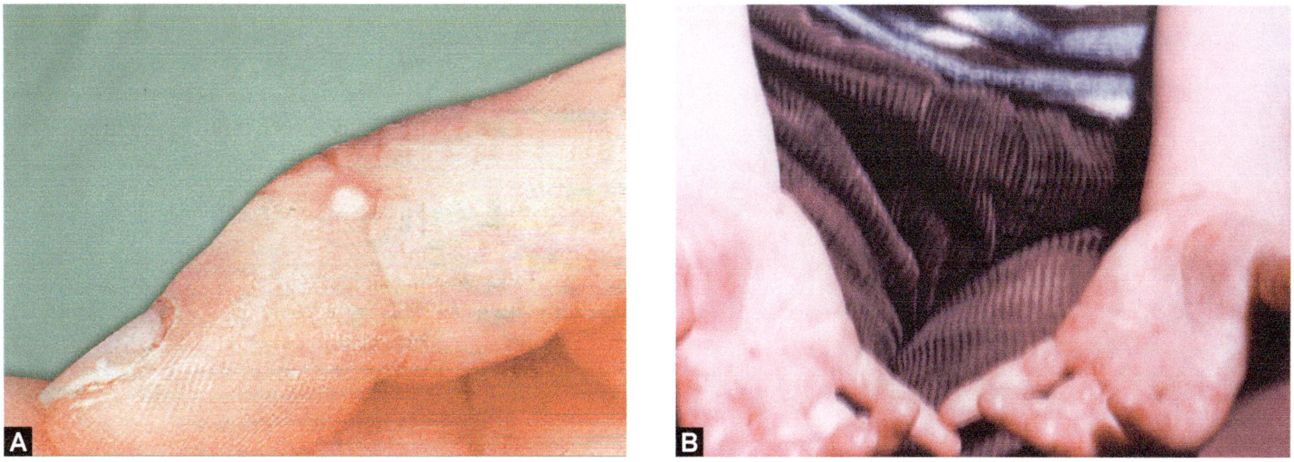

Figures 21.33A and B Hand, foot and mouth disease. (A) A vesicle on the thumb; (B) On the palms.

INFECTIOUS MONONUCLEOSIS

Infectious mononucleosis (IM) is usually a benign febrile illness caused by the Epstein-Barr virus (EBV), a herpes virus, which has a worldwide distribution. It is now generally accepted that IM is caused by EBV; however, most patients with EBV infection are asymptomatic and do not develop IM.

Epidemiology

The exact mode of spread of IM is uncertain, but there is evidence that the agent is transmitted in saliva by activities such as kissing or the sharing of drinking vessels. Spread may also occur via blood transfusion to susceptible recipients. The period of communicability of the disease may be prolonged, and pharyngeal excretion may persist for a year after infection. Infection confers a high degree of protection with lifelong persistence of antibody.

Clinical Features

While most EBV infections are unrecognised events in the childhood years, about 25% of those meeting the virus in young adult life will respond with symptoms and signs of varying severity. It is convenient to describe three main forms of illness: (1) the anginose type, where sore throat predominates; (2) the glandular type, in which lymphadenopathy, especially of the cervical region, is the main finding and (3) the febrile type in which the patient presents with a pyrexia. The clinical reality is, however, less precise and every combination of these features is encountered. The most common presentation is with febrile malaise accompanied by sore throat and cervical lymphadenopathy. The possibility of streptococcal infection will be considered and an appropriate antibiotic may well be prescribed. Failure to respond to an antibiotic after a few days is often the first genuine clue to the diagnosis of IM, by which time inspection of the mouth and throat may show facial oedema with characteristic creamy exudate spread generously over the tonsils and soft palate **(Fig. 21.34)** and occasionally petechial spots on the palate **(Fig. 21.35)**. The voice often has a nasal quality and fetor may be pronounced. Other evidence of a systemic rather than a local infection includes enlargement of other lymph node groups, a palpable spleen, and in a few cases, a macular, non-irritating rash. The duration of acute symptoms is variable but most patients substantially recover within 3 weeks.

A modern feature of IM is the occurrence of a widespread itching eruption in a high proportion of patients given ampicillin **(Figs. 21.36A and B)**.

Diagnosis

The main differential diagnosis is from other causes of exudative tonsillitis, in particular streptococcal infection, which is more common, more painful, yields positive bacteriology and responds to antibiotic therapy. Diphtheria is rare in the developed world but merits continued vigilance. The diphtheritic throat does not have the persistent white exudate of IM but a grey-green membrane becoming darker over a few days, and is accompanied by a more marked toxic state.

Presentation with a persisting pyrexia requires the systematic approach to this recurring medical problem, with chest X-ray, blood culture, differential blood count and a wide-ranging serological screen. This will readily encompass the essential laboratory tests required to confirm a diagnosis of IM.

Laboratory Diagnosis

Until recently, the diagnosis of IM was made from the characteristic triad of clinical, haematological and serological findings. Since the discovery of the aetiological agent, it is now possible to test specifically for EBV antibodies.

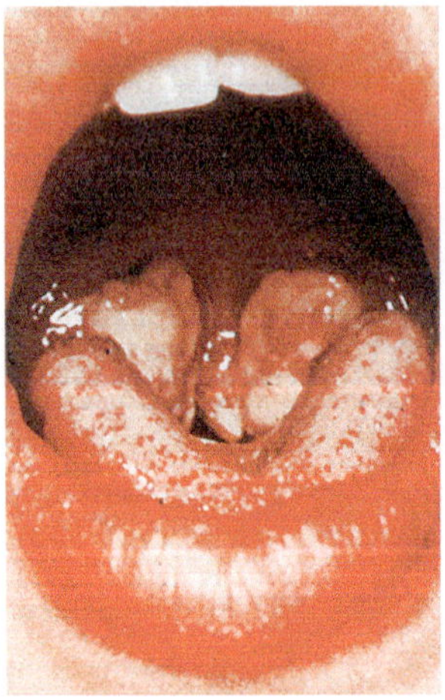

Figure 21.34 Exudate on the tonsils and soft palate of a patient with infectious mononucleosis.

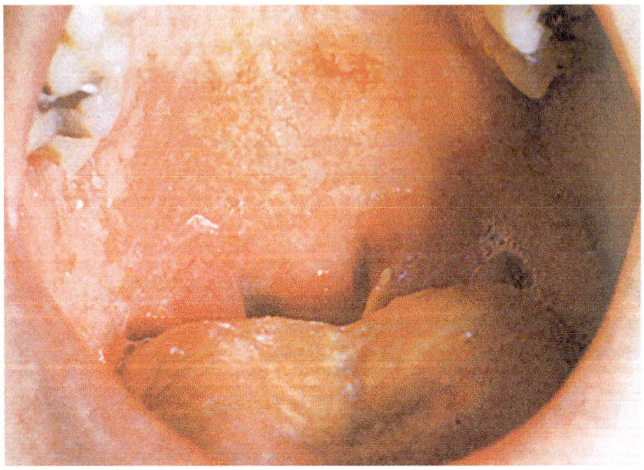

Figure 21.35 Petechial spots on the palate of a patient with infectious mononucleosis.

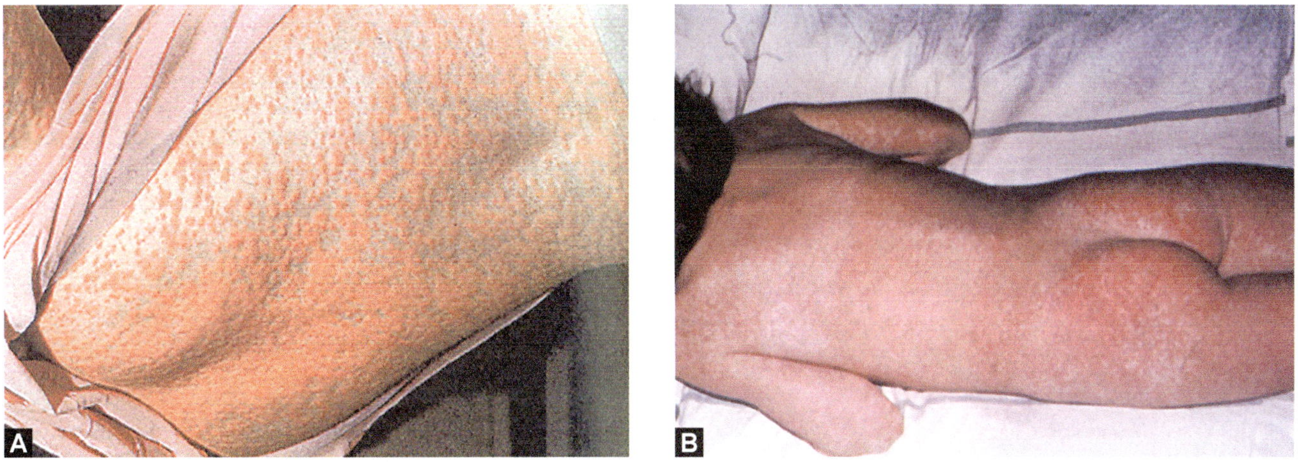

Figures 21.36A and B (A) Widespread itching eruption in a patient with infectious mononucleosis, who had been given ampicillin; (B) Widespread eruption in a child with infectious mononucleosis, who did not receive ampicillin.

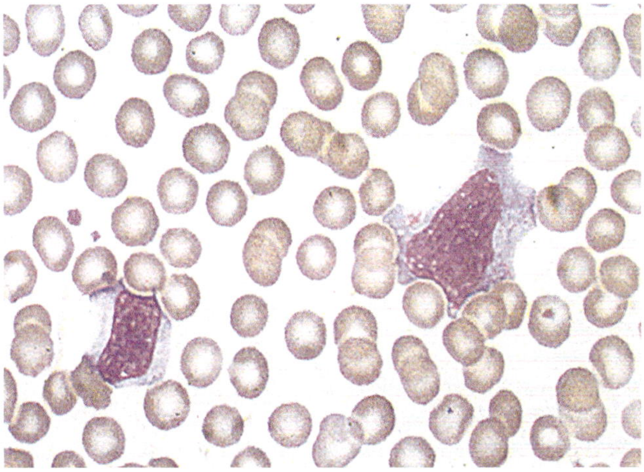

Figure 21.37 Blood film showing 'Downey lymphocytes'.

The distinctive white cells are 'atypical lymphocytes' or 'Downey lymphocytes' **(Fig. 21.37)**. In IM between 1 and 3 weeks after the onset of illness, there is an increase in the number of Downey lymphocytes (more than 20% of all white cells) together with an absolute lymphocytosis (>4.5 × 10^9/L). Thus, a patient may have no positive haematological findings in the first week of illness but will develop them 2 weeks later. Mild neutropaenia and thrombocytopaenia are common. Patients with IM form a wide variety of antibodies, of which two kinds are used for diagnosis: (1) heterophilic antibodies (to other species) (Paul-Bunnell-Davidson test and Monospot/Monotest) and (2) antibodies to EBV. EBV can be isolated in lymphocyte cultures from throat washings of patients. However, this method is not used for routine diagnosis. Moreover, there is a high prevalence of oropharyngeal EBV excretors among healthy people, and thus interpretation of results can be difficult.

FOOD POISONING

Food poisoning is an inexact term medically, but may be defined as an acute gastrointestinal illness, usually developing within 1–48 hours of ingesting contaminated food or drink. Staphylococcal enterotoxin or chemical contamination may cause symptoms within a few hours or even minutes, whereas *Salmonella* food poisoning may have an incubation period of up to 3 or 4 days. Although gastrointestinal symptoms are most typical, salmonellosis may be invasive, and botulism affects the CNS.

Causes

Many bacterial, viral, toxic and chemical agents may cause food poisoning with bacteria predominating, particularly salmonellae, campylobacters and *C. perfringens* (*C. welchii*). Food poisoning bacteria usually need to multiply on food in order to cause clinical illness, with conditions suitable for growth readily provided overnight in a warm kitchen.

Epidemiology

Despite advances in food technology and legislative controls, bacterial food poisoning remains a major health problem in most countries. Salmonellae and *C. perfringens* are present in the intestinal tract of many animals used for food and poultry, and contamination of carcases may readily occur in the abattoir or processing factory. Staphylococcal food poisoning is primarily of human origin, derived from the upper respiratory tract and skin of people preparing food. Food poisoning bacteria have preferences for different foods favourable for their multiplication and toxin production.

Symptoms of nausea, vomiting, fever, myalgia and headache begin 12–72 hours after eating contaminated food, followed by diarrhoea, which thereafter dominates the illness. Abdominal pain varies from mild cramps

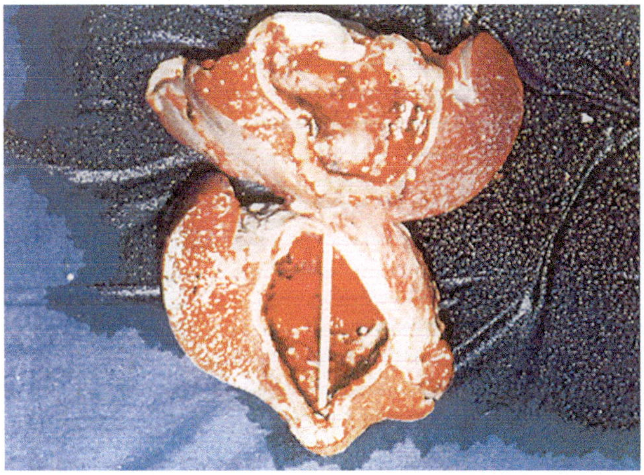

Figure 21.38 Splenic abscess caused by Salmonella infection.

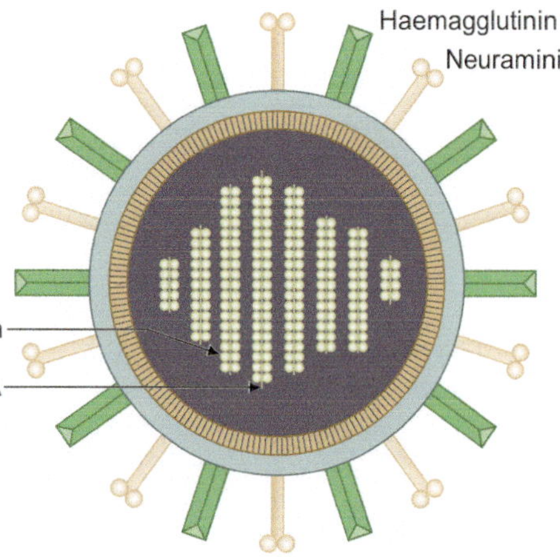

Figure 21.39 Influenza virus.

to severe pain accompanied by features suggestive of an acute abdomen. Diarrhoea usually stops within 7–10 days, but where colitis is severe, may last for several weeks. Localisation of infection, particularly in neonates and immunosuppressed persons, may result in meningitis, osteitis, septic arthritis or abscess formation in soft tissue, muscle or viscera (Fig. 21.38).

Diagnosis

Food poisoning should be considered when acute illness with gastrointestinal or neurological manifestations affects two or more people within 48 hours of sharing a meal. The pattern of symptoms and the incubation period provide important clues as to the likely aetiology.

Appropriate specimens include any 'left-over' food, vomitus, faeces and blood for culture where indicated by the presence of fever. Serological tests may be useful, particularly where typhoid, salmonellosis or certain virus infections are suspected.

INFLUENZA

In the developed world, influenza has taken over from TB as 'Captain of all the men of death'. Easy to recognise in its classical epidemic form, the diagnosis can be elusive, especially outside epidemics and in its common minor and occasional complicated presentations.

Epidemiology

Influenza occurs nearly every year, often in outbreaks which sometimes reach epidemic proportions. These episodes are usually caused by influenza viruses A or B. Influenza virus C causes minor respiratory disease mainly in children. Influenza A outbreaks occur almost every year while those caused by influenza B virus occur with intervals of 1–5 years. Because influenza B viruses do not show major variations, their appearance in the community affects mainly school aged and younger children. No major change in influenza A virus has been detected since the appearance of the H1N1 strain in 1977.

Influenza viruses are of medium size and variable shape. Their genetic information is carried in eight distinct RNA fragments existing as separate nucleoprotein particles, all contained within a complex outer membrane. Antigenically different nucleoproteins distinguish types A, B and C (Fig. 21.39).

Clinical Features

After an incubation period of 1–3 days, the onset of typical clinical 'flu' is characteristically sudden with chills and shivering, followed by headache, weakness and myalgia and a sharp rise in temperature. The clinical syndrome can be mimicked in the individual case by many other infectious agents. The probability of the cause being influenza is high during epidemics, but accurate diagnosis requires laboratory help. Pneumonia is the main complication, usually pneumococcal. Less severe complications caused by secondary bacterial infection of the respiratory system include sinusitis and otitis media. Influenza A is one of the more serious causes of viral croup.

Early rapid diagnosis can be made by immunefluorescence tests for viral antigen in cells deposited from nasopharyngeal secretions. Serological diagnosis can be made by testing paired sera which have been collected in the 'acute' (within first week) and 'convalescent' (second or third week) stages of illness. A fourfold or greater rise in antibody titre is diagnostic.

ERYTHEMA INFECTIOSUM (FIFTH DISEASE, SLAPPED CHEEK DISEASE)

Erythema infectiosum is caused by parvovirus B19. In children, the first sign of infection is usually marked erythema of the cheeks or slapped cheek appearance

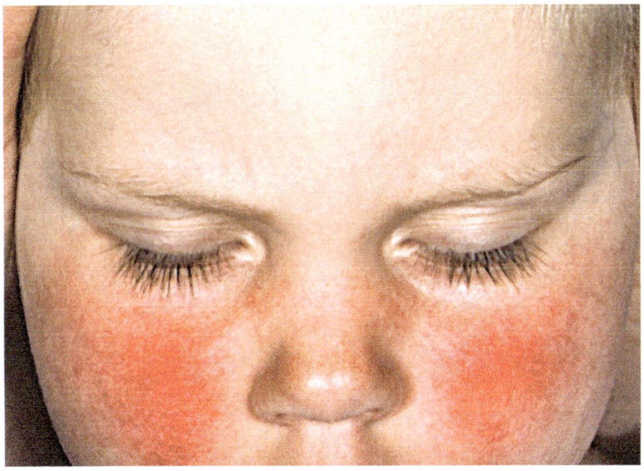

Figure 21.40 Erythema infectiosum: the characteristic 'slapped cheeks' appearance.

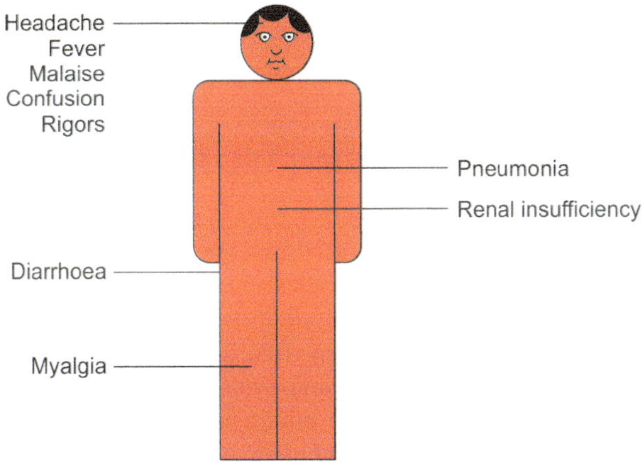

Figure 21.42 Clinical features associated with Legionnaires' disease.

often with relative circumoral pallor **(Fig. 21.40)**. One to four days after the slapped cheeks an itchy, erythematous, maculopapular rash develops on the trunk and limbs.

The slapped cheek appearance with circumoral pallor can be mistaken for scarlet fever. The diagnosis can be made serologically by demonstrating B19, specific IgM on an acute serum sample, although it is always better to get a paired sample in case there is a late rise in antibody.

LEGIONELLOSIS

Epidemiology

Although Legionnaires' disease came to light as the result of spectacular outbreaks, mainly involving people staying in hotels, sporadic, unpredictable cases are more common. Legionellosis is caused by *Legionella pneumophila*, of which serogroup 1 is most commonly associated with human disease **(Fig. 21.41)**.

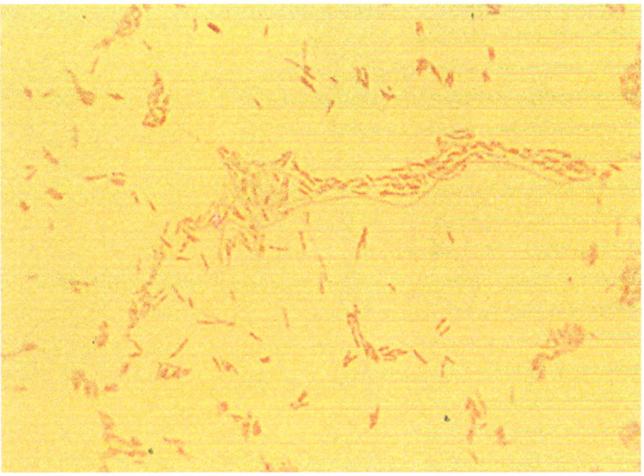

Figure 21.41 *Legionella pneumophila*—Gram-stained, showing gram-negative rods.

Clinical Features

The initial presentation is with malaise, myalgia, headache, a rapidly rising fever with rigors, and a dry and unproductive cough. Progressively severe symptoms occurring within a few days include chest pain (often pleuritic in type), vomiting, diarrhoea, abdominal pain and distension **(Fig. 21.42)**.

In practice, diagnosis in life is usually made by the demonstration of specific antibody, preferably with paired sera so that a diagnostic rise of antibody may be demonstrated. The main antibody detection test used is the indirect fluorescent antibody test, where a rise in titre to the level of at least 128, or a static titre of at least 256, in the presence of compatible clinical disease is regarded as being diagnostic.

ANTHRAX

Anthrax is an acute febrile disease occurring worldwide and may affect virtually all mammals including man. Anthrax is caused by *Bacillus anthracis*, a non-motile spore-bearing gram-positive rod. Anthrax usually presents as a cutaneous disease, but more fulminating pulmonary, intestinal and meningeal forms can occur.

Bacillusanthracis is normally found in the vesicle fluid or pus obtained from the lesion of cutaneous anthrax, and may also be obtained from the sputum of cases of pulmonary anthrax. Commonly, the organism can be isolated from blood culture in pulmonary anthrax and untreated cutaneous anthrax, and from CSF in meningeal cases **(Figs. 21.43A to D)**.

FUNGAL INFECTIONS

Candidiasis (Moniliasis)

Candida albicans causes candidosis in children: Intensely erythematous confluent plaque with a sharply demarcated

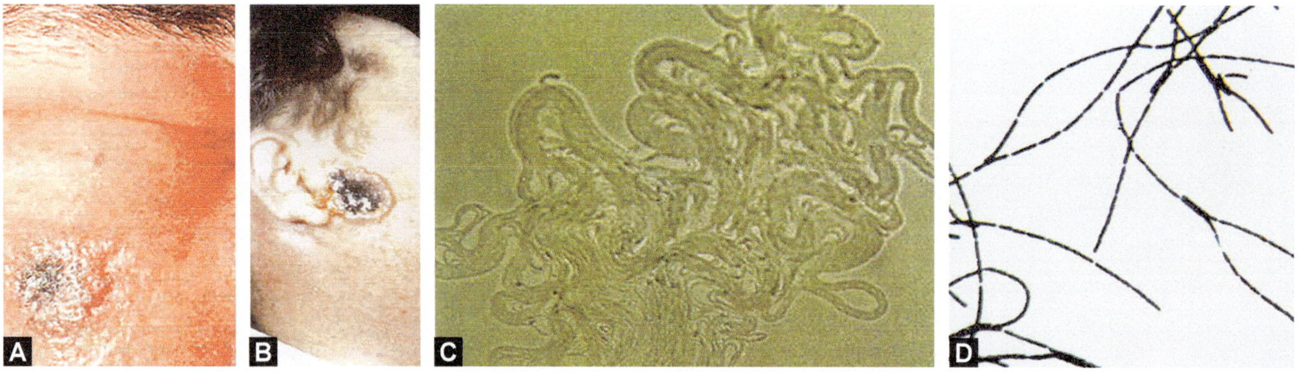

Figures 21.43A to D (A) Anthrax lesion beneath the eye; (B) lesion of the pre-auricular region showing the characteristic black appearance; (C) 'medusa head' appearance of a colony; (D) Chains of *Bacillusanthracis*.

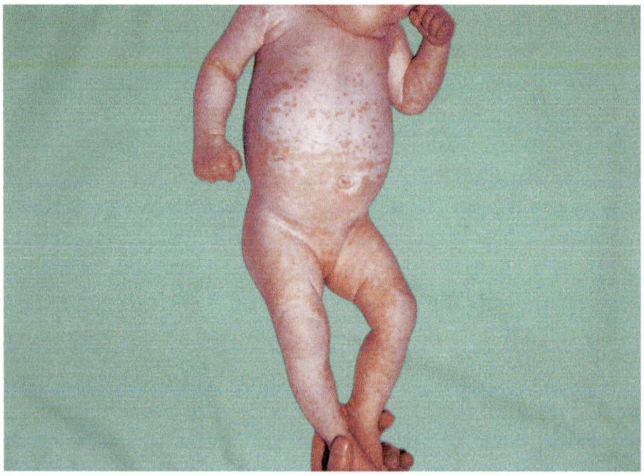

Figure 21.44 Monilial dermatitis.

edge. Usually the inguinal folds, lower abdomen and perineum are affected **(Fig. 21.44)**.

Candida onychomycosis: Candida onychomycosis produces destruction of the nail and massive nailbed hyperkeratosis. It is seen in patients with chronic mucocutaneous candidiasis **(Figs. 21.45A to C)**.

Tinea

This is an infection due to dermatophyte fungi; the source of the fungus is an animal (e.g. dog, cat and cattle), the soil or another human. Tinea occurs on any part of the skin surface and can involve hair and nails **(Figs. 21.46A and B)**.

SEXUALLY TRANSMITTED INFECTIONS/ DISEASES

The term sexually transmitted diseases (STDs) refers to a variety of clinical syndromes and infections caused by pathogens that can be acquired and transmitted through sexual activity. The organisms that cause sexually transmitted diseases may pass from person to person in blood, semen, or vaginal and other bodily fluids. The age group of 15–19 years has the second highest prevalence of sexually transmitted diseases. In the paediatric age group, the modes of transmission can be different.

Neonates: Perinatal transmission

Young children: Sexual abuse

Adolescents: Sexual abuse and voluntary sex, fomites, IV drug use.

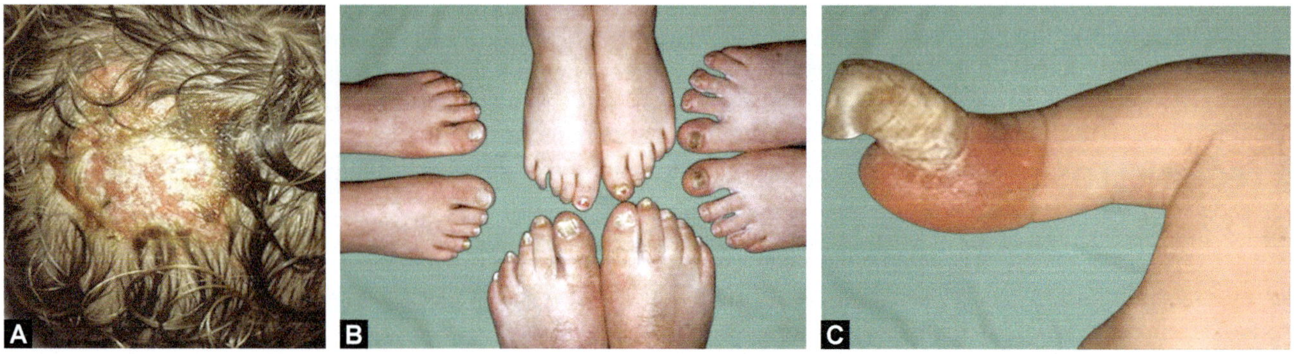

Figures 21.45A to C *Candida onychomycosis:* A family (including two children) with onychomycosis lesion of the scalp and a thumb of a child with chronic mucocutaneouscandidosis.

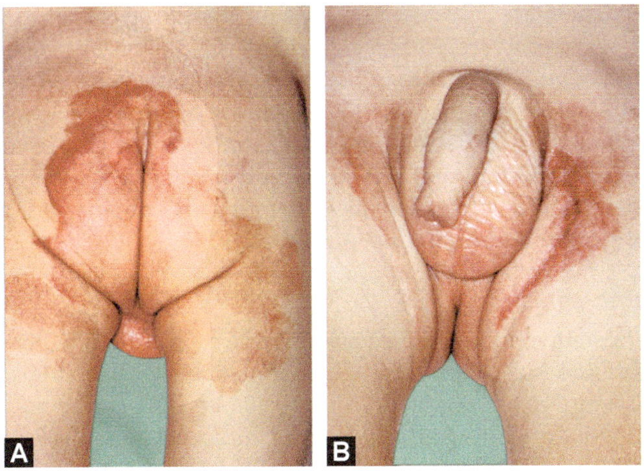

Figures 21.46A and B Tinea. (A) Tinea cruris buttocks; (B) Groins.

The factors that influence the occurrence of STDs in young persons are, viz. gender, number and characteristics of sexual partners, frequency and type of intercourse, rates of condom use and local STI epidemiology.

Modes of Transmission and Causative Organisms

Transplacental

Intrauterine infection/ascending infection: HIV, HBV, HCV, syphilis, HPV

Perinatal

i. Transmission via the birth canal: *Chlamydia trachomatis*, Gonococcal, *Trichomonas vaginalis*, *Herpes simplex*, *Human papilloma*, *Hepatitis B*, *Hepatitis C*, HIV
ii. Transmission via the breast milk: HIV (syphilis, HBV, HCV: risk unknown)

Direct contact

i. Non-sexual/autoinoculation: HPV, HSV
ii. Fomite transmission: ?TV, ?HPV
iii. Consensual sexual contact: All STIs
iv. Sexual assault: All STIs:
v. Injecting drug use or blood transfusion/blood products: HIV, HBV, HCV

Symptoms

Perinatal transmission of gonorrhoea and chlamydia can lead to conjunctivitis, pneumonia, and rarely, disseminated gonococcal infections in neonates. HSV infection in the newborn can be limited or present as encephalitis or disseminated disease. Perinatal HPV transmission can lead to cutaneous or laryngeal papillomas in infants or children. Congenital syphilis can cause stillbirth, premature delivery, and a wide spectrum of clinical manifestations, including developmental delay and seizures.

TABLE 21.6 Diagnosis and treatment of a few common STIs.

S. no	Name	Diagnosis	Treatment
1.	*Chlamydia trachomatis*	Culture, Antigen or Nucleic acid detection in specimen	Oral Erythromycin/ Azithromycin/ Doxycycline
2.	Gonorrhea	Gram-negative intracellular diplococci in smear/ culture, Antigen or Nucleic acid detection in specimen	Parenteral 3rd Generation Cephalosporins,
3.	Syphilis	*T. pallidum* on darkfield microscopy, PCR, other molecular methods	Inj Benzyl Penicillin
4.	*Trichomonas*	Microscopy or culture for *T. vaginalis*	Metronidazole
5.	Herpes simplex	HSV serology, PCR	Aciclovir

In young children and adolescents, sexually transmitted infections (STIs) can have a range of signs and symptoms, including no symptoms. Signs and symptoms may appear a few days after urination, discharge from the penis, unusual or odd-smelling vaginal discharge, unusual vaginal bleeding, pain during sex, sore, swollen lymph nodes, particularly in the groin, lower abdominal pain, fever, rash over the trunk, hands or feet. Untreated STIs can cause pelvic inflammatory disease (PID) which can lead to infertility, ectopic pregnancy, adverse pregnancy outcomes, anogenital and cervical cancers **(Table 21.6)**.

ZIKA VIRUS INFECTION

Zika is a mosquito borne disease, which is currently spreading to various parts of the world. Zika virus belongs to the family of Flaviviruses such as Yellow fever and Dengue viruses. It is transmitted primarily via the bite of the *Aedes* mosquito, although persons may also acquire the infection through sexual intercourse or blood transfusion. Only about 20% of patients infected with the Zika virus develop typical symptoms of fever, arthralgia, maculopapular rash, and conjunctivitis. There may be myalgia and headache also. Symptoms may be very transient or last days to weeks. Zika virus infection during pregnancy can be transmitted to the foetus and cause birth defects.

Congenital Zika Virus Syndrome

Congenital microcephaly was the sign that first raised attention to the effect of Zika virus on the developing fetus, in up to one in five cases. Later certain other neurological abnormalities have also been noted to occur with or without associated microcephaly. The abnormalities consistently reported in these infants, including abnormal neuroimaging findings, suggest that a congenital syndrome, akin to congenital rubella or cytomegalovirus (CMV) infection, is attributable to in utero Zika virus infection. In addition to congenital microcephaly, a range of manifestations including craniofacial disproportion, spasticity, seizures, irritability, brainstem dysfunction such as swallowing problems, limb contractures, hearing and ocular abnormalities, and brain anomalies detected by neuroimaging have been reported among neonates where there has been in utero exposure to Zika virus. Reported neuroimaging findings include cortical/subcortical calcifications, cortical malformations, simplified gyral pattern/migrational abnormalities, brainstem/cerebellar hypoplasia, and ventriculomegaly.

There are currently no validated laboratory diagnostic test or commercial assay to confirm congenital Zika virus infection or exposure in neonates. Diagnosis is based on clinical assessment and supported by neuroradiological evidence. RT-PCR and IgM testing on serum or CSF have been done but their sensitivity and specificity are yet to be established. Management is primarily supportive for the neurodevelopmental problems.

Prevention

Presently, no vaccine against Zika virus is available. Prevention is primarily aimed at preventing mosquito bites. Mosquitoes that spread Zika virus bite during day and night. Condoms can help in reducing sexual transmission of Zika infection.

CHAPTER 22

Paediatric Ophthalmology

Sarada David, Kirsteen J. Thompson, Gordon N. Dutton, Richard Bowman

VISUAL ASSESSMENT IN CHILDREN

A child's eye is different from that of an adult. It is a growing eye, with the most rapid growth taking place within the first 2 years of life. Astigmatism is often present during the first few months of life, and most infants are hypermetropic, becoming normal sighted (emmetropic) during the first few years of life.

- The developing immune system results in children responding to inflammation and to other disease conditions differently from adults.
- Myelination of the optic nerve and maturation of the fovea continue after birth, as does pigment deposition in the anterior iris stroma.

VISUAL ACUITY

Visual acuity is a measure of the clarity of central vision. It is defined as the measurement of the resolution of the visual system in terms of the angle subtended at the fovea by an object at a distance of 6 m from the eye, tested at maximum contrast (black on white).

- In clinical practice, quantification of visual acuity is required to diagnose abnormality, to chart progress of disease and to determine the results of treatment.
- Standard visual acuity measurement in ophthalmology has traditionally been performed using the Snellen chart. 6/6 is a normal visual acuity. The numerator of this fraction is the distance in metres at which the letters are shown to the patient, and the denominator is the distance at which that letter being read subtends 5 minutes of arc at the eye. The 6/60 letter at the top of the chart therefore subtends 5 minutes of arc at a distance of 60 m. In the USA, the numbers used refer to feet, so that 6/6 acuity is the same as 20/20 acuity.
- An alternative and arguably more logical way to record visual acuity is the logarithm of the minimum angle of resolution (LogMAR) notation in which 6/6 is an acuity of 0.1 and 6/60 becomes 1.0 with eight intervening steps.
- In infants and young children, such methods are not feasible, but quantification of visual acuity is obtained using different methods (below), and equivalent scales of measurement.

AMBLYOPIA

Visual development takes place from birth until the age of 6–7 years, and requires clear visual images to be formed on the retina of each eye.

Amblyopia occurs when there is deficient development of the visual brain due to impaired stimulation of the fovea during the first few years of life (**Box 22.1**). This may occur due to the presence of uncorrected refractive error, squint (deviation of the eye such that the image formed on the retina is extrafoveal, i.e. falls on an area of retina other than the fovea), or any type of occlusion in front of the retina including media opacities (cataract, vitreous opacity, blood or inflammatory cells in the anterior chamber), corneal opacity or abnormal eyelid position (ptosis) causing stimulus deprivation.

Iatrogenic causes of amblyopia may include prolonged use of eye ointment, or of eye padding following injury or surgery to an eye. Prolonged pupil dilatation may also be amblyogenic. The retina appears normal, but visual acuity is reduced. If detected before the age of 7–8 years, amblyopia may be partially or wholly reversible by treating the underlying cause. Amblyopia is usually unilateral or asymmetrical, and occlusion of the better eye (taking care not to induce amblyopia in that eye!) is used to bring about adequate retinal stimulation of the eye with poorer vision (once the refractive error or media opacities, etc. have been dealt with) in order to overcome amblyopia. It is, therefore, important to be aware of, and to use, accurate methods for determining vision in young children of different age groups. Appropriate measures for treatment of amblyopia can then be instituted promptly.

BOX 22.1	Types of amblyopia.
Refractive	
Strabismic	
Stimulus deprivation	

ASSESSING VISION

There are several key factors to be considered when assessing vision in young children.

Young children are neither in a position to understand "normality" of visual ability, nor can they articulate what they can or cannot see.

- A "difficult" examination of a child is usually due to a "difficult" examiner rather than a "difficult" child. Entering a child's mind-set, setting them at their ease, and maintaining patience and respect throughout the examination may be a daunting thought for some of us, particularly in the presence of anxious parents. However, it is a skill we ignore at our peril. Once the skill is mastered, or even haltingly attempted, clinic appointments can become something child and examiner alike, look forward to, though fewer are likely to be required, and the final outcome has a much greater likelihood of being successful and satisfying for all parties involved.
- A child's general demeanour and ability to move around and to communicate is not necessarily a guide to the level of their visual function, as different aspects of general development as well as of visual development, may be impaired in different disease states. A child can have very poor clarity of visual acuity and yet have practically normal mobility.
- Accommodation of the lens is easily stimulated in children and resting accommodative tone is high. Thus, accurate assessment of refractive error must always be performed after full cycloplegia using cyclopentolate or atropine drops.

ASSESSMENT OF VISUAL FUNCTION

Formal visual acuity assessment in children is carried out in the following ways:

- Infants (0–6 months):
  - Preferential looking
  - Visual evoked potentials (VEPs)
  - Watching the child's visual behaviour, whether she returns a smile and at what distance
  - Vestibulo-ocular reflex (VOR): Spinning the child gently to find out what speed is required to make the eyes move to and fro, giving an index of central visual function. Good vision suppresses VOR
- Toddlers (7 months–3 years)—Cardiff acuity cards:
- Preschool children (3–5 years): Kay's pictures.
- Primary school children (5–7 years): Sheridan-Gardiner acuity cards or Glasgow Acuity cards, with a card of letters to point to.
- Over 7 years: LogMAR chart or Snellen's chart **(Figs. 22.1 and 22.2)**

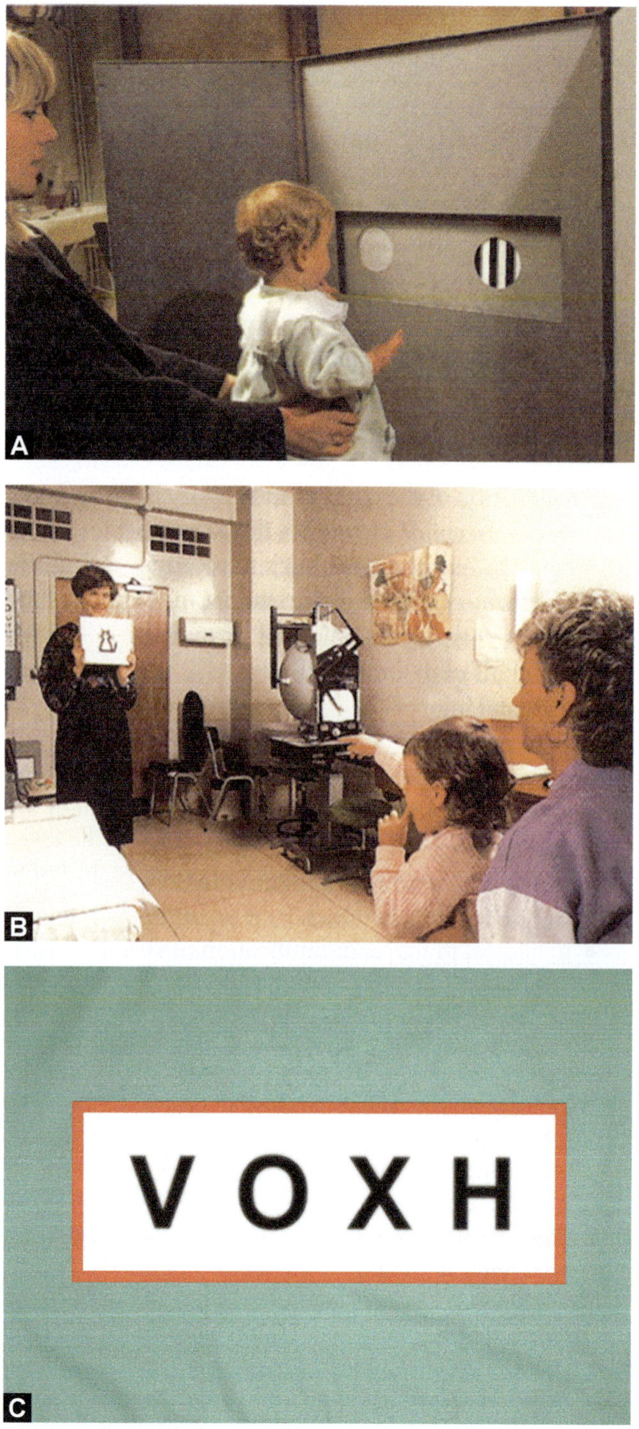

Figures 22.1A to C (A) Forced preferential looking; (B) Kay's pictures; (C) Logarithm of the minimum angle of resolution (LogMAR) crowded test.

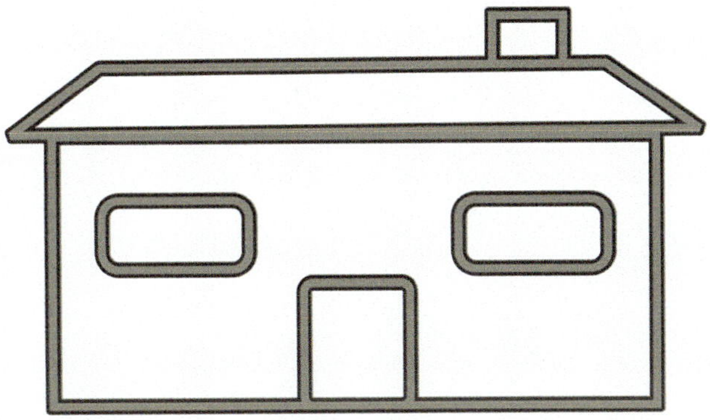

Figure 22.2 Example of a Cardiff card.

ASSESSMENT OF EYE MOVEMENTS

Orthoptic assessment of ocular muscle balance and the presence or absence of latent or manifest squint is assessed using the cover test (Box 22.2) and an uncover or an alternate cover test (Box 22.3). A target of interest or a light moved into the nine directions of gaze, brought about by the action of the six extraocular muscles, is then used to examine the adequacy of the muscle actions. Further tests using prism bars are used to record the magnitude and precise type of squint present, and the ability to fuse disparate images.

If both eyes see well, the brain can join the images by fusing them (fusion), and this keeps the eyes straight. When an eye is covered, fusion is lost. If that eye has a position of rest which is turned out (exophoria), turned in (esophoria), turned up (hyperphoria) or turned down (hypophoria), then it will do so when covered, but will be seen to straighten up when uncovered.

BOX 22.2 Cover test.

One eye is covered and the other eye is observed to see if it moves to look at a target (in the absence of squint, no movement takes place)

In children who look as if they have a squint, the cover test shows:

- A fixation movement occurs if a true squint is present and the eye can see
- No fixation movement occurs if:
  - There is a true squint and the eye is blind, e.g. due to cataract or retinoblastoma
  - The squinting eye is an artificial eye
  - The macula is displaced. This causes the eye to appear to have a squint despite "fixing" with the macula
  - The image is being viewed with eccentric retina (extrafoveal fixation)
  - The eye is tethered and cannot move. When the eye is uncovered, the other eye is observed, if it moved in the first instance
  - If it moves back immediately, it has poor vision
  - If it keeps looking, but moves back after blinking, it has reduced vision
  - If it keeps looking, and does not move back, it has equal vision to the other eye.

In children who look as if their eyes are straight, the cover test may reveal:

- A very small angle squint (the uncovered eye moves slightly to take up fixation)
- Latent nystagmus (a to-and-fro movement of the eyes which only occurs when one eye is covered)

BOX 22.3 The uncover or alternate cover test.

- The test is done when the eyes have been shown to be straight by the cover test
- One eye is covered and then observed when it is uncovered. The test is repeated for the other eye. If either eye moves when uncovered a latent squint (a phoria) is present

OTHER VISUAL FUNCTIONS

Colour vision is tested using Ishihara plates for red-green defects, Lanthony plates for blue-yellow defects or the City University test. The child is asked to trace along, or to point to a particular colour.

Central and peripheral visual fields are assessed manually using a target, a light or a variable number of fingers held up, in the four quadrants of each visual field, while watching the child's attentiveness to the target. The target may be moved in order to map the point at which it comes into view. Older children are able to cooperate with Goldmann perimetry or with automated perimetry. Lesions of the occipital cortex or posterior visual pathways cause homonymous visual field defects in both eyes. Lesions affecting the optic chiasm typically cause a bitemporal hemianopia, while lesions of the anterior visual pathways or the retina, cause non-homonymous or unilateral field defects.

Binocular depth perception or stereopsis, measured in seconds of arc, is tested using the Titmus fly and Randot test, where superimposed images, displaced by varying degrees are viewed through polarised lenses, and, with adequate levels of stereopsis, are identified as three-dimensional. In children younger than 5 years old, the Lang or Frisby tests, where the child identifies an elevated image in a group of otherwise identical images, are used. As in the Titmus test, image disparity is graded in order to quantify the level of stereopsis achieved.

Refractive error is measured using retinoscopy and trial lenses (spherical and cylindrical), while singing (at least, the budding performers among us!), or holding up an interesting target, to hold the child's attention.

Contrast sensitivity is not routinely tested in children, but can be useful for monitoring amblyopia and to quantify visual dysfunction.

BOX 22.4 Checklist of visual problems.

Features

Dorsal stream dysfunction

Impaired ability to handle complex visual scenes can cause difficulties with:

Finding a toy in a toy box

Finding an object on a patterned background **(Fig. 22.3A)**

Finding an item of clothing in a pile of clothes

Seeing a distant object (despite adequate acuity)

Identifying someone in a group

Tendency to get lost in crowded locations

Distress in busy shops and crowded places

Reading

Impaired visually guided movement (optic ataxia)

Upper limbs: Inaccurate visually guided reach, which may be compensated for by reaching beyond an object then gathering it up

Lower limbs: Feeling with the foot for the height of the ground ahead at floor boundaries. Difficulty walking over uneven surfaces (despite full visual field, and looking down)

Impaired attention

Difficulty "seeing" when talking at the same time, which may cause a child to trip or bump into obstacles

Marked frustration at being distracted

Ventral stream dysfunction

Impaired recognition

Difficulty recognising people and photographs

Difficulty recognising shapes and objects

Impaired orientation

Tendency to easily get lost in known locations

Recommendations

Dorsal stream dysfunction

Store toys separately **(Figs. 22.3B and C)**

Use plain carpets, bedspreads and decoration **(Fig. 22.3D)**

Store clothes separately in clear compartments. Get close

Share a zoom video or digital camera view

Identify through waving and speaking

Training in seeking and identifying landmarks

Visit shops when they are quiet

Determine whether masking surrounding text improves reading ability

Occupational therapy training

Provision of tactile guides to the height of the ground ahead, e.g., pushing a toy pram or holding onto the belt pocket or elbow of an accompanying person.

Limit conversation when walking.

Limit distraction by reducing background clutter and background activity. (Performance may be enhanced at the "quiet table" at school)

Ventral stream dysfunction

Family and friends introduce themselves and wear consistent identifiers

Training to identify and recognise identifiers

Training in tactile as well as visual recognition

Training in orientation

Source: Dutton GN, McKillop EC, Saidkasimova S. *Visual problems as a result of brain damage in children*. Br J Ophthalmol. 2006;90:932–3.

A child may perform well in all the above tests and yet have significant visual problems in daily life such as difficulty identifying an object in a crowded scene, difficulty recognising faces or route finding, due to impaired visual integration processes at a cerebral level. Such problems occur more commonly than hitherto acknowledged. They are commonly associated with periventricular leucomalacia, which may occur as a consequence of premature birth, antenatal or postnatal cerebral hypoxic episodes, meningitis or head injury. Typical features can usually be elicited by detailed history taking (*see* checklist in **Box 22.4**), and by an awareness of the typical patterns of disorder, often suggested by symptoms described by a child or their care takers.

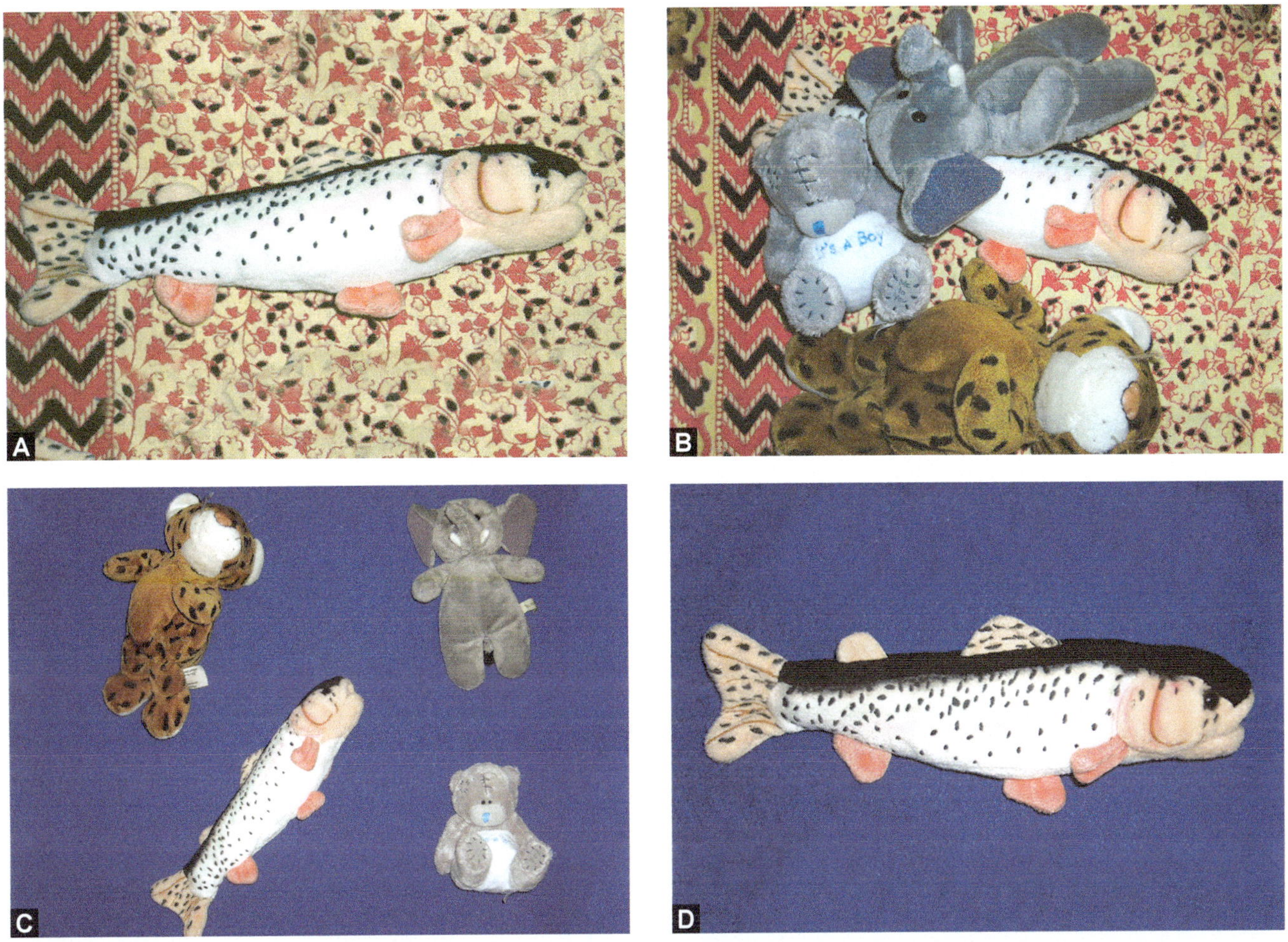

Figures 22.3A to D (A) Single toy on patterned background: Visual information too complex; (B) Group of toys on patterned background: Visual information too complex; (C) Toys spaced out on plain background to simplify visual information; (D) Single toy on plain background: Good contrast.

STRABISMUS

Strabismus, or squint, refers to a deviation of an eye due to an imbalance of function of the extraocular muscles such that both eyes do not function together. There may be eso- or exo-, hyper- or hypodeviation, representing convergence, divergence, depression and elevation of the eye respectively. Occasionally, a torsional abnormality is present. Most strabismus in children is concomitant, i.e. similar in magnitude in all positions of gaze. Incomitant strabismus varies in magnitude with gaze in different directions and is associated with paresis or palsy of the third, fourth or sixth cranial nerves. The commonest type of strabismus encountered in paediatric practice is a concomitant congenital esotropia, which may not present until 2–3 years of age **(Figs. 22.4 to 22.6)**.

Strabismus may be latent (termed a "phoria") and brought out only by dissociating the two eyes by alternate cover testing, or manifest (a "tropia") even before testing. It may be intermittent or constant, and there may alternate fixation of each eye or, in large angle esotropia, cross-fixation (in which the child uses the right eye to look to the left and the left eye to look to the right).

Amblyopia is both a cause and a consequence of strabismus and should therefore be identified and treated as early as possible.

Uncorrected refractive error, particularly hypermetropia in young children, may cause strabismus.

A red reflex should be sought in every child with a squint because conditions such as cataract or retinoblastoma with reduced acuity (with or without amblyopia) can present with squint and may cause a white pupil (leucocoria) **(Figs. 22.7A and B)**.

There is a higher incidence of strabismus following premature birth, in individuals with a positive family history of strabismus and in children with other developmental abnormalities.

Management

On diagnosing strabismus, findings on base-line examination are documented, including the magnitude of the deviation (measured in prism Dioptres), enabling comparison with future tests. The degree of stereopsis present is also noted as this affects the final prognosis of treatment.

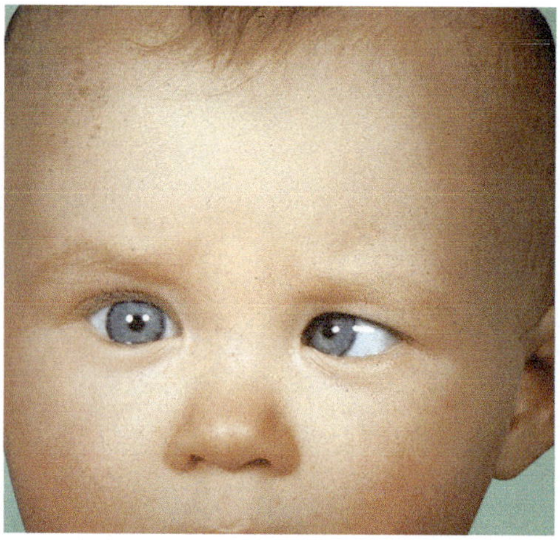

Figure 22.4 Left esotropia.

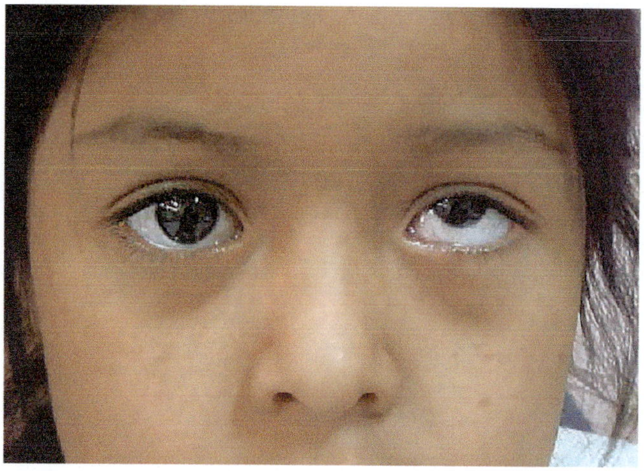

Figure 22.5 Left hypertropia: Orbis.

(*Courtesy*: Photograph published in Community Eye Health Journal, www.cehjournal.org).

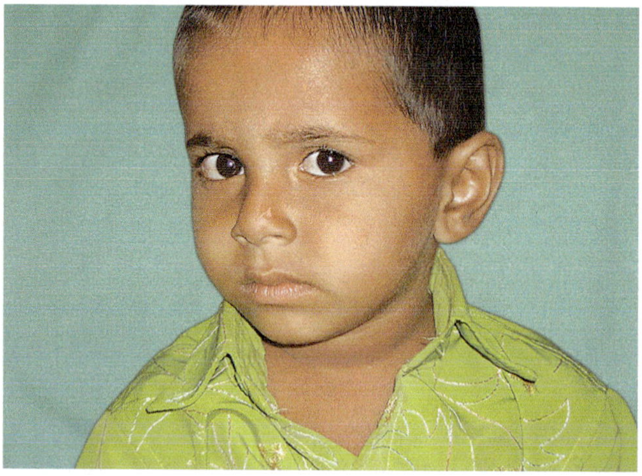

Figure 22.6 Abnormal head posture due to paralytic squint.

(*Courtesy*: Photograph published in Community Eye Health Journal, www.cehjournal.org).

Treatment of strabismus includes the following measures as indicated:

- Accurate refractive correction and ensuring that spectacles fit well and are worn
- Treatment of underlying causes of amblyopia such as refractive error (as above) or cataract
- Treatment of amblyopia itself (in children under 7–8 years), by occlusion of the other eye, and detailed visual tasks given, such as drawing or reading
- Exercises to strengthen accommodative convergence and fusional range
- Surgery to realign the visual axes by weakening and/or strengthening the appropriate extraocular muscles by recession or resection of the muscle insertions. Due to the dynamic nature of

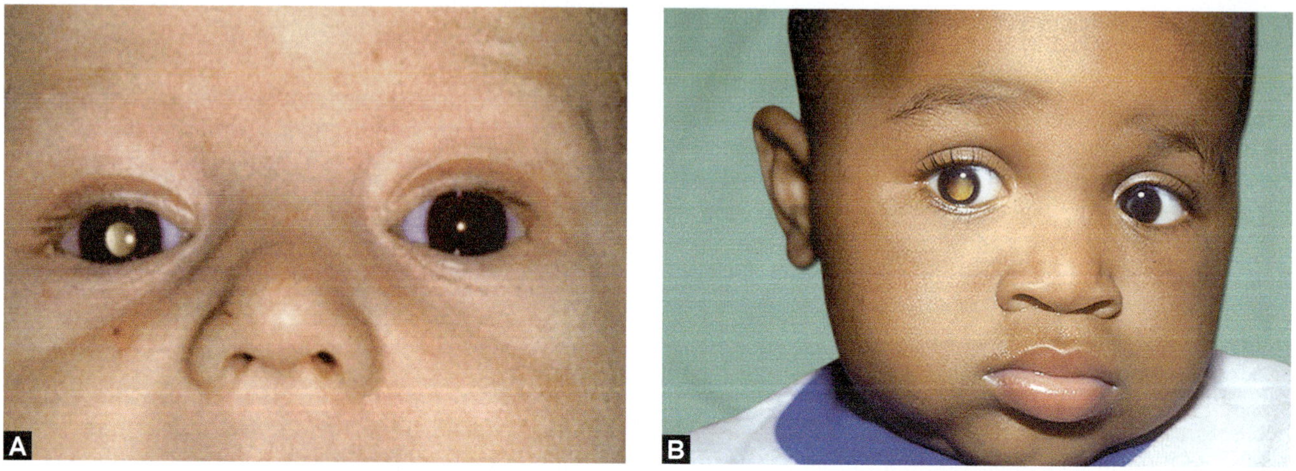

Figures 22.7A and B (A) Leucocoria: a white pupillary reflex. Retinoblastoma must be excluded; (B) Impaired red reflex due to retinoblastoma.

(A) (*Courtesy*: Photograph published in Community Eye Health Journal, www.cehjournal.org); (B) (*Courtesy*: Pak Sang Lee. Photograph published in Community Eye Health Journal, www.cehjournal.org).

extraocular muscle imbalance, a single surgical procedure may not suffice. Patients and their carers should always be prepared for the possibility of further surgery

NYSTAGMUS

Nystagmus in children can be congenital or acquired.

Congenital nystagmus has the following features:

- Onset during the first month of life
- The meridian of the nystagmus is the same in each position of gaze (it is uniplanar)
- The nystagmus tends to be greater on distance fixation and least on near fixation
- There is a position in which the nystagmus is least (the null position)
- There may be a head posture to place the eyes in the null position to optimise vision
- Compensatory head nodding to stabilise the eyes can occur

The causes of congenital nystagmus include:

- Idiopathic motor nystagmus, which may be idiopathic or inherited with dominant or recessive inheritance
- Albinism (look for fair hair, pale complexion, iris transillumination and macular hypoplasia)
- X-linked ocular albinism (most commonly in boys) (in this condition there is patchy iris transillumination, but the hair may be dark coloured and the skin pigmented)
- Congenital stationary night blindness in which there is poor rod photoreceptor function (ask whether the child can see in dark conditions)
- Achromatopsia in which there is rapid fine horizontal nystagmus (ask whether the child is photophobic and sees better in dark conditions than in daylight)
- Optic nerve hypoplasia (look for small optic nerve heads)
- Achiasmia (look for bitemporal visual field impairment)
- Damage in the occipital area of the brain, in particular damage to the white matter (posterior periventricular leucomalacia)
- Methadone use during pregnancy

Acquired nystagmus has the following features:

- The key feature is that the pattern of nystagmus is not uniplanar and is different in different positions of gaze
- The causes of acquired nystagmus include loss of vision, tumours in the region of the chiasm and posterior fossa tumours

Clinical Assessment of Patients with Nystagmus

History taking seeks a family history and determines whether vision is worse in dark or daylight conditions. A history of premature birth may suggest periventricular leucomalacia.

As in all patients with an eye problem vision is assessed.

The pattern of nystagmus is assessed in each position of gaze. If the nystagmus is uniplanar then it is very likely to be congenital in origin. If it is not, and the pattern of nystagmus is different in different positions of gaze, imaging of the brain must be carried out to seek evidence of organic pathology such as tumours in the region of the chiasm or brainstem.

Eye examination seeks evidence of blinding pathology such as cataract, iris transillumination, macular hypoplasia, optic nerve hypoplasia and optic atrophy.

Investigation by electroretinography detects rod and cone photoreceptor dysfunction. Visual evoked potentials may be delayed and reduced in amplitude if there is pathology affecting the visual pathways or the brain. Brain imaging is carried out if pathology is suspected.

Management

Vision is optimised by spectacle correction if required for refractive error. Treatable blinding pathology is identified and treated (e.g. cataract). Nystagmus reduces visual function, which may require appropriate action to be taken to ensure that school material is enlarged or magnified.

INTRAUTERINE INFECTIOUS DISEASES

Maternally transmitted infections can be remembered by the acronym TORCHES (toxoplasmosis, rubella, cytomegalovirus, herpes viruses including the Epstein Barr virus and syphilis). These infections have a broad range of presentations, from subclinical forms to severe organ damage. Continuing tissue damage can occur throughout life; therefore, long-term follow-up is necessary.

TOXOPLASMOSIS

Toxoplasma gondii is an obligate intracellular protozoan parasite. Feline animals are the definitive hosts. Infected rodents, farm animals, birds, and humans serve as the intermediate hosts. Cats shed millions of oocysts in their faeces, and when these oocysts are then ingested by the intermediate host, the cyst wall dissolves releasing actively dividing tachyzoites. These are transported via intestinal lymphatics to various organs. Dissemination occurs to liver, lung, heart muscles and eyes. Once host immunity is established, the organisms transform to bradyzoites contained within tissue cysts. Bradyzoites lie dormant within the tissues of the intermediate host and when conditions are favourable, cause reactivated infection. The stimulus for local reactivation of an infected cyst is unknown. Humans are infected when they ingest oocysts or contaminated meat containing tissue cysts. Other modes of infection are transplacental transmission, organ transplantation and blood product transfusion.

Clinical Features

Systemic infection is mild and usually goes undiagnosed. Clinical features include fever, headache, sore throat and diffuse lymphadenopathy. If the mother is acutely infected during pregnancy, transplacental transmission can occur. Congenital toxoplasmosis is described as a triad of convulsions, cerebral calcification and retinochoroiditis. If the foetus is infected in the first trimester, the resultant illness may be severe, with microcephaly, seizures and hepatosplenomegaly. Ocular manifestations include retinochoroiditis, often involving the macula, iritis, anterior and posterior uveitis, optic atrophy, strabismus and nystagmus. Infections acquired later in gestation are less severe and may be asymptomatic. Strabismus and poor vision are due to macular scarring, which can be bilateral. Many cases of "acquired" toxoplasma retinochoroiditis are due to reactivation of a congenitally acquired infection. The active area of retinochoroiditis is often at the edge of an old flat atrophic scar, a so-called satellite lesion.

Diagnosis

Diagnosis is primarily clinical, based on characteristic retinal lesions. The presence of immunoglobulin G (IgG) or IgM antibodies in serum can be detected by enzyme-linked immunosorbent assay (ELISA). Any positive testing, even undiluted, is significant. The presence of IgM in the infant serum is evidence of congenital infection because maternal IgM does not cross the placenta. Indications for treatment include a lesion threatening the macula or optic nerve head and severe vitritis. All immunocompromised patients should be treated.

Treatment

Triple drug therapy is commonly used and care should be taken to correct folate deficiency caused by some drugs used. Weekly blood counts are required during therapy. Alternative treatment may be required for immunocompromised patients (**Figs. 22.8 and 22.9**).

RUBELLA (GERMAN MEASLES)

Rubella is a relatively mild illness in the postnatal period, but results in a variety of abnormalities when acquired congenitally. Maternal infection acquired in the first trimester carries the greatest risk of complications. Systemic manifestations include congenital heart diseases, deafness, dental deformities, mental retardation, hydrocephalus, spina bifida, seizures and spasticity. Ocular abnormalities from rubella are microphthalmos, nuclear cataract, glaucoma, optic nerve abnormalities and retinopathy, which vary from salt and pepper retinal pigment epithelial disturbance to an appearance of pseudoretinitis pigmentosa (**Figs. 22.10A and B**). The incidence of the disease has come down worldwide with the institution of routine vaccination.

Diagnosis

Diagnosis is based on a characteristic clinical picture, which may include any of the above features, and is supported by positive serum titres of antibody against the rubella virus. However, a negative antibody titre does not rule out rubella as antibodies may disappear with time.

Treatment

Rubella cataract is managed by lensectomy. Intense postoperative inflammation may follow and requires adequate control with topical steroids (**Fig. 22.11**).

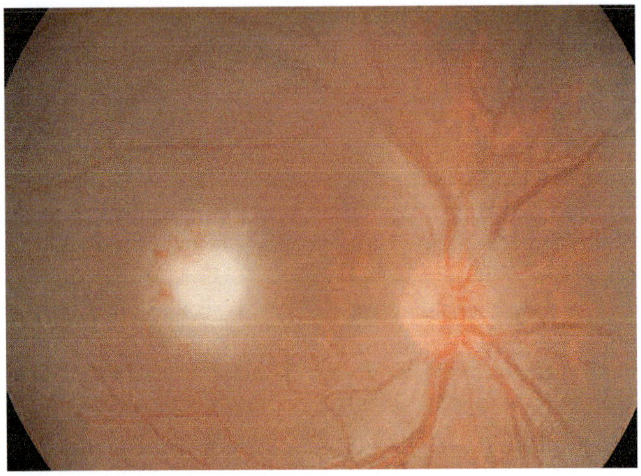

Figure 22.8 Active toxoplasma retinochoroiditis.

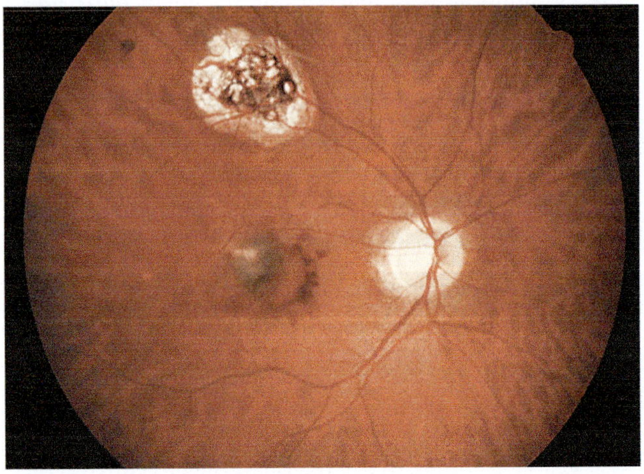

Figure 22.9 Toxoplasma retinochoroiditis showing active and inactive lesions.

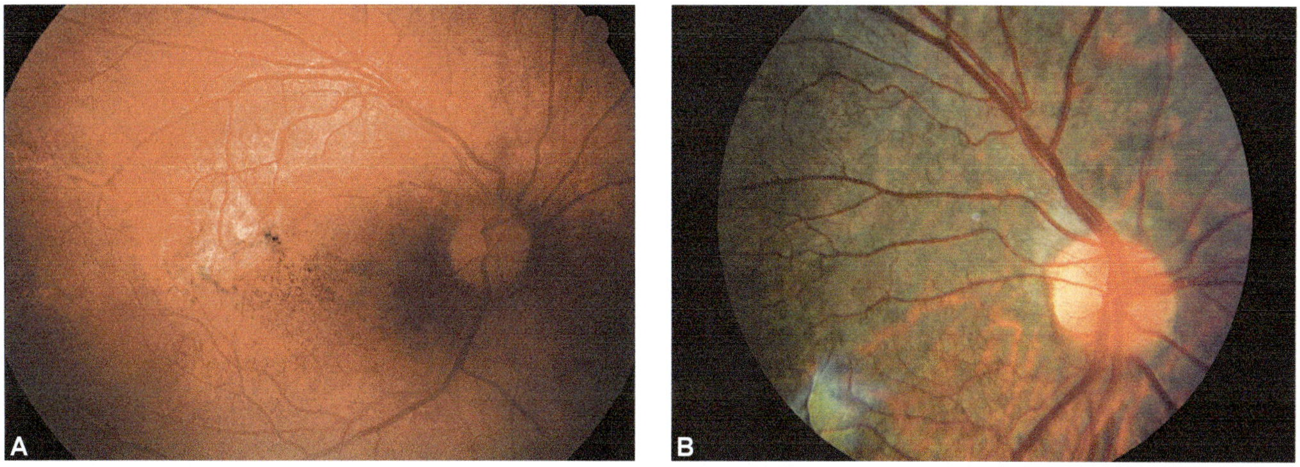

Figures 22.10A and B (A) Rubella "salt and pepper" retinopathy; (B) may also be evident in the mid-peripheral retina.
(*Photograph Courtesy:* David Taylor).

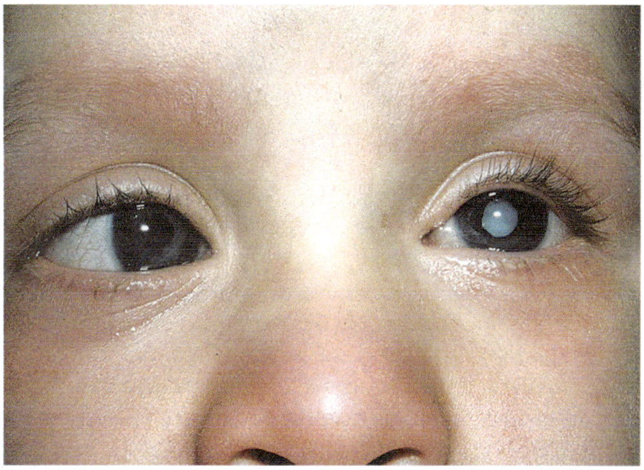

Figure 22.11 Cataract due to congenital rubella.
(*Photograph Courtesy:* David Taylor).

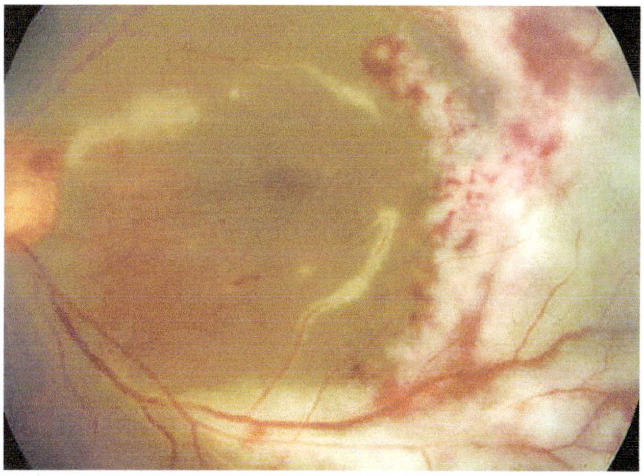

Figure 22.12 Cytomegalovirus (CMV) retinitis.

CYTOMEGALOVIRUS

Cytomegalovirus (CMV) belongs to the herpes family. Infections may occur transplacentally, during birth, through breastfeeding or from other infected children who continue asymptomatic secretion of the virus. Immunocompromised children may acquire the infection through blood transfusion, chemotherapy or organ transplantation.

Congenital CMV presents with jaundice, hepatosplenomegaly, thrombocytopenia and anaemia. Typically, there is microcephaly or hydrocephalus. Ocular manifestations include keratitis, uveitis, cataract, retinochoroiditis, optic nerve abnormalities and microphthalmos. The keratitis may manifest as punctate epithelial lesions, or as a dendritic, or geographical ulcer. Stromal keratitis presents as a zone of epithelial oedema with stromal thickening and keratic precipitates. Retinal involvement consists of bilateral progressive white areas of retinitis, exudates associated with haemorrhage, vasculitis, vitritis and necrosis (Fig. 22.12).

Diagnosis

It is based on clinical presentation, confirmed with viral cultures and polymerase chain reaction (PCR) based assays.

Treatment

The treatment of epithelial keratitis is with topical antiviral agents. Stromal keratitis requires combined therapy with topical steroids and antiviral agents. Disseminated disease and posterior segment involvement require intravenous (IV) antiviral agents.

SYPHILIS

Syphilis is a sexually transmitted infection caused by a Spirochaete, *Treponema pallidum*. Transplacental infection occurs following maternal spirochaetaemia.

Ocular manifestations are anterior uveitis, interstitial keratitis and pigmentary retinopathy. Malformed

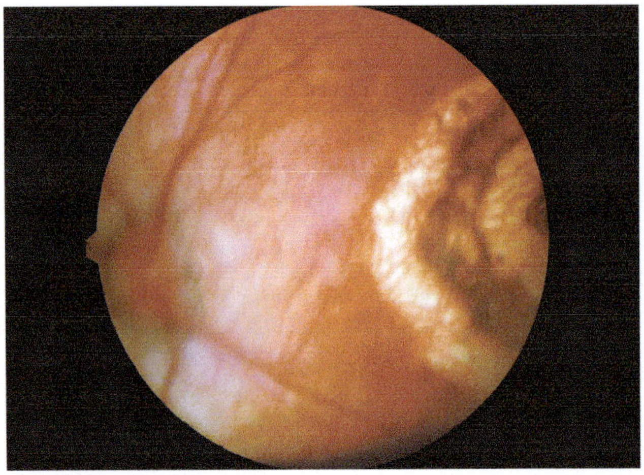

Figure 22.13 Syphilitic retinopathy.
(*Photograph Courtesy*: David Taylor).

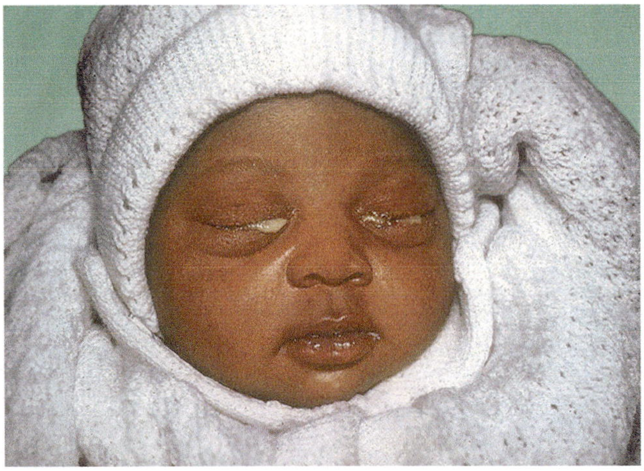

Figure 22.14 Ophthalmia neonatorum.
(*Courtesy*: Pak Sang Lee. Photograph published in Community Eye Health Journal, www.cehjournal.org).

peg-shaped incisors, with nerve deafness and interstitial keratitis constitute Hutchinson's triad. Other signs include frontal bossing, a short maxilla, prognathism, a high arched palate, a saddle-shaped nose and linear scars around body orifices **(Fig. 22.13)**.

Diagnosis

It is done by the venereal disease research laboratory test (VDRL), the fluorescent treponemal antibody absorption (FTA-ABS) test or a microhaemagglutination assay with *Treponema pallidum* antigen (MHA-TP).

Treatment

The treatment of congenital syphilis consists of intravenous antibiotics. Serological tests should be repeated and persistent positive titres at 6 months require re-treatment.

OPHTHALMIA NEONATORUM (NEONATAL CONJUNCTIVITIS)

Ophthalmia neonatorum is a conjunctivitis that occurs within the first month of life. Chemical conjunctivitis due to treatment with silver nitrate used to be the most common cause. However, prophylaxis with silver nitrate is now almost obsolete.

Neonatal conjunctivitis is caused by exposure to organisms in the birth canal. The common pathogens causing this condition are *Gonococcus*, *Chlamydia* and herpes simplex. Other infectious agents include *Streptococcus*, *Staphylococcus*, *Haemophilus*, etc. Any discharge from a newborn infant's eye is pathological and should be taken seriously. Tear production is present from birth but does not become obvious until the infant is a few weeks of age **(Fig. 22.14)**.

GONOCOCCAL CONJUNCTIVITIS

Because of effective antenatal screening and prophylaxis, the incidence of gonococcal conjunctivitis has decreased markedly in affluent countries. In developing countries, however, gonococcal conjunctivitis continues to be a significant problem. Most serious gonococcal conjunctivitis is caused by *Neisseria gonorrhoeae* and presents within 48 hours of birth. There is marked lid oedema, mucopurulent discharge, severe chemosis and intense conjunctival congestion. *Gonococcus* has the power to invade intact corneal epithelium and cause corneal ulceration. Unless effectively treated, ulceration can progress rapidly leading to perforation of the cornea, iris prolapse and lens extrusion. If the corneal ulceration heals with or without perforation, corneal scarring and opacification occur, causing reduced vision or loss of vision.

Diagnosis

Gram staining of conjunctival scrapings reveals Gram-negative intracellular diplococci.

Treatment

Topical and intravenous or intramuscular antibiotics are necessary. Penicillin-resistant gonococci may be involved.

CHLAMYDIA CONJUNCTIVITIS

Chlamydiae are a relatively common cause of ophthalmia neonatorum. Onset is usually at age 4–10 days. Causative agents are *Chlamydia trachomatis* and *Chlamydia oculogenitalis* [called trachoma-inclusion conjunctivitis (TRIC)]. Lid oedema, chemosis and conjunctival congestion are less severe than in gonococcal conjunctivitis. Since infants do not have a subconjunctival adenoid layer, follicles do not appear. Pseudomembranes and superficial keratitis occur **(Figs. 22.15A and B)**.

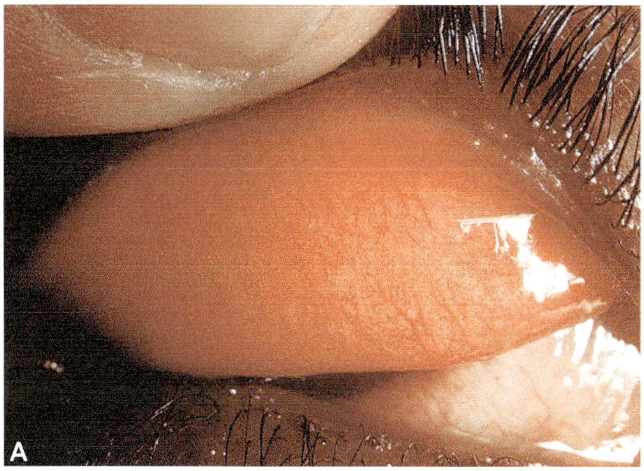
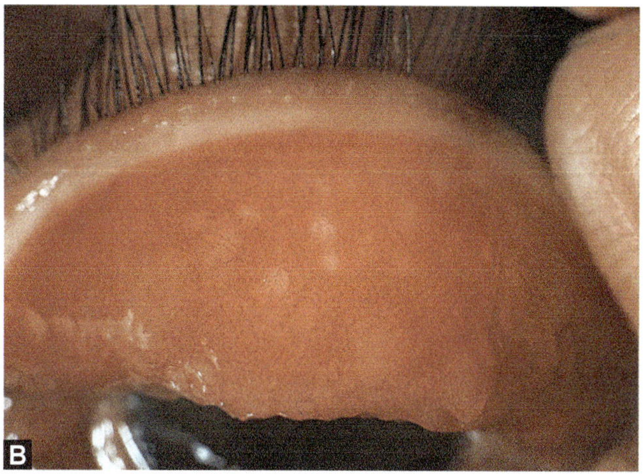

Figures 22.15A and B (A) Trachomatous infiltration, follicular (TF); (B) Trachomatous inflammation, intense (TI).

(A) (*Photograph Courtesy*: John Anderson); (B) (*Photograph courtesy*: Allen Foster. Photographs published in Community Eye Health Journal, www.cehjournal.org).

Diagnosis

Conjunctival scrapings, stained with Giemsa's stain, show intracytoplasmic inclusion bodies. ELISA and direct immunofluorescent antibody tests are available.

Treatment

The treatment of chlamydial conjunctivitis includes topical and oral antibiotics.

HERPES SIMPLEX

Most cases of neonatal herpetic conjunctivitis are due to Herpes simplex type II, but approximately one-third are caused by Herpes simplex type I. The onset is usually between 1 week and 2 weeks after birth. Presenting signs are a watery discharge and conjunctival injection. Fluorescein staining of the cornea shows punctate keratitis or dendritic ulceration.

Diagnosis

Diagnosis is clinical, with conjunctival scrapings taken for viral culture and PCR in the absence of dendritic corneal ulceration.

Treatment

Acyclovir 3% eye ointment is instilled five times a day. Systemic acyclovir is advised for recurrent viral keratitis and when there is systemic involvement.

Prophylaxis for ophthalmia neonatorum: Agents effective against both gonococci and TRIC can be used as preventative agents where risk of infection is significant.

ORBITAL CELLULITIS

The orbit is a pear-shaped cavity surrounded by bony walls, tapering posteriorly into the orbital apex and the optic canal, which contains the optic nerve. The cavity contains the globe, extraocular muscles, nerves, blood vessels, fibrous tissue and fat. The orbit is surrounded by the paranasal sinuses. The ethmoid air cells begin to develop in the second trimester and maxillary sinuses by 2 years of life. The frontal sinus develops between the 15th year and 17th year. Infection from the sinuses spreads easily to the orbit through incomplete bony walls and the valveless veins of the orbit and sinuses.

Other sources of infection are facial skin, ear, teeth, direct inoculations after trauma and bacteraemic spread from a distant focus. Since the orbit is surrounded by bony walls, infection and inflammation cause increase in intraorbital pressure leading to compromise of ocular and optic nerve function. Severe complications may result including cavernous sinus thromboses and intracranial abscess. Therefore, orbital cellulitis must be promptly recognised and aggressively treated.

Classification

Orbital cellulitis can be classified into five stages as described by Chandler.

1. *Preseptal cellulitis:* Inflammation confined to the eyelids with mild anterior orbital involvement. Ocular motility and visual function are normal.
2. *Orbital cellulitis:* The four cardinal signs of orbital involvement are: (I) eyelid oedema, (II) chemosis, (III) proptosis and (IV) loss of motility. Visual impairment may occur.
3. *Subperiosteal abscess:* Collection of pus within the subperiosteal space causes local tenderness, fluctuation and nonaxial proptosis.
4. *Orbital abscess:* Progression of cellulitis leads to intraconal and extraconal loculation of pus. Proptosis, inflammatory signs, ophthalmoplegia, visual deficit and systemic toxicity are increased at this stage.

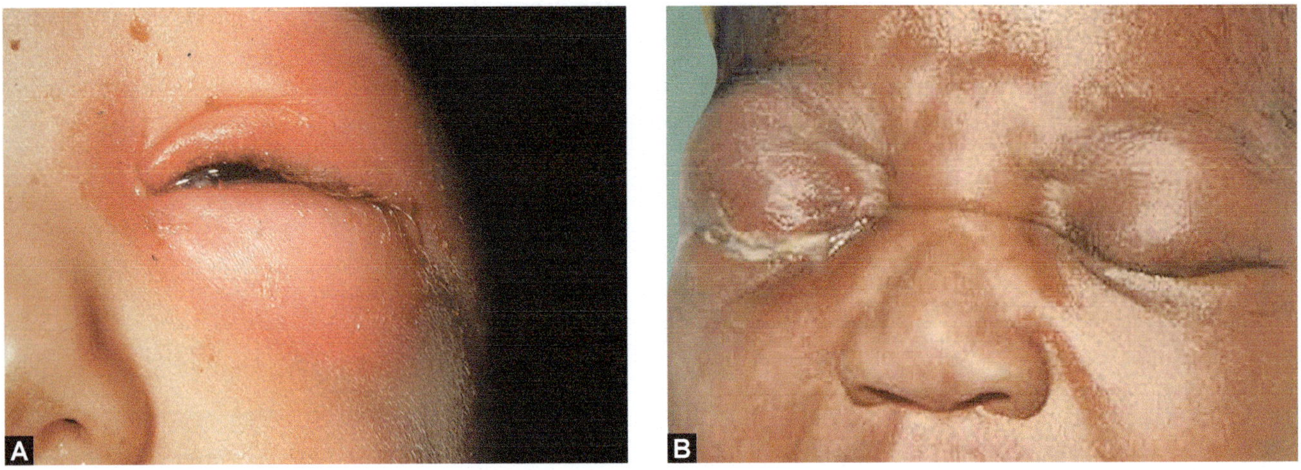

Figures 22.16A and B Preseptal cellulitis.

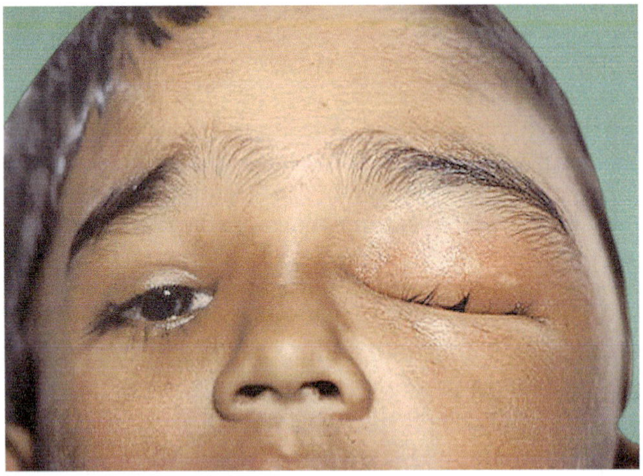

Figure 22.17 Left orbital cellulitis.

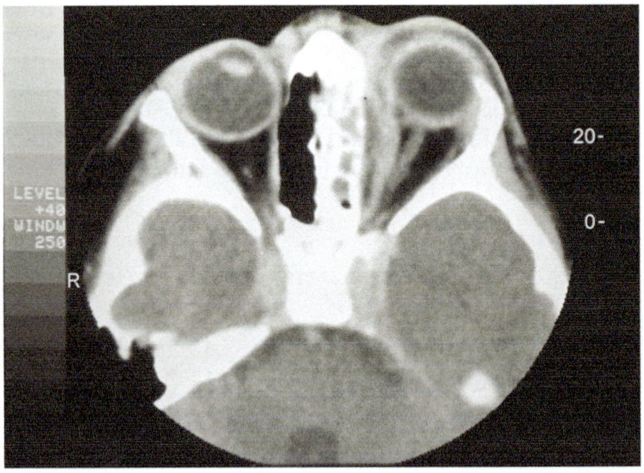

Figure 22.18 Left subperiosteal abscess of medial orbital wall. (*Photograph Courtesy*: David Taylor).

5. *Cavernous sinus thrombosis:* Proptosis progresses rapidly and frequently becomes bilateral, and changes in mental state occur. Meningitis or intracranial abscess may follow. Inflammatory cells are present on lumbar puncture **(Figs. 22.16 to 22.18)**.

Diagnosis

The most common organism causing orbital cellulitis is *Staphylococcus aureus*, followed by *H. influenzae* and *Moraxella catarrhalis*.

Management

All children with orbital cellulitis (any stage) must be admitted to hospital and investigations performed to identify the source of infection. Material for culture and Gram stained smear should be taken from the abscesses or nasopharynx. Signs of central nervous system (CNS) involvement warrant lumbar puncture. Blood cultures are taken if leucocytosis and fever are present.

Treatment

Parenteral antibiotics are required. If there is no response within 24 hours, the plan of management should quickly proceed to computed tomography (CT) scan of the orbit and sinuses. If there is no direct site of inoculation seen, adequate drainage of sinusitis abscess should be performed to prevent complications. The condition should be managed jointly by the ophthalmologist, paediatrician and neurologist, if necessary.

ALLERGIC CONJUNCTIVITIS

Allergic conjunctivitis is a type I hypersensitivity reaction caused by interaction between allergens and IgE antibodies on the surface of mast cells in the conjunctiva. This interaction causes degranulation of mast cells and release of mast cell mediators. The mediators that are implicated in allergic ocular disease include histamine, leucotrienes, eosinophilic chemotactic factors (ECF), eosinophilic granule major basic protein (EMBP), platelet-activating

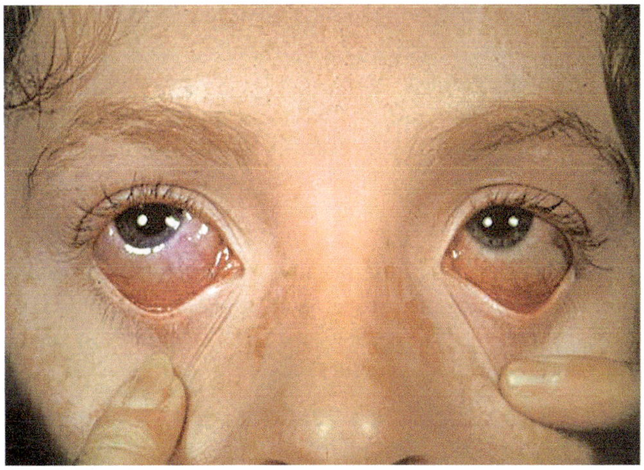

Figure 22.19 Acute allergic conjunctivitis.

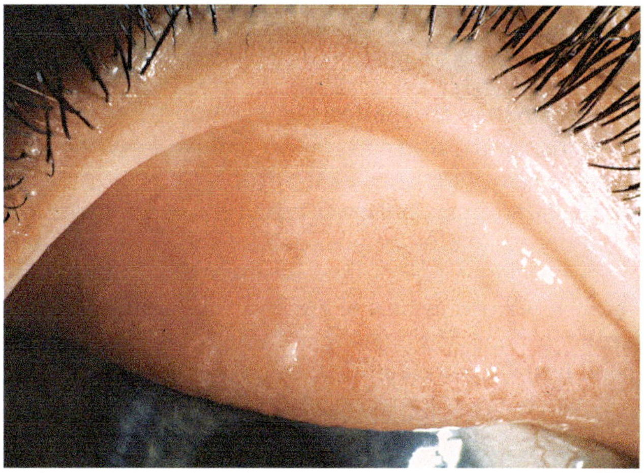

Figure 22.20 Allergic conjunctivitis.

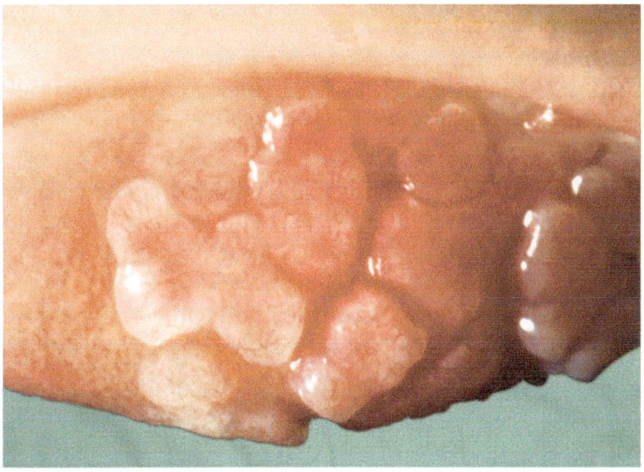

Figure 22.21 Giant papillae in vernal conjunctivitis.

factor (PAF), prostaglandin D2 (PGD2) and several other less well-defined factors. The hallmark of allergic ocular disease is itching and hyperaemia. The chronic, recurrent and seasonal nature of the disease is characteristic. Affected children often have a history of asthma, allergic rhinitis and atopic dermatitis.

Types

Seasonal Allergic Conjunctivitis (Hay Fever Conjunctivitis)

Airborne allergens such as pollen, moulds, dander, grasses and weeds trigger a hypersensitivity reaction. As the name suggests the conjunctivitis is seasonal. Patients present with watering, conjunctival hyperaemia and chemosis.

Vernal Keratoconjunctivitis

Vernal keratoconjunctivitis is a severe form of IgE-mediated mast cell dependent, type I hypersensitivity reaction. The onset of the disease is usually between 3 years and 4 years of age. It can last 4–10 years with exacerbations and remissions. Symptoms include photophobia, severe itching, foreign body sensation and watering of the eyes. Vernal conjunctivitis is divided into two types: (1) palpebral and (2) bulbar. Both types can coexist. The palpebral form has hypertrophied papillae, most prominently over the upper palpebral conjunctiva, the so-called cobblestone appearance. The conjunctiva has a milky hue and thick, ropy, white discharge. The bulbar form has nodules or gelatinous thickening of the conjunctiva along the limbus. Corneal involvement in vernal conjunctivitis includes punctate epithelial erosions, which can progress to form a sterile ulcer, called a shield ulcer, on the upper part of the cornea.

Atopic Keratoconjunctivitis

Atopic keratoconjunctivitis is relatively rare in children, usually affecting young men with atopic dermatitis. Ocular symptoms and signs are similar to vernal keratocojunctivitis. Unlike vernal keratoconjunctivitis, the inferior palpebral conjunctiva can be involved **(Figs. 22.19 to 22.21)**.

Treatment

Treatment of all ocular allergic diseases is basically similar. It is often impossible to identify and remove the allergens. Therefore, therapy is directed towards relief of symptoms. Topical eye drops are the mainstay of therapy. The therapeutic agents employed are as follows:

- Mast cell stabilisers
- H_1-reception antagonists
- Agents with both mast cell stabiliser activity and H_1-receptor blocking activity.

Other useful agents include nonsteroidal anti-inflammatory agents (NSAIDs) and topical steroids, although the risk of steroid-induced glaucoma and cataract limits the use of steroids to short intervals.

LACRIMAL SYSTEM

Anatomy

The lacrimal system consists of epithelium-lined passages that drain tears from each eye to the nasal cavity. Tears enter a punctum at the medial end of each eyelid, proceed through the upper- and lower-canaliculi, which then form a common canaliculus on each side, and enter the lacrimal sac. This leads to the nasolacrimal duct, which opens into the inferior meatus of the nose beneath the inferior turbinate bone. The opening of the upper and lower canaliculi into the common canaliculus is guarded by a one-way valve, the valve of Rosenmüller. The membranous opening into the nose is called the valve of Hasner.

Congenital Abnormalities of the Lacrimal Drainage System

Puncta: The puncta may be absent (atresia), rudimentary, or covered by epithelium.

Canaliculi: The canaliculi may be rudimentary or anomalous in position and number.

Amniocele (Dacryocystocele): If there is obstruction at the valve of Rosenmüller and also inferiorly at the nasolacrimal duct, the lacrimal sac becomes distended. This condition may be present at birth or in early infancy and is termed an amniocele or dacryocystocele. The distended sac may become secondarily infected, causing dacryocystitis **(Fig. 22.22)**.

Management

Hydrostatic massage and topical antibiotics may resolve the condition. If the condition persists lacrimal probing should be done no later than 1 month.

Congenital Nasolacrimal Duct Obstruction

Nasolacrimal duct (NLD) obstruction may occur, most often due to delayed canalisation at the valve of Hasner. The clinician can elicit regurgitation of mucopurulent discharge with pressure over lacrimal sac area. The differential diagnosis of congenital NLD obstruction includes conditions which present with epiphora: punctal atresia, conjunctivitis, blepharitis, keratitis and congenital glaucoma.

Management

Conservative management includes lacrimal sac massage and administration of topical antibiotics. NLD obstruction resolves spontaneously in the majority of the cases. Beyond 1 year of age, the rate of spontaneous resolution is significantly reduced.

Surgical Treatment

Early probing reduces the burden of conservative management and the potential for infection. However, delaying probing until 1 year age may avoid surgery altogether in many cases. The success rate of properly performed probing exceeds 90%. There is no convincing evidence that delaying probing until 1–2 years of age is harmful. However, after 2 years of age, simple probing may fail in as many as 30% of the cases.

Balloon catheter dilation: A lacrimal drainage system that appears to be blocked by scarring or constriction can be dilated by an inflatable balloon carried on a probe.

Intubation: Silicone tube intubation of the lacrimal system is usually recommended when one or more probing fail. The silicone tube should be left in situ for 3–6 months.

Dacryo-cysto-rhinostomy: Dacryo-cysto-rhinostomy (DCR) is indicated when repeated probing fail, when intubation cannot be accomplished and when significant symptoms recur after tube removal **(Fig. 22.23)**.

In this procedure, the sac wall is anastomosed to the nasal mucosa after creating a bony osteum, or hole, in the lacrimal fossa. The new passage thus opens from the lacrimal sac into the middle meatus of the nose

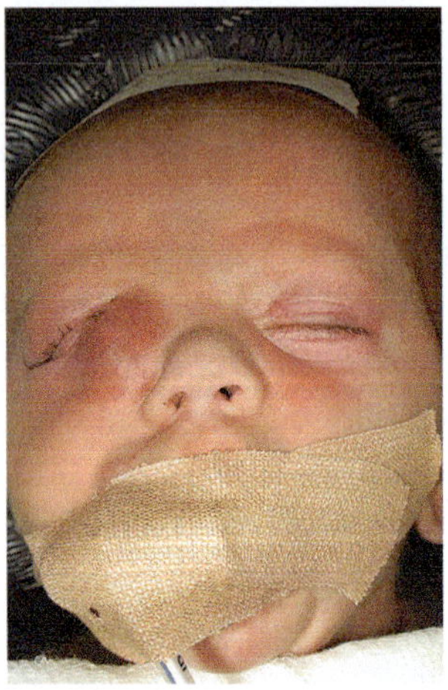

Figure 22.22 Acute dacryocystitis.
(*Photograph Courtesy*: David Taylor).

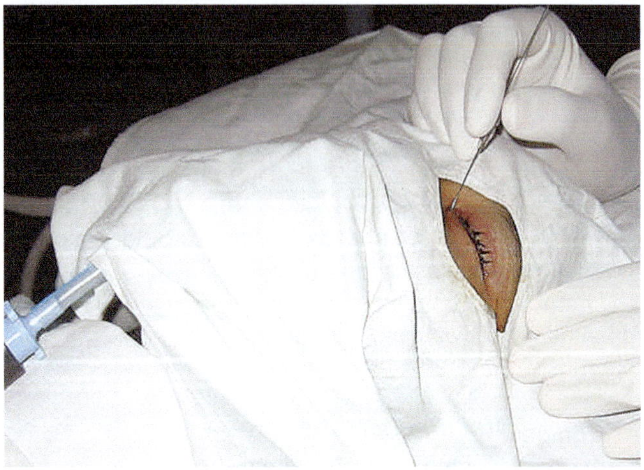

Figure 22.23 Nasolacrimal probing.

CORNEA

Embryology

The primitive cornea develops from surface ectoderm of the optic vesicle, and from neural crest cells, which migrate in waves over the surface of the primitive lens. The lens vesicle separates from surface ectoderm by 6 weeks gestation, and by 4 months gestation, the corneal endothelial layer is complete. However, the iris insertion at this stage is anterior to the primitive trabecular meshwork (neural crest cells), and gradual posterior migration continues until the end of the first year of life.

Abnormalities of neural crest cell migration, proliferation or differentiation may occur and present as a spectrum of anterior dysgenesis syndromes.

Corneal Size and Shape in Childhood

In the neonate, the normal horizontal corneal diameter is 9.5–10.5 mm, which grows to reach 12 mm, the average adult corneal diameter, by the age of 2 years. Abnormalities of corneal size or shape may be evident at birth, and may show a characteristic inheritance pattern, or may occur sporadically. They may be associated with other abnormalities of the eye and may be part of a syndrome affecting other systems of the body also (**Table 22.1**).

Causes of Corneal Opacity in Childhood

Corneal disease remains the most common cause of childhood blindness in the world today.

In the developing world, poor nutrition and the inadequacy of public health measures such as the provision of sanitation and immunisation remain key factors. In more affluent countries, congenital anomalies of the cornea form a small but significant proportion of the blinding conditions in childhood.

The normal cornea is avascular and transparent, and the cause of any opacity, which may interfere with vision, must be diagnosed, and if possible, treated, at the earliest possible opportunity, to avoid irreversible damage and visual loss, or the development of amblyopia.

XEROPHTHALMIA AND NUTRITIONAL CORNEAL ULCERATION OR KERATOMALACIA

Xerophthalmia describes a dry ocular surface due to vitamin A deficiency, which may progress to keratomalacia, an acute keratitis due to untreated vitamin A deficiency, which in-turn, if not treated urgently and adequately, progresses rapidly to corneal melting and perforation.

The earliest symptom of vitamin A deficiency is night blindness. This should be specifically asked about in consultations or in paediatric eye screening programmes, in developing countries. If vitamin A remains deficient, the conjunctiva becomes dry, with a wrinkled, reddened or pigmented appearance. Bitot's spots may form on the exposed conjunctiva, lateral, and sometimes medial, to the cornea. They appear like a triangular or irregular area of froth or tiny bubbles on the conjunctiva, sometimes with underlying pigmentation. Adequate treatment with vitamin A at this stage, and ensuring that inadequate dietary intake as well as conditions causing diarrhoea and vomiting are properly managed, can prevent the occurrence of keratomalacia and blindness. Conversely, neglect of early signs of vitamin A deficiency results in a high risk of adherent leucoma formation. A dense corneal scar develops, due to corneal perforation with adherence to the iris and lens, causing cataract. Secondary infection may result in endophthalmitis. The latter may be life-threatening,

TABLE 22.1 Corneal size and shape in childhood.

	Megalocornea	*Keratoglobus*	*Keratoconus*	*Microcornea*
Typical features	Horizontal corneal diameter >12 mm in neonate, or 13 mm in an older child usually bilateral	Thinned, globular shaped cornea, with deep anterior chamber. Episodes of corneal oedema. Risk of corneal rupture with minor trauma	Coning of the central or paracentral cornea due to progressive thinning. Often presents in adolescence, with gradual or rapid progression	Horizontal corneal diameter <9 mm in the neonate, or 10 mm in an older child. In nanophthalmos, other ocular structures as the cornea, are smaller than normal
Inheritance pattern	X-linked recessive	Autosomal recessive	Undetermined	Sporadic or autosomal dominant
Associations	Glaucoma, lens subluxation, iris hypoplasia and ectopic pupil	Ehlers–Danlos type IV syndrome	Down syndrome, other types of mental retardation Atopy	Cataract, coloboma, high myopia, persistent hyperplastic primary vitreous, oculo-dento-digital dysplasia syndrome

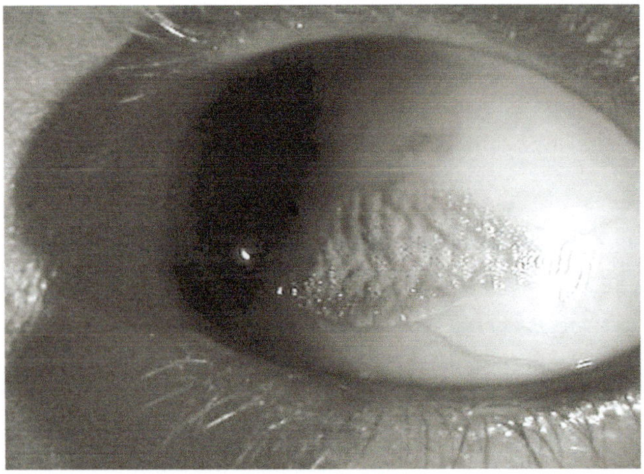

Figure 22.24 Bitot's spots in vitamin A deficiency.

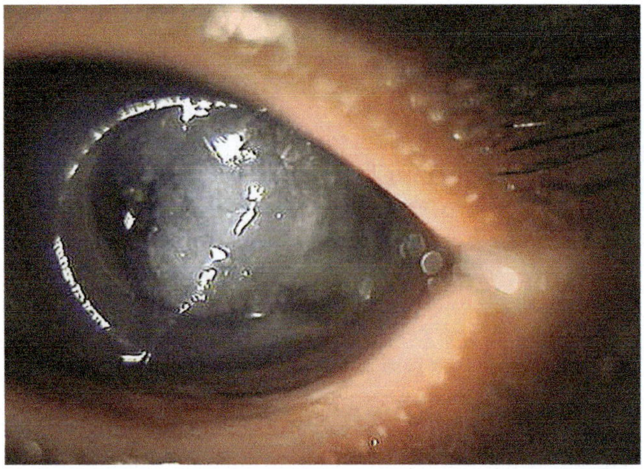

Figure 22.25 Keratomalacia with corneal melt due to vitamin A deficiency.

as is continuing, untreated vitamin A deficiency **(Figs. 22.24 and 22.25)**.

World Health Organization (WHO) Classification of Xerophthalmia

- XN Night blindness
- X1A Conjunctival xerosis
- X1B Bitot's spots
- X2 Corneal xerosis
- X3A Corneal ulcer less than one-third of corneal surface
- X3B Corneal ulcer more than-third of corneal surface
- XS Corneal scar
- XF Xerophthalmic fundus

If the deficiency is progressive, children may go through this spectrum of clinical signs. When there is a sudden increase in metabolic demand, as in the case of infections such as measles or diarrhoea, vitamin A deficiency may rapidly progress to keratomalacia without passing through the whole spectrum of clinical signs. Severe keratomalacia is usually seen in children below 5 years of age. Children between 6 months and 3 years are particularly at risk.

Prevention: 200,000 IU of vitamin A should be administered orally every 6 months to children from 1 to 6 years of age. The first dose can be given at the time of measles, mumps and rubella (MMR) vaccination. Measles vaccination has played an important role in the prevention of vitamin A related blindness. Vitamin A is teratogenic; therefore, administration is not advised in early pregnancy. It can be administered to women at delivery or within 1 month of delivery, and breastfeeding should be encouraged. Health education and improved nutrition, particularly with foods rich in vitamin A, contribute significantly to prevention of deficiency.

Keratomalacia: Keratomalacia is a medical emergency. The affected child requires hospitalization for adequate treatment.

Treatment schedule for vitamin A deficiency in keratomalacia **(Table 22.2)**.

In addition, secondary bacterial infection should be treated with combination antibiotic therapy (e.g., gentamicin drops + cefazolin drops), and protein-calorie malnutrition and diarrhoea should be treated. Small punched out corneal ulcers which occur, usually heal well, but residual scarring may persist.

OTHER DISORDERS AFFECTING THE CORNEA

Infection of the Cornea

Ophthalmia neonatorum refers to neonatal conjunctivitis. If untreated, corneal infection and scarring may be a complication.

In older children, minor corneal trauma or untreated conjunctivitis, particularly in the presence of malnutrition or other systemic illness, may cause corneal infection and ulceration, with subsequent corneal opacity **(Fig. 22.26)**.

Measles keratitis remains a significant cause of corneal scarring and blindness in some regions, although measles immunisation and improved childhood nutrition have markedly reduced the incidence of measles and its complications.

Trachoma, primarily an infection of the conjunctiva, can result in scarring of the tarsal conjunctiva, with consequent misdirected eyelashes or trichiasis, which constantly rub against the cornea. This causes chronic irritation, sometimes with corneal ulceration and scarring.

TABLE 22.2 Treatment schedule for vitamin A deficiency in keratomalacia.

Timing	*<1 year of age*	*>1 year of age*
On diagnosis	100, 000 IU	200,000 IU
Following day	100,000 IU	200,000 IU
2–4 weeks later	100,000 IU	200,000 IU

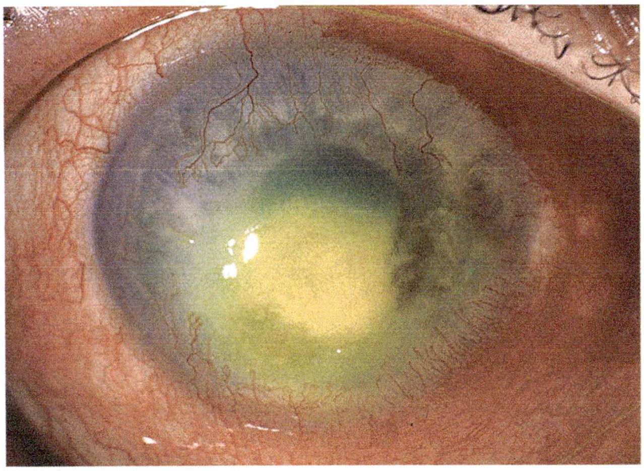

Figure 22.26 Corneal ulcer.

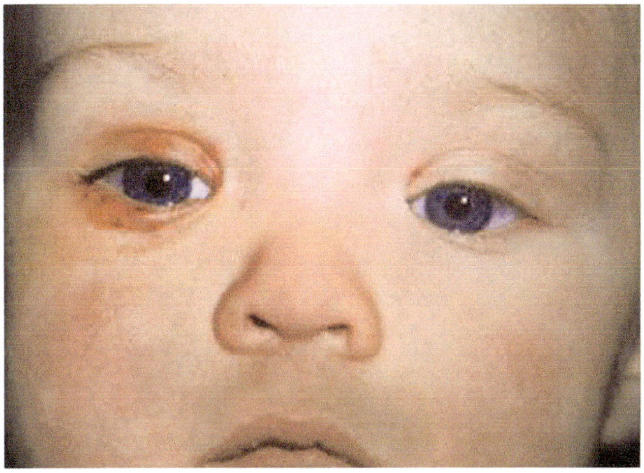

Figure 22.27 Primary herpes simplex of the eyelids with secondary impetigo due to *Staphylococcus aureus* in an atopic individual.

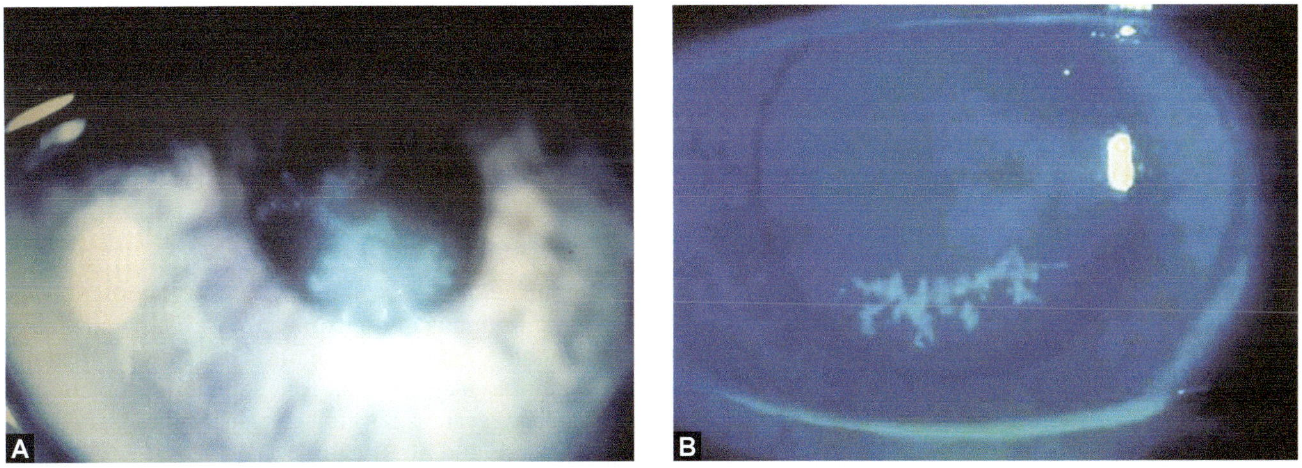

Figures 22.28A and B Dendritic corneal ulcer due to herpes simplex.

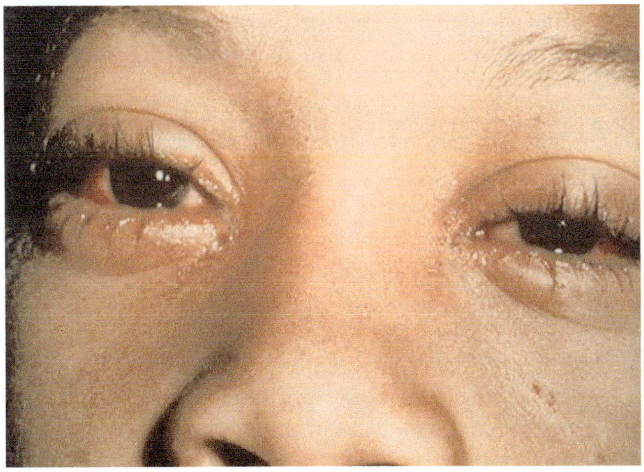

Figure 22.29 Adenoviral conjunctivitis.

Herpes simplex keratitis is more commonly seen in young adults, but can occur in childhood, particularly in atopic individuals **(Figs. 22.27 and 22.28)**.

Adenovirus infection is usually bilateral and self-limiting, but is highly contagious and can cause significant morbidity **(Fig. 22.29)**.

Injury due to birth trauma, which usually involves Descemet membrane (the protective layer of the cornea, adjacent to the endothelium), may resolve spontaneously, or with simple measures to avoid infection if the epithelium is damaged, but may require subsequent correction of astigmatism and patching of the other eye, to overcome amblyopia.

Injury due to Accidental Trauma

Injury due to accidental trauma may also cause corneal scarring in childhood. Delayed treatment is likely to be associated with secondary infection and a worsening of prognosis. Agricultural injuries with secondary fungal infection and injuries (often Gram-negative or anaerobic infections) from pet animals may be particularly severe. In penetrating injuries, adequate tetanus immunisation should always be ensured **(Fig. 22.30)**.

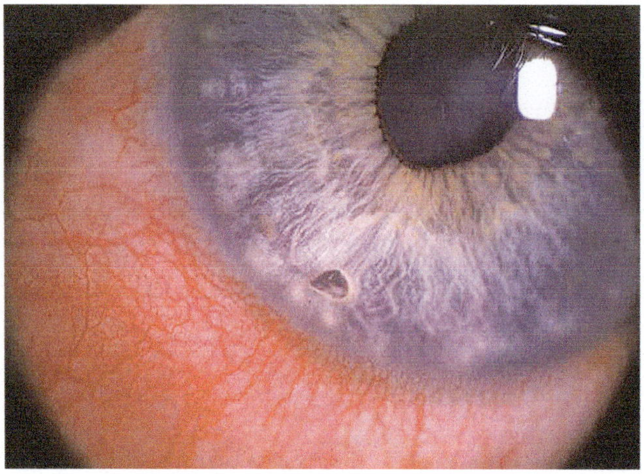

Figure 22.30 Penetrating injury of the cornea.

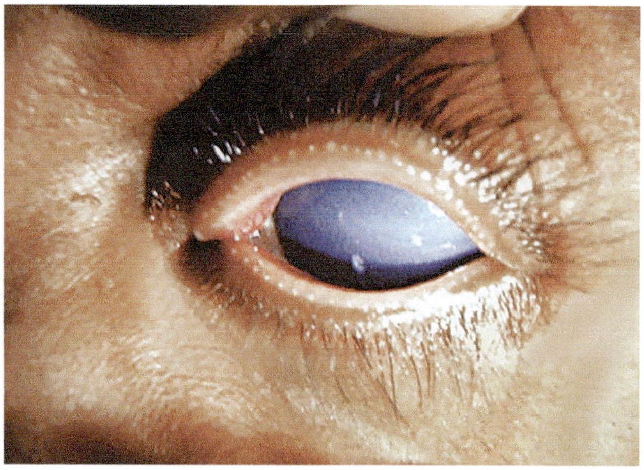

Figure 22.31 Enlarged, hazy cornea due to congenital glaucoma.

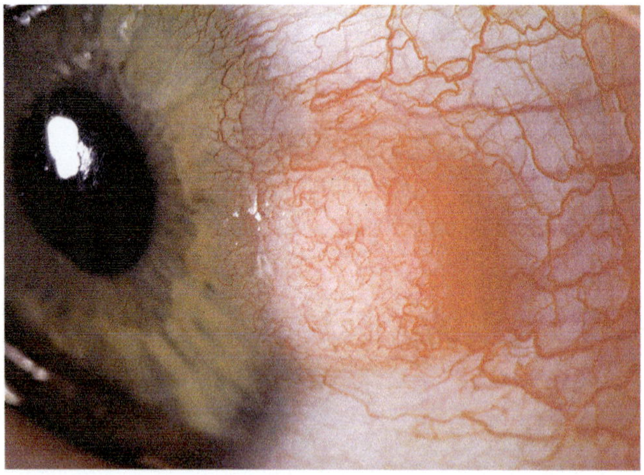

Figure 22.32 Limbal lipodermoid.

CHEMICAL INJURIES

Chemical injuries constitute an emergency where time is of essence. Immediate, copious irrigation of the injured eye, including the upper conjunctival fornix (the area under the upper eyelid) with buffered saline or Ringer's lactate where possible, but with clean water if that is all that is available, can save an eye and its sight, which may otherwise be lost. Acids cause coagulation of surface proteins on the cornea with rapid scarring, whereas alkalis penetrate rapidly into the eye causing widespread destruction of intraocular tissues as well as of the ocular surface. Prompt and prolonged irrigation of the eye dilutes and removes such chemicals from the ocular surface, thereby preventing or minimising these types of destruction.

CONGENITAL GLAUCOMA

Congenital glaucoma can present with cloudy or opaque corneas, which are usually also enlarged. The raised intraocular pressure initially causes enlargement of the globe, which, in infants, is relatively elastic. Without treatment, however, the disease progresses causing atrophy of the optic nerve, and irreversible visual loss. This condition must always be considered, therefore, in the presence of hazy or opaque corneas, in order that early treatment can be instituted, and blindness prevented **(Fig. 22.31)**.

DERMOIDS ON THE CORNEA

Dermoids on the cornea, usually extending from across the rim, or limbus of the cornea (most commonly inferotemporally), consist of hamartomatous fibrofatty tissue and keratinised epithelium. They sometimes contain skin appendages such as hair follicles, sebaceous glands and sweat glands and may be up to a centimetre in diameter. They may involve the corneal stroma, but not usually the whole thickness of the cornea. Large dermoids may cover the visual axis, thereby occluding vision. Smaller ones may result in astigmatism (as may surgical excision), which, uncorrected can cause amblyopia **(Fig. 22.32)**.

ANTERIOR SEGMENT DYSGENESIS

Anterior segment dysgenesis includes a spectrum of developmental genetic anomalies of peripheral and central anterior segment structures, the more severe of which include corneal scarring. The peripheral developmental anomalies include posterior embryotoxon and Axenfeld–Rieger syndrome **(Fig. 22.33)**. The central developmental anomalies include posterior corneal depression and Peter's anomaly. In Peter's anomaly, there is a posterior corneal defect with a central stromal opacity, with iris strands often adherent to its posterior surface. The opacity may lessen with time.

SCLEROCORNEA

Sclerocornea is a congenital condition in which, as its name suggests, the cornea is opaque and appears undifferentiated from the sclera. Flattening of the cornea may

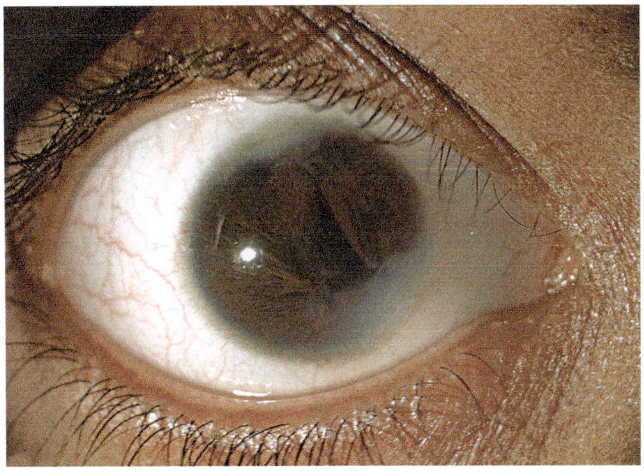

Figure 22.33 Rieger's anomaly.

also occur. The condition is often associated with other ocular or systemic abnormalities.

MUCOPOLYSACCHARIDOSIS AND MUCOLIPIDOSIS

Mucopolysaccharidoses and mucolipidoses constitute a varied group of conditions with lysosomal disorders, resulting in a range of mucopolysaccharides or mucolipids not being broken down and therefore accumulating in the tissues. Some of these conditions manifest ocular abnormalities. In Hurler syndrome (mucopolysaccharidosis Type 1) and in Scheie syndrome (mucopolysaccharidosis Type I-S-previously Type 5), corneal clouding occurs within the first 6 months–2 years of life. In mucolipidosis IV, corneal clouding may occur in the first few weeks of life. In these conditions, electron microscopy on conjunctival biopsies reveals abnormal cytoplasmic inclusions.

CONGENITAL HEREDITARY ENDOTHELIAL DYSTROPHY

Congenital hereditary endothelial dystrophy (CHED) manifests in the early days of life. It is a defect of the endothelial layer of the cornea and of the adjacent Descemet layer, resulting in diffuse oedema of the epithelial and stromal layers of the cornea. The cornea is, therefore, thickened and hazy and must be differentiated from congenital glaucoma, where the corneal diameter is usually increased and the intraocular pressure is elevated. CHED is a rare inherited condition, which may be autosomal dominant or autosomal recessive.

TREATMENT OF CORNEAL OPACITIES IN CHILDHOOD

Treatment of corneal injuries, infections and damage due to vitamin A deficiency must be prompt and adequate in order to preserve or restore sight. In many situations, there may be astigmatism or corneal scarring despite repair, resolution of infection or restoration of adequate levels of vitamin A in the body. Refractive correction of astigmatism can then be undertaken, or corneal grafting if appropriate.

Corneal grafting requires special care and expertise in children, and the final visual outcome may be poorer than one would hope. Furthermore, since deprivation amblyopia has been found to be best reversed by treatment of the underlying cause within the first 3 months of life, the surgery, and the anaesthesia required, may be more complex than if performed later. Some studies have shown less corneal rejection and a better final visual outcome if surgery is delayed until approximately 1 year after birth **(Figs. 22.34 and 22.35)**.

Where treatment of corneal opacities is not possible, support of the child and the family is essential, with appropriate advice and information given, and all possible

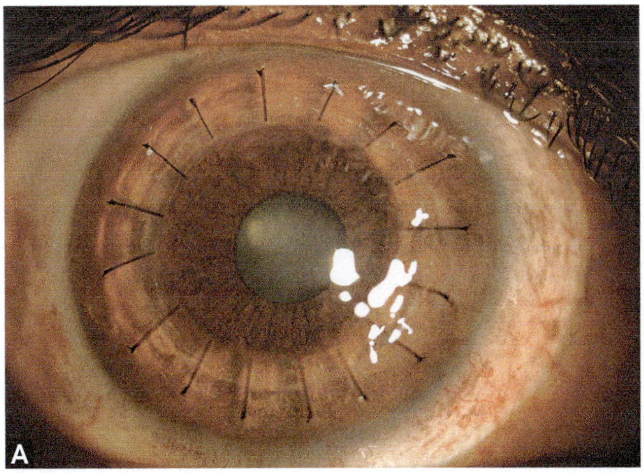

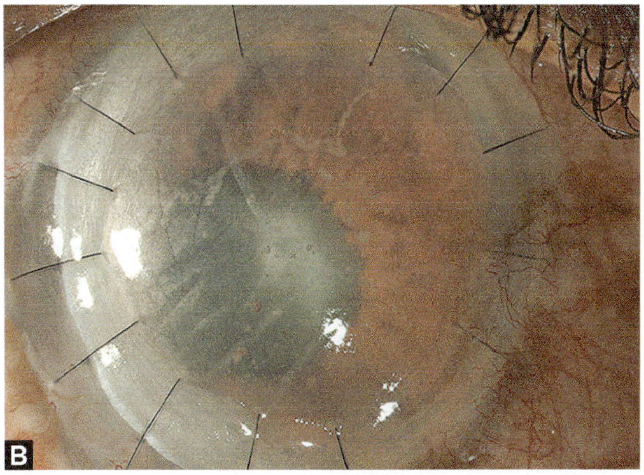

Figures 22.34A and B (A) Penetrating keratoplasty; (B) Corneal graft rejection.

(*Courtesy:* David Yorston. Photograph published in Community Eye Health Journal, www.cehjournal.org).

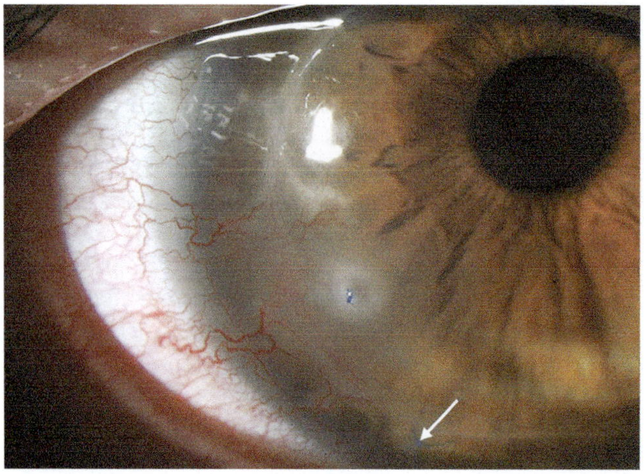

Figure 22.35 A broken stitch has caused blood vessels to grow into the cornea.

(*Courtesy:* David Yorston. Photograph published in Community Eye Health Journal, www.cehjournal.org).

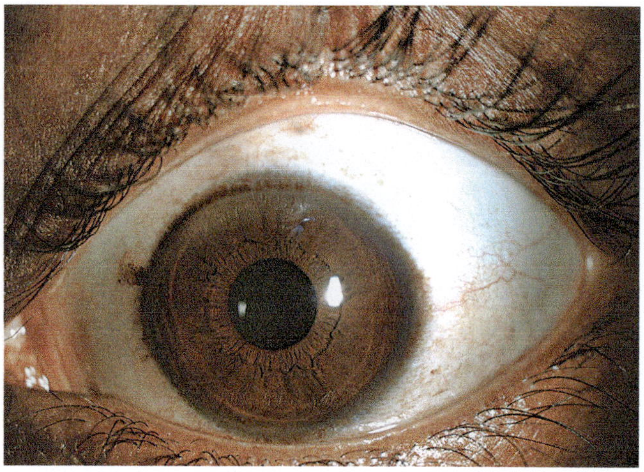

Figure 22.36 Kayser–Fleischer ring.

rehabilitation measures put in place to enable the child to live as full a life as possible, and to avoid the additional risks and possible harm associated with poor sight.

SYSTEMIC DISEASES WITH CORNEAL MANIFESTATIONS IN CHILDHOOD

Congenital Syphilis

Interstitial keratitis secondary to congenital syphilis may present during the first 10 years of life, with corneal oedema and aggressive vascularisation of the deep stromal layer of the cornea, giving it a pink appearance ("salmon patch"). Blood flow through these vessels gradually stops over a period of weeks to months, leaving greyish white "ghost" vessels visible deep in the stroma, which are evident throughout life.

Leprosy

Although the prevalence of leprosy has diminished dramatically over the past 15 years, new cases continue to be diagnosed in children, and may result in impairments such as lagophthalmos and impaired corneal sensation. Neurotrophic keratitis, and exposure keratitis may both result in corneal opacity, and secondary infective keratitis can cause more severe corneal damage or corneal perforation and endophthalmitis. Corneal lepromas (granulomatous lesions which develop as a response to the presence of *Mycobacterium leprae*) are now rare, but chronic iritis my result in band keratopathy—a condition that occurs in eyes with chronic inflammation, in which calcific material is deposited in a band-shaped area across the cornea.

Mucopolysaccharidoses

All of the mucopolysaccharidoses cause varying degrees of corneal haziness due to deposits in the cornea, except for Hunter's syndrome (mucopolysaccharidosis type II) (see previous section).

Hepatolenticular Degeneration (Wilson Disease)

Wilson disease is an inborn error of metabolism in which excess copper deposition occurs in the liver, kidney and basal ganglia of the brain. Inheritance is autosomal recessive, and clinical features include cirrhosis of the liver, renal tubular damage, and a type of Parkinsonism. A copper coloured ring (the Kayser–Fleischer ring) in Descemet layer of the cornea is a diagnostic feature of established disease but may not be present in the early stages. Copper deposits are first seen in the 12 and 6 O'clock positions and then form a complete ring **(Fig. 22.36)**.

Cystinosis

Cystinosis is a rare, metabolic disease in which intracellular cysteine levels are elevated, resulting in the deposition of cysteine crystals in various parts of the body. In infants, failure to thrive, rickets and progressive renal failure occur, and are known as Fanconi syndrome. Ocular features develop in the first year of life, and include the deposition of crystals in the peripheral cornea and throughout Descemet layer, as well as on the anterior iris surface and in the conjunctiva. Photophobia occurs. Oral cysteamine reduces systemic crystal deposition and is more effective than topical cysteamine, which is also difficult to obtain **(Fig. 22.37)**.

Familial Dysautonomia (Riley–Day Syndrome)

This is an autosomal recessive condition seen largely in Ashkenazi Jews. There is autonomic dysfunction with relative insensitivity to pain and temperature instability.

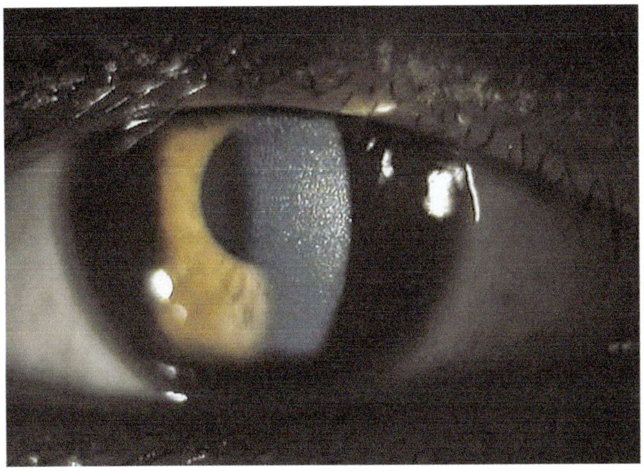

Figure 22.37 Deposition of cysteine crystals in the cornea in cystinosis.

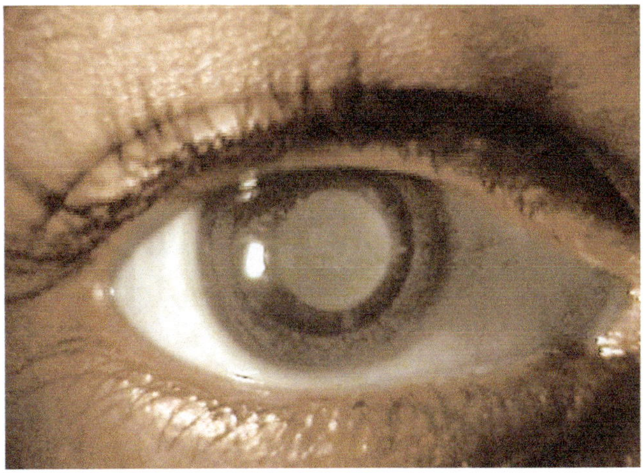

Figure 22.38 Lamellar cataract.

Abnormal lacrimation and decreased corneal sensation result in exposure keratitis and frequent corneal ulceration with secondary opacity. Topical artificial tear preparations and tarsorrhaphies may protect the corneas to some extent.

Childhood Lens Disorders

Childhood lens abnormalities include cataract, subluxation, and abnormal lens shape and development. These abnormalities continue to be an important cause of visual impairment. Lens disorders can be the presenting sign of systemic abnormalities involving the CNS, the urinary tract and the skin.

Paediatric Cataracts

The cause of most cataracts is unknown. They are most commonly inherited in an autosomal dominant pattern, but X-linked and autosomal recessive types have been reported. Trisomy 13, 18 and 21 are associated with cataracts. The onset, location and morphology of cataracts provide important information regarding their cause and likely visual outcome following surgery. Cataracts that present at birth are most serious because the visual system is still immature. Amblyopia is inevitable unless the visual axis is rendered clear by 6–8 weeks of age. Unilateral cataracts tend to cause denser amblyopia because of the rivalry between the two eyes.

MORPHOLOGICAL CLASSIFICATION OF CATARACTS

Cataracts can be classified as:

- Anterior
  - Anterior polar cataract
  - Anterior subcapsular and
  - Anterior lenticonus
- Lamellar
- Nuclear
- Posterior
  - Posterior lenticonus
  - Persistent hyperplastic primary vitreous (PHPV)
  - Posterior subcapsular cataract.

Anterior Cataract

Anterior polar cataract is a small white discrete opacity at the centre of the anterior capsule. These opacities are usually non-progressive and visually insignificant. One-third of them are bilateral. Most of them can be managed conservatively. However, because they can be associated with strabismus, anisometropia and amblyopia, follow-up is necessary.

Anterior pyramidal cataract is a white conical opacity at the anterior pole. These cataracts are usually bilateral and are not associated with any systemic disease.

Anterior subcapsular cataract lies immediately under the anterior capsule of the lens in the anterior cortex. Such cataracts are usually idiopathic. However, the possibility of trauma or Alport syndrome should be considered. Lens changes in Alport syndrome consist of bilateral anterior subcapsular cataract and bilateral anterior lenticonus.

Lamellar Cataract

Lamellar cataracts occupy specific zones in the lens cortex and have spoke-like radial opacities. Most lamellar cataracts progress and require surgery. These may be unilateral or bilateral. Bilateral lamellar cataracts are frequently inherited in an autosomal dominant manner. Metabolic diseases such as neonatal hypoglycaemia and galactosaemia can cause bilateral lamellar cataracts (Fig. 22.38).

Nuclear Cataract

Nuclear cataract is an opacity located within the embryonic or foetal nucleus. These cataracts can be unilateral or bilateral. Bilateral nuclear cataracts are often inherited

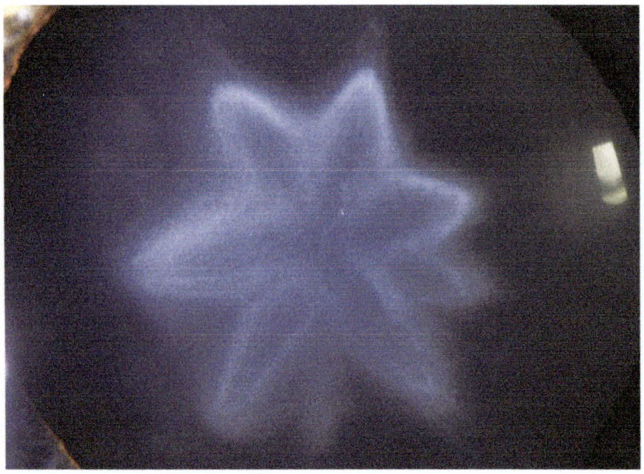

Figure 22.39 Stellate cataract.

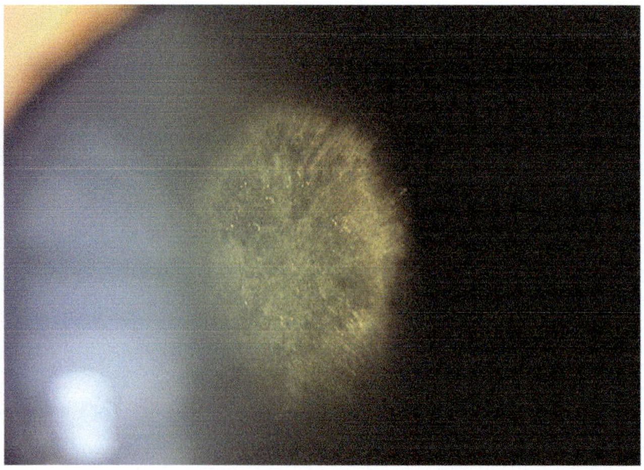

Figure 22.40 Steroid-induced cataract.

according to an autosomal dominant pattern. Intrauterine rubella infection causes a distinctive nuclear cataract with a "shaggy" appearance. Visual prognosis in these cataracts is only fair, even after early surgery.

Posterior Cataract

Posterior lenticonus is almost always unilateral and can cause myopia and astigmatism. Therefore, it is important to monitor vision and prescribe appropriate optical correction to prevent amblyopia.

Persistent hyperplastic primary vitreous is caused by failure of regression of the primitive hyaloid vascular system. PHPV occurs sporadically, is almost always unilateral and is associated with microphthalmia. Clinically there is a retrolenticular fibrovascular membrane, which extends to the optic disc as a stalk. The membrane may contract, push the lens-iris diaphragm anteriorly and cause glaucoma.

Posterior subcapsular cataracts in children are often stellate, or rosette-shaped, and secondary to trauma or steroid-induced. They affect vision significantly and require surgery, for which the visual prognosis is excellent **(Figs. 22.39 and 22.40)**.

EVALUATION OF CATARACT

Examination in a darkened room is performed by shining the light of a direct ophthalmoscope into both eyes simultaneously, in order to detect normal, symmetrical red reflexes. This test is called Bruckner test. Any central opacity or surrounding cortical distortion more than 3 mm is considered to have a significant effect on vision. Taking a family history is important in order to elicit whether there is an autosomal dominant or X-linked pattern of inherited cataract. General physical examination in addition to examination of the anterior and posterior segments of the eye is required. Unilateral cataracts are generally not metabolic or genetic in origin, and therefore laboratory tests are not helpful, except a TORCHES titre (see intrauterine infectious disease). Laboratory tests, however, can provide valuable information in bilateral cataracts, particularly is Lowe syndrome and galactosaemia. Recommended tests include a urine test for reducing substances after milk feeding, TORCH titre and VDRL test. Other optional tests include a urine test for amino acids, and blood tests for calcium, phosphorus and red-cell galactokinase level.

Surgery

The principal surgical options are removal of lens matter through an anterior capsulorhexis (i.e. a hole made in the anterior capsule), or lensectomy with a posterior approach. Intraocular lens implantation (IOL) at the same time in infants remains controversial. IOL is recommended in children above age 2 years. Because rapid posterior capsule opacification occurs, a controlled moderate posterior capsulotomy and anterior vitrectomy should be performed at the time of surgery. This allows establishment of a clear visual axis, facilitating accurate retinoscopy and subsequent fitting of an appropriate optical correction. Optical rehabilitation is important to avoid amblyopia. If an IOL is not inserted at surgery, aphakic spectacles or contact lenses are required. Aphakic spectacles are the safest and can be easily changed according to the refractive requirement. Contact lenses provide more constant refractive correction but are less easily changed, may be displaced by eye rubbing and can pose a risk of infection and corneal ulcer. If an intraocular lens is inserted, it is important to ensure that it is placed within the lens capsule ("in the bag"). Children often require spectacle correction, especially for reading in spite of the intraocular lens. All children need long-term follow-up for changes in refractive status, amblyopia management, intraocular pressure monitoring and posterior segment evaluation.

A good visual outcome depends on the timing of surgery, appropriate optical correction and adequate

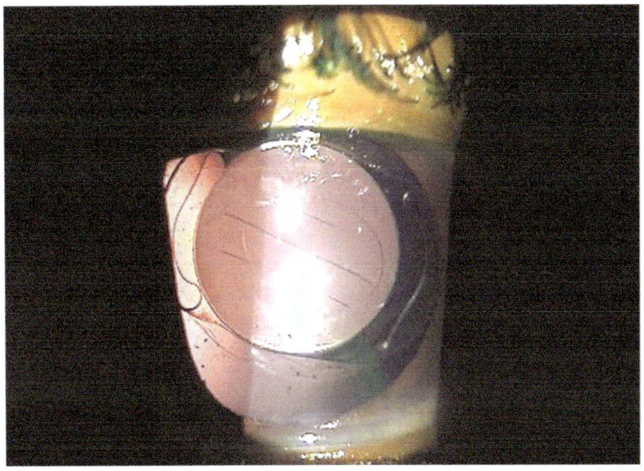

Figure 22.41 Intraocular lens in capsular bag

(*Courtesy:* David Yorston. Photograph published in Community Eye Health Journal, www.cehjournal.org).

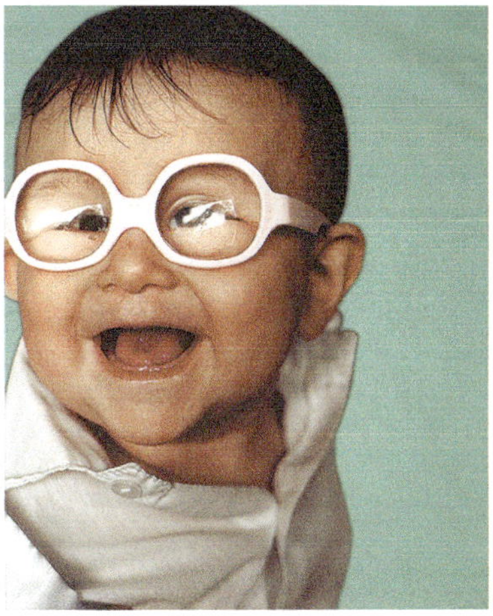

Figure 22.42 Child wearing aphakic spectacles.

(*Courtesy:* Photograph published in Community Eye Health Journal, www.cehjournal.org).

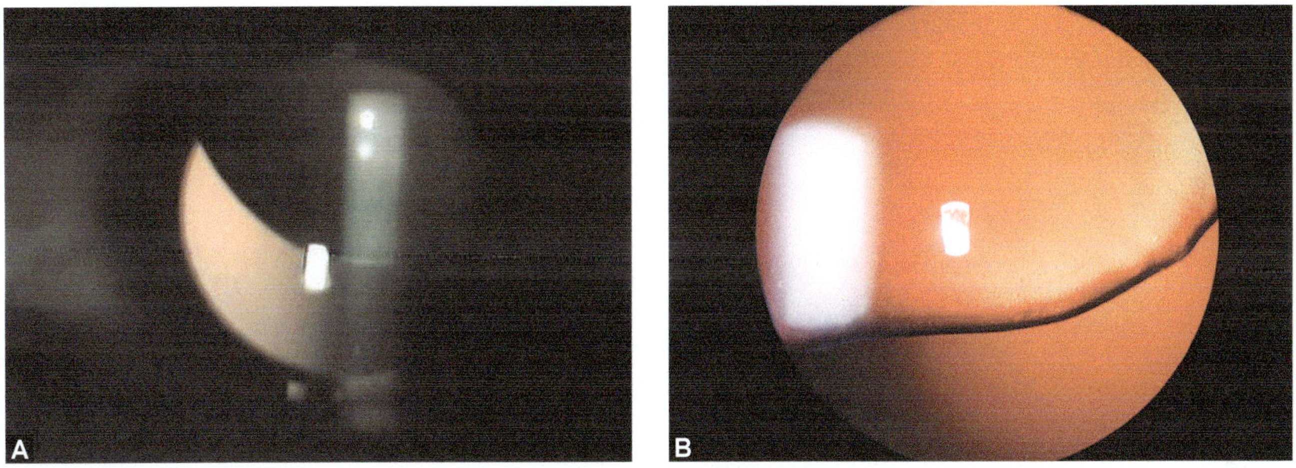

Figures 22.43A and B Marfan syndrome. (A) Lens subluxed upwards; (B) Upward subluxation of lens seen against red reflex.

treatment of amblyopia. In general, children with bilateral cataracts achieve a better final visual outcome than those with a unilateral cataract **(Figs. 22.41 and 22.42)**.

DISLOCATION OF THE LENS

When the lens is not in the normal position, it is said to be subluxated or dislocated (if completely dislodged). The signs of lens subluxation are iridodonesis (a shimmering movement of the iris due to lens movement posterior to it), phacodonesis (a shimmering movement of the lens) and visibility of the lens edge within the pupil. Important systemic conditions associated with subluxated lenses are:

- Marfan syndrome
- Homocystinuria
- Weill-Marchesani syndrome
- Hyperlysinaemia
- Sulphite oxidase deficiency
- Ehlers-Danlos syndrome.

Subluxated lenses may remain stable, and satisfactory vision can be achieved with an appropriate astigmatic, or hypermetropic (aphakic) spectacle correction. In other situations, where the subluxation is unstable or progressive, lens extraction may be indicated to avoid complications such as dislocation into the anterior chamber and secondary glaucoma **(Figs. 22.43 to 22.45)**.

PAEDIATRIC GLAUCOMA

Childhood glaucomas may be classified into two groups:

1. Primary congenital glaucoma
2. Secondary congenital glaucoma

Primary Congenital Glaucoma

This condition is bilateral in almost two-thirds of patients, occurs more frequently in males and has no racial predilection. Inheritance is mostly sporadic or autosomal recessive with variable penetrance.

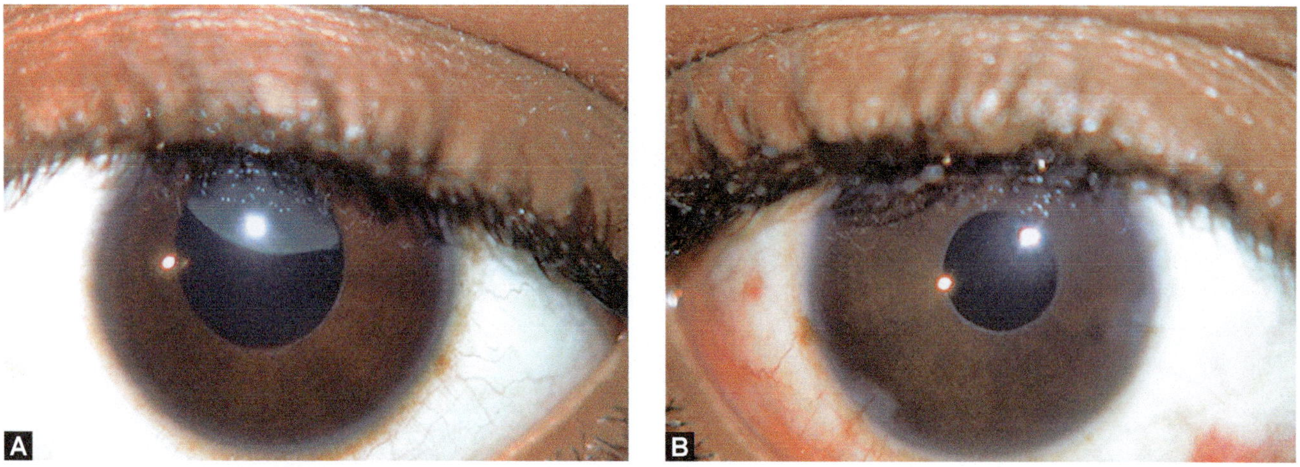

Figures 22.44A and B Marfan syndrome. (A) Upward lens dislocation; (B) Post-lens extraction.
(*Courtesy:* Photographs published in Community Eye Health Journal, www.cehjournal.org).

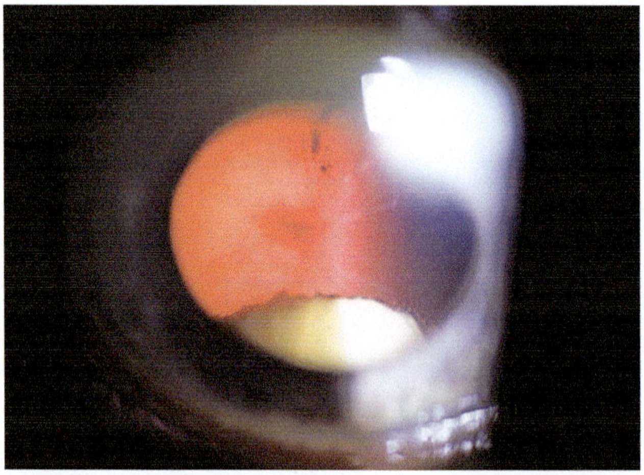

Figure 22.45 Homocystinuria: Lens subluxed downwards.

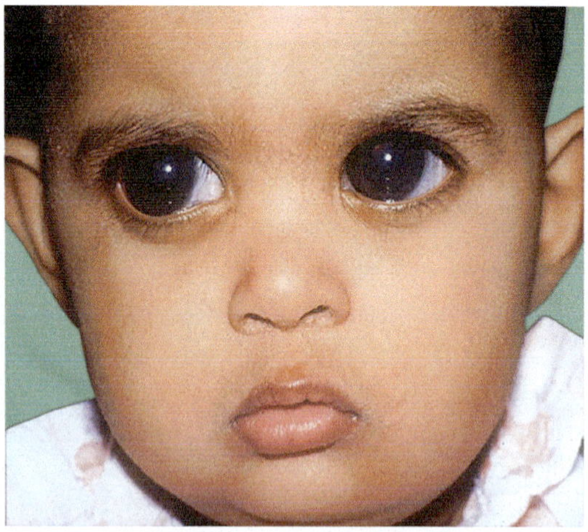

Figure 22.46 Buphthalmos due to congenital glaucoma.
(*Courtesy:* P Khaw. Photograph published in Community Eye Health Journal, www.cehjournal.org).

The cause of this type of glaucoma is abnormal development of the anterior chamber angle which causes obstruction to outflow of the aqueous. This in turn causes increased intraocular pressure and the relatively elastic sclera of the infant eye responds with stretching and enlargement of the globe (Fig. 22.46).

Clinical Features

The classic triad of symptoms comprises:

- Epiphora
- Photophobhia
- Blepharospasm.

Signs

A hazy cornea. Corneal oedema is the presenting sign in most infants, often accompanied by breaks in Descemet membrane called Haab's striae.

Increased corneal diameter. The normal horizontal corneal diameter is 9.5–10.5 mm at birth and 10.5–11.5 mm at 1 year. A diameter of more than 12.5 mm is suggestive of glaucoma.

- Deep anterior chamber.
- Increased intraocular pressure.
- Optic disc changes (pallor, atrophy).

Diagnosis

A detailed ocular examination under anaesthesia should be done. The following tests are required.

- Measurement of corneal diameter
- Intraocular pressure recording
- Gonioscopy
- Ophthalmoscopy.

Differential Diagnosis

- Megalocornea
- Nasolacrimal duct obstruction

- Keratitis
- Trauma
- Metabolic disorders.

Secondary Congenital Glaucoma

Ophthalmologist and paediatrician must be aware of associated systemic and ocular anomalies in an infant with glaucoma. Example of associated systemic abnormalities includes:

- Sturge–Weber syndrome
- Neurofibromatosis
- Oculocerebrorenal syndrome (Lowe's syndrome)
- Congenital rubella.

Treatment

Medical Therapeutic Agents:

- Carbonic anhydrase inhibitors
- Topical beta-blockers
- Prostaglandin derivatives.

Surgical Therapy:

- Goniotomy
- Trabeculotomy
- Trabeculectomy
- Glaucoma implants
- Cycloablation

All cases of childhood glaucoma require careful, long-term follow-up. Visual loss is not only due to corneal scarring and optic nerve damage, but may also be due to significant astigmatism and amblyopia. Glaucoma that presents at birth has a poor visual prognosis. Presentation at 3–12 months age is associated with a better visual prognosis.

UVEITIS IN CHILDREN

Introduction

Uveitis is an inflammatory response to a physical or biological insult, involving part of, or the whole uveal tract. Polymorphonuclear leucocytes and monocytes accumulate in the uvea and stimulate the release of chemical mediators. These may remove the offending stimulant as well as creating further inflammation. Approximately 50% of children presenting with anterior uveitis manifest no obvious cause of the condition. The most common identifiable cause, however, of anterior uveitis in the paediatric age group, is juvenile idiopathic arthritis (JIA), particularly the pauciarticular type (oligoarticular type).

Uveitis in children accounts for 2–8% of uveitis occurring at all ages. It presents particular challenges to the clinician:

- Late presentation is common, because children may not be able to express their symptoms
- Potential side effects and poor compliance may limit the effectiveness of treatment
- Steroid-induced glaucoma, secondary cataract and band keratopathy have a higher incidence rate in children than in adults.

Causes of Uveitis in Children

The majority of uveitis cases in children are bilateral, non-granulomatous and anterior. Intermediate and pan-uveitis are seen less commonly, and posterior uveitis, least of all.

Causes of each type of uveitis are listed in **Table 22.3**.

TABLE 22.3 Causes of uveitis.

Anterior uveitis	*Intermediate uveitis*	*Posterior uveitis*	*Panuveitis*
Juvenile rheumatoid arthritis	Pars planitis Sarcoidosis	Toxoplasmosis Ocular histoplasmosis	Sarcoidosis Vogt–Koyanagi–Harada syndrome
Trauma	Tuberculosis	Herpetic disease Cytomegalovirus (in the immunosuppressed)	
Sarcoidosis	Toxocariasis	Syphilis	Behcet syndrome
HLA B27-related	Lyme disease	Sympathetic ophthalmia	Idiopathic
Herpetic disease	Idiopathic	Lyme disease	
Sympathetic ophthalmia		Idiopathic	
Syphilis			
Lyme disease			
Fuchs' heterochromic cyclitis			
Viral syndromes			
Idiopathic			

Abbreviation: HLA, human leukocyte antigen.

Clinical Features

The symptoms of acute anterior uveitis include pain, redness of the eye and photophobia. There may be watering of the eye. In chronic uveitis, it may be anterior, intermediate or posterior. There is often little in the way of pain or redness, but vision may be blurred, or there may be an awareness of 'floaters' in the eye. On examination, in acute anterior uveitis the redness is found to be maximal around the limbus of the cornea. Keratic precipitates (KP), which may be large and clumped together ("mutton fat" KP), or fine and diffuse, are usually present on the corneal endothelium, and cells (inflammatory cells), and flare (protein exudate) are seen on slit lamp examination of the aqueous fluid, and/or the vitreous (when the posterior segment of the eye is involved). In acute anterior uveitis, the pupil may be miosed (constricted), or irregular, due to adhesions of the iris to the anterior lens surface, known as posterior synechiae (anterior synechiae refer to adhesions of the peripheral iris to the corneal endothelial surface, which may occur in conditions with severe inflammation or in prolonged shallowing of the anterior chamber) **(Figs. 22.47 and 22.48)**.

In intermediate uveitis, creamy, inflammatory exudates are evident in the pars plana of the ciliary body, at the anterior periphery of the retina, and in posterior uveitis, similar lesions may be present elsewhere on the retina or in the vitreous.

Management

Anterior Uveitis

Investigation for an underlying cause of anterior uveitis in children is usually undertaken when the uveitis is bilateral, or recurrent, or does not respond to initial therapy.

Topical steroid and mydriatic drops are usually effective, and the minimum effective doses are used to prevent posterior synechiae and reduce the number of cells in the anterior chamber, while minimising side effects: such as visual blurring in the case of mydriatics, and secondary cataract or glaucoma in the case of steroids.

Periocular depot injections of steroid, oral steroids and systemic immunosuppressives are all reserved for patients in whom topical therapy yields an inadequate response, and they should be used with care due to the occurrence of significant side effects in children.

Surgery for secondary cataracts may be necessary, and corneal epithelial debridement is combined with chelation therapy, for removal of band keratopathy.

Children who present with juvenile idiopathic arthritis should have regular eye screening, as the associated uveitis is often symptom free in its early stages.

Blunt trauma to the eye may present as a mild self-limiting anterior uveitis. More severe blunt trauma, or trauma involving damage to the eye by a sharp object, presents with more severe disruption to the globe, including lens dislocation, retinal detachment or perforation of the globe. In these situations, surgical intervention is required. In penetrating injuries, both infectious and sympathetic endophthalmitis are major risks, particularly if treatment is delayed. Tetanus prophylaxis must also be ensured in all such cases.

Intermediate Uveitis (Pars Planitis)

Due to its chronic nature, treatment is initiated in situations of moderate reduction in visual acuity. Topical or periocular steroids should be tried first, and systemic steroids used only if these do not prove effective. Systemic immunosuppressive therapy is considered if therapy is prolonged to avert steroid-induced cataract and systemic side effects. Other measures including vitrectomy may be indicated in severe, refractory intermediate uveitis.

Posterior Uveitis

Inflammation of the posterior segment occurs in over 50% of childhood uveitis cases. Approximately one-third of these are idiopathic, and on exclusion of conditions requiring

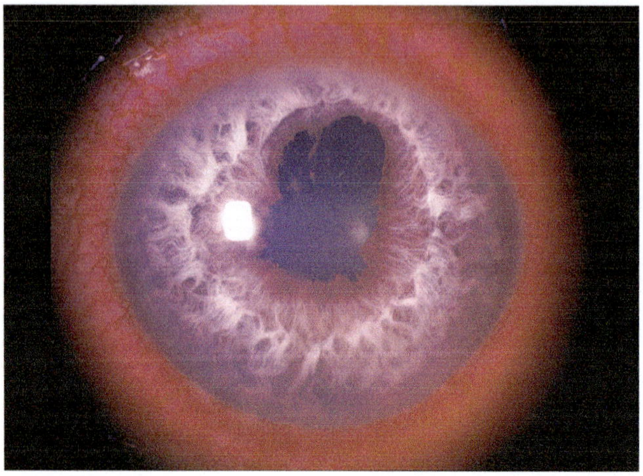

Figure 22.47 Acute anterior uveitis with posterior synechiae.

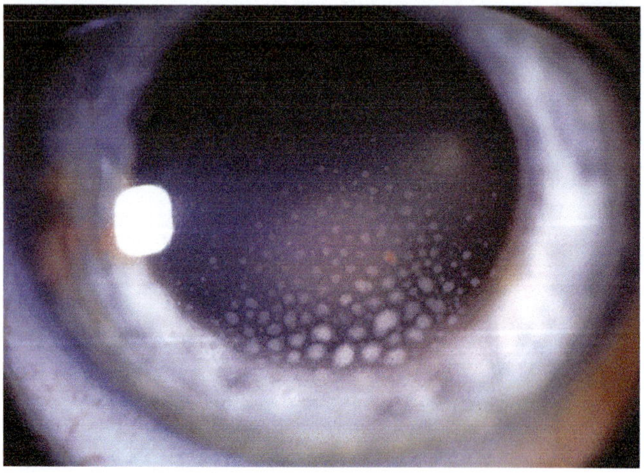

Figure 22.48 Mutton fat keratic precipitates.

more specific measures, treatment is administered as for intermediate uveitis. Almost half the cases of posterior uveitis seen in children are caused by toxoplasmosis. The standard treatment for this has hitherto been a combination of sulphadiazine and pyrimethamine, although more recently, azithromycin has also proved to be effective. Additional systemic steroids are sometimes required.

Systemic Infections and Uveitis

Systemic infections, which may include, or may initially present with uveitis include candidiasis, tuberculosis, syphilis and leprosy.

Systemic candidiasis occurs in drug addicts and in individuals with immunosuppression due to diseases such as cancer or other diseases associated with immunosuppression, or to immunosuppressive therapy. When the eye is involved, typical findings include cells, fibrinous strands and "puff balls" in the vitreous; discrete, and sometimes confluent haemorrhages and creamy exudative lesions on the retina. Diagnosis is confirmed by vitreous biopsy, and intravitreal and intravenous antifungal agents are required.

Herpes Zoster in the ophthalmic division of the trigeminal nerve may be associated with anterior uveitis, where there is involvement of the nasociliary branch, with skin lesions extending to the tip of the nose (Fig. 22.49).

Tuberculosis may affect any part of the uvea, and may manifest as a localised mass with surrounding inflammatory reaction, and mutton fat KP on the corneal endothelium. In miliary tuberculosis, discrete miliary choroidal tubercles or peripheral exudative "candle wax drippings" may be visible on fundoscopy. Focal retinopathy resembling toxoplasmic retinochoroidopathy may also be seen. Antituberculous treatment is mandatory and topical steroids should be used with care, only if systemic antituberculous treatment is also given.

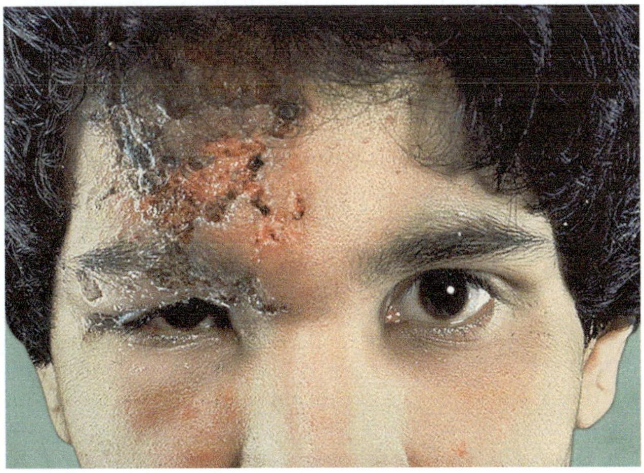

Figure 22.49 Herpes zoster skin rash in ophthalmic division of trigeminal nerve dermatome, with no nasociliary involvement.

(*Photograph Courtesy:* John Sandford-Smith).

Syphilis may cause localised or diffuse uveitis or choroiditis, which resolve leaving areas of iris or choroidal atrophy.

Multibacillary leprosy often causes an acute anterior iritis, particularly as part of a Type II, or erythema nodosum leprosum (ENL) reaction. Chronic, low-grade uveitis is also seen in multibacillary leprosy, and as in juvenile idiopathic arthritis, may present with secondary features such as cataract, iris atrophy, ocular hypotony or band keratopathy. Thus, regular ocular screening of such patients is recommended. Along with anti-leprosy multidrug therapy, topical steroids and cycloplegics are indicated. Where the corneal epithelial surface is compromised due to impaired corneal sensation or weakness of orbicularis oculi, topical steroids must be used with care, and topical non-steroidal anti-inflammatory agents may be preferable.

Systemic viral illnesses including chickenpox and CMV infection are occasionally associated with a posterior uveitis and retinochoroiditis. Inflammatory cells in the vitreous are seen, with foci of exudate and haemorrhage on the retina and sheathing of peripheral retinal vessels.

Onchocerciasis is a parasitic disease caused by onchocerca volvulus, a filarial worm. The geographical distribution of this disease includes West Africa, Central Africa and Yemen, as well as parts of Central America.

The life cycle of the worm includes human hosts in whom the microfilaria mature into adult worms, and a second vector, the Simulium fly; in which young microfilaria develop into mature ones. The larval microfilariae are found all over the body, and accumulate in the eye in large numbers. Microfilaria may be seen under the conjunctiva, or in the anterior chamber on slit-lamp examination. Symptoms occur largely as a result of an inflammatory response to dead or dying microfilaria. A sclerosing keratitis, typically starts peripherally, and spreads to include the whole cornea. Uveitis occurs, with pigmented KP and posterior synechiae. Optic atrophy and chorioretinal atrophy are often observed, and glaucoma may occur in the absence of obvious infection, possibly due to obstruction to aqueous outflow by the microfilaria.

Since the ocular changes due to onchocerciasis are by and large irreversible, early treatment of the disease is required to prevent these changes and the resulting sight impairment or blindness. Ivermectin is now the treatment of choice for onchocerciasis.

Loaiasis, which is caused by the Loa loa filarial worm, occurs in West and Central Africa.

The worm has a similar life cycle to *Onchocerca volvulus*, and often causes inflammation involving the eye, although not usually uveitis. Loa loa worms are often seen under the conjunctiva and may be removed with forceps after instilling local anaesthetic and incising the conjunctiva at the appropriate site. An acute localised inflammatory response to the worms is recognised, and has been called "Calabar swelling." This commonly occurs in the orbit or eyelids, with a dramatic presentation, but with

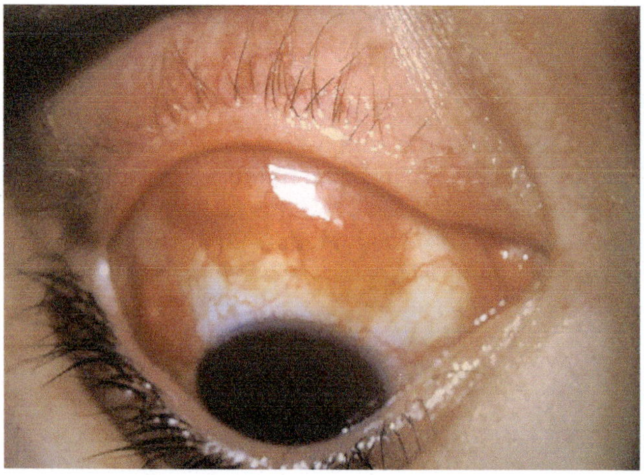

Figure 22.50 Anterior scleritis.

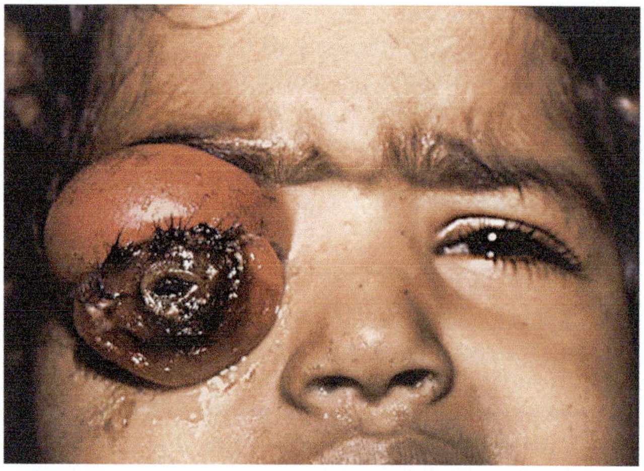

Figure 22.51 Retinoblastoma with orbital extension.

BOX 22.5 Differential diagnosis of a white pupil.
Retinoblastoma
Cataract
Retinal detachment
Severe posterior uveitis
Retinopathy of prematurity
Persistent hyperplastic primary vitreous
Retinal dysplasia (Norrie disease)
Coats disease

resolution to normal in a few days. Treatment is with diethylcarbamazine.

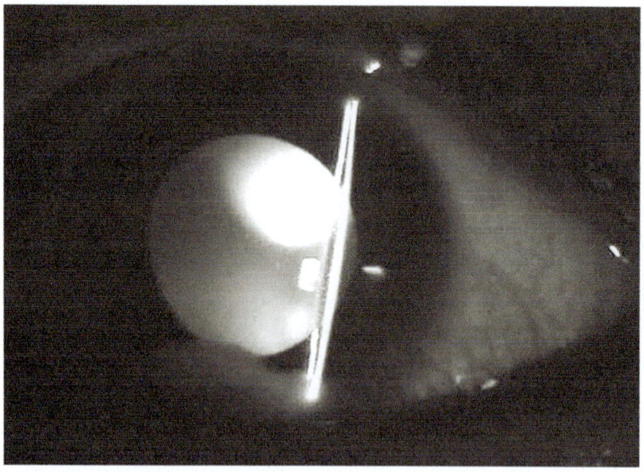

Figure 22.52 Leucocoria and hypopyon due to retinoblastoma.

SCLERITIS AND EPISCLERITIS

Scleritis may rarely occur in infections such as tuberculosis and leprosy, and in autoimmune disease such as rheumatoid arthritis. It may be anterior or posterior and causes severe pain and tenderness. Treatment comprises NSAIDs, systemic steroids or occasionally more powerful immunosuppressive agents **(Fig. 22.50)**.

Episcleritis, affecting the connective tissue overlying the sclera is commoner, usually causes minimal discomfort and is often self-limiting, or resolves with a short course of topical steroids. It may be triggered by helminthic bowel infestations or by skin infestations such as scabies.

RETINOBLASTOMA

Retinoblastoma is the most common primary, malignant intraocular tumour of childhood. If left untreated it is lethal. The long-term survival rate for retinoblastoma is over 90% in the developed world. The prognosis in developing countries continues to be poor because of late diagnosis and intervention **(Fig. 22.51)**.

Epidemiology

Retinoblastoma occurs equally in males and females. There is no racial predilection.

Sixty to seventy percent of tumours are unilateral and the mean age at diagnosis is 24 months. 30–40% are bilateral, with a mean age at diagnosis of 14 months. Only 6% of patients have a family history of retinoblastoma. Inheritance is autosomal dominant. The predisposing gene (RPE1) is at 13q14. Sporadic cases constitute about 94% of all patients with retinoblastoma.

Clinical Presentation

The possibility of retinoblastoma should be considered with any lesion in the posterior segment of a child less than 5 years of age. Presenting features include:

- Leucocoria (a white pupil reflex)—most common **(Box 22.5 and Fig. 22.52)**
- Strabismus—due to a macular lesion causing reduced vision

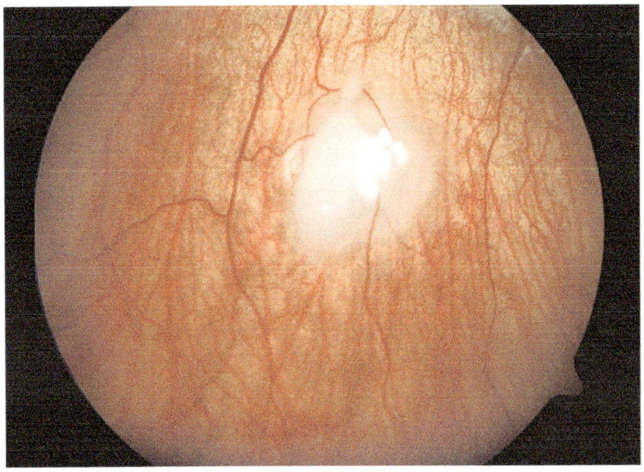

Figure 22.53 Early retinoblastoma.

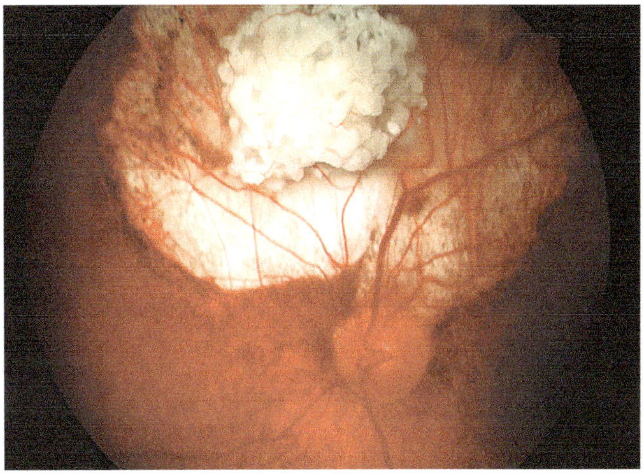

Figure 22.54 Exophytic retinoblastoma with surrounding chorioretinal atrophy.

- Uveitis—with a tumour hypopyon (tumour cells or white blood cells in the anterior chamber)
- Glaucoma—where an eye filled by tumour has raised intraocular pressure
- Hyphaema (red blood cells in the anterior chamber)
- Orbital cellulitis—due to tumour necrosis and inflammation
- Nystagmus
- Proptosis on routine examination—least common

Diagnosis

Indirect ophthalmoscopy with scleral indentation must be done on both eyes after full mydriasis. Appearances depend on the size of the tumour and on its pattern of growth. Multiple tumours may be present in the same eye.

Clinical Findings

An intraretinal tumour is a flat or round grey to white lesion, fed and drained by dilated tortuous retinal vessels.

An endophytic tumour projects from the retinal surface as a white, friable mass and may have vitreous seeding.

An exophytic tumour grows into a cauliflower-like white mass, often associated with a retinal detachment and vitreous haemorrhage.

As the tumour expands, it undergoes necrosis with areas of calcification **(Figs. 22.53 and 22.54)**.

Special Investigations

- *Ultrasonography:* Detects calcification and enables measurement of the tumour dimensions.
- *CT scan:* Detects calcification, gross involvement of the optic nerve, extension to the orbit or CNS and the presence or absence of pinealoblastoma.
- *Magnetic resonance imaging (MRI):* Provides the optimum means of evaluation of the optic nerve and of the detection of pinealoblastoma.
- *Differential diagnosis:* This includes persistent hyperplastic primary vitreous, toxocara granuloma, Coats disease, retinopathy of prematurity, retinal dysplasia.
- *Natural history:* As the tumour grows, the globe is gradually filled with tumour, which then expands further and involves the periocular tissues. It then extends intracranially. Blood-borne metastases to distant sites can occur.

Histologic Features

Retinoblastoma consists of cells with round, oval or spindle-shaped nuclei, which are hyperchromatic and surrounded by scanty cytoplasm.

- *Flexner–Wintersteiner rosettes:* These are a characteristic feature of retinoblastoma. A single layer of columnar cells surrounds a central lumen lined by a retractile structure, corresponding to the external limiting membrane of the retina.
- *Homer–Wright rosettes:* These do not show features of retinal differentiation and are found in other neuroblastic tumours also.
- *Fleurettes:* Are curvilinear clusters of cells composed of rod and cone inner segments that are frequently attached to abortive outer segments.
- *Trilateral retinoblastoma:* This term refers to bilateral retinoblastoma with ectopic intracranial retinoblastoma, usually located in the pineal gland or the parasellar region.

Treatment

Management of retinoblastoma is highly individualised and is based on age at presentation, laterality, tumour location, tumour staging, visual prognosis, systemic involvement and cost-effectiveness. Decisions regarding treatment should be made after detailed discussion with the child's family, who should be involved at all stages of management.

- *Focal therapy:* Laser photocoagulation, transpupillary thermo-therapy (TTT), cryotherapy and plaque brachytherapy.
- *Local therapy:* External beam radiotherapy (EBRT), enucleation.
- *Chemotherapy:* It reduces tumour size and makes it more amenable to laser, cryotherapy, TTT or radiotherapy. Chemotherapy followed by focal treatment is the primary treatment of choice for intraocular retinoblastoma.
- *Primary enucleation:* It is still indicated for advanced intraocular retinoblastoma, especially in unilateral cases.

On histopathological examination, infiltration of the uvea, sclera and optic nerve behind the lamina cribrosa imply a high risk of metastasis. Such patients need chemotherapy or radiotherapy. Various combinations of chemotherapeutic drugs are used, the most frequently used agents being vincristine, etoposide and carboplatin.

Genetic counselling is an important part of the management of retinoblastoma.

Follow-up: Children with unilateral disease should be followed up at least until 5 years of age. Those with familial or genetically transmitted disease should undergo lifelong follow-up.

RETINOPATHY OF PREMATURITY

Retinopathy of prematurity (ROP) is a proliferative retinopathy affecting premature infants of low-birth weight and young gestational age. Despite improvements in detection and treatment, ROP remains a leading cause of lifelong visual impairment among premature children.

The International Classification of Retinopathy of Prematurity (ICROP) provides standards for the clinical assessment of ROP on the basis of severity (stage) and anatomical location (zone) of disease.

Location

- Zone I: Posterior retina within a 60° circle centered on the optic nerve.
- Zone II: From the posterior circle (Zone I) to the nasal ora serrata anteriorly.
- Zone III: The remaining temporal peripheral retina.
- *Extent:* Number of clock hours involved.

Severity

- Stage 1: A demarcation line between vascularised and nonvascularised retina.
- Stage 2: The presence of a demarcation line that has height, width, and volume (ridge).
- Stage 3: A ridge with extraretinal fibrovascular proliferation.
- Stage 4: Subtotal retinal detachment, e.g. extrafoveal, retinal detachment including the fovea.
- Stage 5: Total retinal detachment.

Ophthalmic evaluation of the premature infant may be performed in the nursery or in the office. Examination of the anterior segment is performed with a hand light, with specific attention to the iris vessels, lens and tunica vasculosa lentis. Ophthalmoscopy is performed with an indirect ophthalmoscope and a 28D or 30D condensing lens with scleral indentation when indicated.

Screening for ROP should be performed in all infants with a birth weight with less than 1,500 g or a gestational age of 28 weeks or less, as well as infants weighing between 1,500 g and 2,000 g with an unstable clinical course and who are believed to be at high risk **(Figs. 22.55 and 22.56)**.

Differential Diagnosis

Retinoblastoma, familial exudative vitreoretinopathy, Norrie's disease, X-linked retinoschisis and incontinentia pigmenti.

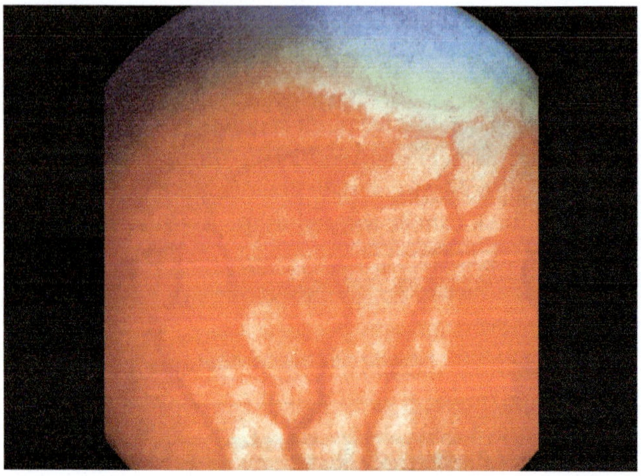

Figure 22.55 Retinopathy of prematurity: Peripheral retinal vessel proliferation and ridge.

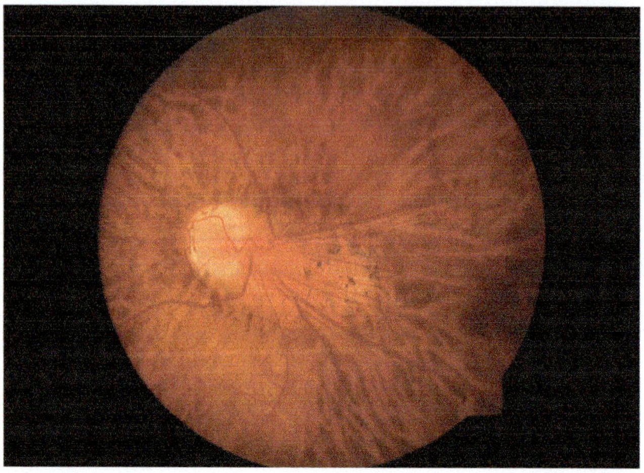

Figure 22.56 Retinopathy of prematurity: Long-term outcome.

Treatment

The ultimate goals of treatment of threshold ROP (stage 3 ROP, zone I or zone II, with at least 5 continuous or 8 total clock hours of disease) are prevention of retinal detachment or of scarring, and optimisation of visual outcome.

Treatment Options

- Cryotherapy
- Laser photocoagulation
- Surgery

Threshold or prethreshold ROP can be treated with laser therapy or retinal cryoablation. Laser therapy is preferred over retinal cryoablation. The treatment is applied in full scatter fashion to the avascular anterior retina with the indirect ophthalmoscope. Laser therapy is believed to be less traumatic systemically than cryoablation; it also appears to yield a better optical and visual outcome.

Surgery may be undertaken for patients with Stage 4 and Stage 5 ROP. The modalities commonly used are scleral buckling and vitrectomy, which relieve the tractional components of the retinal detachment.

Certain problems are more likely to occur in eyes with regressed ROP, including myopia with astigmatism, anisometropia, strabismus, amblyopia, cataract, glaucoma and retinal detachment.

It is important to remember that the sequelae of advanced ROP can cause problems throughout the patient's life, and long-term follow-up is warranted.

TRAUMATIC RETINOPATHY

Retinal haemorrhages concentrated at the macula, or spread extensively over the whole retina, sometimes with the presence of Roth's spots (circular haemorrhages with white centres) can be caused in the first 2 years of life by head injury, e.g. following road traffic accident. However, such retinal haemorrhages are characteristically seen, sometimes accompanied by subdural haematoma and bruising or injuries elsewhere, in what has been termed the shaken baby syndrome. This terminology is best reserved for instances where the aetiology of the injuries has been proved beyond doubt, and the term "traumatic retinopathy" used at all other times, as a descriptor, as other causes such as a coagulation defect must be considered and ruled out. Retinal haemorrhages due to birth injury seldom persist for longer than 1 month **(Figs. 22.57 and 22.58)**.

PREVENTIVE OPHTHALMOLOGY

Childhood Blindness

The WHO definition of blindness is a best-corrected visual acuity of less than 3/60 in the better eye or a field of vision less than 10 degrees. Visual impairment is graded according to intermediate levels of visual acuity less than 6/18. It is estimated that there are about 5 million visually impaired children in the world. Of these, approximately 1.5 million are blind or severely visually impaired, and approximately 1 million of them live in Asia.

Causes of Childhood Blindness

The important causes of preventable childhood blindness in the developing world are vitamin A deficiency, measles, ophthalmia neonatorum, glaucoma, cataract, refractive error, squint, retinopathy of prematurity, trachoma and rubella. Onchocerciasis continues to be a problem in Africa and in parts of the Middle East.

Timely and appropriate intervention in vitamin A deficiency is crucially important in the prevention of blindness in individual patients and, since the condition remains a major public health problem in children (with potentially many years of life ahead) in the developing world, widespread measures of prevention could significantly reduce the burden of blindness, in terms of blind person-years, in these societies.

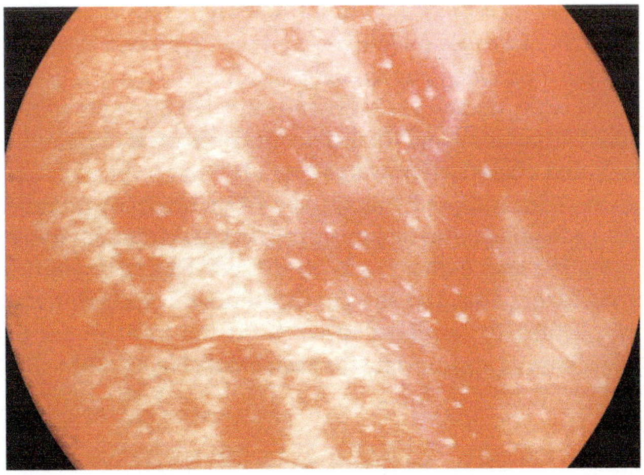

Figure 22.57 Retinal haemorrhages in traumatic retinopathy.

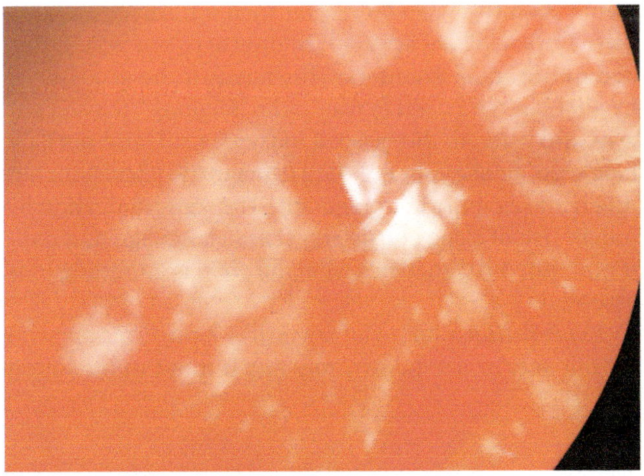

Figure 22.58 Posterior pole in traumatic retinopathy.

THE CHILD WITH VISUAL IMPAIRMENT

Vision is required for:

- Accessing 'information' in the distance. (It is largely through vision that we learn about the environment.)
- Access to near information. (E.g., playing with toys and looking at and reading books.)
- Interacting socially. (Recognising people and their facial expressions and gestures.)
- Guiding movement of the upper limbs. (Picking anything up is usually by means of vision in the sighted person.)
- Guiding movement of the body. (Walking over steps or in a crowd is mediated through vision to give visual guidance.)
- In children, vision is required to learn these attributes.
- Visual impairment can restrict such learning because it imposes limitations on performance.

It is, therefore, essential to measure all aspects of vision and to understand how each child's visual impairment is impacting upon their development. This knowledge is then employed to implement appropriate strategies to minimise the adverse impact of poor vision.

Poor acuity may not impede mobility but can profoundly affect learning if educational material is not enlarged and can limit social interaction, if friends and relatives are not aware of this.

Visual field impairment may not significantly impair access to information and social interaction but can significantly impair mobility.

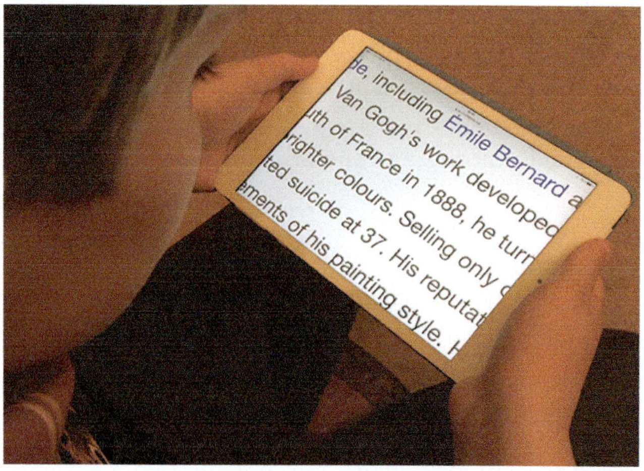

Figure 22.59 Tablets and mobile phones offer multiple resources, including photography and text magnification, as well as a wide range of Apps designed to meet the needs of children with low or absent vision.

Intervention for Visual Impairment in Children

Vision plays a major part in child development. Absent or reduced vision places a child at risk of developmental disorder.

Communication has a large visual component. Facial expressions convey emotion, agreement and disagreement, likewise gesture and body language. Lack of sufficient vision to see and interpret such information and to learn from it, places affected children at risk of developing communication disorders. This needs to be recognised by all those who need to use "radio language" (close your eyes and listen to the radio; it makes sense), and not "TV language" (close your eyes and listen to the television; not much makes sense), supplemented by communication by touch. Use of clear, consistent, simple language that contemporaneously matches what the child is attending to is essential.

Exploration tends to be driven by vision. Children who do not see, or see poorly, rely much more upon sound and touch. They reach out for and explore toys that make sound. A tactile cane that facilitates safe exploration from an early age has a place. Reaching along a parent's hand that is withdrawn to reveal a safe item to explore and learn from encourages exploration, while pain or injury during early exploration can inhibit exploration known as tactile defensiveness, which needs to be avoided.

Learning about the world is greatly facilitated by vision. One needs to fully understand each affected child's vision and to imagine what is not seen and cannot be learned from, and to take appropriate alternative action to ensure that no child with low or absent vision, is not educationally disadvantaged as a result.

More is learned during early life than at any time thereafter. Lack of vision is a developmental emergency necessitating skilled appropriate training for parents, carers and teachers.

Explaining Poor Vision to Parents and Carers

The diagnosis of visual impairment in a child is distressing. The information is conveyed with care and sensitivity, making and giving the requisite time.

Not only do parents and carers need to understand the child's diagnosis and treatment, but if vision is impaired a detailed analysis of how this can adversely impact on day to day life is required, followed by a structured programme for each child, aimed at ensuring that development is not impaired and education is optimised. This may require magnifying aids and the provision of educational material, which is designed either for visual impairment or blindness as appropriate for each child **(Fig. 22.59)**.

CHAPTER 23

Haematological Investigations in Children

Christina Halsey, Elizabeth A. Chalmers

INTRODUCTION

The haematology laboratory is able to perform a number of tests to help establish the cause of illness in children. The full blood count (FBC, also known as a complete blood count—CBC) is one of the most basic blood tests performed on children attending hospital, or a primary care clinic. All doctors should, therefore, have an understanding of how the test is performed, possible pitfalls, be able to interpret results and know when more specialised testing or advice is required. Other haematological investigations in routine use include coagulation screens, blood film examination, reticulocyte counts and methods for estimation of iron stores and detection of abnormal haemoglobins. This section will focus on these basic tests and simple algorithms for the subsequent investigation and differential diagnosis of the commonest haematological abnormalities encountered in general paediatric practice. The reader is referred to Chapter 11 for an account of the clinical presentation and management of primary haematological disorders in children.

FULL BLOOD COUNT

The FBC is a numerical estimate of the number of red cells, platelets and white cells in a given sample of blood along with measurement of the haemoglobin concentration and various red cell indices some of which are directly measured and others derived. Blood is collected into an anticoagulant solution (usually EDTA) and transported to the laboratory. Although counting of each component can be done manually, it is now routine using automated counters in almost all haematology laboratories. These counters recognise cells on the basis of size and physical characteristics. There are two main methods (often used in conjunction). Electrical impedance measurement is based on the fact that blood cells are very poor conductors of electricity. Therefore, when cells in a conducting medium are made to flow in single file through an aperture across which an electric current flows, there is a measurable increase in electrical impedance which is proportional to the volume of the cell. In this way, cells can be both counted and sized. The second method relies on characteristic patterns of light scatter and absorbance as cells pass through a laser beam; this is particularly useful for the recognition and counting of the different types of white blood cell (to produce a white cell differential count). In addition, counters estimate haemoglobin by lysing the red blood cells and measuring the optical density of the resulting solution at an appropriate wavelength. A typical readout from an automated counter is shown in **Figure 23.1**.

RED CELL INDICES

In addition to the red cell count and haemoglobin concentration, it is clinically useful to know the size of red cells (mean cell volume, MCV); the amount of haemoglobin per cell (mean cell haemoglobin) and a measure of the variation in size of individual red cells (red cell distribution width, RDW). Collectively, these values are known as red cell indices. They are particularly useful in the assessment of likely causes of anaemia.

BLOOD FILM

Examination of a stained blood film is an essential part of the assessment of most haematological disorders. Many haematological diseases have characteristic changes. In some cases, it is possible to diagnose a disorder purely from the blood film (e.g. hereditary elliptocytosis); in most cases, other confirmatory tests are needed. The blood film may be very useful in identifying artefactual results, such as thrombocytopaenia caused by platelet clumping. Systemic disease may also produce blood film changes, e.g. sepsis may be accompanied by an increase

WBC	5.65	$[10^9/L]$		
RBC	4.88	$[10^{12}/L]$		
HGB	14.2	[g/dL]		
HCT	41.5	[%]		
MCV	85.0–	[fL]		
MCH	29.1	[pg]		
MCHC	34.2	[g/dL]		
PLT	303	$[10^9/L]$		
RDW-SD	38.5	[fL]		
RDW-CV	12.7	[%]		
RDW	10.8	[fL]		
MPV	9.4	[fL]		
P-LCR	21.2	[%]		
PCT	0.25	[%]		
NEUT	2.73	$[10^9/L]$	48.4	[%]
LYMPH	2.33	$[10^9/L]$	41.2	[%]
MONO	0.45	$[10^9/L]$	8.0	[%]
EO	0.11	$[10^9/L]$	1.9	[%]
BASO	0.03	$[10^9/L]$	0.5	[%]
RET	0.60	[%]	29.3	$[10^9/L]$
IRF	1.4	[%]		
LFR	98.6	[%]		
MFR	0.7	[%]		
HFR	0.7	[%]		

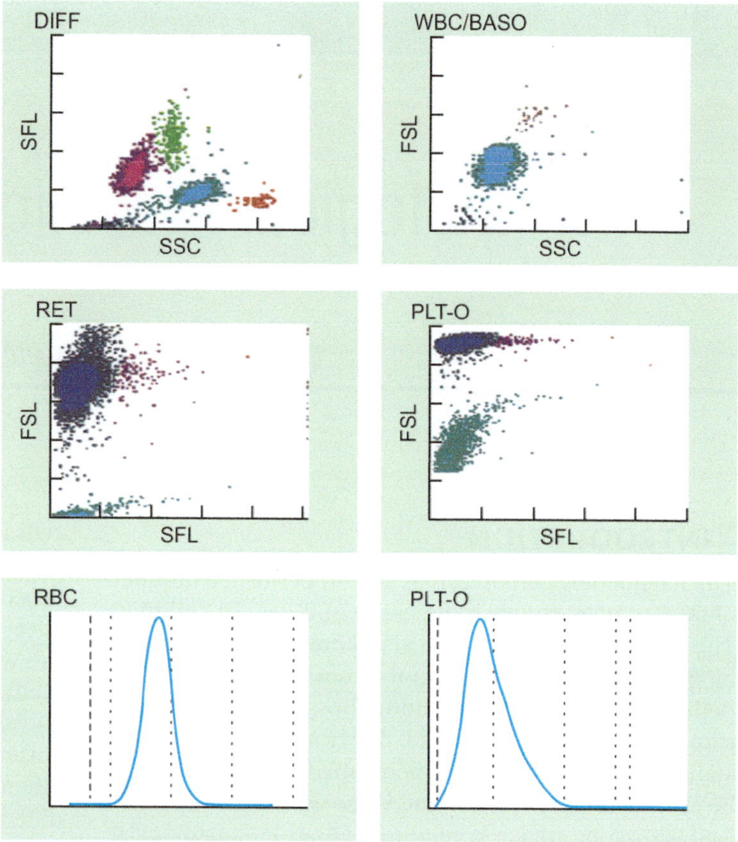

Figure 23.1 A typical computer-generated readout from an automated blood cell analyser. (*Source:* Sysmex XT2000i).

in immature neutrophils (left shift or band forms), toxic granulation and formation of Döhle bodies (pale blue cytoplasmic inclusions) within neutrophils. These latter changes are particularly useful in the assessment of neonates. **Figures 23.2A to G** show some of the characteristic red cell changes seen on the blood film along with common causes for these appearances.

RETICULOCYTE COUNT

Reticulocytes are young red cells that have lost their nucleus, but still contain substantial amounts of ribosomal RNA leading to their characteristic bluish purple colour on standard haematoxylin and eosin (H&E) staining of blood films. They can be more easily identified using special stains, such as new methylene blue, and can be counted manually or on some automated counters. They can be expressed as a percentage of the total red cells, or an absolute count. Reticulocyte numbers are very useful in the evaluation of anaemia, as they allow a distinction to be made between inadequate marrow production of red cells (associated with a low reticulocyte count) and excessive destruction or loss of red cells in the periphery (usually associated with increased reticulocyte release from the marrow).

NORMAL RANGES

The synthesis of blood cells and coagulation proteins go through various changes during development (discussed further in Chapter 11). This is particularly marked in the neonatal period and early infancy because of adaptive changes needed for the transition between the uterine microenvironment and the outside world. Therefore, when interpreting any haematological value, it is important to be aware of age appropriate normal ranges. **Table 23.1** gives approximate values for the FBC from birth to adulthood. Normal ranges should ideally be determined using the local population and the actual instruments in everyday use in the laboratory. In paediatrics, it is difficult to obtain sufficient numbers of samples from healthy controls, and therefore, estimates are usually made using published normal ranges.

KEY LEARNING POINTS

- Normal ranges vary with age, especially in infants. Always interpret results in light of age appropriate normal ranges.
- Haemoglobin values are high at birth, then fall to a nadir at around 3 months of age before slowly rising again.
- Infants and children up to the age of 4 years have a relative lymphocytosis.

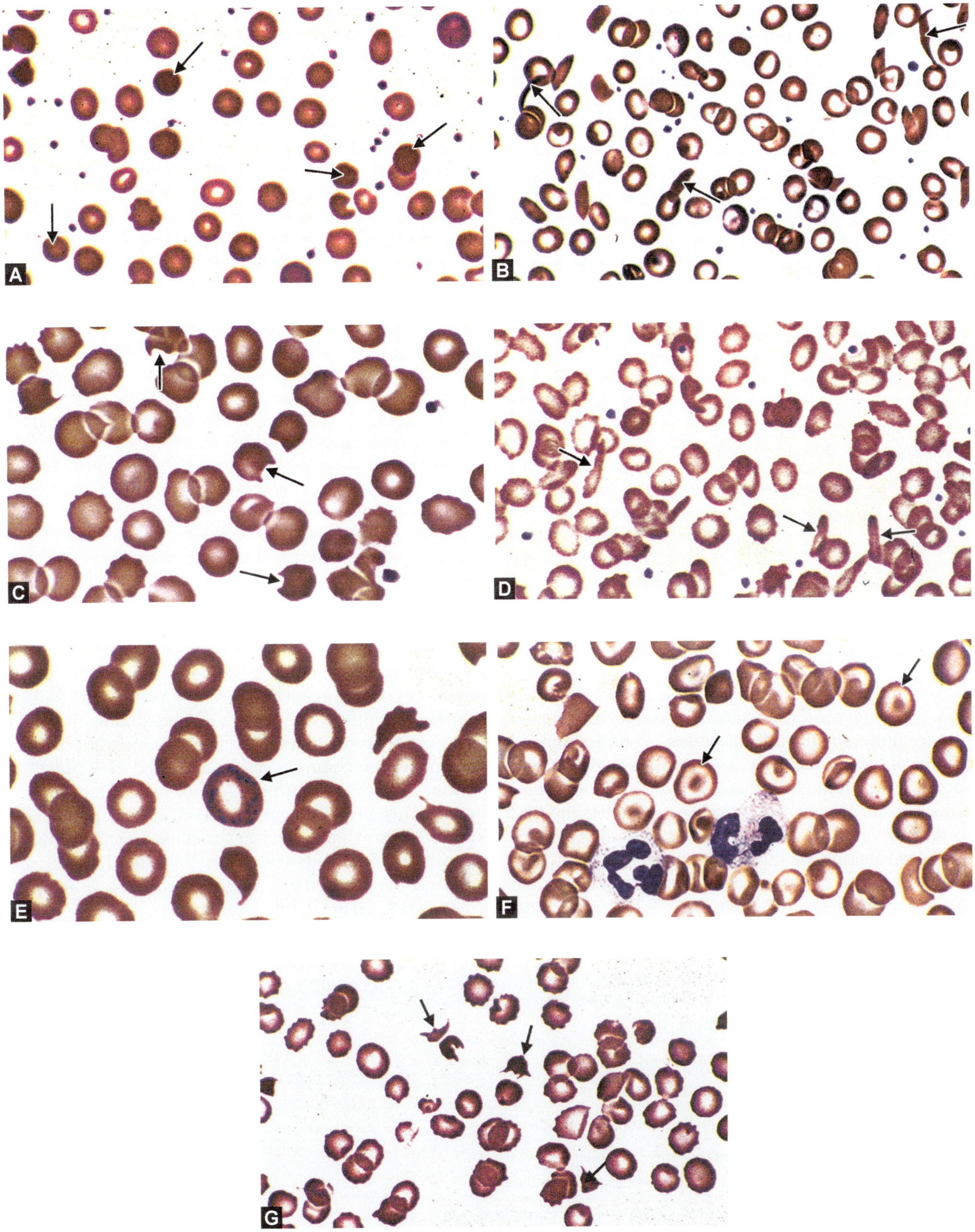

Figures 23.2A to G Red cell changes seen on blood films and their common causes. (A) Spherocytes; (B) Sickle cells; (C) Bite cells; (D) A pencil cell; (E) Basophilic stippling; (F) Target cells; (G) Red cell fragments. Arrows point to the abnormal cell type.

TABLE 23.1 Normal ranges for the full blood count in infancy and childhood.

Age	Haemoglobin (g/dL)	Hct	MCV (fL)	WBC (×10⁹/L)	Neutrophils (×10⁹/L)	Lymphocytes (×10⁹/L)	Monocytes (×10⁹/L)	Eosinophils (×10⁹/L)	Basophils (×10⁹/L)	Platelets (×10⁹/L)
Birth (term infants)	14.9–23.7	0.47–0.75	100–128	10–26	2.7–14.4	2.0–7.3	0–1.9	0–0.85	0–0.1	150–450
2 weeks	13.4–19.8	0.41–0.65	88–110	6–21	1.5–5.4	2.8–9.1	0.1–1.7	0–0.85	0–0.1	170–500
2 months	9.4–13.0	0.28–0.42	84–98	5–15	0.7–4.8	3.3–10.3	0.4–1.2	0.05–0.9	0.02–0.13	210–650
6 months	10.0–13.0	0.3–0.38	73–84	6–17	1–6	3.3–11.5	0.2–1.3	0.1–1.1	0.02–0.2	210–560
1 year	10.1–13.0	0.3–0.38	70–82	6–16	1–8	3.4–10.5	0.2–0.9	0.05–0.9	0.02–0.13	200–550
2–6 years	11.0–13.8	0.32–0.4	72–87	6–17	1.5–8.5	1.8–8.4	0.15–1.3	0.05–1.1	0.02–0.12	210–490
6–12 years	11.1–14.7	0.32–0.43	76–90	4.5–14.5	1.5–8.0	1.5–5.0	0.15–1.3	0.05–1.0	0.02–0.12	170–450
12–18 years female	12.1–15.1	0.35–0.44	77–94							
				4.5–13	1.5–6	1.5–4.5	0.15–1.3	0.05–0.8	0.02–0.12	180–430
12–18 years male	12.1–16.6	0.35–0.49	77–92							

(*Source:* Reproduced from: Arceci, Hann, Smith (Eds). Paediatric Haematology, 3rd edition. Blackwell Publishing; 2006).
Abbreviations: Hct, haematocrit; MCV, mean cell volume; WBC, white blood cells.

INVESTIGATION OF LOW HAEMOGLOBIN IN INFANCY AND CHILDHOOD

Although there are a multitude of causes for anaemia in this age range, the majority of causes can be ascertained by logical use of relatively few tests. An initial history should focus on the length and speed of onset of symptoms, dietary history, ethnic origin, any other medical conditions and any family history of blood disorders. When considering the differential diagnosis for any haematological disorder, it is useful to divide the causes into those due to underproduction of cells from the bone marrow, those due to peripheral destruction of cells and those due to loss of cells from the circulation (haemorrhage or sequestration). A simple way to narrow down the list of differential diagnoses for anaemia is to look at the red cell indices. There are a limited number of causes of a hypochromic microcytic anaemia, or a macrocytic anaemia—the common causes are listed in **Table 23.2**. When assessing a normocytic anaemia, a reticulocyte count is useful to distinguish between marrow production problems and peripheral destruction or haemorrhage. The blood film may also be useful with characteristic changes seen in some red cell haemoglobin or enzyme disorders **(*see* Figs. 23.2A to G)**.

TABLE 23.2 Causes of anaemia classified on red cell indices.

Microcytic	Normocytic	Macrocytic
Iron deficiency	Haemorrhage (acute)	Vitamin B_{12}/folate deficiency
Thalassaemia	Haemolysis—AIHA	Reticulocytosis
Sideroblastic anaemia	Haemoglobinopathy—sickle cell disease	Myelodysplasia
Chronic disease	Red cell membrane defect—hereditary, spherocytosis	Hypothyroidism
Lead poisoning	Red cell enzyme—G6PD, pyruvate kinase	Drugs
	Marrow infiltration—malignancy, aplastic anaemia, Transient erythroblastopenia of childhood Bone marrow failure syndromes—anaemia of chronic disease	Liver disease Scurvy

KEY LEARNING POINTS

When formulating a differential diagnosis for low blood counts (red cells, white cells or platelets), always consider the following mechanisms:

- Reduced production of cells.
- Disorders interfering with normal haemopoiesis, such as nutritional deficiency or aplastic anaemia.
- Primary bone marrow failure syndromes.
- Secondary marrow infiltration.
- Peripheral destruction of cells.
- Loss from the body (e.g. haemorrhage) or sequestration within the tissues or organs.

HYPOCHROMIC MICROCYTIC ANAEMIA

The main differential diagnosis is between iron deficiency and thalassaemia. Thalassaemia major presents in early infancy with a transfusion-dependent anaemia, and characteristic blood film and electrophoretic findings (absent haemoglobin A), and usually presents little diagnostic difficulty. Thalassaemia trait does not produce significant anaemia alone, but does give hypochromic microcytic indices often in association with a raised red cell count but relatively normal RDW. In contrast, iron deficiency usually gives a low red cell count but a raised RDW (this being a measure of variation in red cell width and therefore, raised in the presence of anisocytosis). The blood film is often helpful.

Beta thalassaemia trait is characterised by basophilic stippling (*see* **Figs. 23.2A to G**). Alpha thalassaemia trait has few characteristic features. Iron deficiency gives marked anisopoikilocytosis with hypochromic red cell fragments, pencil and teardrop cells, and frequent accompanying thrombocytosis (*see* **Figs. 23.2A to G**).

TESTS TO DIAGNOSE IRON DEFICIENCY

An inadequate iron supply will initially lead to depletion of iron stores followed by iron deficient erythropoiesis, and finally the development of anaemia **(Fig. 23.3)**. Serum ferritin is the first marker of depleted iron stores in the body. It is diagnostic if low, but false negative results can be seen because ferritin is an acute phase reactant and therefore, can be elevated with acute inflammation or infection even in the presence of iron deficiency. As iron deficiency progresses, the transferrin (measured as total iron binding capacity) becomes elevated with reduced serum iron. The ratio of these two results can be expressed as the transferrin saturation. Immediate precursors of haem accumulate zinc (free erythrocyte) protoporphyrin. Finally, a hypochromic microcytic anaemia develops. Other tests include measurement of soluble transferrin receptors (increased in iron deficiency). The gold standard test remains Perls staining of a particulate bone marrow biopsy specimen for iron but this is rarely necessary.

TESTS TO DIAGNOSE THALASSAEMIA

In order to understand tests for thalassaemia properly, it is necessary to be aware of the composition of haemoglobin and the developmental changes that occur in the use of various globin chains; these are discussed in Chapter 11. Diagnosis of thalassaemia is usually made by tests that separate the haemoglobin molecules on the basis of electrical charge; this allows quantitation of the normal haemoglobins HbA ($\alpha_2\beta_2$), HbA$_2$ ($\alpha_2\delta_2$) and HbF ($\alpha_2\gamma_2$), and also detection of abnormal haemoglobins that contain amino acid changes which alter charge (such as sickle cell HbS). The two main methods in use are haemoglobin electrophoresis and high performance liquid chromatography. Beta thalassaemia major can be diagnosed by the complete absence of haemoglobin A on haemoglobin electrophoresis, provided the test is performed before transfusion of the patient. Beta thalassaemia trait usually shows an elevated HbA$_2$ level above 3.5% (normal ranges will vary from lab to lab); care should be taken in the presence of iron deficiency as this may reduce the HbA$_2$ level back into the normal range—results should be repeated after iron replacement in any iron-deficient individual. Alpha thalassaemia major is usually diagnosed antenatally, or at the time of birth of a severely hydropic infant, since all the normal haemoglobins present at birth contain α-chains. Three α gene deletions, so called haemoglobin H (HbH) disease can be diagnosed by electrophoretic

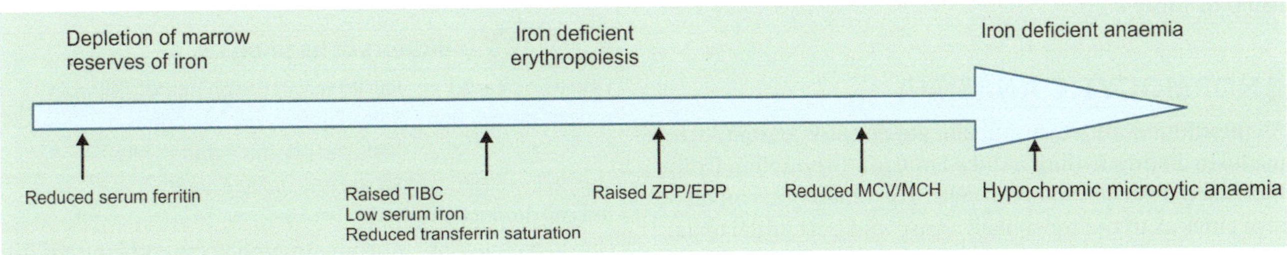

Figure 23.3 Stages of iron deficiency.

Abbreviations: MCV, mean cell volume; MCH, mean cell haemoglobin; ZPP, zinc protoporphyrin; EPP, erythrocyte protoporphyrin; TIBC, total iron binding capacity.

TABLE 23.3 Investigation results in thalassaemia.

Diagnosis	*Genetic defect*	*Blood film*	*Haemoglobin electrophoresis*
Beta thalassaemia major	2 β gene mutations	Severe hypochromic microcytic anaemia, nucleated red cells, target cells	Absent HbA (pretransfusion), high HbF
Beta thalassaemia trait	1 β gene mutation	Basophilic stippling, hypochromia and microcytosis but normal or borderline low haemoglobin	Raised HbA_2 >3.5%
Alpha thalassaemia major (incompatible with survival beyond embryonic period)	4 α gene deletions	Very severe anaemia, nucleated red cells	Absent HbA, A2 and HbF Presence of embryonic haemoglobin Hb Portland and Hb Bart's and HbH
Haemoglobin H disease	3 α gene deletions	Anaemia, target cells, teardrop cells and fragments HbH bodies on special staining of film	HbH
Alpha thalassaemia trait	1 or 2 α gene deletions	Hypochromia, microcytosis	2–8% Hb Bart's at birth (may be detected on neonatal screening programmes)

detection of HbH (β_4 tetramers), or by staining a blood film with brilliant cresyl blue—the β_4 tetramers in the red cells are stained dark blue, and produce a golf-ball like appearance. The diagnosis of alpha thalassaemia trait (one or two gene deletions) is suspected by the presence of hypochromia and microcytosis in the absence of iron deficiency, and with a normal HbA_2 measurement. As it does not produce clinically significant disease, definitive diagnostic investigations (genetic testing for individual mutations) are usually reserved for antenatal patients at significant risk of alpha thalassaemia major in their offspring. Diagnostic investigations for thalassaemia are summarised in Table 23.3.

MACROCYTIC ANAEMIA

The cause of a macrocytic anaemia in children is often obvious from the history. History of concurrent or past illnesses, symptoms and signs of malabsorption and a detailed drug history are important. B_{12} and folate, liver function tests, a reticulocyte count and thyroid function should be measured in unexplained cases. Causes are listed in Table 23.2.

NORMOCYTIC ANAEMIA

As mentioned above, a reticulocyte count is particularly useful in distinguishing reduced marrow production from increased destruction of red cells. The blood film can also give clues as to the most likely cause and best initial tests. A simple algorithm is given in Flow chart 23.1.

Haemolytic anaemias are a large subgroup of normocytic anaemias. The combination of jaundice (unconjugated hyperbilrubinaemia), reticulocytosis and anaemia suggests a haemolytic process. Further tests for haemolysis include serum haptoglobin measurement (proteins present in normal plasma, which can bind free haemoglobin, and are then removed from the circulation by the reticuloendothelial system), urinary haemosiderin (an iron storage protein derived from the breakdown of free haemoglobin in the renal tubular system) and urobilinogen (a natural breakdown product of bilirubin excreted in the urine). These are summarised in Box 23.1. A key test in establishing the cause of haemolysis is the direct Coombs test (DCT), also called the direct antiglobulin test. This test detects the presence of antibody bound to the red cell surface by the use of reagents containing anti-IgG, and anticomplement that cause agglutination of cells, as shown in Figure 23.4. A positive DCT indicates a likely immune cause for the anaemia. If the DCT is negative, then tests for red cell enzyme defects [glucose-6-phosphate dehydrogenase deficiency (G6PD) and pyruvate kinase assays], haemoglobinopathies (haemoglobin electrophoresis and sickle solubility test) and membrane disorders (demonstration of increased

BOX 23.1 Indicators of haemolysis.

Due to increased red cell destruction	Raised serum unconjugated bilirubin Raised urinary urobilinogen Reduced plasma haptoglobins
Due to increased red cell production	Raised reticulocyte count
Due to presence of damaged red cells	Abnormal morphology—spherocytes, bite cells, fragments increased osmotic fragility

Flow chart 23.1 Investigation and causes of normocytic anaemias.

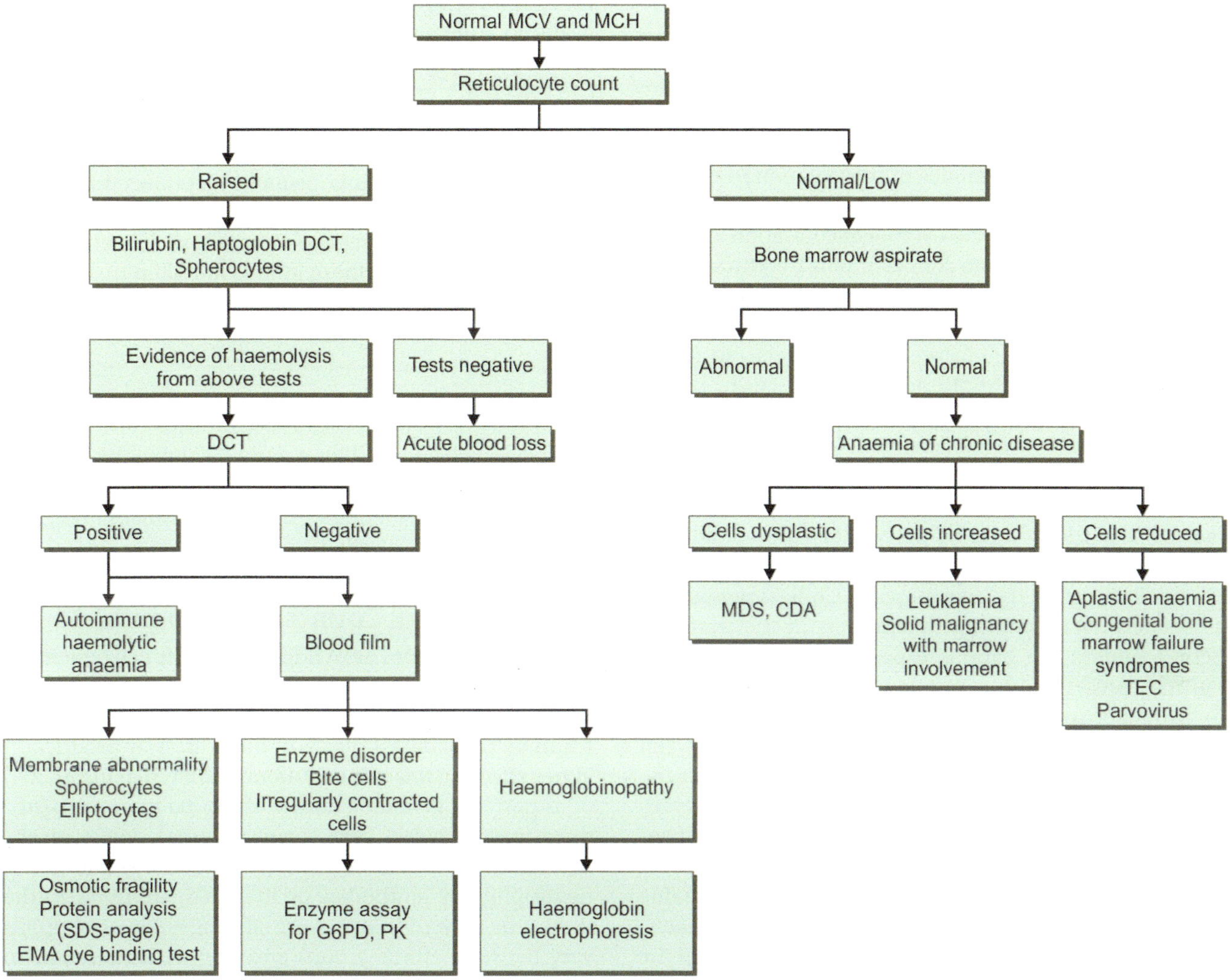

Abbreviations: DCT, direct Coomb test; MDS, myelodysplasia; CDA, congenital dyserythropoietic anaemia; TEC, transient erythroblastopenia of childhood; MCV, mean cell volume; MCH, mean cell haemoglobin; EMA, eosin-5-maleimide; SDS, sodium dodecyl sulphate; G6PD; glucose-6-phosphate dehydrogenase deficiency; PK, pyruvate kinase.

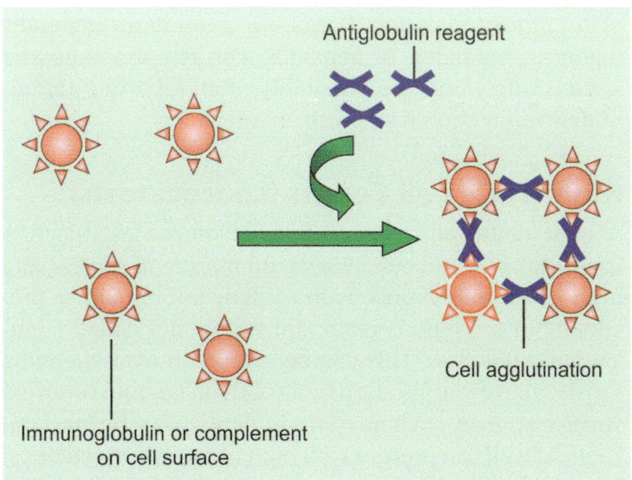

Figure 23.4 Direct Coombs test.

osmotic fragility of cells, protein analysis by sodium dodecylsulphate-polyacrylamide gel electrophoresis, or more recent eosin-5-maleimide dye binding tests) may need to be performed.

If the reticulocyte count is normal or low, it is likely that the anaemia is due to a problem with red cell production in the marrow. A bone marrow aspirate and trephine (see section on white cell disorders below) may be needed to help establish the cause. Lack of red cell precursors in the marrow can be seen as an isolated phenomenon in transient erythroblastopenia of childhood, acute parvovirus B19 infection or inherited red cell aplasia (Diamond-Blackfan anaemia). If part of a pancytopaenia, then aplastic anaemia or hypoplastic myelodysplastic syndrome may be the cause. Occasionally, acute leukaemias can present with an aplastic phase followed several weeks to months later by the development of ALL.

INVESTIGATION OF ANAEMIA IN NEONATES

Anaemia is the commonest haematological abnormality seen in neonates. The spectrum and causes of disease are somewhat different than in older children. There are key differences in red cell physiology in neonates that contribute to the different modes of presentation in this age group. Although the haemoglobin tends to be high initially (due at least in part to haemoconcentration and placental transfusion prior to cord clamping), erythropoiesis is then switched off at the time of birth and haemoglobin falls to a nadir of around 10 g/dL by the age of 8 weeks. This fall is exaggerated in premature infants—so called anaemia of prematurity. In addition, premature babies are particularly vulnerable to iatrogenic anaemia; secondary to blood loss associated with frequent blood testing. The MCV is high in neonates, and differences in red cell membrane composition can make some haemolytic red cell disorders, such as hereditary pyropoikilocytosis and hereditary spherocytosis—worse in the neonatal period. In contrast, the enzymopathy G6PD is not usually associated with significant haemolysis in the newborn period (unless the baby is exposed to oxidant stress), but may present with severe jaundice which is thought to be hepatic in origin. Haemolysis may also be antibody mediated due to Rhesus or ABO incompatibility between mother and infant. Increased red cell destruction puts the baby at risk of kernicterus caused by high bilirubin levels. Hence, it is important to be aware of the possibility of haemolysis in all newborn babies.

Anaemia presenting soon after birth may also be due to haemorrhage pre, during or post-delivery. Fetomaternal haemorrhage can be diagnosed by estimation of the number of HbF-positive cells by flow cytometry on the mother—this test looks for the presence of fetal haemoglobin containing cells in the maternal circulation by virtue of their ability to resist acid elution of haemoglobin. In multiple pregnancies that share a placental circulation, twin-to-twin transfusion may also occur to produce one polycythaemic twin and one anaemic one. An algorithm for the diagnosis of neonatal anaemia is given in **Flow chart 23.2**.

KEY LEARNING POINT

The causes and presentation of anaemia are different in neonates due to differences in red cell physiology. It is important to diagnose haemolytic disorders early to reduce the risk of kernicterus.

POLYCYTHAEMIA

High haemoglobins and haematocrits can be due to increased numbers of red cells (true polycythaemia) or dehydration, leading to a decreased plasma volume (relative polycythaemia). In children, true polycythaemia is usually due to a secondary cause, such as hypoxia from cyanotic congenital heart disease leading to increased erythropoietin production. Occasionally, kidney tumours can secrete erythropoietin. Primary erythrocytosis (a myeloproliferative disease relatively common in adults) is extremely rare in children. Neonates have higher incidences of polycythaemia, usually secondary to placental insufficiency or delayed clamping of the cord. The blood viscosity increases exponentially with haematocrits above 0.65; therefore, these infants are often treated with exchange transfusion—the evidence for benefit from this is lacking.

WHITE CELL DISORDERS

The white cells in the blood can be subdivided into different subpopulations with distinct functions. These are listed in **Table 23.4** along with the main causes of high or low counts for these cells.

Low White Cell Counts (Leucopenia)

The commonest and most important white cell deficiency is that involving neutrophils (neutropenia) since this can be associated with an increased risk of serious infection. It can be caused by a defect in bone marrow production either affecting this cell type alone (isolated neutropenia) or as part of a general failure of the bone marrow to produce mature blood cells (pancytopenia). Alternatively, neutropenia can result from peripheral destruction of neutrophils by antibodies or their redistribution to the tissues or sites of injury. Normal ranges for neutrophils vary between ethnic groups and are particularly low in black Africans. This is thought to represent a different distribution of neutrophils between the tissues and the circulation, rather than an overall lower total body count. Neutrophil numbers circulating in the bloodstream rise after exercise and as a stress response.

Lymphopenia can follow acute infections, or periods of immunosuppression. Lymphocyte counts are generally higher in neonates. In neonates with lymphopenia and serious infections, the possibility of an inherited immunodeficiency should be borne in mind.

High White Cell Counts (Leucocytosis)

A high neutrophil count often accompanies infection (neutrophilia) and can be a useful marker of sepsis. Very high neutrophil counts, with evidence of immature precursors in the bloodstream, are sometimes called a leukaemoid reaction. This can be seen with overwhelming sepsis, marrow infiltration by a solid malignancy, a severe stress response, such as status epilepticus or burns. Leukaemia itself can present with high or low white cell numbers, and is usually suspected by the combination of an abnormal blood count (white cells high or low, usually

Flow chart 23.2 Investigation and causes of neonatal anaemia.

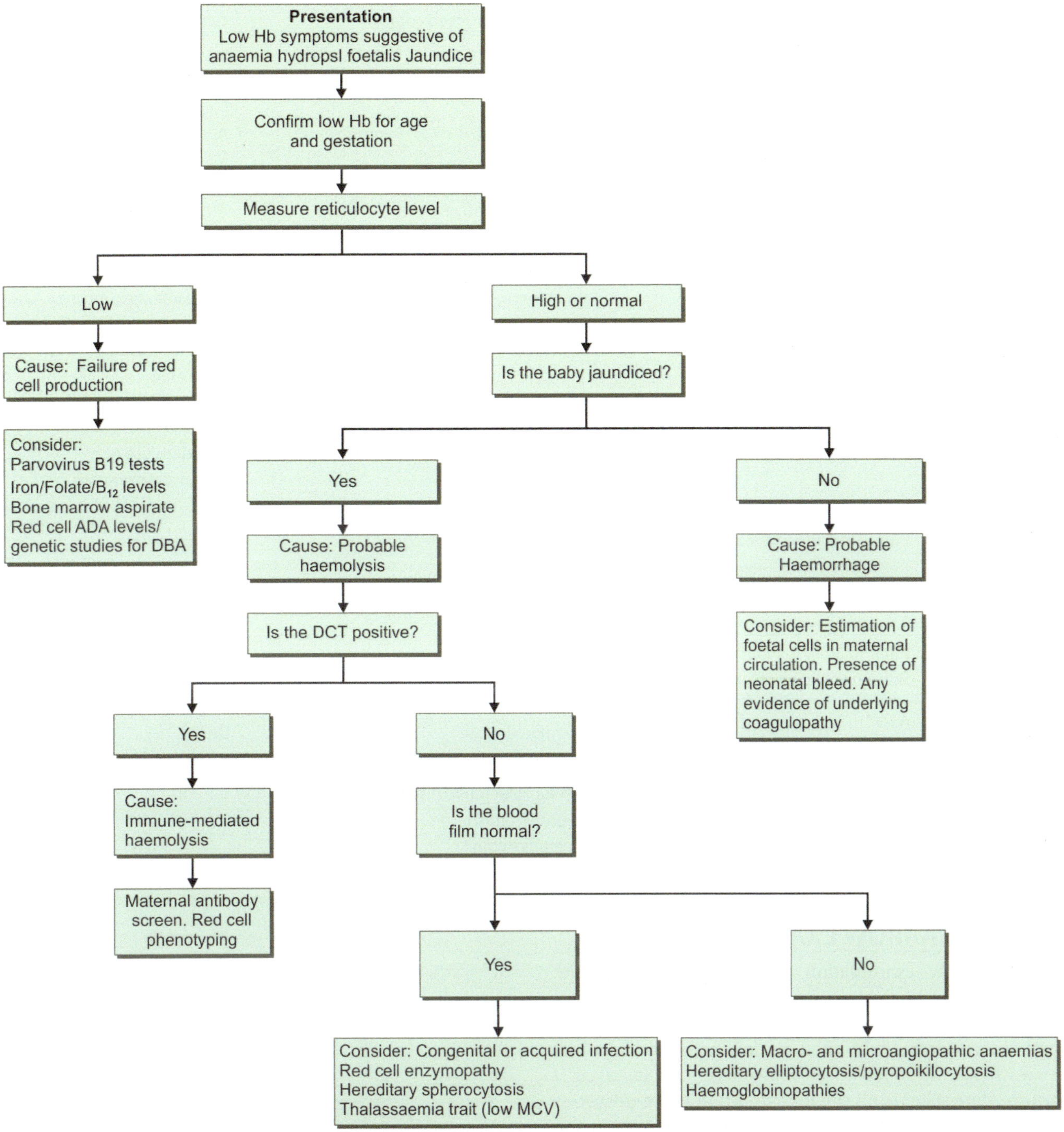

with accompanying anaemia and thrombocytopenia) with a blood film that shows a population of immature precursors (blast cells). Blast cells vary in appearance with the different subtypes of leukaemia, but are generally larger than normal cells with a large nuclei and open chromatin (*see* Figs. 11.27 and 11.28). Myeloid blast cells may have rod-like inclusions in their cytoplasm called Auer rods.

The definitive diagnosis of leukaemia usually requires bone marrow examination; this allows detailed study of the appearance of the cells (morphology) as well as analysis of various specific proteins expressed by the cells (immunophenotyping), and genetic abnormalities (molecular genetics and cytogenetics), which help classify the leukaemia further and guide treatment.

TABLE 23.4 White cell types and their disorders.

Cell type	*Function*	*Causes of increased count*	*Causes of decreased count*
Neutrophil	Innate immunity, control of bacterial and fungal infection, Role in phagocytosis of dead and damaged cells as part of inflammation	Bacterial infection Inflammatory disorders and tissue necrosis Severe marrow stress—haemorrhage or haemolysis Steroid therapy Myeloproliferative disorder (rare in children)	Infection—viral or fulminant bacterial Autoimmune Marrow failure Drugs African race
Lymphocyte	Adaptive immunity Control of viral infection	Acute infection especially viral, e.g. Epstein Barr virus (glandular fever) Chronic infection—TB, toxoplasmosis Acute leukaemia	Acute stress including acute infection, burns, surgery, trauma Steroids, Cushing syndrome Immunodeficiency—congenital and acquired including use of immunosuppressive drugs
Monocytes	Part of reticuloendothelial system macrophage precursors in transit	Chronic bacterial infections (TB) Lymphoma Juvenile myelomonocytic leukaemia Associated with neutropenia	Marrow failure Drugs
Eosinophil	Inflammatory responses Response to parasitic infection	Parasitic infection Allergy, atopy Skin diseases Hodgkin disease	Marrow failure Cushing syndrome Acute stress, e.g. burns Drugs
Basophil	Largely unknown, blood counterpart to tissue mast cell	Chickenpox Myeloproliferative diseases Hypothyroidism Ulcerative colitis	As above

BONE MARROW EXAMINATION

Bone marrow examination is performed for further assessment of haematological disorders where production of cells from the bone marrow is thought to be abnormal. In children, it is often performed under general anaesthesia, although local anaesthetic can be used if appropriate. The usual site for aspiration is the posterior iliac crest. A large bore needle is used to penetrate the bony cortex and enter the marrow cavity. Bone marrow is then aspirated and spread on glass slides, preferably immediately after. If a good specimen is obtained, then a granular appearance should be seen **(Fig. 23.5)**. Further samples can be taken in appropriate anticoagulant or medium for cytogenetics, immunophenotyping and molecular genetic tests. In many cases, a bone marrow trephine can also be taken—this involves introducing a longer needle below the cortex, and taking a core of tissue that can then be fixed and sectioned for pathological examination.

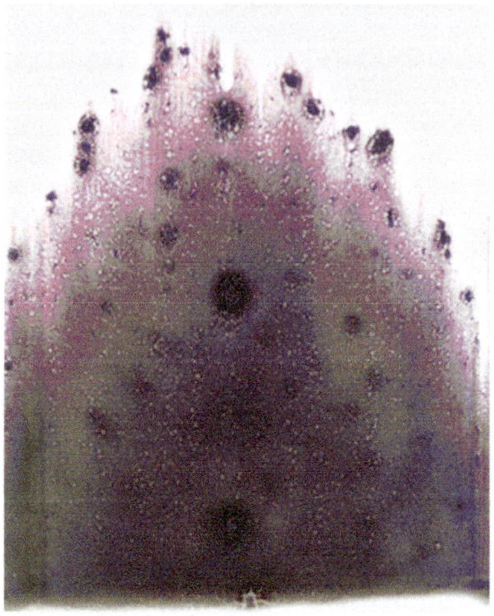

Figure 23.5 Example of bone marrow aspirate specimen spread on a slide and stained with H&E; *Note* the granular appearance at the top of the smear.

PLATELET DISORDERS

Platelets are small cytoplasmic fragments produced from megakaryocytes in the bone marrow and are important for the initiation of haemostasis and may have as yet poorly understood roles in inflammation. As with white and red cells, platelet disorders can be subdivided on the basis of high and low numbers.

High Platelet Counts (Thrombocytosis)

High platelet counts are usually reactive, i.e. not primary bone marrow disorders, but secondary to iron deficiency, ongoing inflammatory processes or infection. Very high platelet counts (>1,500 × 10^9/L) can be associated with an increased risk of thrombosis. Primary thrombocytosis (essential thrombocythemia) is rare in children.

Low Platelet Counts (Thrombocytopenia)

Again, these can be classified according to the underlying problem, i.e. inadequate bone marrow production or peripheral destruction/consumption (*see* Table 11.3). Unexpectedly low platelet counts should always be confirmed by examination of a blood film as artefactually low platelet counts are not uncommon either due to partial clotting of the sample or platelet clumping; the latter is often an in vitro phenomenon due to EDTA dependent antibodies. The commonest cause of true thrombocytopenia in children is immune-mediated peripheral destruction—idiopathic thrombocytopenic purpura (ITP). Unfortunately, there is no diagnostic test for this condition; so, it remains a diagnosis of exclusion. It is characterised by the sudden onset of bruising and/or bleeding in an otherwise well child, often with a history of an antecedent viral infection, or more rarely post immunisation. There should be no other abnormalities in the blood count, and no lymphadenopathy or organomegaly on examination. In these cases, careful examination of a peripheral blood film is sufficient but in the presence of any abnormal or suspicious features, a bone marrow examination should be performed to exclude leukaemia. The bone marrow in ITP shows increased numbers of normal megakaryocytes (*see* Fig. 11.20). Although the disease is immune mediated, platelet-associated antibodies show high false positive and negative results and are therefore, not useful in making or excluding the diagnosis.

Platelets may also be consumed in the periphery, and a low platelet count almost always accompanies established disseminated intravascular coagulation (Box 23.2). Giant haemangiomas (Kasabach-Merritt syndrome) or an enlarged spleen may also sequester and destroy platelets.

Lack of marrow production of platelets often accompanies marrow infiltration by diseases, such as leukaemia. Other bone marrow failure syndromes, such as Fanconi anaemia, can also present initially with low platelets.

It is also possible to have a platelet function disorder. The commonest of these are Glanzmann thrombaesthenia, usually associated with a normal platelet count, and Bernard-Soulier syndrome, associated with a moderate to severe thrombocytopenia. Both are due to different platelet glycoprotein defects, and can be diagnosed by platelet function testing and flow cytometry.

BOX 23.2 Haematological findings in disseminated intravascular coagulation.

1. Prolonged APTT
2. Prolonged PT
3. Prolonged thrombin time
4. Low fibrinogen
5. Low platelet count
6. Raised fibrin degradation products or D-dimers
7. Red cell fragmentation on the blood film

In neonates, causes of thrombocytopenia vary depending on the gestation and clinical condition of the baby. In well-term neonates, alloimmune thrombocytopenia, due to the transplacental passage of maternal antiplatelet antibodies directed against foreign paternal antigens on the babies platelets (akin to the red cell disorder Rhesus haemolytic disease of the newborn), needs to be excluded. In preterm neonates, benign gestational thrombocytopenia may be seen soon after birth, but later appearance of thrombocytopenia often heralds sepsis.

Coagulation Testing in Infants and Children

Interpreting the results of coagulation screening require some basic knowledge of the coagulation cascade. Coagulation tests are performed in the laboratory (in vitro) and do not faithfully replicate the circumstances seen in the body (in vivo). The interpretation of laboratory tests often places a lot of emphasis on extrinsic and intrinsic pathways, but these sequences of activation probably do not play a major role in the initiation of clotting in vivo. Despite this, the concept of extrinsic and intrinsic pathways is useful to be aware of when faced with an abnormal coagulation screen, and is shown in Figure 11.23.

It is now thought that the key initiating event in vivo is exposure of tissue factor in response to endothelial damage. Tissue factor activates factor VII to form a complex, TF-VIIa, which cleaves factor X to its active form Xa. Xa can convert prothrombin to thrombin with low efficiency but this generation of small amounts of thrombin then activates feedback loops to increase coagulation factor activation. Factor VIII (activated by thrombin) and factor IX (activated by TF-VIIa and factor XI) form a complex VIIIa-IXa known as tenase. Tenase generates activated factor X with great efficiency. Thrombin also activates factor V, and a Xa-Va complex is formed which cleaves prothrombin to form thrombin. Thrombin generation leads to conversion of fibrinogen to fibrin with subsequent

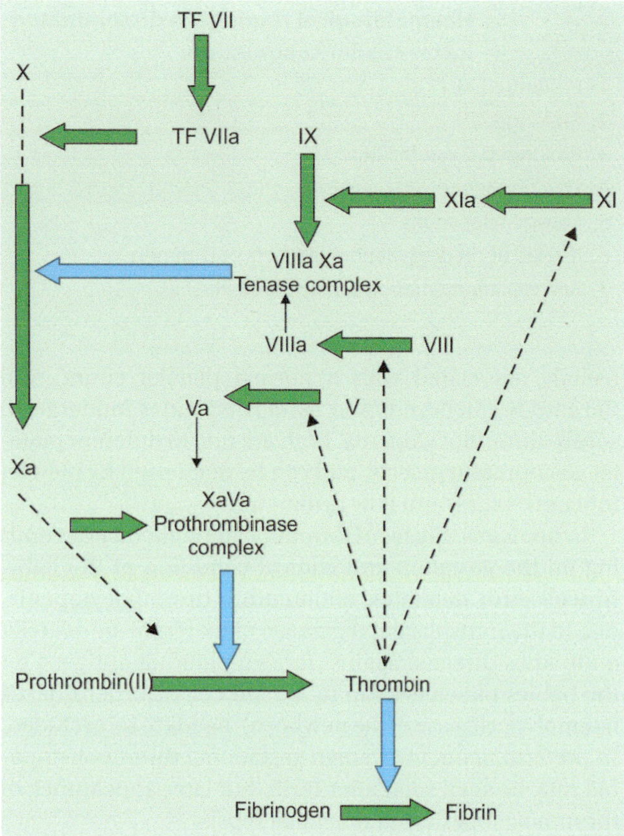

Figure 23.6 A revised coagulation cascade. Thick arrows indicate low efficiency pathways. Thin dashed arrows indicate feedback activation loops. Boxes indicate complexes formed on phospholipid surfaces.

crosslinking by factor XIII. This pathway is summarised in Figure 23.6.

WHEN TO PERFORM A COAGULATION SCREEN

Coagulation screens should not be a routine blood test. They should be performed in any child with unusually severe or unexplained bleeding, or in very unwell children with suspected disseminated intravascular coagulation. They can also be performed prior to high-risk invasive interventions. A good bleeding history needs to be taken to determine the need for investigation and to help guide appropriate tests. This includes a history of abnormal bleeding in the patient or relatives in response to haemostatic challenges, such as tooth extraction, cuts and minor operations, as well as a history of menorrhagia in older females. Some clinically significant bleeding disorders can have a normal coagulation screen (in particular, some von Willebrand disease and Factor XIII deficiency; Box 23.3), and some abnormal coagulation screens do not lead to a clinical risk of bleeding (e.g. Factor XII deficiency or lupus anticoagulant). Therefore, the results of testing always need to be interpreted in the light of a clinical history.

BOX 23.3	**Bleeding disorders that may present with a normal coagulation screen and platelet count.**
Factor XIII deficiency	
Glanzmann thrombasthenia/other platelet function disorders	
von Willebrand disease	
Vascular disorders	

KEY LEARNING POINT

Do not rely on coagulation screening as the sole indicator of bleeding risk. History of bleeding in response to a haemostatic challenge is just as important.

COAGULATION TESTS

When performing a clotting screen, care should be taken during venepuncture to avoid activation of clotting as this can produce artefactually low results. Samples should be from a free flowing vein; in particular, heel prick samples are unsuitable in neonates. Care should be taken to avoid contamination with heparin—a particular problem when sampling is from an indwelling venous catheter. Like the FBC, it is very important to be aware of normal ranges for the clotting screen, especially in neonates who tend to have significantly prolonged values compared to older children. In addition, values vary considerably between different automated analysers and may, therefore, vary between hospitals; local normal ranges should always be used.

Initial screening tests should comprise of:

- *Prothrombin time:* This is a test of the overall activity of the extrinsic pathway. It measures the activity of factors II, V, VII and X and is also dependent on adequate fibrinogen levels.
- *Activated partial thromboplastin time:* This is a test for the overall activity of the intrinsic pathway and measures factors II, V, VIII, IX, X, XI and XII; it also requires adequate fibrinogen levels.
- *Thrombin time:* Prolonged by quantitative and qualitative disorders of fibrinogen, the presence of inhibitory factors, such as fibrin/fibrin degradation products and the presence of heparin.
- Fibrinogen level.
- Platelet count.

Results of these tests along with clinical history can guide subsequent investigation. Bleeding times are generally unhelpful. A diagnostic algorithm is shown in Table 23.5.

TABLE 23.5 Causes of abnormal coagulation tests.

APTT	*PT*	*TT*	*Fibrinogen*	*Platelets*	*Possible diagnosis*
Prolonged	Normal	Normal	Normal	Normal	Factor VIII, IX, XI deficiency (haemophilia A, B or C), von Willebrand disease, lupus anticoagulant factor XII/ contact factor deficiency
Prolonged	Prolonged	Prolonged	Normal or low	Normal or low	Heparin Liver disease Fibrinogen deficiency Vitamin K deficiency DIC
Prolonged	Prolonged	Normal	Normal	Normal	Vitamin K deficiency Warfarin Factor II, V, VII, X deficiency
Normal	Prolonged	Normal	Normal	Normal	Warfarin therapy Factor VII deficiency

Abbreviations: APTT, activated partial thromboplastin time; PT, prothrombin time; TT, thromboplastin time.

The typical findings in disseminated intravascular coagulation are shown in **Box 23.2**; although coagulation screening is useful in this disorder, the primary therapy for DIC is treatment of the underlying cause. Replacement of coagulation factors with fresh frozen plasma or cryoprecipitate should be guided by the patient's clinical condition and presence of other risk factors for bleeding rather than treating the abnormal clotting screen per se.

Factor Assays

Clinical aspects of inherited coagulation disorders are discussed in Chapter 11. Inherited factor deficiencies may initially be suspected on the coagulation screen and confirmed by direct assay of the clotting factor. In the case of suspected von willebrand disease, von Willebrand factor (vWF) should be measured both quantitatively (vWF antigen) and qualitatively (a functional test, such as a ristocetin cofactor assay). This is because low levels of vWF or normal levels of dysfunctional vWF can cause the disease. vWF can also rise with stress and therefore, repeated testing may be needed to exclude disease, especially in young children who are difficult to venepuncture.

Platelet Function Testing

Besides a platelet count and assessment of platelet morphology by light microscopy, it is possible to assess platelet function in a number of ways. Historically, a bleeding time has been used as a global test of platelet function but it is difficult to standardize, and not very predictive of bleeding risk. Currently, the three commonest techniques in use are platelet aggregation studies (looking at aggregation in response to various stimulants, such as epinephrine), flow cytometry (to assess expression of glycoproteins on the platelet surface) and use of a platelet function analyzer (PFA-100, an automated machine that measures the ability of platelets to form a plug under shear stress).

Heparin

The presence of contaminating heparin in a sample is often initially suspected by the combination of a prolonged activated partial thromboplastin time (APTT) with a significantly prolonged thrombin time (this test is exquisitely sensitive to heparin). A number of methods exist to try and confirm whether the abnormal result is due to heparin or not. These include a reptilase time (which measures the same pathway as the TT, but is unaffected by heparin), or methods to neutralize the heparin using protamine sulphate.

MONITORING OF ANTICOAGULANT THERAPY

Therapeutic anticoagulation in children is used to prevent or treat thrombosis. Heparin and warfarin are the two main agents in use. Heparin comes in two main formulations—standard unfractionated heparin and low-molecular-weight heparin. The former is monitored by the APTT with a therapeutic range of 1.5–2.5 times normal control values. Low-molecular-weight heparin therapy does not prolong the APTT and needs to be monitored by anti-Xa levels. Warfarin therapy prolongs the prothrombin time but in order to standardize results between laboratories, this level is converted into an international normalized ratio (INR); the target INR varies depending on the indication for anticoagulation.

CHAPTER 24

Biochemical and Microbiological Investigations in Paediatrics

Peter Galloway, Alison E. Balfour

INTRODUCTION

Most laboratory work is undertaken in laboratories whose principal workload is adult patients. There are specific issues that can arise when the unwary consider children as small adults, e.g. inappropriate reference ranges and how the age of the child may change the nature of the sample submitted. This chapter aims to simply review key issues present in each of the core laboratory disciplines.

With the increasing range of laboratory tests, it is now estimated by the Royal College of Pathologists (UK) that 70% of all diagnoses depend upon laboratory results.

Before undertaking a clinical investigation, the clinician must consider two questions:

Will the chosen test confirm (or refute) a clinical suspicion, affecting alteration of management of the patient to obtain a clinical benefit (or avoid a problem), e.g. why identify hypercholesterolaemia in patients over 85?

If the natural evolution of the condition is trivial or self-limiting, what additional information is obtained, e.g. stool culture in acute diarrhoeal illness?

This concept is best summarised in the quote: 'Before ordering a test, decide what you will do if it is either positive or negative and if both answers are the same and then don't do the test!'

WHAT ARE THE ROLES OF DIAGNOSTIC TESTS?

There are only four specific reasons for doing a test. These are as follows:

Screening

To take a population and pick out those with a disease with few false-positive diagnosis. In certain circumstances, we demand 100% sensitivity, i.e. all cases will be diagnosed, allowing a few false positives through and using a more specific confirmatory assay, e.g. neonatal thyroid stimulating hormone screening using a cut off 30 mU/L on day 6 will identify all congenital hypothyroid cases and a number whose thyroid axis matures over first few weeks. This is necessary to avoid any missed cases.

Down screening in pregnancy uses markers and maternal age to identify women at high enough risk (1 in 220) to justify amniocentesis with its concomitant 1% pregnancy loss. It fails to identify approximately a third of cases.

Diagnosis

While some tests can specifically identify the illness (e.g. abnormal blood film in leukaemia), others may be less specific, e.g. aspartate amino transferase (AST) commonly used as a marker of liver disease is raised in muscle disease, thus all 1–3 years old with a raised AST need a creatine kinase done concomitantly to exclude Duchenne muscular dystrophy.

Prognosis

This allows estimates of the likely outcome. E.g. creatinine in renal impairment can act as a marker of degree of renal damage in an individual, or levels of α-fetoprotein (AFP)/HCG are inversely proportional to outcome in non-seminomatous testicular tumours.

Detection of Complications/Monitoring

With increasing laboratory use, there is routine monitoring such as looking for side-effects from drugs. Identifying those with marrow suppression on immunosuppressants, e.g. azathioprine.

WHAT ARE IMPORTANT FACTORS IN INTERPRETING DATA?

Quality of Information

The laboratory's role is to maximise accuracy and precision of a result (accuracy is an indication of how close to

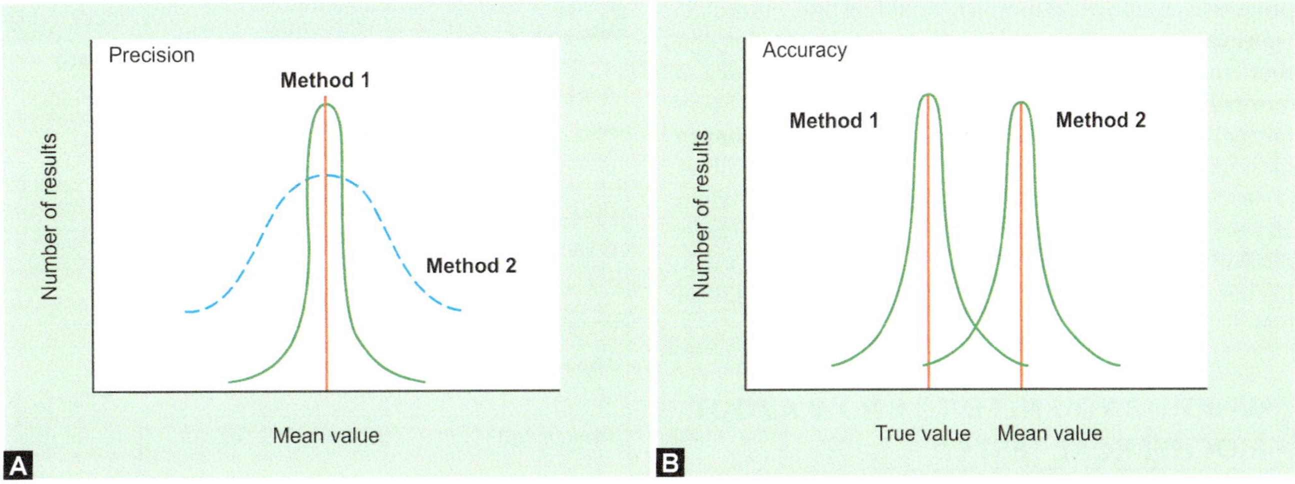

Figures 24.1A and B (A) Precision is a measure of reproducibility with method 1 being more precise than method 2; (B) Both methods 1 and 2 are equally precise but method 1 is more accurate.

the correct value; while precision is how reproducible a result is). To achieve this, laboratories carefully control as many factors as they can. They run quality controls, both internal (allowing regular precision) and intermittent external (to confirm accuracy) **(Figs. 24.1A and B)**.

The expansion of external quality control into rarer analytes has allowed laboratories to improve, particularly inborn errors of metabolism investigations.

Factors Occurring before the Laboratory

Samples must always be collected under appropriate conditions. If the analyte is unstable, then appropriate preservative or rapid handling is required, e.g. fluoride oxalate tubes for glucose. They must be properly identified especially with multiple births.

More specific factors that can affect the result is to consider the biological diurnal variation in an analyte such as cortisol being higher in morning and lower in evening or over longer periods, such as gonadotropin changes postpuberty over a month in a female. Without considering the clinical features, interpretation is impossible.

A major effect on many analytes is the acute phase response to any illness. This physiological process identified by simple measures such as elevated C-reactive protein is associated with widespread changes. There is vascular leakage of albumin into the extravascular space evident by reduced albumin levels and many micronutrient measurements, such as iron and zinc fall rapidly as the body sequesters them to prevent them being available to bacteria. Prolonged inflammatory responses result in altered endocrine disturbances with, e.g. suppression of thyroid function (Euthyroid sick syndrome).

Before being able to interpret a result, we need to be able to compare it to the normal homeostatic levels.

WHAT IS 'NORMAL'?

'Normal' is a term that is often used to include only 'healthy' individuals. The term 'normal range' encompasses a range from two standard deviations more and less than the median in a 'healthy' population. This assumes the population data are Gaussian distributed (or mathematically transformed into Gaussian distributed) and encompass 95% of these individuals.

Interpretation of laboratory data is then made against this healthy group of individuals. But they must be comparable if affected by sex, age and so on. But 2.5% lie above or below that range and are still healthy. The further they lie from the mean, the more likely they are to be ill.

The second problem is best illustrated by cholesterol **(Fig. 24.2)**. The normal UK range is 3.5–6.7 mmol/L. However, the risk of coronary heart disease increases

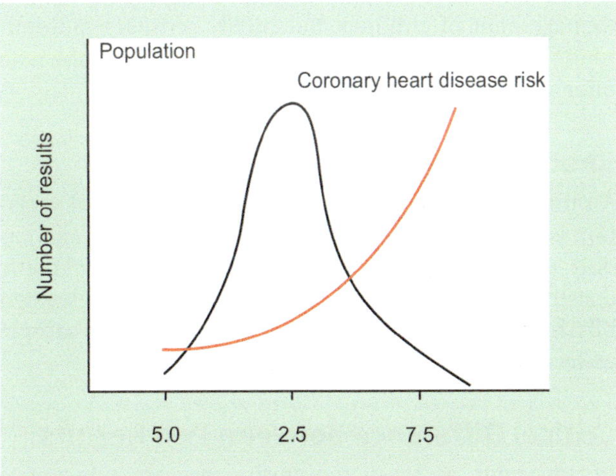

Figure 24.2 Graphic interpretation of cholesterol level against healthy group of individuals.

progressively above 5.2 mmol/L, doubling by 6.7 mmol/L. However, below 5.2 mmol/L, the curve is not flat and there remains a shallow gradient of risk. Thus the idea of 'normal' range may be less helpful. It follows that if 5% of normal results are outside the 'normal' range, the chance of a healthy individual having one abnormal result is ($1-0.95^n$) where n is number of tests performed. When 20 tests are done, two-thirds will have one or more results out with the 'normal range'. In healthy individuals, chasing perceived abnormalities may not result in any clinical benefit.

WHAT DO YOU NEED TO KNOW ABOUT BIOCHEMICAL TESTS?

Analytical

Major analytical advances occurred during the 1970s from manual testing to automated analysers for common tests. The resulting reduction in sample volume requirements allowed biochemistry to support neonatal care.

Problems still remain, particularly in premature neonates where blood volume is more critical. Specific issues that can occur are excessive evaporation from small samples; concentrating the sample; problems if inadequate volume added to tubes containing liquid anticoagulant where there may be a direct dilution effect. With small sample volumes, it is important to discuss ones priorities with the lab to maximise the number of tests, which will impact on that child/ neonates care.

The Assay Detection Limits

In paediatrics, different normal ranges are expected physiologically. A child with Thelarche will have an oestrogen level less than 100 pmol/L. The normal adult postpubertal range being 150–1,000 pmol/L (depending upon day of cycle). Truly prepubertal children are less than 12 pmol/L. Most routine assay, therefore, fails to help in the clinical management of children, but highly sensitive radioimmunoassay with detection limit of less than 10 pmol/L do offer advantages.

Specific Sample Timing

An understanding of analyte stability and diurnal variation is required. Consideration of specific issues, such as only measuring drugs, after adequate pharmacokinetic distribution has occurred, e.g. digoxin remains elevated till 6 hours postdose, should be addressed prior to sample collection.

Critical Difference between Two Results

In particular, as more monitoring occurs, it becomes important to be truly certain that a result has statistically changed. For this, the result must vary by 2.8 times the total variance [i.e. (SD Biological)^2 + (SD Analytical)^2] where biological differences are the physiological variability in an analyte during the day and analytical refers to the imprecision in measurement (Table 24.1).

TABLE 24.1 Clinical difference between two results.

Analyte	*Biological variance (%)*	*Level (mmol/L)*	*Critical difference*
Na	0.7	140	5
K^+	5.1	4.2	0.6
Urea	13.6	5	1.9
Creatinine	4.6	60	14
Calcium	1.7	2.4	0.21
Phosphate	5.1	1.2	0.3
Alkaline phosphatase (IU/L)	6.7	60	20
Albumin (g/L)	3.1	40	4

With increasing automation of analyses, the analytical imprecision has decreased. At present, typical critical differences for routine analytes are given at midpoint of adult reference range.

Neonatal Reference Ranges

With modern ethical considerations, collecting blood to perform reference ranges in children is not possible. In premature neonates, one could even question if this is a pathophysiological state, so that there are no 'healthy' comparable controls.

The ongoing maturation processes will affect the interpretation of results such as the progressive rise in glomerular filtration rate. Other physiological processes must be remembered such as the normal testosterone rise following birth in male infants, which disappears by 4 months of age.

Unfortunately most laboratories offer 'adult reference ranges'. The tables (Appendix A) demonstrate where this can cause particular issues in children. For simplicity, exact data for specific age ranges are not given. When interpreting an analyte, the pathophysiological process needs to be considered; particularly inflammation and the acute phase response such that some analytes increase, e.g. α-1-antitrypsin and others decrease, e.g. zinc.

WHAT DO YOU NEED TO KNOW ABOUT MICROBIOLOGY TESTS?

The aetiology and presentation of infection in the paediatric patient are often different from that in adults; therefore, the clinical microbiology laboratory, and its users, must be aware of this for analysis and interpretation of results.

Urine

There are three major aspects to the microbiological analysis of urine:

- Microscopy
- Culture
- Dipstick testing for leucocyte esterase (a surrogate for the presence of white cells) and nitrite (a bacterial product)

Urine can be collected from children at a variety of ages and in a number of ways. The age of the child and the method of collection and storage may affect the interpretation of the result.

Methods of Urine Collection

Types of Sample

- Suprapubic aspirate: Urine is collected directly via a needle inserted through the skin into the bladder
- Clean-catch urine
- Mid-stream specimen of urine
- Bag specimen of urine
- Catheter specimen of urine

Microscopy of Urine

Microscopy is performed to identify formed elements present within the urine; these include white cells (pyuria), red blood cells (RBC; haematuria), bacteria (bacteriuria) and casts.

Pyuria The excretion of 400,000 leucocytes/hour, which corresponds to more than 10 white cells/mm^3, correlates with the presence of urinary tract infection (UTI). However, pyuria in the absence of bacteriuria is not a reliable guide to infection as leucocytes can be found in all types of inflammation and in older females pus cells may come from the vagina. The amount of pyuria also varies with urine flow and pH.

Bacteriuria The presence of organisms in unspun urine is highly suggestive of significant bacteriuria. Bacteriuria is demonstrable in unspun urine in over 90% of cases when 10^5 bacteria/mL or higher is present. However, a negative result does not rule out infection and has poor sensitivity at lower colony counts.

Culture of Urine

Most UTI are due to a single organism. Common organisms causing UTI in children include: *Escherichia coli*, which probably causes 75% or more of cases, *Klebsiella* spp., *Proteus* spp., and *Staphylococcus saprophyticus*. Less common causative organisms include *Enterobacter* spp., *Citrobacter* spp., *Serratia marcescens*, *Acinetobacter species*, *Pseudomonas* spp., and *Staphylococcus aureus*. The number of bacteria taken as significant bacteriuria varies depending upon the type of sample:

- Suprapubic aspiration of the bladder; significant culture if more than 10^2 colony-forming units per mL (CFU/mL)
- In-out catheterization of the bladder; significant culture if more than 10^3 CFU/mL
- Clean-voided urine; significant culture if more than 10^4 CFU/mL
- Carefully collected bag, nappy or pad specimen; significant culture if more than 10^5 CFU/mL

A false-positive result due to contamination should be suspected when:

- Bacteria, but no leucocytes (except in immunocompromised patients)
- Multiple organisms cultured
- Blood and the specimen is from a menstruating girl
- Prolonged storage more than 8 hours at room temperature.

A false-negative result may be due to:

- Inadequate filling of a specimen bottle containing boric acid (the preservative is bactericidal at high concentrations)
- Antibiotics excreted in the urine
- Prolonged storage, i.e. more than 48 hours at fridge temperature.

Dipstick Testing

Dipstick testing can be performed for a number of analytes. In UTI, the most useful are leucocyte esterase and nitrite. Overall dipstick testing is less reliable in children under 2 years of age; in children over two if both leucocyte esterase and nitrite are positive it is suggestive of the presence of UTI; if both leucocyte esterase and nitrite are negative it is useful to rule out a diagnosis of UTI **(Fig. 24.3)**.

Cerebrospinal Fluid (CSF)

Cerebrospinal fluid is examined microscopically then cultured. Examination for bacterial antigens and polymerase chain reaction (PCR) may also be performed. Meningitis can occur in children with normal CSF microscopy. If it is clinically indicated, children who have a 'normal' CSF should still be treated with IV antibiotics pending cultures.

Microscopy

Cerebrospinal fluid white cell count is higher at birth than in later infancy and falls fairly rapidly in the first 2 weeks of life. In the first week, 90% of normal neonates have a white cell count less than 18.

The presence of any neutrophils in the CSF is unusual in normal children and should raise concern about

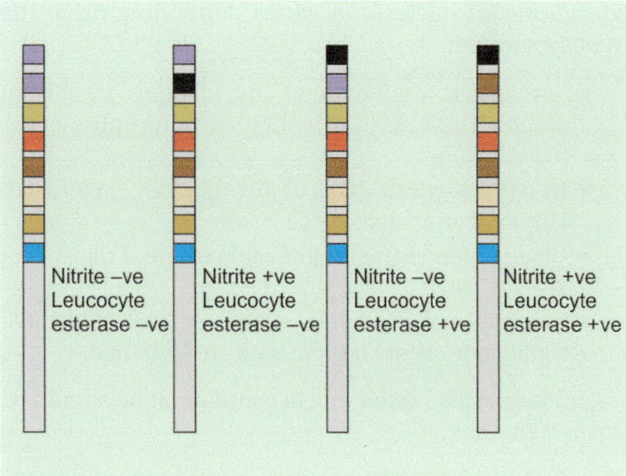

Figure 24.3 Dipstick testing.

bacterial meningitis. Neither a normal Gram stain or lack of white cells excludes bacterial meningitis, in fact a Gram stain may be negative in up to 60% of cases of bacterial meningitis even without prior antibiotics.

Cerebrospinal fluid findings in bacterial meningitis may mimic those found in viral meningitis, particularly early in disease process, and neutrophils may predominate in viral meningitis even after the first 24 hours. Antibiotics are unlikely to significantly affect the CSF cell count in samples taken less than 24 hours after antibiotics. **Table 24.2** shows normal CSF biochemistry and microscopy findings, and those for bacterial and viral meningitis.

Traumatic Tap

In traumatic taps, one can allow one white blood cell for every 500–700 RBC; however, this is not entirely reliable and in order to not to miss any patients with meningitis, the safest way to interpret a traumatic tap is to count the total number of white cells and disregard the red cell count. If there are more white cells than the normal range for age, then the patient should be treated.

Polymerase Chain Reaction

Polymerase chain reaction is routinely available for *Neisseria meningitidis*, herpes simplex (HSV) and enterovirus, but results are not usually available in a timescale which informs immediate management decisions. Meningococcal PCR is particularly useful in patients with a clinical picture consistent with meningococcal meningitis, but who have received prior antibiotics. Enterovirus PCR should be requested on CSF from patients with clinical and/or CSF features of viral meningitis. HSV PCR should be requested for patients with clinical features of encephalitis.

Bacterial Antigens

Cerebrospinal fluid bacterial antigen tests have low sensitivity and specificity, and have little role if any in management.

Blood Culture

The usual organisms causing bacterial meningitis in children over 2 months of age are *Neisseria meningitidis* and *Streptococcus pneumoniae* **(Figs. 24.4 and 24.5)**. *Haemophilus influenzae* type b (Hib) is much less common since the onset of vaccination for Hib.

In infants less than 2 months of age Group B *Streptococcus*, *E. coli* and other gram-negative organisms and *Listeria monocytogenes* should also be considered

To maximize the recovery of bacteria from blood it is important to collect the correct volume of blood to blood culture broth ratio, e.g. specific paediatric blood culture bottles can be used for optimal recovery of organisms from neonates from whom only a small volume of blood can be obtained.

Serology

Most blood tests performed in microbiology measure the immune response to infection and the normal ranges are broadly the same as in adults. The major exception to this is streptococcal serology. Infection with group A Streptococcus (GAS) results in the production of specific

TABLE 24.2 Interpretation of cerebrospinal fluid findings.

	White cell count		*Biochemistry*	
	Neutrophils	***Lymphocytes***	***Protein***	***Glucose***
	(×10⁶/L)	(×10⁶/L)	(g/L)	(CSF: blood ratio)
Normal	0	≤5	<0.4	≥0.6 (or 2.5 mmol/L)
Normal term neonate	0	≤11	<1.0	≥0.6 (or ≥2.1 mmol/L)
Bacterial meningitis	100–10,000 (but may be normal)	Usually <100	>1.0 (but may be normal)	<0.4 (but may be normal)
Viral meningitis	Usually <100	10–1,000 (but may be normal)	0.4–1 (but may be normal)	Usually normal

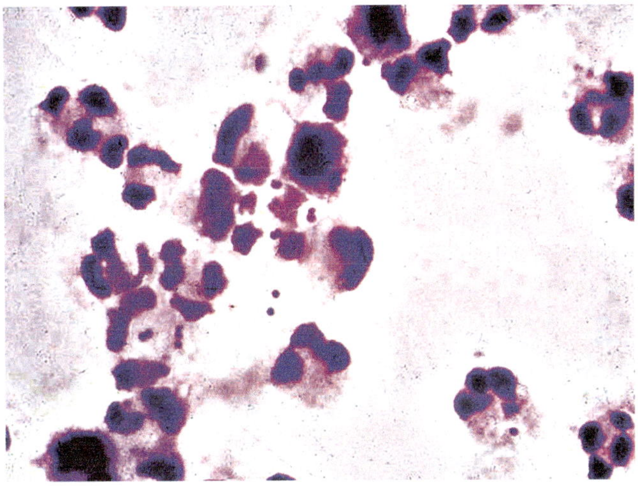

Figure 24.4 Cerebrospinal fluid with pus cells and *Neisseria meningitidis.*

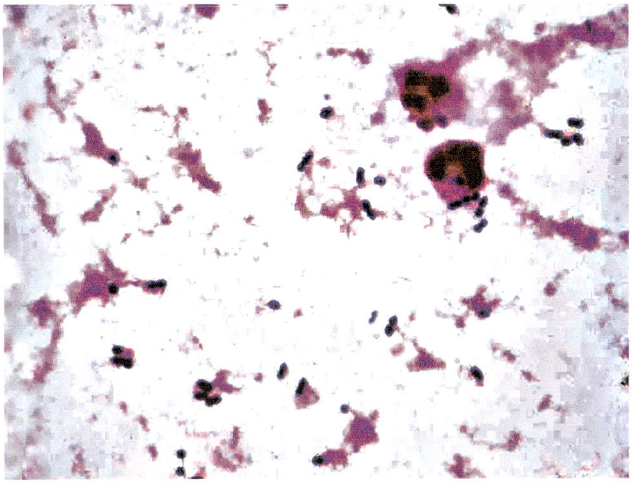

Figure 24.5 Cerebrospinal fluid with pus cells and *Streptococcus pneumoniae.*

antibodies against streptococcal exoenzymes, the most important of which are antistreptolysin O (ASO) and antideoxyribonuclease-B (ADB).

The ASO response is generally good in pharyngitis and tonsillitis but will not distinguish between infections with groups A, C and G streptococci, and the response is generally poor in impetigo and pyoderma. The mean ASO normal levels are age dependent:

- Preschool: Less than 1:200 u/mL
- School age: Less than 1:320 u/mL
- Adult: Less than 1:200 u/mL

The ADB response is good in skin as well as throat infections and may be more specific for GAS infection. The ADB test shows elevated titres in more than 90% of clinically diagnosed cases of pyoderma, acute glomerulonephritis and acute rheumatic fever. ADB titres peak later than ASO levels and remain elevated for several months. The ADB can, therefore, be of value if there is a delay in diagnosis.

The mean normal ADB levels are age dependent:

Preschool: 1:60 u/mL
School age: 1:170 u/mL
Adult: 1:85 u/mL

Examination of Faeces

Gastroenteritis can be caused by bacteria (e.g. *Salmonella*), parasites (e.g. Cryptosporidium) and viruses (e.g. Norovirus). Viral gastroenteritis is the commonest cause of vomiting and diarrhoea in children, causing significant morbidity and mortality.

Pathogens found in the stools of children are broadly the same as those found in adults; however, the age of acquisition of certain pathogens varies between developed and developing countries. In developing countries, *Campylobacter* is the most commonly isolated bacterial pathogen from children less than 2 years old with diarrhoea. The disease does not appear to be as prevalent in adults. In contrast, in developed countries, infection may occur in adults and children. The age of acquisition of *Campylobacter* in a number of countries is illustrated in the Table 24.3.

Thus, the spectrum of pathogens sought in the microbiology laboratory for children of different ages will need to be determined by the knowledge of local epidemiology.

TABLE 24.3 Age of acquisition of *Campylobacter* in different countries.

Countries (ref.)	*Age of infection (months)*
Nigeria	24
Tanzania	18
China	12–24
Thailand	<12 (18.8%) 12–23 (12.3%) 24–59 (10.3%)
Bangladesh	≤12 (38.8%) >12 (15.9%)
Egypt	0–5 (8%) 6–11 (14%) 12–23 (4%)

Source: Adapted from Emerg Infect Dis. 2002;8(3).

Respiratory Viruses

Bronchiolitis is a serious lower respiratory tract infection that occurs predominantly in children aged less than 2 years, principally caused by Respiratory Synctial Virus (RSV). Diagnosis is by PCR and some centres use Point of Care Testing (POCT) to aid diagnosis and for infection prevention control. Multiplex PCR, whereby multiple targets can be amplified in a single PCR assay, is now commonly available to provide sensitive and prompt diagnosis of multiple respiratory pathogens, including *Bordetella pertussis* and *Mycoplasma pneumoniae.*

Antibiotic Monitoring and Interpretation

It is necessary to monitor the levels of antibiotic for two major reasons. Some antibiotics have a narrow therapeutic range, i.e. the ratio between therapeutic levels and toxic levels, so antibiotic levels are measured to reduce the potential for toxicity. For other antibiotics, it may not always be possible to predict serum levels; in this case, antibiotic levels are monitored to ensure efficacy. The antibiotics whose levels are most commonly measured are the aminoglycosides (gentamicin, tobramycin and amikacin) and the glycopeptide antibiotic vancomycin.

CHAPTER 25

Paediatric Emergencies

Sarah Coles, Andrew Carachi

INTRODUCTION

Paediatric patients who present to the emergency department pose extraordinary challenges to healthcare personnel. Faced with such a patient, the situation can at first appear frightening and overwhelming. The purpose of this chapter is to give a brief account of common emergencies seen in the paediatric population and in the process provide a simplified, structured approach to the management of these children that can be applied to any situation. The process outcomes for these patients can be improved, and a stressful situation can be transformed into ultimately one of the most satisfying areas of paediatric medicine.

DIFFERENCES BETWEEN ADULTS AND CHILDREN IN THE EMERGENCY DEPARTMENT

Children are not small adults. They demonstrate important differences in their size, anatomy, physiology and psychology that impact on management in the emergency setting.

Size

Children are obviously smaller than adults and their weight changes as they become older. This is important as almost all drug and fluid calculations in paediatrics are calculated on a per weight basis. It is, therefore, essential to have a relatively accurate weight for any child presenting to the emergency department. Occasionally a parent or guardian may know the child's weight but this tends to be the exception. The most accurate means to assess the child's weight is to simply weigh the child (either on their own or whilst being held by a parent); however, this is often impractical in the emergency setting. Other methods are, therefore, required.

The Broselow tape is a tape measure that is laid alongside the child and gives an estimate of the child's weight based on their height. It is easy to use, relatively accurate and requires minimal training in its use.

An alternative, if the child's age is known, is to use the following formula:

$$\text{Weight (in kg)} = (\text{Age} + 4) \times 2$$

This formula is relatively accurate for children between the ages of 1 year and 10 years and has the advantage that it can be used to plan drug and fluid doses before the child's arrival. For children less than 1 year, in general, the birth weight becomes double at 6 months and triple at 12 months of age. If birth weight is not known, full-term neonate can be considered to weigh 3–4 kg and 12-month-old infant as 10 kg.

Anatomy and Physiology

Children have important differences in their anatomy and physiology to adults that impact on their emergency care.

Airway and Breathing

Young children have relatively larger heads and shorter necks than adults and this can result in relative neck flexion. The face, mouth and jaw are small and the tongue large. The trachea is short and easily compressible. In combination, this can result in an increased risk of airway obstruction and means that great care must be taken during airway positioning manoeuvres. In addition, children's lower airways are also small resulting in a greater propensity to obstruction even to relatively minor stimuli such as viral infections. Additionally, infants rely mainly on diaphragmatic breathing that tends to fatigue more easily than adults. Children's lungs are smaller and their respiratory rates faster—a respiratory rate of 40/minute may be normal in an infant but signify severe respiratory distress in a 12 years old.

Circulation

Infants have a relatively small, fixed stroke volume that relies on a tachycardic response to increase cardiac

TABLE 25.1 Normal range of respiratory rate, heart rate and blood pressure according to ages.

Age in years	*Respiratory rate*	*Heart/pulse rate*	*Systolic BP*
<1	30–40	110–160	70–90
1–2	25–35	100–150	80–95
2–5	25–30	95–140	80–100
5–12	20–25	80–120	90–110
>12	15–20	60–100	100–120

output. This means they tolerate bradycardia poorly. Stroke volume increases with age as the heart enlarges. This results in babies and young children having faster resting heart rates than older children and adults. It is, therefore, important to have an appreciation of the normal range of age-specific heart rates (**Table 25.1**). A heart rate of 60/minute in an adult can be normal; in an infant, it is considered as a cardiac arrest. Young children have a relatively higher circulating blood volume per bodyweight (newborn 85 mL/kg, 1 year old 80 mL/kg, 10 year old 75 mL/kg) than adults (70 mL/kg), but the actual total blood volume is small. The young child does, therefore, not tolerate blood loss well, even when the amount appears to be relatively small. Similarly, even relatively small amounts of fluid loss, such as diarrhoea, can result in significant dehydration.

Psychology

Children are often very frightened in the emergency department. The appearance of a large number of adults they do not know, no matter how well-intentioned, can at times be overwhelming and make the assessment of a child difficult. Young children are often non-verbal and find it difficult to express their emotions. In these settings, the presence of tachycardia and tachypnoea can be difficult to distinguish between pathology and emotional distress. It is important, therefore, to attempt to minimise the distress caused to the child. The child should always be accompanied by their parents except in the most exceptional circumstances. The number of staff around the child and the background noise should be kept to a safe minimum whenever possible and a caring, gentle approach taken at all times.

BASIC STRUCTURED APPROACH TO MANAGEMENT

A structured approach to any seriously ill patient allows appropriate early resuscitation and stabilisation to occur, even if the definitive diagnosis is complex or not known. It is highly reliant on adequate preparation and teamwork is essential. It is the approach recommended by resuscitation organisations such as the Advanced Paediatric Life Support (APLS) Group. Any emergency can be approached in this manner.

'Problem Recognition and Treatment have Higher Priority than Definite Diagnosis'.

The structured approach relies on four basic principles:

1. *Preparation and teamwork:* It is of great benefit when a dedicated communication line from and to the Ambulance Service and the Emergency Medicine Department is available. Basic information can be gathered such as the patient's age and current problems. This allows the team to develop a state of readiness. In particular two key areas can be prepared:
   a. Calling for relevant help in advance, e.g. anaesthetic or intensive care support. Resuscitation is reliant on a team approach.
   'Blow the whistle first and assemble the players before starting the game'.
   b. Prepare appropriate equipment, drugs and fluids. In a resuscitation situation, even simple calculations can prove challenging. Spending a few minutes before the arrival of the patient calculating the likely weight, drug doses, defibrillation charge, endotracheal tube size, etc. can prove extremely valuable and make any resuscitation run more smoothly. A useful mnemonic is **WET FLAG**
   Weight = (age in years +4) × 2 kg
   Energy = 4 J/kg
   T endotracheal tube diameter = (age in years/4) + 4 mm
   Fluids = 10 mL/kg 0.9% sodium chloride
   Lorazepam = 0.1 mg/kg
   Adrenaline = 0.1 mL/kg of 1:10,000 adrenaline
   Glucose = 2 mL/kg of 10% glucose
2. *Recognise and treat immediate life-threatening situations (resuscitation):* This should be approached via a systematic Airway, Breathing, and Circulation (ABC) approach. Examples include obstructed airway requiring airway opening manoeuvres or suction, apnoea or severely compromised breathing requiring oxygen or assisted ventilation and circulatory collapse or cardiorespiratory arrest requiring fluid administration or cardiopulmonary resuscitation (CPR). At this stage, recognition and management of the initial problem is more important than the underlying diagnosis.
3. *Identify key features that point to a likely working diagnosis so that early emergency treatment can be started:* For example, the presence of a rash and fever may point to the provisional diagnosis of sepsis and allow early use of appropriate antimicrobials. Recognition of a heart murmur in a collapsed infant may point to a diagnosis of a duct-dependent cardiac lesion and the initiation of a prostaglandin infusion.

In both of these situations, emergency treatments can be initiated before an absolute definitive diagnosis is arrived at.

4. *Stabilisation and transfer:* Once the patient has been resuscitated and emergency treatment has been started the next aim is to optimise the patient's condition. This involves a thorough reassessment of the patient's physiology and response to resuscitation, repeating the ABC approach, and may involve additional treatment. Examples include optimising electrolytes in a patient post-cardiac arrest or splinting a femoral fracture in a patient post-trauma. Arrangements can then be made for the safe transfer of the patient to an area where definitive treatment can be offered or ongoing resuscitation provided, e.g. operating theatre, ward or intensive care unit (ICU).

With practice, this structured approach can be used quickly and effectively and allows a hierarchical approach to serious problems encountered rather than relying on establishing a definitive diagnosis before treatment is initiated. It can, therefore, be applied to any condition or situation and does not rely on specialist knowledge of at times complex conditions.

KEY LEARNING POINTS

- Problem recognition is more important than establishing a definitive diagnosis.
- Always manage problems in an Airway, Breathing, and Circulation approach. Life-threatening problems must be recognised and treated first.
- Be aware of age-specific normal ranges.
- Team work is essential in the emergency management of unwell children.

CARDIAC ARREST

The science underpinning guidelines on the management of cardiac arrest in children is constantly evolving. In response to this, APLS guidelines are constantly being updated. References are provided at the end of the chapter for interested readers who wish to explore these guidelines in greater depth. Full proficiency at these skills is best achieved by attending a course provided by organisations such as APLS or similar national resuscitation organisations within one's own country. In addition, hospitals and emergency departments can run their own in-house mock resuscitation-based scenarios where staff can practice their skills on resuscitation mannequins on a regular basis.

Mechanisms of Cardiac Arrest in Children

Children are usually healthy with excellent cardiac function, normal heart valves and patent coronary arteries that are not compromised by atherosclerosis. The mechanisms of cardiac arrest in children are, therefore, different from those of adults. In children, cardiac arrest usually occurs secondary to either respiratory or circulatory failure (e.g. severe asthma, airway obstruction or septic shock) rather than a primary cardiac event such as arrhythmia due to myocardial infarction. This means that there may be a period pre-arrest in children that is amenable to intervention to prevent progression to cardiac arrest. It also means that when a cardiac arrest does occur the arresting rhythm is often asystole and the outcome is often poor. It is, therefore, important to realise the importance of recognition of the sick child to prevent cardiac arrest and the importance of following standard treatment algorithms when a cardiac arrest has occurred.

The main aim during basic life support (BLS) is to deliver oxygen, this is the critical step.

Flow chart 25.1 Basic life-support algorithm.
(*Source:* From APLS manual).

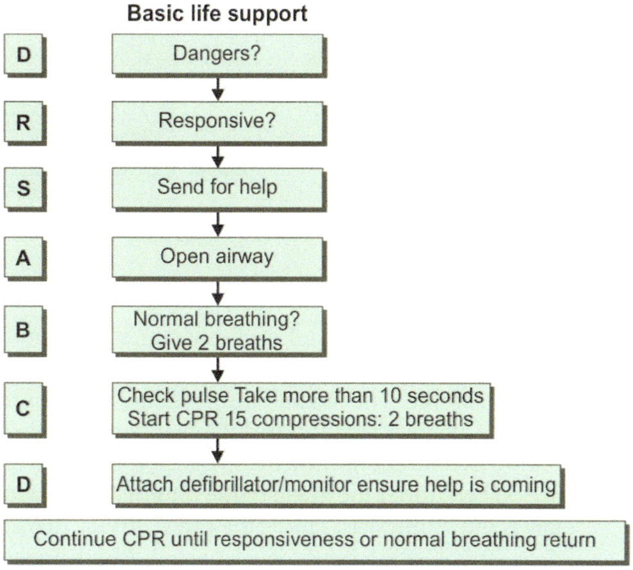

Paediatric Basic Life Support

Initial approach: Safety, Stimulate, Shout (SSS) (**Flow chart 25.1**)

S: Check for danger. It is essential that the rescuer does not become a second victim and these precautions should precede airway management.

S: Check for responsiveness. Gently stimulate and ask the child "are you alright?". Stimulus should be gentle thus to avoid exacerbating possible cervical spine injury.

S: Send for help. In the case of a baby/small child and lone rescuer, the victim can often be taken to the phone while the rescuer attempts to continue CPR.

A: Check for airway patency. Head tilt, chin lift manoeuvres can be used to correct an obstructed

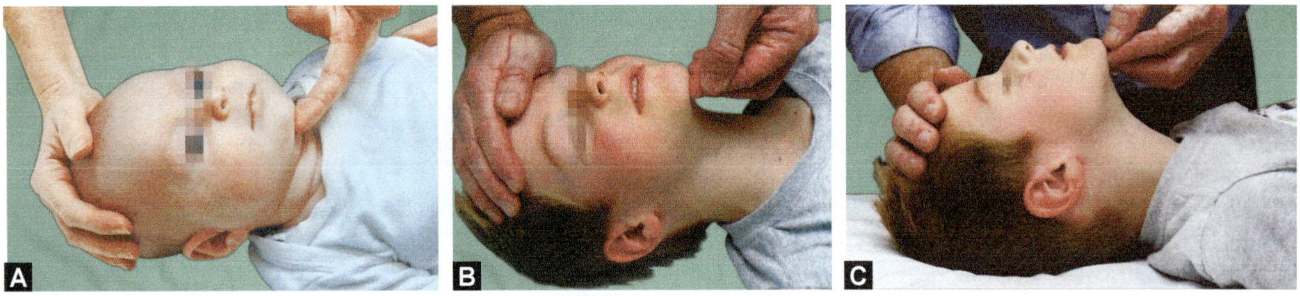

Figures 25.1A to C Neutral and stiffing position from Advanced Paediatric Life Support (APLS) manual.

airway. A hand is placed on the victim's head and two fingers under the chin to achieve the desired degree of tilt. This being the "sniffing" position and the neutral position in infants. An alternative manoeuvre is the jaw thrust—two or three fingers are placed under the angle of the mandible and the jaw is lifted upwards. This is the safest airway to use if a cervical spine injury is suspected. Blind finger sweep should NOT be attempted.

B: Look, listen and feel for chest wall movement for no longer than 10 seconds. If the child is not breathing, five rescue breaths should be administered. These are delivered by covering either nose and mouth in smaller children or occluding the child's nose to administer breaths into the mouth. A bag valve mask should be used if available.

C: Once the resuscitation breaths have been given, a pulse should be felt centrally at either brachial, femoral or carotid arteries. If no pulse felt for 10 seconds or the pulse in less than 60 bpm, CPR should be initiated. The heel of the hand is placed on the lower half of the child's sternum and the chest should be compressed to at least one-third of the depth of the chest. In infants, two fingers or a hand-encirculating technique should be used instead of the heel of the hand. Chest compressions should be at a rate of 100/minute. Chest compressions and ventilation breaths are given at a ratio of 15:2 **(Figs. 25.1A to C)**.

If no help has arrived after 1 minute, the emergency services should be contacted. CPR should be continued until emergency services arrive or responsiveness or normal breathing returns.

Choking Child/Foreign Body in Airway

The algorithm for the management of the choking child is shown in **Flow chart 25.2**. Foreign body obstruction of the airway most commonly occurs in younger children when eating or playing with small toys. The onset of choking or stridor is usually very suddenly and the child is usually otherwise well with no prodrome. This distinguishes

Flow chart 25.2 Choking child algorithm.

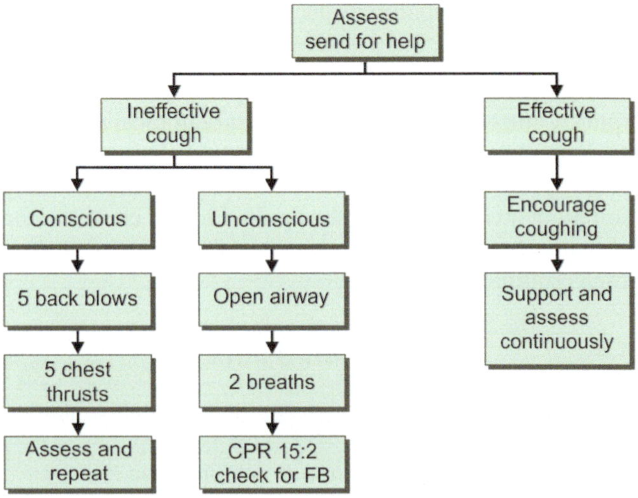

it from other causes of upper airway obstruction such as croup or epiglottitis in which the child usually has a prodromal illness. The treatment of airway obstruction due to other causes, e.g. croup or epiglottitis is different from that of foreign body obstruction.

The main feature of the algorithm is distinguishing between an effective and ineffective cough. The child who is alert and coughing effectively (loud cough, crying, fully responsive, able to take breaths) should be carefully observed until the foreign body is expelled or the child deteriorates. If the cough is ineffective (unable to vocalise, unable to breath, cyanosed, quiet or silent cough) then the child should be placed in a head down position over the rescuer's knee and back blows given (heel of one hand, blow directed between the scapulae). If the foreign body has not been expelled after five back blows then chest thrusts (same landmarks as for CPR) should be used in infants, and abdominal thrusts in children over 1 year old. Abdominal thrusts should not be used in infants due to the high risk of abdominal injury in this age group. If at any point the child loses consciousness, then the rescuer should revert to the Basic Paediatric Life Support algorithm **(Figs. 25.2A and B)**.

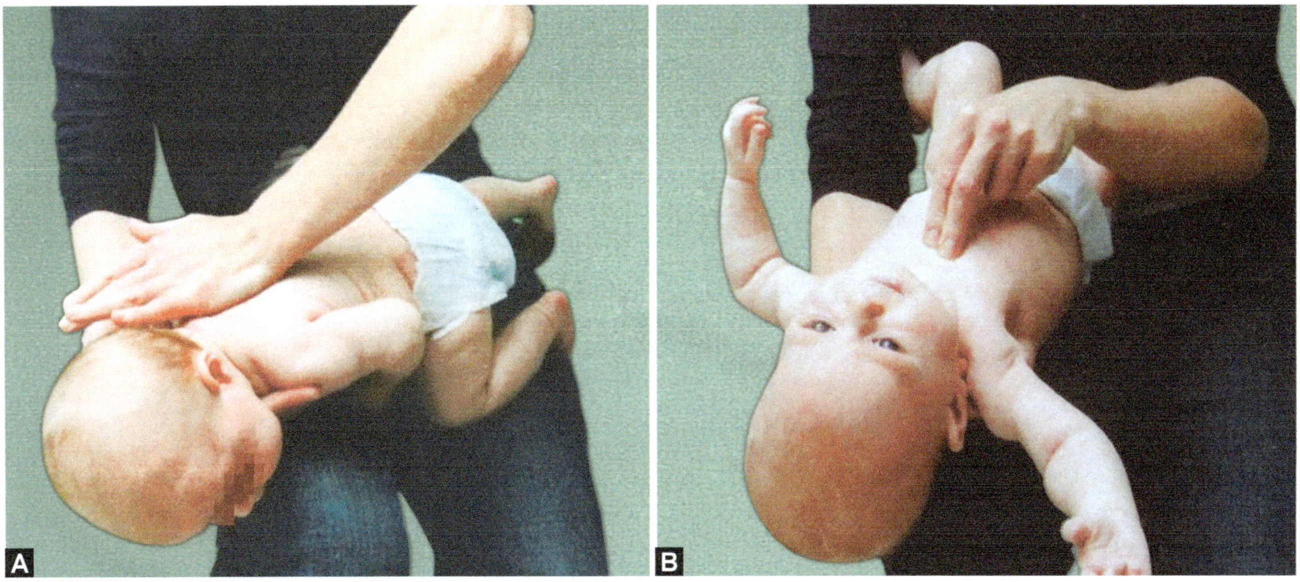

Figures 25.2A and B Back blows and chest thrusts. From Advanced Paediatric Life Support (APLS) manual.

Advanced Management of Cardiopulmonary Arrest

The key difference between BLS and advanced life support is the early assessment of underlying cardiac rhythm to identify whether defibrillation may be of benefit. Shockable rhythms are pulseless ventricular tachycardia (pVT) and ventricular fibrillation (VF). They are most likely to occur in the context of a sudden, witnessed collapse and account for approximately 5–20% of paediatric cardiac arrests and are more likely the older the child. Non-shockable rhythms are pulseless electrical activity [previously known as electromechanical dissociation (EMD)], bradycardia less than 60 beats/minute and asystole. They account for the majority of paediatric cardiac arrests and are the usual arresting rhythm in cardiac arrest in children secondary to hypoxia of whatever cause. The algorithm for APLS is demonstrated in **Flow chart 25.3**. It is important to note that BLS is initiated at the start of advanced resuscitation until monitoring has been established and the underlying rhythm analysed and as such it is important to emphasise that even advanced resuscitation practitioners should be fully competent in BLS.

During cardiopulmonary resuscitation, consideration should be given to possible reversible causes of cardiopulmonary arrest. These can be remembered by using the 4 Hs and 4 Ts approach **(Table 25.2)**:

The sequence of action in APLS is as follows:

- Commence BLS as above, providing a compression: ventilation ratio of 15:2.
- *Establish cardiac monitoring and assess cardiac rhythm:* This should be done as soon as possible and can be done by the attachment of defibrillation pads that also assess rhythm.

TABLE 25.2 4 Hs and 4 Ts approach.

4 Hs	*4 Ts*
Hypoxia	Tension pneumothorax
Hypovolemia	Toxins
Hyper/hypokalaemia	Tamponade (cardiac or pulmonary)
Hypothermia	Thrombosis (cardiac or pulmonary)

- Identify whether arrest rhythm is shockable (pulseless VT, VF) or non-shockable (pulseless electrical activity, bradycardia or asystole).
- *Shockable rhythms:* The main determinant of outcome in cardiac arrest secondary to a shockable rhythm is the time to defibrillation. For every minute delay in defibrillation, survival decreases. Defibrillation should, therefore, be attempted immediately upon identification. The defibrillation charge should be 4 J/kg for all shocks and the dose chosen should be rounded upwards in the event that the deliverable dose is not identical to that available on the defibrillator. Give one shock then immediately recommence CPR for 2 minutes before assessing rhythm on the cardiac monitor. If still in pulseless VT/VF, then give a second shock and recommence another 2 minutes CPR. Following the second shock give IV/IO adrenaline 10 μg/kg (0.1 mL/kg of 1:10,000). Recheck the rhythm again after completing 2 minutes CPR, if still in pulseless VT/VF give a third shock and recommence CPR. Following the third shock, an IV/IO dose of amiodarone 5 mg/kg should be given. Cycles of 2 minutes CPR followed by defibrillation should continue until an organised rhythm is established.

Flow chart 25.3 Advanced Paediatric Life Support algorithm.

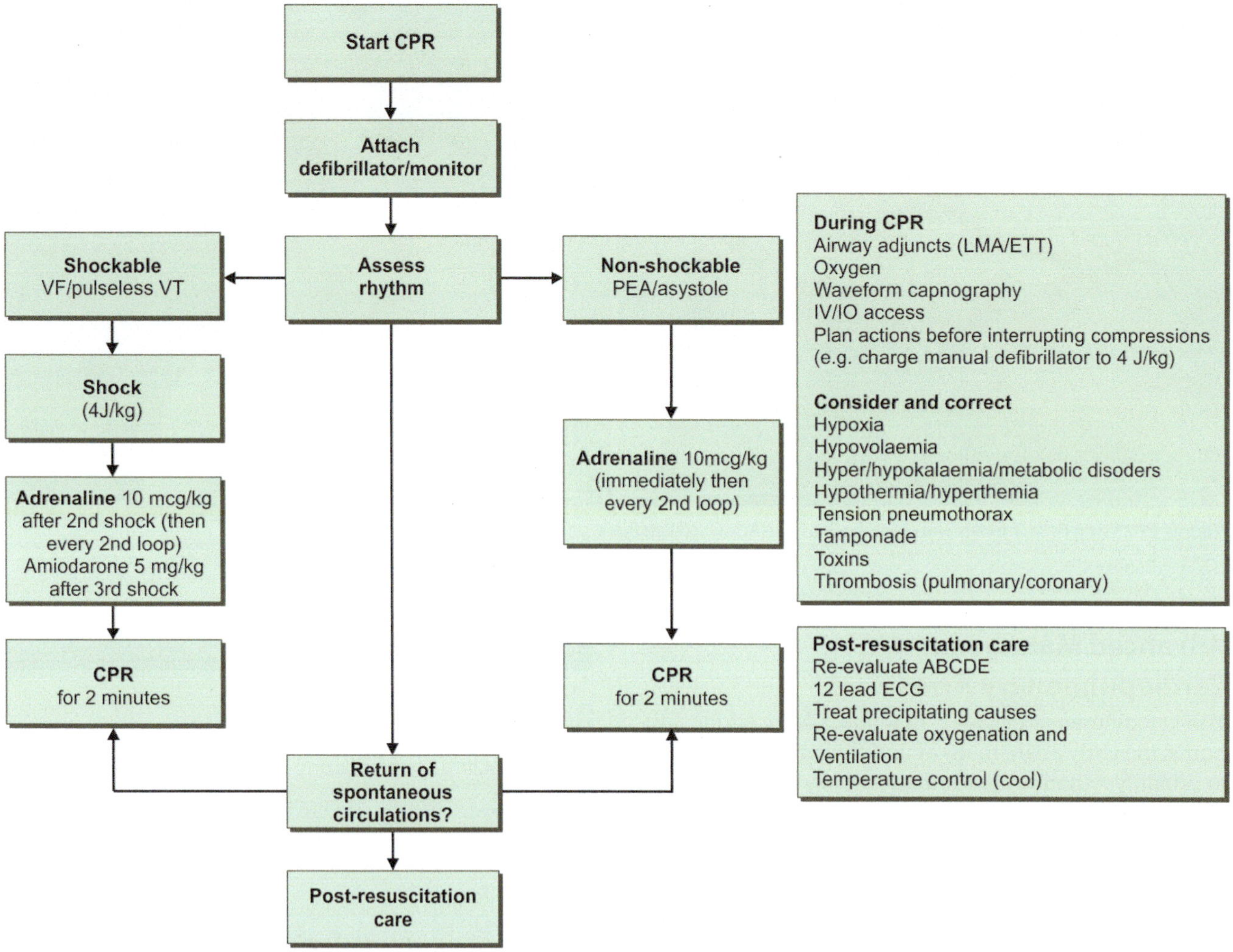

Further doses of adrenaline should be given every alternate cycle (every 3–5 minutes).

- *Non-shockable rhythm:* Continue CPR. Give adrenaline IV/IO [10 µg/kg (0.1 mL/kg of 1 in 10,000 adrenaline)] and repeat every 3–5 minutes.
- Consider the reversible causes of cardiac arrest and treat if present
- Monitor blood sugar frequently and correct any hypoglycaemia.

Newborn Life Support

More information on the management of newborns is given in Chapter 3 'Neonatal Paediatrics'. There are a number of key differences between resuscitating newborn babies and children. When born the newborn baby is small, wet and naked, this means he is prone to hypothermia very quickly, even in warm climates. It is important, therefore, to dry and warm the baby as soon as possible as it is difficult to resuscitate a baby that is hypothermic. Additionally, the main mechanism of cardiac arrest in newborn babies is usually asphyxia. The newborn infant's lungs are usually small and fluid filled. The emphasis is, therefore, upon delivering effective prolonged rescue breaths to allow adequate lung inflation thus permitting gas exchange and oxygenation to the oxygen starved brain and myocardium. The algorithm for newborn life support is shown in Flow chart 25.4.

Post-arrest Management

Following cardiac arrest the patient should be referred to the ICU for ongoing care. The key aims of management at this point are prevention of further cardiac arrest and minimisation of other end-organ damage, primarily protection of the brain. Cardiac dysfunction following cardiac arrest is common and is best managed by the use of vasoactive infusions of inotropes such dopamine, adrenaline, noradrenaline and milrinone. The risk of further cardiac arrest in the setting of arrhythmia can be minimised by optimising serum electrolyte levels and possibly the addition of antiarrhythmics such as an amiodarone infusion. Maintaining an adequate blood pressure is important in ensuring an adequate cerebral perfusion pressure in a patient group that has experienced a period of compromised cerebral blood flow during the arrest period. In patients who remain comatose there is some evidence

Flow chart 25.4 Algorithm for newborn life support from Advanced Paediatric Life Support. New Zealand Resuscitation Council and Australian Council Neonatal Resuscitation algorithm.

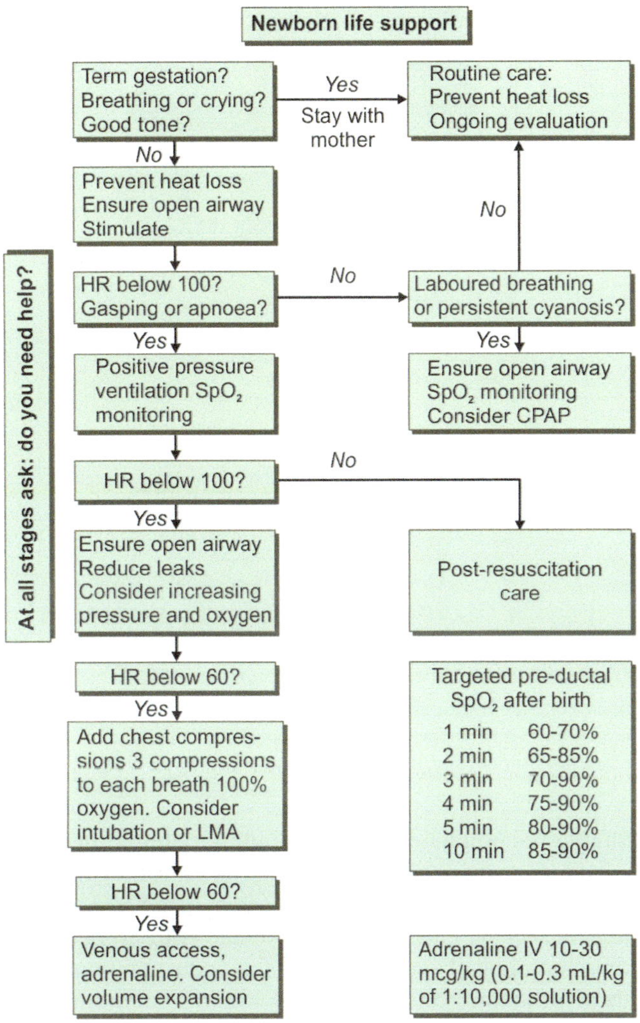

that a degree of neuroprotection may be afforded by avoiding hyperthermia and possibly inducing mild therapeutic hypothermia (32–34°C) for at least 24 hours with the use of external cooling combined with adequate sedation and muscle relaxants. Blood sugar should be monitored frequently and hypoglycaemia treated.

When to Stop Resuscitation?

The outcome following cardiac arrest in children is generally poor but is influenced by the situation of the arrest. A witnessed in-hospital VF arrest that is rapidly defibrillated may have a good outcome; an asystolic arrest out-of-hospital due to an obstructed airway generally has a poor outcome. When undertaking resuscitation, it is important to be aware that longer the resuscitation continues the less likely a favourable outcome becomes. In addition, it should be noted that survivors of prolonged resuscitations may be left with severe brain injury and significant neurodisability. Whilst every cardiopulmonary arrest is different consideration should be given to discontinuing ongoing resuscitation if the child is still requiring CPR beyond 20 minutes. The only situation in which this does not necessarily apply is that of profoundly hypothermic children who have drowned in very cold water in which favourable outcomes have been documented in prolonged resuscitations.

KEY LEARNING POINTS

- Most cardiac arrests in children are due to respiratory failure/hypoxia or cardiovascular collapse rather than primary arrhythmia.
- The Airway, Breathing and Circulation approach should be used in the management of cardiac arrest and a team approach is essential.
- Five rescue breaths should be given to any child not breathing following airway opening manoeuvres.
- Bradycardia less than 60 beats/minutes is considered a cardiac arrest in children.
- Chest compressions should be commenced within 10 seconds of recognition of cardiac arrest—if in doubt, start chest compressions.
- Chest compressions should be 'hard and fast' and the importance of full release or 'recoil' noted following each compression.
- The compression ventilation ratio should be 15:2 in all age groups, except the newborn where it is 3:1.
- Early defibrillation is critical in children with ventricular fibrillation or pulseless ventricular tachycardia.
- Practice using resuscitation mannequins and mock scenarios is important for any clinician involved in the resuscitation of sick children.

Recognition of the Sick Child and Prevention of Cardiac Arrest

It is important to be able to recognise when a child is seriously ill and therefore initiate appropriate therapy that may help prevent deterioration to the cardiac arrest situation. The process involved follows the 'Basic Structured Approach to Management' method outlined at the starting of the chapter and follows the principles of ABC. Once again it is emphasised that the key method is to identify and treat life-threatening abnormalities as they are recognised, using the ABC approach, rather than using precious time trying to identify the definitive diagnosis that can be established after the patient has been stabilised.

Airway, Breathing, and Circulation approach is carried out in the standard format as in resuscitation manuals. D for dextrose and disability and E for exposure are also added. For trauma, assessment and resuscitation are done as a primary and secondary survey.

If there are enough persons available, several procedures can be done simultaneously. In the event that only one medical officer is available, it is vital to go through ABCDE in order and correct deficits as the problems are recognised (e.g. A should be satisfactorily corrected/completed before attempting to improve B and so on). Repeated assessments should be done after performing any action to note the desired effect and if no/poor response, further treatment should be considered before proceeding to the next letter—all are recorded *in seriatum* and time oriented.

Airway

The airway is corrected with the patient in a neutral (infant) or sniffing position (children) with head tilt and chin lift (jaw thrust, without tilting, for trauma). Removal of secretions can be performed using a Yankauer sucker and visible foreign bodies in the mouth should be removed using Magill or similar forceps. Additional airway support, if necessary, can be given by the use of an oropharyngeal airway (Guedel airway) or nasopharyngeal airway. Nasopharyngeal airways should not be used in head-injured children who may have a basal skull fracture. If it is difficult to establish an airway despite these measures consideration should be given to either Laryngeal Mask Airway placement or endotracheal intubation.

Breathing

Oxygen should be delivered to all patients at maximum flow (15 L/minute) via a face mask with a non-rebreathing reservoir bag until resuscitation is complete. The addition of an inflated reservoir bag allows oxygen concentrations close to 100% to be achieved. It is important to note that simple face masks and nasal cannulae can only deliver oxygen concentrations of between 24 and 50%, irrespective of oxygen flow rate and should not be used in the resuscitation environment. Continuous monitoring of oxygen saturation (SpO_2) using a pulse oximeter applied to the finger or toe is useful to assess the severity of hypoxia and monitor response to treatment.

Air entry should be equal and adequate on both sides. Respiratory rate should be assessed as to whether it is within the normal range for a child of that age. Added sounds should be noted. Stridor suggests upper airway obstruction, wheeze suggests lower airway obstruction. Stridor should be managed with nebulised adrenaline and oral or IV dexamethasone if due to croup or antibiotics and nebulised adrenaline if due to epiglottitis. Stridor due to foreign body aspiration should be managed following the protocol documented above for Foreign Body Airway Obstruction and discussed with anaesthetic and ENT colleagues as a matter of urgency. Wheeze due to asthma should be treated with bronchodilators such as salbutamol and ipratropium with the addition of oral or IV steroids. Grunting suggests significant respiratory distress in an infant and its presence should alert the team that additional respiratory support may be required such as nasal continuous positive airway pressure (CPAP) or ventilation. Other signs suggesting significant respiratory distress include nasal flaring and subcostal, intercostal and suprasternal recession.

In the trauma patient if breathing is inadequate on one side, intra-thoracic obstruction should be considered and corrected. Tension pneumothorax should be managed with emergency needle thoracocentesis just under the midpoint of the clavicle followed by an intercostal drain (Fig. 25.3).

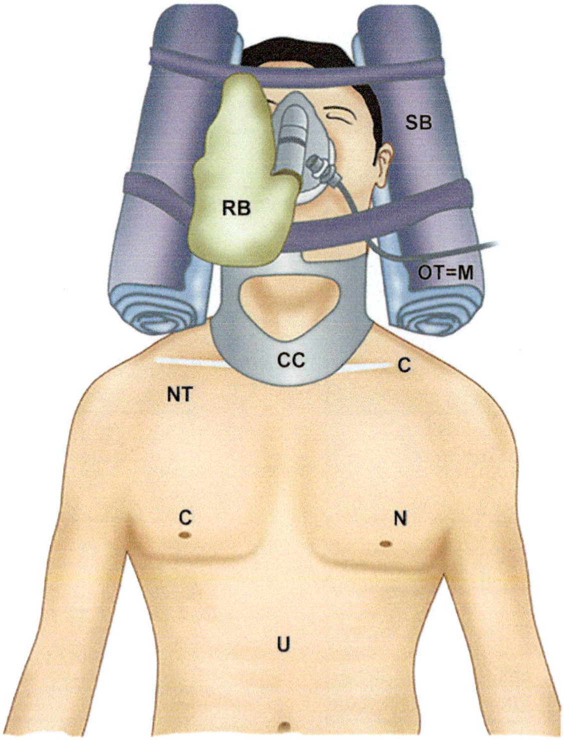

Figure 25.3 Resuscitation, needle thoracocentesis and intercostal drain.

Abbreviations: SB, sand bag; C, clavicle; CC, cervical collar; ID, intercostal drain; NT, needle thoracocentesis; N, nipple; OT=M, oxygen tube and mask; RB, reservoir bag; U, umbilicus.

Simple pneumothorax and haemothorax should be managed with an intercostal drainage placed in the fifth intercostal space (approximately the nipple line) in the mid-axillary line. A sucking effect can be prevented with an occlusive dressing applied on three sides for open pneumothorax thus preventing progression to a tension pneumothorax. Endotracheal tube ventilation may be required for a flail segment when oxygen saturation cannot be improved.

Circulation

Assessment of the circulation is based on heart rate, capillary refill time and blood pressure. Heart rate and capillary refill time are the most important of these variables. Tachycardia in children is an early sign of pending circulatory collapse and bradycardia should be treated as per cardiac arrest protocols. Unfortunately, the heart rate is also influenced by other variables such as pain, anxiety and pyrexia making its use in isolation problematic. Capillary refill time is another useful measure of circulatory adequacy. Refill times greater than 2–3 seconds are suggestive of poor tissue perfusion, particularly if associated with tachycardia or bradycardia. Blood pressure is usually maintained in children until immediately prior to circulatory collapse, and therefore the presence of a normal blood pressure does not exclude circulatory insufficiency. A dropping blood pressure is a late sign of shock and its presence requires immediate intervention.

Circulatory failure is initially treated with volume expansion. Venous access may prove difficult and if there is any delay in establishing venous access then the intraosseous route can be accessed easily and rapidly with an intraosseous needle. The fluid of choice for initial resuscitation is an isotonic crystalloid solution, e.g. 0.9% saline solution. Dextrose-containing solutions should be avoided in the resuscitation phase unless hypoglycaemia is present as they fail to remain in the circulation and can cause hyponatremia and cerebral oedema. Boluses of 0.9% saline (20 mL/kg) should be given rapidly over 5–10 minutes and response to treatment assessed after each bolus by assessing heart rate, refill time and blood pressure. Further, boluses should be administered up to 60 mL/kg total volume if necessary. If signs of circulatory failure persist despite 60 mL/kg of volume resuscitation, then inotropic drug infusions should be commenced. Dopamine, dobutamine or adrenaline infusions should be considered in the first instance. Dopamine and dobutamine have the advantage of being safely given via a peripheral line. Adrenaline should ideally be given via a central venous line, but weak concentrations can be given peripherally in the resuscitation scenario. In the case of vasodilated septic shock, the addition of noradrenaline may be useful. If more than 60 mL/kg volume replacement is required then the child should be intubated and ventilated. This is for several reasons. The administration of large volumes of fluid frequently results in pulmonary oedema, which can be easily managed with mechanical ventilation. Positive pressure ventilation also provides additional inotropic support to a failing left ventricle by reducing after load. In addition, by removing the work of breathing positive pressure ventilation reduces the metabolic demand on the body and allows the cardiac output to redistribute to other organs such as the brain, kidneys and heart. If further fluid is required, it can be administered as blood to increase the oxygen carrying capacity in addition to filling the vascular compartment. In the trauma patient, attempts should be made to control any obvious source of ongoing haemorrhage.

Do Not Ever Forget Glucose

All patients should have a blood glucose level checked. This can usually be done quickly and accurately with a near-patient glucometer machine. Children have small livers and limited glycogen stores that are rapidly depleted when unwell and as such are prone to hypoglycaemia. Additionally, infants can present collapsed with hypoglycaemia as part of a metabolic disorder. If the finger prick blood monitoring and/or laboratory blood sugar is below 3 mmol/L, a bolus injection of glucose should be administered. The dose is as follows:

2 mL/kg of 10% dextrose (0.2 g/kg)

Maintenance fluids should contain dextrose (e.g. 0.45% saline + 5% dextrose) to avoid hypoglycaemia and should be commenced as soon as possible if the child is not able to eat or drink.

Disability

It can be assessed using Glasgow coma score (GCS) and/or alert, response to voice/pain or unresponsive (AVPU), size, reaction and equality of both pupils and neurological examination, including the position of the patient (decorticate or decerebrate). Though many are important, oxygen and blood sugar are the two most vital elements to sustain some basic cerebral functions. The brain can be insulted by many different ways, but reduced oxygen and sugar will derange the brain sufficiently to disturb all other functions. Sufficient oxygen should be made available to the brain, by effective oxygenation and oxygen delivery using the ABC approach. Fixed pupils and abnormal posturing are ominous signs that suggest raised intracranial pressure. In their presence, mannitol should be given and arrangements should be made for urgent transfer to the CT scanner whilst the neurosurgical team is contacted.

Exposure

The team can cut the clothes and remove the footwear so that ABCD can be assessed better. When the patient is lying, supine examination can be done for only 50% of the body. It should be remembered that there is another 50% to be examined on the dorsal aspect in case other significant injuries are missed. Coordinated effort to turn the patient as 'log roll' (three or four persons according to the size of the patient) allow safe examination of the patients back and preserve the existing neurological function even in the presence of vertebral injury.

KEY LEARNING POINTS

- Recognition of the sick child is a critical component of emergency paediatric care.
- Management should be based on an Airway, Breathing, and Circulation approach and problems dealt with as they are encountered.
- High-flow oxygen should be given via a face mask with an inflated reservoir bag.
- A normal blood pressure does not mean that the circulation is adequate.
- Hypotension is a late, pre-terminal sign and needs immediate treatment.
- Volume resuscitation should be given with 0.9% saline or other isotonic fluid.
- Dextrose-containing fluids should not be given for volume resuscitation.
- Bolus IV dextrose should only be given if the child is hypoglycaemic.
- Hypoglycaemia is common in sick children. Blood sugar should be monitored frequently and treated if found to be low.
- Commence inotropes if >60 mL/kg volume resuscitation is required and consider intubation and ventilation early if no response to therapy.
- An urgent CT head scan and neurosurgical referral is important in children.

PAEDIATRIC EMERGENCIES

Sepsis

Infection and septicaemia are one of the leading causes of death in childhood. The range of organisms that cause septicaemia is wide and the initial presentation is often non-specific with parents reporting symptoms such as poor feeding, lethargy or irritability, fever and rash **(Fig. 25.4)**. The onset may be very rapid over the space of a few hours or more insidious over several days. Some organisms have a distinctive pattern of presentation, e.g. meningococcal sepsis due to *Neisseria meningitidis* frequently presents with the rapid onset of a spreading, non-blanching purpuric rash making diagnosis relatively simple. Other organisms, particularly in young children, often present in a more non-specific manner, e.g. Group B streptococcal infection in a newborn may present simply with poor feeding and lethargy. Fever in infants less than 3 months old should be assumed to be due to bacterial sepsis until proven otherwise. This means that the early initiation of a broad spectrum antimicrobial agent (e.g. a third-generation cephalosporin) is essential until culture results are available **(Table 25.3)**.

The approach to resuscitation in sepsis follows the ABC approach outlined above and is identical irrespective of the organism. The main system involved is often circulatory collapse and as such large volumes of isotonic fluid resuscitation are often required. Early, aggressive fluid resuscitation has been demonstrated to improve outcomes and is a priority. A low threshold for the early use of inotropes (if requiring more than 60 mL/kg fluid resuscitation) and referral to intensive care for mechanical ventilation is important as patients with sepsis can frequently deteriorate rapidly. Resuscitation efforts can be assessed by looking at factors such as heart rate, capillary refill time, blood pressure, urine output and blood parameters such as blood lactate levels and mixed venous saturation **(Figs. 25.5A to D)**. The strategy of aggressive fluid

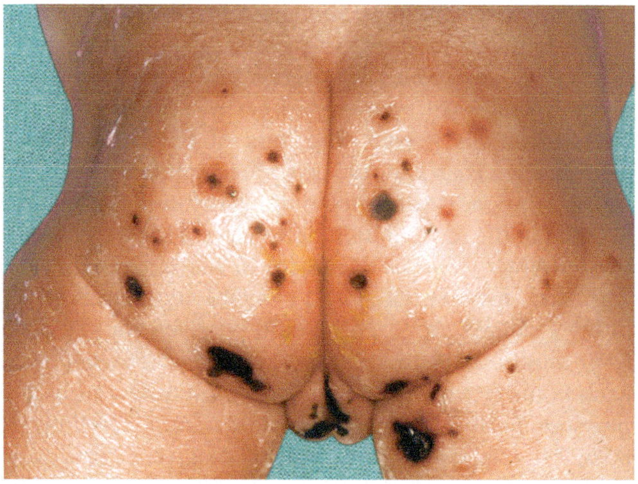

Figure 25.4 Meningococcal septicaemia.

resuscitation combined with the use of inotropes and mechanical ventilation if required is known as 'Early goal-directed therapy'. As mentioned earlier, antibiotics should be given early (within minutes of arrival in the emergency department and absolutely within 1 hour) as any delay in their administration is associated with increased mortality. If possible blood cultures should be obtained prior to administration of antibiotics to guide later therapy although antibiotics should not be delayed if obtaining cultures is difficult. If the patient is first seen in the community, antibiotics (e.g. intramuscular benzyl penicillin) should be administered whilst waiting for the ambulance service.

A raised white cell count and C-reactive protein (CRP) level are often seen in sepsis, although in patients with severe sepsis the white cell count is frequently depressed and the CRP level may be unremarkable. If the focus of infection is unclear, particularly in infants, a septic screen including urine culture and lumbar puncture should be performed. In patients presenting unwell with shock, antibiotics should be given early, and lumbar puncture should be delayed until they are stable. In addition to the blood

TABLE 25.3 Common organisms and antibiotic cover related to age.

Age group	*Common organisms*	*Antibiotic*	*Dose*
0–3 months	Group B *Streptococcus*, *Escherichia coli*, *Listeria monocytogenes*	Ampicillin or benzylpenicillin PLUS cefotaxime	50 mg/kg (maximum 2 g) 4 hourly 60 mg/kg (maximum 2.4 g) * 50 mg/kg (maximum 2 g) 6 hourly
3 month–16 years	*Neisseria meningitidis* *Haemophilus influenzae*	Cefotaxime or ceftriaxone	50 mg/kg (maximum 2 g) 6 hourly 100 mg/kg (maximum 4 g) 12 hourly
Any age	*Streptococcus pneumoniae*	ADD vancomycin to above regime if *Streptococcus pneumoniae* is suspected	15 mg/kg (maximum 500 mg) 6 hourly
	Herpes simplex infection suspected	ADD acyclovir to above regime if HSV suspected	20 mg/kg

*Rate dependent of age first week of life 12 hourly, 2–4 weeks 6–8 hourly, greater than 4 weeks 4 hourly.

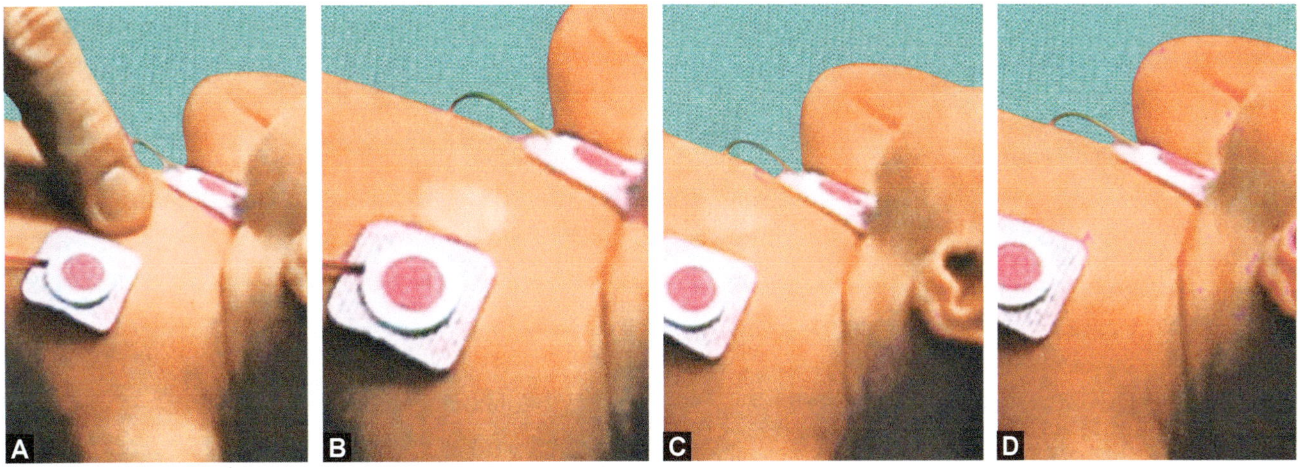

Figures 25.5A to D Capillary refill assessment from Advanced Paediatric Life Support manual.

test taken during resuscitation, the following blood tests are needed in the septic child: calcium, magnesium, phosphate, coagulation screen. Electrolyte and acid base abnormalities can have deleterious effect on myocardial function.

It is difficult to manage a serious ill-patient requiring mechanical ventilation and inotropic support without intensive care facilities and invasive monitoring. Therefore, a paediatric ICU must be involved early to give advice and retrieve the patient, if these treatments are required.

KEY LEARNING POINTS

- Presentation of sepsis in children is often non-specific.
- Fever in an infant less than 3 months old should be treated as bacterial sepsis until proven otherwise.
- Broad-spectrum antibiotics should be given as soon as possible—do not delay therapy waiting for laboratory results.
- Resuscitation should follow the Airway, Breathing, and Circulation approach.
- Early aggressive fluid resuscitation is critical in children with septic shock.
- A low threshold should exist for the use of inotropic drugs and early referral to intensive care.
- Once the definitive diagnosis has been established the antibiotics should be altered to a narrower spectrum.

Diabetes

Hypoglycaemia

Symptomatic hypoglycaemia (confusion, jitteriness, seizures and coma) should be corrected when the glucose stick test [finger/heel prick blood sugar level (BSL)] indicates blood sugar less than 4mmol/L.

When treating hypoglycaemia, if the child is conscious and cooperative use

- 1 glass of oral glucose solution.
- If the child is unconscious use
- Glucagon 0.5 mg subcutaneous or intramuscular (if weight <25 kg) or 1 mg (weight >25 kg)
- Followed by oral feeding ONLY when conscious
- If the child is unconscious and in hospital:
- Bolus of glucose 2 mL/kg of 10% dextrose IV.
- Followed by a glucose infusion 3–5 mL/kg/hour of 10% dextrose to maintain BSL greater than 4.0
- Maintain BSL 4–8

Blood sugar levels should be checked every 30 minutes initially and then every 60 minutes until BSL greater than 5 for two consecutive hours. They check BSL every 2–4 hours. Do not use glucose 50% as this has caused deaths in children due to hyperosmolality.

Diabetic Ketoacidosis

The risk of diabetic ketoacidosis (DKA) in patients with known diabetes mellitus is 1–10% per patient per year. This risk is increased in patients with poor diabetic control. DKA at initial diagnosis of diabetes is more common in children less than 5 years old. The mortality rate in the developed world is approximately 0.13–0.15% and cerebral oedema is the mode of death in most instances. DKA is a condition in which a relative or absolute lack of insulin leads to the inability to metabolise insulin. This leads to hyperglycaemia and osmotic diuresis. Once urine output exceeds the ability of the patient to drink, dehydration occurs. In addition without insulin, fat is used as a source of energy, resulting in the production of large quantities of ketones and metabolic acidosis.

The biochemical criteria for DKA are as follows:

- Hyperglycaemia greater than 11 mmol/L
- Venous pH less than 7.3 or plasma bicarbonate less than 15 mmol/L
- Ketonaemia or ketonuria.

Assessment

- Degree of dehydration:
  - Mild less than 4%: no signs
  - Moderate 4–7%: reduced skin turgor, poor capillary return (*see* **Figs. 25.5A to D**)
  - Severe greater than 7%: poor perfusion, rapid pulse, reduced blood pressure
- Level of consciousness
- Insert IV lines to obtain blood for:
  - Blood glucose
  - Venous blood gas including bicarbonate
  - Urea and electrolytes (sodium, potassium, magnesium, phosphate, calcium)
  - Glucose (laboratory and bedside)
  - Ketones
  - Haemoglobin and WCC differential

Urine

Ketones and cultures: The basic goals of therapy are to correct dehydration, correct acidosis and reverse ketosis, restore blood glucose to near normal and avoid complications of therapy. It is important to recognise that correction of DKA should be a gradual process over approximately 48 hours as rapid correction of blood glucose and excessive fluid administration is associated with an increased risk of cerebral oedema. National and international guidelines exist to aid the management of DKA.

The key features of the management of DKA are as follows:

- *Airway:* Secure airway, if unconscious/severely obtunded, consider NG tube to avoid aspiration
- *Breathing:* Oxygen if peripherally shutdown
- *Circulation:* Cardiac monitoring watch for signs of electrolyte abnormalities

Fluids

Fluid Bolus

Fluid boluses are only given to reverse signs of shock. If shocked: Give 10 mL/kg 0.9% saline fluid bolus slowly and then reassess.

Commence Rehydration

Rehydration after reversal of signs of shock should be given with replacement fluids over 48 hours. Resuscitation fluids up to 20 mL/kg are given in addition to replacement fluids, anything over 20 mL/kg should be subtracted from the total fluid replacement volume.

When calculating fluid replacement, assume 5% (mild to moderate) dehydration/deficit in patients with a pH of equal to or greater than 7.1 and 10% (severe) dehydration in patients who have a pH of <7.1. The deficit volume equals the percentage dehydration times the child's bodyweight.

To calculate the maintenance fluid in DKA, you should use these "reduced volume" rules. This is to help prevent cerebral oedema in these patients.

- Weight less than 10 kg, give 2 mL/kg/h
- Weight between 10 and 40 kg, give 1 mL/kg/h
- Weight greater than 40 kg, give a fixed volume of 40 mL/h

Therefore, the total replacement fluid to be given over 48 hours:

Hourly rate = (deficit/48 hours) + maintenance per hour

Further Management

Insulin: Do not start insulin until IV fluids have been running for at least 1 hour.

This is because restoration of circulating blood volume often results in a significant reduction in blood glucose due to a combination of improved glomerular filtration rate and dilution. Commencing insulin early may accelerate the rapid drop in blood sugar and increase the risk of cerebral oedema. The aim is to reduce the blood sugar slowly and to prevent drops of greater than 5 mmol/L per hour.

- *Commence Insulin at a dosage between 0.05 and 0.1 units/kg/hour:* The insulin infusion should normally remain at 0.1 units/kg/hour to slowly normalise blood sugar and suppress lipolysis, ketogenesis and acidosis.
- *50 units soluble insulin added to 50 mL 0.9% saline = 1 unit/mL.*
- *Run infusion at 0.1 units/kg per hour (equivalent to 0.1 mL/kg per hour)*
- *Ongoing management:*
- Recheck biochemistry, blood pH, laboratory glucose 2 hours after the start of resuscitation and then every 4 hours.
- Accurate documentation of fluid balance is important. All urine needs to be measured and all fluid input must be charted (even oral fluids).
- Continuing cardiac monitoring to check for electrolyte-induced arrhythmias.
- *Avoid bicarbonate:* The acidosis seen in DKA is as a result of ketoacid production and dehydration. It slowly resolves with the administration of insulin and fluid. There is no clinical benefit from the use of bicarbonate and its use may be associated with an increased risk of cerebral oedema. The only occasion when bicarbonate may be useful is in selected patients with severe acidosis (pH <6.9) with resulting haemodynamic compromise.
- *Monitor for signs of complications*
- *Cerebral Oedema:* The mechanism of cerebral oedema in DKA is complex and not fully understood. It is associated with excessive fluid administration, rapid changes in blood glucose and effective

osmolality, although it is also seen in patients who have received no therapy. Cerebral oedema usually presents clinically 4–12 hours after starting treatment but can be seen at any time from diagnosis up to 48 hours later. Clinical features include headache, vomiting, altered level of consciousness, cranial nerve palsies and abnormal posturing. Management is with mannitol and referral to intensive care for intubation and ventilation.

- *Hypoglycaemia and hypokalaemia:* Avoid by careful monitoring and adjustment of infusion rates. Consideration should be given to adding more glucose if blood glucose falling quickly even if still above 4 mmol/L.
- *Systemic infections:* Antibiotics are not given as a routine unless a severe bacterial infection is suspected.
- *Aspiration pneumonia:* Avoid by nasogastric tube in vomiting child with impaired consciousness.
- *Treat underlying cause:* In some cases, DKA may be precipitated by an underlying condition such as an infection. If such a cause is identified it should be treated.

KEY LEARNING POINTS

- The aim is to correct blood sugar and dehydration slowly over 48 hours.
- Insulin should be run at 0.1 units/kg/hour.
- Avoid hypotonic fluids.
- Be aware of hypokalaemia.
- Do not routinely use bicarbonate therapy.
- The biggest risk of death is cerebral oedema.
- Look for and treat underlying precipitating reasons for diabetic ketoacidosis such as infection.

Poisoning

Iron, tricyclic antidepressants, opiates, paracetamol, salicylates, etc. are some of the commonly ingested medications with high fatality rates. In any unconscious child without a clear history suggestive of illness ingestions of medications or toxins should be considered.

The patient should be stabilised and deficits of A, B, C, D, E addressed while waiting for the results of poison profile tests in blood and urine when the medications or toxins are unknown. Specific antidotes should be given in appropriate doses when the substance is identified. E.g. *N*-acetylcysteine in paracetamol overdose. Charcoal should be used carefully in certain indications and not as routine. It must not be used unless the airway is secure as aspiration of charcoal can result in significant lung injury. Whole bowel irrigation has a limited role in treatment of some slow release preparations. Gastric lavage has a very limited role in treatment and should not be used without consultation. Specific antidotes may be available and serum drug levels may help in treatment decisions.

Accidental ingestion is more common in infants and young children although deliberate ingestions are not uncommon in older/teenage children (Chapter 15 "Accidental Poisoning in Childhood").

Seizures

Seizures are common in childhood and a common cause of presentation to the emergency department. The commonest cause of seizures in childhood is a simple febrile convulsion, which often resolves spontaneous without intervention. The differential diagnosis, however, includes hypoglycaemia, meningitis or encephalitis, epilepsy, hypertensive encephalopathy and raised intracranial pressure. It is important to note that whilst the differential may be diverse, the initial management is identical in all cases and involves following the ABC approach outlined earlier and the Emergency Treatment of Convulsion protocol outlined in **(Flow chart 25.5)**.

The key components of the Emergency Treatment of Convulsion protocol are as follows:

- Commence high-flow oxygen and check blood sugar as soon as possible. Treat any hypoglycaemia.
- Insert an IV cannula and give IV lorazepam (0.1 mg/kg). If IV access is not possible, then rectal diazepam (0.5 mg/kg) or buccal midazolam (0.5 mg/kg) can be given. Lorazepam is the initial drug of choice if an IV line is available as it is equally efficacious as diazepam at terminating seizures but has a longer duration of action and causes less respiratory depression than diazepam. Buccal midazolam is fast acting and effective but its duration of action is less than lorazepam. The correct dose can be drawn up from the IV preparation and injected (without an attached needle) into the buccal mucosa between the gum and bottom lip. This method of administration is easier and more socially acceptable than the rectal route for diazepam, although rectal diazepam remains an effective alternative.
- *Wait for 10 minutes:* This is important as in many cases the seizure will terminate if the drugs are given time to work. If further doses of benzodiazepine are given before 10 minutes the chance of respiratory depression is increased. If this occurs, it can usually be managed with simple airway opening manoeuvres and bag or mask ventilation.
- If vascular access is still not available, give another dose or Midazolam IM, buccal or intranasally a dose of rectal paraldehyde should be given. This should be made up in equal volumes of saline or olive oil. It is frequently stated that paraldehyde needs to be given in a glass syringe. This is not necessary and paraldehyde can be drawn up in a plastic syringe so long as it is not allowed to stand in the plastic syringe for more than a few minutes.

Flow chart 25.5 Status epilepticus algorithm from APLS manual.

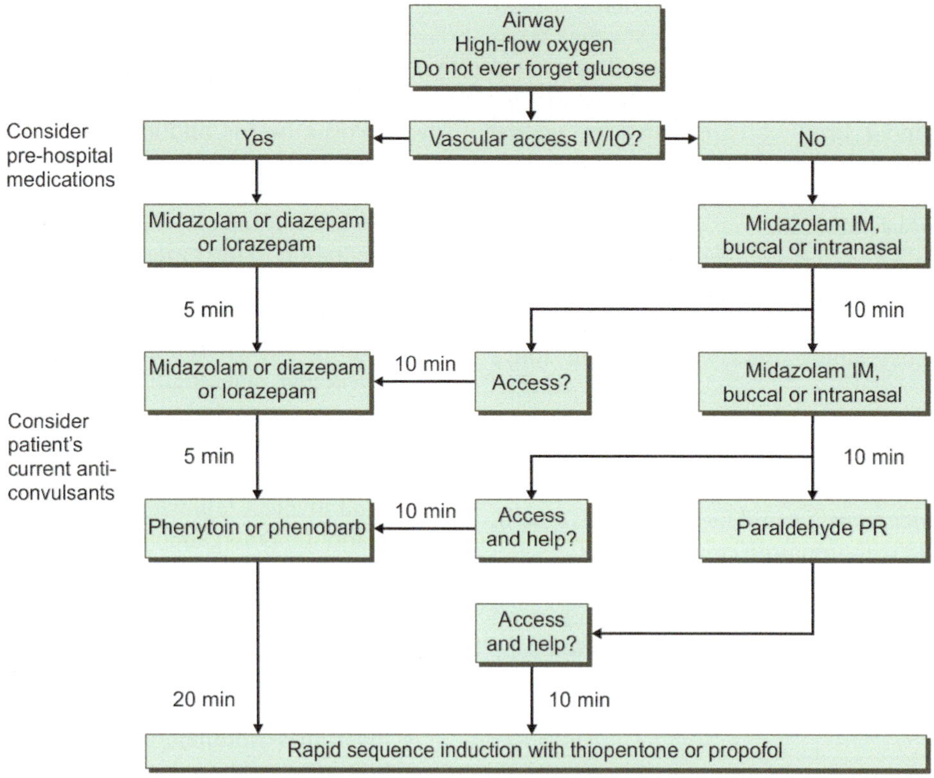

- If venous access is available, then a second dose of lorazepam should be given after 10 minutes.
- If still seizing after another 10 minutes (total 20 minutes since first dose of lorazepam or midazolam/diazepam), then an IV loading dose of phenytoin should be given over 30 minutes. If paraldehyde has not been given at this stage, it should be given whilst the phenytoin is being prepared.
- If after administration of phenytoin the child is still fitting, then the child will required to be intubated and ventilated using thiopentone as an induction agent. Normally, this would not be done until approximately 40–50 minutes after the first dose of benzodiazepine as time must be given for subsequent doses of lorazepam, paraldehyde and phenytoin to work. An anaesthetist or intensivist should be involved at this stage as ongoing care will be required in the ICU.
- Treat the underlying cause, e.g. antibiotics in meningitis (do not do a lumbar puncture in a fitting child or child with reduced level of consciousness!). Most cases of simple febrile convulsion require no further treatment once the seizure has been terminated.

It is important to recognise the difference between seizures and abnormal posturing (decorticate or decerebrate) due to raised intracranial pressure. In the event of raised intracranial pressure management should be directed towards reducing the intracranial pressure with intravenous mannitol, intubation or ventilation, urgent CT brain imaging and neurosurgical intervention.

The medications for seizing child have been mentioned in **Table 25.4**.

KEY LEARNING POINTS

- Approach the convulsing child with the usual Airway, Breathing, and Circulation approach.
- Check blood sugar early as hypoglycaemia can result in seizures.
- Allow anticonvulsant drugs time to work—too rapid administration of further doses of benzodiazepines are likely to cause respiratory depression.
- Be aware that abnormal posturing with reduced level of consciousness may result from raised intracranial pressure and may be confused with a simple seizure.
- Treat the underlying cause.

Respiratory Distress

Reduction in the diameter of the airway is a common reason for acute respiratory distress in the paediatric age. Larger airways like the trachea and bronchi may be narrowed due to infection such as croup (laryngotracheobronchitis), epiglottitis or bacterial tracheitis as well as foreign bodies or tumours. Smaller airways may be narrowed in conditions such as asthma or bronchiolitis. It is

TABLE 25.4 Medications for seizing child.

Drug	Route	Dose	Comments
Midazolam	IV/IO IM Buccal Intranasal	0.15 mg/kg 0.2 mg/kg 0.5 mg/kg 0.5 mg/kg	Maximum 10 mg. Takes affect within minutes but shorter duration of affect than lorazepam. Can depress respiration, particularly if repeated dosing. Is usually short lived and is usually easily managed with bag-mask-valve ventilatory support. IM midazolam more effective than buccal or intranasal routes
Diazepam	IV/IO PR	0.25 mg/kg 0.5 mg/kg	Maximum 10 mg. Rapid onset, duration less than 1 hour. Well-absorbed rectally. Widely used but may now be superseded by the more effective midazolam or lorazepam
Lorazepam	IV/IO	0.1 mg/kg	Maximum 4 mg, equally or more effective than midazolam and diazepam, possibly less respiratory depression. Longer duration of action (12–24 hours)
Phenytoin	IV/IO	20 mg/kg	Maximum 1 g. Gives over 20 minutes, made up in 0.9% NaCl to a maximum concentration of 10 mg in 1 mL. Can cause dysrhythmias and hypotension, therefore monitor blood pressure and electrocardiography. Little depressant effect on respiration
Phenobarbitone	IV/IO	20 mg/kg	Maximum 1 g. Give over 20 minutes. Ensure airway support available, often causes respiratory depression, monitor blood pressure
Paraldehyde	PR	0.4 mL/kg	Maximum 10 mL. Make up as 50:550 solution in olive oil to 0.9% NaCl. Avoid intramuscular use as it causes severe pain and can lead to abscess formation. Avoid in liver disease. Takes 10–15 minutes to act, sustained for 2–4 hours. Do not leave paraldehyde standing in plastic syringes for longer than a few minutes
Thiopentone	IV/IO	3–5 mg/kg	Suitable for anaesthetic option for RSI
Propofol	IV/IO	2–4 mg/kg	Suitable for anaesthetic option for RSI
Suxomethonium	IV/IO	1–2 mg/kg	Short acting muscle relaxation in RSI

Abbreviation: RSI, rapid sequence intubation.

important to remember that resistance to gas flow in the airway is inversely proportional to the airway radius to the power of 4 ($1/r^4$) and as such even small reductions in radius can result in a significant reduction in gas flow. As a general rule, upper airway obstruction results in stridor and lower airway obstruction in wheeze. Severe infection such as pneumonia affects the parenchymal function and reduces the airspace available for gas exchange (**Fig. 25.6**).

Epiglottitis

Due to compulsory vaccination against *Haemophilus influenza* B, the incidence of epiglottitis is declining in many countries, but this remains a life-threatening disease in the unvaccinated childhood population. Acute respiratory distress not settling or rapidly progressing over a few hours accompanied by stridor should alert the practitioner as to the possibility of epiglottitis. Other features such as a sick 'toxic looking' child, high fever and the inability to speak or whisper, especially if accompanied by drooling due to inability to swallow secretions should help differentiate epiglottitis from croup. In such a compromised airway, care needs to be taken to prevent progression to complete airway obstruction. As such, it is important to avoid upsetting the child. For example, no attempt should be made to examine the child's throat or remove the child from their parent. Immediate explanation and oxygen by mask, held by mother, whilst administering nebulised adrenaline should be attempted while awaiting arrival of an anaesthetist and ENT surgeon to secure the airway with intubation or possibly

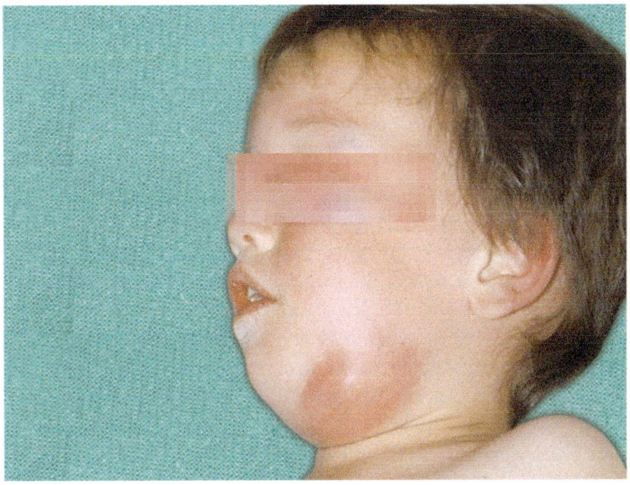

Figure 25.6 Child in respiratory distress from acute lymphadenitis of the neck.

tracheostomy or needle cricothyroidotomy. A cephalosporin, such as cefotaxime and steroids, should be given when the airway is controlled.

KEY LEARNING POINTS

- Epiglottitis is a medical emergency.
- Give high-flow oxygen and nebulised adrenaline.
- Do not examine the child's throat.
- Call anaesthesia and ENT as an emergency.
- Start IV cefotaxime.

Croup (Laryngotracheobronchitis)

Croup typically presents with barking cough, hoarseness and respiratory distress. It affects the upper airways where the proximal air passages become narrowed due to inflammation and oedema of the mucosa. It is either spasmodic or viral (laryngotracheobronchitis). Viral croup can be caused by many viruses but most commonly: parainfluenza 1/2, respiratory syncytial virus (RSV) and adenoviruses. Most hospital admissions are in children aged 6 months to 5 years. Viral croup presents as above but is usually preceded by fever and coryzal symptoms for 1–3 days. The severity of the disease can be split into mild/moderate/severe depending on the presence of stridor and respiratory distress. Hypoxia is an indicator of pending complete obstruction of the airway.

Management

- STAT dose of dexamethasone (oral 0.15 mg/kg). Prednisolone can be used as an alternative, however not as effective. Steroids alter the natural history of croup and lead to less hospital admissions and decreased numbers of intubations. They can have an effect after 30 minutes. Nebulised budesonide 2 mg can be used as an alternative if oral treatment not tolerated.
- If harsh stridor present, nebulised adrenaline 0.5 mL/kg 1:1,000 (up to 5 mL) should be administered. This will provide some short-term relief as it reduces the clinical severity of the obstruction.
- High-flow oxygen via face mask, monitor saturations
- In severe disease, senior help should be sought quickly, especially if child not improving quickly.

KEY LEARNING POINTS

- Treat croup with oral, IV or nebulised steroids. If respiratory distress is present, nebulised adrenaline may be useful.
- The presence of hypoxia is an emergency as it suggests pending complete airway obstruction.

Asthma

Acute exacerbation of asthma is one of the commonest respiratory presentations to the emergency department.

TABLE 25.5 Assessment of asthma.

Acute severe	*Life threatening*
Too breathless to talk/feed	Exhaustion (pre-terminal event)
RR	Poor respiratory effort
>30 breaths/minute (>5 years)	Silent chest
>50 breaths/minute (2–5 years)	Hypotension
Heart rate	Decreased Glasgow coma score or agitated
>120 bpm (>5 years)	
>130 bpm (2–5 years)	

Upper respiratory viral illness is the biggest precipitant. It is approached using the usual ABC approach.
Those at high risk of serious illness are indicated below:

- Long duration of symptoms
- Poor response to treatment
- Previous ICU admissions/intubation
- Poor compliance with therapy

Symptoms of severe/life-threatening asthma are outline in (Table 25.5).

It is important to initiate early, aggressive therapy. If the patient responds favourably, then treatment can be reduced. The key features of the management of asthma are as follows:

- High-flow oxygen via face mask and reservoir bag if saturation is less than 92%
- Give short-acting beta-agonist (salbutamol). If well and maintaining SpO_2 greater than 92%:
- Ten puffs via metered dose inhaler (MDI) with spacer. If the child is unwell and requires oxygen, salbutamol should be given via an oxygen-driven nebuliser (2.5 mg in </=5 year olds, 5 mg in >5 year olds). The nebuliser or MDI is given as required depending on response to treatment
- Give oral prednisolone (1–2 mg/kg) or IV hydrocortisone (4 mg/kg) if unable to use the oral route.
- Add nebulised ipratropium bromide (250 µg </= 5 years, 500 µg >5 years) if not responding to treatment. This can be repeated at 20 minute intervals, to a total of three doses.

If poor response to therapy or deterioration considers the following:

- Bolus IV salbutamol followed by continuous infusion salbutamol 1–5 µg/kg/minute
- Bolus IV aminophylline 10 mg/kg followed by continuous infusion
- Bolus IV magnesium sulphate 50 mg/kg over 20 minutes
- Ensure constant electrocardiography monitoring, contact paediatric ICU and senior anaesthetic support.

- If not responding or deteriorating then refer to intensive care for trial of either non-invasive mask ventilation (CPAP) or intubation and invasive ventilation.

Investigations such as chest X-ray are rarely helpful in mild/moderate asthma unless pneumothorax is suspected. Likewise, antibiotics are rarely indicated unless it is felt that the exacerbation has been triggered by a bacterial infection.

KEY LEARNING POINTS

- The asthmatic child unable to talk in an emergency. Exhaustion is a pre-terminal event.
- Treat acute exacerbations of asthma aggressively then de-escalate therapy as the child improves.
- Salbutamol administration via an inhaler and spacer is the delivery mechanism of choice in the non-oxygen-dependent child. If the child is oxygen-dependent, salbutamol should be given via an oxygen-driven nebuliser.
- Start steroids early.
- Consider IV therapy if the child is not improving.

Bronchiolitis

Bronchiolitis occurs in 10% of all infants and 2–3% are admitted to hospital. It is rare after 1 year of age with the most common age group being 1–9 months. The most common cause is RSV, but it can also be caused by parainfluenza and adenovirus. Low-grade fever and coryzal symptoms are the prodrome for dry cough and increasing work of breathing.

Hypoxia can be resulted when the small air passages are further narrowed due to inflammation in young babies and infants. Most of the patients can be managed at home but may require hospitalisation if hypoxia and/or feeding is sufficiently interfered. Risk factors for severe bronchiolitis are as follows:

- Less than 6 weeks of age
- Premature birth
- Chronic lung disease
- Immunodeficiency

Management is supportive:

- Assess ABC
- Clear airway; suction can be used gently to clear nasal passages.
- High-flow oxygen. Maintain SpO_2 at 94–98%. If mild/moderate illness, nasal cannulae can be used
- Humidified oxygen should be considered
- Hydration should be maintained in NG tube if not tolerating feeds. Intravenous hydration should be kept at two-thirds of maintenance; infants with broncholitis are prone to SIADH (raised levels of antidiuretic hormone).

Monitor:

- SpO_2 levels
- Apnoeic episodes (especially in those <2 months old)

Non-invasive ventilation (CPAP) can be used in those infants failing to improve on oxygen. Mechanical ventilation with intubation may be required in infants with the following:

- Recurrent apnoea
- Exhaustion
- Severe hypercapnia/hypoxia
- There is no evidence for the use of bronchodilators, steroids or antibiotics.

Moderately, ill infants can be treated with high-flow oxygen (mask and reservoir bag) until stabilised when nasal prong oxygen usually suffices. Fluid and nutrition is best managed with nasogastric tube feeding, if too breathless to feed. Intravenous fluids are rarely required. It is important to realise that unwell infants with bronchiolitis tend to have raised levels of antidiuretic hormone (SIADH) and are, therefore, at risk of hyponatremia. Once any element of shock has been reversed, it is important to moderately restrict fluid input (approximately 75–80% normal maintenance) until the child is well enough to feed themselves and thus regulate their own fluid balance. If the infant fails to respond to nasal prong oxygen the use of nasal CPAP is often useful. Patients who fail to respond to nasal CPAP should be treated with endotracheal tube ventilation and transferred to ICU after stabilising. Disappointingly, there is little evidence to suggest benefit of any other therapies. Antibiotics and steroids are not considered beneficial, although there is some emerging evidence that the combination of nebulised adrenaline plus oral dexamethasone may help reduce in-patient admissions from the emergency department.

Anaphylaxis

Anaphylaxis is a life-threatening allergic reaction that can occur to a wide variety of stimuli and may occur at any age. Common allergens that may precipitate anaphylaxis include nuts, milk, other foods and some common medications, e.g. penicillin. The management remains the same irrespective of the precipitating allergen and is shown in Figure 30.8.

The key factors involved in any anaphylactic reaction are as follows:

- Airway swelling and obstruction
- Circulatory collapse

Airway swelling can occur at any level of the respiratory tract from the lips to the larynx (causing laryngeal oedema, stridor and airway obstruction) to the distal airways causing wheeze identical to asthma. Circulatory collapse and shock occur secondary to profound vasodilatation, resulting from the release of histamine and other vasoactive inflammatory mediators.

Flow chart 25.6 Anaphylaxis algorithm.

(*Source:* From NSW health)

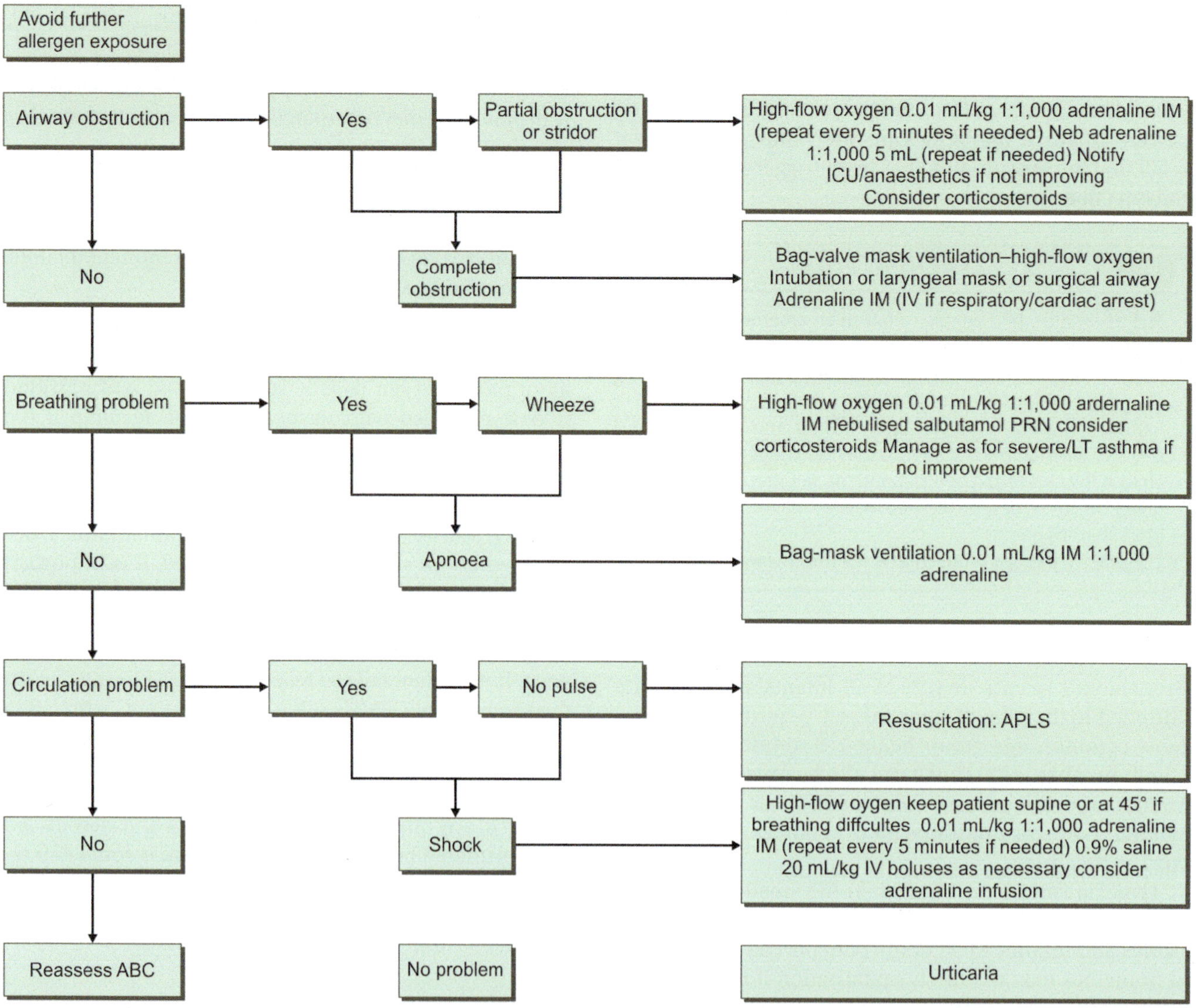

Treatment of anaphylaxis follows the standard ABC approach. Intramuscular adrenaline should be given early and can be repeated after 5 minutes if there has not been significant improvement. Antihistamines (IM or slow IV chlorpheniramine) and steroids (IM or slow IV hydrocortisone) should be given once IM adrenaline has been administered but they have a delayed onset. Stridor should be treated with nebulised adrenaline and steroids. Wheeze should be treated as per asthma. Shock should be treated with volume resuscitation and IM adrenaline. An adrenaline infusion may be required if the patient remains unstable despite these measures (Flow chart 25.6).

- Posture: Treat in supine position or left lateral position if patient vomiting. If patient has breathing difficulties, nurse at 45°. Legs should be elevated if hypotensive.
- Adrenaline: IM 0.01 mL/kg 1:1,000, repeated every 5 minutes if needed

Greater than 12 years	500 µg (0.5 mL)
6–12 years	300 µg (0.3 mL)
Less than 6 years	150 µg (0.15 mL)

Considered adrenaline infusion (0.05 µg–1 µg/kg/minute) if multiple IM doses required. Nebulised adrenaline (5 mL) if upper respiratory obstruction present. Early intubation must be considered if the child if not improving.

- IV Fluids:
  - 20 mL/kg 0.9% saline IV should be administered if shock is present.
  - Other treatments to consider are salbutamol and antihistamines if wheeze or pruritus present.

All children with anaphylaxis should be monitored for at least 4 hours. Children with anaphylaxis require admission to hospital if they require any of the following:

- More than 1 dose of adrenaline (IM or nebulized)
- A fluid bolus
- Inadequate response to treatment
- Live a long distance from hospital

Collapsed Neonate

Infants presenting collapsed in the first few days of life provide a unique challenge to the paediatrician. Common aetiologies in this age group include sepsis, duct-dependent cardiac lesions and inborn errors of metabolism. All can present in a similar fashion making early diagnosis challenging. It is, therefore, important to have a structured approach concentrating on ABC that covers the most likely diagnoses.

Sepsis

Sepsis causing organisms include Group B *Streptococcus*, *E Coli*, *Klebsiella* and *Listeria*. Antibiotics that cover these organisms should be given early to any collapsed neonate, e.g. cefotaxime plus amoxicillin.

Duct-dependent Cardiac Lesion

Pulmonary obstructive lesions, such as pulmonary atresia, critical pulmonary stenosis, tricuspid atresia and transposition of the great arteries, can present collapsed with severe cyanosis when the ductus arteriosus closes after a few days of life. Systemic obstructive lesions, such as coarctation of the aorta, critical aortic stenosis and hypoplastic left heart syndrome, can also present with collapse and may or may not be cyanosed depending on the general state of the child. Classically, infants with systemic obstructions present with absent femoral pulses, but it should be noted that in any collapsed neonate palpation of any pulse is often difficult if the patient is shocked. Infants with heart failure also frequently have a heart murmur and enlarged liver.

The treatment of a duct-dependent cardiac lesion follows the standard ABC approach. In addition, an infusion of prostaglandin should be started in any collapsed neonate in which a duct-dependent lesion is suspected. Inotropic support is also frequently required.

Maintenance of Ductal Patency Alprostadil (Prostin VR)—to open duct commence at 5 nanograms/kg/minute, this may be increased to 20 nanograms/kg/minute. Aim to decrease to the lowest effective dose.

The most significant side effect of prostaglandin is the occurrence of apnoea. This tends to be dose-dependent. If apnoea is troublesome, intubation and ventilation may be required.

Inborn Error of Metabolism

These children may present after a period of apparent normality after feeding on breast milk or standard formula at home. They may present collapsed with a profound metabolic acidosis and hypoglycaemia. Management is with the ABC approach. Bicarbonate infusions may be required. The key is to properly resuscitate the infant and provide a source of glucose in the short term whilst feeds are stopped pending further investigations.

KEY LEARNING POINTS

- In any collapsed neonate the possibility of sepsis, duct-dependent congenital heart disease or an inborn error of metabolism should be considered.
- Commence broad spectrum antibiotics in any collapsed neonate.
- Have a low threshold for commencing a prostaglandin infusion.
- Note that the dose of prostaglandin is in nanograms/kg per minute.
- Stop feeds and provide a glucose source if a metabolic disorder is thought likely.

Trauma

The child with trauma should be approached. Following the same ABC approach as described earlier. The only difference is that cervical spine control should be assessed and managed at the same time as the airway.

Radiological Investigations

The primary cause of death in significant trauma, particularly if they have a reduced level of consciousness or distracting painful injury is bleeding. CT is used to accurately detect bleeding in the trauma patient. The use of CT in children has to weigh the benefits of finding injuries against the real risk of significant radiation doses.

A primary survey routine ordering of C-spine, chest and pelvis X-ray is no longer considered appropriate. Primary survey imaging should consist of a chest X-ray and a C-spine X-ray if the injury is unable to be cleared clinically and there is no upfront indication for C-spine CT. Time should not be wasted for X-ray chest, if tension pneumothorax is suspected and treatment (needle thoracocentesis, at the lower border of the midpoint of clavicle) should be carried out immediately. The need for a pelvic X-ray should be considered carefully.

Head and Neck Injuries

In the head injured patient cerebral functions may be depressed due to raised intracranial compression secondary to oedema and/or bleeding. This can result from both localised injury and bleeding as well as more diffuse head injury resulting in diffuse axonal injury. In head injuries with raised intracranial pressure and subsequent compression of the brain, Cushing triad (altered consciousness, slow pulse rate and increased blood pressure) is often noted. Therefore, increased pulse rate and/or low

BOX 25.1 Indications for urgent computed tomography head scan.

Witnessed loss of consciousness lasting greater than 5 minutes
Amnesia lasting greater than 5 minutes
Abnormal drowsiness
Three or more discrete episodes of vomiting
Dangerous mechanism of injury
Clinical suspicion of non-accidental injury
Post-traumatic seizure with no history of epilepsy
Age greater than 1 year with GCS less than 14; age less than 1 year with GCS less than 15
Suspicion of open or depressed skull fracture or tense fontanelle
Any sign of basal skull fracture
Focal neurological deficit
Age less than 1 year with presence of bruising, swelling or laceration greater than 5 cm on the head

blood pressure should raise the suspicion of trauma and bleeding elsewhere in chest, abdomen, pelvis or major bony injuries rather than concentrating on the head injury in isolation. The mechanism of injury may also indicate the potential severity of the injury. High speed impacts and road traffic accidents (RTAs) with fatalities point to a high likelihood of significant injury as do fall from a reasonable height. If there is any suspicion of head injury then an urgent CT head scan should be performed. A CT scan of the cervical spine may be done at the same time if there is a severe head injury (GCS <8) or if the plain films are inadequate or there remains strong suspicion of injury despite normal plain films.

Patients who should undergo a CT head scan have been identified in the UK National Institute of Clinical Excellence Head Injury guidelines **(Box 25.1)**. They are as follows:

The key aspects of head injury management are as follows:

- *Cervical spine control:* The head and neck should be stabilised initially by manual in-line immobilisation. An injured child maybe uncooperative and too rigid immobilisation of the head in cases may increase leverage on the neck as the child struggles. If the patient is unconscious, head block and tape should be considered to assist with stabilisation of the neck and to provide staff with a visual indicator that the neck has not been cleared. Cervical spine injuries are rare in children and usually involve the upper three vertebrae. Manual in-line immobilisation should be maintained until spinal injury has been excluded. If there is a high index of spinal cord injury despite a negative CT an MRI is indicated.
- *Rapid assessment of mental state if GCS less than 8:* Intubate and ventilate
- *Urgent imaging of brain:* Identify any surgically amenable lesion early
- Involve neurosurgeons early
- Secondary survey and treat any other injuries

Secondary survey:

- Perform a formal GCS
- Neck and cervical spine:
  - Deformity
  - Tenderness
  - Muscle spasm
- Head
  - Scalp bruising
  - Lacerations
  - Swelling
  - Tenderness
  - Raccoon eyes
  - Bruising behind the ear (Battles sign)
- Eyes
  - Pupil size
  - Equality
  - Reactivity
  - Fundoscopy for retinal haemorrhage (may indicate non-accidental injury)
- Ears
  - Blood behind the ear drum
  - CSF leak
- Nose
  - Deformity
  - Swelling
  - Bleeding
  - CSF leak
- Mouth
  - Dental trauma
  - Soft tissue injuries
- Face
  - Focal tenderness
  - Crepitus
- Motor function
  - Reflexes present
  - Lateralising signs

All patients with significant abnormalities on CT scanning should be referred urgently to a neurosurgeon. In addition, regardless of the imaging findings, patients should be discussed with a neurosurgeon if significant clinical concerns continue despite adequate resuscitation **(Box 25.2)**.

When a head injury is severe enough to result in a depressed conscious level (GCS <13), injury to the cervical vertebra should be presumed to be present until later neurological and radiological investigations (plain X-rays and, if necessary, CT or MRI) are proven to be normal. It is important to be aware that children are at risk of spinal cord injury without any apparent radiological abnormality (SCIWORA), and therefore the cervical spine cannot be cleared until neurological examination is normal even

BOX 25.2 Indications for referral to a neurosurgeon.

Persisting coma (Glasgow coma score < 8) after initial resuscitation
Unexplained confusion lasting more than 4 hours
Deteriorating conscious level (especially motor changes)
Focal neurological signs
Seizure without full recovery
Definite suspecting penetrating injury
A cerebrospinal fluid leak

BOX 25.3 Measures to increase cerebral perfusion temporarily.

Nurse in the 20° head-up position and head in midline to help venous drainage
Ventilation to $PaCO_2$ of 4.0–4.5 kPa
Combat hypotension if present with colloid infusion or inotropes
Consider infusion of IV mannitol 0.25–0.5 g/kg or hypertonic saline
Consider phenytoin loading

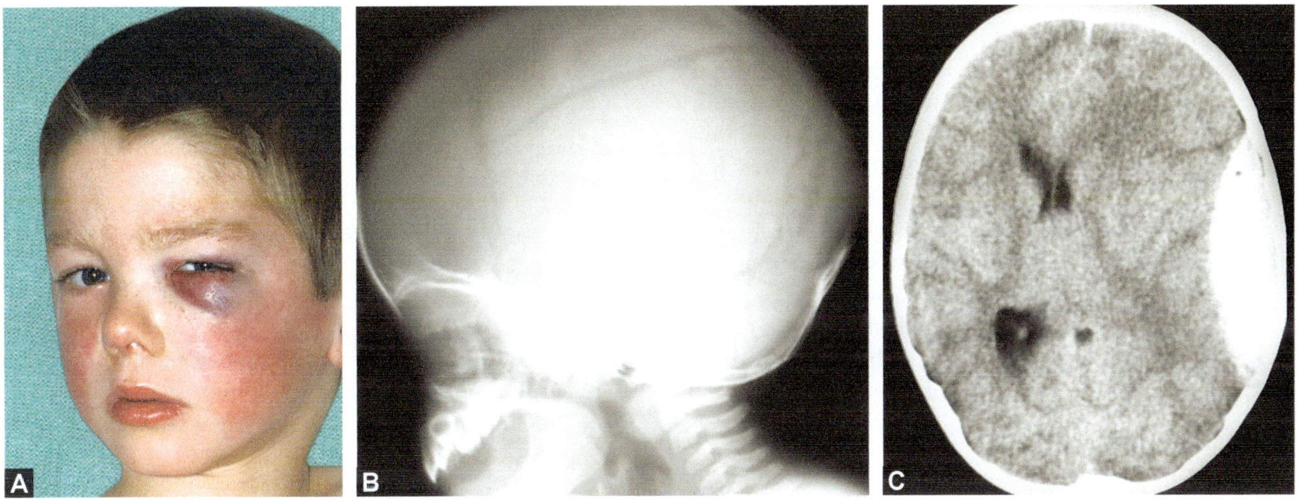

Figures 25.7A to C (A) Clinical photograph with periorbital haematoma in a base of skull fracture, (B) plain X-ray showing a fractured skull and (C) computed tomography scan showing an extra dural haemorrhage.

in the presence of normal radiological imaging. Therefore, it is important to immobilise the neck with a cervical collar, spinal board and sandbags on either side of the neck (the Ambulance Service personnel are trained to apply, from the initial scene). Controlled "log rolling" (with three or four persons according to age) under the orders of the leader who stabilises head and neck, for any examination or procedure at the back, will minimise the risk of iatrogenic cord/nerve injury. It should be noted that any agitated child who struggles should not be head-blocked or sandbagged as the risk of the body struggling against a fixed head may increase the chances of a spinal cord injury.

Blood loss can be considerable due to cut injuries of scalp, especially in neonates and infants, as the blood supply to a unit area of scalp is similar to tongue and heart and considerably greater than many parts of the body. Hypovolemic shock may result especially in babies, even with a haematoma (scalp, fracture femur) with loss of considerable amount of blood **(Figs. 25.7A to C)**.

Consciousness should be assessed by GCS or quickly with AVPU scale. GCS of less than 14 indicates a serious problem, and head injury should be considered if the mechanism of injury is suspicious. Pupils are windows of the brain. Size, reaction equality are under the control of sympathetic and parasympathetic fibres (in Oculomotor nerve). Alteration (Hutchinson pupils) indicates intracranial compression and the side of the problem clinically, though CT scan is required to confirm and for further management.

If a significant brain injury has occurred that is surgically remedial, then the patient should be intubated and ventilated and nursed in a head-up position. If there are signs of raised intracranial pressure, a dose of mannitol may be given whilst awaiting surgical decompression.

In consultation with neurosurgeon consider measures to decrease intracranial pressure **(Box 25.3)**.

KEY LEARNING POINTS

- Airway and cervical spine control take precedence in the trauma or head injured patient.
- Airway, breathing and circulation should be managed as normal to ensure adequate oxygenation and circulation to the injured brain.
- If Glasgow coma score <8 then involve anaesthetist or intensivist, and intubate and ventilate.
- Have a low threshold for CT brain imaging
- Involve neurosurgeons early

Chest Injuries

Isolated chest injuries are rare in paediatrics but are usually a consequence of blunt trauma to the chest, e.g. RTA. Penetrating injury accounts for less than 10% of chest trauma.

There are important differences between adult and children:

- Children's tissues are relatively elastic; they have a compliant chest wall which allows a great deformation of the chest wall before fracture occurs. Therefore, there can be significant internal injury without an obvious external injury.
- Hypoxia is the best indication of chest injury. Hypotension is a late sign due to the greater compensatory mechanisms that mask hypovolemia and respiratory distress. Due to their underdeveloped musculature, children do not tolerate a disruption of the chest wall, e.g. flail chest and tend to decompensate rapidly.
- Infants are diaphragmatic breathers and therefore any increase in gastric dilation/pressure will increase respiratory distress. A nasogastric tube should be placed in these infants unless a head injury is suspected (where an orogastric tube should be considered).

Significant chest injuries include:

- *Tension Pneumothorax*
- Life threatening: Progressive accumulation of air in the pleural space under pressure causes impaired venous return and impaired cardiac output
- Signs hypoxia, distended neck veins, mediastinal shift, shock decreased air entry on affected side
- Diagnosis should be clinical and Chest X-ray should never be taken
- Immediate needle thoracocentesis of the affected side in the second intercostal space mid clavicular line **(Flow chart 25.7)**.

Flow chart 25.7 Head injury chart: initial management.

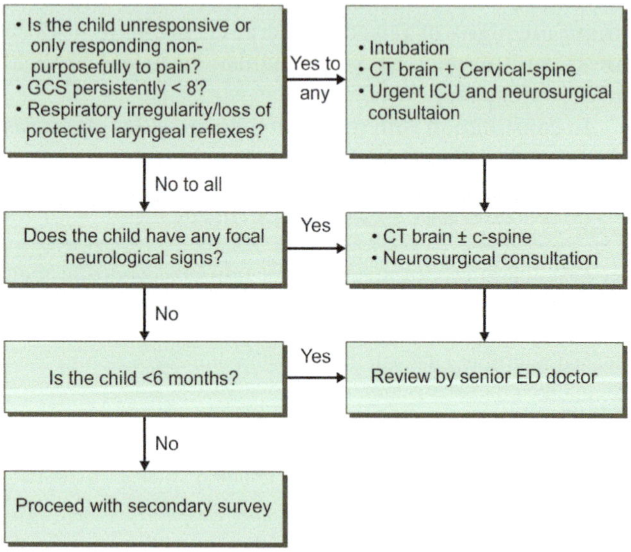

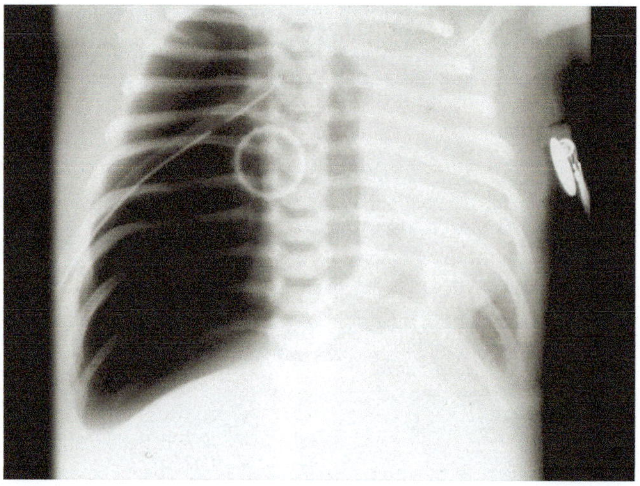

Figure 25.8 Chest X-ray showing a traumatic tension pneumothorax with a malpositioned chest drain.

This should be followed by an urgent chest drain to prevent recurrence

Open Pneumothorax

- Pneumothorax secondary to penetrating wound
- Parietal pleura is penetrated, this creates a sucking effect in inspiration and air is drawn into the pleural cavity
- Occlusive dressing sealed on three sides allows air to escape from the chest and prevents sucking air from the atmosphere, thus preventing tension pneumothorax until a definite action is planned **(Fig. 25.8)**.

Lung injuries Injury to the parenchyma of lung (contusion) should be suspected in any child experiencing blunt or penetrating trauma to the chest.

Lung contusion is managed in the same way as any trauma using an ABC approach.

Significant lung contusion may cause considerable respiratory distress and may require intubation and mechanical ventilation.

Flail chest When two or more adjacent ribs are fractured in two or more places, which will lead to a floating rib section which moves paradoxically with respiration:

- Resulting poor oxygenation and ventilation
- Endotracheal intubation may be required if ventilation is inadequate.

Abdominal Injuries

The majority of abdominal injuries are caused by blunt trauma and a high index of suspicion is required when the trauma is related to high speed acceleration/deceleration.

The important differences are as follows:

- Less adipose and muscle tissue. Children's organs lie closer to the surface and therefore are less protective.

- The diaphragm lies lower and therefore the liver and spleen lie lower in the abdomen making them more vulnerable to trauma.
- The bladder lies in the abdomen rather than the pelvis, making it more exposed when full.

Assessment

- History of mechanism
- Examination of the abdomen
- Abdominal tenderness, bruising, distension, rigidity, guarding, haematuria, examination of external genitalia, blood at the external meatus

Investigations

- Focus abdominal sonography for trauma (FAST scan) looking for free fluid
- Radiographs
  - CXR looking for air under the diaphragm
  - AXR—rarely useful
  - Abdominal CT is radiological investigation of choice
  - Blood at the external urethral meatus may require investigation using retrograde urethrography
- A surgical consult for further management is essential although the vast majority of solid organ injuries can be managed conservatively with frequent observation and fluid management.

Indications for emergency laparotomy are:

- There is refractory shock with suspicion of intra-abdominal bleeding
- Penetrating injuries
- Signs of bowel perforation
- Children with a significant history of trauma without any injuries should be admitted and monitored in hospital.

Pelvic Injuries

Run-over injuries typically result in pelvic injuries and genitourinary and other hollow visceral injuries may accompany. Immediate management is on general principles of standard resuscitation. Urethral catheterisation should be performed only after discussion with the surgical team. Stabilisation with a pelvic binder is useful till orthopaedic team takes over the management.

Limb Injuries

Blood loss can be considerable for long bone injuries, and circulation should be taken care of once A and B are satisfactory. Emergency action is required for neurovascular compromise in conditions such as angulated or displaced fractures, compound fractures and compartment syndromes. Immediate manipulation and reduction may restore blood supply, but exploration or adequate incisional release for compartment syndrome should not be delayed if there is no adequate improvement. When delay is anticipated to gain access to operation theatre, incisions deep enough to release acute compression should be done in the emergency room. Immobilisation and parental analgesia and/or nerve blocks (e.g. femoral nerve block for fracture femur) result in comfort for the child.

KEY LEARNING POINTS

- The general approach to trauma follows the ABC approach.
- Tension pneumothorax should be managed with immediate needle thoracocentesis—do not wait for radiological confirmation.
- Small volumes of blood loss may result in significant haemodynamic compromise.
- Abdominal ultrasound followed by CT abdomen is the imaging modality of choice in abdominal trauma **(Figs. 25.9A and B)**.

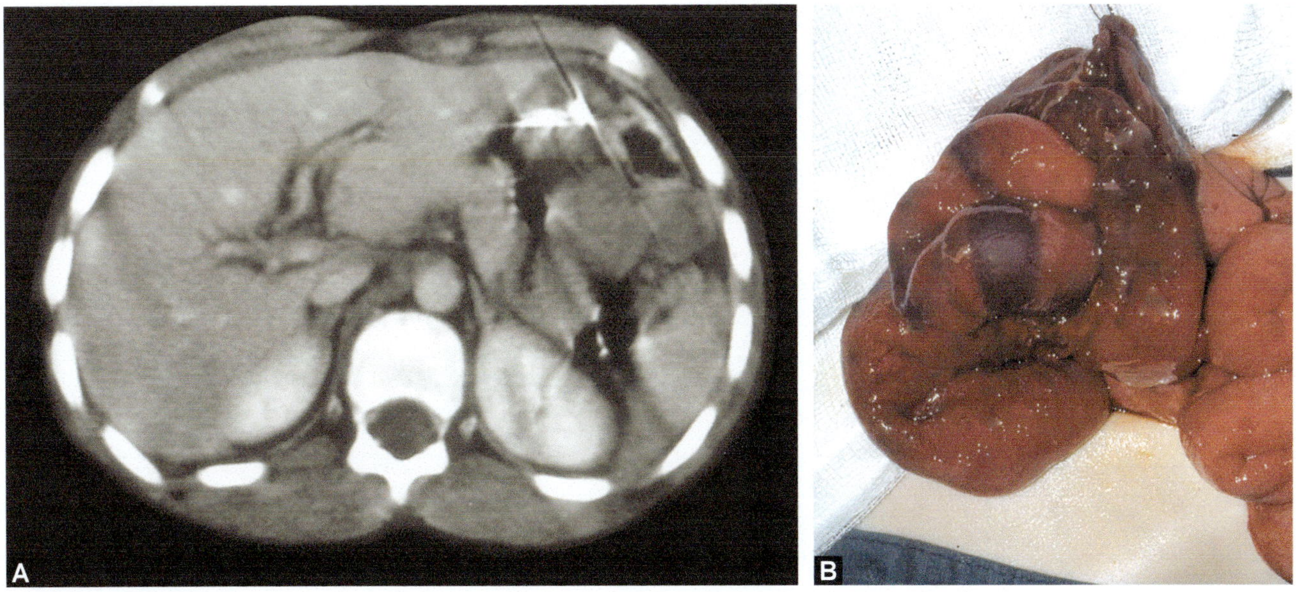

Figures 25.9A and B (A) Computed tomography scan of abdominal trauma showing a fractured liver and (B) operative picture of abdominal trauma showing a mesenteric tear.

Thermal Injuries

The majority of burns (70%) in children occur in the under 4, the most common age being between 1 and 2 years. Boys are more likely to suffer from burns/serious scalds than girls. Most fatal burns occur in house fires, whereas scalds usually occur from contact with hot liquids.

The depth of the burn is dependent on the heat from the source and the duration of contact with subject. Children who are unable to minimize contact time with source result in having deeper burns (e.g. infants).

Burns should be treated as any multi-trauma with an ABC approach. It is important to remember that a burn is often accompanied by other injuries and a formal primary and secondary survey approach is essential. The size of the burn is best assessed in relation to body surface area. In children, the most accurate method to assess the burn area is by using a chart such as the Lund-Browder chart **(Figs. 25.10A and B)**. Other methods such as "the rule of nines" tend not to be accurate in children until the age of 15.

Initial Management

First aid

- Run under cold water for 20 minutes, avoid hypothermia. This is effective up to 3 hours after thermal injury
- Cold compress can be applied to localized burns, ensuring that this is reapplied. This advice should not be applied to extensive burns as it may result in hypothermia
- Do not use ice
- Chemical burns and burns to eyes should be irrigated with copious amounts and saline
- Cling-film wrap should be applied to area to avoid evaporation/loss of heat

Pain relief

- Oral analgesia should be given immediately unless oral burns suspected
- IN fentanyl 0.15 µg/kg
- IV morphine 0.1 mg/kg
- Nitrous oxide

Assessment

- *Airway:* Inhalation of hot gases can result in airway swelling and compromise breathing. Any suspicion that the airway may be compromised should lead to prompt intubation to protect the airway rather than allowing hypoxia to intervene.
- Indications of inhalational injury include:
- Burns around mouth
- Cough
- Stridor
- Hoarseness
- Weak voice

Breathing

Burns can affect the lower airways in a number of ways. Smoke inhalation can result in bronchospasm and acute lung injury. Circumferential burns to the chest/abdomen can result in a restrictive lung defect. If there are any signs of breathing problems, high-flow oxygen should be applied and early intubation and ventilation should be considered **(Fig. 25.11)**.

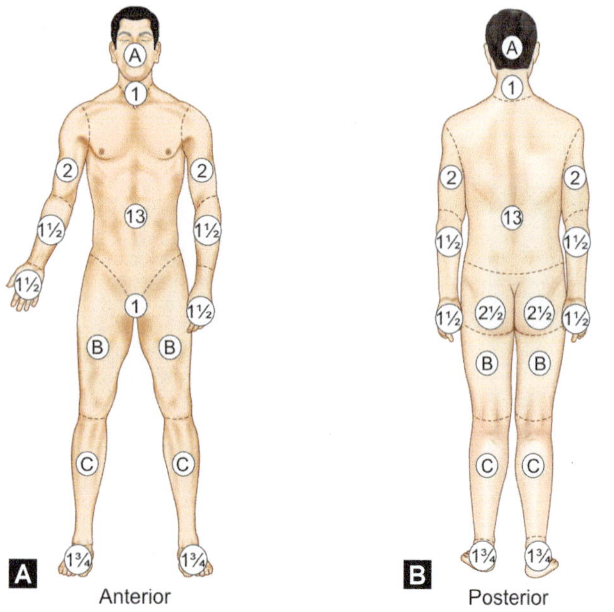

Area indicated	Surface area at 0 year	1 year	5 years	10 years	15 years
A	9.5	8.5	6.5	5.5	4.5
B	2.75	3.25	4	4.25	4.5
C	2.5	2.5	2.75	3.75	3.25

Figures 25.10A and B (A) Rule of nines; (B) Lund–Browder chart. (*Source:* Chemical Hazards Emergency Medical Management (CHEMM))

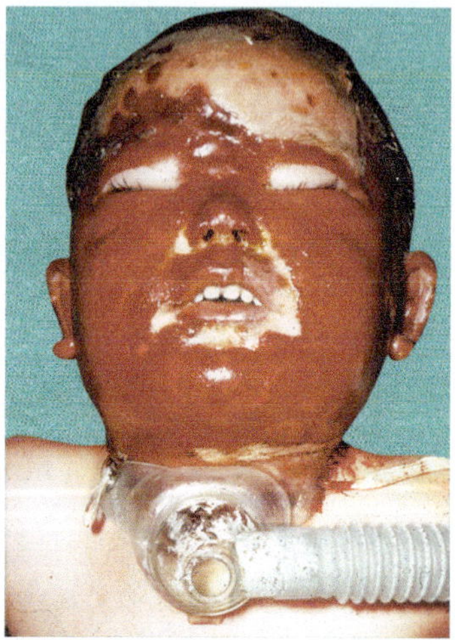

Figure 25.11 Fifty per cent burns to body and face with acute lung injury from smoke inhalation. Patient has a tracheostomy.

Circulation

Fluid management is critical as significant fluid losses occur and must be replaced to maintain adequate tissue perfusion. IV or IO access should be obtained and bloods sent including haemoglobin, electrolytes and urea, blood glucose and carboxyhaemoglobin. Signs of hypovolemic shock in the early hours after thermal injury are rarely due to burns and therefore other sources of fluid loss should be sought. Shock should be treated appropriately with fluid bolus (20 mL/kg). Children with greater than 10% burns will require further IV fluid, in addition to their normal fluid requirements. The additional fluid (mL) in the first 24 hours can be calculated as follows:

$$\text{Percentage burn} \times \text{weight (kg)} \times 4$$

Half of this fluid is given in the first 8 hours and the second half given over the following 16 hours.

Assessing the burnseverity of the thermal injury depends on the depth and area of the burn.

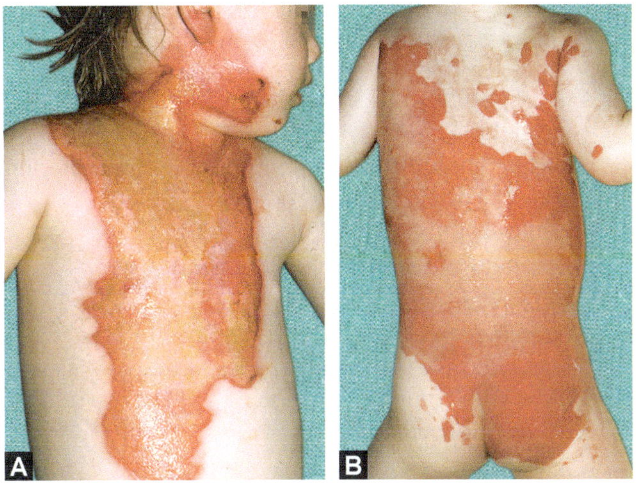

Figures 25.12A and B (A) Scald involving most of head, neck and front of chest wall; (B) Scald involving most of the back and buttocks.

Surface Area

The surface area of the burn is usually estimated using burns charts. The patient's palm approximates 1% of their total body surface area and may be used when burn charts are unavailable **(Figs. 25.12A and B)**.

Depth

The depth of the burn is classified as being superficial, partial thickness or full thickness **(Figs. 25.13A and B)**. **Table 25.6** summarises the appearance of each class.

Definitive care of severe burns requires transfer to a burns unit. Examples of burns that require transfer are:

- 10% partial thickness burns
- 5% full thickness burns
- Suspicion of non-accidental injury

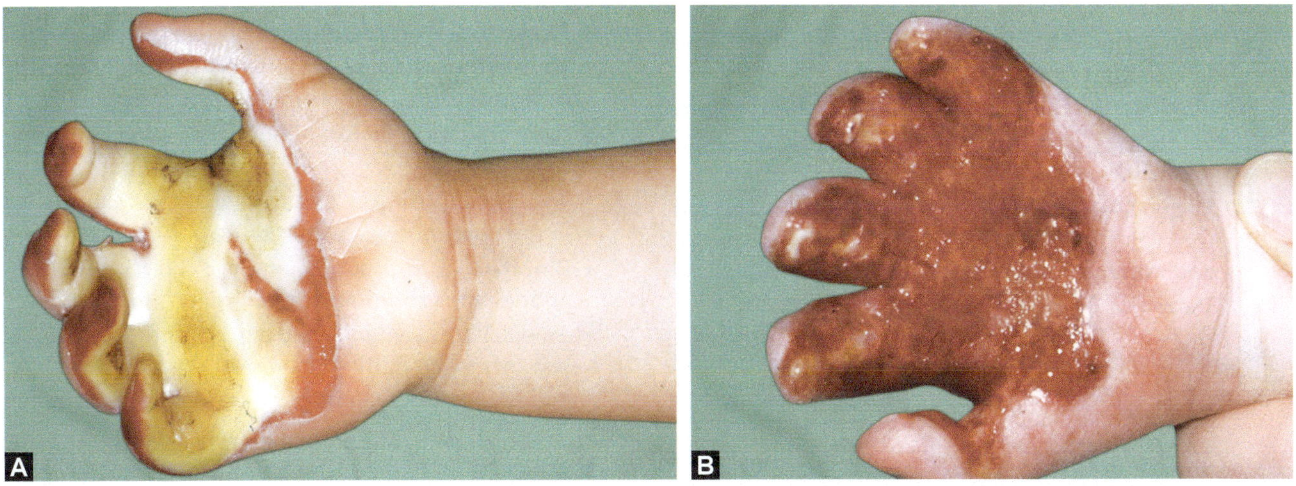

Figures 25.13A and B (A) Full thickness burn on the palm of the hand caused by an electric appliance; (B) Same patient after debridement.

TABLE 25.6 Classification of depth of burn.

Depth	*Colour/appearance*	*Pain sensation*
Superficial	Dry, minor blisters, erythema, brisk capillary refill	Painful
Partial thickness—superficial (superficial dermal)	Moist, reddened with broken blisters, brisk capillary refill	Painful
Partial thickness—deep (deep dermal)	Moist white slough, red mottled, sluggish capillary refill	Painless
Full thickness	Dry, charred whitish, absent capillary refill	Painless

Source: Adapted from Melbourne's Royal Children's Hospital, Burns guideline.

Burns to special areas (e.g. face, hands, feet, perineum)
Circumferential burns
Chemical burns

KEY LEARNING POINTS

- Approach a major burn as a multi-trauma using the Airway, Breathing, and Circulation approach.
- First aid should be initiated immediately.
- Fluid resuscitation is an essential part of burns resuscitation.

Bites

Animal and human bites cause contaminated puncture wounds and possible crush injuries. This means there is a much higher risk of the wound being infected by either bacterial or viral infections. Eighty five percent of all bites harbour bacterial infection.
Bacterial organisms responsible include:

- Human bites:
  - Fifty four percent of all human bites will be contaminated with a mixture of aerobic and anaerobic organisms.
  - Aerobes: Streptococci, *S. aureus.*
  - Anaerobes: *Eikenella, Fusobacterium, Peptostreptococcus, Porphyromonas* and Prevotella.
- Animal bites:
  - Sixty percent harbour aerobic and anaerobic bacteria.
  - Pasteurella—50% dog bite wounds and 75% cat bite wounds (Fig. 25.14).
  - Staphylococci and streptococci are isolated in 40% of bites.
  - Anaerobes.
  - *Capnocytophagacanimorsus*—gram-negative rod that can cause fatal sepsis, especially in asplenic and immunocompromised patients.
  - *Bartonellahenselae*—transmitted by cats.

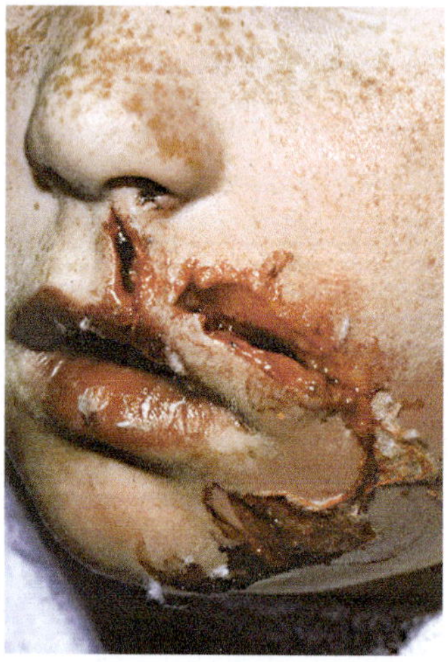

Figure 25.14 Multiple facial lacerations caused by dog bite.

Initial Management

Direct pressure to achieve haemostasis. Deep wounds should be treated as penetrating injuries.

Thorough wound cleaning:

- Ensure wound is adequately anaesthetised
- Clean using 1% povidone iodine and copious amounts of saline
- Thorough wound exploration, especially if wound is on the scalp or near a joint. Remove foreign bodies or wound contaminants.
- Primary closure should only be undertaken by an experienced clinician and is usually only performed for cosmetic purposes. Wounds are often left open for drainage and possible delayed closure. Primary closure should only be attempted if the laceration meets all of the following criteria:
- Clinically uninfected
- Less than 12 hours old (<24 hours on face)
- Not located on hand or foot
- Bites that are deep to bone/joints, complex facial bites, wounds with neurovascular compromise and those with complex infections should be referred for surgical consultation.

Prophylactic antibiotics are shown to reduce the rate of infection in animal/human bites and should be considered for the following:

- Deep puncture wounds
- Moderate-severe wounds with crush injury
- Wounds in areas of underlying venous/lymphatic compromise
- Bites on hands, face, genitalia or in close proximity to joints
- Wounds requiring closure
- In the immunocompromised host
- Prophylactic antibiotic therapy for both human and animal bites should be broad-spectrum as follows:
- Amoxicillin-clavulanate 20 mg/kg (amoxicillin component) twice daily (maximum 875 mg amoxicillin and 125 mg clavulanate per dose)
- Alternatively (e.g. in penicillin allergy):
- Cefuroxime 10 mg/kg twice daily (maximum 500 mg per dose)

PLUS

- Metronidazole 10 mg/kg three times daily (maximum 400 mg per dose)
- In high-risk wounds, or those severely infected, IV antibiotic therapy should be used.

If the bite is minor and superficial, a tetanus booster should be given to those children who have not been immunised for more than 10 years. If the bite is severe or high-risk, a tetanus booster should be given to those who have not been immunised for more than 5 years.

Pain Management

Assessing pain in paediatric patients is very challenging. The best tool for subjective pain measurement must take into account the patients developmental and verbal abilities. The numerical pain rating scale is suitable for patients who have a developmental age of at least 7 years. The "FACES" pain scale is typically used for patients who function at the level of a 3 year old. This correlates symbolic facial expressions with pain severity. There is also the FLACC (faces, legs, activity, cry and consolability) scale.

The next challenge is interpreting the pain score. It is not uncommon for children to report pain scores out of proportion to their affect. When a child reports that pain from a sore finger is a "10" while completely engrossed in a video game, it is not surprising that the clinicians disbelieve the report and treat the pain more to the level of the child's affect rather than reported score, undermining the credibility of the pain score.

There are pharmacological and non-pharmacological approaches to dealing with pain in children. A combination of both of these is the best approach to manage paediatric pain effectively.

Non-pharmacological Interventions

- Hypnosis
- Distraction
- Music
- Parental involvement
- Vibration
- Cold spray

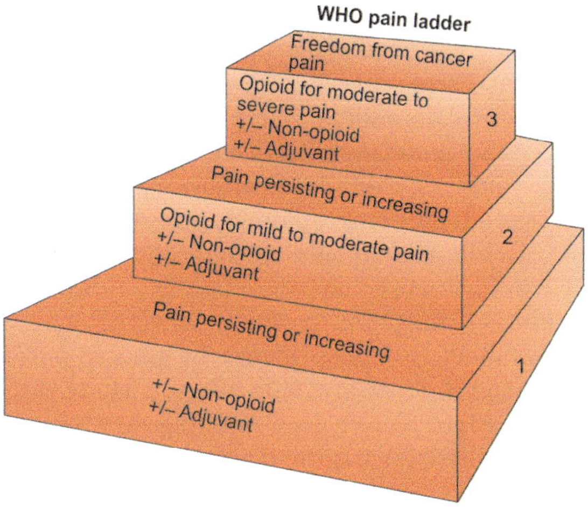

Figure 25.15 WHO pain ladder.
(*Source:* WHO)

Pharmacological As with management in adults, pain in children is based on the World Health Organisation (WHO) stepwise approach according to pain severity **(Fig. 25.15)**.

Oral analgesics: Paracetamol is the most commonly used analgesia for paediatric practice. It can be administered orally, rectally and intravenously. It is thought to work by inhibiting cycloxygenase in the central nervous system. It provides analgesia without anti-inflammatory affect **(Table 25.7)**.

Non-steroidal anti-inflammatories have anti-inflammatory, antipyretic and moderate analgesic properties.

TABLE 25.7 Analgesia.

Analgesic	*Pain severity*	*Single dose*	*Duration of affect*	*Common side effects*	*Comments*
Paracetamol	Mild	15 mg/kg orally 4–6 hourly	4–6 hours		Avoid in liver disease
Ibuprofen	Mild-moderate	10 mg/kg	4–6 hours		Caution with asthmatics
Diclofenac	Moderate	300 µg to 1 mg/kg orally or rectally	4–6 hours		
Codeine	Mild to moderate	0.5–1 mg/kg	4 hours	Respiratory depression hypotension	Avoid in patients <1 year. Do not give IV
Morphine oral	Moderate	0.2 mg/kg dose *max 10 mg*	3–6 hours	Respiratory depression hypotension	Observe respiration
Fentanyl intranasally	Moderate to severe	1.5 µg/kg/dose *max dose 90 mcg*	30–60 minutes	Respiratory depression hypotension	Use an atomise device. Age >1 year old
Morphine IV	Severe	Initial dose 0.05 mg/kg/dose under 1 year 0.1 mg/kg/dose over 1 year subsequent dose	2–4 hours	Respiratory depression hypotension	Cardiorespiratory and pulse oximetry monitoring
Sucrose	Mild to moderate procedural pain	24% solution 0.5 mL <1,500 g 1 mL >1,500 g 2 mL older than 4 months	2 hours		

Source: Adapted from APLS manual.

They are less well tolerated than paracetamol causing gastric irritation, platelet disorders, bronchospasm and renal impairment. These are especially useful for post-traumatic pain because of the additional anti-inflammatory affect.

Opioids are generally used in children with moderate to severe pain, or pain that is refractory to non-opioid analgesics. Opioids have opium or morphine like properties. In children, opioids are typically administered orally, intravenously or intranasally. Administered intavenously, morphine produces a rapid onset and excellent analgesic effect. It may be titrated to effect and reversed if necessary. Side effects include respiratory depression, nausea and vomiting. The intranasal route for the administration of opiates such as fentanyl has been shown to be a safe and effective route and is becoming increasingly popular for children. It also has the advantage of being quick and easy, avoiding the trauma of intravenous cannulation.

Inhalation analgesia: Nitrous oxide is a colourless, odourless gas that provides analgesia at a subanaesthetic level. During nitrous oxide therapy, the patient needs to be awake and cooperative to inhale the gas. The onset is very rapid, reaching peak affect in 2–3 minutes and has a short half-life. Nitrous oxide is most suitable for procedures where short-lived intense analgesia is required, e.g. dressing changes, suturing, pain relief during splinting or immediate pain relief on presentation until definitive analgesia is effective.

CHAPTER 26

Paediatric Otolaryngology

W. Andrew Clement, Ameet Kishore

INTRODUCTION

Ear nose and throat conditions are reported to make up approximately half of the attendances to paediatricians in the North America with the majority of these being otology related. Most of these conditions can be managed by primary care physicians and paediatricians. In cases where children have more complex problems or where surgery may be considered, referral to a paediatric otolaryngologist should be considered. The aim of this chapter is to assist paediatricians in clinical decision-making and identify where the paediatric otolaryngologist may be able to assist in the ongoing care and management for these children.

EAR, NOSE AND THROAT EXAMINATION IN CHILDREN

Prior to examination, it should be ascertained if there is any pain or discomfort in the area. Examination of the ear should be undertaken with the child sitting comfortably on their parent's knee. The child should be then cuddled into their parent who will place one arm around their head and another around their body and arms. The external ear and canal should be inspected prior to insertion of the otoscope speculum. The pinna should be gently pulled down and backwards to allow visualisation of the tympanic membrane (Fig. 26.1). Pneumatic otoscopy will allow assessment of tympanic mobility.

Examination of the pharynx is most easily undertaken with the child sitting upright,where possible tongue depressors are not used as the use of these will often distress the child. Tricks to help with visualisation of the pharynx include asking the child to stick their tongue out and make a noise at the same time and/or asking the child to pant or huff (as this suppresses the gag reflex) with their mouth open. Where the child is finding it difficult, the child should be sat on their parent's knee, whereby the parent puts one arm around the child's body and arms and another around the child's head, which is then tilted slightly upwards, and a tongue depressor used.

Examination of the nose can be undertaken by gently lifting the tip of the nose up with the examiners thumb. In cases where there is a suspected foreign body, illumination in the form of an otoscope may aid the clinician. An otoscope with a large speculum may be used for a well-illuminated and slightly magnified view into the nasal cavity. A Thudicum's nasal speculum is rarely required. Airflow may be assessed using a metal tongue depressor to look for frosting.

Examination of neck should be undertaken visually from both the front and the back. Palpation of the neck is most easily and effectively performed from behind. If a thyroglossal cyst or thyroid mass is suspected, asking the child to swallow or stick out their tongue and assessing if there is movement may aid with the diagnosis.

Further examination, including examination of the larynx and post-nasal space, is most easily undertaken by a paediatric otolaryngologist using fibre-optic endoscopes (Fig. 26.2).

HEARING TESTS IN CHILDREN

Hearing Screening

Early identification and intervention for children with hearing loss is associated with improved outcomes as well as being proven to be cost-effective. Universal newborn hearing screening is now the norm in most Western countries with some later targeted screening reserved for high-risk infants and children (see congenital hearing loss section). Two methods of hearing screening are used in newborns, otoacoustic emissions (OAE) and automated auditory brainstem responses (AABR). There are several types of OAE with transient evoked OAEs being the type used for screening. Transient evoked OAEs are sounds generated by the outer cells in the cochlea in response to a received auditory input (please see below

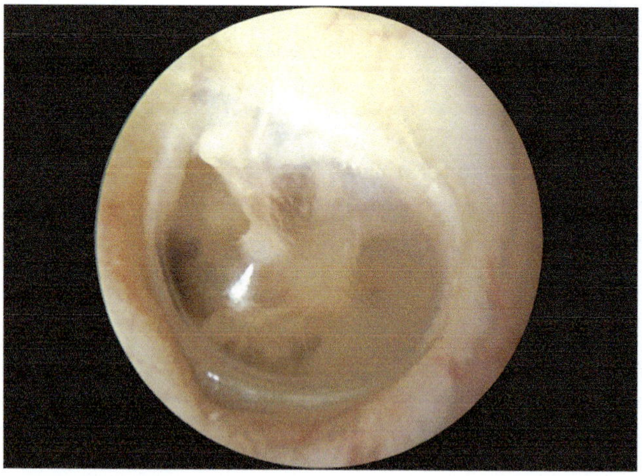

Figure 26.1 Normal left tympanic membrane.

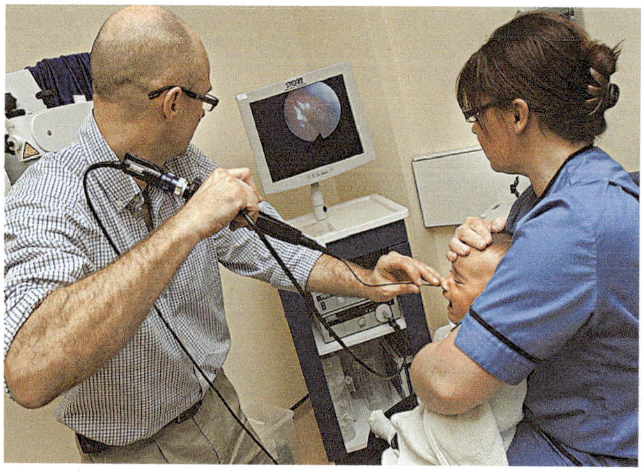

Figure 26.2 Fiberoptic laryngoscopy.

for details). If there is a hearing loss of 30 dB or greater this response is generally absent. AABR relies on an intact auditory pathway and measures the effect of auditory stimuli by measuring electrical activity at the level of the lateral lemniscus/inferior colliculus in the brainstem. This is detected as a wave (wave V) on the AABR and is given as a pass/fail result. Screening is usually performed at 40 dB. The choice of which, screening programme to institute, should be determined by local services. OAEs carry a lower sensitivity and specificity than AABR but are quicker to do. Many programmes that use OAEs have a two-stage programme with AABR being used at the second stage for those newborns that have failed OAE testing at the first stage. Two-stage programmes carry the disadvantages of higher levels of parental anxiety due to failed tests, and also the added difficulty of parental compliance, as they have to return for the second test (AABR). Both programmes are now similar in cost. The disadvantages of screening programmes include the cost of set-up, diagnosis, counselling, intervention and follow-up along with the anxiety generated by a failed test, but these are far outweighed by the potential benefits. It should be noted that screening will not identify some children with mild and/or progressive hearing losses.

Age and Developmentally Appropriate Levels of Testing

Various different hearing tests can be utilised for differing ages of children. The ages stated below are a guide only. The type of tests used will depend upon the experience and familiarity of the tester/s and the equipment available as well the level of understanding and cooperation of the child. All testing should be performed in appropriately soundproofed testing booths with standardised acceptable levels of ambient noise and equipment. Testing is carried out using the principle of initial presentation of suprathreshold stimuli and utilising the 10 dB down/5 dB up rule to establish accurate hearing levels. Testing is carried out at a minimum of 500 Hz, 1 kHz, 2 kHz and 4 kHz frequencies, as these cover the range of speech frequencies. Where possible each ear is tested individually, but in younger children where headphones will not be tolerated, the sounds are presented in other ways, as described below. These are known as free-field tests and these techniques may miss a hearing loss if a mild single sided hearing loss is present.

Behavioural Techniques

Behavioural hearing testing techniques can be used for infants from birth to the age of 6 months. This type of testing involves providing an auditory stimulus to the infant and assessing if a response is present. The test is very reliant on the tester's interpretation. Behavioural techniques are now rarely employed as these have now largely been replaced by newborn screening tests, as discussed above, which are far more reliable.

Distraction Testing

Distraction testing is carried on infants and children between the ages of 6 and 18 months. This requires a tester and an observer/distracter. The child sits on their parent's knee. This test utilises special frequency rattles and frequency specific warbler devices. The observer/distracter gets the child's attention by the use of a toy. Standardised different frequencies and intensities of sound are then presented slightly behind and to either side of the child in an attempt to test each ear. The distracter/observer will confirm to the tester if there has been an indication that the child has heard, such as turning, blinking or eye movement.

Visual Reinforcement Audiometry

This test is useful for children aged 9 months to 3 years. It requires a loudspeaker system and specialised lightboxes.

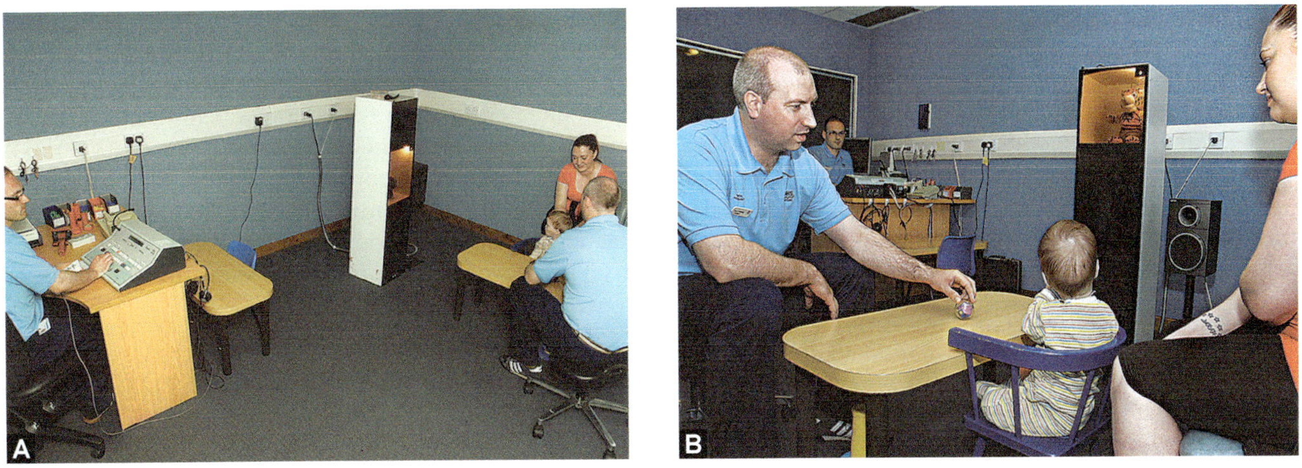

Figures 26.3A and B Visual response audiometry.

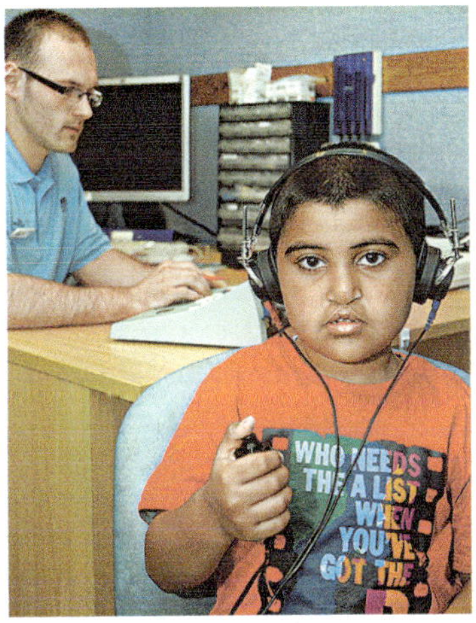

Figure 26.4 Pure tone audiometry.

It works on the principle of positive reinforcement. The lightboxes contain a toy, which is illuminated if a positive response is identified. This again is a type of free field hearing test. It requires two testers. The sound field generators/loudspeakers are positioned at least 1 m and directly to either side from where the test subject will be as are the lightboxes. The first tester sits directly in front of the child with a table between them. The second tester controls the presentation of the test stimuli. Younger children will sit on their parent's knee whereas older children can sit by themselves. Standardised different frequencies and intensities of sound are then presented from the loudspeakers. If the child responds to the presented sound, their behaviour is reinforced/rewarded by illumination of a toy in one of the lightboxes **(Figs. 26.3A and B)**.

Play Audiometry/Conditioned Reflex Audiology

This test is useful for children aged 2–5 years. This again is a free-field hearing test. Usually for this test, the same set up for visual reinforcement audiometry is used with the only difference being that lightboxes are not required. Stimuli can also be presented as with distraction testing. The child is conditioned to place a marble or peg into a box every time they hear a sound thereby creating a game out of the test.

Speech Discrimination Tests

This test is also useful for children aged 2–5 years. The most commonly used speech discrimination test used for children in the United Kingdom is the McCormick toy test. This uses seven paired toys with names that are acoustically similar. The name of the toy is presented to the child at a minimal level of 40 dB, and they are asked to identify the named toy by pointing at a picture of it.

Pure Tone Audiometry

This test is useful for children aged 4 years and upwards. The child wears headphones so each ear can be tested individually. Each ear is presented with pure tones at 500 Hz, 1 kHz, 2 kHz and 4 kHz frequencies as a minimum. If a hearing loss is identified, bone conduction can also be assessed as part of this test to identify if the loss is sensorineural or conductive **(Fig. 26.4)**.

Auditory Brainstem Response/Brainstem-evoked Response Audiometry Testing

For children who have communication and/or comprehension difficulties and where other forms of testing are unable to identify accurately the level of hearing, auditory brainstem response (ABR) testing may be required. This test is also used for children who fail their newborn screening testing, as this test will allow hearing levels to be ascertained. The test requires the child to be asleep using either sedation or a general anaesthetic. Headphones are placed on both ears and stimuli played through each headphone individually. Standard speech range frequencies are used as described above. This test is done at various intensity levels with various stimuli to choose from, thus allowing for a differential diagnosis and differentiating conductive, sensorineural or retrocochlear lesions. Typically five waves could be seen with the third and fifth being most robust. The mechanism of ABR is described in the screening section above.

Otoacoustic Emissions (OAE)

This test is done to check the functioning of the outer hair cells (OHC) inside the cochlea. OHC are known to produce very small emissions which could be spontaneous as well as evoked. The evoked responses are described as either Transient Evoked or Distortion Product. Clinically we record evoked emissions through sophisticated instruments to record the minute responses. It could be done clinically for screening and diagnostic purpose. Clinically we find that emissions are very decreased or absent in hearing loss above 30–40 dBHL.

Auditory Steady-state Response (ASSR)

These are Auditorily Evoked Steady-state Potentials that arise from the auditory nerve, brainstem and auditory cortex in response to regularly varying stimuli such as sinusoidal amplitude and/or frequency modulated tones. It allows objective frequency-specific measurements (250–4,000 Hz in octave steps). The responses are unaffected by sleep/sedation. This test is a fast objective estimation of audiograms and thus allows for more accurate estimation of behavioural threshold (within 5 dB). This can be also used for fitting of hearing aids in young infants.

Tympanograms

Tympanograms allow assessment of the compliance of the tympanic membrane, i.e. how much energy is absorbed by this structure. These are graded as A, B or C. Type Atympanograms have a peak between –100 and +100 daPa, type C tympanograms peak at less than –100 daPa and type B tympanograms have no peak and are flat. Type A tympanograms occur in ears with normal tympanic membrane compliance, type C tympanograms occur with reduced compliance and are most commonly seen with resolving otitis media with effusion (OME) and type B tympanograms are associated with either OME or a perforation (Fig. 26.5).

ACQUIRED CONDITIONS OF THE EAR

Acute Otitis Media

Acute infections of the middle ear in children are common. Acute otitis media (AOM) usually presents between the ages of 3 months and 3 years with a peak between the ages of 6 and 9 months. The older child will complain of severe otalgia and general unwellness; whereas infants and younger children who are less able to communicate may not be able to articulate their symptoms. Where possible direct questioning with regards to fever, disturbed sleep pattern and hearing loss may direct the clinician to the diagnosis. In the case of these younger children, as their primary and only presenting symptom may be that they are systemically unwell, examination of ears is mandatory. Anecdotally infants with AOM are often reported to rub or bang their ears. In most cases, a history of a preceding upper respiratory tract infection will be identified. In some cases, the tympanic membrane will have already ruptured leading to pus discharge and a rapid improvement in symptoms. Examination of the ear will demonstrate a bulging tympanic membrane with prominent blood vessels on its surface, or the tympanic membrane will be obscured by pus in the canal (Fig. 26.6). Risk factors for developing AOM include day care/nursery attendance, exposure to environmental tobacco smoke, not being breastfed and having older siblings. Pacifier

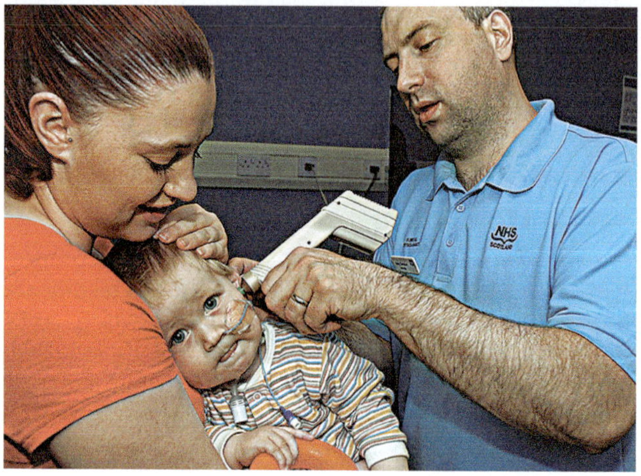

Figure 26.5 Tympanogram—use of tympanometer.

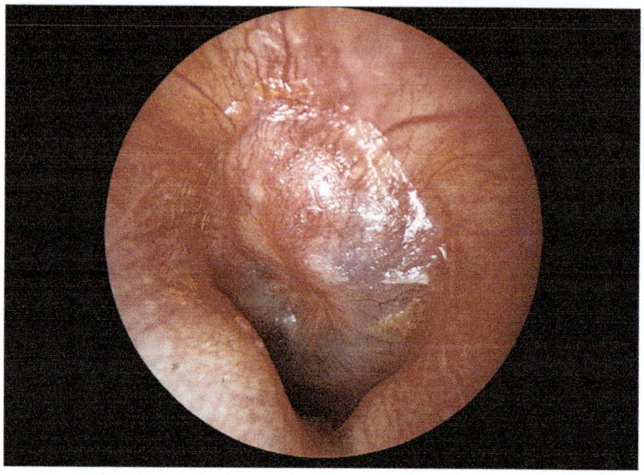

Figure 26.6 Acute otitis media.

usage, poor sanitation, allergy, overcrowding and malnutrition have also been implicated. *Streptococcus pneumo niae,Haemophilusinfluenzae*and *Moraxella catarrhalis* are the most frequent bacterial organisms identified on tympanocentesis. Bacterial co-infections with viruses are common, whereas isolated viral infections are reported to make up only 20% of AOM infections. Overall rates of AOM appear to be falling in North America. The reason for this remains unknown. Vaccination for *Pneumococcus* serotypes has been reported to have a significant impact in decreasing the incidence of pneumococcal AOMand its complications. Vaccination against *Influenza* is also recommended by some authorities as this may decrease the incidence of AOM and has also been implicated in its declining incidence.

For the majority of children, AOM is usually a self-resolving condition. First-line treatment for all children with AOM remains adequate analgesia and effective control of fever. Antibiotic usage in the management of children with AOM remains debated with some advocating a 24–72-hour period of watchful waiting. Antibiotic treatment has been proven to reduce pain, rate of tympanic membrane perforation and episodes of contralateral AOM, but this must be considered against the potential adverse events of antibiotic usage such as vomiting, diarrhoea or rash. The majority of published guidelines for AOM recommend that routine antibiotic prescription should be avoided in mild to moderate cases and when there is a diagnostic uncertainty in patients who are 2 years of age or older. Antibiotics are reported to be most beneficial in children who are aged 2 years and younger and that have bilateral disease. A 5-day course of amoxicillin or a macrolide in patients allergic to penicillin is recommended. Rare complications of AOM include mastoiditis, meningitis and intra-cranial abscesses. Population based studies in the Netherlands, where antibiotic usage for AOM is less common have demonstrated an increase in the incidence of mastoiditis. In the United Kingdom, it has been estimated that for children with AOM although antibiotic usage is likely to have reduced the incidence by half, that is approximately 4,800 children still need to be treated to prevent one episode of mastoiditis. Many of the large trials looking at antibiotic usage for AOM excluded children who were systemically unwell. It should also be noted that the majority of evidence in these reviews is derived from research in first world countries, and it is not known whether these management protocols are appropriate for populations outwith this group of countries and/or populations that have a higher risks of complications. Evidence based guidelines must therefore be interpreted with this in mind.

Recurrent AOM may be managed either expectantly with a long-term course of antibiotics, such as amoxicillin for 6 weeks, or surgically with ventilation tubes and/or adenoidectomy. Studies have identified those children who are diagnosed with AOM before the age of 2 years as being at higher risk of recurrence. The Scottish Intercollegiate Guidelines Network recommends that any child with four or more episodes of AOM over a period of 6 months may be considered for ventilation tube insertion. Factors such as frequency, severity, and impact on activities of daily living of the effects of recurrent AOM should be taken into account when considering ongoing management, as should associated factors such as the occurrence of febrile convulsions, mastoiditis and the presence of ventriculoperitoneal shunts.

Chronic Suppurative Otitis Media

For most tympanic membrane, perforations associated with AOM, the discharge will settle spontaneously and the underlying perforation will heal without any intervention being required. However, in a small number of children, the perforation will not heal, and they can end up with a chronically or intermittently discharging ear **(Figs. 26.7 and 26.8)**. Chronic otorrhoea can also occur

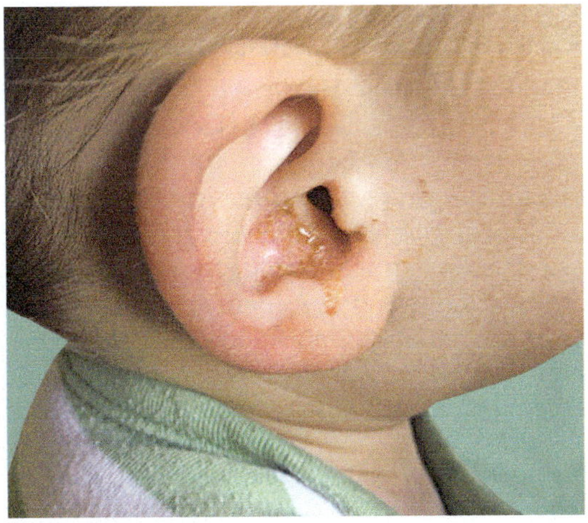

Figure 26.7 Right ear with otorrhoea.

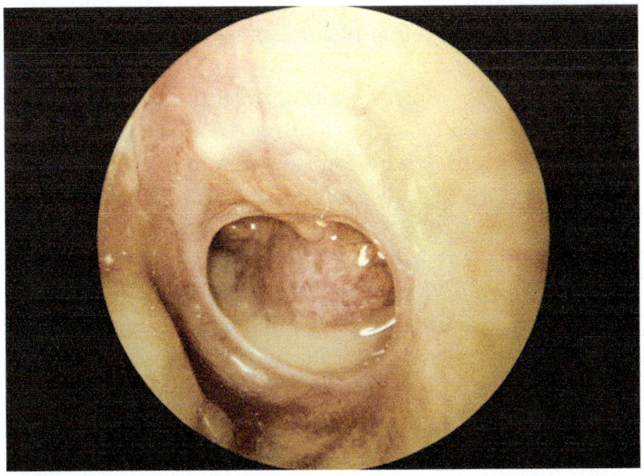

Figure 26.8 Tympanic membrane showing large central perforation and discharge.

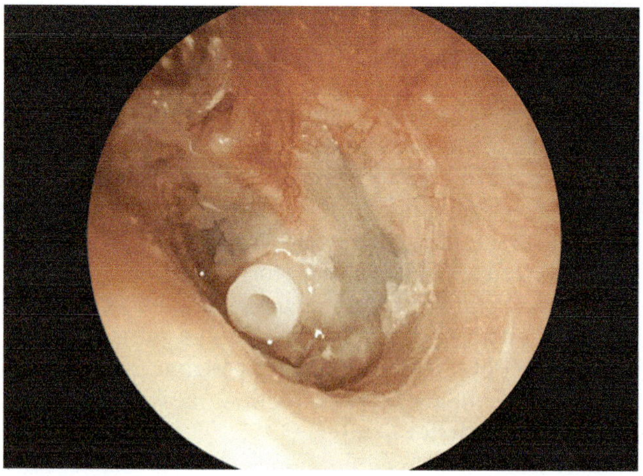

Figure 26.9 Left tympanic membrane showing ventilation tube in situ with discharge.

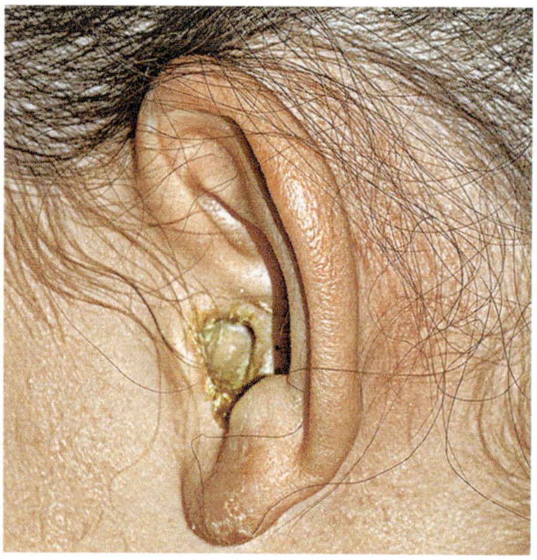

Figure 26.10 Post-auricular oedema, erythema—mastoiditis.

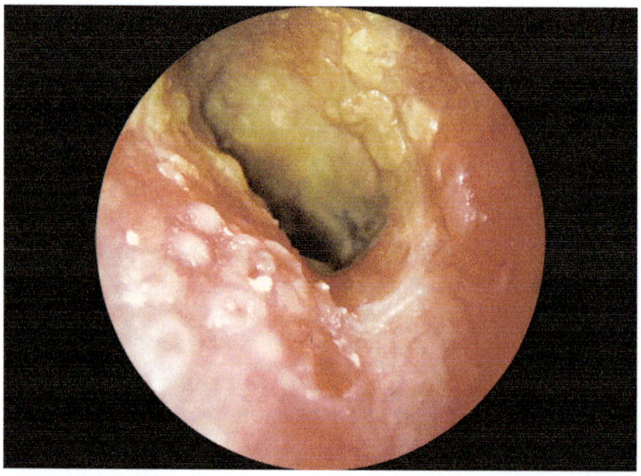

Figure 26.11 Otitis externa.

following ventilation tube insertion (Fig. 26.9). The management for both remains the same with treatment with either topical or oral antibiotics. Recent Cochrane reviews show the use of topical quinolone eardrops to be superior to oral antibiotics in clearing the discharge. In the United Kingdom, where topical quinolone eardrops are not licensed ENT UK recommends the use of topical antibiotic/steroid eardrops (such as gentamicin with hydrocortisone). In cases where topical aminoglycosides are used, these should be used for no longer than 2 weeks. Chronically discharging ears put patients at greater of risk of developing intracranial infections and abscesses. Where the discharge fails to respond to appropriate antibiotic therapy onward referral to exclude an underlying cholesteatoma or for surgery to repair the perforation or remove the ventilation tube is advised. In the case of an asymptomatic tympanic membrane perforation, no treatment is required.

Mastoiditis

Mastoiditis is infection in the air cells in the mastoid process of the temporal bone. The infection is preceded by AOM and caused by the same organisms. Swelling will be identified in the post auricular sulcus due to the occurrence of a cellulitis or subperiosteal abscess (Fig. 26.10). Urgent referral is required for intravenous antibiotics and possible surgery. Associated complications include facial palsy, sigmoid sinus thrombosis, meningitis and extradural, temporal lobe and posterior fossa abscesses.

Cholesteatoma

Cholesteatoma is a process whereby squamous epithelium that would normally migrate out via the external auditory canal fails to do so and is caught in the middle ear cleft. This may be either a congenital process where a keratin pearl has become entrapped behind the tympanic membrane during development or an acquired process where the middle ear respiratory epithelium changes to become squamous epithelium, or a retraction pocket develops in the tympanic membrane that is unable to effectively clear itself. The mechanisms of the development of acquired cholesteatomas are poorly understood and probably multifactorial. Clinically cholesteatomas present with recurrent intermittent or chronic foul smelling otorrhoea with or without hearing loss. There is an associated risk of developing permanent hearing loss due to damage to the ossicles as well as intracranial complications as discussed above. Any patient with a suspected cholesteatoma should be referred.

Otitis Externa

Otitis externa is inflammation of the skin of the external auditory canal (Fig. 26.11). This can be either primary or secondary to AOM. Primary otitis externa is often associated with underlying dermatological problems such as eczema, psoriasis and other dermatitides. Treatment includes dry mopping of the ear with cotton wool, syringing with body temperature saline and topical antibiotic eardrops. Patients should be advised not to go swimming whilst the infection is active. Microbial swabs are not required routinely for simple otitis externa. In recurrent cases where swimming is involved, ear protection in the form of ear plugs can be recommended. For cases of recalcitrant otitis externa not settling with the above measures, a microbial swab should be sent to exclude a fungal infection and skin patch testing to common carrier agents (such as benzylalkalonium) should be undertaken to exclude an allergy to eardrops.

Otitis Media with Effusion, Glue Ear, Serous Otitis Media

Otitis media with effusion is defined as the accumulation of fluid in the middle ear cleft without the symptoms and signs of acute inflammation. It is common with up to 80% children having OME before the age of 10 years. Risk factors for the development of OME include being male, attending day care/nursery, having older siblings, seasonal (winter), having frequent respiratory tract infections, exposure to tobacco smoke, prematurity, trisomy 21, having a cleft palate and ethnicity (New Zealand Māori, Australian Aboriginals and North America Inuits). The role of allergy is implicated but not proven. Children with OME may present with any or all of the following symptoms including hearing loss, poor attention and/or behaviour, concerns with speech/language, and delayed educational progress. Earache and balance problems are both uncommon. Clinically on examination, the tympanic membrane will appear opaque with a yellow or brown hue (Fig. 26.12). For the majority of children, this is a self-limiting process with the effusion/s clearing spontaneously in 50–90% of children within 3 months. Predictors that the effusion is more likely to resolve spontaneously include being 4 years of age or older, being female, having a hearing loss less than 40 dB through speech frequencies and summer coming up. These factors should be considered in the ongoing management for these children. Advice to parents should include smoking cessation, and where appropriate and possible, encouraging breastfeeding. On a practical level people involved in the care of a child with OME should be instructed to speak facing the child directly (to allow for pick-up of visual cues), to speak slowly and clearly (not shouting) and to minimise background noise. Placement in the classroom should be optimised so that the child's better hearing ear is always facing towards the teacher. Most guidelines recommend that if the effusion has been present for greater than 3 months, and there is an associated disability in the form of a hearing loss of greater than 25–30 dB on average through speech frequencies proven on audiogram, then either surgery in the form of ventilation tube insertion with or without adjuvant adenoidectomy or a trial of hearing aids is appropriate. In the interim, the use of devices to encourage autoinflation (ear popping) have been advocated. As with all guideline interpretation the clinician should consider other factors that may impact on the child's overall well-being, which may well prompt earlier referral for these children. These factors include severity of hearing loss, impact on quality of life, developmental concerns/problems, speech and language delay. Ongoing debate remains around adjuvant adenoidectomy at the first set of ventilation tube insertion with its proponents citing the TARGET study that demonstrated that adjuvant adenoidectomy conferred benefit in hearing for up to 2 years. The NICE Clinical Guideline recommends adenoidectomy only if a second set of ventilation tubes are required whereas the more recently updated AAP/AAOHNS clinical guideline recommends adenoidectomy routinely be undertaken by itself or combination with ventilation tube insertion in children aged 4 years or older and in those aged 4 years if there are nasal symptoms. No other treatments have been shown to provide effective treatment, including homeopathy, nasal decongestants, antibiotics, antihistamines, mucolytics and steroids.

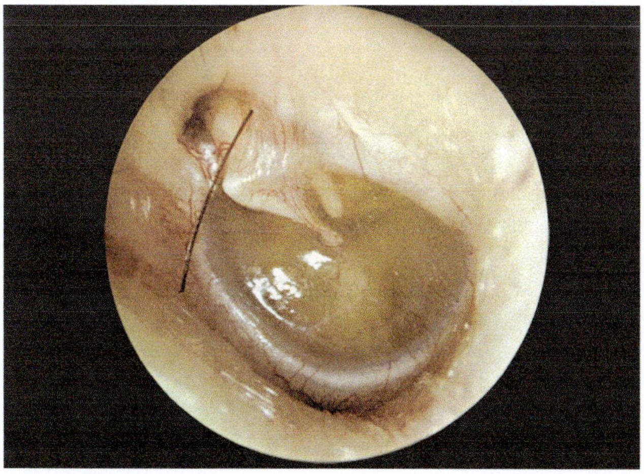

Figure 26.12 Otitis media with effusion.

Two groups of children who are at higher risk of OME and ear complications warrant further mention. First children with trisomy 21, as these children are reported to do less well with ventilation tube insertion with poorer hearing outcomes and higher rates of complications. A trial of hearing aids may be a more appropriate way of managing these children's hearing loss and is recommended as first line treatment by NICE, with ventilation tube insertion being recommended only if children and families are aware of potential poorer outcomes. This was also thought to be so for children with cleft lip and palate (CLP).However, there is now a growing body of evidence that demonstrates the benefits of ventilation tube insertion in the development of speech and language in children with cleft palate and OME and that complication rates for ventilation tube insertion among these children are not any higher than those among patients without CLP.

Trauma to the Tympanic Membrane

Following blunt trauma to the pinna or side of the head, some patients will experience bleeding from the ear canal and hearing loss. In the cases where there is a suspected tympanic membrane perforation, the patient should be advised to keep the ear dry and be reviewed in around 6 weeks. The majority of tympanic membrane perforations will heal spontaneously during this time. No attempt should be made during this time to try and remove any clot from the ear canal mechanically or with drops as removal of the clot may prevent normal healing of the tympanic membrane. If the patient has a haemotympanum (blood in the middle ear), this should resolve spontaneously over a similar time period. In cases of high velocity trauma, remember to consider a basal skull fracture, in particular, if there is cerebrospinal fluid (CSF) leakage from the ear canal, Battle's sign (mastoid ecchymoses) or a facial palsy. If the facial palsy occurs immediately at the time of trauma, surgical decompression and repair of the nerve should be considered urgently. In cases where a neurological injury is suspected referral to a paediatric neurosurgeon should be sought. Hearing testing, once the tympanic membrane has healed or haemotympanumresolved, should be undertaken to exclude an ossicular dislocation or a dead ear due to temporal bone fracture through the cochlea.

Foreign Bodies in the Ear

Children will frequently put things into their ears. Non-organic foreign bodies, excluding batteries, will often be able to be removed with gentle syringing. In cases where the foreign body is unable to be removed, referral to a paediatric otolaryngologist should be sought.

CONGENITAL CONDITIONS OF THE EAR

Congenital Hearing Loss in Children

The reported incidence of congenital hearing loss in children is 1–2:1,000 live births. This increases up to around 3:1,000 children within the first 5 years of life. Around 50% of these children will have a hearing loss due to genetic causes including some syndromes, 30% will be due to post-natal causes such as childhood infections, 12% due to perinatal causes, 8% due to intrauterine causes, and in 20–30%, there will be no identifiable cause. The majority of children will have a sensorineural hearing loss. Universal screening for congenital hearing loss is now undertaken routinely in most Western countries using automated auditory brainstem reflex (AABR) testing or transient evoked OAE. It should still be remembered that half of the children who have a hearing loss in the first 5 years of life will not be identified by universal hearing screening as these children will have a loss that develops after the first few weeks of life. Risk factors for developing a hearing loss include low birth weight (<1,500 g), Apgar Scores less than 6 at 5 minutes, kernicterus, family history of hearing loss, meningitis, encephalitis, ototoxic drug exposure, craniofacial syndrome, maternal diabetes mellitus and intrauterine exposure to any of the TORCH agents (toxoplasmosis, syphilis, rubella, cytomegalovirus, herpes simplex virus). Children who have any of the above risk factors require ongoingaudiological review. Hearing loss may present with any of the symptoms already discussed in the OME section above. Where an anomaly of the pinna or external auditory canal is noted **(Fig. 26.13)**, a hearing loss should also be suspected and appropriate testing undertaken. It is most likely that any associated hearing loss will be conductive in nature although these children can also have either mixed or sensorineural hearing losses. Genetic causes for hearing loss are most easily thought of as syndromal or non-syndromal and autosomal dominant, autosomal recessive, X linked or de novo. The majority of children with prelingual hearing loss (hearing loss occurring prior to the development of speech and language) of genetic origin will have a hearing loss due to autosomal recessive traits with the most common of these being mutations in *GJB2* gene encoding connexin 26. Syndromes associated with autosomal recessive hearing loss include Pendreds syndrome, Ushers syndrome, Jervell and Lange-Nielsen syndrome and branchio-otorenal syndrome. Autosomal dominant causes associated with congenital hearing loss include Treacher Collins syndrome, Waardenburg syndrome, Pierre-Robin syndrome, Crouzons syndrome and Aperts syndrome. Many children will have genetic syndromic hearing loss due to de novo mutations with the most common being children with trisomy 21.

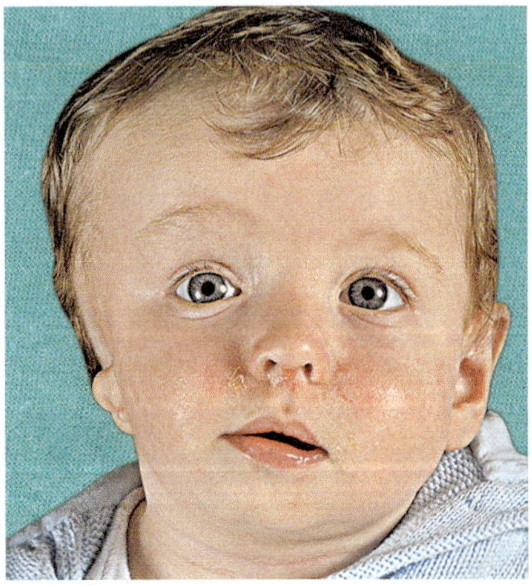

Figure 26.13 Child with right hemifacial microsomia (Goldenhar syndrome).

Management of Hearing Loss in Children

Once a hearing loss has been identified, it is important to assess the degree and type of loss. For this it is recommended to carry out a battery of tests which includes ABR, ASSR. Tympanograms, Diagnostic Oto Acoustic Emissions and the age appropriate behavioural hearing test/ pure tone audiogram (see above for details of each test).

The hearing loss is then categorised as conductive, sensorineural or mixed (both conductive and sensorineural). Based on the threshold of hearing, the severity is classified as mild, moderate, severe or profound.

Conductive Hearing Loss

A conductive hearing loss occurs when there is a problem with the outer or middle ear. The most common cause of a conductive hearing loss in children is Otitis Media with Effusion (OME). Other conditions are Chronic Otitis Media and Cholesteatoma. Atresia of the ear canals with/without a Microtia (underdevelopment or absence of the pinna) will also result in a conductive hearing loss. Rarely it may be due to a congenital fixation of the ossicular chain. The management of OME, CSOM and Cholesteatoma is described above. Congenital ossicular chain fixation is best managed with conventional hearing aids. If the wearing of conventional hearing aids is not possible (such as in the case of atretic ear canals) and the hearing loss is of a conductive nature, a bone conduction hearing aid is more appropriate.

Sensorineural Hearing Loss

Sensorineural hearing loss, often called 'nerve deafness' is caused by damage to the cochlea, or the nerve pathways between the cochlea and the brain and is usually permanent.

For children with mild to moderate hearing loss, the clinician should consider the best form of hearing aids for that individual child. Where possible appropriately programmed, bilateral, behind the ear hearing digital aids are the first line of treatment. In the classroom setting, the use of loop systems or FM devices to assist amplification have been found to be helpful. If the hearing loss is severe or profound (greater than 70dB through speech frequencies), then cochlear implantation should be considered and referral to the Cochlear Implant team should be undertaken.

Once the child is referred to the Cochlear Implant team, they undergo a series of assessments to assess eligibility for cochlear implantation. The information gathered also enables to cochlea implant team to identify any additional conditions or needs and helps candidates establish appropriate expectations.

- *Audiological*
  - Hearing levels with and without hearing aids.
  - Speech understanding with hearing aids.
  - Auditory nerve function.
- *Medical*
  - Evaluation of cause of hearing loss
  - General health.
- *Radiological*
  - CT and/or MRI studies of the brain and ears
- *Speech and Language*
  - Assessment of stage of speech and language development.
- *Psychological*
  - Ability to cope with surgery.
  - Ability to participate in follow up programme.
- *Educational*
  - Assessment of educational needs.

When the team has gathered all the information they need, they may decide either that an implant is unlikely to help the child, or that an implant might help the child.

Sometimes this is a complex decision. Parents are usually involved in discussion leading up to the decision.

Cochlear Implant

Cochlear implants differ from hearing aids in that hearing aids simply amplify sounds. A cochlear implant, on the other hand, transforms speech and other sounds into electrical energy that is used to stimulate the spiral ganglion in the cochlea.

Cochlear implants have both internal and external components. The implant system consists of an external speech processor and an internal, surgically implanted receiver/stimulator package with an electrode array.

Sound is picked up by a microphone placed on the ear. The microphone converts the sound into electrical energy. This electrical signal is transmitted through a cable to the speech processor.

The speech processor, an ear level device analyses and digitises the sound into coded signals. This coding is done by the processor depending on how it is programmed/ mapped. The speech processor decides how much current is to be sent into the cochlea so that the wearer will hear the sound. The coded signal from the speech processor is sent to the transmitting coil worn on the head. This coil is held in place with a magnet. The transmitting coil sends the coded signal across the skin via radio frequency link, to the receiver stimulator package.

The receiver-stimulator package is surgically fitted in the mastoid bone of the skull just behind the ear. The receiver stimulator package contains a magnet so that the transmitting coil and receiver are aligned with each other without any direct contact through the skin. The signal from the receiver stimulator package is sent to the electrode array which has been surgically placed into the scala tympani of the cochlea. Stimulation of the electrode array leads to stimulation of the nerve endings of the spiral ganglion in the cochlea. This results in a sensation of sound.

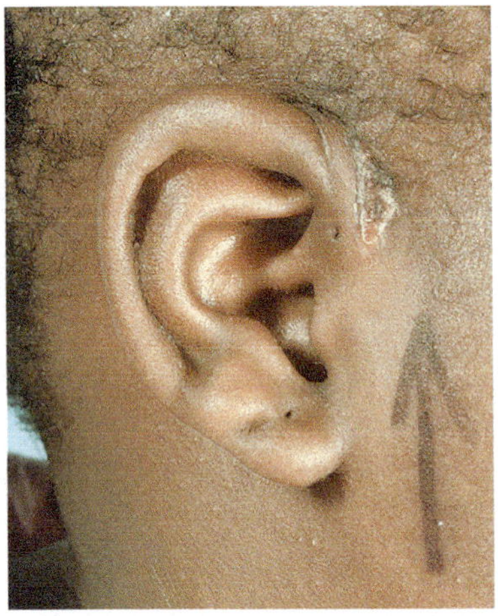

Figure 26.14 Right pre-auricular sinus with area of previous infection.

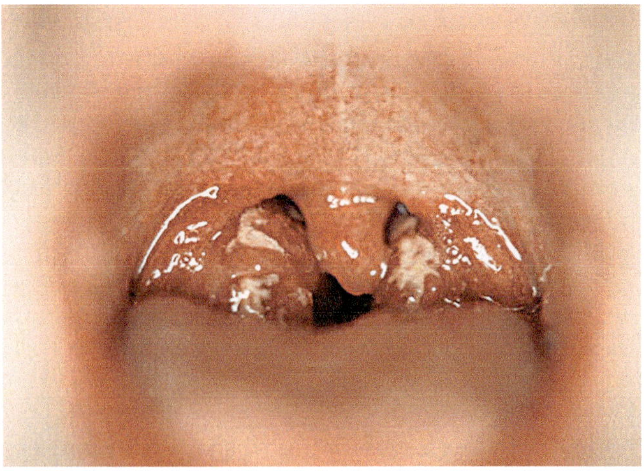

Figure 26.15 Acute tonsillitis.

Early Intervention for Hearing Loss in Children

Babies start to develop language from the moment they are born. If a child has a hearing loss, the basic development of language will often by delayed. The phenomenon of neural plasticity allows the younger child's brain process new information better than that of older children. The first 2 years are especially important for language acquisition. The younger a child's age when receiving a hearing device, the easier it will be for him/ her to learn to hear and speak.

Habilitation is the learning phase following fitting of hearing aids or cochlear implantation and is essential to good hearing and communication outcomes. Babies have to learn to understand the sounds they now hear and to communicate with the people around them. A comprehensive educational and habilitation programme of speech and language therapy will increase the child's ability to benefit from their hearing aid or cochlear implant.

Pre-auricular Sinus

This a common congenital anomaly with the incidence being reported as between 0.1 and 0.9% in European and North American populations, 2.5% in Taiwan and increasing to up to 10% in some African regions. They can occur bilaterally. They have been associated with hearing loss and renal anomalies, but these associations as yet remain unproven. Surgery is only recommended if any infections have occurred, or the patient is troubled by unpleasant discharge. The lifetime incidence of infection is reported at around one in every three **(Fig. 26.14)**.

ACQUIRED CONDITIONS OF THE PHARYNX

Acute Tonsillitis

Sore throats are a common presenting complaint in children. The majority of these sore throats are of viral origin. Bacterial infections are less common with group A beta-haemolytic *Streptococcus*, the most common bacterial infection, being identified as causing only 5–36% of all throat infections. Tonsillar exudate, tender anterior cervical lymph nodes, a history of fever and absence of cough should all alert the clinician to the diagnosis of acute tonsillitis. The likelihood of streptococcal infection is greatest in the 5–15-year-old age group. If there is any stridor, stertor or other breathing difficulties admission to hospital should be considered.

The keystones to treating children with acute tonsillitis are adequate analgesia and rehydration. Paracetamol/ acetaminophen is most appropriate first-line analgesic for children. Ibuprofen can be used in combination with paracetamol/acetaminophen or separately as long as the child is well hydrated. Oral rehydration is the preferred route; however, in severe cases, intravenous fluids may be required. Where a diagnosis of acute tonsillitis has been made, the antibiotic of choice is penicillin. A macrolide antibiotic should be considered where a penicillin allergy exists. It should be remembered that Epstein-Barr virus (glandular fever/infectious mononucleosis) will also commonly present with a tonsillar exudate. As some children diagnosed with bacterial tonsillitis will later be found to have tonsillitis due to the Epstein-Barr virus; ampicillin-based antibiotics are not recommended, as these have been noted to cause a rash in up to 10% of these children **(Fig. 26.15)**.

Recurrent Tonsillitis

The aetiology of recurrent tonsillitis is poorly understood. Over time, in the majority of children, the frequency and severity of episodes of tonsillitis usually improve spontaneously. There are no useful clinical or laboratory predictors to assist in predicting which child is going to progress with chronic symptoms.

Both the AAO-HNS/AAP and Scottish Intercollegiate Guidelines Network (SIGN) clinical guidelines recommend the following as basis for referral to a paediatric otolaryngologist for consideration for tonsillectomy.

- Sore throats are due to acute tonsillitis
- The episodes of sore throat are disabling and prevent normal functioning
- Seven or more well documented, clinically significant, adequately treated sore throats in the preceding year or
- Five or more such episodes in each of the preceding 2 years or
- Three or more such episodes in each of the preceding 3 years.

The clinician should also take into account the individual patients overall condition as well as the frequency, severity and trends of these infections as well as their complications.

Following surgery, many patients will present with increasing pain and halitosis. This is rarely a sign of infection, unless there are associated fevers and antibiotics are not recommended routinely rather an improved analgesic regime should be instituted.

Drooling

In children with no neurodevelopmental problems, drooling is normal up to the age of 5 years of age. All that is required is to increase oral awareness, which should be encouraged by simple measures, such as reminding the child to wipe their mouth and swallow. The use of play in the form of using a toothbrush may be found to help with oral awareness. Some clinicians recommend the use of sweatbands around the wrist for the child to wipe their mouth with. Drooling is more common and will often take longer to resolve in boys and/or if there is nasal obstruction. In severe cases, where the drooling is failing to resolve within the normal time parameters or there is severe excoriation, referral to a paediatric otolaryngologist should be considered. Adenoidectomy or adenotonsillectomy may prove beneficial for these children.

For children with identified neurodevelopmental problems drooling can be a major problem not only with skin breakdown but also as obstacle to normal social interactions. For the majority of these children, this is not a problem of hypersalivation but inability to swallow their own normal saliva. This can be made worse by poor posture and mouth control as well as a dyskinetic swallow. Factors that may potentiate drooling by increasing salivation include gastro-oesophageal reflux disease, dental caries and some medications including the benzodiazepine group. Positioning should be assessed as effective support to sit the child in an upright position, such as in a customised chair, may help. Where conservative measures have failed, review by a saliva control multi-disciplinary team should be undertaken. The multidisciplinary team (MDT) should include speech and language therapy and physiotherapy review in the first instance. Where these interventions have failed other treatment options can be considered. The use of oral or transcutaneous anticholinergic medications and/or botulinum toxin injections to the major salivary glands can prove effective. Where all other options have failed, surgery may be considered in the form of adenoidectomy, adenotonsillectomy or salivary gland surgery. Salivary gland surgery may include either ligation of some or most of the major salivary gland ducts, transposition of the submandibular ducts to the tonsillar fossa or submandibular gland excision.

Snoring/Obstructive Sleep Apnoea Hypopnoea Syndrome/Sleep-related Breathing Disorder

Most children will snore at some time during their childhood. Habitual snoring is common and is reported to occur in 5–12% of general paediatric populations with disruptive sleeping occurring in 4–11% and obstructive sleep apnoea hypopnoea syndrome (OSAHS) in 1–4%. The diagnosis is often not straightforward as there are no single or combined symptoms and/or signs that can satisfactorily predict the presence of OSAHS. Nocturnal symptoms that are suggestive of OSAHS include snoring, witnessed apnoeas, restlessness, frequent awakening, enuresis, sweating and positioning with neck extended. Daytime symptoms can include hypersomnolence, hyperactivity, poor concentration/neurocognitive changes, low-energy levels, failure to thrive, behavioural concerns (becoming withdrawn/shy or aggressive/disruptive) and symptoms of pulmonary hypertension (rare). The peak incidence of OSAHS is reported in the 2–4-year-old age group. Risk factors for developing OSAHS include being male, deprivation, obesity, ethnicity, generalized low motor tone (cerebral palsy) and processes, which affect normal mandibular or maxillary development. Other factors implicated include exposure to tobacco smoke, atopic disorders and viral infections. Syndromes associated with OSAHS include Pierre Robin/cleft palate, craniofacial syndromes (Apert syndrome, Crouzons syndrome, Treacher–Collins syndrome), the achondroplasia group, children with mucopolysaccharidoses and Downs syndrome.

Examination should include assessment of the size of the tonsils, presence or absence of mouth breathing (adenoidal facies), listening for stertor, assessing nasal airflow (spatula test) and the chest for associated deformities (pectusexcavatum or carinatum) **(Fig. 26.16)**. Parents will often attend with a recording of their child sleeping on a camera phone, which may also assist with the diagnosis. Polysomnography is the gold standard investigation, but its routine use in most centres is limited due to resource availability. Overnight home pulse oximetry

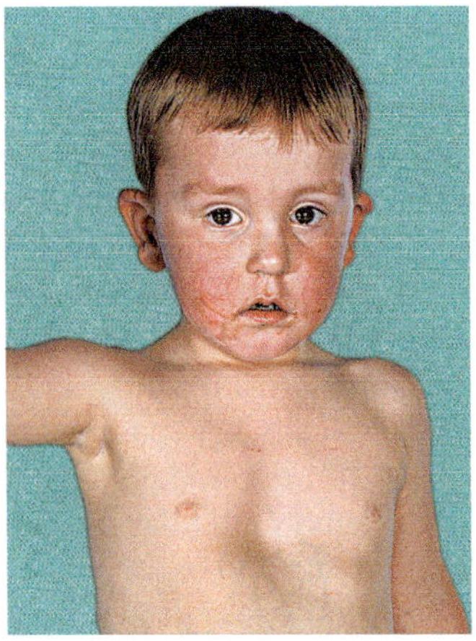

Figure 26.16 Child demonstrating adenoidal facies and pectusexcavatum.

(Fig. 26.17) is now used by many clinicians as it has a reasonable correlation with polysomnography but this will fail to identify some of the children with moderate to mild OSAHS. A consensus statement drafted by an ENT UK multi-disciplinary working group suggested formal investigation should be undertakenwhere:

- Diagnosis of OSA unclear or inconsistent
- Age less than 2 years
- Weight less than 15 kg
- Downs syndrome
- Cerebral palsy
- Hypotonia or neuromuscular disorders
- Craniofacial anomalies
- Mucopolysaccharidosis
- Obesity (body mass index >2.5 standard deviation scores or >99th centile for age and gender)
- Significant co-morbidity such as congenital heart disease, chronic lung disease
- Residual symptoms after adenotonsillectomy

X-ray of the post-nasal space does not assist with diagnosis, and therefore is not required as it exposes the child to unnecessary radiation. Although there has been a poor correlation reported between symptomatology

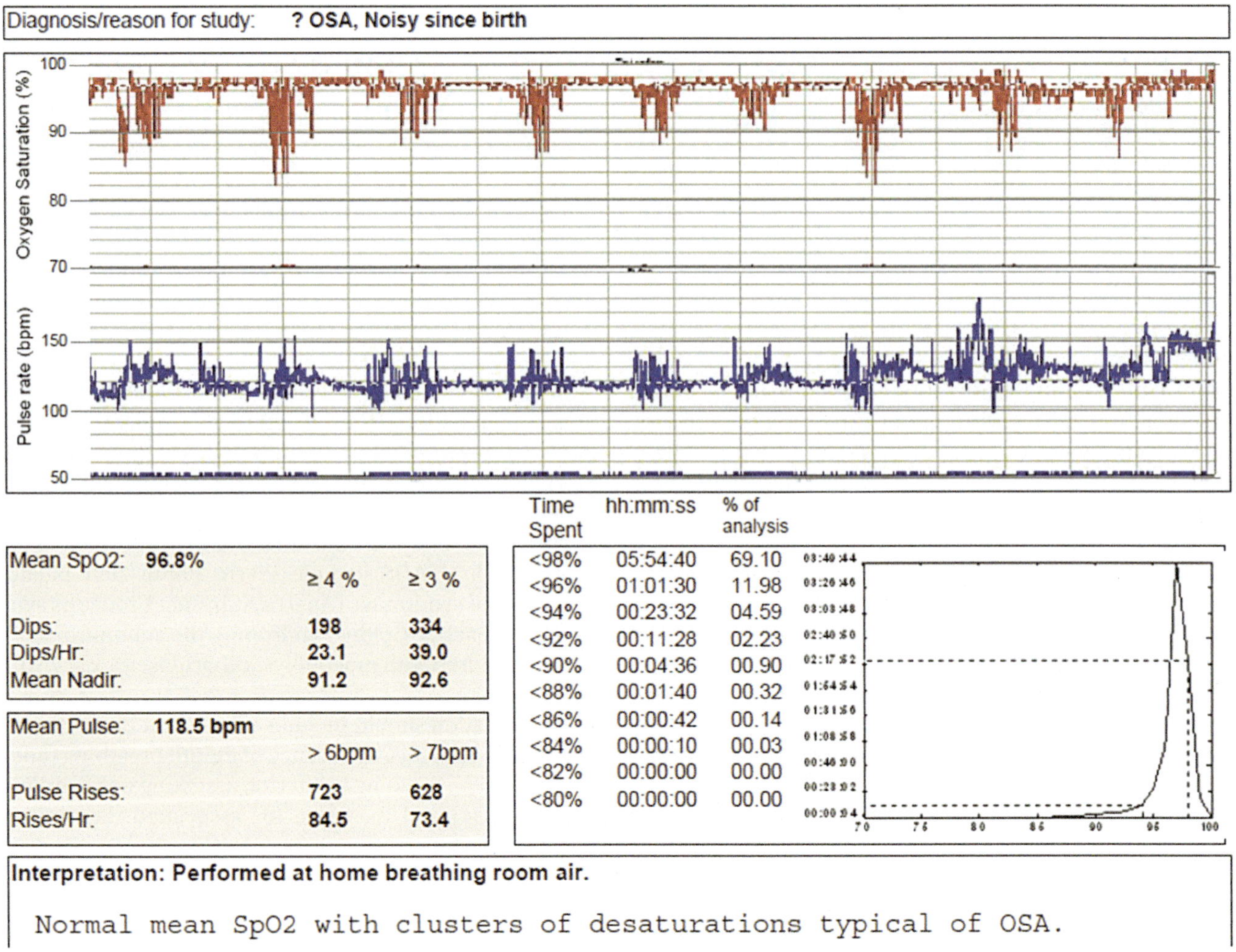

Figure 26.17 Overnight pulse oximetry demonstrating obstructive sleep apnoea syndrome.

and polysomnography; many clinicians continue to rely on symptoms as their sole means of diagnosis. For children with craniofacial syndromes, in particular those with craniosynostoses, that have the potential for raised intracranial pressure, full polysomnography is essential, as this will allow differentiation between central and obstructive events.

The main thrust in diagnosing and treating OSAHS is to prevent its more severe long-term effects in the areas of neurocognitive development, growth and pulmonary hypertension. The treatment of OSAHS is dependent upon the underlying cause/s. For children with craniofacial syndromes corrective surgery to the mid face and mandible may expedite the resolution of OSAHS. Children with low motor tone may benefit more from positive pressure ventilation. Obese children will benefit from weight loss and where appropriate onward referral to a dietician and paediatric endocrinologist. For the majority of children however, adenoidectomy or adenotonsillectomy remains the first line in treatment of OSAHS. Using polysomnography as an outcome the success rate of adenotonsillectomy is reported to range from 79 to 92%. Quality of life improvements following adenotonsillectomy have also been demonstrated in a number of studies as have improvements in behavioural and neurocognitive parameters. For some children where an allergic component is thought to be significant, treatment with topical nasal steroids have been reported to lead to improvement. For children with more complex airway problems, the placement of a nasopharyngeal airway or tracheostomy or positive pressure ventilation may be required as a short term or permanent treatment. Where symptoms/investigations are inconclusive or the child has failed to simple treatment measures, referral to paediatric pulmonologist/respiratory paediatrician with an interest in sleep should be considered.

CONDITIONS OF THE AIRWAY

Neonatal/Infantile Stridor

Stridor is an inspiratory or biphasic sound created by turbulent airflow from the level of larynx to the thoracic inlet. Its likely aetiology **(Flow chart 26.1)** will vary with the age of the child. A good history will alert the clinician to any atypical features, which would warrant onward referral. In infants or neonates presenting with stridor the history should include the age of onset, quality, severity, if it is worsening or improving with time and if there are any feeding, sleep or growth concerns. Associated symptoms of apnoeic or cyanotic events as well as the presence and/or severity of gastro-oesophageal reflux should be enquired about. Intubation history, previous surgery, cardiac conditions along with any birthmarks also should be ascertained. The examination should include determining if it is definitely stridor, the phasess of the stridor, looking for other signs of

Flow chart 26.1 Aetiology of stridor in children and infants.

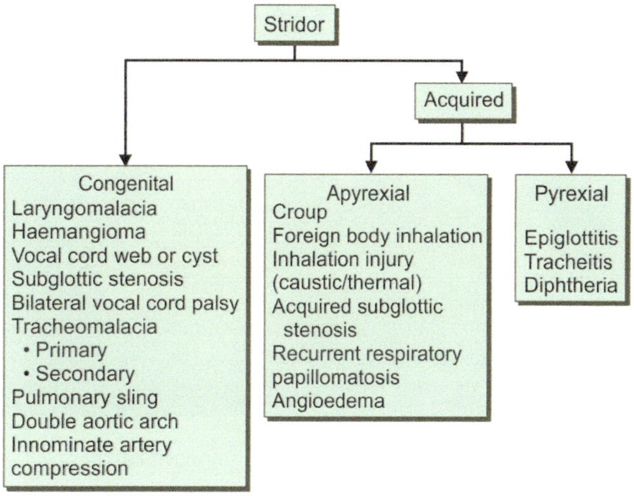

increasing work of breathing including head bobbing, indrawing/recession, chest changes (most commonly pectusexcavatum) and tracheal tug. If the stridor is biphasic then it is likely that the child has a subglottic lesion and immediate referral for further investigation should be undertaken. The strength and quality of the baby's cry, in particular, if it has a weak or hoarse cry should also be assessed as these can be signs of unilateral vocal cord paralysis, tracheomalacia or laryngeal papillomatosis. The baby should be checked for birthmarks in particular cutaneous haemangiomas as these can be associated with similar airway lesions. Where possible the baby should be observed during feeding and growth charts assessed. The following should alert the clinician to consider onward referral.

Warning Signs

- Biphasic stridor
- Failure to thrive
- Feeding difficulties
- Stridor severity or frequency worsening over time
- Severe gastro-oesophageal reflux (GORD)
- Work of breathing—high rate
- Chest anatomical changes (pectusexcavatum/carinatum)
- Hoarseness
- Cyanotic episodes
- Apnoeic episodes

Congenital Conditions of the Airway

Laryngomalacia

Laryngomalacia is the process where there is collapse of the airway at the level of the laryngeal inlet due to the structures of supraglottis (epiglottis, aryepiglottic folds and arytenoids) being drawn in on inspiration **(Fig. 26.18)**. It is

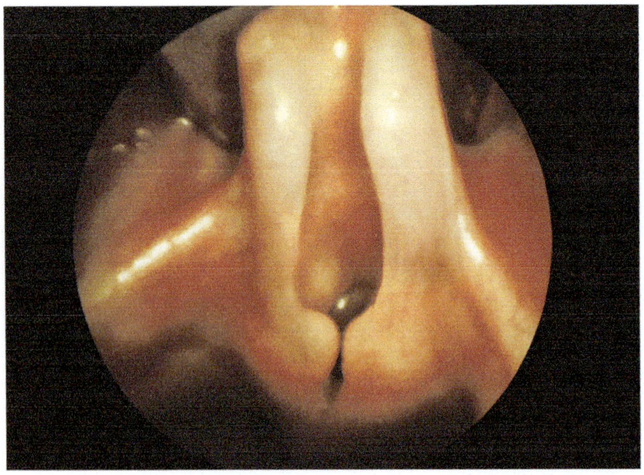

Figure 26.18 Omega-shaped epiglottitis with laryngomalacia.

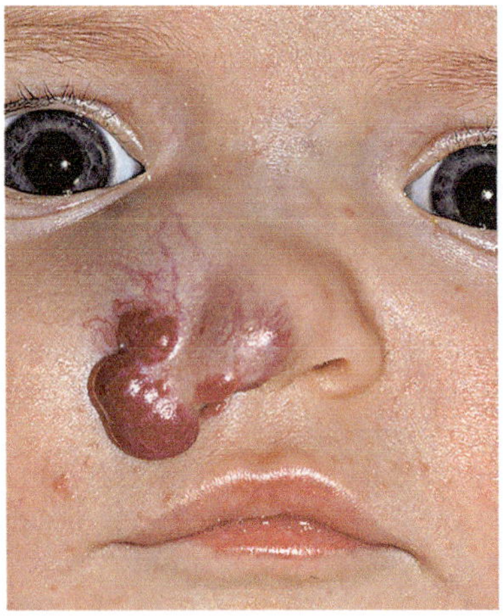

Figure 26.19 Nasal haemangioma.

reported to cause 80–90% of neonatal/infantile stridor. In the majority of children, this is a self-resolving condition. The aetiology of laryngomalacia is poorly understood, but there is a reported association with gastro-oesophageal reflux disease. The onset of stridor is classically described from around 1–2 weeks of age, but this is now debated with the onset of stridor not infrequently being heard earlier from around birth. Symptoms may worsen with feeding, lying prone or at night. Where the child is growing and feeding well, and there are no atypical features, reassurance and routine review of growth parameters is all that is required. If there are concerns regarding frequent or severe vomiting, slow or prolonged feeding or poor weight gain, a trial of thickeners and/or anti-reflux medications may prove beneficial. Cyanotic/apnoeic events are occasionally reported and are also most likely related to reflux. Where there is uncertainty regarding the diagnosis, fibre-optic laryngoscopy is helpful. If any of the above symptoms fail to resolve with optimal medical management then surgical review is warranted. Surgery involves procedures to widen the laryngeal inlet, debulk any prolapsing mucosa and stiffen the epiglottis. Surgery, when required, is successful in over 95% of infants with simple laryngomalacia.

Haemangiomas of the Airways

These are an uncommon cause of airway obstruction in infants. Fifty per cent of children with airway haemangiomas will have an associated cutaneous lesion **(Fig. 26.19)**. The most common site for these to occur in the airway is the subglottis, and they therefore present with biphasic stridor. The natural history of the airway lesions is the same as that of cutaneous infantile haemangiomas with a prolific growth phase up to the first 18 months of life followed by a gradual spontaneous regression. Management involves early confirmation of diagnosis by airway endoscopy. The majority of haemangiomas will respond to regular beta-blockers. Where the lesion proves to be resistant to beta-blockers, or it is small and isolated to the subglottis, surgical resection should be considered. CO_2 lasering has been employed in the past with limited success. Other medical treatments that have been used with reported success, include vincristine and interferon. Exacerbations of airway symptoms may be managed with short courses of oral steroids. Rarely in severe cases with extensive disease unresponsive to medical or local surgical treatment tracheostomy may still be required.

Acquired Conditions of the Airway

The most common acquired condition of the airway presenting with stridor is croup. **Table 26.1** demonstrates differences and similarities between the more common causes of acquired stridor.

Voice/Hoarseness

Hoarseness in children is uncommon. Where this occurs, the majority of children will be found to have vocal cord nodules or cysts. Infrequently hoarseness arises due to laryngeal papilloma. Hoarseness following cardiac surgery or patent ductusarteriosus surgery may be caused by the damage to the left recurrent laryngeal nerve. If constant hoarseness is present for more than 6 weeks, or there are feeding issues, stridor or concerns with regards to potential aspiration events awake laryngoscopy alone will allow for a diagnosis and decisions for appropriate management in most cases. Vocal cord nodules respond well to speech and language therapy exercises.

Recurrent Respiratory Papillomatosis

Recurrent respiratory papillomatosis (RRP) is caused by human papilloma virus (HPV) infection with subtypes 6 and 11 being the most commonly identified subtypes. The infection is acquired whilst in utero. It is uncommon

TABLE 26.1 Acquired stridor differential.

	Group	*Inhaled foreign body*	*Epiglottitis*	*Bacterial tracheitis*
Age range	3/12 months to 6 years	6/12 months to 5 years	2–6 years	3/12 months to 12 years
Peak ages	3/12 months to 3 years	1–3 years	3–4 years	5 years
Key symptoms	Upper respiratory tract infection prodrome Cough—seal bark Hoarseness	Witnessed event Choking episode	Drooling Dysphagia Toxic Aphonia	Upper respiratory tract infection prodrome Toxic Hoarseness
Key signs	Stridor Cough	± Stridor ± Cough	Stridor Prefer to sit Tripod Fever	Stridor Cough—frequent Fever
Chest X-ray	Non-diagnostic	Can be diagnostic	Non-diagnostic	Non-diagnostic
White cell count	Usually normal	Usually normal	Raised	Usually raised
Response to steroids ± adrenaline	Yes	Sometimes but less likely	Yes	Sometimes but less likely
Incidence	Common	Less common	Rare	Very rare

with its incidence in children being reported between 0.24 and 4.3 per 100,000. RRP most commonly presents between the ages 0–5 years. Risk factors for developing RRP include young mothers, primigravida mothers, vaginal delivery birth, genital condylomata and lower socioeconomic status. Symptoms include hoarseness, voice change, stridor, and in severe cases respiratory distress. Treatment involves maintaining an adequate airway by intermittent surgical debridement. In severe cases, tracheostomy may be required, but where possible, it should be avoided as it may seed papillomata further down the airway. In severe cases, adjuvant treatments may be considered with intralesional injection with the virostatic agent cidofovir, intravenous interferon and oral indole-3-carbinol being most commonly used. For the majority of children, the disease activity will decrease and eventually cease over time. In some children with more aggressive disease, however the picture is one of seeding of papilloma throughout the airway and lungs with death from respiratory failure or malignant transformation. The introduction of universal or targeted vaccination with the quadrivalentHPV vaccine in some countries has the potential to significantly reduce the burden of this disease (Fig. 26.20).

Epiglottitis

This is acute inflammation of the epiglottis. The majority of cases are caused by *H. influenzae* type b. This usually affects children between the ages of 2 and 6 years. Clinically the child will look unwell, be stridulous, have a fever, be drooling and frequently sits in an upright position often using their arms to support himself (tripod position). If epiglottitis is suspected no further attempt should be made to examine the child without intensive care or anaesthetic back up. The child should be maintained in an upright position in a calm environment preferably on their parent's knee. Nebulised adrenaline may be given if this does not significantly distress the child. No attempt should be made to put in a cannula, examine the oropharynx or undertake an X-ray. The child should have a gaseous induction anaesthetic and intubated. Following this an appropriate antibiotic, such as co-amoxiclav and steroid therapy should be introduced. In countries where universal *H. influenzae* type b vaccination has been undertaken this disease has all but been eliminated (Fig. 26.21).

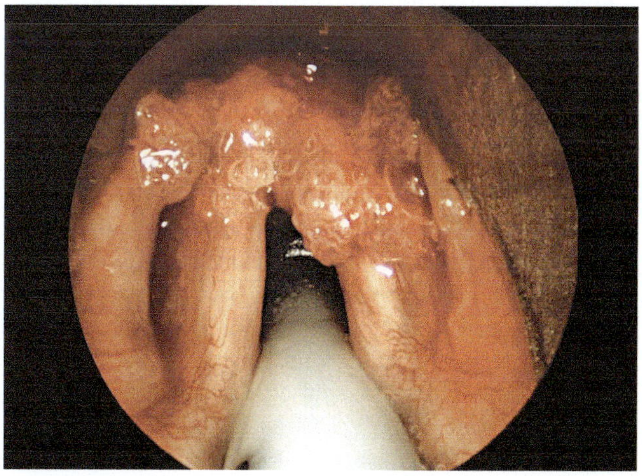

Figure 26.20 Laryngeal papillomatosis.

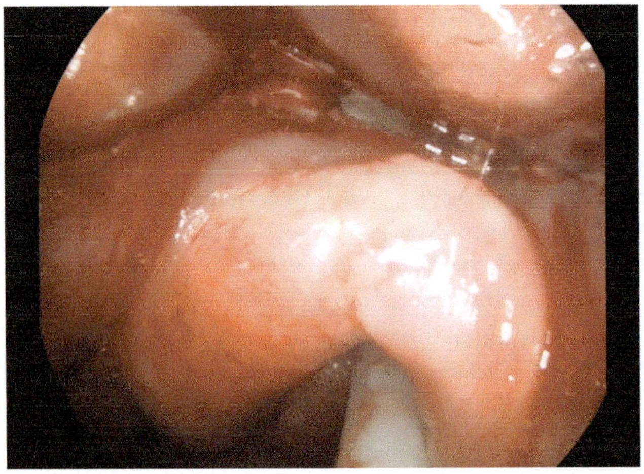

Figure 26.21 *Haemophilus influenzae* type B epiglottitis.

Bacterial Tracheitis

Bacterial tracheitis is an uncommon cause of stridor in children. It is caused by *Staphylococcus aureus* infection that leads to crusting and inflammation throughout the trachea. It occurs between the ages 3 months and 12 years with a peak age of 5 years. The child will usually have a preceding upper respiratory tract infection then subsequently develop a high fever, stridor, cough and hoarseness. Similar to epiglottitis, this can be a life threatening condition as the crusts that form in the trachea can consolidate to occlude the airway. Milder cases can be managed with intravenous flucloxacillin, steroids and nebulised adrenaline and saline. More severe cases will require intubation and/or rigid bronchoscopy with sequential debridement of the tracheal crusts.

Subglottic Stenosis

Subglottic stenosis can either be a congenital or acquired condition with the acquired forms occurring more commonly. Most often children with this condition will present with repeated failed attempts at extubation with associated stridor in the paediatric intensive care unit (PICU) or neonatal intensive care unit (NICU). More rarely, it will present with stridor on exertion or with repeated upper respiratory tract infections. Acquired subglottic stenosis is associated with intubation injuries, in particular too large an endotracheal tube being used, traumatic intubation or significant movement of this tube once in place. Nasotracheal rather than orotracheal intubation appears to be protective against the development of this condition. Subglottic stenosis occurs due to the cricoid cartilage being the only complete ring of cartilage in the airway so if there is damage in this area a circumferential scar occurs leading to a narrowing of the airway. Subglottic stenosis is graded using the Cotton-Myer grading system with grade 1 (<50% stenosis) being mild and grade 4 being complete occlusion of airway. It should be remembered that mild subglottic stenosis may require no treatment at all. If symptomatic and identified early, ballooning using specially designed airway balloons have been reported to give good results. In more severe cases or where ballooning has failed, grafting using a piece of rib cartilage may be required. This is known as laryngotracheal reconstruction. Tracheostomy can be used to temporise the patients' airway, but laryngotracheal reconstruction is the definitive treatment.

Foreign Bodies of the Airway

Children frequently inhale foreign bodies with the peak incidence occurring between 1 and 3 years of age. In extreme cases, the child will present with signs of respiratory distress, often however there is only a history of a choking or coughing event. Clinically, there may be increased work of breathing, stridor, cough or decreased air entry on auscultation. Chest X-ray is helpful if positive for the radio-opaque foreign body, mediastinal shift or focal hyperinflation, but carries a low sensitivity. Children who require immediate attention with urgent formal rigid bronchoscopy include those with airway compromise, suspected battery ingestion, suspected sharp foreign body, suspected nut aspiration and those with a suspected caustic burn. Those children with positive clinical signs or X-ray findings warrant bronchoscopy. In one series, a witnessed choking event was reported to carry a positive predictive value of around 97% of identifying a foreign body at bronchoscopy. However, debate still remains over the management of other children with a suspected foreign body inhalation although consideration of bronchoscopy for all children with suspected airway foreign bodies should be undertaken as the seriousness of the complications far outweighs the risks of anaesthesia in the majority of children. Complications of inhaled foreign bodies include pneumothorax, mediastinitis, pneumonia and empyema.

ACQUIRED CONDITIONS OF THE HEAD AND NECK

Cervical Lymphadenopathy

Neck masses in children are common with the most common cause being reactive cervical lymph nodes. Palpable lymphadenopathy is common in children. The majority of palpable nodes are reactive, and serious pathology is rare. Reactive nodes will frequently fluctuate in size and will often increase in size with subsequent upper respiratory tract infections.

Warning Signs

- Nodes greater than 2–3 cm in size
- Nodes in the supraclavicular region

- Associated groin or axillary lymphadenopathy
- Hepatosplenomegaly
- Nodes increasing rapidly in size over time
- Night sweats
- Weight loss
- Recurrent fevers

Biopsy in these cases should be considered to exclude other underlying pathology. Other investigations should be tailored to the clinical presentation along with consideration of local epidemiological factors such as in areas of endemic tuberculosis or human immunodeficiency virus (HIV).

Neck Abscesses

Neck abscesses can occur following cervical lymphadenopathy. Usually the initial infection is in the skin and soft tissues. Most are caused by *S. aureus* or streptococcal species. Dental abscesses can also cause this. Ultrasound or computed tomographic (CT) scanning may aid with the diagnosis but often clinical examination is all that is required. In patients where the child is not systemically unwell, consider mycobacterial infection from both *Mycobacterium tuberculosis* as well atypical infections such as *M. Avium* **(Fig. 26.22)**. The management of atypical mycobacterial infections is conservative, as this will resolve spontaneously in the majority of cases. In some cases of atypical mycobacterial infections, surgery or anti-tubercular medication may be considered.

Acute deep space neck abscesses can occur in the retropharyngeal and parapharyngeal spaces. The child will present systemically unwell with fever, symptoms of airway obstruction and often with torticollis and limited neck movement. The airway should be maintained throughout, and endotracheal intubation is frequently required. Diagnostic imaging in the form of CT scanning is the modality of choice. Intravenous antibiotic cover should be initiated which should include a broad-spectrum antibiotic along with anaerobic cover. In children with retropharyngeal pharyngeal abscesses that are well or there is significant bony erosion on CT scanning *M. tuberculosis* infections should always be considered.

Parotitis

This is an uncommon condition in children. Infantile parotitis is usually caused by a bacterial infection of the parotid gland. It usually affects babies 6 months and under and is thought to be more common if the infant is dehydrated. *S. aureus* is the most commonly isolated organism. The facial swelling will be of rapid onset and the gland will be hot tender and painful. Management involves adequate rehydration, analgesia and antibiotics. Parotitis in older children is also uncommon. Where it occurs, it is usually caused by the mumps virus. Examination should always involve checking both parotid glands for symmetry, and also checking the parotid duct for stones. The management of mumps is symptomatic. Where enlargement of the parotid glands without any systemic symptoms occurs ultrasound of the glands and checking for antibodies (SSro, SSla, antinuclear antibody) may prove helpful. Cysts within the body of the parotid should alert the clinician to the possibility of an HIV infection **(Fig. 26.23)**.

Recurrent juvenile parotitis is a rare and poorly understood entity. The management is symptomatic in the first instance with disease usually burning itself out over time. In recalcitrant cases and where other causes have been ruled out, a prophylactic course of antibiotics may prove helpful. The field of sialoendoscopy is a developing area and appears promising in the future management of this condition. Very rarely surgical excision of the affected gland is required.

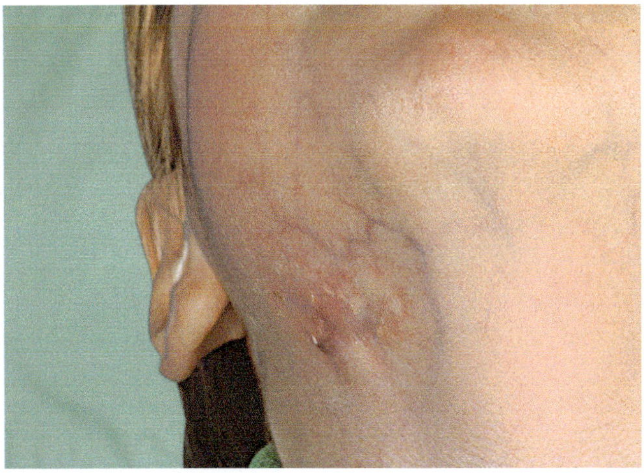

Figure 26.22 Right resolving neck abscess of atypical mycobacterial infection.

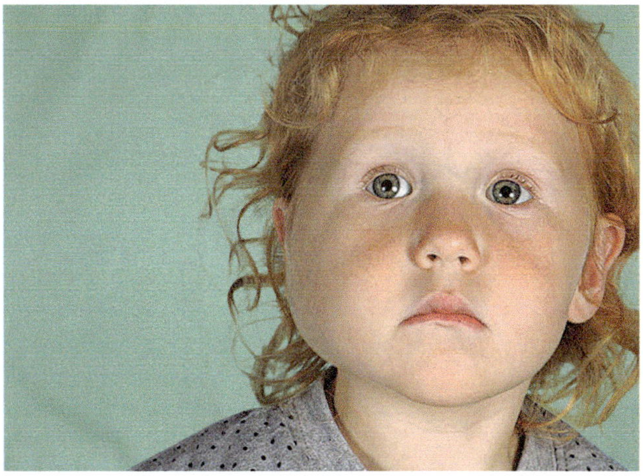

Figure 26.23 Child with acute right parotitis.

CONGENITAL CONDITIONS OF THE HEAD AND NECK

Infantile Haemangioma

Infantilehaemangiomas are the most common tumour of infancy occurring in up to 5% of infants. The most common site in the head and neck region outwith the skin is the parotid. Diagnosis is easily confirmed by ultrasound. Management is expectant as the natural history is one of spontaneous regression **(Fig. 26.24)**.

Lymphangiomas (Cystic Hygroma)

Lymphangiomas are rare congenital malformations due to an abnormal development of the lymphatic system. These lesions have a predilection for the head and neck region. They are often present from birth but can develop in the first few years of life, and frequently coming to light following an upper respiratory tract infection. Clinically, these are soft compressible lesion/s, but rapid enlargement with an associated tense painful swelling can be caused by infection or haemorrhage into the cysts. Diagnosis is confirmed initially by ultrasonography or magnetic resonance imaging (MRI). As these lesions can be extensive, if any intervention is considered MRI should be undertaken. Overall there is now a growing body of evidence that there is a much higher rate of spontaneous regression of these lesions than previously thought. A recent study has reported that in lymphangiomas, deemed to not require any intervention, that the rate of spontaneous regression is around 45%. Cosmetic improvement with or without spontaneous regression can also occur over time. This suggests that in the initial phases in appropriately selected patients, conservative management has a significant role to play. In cases where the disease is life or organ threatening or there is a significant cosmetic component which is not improving spontaneously then active treatment should be considered. The use of interventional management will depend upon how extensive the disease is, if it has a functional impact on breathing, swallowing or feeding, the likelihood of complete resection, cosmesis and the site of the lesion/s in particular the potential risk of significant complications. In cases where airway obstruction occurs or is anticipated, tracheostomy is likely to be required. Commonly employed management modalities include surgery or sclerotherapy with these being used individually or as a combined treatment. The aims and risks of any procedure must be discussed with the child and their family and agreed and understood pre-operatively. Clinically, isolated infrahyoid supraclavicular macrocystic disease has the best prognosis, with microcystic disease extending into the tongue, floor of mouth and/or palate carrying the poorest prognosis. Interventional debulking of these lesions for cosmetic reasons should only be undertaken with all involved fully understanding the aims of the treatment and being aware of the risk of recurrence. Recently there has been a move towards the use of medications such as sirolimus, sildenafil and propranolol to try to treat these lesions. There is however only limited evidence in the form of case reports to support the use of these medications as it is difficult to ascertain whether or not the reported effects were due to the treatment or to spontaneous regression. Larger studies are required to assess the clinical efficacies of these treatments **(Fig. 26.25)**.

Sternocleidomastoid Tumours (Sternomastoid Tumours, Fibromatosis Colli)

Sternocleidomastoid tumours (SCMT) are benign fibrous lesions that occur within the sternocleidomastoid muscle. The term tumour applies to the classical Latin definition as a swelling. Histologically, these lesions are made up of spindle fibroblasts and collagen depositions around decomposing multinuclear muscle fibres. They are usually

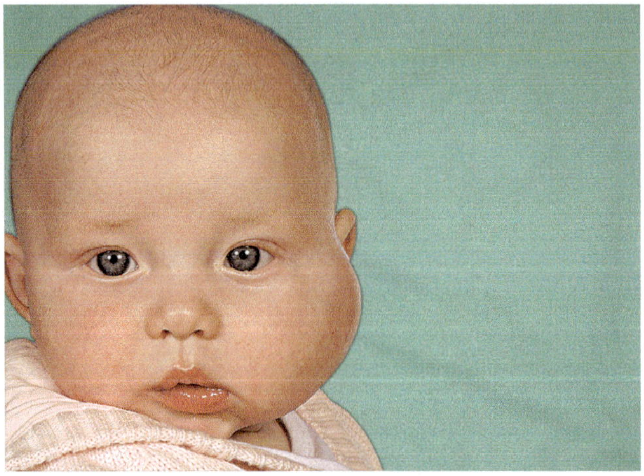

Figure 26.24 Child demonstrating left parotid haemangioma.

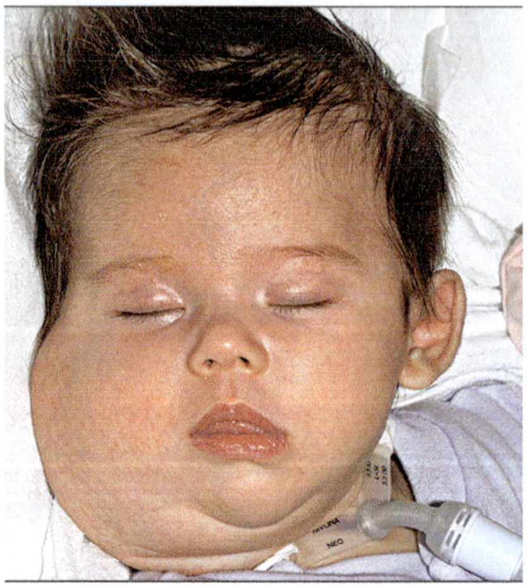

Figure 26.25 Child with large cystic hygroma with associated airway compromise requiring tracheostomy.

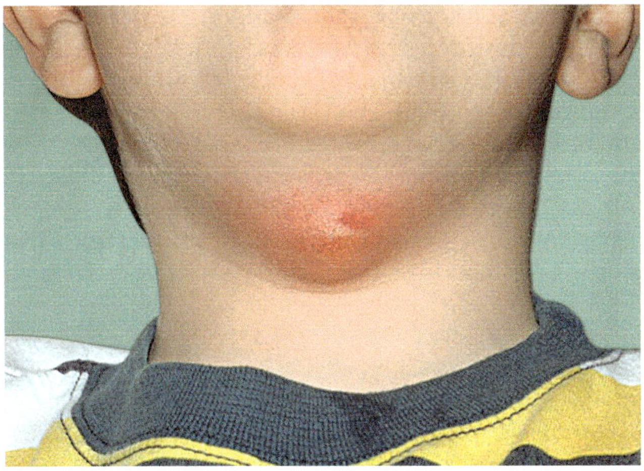

Figure 26.26 Infected thyroglossal duct cyst.

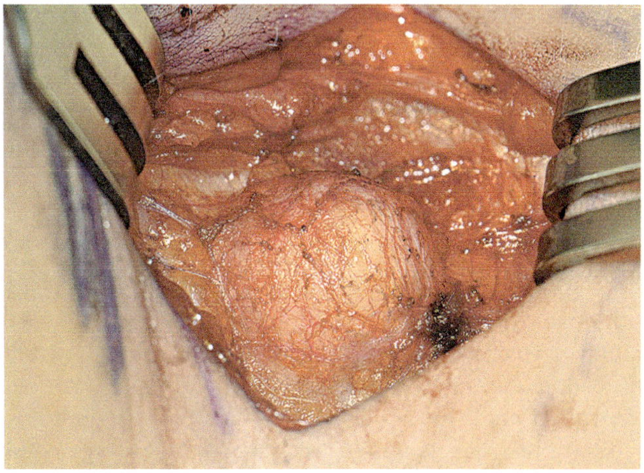

Figure 26.27 Dissection of thyroglossal duct cyst at surgery.

identified in the first few weeks to months of life as a smooth non-tender mass usually in the lower third of the muscle. Often there is a torticollis with head turning away from the affected side. The aetiology is unknown, but there is an association with birth trauma with an increased incidence reported infants born by breech or forceps delivery. Other associations include primiparous birth and congenital dysplasia of the hip. It recommended that all children with SCMT have an ultrasound of their hips to exclude the latter condition. Ultrasound can also be used to confirm the diagnosis of SCMT in cases if there is any clinical uncertainty with MRI and computed tomography reserved for more complex cases. Massage and head positioning in the early stages will often lead to complete resolution without any requirement for further intervention. If any concerns remain about head movement after first few months physiotherapy may be beneficial. The torticollis should be investigated more extensively if has not resolved or improved significantly within the first year of life with imaging and orthopaedic and ophthalmological review, as in the long term this can lead to facial asymmetry. Surgical intervention with muscle releases in progressive cases or those failing to respond to physiotherapy is only very rarely required.

Thyroglossal Duct Cysts

Thyroglossal duct cysts (TGDC) are rare congenital midline neck swellings that occur anywhere from the submental region to sternal notch (Fig. 26.26). These constitute the most common congenital neck lesion. TGDC have a peak incidence at around 7 years of age. These occur due to failure of resolution of the thyroglossal tract. This being an embryological remnant of the descent of the thyroid gland from the foramen caecum in the tongue base from around third to fourth week of gestation. Clinically, these lesions present as midline neck swellings that move with tongue protrusion and swallowing. Sudden enlargement can occur if they become infected. TGDC can also rupture and have purulent or mucinous discharge with subsequent sinus or fistula as the tract is lined with respiratory epithelium. Ultrasound scan is helpful in the diagnosis of TGDC and is often able to differentiate between this lesion and other midline lesions such as dermoid cysts and lymph nodes. It is also useful in determining the presence of a normal thyroid gland because very rarely TGDC represent the only thyroid tissue in the body. Management is by surgical excision with an en bloc dissection taking a cuff of strap muscles down to the thyroid gland, the mid-portion of the hyoid bone and core of muscle into the tongue base (extended Sistrunk Procedure) (Fig. 26.27).

Branchial Arch Sinuses

Branchial arch lesions are the second most common congenital lesion of the neck. These present most commonly as sinuses but also rarely as cysts or fistulas. They are caused by the failure of normal fusion of two adjacent branchial arches. The most common level for this to occur is between the second and third arches and these are known as second branchial arch sinuses. The anatomical course of the sinus is determined by its embryological level with second arch lesion usually presenting with a sinus on the anterior border of sternocleidomastoid at the junction of its lower third and upper two-thirds. Clinically the sinus will either discharge mucous, but occasionally, it may also become infected. Branchial sinuses can be associated with hearing loss and renal anomalies, which can also be familial as in branchio-oto-renal syndrome. Surgical excision is the management of choice.

ACQUIRED CONDITIONS OF THE NOSE AND PARANASAL SINUSES

Nasal Obstruction

Nasal obstruction in children is common. After recurrent upper respiratory tract infections, the most frequent causes of this are either adenoidal hypertrophy (usually

<6 years of age) or allergic rhinitis (usually >6 years of age). The natural history of adenoidal tissue is that it will atrophy over time, and with it, the symptoms should abate. Warning signs that should alert the clinician to other significant underlying pathology include bloody nasal discharge, unilateral nasal discharge, foul smell, facial swelling or a polyp protruding from the nose.

Chronic Rhinosinusitis

Rhinosinusitis in children is common and will usually last a few days to weeks following an upper respiratory tract infection. Parents will frequently complain that they feel that their child has a constant cold during the first few years of life. This is understandable as the average child under the aged 5 years or under will have approximately 6–8 upper respiratory tract infections every year. Reassurance is frequently all that is required. Where the discharge is extremely problematic and is affecting the child's every day quality of life the use of topical saline spray or drops may prove helpful. In more prolonged courses, some clinicians recommend a 2-week course of oral antibiotics or short course of steroid nasal drops or spray. In older children, the clinician should always consider the diagnosis of allergic rhinitis and a full history including individual and family history of atopy should be explored. Where medical and conservative measures have failed surgery may be considered. Usually this is in the form of adenoidectomy. Paranasal sinus surgery is very rarely required for children.

Epistaxis/Nose Bleeds

Epistaxes are common in children and are usually self-limiting. There is a growing body of evidence to implicate low grade *S. aureus* infection as a contributory factor to ongoing epistaxis, and treatments designed to reduce carriage of this organism lead to resolution of symptoms. A full history should be undertaken including the frequency, periodicity, length of bleeds as well any previous history of bruising or bleeding tendency in the individual or family. Where bleeding is prolonged, a full blood count and coagulation screen should be obtained. Management along with advice on first aid in the first instance is a trial of a topical antiseptic or antibiotic cream or ointment with anti-staphylococcal properties for 1 month. Studies examining the effectiveness of petroleum jelly alone have shown this to be no more effective than no treatment. Where conservative and medical management have failed cautery to the nasal septum may be considered.

Peri-orbital and Orbital Cellulitis

The orbit is divided anatomically into pre-septal and post-septal components by the orbital septum. This is a fibrous layer attached around the margin of the orbit where it is contiguous with the periosteum fusing centrally with the tarsal plates. Clinically, this is important as the defining boundary for peri-orbital and orbital cellulitis. Peri-orbital cellulitis is an infection of the soft tissues of the eye anterior to the orbital septum. Orbital cellulitis is defined any infection that involves the orbit and has a post-septal component. Peri-orbital cellulitis has the potential to progress on to cause orbital cellulitis. Clinically, the two conditions can be difficult to distinguish. Either can occur as extensions of an extra-ocular infection, such as skin and/or soft tissue infection, which may be either primary (erysipelas, *S. aureus*) or secondary (herpes zoster infection, eczema, trauma, a stye, dacryocystitis or a dental abscess). Infections of the paranasal sinuses (acute rhinosinusitis) may also progress on to orbital cellulitis. There is a similar spectrum of microbiological organisms causing both conditions with *S. aureus, S. pneumoniae* and *S. epidermidis* causing the majority of infections. However, anaerobic organisms are now more commonly being identified in orbital cellulitis. Peri-orbital cellulitis more common usually affects younger children (less than 5 years of age) and has an equal sex distribution. Orbital cellulitis affects older children (average age 7 years) and is common in boys and during the winter months. Overall the incidence of periorbital cellulitis and its complications appears to be decreasing. However in those children requiring hospital admission it has been found that they are more unwell, have higher complication rates and longer lengths of inpatient stay than previously seen. Children who are aged 3 years or younger, who have previously been treated with antibiotics and/or who have a white cell count of greater than 10 are reported to be at higher risk of developing abscesses. Clinical signs that are helpful in predicting if there is an orbital abscess include decreased or painful eye movement, spread of cellulitis beyond the margins of the eyelid, loss of red-green colour vision and proptosis, with loss of vision and papilloedema being late signs. Management (see diagram 2) involves intravenous antibiotics and regular topical nasal decongestants as well as having a high level of suspicion of intra-orbital and intra-cranial complications. Early referral to a Paediatric Ophthalmology and Otolaryngology services should be sought. Full blood, blood cultures and eye swabs for microbiology may prove helpful. X-rays of the paranasal sinuses and nasal swabs have been proven to be of no clinical benefit. CT scanning of the orbit is the most useful investigation to identify if an abscess has occurred within the orbit, intracranially or if a cavernous sinus thrombosis is present. Indications for CT scanning include, any central signs, inability to adequately assess vision, proptosis, ophthalmoplegia, deteriorating vision, loss of red-green colour vision, no significant improvement to IV antibiotics at 24 hours and/or a swinging pyrexia at 36 hours. Where an intra-orbital abscess is identified the management is surgical drainage. In small abscesses, less than 1 cm^3, there is some debate as there is a body of evidence to support conservative management

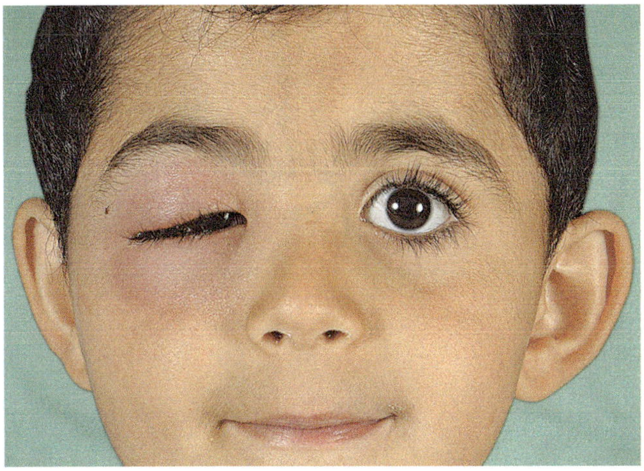

Figure 26.28 Child demonstrating right orbital cellulitis.

in these cases. Complications of orbital cellulitis include visual loss, septicaemia and intracranial infections (Fig. 26.28 and Flow chart 26.2).

Foreign Bodies of the Nose

Nasal foreign bodies are frequently encountered in children. In the early stages, there may only be a history of seeing the child put something up their nose. Otherwise, these usually present with foul smelling intermittent unilateral nasal discharge. In some cases, the discharge or history of discharge may not be present. Adequate illumination and examination of the nose should identify most foreign bodies. Management options include the use of the 'parental kiss,' blanketing and removal or removal under general anaesthesia. The 'parental kiss' involves the parent occluding the nostril which does not have the foreign body in it, forming a seal with their own mouth around the child's and blowing gently. If this fails and the parent is amenable then removal by the clinician with the child blanketed/restrained and sitting upright may be attempted. This is only recommended if a JobsonHorne probe is used with adequate head lighting and if the clinician has been trained in this technique. If all else fails, removal under a general anaesthetic may be required. Special mention of the importance of batteries as foreign bodies in the nasal cavity should be mentioned as these set up an electric current which is extremely damaging to the surrounding tissues and can cause a septal perforation if not removed expediently.

CONGENITAL CONDITIONS OF THE NOSE

Choanal Atresia

Choanal atresia is thought to be caused by the failure of resolution of the bucco-pharyngeal membrane, which is an embryological remnant at the junction of nose and nasopharynx. Effectively this leads to an occlusion of the choanae or posterior nasal aperture. It occurs in 1 in 8,000–10,000 live births is frequently associated with syndromal children; the most common being CHARGE syndrome and is usually bilateral. It is of significant clinical importance as neonates are obligate mouth breathers. Clinically, these babies are reported to have a cyclical breathing pattern where they have a period of obstructed

Flow chart 26.2 Periorbital/orbital cellulitis protocol.

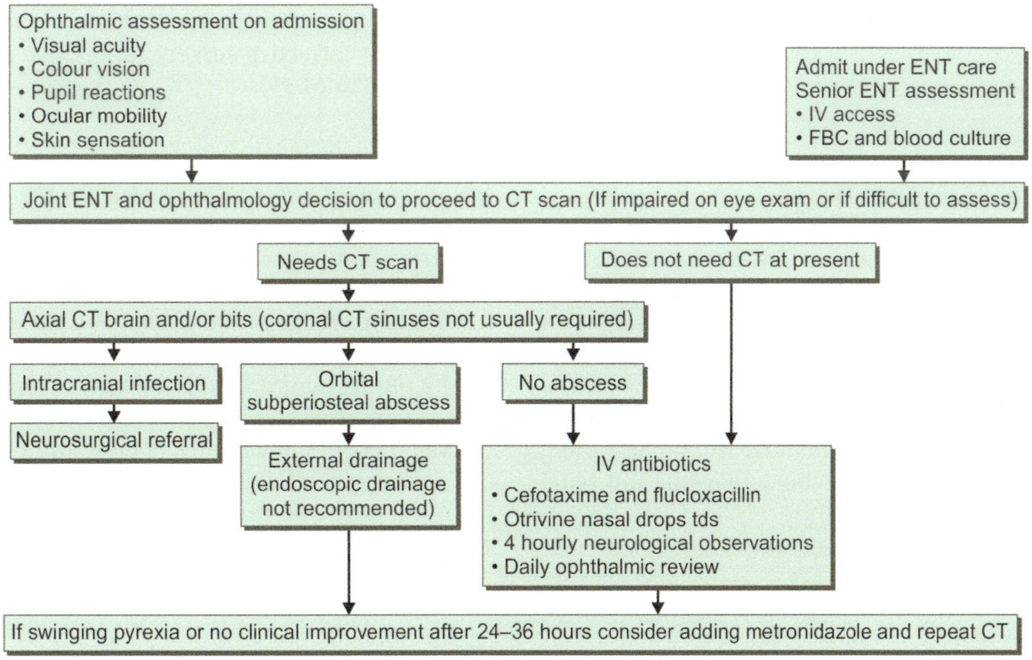

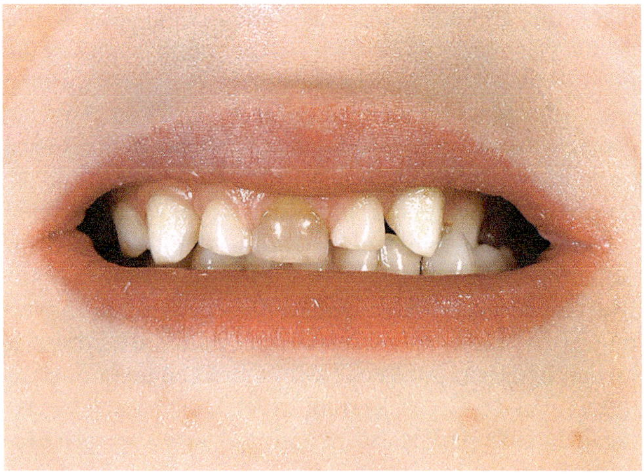

Figure 26.29 Single central incisor associated with pyriform aperture stenosis.

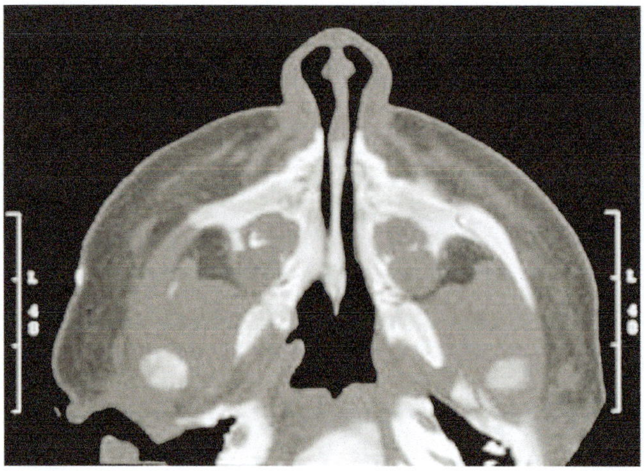

Figure 26.30 Computed tomographic scan demonstrating pyriform aperture stenosis—*note* also right choanal atresia.

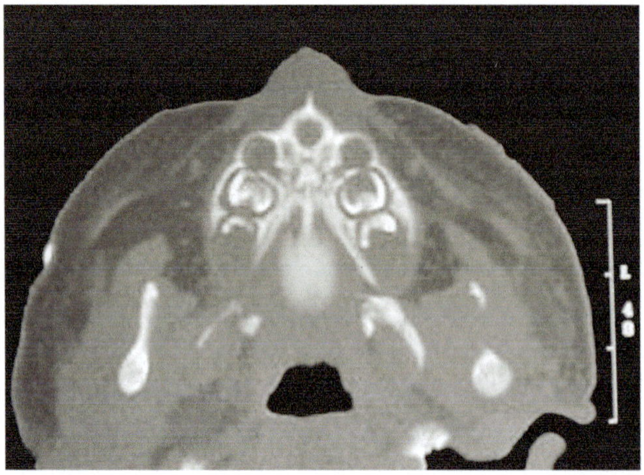

Figure 26.31 Computed tomographic scan demonstrating single central incisor associated with pyriform aperture stenosis.

looking breathing pattern with eventual cyanosis followed by a cry then a gasp. Diagnosis may be supported attempting to pass catheters through each nostril. The baby's airway may be maintained by the use Guedel airway or endotracheal intubation. Care should be taken when using a Guedel as this should only be used as a short-term means of maintaining an airway as this artificial airway has the potential to cause erosions on the palate. Management is surgical repair following endotracheal intubation with the preoperative workup including CT imaging of the choanae, echocardiogram and renal ultrasound.

Pyriform Aperture Stenosis

Pyriform aperture stenosis (PAS) is caused by bony overgrowth of the nasal process of maxilla leading to nasal obstruction. This is again important as infants are obligate nasal breathers. The aetiology is poorly understood but may relate to problems with midline fusion as associations include holoprosencephaly, pituitary abnormalities and a single central incisor. Other frequently associated anomalies include vertebral, limb, cardiac and genitourinary anomalies. Both VACTERL and CHARGE syndromes have also been associated with PAS. Familial cases have also been reported. Clinically PAS presents with symptoms of airway obstruction in particular respiratory distress, cyanotic events, poor feeding, apnoeic events, failure to thrive and sleep apnoea. Around half of the children identified with this condition at birth will require corrective surgery to improve nasal airflow **(Figs. 26.29 to 26.31)**.

Nasal Dermoids

Nasal dermoid cysts and sinuses are rare (1 in every 20,000–40,000 live births) congenital midline facial lesions. Histologically, they are lined by stratified squamous epithelium, with normal dermal appendages, including hairs and sebaceous glands. They can occur anywhere in the midline from a punctum or cyst on the philtrum or dorsum of the nose and can extend into the anterior cranial fossa. Clinically, these lesions usually present with a midline punctum that has caseous debris extruding from it intermittently, hairs growing out if it or with infection.Infection in these lesions

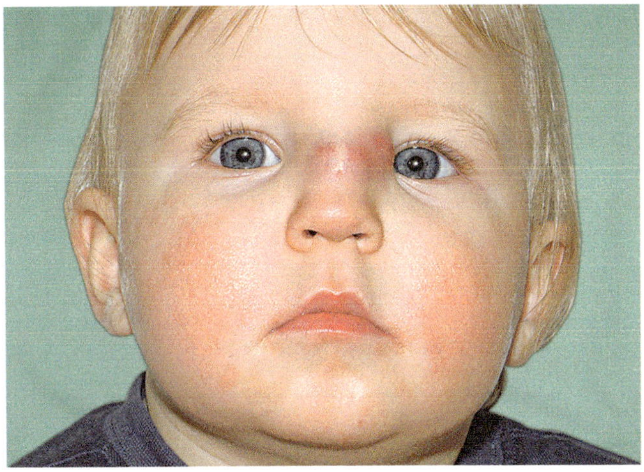

Figure 26.32 Child demonstrating infected nasal dermoid cyst—*note* punctum on dorsum of nose.

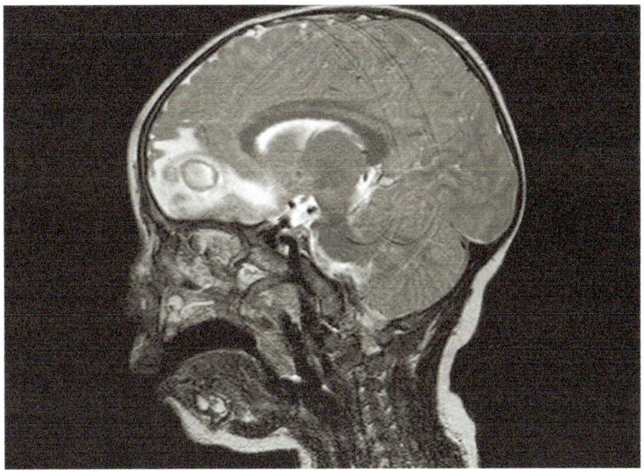

Figure 26.33 Computed tomographic scan demonstrating intra-cranial extension of nasal dermoid sinus with intracranial cyst—compressing frontal lobes.

can be extremely serious as if the tract traverses the cribriform plate the infection has the potential to track intracranially and can present with meningitis, seizures and/or other symptoms associated with intracranial abscesses. Chronic infection can occur in form of osteomyelitis. MRI is the imaging modality of choice to identify the extension of the lesion and confirm diagnosis. Early identification and surgery is essential in preventing potential infections. Surgery in cases where previous infection has occurred is associated with higher complication and recurrence rates **(Figs. 26.32 and 26.33)**.

CHAPTER 27

Paediatric and Adolescent Gynaecology

Kevin P. Hanretty, Paul L. Wood

INTRODUCTION

As a speciality, paediatric and adolescent gynaecology is a relative newcomer; the North American Society for Pediatric and Adolescent Gynecology[1] was founded in 1986. The British Society for Paediatric Gynaecology[2] was founded in 2000, and the European Association of Paediatric and Adolescent Gynaecology[3] was founded in 2008.

These various societies developed in recognition of the complex needs of the young female, and these different associations reflect the relatively recent identification of the importance of mutual collaboration and sharing of specific expertise in dealing with and developing the optimal management of gynaecological issues affecting children and adolescents.

The nature of gynaecological problems in this particular population is such that there is complex interplay between various disciplines and some of these are highlighted in **Box 27.1**. The need for interdisciplinary and multidisciplinary team working in paediatric and adolescent gynaecology is essential and cannot be overstated.

NEONATAL PERIOD

Gynaecological anatomy in the newborn is influenced inevitably by in utero exposure to oestrogen levels, notably oestradiol, derived from the foetal ovaries, placenta and in terms of magnitude, from the maternal circulation. This results in the labia majora and minora, appearing somewhat oedematous, more so if the baby is delivered vaginally by the breech.

These circulating oestrogen levels may be sufficient to induce endometrial proliferation resulting in a withdrawal bleed some days after delivery. Some milky discharge from the nipple and a mucous vaginal discharge are also not rare in association with neonatal ovarian activity following a temporary rise in neonatal gonadotrophins and endogenous oestrogen levels which however rapidly decline until the onset of puberty.

At puberty, there is reactivation of the hypothalamic gonadotrophin-releasing hormone system. Puberty normally begins between 8 years and 13 years in girls and describes all of those morphological, psychological and physiological changes in human development from prereproductive to potentially reproductive. Thelarche or breast development precedes the onset of menarche by a couple of years on average. Median age of menarche has not altered dramatically in recent years, but over the last 40 years, menarche has become on average 4–5 months earlier but breast development now occurs on average 2 years earlier than in the 1960s.[4,5]

A number of studies have demonstrated that an increase in childhood body mass index (BMI) results in earlier onset of puberty and this is becoming a cause for concern gynaecologically as well as in the general paediatric sense.[6,7]

Thus puberty is said to be precocious if changes occur before the age of 8 years and if the menarche occurs before 10 years.

The normal stages of breast and pubic hair development (pubarche) are described in the Tanner classification **(Fig. 27.1)**.

DEVELOPMENTAL ABNORMALITIES IN THE GENITAL TRACT

Whilst developmental abnormalities in the female genital tract are unlikely to be a frequent source of clinical concern to the paediatrician, such abnormalities may be diagnosed as part of the investigation of a child with a number of different symptoms. Thus, between 2 and 4% of women who subsequently have a normal reproductive outcome have some form of gynaecological developmental abnormality. The data in those who have not achieved a pregnancy are even more problematic. A significant proportion of these women will have associated renal abnormalities. Twelve percent of women with uterovaginal agenesis have unilateral renal agenesis.[8]

BOX 27.1 Specialists interacting in multidisciplinary team working in paediatric gynaecology.

- General paediatricians
- Paediatric surgeons/urologists
- Geneticists
- Paediatric endocrinologists
- Psychologists
- Microbiologists
- Plastic surgeons
- Gynaecologists
- Dermatologists
- Paediatric nurse specialists
- Sexual health practitioners
- Forensic practitioners

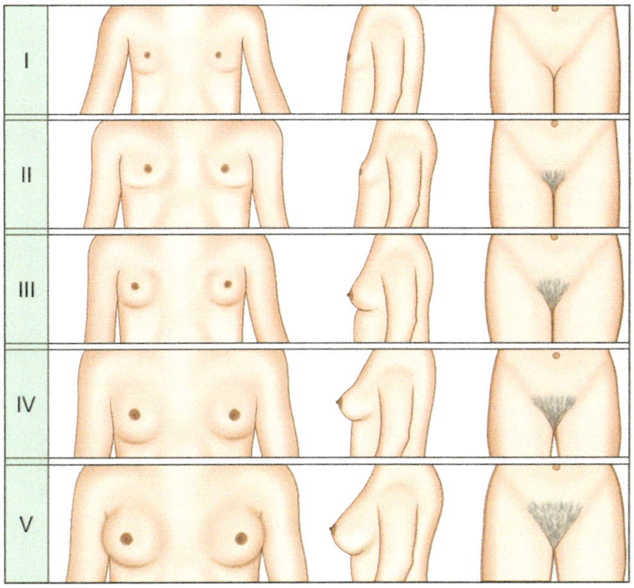

Figure 27.1 Tanner classification.

The majority of developmental abnormalities result from defects in development of the Müllerian system, and these have been categorised and described by the American Fertility Society (American Society for Reproductive Medicine) **(Fig. 27.2)**.[9]

Müllerian malformations rarely present in childhood but when there is an outflow blockage then at puberty a girl may present with amenorrhoea and a pelvi-abdominal mass caused by a complete transverse vaginal septum or imperforate hymen in which menstrual blood accumulates in the vagina and uterus causing a haematocolpos leading to a haematometra **(Fig. 27.3)**. This may present as urinary retention or apparent delayed menarche because of so-called cryptomenorrhoea.

Whilst the management of Müllerian malformations is out with the scope of this chapter, it should be remembered that the management of the imperforate hymen is simple, involving a cruciate incision into the membrane, which will permit free drainage and resolution of the presenting problem. Management of transverse septa is more challenging since these require excision to prevent undue scarring and a recurrence of the obstruction.

It is noteworthy that the diagnosis of potential/later fertility problems associated with Müllerian abnormalities and conditions such as X-linked complete androgen insensitivity syndrome (CAIS) (formerly testicular feminisation syndrome) may now be made in childhood, and indeed in infancy. The management of parents in this situation is complex and issues relating to sex and sexuality for the child require multidisciplinary input and can be challenging.

The management of intersex disorders is beyond the scope of this chapter and the interested reader is referred to the 2006 Consensus Statement on Management of Intersex disorders.[10]

OVARIAN CYSTS

The advent of widespread prenatal ultrasound diagnosis led to a recognition that foetal and hence neonatal ovarian cysts are not uncommon and may occur in around one newborn girl in 2500.

Ovarian cysts in childhood are relatively rare and may present with acute abdominal pain resulting from torsion or rupture. These are discussed later.

Cysts of up to 4 cm usually regress and the management of larger or sonographically complex cysts remains controversial. Surgery is often recommended in order to prevent subsequent torsion of the ovary leading to infarction but in most series the surgery undertaken includes oophorectomy![11] However, even in cases of torsion it is usually possible to salvage ovarian tissue which regains viability thus avoiding oophorectomy.

Some medical disorders including hypothyroidism and McCune Albright Syndrome are associated with simple ovarian cysts.

GYNAECOLOGICAL PROBLEMS IN PAEDIATRIC CARE

Vulvovaginitis

This is the commonest gynaecological presentation in this age group to the primary care physician and paediatrician and describes inflammation of the vulva and vagina most commonly related to poor vulval hygiene and perianal care.

Vulvovaginitis occasionally may present as blood stained vaginal discharge but in such cases foreign bodies should be excluded by vaginoscopy under anaesthesia. Very rarely vaginal rhabdomyosarcoma presents as vaginal bleeding in a prepubertal girl (see later).

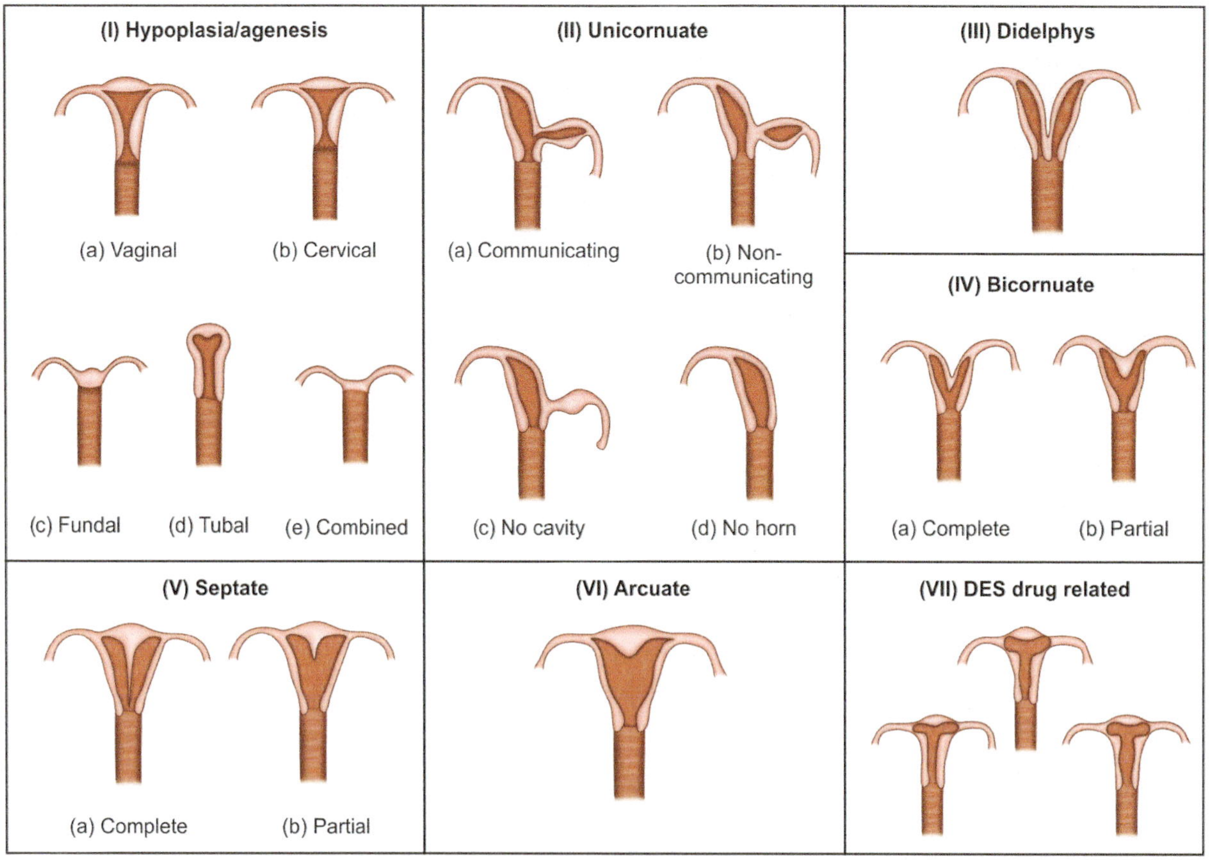

Figure 27.2 American Fertility Society classification of congenital abnormalities of the genital tract.

(Source: Reprinted from Journal of Pediatric Surgery. Gholoum S, Puligandla PS, Hui T, et al. Management and outcome of patients with combined vaginal septum, bifid uterus, and ipsilateral renal agenesis (Herlyn–Werner–Wunderlich syndrome). J Pediatr Surg. 2006;41(5):987-92).

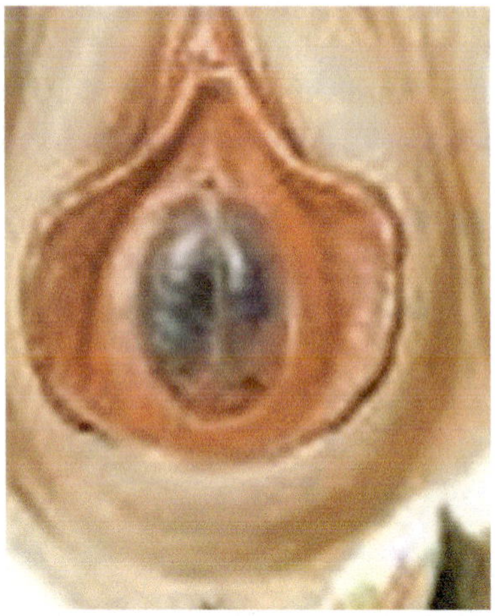

Figure 27.3 Showing imperforate hymen with haematocolpos.

The prepubertal vagina does not have the relatively acid environment necessary for lactobacilli to colonise and this lends itself to a condition which in the postmenopausal women is best described as atrophic vaginitis. Nevertheless, there is no role for oestrogen in this situation. Consequently, in early childhood infection with faecal organisms is not uncommon and appropriate antibiotic therapy may be indicated. Repeat infection with different organisms makes rational antibiotic prescribing problematic.

Fungal infection with candida is relatively uncommon in paediatric gynaecology and antifungal agents should be used rarely.

Pinworm (Threadworm) infestation is common in early childhood and although it usually causes perianal itch it can manifest with vulval itch. Treatment under 3 months of age is usually not recommended but thereafter piperazine and mebendazole may be used in association with the usual hygiene measures and recommendations on treating family members.

Non-infectious causes include the use of topical cleansing agents and in particular perfumed soaps, laundry detergents and the use of biological soap powders for washing underwear.

These should be avoided and if necessary soap substitutes used. Where persistent vulvitis occurs and the usual hygiene message methods have been employed, other aetiologies should be considered. It is rarely necessary to take bacteriological swabs unless there is suspicion of sexual abuse or sexually transmitted infection.

Consideration should therefore be given to dermatological conditions.

Eczema

Atopic eczema/dermatitis may manifest as vulval itch although lesions elsewhere usually make the diagnosis relatively straightforward. A satisfactory response is often obtained using the hygiene measures mentioned above, but occasionally emollients or even hydrocortisone topically may be required.

Psoriasis

Psoriasis may also present with vaginal itch. The diagnosis is generally based on clinical findings and family history. Topical corticosteroids can be used, preferably under the direction of a dermatologist.

Lichen Sclerosus

Lichen sclerosus is a chronic mucocutaneous disorder of unknown aetiology occurring at either end of the age spectrum. There may be a genetic component because of a recognised familial distribution.

Symptoms can be very severe and characterised by intense itch. As skin can be involved anywhere from the perianal region to the mons pubis, presentation with constipation is well recognised, and may require laxative therapy in addition to specific treatments.

The clinical features are of a characteristic appearance described as "pearly white" macular or papular areas, which may combine to give an overall plaque like appearance.

In contrast with the postmenopausal manifestation of lichen sclerosus, there appears to be no association with malignant change although the appearances can be quite alarming.

The ulceration and bruising sometimes associated with the condition can give a misleading impression of sexual abuse and unwarranted diagnoses should be avoided.

Often symptomatic control with emollients may be sufficient, but there is a place for topical treatment with steroids. The condition can be self-limiting but repeated courses of steroids may well be required until usually complete resolution around about puberty.

ASYMPTOMATIC VULVAL CONDITIONS

Labial Adhesions

Labial adhesions are relatively common in girls under the age of three and are almost entirely asymptomatic. The exception may be in the older girl when poor urinary flow is associated with entrapment of urine behind the adherent labia. This then presents as urinary incontinence when the girl stands up and can predispose to urinary infections.

In the absence of symptoms this condition does not require any treatment as it is self-limiting and spontaneous resolution is the norm. Occasionally, in the presence of urinary problems there may be a role for twice daily topical oestrogen cream for a few weeks, although it may well be that the manipulation during application of the cream alone is the effective treatment.

Perceived Vulval Dysmorphism

Labial adhesions and vulval asymmetry may present to the paediatrician as a source of considerable parental anxiety. As mentioned earlier, labial adhesions are rarely problematic. Occasionally the parental interpretation is of some form of vaginal agenesis.

- Reassurance is required only
- Asymmetry of the labia minora is common.

Increasingly, mothers and even adolescent females may present with concern regarding vulval asymmetry and indeed labial dimensions. There is considerable professional concern regarding the increasing numbers of labioplasty procedures for perceived, but otherwise normal variations, of vulval anatomy. There is increasing recognition that access to the internet and widespread availability of images of 'desirable anatomy' is contributing to this. The long-term consequences for these young women are unknown, although the immediate complications of surgery including haemorrhage, infection, scarring and neuropathic pain are significant and surgery is best avoided in the formative years through to the end of adolescence. Labioplasty as a procedure should therefore be restricted to those (rare) situations when it could be said to be clinically justified.

Female Genital Cutting (Mutilation)

According to the World Health Organisation approximately 140,000,000 women are dealing with the consequences of female genital mutilation, usually undertaken in childhood or adolescence. In Africa, more than 3 million women are at risk annually.

Whilst commonly undertaken without specific malice to the child there is no doubt that these procedures represent a violation of the rights of females.

There are no health benefits to any form of female genital cutting. The immediate consequences may well present to physicians in the form of haemorrhage and infection. The later sequelae are not inconsiderable and include apareunia, dyspareunia and problems in childbirth.[12] Despite legislation banning this practice in the UK there have not to date been any convictions for female genital cutting (Box 27.2).

MENSTRUAL DISORDERS IN CHILDHOOD AND ADOLESCENCE

Delayed Puberty

This describes absence of breast development in girls beyond 13 years of age.

The majority of cases result from simple constitutional delay and there may be a familial element to this.

BOX 27.2 Female genital mutilation: Classification.

Type I: Partial or total removal of the clitoris and/or the prepuce (clitoridectomy)

Type II: Partial or total removal of the clitoris and the labia minora, with or without excision of the labia majora (excision)

Type III: Narrowing of the vaginal orifice with creation of a covering seal by cutting and appositioning the labia minora and/or the labia majora, with or without excision of the clitoris (infibulation)

Type IIIa: Removal and apposition of the labia minora; Type IIIb, removal and apposition of the labia majora

Type IV: All other harmful procedures to the female genitalia for non-medical purposes, e.g.: pricking, piercing, incising, scraping and cauterization.

Other causes include chronic conditions, notably chronic renal disease, cystic fibrosis and inflammatory bowel disease.

Malnutrition/eating disorders and excessive physical exercise as seen in young gymnasts and ballet dancers are also associated with a delay in puberty.

Hypothalamic/pituitary disorders may result in delayed puberty, notably prolactinomas but other conditions such as primary hypothyroidism, independent of pituitary function may be seen as a cause, although hypothyroidism is also associated with peripheral precocious puberty with vaginal bleeding and ovarian cysts linked to production of, and stimulation by thyroid-stimulating hormone (TSH).

Rare causes include craniopharyngiomas and other central nervous system (CNS) lesions.

Chemotherapy or radiotherapy in childhood may also be associated with a delay in puberty.

Gonadal dysgenesis is associated with delayed puberty although may present more specifically with primary amenorrhoea such as with Swyer syndrome. The majority of cases are chromosomally XO, i.e. Turner syndrome, but a variety of sex chromosomal constitutions may be seen. In XY gonadal dysgenesis (Swyer syndrome) normal female pelvic organs exist but with no functional ovarian tissue. The gonadal tissue has a high malignant potential and gonadectomy is indicated.

Primary Amenorrhoea (Including Polycystic Ovarian Syndrome)

This term describes the absence of menstruation by the age of 16 years. It is important to distinguish the difference between amenorrhoea and delayed puberty with failure of breast development by the age of 14 years prompting investigation.

The causes of delayed (or absent) puberty are also causes of primary amenorrhoea. Secondary sexual characteristics can develop independently of the onset of menstruation.

Complete androgen insensitivity syndrome may present as primary amenorrhoea and uterine agenesis.

Although commonly a cause of secondary amenorrhoea, it is important to note that polycystic ovarian syndrome (PCOS) may present as primary amenorrhoea.

The evaluation of primary amenorrhoea involves identification of Müllerian abnormalities or congenital absence of the uterus, vagina or both. Uterine agenesis, the commonest form of which is Mayer–Rokitansky–Kuster–Hauser syndrome (MRKH or Rokitansky syndrome), is found in phenotypically normal females with normal ovarian function and pubertal development but isolated primary amenorrhoea.

These young women can become genetic mothers insofar as their eggs may be retrieved for in vitro fertilization (IVF) and incubation in a surrogate.

In contrast, females with CAIS have no functional ovarian tissue though they are phenotypically female. There should be no doubt on the part of their physicians regarding their female sexuality but they may require surgical intervention if the vaginal length is too short for satisfactory intercourse. Psychological input is often helpful for the patient faced with the need to understand the chromosomal background of the condition.

Minimally invasive approaches such as the Vecchietti approach as used for vaginal agenesis, are highly effective in producing anatomically and functionally appropriate vaginal anatomy.[13] As they do not possess ovarian tissue or a uterus, motherhood, genetic or otherwise is not possible.

Rarely congenital disorders of the outflow tract may present as a primary amenorrhoea but more correctly have cryptomenorrhoea. The commonest manifestation of this is imperforate hymen, which is easily treated surgically although, as with similar obstructive conditions, delayed treatment may be associated with endometriosis.

The haematocolpos (and/or haematometra) in these cases may present as primary amenorrhoea with a pelvic mass and urinary retention, so that accurate imaging is essential in order to ensure the correct diagnosis, especially with hemiobstructive congenital abnormalities linked to uterus didelphys (when a double genital tract develops).

Menorrhagia/Dysmenorrhoea

After the menarche, menstrual cycles are often irregular until the onset of regular ovulation. The irregular cycles may initially be heavy in association with proliferative endometrium until ovulation is established although young patients and their parents have difficulty assessing the normality or otherwise of their menstrual cycles.

Some young women will seek medical attention for cycles which fall with the normal degree of variation. A median cycle length of 34 days in first cycles is recognized but almost 40% of young women had cycle lengths exceeding 40 days.

TABLE 27.1 Descriptors of normal menstrual cycles in young females.

Menarche (median age)	12.43 years
Mean cycle interval	32.2 days in the first year
Menstrual cycle interval	Typically 21–45 days
Menstrual flow length	7 days or less
Menstrual product use	Three to six pads/tampons per day

The variation in perceived normality has prompted the American College of Obstetricians and Gynecologists to produce the following descriptors of normal menstrual cycles in young females (**Table 27.1**).[13]

While the majority of adolescents with heavy periods have no underlying pathology around 1% will have Von Willebrand disease. Such cases account for around 1 in 6 referrals for emergency management of heavy periods in girls.

However, the majority of young women with painful heavy periods who are not sexually active need little in the way of investigation and clinical examination (vaginal or rectal) is unnecessary. When evaluation of the pelvic organs is required, this should be done using ultrasound.

Anaemia is not common, but where clinical suspicion arises a full blood count should be taken. There is little place for endocrine evaluation, although clinical features of thyroid disease merit measurement of TSH. Anti-fibrinolytics such as tranexamic acid and prostaglandin synthetase inhibitors such as mefenamic acid form the mainstay of the management of heavier painful periods in this population.

Dysmenorrhoea can occasionally be incapacitating in this group and where there is significant impact on the quality of life or on school performance then there is an undoubted role for the oral contraceptive pill. Treatment may be continued for up to a year, either using the standard protocol or else on a continuous basis, and the situation reassessed. The adverse effects of significant school absence outweigh concerns about potential side-effects of the oral contraceptive pill for the vast majority of young women.

In those rare situations in which the oral contraceptive is not effective, then underlying pathology, namely, endometriosis, should be considered and laparoscopy offered. If gonadotrophin analogues are administered best deferred until after the age of 16 years and the risks of osteoporosis associated with these merit 'add back' oestrogen.

In severe or incapacitating resistant dysmenorrhoea and/or menorrhagia, there is a place for the use of the Mirena intrauterine system, which is a levonorgestrel releasing intrauterine device and which is associated with considerable symptomatic improvement.

This can be of particular value in managing young women with special needs /learning disability when menstruation can be distressing or challenging.

Rarely, the pain can be caused by a non-communicating rudimentary uterine horn (Müllerian abnormality 2B), effectively a localised haematometra. This requires excisional surgery that ideally should be performed using minimal access techniques.

The indications for evaluation of abnormal menstruation in young women is given in **Box 27.3**.[5]

BOX 27.3 The indications for evaluation of abnormal menstruation in young women.

Menstrual conditions requiring evaluation

Menstrual periods that:

- Have not started within 3 years of the thelarche
- Have not started by 13 years of age with no signs of pubertal development
- Have not started by 14 years of age with signs of hirsutism
- Have not started by 14 years of age with a history or examination suggestive of excessive exercise or eating disorder
- Have not started by 14 years of age with concerns about genital outflow tract obstruction or anomaly
- Have not started by 15 years of age
- Are regular, occurring monthly, and then become markedly irregular
- Occur more frequently than every 21 days or less frequently than every 45 days
- Occur 90 days apart even for one cycle
- Last more than 7 days
- Require frequent pad or tampon changes (soaking more than one every 1–2 hours)

GYNAECOLOGICAL MALIGNANCY IN CHILDHOOD AND ADOLESCENCE

Gynaecological malignancy in childhood is rare, with around 2:1,000,000 girls under 15 years being affected by a solid ovarian mass. The majority of these are germ cell in origin and approximately 60% of these are malignant.

Vaginal malignancy, and in particular rhabdomyosarcoma, is the second commonest gynaecological cancer in this age group and may present with vaginal bleeding before puberty.

Management of these conditions should be centralised in tertiary centres with multidisciplinary team care and in the absence of major life threatening complications, there is no place for primary management by the generalist (or even paediatric) gynaecologist.

SEX AND SEXUALITY IN THE ADOLESCENT POPULATION

Whilst paediatricians may be understandably hesitant to discuss sex and sexuality with their patients, there is undoubtedly a role for all of those involved in the care of adolescents in advising on these issues with a view to reducing the incidence of adverse outcomes related to developing sexuality and sexual expression. Screening for sexually transmitted infections is important, as is recognition of cases of sexual abuse. The adoption of vaccination for Human Papilloma Virus in teenagers should be actively encouraged.

Prevention of adverse outcomes related to advising on risk avoidance in terms of sexually transmitted infections, and later consequences, e.g. cervical carcinoma and pregnancy.

Prevention of Cervical Cancer

The recognition that the vast majority of squamous carcinomas of the cervix are associated with oncogenic strains of human papilloma virus has led to the development of vaccination protocols. Human papillomavirus (HPV) vaccination is highly effective in the prevention of cervical intraepithelial neoplasia.

Two vaccines are currently available and both vaccines protect against the two main HPV types (HPV-16 and HPV-18) that cause 70% of cervical cancers, 80% of anal cancers, 60% of vaginal cancers and 40% of vulval cancers. A quadrivalent vaccine also protects against the two HPV types (HPV-6 and HPV-11) that cause 90% of genital warts and is the preferred approach to vaccination.

Teenage and Adolescent Pregnancy

Worldwide, the proportion of adolescents having sexual intercourse has increased steadily over the last 30 years. In the US, 18% of adolescents have intercourse before reaching age 15.

This probably reflects mass and social media influences on behavioural norms.

In the third world, issues such as child marriage remain major contributors to poor obstetric outcomes in female adolescents. This is particularly the case in sub-Saharan Africa.

Thus, the factors involved in teenage pregnancy are complex and depend on the perceived societal norms.

In Europe and North America, high teenage pregnancy rates are associated with poor educational achievement, poor social circumstances and substance abuse.

Improved education about avoidance of risk behaviour and about contraception improves long-term outcomes.

Advising on provision of contraceptive, sexual and reproductive health issues in adolescents should be patient/client centred but legal ethical constraints in the population need to be considered. This is particularly the case for young women with special needs and learning disabilities.

The adverse sequelae of unplanned pregnancy almost always outweigh any disadvantages or side effects of contraception.

Whilst the various methods of hormonal contraception all have higher efficacy ratings than barrier methods, all teenagers should be advised on the desirability of the use of barrier methods in addition to these in order to protect against sexually transmitted infections.

Long-acting reversible contraception, [the levonorgestrel-releasing intrauterine system, injectable and implantable progestogen preparations and copper intrauterine contraceptive devices (IUCDs)] all have a role in preventing unwanted pregnancy.

These have advantages for this population in terms of (relative) confidentiality, low requirement for daily compliance and relatively low economic cost.

GYNAECOLOGICAL EMERGENCIES IN PAEDIATRIC CARE

Urinary Retention

Young females may present with urinary retention secondary to a haematocolpos causing urethral blockage. Treatment is catheterisation, recognition of the underlying diagnosis and a plan for definitive surgery by an appropriate clinician.

Abdominal Pain

A gynaecological cause of abdominal pain is uncommon in routine practice, but occasionally young females may present with abdominal pain caused by torsion, haemorrhage or rupture of an ovarian cyst.

Management of an asymptomatic simple ovarian cyst as an incidental finding can be problematic but should be guided by the clinical picture, age of the patient and ultrasound features. Treatment should be primarily conservative.

Torsion of an apparently simple ovarian cyst is more likely if the cyst is larger than 70 mm in diameter and surgery is required. This should preferably be carried out by laparoscopy.

Longstanding clinical opinion has held that a torted cyst showing apparent features of infarction should be managed by oophorectomy but there is accumulating evidence that ovarian cystectomy and stabilisation by oophoropexy should salvage a functional ovary. Salvage and retention of reproductive function is essential in this population.

Trauma

Common trauma encountered in paediatric practice tends to result from falls involving the vulva. Vulval haematomas are, if large, best treated by incision and drainage. The potential for underlying sexual abuse needs to be considered. And finally, gynaecological problems in paediatric practice are not rare and their proper management requires interactions between many specialties and disciplines. The adverse consequences of poor management can be profound and impact on the young female's capacity to enjoy a healthy and productive life.

REFERENCES

1. North American Society for Pediatric and Adolescent Gynecology. Health professionals committed to the reproductive needs of children and adolescents. [online] Available from *http://www.naspag.org/*. [Accessed November, 2013].
2. BritSPAG.org. [online] *http://www.britspag.org*. [Accessed November 2013].
3. European Association of Paediatric and Adolescent Gynaecology. [online] Available from *http://www.eurapag.com/*. [Accessed November 2013].
4. Whincup PH, Gilg JA, Odoki K, Taylor SJC, Cook DJ. Age of menarche in contemporary British teenagers: survey of girls born between 1982 and 1986. BMJ. 2001;322:1095-6.
5. American Academy of Pediatrics, Committee on Adolescence, American College of Obstetricians and Gynecologists, Committee on Adolescent Health Care, Diaz A, Laufer MR, et al. Menstruation in girls and adolescents: using the menstrual cycle as a vital sign. Pediatrics. 2006;118:2245-50.
6. Oh CM, Oh IH, Choi KS, Choi J-M. Relationship between body mass index and early menarche of adolescent girls in Seoul. J Prev Med Public Health. 2012;45(4):227-34.
7. Trikudanathan S, Pedley A, Massaro JM, Hoffmann U, Seely EW, Murabito JM, et al. Association of Female Reproductive Factors with Body Composition: The Framingham Heart Study. J Clin Endocrinol Metab. 2013;98(1):236-44.
8. Edmonds DK, Rose GL. Outflow tract disorders of the female genital tract. Obstetr Gynaecol. 2013;15(1):11-7.
9. Gholoum S, Puligandla PS, Hui T, Su W, Quiros E, Laberge JM. Management and outcome of patients with combined vaginal septum, bifid uterus, and ipsilateral renal agenesis (Herlyn-Werner-Wunderlich syndrome). J Pediar Surg. 2006;41(5):987-92.
10. Hughes IA, Houk C, Ahmed SF, Lee PA, L WPES1/ESPE2 Consensus Group. Consensus statement on management of intersex disorders. Arch Dis Child. 2006;91(7):554-63.
11. Brandt LM, Helmrath MA. Ovarian cysts in infants and children. Seminars in Pediatr Surg. 2005;14:78-85.
12. Classification of female genital mutilation. [online] Available from www.who.int/reproductivehealth/topics/fgm/overview/en/http://www.who.int/reproductivehealth/topics/fgm/overview/en/. [Accessed November, 2013].
13. Veronikis DK, McClure GB, Nichols DH. The Vecchietti operation for constructing a neovagina: indications, instrumentation, and techniques. Obstet Gynecol. 1997;199;90(2):301-4.

CHAPTER 28

Disorders of Emotion and Behaviour

Michael Morton, David James

AN INTRODUCTION TO CHILD AND ADOLESCENT PSYCHIATRY

Perhaps knowledge of the emotional process of child development within a family, social and cultural context is essential in paediatric practice. This chapter may differ in many ways from others in this book. Effort has been made to illustrate key points visually in a way that reflects the creativity required to engage with the complexity of child development. The disturbances discussed are generally not based upon easily defined 'organic disease'. Although advances in brain scanning and neurochemistry are becoming more relevant, it is only in a minority of these disorders that laboratory investigations yield useful information. While there is a scientific basis to the measurement of psychiatric symptoms and there are real advances in quantifying parameters of family and social disturbance, the questionnaires or rating scales used may appear less objective than many clinical investigations. In organic disease, there is usually a primary cause such as an infective agent or a mutant gene. In psychological disorders, there is an interplay of heredity and environment. Interaction within a culture, between the patient, the family and the school contributes to the clinical presentation. When a diagnostic formulation is reached, although there is a good evidence base for some treatments, the management of disorder may vary in the hands of different physicians or psychiatrists and some factors are beyond the reach of medical intervention. The range of knowledge that contributes to an understanding of emotional and cognitive development goes beyond the scope of this chapter. Some discussion of development is given in the context of an overview of the mental health problems and psychiatric disorders that may present in paediatric practice **(Box 28.1)**.

BOX 28.1 Childhood disorders that require psychological understanding.

Problems in early childhood: Feeding, sleeping and crying

Problems in physical illness: Problems with adjustment to illness and treatment adherence, procedural anxiety

Disorders with physical presentations: Pain and fatigue, conversion disorder and medically unexplained symptoms

Emotional disorders: Separation anxiety, fears and phobias, school refusal, depression, self-harm, attempted suicide, phobic anxiety, obsessive-compulsive disorder

Elimination disorders: Wetting and soiling

Behaviour disorders: Oppositional defiant and conduct disorders, attention deficit hyperkinetic disorder (ADHD)

Eating disorders: Anorexia, bulimia and food avoidant emotional disorder

Psychotic disorders: Schizophrenia, bipolar disorder

Communication disorders: Autism spectrum disorders, language disorder

Disorders with motor presentations: Developmental coordination disorder, tic disorders

Problems of learning: Scholastic skills disorders, learning disability

Problems associated with abuse and neglect: attachment disorders and stress

There are difficulties in making a diagnosis of a behavioural/emotional disorder using the medical model. Diagnosis in medicine depends on symptoms and physical signs fitting a recognised pattern, but the quality of diagnosis improves when aetiology can be proved. For example there may be disagreement about a pain of acute onset in the left upper abdomen or lower chest with a patient in a state of collapse. This may be a myocardial infarct or an exacerbation of a peptic ulcer. Once the abdomen is examined and the electrocardiogram (ECG) done, the diagnosis may be clear. With emotional and behavioural difficulties, it is often difficult to get beyond grouping signs and symptoms to make a descriptive diagnosis that does not generally include an assumption of causation.

Some attempt to deal with this complexity is found in classification systems using different axes for different

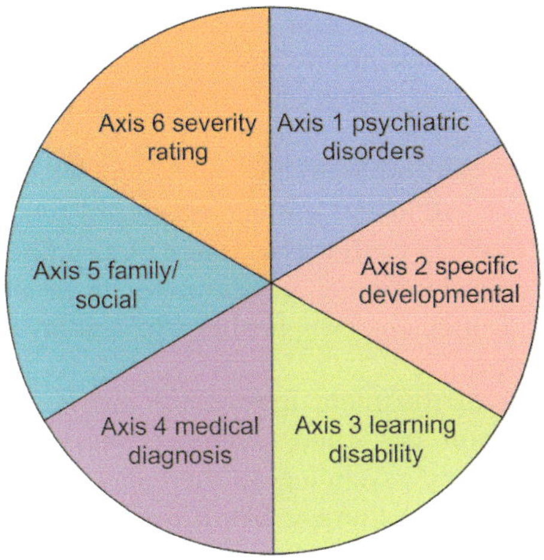

Figure 28.1 Multiaxial classification.

aspects of a presentation, such as the International Classification of Diseases, 10th Revision (ICD-10) Multiaxial Classification. The first axis in ICD-10 is generally related to the presenting symptoms, e.g. encopresis or hyperkinesis. The second axis offers a range of specific developmental delays, e.g. reading retardation, developmental speech/language disorder. The third axis deals with grades of generalized learning disability, labelled as 'mental retardation'. The fourth axis labels any associated physical disorder in the child, e.g. asthma or epilepsy. The fifth axis lists categories of psychosocial difficulty including mental disturbances in other family members, discordant intrafamilial relationships, inadequate or inconsistent parental control and familial over involvement. This axis also includes social transplantation, stresses in school or work environment and other problems including persecution or discrimination. A sixth axis enables a rating of the degree of disability. When all of these axes have been accounted, a meaningful diagnostic formulation is produced. The skill of the clinician then lies in deciding which factors are amenable to change **(Fig. 28.1)**.

The complexity of presentations to specialist child and adolescent mental health service (CAMHS) clinics requires a range of approaches to understand them fully. The CAMHS team usually includes psychiatric nurses, psychiatrists and psychologists and may include occupational therapists, social workers, teachers, child psychotherapists, family therapists, speech and language therapists and dietitians.

The style of history taking should allow a shift from the presenting symptom towards finding out what has actually gone wrong in the family. Allowing for age, the child may be seen on their own or with parents/carers, but the adult, who has usually initiated the consultation, will require time to express their concern. It is important to begin with clarity about the reasons for consultation and the approach to be taken. Sometimes, youngsters have been threatened with the clinic as a response to bad behaviour; they may sit in trepidation awaiting some imagined distressing intervention. A child will usually talk readily about his or her interests, friends, school and relationships at home. A more direct discussion of the child's difficulties may be achieved once a shared understanding is established between interviewer and family.

An attitude of non-judgemental empathy may enable a child or parent to move from describing the complaint to express feelings of despair and anger and then perhaps state how unhelpful other members of the family can be. For example it is not uncommon for a parent of a child with unexplained pain to move on to their own feelings of depression. In due course, there may be tears, perhaps about marital difficulties. Although the first part of the initial interview can be time-consuming, it may save hours later on. The interviewer may then ask a wide range of questions, perhaps including details of the child's eating, problems with elimination, sleep, pain, levels of activity, details about temperament and relationships, antisocial behaviour, sexual difficulties, episodic disorders and school progress. The usual run through of systems, cardiovascular, respiratory, gastrointestinal, neurological and urogenital are included as appropriate. The personal history pays particular attention to pregnancy, birth and post-natal period, with details of personal and social development and the relationship between child and parents during these stages. The family and social history may take more than one interview to complete. It is important to know about parents or carers and also to obtain details about grandparents. Information about cultural factors, parents' childhood experiences, social values and models from families of origin leads to an understanding of the child's problem within the extended family context. Social inquiry includes details of peer group, education, housing, neighbourhood and finance. The potential impact of drug and alcohol use by the patient or family members in the recent past and also during pregnancy should be explored.

Apart from any physical examination determined by the complaint, it is important to assess the child's emotional state. One notes the child's appearance, communication, mood and self-esteem. The content and nature of the child's free play or creative behaviour during the assessment may be informative. More detailed approaches to observation may be indicated, e.g. one might make a modified mental state examination or use structured observations, e.g. looking at behaviours suggestive of hyperactivity in the classroom.

Psychopathology in youngsters is often heightened by family conflict. Adult disharmony leads to inconsistent methods of discipline, which predispose to behavioural difficulty in the children. Children and adolescents can so easily be blamed or blame themselves for a parent's unhappiness. This can lead to anxiety and depression, school phobia and other psychogenic symptoms. As there are so often difficulties in family relationships even when

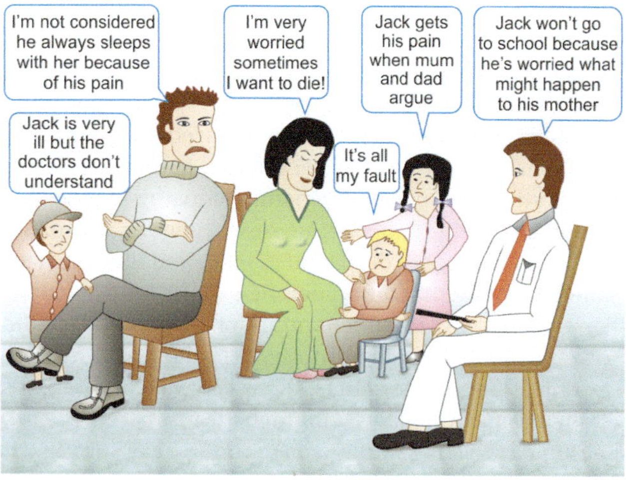
I'm not considered he always sleeps with her because of his pain
Jack is very ill but the doctors don't understand
I'm very worried sometimes I want to die!
It's all my fault
Jack gets his pain when mum and dad argue
Jack won't go to school because he's worried what might happen to his mother

Figure 28.2 Family therapy may resolve abdominal pain.

there is an obvious biological component to the disorder; some CAMHS clinics begin with a family assessment. In this situation, all members of the family living at home are invited to a first appointment. The therapist joins the family, occupying one of a circle of easy chairs. The initial explanation involves an acceptance that the problem with the child or adolescent involves all members of the family. The aim is to help the family discover where difficulties are so that, with the therapist, they can plan the changes needed to bring about a resolution **(Fig. 28.2)**. While family therapy techniques require special training, it is worth bearing in mind that involving more than just one parent in the interview can yield here and now information about the family's style of communication and the degree of mutual support available.

To complete an assessment, consent may be obtained to seek information from third parties such as teachers or social workers. When all is drawn together, a multiaxial classification can be completed. This should lead to a formulation summarising the factors leading to the child's presentation and leading to a plan of action. There may be a need for further assessment that could be medical, neurodevelopmental, psychometric or psychotherapeutic and often involves further exploration of family relationships.

A range of treatment approaches exists. Some are focussed upon the child, such as pharmacotherapy **(Table 28.1)** and psychological therapies, of which cognitive behavioural therapy has the strongest evidence base. Family interventions are common, and the power of group-based therapeutic interventions, especially in adolescence, is well recognized. Schools provide an opportunity for environmental management and specific supports for learning. Community projects are often geared to prevention and early intervention in support of parenting. At the other extreme, in-patient care, intensive outreach or day services are used in the most severe and complex disorders.

There are social benefits arising from effective mental health interventions in childhood. Cycles of abuse and parental mismanagement may be broken, and there is a prospect of reducing the progression of childhood disturbance into adult disorder. For example vulnerable children who present with antisocial behaviour may benefit from the collaboration of health and social agencies in a co-coordinated approach to reducing the risk of adult offending.

Most people understand the bodily changes as children grow. The changes involved in intellectual and emotional

TABLE 28.1 Medications used in treatment of child psychiatric disorders (UK Practice).

Medication group	*Indications (not all drug groups are used under UK licence)*	*Principal side effects*	*Strength of evidence base in children*
Antidepressants (SSRIs)	Depression, OCD, anxiety disorders	Nausea, arousal, sedation, cardiac risks, suicide risk	Moderate (strongest for OCD)
Stimulants	ADHD	Appetite loss, weight loss, anxiety, insomnia, tachycardia	Strong
Adrenergic and noradrenergic drugs	ADHD, tics, Tourette	Sedation, dizziness, appetite loss, mood swings, suicidal ideation	Moderate
Neuroleptics (antipsychotics)	Tics/Tourette, psychosis, behaviour problems in neuro-developmental disorder	Sedation, weight gain, diabetes, cardiac risks, *First-generation neuroleptics have high risk of motor side effects	Moderate
Melatonin	Sleep disorders	Minimal	Limited
Mood stabilisers (antiepileptic drugs)	Bipolar disorder	Various	Limited

Abbreviations: SSRIs, selective serotonin reuptake inhibitors; OCD, obsessive–compulsive disorder; ADHD, attention deficit hyperkinetic disorder.

development are less easily comprehended. The development of speech and language amongst the complex skills of social communication is crucial for further learning and social interaction. A massive amount of learning takes place during the toddler years. A normal child enters school with a good grasp of language that underpins the development of social and emotional behaviour.

Adverse environmental circumstances can retard physical growth and cause children to function intellectually below their potential, but the greatest effects of adverse family relationships and social difficulties are generally upon children's feelings and behaviour. The first year of life is largely to do with the relationship between the caring adult or adults and the child. The infant needs to be kept warm, fed, clean, cuddled and interacted with. The beginning of shaping up vocalisation into speech involves eye-to-eye contact and social communication grows. A child should begin to feel secure in the knowledge of adult care and understanding of his or her needs. Important problems can arise during early development. The initial attachment of infant and caregiver may be adversely affected by maternal depression or illness in the child requiring long hospitalisation.

PROBLEMS IN EARLY CHILDHOOD

Preschool behaviour problems usually start during the next phase of emotional development, when children may appear defiant and demanding. The toddler thinks as if he/she is at the centre of everything and has little awareness of the needs of others. The toddler's timescale is poorly developed, and there is little ability to tolerate frustration or wait until later. Temper tantrums are common and may be intolerable for parents who lack awareness of what is normal in this developmental stage.

A baby can be put in a cot for periods of time, but a toddler is mobile. Rapid cognitive development makes for a huge interest in exploring an environment that was previously inaccessible. It is often a full-time job for the mother to keep the toddler safe and involved in learning. Tables are pulled over, taps left running and electrical sockets interfered with. As speech develops, there can be constant unanswerable questions, loud singing or protests if visitors or siblings interfere with activities or social discourse with the parent. Where a parent is feeling below par, perhaps living in a high flat where there is nowhere safe to go out to play, the tension mounts. Where two or three youngsters are vying for attention in a family, the parent may be reduced to shouting, smacking or ignoring behaviour that requires attention or correction. In such circumstances, social programmes and parent support groups may be effective interventions. Although early childhood problems are often understandable in this way, a significant proportion of children presenting at this age will have temperamental characteristics or developmental disorders contributing to their difficulties.

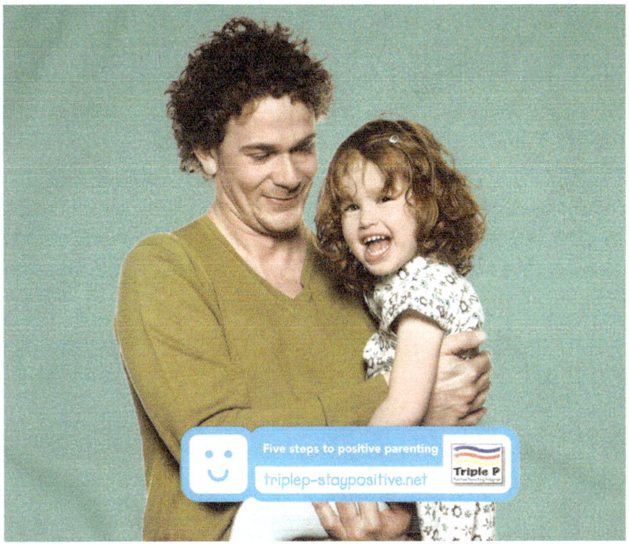

Figure 28.3 Triple P-positive parenting programme.
(*Source:* Reproduced with permission from Triple P International Pvt Ltd).

Expectations of behaviour should be clear and consistent but also reasonable. They should relate to the child's developmental stage and understanding. A child learns most easily when feeling secure with a parent or carer. Prompt positive reinforcement with respect, praise and love is the best way to modify behaviour. Nurturing creativity through the developmental path of shared play enriches the parent child bond and supports prosocial behaviour. Punishment is not recommended but, if carefully considered and quickly carried through, the withdrawal of positive experiences helps to emphasise the cause and effect relationship between antisocial behaviour and undesirable outcomes. The more frequent the punishment the less its effect and too often threats are postponed until behaviour causes damage or an accident. Most importantly, parents must not be split, with one colluding with behaviour, which the other is trying to correct. Parenting advice and training may be offered individually or through group work as well as in books and on-line **(Fig. 28.3)**.

A number of problems arise with failures of parenting. These may include feeding problems, temper tantrums, difficulty going to sleep and battles over toilet training. Sometimes a child has particular temperamental difficulties that challenge the most competent parent but by the time professional help is sought, parents have become inconsistent in their management of the problem. Parents often claim to have 'tried everything'. Similar themes are found in most discipline problems, but each type has particular features (*see* Case examples 1 and 2).

Case Example 1

A child of 4 years who will not go to sleep is told a story. Then he calls out, a reprimand is given and a testing cry tinged with uncertainty follows. Perhaps he will be given a drink and put back to bed. Opportunistically he cries again only to be given a severe telling-off by a mother who is beginning to be irate and exhausted. She says that she will leave him if he is not good, so he cries again. Eventually after further loss of temper, the mother feels guilty and upset that the child's shrieking will invite criticism. She brings the child back into the living area to watch the television. Another attempt is made to go to bed and the crying starts again. Night after night the situation worsens. Mother confides that she once put a pillow over the child's head momentarily and then became overwhelmed with guilt and took the child to bed with her.

Case Example 2

A 2-year-old child with food fads raises parental anxiety by refusing to eat and thus manipulates the situation so that their favourite baked beans or biscuits have to be eaten for breakfast, lunch and tea. All kinds of bribes, punishments and ultimata are given while the toddler resolutely refuses to comply with normal meals. There is inconsistency between anxiety that the child may become ill or even not survive, and the adults' temper loss with sometimes severe smacking and episodes of rejection.

Distraught parents require a sympathetic ear with some exploration of why this stage of development is difficult. Reassurance is important (e.g. a parent may fear that the child will grow up delinquent or anorexic). Where possible good parenting principles should be reinforced but some parents need referral to social services for support and guidance.

WORKING WITH PHYSICALLY ILL CHILDREN

If a child becomes unwell for significant periods of time, the task is not only to get them well but also to enable them achieve their developmental potential. Children grow in three ways: (1) They become physically larger and sexually mature, (2) they increase in cognitive abilities and (3) they achieve social and emotional development. As children become more mature, they are better able to handle extremes of feeling and to give and take in interpersonal relationships. The tasks of adolescence involve issues of separation and dependency as well as coping with adult values and sexual maturation.

CAMHS can work with the pathology of interpersonal relationships and any disability, inborn or acquired, increases the risk of harmful attitudes in other family members, e.g. overprotection and rejection. Sometimes, a parent's need to overindulge the child is based on (usually) irrational feelings of guilt about their disorder. It is also important to note that hospitals, like families, sometimes contain 'sick systems' where anxieties, frustrations and interpersonal difficulties of doctors, nurses and other therapists damage the effectiveness of professional networks.

Physical illnesses make children more vulnerable to psychological disorder and this effect is magnified in diseases affecting the brain such as epilepsy. Technical advances in treatment subject children to stressful situations. Family disruption with frequent hospital attendances, transport problems, boredom, pain and tiredness take their toll. Such stresses are particularly damaging for vulnerable families. Preschool children do not always understand why they are being hurt or why their parents sometimes leave when they are scared and in pain. The sequence of protest followed by despair and then emotional detachment from parents is well recognised in association with hospitalisation of younger children without their parents. Children's hospitals encourage parents to stay with their children, but mothers sometimes have to leave to look after the rest of the family. This kind of separation can have harmful, albeit temporary, effects. Thus, a young child perplexed when mother visited, turned to run towards her, halted and then ran to the comfort of the ward sister.

A child can accept handicaps or painful treatments as long as all is explained honestly and at a level that can be understood. Distraction and play can reduce the pain associated with procedures **(Fig. 28.4)**.

Anxiety increases if parents do not appear at ease and when a child realises that they have been told untruths. It is helpful to listen to the child's worries and questions and then discuss with parents how these should be answered. Children think in concrete terms and can be confused about illness and the possibility of dying. Death is seen as a reversible phenomenon by the very young. An older child may personify death and can express fears through play **(Fig. 28.5)**.

While it may be unnecessary to trouble a child with details of a poor prognosis, it is not helpful to ignore a child's concerns. When distressed children are told not to

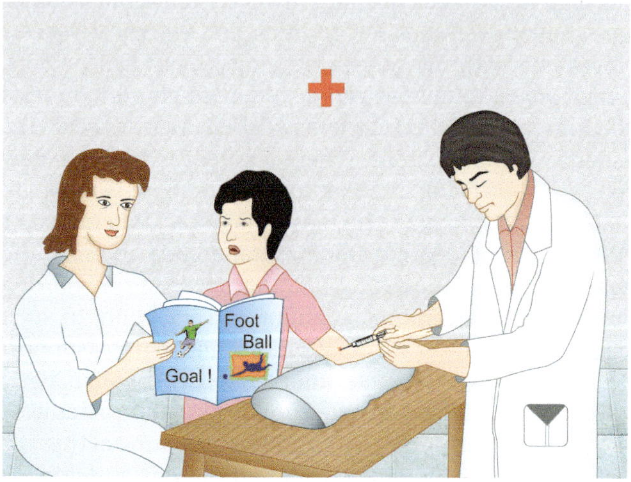

Figure 28.4 Distraction helps in venepuncture.

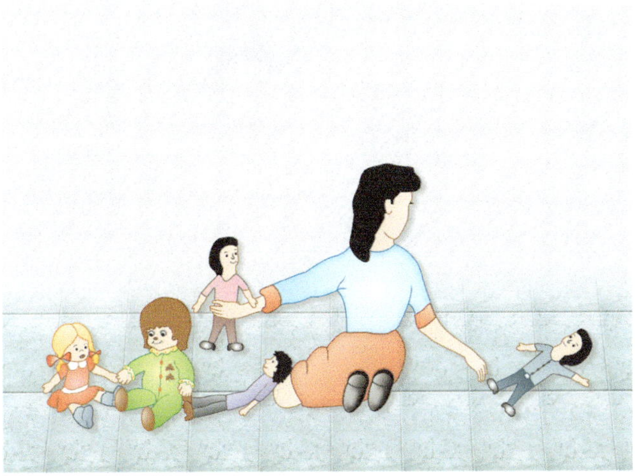

Figure 28.5 In play therapy, a doll may represent family members on even illness or death.

'be silly' or 'let's see a smile', anxieties are deflected and not dealt with.

Case Example 3

One young child almost died from a deliberate overdose. A much-loved relative had died, it appeared the only way to visit him was to go to heaven, and the only way to heaven was to become dead. Having been told that medicine cupboard contained poison he carefully consumed some of its contents and waited for a 'sort of aeroplane ride' to get to heaven. When it was explained that there was no way back and he would not see his friends and relatives again, he decided that he had been unwise.

Coping

There are predictable patterns in coping with bad news, e.g. when mild malaise is found to be a symptom of a renal failure or even a leukaemia. *Denial* is a common mental mechanism, characterised by disbelief. This may be helpful at times, but sometimes its effect is that treatment regimes are not adhered to, particularly in adolescence. Thus, denial becomes unhelpful when insulin injections penetrate the arm of the chair rather than the skin. *Reaction formation* occurs where the underlying feeling is intolerable, and an ill child may seek to take control when this is not safe for them to do so. Small vulnerable children may need to feel big and tough. Others may *regress* to infantile and dependent behaviour. Some youngsters develop *rituals* before treatment regimes and others dispel anxiety in *fantasy*. In children's hospitals, there are a lot of bandaged teddies. Adolescents sometimes identify with medical staff, taking an *intellectualised* interest in their disorder **(Figs. 28.6A to D)**.

All of these defence mechanisms can be helpful as well as destructive and if defences fail too rapidly the youngster may be overcome with anxiety, become severely depressed or on occasion curl up in a foetal position and withdraw from treatment or refuse to eat. *Guilt* is anger turned inwards with soul searching as to how the disease or accident could have been avoided. Sometimes, parents become depressed with an escalation of guilt, morbid thoughts, sleep and appetite disturbance. The *marital situation* can deteriorate and where one parent spends a long time in hospital with the child, the other may be marginalised. Exhaustion and disruption of routine cause irritability and disagreements about the way the child is managed. The *siblings* are also compromised if parents cannot always meet their basic emotional needs.

Case Example 4

A young child with a urinary infection was reassured that he would not need dialysis like his sister. In a temper, he slammed out of the room, saying, 'Does that mean I am not getting the machine as well then.'

The predicament of a sick child involves the whole family. All should benefit from a realistic acceptance of difficulties so that the child is neither overprotected nor expected to do more than he is able. To achieve such adjustment, it helps to see both parents together. If the same person sees the parents on a number of occasions, it is possible to check out what they took from previous interviews. However bad the reality, a child's fantasy may be worse. In general, questions should be answered directly, honestly and in a way that is understandable. Schooling is important as educational achievement is a major determinant of adult outcome in chronic childhood disease. Sick children need discipline and structure as well as care. A team approach ensures that communication is strong enough to avoid anxious parents inadvertently setting one professional against another. Anxious parents may make staff feel ill at ease but should be given their place. Close relationships may develop with some staff, but all members of the team should feel valued. Work will be stressful, especially when children do not recover. Morale is helped by regular discussion both case centred and more informally so that anxieties are shared and treatment goals sustained.

EMOTIONAL DISORDERS AND MEDICALLY UNEXPLAINED SYMPTOMS

Children express themselves in physical as well as psychological ways, and it is helpful to understand the language used about such presentations. Various terms may be found in the literature and the confusion of terminology reflects the complexity of the topic.

Neurosis is a term used to describe predominantly psychiatric disorders that nevertheless may cause a number of worrying and apparently 'physical' symptoms including abdominal pain, headaches and limb pains, which can be severe and disabling. Thus, appetite disturbance, nausea and vomiting can be symptoms of anxiety.

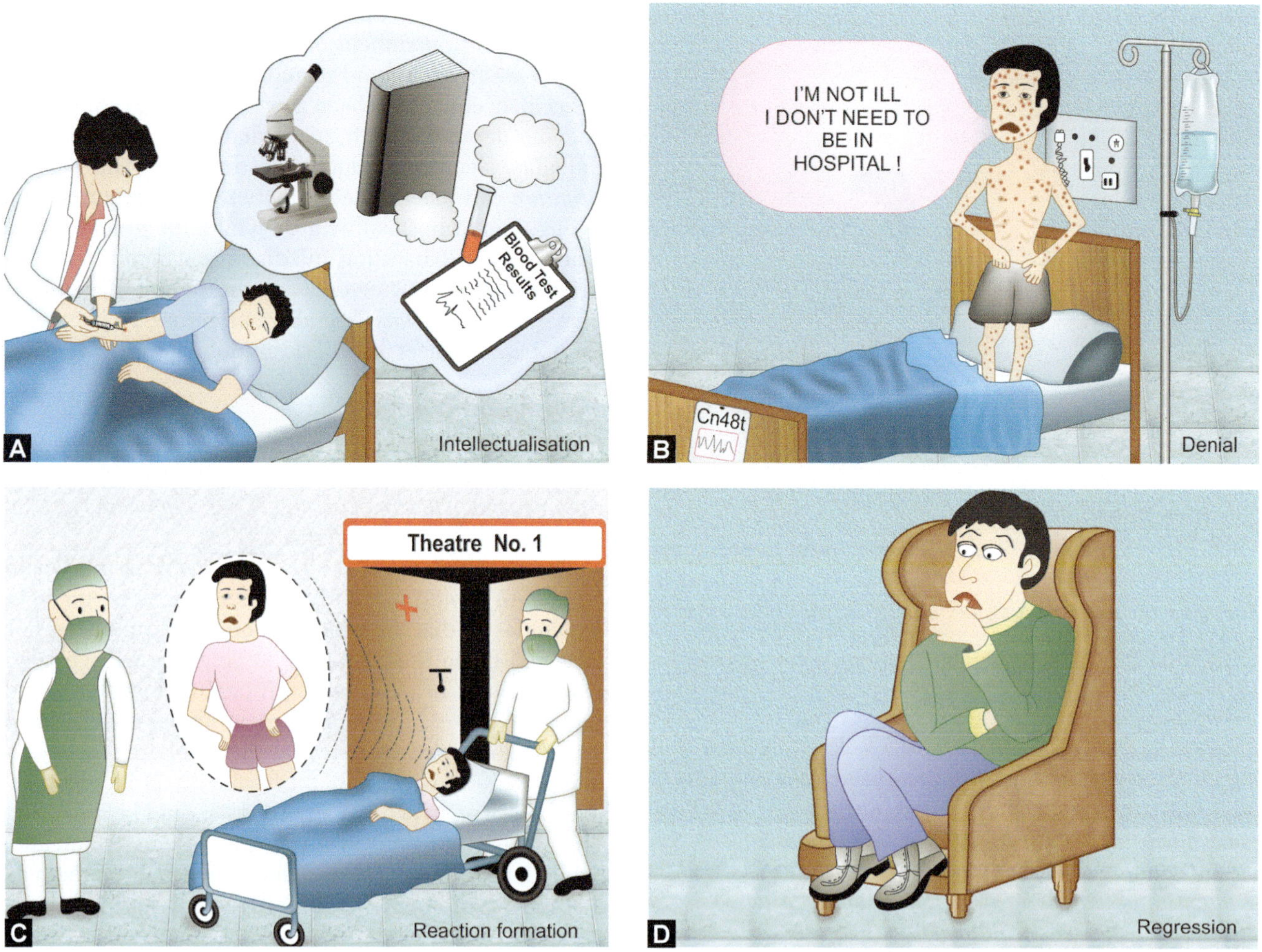

Figures 28.6A to D Psychological defence mechanisms.

Somatoform disorders include a range of stress-linked physical symptoms that may be the main presentation of emotional disturbance. For example somatoform abdominal pain can be severe and although there is no real guarding or tenderness, some children appear exquisitely tender or find it difficult to relax to have their abdomens palpated. It is surprising how such pain can become localised to the right iliac fossa or epigastrium when various doctors have made repeated examinations querying acute appendicitis or peptic ulceration.

Psychosomatic disorder is a term sometimes used in illnesses where there are changes in tissue structure or function, but where the disorder or exacerbations of the disorder are partly or mainly induced by stress. A number of illnesses can be included in this category, e.g. some cases of asthma, migraine, skin disorders or bowel problems. Cyclical vomiting syndrome, where attacks of prostrating vomiting occasionally needing intravenous fluids can last for one or two days, is a complex example, linked to migraine. As the child gets older, visual disturbance, photophobia and pulsating headache become more apparent and vomiting less obvious. In some cases, episodes are triggered or maintained by stress. Children with migraine disorders are often normal between episodes and these are clearly organic conditions, they often have a psychosomatic element, but they are not neurotic disorders.

Conversion disorders are thought to involve the psychological mechanism of dissociation, whereby a patient is not connecting emotion with experience and is unaware that the symptom is other than organic. Conversion symptoms include some disorders of movement, apparent paralysis of limbs and psychological seizures. Children presenting with these disorders may be in some kind of an emotional trap or predicament. Where dissociation is suspected one should look at all aspects of the situation and check if the symptom is serving a purpose, perhaps protecting the child from what happens if the symptom goes away. Episodes of vomiting may keep together parents who are on the verge of separating. A girl's sore tummy may be stopping her highly esteemed father from trying to have sexual intercourse with her. The astute clinician sometimes sees something symbolic in the presenting complaint, as it is not just chance that certain symptoms are unconsciously selected **(Fig. 28.2)**.

'Medically unexplained symptom' is a description that helps to avoid problems in categorising such disorders, avoiding pitfalls in attempts to determine the cause of symptoms. Some symptoms can be frankly goal directed with conscious awareness of the gain involved, but the diagnosis of conversion disorder implies an element of dissociation or unawareness. A diagnosis of conversion requires a satisfactory formulation of the child's difficulty and is confirmed when attempts to ameliorate that situation bring about improvement. Children and families may resist a conversion diagnosis for many reasons and many find it hard to understand psychosomatic causation. Often there is dual pathology, e.g. psychological seizures are often found in children with epilepsy. Some cases of so-called psychogenic disorder turn out to have an organic basis when followed up. Unusual presentations of common disorder and sometimes extremely unusual disorders can emerge over time. For example peptic ulcers are a not uncommon cause of intermittent abdominal pain and very rarely, peculiar panic attacks are due to cerebral tumours. Where there is doubt, a decision about diagnosis is best made using both paediatric and psychiatric expertise with joint review when there is continuing uncertainty. Even with organic disease, it is possible to make progress through psychological interventions geared to the individual without requiring precision on the mechanism of symptom causation.

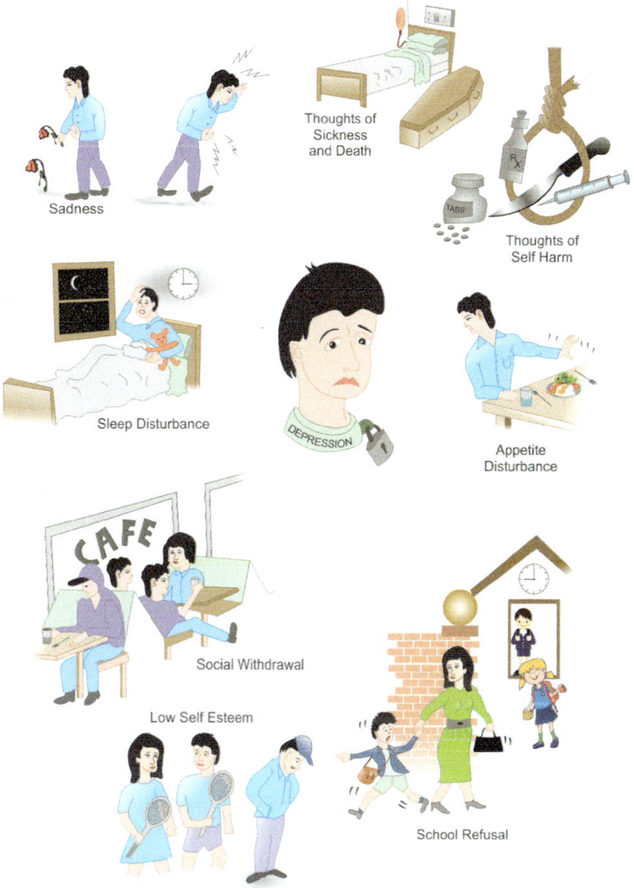

Figure 28.7 Symptoms of depression.

Emotional Disorders

Anxiety and depression often coexist and may be missed when they present in children, especially when expressed through somatic symptoms. More psychological signs of emotional disorder include sleep difficulties with anxious or depressing thoughts keeping the child awake or preventing him/her going to bed. Early wakening, usually regarded as a symptom of endogenous depression can also occur, especially in older children. Poor concentration is frequently present and may have gone unnoticed in school, as children with emotional disorders do not usually present a behavioural problem in the classroom. Tearfulness, oversensitivity, agitation and irritability are common. Anxious toddlers and young children are unsettled and on the go and may be thought to be hyperkinetic. Where depression predominates, the youngster will admit to feeling bad and guilty and sometimes overwhelming feelings of wretchedness can be associated with stealing, tearing up promising work, being unable to accept praise and wanting to die. In preschool and young primary children, the ultimate depressive thought seems to be separation and abandonment from the parents or those looking after them. Emotional disorders occur in at least 2% of the population of late primary school children. Feelings of guilt and suicidal ideas have to be checked out in the older primary school child and certainly in the adolescent. One might ask, 'Do you sometimes feel so bad or unhappy that you would like to run away from home or have a bad accident or die'. A reply in the affirmative must be taken seriously and it is a myth that children who talk about harming themselves would not do so **(Fig. 28.7)**.

Self-harming behaviour and attempted suicide are common in adolescent populations although sociocultural factors led to varying prevalence across communities. Such presentations require urgent and careful attention to the range of individual and family factors that may have preceded the event. It is important to look for treatable disorders such as depression. Specific interventions may reduce the risk of recurrence and address the underlying difficulties revealed in the crisis. Sometimes young people can benefit from direction to on-line resources (e.g. www.depressioninteenagers.com) **(Fig. 28.8)**.

Phobic anxiety presents with specific anxiety in certain situations, e.g. thunderstorms, fear of dogs and being upset by insects. Often these fears are not generalised into other situations and the youngsters may in other ways be quite emotionally robust. Specific psychological intervention with the child can be most helpful. Phobias in children may be learnt from a parent, friend or relative. This is not always volunteered until asked about during history

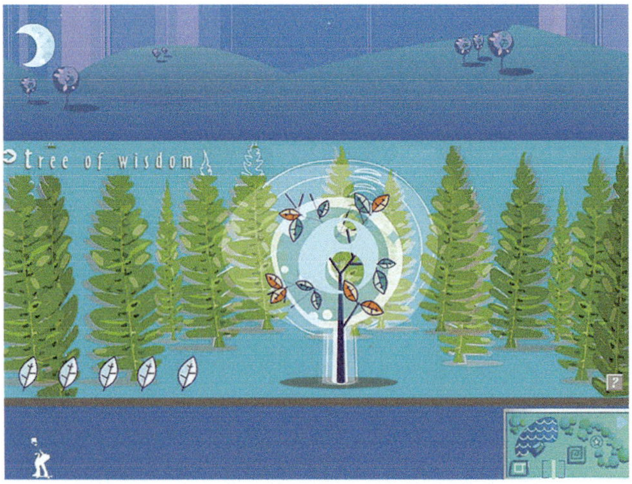

Figure 28.8 Websites aim to help young people with depression.

(*Source:* Reproduced with permission from NHS Lothian Child and Adolescent Mental Health Service, Scotland, United Kingdom).

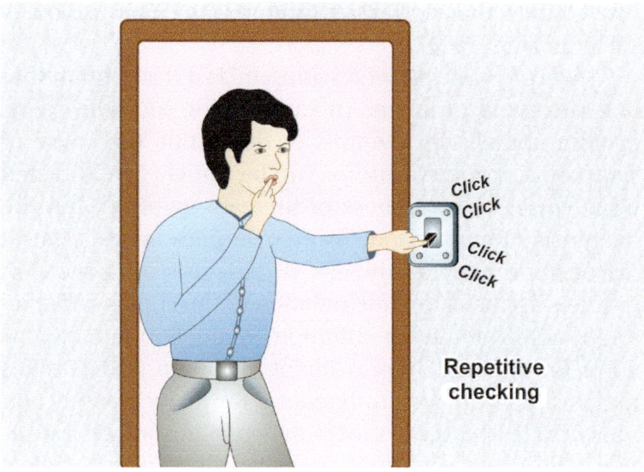

Figure 28.9 Repetitive checking is common in obsessive-compulsive disorder.

taking but it is useful to try and help the affected parent to overcome their own difficulties.

Obsessive-compulsive disorder is characterised by feelings of compulsion to carry out some action or repeatedly dwell on an idea that is difficult to resist **(Fig. 28.9)**. This leads to repetitive rituals, e.g. hand washing which has to be performed time and time again, despite the child and the parent wishing this not to happen. Obsessive-compulsive disorders are more common in children with neurodevelopmental impairments and there is a genetic contribution to aetiology. In younger children, however, rituals can sometimes be a way of reducing anxiety. Anxiety may have its roots in disturbed family relationships, schoolwork that is too hard or pressure from friends. Toddlers and young children love repetitive games and songs. They can exhibit ritualistic behaviour as part of normal development, e.g. needing to go round every lamp-post twice. These preoccupations are usually short-lived unless re-enforced by an anxious parent; nevertheless, it is important to remember that obsessive-compulsive disorders are treatable and not rare.

School phobia and school refusal are terms used for children who develop emotional or unexplained physical symptoms in the morning before school. The symptoms ameliorate either when they have been at school for a while or when the decision is made that they are too ill to attend. Often symptoms are not due to a true phobia of school but are caused by separation anxiety about leaving home and parents. Some school phobic children are depressed. Such children are often good achievers, and although they may try to go to school, symptoms occur to prevent this happening. Their parent or parents are much in evidence, worrying about the child's pains and vomiting, or else being angry that he/she has failed to leave the home for school. These patterns of behaviour are totally different from truancy (see following text, Behaviour Disorders).

Aetiology of childhood emotional disorder is often multifactorial and is frequently bound up with family relationships, which may include elements that are genetically inherited. In some cases, the mother of the affected child is frankly depressed or very anxious. In the seclusion of a one-to-one interview, mothers will often begin to cry and disclose morbid ideas. Doctors are thought to be missing a fatal disorder in the child and depressive thoughts become unwittingly projected onto the youngster. In school phobia, the parent feels worn out by the daily decision whether to send the child to school after being reassured he is physically well. Sometimes when asked 'Have you ever felt that you could not go any longer?' mothers will disclose feelings of total hopelessness and frustration. If the child is asked if he/she worries that their illness upsets the mother, they may burst into tears. On questioning it emerges that he/she is worried that mother cannot cope. Occasionally, the mother has said she can go on no longer and she may leave home or try to 'end it all'. Separation anxiety is then only too real, the child is scared to allow the depressed parent out of their sight, and the parent requires the child to be around to help her get through the day. Frequently there are associated marital problems and the father may resent the overcloseness of the child and his spouse.

Emotional disorders can be triggered or maintained by stresses affecting the child, especially in school or with friends. Bullying is often a hidden problem in schools, and stress may also arise if a child with specific learning difficulties is seen as lazy and ridiculed or punished when trying to do his/her best. Losses and separations can trigger depression. Illness or death of an important family member may cause a bereavement reaction in a parent for many months. The parent is reluctant to discuss this and the child patient feels blamed when his carer is irritable and unresponsive.

Many children are resilient and can adjust well to stress, but some are more vulnerable due to constitutional factors and past experience. Stress may trigger a range of problems including *adjustment disorders* with conduct and/or emotional symptoms. Extreme stress can lead to *post-traumatic stress disorders* with characteristic avoidance of possible reminders of stress, nightmares and sleep disturbance and some re-experiencing of stress or 'flashback' phenomena.

Classical adult presentations of *depressive illness* occur particularly in older children and young people. *Bipolar affective disorder* may have onset in adolescence, but great care should be taken in the interpretation of symptoms in making this diagnosis. There is an international debate about the diagnosis of bipolar affective disorder in younger children.

A proportion of children have *mixed conduct and emotional disorder.* These children are often brought up in disorganised, delinquent and socially deprived families with patterns of antisocial behaviour. If they become depressed, the symptoms are more likely to be difficult to contain and control. Children exhibit outbursts of self-destructive behaviour and anger with extreme sadness, guilt and feelings of hopelessness. Sometimes, such a youngster will have trouble in trusting adults and needs to be contained and controlled because of the disturbed risk-taking aspects of their behaviour. While it may be difficult to understand such emotional symptoms, some children are so frequently undermined and put down by their parents, teachers and potential friends that they can only see themselves as inadequate and hopeless. Anyone trying to be nice to them feels like a phony. Children often exhibit their feelings in the way they behave. A happy child will be spontaneously bright, but a child who is feeling bad will sometimes be unable to stop itself from doing bad things.

First-line treatment of emotional disorders will generally be psychological and family based for the younger child. In older children and adolescents, adult forms of treatment are more likely to be used. There is good evidence for the benefits of individual treatments, particularly cognitive behavioural therapy, which combines behavioural principles with strategies designed to alter thought content presented in age appropriate fashion **(Fig. 28.10)**. Medication with specific serotonin reuptake inhibitors may be considered. The risks of heightened arousal and increased suicidality may outweigh the benefits of such antidepressants especially in less severe disorders. Rarely treatment resistance in this group of disorders can lead to complex interventions including in-patient care.

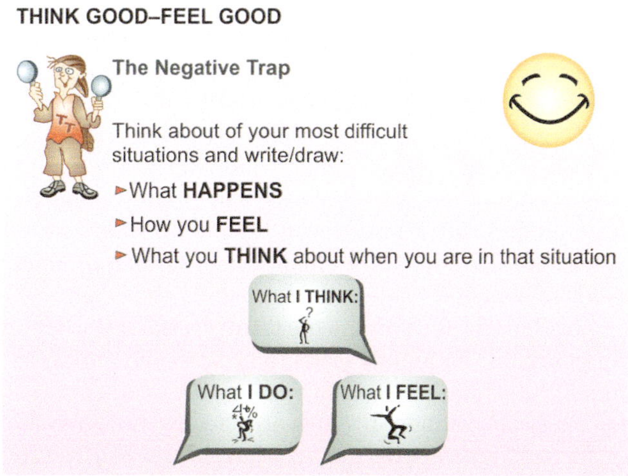

Figure 28.10 Cognitive behavioural therapy can be presented in a child-friendly way.

(*Source:* Reproduced with permission from Wiley UK: Paul Stallard's Book, A Clinician's Guide to Think Good Feel Good Using CBT with Children and Young People, 2005. p. 47.)

ELIMINATION DISORDERS

Enuresis

Enuresis refers to the persistent involuntary or inappropriate voiding of urine. This can occur while the child is asleep (nocturnal) or during the day (diurnal). The disorder may be lifelong (primary) or come on at a later stage (secondary). It is useful to think of primary enuresis as a developmental delay but like secondary enuresis it may have many physical causes. Nocturnal enuresis is common affecting approximately 10% of UK children at the age of 5 and 5% at the age of 10, with 1 or 2% continuing to wet throughout the teens. There is frequently a family history, and it is usually a mono-symptom with emotional factors being secondary. There is an increased incidence of wetting amongst children with child psychiatric problems, but no correlation with any specific emotional disorder. Enuresis more often occurs in children in poor social circumstances where early training has not been established. Some children have had disturbing life events at the time when night-time bladder control should be acquired and the symptom is more frequent in children with other developmental delays and with encopresis. Nocturnal enuresis is not primarily a child psychiatric problem and is generally managed by families with primary care support or in nurse led clinics, with referral to CAMHS restricted to cases where more complex problems are suspected. Associated urinary tract problems and other medical problems are unusual but should be borne in mind and investigated as necessary.

The simple technique of uplifting a child when the parents go to bed sometimes solves the problem at a practical level. The use of star charts should be reserved for children who wish to fill them in. All too often there is an expectation that the star chart will work and if it does not there is loss of face for child, parent and doctor. Where angry feelings exacerbate the problem the chart will merely emphasise difficulties, which may or may not please the youngster. If the child has regressed, the chart will be meaningless. The chart can imply that the child has voluntary control; to be dry is 'good' and to have accidents is 'bad'. Some children who wet are depressed and for them it feels appropriate to be smelly, damp and chastised; the chart may reinforce these feelings.

The enuresis alarm is a behavioural treatment designed to wake the child when voiding commences. Attention to detail is important as false alarms can be caused. If there is no progress after 3 months, it is better to withdraw the apparatus assuming the child is not developmentally ready to benefit.

Antidiuretic hormone, in the form of nasal spray or oral preparations, frequently leads to symptomatic improvement, but caution is needed with renal or cardiac problems. Tricyclic antidepressants are effective but have side effects and are very dangerous in overdose. Bed-wetting often recurs when drugs are stopped, unless the child grows out of the problem during the time of treatment.

Encopresis

Faecal soiling without physical cause is known as encopresis, and like enuresis is sometimes helpfully understood as a developmental delay. Soiling may be continuous or discontinuous. *Continuous soiling* occurs where the problem has always been present. Affected children may come from families with low expectation, poor motivation and inconsistent attempts to start toilet training. Such families have other social difficulties and the carer may have a background with poor models of parenting or be depressed and preoccupied with problems in the family. *Discontinuous soilers* may have been satisfactorily trained or sometimes especially early trained in bowel control.

A way of looking at the mechanisms and family attitudes of children with discontinuous soiling is to look for signs of *regressive behaviour* or an *aggressive toileting situation*.

Regressive soilers are usually reacting to stress and anxiety. Stresses arise within the family and may be made worse by the effects of soiling leading to a vicious cycle. Children feel criticised and scapegoated and some have been harshly disciplined when soiled. The soiling may not be the only developmental milestone that has slipped back. The child may be clingy, withdrawn and exhibit toddler-like temper tantrums. Such children are often difficult to engage in play and sit dull, poorly motivated and emotionally flat. Discussion about the bowel problem is useless at first as the mental mechanism of regression switches off understanding.

Aggressive soiling presents with an account of reasonable attempts to toilet train in the past, but if sufficient interview time is allowed, one becomes aware of considerable tension and anger regarding soiling. All too often a youngster is expected to perform by a harassed mother in a setting where relaxed toilet training cannot occur. The child may respond negatively and, either voluntarily or involuntarily, retains faeces. Megacolon is associated with this situation.

Megacolon is a physical disorder that must be suspected in any child with a history of intermittent, runny stools often with a fusty acrid smell, with overflow incontinence, especially if there is an intermittent history of extremely large bowel evacuations. The condition is frequently chronic with impaction of large faecal masses associated with dilatation of the rectum and colon. The bowel becomes flaccid and unable to pass stools in the normal way. As the situation progresses, the child completely loses any sensation of needing the toilet. It is often difficult to weight the physical and emotional maintaining factors. Children with lack of continence are not always treated sympathetically, because adults think the cause is behavioural whereas the child has no bowel control. Occasionally, an anal fissure compounds the problem. Often family psychopathology appears secondary to physical problems and careful medical assessment is required. Dietary advice to increase fibre and fluids may be helpful. Laxatives are the mainstay of management, but enemata and/or suppositories may be needed and rarely surgical intervention is required.

Case Example 5

A 9-year-old boy, sexually abused as an infant, lived with adoptive parents. His discontinuous soiling had become entrenched and he developed a megacolon. Attempts at paediatric treatment were complicated by his emotional reactions and adoptive parents feelings of failure. The family benefited from an approach that carefully presented the problem of megacolon in a cartoon form that the child could understand. As the child engaged with therapist and adoptive parents in the task of 'Beating Sneaky Poo' his adherence to a laxative regime and toileting programme led to slow bowel retraining taking around 6 months **(Figs. 28.11A and B)**.

In encopresis where there is no megacolon and where the child passes a normal consistency stool at regular intervals, there is little value in using laxatives. Excessive use of laxatives impairs function of a healthy bowel. A behavioural approach with the use of a star chart and simple educative advice may help a child who has not received basic toilet training. Positive reinforcement is more acceptable than a programme that increases parents' anger or discourages the child especially where there is no voluntary bowel control. If possible, the child and family should be brought together as allies with the therapist in tackling the problem of soiling, which is helpfully thought of as a problem external to the child and family and nobody's fault. Where the child is under considerable stress, or where there is too much anger for co-operation with treatment, it may be helpful to review family relationships. Psychotherapy often in the form of play therapy for the child can be helpful in selected cases.

Where ongoing psychological treatment for soiling is needed it may be best to delegate physical treatment to a separate paediatric clinic. Therapy is undermined if the

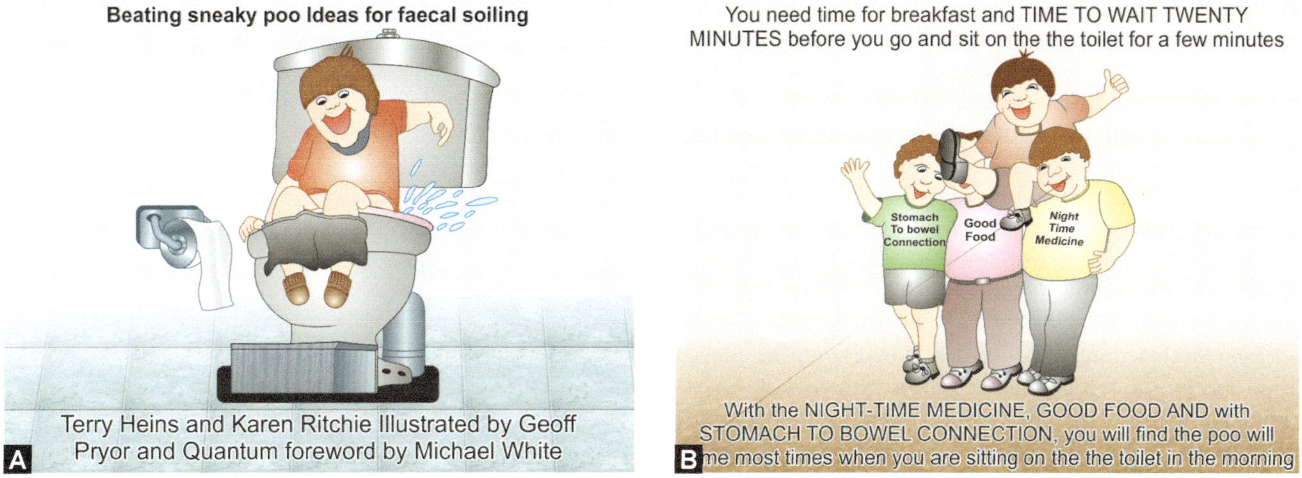

Figures 28.11A and B 'Beating Sneaky Poo'.
(*Source:* Reproduced with permission from Dulwich Centre in Adelaide, Australia.)

therapist plays the dual role of doctor and psychotherapist. A preschool toddler, who soiled in anger, attacked a Daddy doll during therapy, buried him in the sand and beat the sand down with a shovel. The Mother doll was also given a hard time for sending the Daddy away. After 30 minutes of this, it would not feel right for the therapist, let alone the child, for the session to be followed by the therapist giving the child an enema.

BEHAVIOUR DISORDERS

Attention Deficit Hyperkinetic Disorder

Attention deficit hyperkinetic disorder (ADHD) **(Figs. 28.12A to E)** is often described as a straightforward condition manifested by motor restlessness, distractibility, poor concentration, impulsivity and labile mood. The simple explanation that this disorder is caused by brain

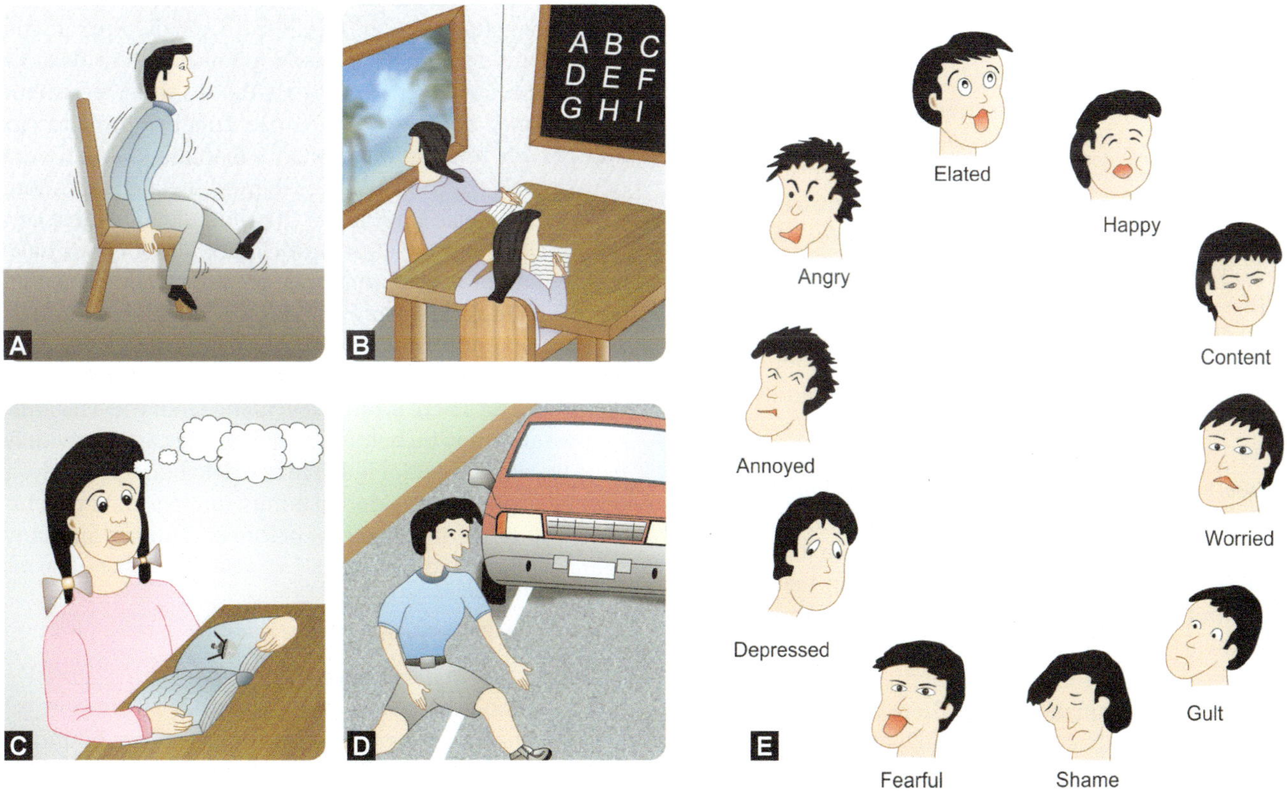

Figures 28.12A to E Attention deficit hyperkinetic disorder (A) Motor restlessness; (B) Distractibility; (C) Poor concentration; (D) Impulsivity; (E) Labile mood.

dysfunction and elegantly responds to methylphenidate is a neat and tidy a concept which bears only a limited relationship to the assessment of badly behaved, inappropriately controlled and understimulated children who are referred to paediatricians and child psychiatrists. As knowledge of developmental neuropsychiatry has increased, so the simple story is seen to be flawed. It is important to realise that hyperactivity is not simply a manifestation of brain impairment. ADHD is not unitary condition and various aetiological theories have been put forward.

Specific learning difficulties not explained by global retardation are common in children with ADHD. Occasionally, ADHD may follow brain damage that is identifiable on scanning. This is a recognized outcome of low birth weight and is found in conditions arising from intrauterine adversity, such as foetal alcohol syndrome. The infant's brain is both vulnerable and plastic with an enormous capacity for function to develop despite damage. Such damage may be generalised e.g. by anoxia rather than localised. The long-term outcome may be that some years on the effects of damage will be manifest by impulsivity and labile mood. The parents of children with ADHD have increased rates of alcoholism and sociopathy when compared with the relatives of normal children. Theories of disorders of monoamine neurotransmission are well supported, and genetic effects have been robustly demonstrated, but the constitutional basis for this disorder remains unclear. While specific factors in heredity, pregnancy, delivery or neonatal period may correlate with dysfunction; it can be difficult to confirm such links when dealing with individuals.

Food allergy is considered important by some, but additive-free diets may be expensive and difficult to follow. If there is evidence that certain foods upset the child, a dietitian can devise a trial of diet that is sensible, within the grasp of the parent and unlikely to deprive the child of essential nutrition. Sometimes, helpful results are obtained, although it is not always clear what is due to support and what is due to diet. It appears reasonable to keep an open mind and carefully accumulate data. There is little doubt that some children are irritable and restless when they are itchy with eczema or frustrated by coryza and nasal stuffiness.

Whatever be the underlying constitutional disturbance, there always needs to be an emphasis on consistent and positive management. Children with ADHD struggle in a classroom, often receiving criticism and negative reinforcements, which alienate them from teachers and sometimes classmates. This leads to over arousal, making distractibility worse and contributing to the development of poor self-esteem. Depressive feelings may further reduce motivation, and there may be a defensive reaction 'that teacher is always bugging me' or 'I am not working for him'. It can be difficult to sort out cause and effect when parents appear tired, angry or depressed. As the cycle of events winds up, parents become inconsistent being either inappropriately angry or at other times too negative and exhausted to intervene. Follow-up of children with ADHD shows a high risk of developing conduct disorder in later childhood and antisocial behaviour and alcoholism in adult life, treatment can reduce these risks.

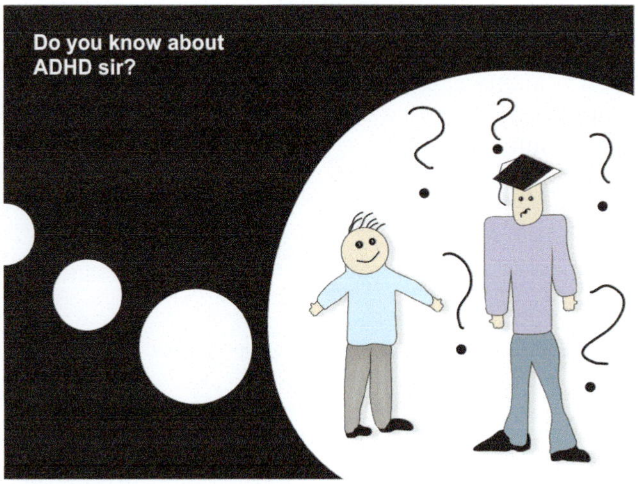

Figure 28.13 A resource to help teachers to manage ADHD.

(*Source:* Reproduced with permission from ADDISS, Edgware, United Kingdom.)

Children with ADHD require a treatment plan. This should include advice on their management, with guidance for teachers (Fig. 28.13), perhaps involving an educational psychologist working with the school and sometimes support to the family from a social worker. The neurostimulants, such as methylphenidate and dexamphetamine, are effective with or without a wider treatment programme. Their use can cause appetite impairment and growth retardation, anxiety, sleeplessness and very occasionally psychosis. Where there is social deprivation, others may abuse stimulants. Other medications that can help include atomoxetine and clonidine. All drugs have a potential for interactions and side effects, in particular, antipsychotics, which are sometimes considered for their benefits in modulating arousal, present serious long-term dangers, e.g. risking tardive dyskinesia and metabolic disturbances. There is limited evidence that tricyclic antidepressants may be helpful, although they are not widely used because of a poor balance of risk to benefit. Rarely, it may be useful to consider an admission to a child psychiatric unit to clarify diagnosis before embarking on many years of pharmacotherapy.

Conduct Disorder

Although the management of children with aggressive and destructive behaviour giving rise to social disapproval usually falls to other professionals, doctors are bound to become involved as such problems are common. The incidence of antisocial disorders varies from around 2 to 10%

in the mid-childhood years, depending on population characteristics.

A well-researched approach to understanding development of social behaviour comes from cognitive and behavioural models of social learning, suggesting that consistent rewards and reprimands, with exposure to prosocial attitudes and behaviours, lead to appropriate responses. The psychodynamic model concentrates on the quality of relationship between child and parent or authority figure. It is generally accepted that problems may arise in the family as well as in other areas of community life, especially in school.

Some family norms may not be acceptable to society: many delinquent children have a parent with a criminal record. Some families have no clear guidelines, being very punitive on occasion and at another time amused when the youngster does something inappropriate. Some families have unclear roles with perhaps the elder sister taking over when the mother is not coping. The impact of personality disorder or substance misuse in a parent must be taken into account with a range of other social factors.

Factors in the community can foster antisocial behaviour. Housing may be allocated so that families with social difficulties are housed together in unpopular areas. Their children are exposed to a peer group with high delinquency rates which potentiates a downward cycle. The culture of school can make or break a youngster who is not well supported at home. Children with conduct disorder often fall behind in reading and other school attainments; conversely children with learning difficulties have an increased rate of conduct problems. If the child is encouraged within school, identification with the school system and certain teachers will exert a positive influence. A child who does not succeed in school is much more likely to get recognition from other antisocial youngsters. If specific learning difficulties are missed, a child of average intelligence is labelled as 'lazy' or 'not trying' in the area of disability and depressive or angry attitudes towards school destroy motivation.

The medical skill lies in identifying conditions within the child that predispose to antisocial difficulties, especially treatable disorders such as ADHD. Children vary in temperament and parents who have successfully reared one or more 'easy' children may find that their methods do not succeed with a more challenging child. Children who are hyperkinetic with poor concentration and sometimes poor coordination are difficult to discipline. They get discouraged with repeated failure and develop habits of opposition. Depression can give rise to stealing and under functioning as the 'I am bad' guilt is enacted or the stolen item held for comfort. Also children with long-term illness or other vulnerability may over-react to show friends and teachers that they are a force to be reckoned with.

Conduct disorder may develop out of *attachment disorders*, when early emotional deprivation (e.g. poor quality institutional care or care by a mentally disordered parent) can lead to profound difficulties in relationships, with striking abnormalities in social contact. Initially such children may be inhibited with 'frozen watchfulness' or disinhibited and indiscriminately friendly. There are continuing rages and toddler-like behaviour sometimes for many years even though a child may be in an improved home situation.

Case Example 6

A 13-year-old boy was brought to the clinic by his social worker and his mother. He had been in trouble with gang-related offences of violence, theft and possession of street drugs. His father, an aggressive man, had left home 4 years ago and his mother was an alcoholic, unable to give consistent care to her children. He lived in a children's home but was not able to relate well to staff, testing their commitment to him. If he began to feel secure, he would do something bad. Thus, if he were moved on it would be on his terms, which he saw as better than being rejected 'for no reason.' Nevertheless, after an incident he hoped to be allowed to stay. Similar testing behaviour occurred in school. Like his father, he had specific learning difficulties as yet unappreciated by teachers who focussed more on his behaviour. Unable to gain satisfaction in lessons, he found it more rewarding to truant and revelled in his role in the gang.

Truancy

This form of school non-attendance is more frequent in underachievers, from families who (rather than being overinvolved with the non-attendance as in school refusal, above) are unconcerned or unaware of the situation until the authorities make contact. It is unusual for psychiatric symptoms to be found in truants who frequently go off to join friends in conduct disordered activity.

EATING DISORDERS

A range of emotional and behavioural disorders lead to abnormal eating in childhood and unusual eating behaviours are commonplace in adolescence. Although eating disorders may be a focus of considerable parental concern, the insidious development of anorexia nervosa is still sometimes overlooked **(Fig. 28.14)**.

Anorexia nervosa has at its core a morbid fear of fatness and a distorted body image. Weight loss leads to a low body mass index, pubertal development and growth may be retarded. The disorder sometimes develops from dieting with selective rejection of calorific food. Various tactics to lose weight are displayed, the most dangerous of which is vomiting, sometimes done quietly and with remarkable ease. Bursts of frantic exercise may occur openly or in secret while increasing quantities of laxatives and purgatives may be consumed. Girls develop amenorrhoea. On examination, there may be bradycardia, hypotension, a growth of fine hair and increased pigmentation.

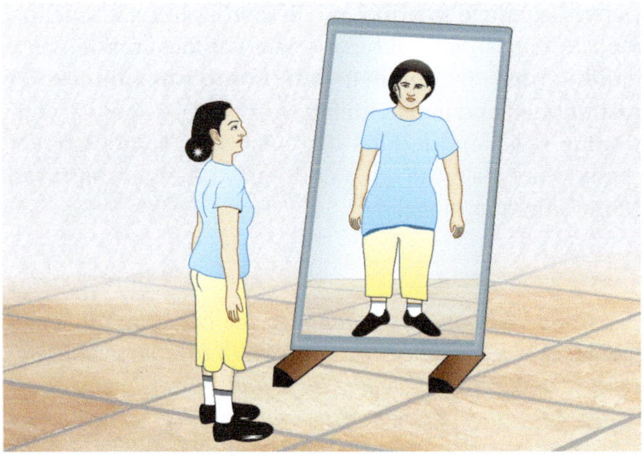

Figure 28.14 Body image distortion is a key feature of anorexia nervosa. An anorexic girl is unable to see herself as she really is.

Sometimes, parotid glands are swollen and the back teeth decayed because of acid reflux from vomiting. Baggy clothes often disguise weight loss. It is only when one has sight of the protruding ribs, scapulae, clavicles and the scaphoid abdomen with prominent iliac crests that the degree of starvation becomes apparent. Emotional state is adversely affected often with obsessive or depressive and suicidal thoughts. Some youngsters show attention seeking and confrontational behaviour, which may involve the family and therapists, who become fearful for the fate of the patient and also angry with them (Box 28.2).

Aetiology remains a topic for debate. The disorder is more common in girls than boys and often appears during adolescence. Cultural factors may reinforce the fear of fatness and evidence suggests that anorexia nervosa is becoming more common in countries where traditional attitudes to weight are replaced by fashionable ideals of thinness. Neurodevelopmental disorders may precede anorexia and, in a small minority, eating disorders follow sexual abuse. Anorexia nervosa still carries a significant mortality. While approximately one-third make a full recovery, many remain vulnerable, psychiatrically disturbed and requiring repeated periods of therapy; some require hospitalisation.

In treatment, prescribed food is taken regularly. This may involve the exhausting task of sitting with the patient until food has been finished and after that for at least another hour. Where the patient is very underweight, diet should be built-up gradually, with dietetic advice. In severe cases, refed too rapidly, acute gastric dilatation can develop and refeeding syndrome can be fatal.

Family therapy approaches involve supporting parents in understanding the disorder and managing mealtimes. Cognitive behavioural approaches to anorexic beliefs are helpful once a patient has recognised their problem and can engage in individual work. Intensive day-patient programmes that involve group dynamics can enable youngsters to enforce their own dietary control. Sometimes, antidepressants or neuroleptics are used, but doses should be gradually built-up if the patient is frail.

Those who pursue a relapsing course often develop *bulimia nervosa*, where there is intermittent bingeing, often with very large amounts eaten, followed by self-induced vomiting or purging. As with anorexia, treatment plans must be clear, often with contracts drawn up so that therapy is underpinned with behavioural objectives.

BOX 28.2 Diagnostic criteria for anorexia nervosa (ICD-10).

Body weight maintained at least 15% below that expected or prepubertal patients show failure to make expected weight gain

Avoidance of 'fattening foods' and one or more of:

- Self-induced vomiting
- Self-induced purging
- Excessive exercise
- Use of appetite suppressants and/or diuretics

Body image distortion with a dread of fatness

Endocrine disorder of the hypothalamic–pituitary–gonadal axis:

- In women, amenorrhoea
- In men, loss of sexual interest and potency
- In prepubertal onset, pubertal delay or arrest

PSYCHOTIC DISORDERS

Symptoms such as hallucination that are suggestive of psychosis require careful assessment in childhood, but true psychoses are very rare in younger children and when they occur an organic cause should be suspected. Careful medical review is required including consideration of a range of disorders such as temporal lobe epilepsy, infectious, inflammatory and degenerative disorder as well as toxic effects of heavy metals and substance misuse. Mental state examination in children requires particular skill. Where children have not established good communication or clear boundaries between fantasy and reality, it is a highly complex task to use diagnostic criteria derived from adult psychiatry. Children with communication disorders and learning disability may present symptoms suggestive of psychosis but are at particular risk of misdiagnosis, as well as being at increased risk of psychosis. Psychoses such as schizophrenia and hypomania become more prevalent in adolescence.

Treatment approaches need to take account of the young person's stage of development. Family involvement is important and, in particular, neuroleptic drugs have higher rates of side effects in younger people and doses need careful consideration.

Case Example 7

A 9-year-old boy living with socially isolated parents is seen by an education officer concerned about non-attendance. He has stopped sleeping at night and plays computer games for hours. He appears distracted by what he describes as 'voices of aliens.' He recovers quickly in a psychiatric unit, where magnetic resonance imaging (MRI) scan shows cortical dysplasia, consistent with his abnormal pattern of cognitive skills. His psychosis is seen as a consequence of abnormal functioning within an abnormal environment and medication is not required.

COMMUNICATION DISORDER

Where there is delay in *expressive* communication, the child clearly understands what is being said and will obey verbal instructions but has difficulty finding words to express himself. Children with this problem may be irritable and demanding, as they live in a frustrating world of adults moving on to the next topic before they have been able to join in. There is frequent gesticulating, pulling parents over to indicate their wishes by body language and general upset. Providing the child is socially aware and develops an understanding of language the problem may resolve with support and possibly speech and language therapy.

Autism spectrum disorder (ASD) is a concept that provides a useful way of thinking about various severe disorders of communication that in ICD-10 are categorised as *pervasive developmental disorders*. The core of the difficulties faced in ASD lies in the *autistic triad* of impairments of communication, social development and behavioural rigidity. The recognition of ASDs is the first step towards ensuring that such children achieve their developmental potential. Specific treatments have a limited evidence base, but early supports for parents, later educational and social interventions, individually tailored, can reduce the impact of a child's impairments (Box 28.3).

The signs of *infantile autism* usually present within the first 30 months with abnormal responses to both auditory and sometimes visual stimuli. Speech is delayed and if it begins to develop it tends to be echolalic and later lacking in ability to use abstract terms. Autistic children appear detached socially and classically there is impairment of eye-to-eye contact and lack of ability to relate meaningfully to parents or age-mates. Autistic children resist change and may have catastrophic rage reactions for minor causes, e.g. if an item in a room has been moved or if their transport to a school goes by an unusual route. Routines, rituals and obsessional behaviour are commonplace and if the disorder improves patterns of logically concrete thinking emerge with a lack of social empathy (Fig. 28.15).

BOX 28.3	Features of autism spectrum disorder (ASD).
ASD is characterised by a triad of impairments:	
Social interaction	
Verbal and non-verbal communication	
Restricted and repetitive interests, behaviours and routines	

There are a number of theories of aetiology. The disorder is male predominant but not X-linked. In the past, family influences were suspected, but it is now clear that genetic factors are highly relevant, with multiple interacting genes and high heritability. Associated medical disorders (e.g. specific disorders of the brain such as tuberous sclerosis) are found in more than 10%. Better prognosis is found where there are no signs of severe learning disability. Many require ongoing family, educational and social support with only a minority achieving more positive adjustment. A few truly gifted individuals achieve great success in areas less dependent upon their areas of difficulty, e.g. as musicians or scientists.

Asperger syndrome has been conceptualised as high-functioning autism, but this may be misleading as the social deficits of this condition can be as disabling as in infantile autism. The criteria for diagnosis of Asperger syndrome are open to debate, but the syndrome differs from infantile autism in that the level of speech and language impairment is much less obvious. Such children will still have marked impairments in language in areas such as semantics (the construction of meaning) and pragmatics (the use of language in social interaction). As more subtle social impairments have been identified clinically, there has been debate over the validity over the subdivision of ASDs and the use of the term Asperger syndrome may be abandoned.

Atypical autism is a term that is sometimes applied to children with marked autistic features who do not fulfil criteria for another diagnosis, especially where there is learning disability.

Rett syndrome is a rare genetic disorder leading to autistic regression with a characteristic pattern of abnormal hand movements.

DISORDERS WITH MOTOR PRESENTATIONS

Children may present in paediatric clinics with a range of motor disturbances that are best managed with the skills of a child psychiatrist. Repetitive stereotyped movements are common features of autism and may need to be distinguished from self-stimulating behaviours, which are also common in developmentally impaired children. *Tics* are rapid repetitive movements that are driven by an internal compulsion that older children may describe as 'like an itch,' they are often self-limiting. Tics are usually motor phenomena but can also be vocal, such as grunting or throat clearing. It can be helpful for children and

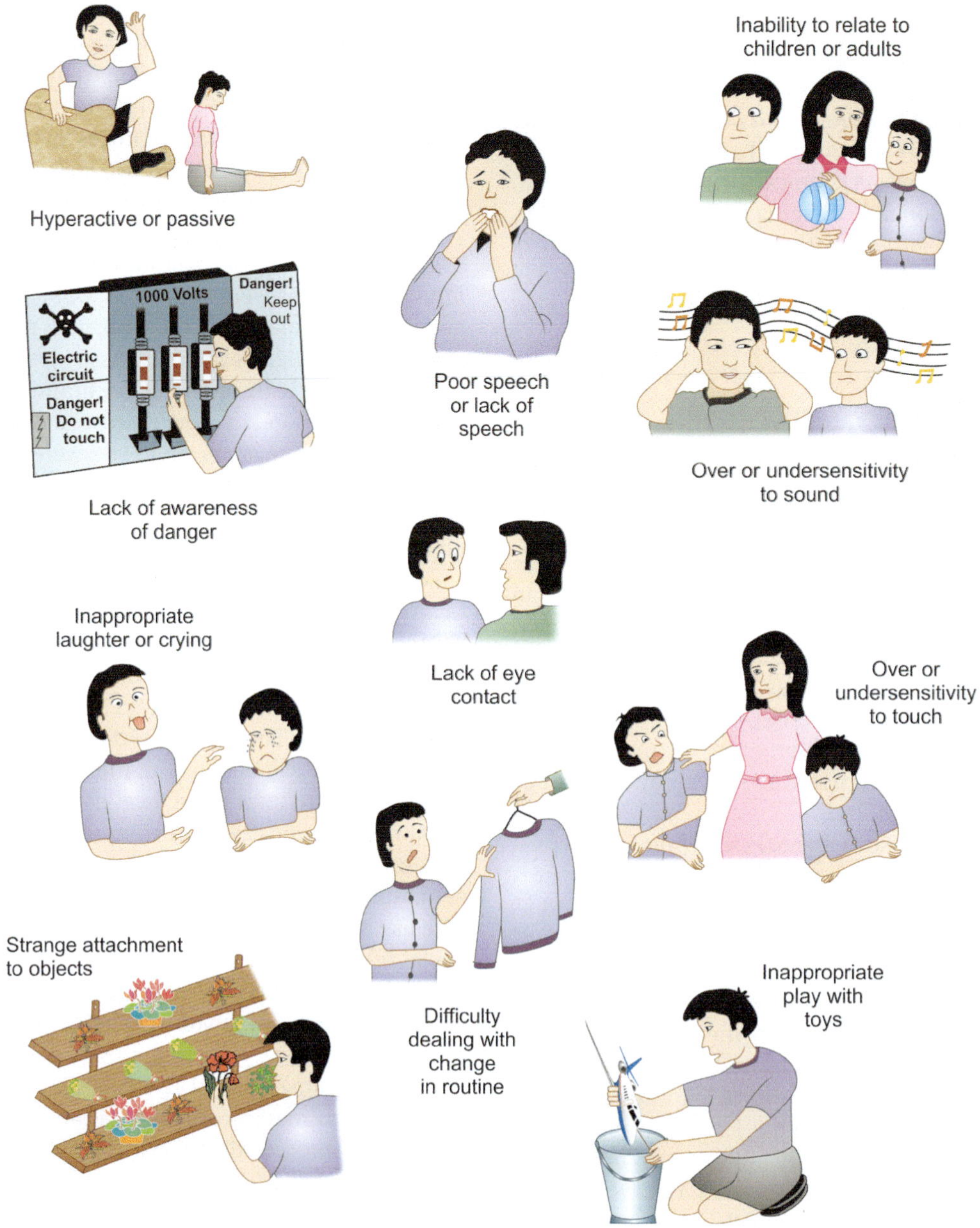

Figure 28.15 Features of autism.

families to understand that tics are basically involuntary although children may learn to control some of their manifestations.

Tourette syndrome is diagnosed when both motor and vocal tics occur for a sustained period; vocal tics may progress to explosive and sometimes culturally unacceptable utterances. In themselves, tics rarely require treatment but when they cause significant impairment a child may benefit from psychological therapies or one of a number of medications, of which clonidine or guanfacine is the least likely to cause harmful long-term side effects. Tourette syndrome often coexists with obsessive-compulsive behaviours or attentional problems and in a few children these difficulties may be triggered by group B streptococcal infection associated with Sydenham chorea. The fascinating hypothesis that a range of psychiatric symptoms may be triggered by streptococcal disease without associated neurological signs reflects increasing interest in autoimmune processes within the nervous system.

Motor overactivity is a core feature of ADHD, but symptoms of motor restlessness or of immobility can more rarely be seen in childhood affective states and psychosis, including rare cases of childhood catatonia. Awareness of the link between specific disorders of motor development (developmental coordination disorder/dyspraxia) and other developmental and psychiatric disorders should lead to careful global assessment when problems in areas such as coordination and visuospatial capacity are identified.

PROBLEMS OF LEARNING

Many disorders can directly or indirectly affect learning. Children with emotional disorders are frequently anxious and depressed. They find it difficult to concentrate in class if preoccupied by feelings of worthlessness or worrying that a parent may be unwell. Their distress and falling off of attainments may be missed by the teacher who is more preoccupied by disruptive behaviourally disturbed children. Somatic symptoms including abdominal pains and headache lead to frequent school absence and the continuity of learning is lost. A child with a chronic or relapsing illness may find learning difficult because of malaise, pain, repeated time-consuming or traumatic medical treatments and time lost from school. The side effects of medications (e.g. anticonvulsants) are important causes of cognitive impairment.

Attainments are frequently poor in conduct disordered children. The causes are multifactorial. In areas of social deprivation, parents' attitude towards education is not always positive, homework is not encouraged, and there is no space to work in overcrowded, noisy, disorganised households. A youngster behind with his attainments is frequently criticised by teachers. If the child believes that he cannot learn, motivation will be adversely affected. A mental process guarding against depression and poor self-esteem is to blame others. It is safer to reject the school and denigrate the teachers than to accept criticism. This attitude can become the group norm and outshining truanting colleagues with antisocial behaviour can preserve self-respect as school attainments fall behind.

In a number of cases, constitutional difficulties with attention, concentration or more specific learning skills precede behavioural difficulties. Where difficulties are not discovered and educational help is not given, a child's self-esteem and motivation worsens and the situation escalates.

Specific learning difficulty is described when children with otherwise normal developmental capacity demonstrate defined problems in one area of learning or development, e.g. dyslexia is specific reading retardation and dyscalculia a similar problem with numbers. Specific learning difficulties may present with depression or conduct disorder. Impressed by a youngster's unhappiness, it is all too easy to miss the underlying stress of a child trying his/her hardest and never being able to succeed at school. If a child does not have the ability to cope with an aspect of learning, it is often wrongly assumed that extensive practice will improve the situation but often the converse is true. It is not surprising that such children may feel despairing and only careful attention to their specific needs will offer a way forward. However, the term 'dyslexia' can give rise to confusion. Worried parents can regard dyslexia as an illness; others may use this as an excuse for school failure that has other causes. The problem is that the label does not describe the nature of the underlying learning difficulty. Many professionals prefer to describe the nature of the problem in functional terms.

Three cognitive processes are often found to be affected in specific reading retardation. The first is a problem of short-term memory or a sequencing difficulty. This may be associated with difficulty of recall of information obtained through the auditory route, or the problem may be in recalling material, which has recently been read from writing or print (e.g. a person can be told a telephone number and not recall it, whereas they can retain the same number read from a book or vice versa). The second major difficulty is with spatial ability, e.g. some children have enormous difficulty in learning left from right. The third problem area may be visuomotor or perceptual difficulties, often associated with problems of putting thoughts into legible writing and decoding information from the written page. A child may acknowledge that his written page is full of mistakes but be unable to correct them.

Severe dyslexic problems may overlap with communication disorders and specific learning difficulties can be found in association with hyperkinesis or in children with poor motor control. ADHD, specific learning difficulty and specific disorder of motor development (dyspraxia) are sometimes grouped together. Aetiological theories are covered above in relation to ADHD.

Severe head trauma, cerebral tumours and other forms of brain injury in childhood may impair learning. Intellectual abilities may appear remarkably intact after marked anatomical damage has occurred, especially if early in the child's life. However, brain-injured children may become more obviously disabled as the demands of development outstrip their capacity.

A child who has problems affecting all aspects of cognitive development is described in ICD-10 as 'Mentally Retarded' although the term 'Learning disabled' is less stigmatising. Stigma is compounded when a child looks dysmorphic or has an associated movement disorder. Learning disability generally does not have an identifiable cause, but various aetiologies are recognised. The commonest single cause is chromosomal disorder, e.g. Down syndrome. There are a number of genetic disorders where an inborn error of metabolism can be proven; e.g. Wilson disease, which is a defect of copper metabolism, and the mucopolysaccharide disorders, which are progressive. Screening at birth allows for intervention to prevent the insidious mental retardation resulting from phenylketonuria and hypothyroidism. Children born with neurological impairments, such as spastic hemiplegia, frequently have learning disability. There are many rare medical causes of deteriorating cognitive capacity or dementia in childhood.

WORKING WITH SOCIAL SERVICES AND POLICE

Professional responsibility in dealing with children includes a responsibility to work within a legal framework governing the acceptable treatment of children as well as attending to the childhood roots of adult criminality. It is important that doctors understand the social arrangements and statutory procedures for working with social services and where necessary with the Police and the Courts or equivalent legal bodies.

In certain circumstances, a professional opinion is sought in relation to severe *offending behaviour in children*. Adult approaches to forensic examination need to be modified to take account of developmental factors and the influence of family and social factors must be acknowledged. Careful notes should be kept of *forensic* interviews and examinations. Cultures vary in their attitude to antisocial behaviour in childhood, but it is generally accepted that the younger the child the more their behaviour must be seen in the context of age. Punishment may then seem less important than attempts to intervene to reduce the risk of further offending.

Psychological signs may arouse suspicion of *abuse or neglect*. Psychogenic pains, often abdominal, and conversion symptoms may indicate that a child is under stress that is too difficult to go on tolerating and too difficult to be disclosed. Abused children may be fearful of adults and appear apprehensive or withdrawn; particularly where circumstances recall the abuse, e.g. a male doctor reminds the child of a male abuser. Children often replicate confusing or worrying incidents in their play. Children's drawings may also indicate fears of sexual objects or sexual knowledge beyond what is age-appropriate. Most of all, it is important to listen to what the child has to say. It is very unusual (but not unknown) for children to disclose abuse that has not actually occurred. They are more likely to remain mute or ill at ease in order to protect their perpetrators.

If sexual abuse is suspected, it is important that arrangements for paediatric examination give due weight to the emotional needs of the child. Provision of special units with quietness and appropriately comfortable furnishing is helpful. In this setting, full explanations can be given and trust built-up between the child and the examining doctor. The skills of being frank and open at a level the child can understand, seeking the child's permission and talking them through the examination go some way to reducing the secondary emotional damage from fear resulting from disclosure. If a parent or relative has been the perpetrator and then doctors remove the child's clothes carelessly and intrude into the child's personal space, it must seem as if no adult can ever be trusted again.

Although dialogue with the child or interpretation of his/her behaviour sometimes leaves little doubt to the clinician that abuse has occurred, the legal process may not progress without physical evidence. A number of cases are not proven with further difficulties resulting for all concerned. Perhaps most difficult of all are the categories of *emotional abuse* and *failure to thrive* where parents may contest the need for intervention. Close cooperation is required across agencies involved.

Fabricated and induced illness (FII), otherwise *medical child abuse*, formerly known as Munchausen syndrome by Proxy or Meadow syndrome, involves children repeatedly brought to doctors with symptoms which tempt the physician or surgeon to subject the child to numerous investigations, sometimes of an increasingly intrusive, traumatic and expensive form. While anxious parents may unwittingly subject their children to the effects of over concern; in FII, the problem is that the parent is usually doing something actively to produce the child's symptoms. Mothers have used their own blood to contaminate a child's urine specimen to precipitate investigations for haematuria and anoxic seizures have been deliberately produced by mothers partially suffocating their children. Such problems may be more likely in medical systems where care is compartmentalised by specialty and consideration of psychosocial mechanisms neglected. Complex treatment regimes may be set up but the problem fails to resolve. Mothers of children with FII often have a lifetime of somatic complaints and a habit of lying. They are often cooperative, adapt well to ward routine and are well acquainted with hospital, where their emotional needs may be met. It is difficult to empathise with their psychopathology and dissociation may be present. The ability to play the competent caring mother and yet behave destructively in order to gain input from doctors and nurses is hard to comprehend. Confrontation is often not met by an admission of guilt and it is important that appropriate child protection orders are sought. Sometimes after confrontation the parent may decompensate. A needy, distraught mother feels she has failed once again. Adult psychiatric intervention may be necessary as depressive feelings emerge when dissociation is broken down.

ACKNOWLEDGEMENTS

The authors wish to acknowledge the published work of RS Illingworth and DW Winnicott, two paediatricians whose influence has shaped medical practice in support of children and young people's mental health. We are extremely grateful to Mr. Duncan Galbraith of Scotland, United Kingdom, for drawing illustrations for this chapter.

CHAPTER 29

Paediatric Radiology

Sanjay V. Maroo, Sandra J. Butler

GENERAL CONSIDERATIONS IN PAEDIATRIC RADIOLOGY

- Imaging has assumed an important role in the diagnosis, understanding and, in certain cases, treatment of paediatric diseases.
- The availability of many imaging modalities [plain film, ultrasound, computed tomography (CT), magnetic resonance imaging (MRI), nuclear medicine, angiography and single photon emission computed tomography scanning] requires problem-oriented decisions to determine which techniques should be used or omitted in any given clinical situation.
- The radiologist plays a central role in the diagnostic imaging process and is actively involved in formulating an appropriate pathway of diagnostic evaluation to maximize the benefits from any imaging examination.
- Adequate clinical information should always be available on the radiology consultation in order to determine, what, if any, imaging modalities are indicated for diagnostic evaluation.
- Open communication between the referring physician and the radiologist improves the quality of patient care.
- There is no place for routine radiological examinations.

RADIATION EFFECTS ON CHILDREN

- The biologic effects of radiation result primarily from damage to DNA and the effects are greatest on fastest growing organisms—the foetus, infant and the young child. All ionising radiations are potentially harmful.
- The consequences of radiation relate to both dose and time of radiation and may appear later in life. There is no existence of a threshold dose.
- The ALARA principle states that radiation dose of exposed individuals should be kept as low as is reasonably achievable, with economic and social factors being taken into account.
- Medical diagnostic X-rays represent the largest source of radiation exposure resulting from human activity. The greatest source of background radiation is radon gas—a decay product in the uranium series.
- Imaging modalities that deliver ionizing radiation are plain films, fluoroscopy, CT and isotope studies. The modality that delivers the highest dose is CT and use of this modality is increasing with children (0–15 years) receiving 11.2% of all CT examinations.
- All effective methodologies to reduce radiation exposure in children should be employed. These include tailoring the examination to the child, adjusting technical factors for plain films using pulsed fluoroscopy, screening of CT examinations and utilizing other modalities that do not involve ionising radiation such as ultrasound and MRI.
- Radiology consultation should be obtained to get a proper test. Factors utilized in determining the best test include sensitivity in diagnosis, cost, timeliness and safety.
- Dose may be decreased by performing only examinations that are clinically indicated.

IMAGING MODALITIES USED IN PAEDIATRIC IMAGING

Plain Film Radiography

Conventional radiography is based on the variable attenuation of an X-ray beam as it passes through tissue.

This modality is frequently a starting point for radiological investigations in a number of conditions. The radiology request should provide adequate clinical information and specify the views.

There are standard views for specific anatomic areas and specific conditions:

- Head: Anteroposterior (AP), Towne and lateral
- Spine: AP and lateral
- Chest: Frontal and lateral
- Abdomen: AP
- Pelvis: AP.

Contrast Media

Contrast media are externally administered agents used to provide positive or negative contrast in certain areas of the body. Areas where contrast media are frequently used include gastrointestinal tract, genitourinary tract and the vascular system. Barium compounds (barium sulphate) are used for routine gastrointestinal studies. Water soluble iodinated compounds are used for assessing the gastrointestinal system in emergency cases or where perforation is suspected, for the genitourinary system, the cardiovascular system and CT scanning. Water soluble contrast agents contain iodine. Low osmolar iodinated contrast media should be used as a routine. High osmolar contrast media can have a profound effect on serum osmolality and the haemodynamics status of infants and children.

Fluoroscopy

Indications include gastrointestinal, genitourinary studies, orthopaedic procedures and diagnostic angiography and during image guided therapeutic (IGT) procedures. Image intensification is necessary for fluoroscopy of children and most procedures usually involve contrast medium administration. Techniques reducing radiation doses in children without any significant loss in image quality include pulsed fluoroscopy, last image hold and collimation.

Ultrasound

Ultrasound is ideal for imaging children for a number of reasons:

- Uses no ionising radiation.
- Sedation is almost never required.

There is no evidence that energy levels of diagnostic ultrasound used in humans are harmful to humans.

Examination can be performed at the bedside in sick children.

Paucity of fat in the paediatric abdomen and the smaller size of the patient allow detailed visualisation of the abdominal anatomy.

Indications include intracranial examinations in neonates, urinary tract infections, abdominal pathology, scrotal conditions, anomalies of soft tissues and certain chest conditions and for interventional procedures.

Computed Tomography

Computed tomography uses a radiation beam that is highly collimated through one cross-sectional slice of tissue from different angles. The data are then computed to record X-ray absorption in a specific volume element, which is then converted to an image. CT has high spatial resolution and demonstrates anatomy as a two-dimensional image, which helps to determine the extent of disease. Recent advances in CT and software technology now allow CT imaging in a volume of tissue such as the abdomen in less than 5 seconds and also enable reconstruction of the image in any plane including three dimensions. A major disadvantage in children is the radiation dose.

Magnetic Resonance Imaging

Magnetic resonance imaging uses a strong magnetic field and radiofrequency energy to generate a synchronised precessional motion of protons in body tissues.

An MRI image reflects the distribution of protons in the section of the body.

Applications of MRI are gradually increasing in paediatrics. Reasons include lack of ionising radiation, multiplanar capabilities, superior contrast resolution and the ability to image blood vessels without using intravenous contrast agents. In addition to illustrating normal and pathologic anatomy, MR is also used to assess chemical composition and tissue perfusion.

Disadvantages include need for sedation or anaesthesia in younger children and the examination is contraindicated in children with pacemakers and certain implants.

Radioisotope Studies (Nuclear Medicine)

The imaging energy source for scintigraphy is the isotope attached to a radiopharmaceutical injected into the body. The detection system, a gamma camera, uses a collimator and photomultiplier tubes to detect the gamma rays emitted from the body to a scintillation crystal. The raw data from the scintillation crystal then yield a raw image after computer reconstruction and signal processing. Most radioisotopes are injected intravenously and the functional information provided by scintigraphy often complements the anatomic information provided by anatomical studies and may provide the only imaging evidence of pathology. Radiopharmaceuticals are given in small doses and are relatively innocuous, i.e. they do not produce significant pharmacologic, haemodynamic, osmotic or toxic effects. Radiation exposures from their use in diagnostic imaging usually fall in the lower range of radiation exposures from common radiological examinations.

The technique has high sensitivity but low specificity. Common radioisotopes include 99mTc dimercaptosuccinic acid (DMSA), 99mTc DTPA and 99Tcm MDP.

Image-guided Therapeutic Procedures

A steady increase in non-vascular and vascular image-guided therapeutic (IGT) procedures has occurred in the last decade. This increase stems from the growing recognition that many paediatric interventional procedures like their counterparts in the adult world can achieve the same results as surgery without being as invasive and usually with less morbidity and more rapid recovery.

Most of the interventional procedures are performed with ultrasound and fluoroscopic guidance. Use of contrast media is made at every stage, if indicated, as an additional safety margin.

Non-vascular IGT procedures include biopsies, drainages of pleural fluid, abscesses, other fluid collections, balloon dilatation of oesophageal strictures, percutaneous nephrostomy, pyeloplasty, percutaneous gastrostomy/gastrojejunostomy.

Vascular interventional procedures include image guided central and peripheral central venous catheter placement, sclerotherapy of vascular malformations, angioplasty, embolisation and transjugular liver biopsy.

RESPIRATORY AND CARDIAC

Child with Cough and Fever

Common Causes

- Acute pneumonias:
  - Viral
  - Bacterial
  - Atypical organism.
- Other pneumonias:
  - Tuberculosis
  - Aspiration
  - Cystic fibrosis
  - Opportunistic organisms.

VIRAL PNEUMONIA (FIG. 29.1)

- Bronchiolitis **(Fig. 29.2)**
- Bacterial Pneumonia **(Fig. 29.3)**
- Round Pneumonia **(Fig. 29.4)**
- Primary Pulmonary Tuberculosis **(Figs. 29.5A and B)**
- Cystic Fibrosis **(Fig. 29.6)**
- Bronchiectasis **(Fig. 29.7)**
- Inhaled Foreign Body **(Figs. 29.8A and B)**
- Complications of Pneumonia

Empyema (Fig. 29.9)

The appearance of pleural fluid in the setting of pneumonia suggests an empyema. Ultrasound and CT scanning reveal helpful information such as depicting whether the effusion is loculated or free, clear or containing debris. Image-guided drainage can be done using ultrasound and fluoroscopy to accurately place the drainage catheter **(Fig. 29.10)**.

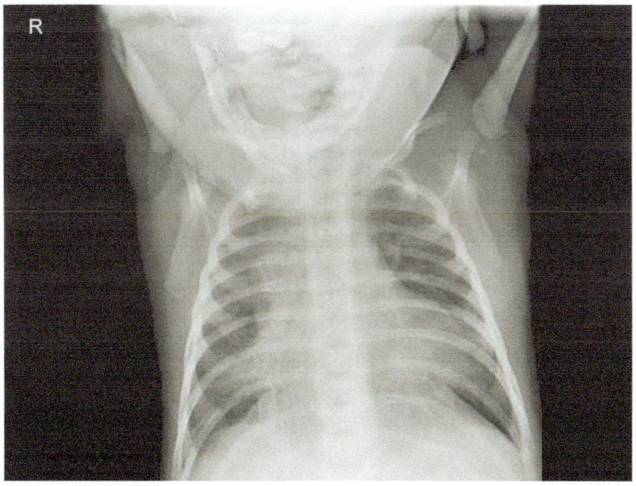

Figure 29.1 Viral pneumonias are mainly small and large airway disorders, and radiological findings are due to partial and complete airway occlusion leading to atelectasis and hyperinflation. Chest radiograph in a 1-month-old baby with viral pneumonia showing hyperinflation and atelectasis of the lingua (seen as effacement of the left heart margin) and the middle lobe (seen as effacement of the right heart lobe).

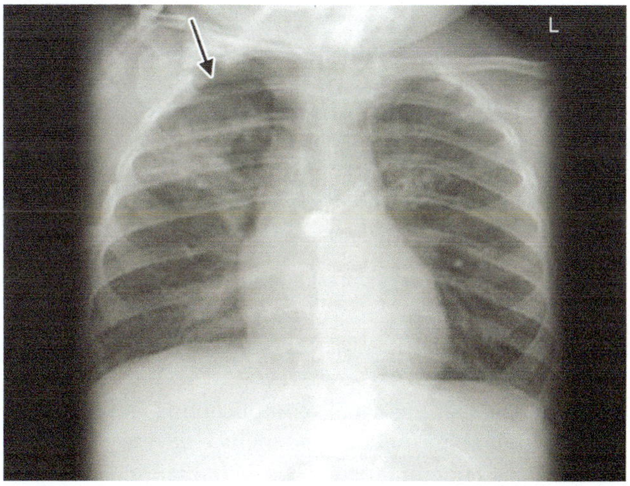

Figure 29.2 Bronchiolitis is a serious manifestation of a lower respiratory infection occurring in infants in the first 2 years of life. Radiologically, air trapping and atelectasis are the common features. The infection is a caused by the respiratory syncytial virus (RSV). Bronchiolitis with air trapping and right apical pneumothorax (arrow). Additional findings include bilateral parahilar infiltrates and atelectases.

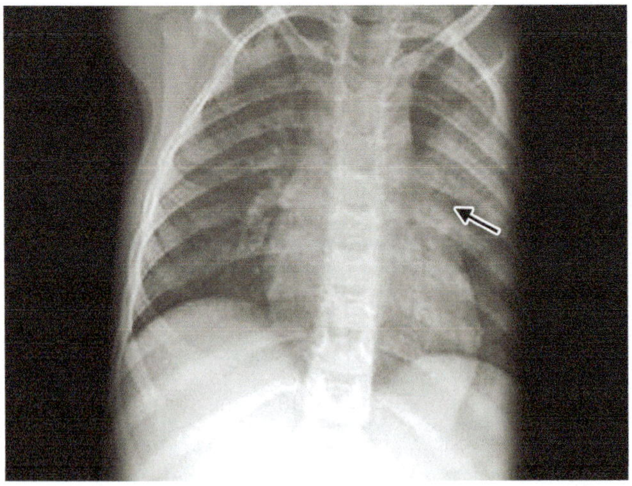

Figure 29.3 Bacterial infections present as lobar or segmental consolidations or fluffy infiltrates. Even though consolidation may be extensive, volume loss may be minimal. The organisms are commonly *Haemophilus influenzae* in infants less than 2 years and *Streptococcus pneumoniae* in older children. Chest X-ray showing segmental consolidation in the left upper lobe with air bronchograms (arrow).

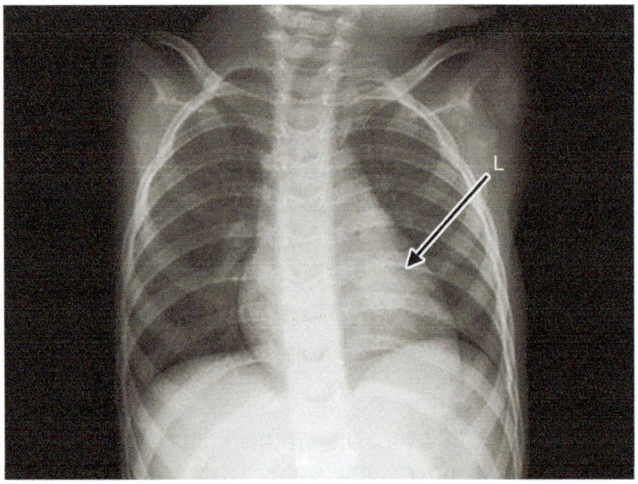

Figure 29.4 A round pneumonia (arrow) is seen exclusively in children, usually in the superior segment of the lower lobes. Consolidations in the early phases may appear rounded and one should not be misled by their appearance which is strictly fortuitous. It can be mistaken for a neoplasm, but a history of an acute illness and the extreme rarity of such neoplastic lung nodules in children should confirm the diagnosis. Causative organism is commonly *Streptococcus pneumonia*.

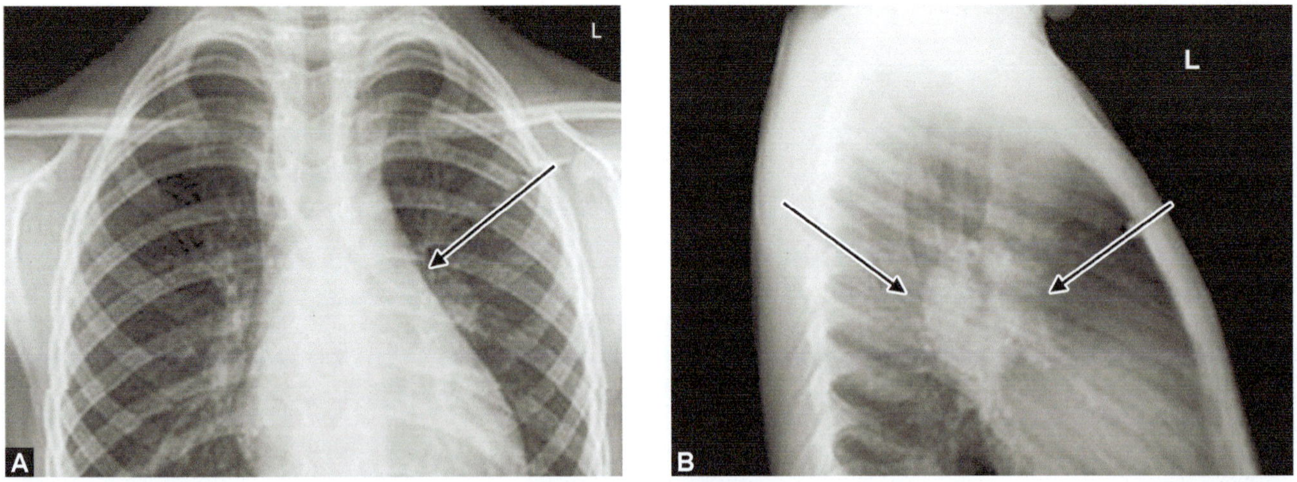

Figures 29.5A and B Primary pulmonary tuberculosis results from inhalation of the organism from an infected individual. The radiologic hallmark is unilateral hilar or paratracheal lymphadenopathy, very often accompanied by atelectasis due to compression of the bronchus by the enlarged nodes. Frontal and lateral chest X-ray showing left hilar adenopathy in a patient with cough and fever (arrows).

Lung Abscess (Fig. 29.11)

Suppurative parenchymal complications represent a spectrum of abnormalities and include cavitary necrosis, lung abscess, pneumatocoele, bronchopleural fistula and pulmonary gangrene. When lung first becomes necrotic, the necrotic tissue liquefies and forms fluid filled cavities. When portions of this necrotic fluid are expectorated via bronchial communications, the cavities may fill with air. CT is more sensitive to earlier detection of lung abscesses, can assess proximity to pleura and plan drainage **(Fig. 29.12)**.

Pneumatocoeles (Fig. 29.13)

Pneumatocoele is a term given to thin-walled cysts seen at imaging and may represent a later stage of healing necrosis.

Bronchopleural Fistula

Bronchopleural fistula is identified on CT when a direct communication is visualised between the air spaces of the lung and the pleural space **(Fig. 29.14)**. There may be a chronic air leak.

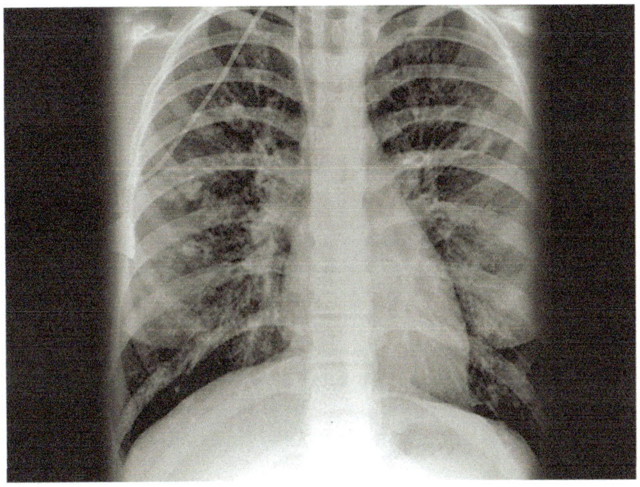

Figure 29.6 An autosomal recessive error in chloride ion transport results in thick tenacious mucous. Clinical manifestations result from bronchiectasis, lung abscesses, air trapping, airway obstruction and right heart failure. On chest radiograph, early CF can be seen as hyperaeration and bronchial wall cuffing. Mucoid impaction is seen as finger-like densities radiating from the hilum. Bronchiectasis is seen as tram tracks radiating from the hilum. Chest radiograph showing lung hyperinflation, patchy infiltrates and peribronchial thickening and dilatation in an 11-year-old patient with cystic fibrosis.

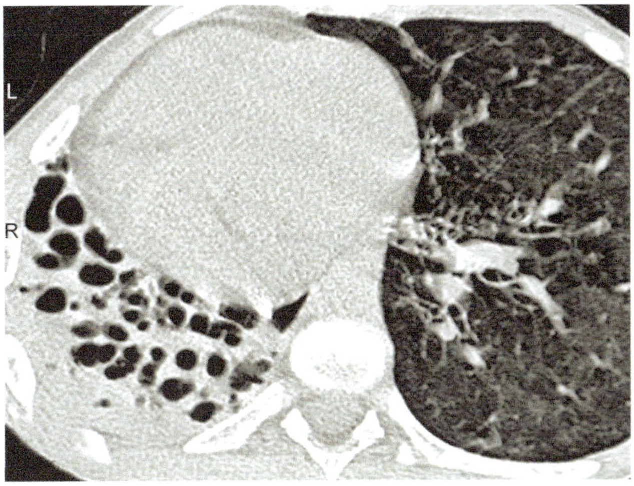

Figure 29.7 High-resolution CT confirms the presence and extent of bronchiectasis. Evaluation of segmental/lobar involvement is important if surgery is contemplated. CT scan shows cystic bronchiectasis in the right lower lobe.

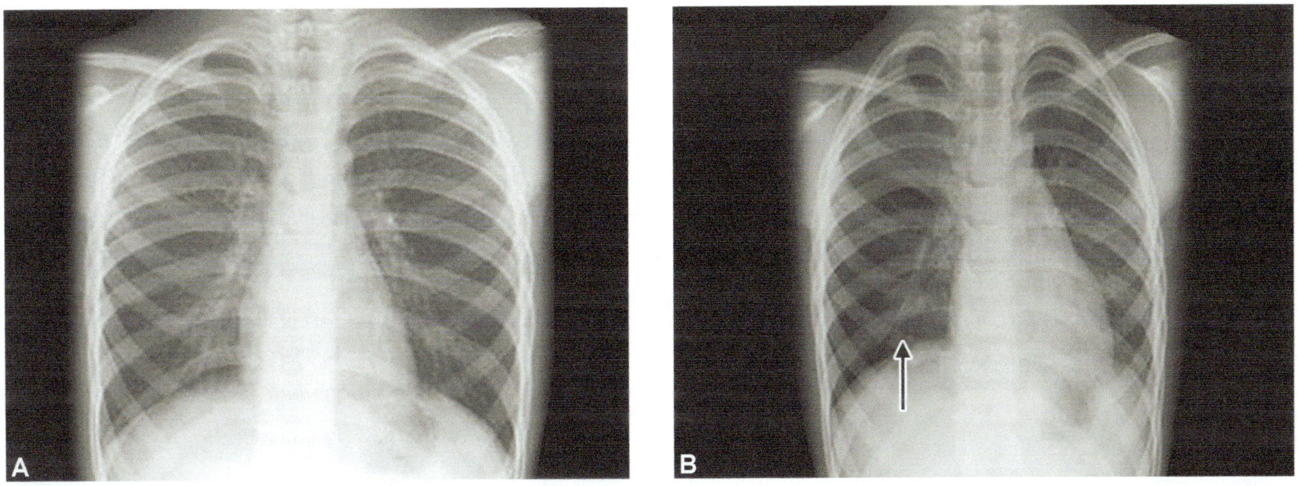

Figures 29.8A and B Airway obstruction by foreign body (FB) usually affects toddlers and presents with stridor, wheezing, cough or pneumonia. The FB, which can be radio-opaque or non-radio-opaque, usually lodges in bronchi (right commoner than left) and can obstruct the airway. Total obstruction can cause collapse. Partial obstruction can cause ball valve effect permitting air to enter but not leave the lungs. The affected side will demonstrate air trapping made prominent on expiration. Inspiratory (A) and expiratory (B) radiographs showing air trapping in the right middle lobe on expiration (arrow).

Neonate in Respiratory Distress

Common causes:

- *Medical:* Respiratory distress syndrome (RDS) (surfactant deficiency disorder), transient tachypnoea of the newborn (TTN) (retained foetal lung fluid), meconium aspiration, neonatal pneumonia.
- *Surgical:* Intrathoracic air leaks, diaphragmatic hernia, intrathoracic masses of the newborn (congenital lobar emphysema, congenital cystic adenomatoid malformation, sequestration, bronchogenic and gut duplication cysts).
- *Imaging:* Chest X-ray, mainly frontal view. Lateral view to localise focal air collections/masses. Ultrasound for solid chest masses. CT/MRI for further assessment of radiologically detected masses.

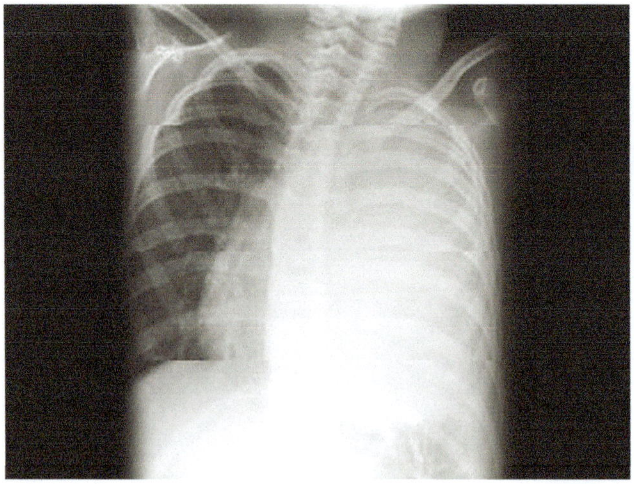

Figure 29.9 Chest X-ray of a 6-year-old girl showing an opaque left hemithorax due to a large empyema. Note the scoliosis concave to the left.

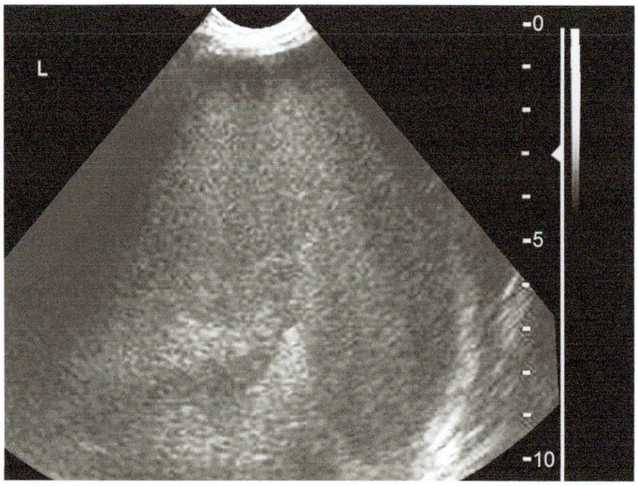

Figure 29.10 Ultrasound scan in the same patient as above shows debris in the pleural fluid.

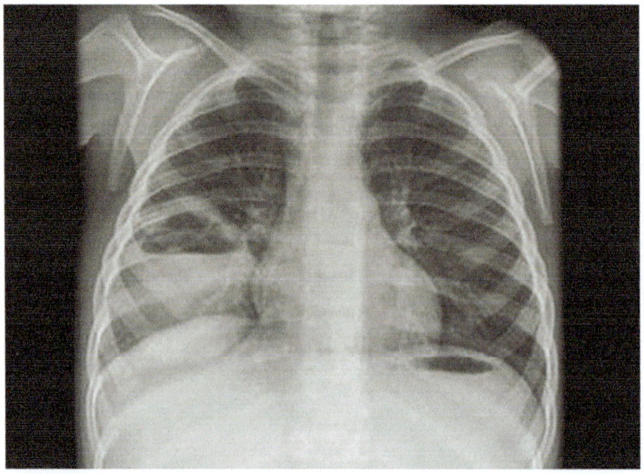

Figure 29.11 Chest X-ray showing an abscess in the right lower lobe containing an air fluid level.

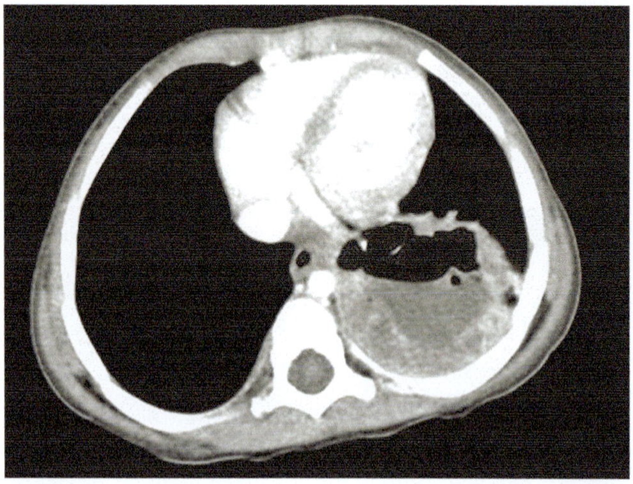

Figure 29.12 CT scan in another patient showing left basal lung abscess.

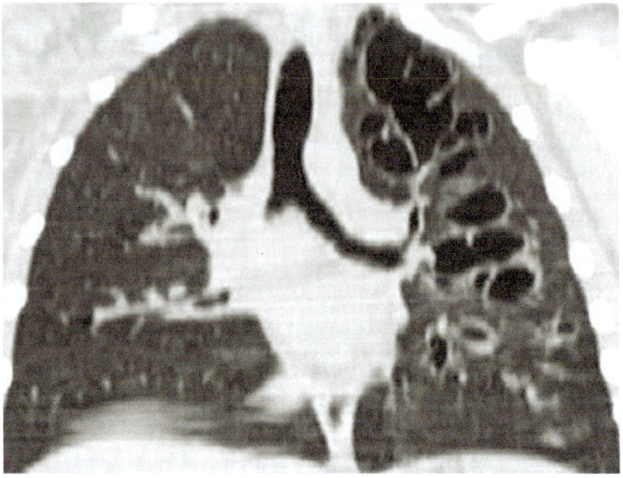

Figure 29.13 Coronal CT reconstruction shows left upper lobe pneumatocoeles as thin-walled cysts containing air.

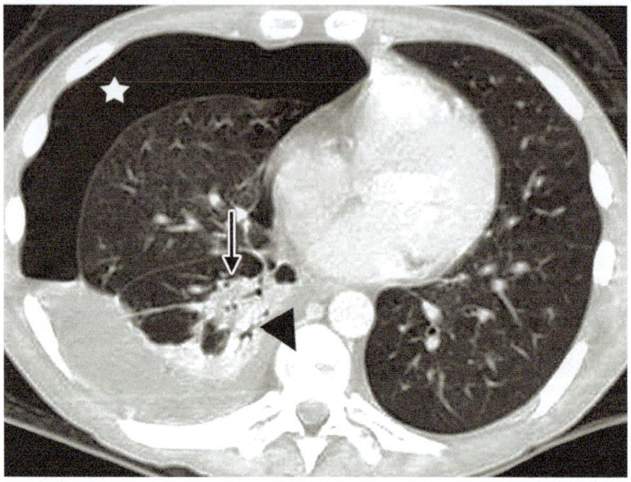

Figure 29.14 CT scan in a patient with necrotising right lower lobe pneumonia shows right basal consolidation (arrow) and a large right tension pneumothorax (asterisk). The site of the fistula is shown by the arrow.

MEDICAL CAUSES

Respiratory Distress Syndrome or Surfactant Deficiency Disorder

Respiratory distress syndrome results from a deficiency of pulmonary surfactant due to prematurity. Surfactant deficiency leads to instability and collapse of the alveoli producing diffuse microatelectasis, stiff lungs and impaired gas exchange with resultant respiratory distress radiologically, the lungs are diffusely involved with a granular pattern of opacification and abnormal air bronchograms **(Fig. 29.15)**.

Surfactant is now administered prophylactically in premature babies and in most infants the lungs clear rapidly.

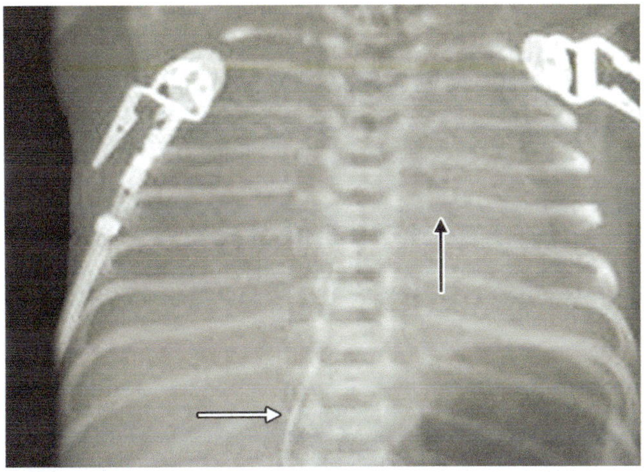

Figure 29.15 Chest X-ray on a premature baby with respiratory distress syndrome done on day one shows generalised under-aeration of the lungs, reticulogranular densities caused by acinar atelectasis and air bronchograms (black arrow). Incidental note is made of the umbilical venous catheter lying at the inferior vena cava and right atrial junction (white arrow).

Since the surfactant is unevenly distributed throughout the lungs, the uneven distribution of surfactant leads to a radiographic appearance, which stimulates pneumonia or meconium aspiration syndrome (MAS) **(Figs. 29.16A and B)**.

Complications of Respiratory Distress Syndrome

Iatrogenic or disease-related complications might occur during the course of RDS. These include air leaks (pulmonary interstitial emphysema, pneumomediastinum and pneumothorax), tube malposition (endotracheal, umbilical catheters), pulmonary haemorrhage and bronchopulmonary dysplasia.

Pulmonary Interstitial Emphysema (Fig. 29.17), Pneumothorax (Figs. 29.18 to 29.20A and B), and Bronchopulmonary Dysplasia

Bronchopulmonary dysplasia is a distinct pulmonary disease affecting the developing lung after prolonged respirator or oxygen therapy of RDS. Also called chronic lung disease of prematurity, the radiological findings include bubbly appearance to the lungs, hyperaeration and cardiomegaly **(Fig. 29.21)**.

Endotracheal Tube Malposition (Fig. 29.22), Umbilical Arterial Catheter and Umbilical Venous Catheter

The umbilical artery catheter (UAC) passes through the umbilicus, umbilical artery, internal iliac artery, common iliac artery and the abdominal aorta. It should ideally be

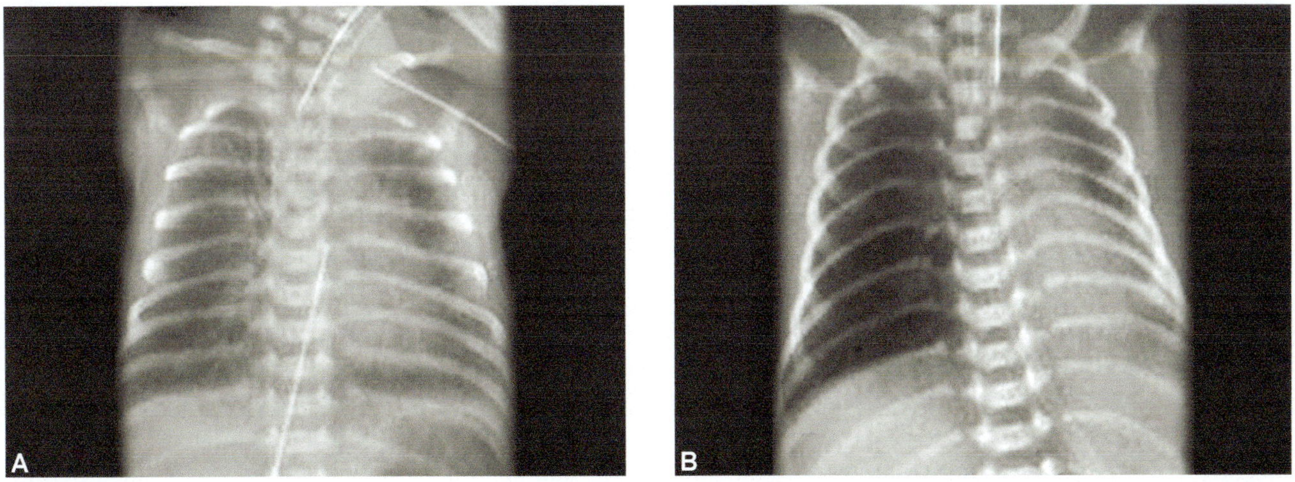

Figures 29.16A and B Asymmetric surfactant deficiency disorder in two patients due to administration of exogenous surfactant. Chest X-rays show asymmetrical opacities in both lungs.

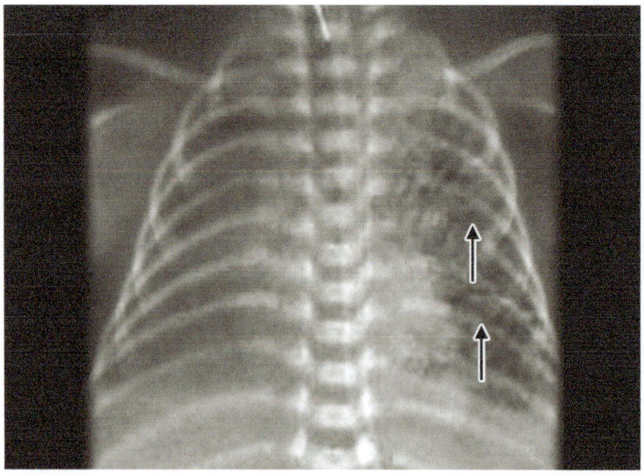

Figure 29.17 Pulmonary interstitial emphysema in the left lung. This often appears as pseudo-clearing of surfactant deficiency disorder. Irregular and tubular densities (arrows) extending to the pleural edge are identified as pulmonary interstitial air. Peripheral pulmonary interstitial emphysema can produce sub-pleural blebs and can often rupture into the pleural space giving a pneumothorax or extend centrally to produce a pneumomediastinum or pneumopericardium.

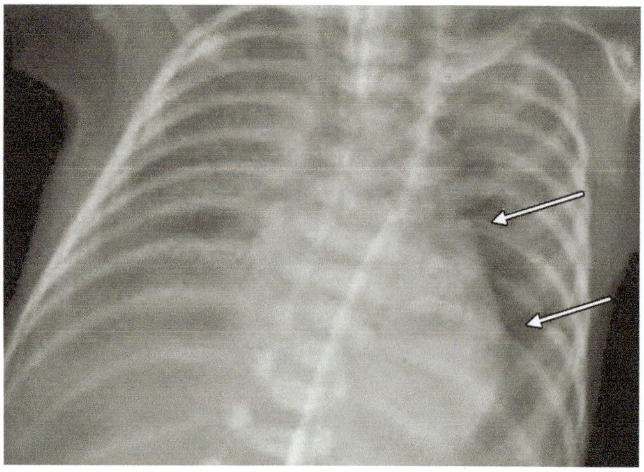

Figure 29.18 Chest X-ray showing an early left medial pneumothorax (arrows) in a 2-day-old infant with respiratory distress syndrome. When a pneumothorax collects medially, the findings must be differentiated from pneumomediastinum or pneumopericardium. Pneumomediastinal air tends to outline the thymus while pneumopericardium surrounds the heart entirely.

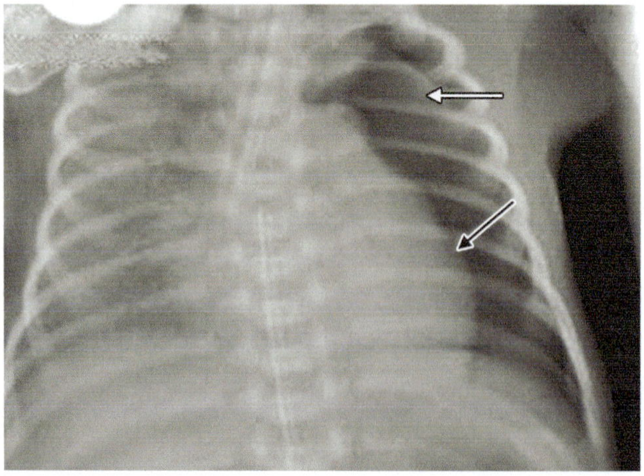

Figure 29.19 Anterior left pneumothorax in the same infant as above in a chest X-ray taken about 10 hours after the above radiograph. In the supine position, air accumulates over the anterior surface of the lung and produces a hyperlucent large hemithorax, increased sharpness of the ipsilateral mediastinal edge (black arrow) with a visible free edge of the left lung (white arrow). The thymus (T) may be compressed to form a pseudomass. Note the endotracheal tube down the right main bronchus.

placed away from the vessels to abdominal and pelvic viscera approximately at L3/L4 or T8/T10. The umbilical venous catheter (UVC) passes through the umbilicus, umbilical vein, medial part of left portal vein, ductus venosus, inferior vena cava (IVC) and right atrium **(Fig. 29.23)**.

Meconium Aspiration Syndrome

Meconium aspiration syndrome (MAS) is caused by the intrauterine or intrapartum aspiration of meconium-stained fluid in term or post-term infants. Aspiration of meconium into the tracheobronchial tree causes complete or partial bronchial obstruction leading to patchy areas of subsegmental atelectasis and compensatory areas of hyperinflation. Meconium also causes chemical pneumonitis, which is complicated by bronchopneumonia.

Radiologically, there are patchy, bilateral asymmetric areas of rounded/linear opacities and marked hyperinflation **(Figs. 29.24A and B)**. Air leaks, such as pneumomediastinum, pneumothorax is seen in 25% of patients.

Transient Tachypnoea of the Newborn

Usually affects full-term infants, often following caesarean section or infants of diabetic mothers and is symptomatic within first 2–4 hours of life. It is caused by retained foetal lung fluid and treatment is supportive. CXR reveals normal lung volumes with interstitial oedema, which clears within 1–2 days **(Figs. 29.25A and B)**.

SURGICAL CAUSES

Congenital Diaphragmatic Hernia

Left-sided hernias, through the foramen of Bochdalek, are commoner than right-sided ones in the newborn. Variable quantities of intestinal contents, stomach and liver enter the chest during foetal life. The CXR shows an abnormal hemithorax, which is opaque initially but later fills with bubbles representing gas-filled bowel and contralateral mediastinal shift **(Fig. 29.26)**. The lungs are hypoplastic. The abdomen is small and narrow. Right-sided hernias are less common in the newborn and usually present later in life.

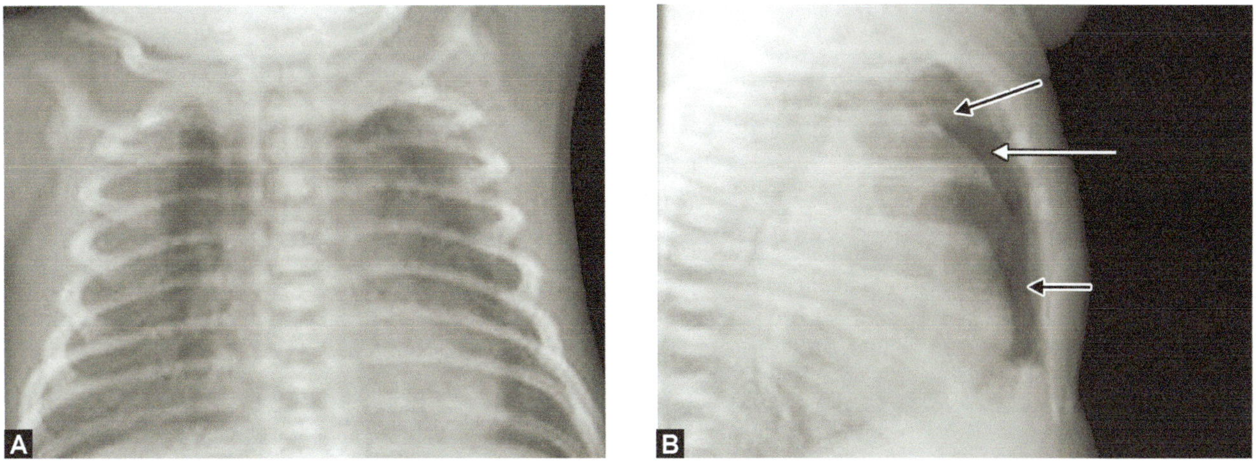

Figures 29.20A and B Pneumomediastinum: (A) Frontal chest X-ray shows a large lucency overlying the mediastinum; (B) Lateral view shows the air collection in the anterior mediastinum (black arrows) lifting and outlining the thymus (white arrow).

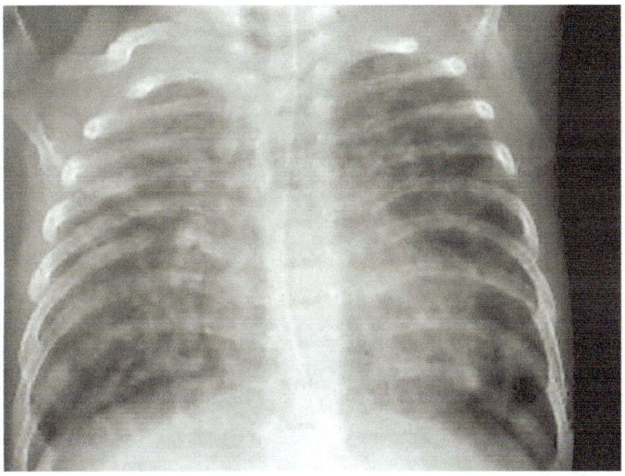

Figure 29.21 Chest X-ray of a 1-month-old infant with bronchopulmonary dysplasia shows bilateral lung hyperinflation, bubbly appearance of the lungs and cardiomegaly.

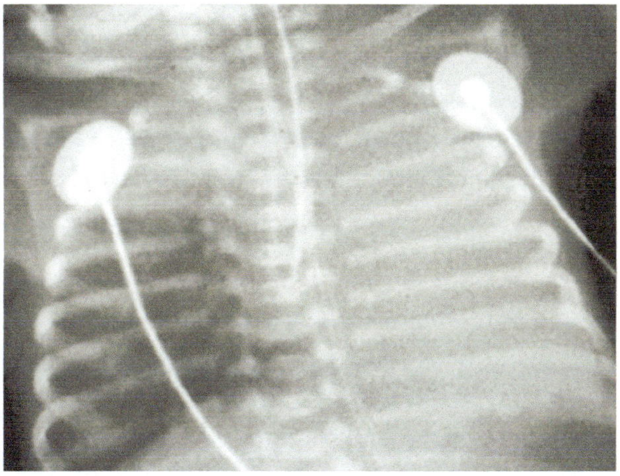

Figure 29.22 The ideal position of the endotracheal tube (ETT) is 2.0 cm above the carina with the neonates head in a neutral position. Chest X-ray showing the ETT down the right mainstem bronchus with total atelectasis of the left lung and right upper lobe.

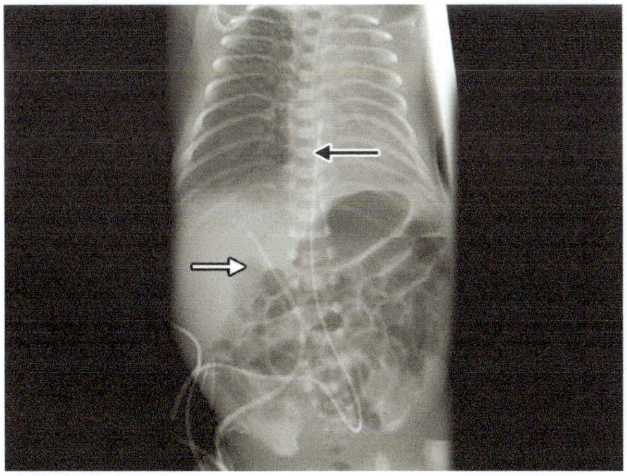

Figure 29.23 Chest and abdominal film showing umbilical artery catheter (black arrow) in distal thoracic aorta and umbilical venous catheter (white arrow) at the level of left portal vein.

Congenital Adenomatoid Malformation

A congenital hamartomatous lesion characterised by proliferation of terminal respiratory bronchioles with no alveolar communication and usually presents in the neonate as respiratory distress. The lesion initially appears radio-opaque due to fluid filled cysts. As lungs aerate, these cysts gradually fill with air giving a 'cystic' appearance (Fig. 29.27). The radiological appearance can mimic diaphragmatic hernia. A helpful differentiating feature is the presence of air filled loops of bowel in the abdomen (Fig. 29.28). Ten per cent of congenital adenomatoid malformations present after first year of life, often with recurrent pneumonias.

Congenital Lobar Emphysema

Congenital lobar emphysema initially appears as an opacification of one lobe or the whole lung due to partial

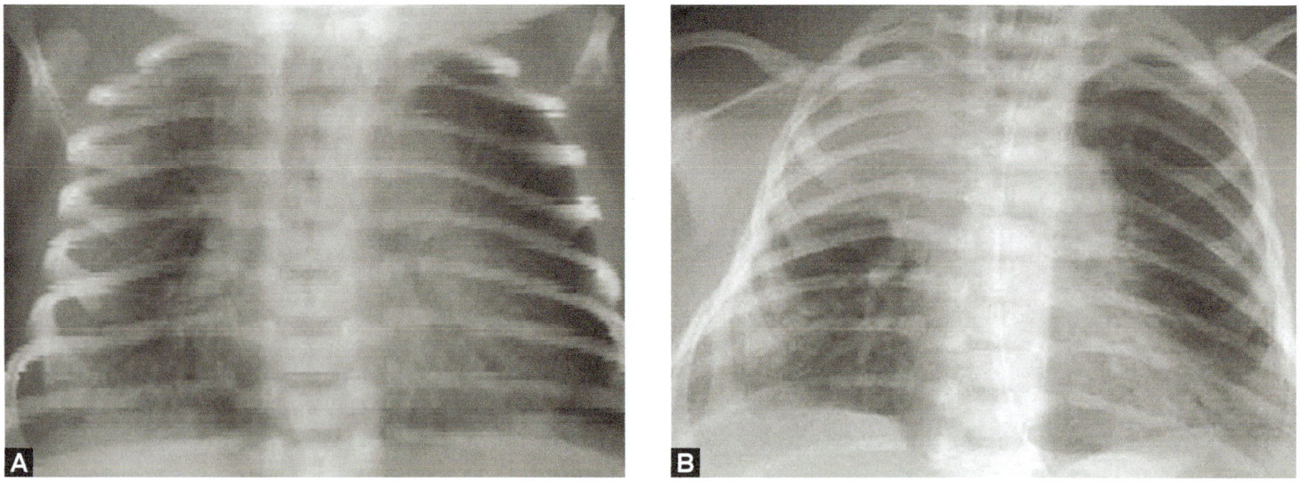

Figures 29.24A and B Term newborns with meconium aspiration syndrome. (A) Chest X-ray shows asymmetrical lung hyperinflation, patchy right basal infiltrates and areas of atelectasis; (B) Chest X-ray showing left and right upper lobe atelectasis and right basal infiltrates.

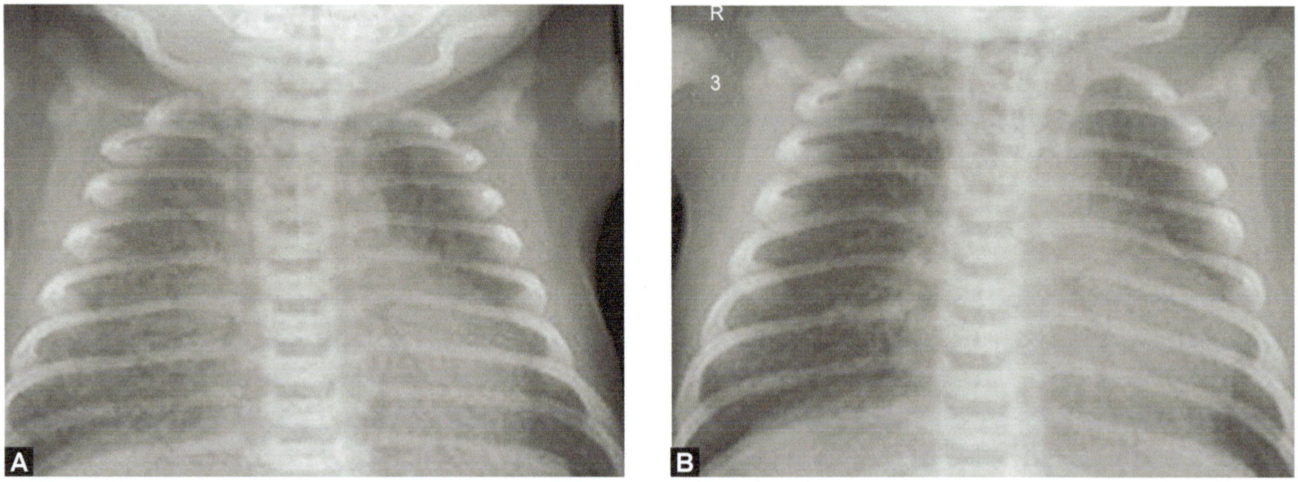

Figures 29.25A and B (A) Chest X-ray in an infant with transient tachypnoea of the newborn taken on day 1 shows cardiomegaly and interstitial pulmonary oedema; (B) Follow-up chest X-ray taken on day 2 shows almost complete clearing of the lungs.

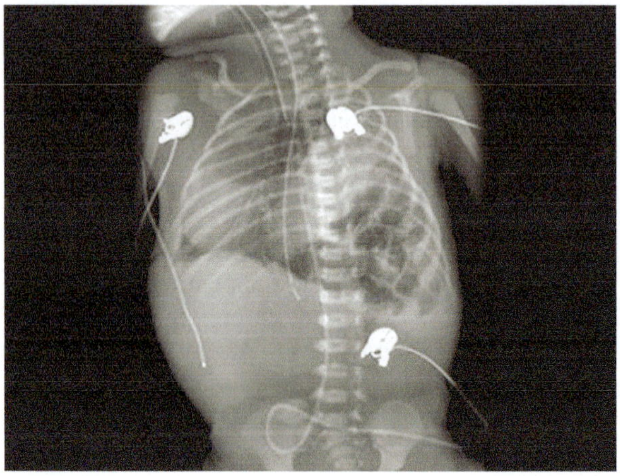

Figure 29.26 Left diaphragmatic hernia: Many intrathoracic air filled loops of bowel and absence of normal amounts of gas in the abdomen are seen in this neonate with severe respiratory distress. The prognosis correlates with the degree of underlying lung hypoplasia.

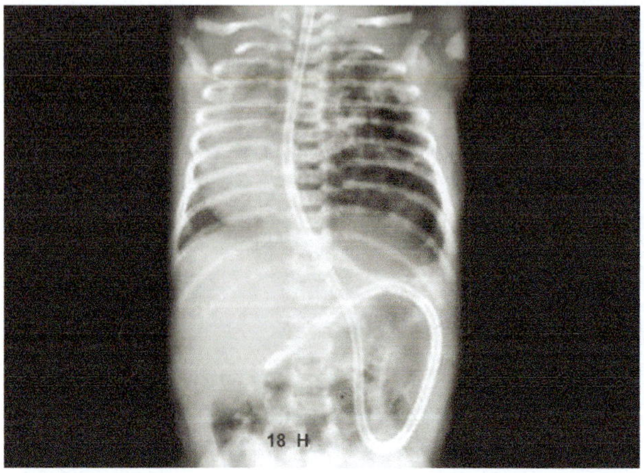

Figure 29.27 Chest X-ray showing multiple cystic lucencies in the left hemithorax. There is mediastinal shift, which can cause progressive pulmonary hypoplasia. Note the multiple air filled loops of bowel in the abdomen and the intra-abdominal nasogastric tube tip.

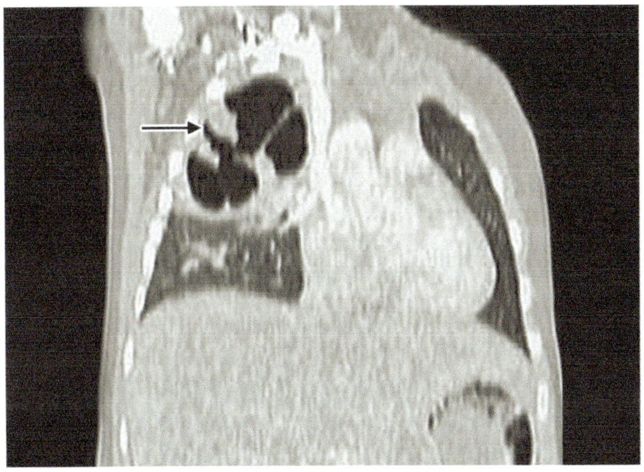

Figure 29.28 Coronal CT reconstruction shows a congenital adenomatoid malformations in the right upper lobe (arrow).

bronchial obstruction causing retention of fluid. Over a period of few days, the fluid is resorbed and replaced by air at which point the diagnosis becomes obvious. Progressive over distension results in air trapping and its consequences, namely, mediastinal shift, compression of normal lung or lobes.

Common sites to be affected are left upper and right upper lobes (Figs. 29.29A to C).

Bronchogenic Cyst

Usually arise from an abnormal lung bud from developing foregut. The mediastinal form is usually asymptomatic but can present with respiratory distress if the major airways are compressed due to gradual expansion over time. The cyst is often subcarinal in location and can be mistaken for a duplication cyst (Figs. 29.30A and B).

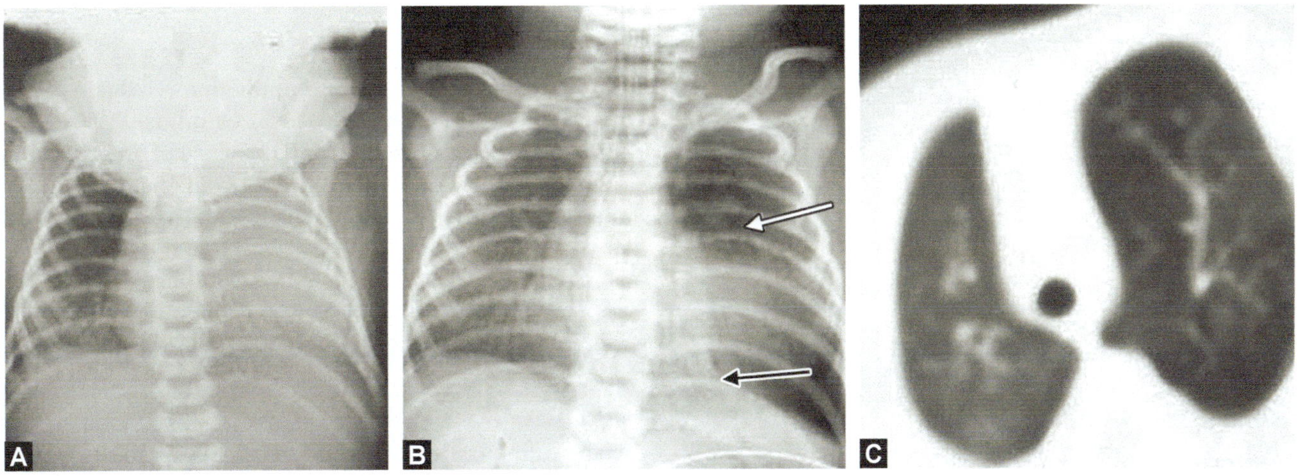

Figures 29.29A to C Chest X-ray (A and B) of a term neonate with respiratory distress. (A) Day 1 shows an opaque left hemithorax; (B) Day 2 shows a hyperinflated left upper lobe (white arrow) and compression collapse of left lower lobe (black arrow); (C) CT scan on day 3 shows an emphysematous left upper lobe and moderate mediastinal shift.

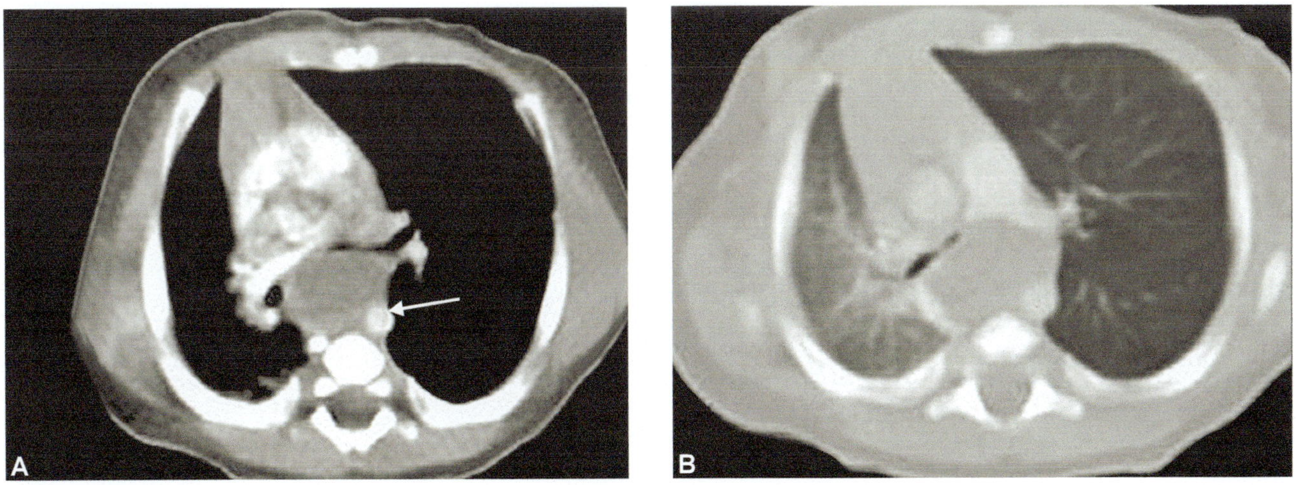

Figures 29.30A and B Computed tomography scans (A) showing a posterior mediastinal cystic lesion (white arrow) causing compression of the left main bronchus (asterisk) and (B) hyperinflation of the left lung. Differential diagnosis includes duplication cyst of the oesophagus.

Neurenteric Cyst

Faulty neural tube closure results in abnormal mesenchyme leading to abnormal vertebral body formation and continued neural connection with endoderm. The abnormality is found most commonly in the thoracic spine with a cystic mass in the mediastinum and segmentation anomalies of the spine (butterfly vertebrae or hemivertebrae) (Fig. 29.31).

A CHILD WITH A MEDIASTINAL MASS

Normal Thymus

The thymus gland is found in the anterior mediastinum and can have a variety of appearances. The two lobes of the thymus are often dense enough to obscure the upper and middle mediastinum. A thymus is recognised by its wavy margin from indentation by the ribs, by a sail configuration and by a notch where the thymic shadow intersects the cardiac margin. A normal thymus can be a notorious source of difficulty when interpreting chest films. Sonography can be useful in thymic imaging, especially to determine if the anterior mediastinal mass is a normal thymus (Figs. 29.32A and B).

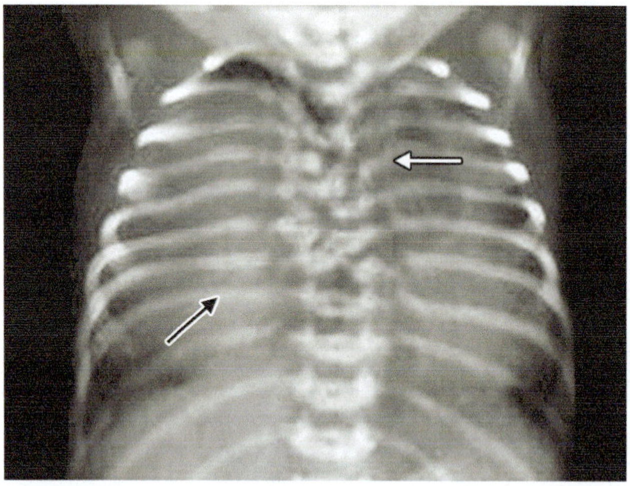

Figure 29.31 Chest X-ray showing a soft-tissue mass in the right hemithorax (black arrow) and multiple segmentation anomalies of the thoracic spine (white arrow). Differentials include a large intrathoracic meningocoele.

Thymic Sonography

Sonographically, the thymus has an echotexture similar to liver with punctate echoes and echogenic lines. Realtime sonography demonstrates normal thymic malleability during the respiratory cycle, helping in differentiating from a thymic mass. In the setting of a mass presence of cysts, calcification or heterogeneity of architecture can suggest thymic pathology (Fig. 29.33).

Lymphoma

Thymic involvement with lymphoma (Hodgkins and non-Hodgkins) can be multifocal or diffuse. With lymphoma, the age of the child and presence of other regions of adenopathy can be helpful in prioritising histology. If the lymphoma is confined to the thymus in an older child or adolescent, a Hodgkin-type lymphoma is likely. Non-Hodgkin lymphoma can occur at any age. On CT, the appearances can be homogenous or heterogeneous with areas of fibrosis, necrosis (Figs. 29.34A and B).

Germ-cell Tumours

These tumours include teratomas, seminomas, dysgerminomas and choriocarcinomas. Second to lymphoma as a cause of mediastinal mass, most are located in the superior mediastinum and can be asymptomatic in up to

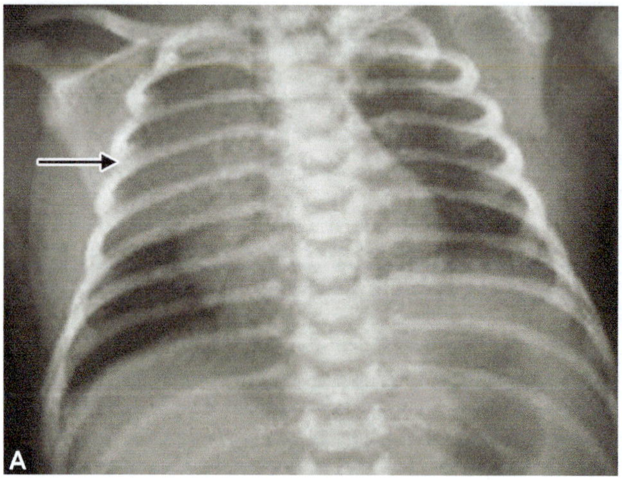

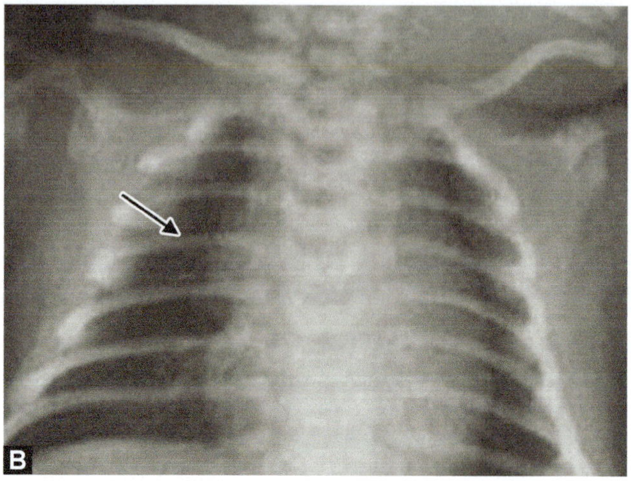

Figures 29.32A and B Radiographs of neonates showing a prominent normal thymus exhibiting the 'sail sign' (arrow in A) or the wave sign (arrow in B). It is often difficult to ascertain true heart size on the frontal radiograph. Mass effect or mediastinal shift is almost never seen with a normal thymus.

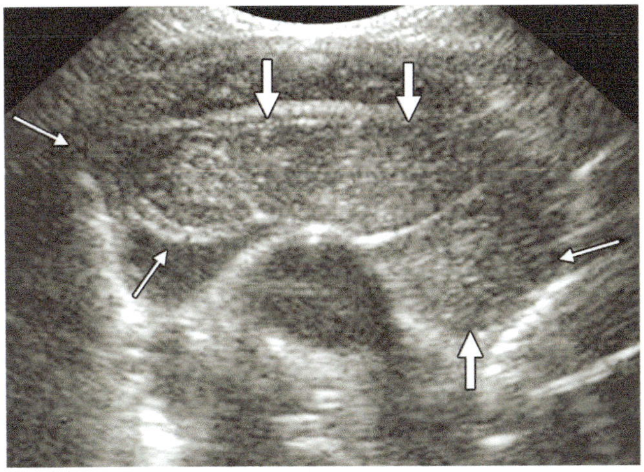

Figure 29.33 Axial ultrasound of the thymus at the level of ascending aorta. The normal thymus (arrows) can have a bilobed appearance, homogenous texture and some echogenic strands.

half of the patients. Large tumours can cause tracheal and superior vena caval compression and are malignant in up to 10% of cases. Teratomas are the most common germ-cell tumours and consist of ectodermal, mesenchymal and endodermal derivatives. On CT/MR they contain variable amounts of fat, calcium or soft tissue. Fat or calcium in an anterior mediastinal mass almost always indicates a germ-cell tumour (Figs. 29.35 and 29.36).

Metastases

Most paediatric malignant tumours are pulmonary metastases, usually found during staging of a known or a new malignancy. Common paediatric tumours associated with lung metastases include Wilms tumour, rhabdomyosarcoma, hepatoblastoma, Ewing and osteosarcoma. CT is more sensitive than plain films in detecting metastases (Figs. 29.37 and 29.38).

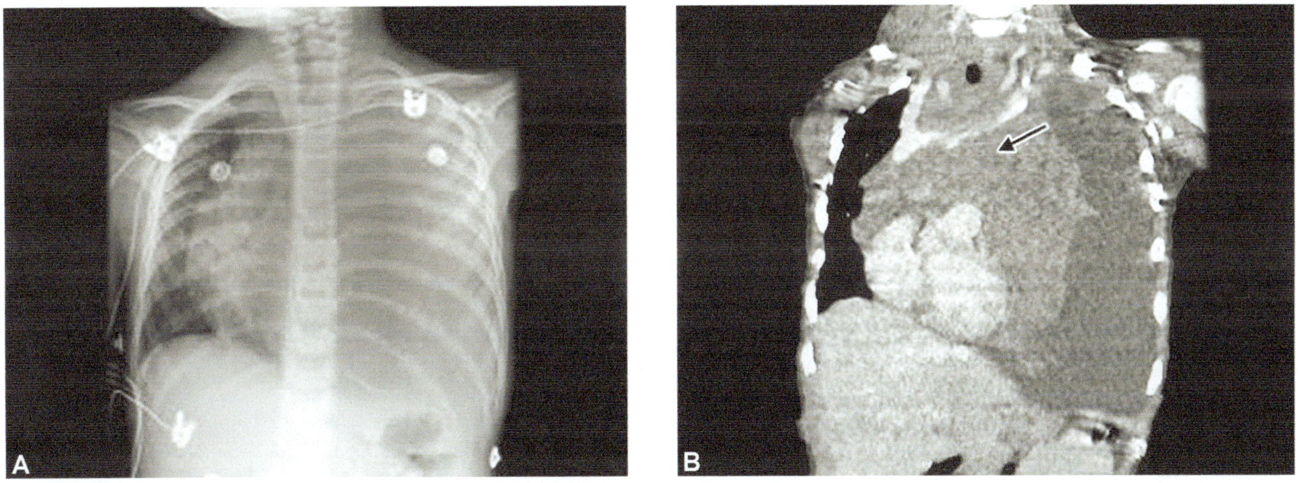

Figures 29.34A and B Chest X-ray (A) and coronal reconstruction of a CT scan (B) of a 5-year-old showing a large mediastinal mass (arrow) midline shift and a left pleural effusion. Diagnosis at biopsy was of a T-cell lymphoma.

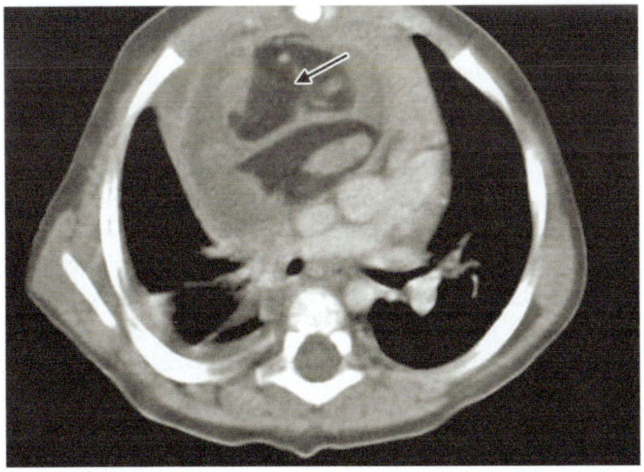

Figure 29.35 Mixed attenuation mass in the anterior mediastinum containing low attenuation areas representing fat (seen as low attenuation areas, arrow), in a child with chronic stridor from was airway compression.

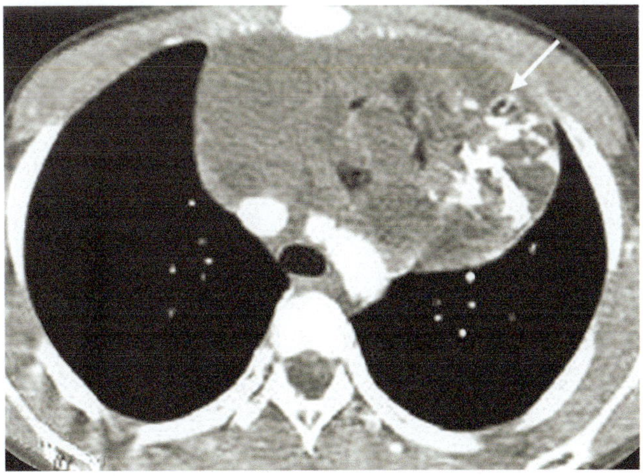

Figure 29.36 CT scan in another patient with stridor shows a calcified anterior mediastinal mass (white arrow). The low attenuation areas within the mass represent fat.

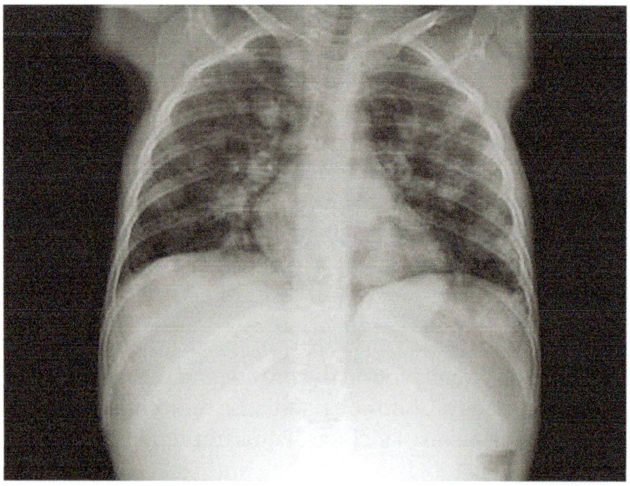

Figure 29.37 Multiple intrapulmonary metastases from hepatoblastoma.

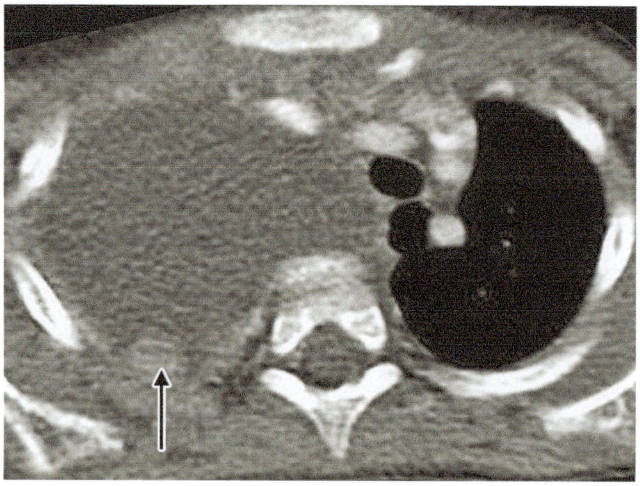

Figure 29.38 Pleural-based metastases (arrow) and effusion in a patient with Wilms tumour.

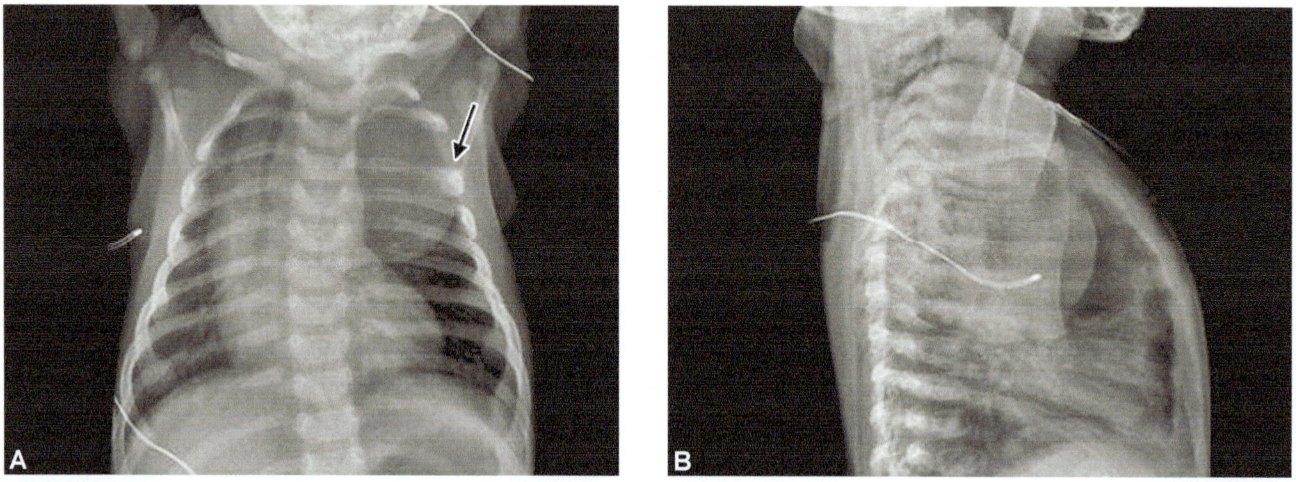

Figures 29.39A and B Chest X-ray in a child showing a well-defined left posterior mediastinal mass (arrow) with erosion, splaying and thinning of the posterior ribs. (A) Antero-posterior view; (B) Lateral view.

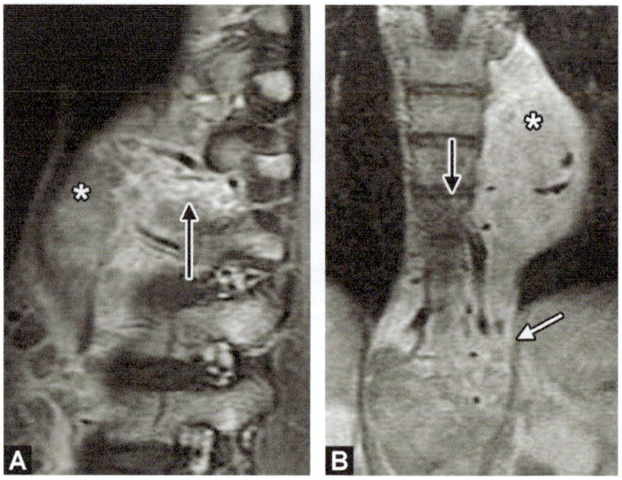

Figures 29.40A and B MR images show a left paraspinal mass (asterisk) with extension into the intervertebral foramina (black arrows) and into the abdomen via the aortic hiatus (white arrow). (A) Sagittal view; (B) Coronal view.

Neuroblastoma

Majority of posterior mediastinal masses in children are of neurogenic origin, namely, neuroblastoma, ganglioneuroblastoma and ganglioneuroma. Thoracic neuroblastoma has a better prognosis than abdominal neuroblastoma. The plain film suggests the diagnosis with posterior rib erosion and a mass, which may have some calcification **(Figs. 29.39A and B)**. At CT, most tumours are well circumscribed fusiform masses in the para-spinal location. Enlargement of the intervertebral neural foramina and spread into the abdomen via the aortic or oesophageal hiatus may be evident **(Figs. 29.40 to 29.42)**.

CHEST WALL MASSES

Ewing Sarcoma

Ewing sarcoma is a malignant round cell tumour and is the most common malignant chest wall mass in children.

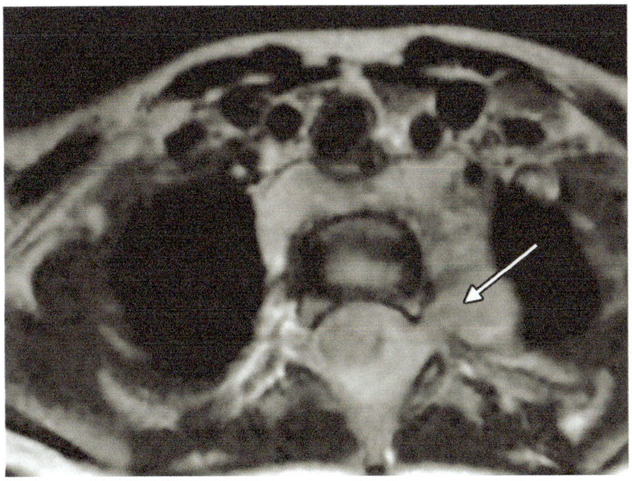

Figure 29.41 Axial MR in a 6-year-old child showing a well-defined left paravertebral mass with extension into the intervertebral foramen (arrow).

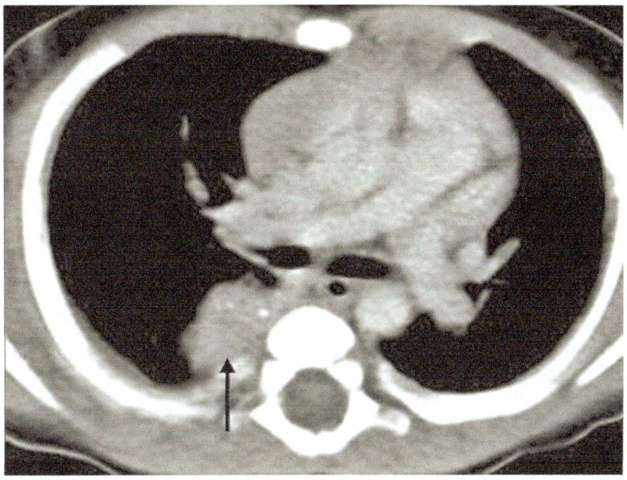

Figure 29.42 Calcified neuroblastoma in the right para-vertebral area (arrow) in a 6-month-old infant.

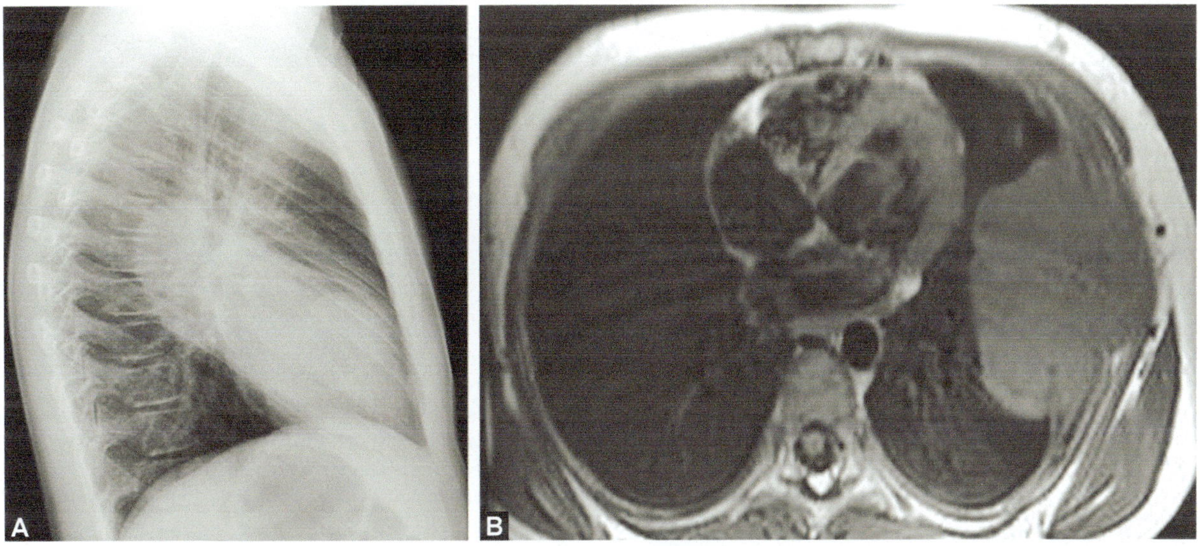

Figures 29.43A and B (A) Lateral chest X-ray and (B) T1 weighted MR showing a left chest wall mass following the rib contours and extending into the thoracic cavity.

It usually manifests as a peripheral chest wall mass with or without rib destruction. The CXR will show a mass with intrathoracic growth, rib and chest wall involvement and accompanying pleural effusion. MRI and CT play complimentary roles in staging these tumours (Figs. 29.43 and 29.44).

Rhabdomyosarcoma

Rhabdomyosarcoma is the most common extrapleural chest wall tumour in children. The radiologic features are difficult to distinguish from Ewing sarcoma.

Osteochondroma of the Ribs

The most common benign tumour of the chest wall, composed of cortical and medullary bone with a cartilaginous cap and usually continuous with the underlying bone (Fig. 29.45).

CONGENITAL HEART DISEASE

Imaging approach:

- Echocardiography
- Chest radiography

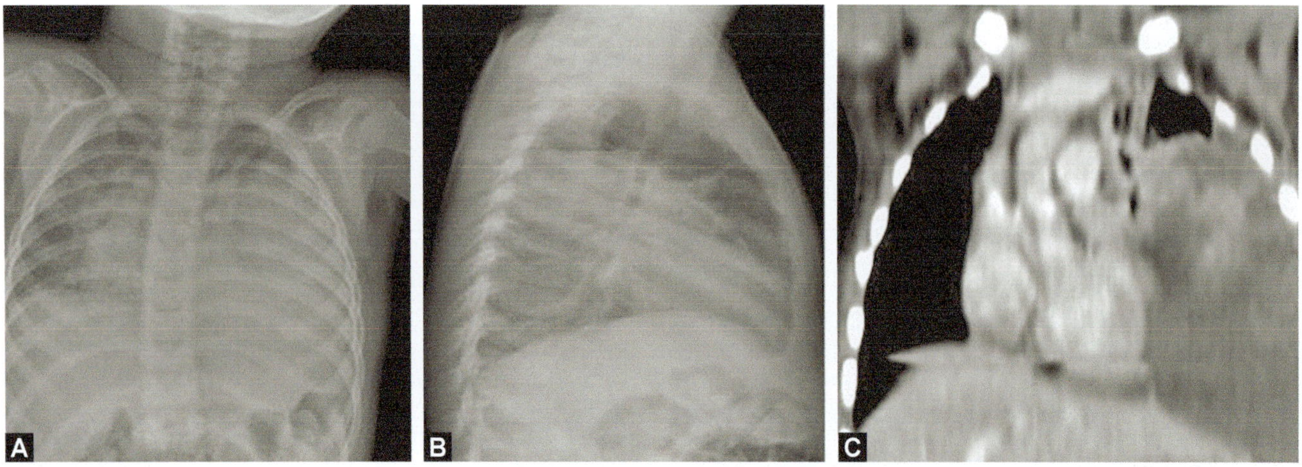

Figures 29.44A to C Chest X-ray showing a left chest soft-tissue mass and mediastinal shift: (A) Antero–posterior view; (B) Lateral view; (C) Coronal CT reconstruction shows a mixed density mass with fluid and solid components. These appearances may be confused with empyema.

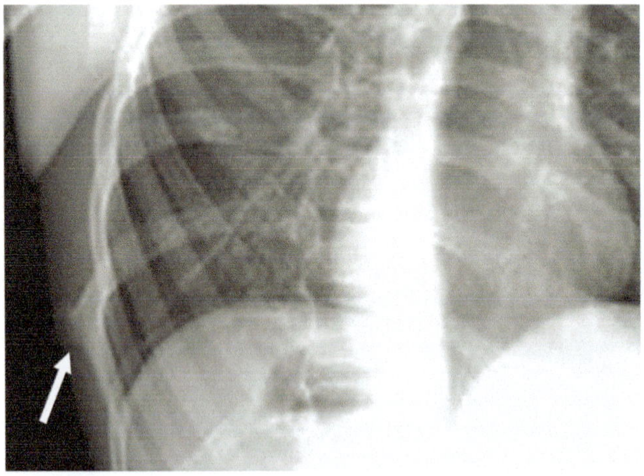

Figure 29.45 Oblique view of the ribs shows bony lesion attached to the ribs by a broad base (arrow).

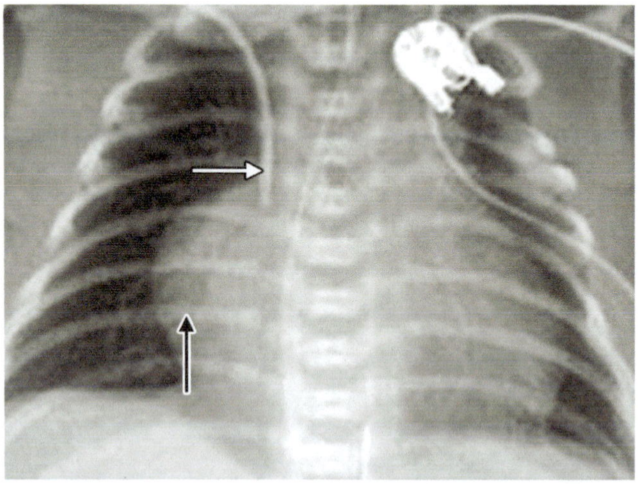

Figure 29.46 The enlarged right atrium displaces the right heart border to the right and increased curvature of the right heart border. A step-like angle (white arrow) between the right atrium and the superior vena cava (SVC) may be seen.

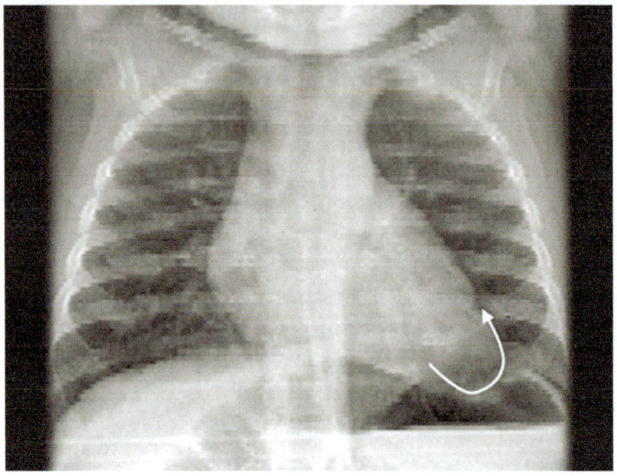

Figure 29.47 The right ventricle occupies the front of the heart and is non-border forming in the frontal view. Enlargement of the right ventricle results in tilting up and posterior displacement of the left ventricle and a triangular configuration of the heart and elevation of the apex (curved arrow).

- Cardiac catheterisation
- Magnetic resonance imaging

Specific Chamber Enlargement on Plain Film

- Right atrium **(Fig. 29.46)**
- Right ventricle **(Fig. 29.47)**
- Left atrium **(Fig. 29.48)**
- Left ventricle **(Fig. 29.49)**

ACYANOTIC CHILD WITH CONGENITAL HEART DISEASE

Left to right shunts account for about half of all forms of congenital heart disease.

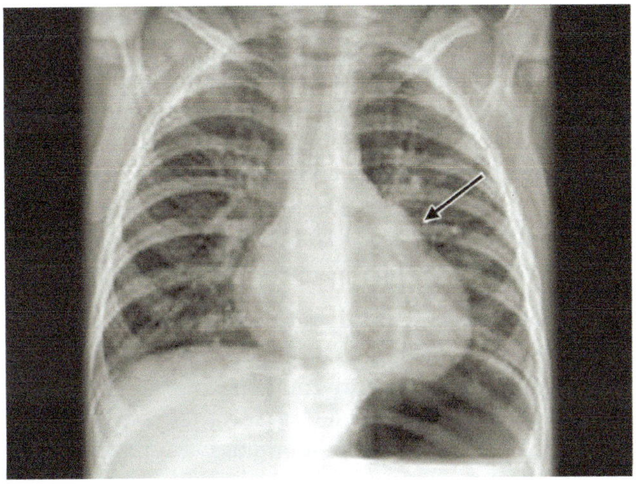

Figure 29.48 An enlarging left atrium may elevate the left main bronchus and cause a bulge in the right heart border producing a double shadow seen through the right heart border. Particularly in rheumatic heart disease, there may be left atrial enlargement seen as a discrete bulge on the left heart border below the pulmonary bay (arrow).

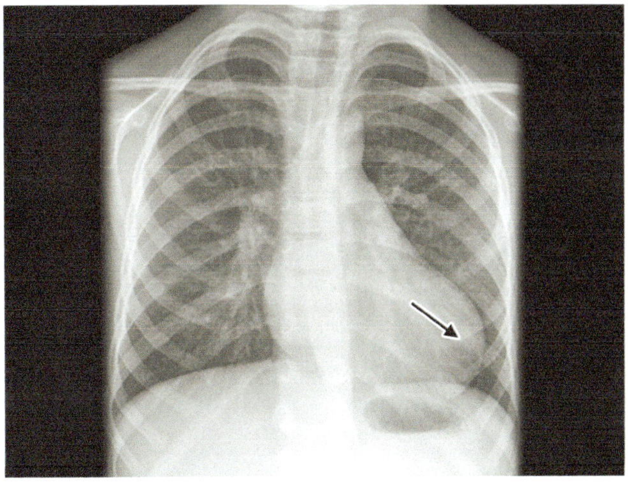

Figure 29.49 The left ventricle forms the left border and the apex of the cardiac shadow on a frontal chest X-ray. Enlargement leads to rounding of the apex of the heart and elongation of long axis of the left ventricle (arrow).

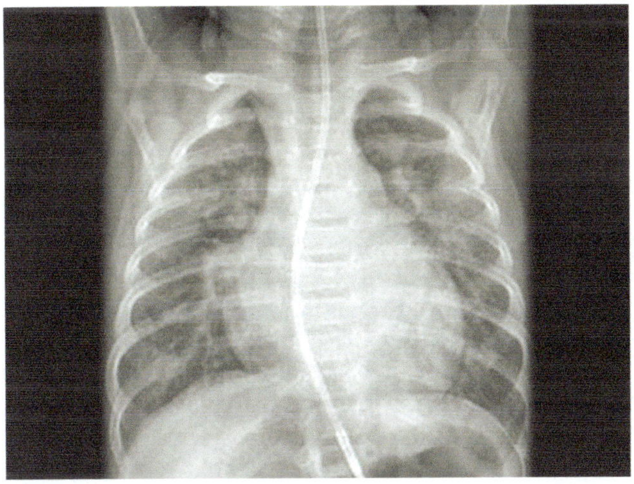

Figure 29.50 Chest radiograph showing cardiomegaly, biventricular enlargement and increased lung vascularity.

Three common diagnoses include:

1. Ventricular septal defect (VSD)
2. Patent ductus arteriosus (PDA)
3. Atrial septal defect (ASD).

Ventricular Septal Defect

Ventricular septal defect is the most common congenital cardiac anomaly, usually presenting in infants and toddlers. It may be isolated or associated with other congenital defects. Defects can occur in any part of the interventricular septum: perimembranous, muscular or trabecular, outlet or inlet. The haemodynamics of the VSD are determined by the size of the defect and the pressure difference between the left and right ventricle. In neonates with a high pulmonary vascular resistance significant left to right shunting is uncommon but in large defects congestive heart failure develops at 1–3 months of age due to normal decrease in pulmonary vascular resistance. The CXR in a VSD with a small left to right shunt is normal. In large shunts, the main branch and the intrapulmonary branches of the pulmonary arteries dilate. There is enlargement of the left atrium and the ventricles **(Fig. 29.50)**.

Patent Ductus Arteriosus

The ductus arteriosus extends from the origin of the left pulmonary artery to the descending aorta just beyond the origin of the left subclavian artery and shunts blood from the main pulmonary artery to the aorta. In newborns, the PDA is a common cause of congestive heart failure. Small premature infants with a PDA and a left to right shunt may have evidence of left ventricular failure. Patients with small PDA have no radiographic abnormalities. Large PDAs show increased lung vascularity and enlarged left atrium and ventricle **(Fig. 29.51)**.

Atrial Septal Defect

Atrial septal defect is commonly an isolated lesion. The shunt is from the left to the right atrium leading to enlargement of the right atrium, ventricle and the pulmonary arteries. Most children are asymptomatic, and it is usually diagnosed in older children or adults. The condition is usually undetected until a murmur is heard. A moderate-sized ASD shows increased lung vascularity, an enlarged heart with prominent right atrium and pulmonary artery. Right ventricular filling may be seen as filling of the retrosternal space on a lateral CXR **(Figs. 29.52A and B)**.

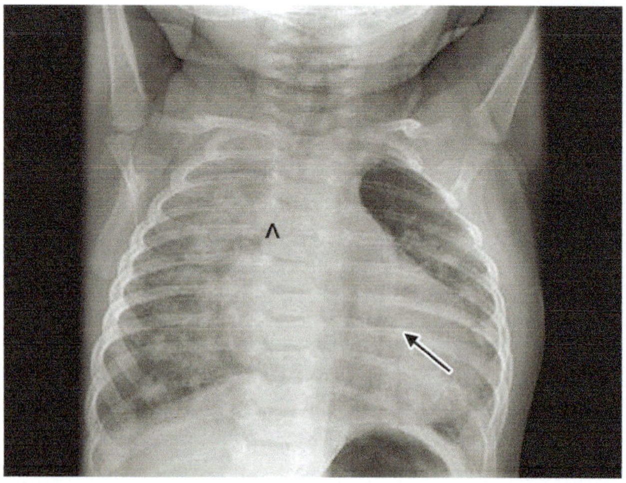

Figure 29.51 Chest radiograph showing marked cardiomegaly with left ventricular enlargement (downward pointing apex, arrow), left atrial enlargement resulting in carinal splaying and areas of atelectasis interspersed with hyperinflation, and pulmonary oedema in a patient with a large patent ductus arteriosus. Atelectasis is due to a large left atrium compressing the airways.

CYANOTIC CHILD WITH CONGENITAL HEART DISEASE

Common causes include tetralogy of Fallot, transposition of great vessels and pulmonary atresia with intact ventricular septum.

Tetralogy of Fallot

Tetralogy of Fallot (TOF) is the most common cyanotic congenital cardiac disease in children. The four components of TOF are right ventricular out flow tract (RVOT) obstruction, subaortic VSD, over-riding aorta and right ventricular hypertrophy. The severity of RVOT obstruction determines the amount of left to right shunting across the VSD. The infundibular stenosis progresses with age and left to right shunting increases proportionately. The CXR shows a mild to moderate cardiomegaly, uplifted apex secondary to right ventricular enlargement and concavity in the region of pulmonary artery segment giving a boot shaped heart **(Fig. 29.53)**. A right-sided aortic arch occurs in 25% of patients with TOF.

Dextro (D)-transposition of Great Vessels

Transposition of great vessels is the most common congenital cardiac disorder causing cyanosis in the first 24 hours of life. The aorta and the pulmonary artery are transposed. The ascending aorta (AA) arises from the right ventricle and the pulmonary artery rises from the left ventricle giving two parallel circuits between the pulmonary and systemic circulations. Communications between the two circulations are vital for survival and include PDA, ASD and VSD. The CXR shows a narrow superior mediastinum due to decrease in thymic tissue and abnormal relations of the great vessels and lack of visualisation of the aortic arch which is malpositioned and lack of normal shadow of the main pulmonary artery **(Fig. 29.54)**. The lung vascularity can be increased, decreased or normal.

Pulmonary Atresia with Ventricular Septal Defect

There is severe hypoplasia or atresia of the main pulmonary artery leading to no forward flow from the right ventricle into the lungs. Blood supply to the lungs is usually via collaterals from the aorta. Most infants are hypoxic and cyanotic. Radiologically the heart is enlarged with an upturned apex secondary to right ventricular hypertrophy **(Fig. 29.55)**. There is marked concavity in the region of the main pulmonary artery because of

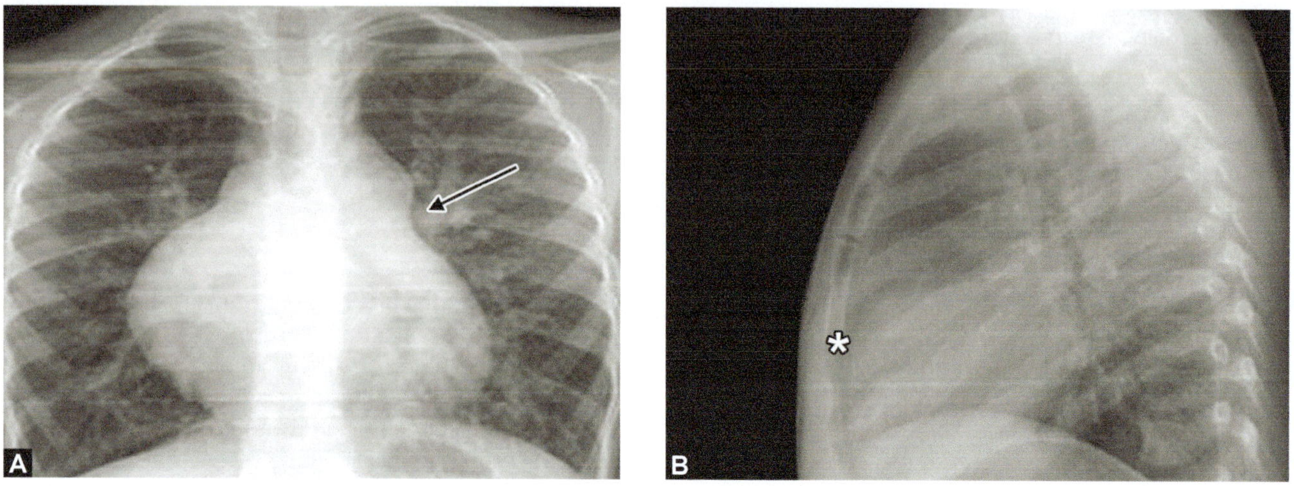

Figures 29.52A and B Chest X-ray showing enlarged right atrium and right ventricle (shown as filling of the retrosternal space on a lateral chest X-ray, (asterisk) main pulmonary artery (arrow) with increased pulmonary flow.

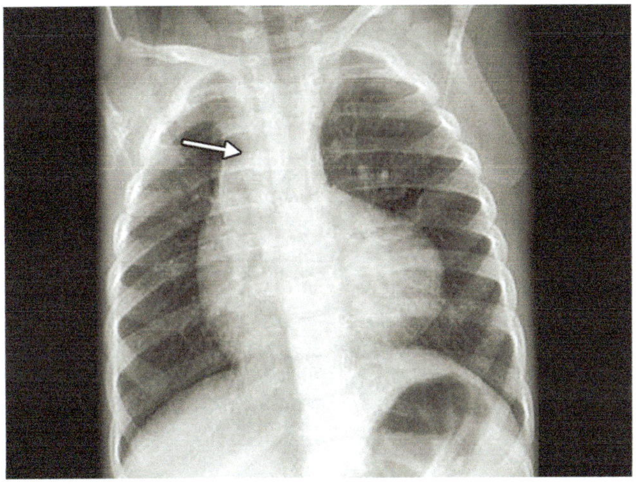

Figure 29.53 Chest X-ray showing a 'boot-shaped heart', due to elevation of the apex secondary to right ventricular hypertrophy, right aortic arch (arrow) and pulmonary oligaemia.

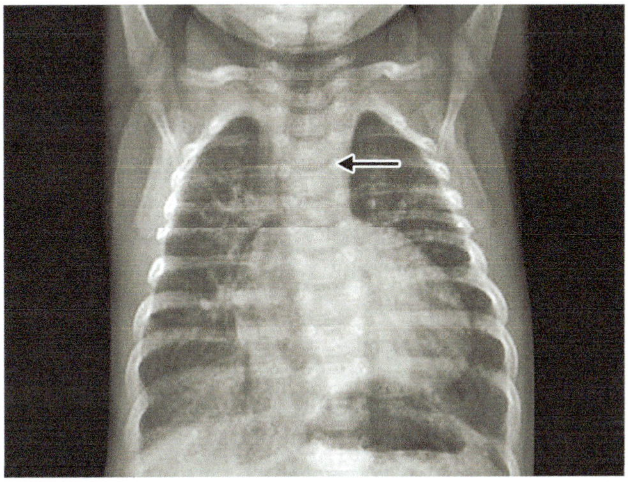

Figure 29.54 D-Transposition of great vessels. Newborn with marked cyanosis. The heart is enlarged and there is a narrow superior mediastinum (arrow). The pulmonary vascularity is increased despite an inconspicuous main pulmonary artery segment.

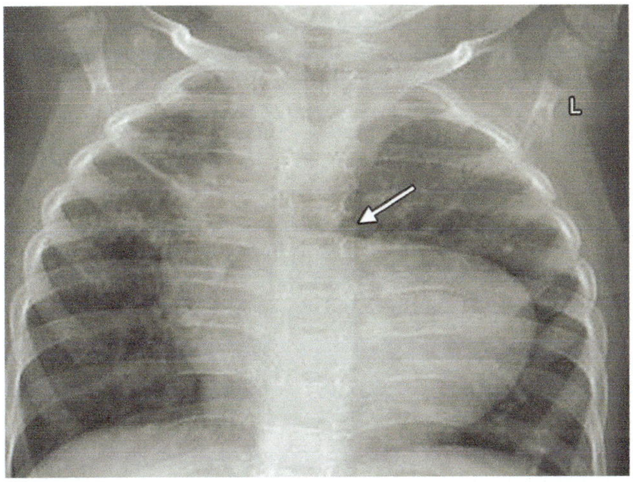

Figure 29.55 Pulmonary atresia with ventricular septal defect. Cardiomegaly with a markedly elevated apex, concavity in the region of the main pulmonary artery (arrow) and a right aortic arch with abnormal lung vascularity.

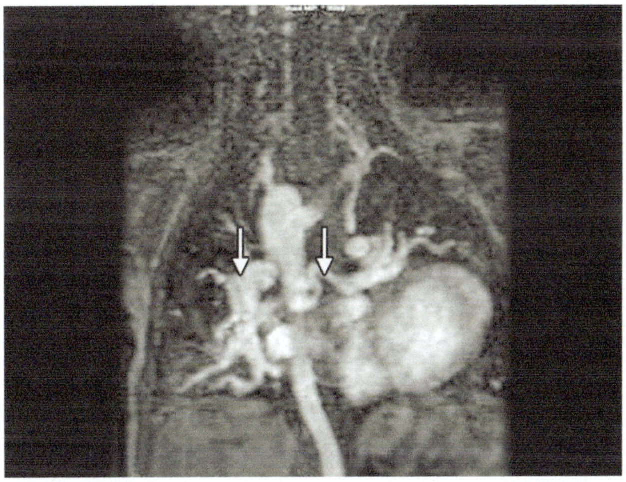

Figure 29.56 Contrast-enhanced MRA shows multiple aortopulmonary collateral arteries (arrows) supplying the lungs.

underdevelopment of the infundibulum and the main pulmonary artery **(Fig. 29.56)**. Pulmonary vascular markings have an unusual reticular appearance due to abnormal.

Truncus Arteriosus

An uncommon anomaly, truncus arteriosus is due to failure of division of the primitive truncus into the aorta and pulmonary artery. One large vessel originates from the heart to supply the systemic, pulmonary and coronary circulations. A large VSD is always present. Several types of truncus are described. Radiologically, cardiomegaly and increased pulmonary flow are seen at birth in a cyanosed infant **(Fig. 29.57)**. There is enlargement of the left atrium, pulmonary oedema and a prominent truncus. The main pulmonary artery segment is concave. The aorta is right sided in one-third of patients.

Total Anomalous Pulmonary Venous Drainage

Total anomalous pulmonary venous drainage (TAPVD) occurs when the common pulmonary vein fails to develop and the branch pulmonary veins connect to other venous structures such as SVC, IVC, right atrium, or portal venous system. TAPVD is divided into four types: supracardiac, cardiac, infracardiac and mixed. The supracardiac type is the most common. All four pulmonary veins converge into a left vertical, which drains into the left innominate

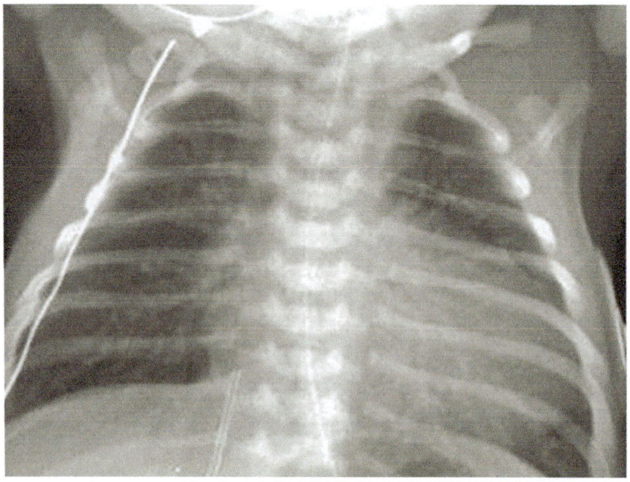

Figure 29.57 A 2-month-old boy with cyanosis. The heart is enlarged, the main pulmonary artery segment is concave and the pulmonary vascularity is increased.

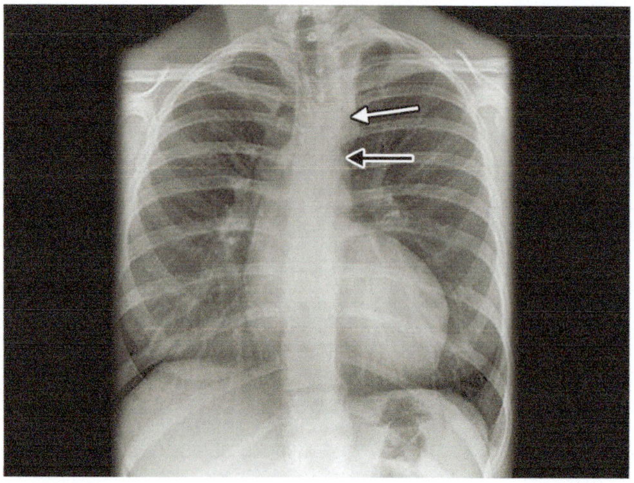

Figure 29.58 Chest X-ray of a 14-year-old patient with a late diagnosis of coarctation shows a high aortic arch (black arrow), a reverse appearance at the coarctation site (white arrow), rib notching (small arrows) and left ventricular hypertrophy.

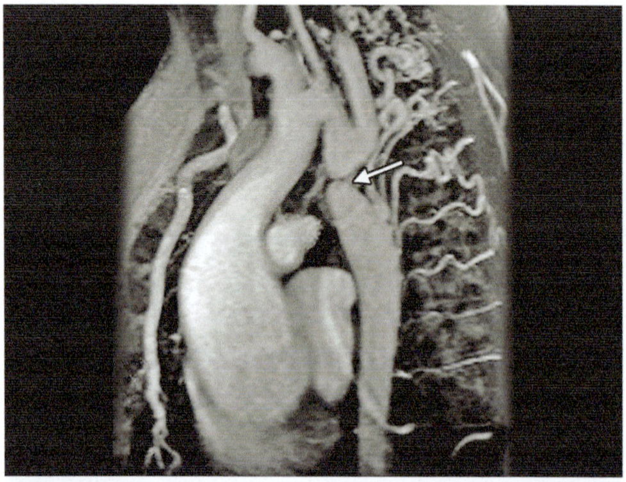

Figure 29.59 Contrast-enhanced MRA of the aorta demonstrates the tight coarctation (arrow) and intercostal, internal mammary and lateral thoracic collaterals.

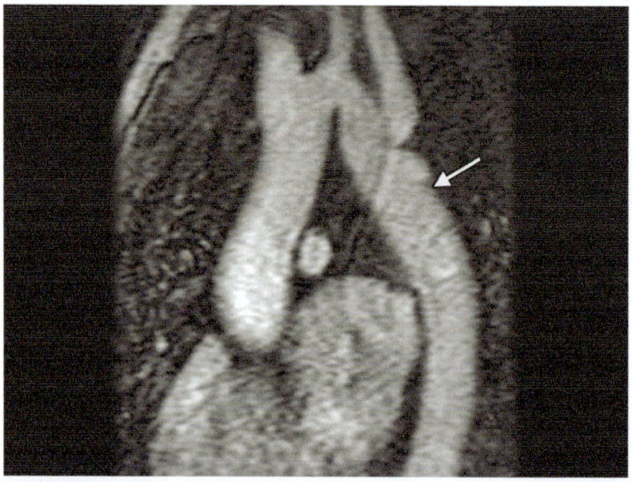

Figure 29.60 Post-balloon angioplasty of another patient with coarctation shows resolution of the stenosis with a small intimal flap from dissection (arrow).

vein. Because both systemic and pulmonary veins drain into the right atrium, there is increased volume overload of the right heart, which enlarges. Radiologically, the appearance of the mediastinum is likened to a snow man with the upper half of the 'snowman' consisting of the vertical vein and the dilated SVC.

OTHER CARDIAC AND RELATED CONDITIONS

Coarctation of Aorta

Coarctation of aorta (CoA) results from membranous infolding of the posterolateral wall of the thoracic aorta at the level of ligamentum or ductus arteriosus causing obstruction to forward blood flow. Post-stenotic dilatation of the proximal descending thoracic aorta is present. Significant coarctation impairs blood flow into the descending thoracic aorta necessitating the presence of collaterals to re-establish blood flow. The intercostal arteries are major collaterals resulting in rib notching along the inferior surface of three to eighth ribs in untreated patients usually by 10 years. Other collaterals arise from internal mammary, lateral thoracic and epigastric arteries. On a frontal CXR, one can identify a high aortic arch, a reverse '3' indentation at the site of coarctation (reflecting pre-coarctation dilatation, the coarctation and post-coarctation dilatation and rib notching **(Figs. 29.58 to 29.60)**. The coarctation can be well demonstrated by MR angiography.

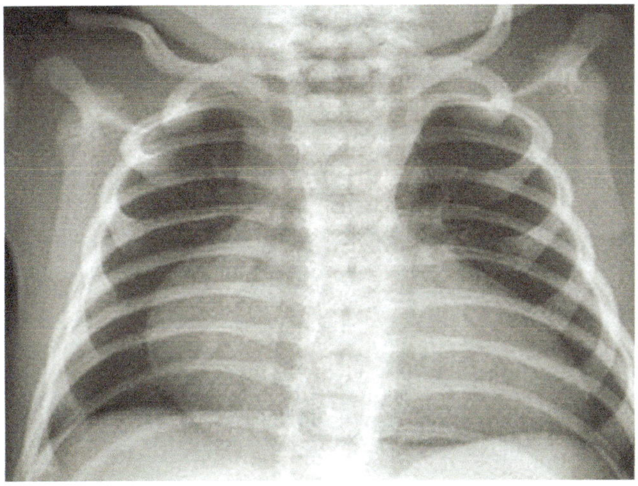

Figure 29.61 Chest X-ray showing a globular cardiomegaly, enlarged right atrium and reduced lung vascularity.

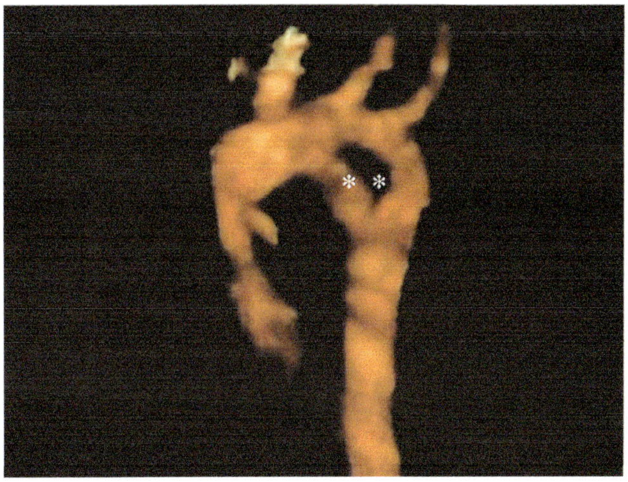

Figure 29.62 Three-dimensional reconstruction of a CT angiogram shows a double aortic arch (asterisks).

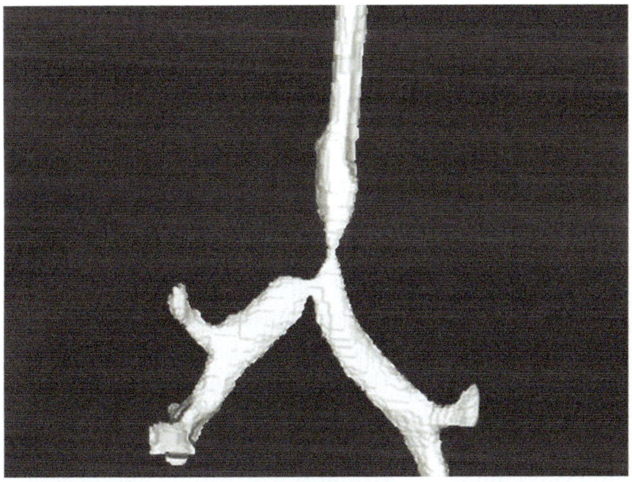

Figure 29.63 Three-dimensional reconstruction of the airway in a patient with double aortic arch and stridor shows tight narrowing of the distal trachea by the complete vascular ring.

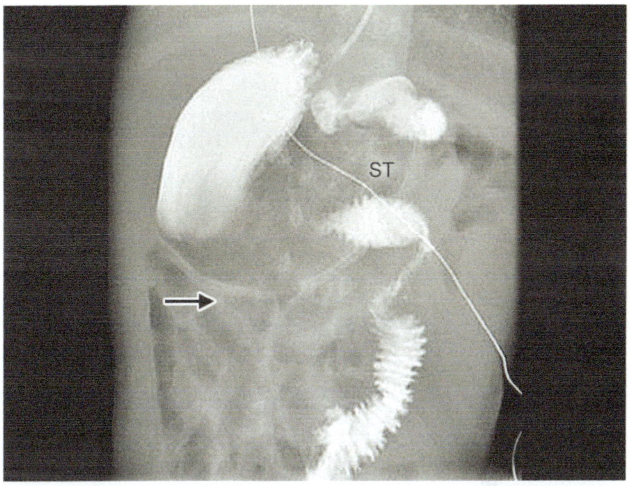

Figure 29.64 Upper gastrointestinal contrast examination in a newborn baby with bilious vomiting shows malrotation of the small bowel with the duodenal jejunal flexure and jejunal loops lying to the right of the spine (arrow).

Ebstein Anomaly

An uncommon congenital abnormality in which the septal and posterior leaflets of the tricuspid valve are attached to the wall of the middle of the right ventricular chamber instead of the valve ring. This results in mild to gross tricuspid regurgitation and marked right atrial enlargement. The foramen ovale is patent and the raised right atrial pressure results in right to left shunt and cyanosis. The frontal CXR shows an enlarged globular or square cardiac silhouette and reduced pulmonary vascularity (Fig. 29.61).

Double Aortic Arch

In this type of anomaly, the AA is anterior to the trachea bifurcating into two arches that pass to the sides of the trachea before joining posterior to the oesophagus to form the descending aorta. The double aortic arch forms a tight vascular ring that may present with severe stridor and requires surgical intervention (Figs. 29.62 and 29.63).

ABDOMEN

A Neonate with Bilious Vomiting

Common causes:

- Malrotation with or without small bowel volvulus
- Duodenal/small bowel atresias and webs
- Meconium ileus.

Malrotation (Figs. 29.64 and 29.65A and B)

Malrotation is a general term for any abnormal variation in intestinal rotation. Any variety of malrotation seen in

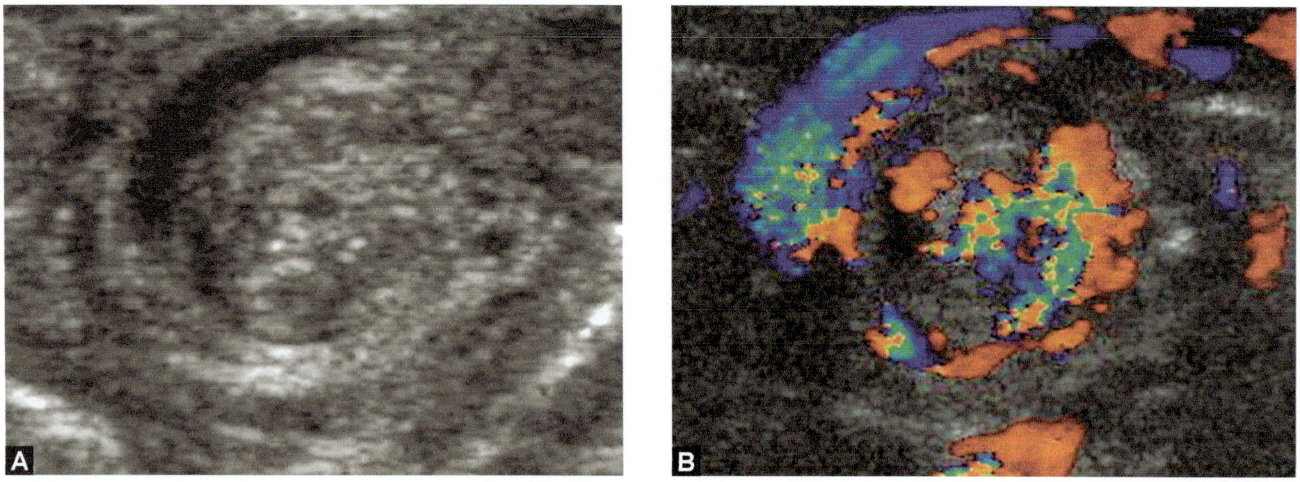

Figures 29.65A and B Malrotation with volvulus in another patient: Sonography with colour Doppler shows (A) a 'whirlpool' appearance of the involved small bowel and (B) twisting of the superior mesenteric artery and vein.

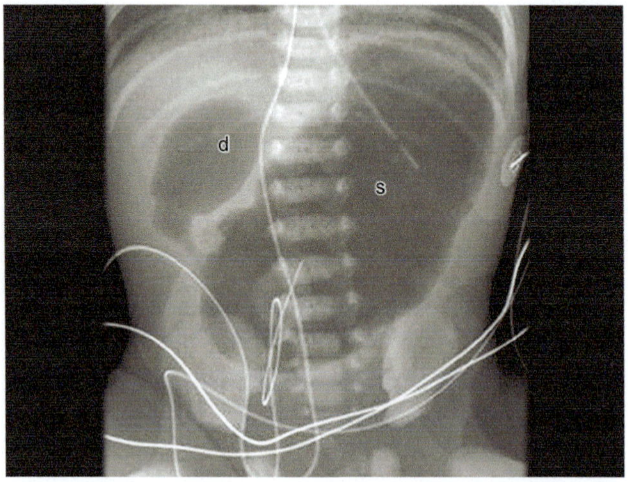

Figure 29.66 Abdominal film in a neonate with bilious vomiting showing a 'double bubble' appearance in duodenal atresia due to a dilated stomach (s) and first part of duodenum (d). No air is present distal to the stomach.

a child with abdominal symptoms should be assumed to be the cause of the symptoms unless proven otherwise. Malrotation of the intestines is accompanied by malfixation of the mesenteric root, which can have catastrophic consequences. The duodenal junction and the ileocaecal junctions are normal points of fixation of the mesentery, which has a broad base and unlikely to twist. When these points of fixation are not in their usual location the mesentery has a narrow base and there is a tendency for the intestines to twist around it. Abnormal peritoneal bands Ladd bands frequently accompany malrotation and can cause duodenal obstruction. Patients with malrotation can present at any age with bilious vomiting but most patients with symptomatic malrotation present in the first month of life.

Radiological investigations should include a plain film of the abdomen, which may show duodenal obstruction and an upper gastrointestinal studies which demonstrate malfixation of bowel, namely, malposition of the duodeno-jejunal flexure (more accurate indicator of malrotation) and the caecum.

Duodenal Atresia

Infants with duodenal atresia present with bilious vomiting in the first few hours of life. The obstruction is usually below the ampulla of Vater. Plain abdominal film shows a characteristic double bubble sign **(Fig. 29.66)**. Once this pattern is seen there is no need for further contrast studies. DA is commoner in infants with trisomy 21.

Duodenal Diaphragm

Duodenal diaphragms usually occur in the descending portion of the duodenum and frequently the common bile duct is incorporated in the diaphragm. Vomiting is bile stained and plain abdominal films show obstruction at the level of descending duodenum **(Figs. 29.67 and 29.68)**. Definitive diagnosis is usually made with barium studies.

Small Bowel Atresia

Small bowel atresia presents with abdominal distension and bilious vomiting condition is often not diagnosed until laparotomy. Radiographs show one or two dilated small bowel loops if the obstruction involves jejunum. If distal small bowel is involved multiple dilated loops of small bowel is seen with air fluid levels **(Figs. 29.69 and 29.70)**. A contrast enema is then necessary to assess for colonic obstruction.

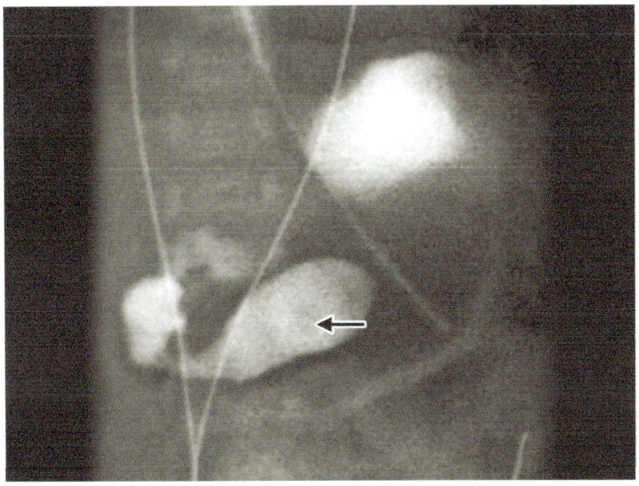

Figure 29.67 Upper gastrointestinal contrast study in a newborn with bilious vomiting shows the duodenal diaphragm (arrow).

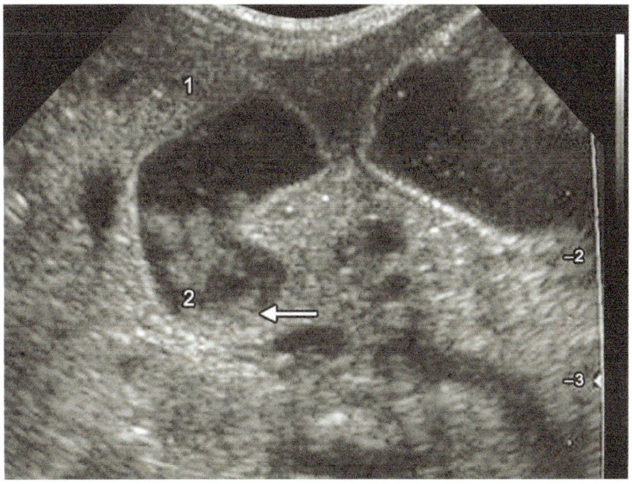

Figure 29.68 Upper abdominal ultrasound in a neonate showing dilated and fluid filled first (1) and second (2) parts of the duodenum due to a web (arrow).

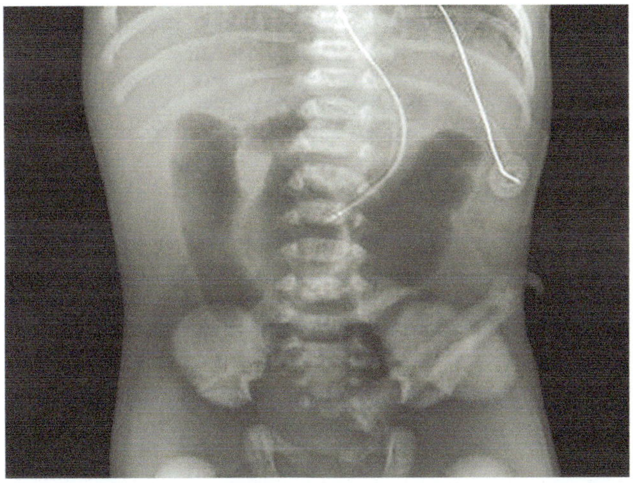

Figure 29.69 Plain radiograph in an infant with jejunal atresia showing dilatation of proximal bowel loops.

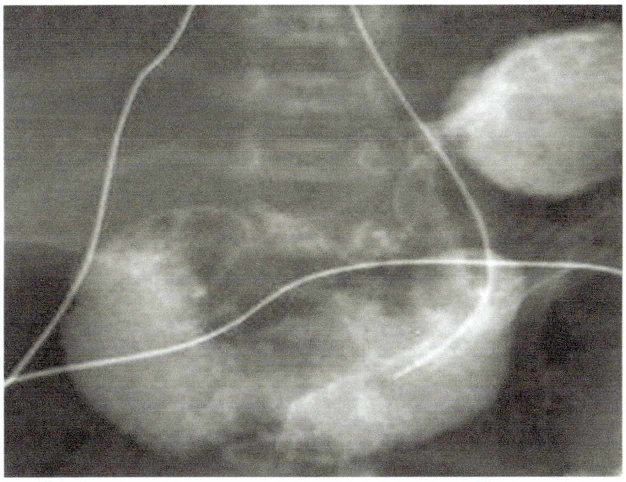

Figure 29.70 Water-soluble contrast study showing a dilated duodenum and failure of passage of contrast beyond the duodenal jejunal flexure in proximal jejunal atresia.

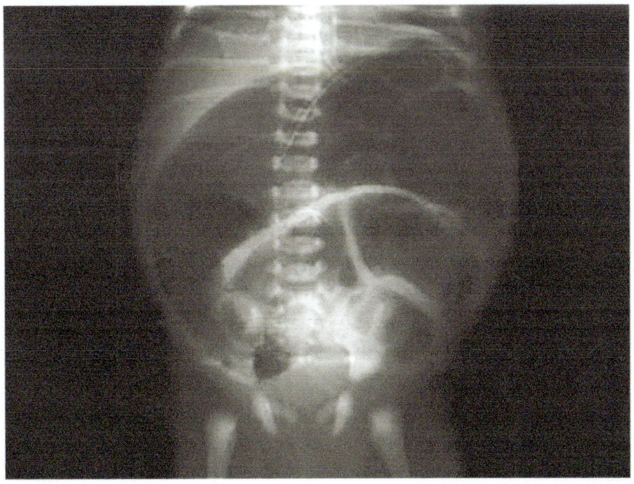

Figure 29.71 Abdominal film in an infant with meconium ileus shows marked small bowel dilatation.

Meconium Ileus

Usually considered a manifestation of cystic fibrosis (CF) in neonates. Obstruction results from impaction of thick tenacious meconium in the distal small bowel and complications such as ileal atresia, stenosis, ileal perforation, meconium peritonitis and volvulus with or without pseudocyst formation are common. Infants present with bile stained vomiting, abdominal distension and failure to pass meconium. Plain films show low small bowel obstruction with marked small bowel dilatation (Fig. 29.71). Air fluid levels are generally absent due to tenacious mucous. A contrast enema demonstrates a microcolon (Fig. 29.72). The enema can also be therapeutic.

OTHER ABDOMINAL CONDITIONS IN CHILDREN

Hypertrophic Pyloric Stenosis (Figs. 29.73A and B)

Hypertrophic pyloric stenosis (HPS) is a common condition presenting between 2 weeks and 6 weeks of life in predominantly male infants with non-bilious projectile vomiting. Severe cases also have weight loss and metabolic alkalosis of varying severity with potassium depletion. A small firm mass—the pseudotumour of HPS may be palpable. Sonography is the modality of choice to diagnose HPS. The stomach is emptied prior to exam by inserting a nasogastric tube and aspirating the contents. Sterile water is then introduced under sonographic guidance. HPS is seen as enlarged hypoechoic pyloric musculature with minimal emptying of the water into the duodenum (Figs. 29.73A and B). A plain film done to assess for other causes of vomiting may show gaseous distension of the stomach with little gas distally.

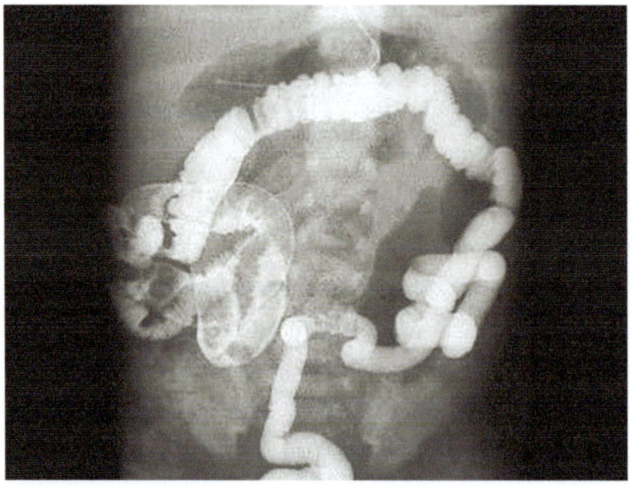

Figure 29.72 A contrast enema shows a microcolon.

Acute Appendicitis

Acute appendicitis is the most common indication for emergency abdominal surgery in children. It is caused by obstruction to the appendiceal lumen commonly by a faecalith. The appendix distends with secondary bacterial inflammation, oedema and vascular engorgement. Compromised blood supply may produce necrosis, gangrene and perforation with peritonitis. Complicated peritonitis can lead to a local walled off abscess or multiple intra-abdominal abscesses. Plain abdominal films may be normal or demonstrate a gasless right iliac fossa and a calcified faecalith (Figs. 29.74 and 29.75). Complicated cases may present with small bowel obstruction from the complex appendiceal mass which comprises of the inflamed appendix, adjacent loops of small bowel and inflamed mesentery. Sonography shows the inflamed appendix, abscess and the complex right lower quadrant mass (Figs. 29.76 and 29.77).

Intussusception

Intussusception is the invagination of the proximal bowel into its distal lumen. Ileocolic intussusceptions are most common (90%) and may or may not have a lead point, which includes Meckel diverticulum, polyps, lymphoma or sub-mucosal haemorrhage. Most intussusceptions are idiopathic and the clinical symptoms include intermittent abdominal pain, vomiting, bloody stools and palpable abdominal mass. The plain film is normal in 25% of patients or may show soft-tissue mass or small bowel obstruction (Fig. 29.78). Ultrasound helps in the

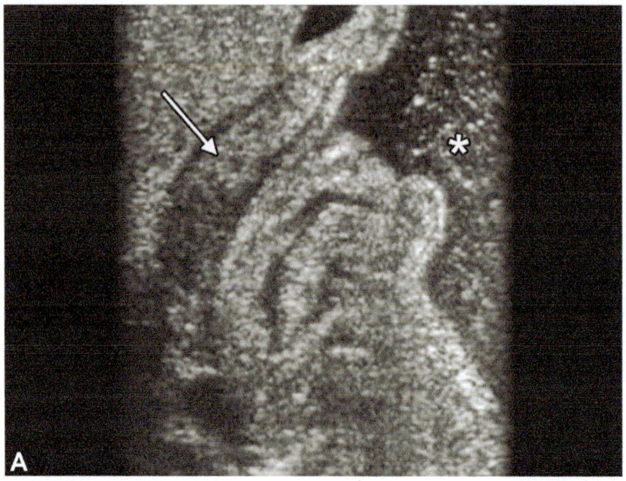

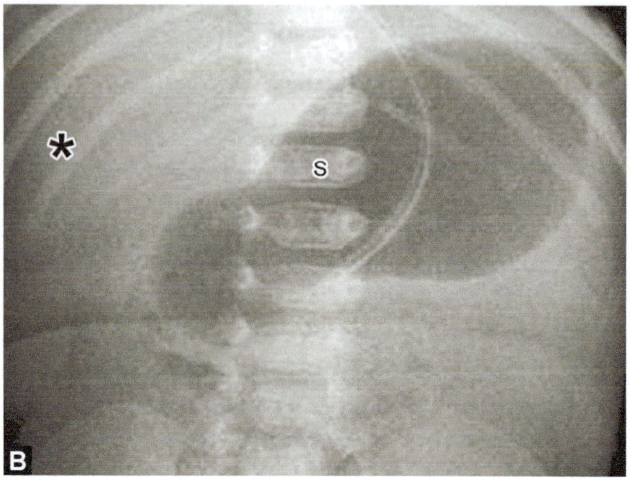

Figures 29.73A and B (A) Ultrasound showing an enlarged pylorus with hypoechoic muscle (arrow). Water introduced through a nasogastric tube is seen in the antrum (asterisk); (B) Plain abdominal film showing a distended stomach (s).

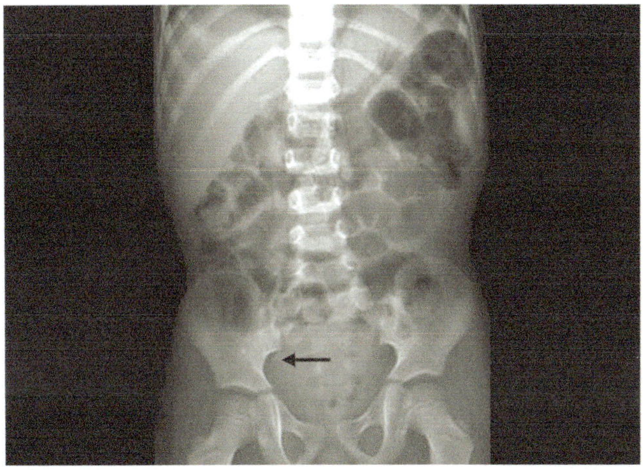

Figure 29.74 Plain abdominal film shows a calcified faecalith (arrow) in the right iliac fossa and small bowel dilatation in a patient with appendicitis.

diagnosis and shows a mass with alternating hypo and hyperechoic concentric rings axially and a 'pseudokidney sign' longitudinally (Figs. 29.79A and B).

Depending on the sonographic appearances and clinical state of the patient radiological reduction using air is attempted (Fig. 29.80).

Abdominal Trauma

Abdominal trauma in children can be penetrating or blunt. Blunt trauma is commoner in children and can cause solid organ or bowel trauma. Various types of solid organ injuries like liver fractures and contusions, splenic fractures, pancreatic and renal injuries can occur. Bowel trauma with contusion and perforation can also occur. The main modality for investigating these surgical emergencies is CT scanning, which should be done with intravenous and gut contract enhancement as far as possible.

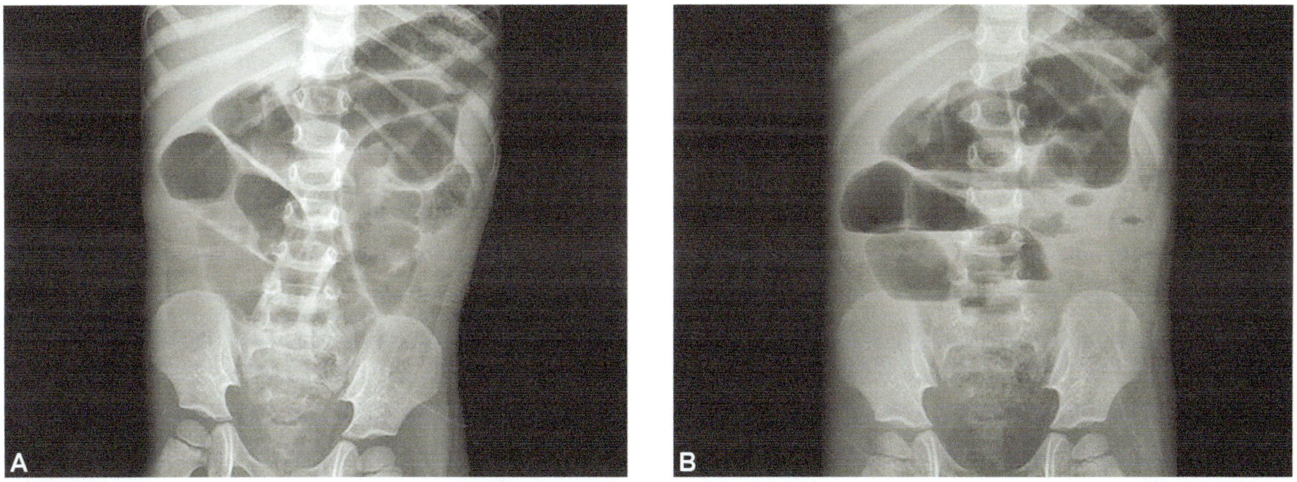

Figures 29.75A and B Appendicitis with obstruction: (A) Supine view of the abdomen shows small bowel dilatation and a gasless right iliac fossa; (B) Erect view demonstrates air-fluid levels in the small bowel.

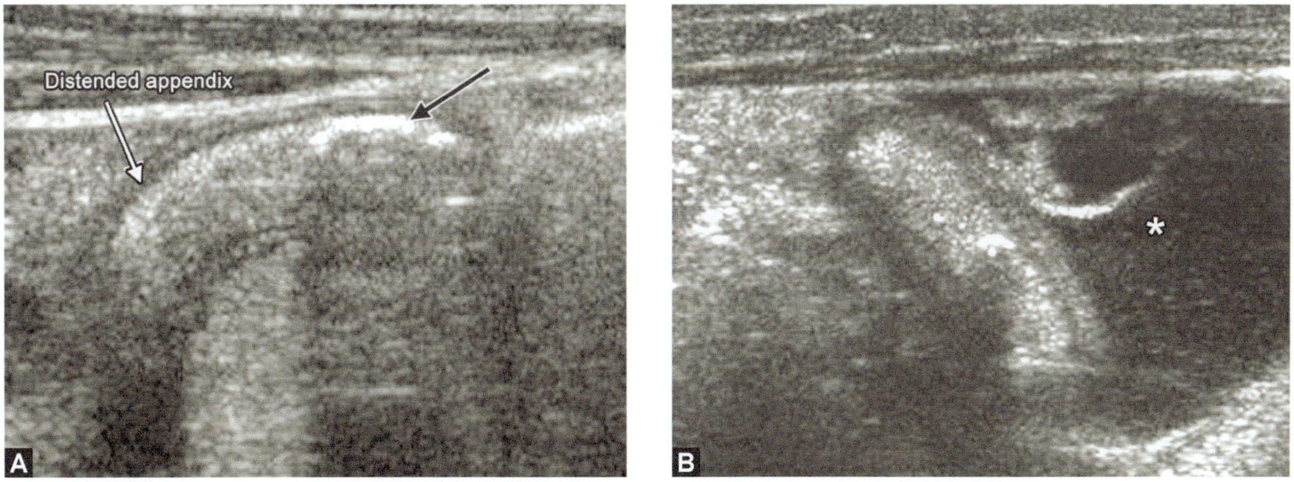

Figures 29.76A and B (A) Ultrasound of a patient with complicated appendicitis shows a distended appendix with a phlebolith (white arrow). The phlebolith is seen as an echogenic curvilinear structure with posterior acoustic shadowing (black arrow; (B) There is a focal fluid collection near the appendix (asterisk).

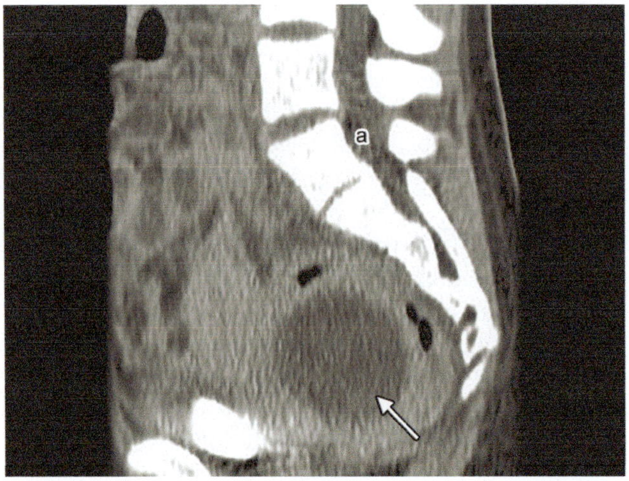

Figure 29.77 Sagittal reconstruction of a CT scan of the abdomen in a patient with complicated appendicitis shows a thick walled abscess (arrow) which was successfully drained transrectally.

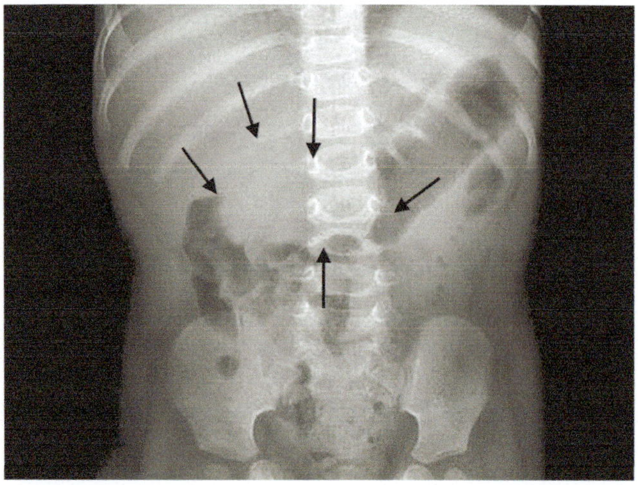

Figure 29.78 Abdominal radiograph in a patient with typical clinical features of an intussusception shows a soft-tissue mass in the right upper quadrant (black arrows).

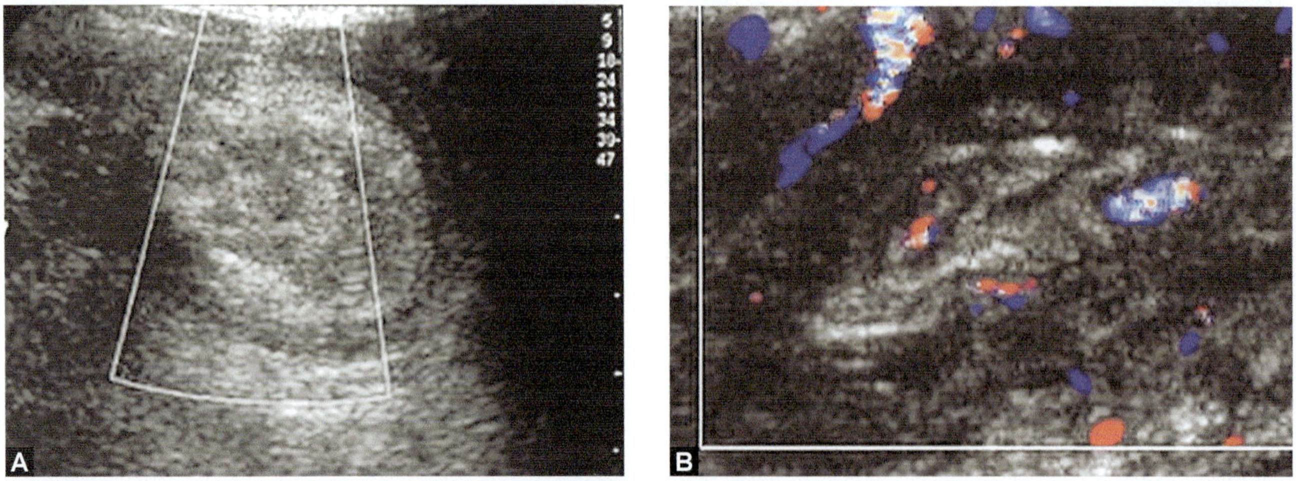

Figures 29.79A and B Air enema reduction shows the intussusception reduced to the caecum (arrow).

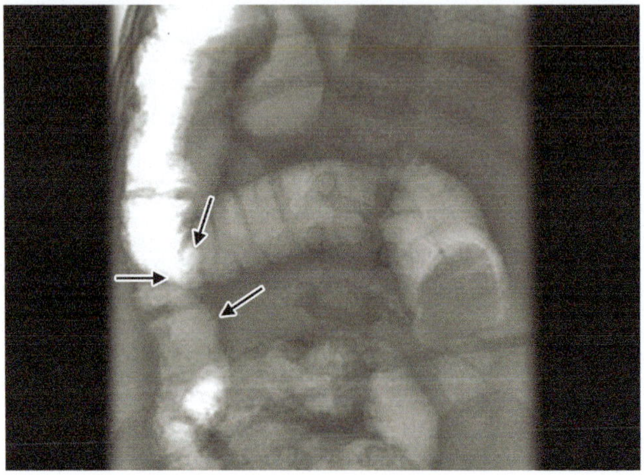

Figure 29.80 Air enema reduction shows the intussusception reduced to the caecum (arrows).

Associated lung trauma such as contusions, pneumothoraces and rib fractures may occur. Vertebral injuries like Chance fractures may also occur **(Figs. 29.81 to 29.85)**.

A CHILD WITH ABDOMINAL MASS

Common masses include:

- Neuroblastoma
- Wilms tumour
- Multicystic dysplastic kidney (MCDK)
- Hepatoblastoma
- Pelviureteric junction obstruction
- Lymphoma

The differential diagnosis varies according to the age. An abdominal mass in the newborn is most commonly benign and of renal origin (neonatal hydronephrosis

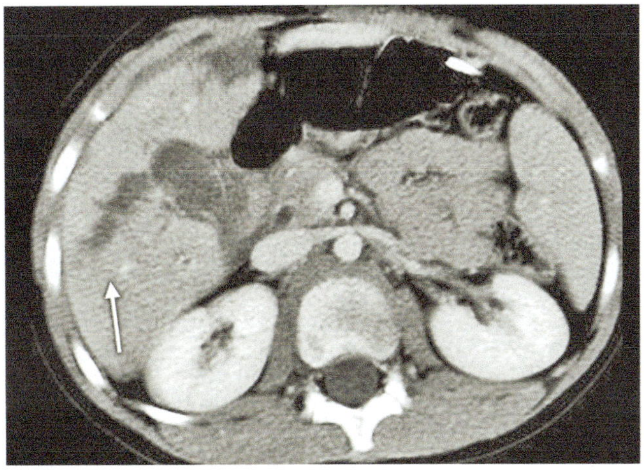

Figure 29.81 CT scan of a child following a fall from a height shows a fracture of the right lobe of the liver (arrow).

due to various causes). Renal, neoplasms are unusual in this group but occasionally mesoblastic nephroma may be seen. Other masses include renal enlargement due to renal vein thrombosis, adrenal haemorrhage, bowel related masses and sacrococcygeal teratoma. In infants and young children, the retroperitoneal masses are common. These include neuroblastomas and Wilms tumour. Other masses include hepatoblastomas, lymphomas, teratomas and lymphangiomas.

Abdominal Neuroblastoma (Figs. 29.86 and 29.87)

It is the most common extracranial solid tumour of childhood and accounts for 10% of all paediatric neoplasms. Presentation is common with an abdominal mass. Other modes of presentation include cord compression,

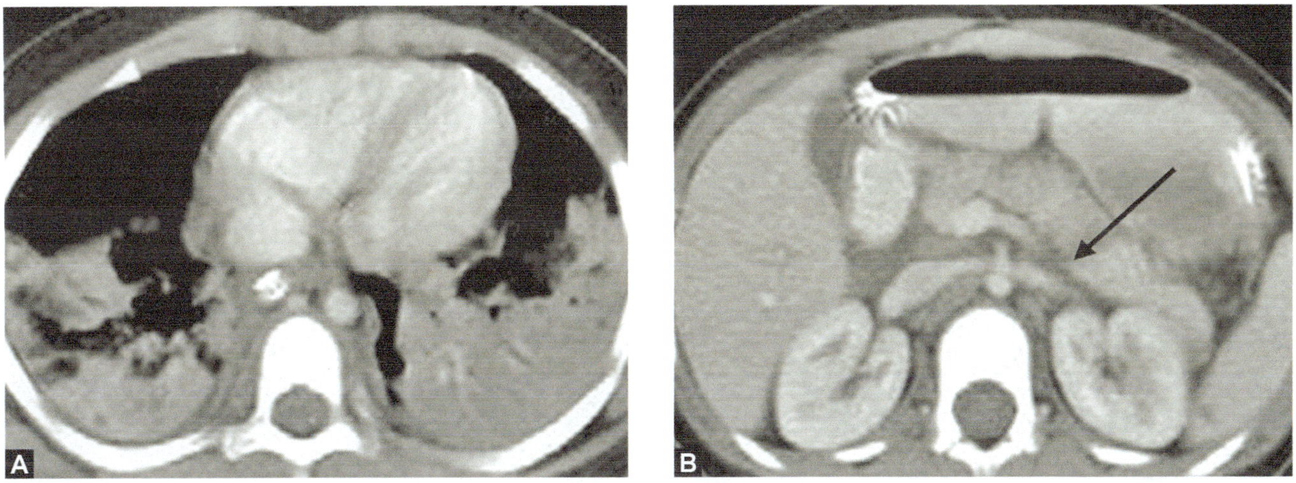

Figures 29.82A and B CT scan of a child with blunt trauma shows: (A) Bilateral lung contusions; (B) Pancreatic fracture (arrow).

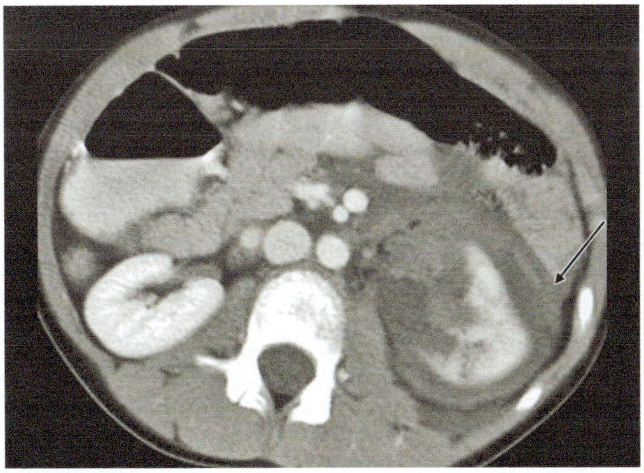

Figure 29.83 Renal trauma: CT scan shows a left renal fracture and contusion with perirenal fluid (arrow). Note the normal right kidney.

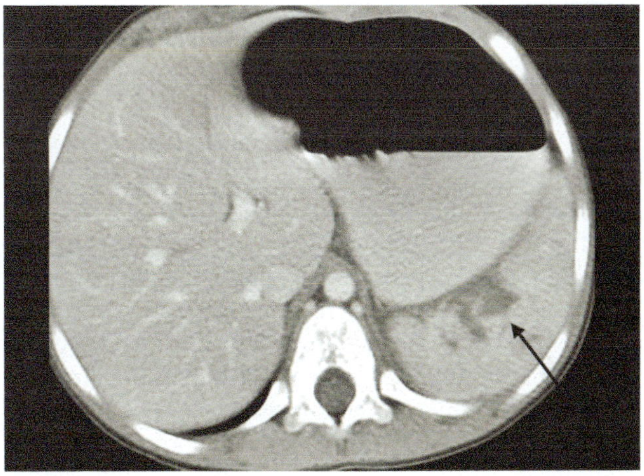

Figure 29.84 Splenic fracture (arrow) seen in a 7-year-old after fall from a horse.

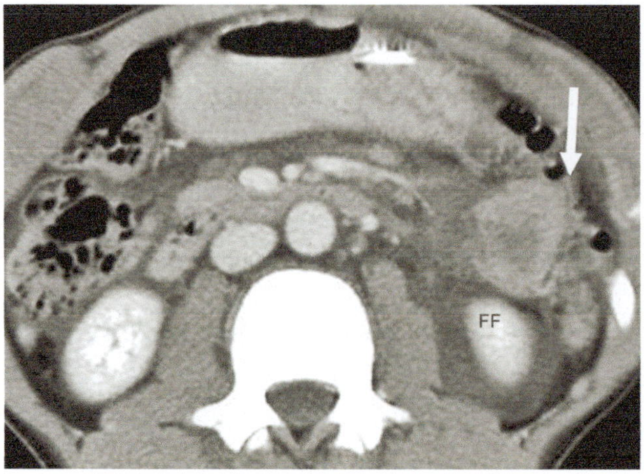

Figure 29.85 Jejunal contusion (arrow) and free fluid in the left flank in a patient with blunt trauma to the abdomen due to fall from a tree.

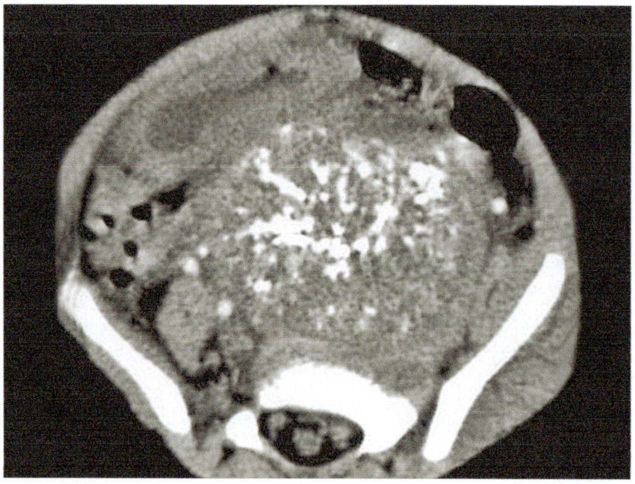

Figure 29.86 Neuroblastoma: CT scan showing a calcified lower abdominal mass with presacral lymphadenopathy.

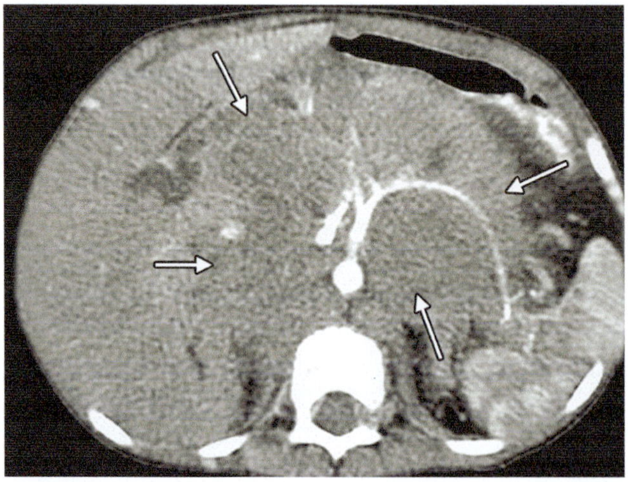

Figure 29.87 Neuroblastoma: 2 years old with neuroblastoma. An enhanced CT image shows a retroperitoneal mass with vascular encasement (arrows).

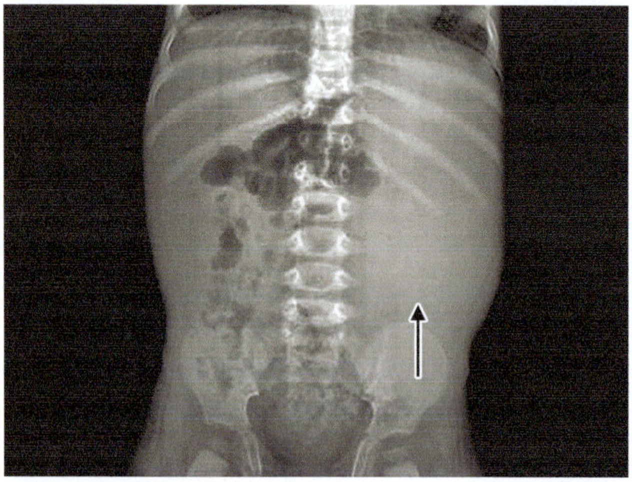

Figure 29.88 Left-sided Wilms tumour. Plain abdominal radiograph shows a left-sided soft-tissue mass (arrow).

constipation or as a paraneoplastic syndrome. Two of these syndromes are recognised, namely, the opsoclonus myoclonus syndrome and the watery diarrhoea, hypokalaemia and achlorhydria syndrome. Radiological evaluation begins with a plain film, which shows a mass with calcification. Sonography shows a tumour, which is in homogenous, echogenic and a poorly defined extrarenal mass. Hypoechoic regions may be due to haemorrhage, necrosis or cyst formation. Areas of calcification are echogenic. CT scanning accurately stages the tumour and demonstrates the primary tumour, contiguous spread, vascular encasement retroperitoneal lymphadenopathy and liver metastases. MRI is the imaging modality of choice and is superior in imaging adenopathy, vascular involvement, bone marrow metastases and intraspinal extension.

Wilms Tumour

Wilms tumour is the most common renal tumour of childhood and presents mostly as an asymptomatic abdominal mass. Other symptoms include abdominal pain and haematuria. Plain abdominal radiography shows a soft-tissue mass with calcification in about 5%. Sonography shows an intrarenal mass which is hyperechoic compared to normal renal parenchyma with areas of necrosis and cysts. Renal vein and inferior caval invasion occurs in 15%. CT scan shows a well-defined intrarenal mass distorting the collecting system and with inhomogeneous enhancement post-contrast. MRI is better than CT in the evaluation of the intrarenal mass, assessment of perinephric extension, contralateral kidney and evaluation of the renal vein and IVC **(Figs. 29.88 to 29.91)**.

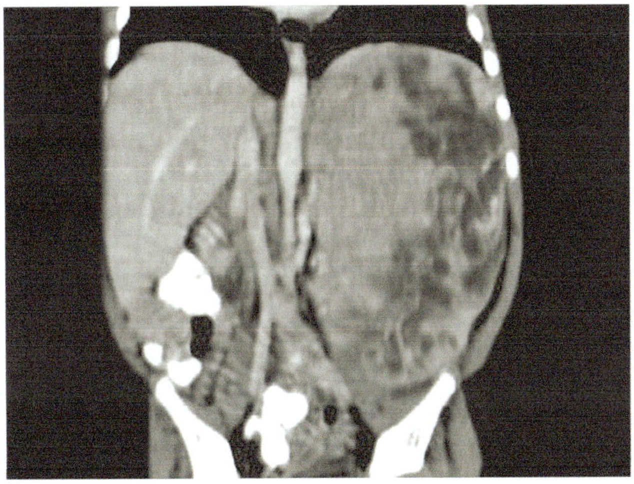

Figure 29.89 Left-sided Wilms tumour (same patient as in Figure 29.88). Coronal CT reconstruction shows a mixed density mass containing areas of necrosis and cysts.

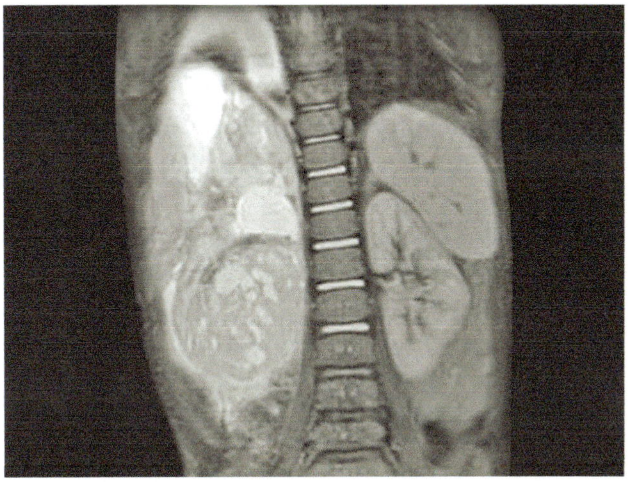

Figure 29.90 Right-sided Wilms tumour: coronal MRI shows a large right-sided mass containing areas of cystic degeneration.

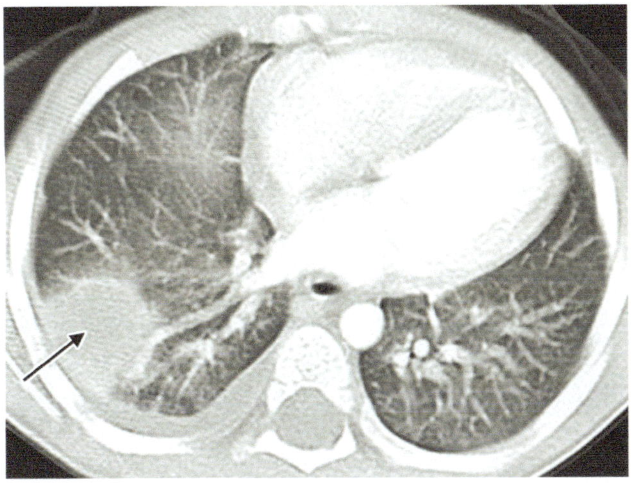

Figure 29.91 Lung metastases from a Wilms tumour. CT image showing a large right-sided lung metastasis (arrow).

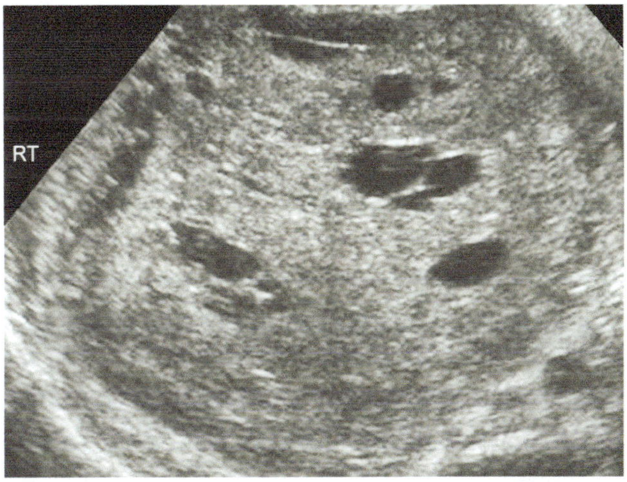

Figure 29.92 Mesoblastic nephroma: Ultrasound shows a hyperechoic mass containing cysts in a newborn.

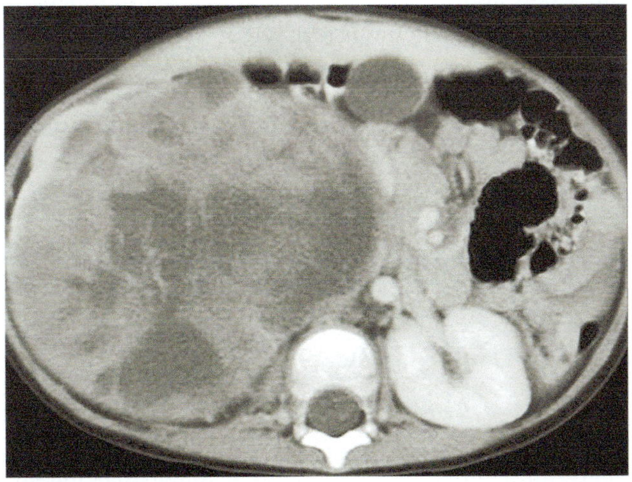

Figure 29.93 Mesoblastic nephroma (same patient as above). CT image shows a right renal mass of mixed attenuation.

Congenital Mesoblastic Nephroma (Figs. 29.92 and 29.93)

Most common renal tumour of neonates and the pathologic spectrum ranges from benign congenital mesoblastic nephroma to malignant spindle cell sarcoma. Plain radiographs show a soft-tissue mass. Sonographically the mass is well defined and hypoechoic or hyperechoic. CT demonstrates the intrarenal location of the mass.

Hepatoblastoma (Figs. 29.94 to 29.98)

Primary liver tumours account for 15% of abdominal neoplasms in children. Most children present with an asymptomatic abdominal mass. Others present with anorexia, weight loss, jaundice and pain. Alpha fetoprotein levels are raised in up to 90% of cases. Plain films reveal a soft-tissue mass in the upper abdomen. Sonographically,

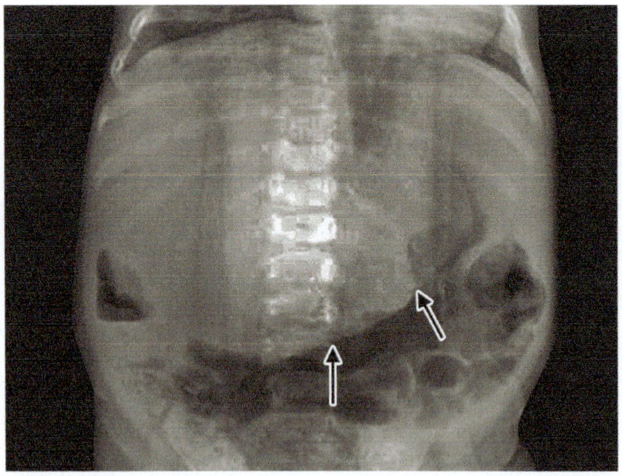

Figure 29.94 Hepatoblastoma: Plain abdominal film shows a large upper abdominal soft-tissue mass in a 3-month-old infant (arrows).

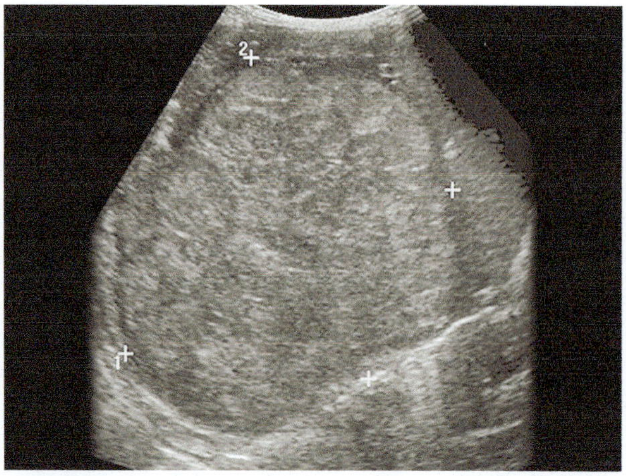

Figure 29.95 Hepatoblastoma: Ultrasound scan of a 1-month-old infant with an abdominal mass shows a large hyperechoic mass.

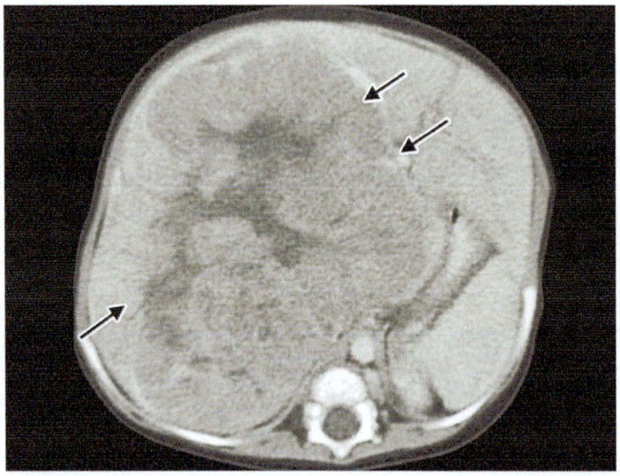

Figure 29.96 Hepatoblastoma: CT image shows a large well-defined homogenous lobulated intrahepatic mass (arrows) with slightly lower attenuation and enhancement than the normal liver. Fibrous bands can be seen as unenhancing linear structures.

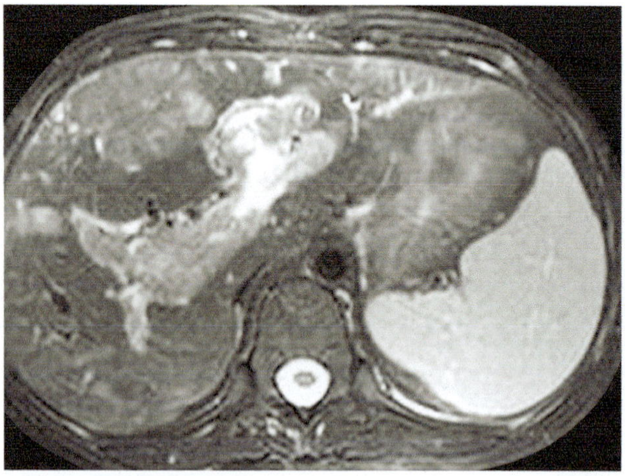

Figure 29.97 Hepatoblastoma with portal vein invasion: Axial MRI (T2 weighted) shows a distended portal venous confluence (arrows) and multiple tumour thrombi.

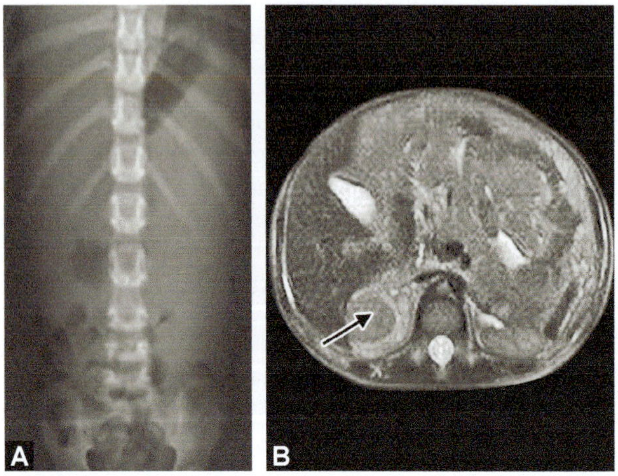

Figures 29.98A and B (A) Plain abdominal film showing upper abdominal fullness due to masses; (B) MRI showing diffuse bowel wall infiltration and a right renal mass (arrow).

the lesion appears as a large, well-defined intrahepatic hyperechoic mass containing areas of cystic degeneration, necrosis and haemorrhage. Hepatic and portal venous invasion may occur. CT and MRI define the intrahepatic extent, extrahepatic spread and vascular invasion.

PAEDIATRIC NEURORADIOLOGY: CONGENITAL BRAIN MALFORMATIONS

Cephalocoele (Figs. 29.99 and 29.100)

A cephalocoele is a defect in the skull and dura, through which intracranial structures (cerebrospinal fluid, meninges and brain tissue) can herniate. MRI is the study of choice for investigating this condition.

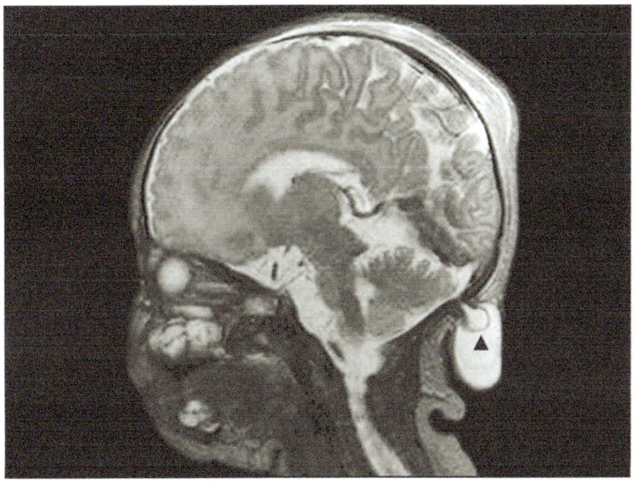

Figure 29.99 Occipital cephalocoele. Sagittal T2 weighted MR image shows a small occipital cephalocoele with herniation of cerebrospinal fluid and meninges (arrowhead).

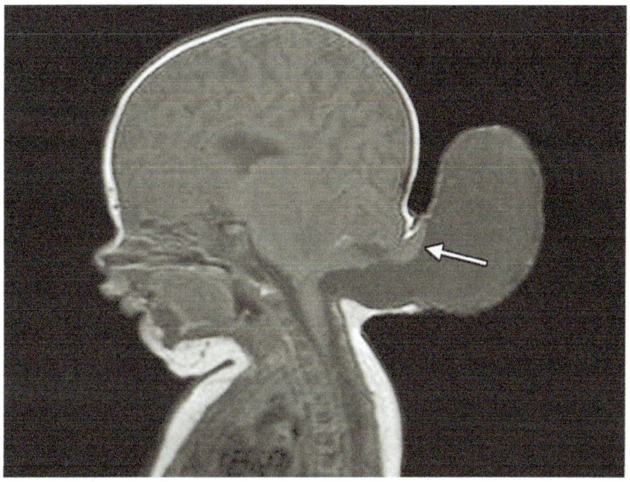

Figure 29.100 Occipital cephalocoele. Sagittal T1 weighted MR image shows a large occipital cephalocoele with herniation of cerebellar tissue (arrow) and cerebrospinal fluid into the cephalocoele.

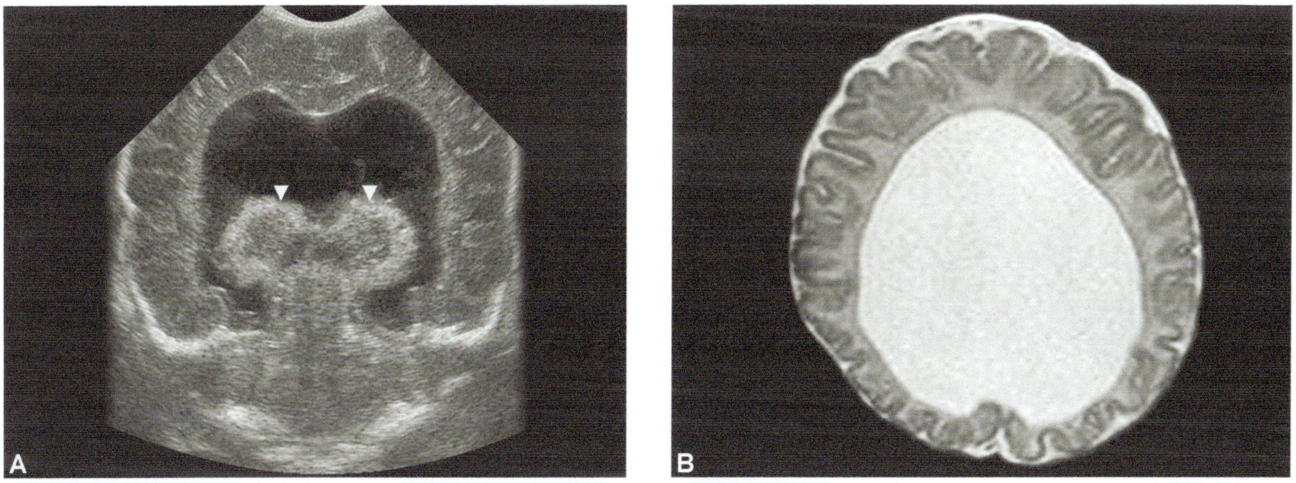

Figures 29.101A and B Holoprosencephaly. (A) Coronal ultrasound scan shows a holoventricle due to the absence of midline structures (septum pellucidum, corpus callosum and falx cerebri). The thalami (arrowheads) are fused in the midline; (B) Axial T2 weighted image shows a holoventricle.

HOLOPROSENCEPHALY (FIGS. 29.101A AND B)

The holoprosencephalies are a group of disorders typified by failure of the embryonic forebrain (prosencephalon) to sufficiently divide into two cerebral hemispheres.

Dandy-Walker Malformation (Figs. 29.102 and 29.103)

The Dandy-Walker malformation consists of complete or partial agenesis of the cerebellar vermis, an enlarged posterior cranial fossa and cystic dilatation of the fourth ventricle, which almost entirely fills the posterior cranial fossa.

Chiari I Malformation (Figs. 29.104 and 29.105)

The Chiari I malformation is defined as caudal (downward) extension of the cerebellar tonsils below the foramen magnum. The cerebellar tonsils are elongated and pointed. There may be mild caudal displacement and flattening or kinking of the medulla. A syrinx is present in the spinal cord in up to 25% of patients.

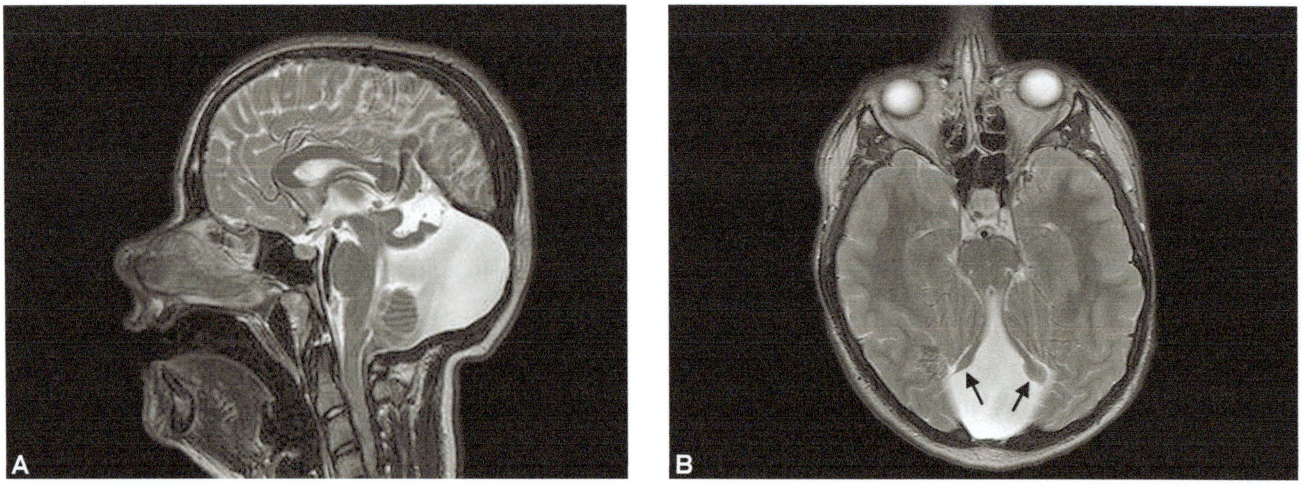

Figures 29.102A and B Dandy–Walker malformation. (A) Sagittal T2 weighted MR image shows a markedly enlarged posterior fossa and cystic dilatation of the fourth ventricle; (B) Axial T2 weighted MR image shows the markedly hypoplastic cerebellar vermis (arrows).

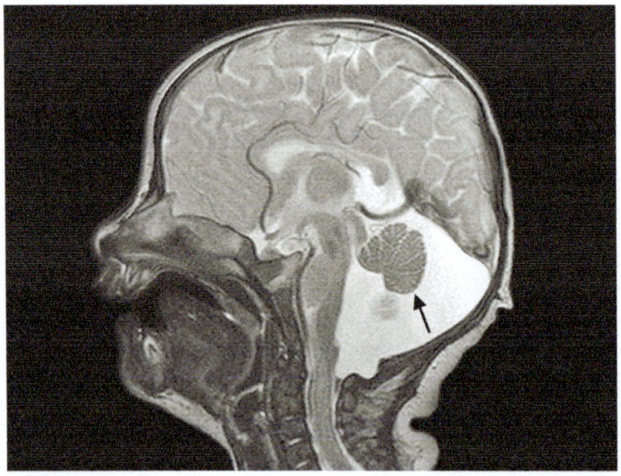

Figure 29.103 Dandy–Walker malformation. Sagittal T2 MR image shows enlarged posterior cranial fossa with mild hypoplasia of the cerebellar vermis (arrow).

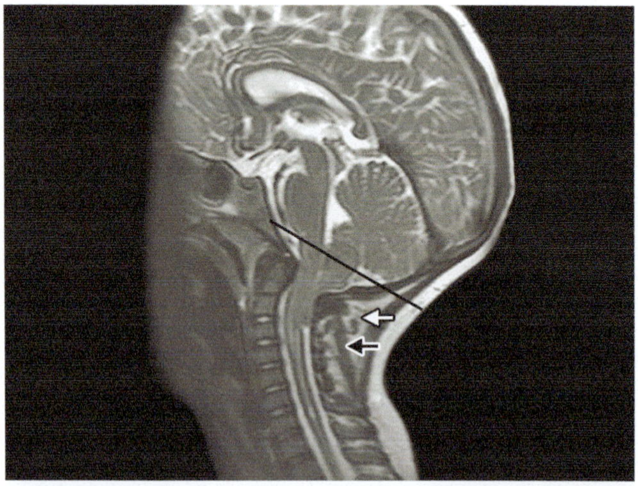

Figure 29.104 Chiari I malformation on sagittal T2 weighted MR image. The cerebellar tonsil (white arrow) extends well below the foramen magnum (black line). The high signal within the cervical cord (black arrow) indicates the presence of a syrinx.

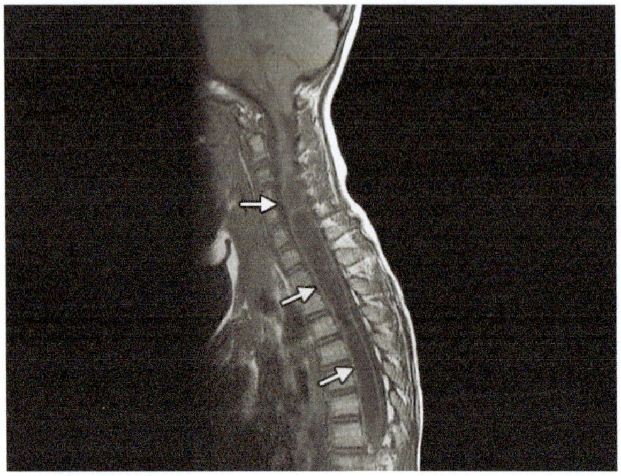

Figure 29.105 Chiari I malformation. Sagittal T1 weighted MR image shows cerebellar tonsillar descent below the foramen magnum. There is a large syrinx in the cervical and thoracic spinal cord (arrows).

Sturge–Weber Syndrome (Figs. 29.106 and 29.107)

The Sturge-Weber syndrome is a neurocutaneous disorder with angiomas involving the leptomeninges and the skin of the face (port wine stain). The syndrome can affect one or both cerebral hemispheres.

Contrast enhanced MRI is the best imaging study for showing the extent of the pial angioma. After IV contrast administration, the angioma is identified as an area of enhancement following the contours of the gyri and sulci. Cortical calcification and cerebral atrophy are seen in long standing cases. The cortical calcification is best demonstrated on CT scanning.

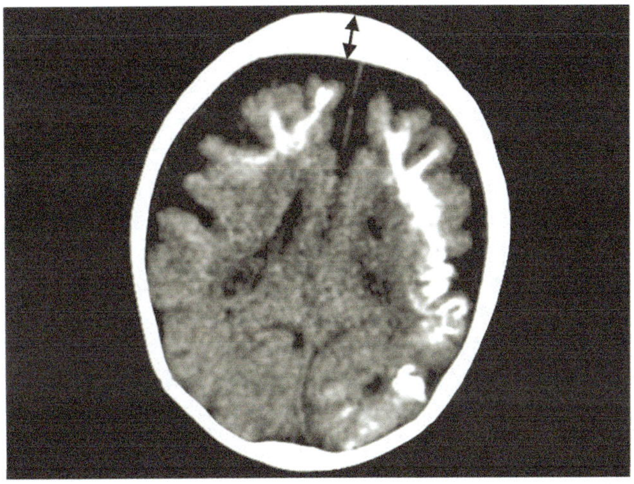

Figure 29.106 Sturge–Weber syndrome. Axial unenhanced CT scan of brain shows marked subcortical and cortical calcification in both cerebral hemispheres in a gyriform pattern. The calcification is more extensive in the left cerebral hemisphere. There is evidence of cerebral atrophy with enlargement of the surrounding cerebrospinal fluid spaces and thickening of the skull vault anteriorly (black arrow).

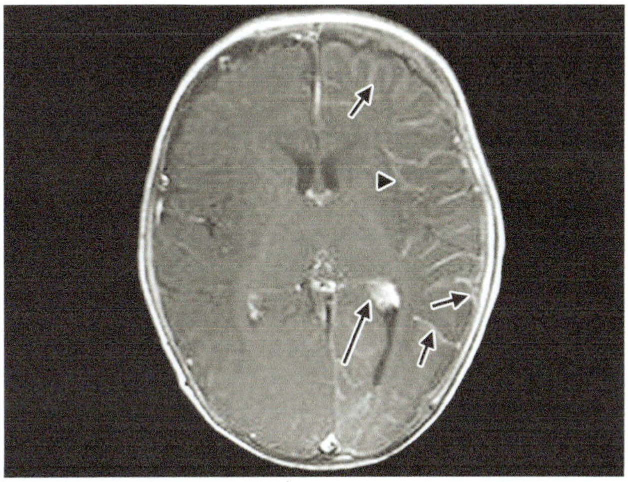

Figure 29.107 Sturge–Weber syndrome. Post-contrast axial T1 weighted MR image shows pial enhancement, which follows the gyral and sulcal contours of the entire left cerebral hemisphere (arrowhead). The choroid plexus in the left lateral ventricle is enlarged (arrows)—another feature of the syndrome.

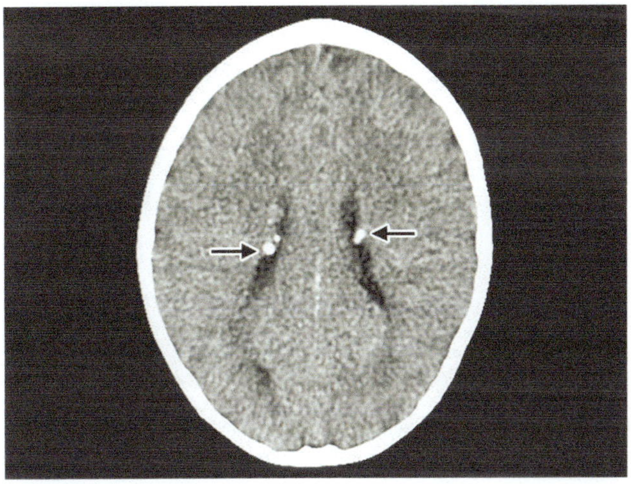

Figure 29.108 Tuberous sclerosis. Axial unenhanced CT scan of brain shows calcified subependymal nodules within both lateral ventricles (arrows).

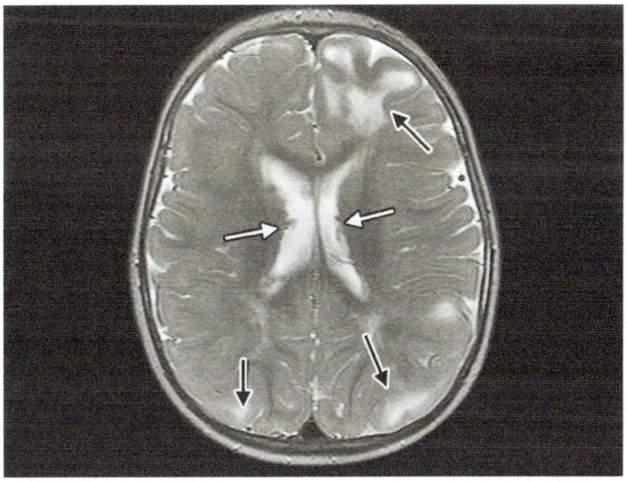

Figure 29.109 Tuberous sclerosis. Axial T2 weighted MR image shows several subependymal nodules within both lateral ventricles (white arrows). The high signal intensity lesions within the cerebral hemispheres represent cortical tubers (black arrows).

Tuberous Sclerosis (Figs. 29.108 and 29.109)

Tuberous sclerosis is a genetic disorder that results in hamartoma formation in many organs, including the brain. Intracranial manifestations include

Subependymal hamartomas: small nodules, which protrude into the ventricles (usually the lateral ventricles). These can be calcified.

Cerebral hamartomas or cortical "tubers": these hamartomas are identified as subcortical areas of abnormal signal intensity associated with adjacent gyral broadening. Cerebral hamartomas can also calcify.

Vein of Galen Malformation (Figs. 29.110 and 29.111)

The malformation occurs because of a congenital connection between intracranial arteries and the vein of Galen or other primitive midline vein. On ultrasound, the malformation is usually identified as a round hypoechoic structure posterior to the third ventricle. Colour Doppler studies can show the rapid blood flow within the malformation. On T2 weighted MR sequences, the malformation is identified as a low signal (black) structure posterior to the third ventricle. Intracranial complications include hydrocephalus and brain ischaemia.

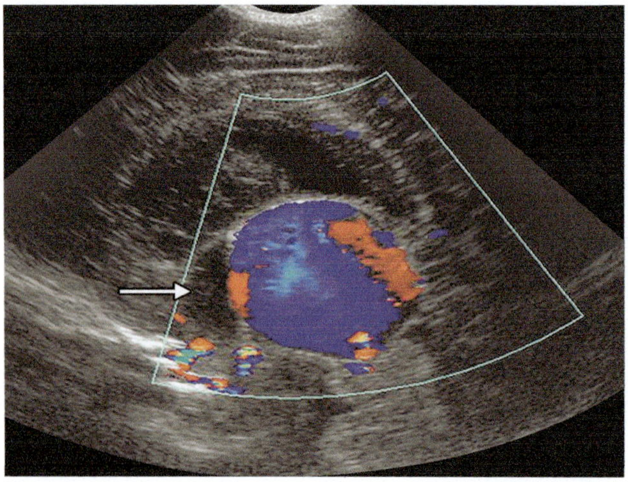

Figure 29.110 Vein of Galen malformation on ultrasound. Midline sagittal image shows blood flow within the malformation which lies posterior to the third ventricle (arrow).

TRAUMA, HYPOXIA–ISCHAEMIA AND HAEMORRHAGE

Head Injury (Figs. 29.112 to 29.114)

As a general rule, CT is the initial study of choice for children who have sustained a head injury. Skull fractures, intracranial haemorrhage and any associated mass effect can be detected with CT.

On CT, an extradural haematoma is a biconvex collection of blood between the brain surface and the skull. The acute haematoma is of increased attenuation (i.e. appears white). A subdural haematoma is identified as a crescentic collection of blood between the brain surface and the skull.

Periventricular and Intraventricular Haemorrhage in Premature Infants

Intracranial haemorrhage in the preterm infant has been divided into four grades:

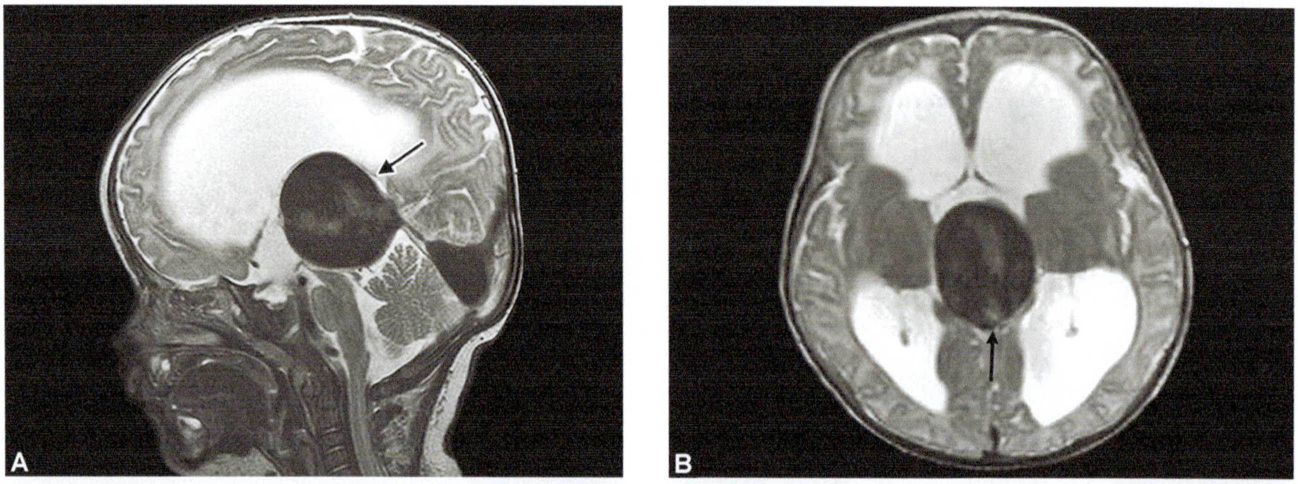

Figures 29.111A and B Vein of Galen malformation. T2 weighted MR sagittal (A) and axial (B) images demonstrating the malformation (black arrows). There is obstructive hydrocephalus involving the lateral and third ventricles.

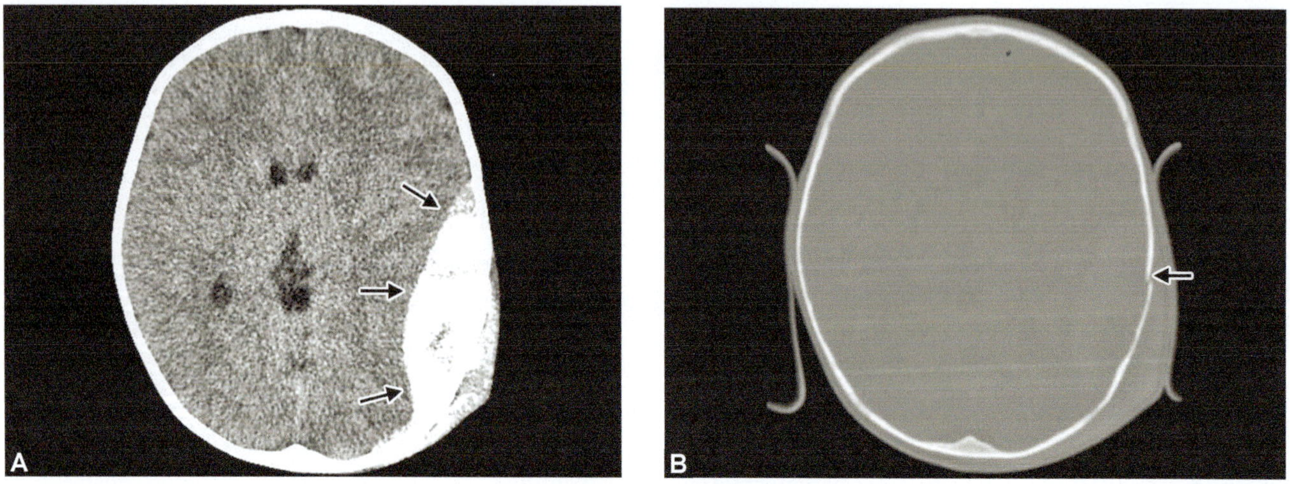

Figures 29.112A and B Left parietal skull fracture and extradural haematoma. (A) Unenhanced CT brain scan shows a large biconvex collection of blood adjacent to the left cerebral hemisphere (arrows); (B) Left parietal skull fracture is demonstrated (arrow).

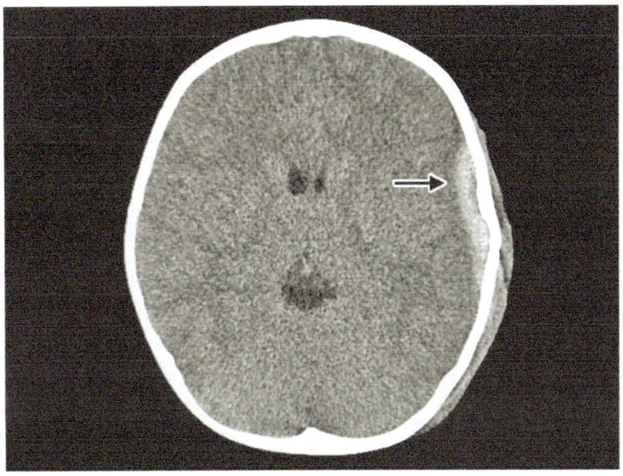

Figure 29.113 Acute left subdural haematoma. Unenhanced CT scan of brain demonstrates a crescentic collection of blood overlying the left cerebral hemisphere (arrow).

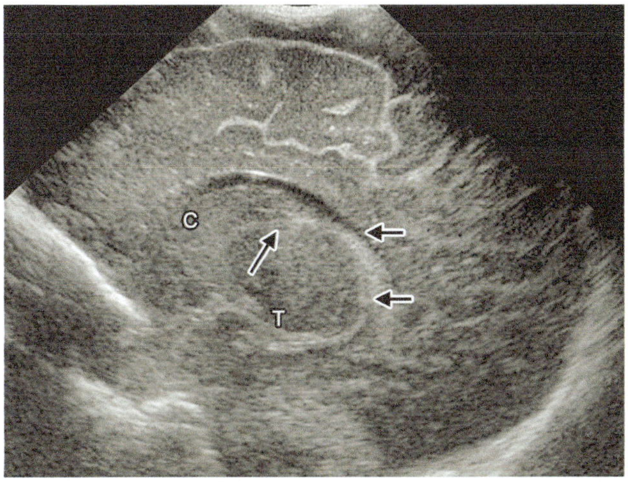

Figure 29.114 Normal parasagittal view of lateral ventricle (left). The head of the caudate nucleus (C) lies inferior to the body of the ventricle anteriorly. The thalamus (T) is located inferior to the body of the ventricle posteriorly. The echogenic choroid plexus (small arrows) is seen within the ventricle. The caudothalamic groove is a small echogenic area, which lies between the head of caudate and the thalamus (arrow).

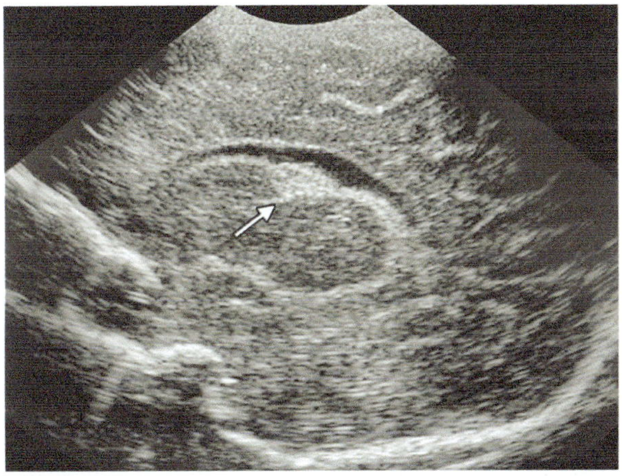

Figure 29.115 Grade 1 haemorrhage. Left parasagittal ultrasound scan shows a focus of increased echogenicity in the caudothalamic groove in keeping with subependymal haemorrhage (arrow).

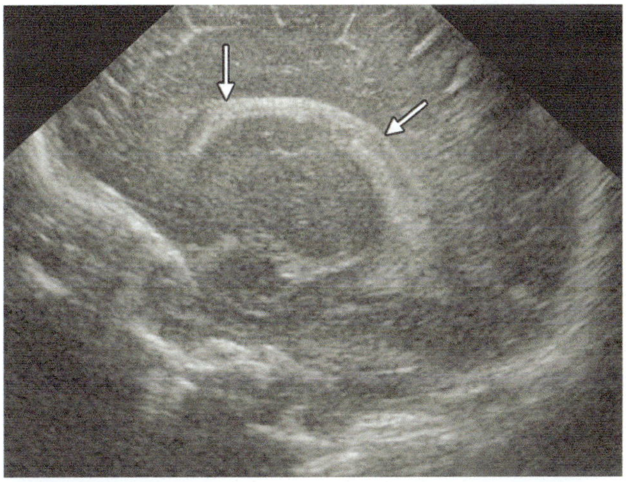

Figure 29.116 Grade 2 intraventricular haemorrhage. Left parasagittal ultrasound scan shows blood within the left lateral ventricle (arrows). The ventricle is not dilated.

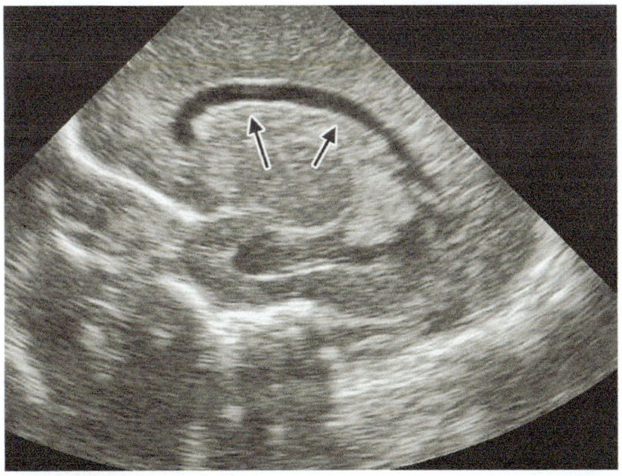

Figure 29.117 Grade 3 intraventricular haemorrhage. Right parasagittal ultrasound scan shows haemorrhage (arrows) in the right lateral ventricle which is dilated.

1. *Grade* 1: Subependymal haemorrhage only **(Fig. 29.115)**
2. *Grade* 2: Extension of subependymal haemorrhage into non-dilated ventricle **(Fig. 29.116)**
3. *Grade* 3: Intraventricular haemorrhage associated with ventricular dilatation **(Fig. 29.117)**
4. *Grade* 4: Periventricular parenchymal haemorrhage associated with intraventricular haemorrhage **(Figs. 29.118A and B)**.

On cranial ultrasound, intraventricular haemorrhage is identified as echogenic material within the ventricle.

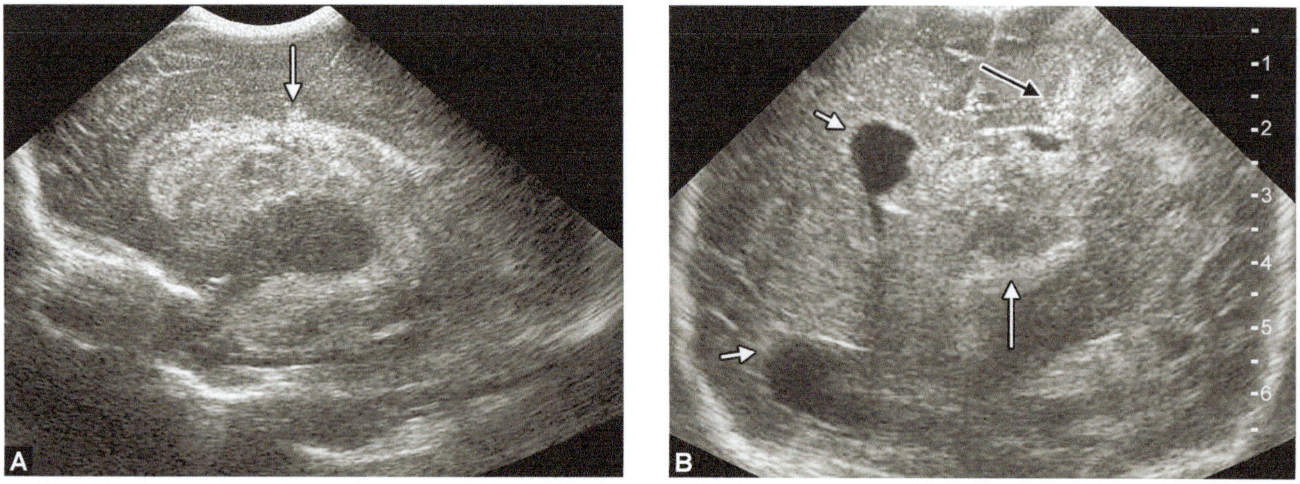

Figures 29.118A and B Grade 4 haemorrhage. (A) Left parasagittal ultrasound scan shows haemorrhage in the parenchyma adjacent to the left lateral ventricle (arrow); (B) Coronal ultrasound scan shows extensive intraventricular haemorrhage (white arrow) and periventricular parenchymal haemorrhage (black arrow). Note the obstructive hydrocephalus of the right lateral ventricle (small arrows).

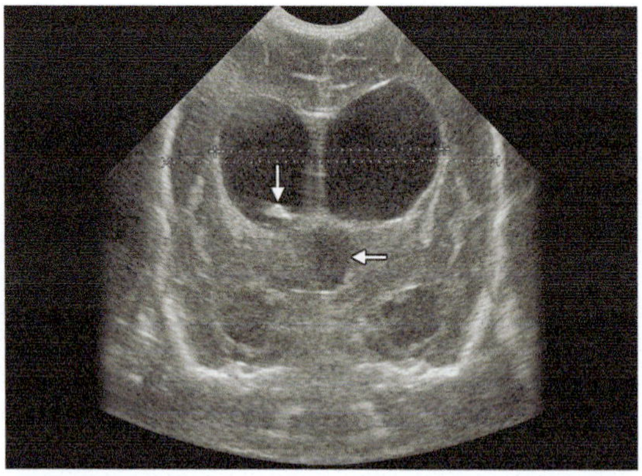

Figure 29.119 Post-haemorrhagic hydrocephalus. Coronal ultrasound scan shows marked dilatation of both lateral ventricles and the third ventricle (thick arrow). Some residual clot is present in the right lateral ventricle (thin arrow).

Post-haemorrhagic Hydrocephalus (Fig. 29.119)

Ventricular dilatation after intraventricular haemorrhage occurs as a result of intraventricular obstruction by clot or septations or because of an obliterative arachnoiditis. The lateral ventricles usually dilate more than the third and fourth ventricles.

Periventricular Leukomalacia (Figs. 29.120 and 29.121)

Periventricular leukomalacia is an ischaemic brain injury in preterm infants affecting the deep white matter in the immediate periventricular region. The earliest sonographic sign is increased echogenicity in the periventricular white matter. Cystic change becomes evident within

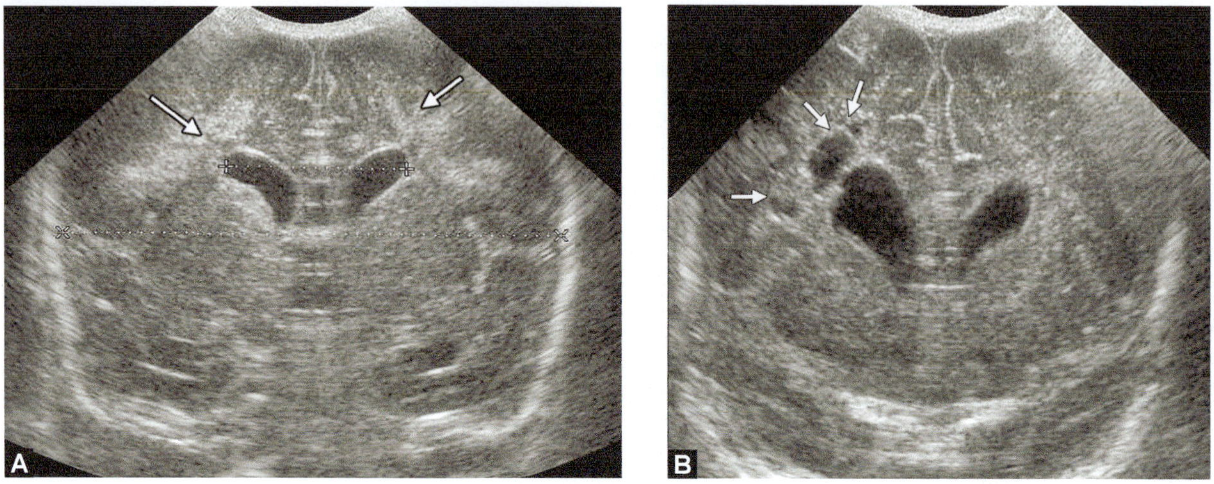

Figures 29.120A and B Progression of periventricular leukomalacia. (A) Coronal ultrasound scan at approximately 1 week of age shows increased periventricular echogenicity around the frontal horns of the lateral ventricles (arrows); (B) A follow-up ultrasound scan shows significant cavitation in the right frontal periventricular white matter (small arrows).

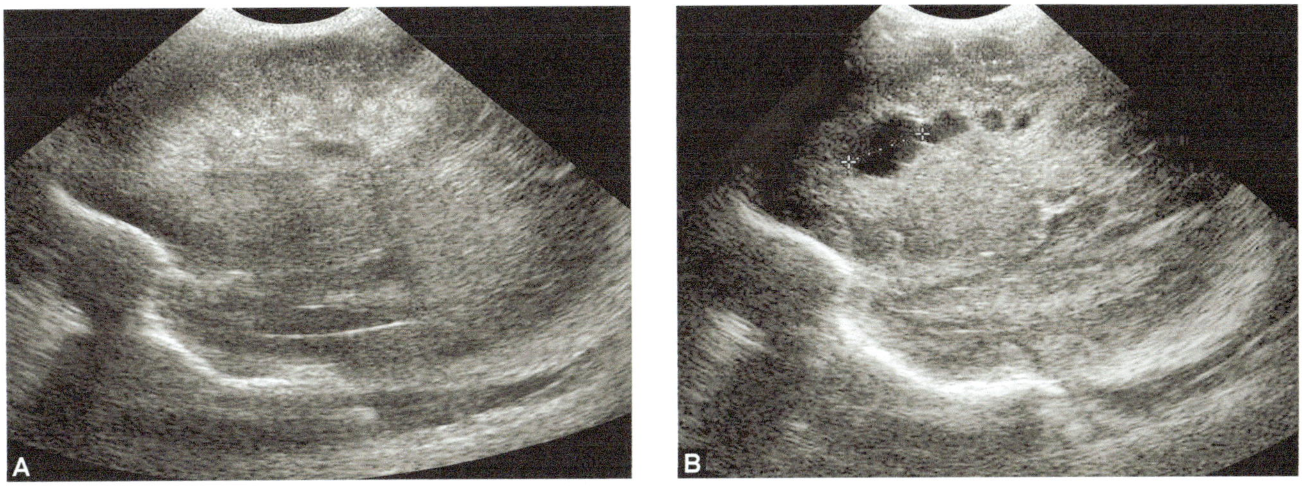

Figures 29.121A and B Periventricular leukomalacia. (A) Parasagittal ultrasound scan shows increased echogenicity in the white matter adjacent to the right lateral ventricle; (B) Follow-up scan shows cavitation in the same area, consistent with cystic periventricular leukomalacia.

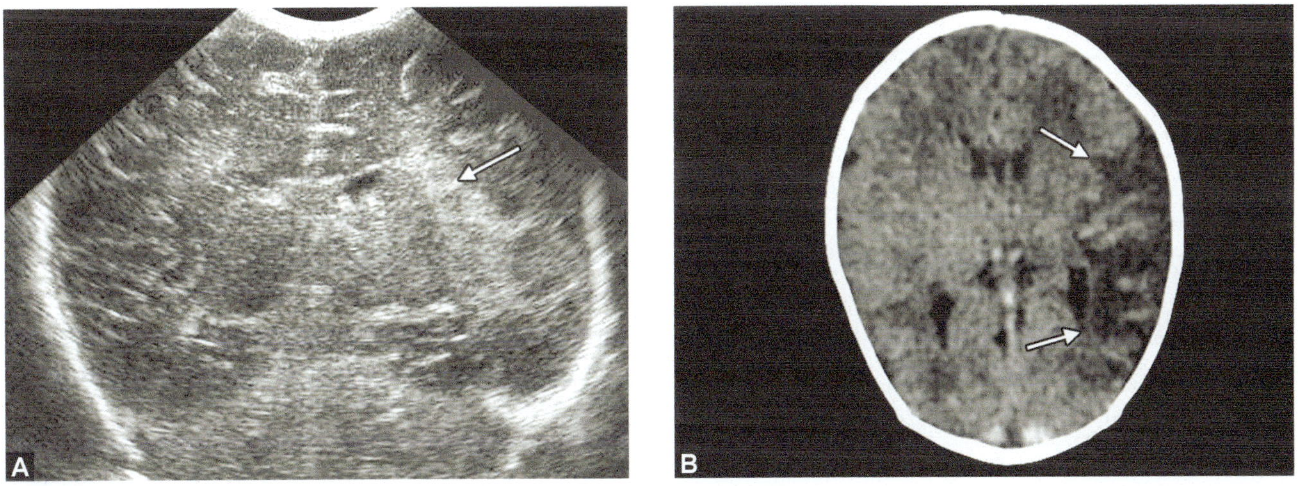

Figures 29.122A and B Left middle cerebral artery (MCA) territory infarct. (A) Coronal ultrasound scan in a neonate shows subtle increased echogenicity in the left MCA territory (arrow); (B) Unenhanced axial CT scan shows decreased attenuation (dark area) in the left MCA territory, consistent with an infarct (arrows).

the injured periventricular white matter approximately 2–3 weeks following the ischaemic insult.

Infarction (Figs. 29.122 to 29.124)

There are a number of causes of hypoxic-ischaemic brain infarction in infants and children. Cardiac causes, thrombotic conditions and metabolic diseases are a few categories of conditions responsible for strokes in the paediatric population.

Cranial ultrasound can be used to investigate neonates and infants in whom cerebral infarction is suspected. It is however less sensitive to CT and MR imaging in the detection of areas of hypoxic-ischaemic brain injury.

INFECTIONS, TUMOURS AND HYDROCEPHALUS

Congenital Brain Infection (Figs. 29.125A and B)

Congenital brain infection can be caused by cytomegalovirus, toxoplasmosis, herpes simplex virus, rubella, syphilis and human immunodeficiency virus. Radiological findings generally depend on the timing of the injury and the degree of brain destruction. Brain patterns identified include abnormal brain formation, periventricular white matter injury and intracranial calcification.

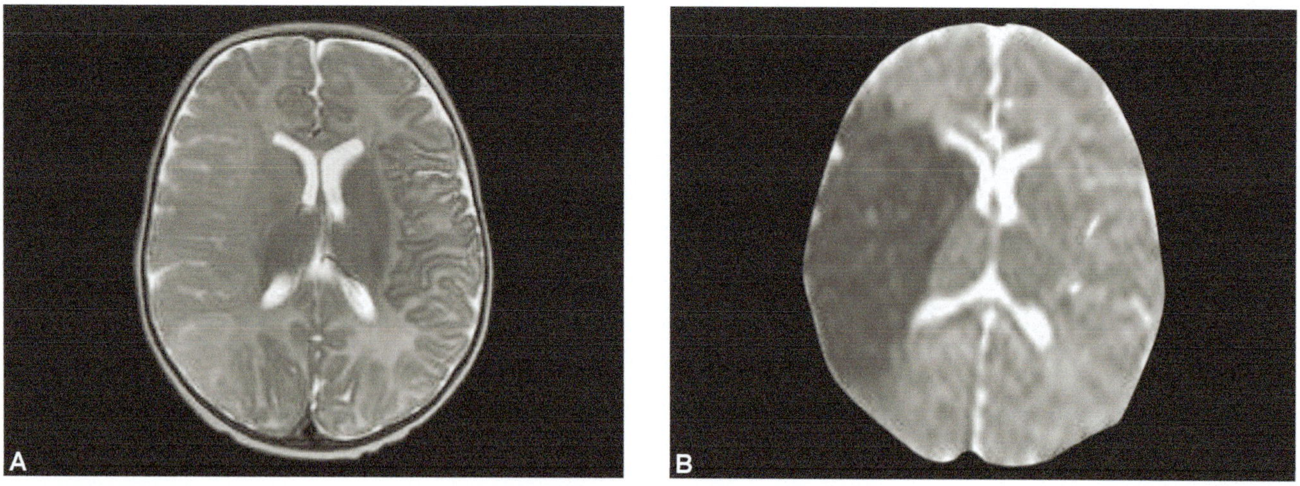

Figures 29.123A and B Right middle cerebral artery (MCA) territory infarct. (A) Axial T2 weighted MR image shows subtle swelling and loss of grey-white matter differentiation in the right MCA territory, consistent with an acute infarct; (B) ADC map of the diffusion sequence best demonstrates the acute infarct.

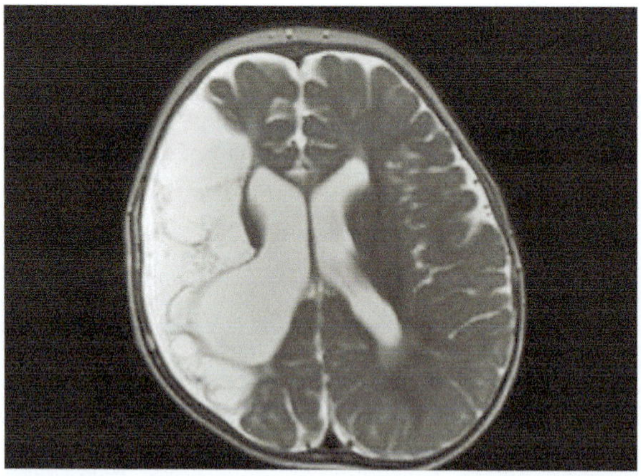

Figure 29.124 Established right middle cerebral artery (MCA) territory infarct. Axial T2 weighted MR image shows cystic change (encephalomalacia) in the right MCA territory, due to loss of brain tissue. The right lateral ventricle is enlarged due to the adjacent brain loss.

Brain Abscess (Fig. 29.126)

Pyogenic organisms causing brain infection can reach the brain by haematogenous spread from a distant infection, extension of infection from adjacent sites (sinus or middle ear infection), as a result of congenital heart disease, or as a complication of a penetrating wound or sinus tract. Cerebritis is the earliest stage of purulent brain infection. If undetected or untreated, it can develop into an abscess.

Tuberculous Meningitis (Figs. 29.127A and B)

Central nervous system manifestations of tuberculous (TB) infection include meningitis, tuberculoma, TB abscess or spinal leptomeningitis.

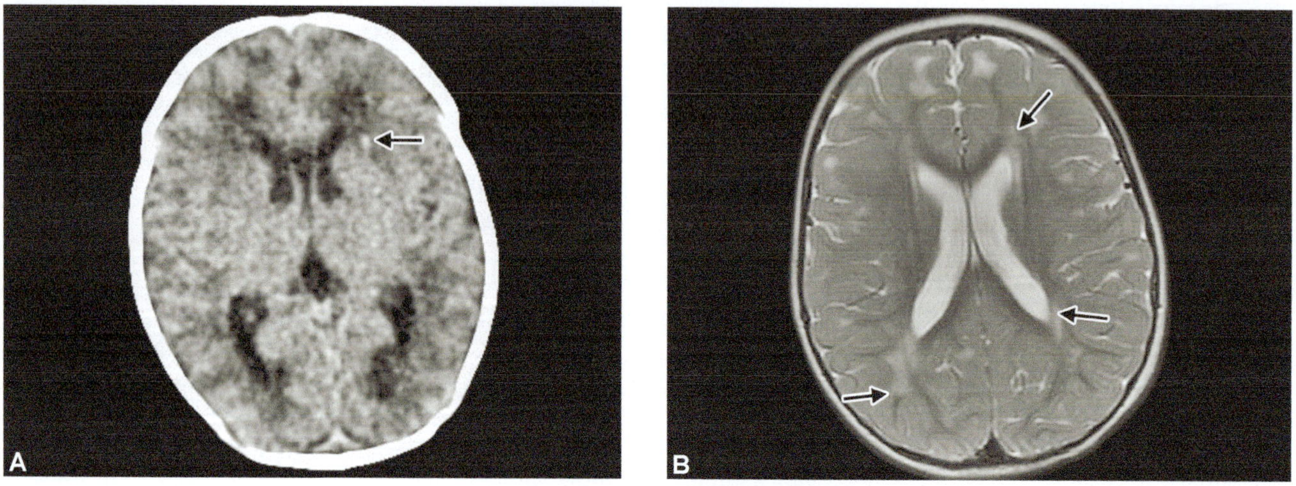

Figures 29.125A and B Congenital cytomegalovirus infection of the brain. (A) Unenhanced axial CT scan of brain shows a tiny area of periventricular calcification (arrow) near the frontal horn of the left lateral ventricle; (B) Axial T2 weighted MR image shows abnormal areas of increased signal in the periventricular and deep white matter (arrows).

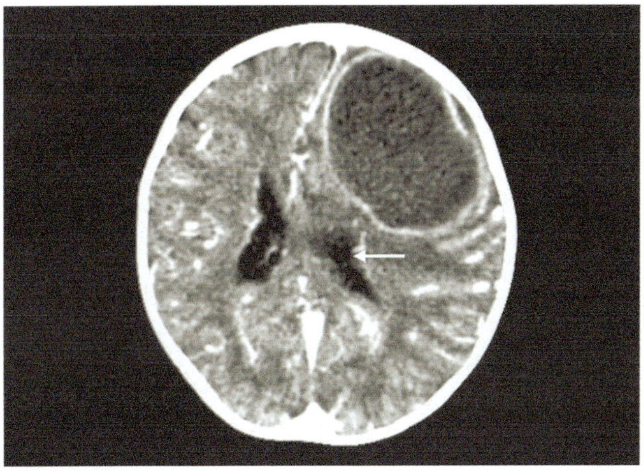

Figure 29.126 Left frontal lobe cerebral abscess in a child with congenital heart disease. Contrast enhanced axial CT scan of brain shows a large low density lesion in the left frontal lobe, with an enhancing rim. Note the distortion of the anterior midline brain structures (arrowheads) and the left lateral ventricle (thin arrow).

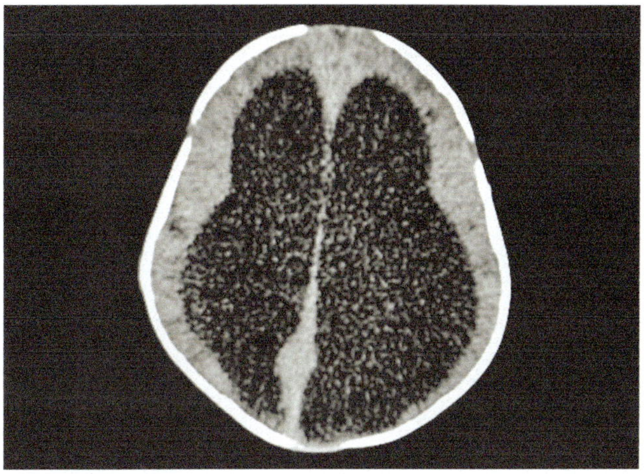

Figure 29.128 Hydrocephalus. Axial CT scan shows marked dilatation of both lateral ventricles.

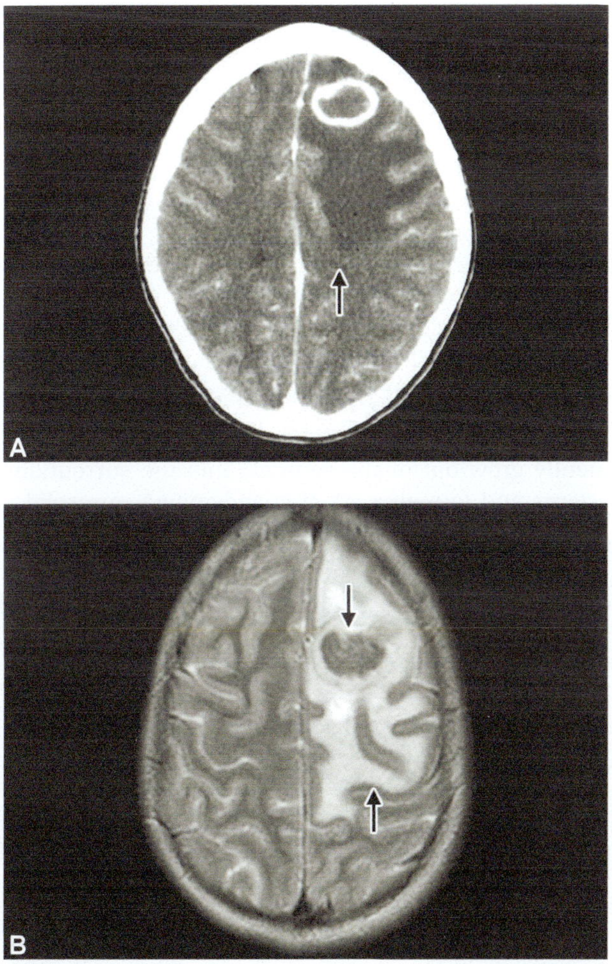

Figures 29.127A and B Left frontal lobe tuberculoma. (A) Contrast enhanced axial CT scan shows a ring enhancing lesion in the left frontal lobe of the brain. There is adjacent white matter oedema (arrow); (B) Axial T2 weighted MR brain image. The tuberculoma (black arrow) is isointense to brain. Note the adjacent white matter oedema (white arrow).

In TB meningitis, a thick exudate fills the basal cisterns. The basal cisterns on contrast enhanced scans. The thick exudate blocks the subarachnoid spaces, causing hydrocephalus. Another complication is small vessel disease which results in basal ganglia and thalamic infarcts.

Tuberculomas are ring enhancing lesions within the brain. They can be single or multiple.

Hydrocephalus (Figs. 29.128 and 29.129)

Hydrocephalus is a disorder where there is disturbance in the production, flow or absorption of cerebrospinal fluid (CSF). Consequently, there is increased CSF volume within the central nervous system, causing distension of the CSF pathways and increased pressure transmitted to the brain parenchyma.

Tumours

CT is usually the imaging modality employed in the initial diagnosis of intracranial tumours. However, MR is becoming the preferred study because of its multiplanar imaging capability, which is useful for surgical planning. Furthermore, it can image the spine. This is a prerequisite for the staging of intracranial neoplasms which metastasise to the spine.

Craniopharyngioma (Fig. 29.130)

On CT scanning, craniopharyngiomas are identified as mass lesions in the suprasellar region, composed of cystic areas and calcification.

Medulloblastoma (Figs. 29.131 to 29.133)

A medulloblastoma on CT scanning is usually a dense neoplasm arising from the cerebellar vermis. Cystic

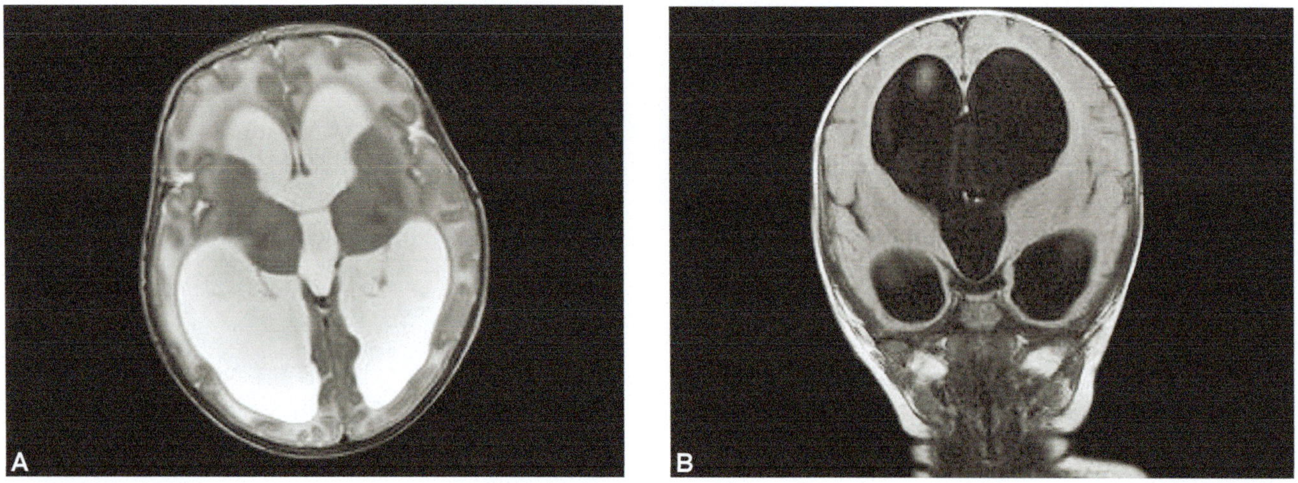

Figures 29.129A and B Examples of hydrocephalus on MR imaging. (A) Axial T2 weighted MR scan demonstrates marked dilatation of both lateral ventricles and the third ventricle (arrow); (B) Coronal MR image from another patient also shows hydrocephalus involving both lateral ventricles and the third ventricle.

change can be seen in approximately 50% of tumours and calcification in up to 20%. The tumours enhance with intravenous contrast. Hydrocephalus is usually present at the time of diagnosis.

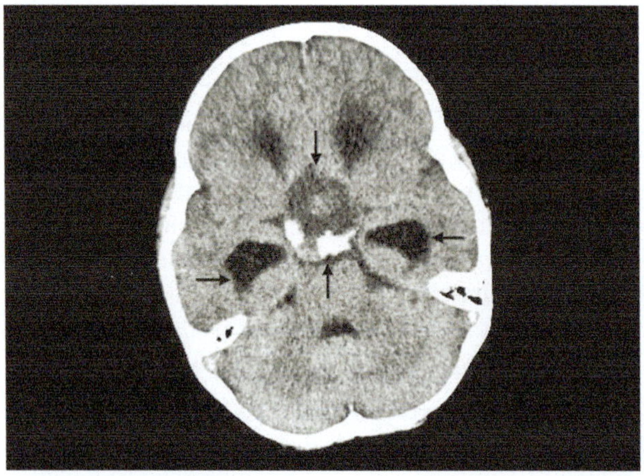

Figure 29.130 Craniopharyngioma. Unenhanced axial CT brain scan shows a cystic (white arrow) and calcified (black arrow) lesion in the suprasellar region. Note the hydrocephalus affecting the lateral ventricles with marked dilatation of the temporal horns (small arrows).

Cerebellar Astrocytoma (Figs. 29.134 and 29.135)

The cerebellar astrocytoma arises from the vermis or the cerebellar hemisphere. Most tumours are cystic with a tumour nodule located in the cyst wall. The mural nodule enhances with contrast. Hydrocephalus is usually present due to compression of the fourth ventricle.

Ependymoma (Figs. 29.136A and B)

Ependymomas arise from the fourth ventricle and frequently grow out of the ventricle into the surrounding cisterns and foramina. Most ependymomas are solid in

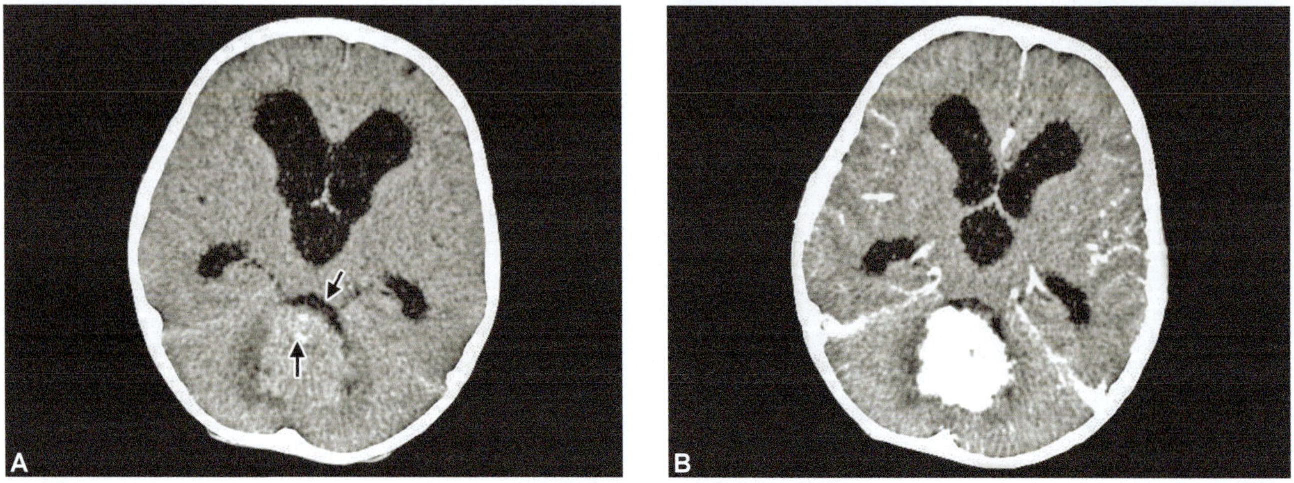

Figures 29.131A and B Medulloblastoma. (A) Unenhanced axial CT scan shows dense mass lesion situated within the cerebellar vermis, containing a small area of calcification (black arrow). The tumour is impinging upon the fourth ventricle (white arrow), restricting CSF flow and consequently there is hydrocephalus of the lateral and third ventricles; (B) After injection of intravenous contrast, there is marked tumour enhancement.

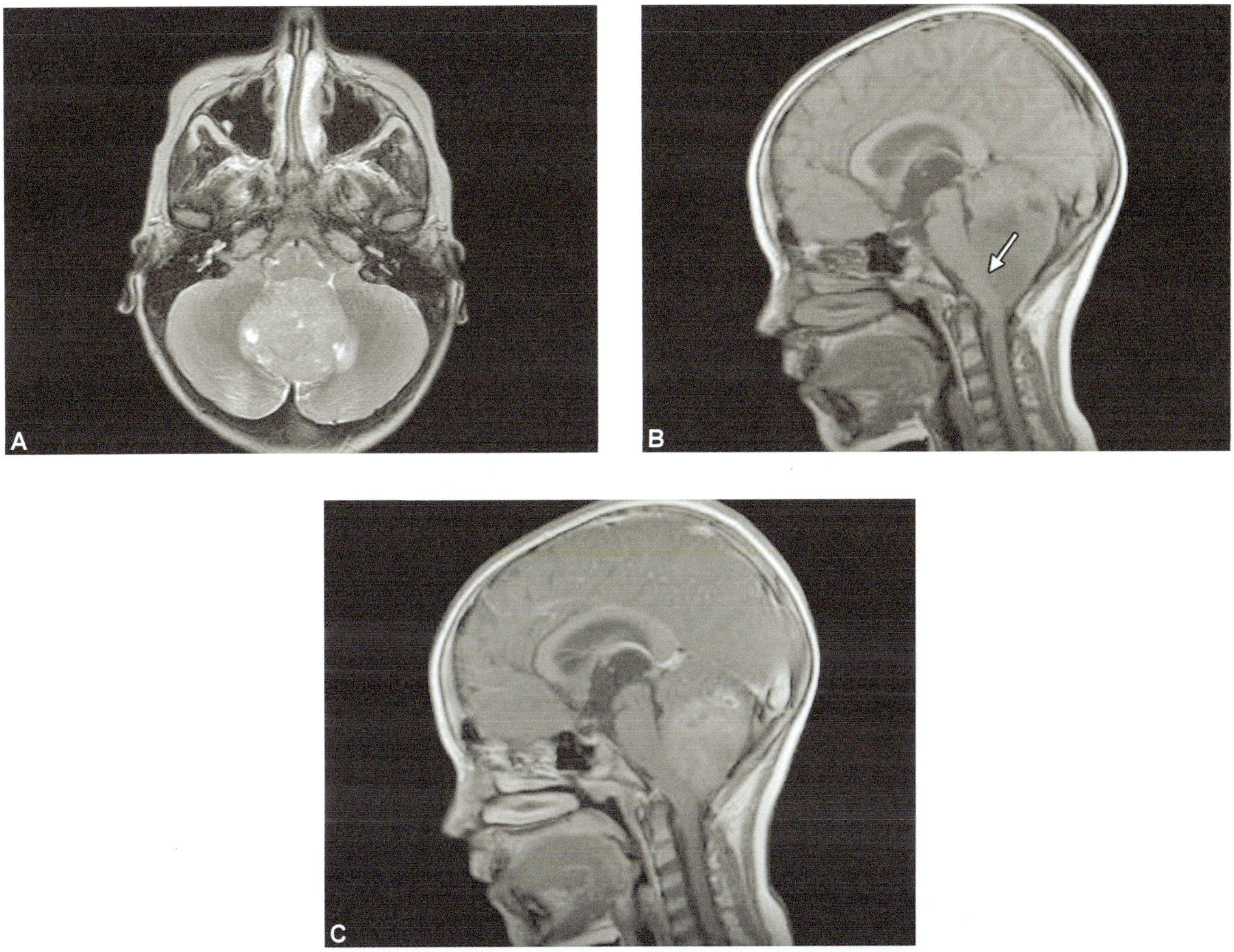

Figures 29.132A to C Medulloblastoma. (A) Axial T2 weighted MR image shows a midline posterior fossa mass which is of increased signal intensity relative to the cerebellum; (B) Sagittal T1 weighted MR image shows the mass to be hypointense on this sequence. The mass is obstructing the fourth ventricle (arrow); (C) Sagittal T1 weighted MR image following intravenous contrast. The tumour demonstrates enhancement with contrast.

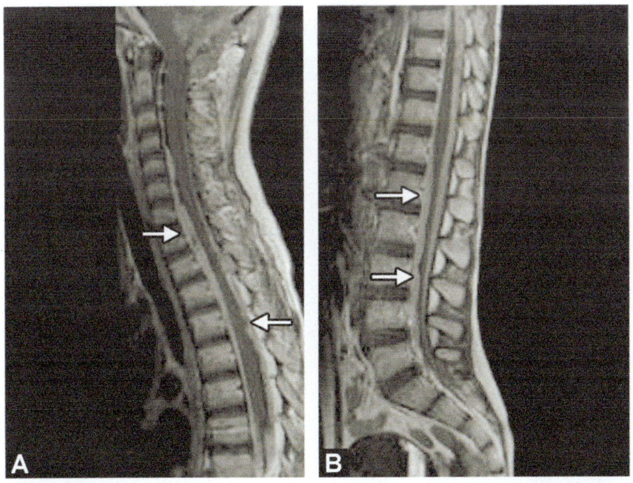

Figures 29.133A and B Medulloblastoma spinal metastatic disease. Post-contrast T1 weighted sagittal MR scans of the whole spine show nodular tumour enhancement along the entire cord (arrows) consistent with spinal metastatic disease.

nature. Calcification is seen in up to 50% of tumours and cystic change in about 20%. Hydrocephalus is usually present at diagnosis.

Brainstem Glioma (Figs. 29.137A to D)

Because of its location, MR is the best imaging modality for assessing the brainstem glioma. It allows multiplanar assessment of the tumour. In contrast to CT scanning, there is no bony artefact from the adjacent skull base.

Most brainstem gliomas arise from the pons. The tumour may be focal or diffuse and typically expands the pons. Tumour enhancement with intravenous contrast agents is variable.

Retinoblastoma (Figs. 29.138 to 29.140)

Retinoblastoma is the most common orbital malignancy and is almost universally a tumour of infancy. The tumour can be unilateral or bilateral. Calcification is present in excess of 90% of tumours.

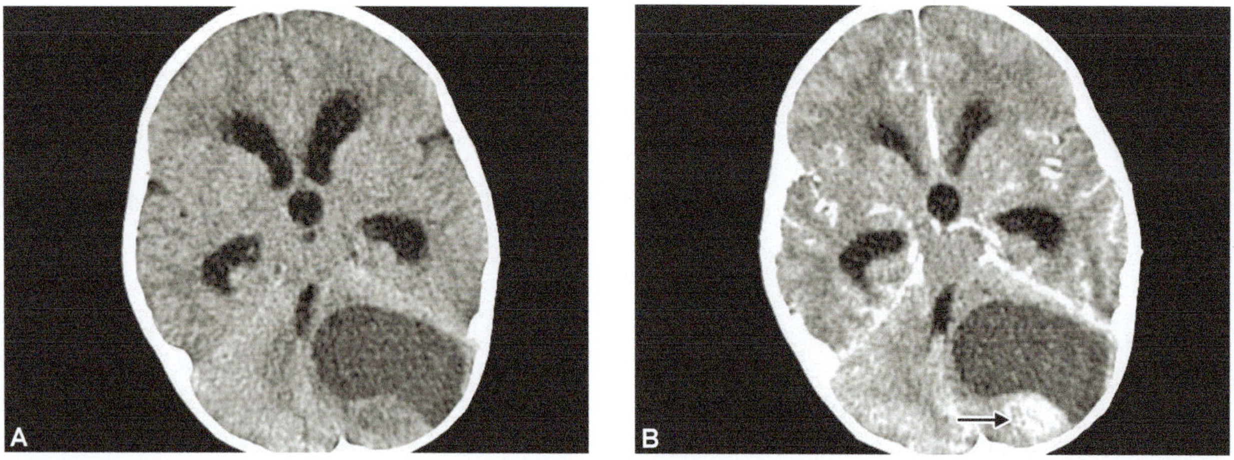

Figures 29.134A and B Pilocytic astrocytoma. (A) Unenhanced axial CT scan shows a cystic mass centred on the left cerebellar hemisphere. It distorts the fourth ventricle and there is hydrocephalus of the third and lateral ventricles; (B) Following intravenous contrast infusion, there is marked enhancement of a mural nodule in the posterior aspect of the cystic tumour (arrow).

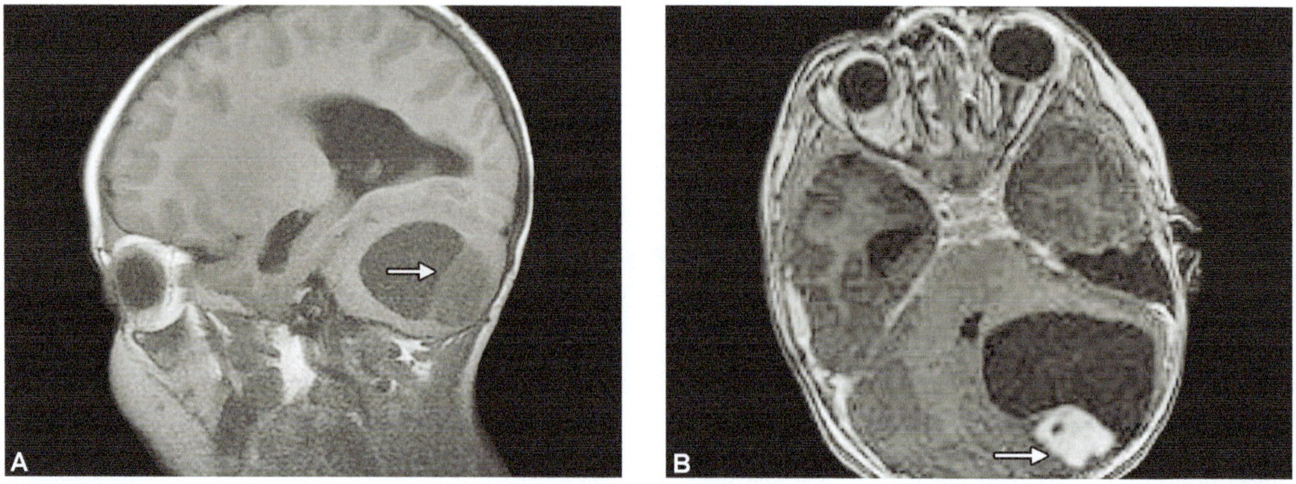

Figures 29.135A and B Pilocytic astrocytoma. (A) Sagittal T1 weighted MR image shows a hypointense cystic tumour in the cerebellum. The mural nodule is situated posteriorly within the tumour (arrow); (B) Axial T1 weighted MR image shows intense enhancement of the tumour nodule following intravenous contrast administration (arrow).

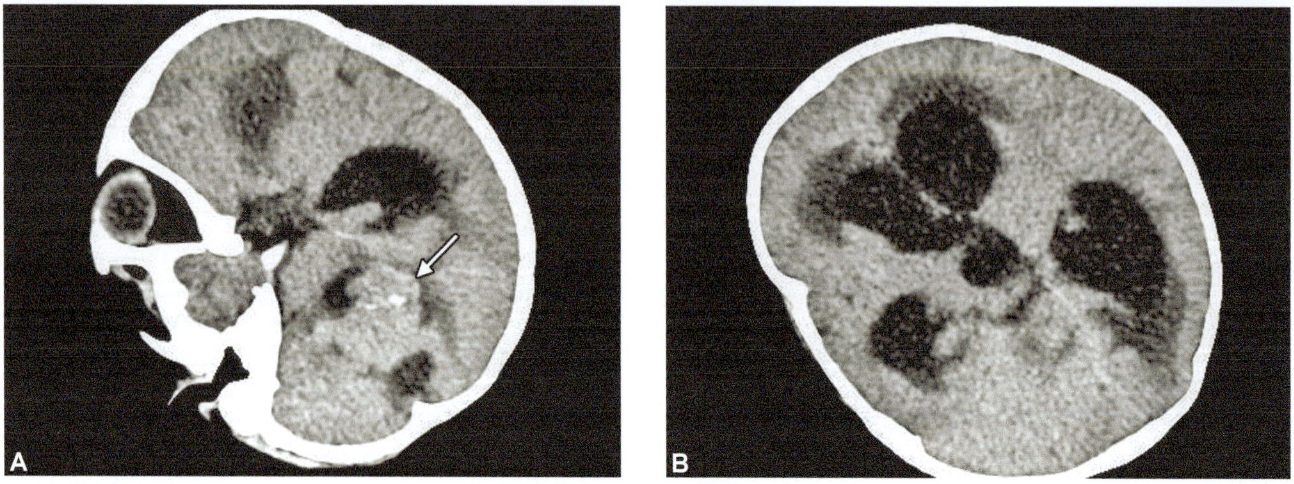

Figures 29.136A and B Ependymoma. (A) Unenhanced axial CT scan through the posterior cranial fossa shows an isodense mass (arrow) containing punctate calcification, arising from the fourth ventricle; (B) Axial image from a higher level shows hydrocephalus affecting the lateral ventricles and the third ventricle.

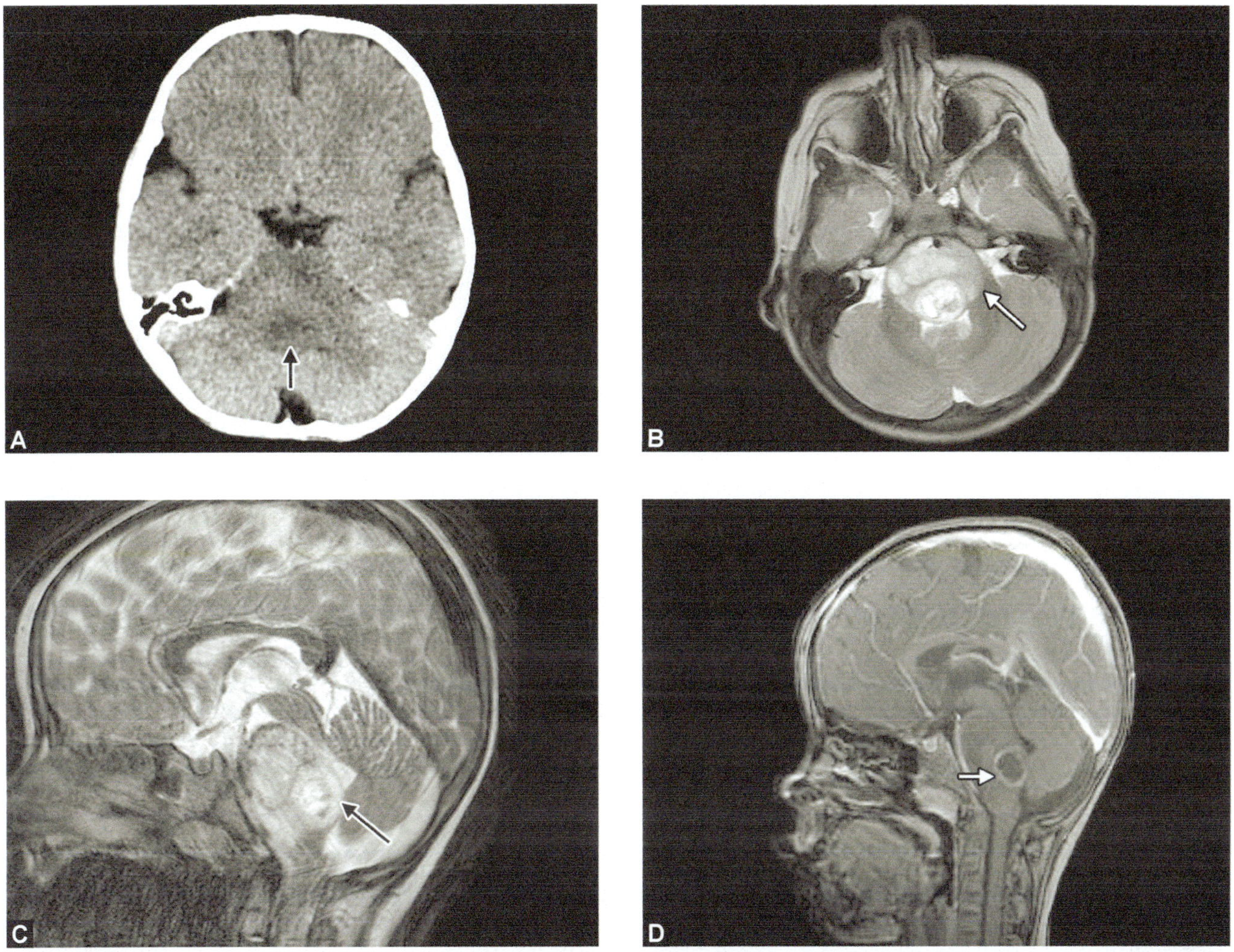

Figures 29.137A to D Brainstem glioma. (A) Axial unenhanced CT scan shows a poorly defined low density mass in the pons (arrow); (B) Axial; (C) Sagittal T2 weighted MR images show a heterogeneous mass of increased signal intensity expanding the pons (arrow). There is minor distortion of the fourth ventricle; (D) T1 weighted sagittal MR scan following intravenous contrast administration. There is peripheral enhancement of a cystic area posteriorly within the tumour (arrow). The remainder of pontine glioma is poorly enhancing.

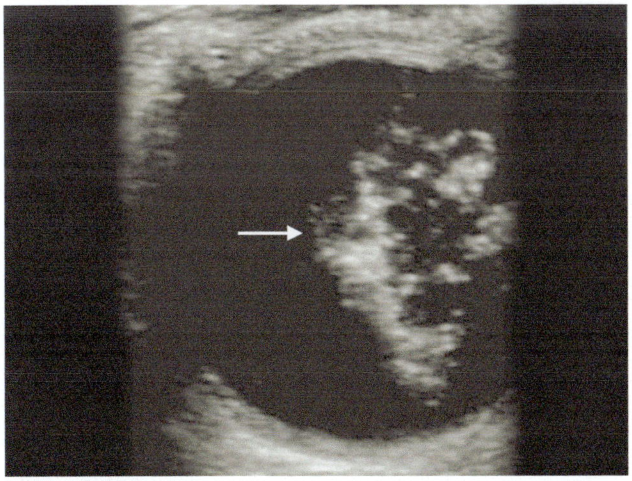

Figure 29.138 Retinoblastoma. Ultrasound scan of right globe reveals an irregular mass (arrow) containing multiple specks of calcification.

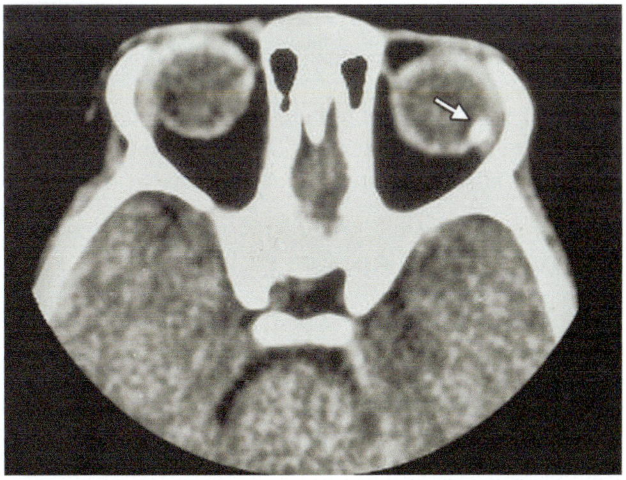

Figure 29.139 Retinoblastoma left orbit. Unenhanced axial CT scan through the orbits shows a small calcified lesion arising from the retina in the temporal aspect of the left globe (arrow).

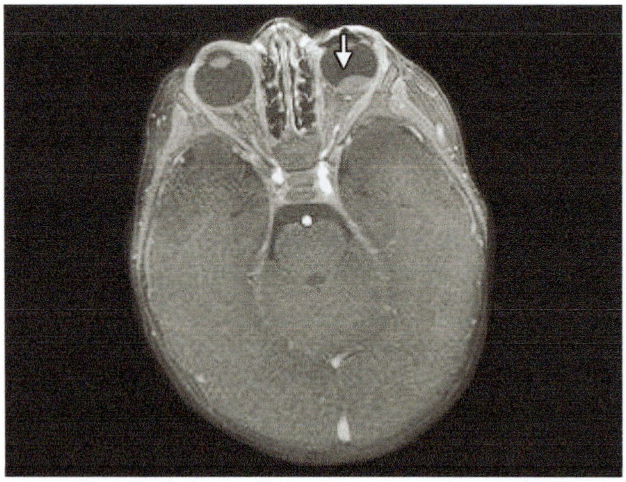

Figure 29.140 Left-sided retinoblastoma, axial T1 weighted MR image (fat saturated and post-contrast administration) shows an enhancing mass lesion situated posteriorly within the left globe (arrow).

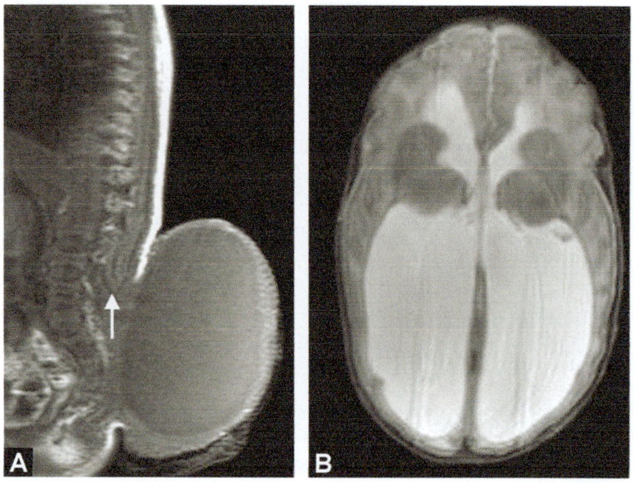

Figures 29.141A and B Myelomeningocoele and hydrocephalus. (A) Sagittal T1 weighted MR image of the lower spine shows a large lumbosacral meningocoele. The spinal cord is stretched and can be identified passing through the posterior spinal defect (arrow); (B) Axial T2 weighted MR image of the brain shows marked dilatation of the lateral ventricles due to hydrocephalus.

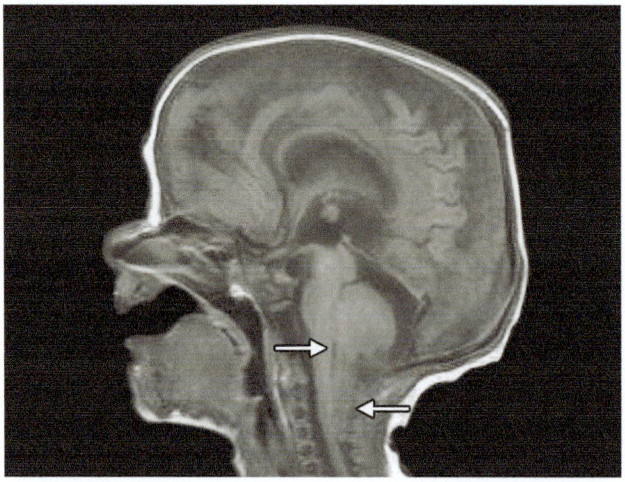

Figure 29.142 Chiari II malformation. Sagittal T1 weighted MR image shows a small posterior cranial fossa and inferior displacement of the cerebellum through the foramen magnum (white arrow). The fourth ventricle is narrow and displaced caudally (white arrow).

On CT scanning, the retinoblastoma is identified as a calcified mass within the globe, arising from the retina. It usually enhances with intravenous contrast.

CONGENITAL SPINE LESIONS

Myelomeningocoele (Figs. 29.141A and B)

Myelomeningocoele results from impaired closure of the caudal end of the neural tube. This results in an open lesion or sac containing abnormal spinal cord, nerve roots and meninges, which herniate through a posterior defect in the vertebral column.

Closure of the spinal defect is usually performed within 48 hours of delivery and consequently imaging studies of the spine are rarely performed preoperatively.

Myelomeningocoele is associated with the Chiari II malformation (Fig. 29.142). The malformation is associated with caudal displacement of the medulla, fourth ventricle and cerebellum into the cervical spinal canal. Consequently, there is elongation of the pons and fourth ventricle. In combination, these features impede the flow and absorption of CSF causing hydrocephalus, usually after surgical closure of the spinal defect.

Diastematomyelia (Figs. 29.143A to C)

Diastematomyelia is the sagittal division of the spinal cord into two hemicords by a bony or cartilaginous spur, or fibrous septum. MRI is the preferred modality for imaging children with suspected diastematomyelia. The defect is most commonly found in the lumbar region.

Sacrococcygeal Teratoma (Figs. 29.144 and 29.145)

This is a rare congenital tumour that develops in the sacrococcygeal region. The tumour usually presents as an external mass protruding from the gluteal cleft or the perineum. The tumour is divided into four types:

Type I: Tumours are predominantly external, situated posteriorly, and have only a minimal presacral component

Type II: Tumours have significant pelvic extension but the external portion predominates

Type III: Tumours have a predominant internal component although the external component is still visible

Type IV: Tumours are entirely presacral without any external component.

Plain films will demonstrate a large soft-tissue mass associated with the lower sacrum and coccyx.

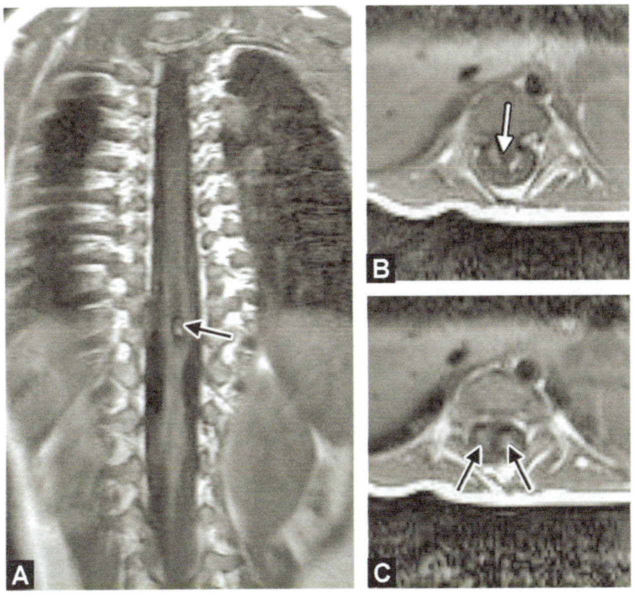

Figures 29.143A to C Diastematomyelia. (A) Coronal and (B) axial T1 weighted MR images show a bony spur (arrow) extending posteriorly from a vertebral body in the lower thoracic spine, splitting the spinal cord into two hemicords; (C) Axial T1 weighted MR image obtained above the level of the bony spur shows the hemicords (arrows).

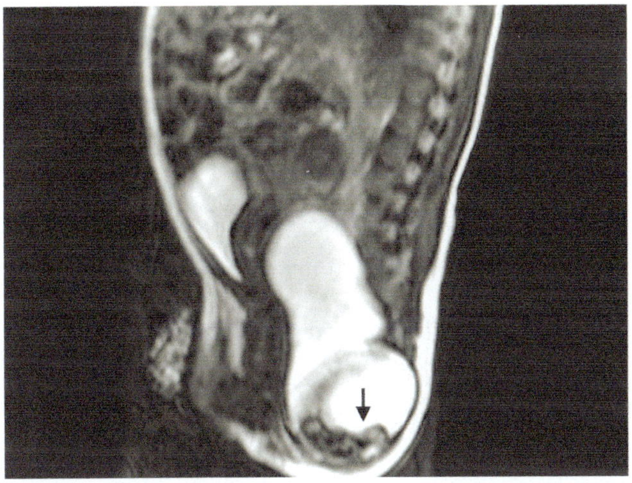

Figure 29.145 Sacrococcygeal teratoma. Sagittal T2 weighted MR image demonstrates a large cystic structure in the presacral region. Some solid elements are present inferiorly within the lesion (arrow). There is significant anterior displacement of the rectum and bladder by the mass. This is a type III tumour since it has a small external component.

Approximately two-thirds of tumours will contain calcification.

PAEDIATRIC SKELETAL RADIOLOGY

Skeletal Dysplasias

Thanatophoric Dysplasia (Figs. 29.146A to C)

Radiographic findings:

- Skull: Proportionately large skull relative to trunk

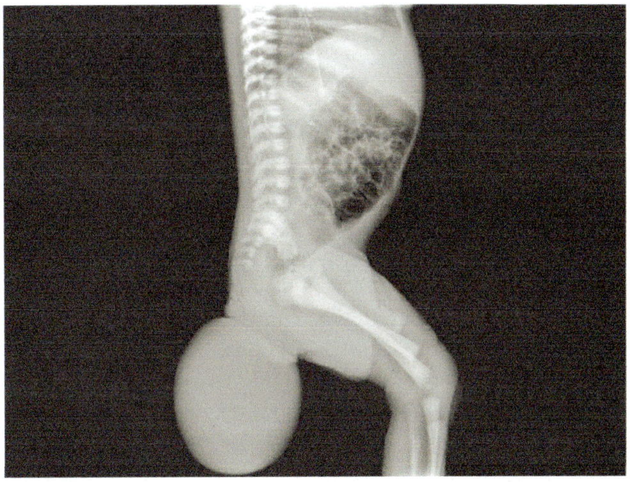

Figure 29.144 Sacrococcygeal teratoma in a neonate. Lateral radiograph shows a large exophytic soft-tissue mass arising from the gluteal region. The lower density area within the lesion represents fat.

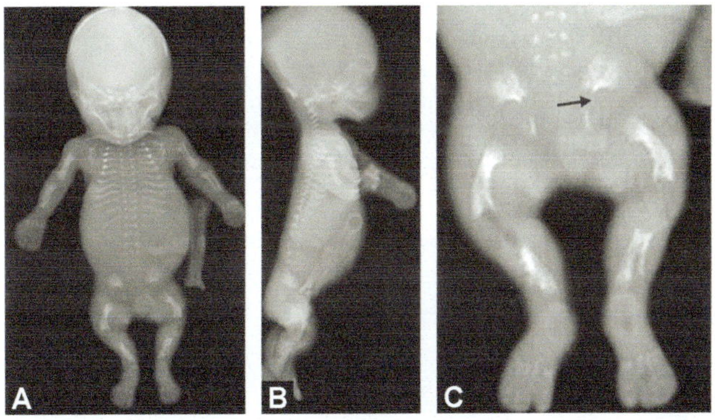

Figures 29.146A to C Thanatophoric dysplasia. (A) The head is proportionately large and the trunk is long and narrow. There is marked rib shortening and the scapulae are small. There is shortening of the long bones of the limbs (micromelia)—note the French telephone receiver femurs. The vertebral bodies are flat and H-shaped; (B) Lateral view shows the flattened vertebrae and the proportionately large skull; (C) Coned view of the pelvis and lower limbs demonstrates small, flared iliac wings, narrowed sacrosciatic notches (black arrow) and horizontal acetabula.

- Thorax: Long narrow trunk with very short ribs, small abnormal scapulae
- Spine: Small, flat vertebrae with U or H shaped vertebrae in the AP projection
- Pelvis: Small flared iliac wings, narrow sacrosciatic notches and flat acetabula
- Limbs: Long bone shortening and bowing; French telephone receiver femurs
- Hands and feet: Marked shortening and broadening of the tubular bones.

Achondroplasia (Figs. 29.147 and 29.148)

Radiographic findings:

- Skull: Large skull with relatively small base and mid face hypoplasia

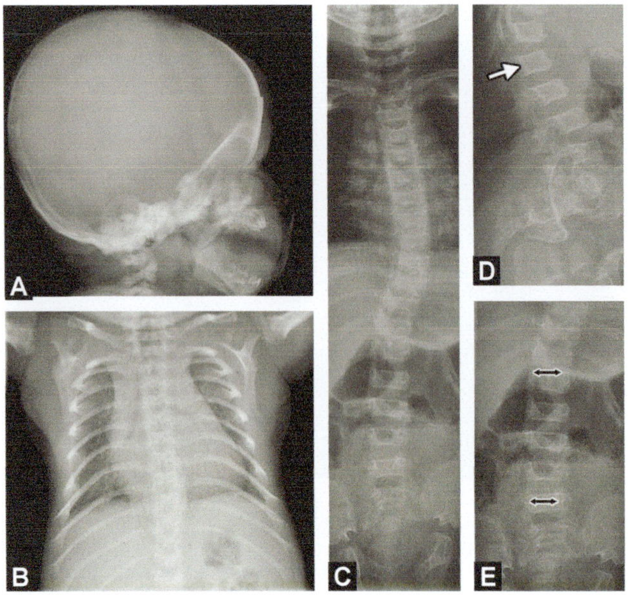

Figures 29.147A to E Achondroplasia in a newborn. (A) Large skull with mid face hypoplasia; (B) Small thorax with short ribs; (C) AP and lateral views of spine show a thoracolumbar kyphoscoliosis. The lateral view shows posterior vertebral body scalloping (arrow) and a horizontal sacrum; (D and E) AP view of lumbar spine demonstrates gradual reduction in interpediculate distance caudally (arrows).

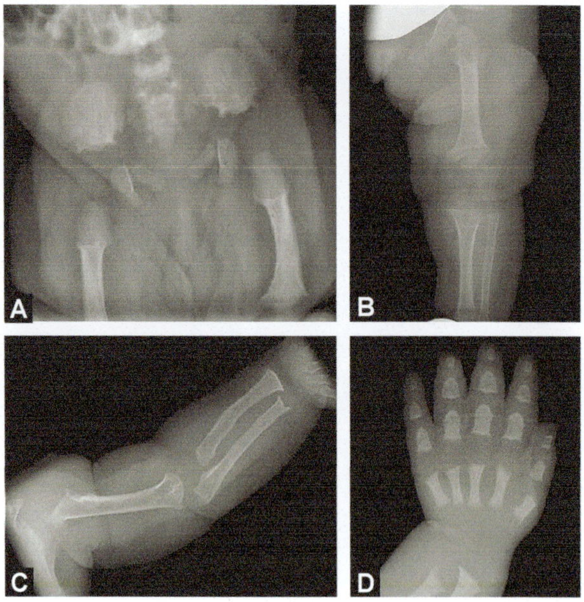

Figures 29.148A to D Achondroplasia in neonate. (A) The pelvis X-ray shows flared iliac bones, flat acetabular roofs and narrow sacrosciatic notches; (B and C) Limb X-rays show shortening of the long bones; (D) Hand: short and broad metacarpal and phalangeal bones.

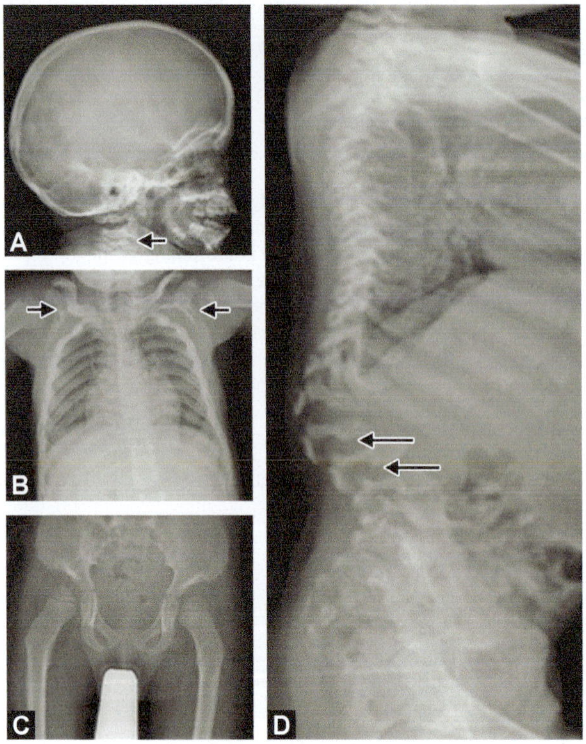

Figures 29.149A to D Hurler syndrome. (A) Lateral radiograph demonstrates an enlarged skull. The dens is hypoplastic (arrow); (B) Frontal chest X-ray shows thickened clavicles and broad ribs. The glenoid fossae are poorly formed (arrows); (C) The pelvic X-ray demonstrates small, flared iliac wings and steep acetabular roofs; (D) The lateral spine film features a thoracolumbar gibbus, and antero-inferior beaking of the vertebrae at the apex of the gibbus (arrows).

- Thorax: Small short ribs which are splayed anteriorly
- Spine: Short flat vertebral bodies. Short pedicles with decreasing interpedicular distance caudally in lumbar spine. Posterior scalloping of vertebral bodies
- Pelvis: Champagne glass appearance of pelvis. Flared iliac wings, narrow sacrosciatic notches and flat acetabular roofs
- Limbs: Short and thick tubular bones, flared metaphyses
- Hands: Shortening and broadening of metacarpal and phalangeal bones.

MUCOPOLYSACCHARIDOSES

Mucopolysaccharidosis 1-H (Hurler Syndrome) (Figs. 29.149 and 29.150)

Radiographic findings:

- Skull: Large skull with abnormal J-shaped sella
- Thorax: Short thick clavicles, broad 'oar-shaped' ribs and hypoplastic glenoid
- Spine: Antero-inferior beaking of thoracolumbar vertebral bodies, atlantoaxial subluxation due to hypoplastic dens
- Pelvis: Small, flared iliac wings; steep
- Limbs: Widening of the midshaft of long bones
- Hands: Widening of the diaphyses of the metacarpals and proximal and middle phalanges; phalangeal shortening; small and irregular carpal bones, pointed proximal ends of the metacarpals.

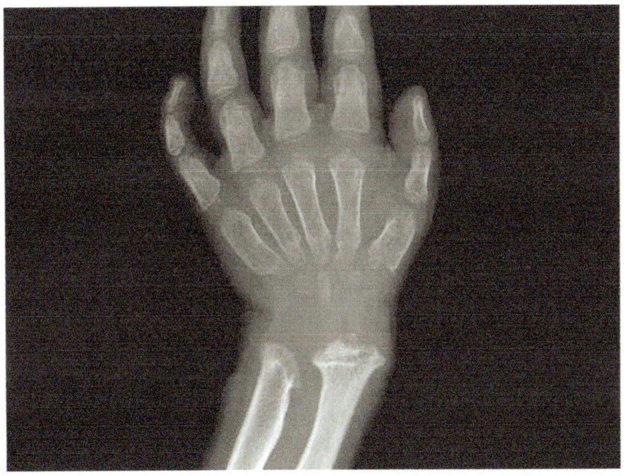

Figure 29.150 Hurler syndrome: Hand radiograph. X-ray of right hand reveals widening of the diaphyses of the metacarpals and proximal and middle phalanges. The phalanges are short. The carpal bones are small and irregular. There is proximal tapering of the metacarpals. The distal radius and ulna tilt towards each other.

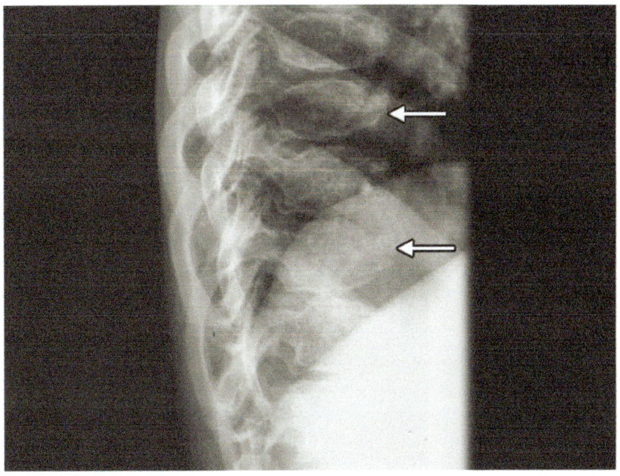

Figure 29.151 Morquio syndrome. Lateral radiograph of lower thoracic spine demonstrates decreased height of the vertebral bodies (platyspondyly). Note the central anterior bony protrusion or breaking of the vertebral bodies (arrows).

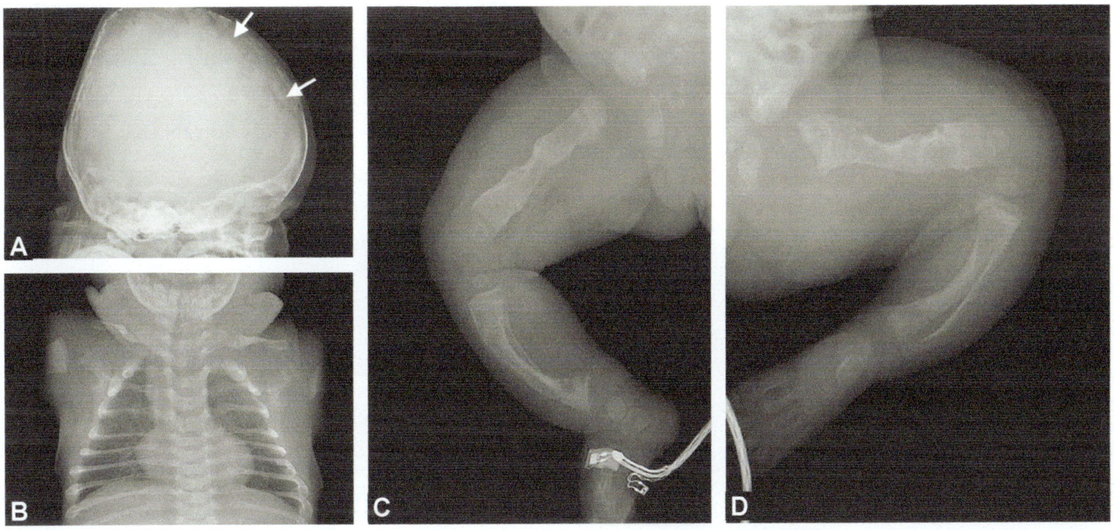

Figures 29.152A to D Osteogenesis imperfecta in a neonate. (A) Lateral skull film shows multiple intrasutural (Wormian) bones (arrows); (B) Chest radiograph demonstrates multiple healing rib fractures giving the ribs a beaded appearance. There is also a healing left clavicular fracture; (C and D) There are multiple fractures within both lower limbs. The femurs are short and crumpled due to healing fractures and there is bowing deformity of the tibia and fibula bilaterally. The bones are osteopenic.

Mucopolysaccharidosis IV (Morquio Syndrome)

Radiographic findings (Fig. 29.151):

- Thorax: Flaring of ribs
- Spine: Platyspondyly within thoracolumbar spine; central anterior bony beaking; odontoid hypoplasia and atlantoaxial instability
- Pelvis: Steeply oblique acetabular roofs; defective irregular ossification of femoral heads (FHs) leading to flattening
- Limbs: Widening of the long bone diaphyses; irregular metaphyses
- Hands: Small, irregular carpal bones; proximal tapering of metacarpals.

Osteogenesis Imperfecta (Figs. 29.152 and 29.153)

There are a several types of osteogenesis imperfecta. The radiographic findings are variable and depend upon the type and severity of the disease.

Radiographic findings:

- Skull: Variable decreased ossification, abnormal number of Wormian bones (small bones within the cranial sutures)

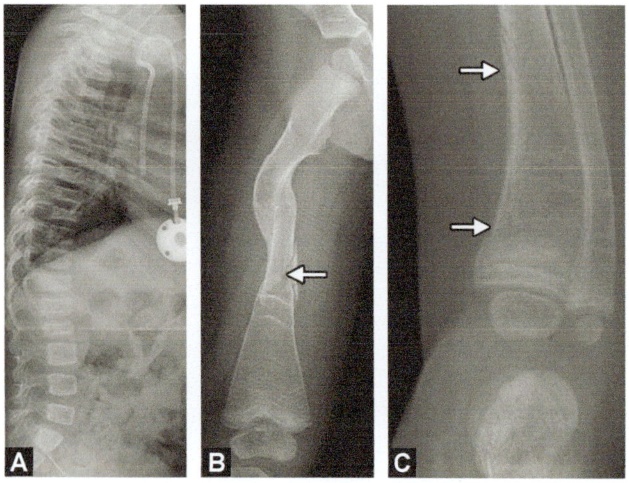

Figures 29.153A to C Osteogenesis imperfecta in an older child. (A) The lateral spine X-ray shows wedging and collapse of several vertebral bodies. The child has a Portacath device in situ for intravenous biphosphonate treatment; (B) Right leg is in a plaster cast due to a recent mid shaft spiral fracture of the right femur (arrow). There is also an older healing fracture in the proximal shaft; (C) There are fractures within the distal left tibia (arrows). Note the osteopenia. There is also lateral bowing of the distal tibia and fibula.

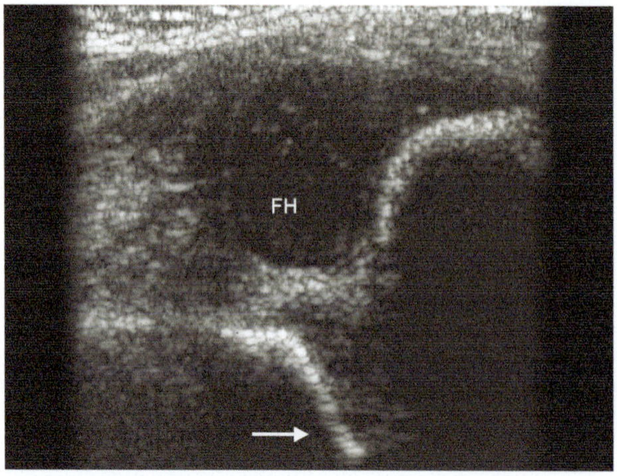

Figure 29.155 Decentered hip. Coronal ultrasound scan shows the cartilaginous femoral head lies out with the bony acetabular roof (arrow).

- Spine: Wedged or collapsed vertebrae, kyphoscoliosis
- Remainder of skeleton: Osteoporosis and fractures

PAEDIATRIC HIP ABNORMALITIES

Developmental Dysplasia of the Hip (Figs. 29.154 to 29.157)

Developmental dysplasia of the hip (DDH) can be diagnosed radiologically using ultrasound or X-ray. Ultrasound is the preferred imaging modality in neonates since the neonatal hip is composed almost entirely of cartilage, thereby making it difficult to establish the relationship of the FH to the acetabulum on radiographs.

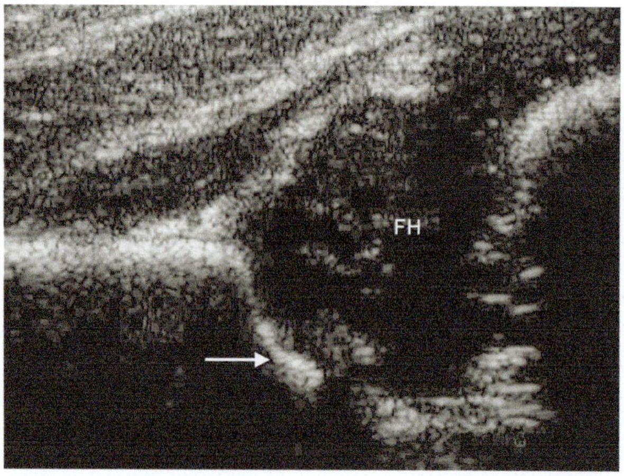

Figure 29.154 Normal hip ultrasound. Coronal ultrasound scan of hip shows the femoral head covered by the bony acetabular roof (arrow) and acetabular labrum (arrowheads).

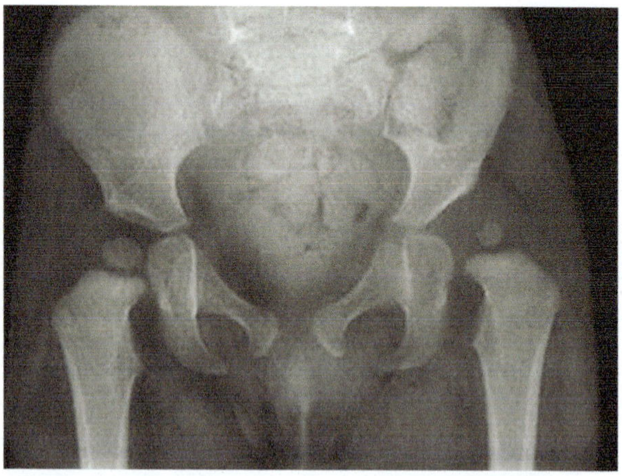

Figure 29.156 Developmental dysplasia of hip and dislocation. There is increased slope of the left bony acetabulum. The left femoral head ossification centre is hypoplastic. The left femoral head is dislocated superiorly and laterally. The right hip is normal.

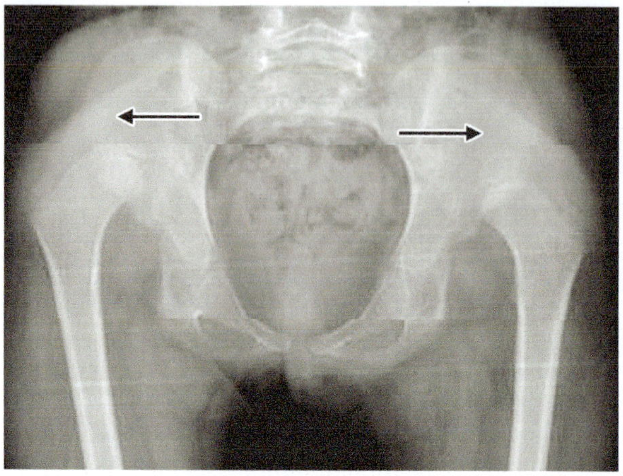

Figure 29.157 Late diagnosis of bilateral developmental dysplasia of the hip in a four-year-old girl. Both hips are dislocated superiorly and laterally and articulate with pseudoacetabula (arrows).

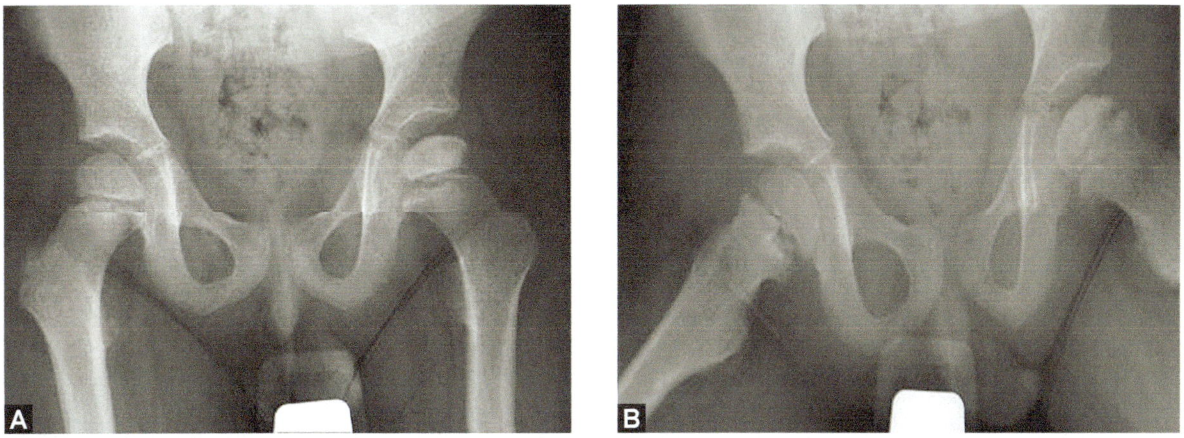

Figures 29:158A and B Legg–Calvé–Perthes disease left hip. (A and B) Frontal and frog-leg lateral radiographs demonstrate flattening, irregularity, fragmentation and sclerosis of the left capital femoral epiphysis. The right capital femoral epiphysis is normal.

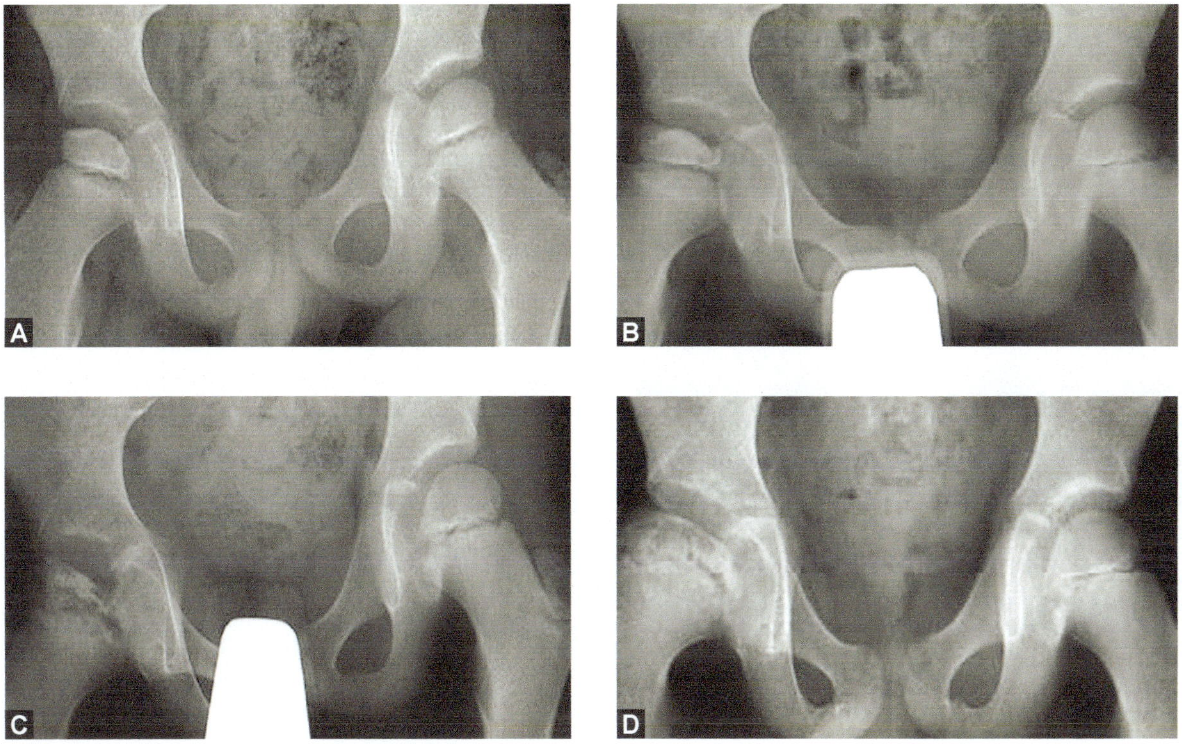

Figures 29.159A to D Serial radiographic changes of Legg–Calvé–Perthes disease of right hip. (A) Radiograph at presentation demonstrates flattening and sclerosis of the right capital femoral epiphysis; (B) Radiograph 5 months later reveals further loss of epiphyseal height; (C) Ten months later, there is marked fragmentation and flattening of the right capital femoral epiphysis; (D) Two and a half years after the onset, the capital femoral epiphysis has healed but is flatter and wider to fit the widened femoral neck.

By 4–6 months of age, the FH ossifies and radiographs are then used to evaluate infants with suspected DDH. The radiographic findings in DDH are as follows:

- Increased slope of bony acetabulum (acetabular dysplasia)
- Delayed growth of the FH ossification centre compared to the normal side
- A pseudoacetabulum, which is a late radiographic sign in DDH.

Legg–Calvé–Perthes Disease (Figs. 29.158 and 29.159)

Legg-Calvé-Perthes disease is avascular necrosis of the proximal (capital) femoral epiphysis. The peak incidence is 6–8 years of age. The disease can be bilateral.

The radiographic findings include flattening, sclerosis and fragmentation of the capital femoral epiphysis. Early subchondral fractures can be detected on frog lateral views as a curvilinear lucency within the epiphysis.

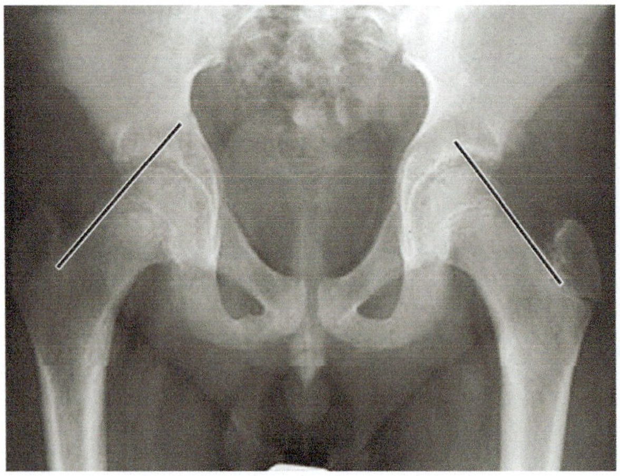

Figure 29.160 Slipped right capital femoral epiphysis. Frontal radiograph of the pelvis demonstrates medial slippage of the right capital femoral epiphysis. A line drawn along the lateral femoral neck on the normal left side intersects a portion of the femoral epiphysis. However, a similar line drawn along the lateral aspect of the right femoral neck just misses the epiphysis.

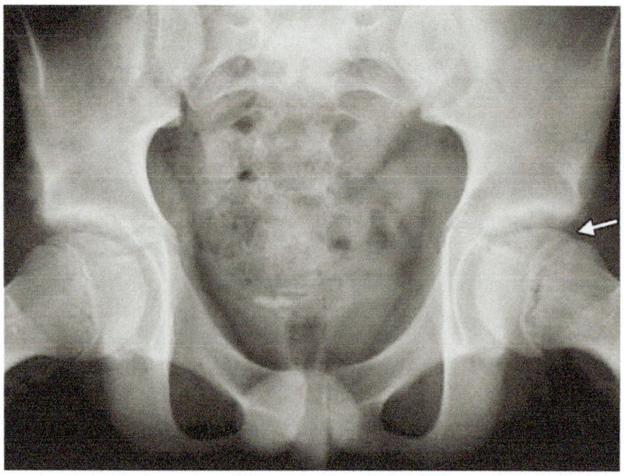

Figure 29.161 Left slipped capital femoral epiphysis. Frog leg lateral view shows mild slippage of the left capital femoral epiphysis (arrow).

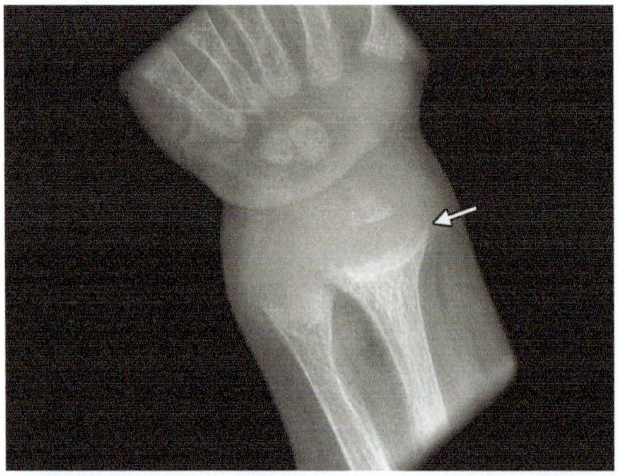

Figure 29.162 Rickets. Radiograph of the left wrist shows a wide distal radial growth plate. Note the cupping, fraying and splaying of the distal radial and ulnar metaphyses. There is a prominent bony spur extending from the distal radial metaphysis (arrow). The distal radial epiphysis is poorly ossified and has an indistinct contour. The forearm bones are demineralised with coarsened trabeculae and indistinct cortices.

With progressive fragmentation and collapse of the femoral head, the femoral neck becomes short and wide. Eventually, the epiphysis remineralises and heals. The healed capital femoral epiphysis is flat and wide.

Slipped Capital Femoral Epiphysis (Figs. 29.160 and 29.161)

Slipped capital femoral epiphysis (SCFE) is a disease of the adolescent hip. The disease can be bilateral.

The radiographic findings of SCFE are as follows:

- Widening of the epiphyseal plate
- Displacement of the femoral head posteriorly and medially

Medial slippage can be identified on a frontal projection of the pelvis. Mild displacement, which may not be immediately apparent on the frontal projection, is best appreciated on the frog leg lateral view.

METABOLIC BONE DISORDERS

Rickets (Fig. 29.162)

There are a number of clinical conditions, which can lead to the development of rickets. The radiographic features of this metabolic disorder are shared, whatever its underlying cause.

Radiographic findings:

- Demineralisation
- Widening of the growth plate
- Cupping, fraying and splaying of the metaphysis, which is of reduced density
- Thin bony spur extending from the metaphysis to surround the uncalcified growth plate
- Indistinct cortex because of uncalcifiedsubperiosteal osteoid
- Poorly ossified epiphyses with faint, indistinct borders.

Scurvy (Fig. 29.163)

Scurvy is the result of vitamin C deficiency.

Radiographic findings:

- Generalised osteopenia
- Dense zone of provisional calcification due to excessive calcification of osteoid
- Metaphyseal lucency
- Metaphyseal corner fractures through the weakened lucent metaphyses (Pelkan spurs)
- Periosteal reaction due to subperiosteal haematoma
- Loss of epiphyseal density with a pencil thin cortex.

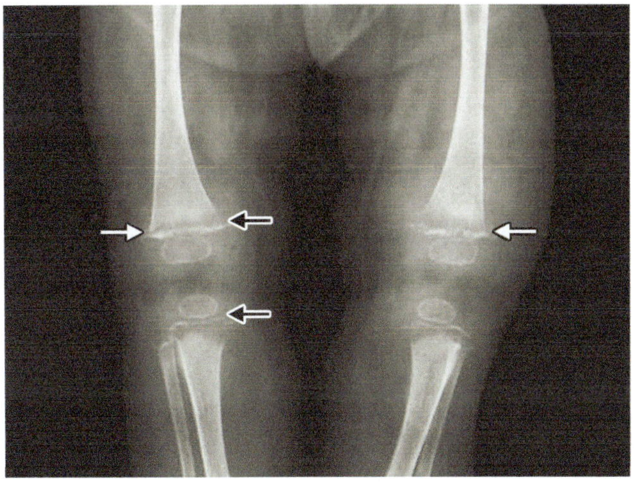

Figure 29.163 Scurvy. AP radiograph of the knees. Transverse bands of metaphyseal lucency lie adjacent to dense zones of provisional calcification (white arrows). There are metaphyseal corner fractures through the weakened metaphyses (white arrows).

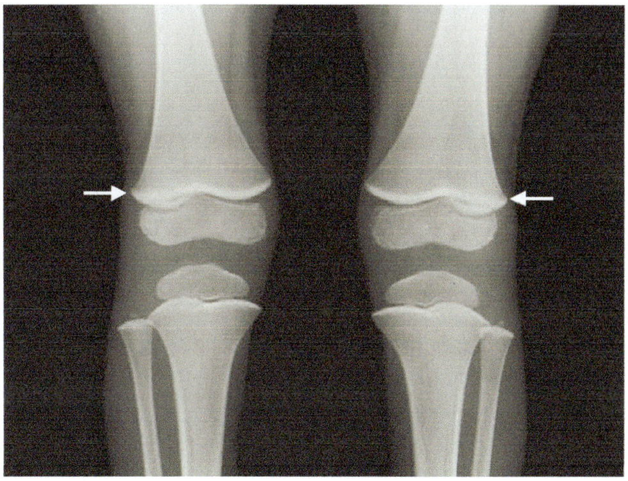

Figure 29.164 Lead poisoning. AP radiograph of the knees reveals transverse bands of increased density in the metaphyses of the long bones (arrows).

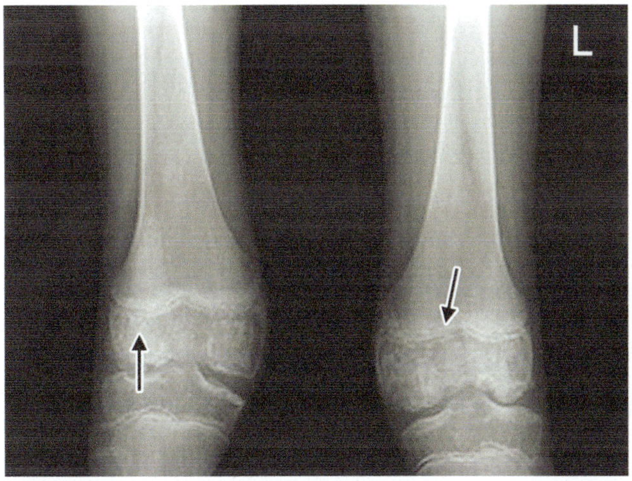

Figure 29.165 Juvenile idiopathic arthritis of both knees. The bones are osteopenic and there is significant joint space loss at the femoro-tibial joints. Subarticular bony erosions are present (arrow). The epiphyses are enlarged (overgrowth). There is slight lateral subluxation of the tibia in relation to the femur bilaterally.

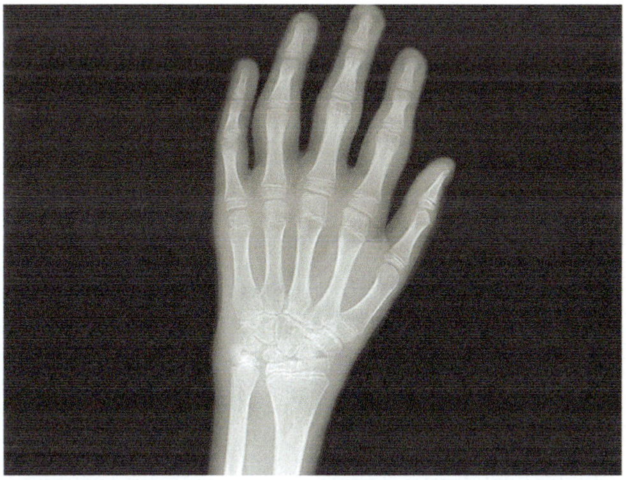

Figure 29.166 Juvenile idiopathic arthritis of the left hand and wrist. There is osteopenia, especially in a periarticular distribution. There is significant joint space loss at the radiocarpal and carpal joints. Note the irregularity of the carpal bones. Joint space loss is also present at the metacarpophalangeal and the interphalangeal joints. There is soft-tissue swelling of the fingers proximally.

Lead Poisoning (Fig. 29.164)

Lead intoxication may occur by ingesting or inhaling the metal. Lead is present in many products including leaded petrol, old water pipes and lead paint. Exposure to lead can lead to anaemia, abdominal symptoms (abdominal pain, vomiting, diarrhoea), a blue line around the gums and encephalopathy. In the skeletal system, lead intoxication causes widening of the cranial sutures (due to increased intracranial pressure) and dense transverse lines in the metaphyses of tubular bones. Opaque lead particles can be seen within bowel on abdominal radiographs.

INFLAMMATORY JOINT AND MUSCLE CONDITIONS

Juvenile Idiopathic Arthritis (Figs. 29.165 and 29.166)

Plain radiography in the early stages of juvenile idiopathic arthritis is usually unhelpful. Soft-tissue swelling and periarticular osteopenia may be visible. Late findings include joint space loss (due to cartilage loss), bony erosions and joint subluxation or dislocation. In children, growth disturbance can occur with epiphyseal overgrowth and premature growth plate fusion.

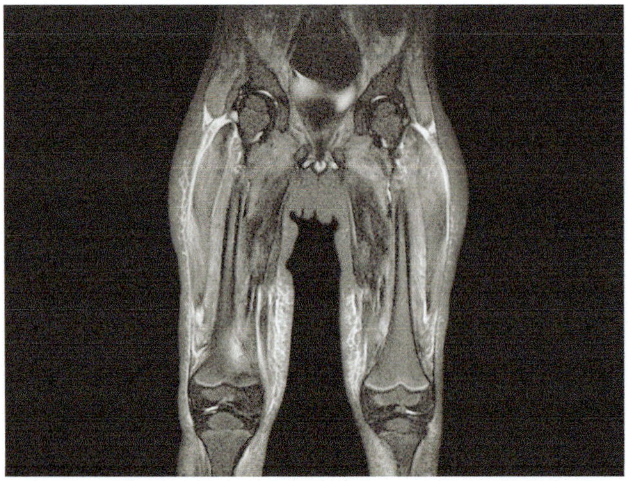

Figure 29.167 Dermatomyositis. Coronal T2 weighted MR sequence through the thighs with fat saturation shows diffusely abnormal increased signal intensity within the muscles of both thighs and also within the subcutaneous tissues.

Dermatomyositis (Figs. 29.167 and 29.168A to C)

Juvenile dermatomyositis is the most common idiopathic inflammatory condition of muscle in children.

Magnetic resonance imaging is helpful in establishing the diagnosis of dermatomyositis and is also useful in assessing the response to treatment.

Soft-tissue calcification is best demonstrated on plain films. Calcium deposition in soft tissues usually occurs around pressure-point sites: the buttocks, knees and elbows. Calcium deposition occurs in the cutaneous and subcutaneous tissues, muscles and fascial planes.

BONE INFECTIONS (FIGS. 29.169 AND 29.170)

Congenital Syphilis

Congenital syphilis is caused by transplacental spread of *Treponema pallidum*.

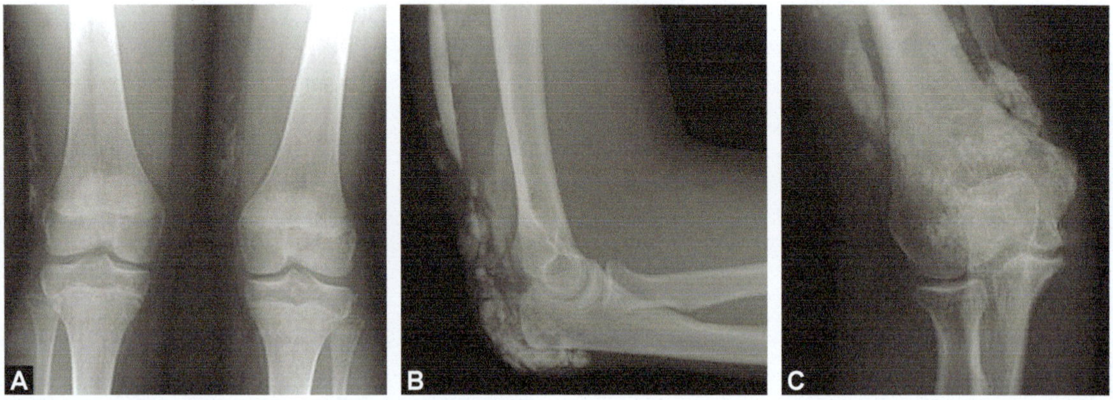

Figures 29.168A to C Dermatomyositis. (A) AP radiograph of both knees shows amorphous calcification mainly in the cutaneous tissues bilaterally; (B and C) AP and lateral radiographs of right elbow. There is extensive calcification in the cutaneous tissues and in the muscles around the elbow joint.

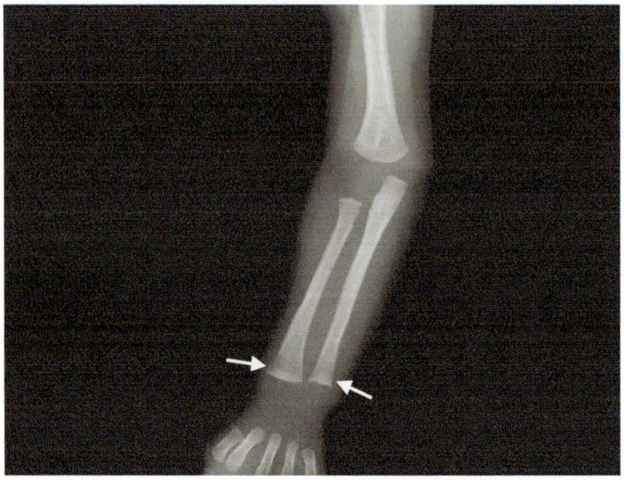

Figure 29.169 Congenital syphilis. Radiograph of left forearm in a neonate shows metaphyseal lucency within the long bones, best demonstrated in the distal radius and ulna (arrows).

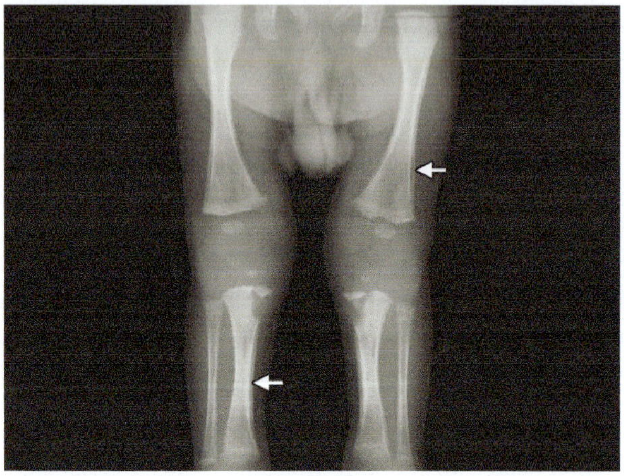

Figure 29.170 Congenital syphilis. There are bilateral symmetric destructive metaphyseal lesions on the medial aspect of the tibiae. There is also significant periosteal reaction along the diaphyses of the femurs and tibiae (arrows).

The radiographic features in infants include the following:

- Metaphyseal lucent bands
- Metaphyseal serration (saw teeth)
- Metaphyseal bony destruction on the medial aspect of the proximal tibia
- Periosteal reaction
- Diaphyseal destructive lesions.

The radiographic features of congenital syphilis in childhood are as follows:

- Periosteal and cortical thickening
- Focal destructive lesions.

Osteomyelitis (Figs. 29.171A and B)

Osteomyelitis is an acute or chronic inflammatory condition of bone and its adjacent structures due to pyogenic organisms. Radiographs often show no bony abnormality in the early stages, although soft-tissue swelling may be evident. Bony involvement is often not detected on radiographs until the second week of the disease. This manifests as radiolucent areas, usually in the metaphysis, where bony destruction has occurred. Periosteal reaction is also evident. If treatment is delayed or ineffective, there is an increase in the amount of periosteal reaction to form an involucrum around the fragments of dead bone (sequestrum).

HAEMOLYTIC ANAEMIAS

Thalassaemia (Figs. 29.172 and 29.173)

Skeletal findings:

- Skull: Osteoporosis; expansion of the diploic space, especially in the frontal bone; thinning of the outer table of the skull; hair-on-end appearance.

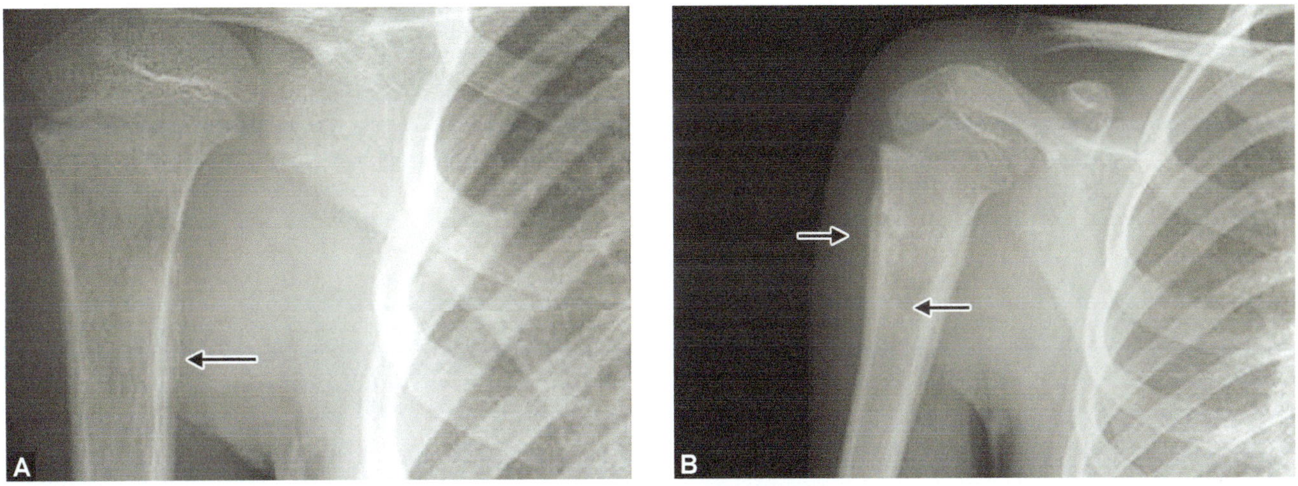

Figures 29.171A and B Osteomyelitis proximal right humerus. (A) AP radiograph at time of presentation shows patchy radiolucency within the proximal right humeral shaft and faint periosteal reaction (arrow); (B) Follow-up radiograph 1 month later with treatment. The lucent area within bone is smaller and well defined. The periosteum has produced new cortical bone (arrows).

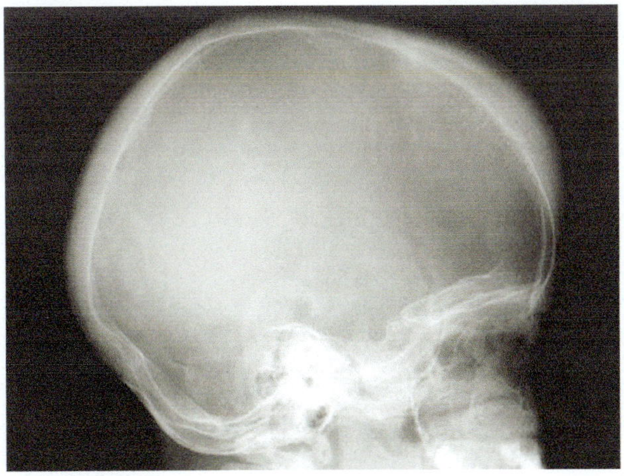

Figure 29.172 Thalassaemia. There is widening of the diploic space and thinning of the outer table of the skull. Note the hair-on-end appearance in the frontal region on this lateral skull radiograph.

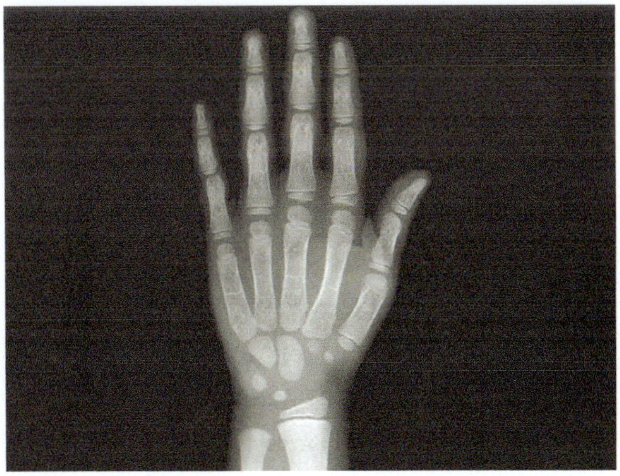

Figure 29.173 Thalassaemia. Radiograph of the left hand demonstrates widening of the medullary cavity and thinning of the cortex within the tubular bones.

Hypoplasia of the paranasal sinuses due to expansion of the facial bones; malocclusion of the jaw
- Trunk: Osteoporosis, coarse bony trabeculae and cortical thinning. Accentuation of vertical trabecular pattern in the vertebrae; biconcave vertebral bodies
- Tubular bones: Widened medullary cavity and cortical thinning.

Sickle Cell Anaemia (Fig. 29.174)

The skeletal findings in sickle cell anaemia are similar to those in thalassaemia. The skull changes are less severe. Compression fractures of the spine can occur due to loss of bony support resulting from marrow hypertrophy. Vertebral fractures, however, can also be due to infarcts involving the blood vessels supplying the central portions of the superior and inferior endplates. This latter feature results in a depression of the central portion of the vertebral endplate.

Vascular occlusion due to sickling also results in osteonecrosis in other bones. Diaphyseal or epiphyseal infarcts can occur in the long bones. In young children, the bones of the hands and feet can be affected. This is known as sickle cell dactylitis or hand-foot syndrome. Patients with sickle cell disease are also at risk of osteomyelitis and pyogenic arthritis.

LANGERHANS CELL HISTIOCYTOSIS (FIGS. 29.175 AND 29.176)

Langerhans cell histiocytosis (LCH) in the skeleton can be unifocal or multifocal. The most common affected site is the skull. Other frequent locations include the femur, ribs mandible, pelvis and spine.

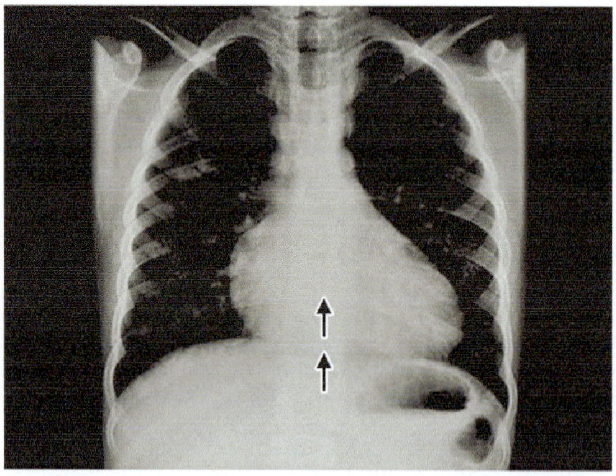

Figure 29.174 Sickle cell disease. There is central endplate depression within some of the thoracic vertebrae (arrows) due to focal fractures resulting from local vascular occlusion. There is also cardiomegaly due to anaemia.

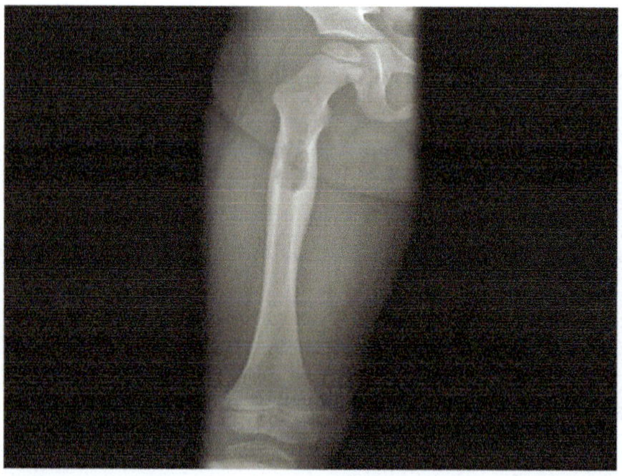

Figure 29.175 Langerhans cell histiocytosis proximal right femur. Anterior posterior radiograph demonstrates a well-defined, ovoid lytic lesion in the proximal right femur. The margins of the lesion are slightly sclerotic. There is cortical expansion and periosteal reaction.

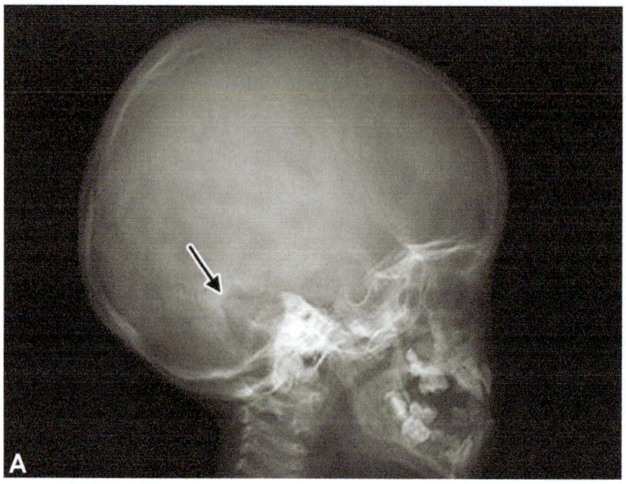

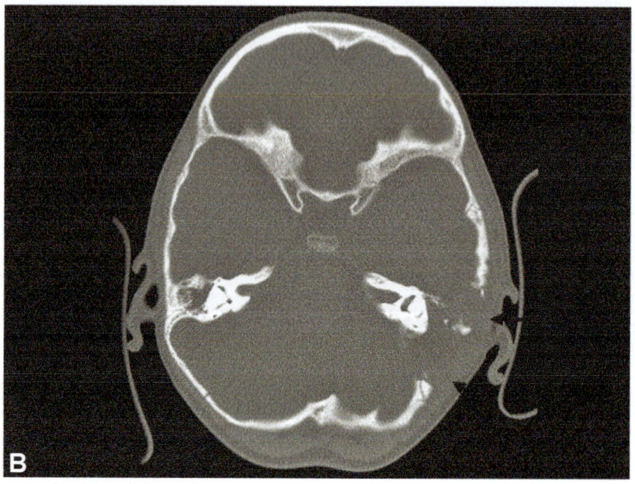

Figures 29.176A and B Langerhans cell histiocytosis of skull. (A) Lateral skull radiograph shows a large, well-defined lytic lesion within the temporal bone region of the skull (arrow); (B) Axial CT scan through the skull on bone window settings. This confirms the presence of an extensive destructive process involving the left petrous temporal bone (arrows).

Langerhans cell histiocytosis lesions in the skull are usually well-defined lytic lesions with sharp margins. In the spine, the disease causes lytic destruction and collapse of the vertebral body. Elsewhere in the skeleton, LCH lesions are usually well defined with minimally sclerotic borders.

PAEDIATRIC BONE TUMOURS

Osteoid Osteoma (Figs. 29.177 and 29.178)

The osteoid osteoma is a painful lesion, with patients classically complaining of night pain. The most common sites for osteoid osteoma are the femur and tibia. The typical radiographic appearance is a cortically based sclerotic lesion in a long bone, which has a small lucent area within it known as the nidus.

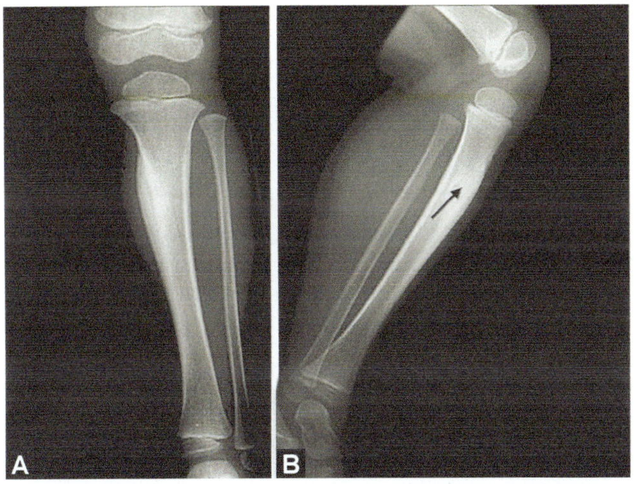

Figures 29.177A and B Osteoid osteoma of the left tibia. (A) AP radiograph of left lower leg demonstrates dense sclerosis and focal cortical thickening along the medial aspect of the proximal left tibia; (B) Lateral radiograph shows the small radiolucent nidus within the bony lesion (arrow).

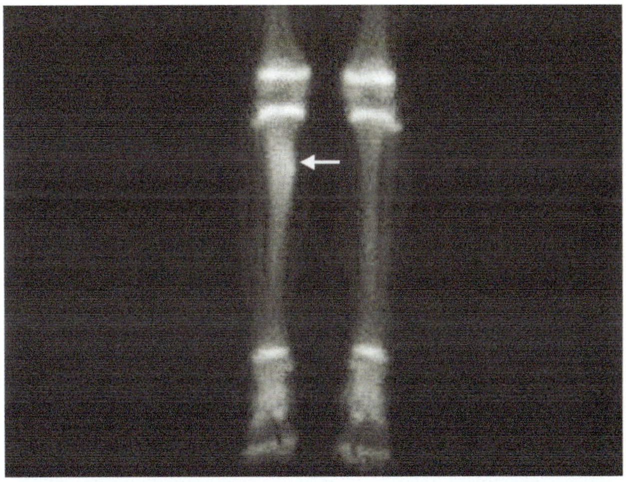

Figure 29.178 Osteoid osteoma on radionuclide bone scan. Image taken from the front shows increased tracer uptake medially within the proximal right tibia, which corresponds to the sclerotic component of the lesion. The smaller more focal area of intense uptake corresponds to the nidus (arrow).

Osteosarcoma (Figs. 29.179 and 29.180)

Osteosarcomas can occur anywhere in the skeleton. Frequently encountered sites are the distal femur, proximal tibia, proximal humerus and pelvis. Long bone tumours usually arise from the metaphysis. On X-ray, a typical osteosarcoma is identified as a mixed lytic and sclerotic lesion involving the long bone metaphysis. There is usually cortical erosion and destruction, often with a spiculated 'sunburst' periosteal reaction. Elevated periosteal reaction is also demonstrated at the tumour extremities (Codman triangle).

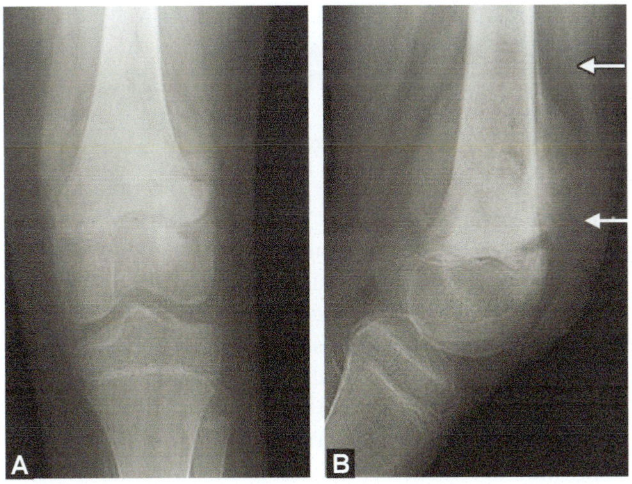

Figures 29.179A and B Osteosarcoma of distal left femur. (A and B) AP and lateral radiographs of left knee show a sclerotic lesion arising from the distal left femoral diametaphysis. Spiculated periosteal reaction is present (white arrow) and there is also elevated periosteal reaction (Codmans triangle) at the superior margin of the lesion (white arrow).

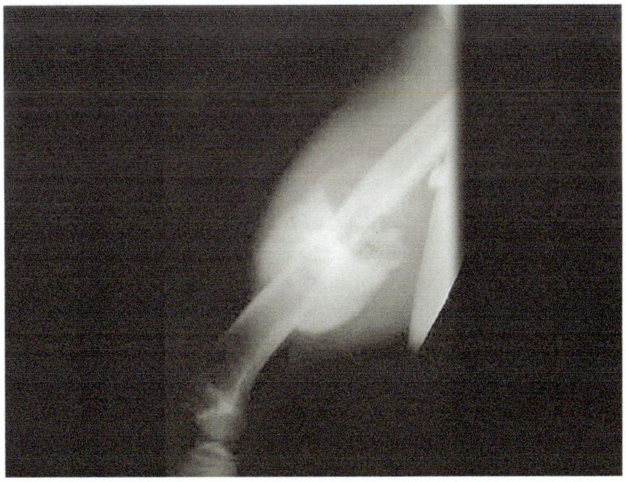

Figure 29.180 Osteosarcoma of femur. Lateral view of the femur shows marked-sunray-periosteal new bone formation associated with the mid femoral shaft tumour. Osteosarcoma was confirmed pathologically at biopsy.

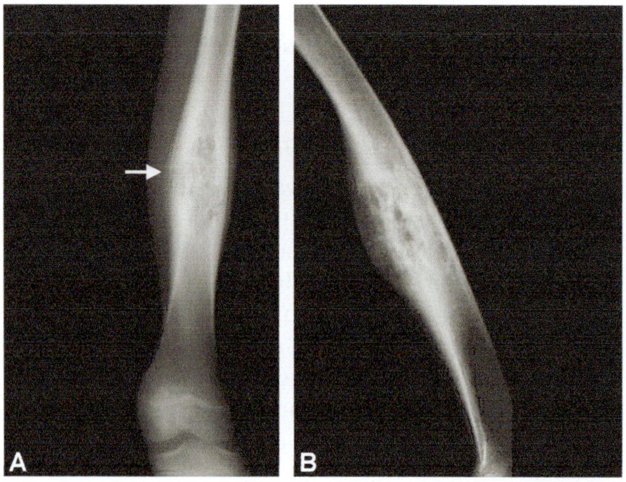

Figures 29.181A and B Ewing sarcoma left femur. AP and lateral radiographs show a mixed lytic and sclerotic lesion in the diaphysis of the left femur resulting in a 'moth-eaten' appearance. There is 'onion-skin' type periosteal reaction (arrow).

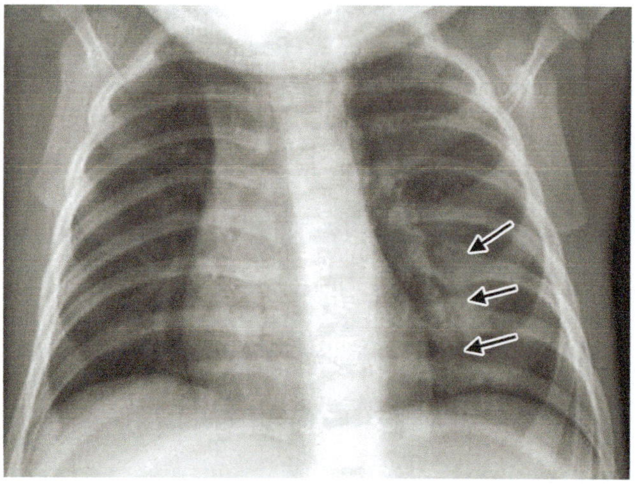

Figure 29.182 Frontal chest radiograph shows healing posterior rib fractures involving the left seventh, eighth and ninth ribs (arrows).

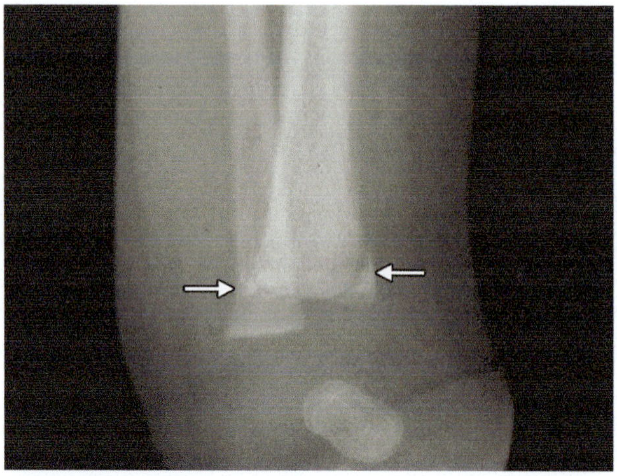

Figure 29.183 Lateral view of ankle demonstrates metaphyseal corner fractures of the distal tibia (arrows).

Ewing Sarcoma (Figs. 29.181A and B)

The most common site for Ewing sarcoma is the long bone diaphysis. Flat bones (pelvis and ribs) are also commonly involved.

The typical radiographic appearance of Ewing sarcoma is a 'moth eaten' lesion (due to multiple small holes) in the diaphysis or, less commonly, the metaphysis of a long bone. There is usually an 'onion skin' type of periosteal reaction.

Non-accidental Injury (Figs. 29.182 and 29.183)

Skeletal findings:

- Multiple fractures in varying stages of healing
- Diaphyseal fractures, especially in the non-ambulatory infant/child
- Metaphyseal fractures: The classic metaphyseal fracture is often described as a corner or bucket-handle fracture
- Rib fractures: Posterior rib fractures have a higher specificity for inflicted injury than antero-lateral fractures
- Scapula fracture: Fracture of the acromion is highly specific for abuse
- Spinal fractures
- Skull fractures.

Other types of injury encountered in this situation include intracranial and visceral trauma.

PAEDIATRIC RENAL IMAGING CONGENITAL ANOMALIES

Ureteral Duplication (Figs. 29.184 to 29.187)

Ureteral duplication may be partial or complete. In partial duplication, the ureters unite anywhere along their course and then continue inferiorly as a single structure. In completely duplicated systems, the two ureters are separate throughout their entire course. The ureter draining the upper moiety usually inserts into the bladder ectopically, below and more medial to the insertion of the ureter, which drains the lower renal moiety. The ectopic ureter is more likely to become obstructed, sometimes due to an associated ureterocoele. The lower-moiety ureter is more prone to reflux. When renal function is adequate, duplication of the pelvicalyceal system and ureter can be visualised on excretion urography. It is sometimes difficult to establish if the ureteric duplication is partial or complete on this study.

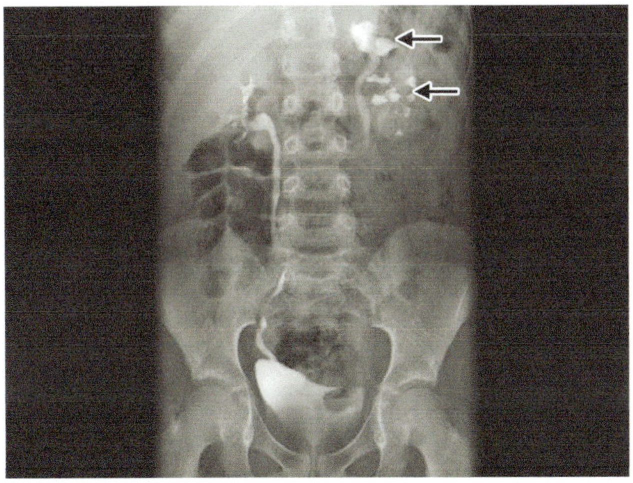

Figure 29.184 Left-sided upper ureteric duplication. Excretory urogram shows two left-sided pelvocalyceal systems (arrows). The separate proximal ureters are visible. There is a filling defect in the left side of the bladder due to a ureterocoele (arrows). This is causing some obstruction to the upper renal moiety which demonstrates clubbing of its calyces.

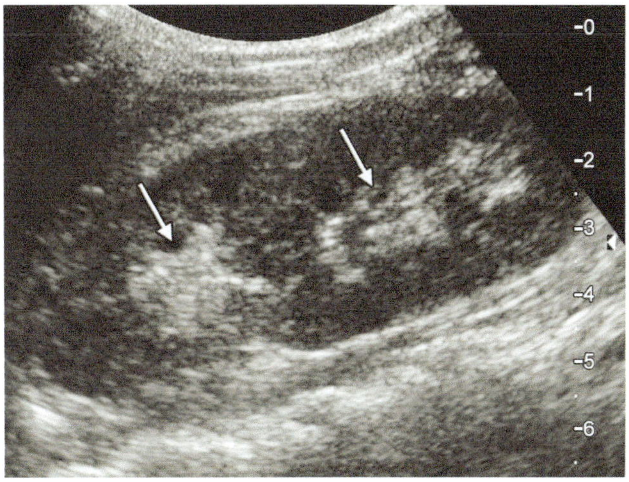

Figure 29.185 Uncomplicated ureteral duplication. Parasagittal ultrasound scan of left kidney shows two echogenic renal sinuses (arrows). The kidney is also enlarged. These findings are typical for an uncomplicated duplex kidney.

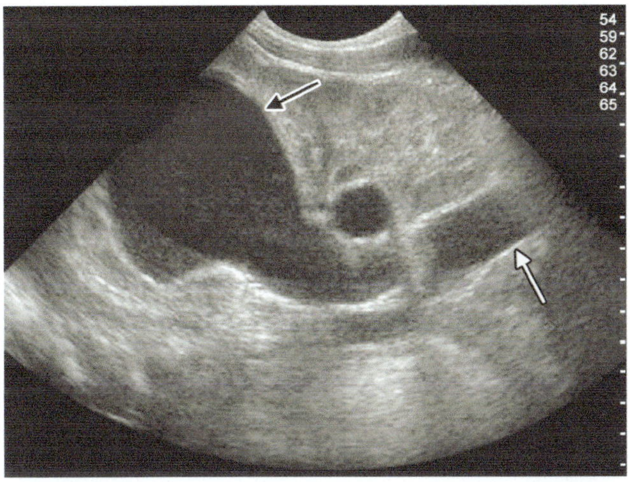

Figure 29.186 Ureteral duplication with obstructed upper renal moiety. Longitudinal ultrasound scan of left kidney shows a hydronephrotic upper moiety renal pelvis (white arrow) and its associated hydroureter (white arrows).

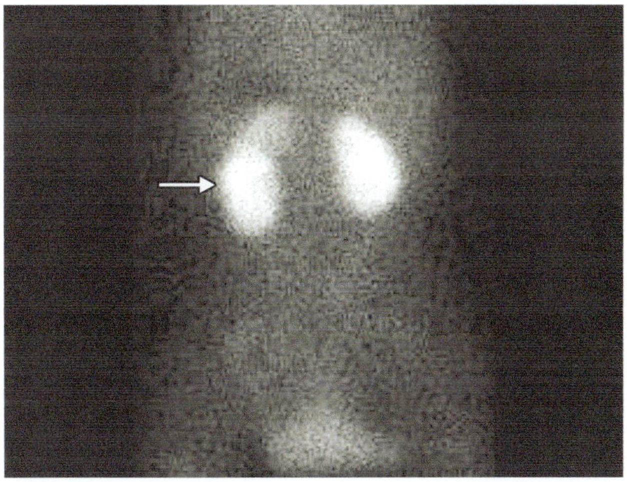

Figure 29.187 Duplex left kidney. Renal radionuclide study using technetium 99 m dimercaptosuccinic acid. This image taken from the back shows an enlarged left kidney consistent with a duplex kidney (arrow).

Horseshoe Kidney (Figs. 29.188 and 29.189)

The horseshoe kidney arises because of fusion of the lower poles of the kidneys across the midline. This fusion produces an abnormal renal axis, which may be detected on ultrasound. The fused portion of the kidney (known as the isthmus) may also be visualised on ultrasound as renal tissue which overlies the spine. The horseshoe kidney is best demonstrated in its entirety on renal scintigraphy (DMSA scan) and abdominal CT or MR scans.

ECTOPIA

Ipsilateral Renal Ectopia (Figs. 29.190 and 29.191)

In the foetus, the normal migration of the kidney from the pelvis to the renal fossa may become interrupted. Consequently, the kidney can be located anywhere along the migrational path. When a kidney cannot be found in its usual position on ultrasound, the pelvis should be closely scrutinised to see if there is an ectopic pelvic kidney. Pelvic kidneys are more prone to vesicoureteric reflux than

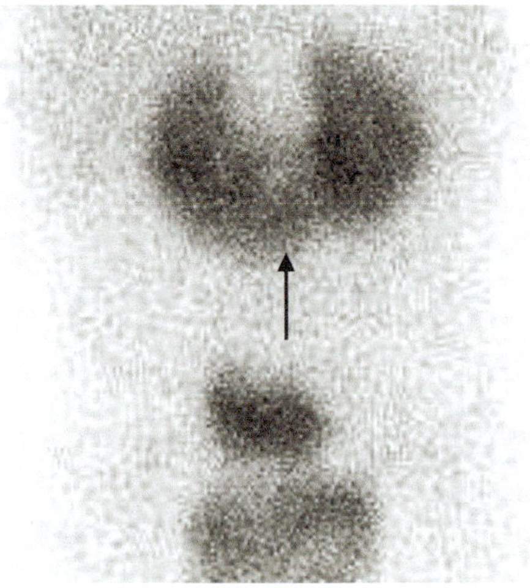

Figure 29.188 Horseshoe kidney. Dimercaptosuccinic acid scan demonstrates uptake within both kidneys and within the renal isthmus (arrow).

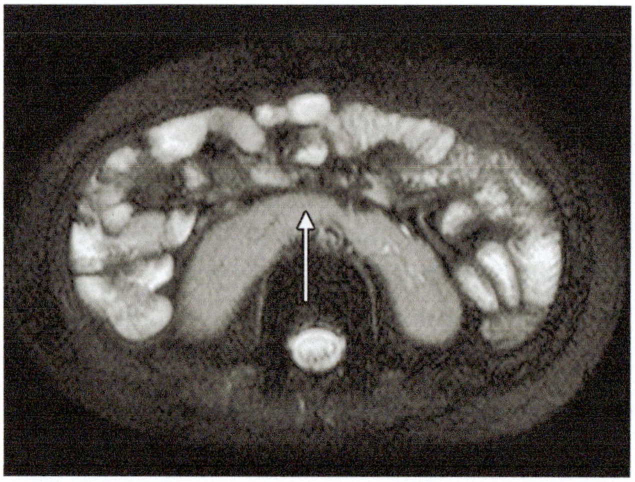

Figure 29.189 Horseshoe kidney on abdominal MR scan. Axial T2 weighted (fat saturated) image demonstrates fusion of the lower poles of the kidneys anterior to the spine (arrow).

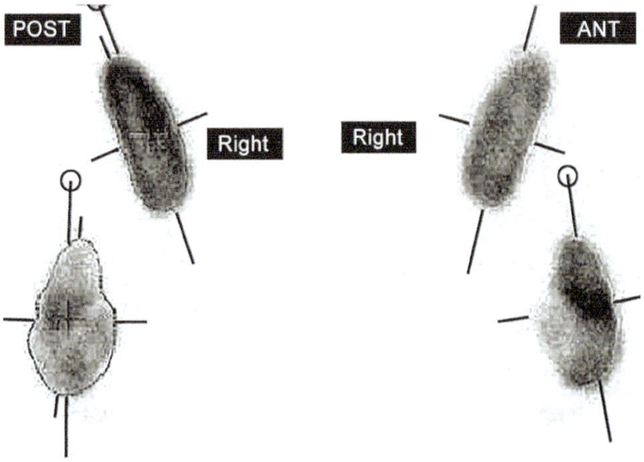

Figure 29.190 Pelvic kidney on dimercaptosuccinic acid scan. The right kidney is located in a normal position. The left kidney is ectopic, lying within the pelvis.

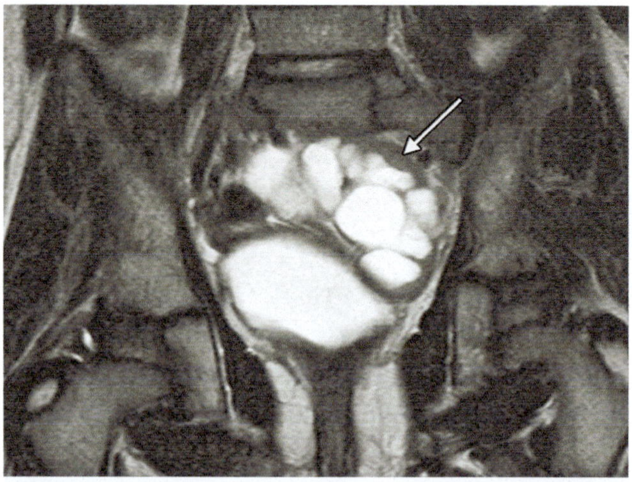

Figure 29.191 Pelvic kidney. Coronal T2 weighted MR scan shows an ectopic left kidney above the bladder (arrow). The renal pelvis and calyces are dilated.

normal kidneys. They have an abnormal rotation and are also more likely to have ureteropelvic junction (UPJ) obstruction.

Crossed Fused Renal Ectopia (Figs. 29.192A to C)

This is a condition where the bulk of both kidneys is on one side of the spine. Part of the ectopic kidney may extend across the spine. The ectopic kidney is usually smaller than normal and malrotated. It usually lies below the normally sited kidney. The kidneys are usually fused and surrounded by a common renal fascia; hence the given term *crossed fused renal ectopia*. The ureter from the ectopic lower kidney usually crosses the midline to insert into the bladder in its normal position.

Abdominal ultrasound will reveal an empty renal fossa on one side and an apparently enlarged kidney on the other side, with two renal sinuses. The ectopic kidney is generally positioned medially, extending anteriorly across the spine. Nuclear scintigraphy can also be used to confirm the presence of crossed fused renal ectopia.

Renal Agenesis (Figs. 29.193 and 29.194)

Bilateral renal agenesis is a lethal anomaly. If the diagnosis is not made until birth, the infant will have features of Potter sequence. A renal ultrasound scan in the early neonatal period usually confirms the diagnosis by showing no renal tissue in the renal flanks or in an ectopic location.

Unilateral renal agenesis is sometimes detected antenatally or on post-natal ultrasound because of anomalies

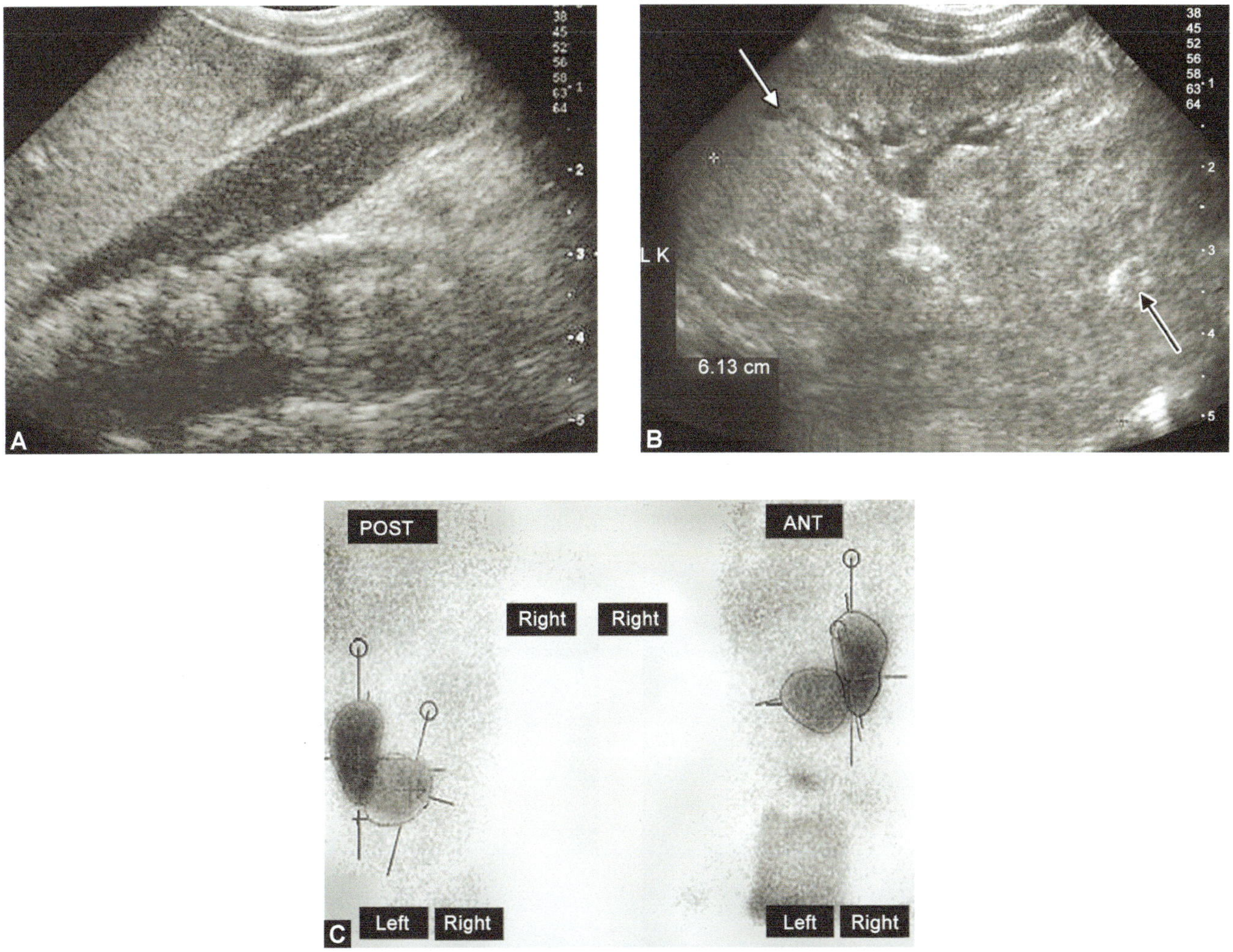

Figures 29.192A to C Crossed-fused renal ectopia. (A) Parasagittal ultrasound scan of right flank shows absent right kidney; (B) Parasagittal scan ultrasound scan of left flank shows a normally positioned left kidney (white arrow) with an apparent mass of renal tissue at its lower pole (black arrow). This is the ectopic right kidney; (C) Dimercaptosuccinic acid renal scan demonstrates the ectopic right kidney lying medially and horizontally, attached to the lower pole of the left kidney.

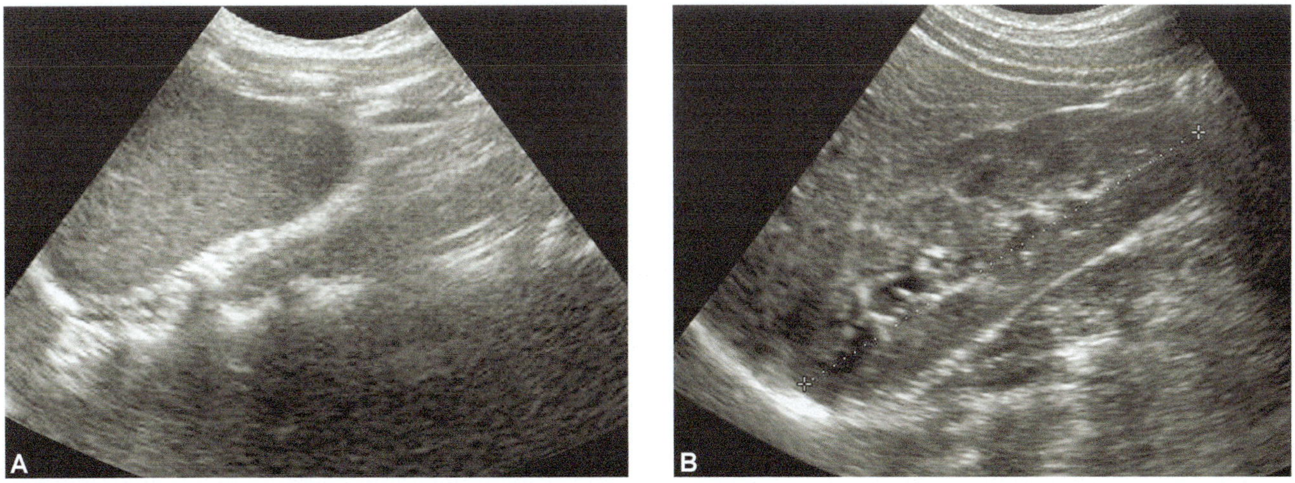

Figures 29.193A and B Agenesis of left kidney. (A) Left parasagittal ultrasound scan shows no kidney in the left flank; (B) Right parasagittal ultrasound scan demonstrates a normal appearing right kidney, which is larger than usual due to compensatory hypertrophy.

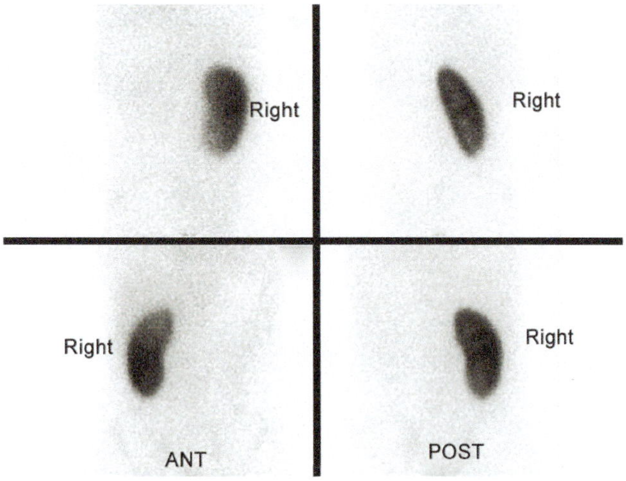

Figure 29.194 Agenesis of left kidney. Radioisotope study (dimercapto-succinic acid) shows a solitary right kidney. No left kidney or ectopic renal tissue is identified.

elsewhere. It is also associated with anomalies of the genital tract.

Autosomal Recessive Polycystic Kidney Disease (Figs. 29.195 and 29.196)

This is a rare disorder involving both kidneys and the liver. The disease causes ectasia of the renal collecting tubules and this is manifest pathologically as numerous tiny cysts in the cortex and medulla.

The ultrasound appearances of autosomal recessive polycystic kidney disease in neonates are bilateral enlarged kidneys, which are diffusely echogenic. Discrete small cysts may be visible.

Multicystic Dysplastic Kidney (Figs. 29.197 and 29.198)

Multicystic dysplastic kidney is a severe form of renal dysplasia, which is associated with obstruction of urinary

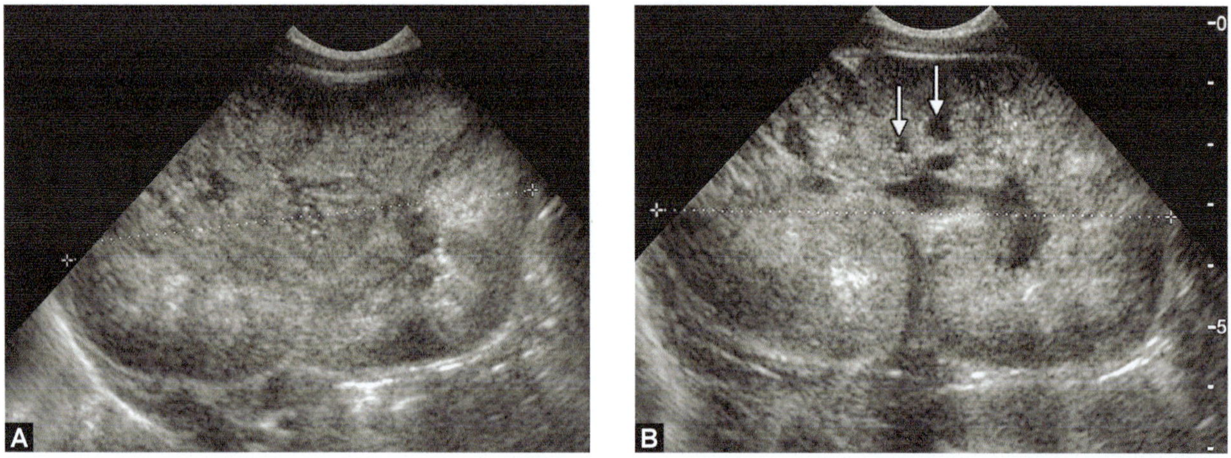

Figures 29.195A and B Autosomal recessive polycystic kidney disease in a newborn infant. (A) Longitudinal ultrasound scan of right kidney demonstrates a markedly enlarged, echogenic kidney; (B) Longitudinal ultrasound scan of the left kidney also shows an enlarged, echogenic kidney. There are a few small discrete cysts within the renal parenchyma (arrows).

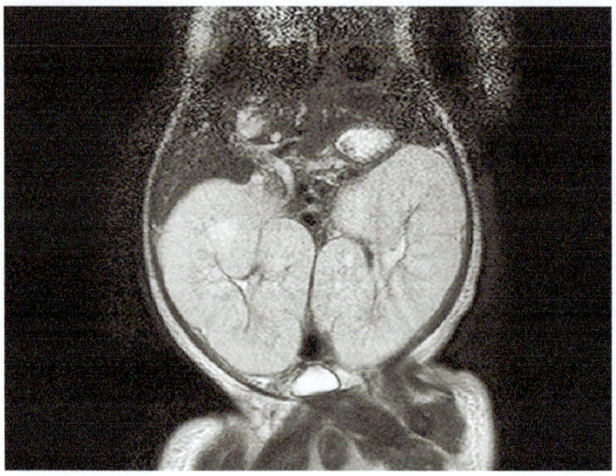

Figure 29.196 Autosomal recessive polycystic kidney disease on abdominal MR scan. Coronal T2 weighted abdominal MR image from the same patient shows the extent of the bilateral nephromegaly.

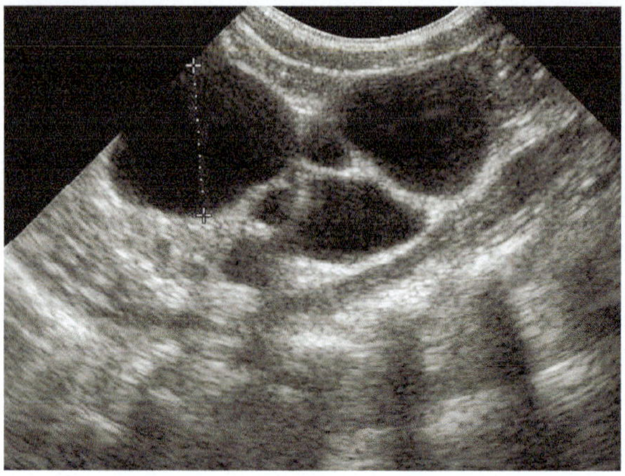

Figure 29.197 Multicystic dysplastic kidney. Longitudinal ultrasound image of the left kidney reveals several cysts of different size within the kidney. The cysts are non-communicating. No normal renal parenchyma is identified.

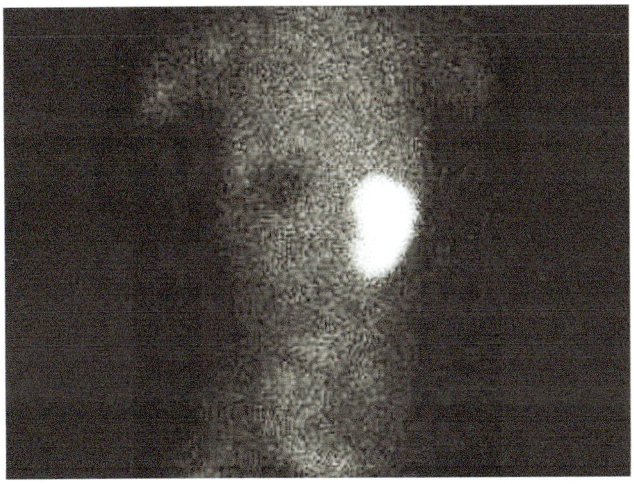

Figure 29.198 Multicystic dysplastic kidney. Dimercaptosuccinic acid study performed in the same patient. This image, taken from behind, shows tracer uptake only in the normal right kidney. There is no uptake in the dysplastic left kidney.

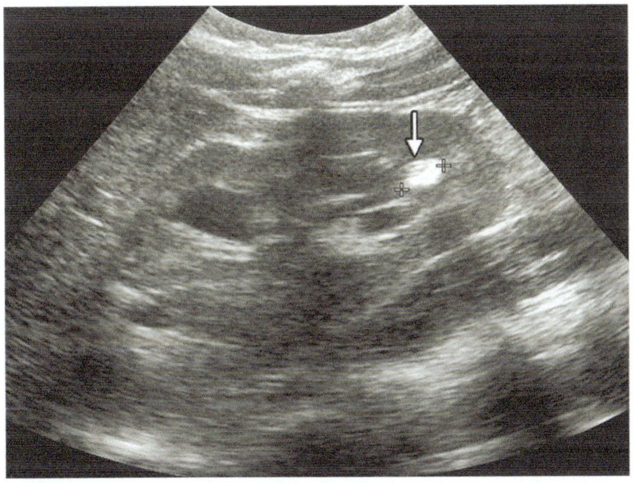

Figure 29.200 Calculus within lower pole of the left kidney. Longitudinal ultrasound scan of left kidney shows a bright (hyperechoic) structure at the lower pole of the kidney (arrow), consistent with a small renal calculus.

drainage on the affected side, probably occurring in utero. The sonographic features of classic MCDK are multiple cysts of variable size, which do not communicate with each other. There is absent or dysplastic renal parenchyma and no renal pelvis is identified. There is no function in a MCDK.

URINARY TRACT STONES AND NEPHROCALCINOSIS

Urinary Tract Stones (Figs. 29.199 and 29.200)

Causes of renal tract stones in children include the following:

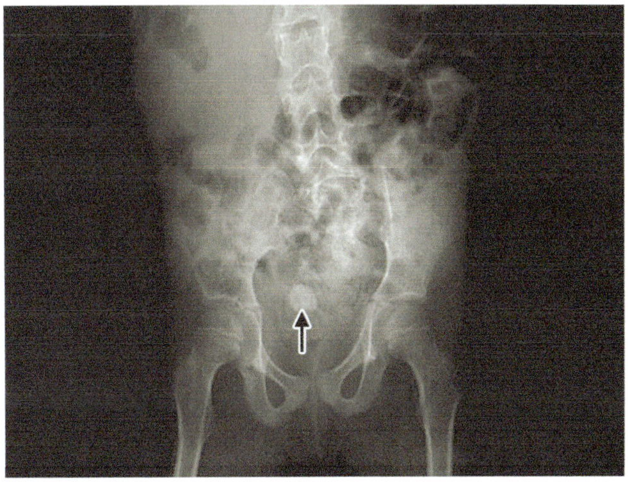

Figure 29.199 Bladder calculus. AP radiograph shows a large, radio-opaque structure projected over the pelvis, consistent with a bladder calculus (arrow).

- Infection
- Developmental anomalies of the urinary tract
- Immobilisation
- Metabolic disorders such as hypercalcaemia and hypercalciuria
- Idiopathic.

Calcium stones are radio-opaque and therefore can be identified on X-ray. Cystine stones are poorly opaque. Uric acid stones are radiolucent.

Nephrocalcinosis (Figs. 29.201A and B)

Nephrocalcinosis is the deposition of calcium in the renal medulla or cortex. Calcium deposition is more common in the medulla than in the cortex.

Causes of medullary nephrocalcinosis include the following:

- Hyperparathyroidism
- Renal tubular acidosis
- Medullary sponge kidney
- Causes of hypercalcaemia or hypercalciuria
- Hyperoxaluria
- Frusemide.

DILATATION OF URINARY TRACT

Dilatation of the urinary tract can be due to one of three general problems:

1. Obstruction
2. Vesicoureteric reflux
3. A combination of both.

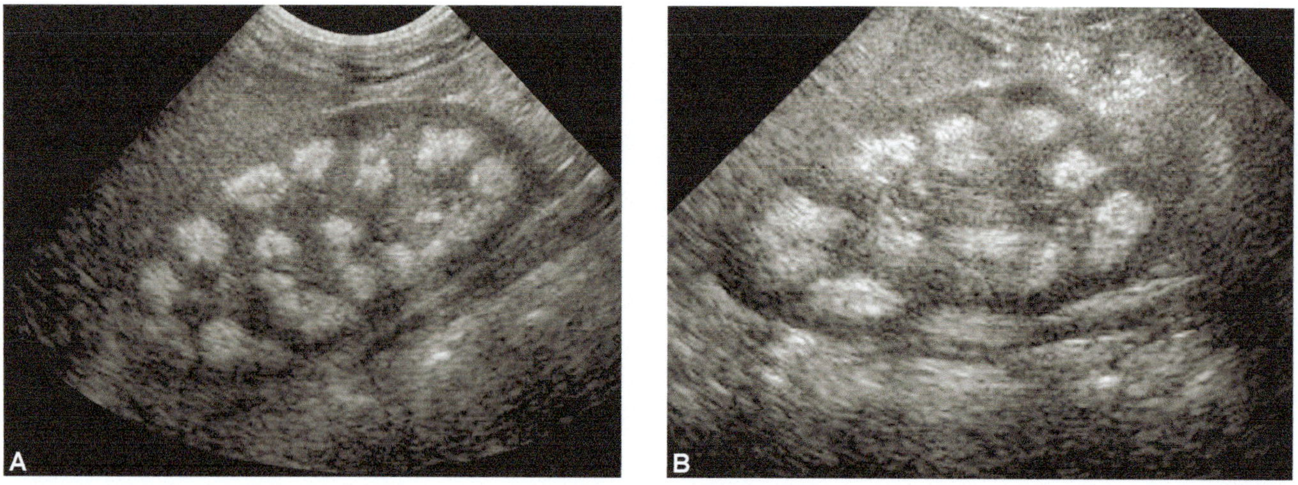

Figures 29.201A and B Medullar nephrocalcinosis. (A and B) Longitudinal ultrasound images of right and left kidneys, respectively. The renal pyramids are markedly hyperechoic due to medullary calcinosis.

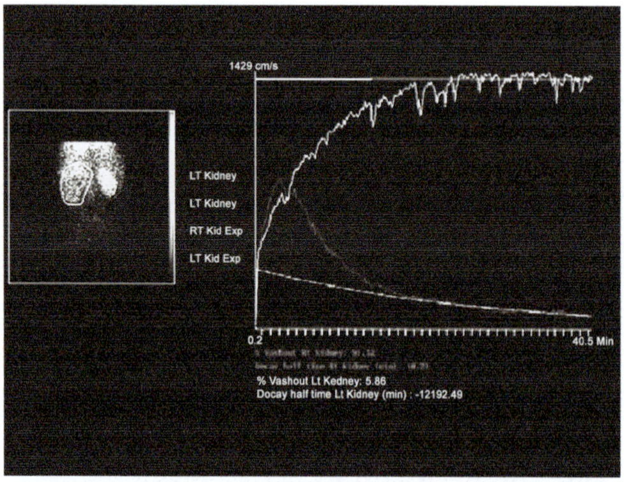

Figure 29.202 Left-sided ureteropelvic obstruction. On this diuretic renogram study using technetium-99 m mercaptoacetyl triglycine (MAG 3), there is normal excretion of radioisotope from the right kidney. There is no excretion of radioisotope from the left kidney, even after the administration of frusemide at 20 minutes.

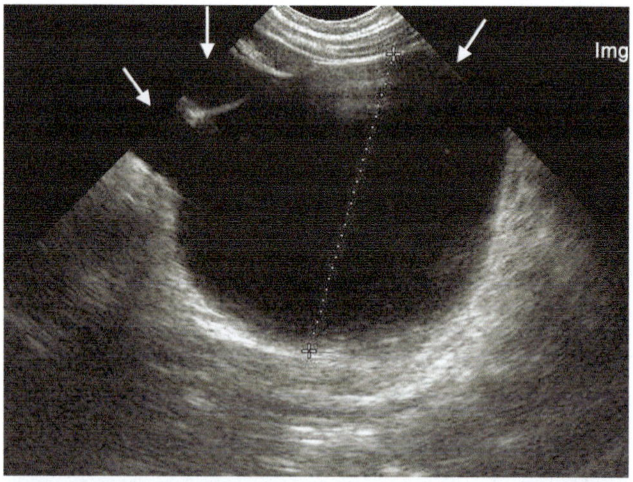

Figure 29.203 Ureteropelvic junction obstruction. Longitudinal ultrasound scan demonstrates markedly dilated renal pelvis and moderately dilated calyces (arrows).

Ureteropelvic Junction Obstruction (Figs. 29.202 and 29.203)

Ureteropelvic junction obstruction is the most common cause of upper urinary tract obstruction in infants and children. The characteristic ultrasound findings include dilated calyces with a moderate or large renal pelvis. The renal parenchyma is of varying thickness depending on the degree of pelvocalyceal dilatation. Diuretic renography is commonly performed to assess UPJ obstruction.

Posterior Urethral Valves (Fig. 29.204)

Posterior urethral valves are the most common cause of urethral obstruction in males and the diagnosis is usually confirmed with a micturating cystourethrogram. The features of posterior urethral valves on this study are as follows:

- Dilated posterior urethra
- Visualisation of valves
- Trabeculated bladder with wide neck
- Usually reflux of contrast into dilated, tortuous ureters.

Vesicoureteric Reflux

The severity of vesicoureteric reflux is graded according to the degree of upper renal tract dilatation on the micturationcystourethrogram:

Grade 1: Reflux into ureter only

Grade 2: Reflux into ureter, renal pelvis and calyces which are preserved (Fig. 29.205)

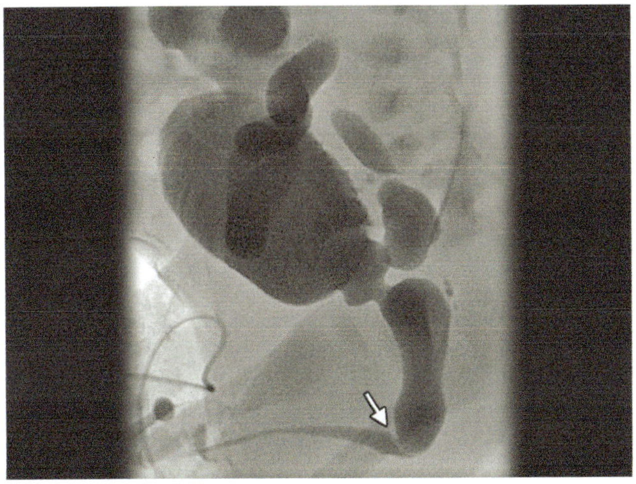

Figure 29.204 Posterior urethral valves. Micturating cystourethrogram study after urinary catheter removed. There is a filling defect in the posterior urethra due to posterior urethral valves (arrow). The posterior urethra proximal to this is dilated and the bladder neck is wide. There is reflux of contrast into both ureters.

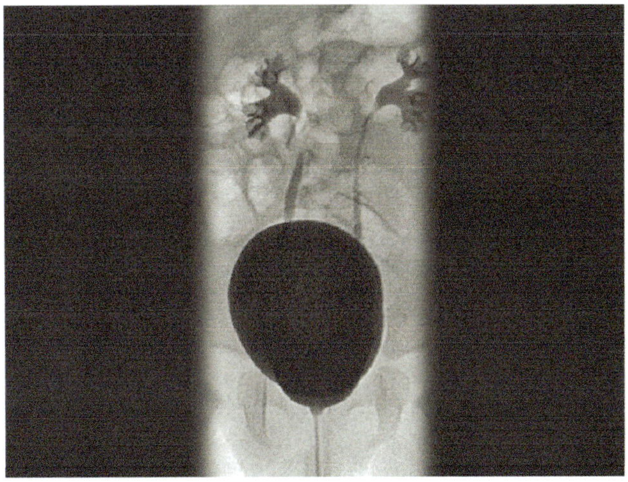

Figure 29.205 Bilateral grade 2 vesicoureteric reflux. Micturating cystourethrogram study demonstrates reflux of contrast into the pelvocalyceal system and ureter bilaterally. The calyces are preserved.

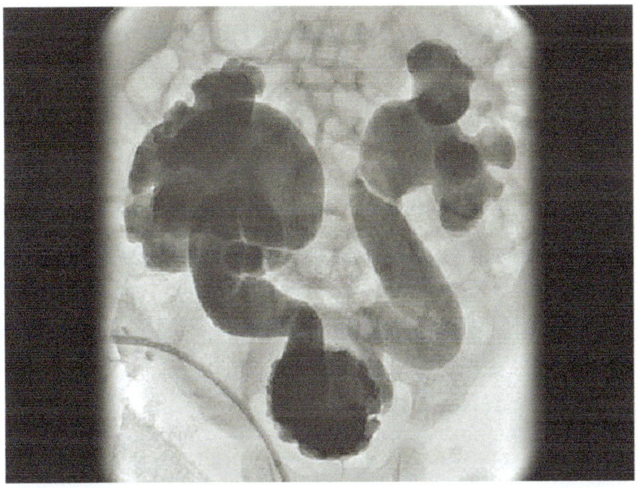

Figure 29.206 Severe bilateral vesicoureteric reflux. There is grade 5 reflux on the right. The right ureter is dilated and tortuous. There is marked dilatation of the right pelvocalyceal system with severe calyceal blunting. The appearances are slightly less marked on the left side and represent grade 4/5 vesicoureteric reflux.

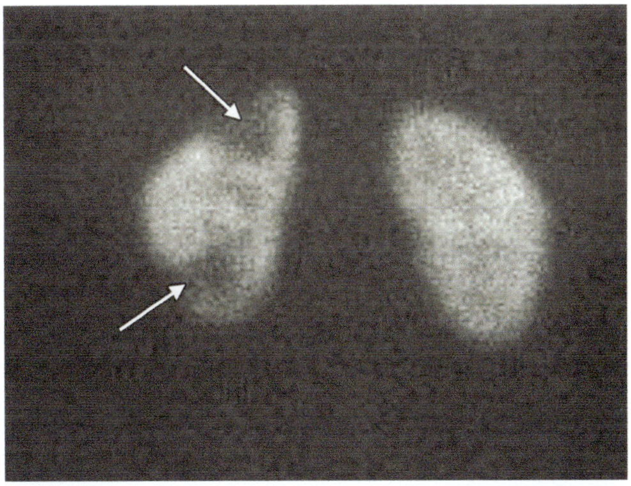

Figure 29.207 Cortical scarring left kidney. This dimercaptosuccinic acid study reveals photopenic areas (arrows) in the upper and lower poles of the left kidney, consistent with renal cortical scarring. The right kidney is normal.

Grade 3: Reflux into mildly dilated ureter and renal pelvis; the calyces are slightly blunted

Grade 4: Reflux into moderately dilated ureter and renal pelvis; moderately blunted calyces

Grade 5: Reflux into tortuous dilated ureter and markedly dilated renal pelvis; severe calyceal blunting (Fig. 29.206).

Renal Tract Infection (Fig. 29.207)

Urinary tract infection can involve the kidney, bladder or both areas. The role of imaging in the child with a proven urinary tract infection is to diagnose underlying conditions, which predispose to infection such as hydronephrosis and reflux, and to detect renal scarring.

The ultrasound scan often appears normal in uncomplicated cases of pyelonephritis. Renal cortical scarring is usually detected using renal scintigraphy.

NEOPLASTIC DISEASES

Wilms Tumour (Figs. 29.208 to 29.210)

Wilms tumour is the most common abdominal malignancy of childhood. Radiologic examinations help to stage the disease in order to assist surgical planning and

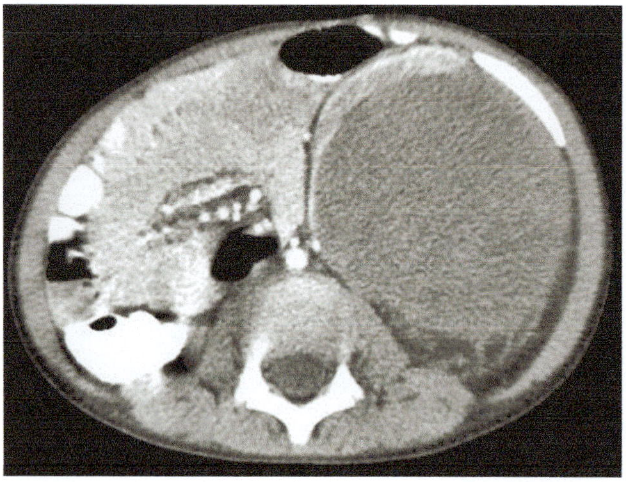

Figure 29.208 Wilms tumour of the left kidney. Contrast-enhanced axial CT scan through the abdomen demonstrates a large mass arising from the left kidney. There is a thin rim of normal renal parenchyma around the tumour anteriorly (arrow).

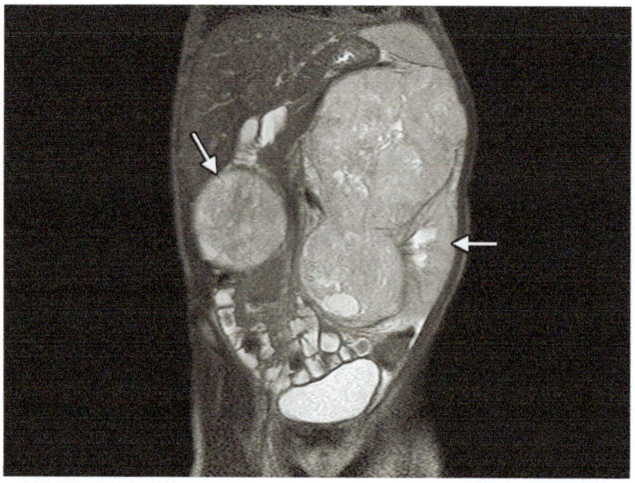

Figure 29.209 Bilateral Wilms tumour (stage V). Coronal T2 weighted scan (fat saturated) shows a bilobed mass within the left kidney. There is normal left renal tissue laterally (arrow). There is a smaller mass within the right kidney (arrow).

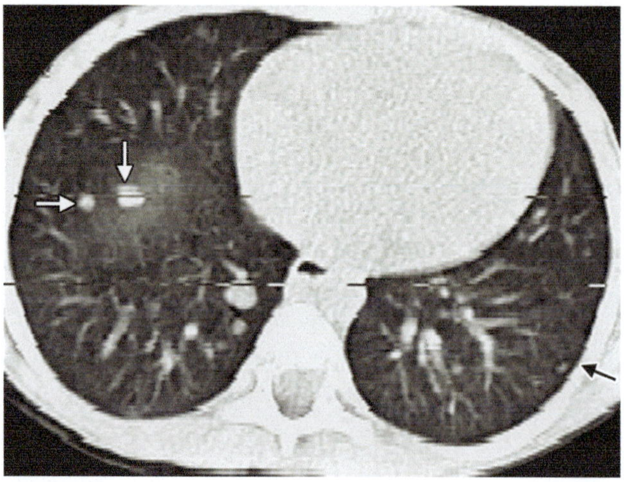

Figure 29.210 Lung metastases from Wilms tumour. Axial CT scan through the chest on lung window settings. There are a number of intrapulmonary nodules within both lungs on this image (some of which are arrowed), consistent with intrapulmonary metastases.

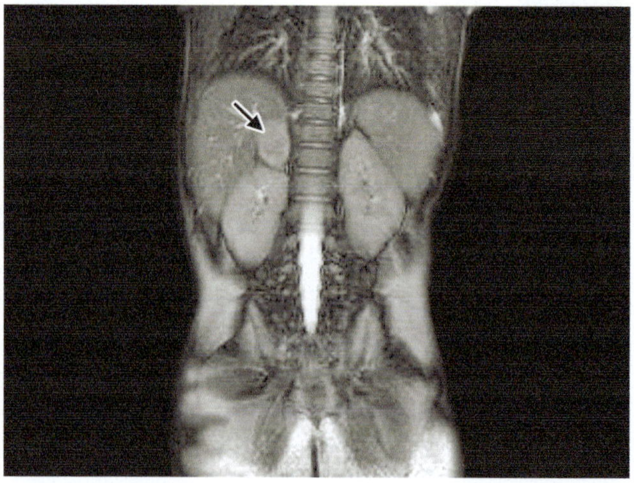

Figure 29.211 Right adrenal neuroblastoma. Coronal T2 weighted (fat saturated) MR scan of abdomen demonstrates an ovoid mass situated above the upper pole of the right kidney in the right adrenal gland (arrow).

treatment and to evaluate response to treatment. The tumour is usually identified as an intrarenal mass. It can extend via the renal vein into the IVC and right atrium and it can metastasise to the lungs. Bilateral Wilms tumours can occur.

Where possible, an MR scan of the abdomen should be used to stage Wilms tumour since this avoids ionising radiation. CT scanning however is required to image the chest.

Neuroblastoma (Figs. 29.111 to 29.113)

Among paediatric abdominal neoplasms, neuroblastoma is the second most common after Wilms tumour. Neuroblastomas, which arise within the abdomen, are staged

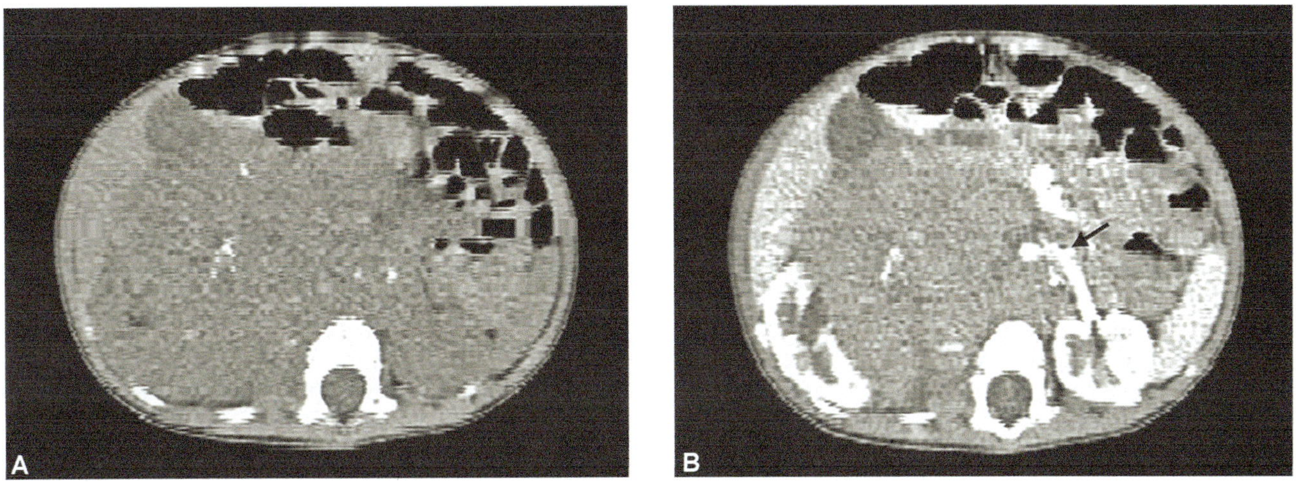

Figures 29.212A and B Right adrenal neuroblastoma with nodal metastases. (A) Unenhanced axial CT scan through the upper abdomen demonstrates a large low density mass in the right flank which crosses the midline. The mass contains small areas of increased density, which are flecks of calcium. This is a feature in up to 90% of tumours on CT scanning; (B) Contrast enhanced axial CT scan through the same region shows the conglomerate mass of tumour and retroperitoneal lymphadenopathy. The lymphadenopathy is displacing the aorta and left renal artery anteriorly (arrow).

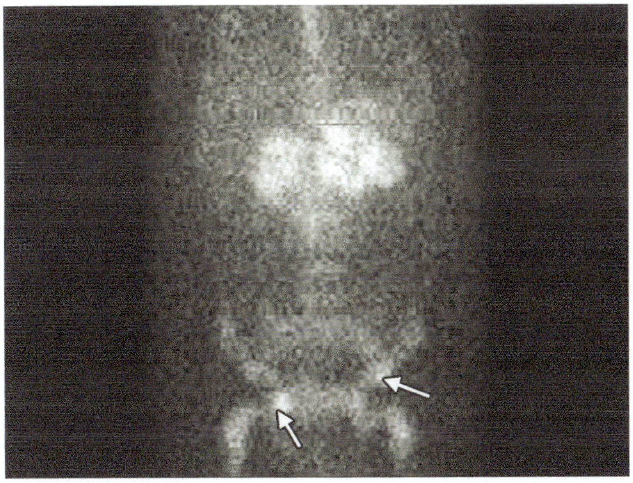

Figure 29.213 Abdominal neuroblastoma with metastases on metaiodobenzylguanidine scan. There is increased tracer uptake in the upper abdomen at the site of the tumour and nodal disease. There are also other areas of increased uptake in the pelvis, consistent with skeletal metastases.

with an abdominal MR scan (where possible) and a CT scan of the chest. Neuroblastomas arising from the adrenal gland can invade the adjacent kidney. The tumour spreads to lymph nodes, bone, bone marrow, liver and skin. Bone metastases are best identified with radionuclide bone studies.

I-131-metaiodobenzylguanidine scintigraphy assesses functional uptake by the tumour and metastases.

ACKNOWLEDGEMENTS

The authors are grateful to Dr Ruth Allen, Consultant Paediatric Radiologist; Dr Greg J Irwin, Consultant Paediatric Radiologist; Dr Andrew J Watt, Consultant Paediatric Radiologist; Mr Rod Duncan, Consultant Orthopaedic Surgeon and Mrs Morag Attaie, Lead Sonographer at Royal Hospital for Sick Children, Glasgow for providing some images.

CHAPTER 30

Prescribing for Children

James Wallace

THE CHALLENGE

Prescribing for children presents a number of challenges. Children are not 'little adults' and should not be treated as such. Their bodies handle medicines differently to adults and the response of young children differs from older ones. Detailed care and attention is needed when making prescribing decisions for children, taking into account their developmental stage. Children can require both specialised care for serious conditions such as cancer or transplantation and general care for more common complaints such as asthma and diarrhoea. The paediatric prescriber requires a sound knowledge of the concepts of care within the whole age range of paediatrics. Neonatology can probably be regarded as a speciality in its own right with different clinical situations and huge differences in pharmacokinetics and dynamics.

Table 30.1 defines the descriptors commonly used for the different age groups, and the key stages, which define the development of a child.

Lack of evidence on the use of medicines in children leads to uncertainty in dosing and increases the risk of medication errors. Even the most appropriate dose may lead to differences in effectiveness and adverse effects to those seen in adults. The evidence suggests that medication safety needs to be improved, particularly in babies and young children. Medication errors occur in children in hospital at similar rates to adults but have three times the potential to cause harm. It is worth remembering that medicines are an important part of treatment strategies but a holistic approach to care of the child is required. Consideration also needs to be given to other approaches where possible including, e.g. psychological management and nutrition. Many changes occur in the way infants and children handle drugs in the period from birth to adulthood. They are important to take into consideration terms of understanding how doses are derived.

PHARMACOKINETICS

Absorption

Absorption of both orally and parenterally administered drugs is similar in children and adults. The exceptions to this are as follows:

- Increased oral absorption of penicillin antibiotics;
- Reduced oral absorptions of phenobarbitone, phenytoin and rifampicin in infants.

This is mainly due to decreased gastric acid secretion and an increased gastric emptying time at birth. Normal emptying times and pH are reached at about the age of 3 years.

TABLE 30.1 Descriptors used for different age groups.

Descriptor	*Age of the child*	*Key stages*
Preterm neonate	23–37 weeks	a. Rapid growth, fully formed gestation b. Most systems not fully developed
Neonate	Birth to 1 month	Normal initial period of human development and growth
Infant	1 month to 1 year	High growth rates and rapid changes
Child	1–12 years	Slower growth and development
Adolescent	12–18 years	Final period growth and puberty, stretching into adulthood

Absorption from intramuscular (IM) administration is erratic, just as it is in adults, and the same types of drugs should be avoided with this route, i.e. phenytoin, digoxin and diazepam. The relatively small amount of muscle in neonates and infants means that IM injections are not only painful but relatively ineffective at achieving adequate drug levels. This route is, therefore, avoided whenever possible.

Fragility of neonatal veins leads to an increased risk of extravasation of intravenous (IV) drugs in this group. Consideration needs to be given to which drugs are likely to cause problems if they leak into surrounding tissue.

Percutaneous absorption is enhanced in infants and children. Their skin is much thinner and better hydrated than adult, and this can lead to problems with topical steroids. This is particularly the case if the skin is broken or burnt. Potent topical steroids should be avoided as systemic adverse effects have been reported in infants. The skin is so thin in neonates (especially preterm) that some substances designed for skin application in adults and older children may actually cause harm. This is true of some skin disinfectants such as chlorhexidine 2% in ethanol which burns a premature baby's skin. Rectal administration is particularly useful in infants and children who are vomiting or are reluctant to take oral medication. However, as in adults, there is considerable variation in individuals' blood supply to the rectum, causing variation in the rate and extent of absorption of rectally administered drugs. Diazepam can be given rectally, and this is often the most convenient route in a child who is fitting. Paracetamol is also given rectally to treat pyrexia usually in children who are too ill to take their medication orally.

Distribution

The two main factors influencing drug distribution are (1) body composition and (2) plasma protein binding.

Body Composition

Extracellular fluid volume is much higher in newborn infants (50%). It decreases gradually with increasing age, 25% at 1 year of age and 20–25% by adulthood. More importantly, total body water is much higher in premature infants (85%) than in term infants (75%) and adults (50–60%). In addition, the body fat content changes dramatically with age, from 3% in a premature newborn to 12% in full-term infants, 30% at 1 year and 18% in adulthood.

This tends to mean greater doses of water-soluble drugs, e.g. penicillin and aminoglycosides on a weight-for-weight basis are required, e.g. the normal dose of IV flucloxacillin for a premature neonate is 25 mg/kg. If you were to give this to a 70 kg adult, the dose would be 1.75 g.

Plasma Protein Binding

In premature babies, plasma protein binding is reduced resulting in higher concentrations of free (active) drug. This is due to reduced levels of circulating proteins and a reduced ability to bind. Thus, these patients have a higher apparent volume of distribution than adults. Phenytoin is an example where the increased proportion of free drug in the overall plasma level means that the therapeutic window in neonates (6–15 mg/L) is lower than in older children (10–20 mg/L).

Elimination

The neonatal liver and kidneys are immature in their capacity to eliminate drugs. Both hepatic metabolism and kidney function are reduced in premature babies resulting in increased plasma half-lives of both hepatically and renally cleared drugs. This leads to longer plasma half-lives and increased plasma concentrations. The more premature the infant, the more depressed is the hepatic metabolism.

Hepatic Metabolism

Enzyme systems in the liver are immature in newborn and preterms infants, particularly oxidation and glucuronidation. In the past, this led to the 'grey baby' syndrome when large doses of chloramphenicol were administered to infants with meningitis. It also accounts for the much longer half-life of diazepam in neonates.

In older children, hepatic function is greater than in adults. Most antiepileptics and theophylline require a larger dose per kilogram than in adults to achieve therapeutic plasma concentrations. This is thought to be due to the fact that, relative to body size, the liver is larger than in adults.

Renal Excretion

Renal excretion is the most important parameter, which affects dosing of children at any age. Renal function is immature in premature infants, leading to extended half-lives of drugs such as aminoglycosides or penicillins. Dosing changes are made in the same way as adults with poor renal function, i.e. increasing the dosing interval or decreasing the dose **(Table 30.2)**.

Conversely, patients with cystic fibrosis are able to clear aminoglycoside at a much higher rate than normal children of the same age. The reasons for this have

TABLE 30.2 Glomerular filtration rate (GFR) at different stages of gestation.

Gestation (weeks)	*GFR (mL/min)*	*GFR (mL/min/m²)*
26	0.6	2
34	1	4
>34 to term	2–4	7–13
Term	4	13
Adult	120–140	70–80

never been fully explained but theories include enhanced tubular secretion, increased extrarenal clearance and increased volume of distribution.

These patients nearly always require much higher doses of aminoglycosides to achieve therapeutic plasma concentrations.

COMPLIANCE AND CONCORDANCE

Medicines should only be prescribed for children when absolutely necessary and always after careful consideration of the benefits of administering the medicine versus the risk involved from side effects and adverse drug reactions. It is important to discuss treatment options carefully with the child and the child's carer.

Compliance

Factors that contribute to poor compliance with prescribed medicines include the following:

- Difficulty in taking the medicine (e.g. inability to swallow tablets)
- Unpalatable formulation (e.g. unpleasant taste or unwillingness to administer medicines rectally)
- Purpose of medicine not clear
- Perceived lack of effectiveness
- Real or perceived side effects
- Difference between the carer's or child's perception of risk and severity of side effects from that of the prescriber
- Unclear instructions for administration.

Concordance

The concept of compliance (the extent to which the prescriber's instructions are followed) is now giving way to that of concordance, where the patient is an active participant in decisions about treatment. Concordance is paramount between the health care professional, the child and the family. Time, effort and understanding are needed to achieve effective use of medicines in children. Children and parents need to be empowered to become active partners in discussions about the risks and benefits of their medicines. Their values and beliefs need to be taken into account as well as the effects of the proposed treatment on daily living.

MAIN ISSUES IN PRACTICE

Dosage Dilemmas

Choosing the most appropriate dose for children is no easy task. Their weight can range from around 0.5 kg for the very young to 120 kg for adolescents. However, adults' weight can also vary from 40 to 120 kg and no prescriber would think twice about giving any adult a 150 mg dose of ranitidine, e.g. even though the plasma concentrations obtained will vary enormously. The difference is that we know this dose is safe and effective for most adults—there is less certainty in prescribing for children.

Most paediatric formularies will state that the ranitidine dose in children is 2 mg/kg, making a 26.4 mg dose for a 13.2-kg child. Ranitidine suspension comes as 15 mg/mL requiring the carer to draw up 1.76 mL. We know that decimal points are a major area of risk so would it be appropriate to give 2 mL (30 mg) to this same child?

The answer in this case is 'yes' as ranitidine has a wide therapeutic range in children just as it does in adults. Good practice would be to round the dose and avoid decimal points. The skill is to know when this is appropriate with individual drugs and how far rounding can be taken.

Although, few drugs are licensed for children, we need to look at what the license really tells us. Let us take the example of aciclovir, which has a licensed dose for children of 10 mg/kg tds for less than 3 months; 500 mg/m^2 tds for 3 months up to 12 years and 10 mg/kg tds for 12 years and over. (Note here that this particular license has different units of measurement for these age groups, depending on how trials were carried out.) There is good evidence that these doses are safe and effective for these age groups. But should an 11-year-old be treated differently than a 12-year-old? How rigidly should these age-related criteria be applied? In practice, an 11-year-old is often given a higher dose than a 12-year-old. It is important to ensure that whatever dose, and whatever source of information is being used, that treatment meets the needs of the individual child.

Information Sources

Prescribers should always use reliable sources of paediatric dose information where these are available. However, the lack of paediatric data means that prescribers are occasionally left to extrapolate information from adult doses. Although, this is plausible, it can also be dangerous. The metabolism and dynamics of babies, for instance, may be totally different to those in adults and may have unpredictable and serious adverse effects.

Dose Calculation

Many methods have developed over the years for calculating doses in paediatrics. The percentage method and the mg/kg method are the only two that should be used.

Percentage Method (Surface Area Method)

The percentage method for estimating doses is calculated as follows:

$$\frac{\text{Surface area of child}(\text{m}^2)}{1.76\text{m}^2} \times 100 = \text{Percentage of adult dose}$$

(1.76 m^2 being the average adult surface area)

TABLE 30.3 Mean values for weight and height by age.

Age	*Weight (kg)*	*Height (cm)*
Full-term neonate	3.5	51
1 month	4.3	55
2 months	5.4	58
3 months	6.1	61
4 months	6.7	63
6 months	7.6	67
1 year	9	75
3 years	14	96
5 years	18	109
7 years	23	122
10 years	32	138
12 years	39	149
14-year-old boy	49	163
14-year-old girl	50	159
Adult male	68	176
Adult female	58	164

Source: Paediatric Formulary Committee. BNF for Children. London: BMJ Publishing Group, RPS Publishing, and RCPCH Publishing Ltd; 2012–13.

Weight, Height and Body Surface Area

Table 30.3 shows the mean values for weight and height by age; these values may be used to calculate doses in the absence of actual measurements. However, the child's actual weight and height might vary considerably from the values in the table and it is important to see the child to ensure that the value chosen is appropriate. In most cases, the child's actual measurement should be obtained as soon as possible and the dose recalculated.

Children are often said to tolerate or require larger doses of drugs than adults based on mg/kg basis. The percentage method helps explain this phenomenon.

Body water (total and extracellular) is known to equate better with surface area than bodyweight. It, therefore, seems appropriate to prescribe drugs by surface area if they are distributed in the extracellular water.

Example

Iain is a 3-month-old baby. He weighs 5.23 kg. His body surface area is 0.31 m^2. Calculate the dose of aciclovir required for him using the percentage method (the adult dose is 800 mg).

$$\frac{0.31}{1.76} \times 100 = 17.6\%$$

Dose is 0.176 × 800 = 140.8 mg
Use 140 mg = 3.5 mL of 200 mg/5 mL aciclovir suspension.

$$\text{Method}: \frac{\text{Adult dose (mg)}}{70\,\text{kg}} = \text{mg / kg}$$

(70 kg being the average adult weight).

This method will give lower doses than the percentage method using surface areas. It is far less accurate in clinical terms but much easier to use since weights are usually more accessible than surface areas. Within limited age bands, it is appropriate to state doses on mg/kg basis. This form of extrapolation from adults is usually inappropriate for accurate therapeutic dosing, although it is unlikely to lead to toxic dosing.

Example

Iain is a 3-month-old baby. He weighs 5.23 kg. His body surface area 0.31 m^2. Calculate the dose of aciclovir required for him using the mg/kg method (the adult dose is 800 mg).

Dose is 11.4 × 5.23 = 59.6 mg
Use 60 mg = 1.5 mL of 200 mg/5 mL aciclovir suspension.

Table 30.4 shows surface area by weight for children. Using body surface area to calculate drug dose is the most accurate method, because it reflects cardiac output, fluid requirements and renal function better than weight-based dosing. In practice, however, it is impractical and necessary for only a limited number of drugs, e.g. cytotoxic agents. Weight-based doses are mainly used. Doses based on age bands may be used for some drugs with a wide therapeutic index.

PRESCRIBING IN PAEDIATRICS

General Issues

Good prescribing is essential in all patients. However, there are key points of good practice in prescribing for children. They can be summarised as follows:

- Always prescribe so that anybody can read it.
- Never prescribe or administer without knowing the allergy status of the child.
- Always be as clear as you can with units: mg, micrograms, nanograms, units are acceptable: μg, ng, ug, iu are not acceptable.
- Decimal points must always have a number in front of them even it is a '0'.
- Try to be logical with doses. There are a few drugs that need precise prescribing on mg/kg basis. Most drugs however can be rounded up or down with no clinical consequences (this reduces the use of decimal points and aids administration).
- Only medication with no strength (e.g. lactulose) or with multiple components (e.g. Abidec) can be prescribed in mL. All others must be in mg, micrograms or mmol for all electrolytes.

Practical Issues

The lack of licensed drugs for children causes practical problems every day for the paediatric pharmacist, doctor,

TABLE 30.4 Body surface area in children.

Body weight (kg)	*Surface area* (m^2)
1	0.10
1.5	0.13
2	0.16
2.5	0.19
3	0.21
3.5	0.24
4	0.26
4.5	0.28
5	0.30
5.5	0.32
6	0.34
6.5	0.36
7	0.38
7.5	0.40
8	0.42
8.5	0.44
9	0.46
9.5	0.47
10	0.49
11	0.53
12	0.56
13	0.59
14	0.62
15	0.65
16	0.68
17	0.71
18	0.74
19	0.77
20	0.79
21	0.82
22	0.85
23	0.87
24	0.90
25	0.92
26	0.95
27	0.97
28	1.0
29	1.0
30	1.1
31	1.1
32	1.1
33	1.1
34	1.1
35	1.2
36	1.2
37	1.2
38	1.2
39	1.3
40	1.3
41	1.3
42	1.3
43	1.3
44	1.4
45	1.4
46	1.4
47	1.4
48	1.4
49	1.5
50	1.5
51	1.5
52	1.5
53	1.5
54	1.6
55	1.6
56	1.6
57	1.6
58	1.6
59	1.7
60	1.7
61	1.7
62	1.7
63	1.7
64	1.7
65	1.8
66	1.8
67	1.8
68	1.8
69	1.8
70	1.9
71	1.9
72	1.9
73	1.9
74	1.9
75	1.9
76	2.0
77	2.0
78	2.0
79	2.0
80	2.0
81	2.0
82	2.1
83	2.1
84	2.1
85	2.1
86	2.1
87	2.1
88	2.2
89	2.2
90	2.2

Values are calculated using the Boyd equation.
Note: Height is not required to estimate body surface area using these tables.
Source: Sharkey I, Boddy AV, Wallace H, Mycroft J, Hollis R, Picton S, et al. Body surface area estimation in children using weight alone. Br J Cancer. 2001;85(1):23-8. (©2001 Macmillan Publishers Ltd.).

nurse, family and patient. These include a lack of dose information. Prescribing too small doses may result in suboptimal therapy, or overdosing may lead to adverse drug reactions. Many paediatric dose reference sources are available but, in some cases, they provide conflicting advice. They tend to be based on local practice and experience rather than hard evidence. A reputable paediatric dose reference source should be used.

Lack of Suitable Formulations

Children are often unable to swallow tablets or capsules and may be in danger of aspiration if they are pushed to do so. Palatable liquid formulations are needed to facilitate administration and accurate measurement of paediatric doses. Often these are not commercially available.

Suitable products such as oral liquid, powders or capsules may therefore have to be prepared extemporaneously. Little information may be available on the bioavailability of the drug or the physical, chemical and microbial stability of the preparation. The result is often unpleasant to take and the preparation will have a short shelf life.

Extemporaneous Dispensing

Extemporaneous dispensing should be seen as a last resort. Standards of extemporaneous dispensing are extremely variable and mistakes have happened with devastating consequences. Currently, there are no common regulations or guidelines to regulate extemporaneous dispensing. It may be performed in a highly equipped laboratory, in a licensed 'specials' manufacturing unit or in a hospital. In such areas, good manufacturing practice guidelines must be met and are enforced by regulatory authorities. This will involve trained personnel who are using strict checking and documentation procedures, suitable equipment and ingredients of a high standard, and are supported by appropriate quality assurance facilities. The whole production process is auditable in terms of ingredients used and personnel involved.

By contrast, extemporaneous dispensing can also be carried out on the dispensary bench in a community pharmacy, often with little equipment and documentation available. There are many variations between these extremes. Although, some countries are developing, or have introduced, guidelines and standards, adherence is usually not a requirement. There needs to be a professional, ethical and legal obligation on practitioners to observe uniformed consistent standards in all areas where extemporaneous dispensing is performed.

Extemporaneous preparation also carries a health risk to pharmacy personnel. An extreme example is infertility and miscarriage in relation to cytotoxic drug handling. Measures are usually taken to ensure the safety of hospital and community pharmacy staff but much better facilities and standards of preparation are required in industry. It would be preferable for all such products to be prepared in a high quality environment to protect the staff involved, the product and the patient.

Alternatives to Extemporaneous Dispensing

A range of options to extemporaneous dispensing is available including the following:

- Choosing an alternative drug that is commercially available in a more suitable form for administration.
- Obtaining a paediatric formulation for a 'specials' manufacturer.
- Using solutions prepared for injections by the oral route. This must be done with care as different formulations may include different salts and therefore have different bioavailability and stability. The pH of some injection solutions can cause problems and other excipients must be checked to be safe. The taste of many injections is problematic and the cost of using an expensive injectable form orally must be considered.
- Cutting tablets to half or quarter size with a tablet cutter. This may help though it is inaccurate and dose equivalence is unlikely to be achieved.
- Dissolving or dispersing tablets in water to make doses of less than a full tablet. Doses can be made up by dissolving a whole tablet in a specified volume and administering an aliquot of the resulting liquid with an oral syringe. Some tablets are soluble or dispersible even if they are not marketed as such. Having a list of such tablets can be helpful. There is a lack of research however to confirm the drug contents of aliquots of liquids when doses are measured in this way.
- Importing licensed formulations from other countries may be a preferable alternative. However, difficulties around importation of free movement of medicines between countries can make this a complicated process. It is also expensive and gaining access to information on such product availability is not always easy.

Excipients

It is important to be aware of inappropriate excipients in some medicine formulations (including some licensed products). The existence of colourings and preservatives has been highlighted in the press. Other examples include the following:

- A commercial formulation of phenobarbital elixir containing 38% alcohol, which is clearly undesirable for children. It has been estimated that if a 5 mL (15 mg) dose was given to a 3 kg baby, this would be equal to an adult swallowing a couple of glasses of wine.

- Phenobarbital injection (200 mg in 1 mL) contains 80–90% propylene glycol that can cause hyperosmolality if the injection is not diluted appropriately. The potential for toxicity is increased with babies and infants.
- Some excipients are undesirable in children with specific disorders. Children with phenylketonuria must avoid aspartame, for instance.

A European Commission (EC) directive issued in 1997 stated that 'benzyl alcohol is contraindicated in infants or young children'. This has implications for formulation of medicines used in children. Summary of product characteristics (SPCs) for amiodarone and lorazepam injections now both state that they contain benzyl alcohol and are contraindicated in infants or young children up to 3 years old. This poses a dilemma given the lack of more appropriate alternatives for these patients.

The sugar content of medicines must also be considered, particularly with long-term treatment. However, it is unlikely to be a major issue in short-term medication.

OTHER ISSUES

Medication Errors

The lack of suitable, licensed formulations for children increases the risk of medication errors by complicating administration. Frequently, a small proportion of the content of an injection vial is required to administer a calculated dose. Miscalculation can lead to a 10-fold or even a 100-fold overdose for a small baby from one vial. Dilution of adult strength injections is also often needed which can involve complex calculations. Fatal errors have indeed occurred.

Other complications are that displacement values must be taken into account and syringes have to be used carefully to avoid administration of the contents of the 'dead space' and overdosing with a concentrated drug.

Different reference sources quote doses in different ways. Some provide dose information as the total daily dose per kg bodyweight, which should then be divided into the appropriate number of doses per day. Others give the individual dose per kg bodyweight and the number of time daily this should be administered. Errors are common due to confusion between these systems. It is therefore essential that prescribers are familiar with the way the reference works to minimise the risk of prescribing errors.

Advanced Formulation

More advanced formulations are becoming increasingly available for adult patients, such as transcutaneous delivery system, fast dissolving drug formulations and multiple unit dose systems, which all offer potential major improvements. Generally, however, this new technology has not benefited children to a major degree so far. It is hoped that recent US and EU legislation will encourage research leading to the development of medicines and formulations designed specifically for children.

ACKNOWLEDGEMENTS

Thanks are due to NES (Pharmacy), the Scottish Neonatal Paediatric Pharmacists Group, and particularly to Steve Tomlin and Sharon Conroy for permission to use and adapt their material for this chapter.

SUGGESTED READING

1. An Introduction to Paediatric Pharmaceutical Care. NHS Education Scotland (Pharmacy); 2009.
2. The British National Formulary for Children. London: BMJ Publishing Group Ltd, RPS Publishing and RCPCH Publications Ltd.; 2012-13.

CHAPTER 31

Child Abuse and Neglect—How do We Protect These Children?

Jean Herbison

"Investigation and management of a case of possible harm to a child must be approached in the same systematic and rigorous manner as would be appropriate to the investigation and management of any other potentially fatal disease".

The Victoria Climbié Inquiry 2003: Report of an Inquiry by Lord Laming, Para 1153

INTRODUCTION

Children, wherever they live, have the right to be protected from all forms of child abuse, neglect and exploitation. This should not be dependent on gender, race or culture. All human beings, including lay persons, professionals, business employees, politicians and governments, have an obligation to ensure that protection.[1] All have a responsibility for the welfare of children and should raise concerns speedily with appropriate persons or authorities should they believe or know that a child is being inappropriately cared for by their parents, carers or others.

VARIOUS FORMS OF ABUSE

Child Neglect

Aspects of neglect include the following:

- Neglect of a child's physical needs, e.g. nutrition or hygiene or clothing.
- Not providing the child with opportunities to socialise with peers. This can be associated with attachment disorders.
- Scapegoating of one child over and above another, e.g. child constantly being unkempt and smelly and being told they are 'useless' whilst other siblings are being complimented and are dressed in clothes acceptable to social norms.

Neglect is usually a chronic or long-term situation, which can have major consequences for the child's self-esteem, development and life chances in general but episodic 'acute' neglect can occur, especially at times of crises in the family or in escalation of parental issues such as mental wellbeing, domestic violence and addiction problems.

Neglect tends to be associated more with poverty and with lower social classes but it certainly occurs also in affluent families, particularly where children are left isolated, unsupported or unsupervised due to parents' work commitments or even resentments at having to look after the children and care for them rather than their priority of life ambition and career.

Recognition of Child Neglect

Health professionals can become concerned or suspicious of child neglect **(Figs. 31.1A to C)** over a range of contacts with children and families, e.g. concern may be raised from:

- A poor uptake of assessment of the child's development at appropriate appointments or parents' attitude to the child's immunisations.
- Leaving diagnosed medical conditions untreated and not responding to sustained medical advice or giving what appears to be essential treatment regularly for a range of health problems.
- Frequent attendance at emergency departments (EDs) with unusual injuries or other presentations which appear to be associated with accidents. These may have been preventable in the household setting or have occurred through a lack of supervision.
- A child being presented either at nursery or school or in other social environments dressed unacceptably, e.g. in a nightie walking outside late at night in cold weather unaccompanied.

Assessment of the Extent of Child Neglect

Many standardised tools can be used but the essential element is to gather all information from professionals surrounding and working with the child and family including the family practitioners, health visitor, school nurse,

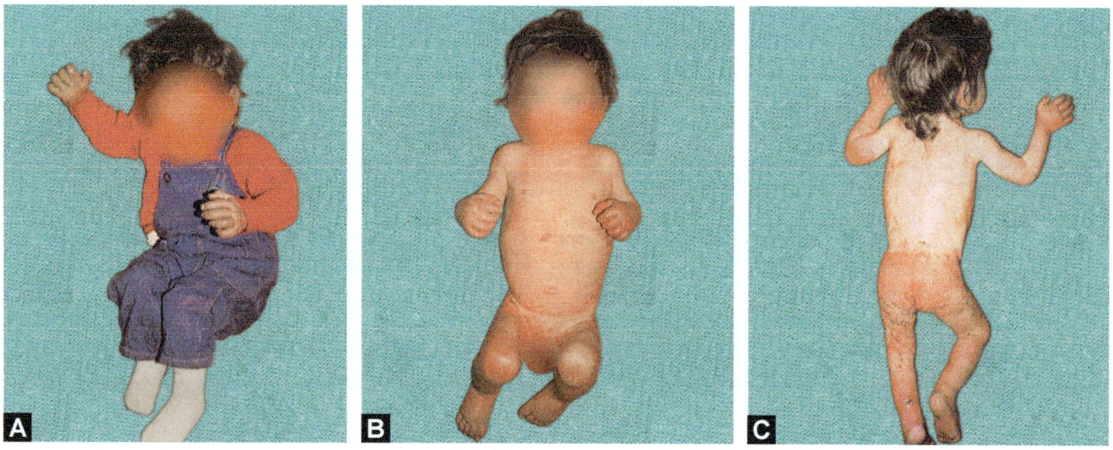

Figures 31.1A to C (A) A small unkempt child in a flexed position with red swollen hands; (B) *Note* that the same posture is maintained when undressed; (C) How the child is emaciated—*note* the wasted buttocks and severe chronic nappy rash extending down the leg. Swollen lower legs are also seen.

(*Source:* Hobbs C. Physical Signs of Child Abuse. London: WB Saunders Co Ltd.)

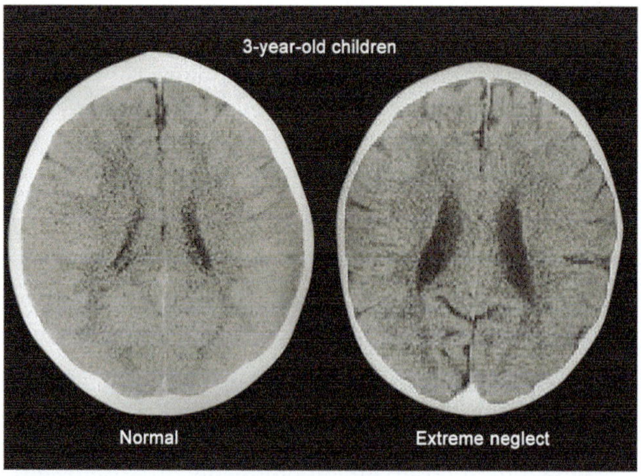

Figure 31.2 Abnormal brain development following sensory neglect in early childhood. The image on the right is from a 3-year-old child suffering from severe sensory-deprivation neglect. This child's brain is significantly smaller than average and has enlarged ventricles and cortical atrophy.

(*Source:* Perry BD. Childhood experience and the expression of genetic potential: what childhood neglect tells us about nature and nurture. Brain and Mind. 2002;3:79–100)

psychologist, school teacher, social worker and sometimes police if they have already been asked to attend due to the family, e.g. the child being left alone or found wandering without supervision at a young age. Other information must also be gathered particularly by social workers and police from neighbours, community volunteer workers or extended family members **(Fig. 31.2)**.

The integrated assessment framework 'triangle' assists all practitioners, including medical practitioners to glean robust detailed information about the individual child's needs, including the child's development, details with regard to parenting and whether there is adequate parenting capacity and/or appropriate standards of care as well as the social environmental circumstances within which the child lives. Key factors, such as poverty, unemployment and overcrowding, can contribute markedly to the chronic neglect of a child. The neglect is not necessarily a deliberate act, but may be the consequence of parental risk factors such as mental health problems or lack of capacity to parent. Other examples or risk factors are parental addiction to drugs or alcohol, domestic violence (gender-based violence) within the home or learning disability in parent or carer. In these situations, the neglect of the child can be by omission (not intended) or by commission. Nevertheless, it is the impact on the child in any case which must be seriously taken into account. Supportive intervention early and/or intervention to remove the child (at the most extreme end of circumstances) can be actioned but the child often lives for years in the context of neglect which has a major detrimental effect on emotional, cognitive and physical development. There is often a future generational impact and if the child has not been parented appropriately or has been abused, they often learn not to parent and the cycle is perpetuated throughout many future generations. That in itself leads to addictions, self-harm, low self-esteem and criminal behaviours. The following diagram shows the importance of the early detection and appropriate intervention in neglect cases **(Figs. 31.3 and 31.4)**.

The sharing of information between professionals involved with the child or families is critical. This should not be obstructed by simply bureaucratic notions of 'confidentiality'. Confidentiality must be in the best interest of the children as our patients. That is between professionals involved in children's services but also professionals involved in adult services, particularly those of mental health learning disability, addictions and where adult practitioners such as the general practitioner may become aware, e.g. that there is violence within the family home. There is substantial evidence that children living within

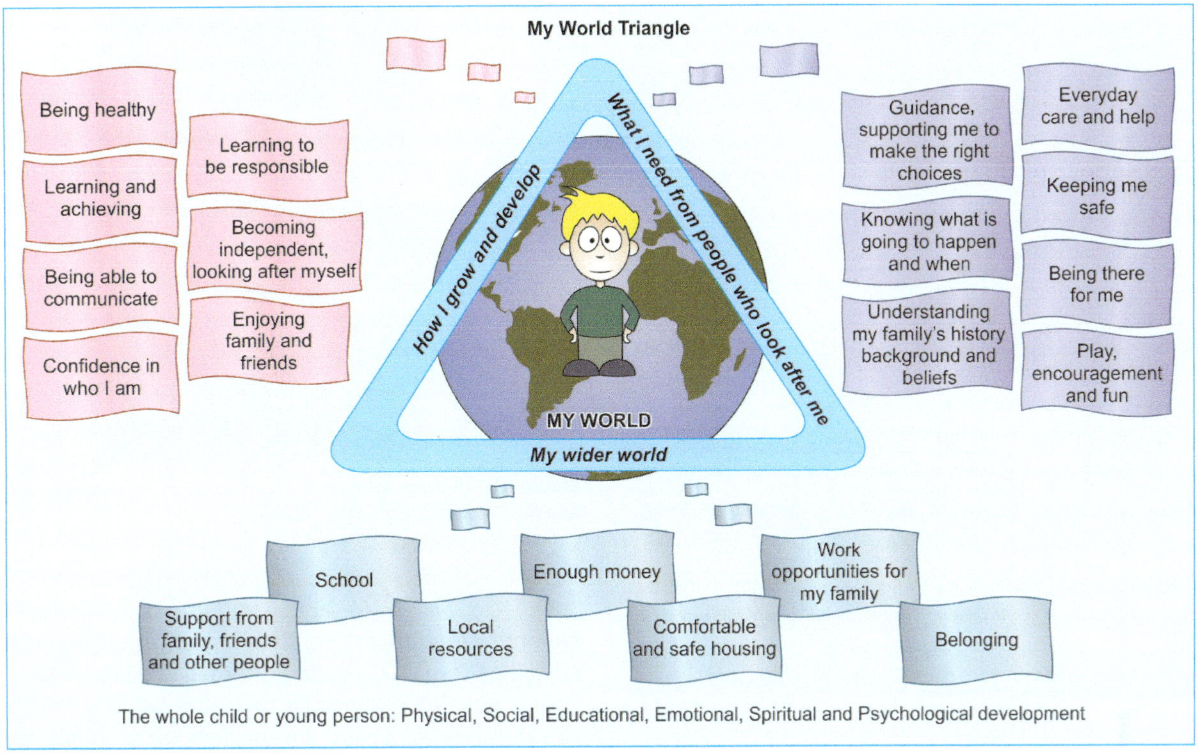

Figure 31.3 My world triangle.

(*Source:* Getting it right for every child (GIRFEC). Scottish Government (2009). Available from www.scotland.gov.uk/Topics/People/Young-people/Childrenservices/Girfec/Practitioners/Tools Resources)

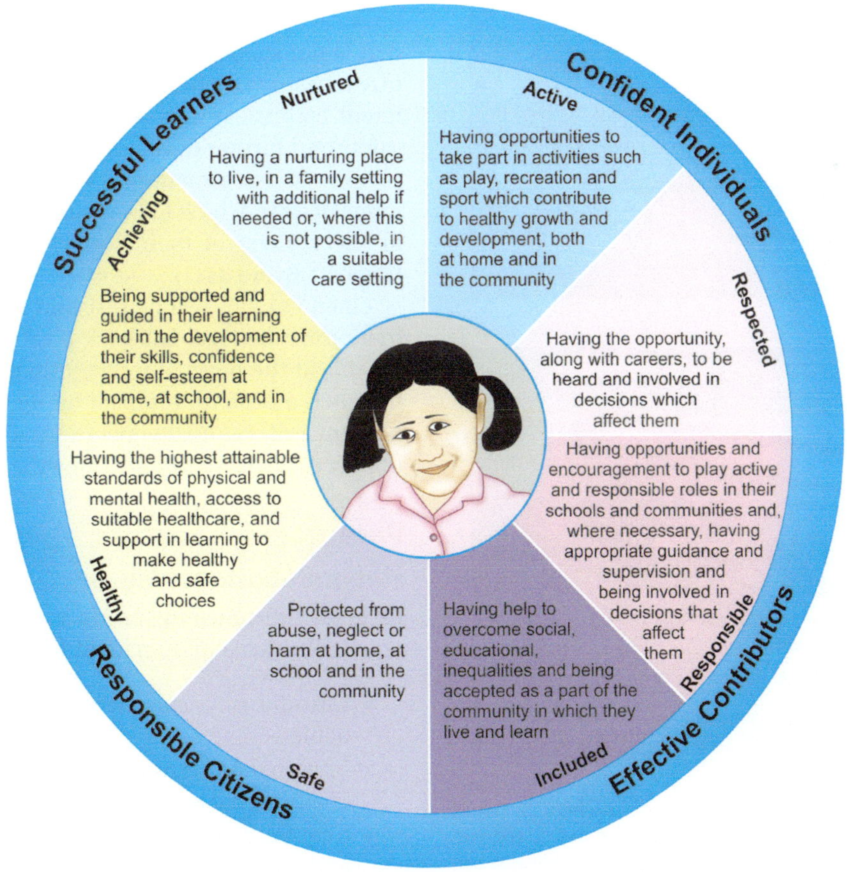

Figure 31.4 Factors that contribute to children developing into successful learners, confident individuals, responsible citizens and effective contributors.

(*Source:* Getting it right for every child (GIRFEC). Practitioner tools and resources; 2008)

Denial of problems by parents (may have learning problems)	History from child—bullied, no friends, aggressive	'Attention-seeking' concern by nursery school of standard of care
Physical symptoms, e.g. pain from dental caries	Poor physical condition—dirty, thin hair, nappy rash	'Growth-stunted/fails, to reach potential height
Development delayed, e.g. language, social skills	Poor compliance with treatment, e.g. asthma	Increased risk of accidents: RTA, fire, drowning
Supportive network, i.e. with family and friends—little effect as share similar problems	Poverty with poor housing, diet, parents, with poor health physical and mental), little education	Large number of involved professionals —health visitor, school nurse, social worker, home care, housing, GP, paediatrician, etc.

Figure 31.5 A range of factors can contribute to the picture of child neglect—often there is accumulative concern with regard to one factor or several.

Abbreviations: RTA, road traffic accident; GP, general practitioner.

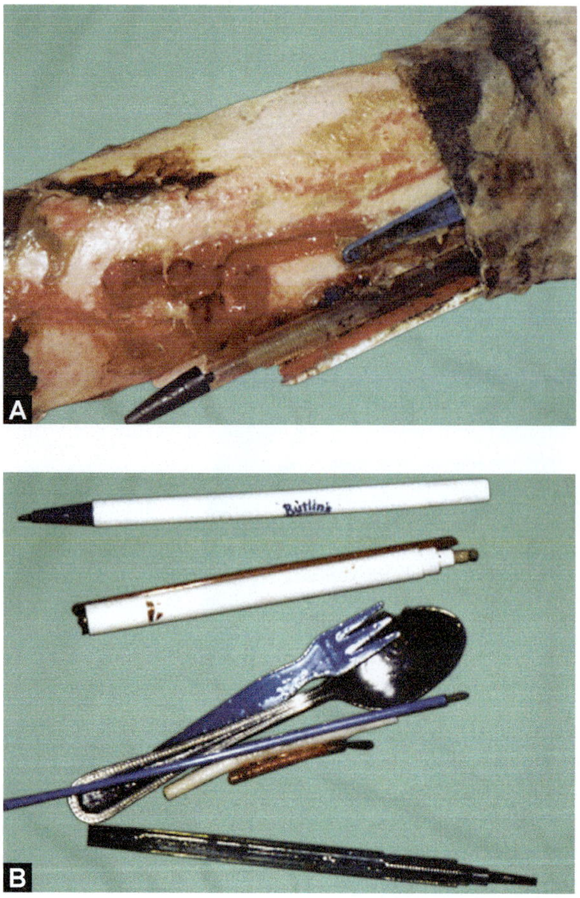

Figures 31.6A and B A 7-year-old boy neglected by parents with mental health problems. Several non-attendances for important medical appointments. Leg plaster not removed found in the house. (A) Implements had to be surgically removed from leg; (B) Implements.

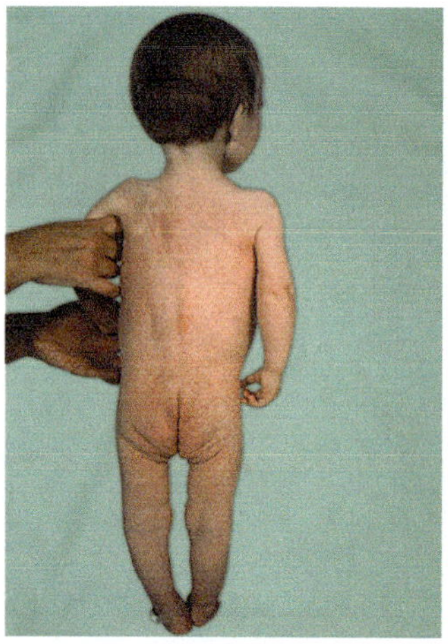

Figure 31.7 Buttock wasting due to starvation. Always consider other organic conditions, e.g. Coeliac disease.

violent homes are at very high risk of physical abuse and sustained impact on their emotional development.

It is absolutely essential that professionals have a low threshold of suspicion for neglect of a child's welfare (**Fig. 31.5**) such that their analysis and assessment can occur and appropriate interventions and support can be implemented early in the child's life to enable the family to encourage nurturance of the child and ensure optimal physical and emotional development in the future. Where that is not sustainable, then local child protection statutory measures (dependent on different procedures in different countries) must be enacted to ensure the child's safety and further development. This requires a dynamic process of assessment and the ability to intervene in a range of ways, which fit every individual and child's needs in the context of their family and community setting (**Figs. 31.6 and 31.7**).

Often families will be resistant to these measures and there must be legal fall-back position to ensure that the child is at the heart of interventions. Continuing neglect has such a profound impact on their longer-term development and on future generations. **Figure 31.8** shows the impact of neglect on child's growth.

Parental Risk Factors

Parental Substance Misuse

Parental substance misuse is associated with a range of potential risk to children including the following:

- Harmful physical effects on unborn and newborn babies.
- Impaired patterns of parental care with a higher risk of emotional and physical neglect or abuse.
- Chaotic lifestyles which disrupt children's routines and relationships, leading to early behavioural and emotional problems.

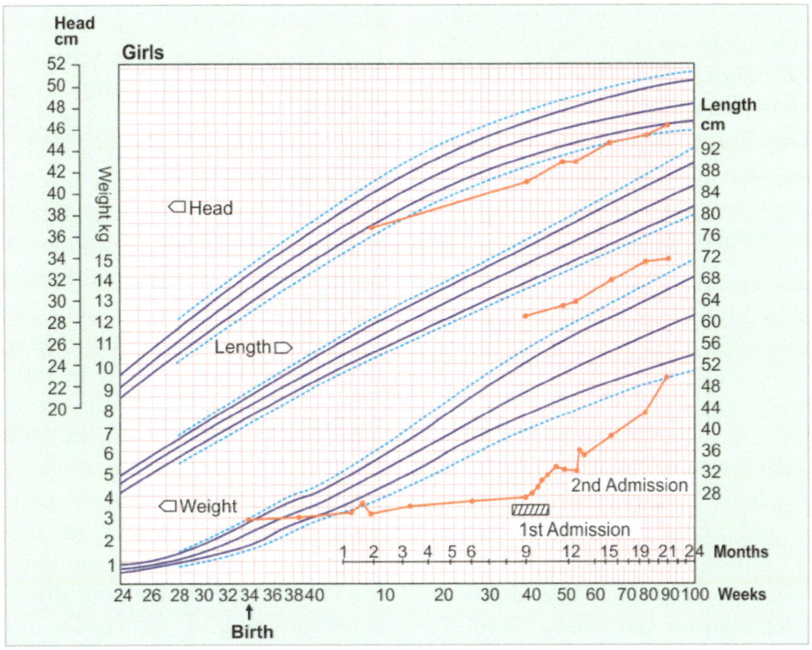

Figure 31.8 The growth chart shows rapid increase in weight of a child following two separate admissions to hospital. Describes clear failure to thrive due to socioenvironmental deprivation.

- Family income may be diverted to buy alcohol or drugs, leading to poverty, debt and material deprivation.
- Unstable accommodation or homelessness as a consequence of antisocial behaviour orders, rent arrears or conviction for alcohol or drugs related offences.
- Children having inappropriately high levels of responsibility for social or personal care of parents with problem substance use, or care of younger siblings.
- Isolation of children and inability to confide in others for fear of the consequences.
- Threat of domestic abuse.
- Disrupted schooling.
- Children's early exposure to and socialisation into, illegal substance misuse and other criminal activity.
- Parents' reduced awareness or loss of consciousness may place children at physical risk in the absence of another adult who is able to supervise and care for them.
- Careless storage of medication and disposal of needles and syringes may cause accident or overdose.
- Repeated separation from parents when parents attend detoxification or rehabilitation facilities, or are in prison, or leave children looked after by multiple or unsuitable carers.
- Multiple episodes of substitute care with extended family or foster carers.

All agencies supporting adult alcohol or drug users should ask new attendees the following:

- Are you a parent?
- How many dependent children live with you?
- Do you have any children who live with others or are in residential care?
- What is your child(ren)'s age and gender?
- Which school or nursery or other preschool facility do they attend?
- Are there any other relatives or support agencies in touch with your family who are supporting the child(ren)?
- Do you need any help looking after children or arranging childcare?

Parental Mental Health

Parental mental health problems have a significant effect on the wellbeing of children and can lead to harm. In a report of 100 cases of fatal child abuse, there was parental psychiatric morbidity in 32% of the cases which included depression, postnatal depression and personality disorder.[2,3]

The crossing bridges family model is a useful framework that can help staff to consider the parent, the child in the family as a whole when assessing the needs of and planning care packages for families with a parent suffering from a mental health problem.[4]

- Parental mental health problems can adversely affect the development and in some cases the safety of children.

- Growing up with a parent who experiences mental health problems can have a negative impact on the young person's adjustment into adulthood including their own transition to parenthood.
- Children, particularly those with emotional, behavioural or chronic physical difficulties, can precipitate or exacerbate the mental ill health in their own parents, therefore, increasing risks.

Public concern has arisen because of a number of high profile cases where children have been directly harmed, sometimes fatally because of the mental health problems of their parents or carers. Common themes emerging from these cases include the following:

- Lack of professional awareness of the impact of parental mental health problems on children.
- Individual agencies and their staff being unaware of, the presence of children within households.
- Lack of any clear assessment of the needs, situation and circumstances of children. In addition, services being too focused on the needs of adults and ignoring or lacking sensitivity to the needs of children and families.
- Ineffective communication between professional staff and between agencies including lack of interpretation of the health information provided with clarity to other agencies.
- Inconsistent recording linked to the issue of poor assessment of children.
- Poor evidence as to why decisions to act or more importantly not to act have been taken.
- Professionals not acting to help children soon enough resulting in crises arising and actual harm or tragedies happening **(Figs. 31.9 and 31.10)**.

Domestic Violence

Domestic violence is a term describing a continuum of violent behaviour within an intimate relationship or close family situation. It can include verbal, financial, sexual, emotional or physical abuse. Domestic violence and child abuse, whether physical or emotional, often coexists. In a National Children's Home (NCH) Charity Study from 1994, 75% of mothers in homes where domestic abuse was occurring said that their children had witnessed violent incidents and 33% of the children had seen their mothers beaten. Ninety per cent of children were present in the same or the next room at the time of the assault.[5] Quite a number of women are abused in pregnancy and in a study by McWilliams et al. in 1993, in relation to 127 women in refuges in Northern Ireland, 60% had been abused in pregnancy, 13% had lost their babies as a result and 22% had threatened miscarriages.[6] There are many effects on the child including lacking in self-confidence, withdrawn, constantly anxious, constantly fearful, difficulties in forming relationships, sleep disturbances, post-traumatic stress disorder, non-attendance or poor attendance at school (NCH, 1994).[7]

Health professionals have a key role in recognising domestic abuse and in referring appropriately to other agencies so optimal and sensitive assistance can be offered to the child and non-abusive parent.

Parental Learning Disability

People with a learning disability need help with everyday living. This means that people with a learning disability need help in at least one of the following skill areas as follows:

- Conceptual skills—receptive and expressive language, reading and writing, money concepts.

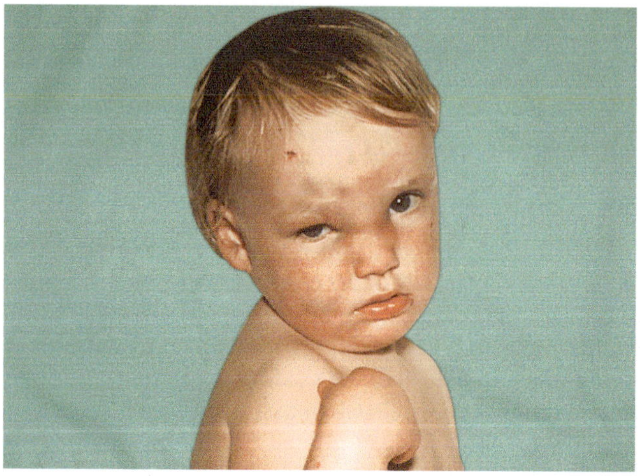

Figure 31.9 Frozen watchfulness. This child also has broken nose and unexplained bruising in context of serious chronic neglect and physical abuse.

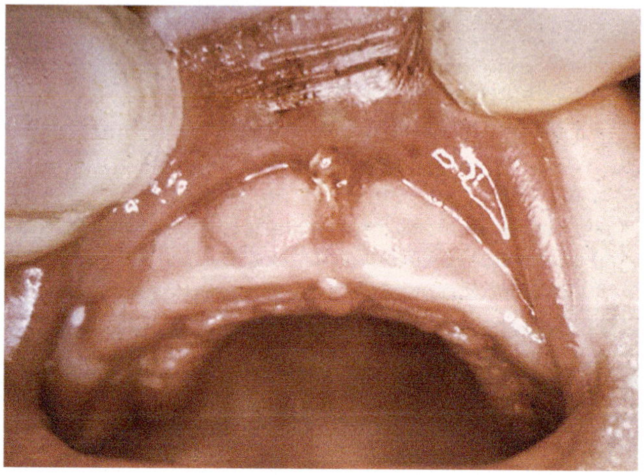

Figure 31.10 Ruptured frenulum in context of inadequate parenting. Clumsy and inappropriately forceful bottle feeding. Can also be caused by direct blows to face.

(*Source:* Hobbs C. Physical Signs of Child Abuse. London: WB Saunders Co Ltd.)

- Social skills—interpersonal, responsibility, self-esteem.
- Practical skills—personal activities of daily living (eating, dressing, mobility and toileting). Instrumental activities of daily living (preparing meals, managing money, housekeeping activities).

The prevalence of communication difficulties is estimated at between 50 and 80% in people with a learning disability.

- Forty per cent to sixty per cent of children born to parents with a learning disability are removed from their care.
- Learning disabled parents are 30–60 times more likely to be subject to a care order application than their numbers in the community would predict.
- Parents with intelligence quotient (IQ) less than 60 experience more difficulty in cognitive functioning and social skills.

What do we know about parents with learning disabilities?

- Purposeful abuse by parents is infrequent.
- Neglect–omission not commission. Family pattern is repeated "I don't know what I'm doing wrong".
- Cognitive functioning and ability to learn
    - Uncertainty in literature regarding the effectiveness of training
    - Input needs to be longer term
    - Maintaining skills, forgetting, failure to generalise, adjusting parenting styles as child grows
- The greater the discrepancy between parents' knowledge, skills and experience and the needs of the children, the higher the degree of risk.[8]
- Vulnerability to psychopathology.[9–11]
- Forty-five per cent depression and anxiety.
- Obsessive compulsive disorder (OCD) in females more severe.
- Study by McGaw looking at high-risk versus low-risk parents found experience of trauma by mothers to be significant for child protection registration for emotional abuse in children (79%).
- Health
    - Mothers with learning disabilities are at particular risk for poor health status.
- Common health problems in learning disability (LD)—department of health (DOH)
    - Mobility problems
    - Respiratory problems
    - Psychiatric disorders
    - Behavioural problems
    - Obesity
    - Eyesight problems
    - Health problems
    - Communication problems.

It has been stated that often the presence of a major medical condition in mother is one of the prime reasons for removal of a child from a family.

The difficulties experienced by parents who have an LD often overlap with those experienced by families of poor economic status.

- Mothers with LDs tend to be isolated from their local communities.

Key risk factors for abuse where parents are learning disabled are as follows:

- Presence of male IQ more than 70. Two LD parents were of less note in terms of risk to child than where male in household had IQ more than 70
- Higher risk are as follows:
    - Previous children on child protection register.
    - Mother had history of trauma (physical, emotional, neglect).
    - Physical or sensory impairment of more than 0.5.
    - Special needs in children.

Improving outcomes for disabled parents and their children:

- Accessible information and communication.
- Clear coordinated referral and assessment procedures, processes, eligibility criteria and care pathways.
- Support designated to meet the needs of parents and children based on assessments of their needs and strengths.
- Long-term support where necessary.
- Access to independent advocacy.

EMOTIONAL ABUSE AND NEGLECT

This must be considered when there is concern that the parent or carer–child interactions may be harmful. Examples include the following:

- Negativity or hostility towards a child or young person.
- Rejection or scapegoating of a child or young person.
- Developmentally inappropriate expectations of or interactions with a child, including inappropriate threats or methods of disciplining.
- Exposure to frightening or traumatic experiences, including domestic abuse.
- Using the child for fulfilment of the adult's needs (e.g. children being used in marital disputes).
- Failure to promote the child's appropriate socialisation (e.g. involving children in unlawful activities, isolation, not providing stimulation or education).

Suspect emotional abuse when persistent harmful parent or carer–child interactions are observed or reported. Consider child maltreatment if parents or carers are seen or reported to punish a child for wetting despite professional advice that the symptom is involuntary. Consider emotional neglect if there is emotional unavailability and unresponsiveness from the parent or carer towards a child and in particular towards an infant.

Consider child maltreatment if a parent or carer refuses to allow a child or young person to speak to a healthcare professional on their own when it is necessary for the assessment of the child or young person.

Additionally, consider child maltreatment if a child or young person displays or is reported to display a marked change in behaviour or emotional state, as per the examples below:

- Behavioural change which is a departure from what would be expected for their age and developmental stage and which is not explained by a known stressful situation, e.g. bereavement or parental separation or a medical cause.

Examples where child maltreatment should be suspected include the following:

Emotional States

- Fearful, withdrawn, low self-esteem.

Behaviour

- Aggressive, oppositional
- Habitual body rocking.

Interpersonal Behaviour

- Indiscriminate contact or affection seeking.
- Over-friendliness to strangers includes healthcare professionals.
- Excessive clinginess.
- Persistently resorting to gaining attention.
- Demonstrating excessively 'good' behaviour to prevent parental or carer disapproval.
- Failure to seek or accept appropriate comfort or affection from an appropriate person when significantly distressed.
- Coercive controlling behaviour towards parents or carers.
- Very young children showing excessive comforting behaviours when witnessing parental or carer distress.[12]

Assessment of Emotional Abuse

Neglected children may present with the following:

- Failure to thrive through lack of understanding of dietary needs of a child or inability to provide an appropriate diet; or they may be present with obesity through inadequate attention to the child's diet.
- Craving attention or ambivalent towards adults, or may be very withdrawn.
- Being too hot or too cold—check hands or feet for cold injury with red swollen and cold hands and feet or they may be dressed in inappropriate clothing.
- Consequences arising from situations of danger—accidents, assaults, poisoning, other hazards (lack of safeguarding).
- Delayed development and failing at school (poor stimulation and opportunity to learn).
- Difficult or challenging behaviour (failure of parenting).
- Unusually severe by preventable conditions owing to lack of awareness of preventive healthcare or failure to treat minor conditions.
- Health problems associated with lack of basic facilities such as heating.

Additional risk of neglect may be present for children with disability and chronic illness. These may be associated with the child's environment, lack of service provision, family circumstances and society's attitude towards disability.

Parenting issues may impact on the parent/carer's ability and motivation to meet the needs of the child. These include the following:

- Learning disabilities
- Mental health problems
- Substance or alcohol abuse, including binge drinking
- Domestic violence
- Disability
- Chronic illness
- Unemployment or poverty
- Homelessness
- Young lone parents.[13]

PHYSICAL ABUSE

Physical abuse (inflicted injury) otherwise known as 'non-accidental injury' (NAI). Types of injuries in infants that may cause concern:

'Those who do not cruise, rarely bruise.'[14] A systematic review of the international literature in infants under the age of 6 months suggests that any bruise in an infant under 6 months must be fully evaluated and a detailed history taken to ascertain consistency with the injury. The under one's in general are a particularly at risk group for various physical injuries. Non-mobile children should not have bruises without a clear and usually observed explanation. Certain areas are rarely (<2%) bruised accidentally at any age including neck, buttocks and hands in children less than 2 years **(Fig. 31.11)**.[13]

Common and important sites for non-accidental bruises are as follows:

- Buttocks and lower back
- Slap marks on side of the face, scalp and ears
- Bruises on external ear
- Neck, eyes and mouth

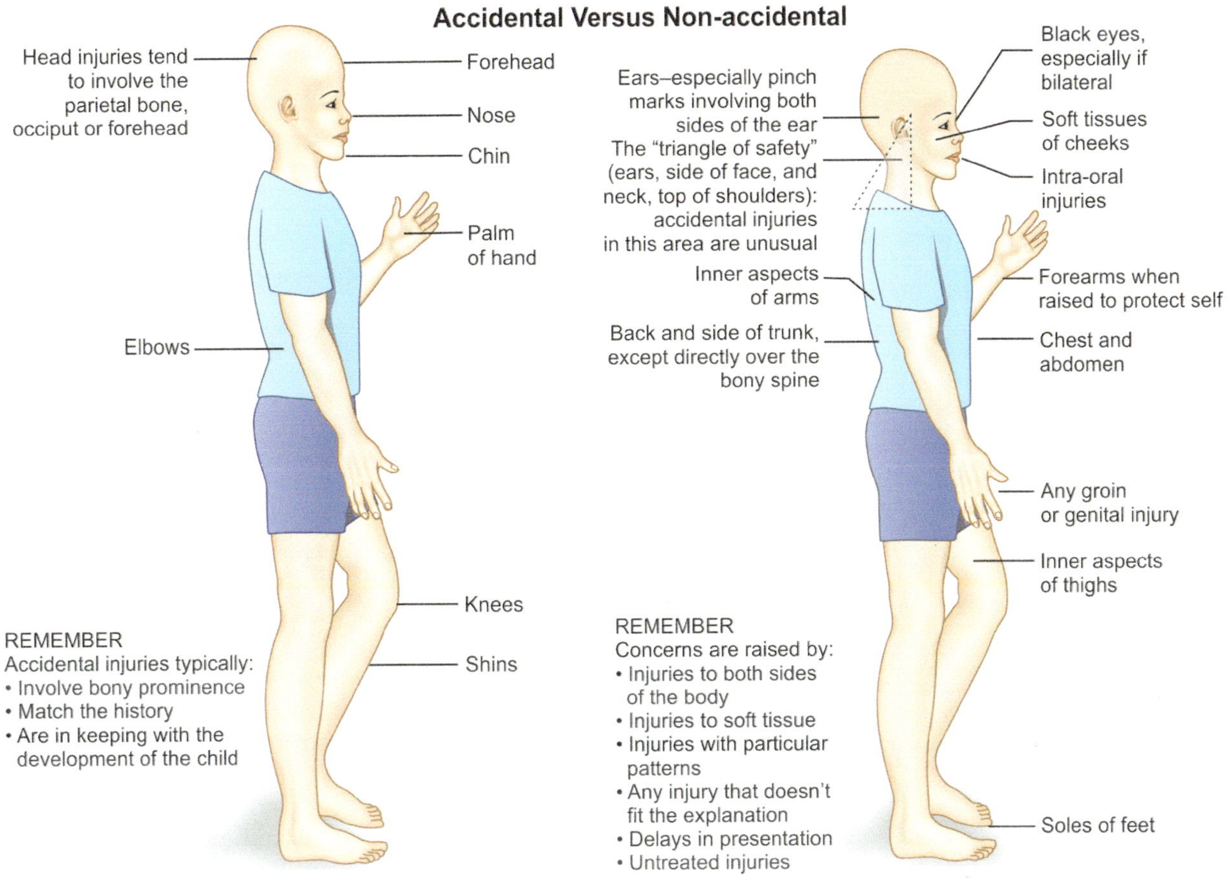

Figure 31.11 Common sites of accidental versus non-accidental bruising.

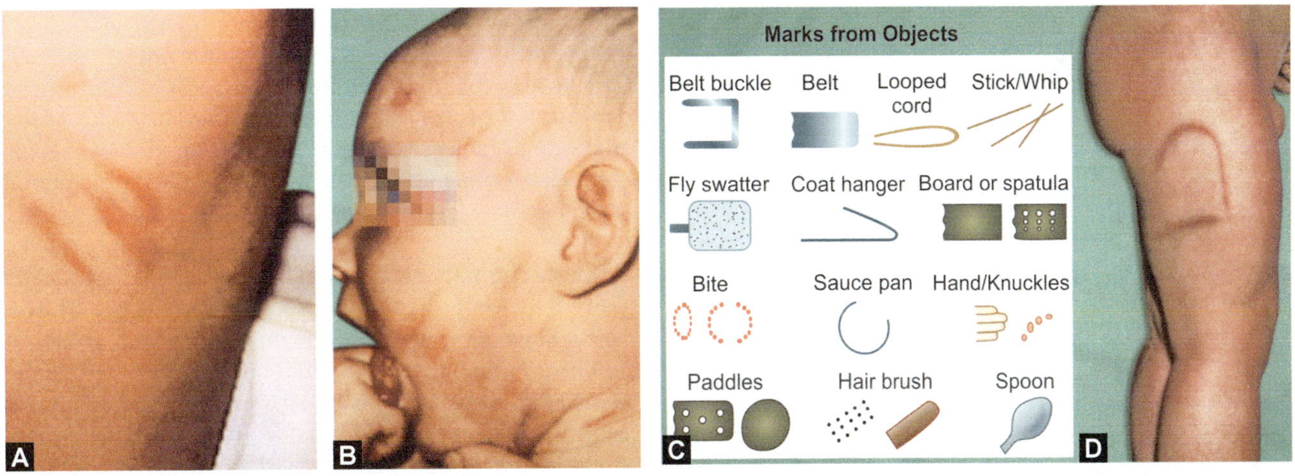

Figures 31.12A to D (A) Well-demarcated bruise demonstrating blunt force trauma by object. On this occasion, the buckle of a belt; (B) Forced hand slap injury (or could have been face forcibly impacting on rigid object). (C) Marks produced by forced trauma using a range of objects; (D) Well-demarcated outline left by object following forced trauma.

- Trunk, including chest and abdomen
- Lower jaw.

The face is the most commonly bruised site in fatally abused children (**Figs. 31.12 to 31.15**). It is important on all parts of the body to look for patterns such as fingertip marks, implement marks, belt, stick or other object marks (**Figs. 31.8 to 31.11**). Obviously differential diagnosis includes bleeding disorder, drug induced bruising either accidentally or deliberate, birth mark including Mongolian blue spot, cultural practices including cupping or coining.

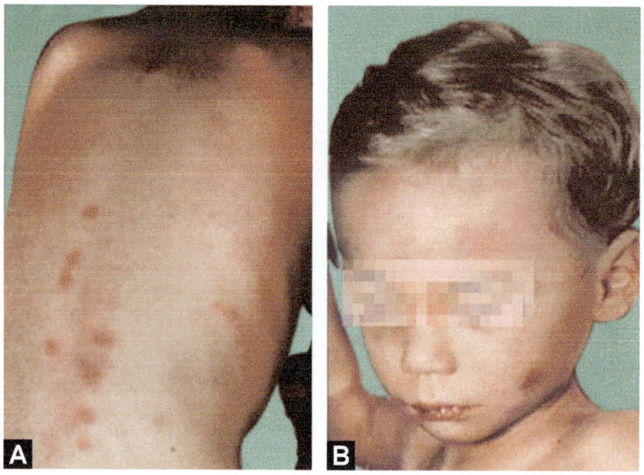

Figures 31.13A and B (A) Fingertip marks due to forceful gripping; (B) Multiple unexplained bruises including fingertip bruises to soft tissue area of left cheek.

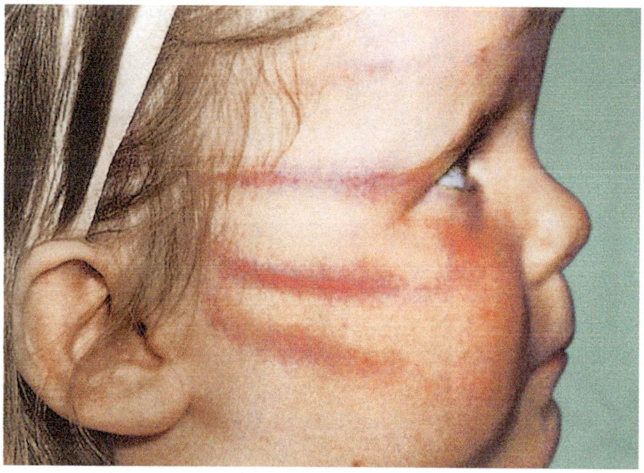

Figure 31.14 Recent horizontal linear bruises extending across the cheek consistent with an adult hand slap.

(*Source:* Hobbs J, Wynne JM. Physical Signs of Child Abuse, 2nd edition. Philadelphia: Saunders Ltd.; 2001)

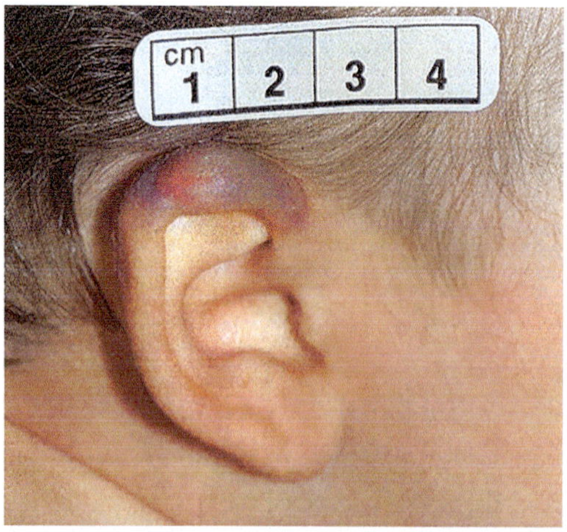

Figure 31.15 Forced impact trauma often includes the upper aspect of the ear—this is rare in accidental trauma but is highly correlated with non-accidental trauma.

Bites

Role of Forensic Odontologist or Forensic Dentist

The recognition and interpretation of the features in the photographs of the bite mark enables the odontologist to prepare a predictor of the dentition that caused the bite mark. The prediction of whether the biter is a child or an adult is particularly relevant in cases involving child victims. The prediction is only possible in bite marks demonstrate a high evidential value in respect of intercanine distance and individual tooth elements.

Examination of Dental Casts

The examination commences with the recognition and interpretation of the features in the upper and lower dental casts of the suspect biter. The general features that are relevant to comparative analysis are the determination of arch size by measuring the intercanine distance and determination of arch shape. The detailed features that form the basis of comparison are the presence or absence, position, rotation and incisal or cuspal anatomy of the individual teeth. The incisal edges of the incisors and the cusps of the canines and first premolars are examined in detail. The incisal and cuspal anatomy may demonstrate a variety of distinctive features; incisal edge tubercles, attrition, fracture, defective incisal restorations, caries, peg-shaped, fixed or removable prosthesis. The level of the incisal edges and cusps is examined and any variations are noted. As the evidential value of the mark diminishes so does the ability to predict the causal dentition; consequently the comparison with the dental casts becomes more limited.

Bites are always non-accidental, though they can be animal or human (adult or child). Human bites are mostly paired crescent shaped arches of bruises **(Figs. 31.16A to F)**. Since a set of crescentic marks are small, it should not be assumed that it is a child bite mark as they can be due to the contact, simply being from the upper and lower incisors of an adult. Individual teeth marks may be seen, the marks may be distorted by the contours of the area bitten.

Fractures

It takes considerable force to produce a fracture in a child. Any explanation must be consistent with the child's developmental age and with the type of fracture. The younger the child with the fracture, the greater the likelihood of abuse. Eighty per cent of abused children with fractures are less than 18 months old, whereas 85% of accidental fractures occur in children over 5 years.

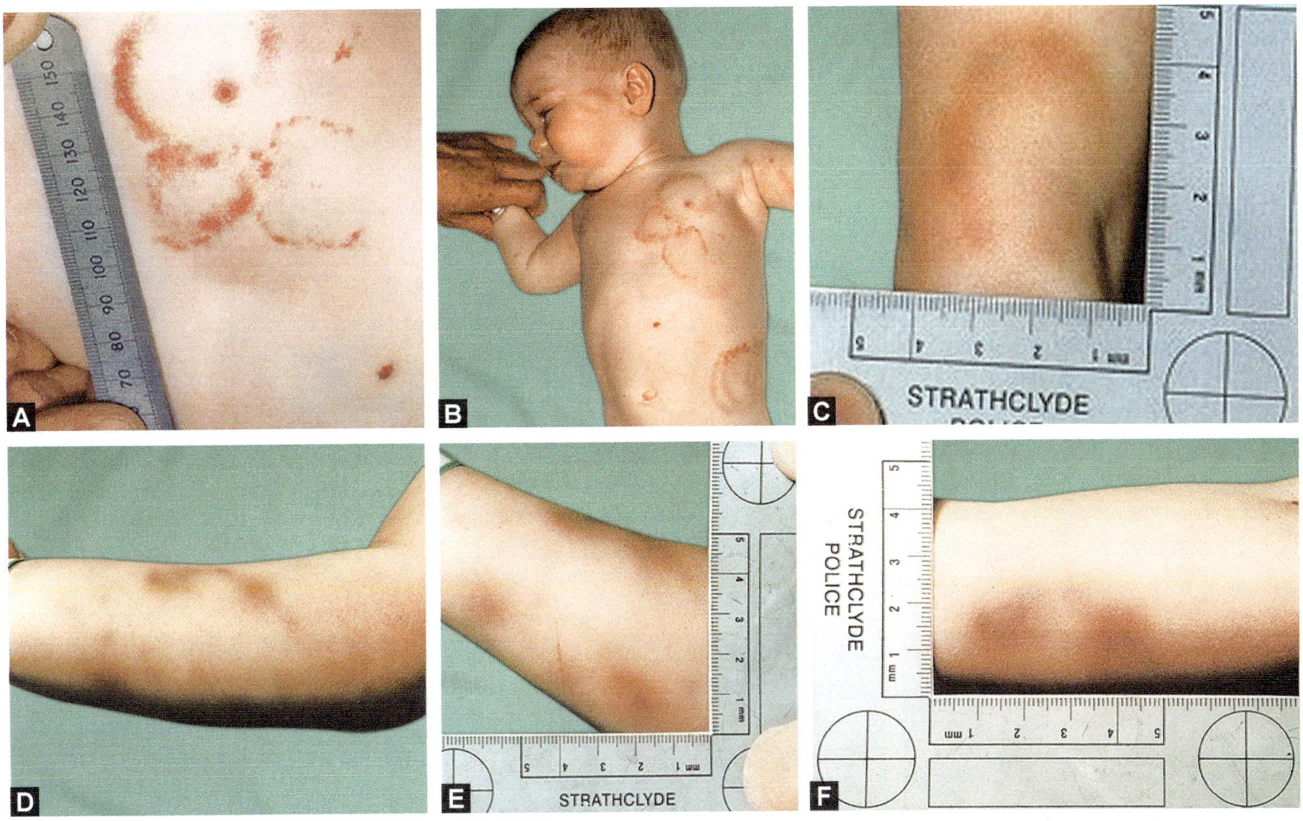

Figures 31.16A to F (A) Adult bite marks on upper left chest of a baby. Teeth marks are also seen. Confirmed by forensic dentistry. The outline of dental arch is evident; (B) Multiple bite marks on thorax, abdomen and axilla; (C) Scaled photograph showing a typical low evidential value human bite mark on the anterior surface of the child's extended right arm. An odontologist holds a rigid, right-angled scale adjacent to the bite mark; to minimise photographic distortion, the planes of the scale and bite mark must be parallel and coincident. In order to record potential posture distortion, the bite mark is photographed with the arm in different degrees of flexion; (D) General photograph showing the location of a low evidential value human bite mark on the opposing surfaces of the child's left forearm. The entire bite mark cannot be viewed from a single direction; to minimise photographic distortion, the opposing surfaces of the forearm are photographed separately; (E) Scaled photograph of the arc of marks on the posterior surface of the left forearm taken under the supervision of an odontologist and (F) Scaled photograph of the arc of marks on the anterior surface of the left forearm taken under the supervision of an odontologist.

(*Courtesy:* Dr Douglas R. Sheasby for Figs. 31.16C to F)

The following types of fracture are more suspicious of abuse in infants:

- Spiral fractures of the humerus are uncommon and strongly linked to abuse. Any humerus fracture other than a supracondylar fracture is suspicious of abuse in children. All humeral fractures in a non-mobile child are suspicious if there is no clear history of an accident.
- Multiple fractures are far commoner in abused children **(Box 31.1)**.

BOX 31.1 Fractures: Suspicious findings.

BOX 31.1 Fractures: Suspicious findings.
Metaphyseal corner or bucket-handle fractures
Major diaphyseal fractures
Rib fractures
Skull fractures
Fractures in unusual sites, e.g. acromion

- Ribs—in the absence of underlying bone disease or major trauma (such as a road traffic accident), rib fractures are highly specific for abuse and may be associated in some cases with shaking **(Figs. 31.17A and B)**. It has been suggested that rib fractures can be caused by the resuscitation process (where there has been an arrest), but posterior rib fractures have never been described following resuscitation. Anterior or costochondral rib fractures have been described extremely rarely in 0.5% in resuscitation.
- Femoral fractures in children who are not independently mobile are extremely suspicious of abuse regardless of the type. Once a child is able to walk, they can sustain a spiral fracture from a fall while running, so once again it is exceptionally important that a clear history is obtained. A transverse fracture of the femur is the most common presentation and can be found in accidental and non-accidental injuries.
- Metaphyseal fractures—these are relatively rare fractures. In the neonatal period, they can be related to

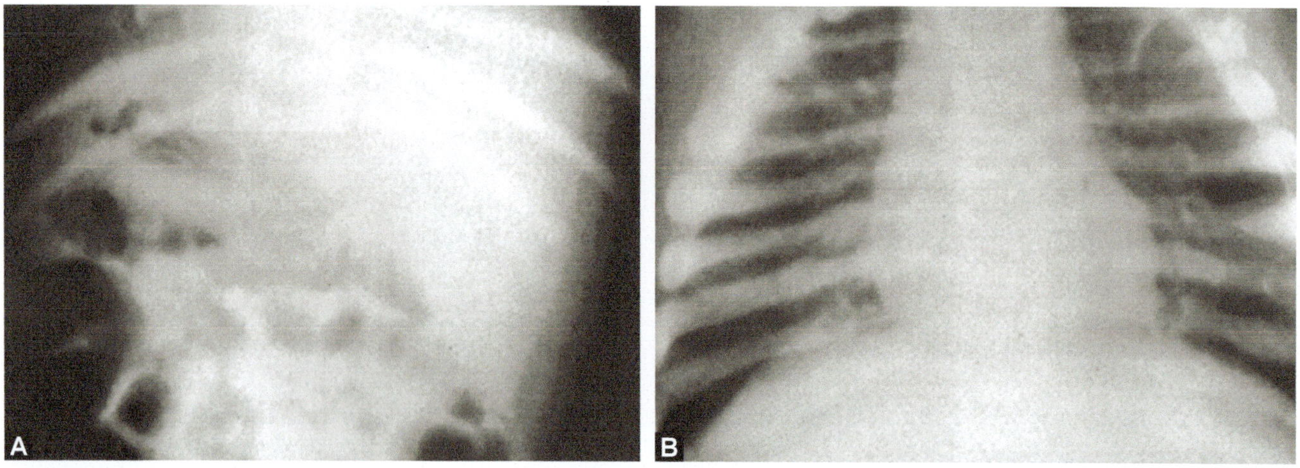

Figures 31.17A and B Multiple rib fractures of different ages—different stages of callous formation—follow several episodes of abuse. Posterior rib fractures are very highly correlated with inflicted trauma in the absence of rare metabolic bone disorders and/or extreme accidental trauma such as road traffic accident (RTA).

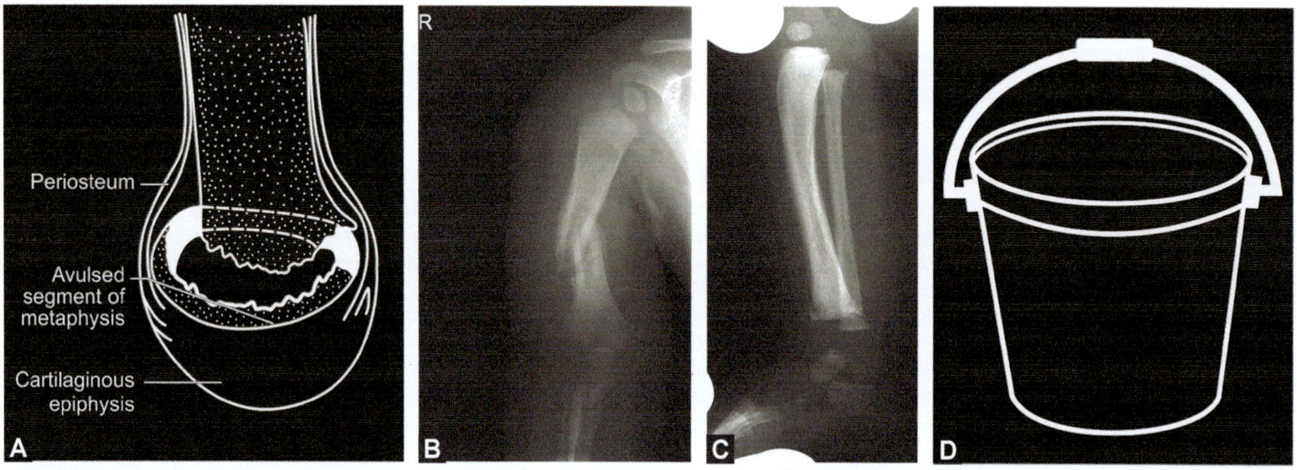

Figures 31.18A to D (A) Metaphyseal fractures in the child under the age of 2 years can be identified during skeletal survey and are highly correlated with twisting or pulling type injuries in the context of abusive trauma; (B) Fractured humerus in a baby girl. Periosteal reaction indicates it is a minimum of 4 days old i.e. delayed presentation; (C) Tibia/fibula of a baby boy; (D) Multiple classic metaphyseal lesions (CMLs) = corner fractures = bucket handle fractures = chip fractures at proximal and distal tibia and proximal fibula. Most obvious is anterior or distal tibia, bottom or left on X-ray

(*Courtesy:* Dr Greg Irwin, Consultant Paediatric Radiologist, Glasgow, Scotland, for Figures 18B and C), and (D) Bucket handle.

birth injury, but outside the neonatal period under the age of 2 years are suggestive of abuse, particularly if femoral. Epiphyseal fractures will only be found if looked for carefully and always require paediatric radiological opinion **(Figs. 31.18A to D)**.

- Skull fractures—a history of a fall less than 3 feet, this rarely produces a fracture.
- A linear parietal fracture is the most common fracture and can be accidental or non-accidental. It is always crucial to obtain a clearly history which has been witnessed **(Fig. 31.19)**. Particularly concerning skull fractures are as follows:
  - Occipital fractures
  - Depressed fractures
  - Growing fractures
  - Fractures complex or multiple in severely injured or fatally injured children. It is twice as likely to be due to abuse
  - Wide fracture (with an X-ray 3.0 mm or more)
  - A fracture which has crossed the suture line or multiple or bilateral
  - A fracture with associated intracranial injury
  - A history of a fall less than 3 feet—this rarely produces a fracture.

Intra-abdominal Injury (Box 31.2)

Intra-abdominal injury is very uncommon and, when abusive, typically occurs in young children, and under

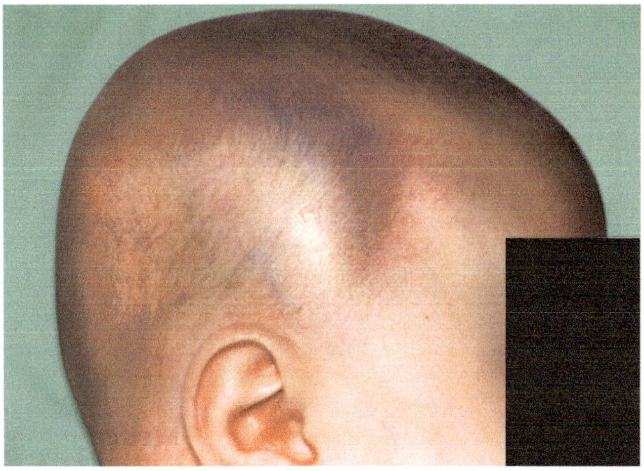

Figure 31.19 Boggy swelling over the right parietal area. X-ray confirmed parietal fracture in this case. An inconsistent history was provided for the injury describing a 4-month infant rolling from a bed which the infant was incapable of doing.

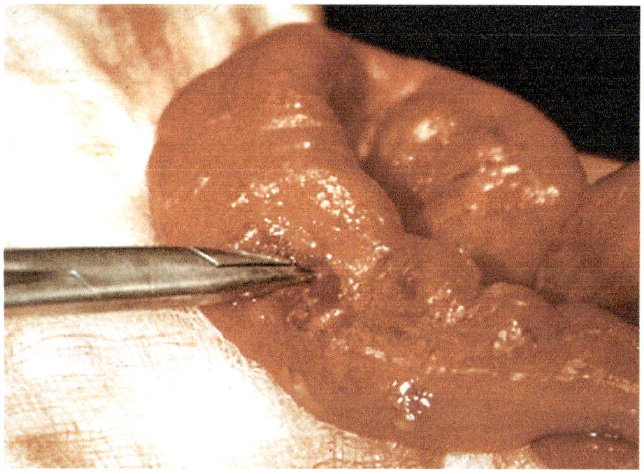

Figure 31.20 Intra-abdominal injury: Direct severe blow to the abdomen resulting in the ruptured small intestine (no external bruising noted).

BOX 31.2 Intra-abdominal injury.

Rare with high mortality rate

Diagnosis can be difficult

Small bowel injury, liver injury or haemorrhage from major blood vessel possible

3 years of age has a high mortality rate, especially if the diagnosis is missed or delayed. Diagnosis can be difficult with delay in presentation and no history of trauma provided by the carer. There may be no signs of external injury and therefore, one must have a low threshold of suspicion particularly if there are any other injuries in a child under 1 year of age. This should always include a search for internal injury (**Fig. 31.20**).

Thermal Injuries

Patterns that suggest abusive burn and scald injuries include the following:

- Glove and stocking circumferential scalds of limbs or buttocks from forced emersion (**Figs. 31.21A to F**)
- Deep cratered circular burns, which heal to leave scars (cigarette burns) (**Figs. 31.22A to C**)
- Clearly outlined brand marked contact burns (hot objects, e.g. clothes, iron, fire grid, cooker/hot plate)
- Poured scald
- Friction or carpet burns (e.g. from dragging child across the floor).

Common sites for abusive burns include the following:

- Feet and hands, especially the backs of hands
- Buttock
- Face
- Multiple sites.

Other Potential Non-accidental Injuries

A variety of other injuries are encountered in abusive circumstances. These include the following:

- Scratches, abrasions, incised wounds
- Mouth injuries, e.g. fractured teeth, lacerations and bruises to lips and tongue, torn labial frenulum in infant or toddler, palatal burns from hot food or lacerations from cutlery or objects forced into the mouth. Needles forced into skull or other tissues in context mainly of induced illness.[13]

Brain injury subsequent to trauma can be due to direct blows angular forces or due to hypoxic ischaemic injury sometimes due to shaking of the child or shaking plus impact injuries (even onto soft surfaces following, e.g. a throw). Retinal haemorrhages can also be associated commonly with inflicted brain injury (IBI) also known as non-accidental head injury involving angular forces. This can be in one or both eyes but classically involves all layers of the retina. It is important that a paediatric ophthalmologist uses indirect ophthalmoscopy to establish the findings (pictures should be taken via RetCam if possible) and provide a specialist opinion in such cases. Inflicted head injury can be accompanied by other injuries on other parts of the body,although only in approximately half of cases, a range of fractures can be found when further investigation is instigated (full skeletal survey) (**Figs. 31.23A to F**).

CHILD SEXUAL ABUSE

Sexual abuse happens when a child or young person under the age of 16 is used for the sexual gratification of an adult. More than 95% of cases present as historical abuse rather than acutely. Child sexual abuse (CSA) is often associated with other forms of abuse including physical abuse, emotional abuse and physical neglect.

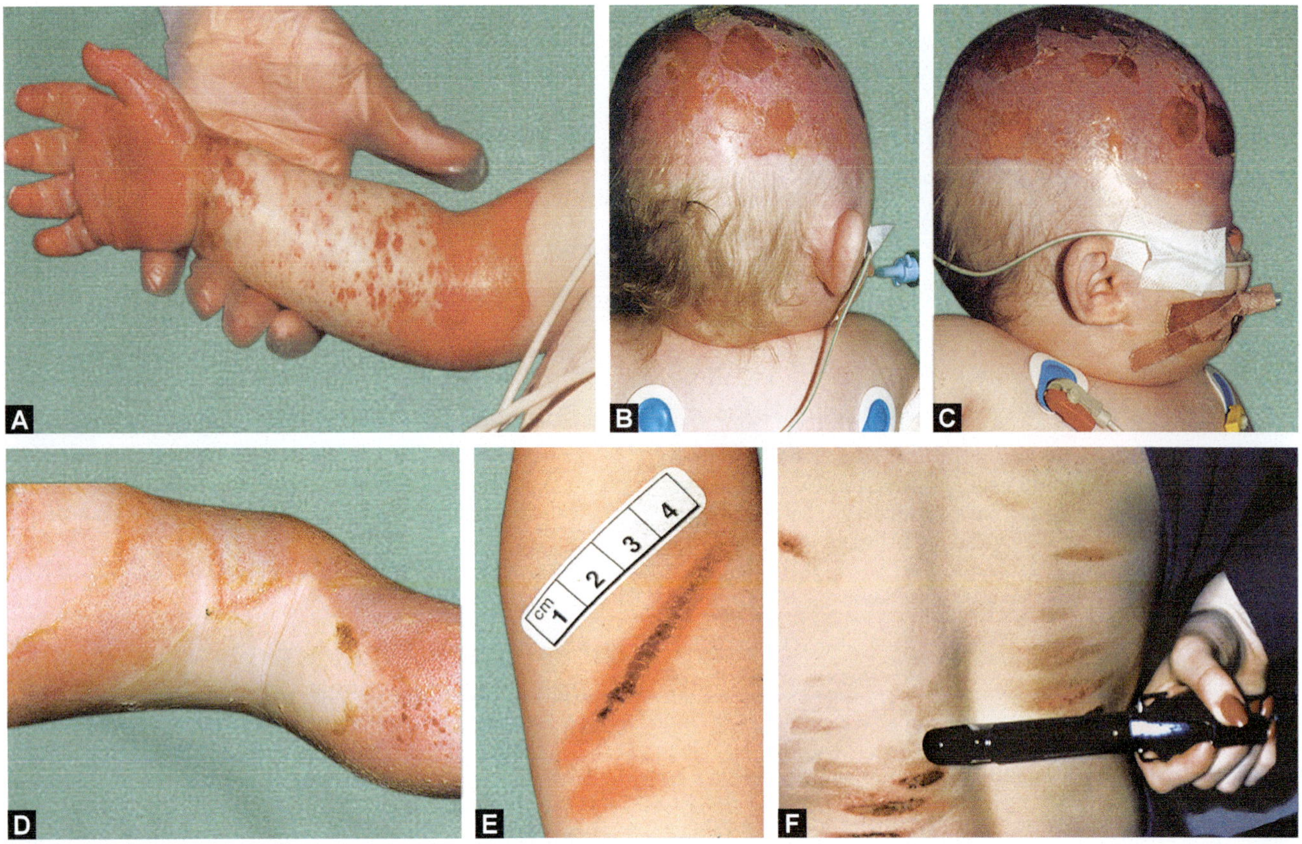

Figures 31.21A to F (A) Forced dipping of arm into hot water of a toddler; (B and C) Forced dipping of scalp in very hot water; (D) Forced dipping with knee fully flexed—clear sparing behind knee; (E) Contact burns—edge of hot iron and; (F) Contact burns: These injuries are due to self-harm inflicted following years of sexual abuse and emotional trauma. Always remember to consider abuse in any self-harm case.

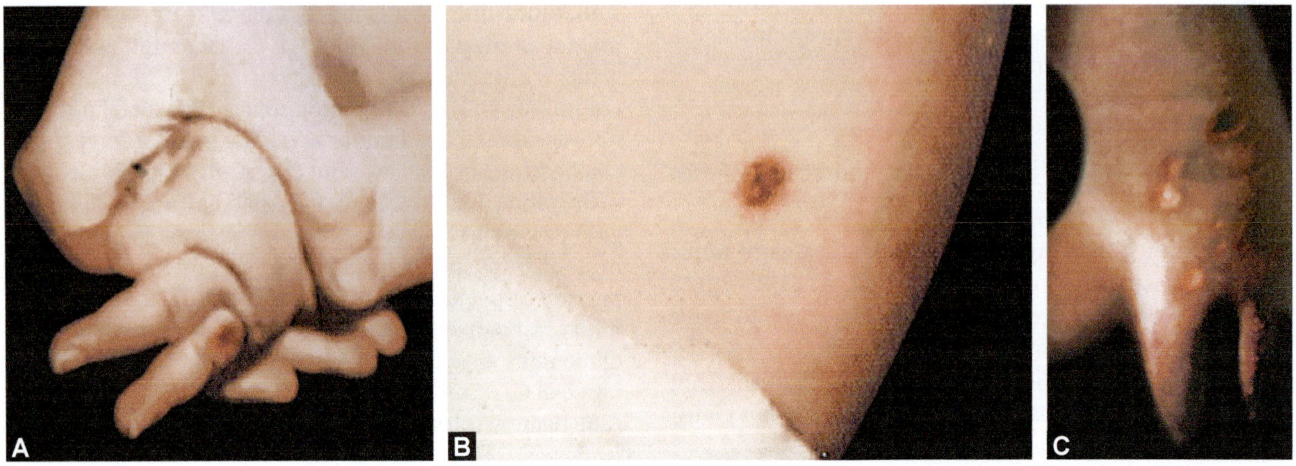

Figures 31.22A to C Contact burns: (A) Punched out 'crater-like' burn 0.8–1.0 cm diameter illustrating inflicted cigarette burn; (B) Cigarette burn healing—can be confused with impetigo at this stage; and (C) Full thickness cigarette burns going onto scar formation.

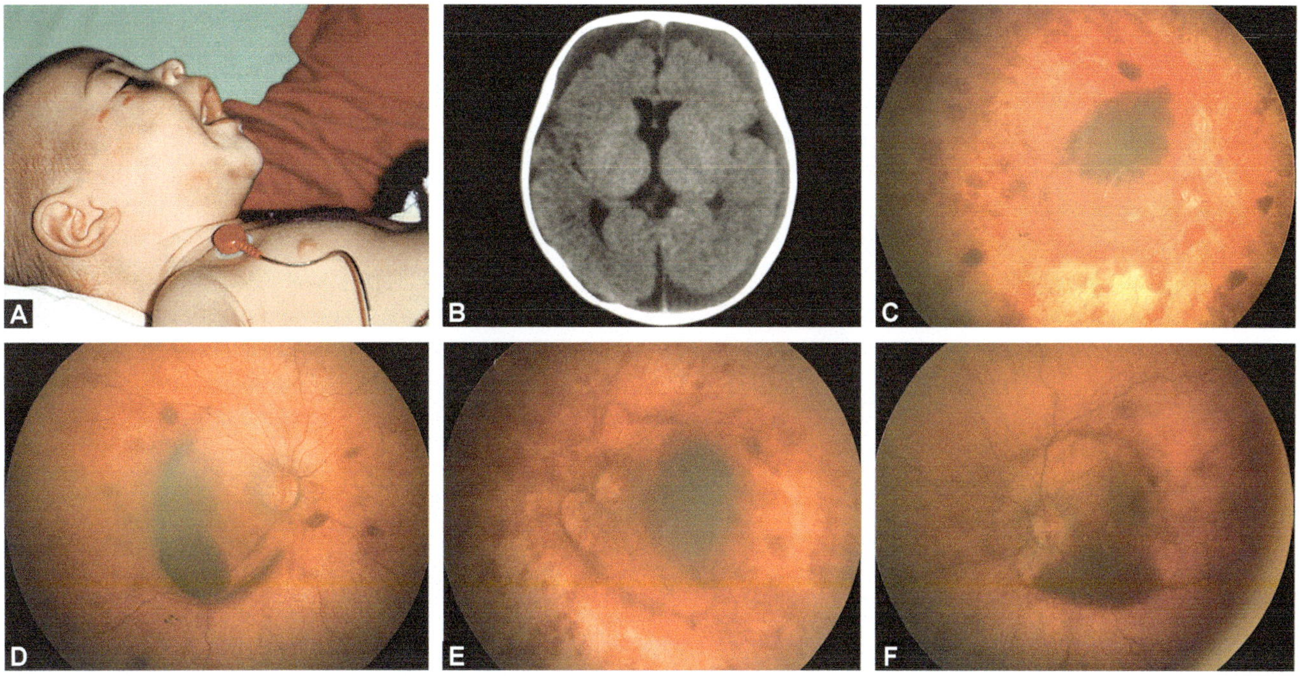

Figures 31.23A to F (A) Facial bruising seen in inflicted brain injury—previously sometimes termed Shaken baby syndrome—often no external bruising is seen despite serious brain injury; (B) Cranial computed tomography (CT) Scan showing bilateral subdural haemorrhages in frontal and occipital region; (C) Right eye: Multiple retinal haemorrhages are seen on ophthalmoscopic examination of an infant who was a victim of inflicted brain injury; (D) Right eye—a week later; (E) Left eye and (F) Left eye—a week later.

The CSA accommodation syndrome, i.e. impact on children of sexual abuse:[15]

- Secrecy
- Helplessness
- Entrapment and accommodation
- Delayed, conflicted and unconvincing disclosure
- Retraction.

Sexual Abuse Recognition

Recognition of sexual molestation of a child is entirely dependent on the individual's inherent willingness to entertain the possibility that the condition may exist. Unfortunately, willingness to consider the diagnosis of suspected child abuse molestation frequently seems to vary in inverse proportion to the individual's level of training.[16]

Behavioural Indicators

None of these are pathognomonic but raise suspicion requiring further detailed enquiry and analysis as follows:

- Regression
- Sleeping disturbances
- Eating disorders
- School problems
- Social or peer problems
- Poor self-esteem
- Sexualised behaviours.

Medical Indicators

- Very few single 'diagnostic' signs
- Sexually transmitted diseases (STDs)
- Bloodstains on underwear
- Bruising or swelling of genital area (history important)
- Grasp marks
- Soiling enuresis
- Anogenital pain
- Various types of penile or vaginal discharge
- Hymenal or anal findings (vulvoscopy).

Further detailed information on the physical signs of CSA can be found in the Royal College of Paediatrics and Child Health (RCPCH) publication 'The Physical Signs of Child Sexual Abuse. An evidence-based review and guidance for best practice, March 2008.'

Sexual Abuse/Medical Evaluation (*see* **Box 31.3** and **Figs. 31.24 to 31.26**).

BOX 31.3 Medical evaluation.

Appraisal of the child's development and emotional status

Expert medical examination for physical signs of child sexual abuse

Full paediatric forensic examination when the case is presenting acutely

'Hymen intact'—this is an unhelpful terminology—it is normal from birth for all children to have hymenal orifice

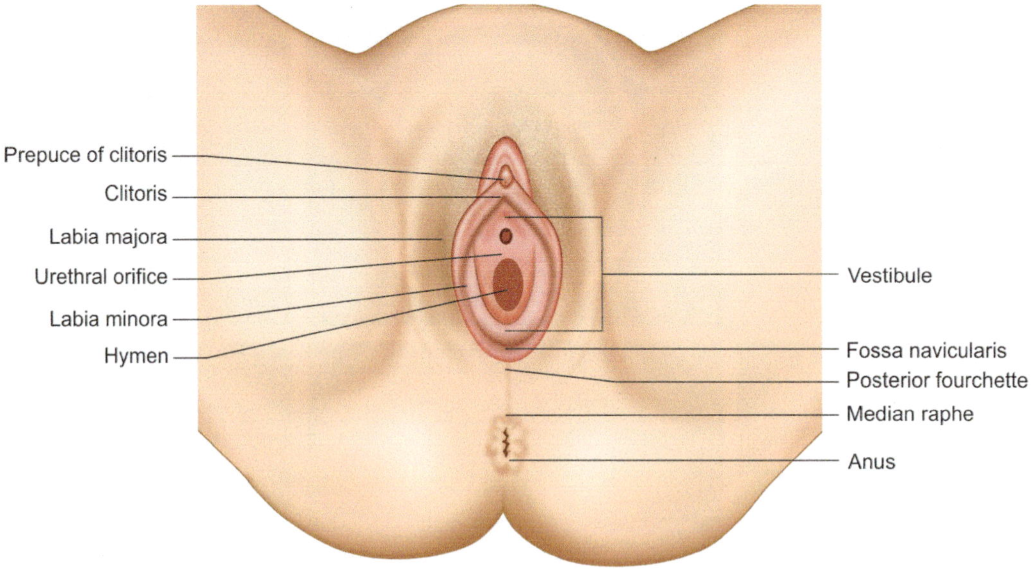

Figure 31.24 Normal anatomy. Location of the genital structures of the prepubescent female.

The jigsaw of sexual abuse		
History from parent	Child's history	Any disclosure
Physical symptoms	Behaviour	Bruises/ injury
Physcial examinations	STDs	Forensic
Police inquiry	Social work assessment	Siblings

Figure 31.25 Many factors require to be considered leading to suspicion and full assessment of sexual abuse.

Abbreviation: STDs, sexually transmitted diseases.

Hymenal Notch (Fig. 31.27)

Hymenal Transection

- Hymenal transections have not been described in a study of 175 prepubertal girls selected for non-abuse
- One study of pubertal girls with a history of vaginal penetration has reported hymenal transections in 8% (17/204)
- A mixed study of prepubertal and pubertal girls has reported complete hymenal transections in 3% (4/155) examined within 72 hours of abuse
- Hymenal transections persist following trauma **(Fig. 31.28)**.

Lacerations or tears to other genital tissues **(Figs. 31.29A and B)**:

- Lacerations are seen more often to the posterior fourchette or fossa navicularis than to any other genital tissues in abused girls

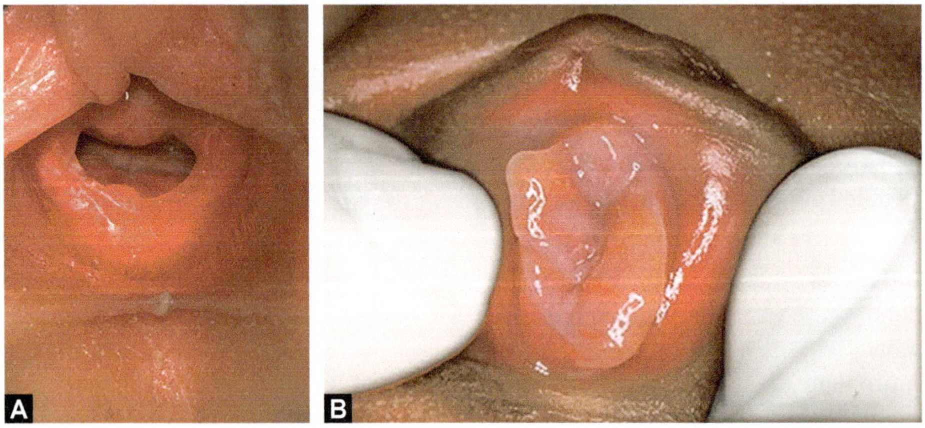

Figures 31.26A and B Variations in normal hymenal configuration crescentic hymen and normal funnel-shaped hymen.

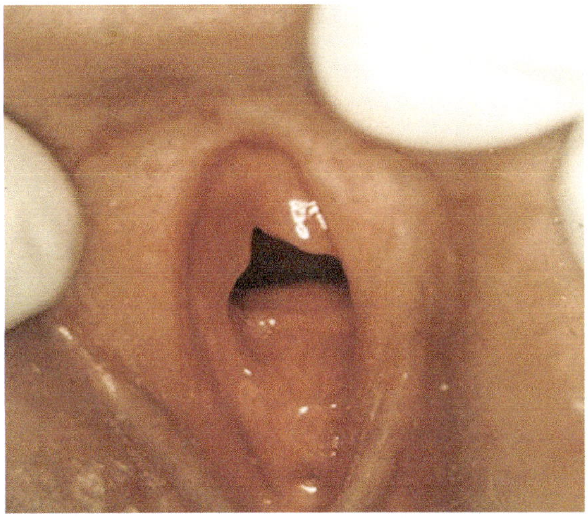

Figure 31.27 The importance of examination using the knee-chest position when a notch is found in the supine position. This is a notch at 5 O'clock position, persisting in the knee-chest position. Sometimes it is beneficial to examine a child in the knee-chest as well as supine position if the child is comfortable. This is a notch in the hymen found in the knee-chest position—this physical finding in its own right is not indicative of sexual abuse but other information should be fully explored.

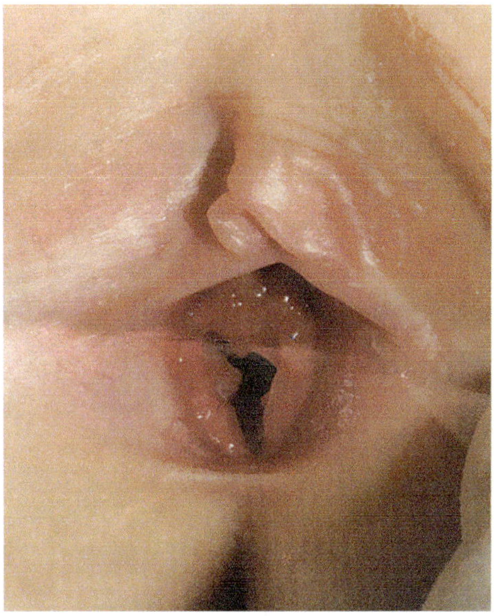

Figure 31.28 There is a fully healed transection (to base of hymen) at 6 O'clock position. This is a highly significant finding and is very suspicious of sexual abuse in a prepubertal child.

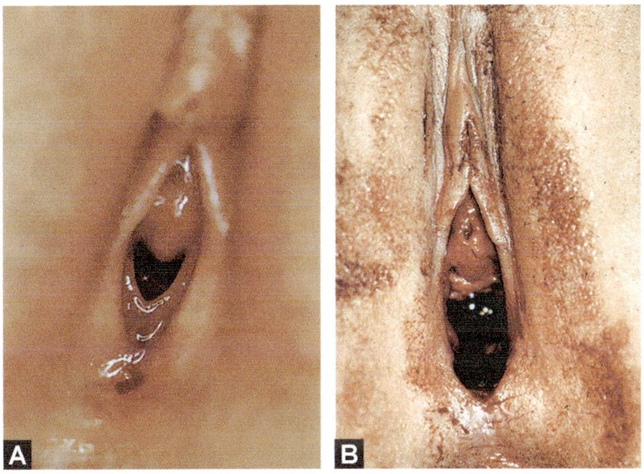

Figures 31.29A and B Acute traumatic findings seen in victims of sexual abuse and assault: (A) Acute lacerations of posterior fourchette; (B) Fresh blood from acute laceration of hymen.

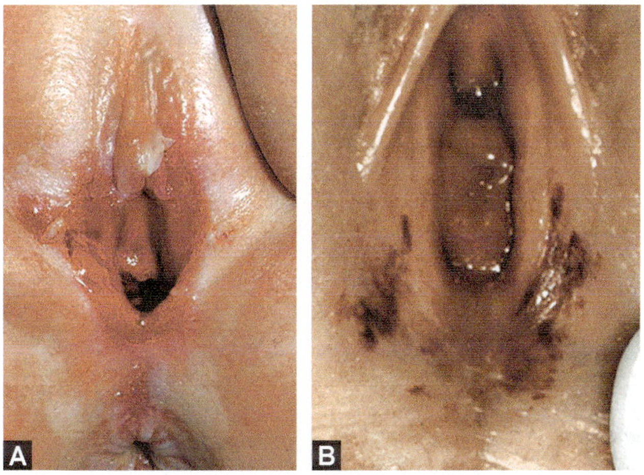

Figures 31.30A and B (A) Lichen sclerosus et atrophicus: *Note* that the pallor on surrounding skin and blood blistering. This child presented with unexplained bleeding on pants and chronic genital itch; (B) This appears as genital bruising but there is associated pallor of skin and blood blistering. In this case, the diagnosis is Lichen sclerosus et atrophicus—can be misdiagnosed as sexual assault.

- Limited evidence suggests that tears are seen more often in pubertal girls when examined within 24 hours of an assault.

Genital Bruising—Issues for Clinical Practice

Early examinations are more likely to detect genital bruising.

If this clinical sign is of concern then the child should be re-examined to assist with diagnosis.

There are many other possible causes of bruising, which should be considered in the differential diagnosis **(Figs. 31.30A and B)**.

When bruising is found on the genitalia, sexual abuse should always be considered **(Fig. 31.31)**.

Other sites of bruising **(Figs. 31.32 and 31.33)**.

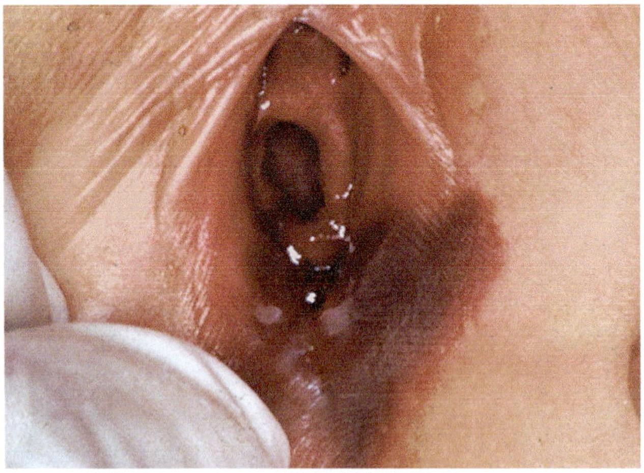

Figure 31.31 Bruising around genitalia. A 1-year-old baby where perpetrator attempted to penetrate with penis. No obvious tear of hymen itself.

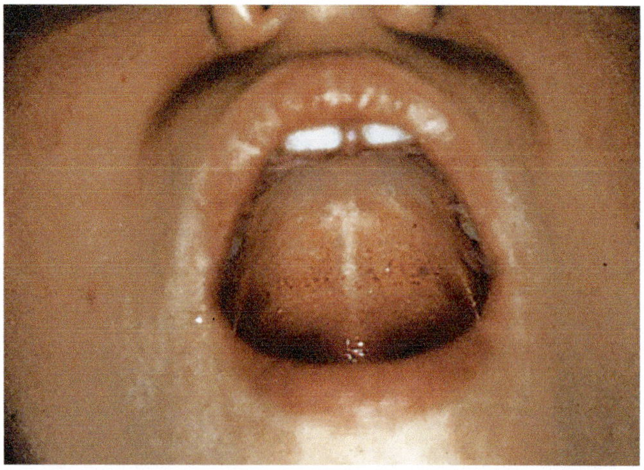

Figure 31.32 Forced to perform oral sex. *Note* palatal contusions. Always remember to inspect carefully the oral cavity when any form of abuse is suspected.

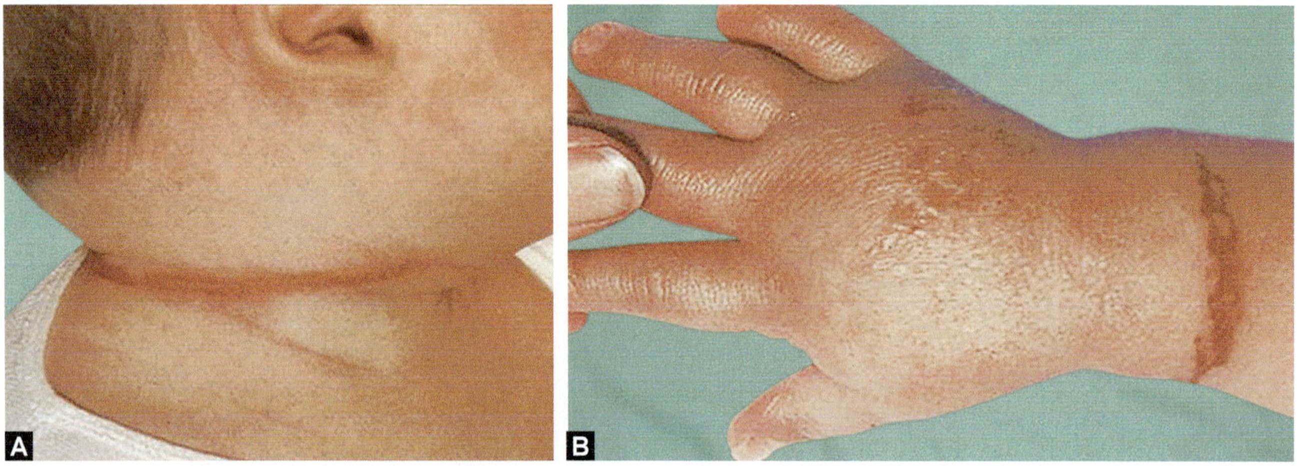

Figures 31.33A and B Ligature marks around wrist and neck of a young child. These can be in the context of physical and or sexual abuse.

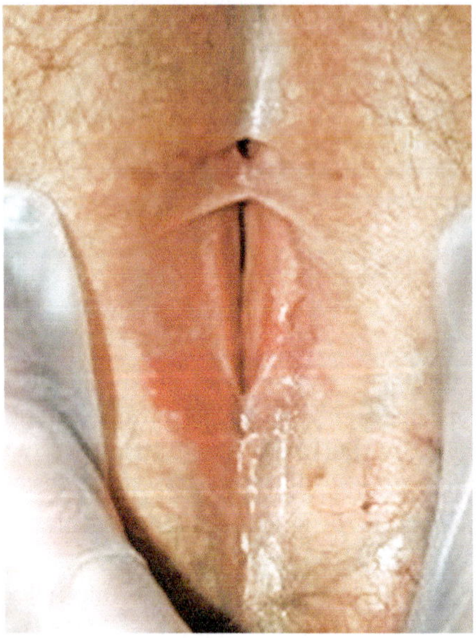

Figure 31.34 Partial labial fusion.

Labial Fusion or Adhesion (Box 31.4 and Fig. 31.34)

BOX 31.4 Labial fusion: evidence statement.

Extensive and partial labial fusion is seen in both prepubertal girls reporting vaginal penetration and girls selected for non-abuse

There is insufficient evidence to determine the significance of labial fusions in pubertal girls

Posterior fourchette tears have been reported to heal with labial fusion

Child Sexual Abuse: Health Consequences in Adulthood

- Gastrointestinal (GI) problems such as ulcers, irritable bowel syndrome and chronic abdominal pain; pelvic pain

- Gynaecological problems
- Chronic headache
- Psychological effects
- Emotional effects
- Physical effects
- Social effects.

Child Pornography

This refers to images or films (also known as child abuse images) and in some cases 'writing' depicting sexually explicit activities involving a child. As such, child pornography is a record of CSA.

Child pornography is among the fastest growing criminal segment on the internet and producers of child pornography try to avoid prosecution by distributing their material across national borders. Prepubescent pornography is viewed and collected by paedophiles for a variety of purposes ranging from private sexual uses, through to trading with other paedophiles. Children of all ages, including young infants, are abused in the production of pornography. The United States Department of Justice estimates that pornographers have recorded the abuse of more than one million children in the United States alone. There is an increasing trend towards younger victims and greater brutality. According to the world congress against commercial sexual exploitation of children while impossible to obtain accurate data, a perusal of the child pornography readily available in the international market indicates that a significant number of children are being sexually exploited through this medium.[17]

Child Sex Tourism

One source of child pornography distributed worldwide is created by 'sex tourists'. Most of the victims of child sex tourism reside in developing countries. Interpol works with its 188-member countries to combat the problem.[18]

FABRICATED AND INDUCED ILLNESS

Fabricated and induced illness (FII) is a form of abuse, not a medical condition. Previously known as Munchausen syndrome by proxy, this label applies to the child, not the perpetrator. The label is used to describe a form of child abuse.

There is a spectrum of fabricated illness behaviour and FII may coexist with other types of child abuse. The range of symptoms and systems involved is very wide and it is usually the parent or caregiver who is the perpetrator. FII includes some cases of suffocation, non-accidental poisoning and sudden infant death.

Features

- A child is presented for medical assessment and care, usually persistently, often resulting in multiple procedures.
- Mismatch or incongruity between symptoms described by parent/carer and those objectively observed by medical attendants.
- The perpetrator denies knowledge of the aetiology of the child's illness.
- Acute symptoms and signs cease when the child is separated from the perpetrator.
- Intention or non-accidental poisoning often presents with bizarre symptomatology—a range of substances are involved (e.g. methadone, salt).

Think of FII, when:

- Inconsistent or unexplained symptoms and signs
- Poor response to treatment
- Unexplained or prolonged illness
- Different symptoms on resolution of previous ones, or over time
- Child's activities inappropriately restricted
- Parents or carers unable to be assured
- Problems only in the presence of parent or carer
- Incongruity between story and actions of parents or carers
- Erroneous or misleading information
- Family history of unexplained illness or death
- Exaggerated catastrophes or fabricated deaths.

The paediatrician is usually the professional who suspects FII. This hinges on taking very detailed histories from all adults who may have information to give, careful checking of aspects of history which can be corroborated and, if necessary, a period of admission or specific tests, constantly weighing up the balance between needing to confirm the abuse and avoiding necessary harm to the child. The production of a detailed chronology is essential in the investigation of this form of abuse (Fig. 31.35).[19]

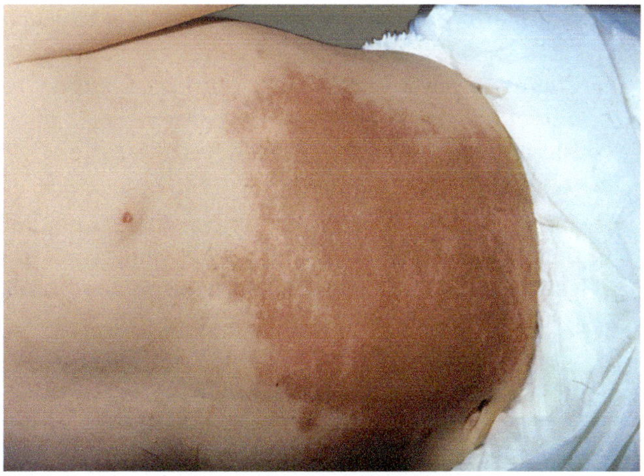

Figure 31.35 Adult applied bleach to the abdomen of a child.

CHILD TRAFFICKING

Theillegal trading of people is a world-wide problem and is thought to be the third largest illegal trade after drugs and weapons trafficking. Globalisation has contributed to the growth of trafficking. The US Department of State estimates that 800,000 people are trafficked across national borders annually, nearly 50% of these being children. That figure is considered to be a minimum with some estimates ranging up to 2 million people. There are no clear estimates about the numbers of children trafficked around the world, but United Nations International Children's Emergency Fund (UNICEF) described the numbers as 'enormous'. Whilst in Western Europe, women are the most numerous victims, globally children constitute the largest numbers.[20-22]

Children are often exploited in relation to the following:

- Child labour, e.g. cannabis farms
- Debt bondage
- Domestic servitude
- Begging
- Benefit fraud
- Drug trafficking or decoys
- Illegal adoptions
- Forced or illegal marriage
- Sexual abuse.

Recognising and Identifying Trafficked Children

High-level Concerns

- Claims to have been exploited through sexual exploitation, criminality (i.e. cannabis farms, petty street crimes, begging, and so on), labour exploitation, domestic servitude, forced marriage, illegal adoption and drug dealing by another person.
- Is located or recovered from a place of exploitation and/or involved in criminality that highlights the involvement of adults, e.g. is recovered from cannabis farm/factory, brothel, street crime, petty theft, pick pocketing, begging.
- Claims to be in debt bondage or 'owes' money to other persons/has to pay off large debts.
- Has entered the country illegally.
- Has no passport or other means of identification.
- Has false documentation or genuine documentation that has been altered or fraudulently obtains' or the child claims that their details [(name, date of birth (DOB)] on the documentation is incorrect.
- Claims to have been in the country for years but has not learned the local language or culture.
- Is unable to confirm the name and address of the person meeting them on arrival.
- Has had their journey or visa arranged by someone other than themselves or their family.
- Is unable, or reluctant to give details of accommodation or other personal details.
- Reports from reliable sources suggesting the likelihood of involvement in sexual exploitation.
- One among a number of unrelated children found at one address.
- Person in control of/with the child has applied for acted as guarantor for visas on behalf of others.
- Person interpreting for the child at interviews and meetings was previously known to them (i.e. not appointed or approved by authorities).

Concerns

- On arrival in the country or when attending meetings or interviews is accompanied by an adult who may not be legal guardian and who insists on remaining with the child at all times.
- Has a prepared story very similar to those that other children have given perhaps hinting they have been coached.
- Leaving home or care setting in clothing unusual for the individual child (inappropriate for age, borrowing clothing from older people).
- Returning after having been missing looks well-cared for despite having no known base.
- In a private fostering arrangement which has not been registered or child being cared for by adult(s) who are not their parents (except those in social work care).
- Is permanently deprived of a large part of their earnings by another person/no control over earnings.
- Goes out the same hours every day (unless legitimate, verified work).
- Works in various locations.
- Has limited freedom of movement.
- Is excessively afraid of being deported.
- Indicators of working (tired in school, condition of hands etc.).
- Does excessive housework around the house.
- Appropriate adult cannot provide photo ID.
- Involved in underage marriage.

General Concerns

- Significantly older boyfriend or girlfriend
- Placement breakdown
- Has gone missing from local authority care
- Is registered at a number of different addresses
- Is malnourished
- Is withdrawn and refuses to talk or appears afraid to talk to a person in authority

- Exhibits self-assurance, maturity and self-confident not expected to be seen in a child of such age
- Does not appear to have money but does have a mobile phone
- Has not been registered with or attended General Physician (GP) practice
- Has not been enrolled in school
- Truancy or disengagement with education
- Receives unexplained or unidentified phone calls whilst in placement/temporary accommodation
- Shows physical or emotional signs of physical or sexual abuse
- Has a history of missing links and unexplained moves
- Evidence of sexually transmitted infection or unwanted pregnancy
- Known to be sexually active
- Evidence of drug, alcohol or substance misuse
- Adults loitering outside the child's usual place of residence
- Accounts of social activities with no plausible explanation of the source of necessary funding
- Pattern of street homelessness
- Acquisition of money, expensive clothes, mobile phones or other possessions without plausible explanation
- Low self-image, low self-esteem, self-harming behaviour including cutting, overdosing, eating disorder, promiscuity
- Entering or leaving vehicles driven by unknown adults
- Possible inappropriate use of the internet and forming online relationships, particularly with adults
- Known to beg for money.[23]

CHILD PROTECTION STANDARDISED PROCEDURES

Roles and responsibilities of various professionals and agencies and that everyone is clear about what everyone does in protecting a child. Where the responsibilities lie and who has responsibility to act often is not clear—so children fall through gaps with professionals thinking it is someone else's job.

Interagency and interprofessional case discussions or planning meetings are essential to ensure that information is shared in detail and the child is helped throughout the whole process of assessment and investigation and that they are not further traumatised throughout this time by the process itself.

Clearly standardised documentation is critical. It must be contemporaneous, i.e. written as soon as is possible on speaking with the child/family or child or with others. It is best to document everything clearly, preferably in typed reports which have adequate analysis and conclusions **(Appendix)**.

LEGAL SYSTEM

There are various legal systems throughout the World. In Scotland, the Child Protection Children's Hearing System is a 'tribunal' system involving lay members of panels deciding on interventions on advice of multiagency assessments. There is also an adversarial criminal process to decide upon whether individuals are culpable specifically for the crime of abuse of children.

ACKNOWLEDGEMENTS

1. Hobbs C. Physical Signs of Child Abuse. London: WB Saunders Co Ltd; 1996.
2. Elsevier Publications.
3. Perry BD.
4. Dr Douglas R Sheasby, Honorary Senior Clinical Lecturer in Forensic Odontology, University of Glasgow, Scotland.
5. Scottish Government, Department of Health.
6. RCPCH Child Companion Document, RCPCH; 2006.
7. The Physical Signs of Child Sexual Abuse, RCPCH; 2008.
8. Elaine Archibald. Personal Assistant to Dr Jean Herbison and to the staff of the Child Protection Unit, NHSGGC.
9. Catherine Martin, Business Manager, Child Protection Unit NHSGGC.

REFERENCES

1. Scottish Executive. (2002). It's everyone's job to make sure I'm alright. [online] Available from www.scotland.gov.uk/Publications/2002/11/15820/14009 [Accessed November, 2013].
2. Falkov A. Study of Working Together 1996, Part and Report. Fatal child abuse and parental psychiatric disorder. An analysis of 100 area Child Protection Committee Case Reviews conducted under the terms of part 8 of the Working Together under Children Act 1989, London, Department of Health. In: Reder P, Duncan S (Eds). Lost Innocents: A Follow Up of Fatal Child Abuse. London: Routledge; 1999. pp. 41-61.
3. Duncan S, Reder P. Adult Psychiatry—a missing link the child protection network. Comments on Falkov's Fatal child abuse and parental psychiatric disorder. Child Abuse Review. 1997;6:35-40.
4. Social Care Institute for Excellence (2009). SCIE Guide 30: Think child, think parent, think family: a guide to parental mental health and child welfare. [online] Available from www.scie.org.uk/publications/guides/guide30 [Accessed November, 2013].
5. Hughes H. Impact of spouse abuse on children of battered women. Violence Update. 1992;1:9-11.

6. McWilliams M, McKiernan J. Bringing it out into the open: domestic violence in Northern Ireland. Belfast: HMSO;1993.
7. National Children's Home. (1994). [online] Available from www.nch.org.uk[Accessed November, 2013].
8. Bakken J, MiltenbergerRG, Schauss S. Teaching parents with mental retardation: knowledge versus skills. Am J Ment Retard. 1993;97(4):405-17.
9. TymchukAJ. Symptoms of psychopathology in mothers with mental handicap. Mental Handicap Research. 1993;6(1)18-35.
10. McGaw S, Newman T. What Works for Parents with Learning Disabilities? Ilford: Barnardo's; 2005.
11. Department of Health and Department for Education and Skills. (2007). Good Practice Guidance on Working with Parents with a learning disability. [online] Available from www.dh.gov.uk [Accessed November, 2013].
12. National Institute for Clinical Excellence (NICE) Guideline. (2009). When to Suspect Child Maltreatment. [online] Available from www.nice.org.uk [Accessed November, 2013].
13. RCPCH. (2006). Child Protection Companion, London. [online] Available from www.core-info.cf.ac.uk [Accessed November, 2013].
14. Sugar NF, Taylor JA, Feldman KW. Bruises in infants and toddlers: those who don't cruise rarely bruise. Arch Paediatr Adolesc Med. 1999;53:399-403.
15. Summit RC. The child sexual abuse accommodation syndrome. Child Abuse Negl. 1983;7(2):177-93.
16. Sgroi SM. Sexual molestation of children: the last frontier in child abuse: Child Today. 1975;4:18-21.
17. Healty MA. Child pornography: an international perspective; 1996.
18. INTERPOL. Crimes against children. [online] Available from www.interpol.int/Public/Children/Default.asp [Accessed November, 2013].
19. RCPCH. (2009). Fabricated or Induced Illness by Carers (FII): a practical guide for paediatricians. [online]. Available from http://www.rcpch.ac.uk/Health-Services/Child-Protection/Child-Protection-Publications [Accessed November, 2013].
20. ILO. (2002). Every Child Counts. New Global Estimates on Child Labour ILO/PEC Geneva. [online] Available from www.ilo.org/ipecinfo/product [Accessed November, 2013].
21. UNICEF. (2005). Combating Child Trafficking: Handbook for Parliamentarians. [online] Available from www.unicef.org/publications [Accessed November, 2013].
22. United Nations Office on Drugs and Crime. (2006). Trafficking in Persons: global pattern. [online] Available from www.unodc.org/documents/human-trafficking/HT/globalpatterns/en_pdf [Accessed November, 2013].
23. Glasgow Child Protection Committee. (2001). Glasgow Child Protection Committee Inter-agency Guidance for Child Trafficking. [online] Available from www.glasgowchildprotection.org.uk/NR/rdonlyres/AADFD622-A183-4B96-9D5E-D6F3C2C31A79/0/GLASGOWCHILDTRAFFICKINGGUIDANCESept09.pdf [Accessed June 2001].

APPENDIX

Child Protection or Child Welfare Documentation

This divider should be inserted into the medical notes once child protection or child welfare concerns are identified and an initial telephone referral to social work has been made. (Yorkhill Child Protection Procedure and Guidance, held in blue folders on all wards or on the Yorkhill Intranet for further guidance).

This section must be retained behind the identification labels at the front of the case notes.

All staff involved in the child's care, who have information related to the child protection concern, must use this section to keep a record of their involvement and concerns, ensuring that a chronological, complete and integrated review is possible. (There can be cross-reference to more complete entries in the medical notes or in locally held files.)

Record keeping must comply with professional standards: All information must be factual, clear, succinct, contemporaneous, dated and timed and the person completing the entry must sign the records and print their name and designation clearly.

WHAT TO FILE IN THIS SECTION

Section 1

Comprehensive health evaluation—this evaluation to be conducted and recorded by paediatrician at specialist registrar (SPR) grade in full collaboration with receiving consultant paediatrician or surgeon. To be signed off by consultant staff only.

All subsequent medical notes for the child must be documented in this section.

Section 2

The standard operating procedure—this is for child protection and should be activated and completed during child's stay as in-patient.

Section 3

Multidisciplinary chronological record and continuation sheets as necessary (Part I).

Action plan(s) as many as necessary should be completed at point of contact or as concerns are identified (Part II).

Conclusion to child protection or child welfare concerns—this should be completed prior to discharge (Part III).

The lead consultant will be responsible for maintaining an overview of this section.

Prior to discharge, agreement for the child to be discharged must be confirmed with the lead consultant and the relevant social worker in the social work department (this may be by fax) and documented in this section. Plans for the protection of the child post-discharge must also be briefly recorded together with the name and designation of the person to contact in the event of a query.

If following assessment, no child protection concerns are substantiated; this should be clearly recorded by the lead consultant and agreed by the social worker involved. However, this section is retained in the notes.

CHILD PROTECTION PROCESS FOR ALL STAFF (FLOW CHART 31.1)

Flow chart 31.1 Child protection process for all staff.

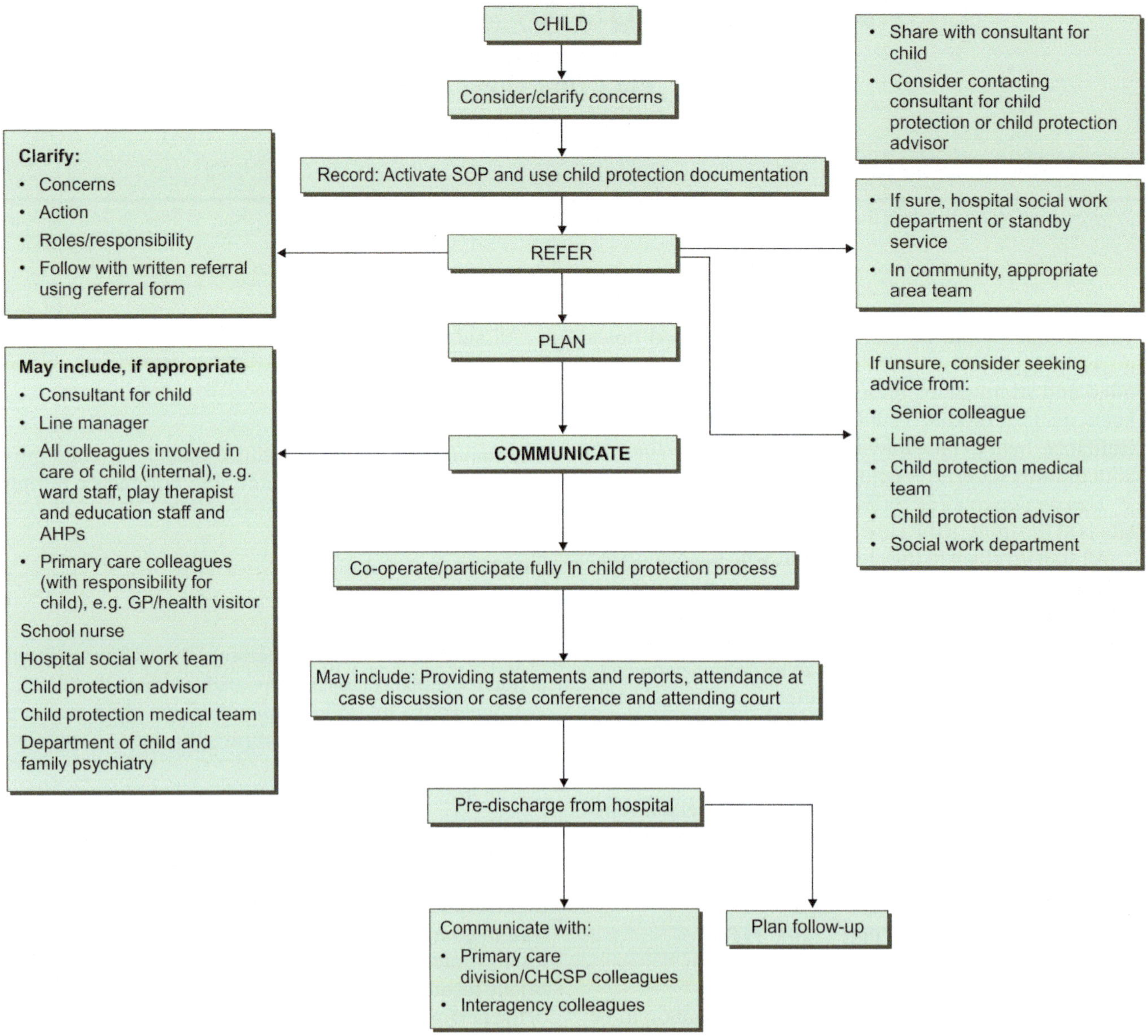

Abbreviations: SOP, standard operating procedure; AHP, alliance health project; GP, general practitioner.

Section 1: Comprehensive Health Evaluation of a Child Where There are Welfare Concerns

Child's surname		***Forename(s)***	
Known As		DOB	Sex:
Address Postcode:			CHI No
Siblings/Unborn Child		DOB	
		DOB	
		DOB	
		DOB	
		DOB	
		DOB	
Mother Name:		Father Name:	
Address (if different)		Address (if different)	
DOB:		DOB:	
GP		Referrer	
Address		Address	
		Home Tel No:	
		Designation:	
School/Nursery Attended:		School Nurse/HV:	

(Contd...)

(Contd...)

Date of Examination:	Time of examination:	Emergency	Planned
Location of Examination: Paediatric Ward GP Surgery Community Paediatric Clinic		Specialist CP Unit Police Medical Suite Other (specify) ______	
Person/s Accompanying Child ______ Relationship to Child Mother in attendance? Yes No		Father in Attendance? Yes No	
Consent to Health Assessment and Information Sharing (source, i.e. parent, young person, person holding parental rights) Parent's signature: ______ Young person's signature: ______ ______ ______ Name Relationship Date Witnessed By: ______ ______ ______ Name Position Date			
Referrer's concern: CSA/Physical Injury/Emotional abuse/Physical neglect/non-organic failure to thrive			

Name:	Date of birth:
Account of circumstances leading to referral (a) From Referrer Name:	Position:
(b) From accompanying adult Name: (c) From Child:	Position:
Background information already available from notes (e.g. previous concerns re-developmental delay, poor growth, possible episodes of NAI)	

Name:	Date of birth:
Concerns Raised by Child/Parent/Carer/Social Worker (Tick box if problem raised and discussed) Illness Diet/Feeding Energy Emotional Health Other (specify) ______ Comments:	Vision Child Substance Abuse Carer's Mental Health Carer's Substance Abuse
Birth Details Antenatal Problems: Maternal drug/alcohol misuse, pregnancy-induced hypertension, limited/no antenatal care. Hospital/Place of Birth: Birth Weight: Gestation: Type of Delivery:	Neonatal Hearing Test: YES /NO PASS/FAIL Guthrie: YES/NO
Any Neonatal Problems: (Give brief description, e.g. SCBU, Jaundice, drug withdrawal, etc.)	
Family History Include any significant family history	

(Contd...)

(Contd...)

Name:	Date of Birth:
Significant Health Problems Include allergies, current medication if known, details of any pharmacy equipment required by the child, e.g. nasogastric tubes, catheters	
Hospital Admissions/A&E Attendances/Appointments Give details if known	

Child Health Surveillance			
	Yes	No	Comments
6–8 weeks			
13 months			
2 years			
3–5 years			
School Entry			
Unscheduled			
Comments:			

Immunisations (Schedule requires to be kept up-to-date)						
	Due	Yes			Date	No
Diphtheria, tetanus, pertussis, Haemophilus influenzae type B (Hib) and Polio	2, 3 and 4 months old	1	2	3		
Meningitis C		1	2	3		
Measles, Mumps and Rubella (German Measles) (MMR)	At around 13 months					
Diphtheria, tetanus, pertussis, hib and polio	3–5 years (pre-school)					
Measles, Mumps and Rubella (German Measles) (MMR)						
Diphtheria, tetanus, pertussis, hib and polio	13–18 years					
Other:						

(Contd...)

(Contd...)

Name:	Date of Birth:
Clinical Examination General physical appearance of child (note especially any evidence of infection, neglect or injury)	
Demeanour/behaviour/impression of developmental/maturation status and emotional health	

Measurements

Weight	kg	Centile
Height	cm	Centile
Head circumference	cm	Centile

Findings on external physical examination

Comment		
Skin and hair		
Teeth		
Eyes		
Ears, nose and throat		
Cardiovascular system		
Blood pressure (if applicable)		
Respiratory system		
Alimentary system		
Genitalia/testes		
Nervous system		
Locomotion/posture		
a) Visual acuity	R	
	L	
b) Hearing	R	
	L	

(Contd...)

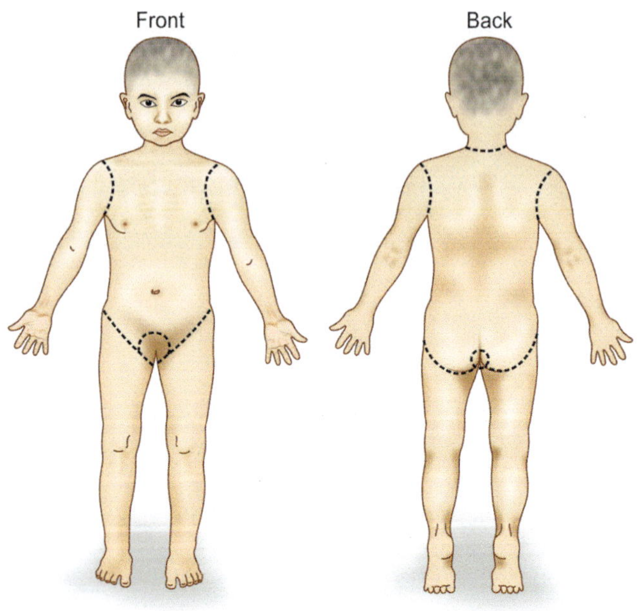

Figure 31.36 Indications on the charts (front and back) any areas of abrasions.

(Contd...)

Name:			Date of Birth:
Involvement with Other Health Professionals			
	Name	Base	Next appointment (if known)
Paediatrician			
S and L Therapy			
Occupational Therapy			
Physiotherapy			
CAMHS			
Other, e.g. eyes, dietician, ENT			
Abbreviations: CAMHS, Child and adolescent mental health services; S and L, Speech and language CONCLUSION/OPINION			

Name:		Date of Birth:	
Summary of Findings (Please report on each item)	Mild (M) Moderate (Mod) Severe (S)	Newly identified at this assessment (tick)	Currently under treatment (tick)
Developmental delay/learning difficulties			
Motor difficulties			
Speech difficulties			
Visual difficulties			
Hearing difficulties			
Missed immunisations (tick if yes)			
Asthma/Allergies			
Epilepsy			
Growth faltering			
Obesity/Overweight			
Tooth decay			
Mental health concerns			
Substance misuse			

(Contd...)

(Contd...)

Enuresis/Encopresis			
Sexual health concerns			
Other (specify)			
ACTION/CARE PLAN			
Further investigation of possible abuse requiring: Joint paediatric/Forensic examination Specialist paediatric examination Need for further assessment/treatment of medical/developmental problems. Refer child to: Child development centre ☐ GP Community paediatrician ☐ Ophthalmology Audiology Dietician ENT Sexual health Speech therapy OT CAMHS Physio Other Action Required: Refer to SWD Refer to Reporter Refer to Special Needs System Signed__________ Date__________ Time__________			
Name in Block Letters	Designation	Review Weeks	
Copy this assessment to:			
File Police School nurse Parents GP Audit office Social work HV Other Paediatrician Please state			

Section 2: Standard Operating Procedure

STANDARD OPERATING PROCEDURE IN RELATION TO CHILD PROTECTION CONCERNS

This standard operating procedure (SOP) is in relation to the management of child protection concerns when a child is in A and E, short stay ward or an inpatient within the general wards in the Royal Hospital for Sick Children (RHSC) Glasgow, Scotland (UK). The general principles can apply to all children in all departments; however, some specialist services may require to develop further guidance.

This has been designed to equip staff with a process to follow, which will support communication both intra- and inter-agency, inform the management of the child in relation to child protection concerns, and ensure prior to discharge, that processes are in place to protect the child. It is not a stand-alone procedure and must form part of a larger framework for all staff in relation to their child protection practice.

This SOP should be activated when child protection concerns are first identified. This may be either at the point of admission to hospital or at a later stage in the child's stay when concerns become apparent. This SOP should be activated when:

- A child is brought to hospital by the police and/or social work in relation to child protection concerns.
- A child is transferred from another hospital with identified child protection concerns.
- Another professional alerts the hospital that the child would be attending with child protection concerns.
- On admission staffs identify child protection concerns.

As an inpatient staff identifies child protection concerns. This may be because of the following:

- There are concerns regarding the child
- Behaviour of the parents
- Other information becoming known
- Child (or adult) discloses abuse.

Parents

Wherever possible we would strive to work in partnership with parents, maintaining an open and honest approach in relation to any concerns noted and subsequent actions taken. This information should be shared with parents (and child if appropriate) at the earliest opportunity. In exceptional circumstances, there would be a delay in sharing information if it was felt that to do so would place the child or staff member (s) at further risk.

Regular updates to the child, if age appropriate and the parents should be made by both social services and the child's consultant as to the progress of any child protection investigation.

Communication is a key in effective child protection work. It is essential to record fully all concerns and assessments and subsequent decisions and actions. This SOP does not replace this process but rather compliments fuller documentation in relation to child protection concerns (comprehensive health evaluation and multidisciplinary record). When referring to social work department, follow-up telephone referral using multiagency referral form.

> *Note:*
> The child protection unit operates Monday to Friday 8.30 am–5.00 pm. Child protection advisors are available within these times to offer information, advice and support in relation to child protection concerns.
> Telephone: Child protection medical team may be contacted at any time for advice, to assist with assessment or to share the clinical management of a child where there are child protection concerns: Monday to Friday 9 am–5 pm.
> Telephone: Out of hours, the on-call consultant can be obtained through hospital switchboard.

In all child protection cases, social work must be informed at the earliest point:

- If Monday–Thursday between 8.45 am and 4.45 pm, and Fridays between 8.45 am and 4 pm. Contact the hospital social work team on Telephone
- If out of hours/weekend/public holiday, contact social work standby services on Telephone
- If a child is brought in by the area social work, or area social work is investigating an incident, please inform the hospital social work team for information only
- Identify the named social worker for the child and record it in the case note.

Who Can Use Standard Operating Procedure?

Any member of staff can activate SOP. This would normally be following discussion with the consultant in charge of the child's care and/or the nurse in charge. The documentation will be widely available in clinical areas and thereafter kept in the child's medical case notes and reviewed on ward round. If SOP is activated, child protection documentation should also be activated to fully record issues.

Inform		Date/time	Signature/initials
Social Work Department informed	Hospital		
	Local (please specify area team)		

If you are referring a child to social work, you should also inform:

Inform	Date/time	Signature/initials
The child's admitting/deputising consultant (Insert name)		
The nurse in-charge of the ward/department (Insert name)		
The child protection unit (Insert name)		
The identified Liaison Health Visitor for the ward/department (Where applicable) (Insert name)		
Inform the child's GP (Insert name)		
If the child is under 5 years, inform the child's health visitor (Insert name)		

This second section addresses issues of the management for the child's care:

Safety	Yes	Date/time achieved	Signature/initials
Place the child's bed in a ward where he/she can be observed by staff. (As appropriate to child's clinical care).			
Have the child's parents been informed (if appropriate) of the actions taken? Consideration must be given to the timing of this, and as to whether it places the child or staff in any danger—usually senior nursing/medical staff will do this.			
Where appropriate ensure staff are aware that the child should not be removed from the ward whilst the child protection investigation is ongoing or if subject to a child protection order without discussion with senior staff and social work colleagues.			

If the child is subject to a child protection order or supervision order requirement, the following procedure must be followed:

	Yes	*Date/time achieved*	*Signature/ initials*
Obtain a copy of the child protection order from social work and place in case notes			
Be aware of and document fully any restrictions on the family regarding contact with the child (either in the ward or in removing the child from the ward).			
Has a discussion with social work taken place as to how restrictions will be managed? And is this recorded in the child's child protection documentation?			

Inter-agency Collaboration and Communication

	Yes	*Date/time achieved*	*Signature/ initials*
Are the names and telephone numbers of key personnel involved with the investigation contained within the child's notes?			
Has a case discussion/conference been arranged?			
Is there a record of the date/time/place of case discussion/conference?			
Names of ward staff attending:			
Has a written report been provided (Medical)?			
Has a written report been provided (Nursing)?			
Inform social work team if child is moving ward/department			
Have medical staff informed social work team of results of medical investigations or change in circumstances			
As early as possible, discussions should have taken place with social work regarding discharge arrangements in relation to the child. Have discussions taken place?			

Once the child is medically fit for discharge–

	Yes	***Date/time***	***Signature/ initials***
Ensure update from social work as to progress of the investigation prior to discharge			
If the child is in receipt of a 'Health Record booklet' ensure this is appropriately completed and returned to child/carer			
Clarify whom the child is being discharged to Name: Address: Relationship to child:			
If the child has identified health needs, is there need to be a direct contact from ward to carer. Is this required?			
Ensure primary care is notified of concerns and actions. (This may differ from the family GP/HV if child is being discharged to other care) Have primary care been informed Carer's GP Name: Carer's GP Address:			
If unable to identify relevant primary care practitioners (GP/HV) contact child protection advisor within Child Protection Unit. Tel: -			
If arranging nursing follow on, inform community nurses of the child protection concerns and actions.			
Has case discussion/conference taken place/been arranged? Date: Time: Place:			
Staff members identified to attend: Names:			
If child is going into foster care, please notify looked after and accommodated children to the health team Contact details:			

Section 3: Child Protection or Child Welfare Multidisciplinary Chronological Record

Part I: Multidisciplinary Chronological Record

All staff involved in the child's care, who have information related to the child protection concern, must record their involvement and concerns, ensuring a chronological, complete and integrated review are possible. This record must include all key points but may also be cross-referenced to more complete entries in the child's medical notes or in locally held files.

Name:	Ward Admitted to:
Hospital No:	Date admitted:
DOB:	

Date and time24 hour clock to be used for all timed entries	***Event/child protection-related information***	***Signature, print name and designation***

Part II: Child Protection or Child Welfare Action Plan

The action plan will be completed by key health professionals and placed into the child protection or child welfare section of the child's medical notes.

Childs Name:		
Hospital Number:		
Allocated	Social Worker:	Date:
Base:	Tel:	Fax:

Key Points/Issues:

Action Plan:	
Lead Consultant/delegated doctor:	
Print Name:	
Signed:	Date:
Senior Nurse:	
Print Name:	
Signed:	Date:
Social Worker:	
Print Name:	
Signed:	Date:

Part III: Conclusion to Child Protection or Child Welfare Concerns

This form to be jointly completed by social worker and lead consultant in all cases where a child about whom there has been child protection concerns is being discharged and where child protection concerns have been investigated and no longer remain. In these circumstances, both the social worker and the lead consultant must be satisfied that the child will be protected or is no longer in need of protection.

Child's Name:	Ward:
Hospital No:	Date:
DOB:	

Please Tick as Appropriate:

Child is being discharged with child protection plan in place.
Please give brief details of plan and local contact number (e.g. follow-up by child's local authority):
Child protection concerns have been investigated and no longer remain:

Please give brief details:

Social Worker:		
Print Name:	Signed:	Date:
Social Work Manager:		
Print Name:	Signed:	Date:
Lead Consultant:		
Print Name:	Signed:	Date:

A copy of this form has to be kept on both the medical notes and in the child's social work file. If further concerns arise in the future, please contact the social work department and refer the case using the multiagency child protection referral form.

CHAPTER 32

Paediatric Rehabilitation

Judy Ann John, Lydia Edward Raj, Debbie Skeil

INTRODUCTION

Disability in childhood can result from multiple conditions. The two main groups of problems that arose before or as the child was born including genetic problems and those acquired after birth. These are listed in **Table 32.1**.

In medicine, doctors are trained to identify the medical problem and to manage that problem. 'Suresh cannot walk very well and so cannot go to school'. Reading this statement it looks like it is Suresh's problem and his fault that he cannot go to school. However, in recent years, there has been a change in how we look at a person. So, Suresh can walk using his walker but needs the ground to be smooth with no steps. Suresh's classroom is on the first floor and the stairs stop him from going to school. Here, we see that Suresh does have a problem. He also has equipment to aid him, but the environment is a major barrier for Suresh.

The International Classification of Functioning, Disability and Health (ICF) was approved by the World Health Organization (WHO) in May 2001. The ICF recognises the complex dynamic interaction between the health of the child and environmental and personal factors **(Flow chart 32.1)**. This has replaced the previous classification of the International Classification of Impairments, Disabilities and Handicaps (ICIDH). The ICF allows the focus to be shifted from 'disability' (cannot do) to 'activity (ability to perform a task appropriate to age)' and from 'handicap' to 'participation'. The emphasis is taken away from the disease to its impact on what the child can do, 'functioning' and the child's ability to take part in everyday activities, in play and school. Both factors, the child's functioning and participation, will determine the goals of rehabilitation. This information is used to determine the extent to which a child's abilities can be improved through therapy and to what extent the environment can be changed to facilitate the child's performance. Hence, disability in the above example does not reside in Suresh but in his environment, which prevents his participation in his community and school.

REHABILITATION PROGRAMME

Multipronged interventions aimed at various components of a child's disability (physical, cognitive, behavioural and psychosocial) can influence the outcome of a rehabilitation programme. Hence, the rehabilitation team consists of the medical doctor (physiatrist/paediatrician), nurse, physiotherapist, occupational therapist, speech orthotist/prosthetist, psychologist, special educator, social worker and orthotic/prosthetic depending on the nature of the condition.

In the *interdisciplinary* model of care, professionals from different disciplines perform evaluations independently and work towards the goals set in collaboration with the parents. In a child with multiple disabilities, various professionals provide therapy in their area of expertise, e.g. speech therapist for communication and swallowing, physiotherapist for head, trunk, limb control and balance, occupational therapist for participation in daily activities and special educator for learning. However, in the *transdisciplinary* approach, each of these members can interact jointly in a way that any one of the therapist can provide the training needed.

The *collaborative* model of service delivery is family centred, integrating services and promoting outcomes that are meaningful to the child and family in daily life. This incorporates therapy into the natural learning environment (in the setting where children live, learn and play), which is based on the assumption that motor learning is optimised by frequent and varied practice within the context of daily activities and routines.

Interventions can be directed towards the child to:

- Optimise the abilities of the child (functional abilities)
- Prevent/reduce the secondary disabilities that occur due to the primary condition such as contractures, dislocation of a hip, pressure sores and behavioural disturbances
- Enable the child to participate in life tasks and interact with his/her environment at home, school and at play

TABLE 32.1 Disability in children can result from the following conditions.

Acquired conditions	***Developmental delay/congenital deficits or deformity***
Traumatic/acquired brain injury (hypoxia, infections)	Cerebral palsy, seizure disorder, hearing, visual, speech, learning deficits
Traumatic/acquired (demyelination/tumours) spinal cord injury (SCI)	Neural tube defects, meningomyelocoele, hydrocephalus
Neuromuscular disease (e.g. poliomyelitis, Guillain–Barré syndrome, myasthenia gravis, polymyositis)	Neuromuscular disorders (e.g. spinal muscular atrophy, Duchenne muscular dystrophy, Becker dystrophy)
Nerve injuries, e.g. Erb palsy	Hereditary sensory motor neuropathy
Juvenile arthritis, haemophiliac arthropathy	Joint deformities, e.g. club feet, arthrogryposis
Amputations due to trauma, tumours, burns	Congenital limb deficiencies—phocomelia

- Provide support and training to the family to continue therapy in the home setting.

Rehabilitation in Brain Injury

An assessment of the child by the various team members helps in planning therapy and making goals for the child. Clinical assessments look at the child's performance in various domains. These include vision, hearing, speech, cognition, behaviour, motor and sensory system. The examination of each system is important, but the main purpose of assessment is to find out what the child can do and not do and the reason for it. Observing a child play by herself, with toys or with people is a quick and pleasant method of evaluating the child's motor control of their head, trunk, upper and lower limbs, hand functions, their eye-hand coordination, cognition and behaviour.

Developmental Delay

Infants with risk factors or history suggestive of developmental delay need to be part of an early intervention programme, which is implemented between birth and 3 years (Chapter 14: Diseases of the Nervous System). This programme focuses on optimising the child's development milestone and includes teaching the family how to help their child become independent, something many parents find very hard to do. Two intervention models described here are activity focussed and impairment focussed intervention.

Flow chart 32.1 The International Classification of Functioning, Disability and Health (ICF).

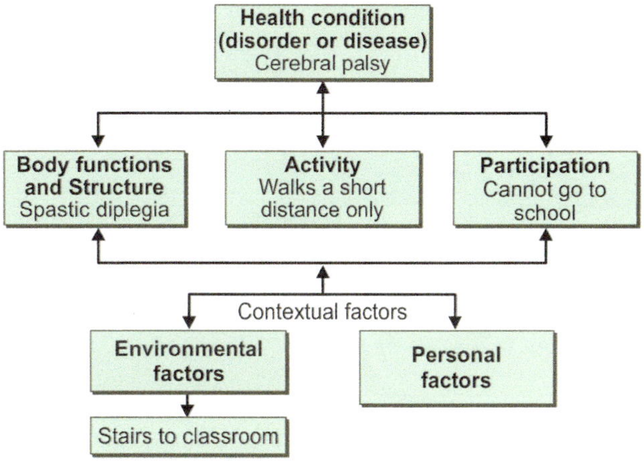

Impairment Focussed Interventions

Impairment focussed intervention includes sensory motor approaches, positioning to prevent contractures, range of motion exercises, strength, endurance and balance training.

Sensory-motor Approaches

The most common physiotherapy approach used in cerebral palsy is the Bobath neurodevelopmental approach. Advances have been made in the Bobath approach, and it is currently regarded as a 'concept' rather than a technique. The basic concept involves the inhibition of abnormal movement patterns and the facilitation of automatic postural reactions (righting and equilibrium reactions). The therapist/mother's hands are used for guided control of body parts along with other stimulation techniques to reduce the abnormal postural tone, improve postural alignment and control. This provides age-appropriate sensorimotor feedback and encourages the appearance of mature reflexes. In turn, this will help in the child develop motor control, usually in this order, including head control, rolling, prone on elbows **(Figs. 32.1A to C)**, sitting, standing and walking **(Figs. 32.2A to C)**. This should be incorporated throughout the day by the parents in the way the child is positioned, carried and assisted for daily activities.

Therapy progresses according to the normal developmental milestone with a focus on functional performance, e.g. trunk control can be facilitated once head control is achieved. Similarly, standing and ambulation can be facilitated once a child has adequate trunk and hip control in sitting **(Fig. 32.2)** and kneeling **(Figs. 32.3A to D)**/half kneeling **(Figs. 32.4A to C)**.

Management of Impaired Motor Control

Deficits in the voluntary muscle contraction in children with cerebral palsy are thought to be due to decreased

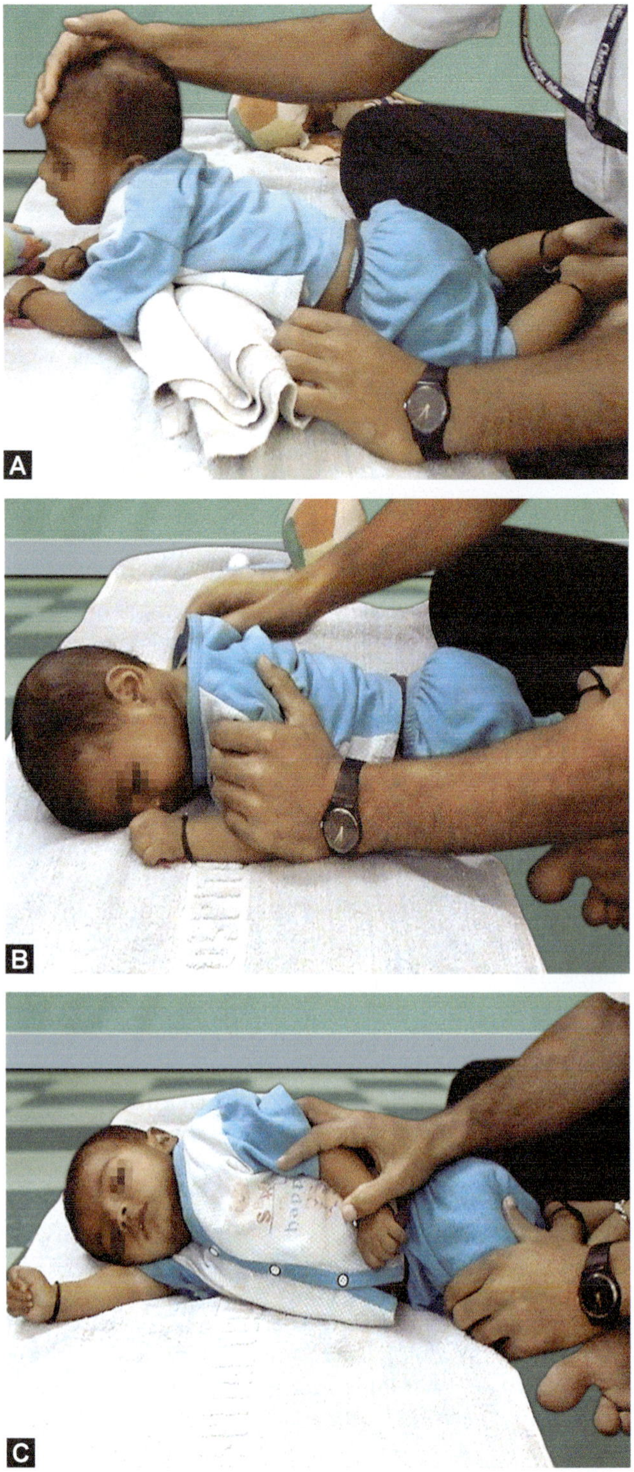

Figures 32.1A to C Early intervention to facilitate head control. (A) A rolled up towel is used to prop up the upper body, and the child's head is supported by the therapist's hand. His mother uses a toy to get the attention of her child; (B) Head control is encouraged by prone lying on the elbows. The therapist helps the child prop himself up on his forearms; (C) Early intervention where rolling is facilitated by the therapist's hand by moving the pelvis and encouraging the child to turn his head and shoulders.

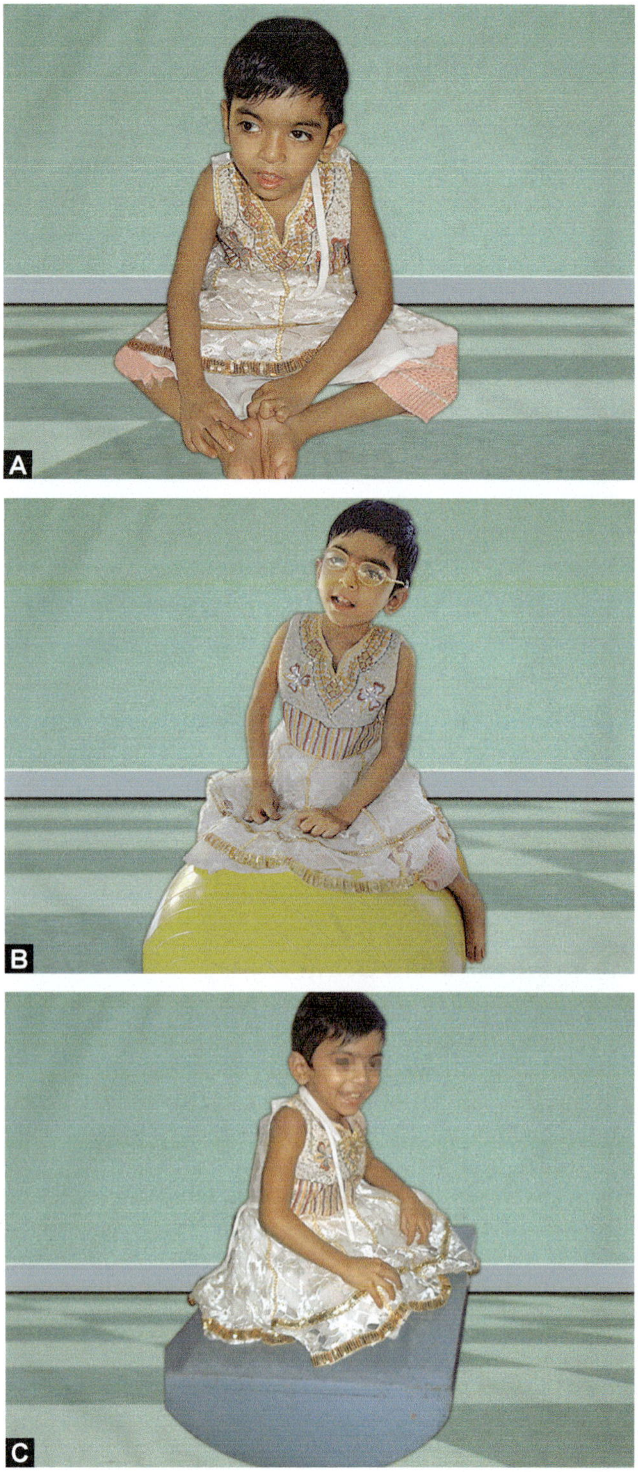

Figures 32.2A to C A 4-year-old child with cerebral palsy. (A) Facilitating a symmetrical sitting position: initially someone will need to hold the child along with verbal and visual (using a mirror) feedback. The legs are positioned to stretch and reduce the tone in the adductors; (B) Using a therapy ball to improve trunk control. A slight movement of the ball will encourage the child to adjust her posture and trunk alignment and thus facilitate equilibrium and righting reactions to improve balance; (C) Therapy on a rocker board to improve trunk control. The child learns to initiate balance strategies by adjusting her position to maintain her centre of gravity over the moving base of support.

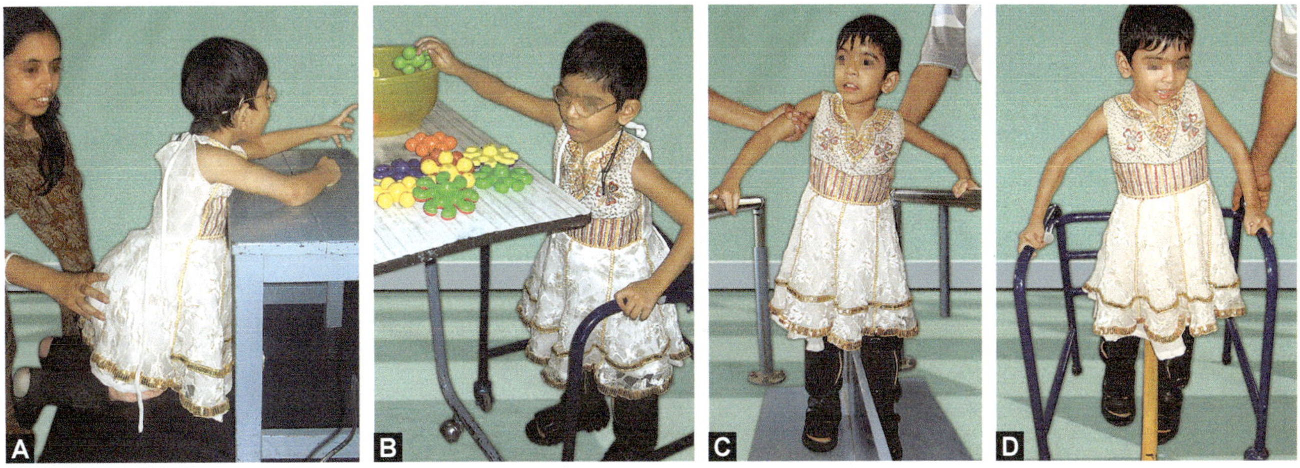

Figures 32.3A to D (A) Kneeling with support helps to improve the control of hip and trunk extensors. The support required to kneel can be gradually reduced as hip and trunk control improves; (B) Activities to improve standing balance with a walker—both ankles are supported with AFOs and knees with braces/gaiters; (C) Gait training in parallel bars with shoulder support; (D) With improvement in her trunk and limb control, this child progressed to gait training with a walker. Ankles and knees are supported with AFOs and knee braces, and now less assistance is needed just to propel the walker. A rod is placed between the legs, during the training period, to reduce scissoring.

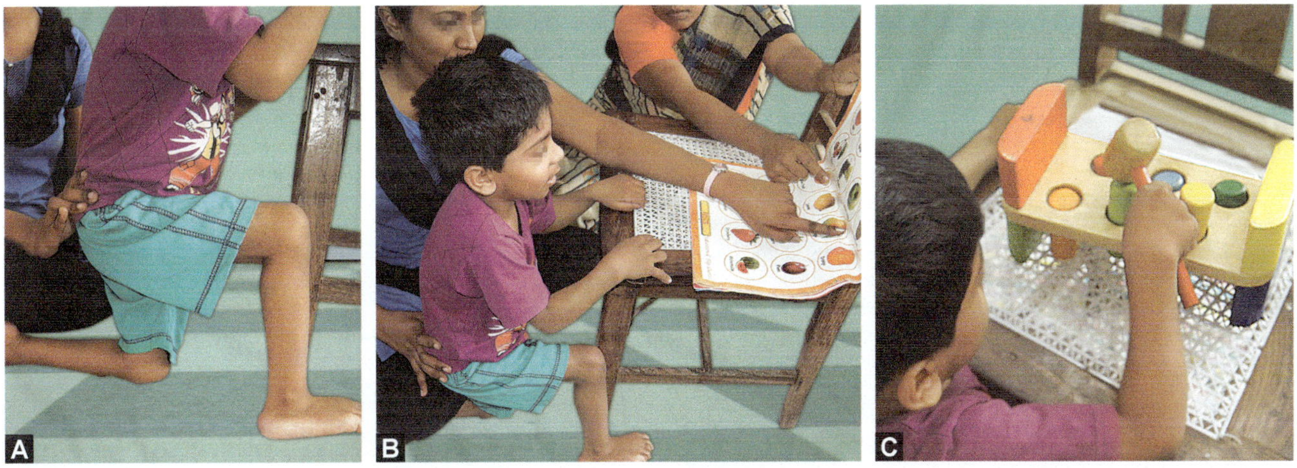

Figures 32.4A to C (A) and (B) The half kneeling position, to develop hip control, can be facilitated while the child is engaged in learning about fruits. Easily available furniture is used for this activity; (C) Other play activities such as hammering pegs onto a stand can be performed to facilitate diagonal grasp while maintaining a kneeling position against a chair. Support is given to the hips as needed by a hand or a strap.

motor recruitment centrally and changes in the muscle morphology. Impaired voluntary control is also seen due to abnormality in central control and motor tone resulting in *spastic* or *dyskinetic* cerebral palsy (also includes *athetoid, choreoathetoid* and *dystonic* cerebral palsies). Goals are made with the family towards improving voluntary control, reducing spasticity and improving functional abilities (what a child can do).

The child must be able to understand the instructions to effectively participate in a programme aimed at improving voluntary control in the weak muscles **(Figs. 32.5 and 32.6)**. A progressive training schedule is planned and this involves initially isolating the contraction of the desired group of muscles and then increasing its strength and endurance **(Figs. 32.7A to D)**. Selective strengthening of antigravity muscles in the lower limb, especially hip **(Fig. 32.7)** and knee extensors **(Fig. 32.8)**, helps to improve the gait pattern and efficiency. Strength training involves exercises against a particular resistance, e.g. free weight **(Figs. 32.8 to 32.11)**, resistance band **(Figs. 32.12A and B)**, which load the muscle. The strength programme can also be carried on through activities like push-ups **(Figs. 32.13A and B)** and play such as ball/toy kicking for hip and knee strengthening **(Figs. 32.14A and B)** and catching and throwing a ball for upper limbs **(Figs. 32.15A to C)**. The endurance of these muscles is improved by increasing the number of repetitions of the activity. A record is made of the progress with therapy.

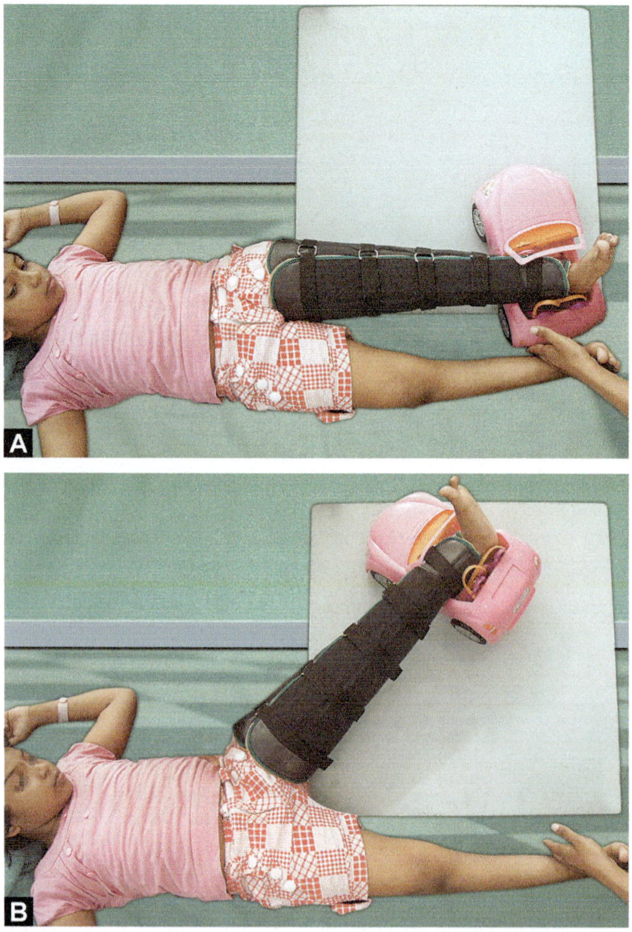

Figures 32.5A and B Strengthening programme for hip abductors in a position where gravity is eliminated in this girl with cerebral palsy. This is done by using a re-education board and a toy on wheels to assist with the movements. These assisted exercises are done when the muscle power is less than grade 3 [Medical Research Council (MRC) grading].

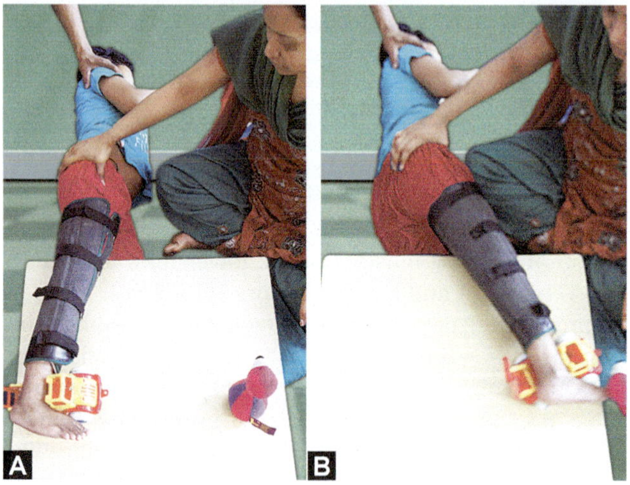

Figures 32.6A and B Strengthening programme for hip flexors and extensors using a re-education board and a toy on wheels to assist with these movements as the muscle power is less than grade 3 (MRC grading). Another toy is used as a target to achieve the full range of the movement and to give positive feedback when it is kicked.

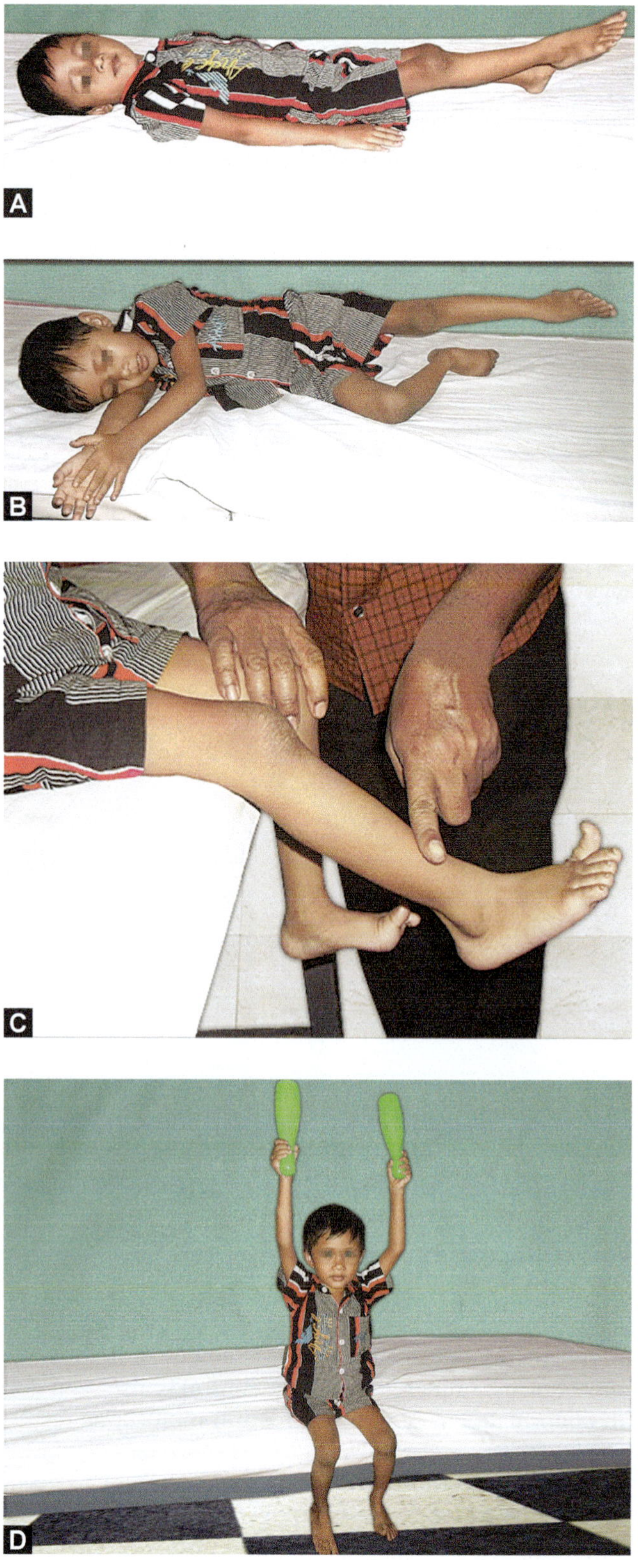

Figures 32.7A to D A boy with muscular dystrophy working on his hip flexors, abductors and upper limb strengthening against gravity. The endurance of these muscles can be improved by increasing the repetitions of these exercises. The recommendations for children are one to three sets of 8–15 repetitions at 50–85% of 1 repetition maximum (1 RM) (maximum weight child can lift once—one RM), with a 1–3 minute rest between the sets.

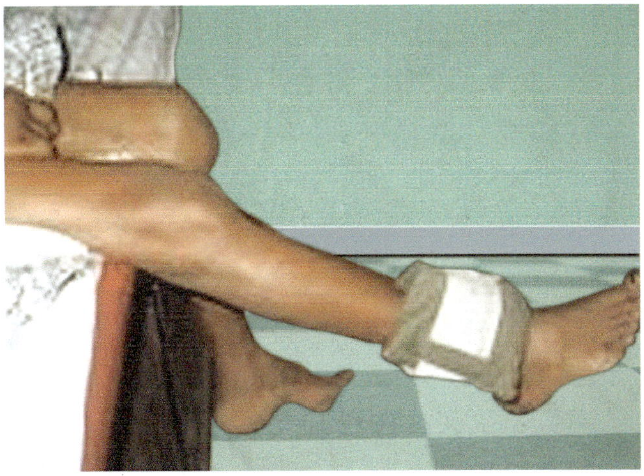

Figure 32.8 A girl with juvenile idiopathic arthritis does resistive quadriceps strengthening exercises using free weights (sandbags).

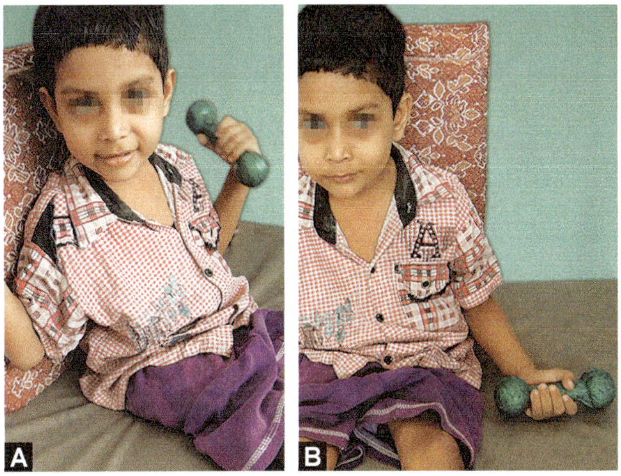

Figures 32.9A and B Elbow flexor strengthening in a 4-year-old boy with T4 traumatic paraplegia (ASIA A) while sitting using free weights (dumbbell). The number of repetitions of elbow flexion is gradually increased to improve the endurance of the muscle.

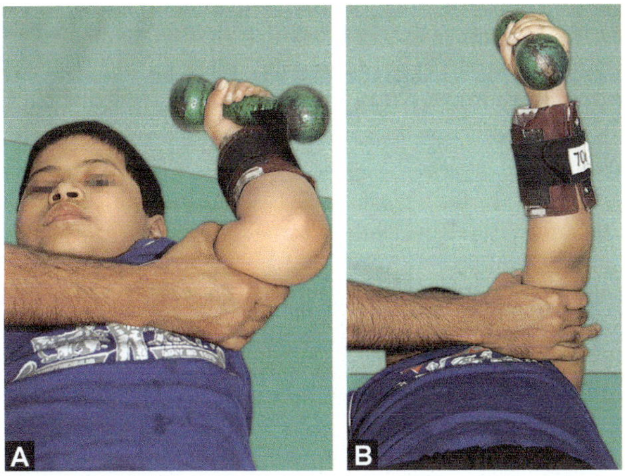

Figures 32.10A and B (A) Elbow extensor strengthening in the supine position using free weights in this 8-year-old boy with T4 ASIA A paraplegia; (B) The arm is positioned to perform this strengthening against gravity.

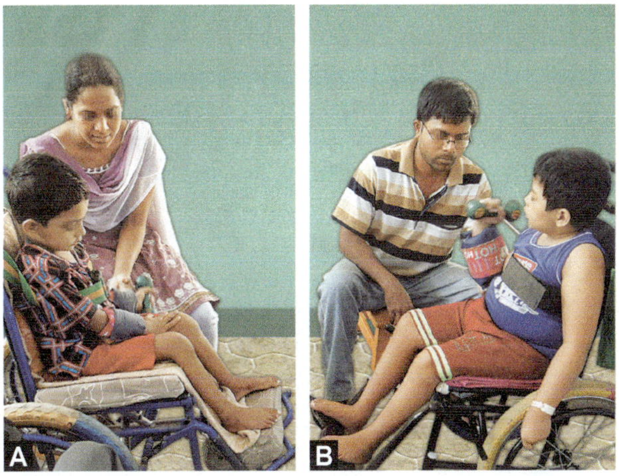

Figures 32.11A and B Group activity for strengthening using free weights.

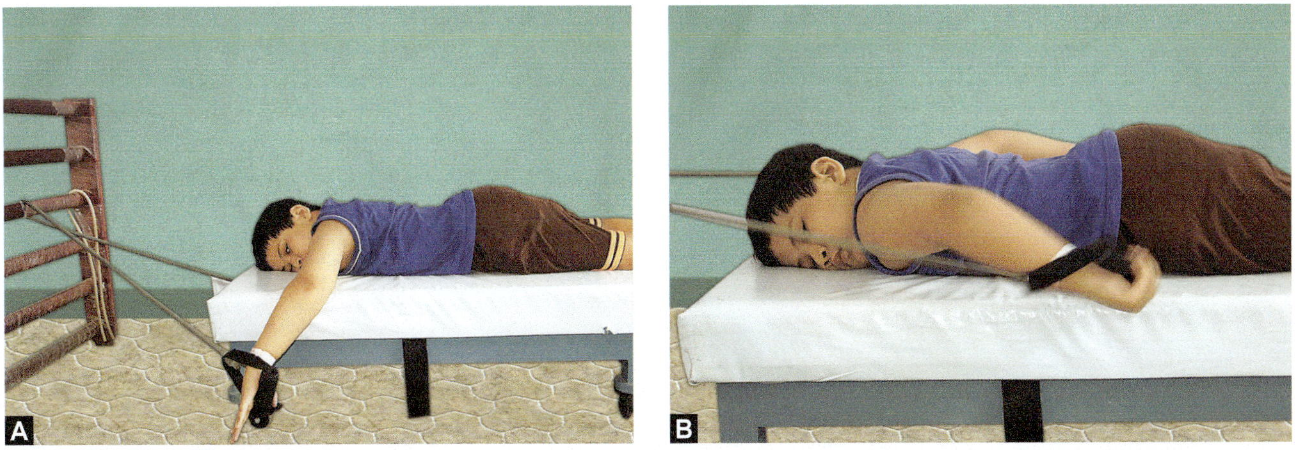

Figures 32.12A and B Latissimus dorsi strengthening by pulling on a Thera-tube (stretchy band) while extending and internally rotating the shoulders. This muscle is supplied by the thoracodorsal nerve (C6, C7 and C8). Elastic bands or tubes of different densities can be used for increasing the resistance of this pull.

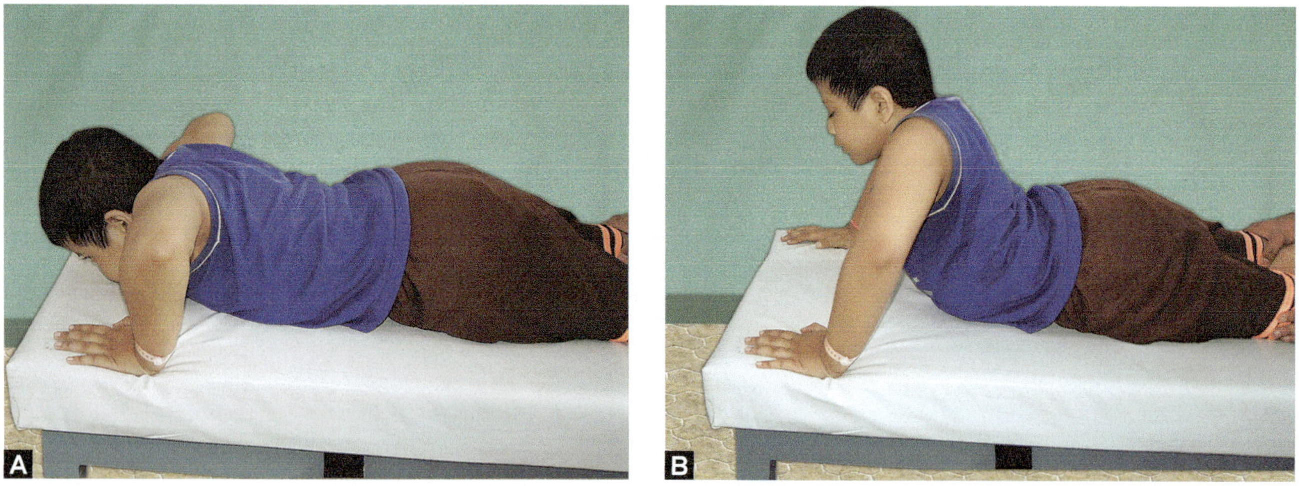

Figures 32.13A and B (A) Prone lying helps prevent hip flexion contractures; (B) Push-ups help with strengthening of the muscles of the shoulder and arm. The number of push-ups has to be progressively increased. This boy with T4 ASIA A paraplegia was able to perform 100 push-ups.

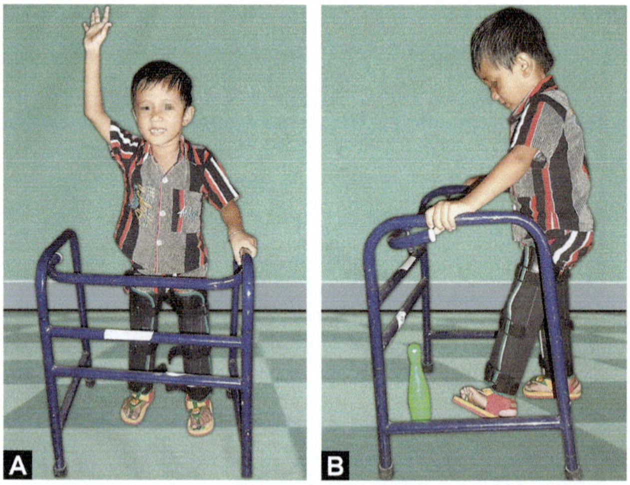

Figures 32.14A and B (A) Working on balance with an anterior walker in a child with congenital myopathy where the child learns to take one hand off. Gaiters//braces are used to support his weak knees; (B) Play activities such as kicking a ball/skittle can be given to improve hip control and single limb stance.

Upper limb strengthening helps with performing transfers **(Fig. 32.16)**, wheelchair propulsion **(Figs. 32.17A and B)** and the use of assistive mobility devices **(Figs. 32.18 and 32.19)**. Strengthening truncal muscles **(Fig. 32.20)** helps with static and dynamic (during activity) postural control in sitting **(Figs. 32.15, 32.21 and 32.22)** and standing **(Fig. 32.14)**.

Neuromuscular electrical stimulation (NMES) is the transcutaneous application of an electrical current to elicit repetitive muscle contractions by stimulating the motor nerves or motor endplates. This helps in maintaining the muscle bulk but is probably particularly effective when the child is able to initiate and enhance the muscle contraction voluntarily during the stimulation.

Management of Impaired Muscle Tone

Hypotonia *This is seen commonly in congenital conditions such as Down syndrome, metabolic syndromes and occasionally in cerebral palsy. Therapy involves*

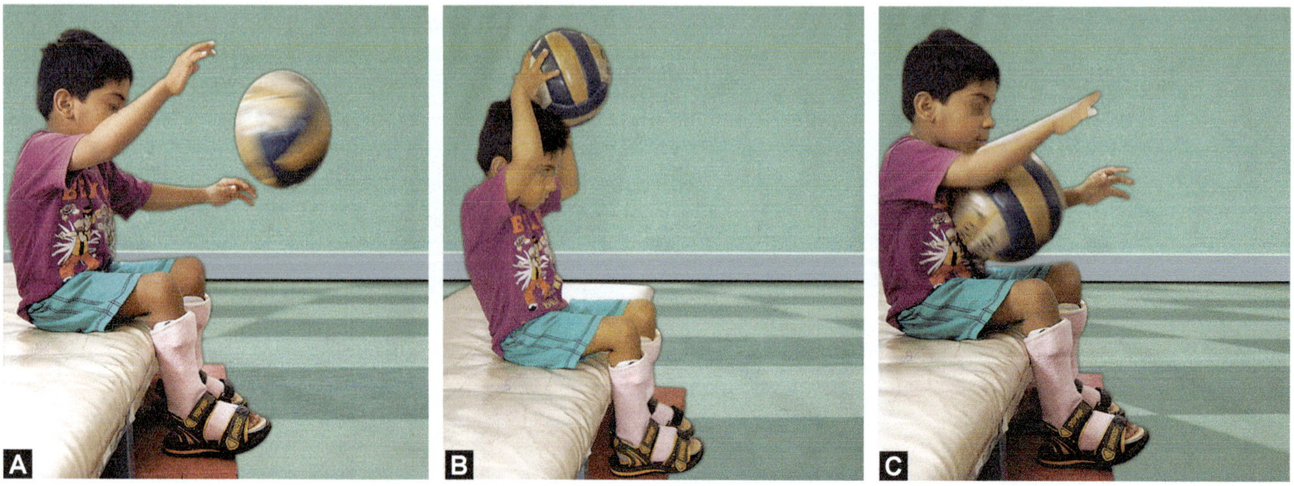

Figures 32.15A to C Throwing a ball and learning to catch it helps improve trunk control, balance in sitting and hand–eye coordination. This can also be a group activity.

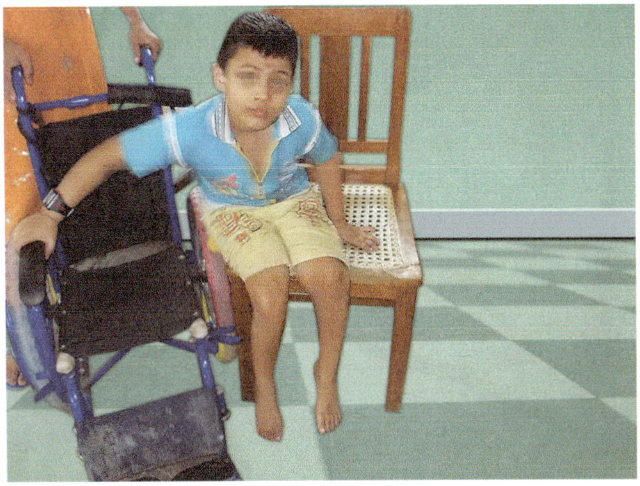

Figure 32.16 Wheelchair transfers on to a chair by a boy with T4 ASIA A paraplegia. The next step is to work on transfers to the bed and toilet stool/western toilet.

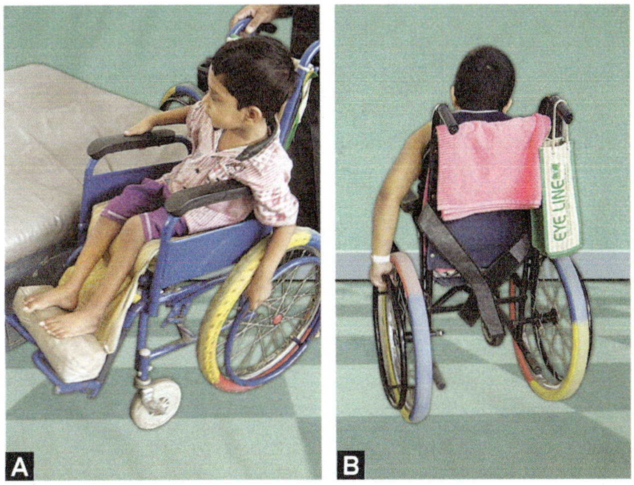

Figures 32.17A and B Learning to manoeuvre the wheelchair using the side rims attached to the wheels to move it in any direction.

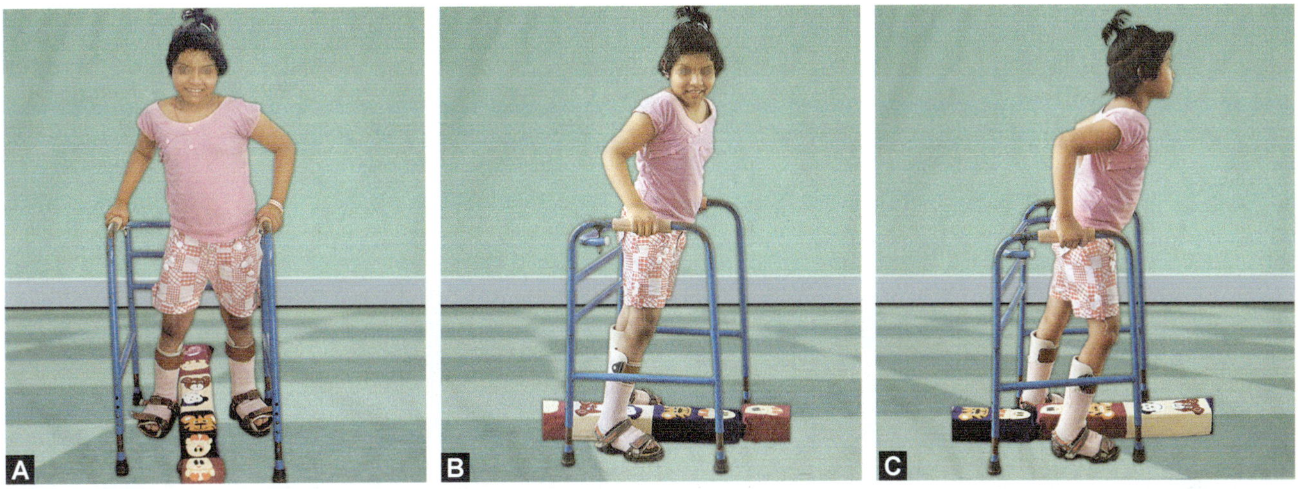

Figures 32.18A to C Gait training with a posterior walker in order to facilitate an upright posture. The use of an adductor bar during gait training reduces scissoring movement of the lower limbs.

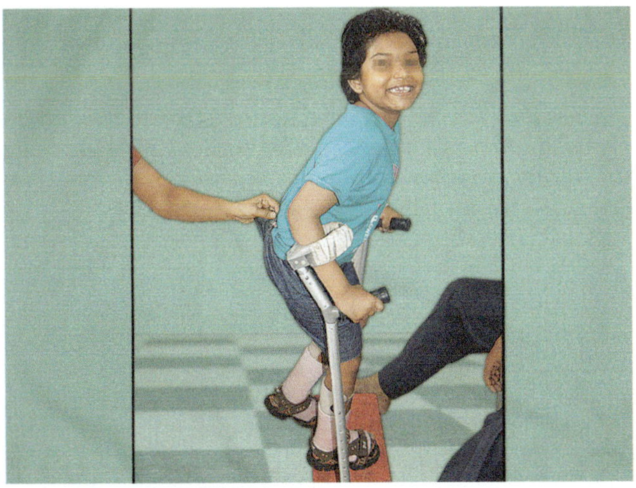

Figure 32.19 Training for step climbing with elbow crutches in a child with cerebral palsy in order to help with the return to school and community ambulation.

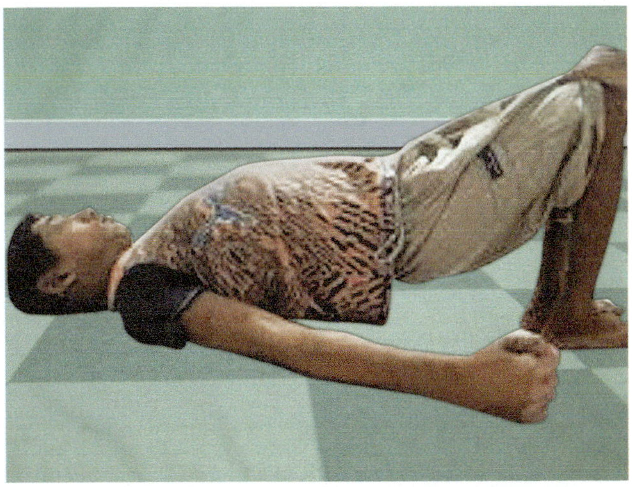

Figure 32.20 Pelvic bridging exercises by a 14-year-old boy with spastic diplegia to improve the strength of his paraspinals and hip extensors. In a younger child, run a toy car underneath as he succeeds as positive feedback.

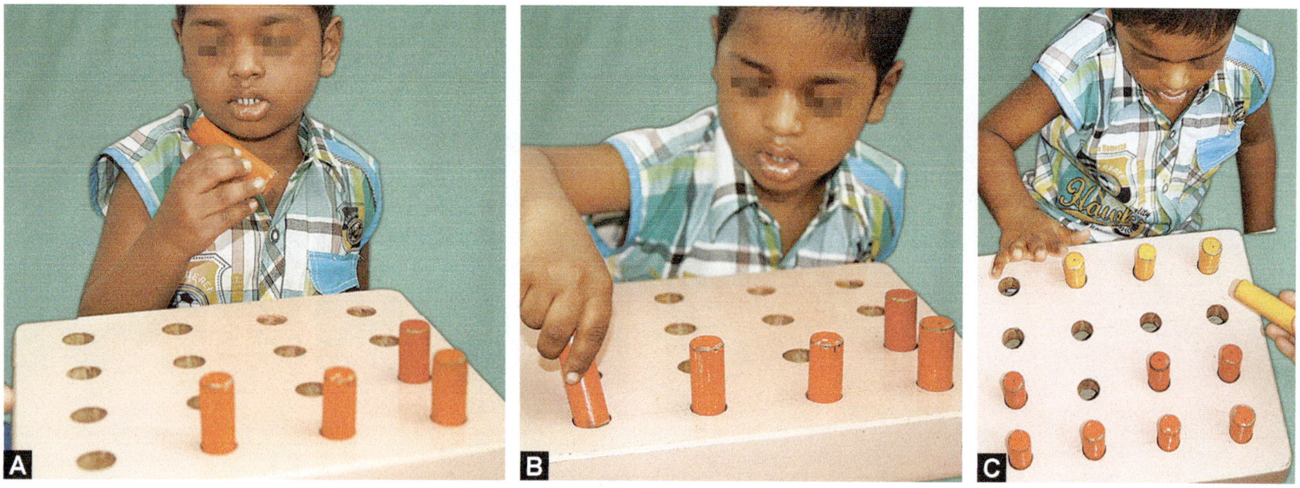

Figures 32.21A to C Cylindrical pegs and a peg board are used to facilitate grasp and precise release. Through this activity, this child with post-encephalitic sequelae, is also given colour concept training.

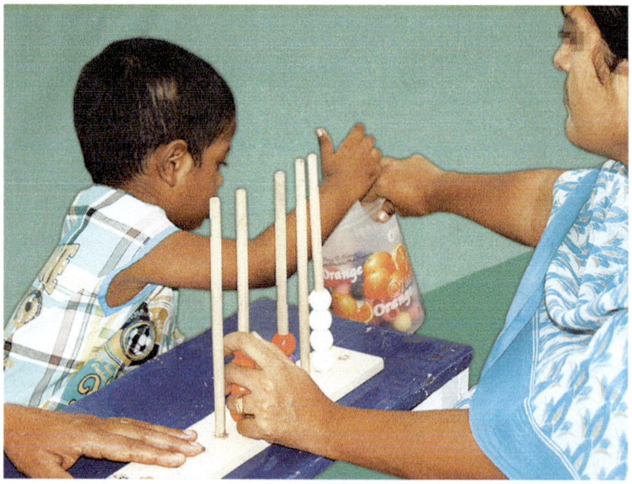

Figure 32.22 Reaching out to take beads from a jar placed across the child at variable distances and positions can help improve visual attention and reach.

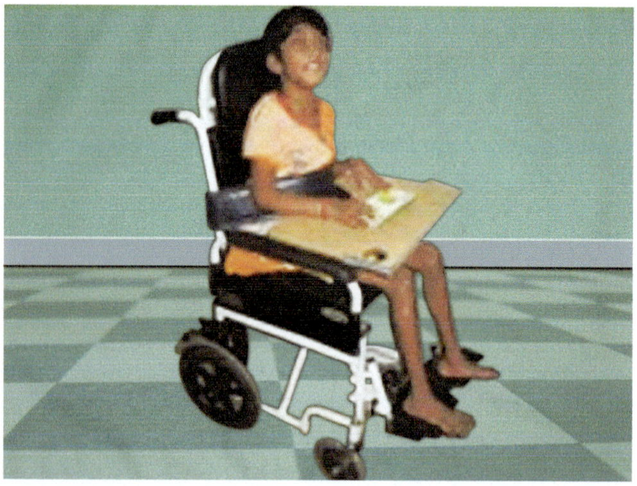

Figure 32.23 A 9-year-old child with cerebral palsy (total body involvement) using a wheelchair (which provides head, trunk and feet support) for mobility in and out of the home. Her upper limbs are well supported on the lapboard and it can be used for placing her food, play or learning activities.

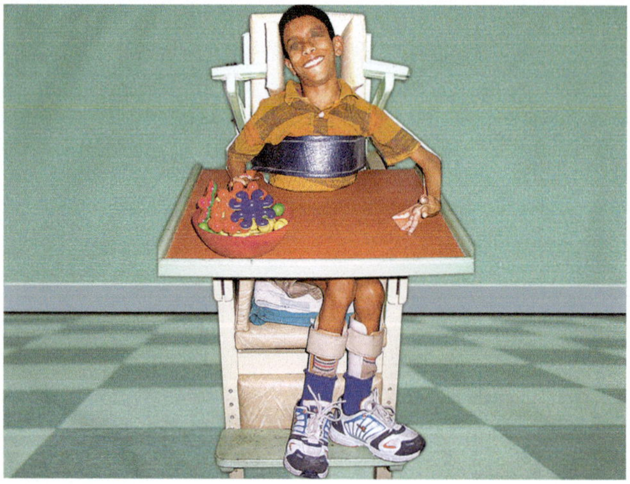

Figure 32.24 Supported seating for a child with generalised dystonia involving the head, neck, trunk and limbs. Supports are given to hold the head, trunk and feet in position. This chair will also require an abductor wedge to keep the legs apart.

encouraging weight bearing and improving muscle power across the joints to help with stability. In cases with severe loss of tone, appropriate seating supports will be needed for head and trunk control **(Figs. 32.23 and 32.24)**.

Spasticity An increase in the tone of muscles can negatively affect the child's functional abilities such as sitting, standing, walking and other activities of daily living (ADL). It can be one of the most difficult aspects to manage and the cause of much disability due to pain, functional limitations, difficulty with maintaining hygiene and resulting complications such as contractures, dislocations and pressure sores. An algorithmic approach to the management of hypertonia is presented in **Flow chart 32.2**. Specific interventions may include the following.

Flow chart 32.2 Components of hand function.

(Adapted from Exner CE. Development of hand skills. In: Case-Smith J. Occupational Therapy for Children, 4th edition, 2001. pp. 289-302)

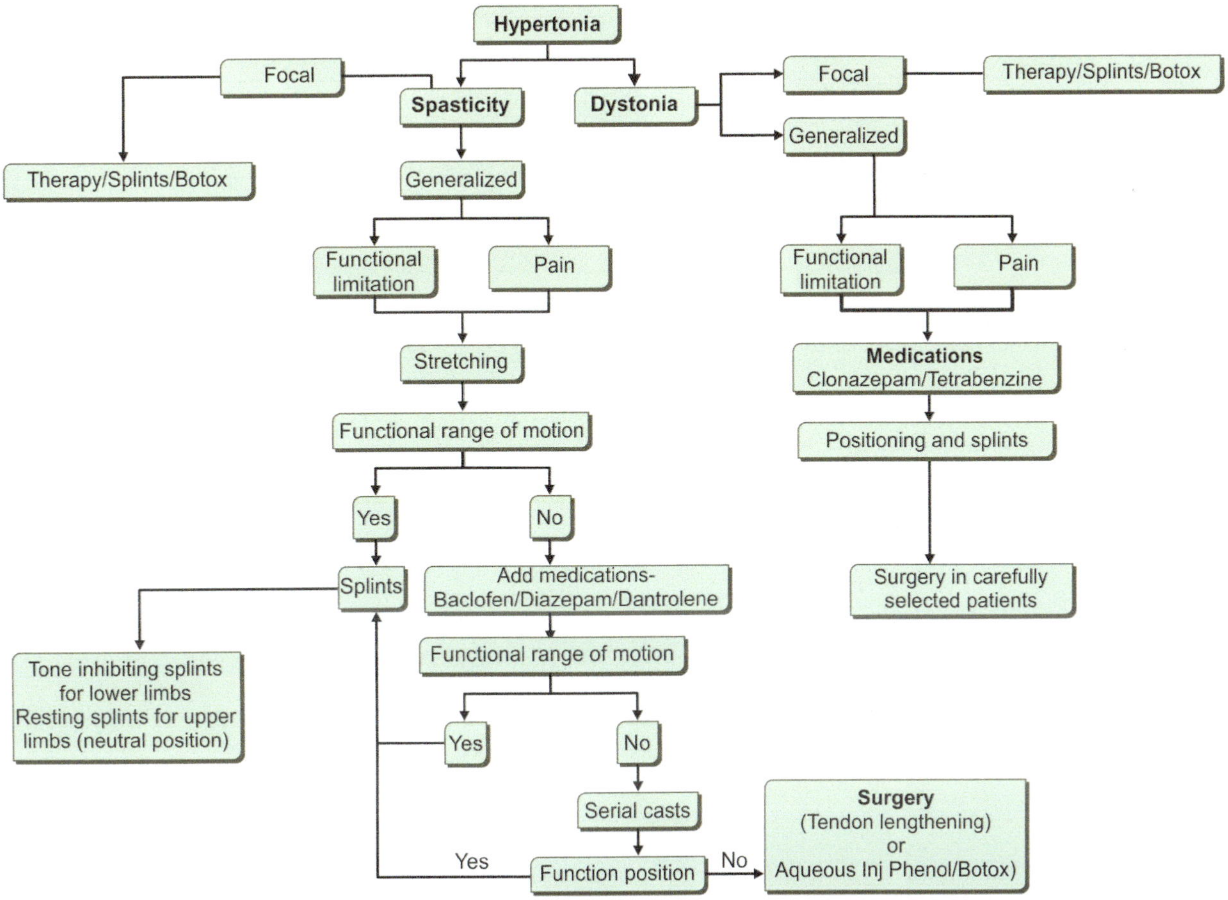

Stretching programme Spasticity in muscles can be reduced by stretching them **(Figs. 32.25A to C)** and strengthening their antagonistic muscles, e.g. strengthening of the hip abductors **(Fig. 32.5)** brings about a reciprocal inhibition in the adductors, so reducing tone in the adductors. Stretching can be maintained with an abduction pillow placed between the knees and used to keep the knees apart. Orthoses on the lower limbs **(Figs. 32.26 and 32.27)** and upper limbs can be used to maintain a good range of movement in the presence of spasticity, e.g. resting splints for the hands provide a continuous stretch to extend the finger and wrist flexors and thus help in reducing tone. A dorsal cock-up splint can be used during the day to stretch the wrist flexors so that the hands are free to use for any activity **(Figs. 32.28A and B)**. Active positioning all day and night is needed but should not inhibit activities.

Serial casting and orthoses Sometimes stretching is not enough to correct the contracture secondary to spasticity. Plaster of Paris casts are used to maintain a continuous stretch on the spastic muscles **(Fig. 32.29)**. Tone inhibition is also facilitated by hyperextension of the toes, pressure under the metatarsal head, medial arch, a stable ankle and neutral position and deep tendon pressure along the tendoachilles, e.g. to stretch the gastrocnemius, a cast is applied below the knee, keeping the ankle as close to a neutral position as possible with the toes in 30° of dorsiflexion with gentle moulding of the cast in the region of the medial arch and tendoachilles, before it sets. This enables the child to have a stable base to work on their standing balance and proximal muscle control. In the presence of hamstring tightness, the next cast should be above the knee cast **(Fig. 32.29)**; this will stretch both the gastrocnemius and the hamstrings. The casts have to be changed every week till the desired correction is obtained or earlier if the child complains of pain which suggests localised pressure. Each new plaster is placed so the contracture is stretched more each time. Once neutral position is achieved, this is replaced by a tone inhibiting ankle-foot orthosis (AFO) with a wedge of microcellular rubber added in the AFO **(Fig. 32.26)** to keep the toes

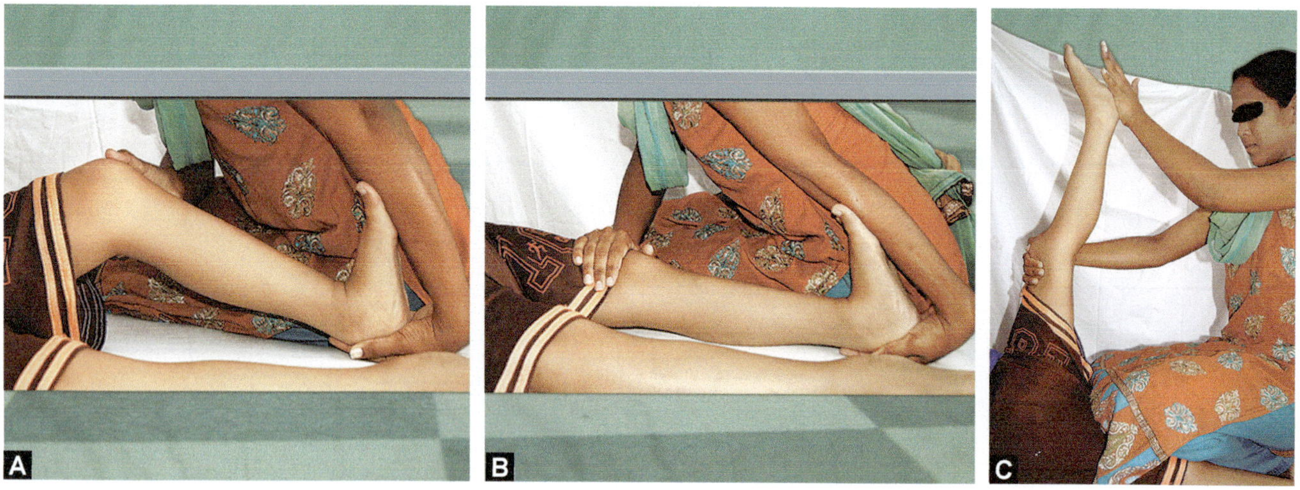

Figures 32.25A to C Assisted gastrosoleus muscle stretches with the knee in flexion (A), and then in extension (B) as this is a two-joint muscle. This is done to prevent an equinus contracture of the ankle. Assisted hamstring stretches where the knee is extended with the hip in a flexed position (C), as this too is a two-joint muscle. This is done to prevent a flexion deformity of the knee.

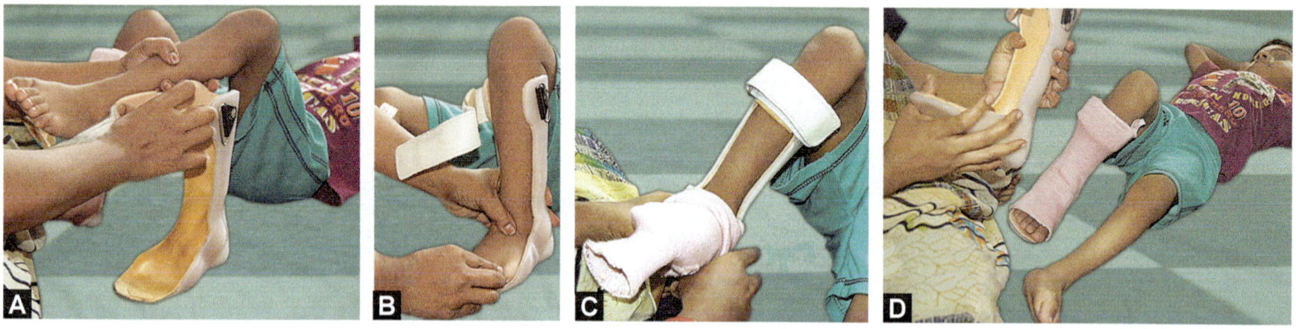

Figures 32.26A to D Putting on (donning) an AFO with the knee bent to relax the gastrosoleus muscle and to keep the ankle in a neutral position. Velcro straps and an anklet are used to stabilise the AFO.

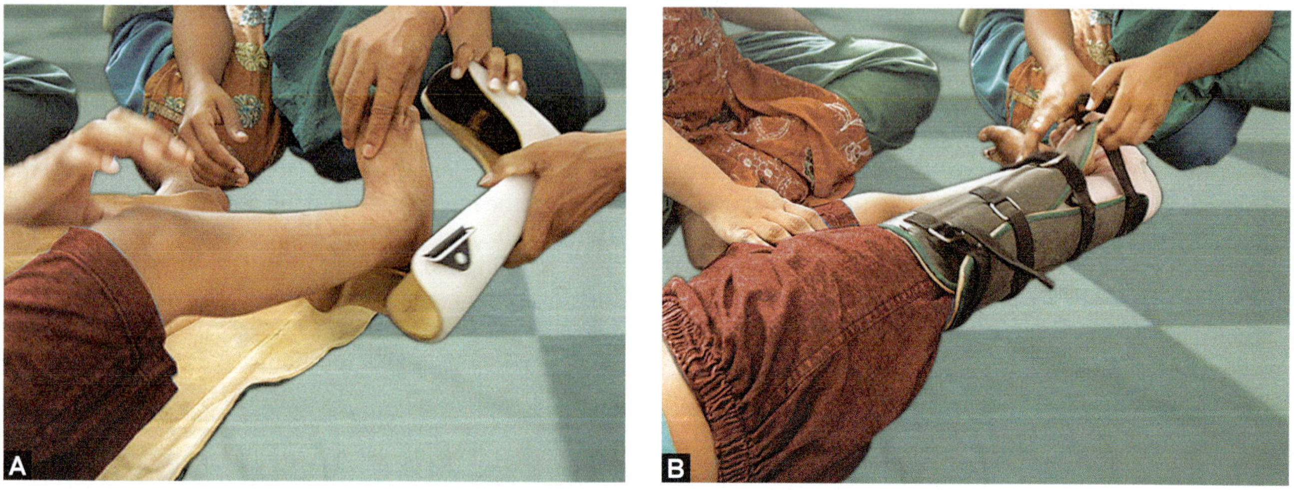

Figures 32.27A and B AFOs along with knee gaiters/braces are used to stretch the gastrosoleus and hamstrings and to keep the knee extended when standing.

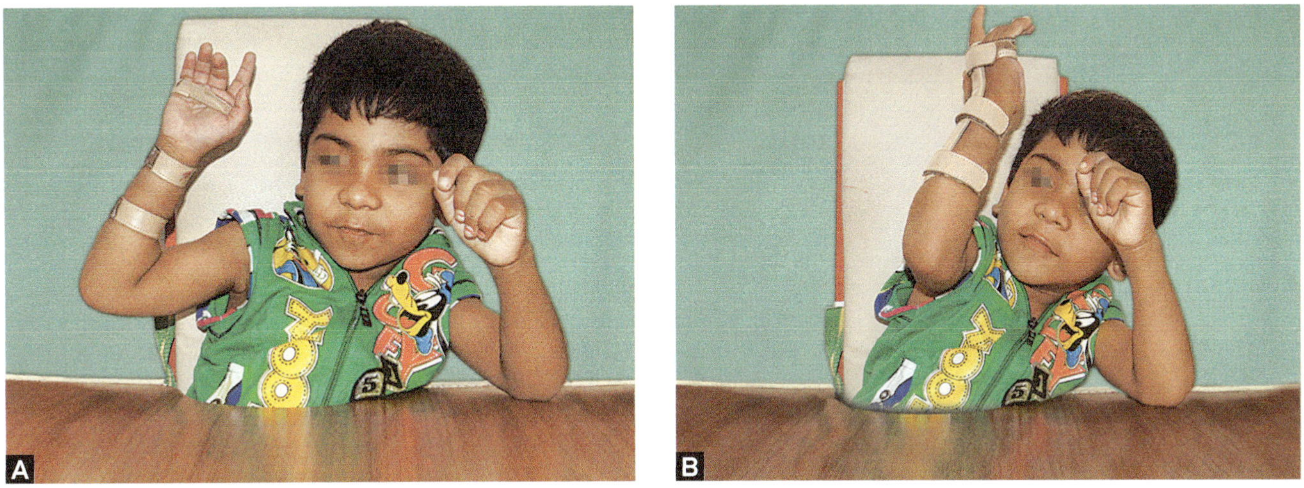

Figures 32.28A and B A dorsal cock-up splint helps to place the wrist in a functional position of 20° of extension and reduce spasticity in the wrist flexors.

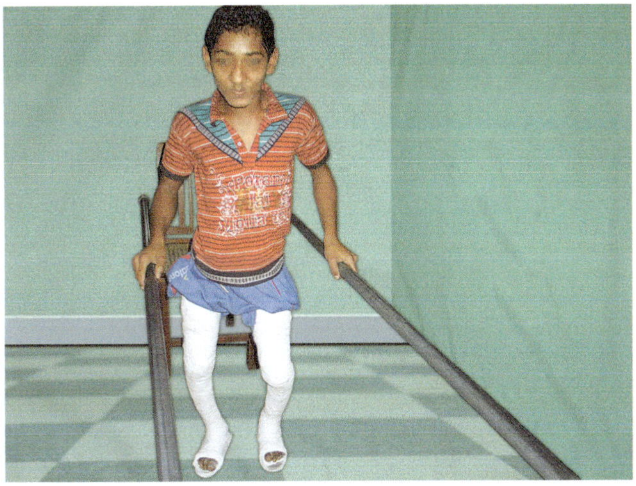

Figure 32.29 Serial above knee casts for correction of knee flexion deformity resulting from uncontrolled spasticity. Ambulation within parallel bars is started once the knee deformities are corrected to below 30°.

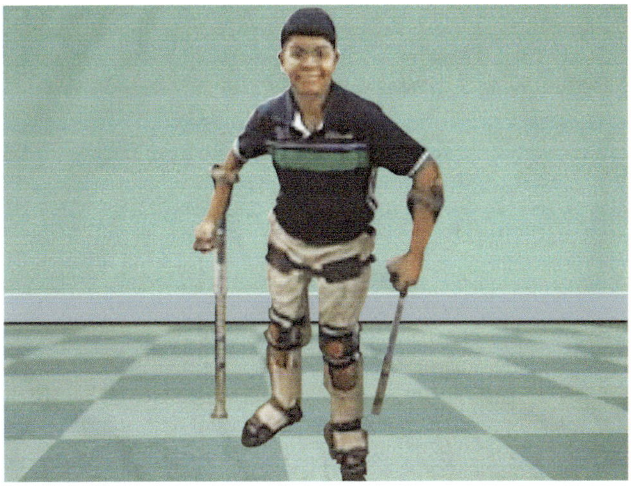

Figure 32.30 Standing balance training with knee-ankle-foot orthoses (KAFOs) and elbow crutches.

dorsiflexed and another wedge to support the medial arch. If the knee extensors are weak, an AFO with a knee gaiter **(Fig. 32.27)** or a knee-ankle-foot orthosis (KAFO) **(Fig. 32.30)** can be used to prevent a crouched gait. Spastic hamstrings often contribute to this gait.

Pharmacological management Oral medications can be given to control spasticity, when a muscle or group of muscles are involved, causing functional limitation, pain or difficulty with skin hygiene, e.g. when the fingers are clenched so the hand cannot be cleaned or the hips are adducted preventing perineal care and dressing. Oral medications are beneficial when a large group of muscles are involved but produce systemic side effect such as fatigue and drowsiness. These drugs can occasionally reduce the useful tone which helps the child in doing activities, e.g. if the tone in the quadriceps is reduced, the child can experience difficulty with standing and walking. At times, children with an abnormal swallow and drooling **(Figs. 32.31A to C)** may develop some worsening in these symptoms on starting antispasticity medications, with risk of aspiration. **Table 32.2** shows a list of commonly used antispastic medications, their mechanism of action, doses and adverse effects.

Often oral medication is inadequate and causes unwanted side effects or seems excessive when only one muscle group is being problematic. Five per cent aqueous phenol can be used for motor point blocks in muscles or for blocking accessible motor nerves by causing chemical denervation. Nerves with no sensory component are preferred to avoid dysesthesia following the injection. This is an economical and effective treatment but the effects are very often permanent so care needs to be taken when deciding who to treat with this modality.

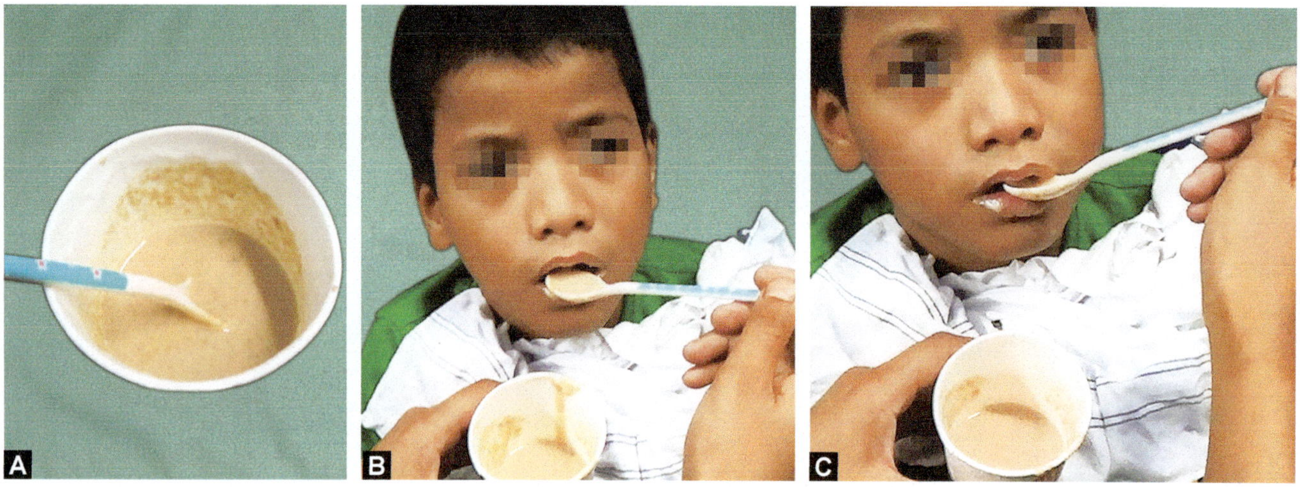

Figures 32.31A to C (A) Swallowing training with paste made from milk and biscuit so there are no lumps and it is all one consistency; (B) and (C) The child is in an upright position and fed small amounts using a plastic spoon with smooth edges.

TABLE 32.2 Pharmacotherapeutic options in the management of spasticity in children.

Medication	*Mechanism of action*	*Dose*	*Side effects*
Dantrolene	Decreases the release of calcium into the sarcoplasmic reticulum of muscles	0.5 mg/kg OD, max: 2 mg/kg QID or 100 mg QID	Drowsiness, dizziness, fatigue, weakness of muscles causing impaired function, e.g. swallow, diarrhoea, hepatotoxicity
Benzodiazepines (a) Diazepam (b) Clonazepam	Facilitates the postsynaptic action of GABA	(a) 0.1–0.8 mg/kg/day in 2–3 divided doses (b) 0.01–0.03 mg/kg/day in 2–3 divided doses	Sedation, ataxia, fatigue, confusion, increased excitement or aggression and dependency Benzodiazepine must be tapered slowly to reduce the chance of withdrawal symptoms, e.g. seizures
Baclofen	Analogue of GABA, binds to GABA B receptors and decreases spinal stretch reflex	2.5 mg to 5 mg/day max: 30 mg/day (2–7years), 60 mg/day (above 8 years)	Muscle weakness, drowsiness, fatigue, confusion, ataxia

Abbreviation: GABA, gamma-aminobutyric acid.

TABLE 32.3 List of commonly done motor nerve blocks.

Nerve block	*Joint effect and spastic muscle (supplied by nerve)*
Obturator nerve block	Hip adduction from adductor spasticity
Sciatic nerve block	Knee flexion and plantar flexion from hamstring and gastrosoleus spasticity
Peroneal nerve block	Ankle equinus from gastrosoleus spasticity
Femoral nerve block	Knee hyperextension or impaired knee flexion from rectus femoris spasticity
Median nerve block	Wrist and finger flexor spasticity (FCR, FCU, FDS, FDP)
Musculocutaneous nerve block	Biceps for elbow flexor spasticity

Abbreviations: FCR, flexor carpi radialis; FCU, flexor carpi ulnaris; FDS, flexor digitorum superficialis; FDP, flexor digitorum profundus.

Commonly employed motor nerve blocks in the treatment of hypertonia are summarised in **Table 32.3**.

Intramuscular botulinum blocks the release of acetylcholine into the neuromuscular junction. This is beneficial in localised muscle group spasticity with the goal of improving a specific function, e.g botulinum injection into the wrist and finger flexors can help improve voluntary release of objects by reducing flexor spasticity. Local anaesthetic cream can be used to numb the skin before the injections and a sedative will be needed for some children. The botulinum can cause local weakness and flu like symptoms, occasionally there are systemic effects with dysphagia, dysphonia and dyspnoea hours to weeks after the injection. These side effects must be clearly explained to the parents. The effects of botulinum toxin injections appear after a few days to 3 weeks and wear off by 6 months. The high cost and need for repeated injections make this option viable only for a selective group of children.

Subdermal implantation of an intrathecal baclofen pump enables direct delivery of the drug avoiding the general effects of sedation. However, this is expensive and at least 5% develop infection or other complications such as pump failure.

Management of Movement Disorders

Dystonia is the abnormal posturing of the any of the limbs, head or trunk due to sustained or intermittent involuntary co-contraction of muscles.

Speech and swallowing Dystonia involving the muscles of the face, mouth and oropharynx may result in dysarthria and/or dysphagia. Speech therapy will teach children how to make the sounds of letters and words and give them exercises to improve oropharyngeal muscle control. In children with dysphagia, optimal positioning in a supported seat with the neck in neutral or slight flexion is required for safe swallowing **(Fig. 32.24)**. The consistency of the food is altered to uniformly soft semisolids/thick fluids, which are easier to swallow as compared to thin fluids **(Fig. 32.31)**. In those with oral hypersensitivity, the material of the spoon/cup should be gentle and smooth **(Fig. 32.31)**.

Positioning Therapy involves looking for body positions and sensory inputs, which can reduce the dystonia. The ataxic arm will show the greatest degree of past pointing when the hand is the greatest distance away from the trunk. Children soon learn this and are very reluctant to stretch their arms far from their trunk! This is because the past pointing of the finger is the sum of the abnormal movements across each of the joints that are moving. So if the shoulder component moves 3 cm, the elbow 3 cm, the wrist 3 cm and so on, so the hand will move 9 cm. Treating ataxia is about providing a stable base of support to reduce the involuntary movements. A child will be made to sit in a chair and given support to the trunk and head, the arm will be supported on a table so the only part moving is the hand itself **(Fig. 32.25)**. Eliminating the need to move parts of the body allows them to do tasks with less shaking and also allows training to control the distal part/hand. As the child learns to control the hand better, less support is given to the wrist and once this is better controlled, support is removed from the elbow.

Therapy for balance and coordination The visual, vestibular and joint proprioception systems provide the sensory feedback required to achieve postural stability. Frenkel exercises are a series of exercises for coordination, which begin as simple movements in the direction where gravity has been eliminated and that gradually progress to more complex movements against gravity. Therapy for balance should also progress in a sequential manner, i.e. once head and trunk control is obtained then sitting balance can be worked on **(Figs. 32.2 and 32.15)**. Therapy is then progressed to balance in kneeling **(Figs. 32.2 and 32.4)** then standing **(Figs. 32.3, 32.14 and 32.18)** then standing on a single leg then walking with a broad base and finally to walking on a straight line.

Pharmacological management Oral medications used to reduce dystonia include tetrabenazine (synthetic benzoquinolizine), trihexiphenidyl hydrochloride (anticholinergic) and clonazepam (benzodiazepine). Tetrabenazine acts by inhibiting the uptake of monoamines into synaptic vesicles and hence diminishes their output at the synapses. Botulinum injections can be used if there is localised dystonia, as in spasticity, with a goal of improving a specific function. Caution should be exercised in the surgical intervention for regional dystonia as it may cause a worsening of deformity in the opposite direction.

Activity-focussed Interventions

This involves structured practice and repetitions of functional actions that increase independence in daily tasks. Functional actions are things that we do every day like sitting, balancing, standing, using your hands to achieve a particular task or parts of the movements needed for a particular actions (**Fig. 32.14** shows a child kicking a skittle—hip flexion is part of the gait cycle).

Self care The things that we do every day to get washed, dressed, comb our hair, shave, eat and walk are called activities of daily living (ADL). It is important to remember the developmental stage of a child to identify and analyse the tasks, which are difficult but meaningful for the child. The components of the task are then improved through specific therapy aimed at reducing impairments and activity based tasks with repetition, physical guidance and feedback **(Fig. 32.32)**.

A child learning to feed himself/herself needs to be able to take the spoon to the plate, angle the wrist to then

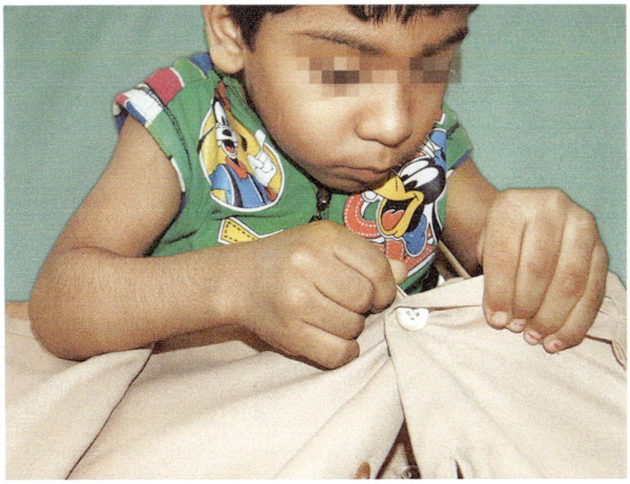

Figure 32.32 Simulated skill training for buttoning in a child with cerebral palsy (spastic quadriparesis) using a jacket with large buttons.

load the spoon, lift the spoon up to the mouth and put the spoon in the mouth. The child may have a problem lifting up the spoon. So, exercises can be given to strengthen the ability to lift the arm. The child can practice feeding using a table that is higher than normal so the hand does not need to be lifted up so high. The child may be given a plate with 'mock food' to practice lifting the spoon without actually eating the food. The challenge with these activities is keeping them interesting. For teaching these skills, each component of the task can be taught through techniques like chaining, modelling and prompting. In chaining, the child is enabled to perform one step of the task and the rest are completed by the caretaker. When the child becomes successful in one step the child is encouraged to attempt the next step in the sequence and so on till the whole task is mastered. Prompting involves use of physical or verbal assistance to help the child to learn a task, e.g. the mother holds the child's hand over the spoon to help him or her to learn to bring food to his/her mouth. In modelling, the parent demonstrates how a task should be done and the child learns though imitation.

For toilet training, the parents can be taught to make a schedule according to the child's frequency or pattern that has been observed over a period of time. The child is taken to the toilet according to this schedule and rewarded appropriately.

Behaviour Modification

Behaviour modification techniques are used for both promoting adaptive behaviour such as learning to dress oneself, feeding, toilet training and for reducing maladaptive behaviour such as head banging, biting or hyperactivity. Rewarding the child according to specific principles helps to develop acceptable behaviour in the child. Therefore, *absence* of maladaptive behaviour should be rewarded, initially at short intervals which can be decided by using a behavioural monitoring chart. Examples of reward include a favourite snack, toy, activities like a trip to the park or lavish praise. Behaviour modification can also be used for teaching the child social skills and communication.

Positioning Appropriate positioning of children with equipment to hold the child's trunk, head and limbs promotes their ability to do things and participate within their surroundings. This improves head control, permits greater freedom in the use of their upper extremities, improves ability to perform ADL, such as eating and dressing, improves postural alignment and decreases fatigue. Seating systems include supportive chairs **(Fig. 32.24)**, strollers, car seats, floor seats and wheelchairs **(Fig. 32.23)**. The components that provide support in any seating system include armrests, foot supports, lap tray, abductor wedge, pelvic belts, calf straps, head rest and cushions which also relieve pressure. The aim is to support the child in a position that makes it easier to do things and/or prevents complications. So, the child is made to sit with the head supported and looking forward so they can see what is going on and to help communication **(Figs. 32.23 and 32.24)**. The legs are held slightly abducted to reduce adductor spasms and reduce the chance of contractures and the feet should be well supported **(Figs. 32.33A to C)**. A child with complex physical disabilities needs their positioning to be controlled 24 hours a day.

Upright standing systems usually have a table or tray attachment that allows the child to play while standing.

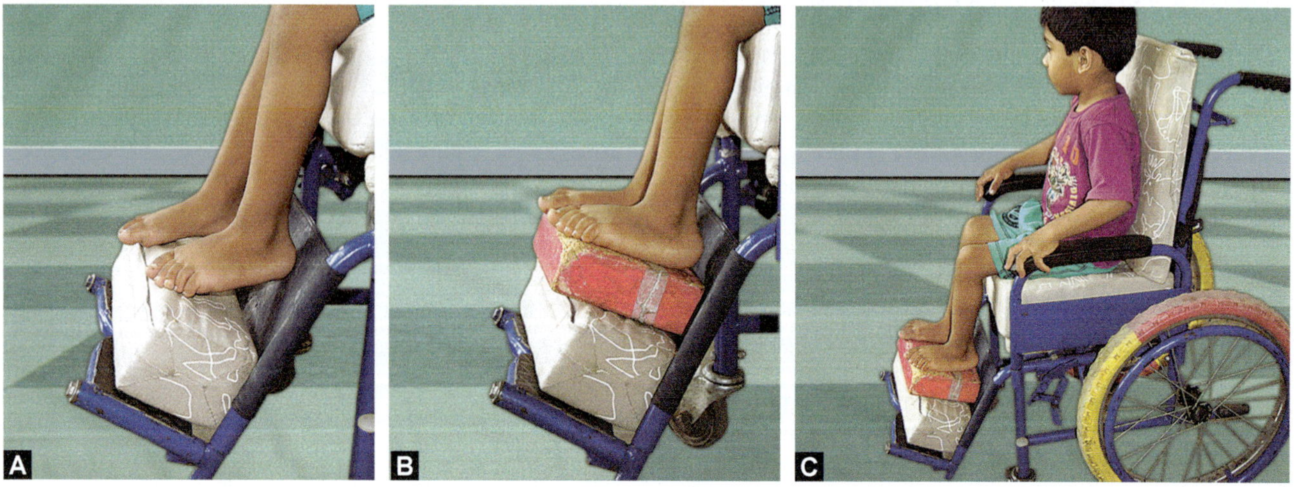

Figures 32.33A to C The forearms and feet have to be well-supported in a wheelchair. If the wheelchair does not have height-adjustable footrests then layers of thermocol/wooden boards/boxes can be attached to the footrest till the ankles are in a neutral position (or as near neutral position as contractures allow).

There are many varieties all with similar components. The feet are held in place with straps or blocks; the child's knees are kept extended with a strap in front of the knees, the hips are kept extended with a strap behind the hips and the body supported with a strap to a table anteriorly. Standing helps reduce tone, prevent contractures, improve bone density, facilitates ankle, knee and hip joint development. Children should be encouraged to experience weight bearing in an upright position as close to the typical age of standing as possible if they have sufficient head and trunk control to be aligned correctly. If the child has KAFO or AFO and knee braces/gaiters, these can be used to facilitate standing.

Hand skills Hand skills are critical for a child to be able to explore his/her surroundings. They are required for self-care, learning, communication and playing. The following are the general methods for intervention:

If a child has poor sitting balance, provide adequate trunk control through appropriate seating devices **(Figs. 32.34A and B)**. Then the child's arms need not support the child and can be free to engage in play, writing, eating and so on.

- Help the child to integrate tactile and proprioceptive stimuli through graded exposure to different shapes, textures, sizes and a variety of objects. Articles that can facilitate grasps are spoons, lids, balls, brushes and so on. Commonly available materials at home that can facilitate pinches are dry pulses, bottle caps, beads, coins and pebbles. The various components of hand function are tabulated in **Flow chart 32.2** with illustrative examples in **Figures 32.21, 32.22 and 32.35 to 32.39**.
- Reduce impairment in tone, range of motion and muscle strength, where possible
- Introduce objects early through play, using objects appropriate to the child's developmental status and in the sequence that parallels how hand function develops
- Constraint-induced therapy can be used in hemiplegics where the child is stopped from using the normal limb so that the child is forced to use the affected limb.

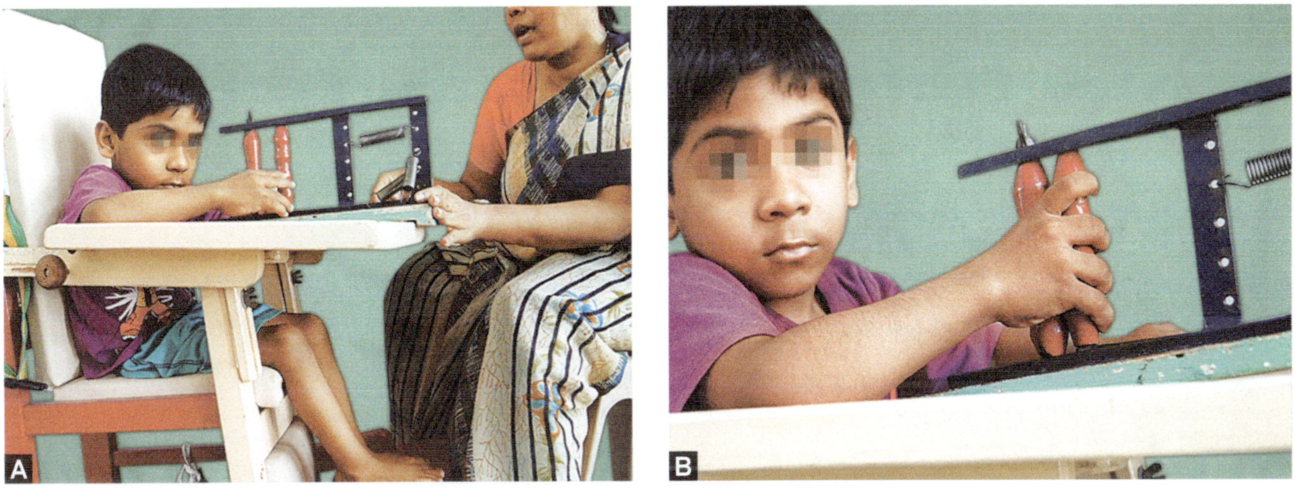

Figures 32.34A and B A cerebral palsy child with spastic quadriparesis on a supported chair, with a lapboard, performing hand grip strengthening exercises using a simple device with springs attached. As the strength improves, the resistance to gripping can be changed by increasing the springs attached.

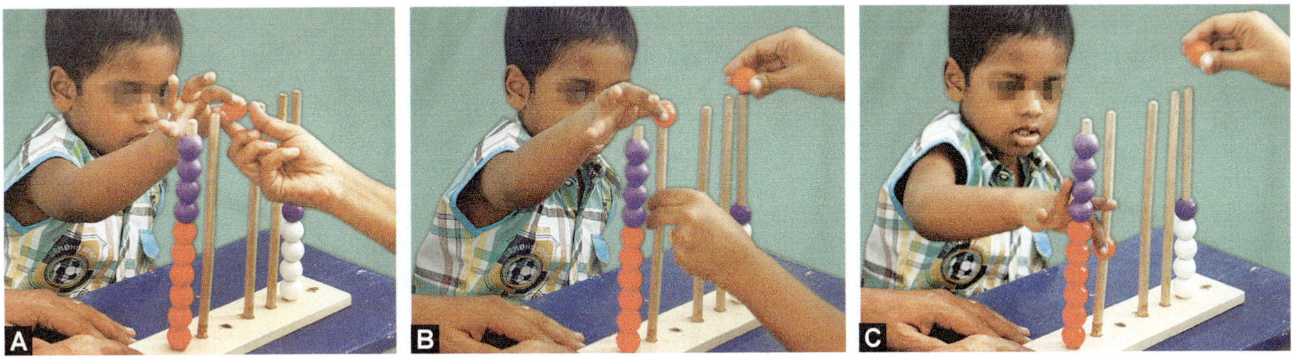

Figures 32.35A to C Large beads and a peg board are used to facilitate the pincer grasp to carry items and then precisely position them, then to release the grip and put them on the peg.

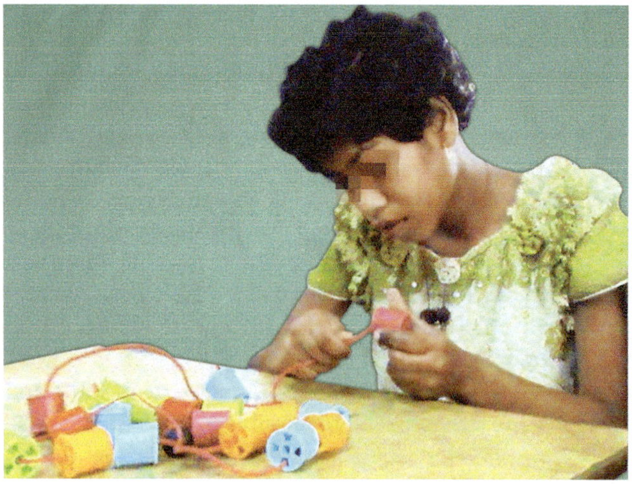

Figure 32.36 A girl with cerebral palsy, practicing bimanual tasks (threading a string through cylindrical blocks/reels).

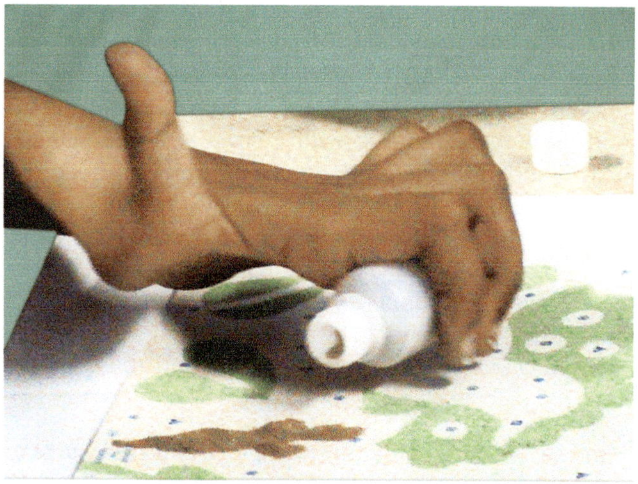

Figure 32.37 A boy with intrinsic muscle weakness of his hand, due to hereditary motor sensory neuropathy, is able to hold objects with a hook grasp.

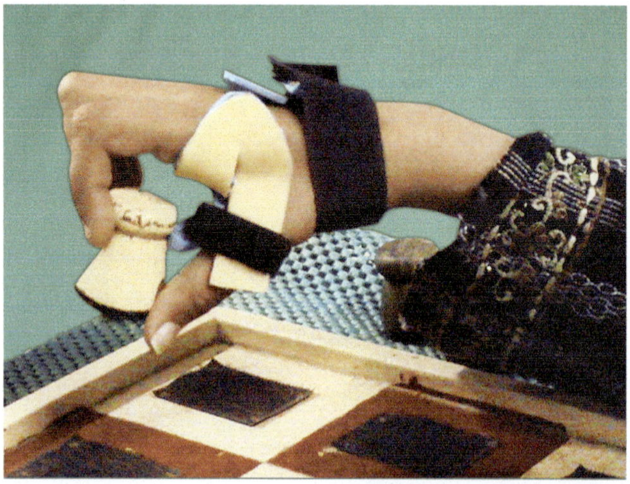

Figure 32.38 A splint which supports the thumb in opposition, helps in achieving the tripod pinch.

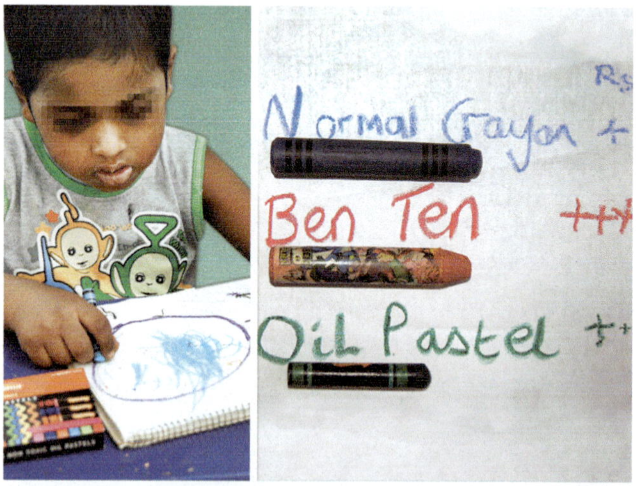

Figure 32.39 A variety of crayons to suit the needs of the child: thicker crayons can make grasping easier for children with hand function problems, brighter crayons can give more visual stimulation. As the grasp improves, the child can progress to using thinner crayons.

Play Play is a powerful therapeutic tool as it is the best way a child learns. Any activity or exercise can be turned to play with some aspect of adventure, surprise and freedom in it. The play activity should be chosen as per the child's level of development with a goal of moving him one step further. Toys provide stimulation for a child to play alone or with others. Play activities such as placing pegs on to a board **(Fig. 32.21)** or picking beads and dropping on to a peg **(Figs. 32.22 and 32.35)**, matching of shapes, sand art **(Figs. 32.40A to D)**, jigsaw and block puzzles also enhance the development of eye-hand coordination and cognitive skills. Play like ball throwing enhances the use of both hands and helps to improve trunk control **(Fig. 32.15)**.

Assistive Mobility

Mobility training is initially done in the parallel bars **(Figs. 32.3 and 32.29)**. An anterior **(Fig. 32.14)** or posterior walker **(Fig. 32.18)** can be used with or without wheels depending on the stability and the ease, with which the child propels the walker. Energy expenditure, as measured by oxygen consumption and oxygen cost, is lower with the posterior walker as compared to the anterior walker. The posterior walker also facilitates a more upright walking posture and decreases the amount of double support time **(Figs. 32.3 and 32.18)**. With improvement in the balance, gait pattern and endurance of walking, the child

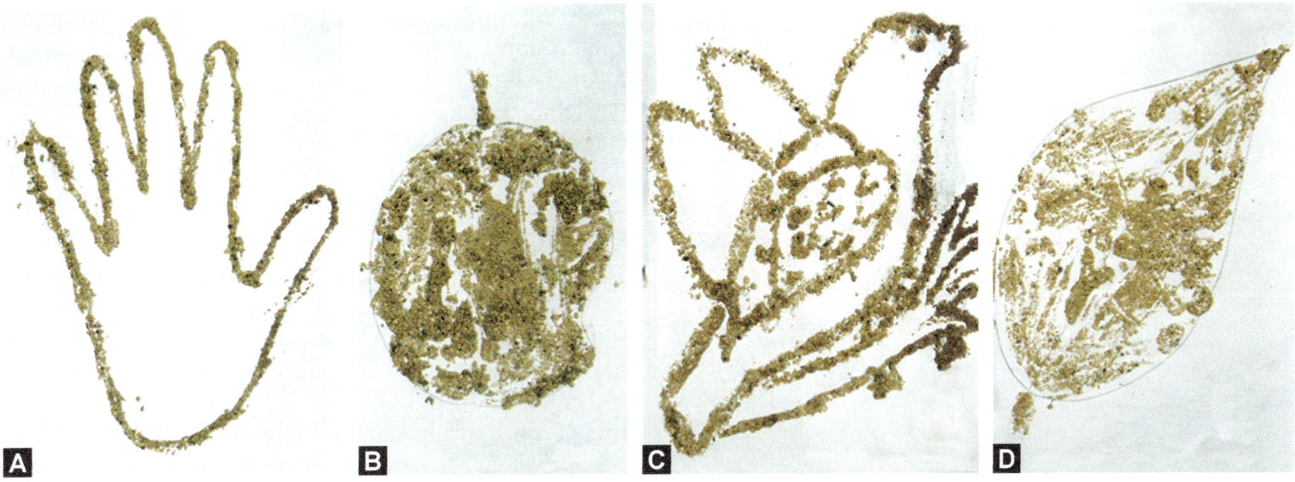

Figures 32.40A to D Sand art can be given to facilitate group play and hand function. Glue is put on the paper outlining the shape. The children then sprinkle sand over this.

can progress to walking with elbow crutches (Figs. 32.19 and 32.30) and subsequently with sticks.

Gait analysis is an important part of rehabilitation as it assists with planning intervention to optimise gait pattern and efficiency. Qualitative gait analysis involves observing the gait pattern in a clinical setting and analysing video in slow motion. Quantitative gait analysis looks at the range of motion (kinematics), moments of force and power generated or absorbed at each major lower limb joint and through the various phases of gait cycle (kinetics). Clinical decisions regarding interventions, e.g. whether AFOs are needed for ambulation, can be taken by comparing the gait parameters with and without AFO. The energy cost of ambulation or the physiological cost index (PCI) calculated from the gait analysis also assists with these decisions. Gait analysis is particularly helpful when planning for surgical intervention in children with spasticity as it helps in identifying the primary and compensatory gait abnormalities.

Acquired or Traumatic Brain Injury

Interventions are decided according to the severity and type of neurological/musculoskeletal involvement. Early intervention is needed to prevent complications which further delay rehabilitation and to promote responses which result from neuroplasticity. The severity of the brain injury is assessed by the Glasgow Coma Scale (GCS), which rates the eye opening, motor and verbal response on a scale of 3–15.

In severe brain injury (GCS ≤ 8), look for small changes over time to various stimuli. A multimodal stimulation programme involves observation of responses to visual, auditory, tactile, olfactory and proprioception, to see if the child has the ability to localise or discriminate any of these stimuli. Movements are categorised as reflexive, spontaneous (without stimuli) or purposeful. The Sensory Modality Assessment and Rehabilitation Technique (SMART) is a tool designed to assess the patient's response on a daily basis. Multiple assessments are done by the family as well as the team to observe the potential for a meaningful response to the stimuli and plan therapy accordingly. If the child is unable to vocalise but has consistent voluntary motor responses, these can be used as a method to communicate with the child, e.g. one blink of the eye can be used to indicate 'Yes' and two blinks as 'No'.

Recovery Continuum

The normal sequence of recovery from brain injury is Coma → Vegetative state → Minimal conscious state → Cognitive impaired states → Normal. The child is said to be in a coma if the eyes are closed all the time and reflexive movements are present only to noxious stimuli. A diagnosis of vegetative state is made if the eyes are open with sleep-wake cycles plus reflexive and/or withdrawal responses are present to stimuli. If there is any awareness of self or the environment, a diagnosis of minimally conscious state is made.

Management of Respiratory System

Positioning for swallowing is crucial for the prevention of aspiration. Elevation of the head end of the bed also reduces the risk of regurgitation at night. Chest physiotherapy, which involves tapping the chest wall beginning laterally going to the midline and from below going up towards the sternum, enables the child to clear his/her secretions. With improvement in cognition, the child can improve his/her respiratory capacity through activities such as blowing a flute, a candle, a party inflatable toy, and so on. Toys or devices that give visual and auditory feedback encourage the child's participation—making this a fun and playful activity (Fig. 32.41).

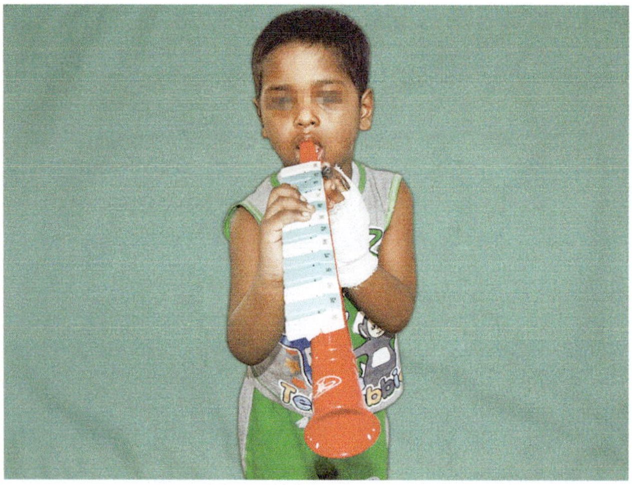

Figure 32.41 Blowing activity with a play pipe for improving respiratory control as this provides auditory feedback with a different frequency of sound when greater effort is applied.

Post-traumatic Seizures

There is an incidence of 20–39% in the development of early seizures (i.e. within the first week of trauma) and the use of anti-epileptics during this period are beneficial but can be stopped after this except in some conditions such a depressed fracture or penetrating brain injuries. Lower GCS and younger children are more prone for early seizures. There is no evidence for using prophylactic anti-epileptics in the prevention of late onset seizures.

Cognitive/Motor Deficits

The impairments following a brain injury will depend on whether the damage is focal or diffuse and the site(s) involved. The goal of rehabilitation is to prevent secondary impairments like contractures **(Fig. 32.25)** and to help the child attain the maximum possible age-appropriate function physically, cognitively and socially. As children become more responsive and interactive, specific therapy is given in the area of cognitive need [speech, attention, memory, executive function, visuospatial functioning **(Fig. 32.35)**] or physical needs (weakness, spasticity, hand functions, balance and gait as shown in **Figures 32.5 to 32.15, 32.18 to 32.30, 32.32 to 32.40** and **Flow chart 32.3**). The concepts for therapy for these deficits are similar to what is practised for children with congenital brain injury as mentioned in Section Developmental Delay.

Flow chart 32.3 Algorithmic approach to the management of hypertonia.

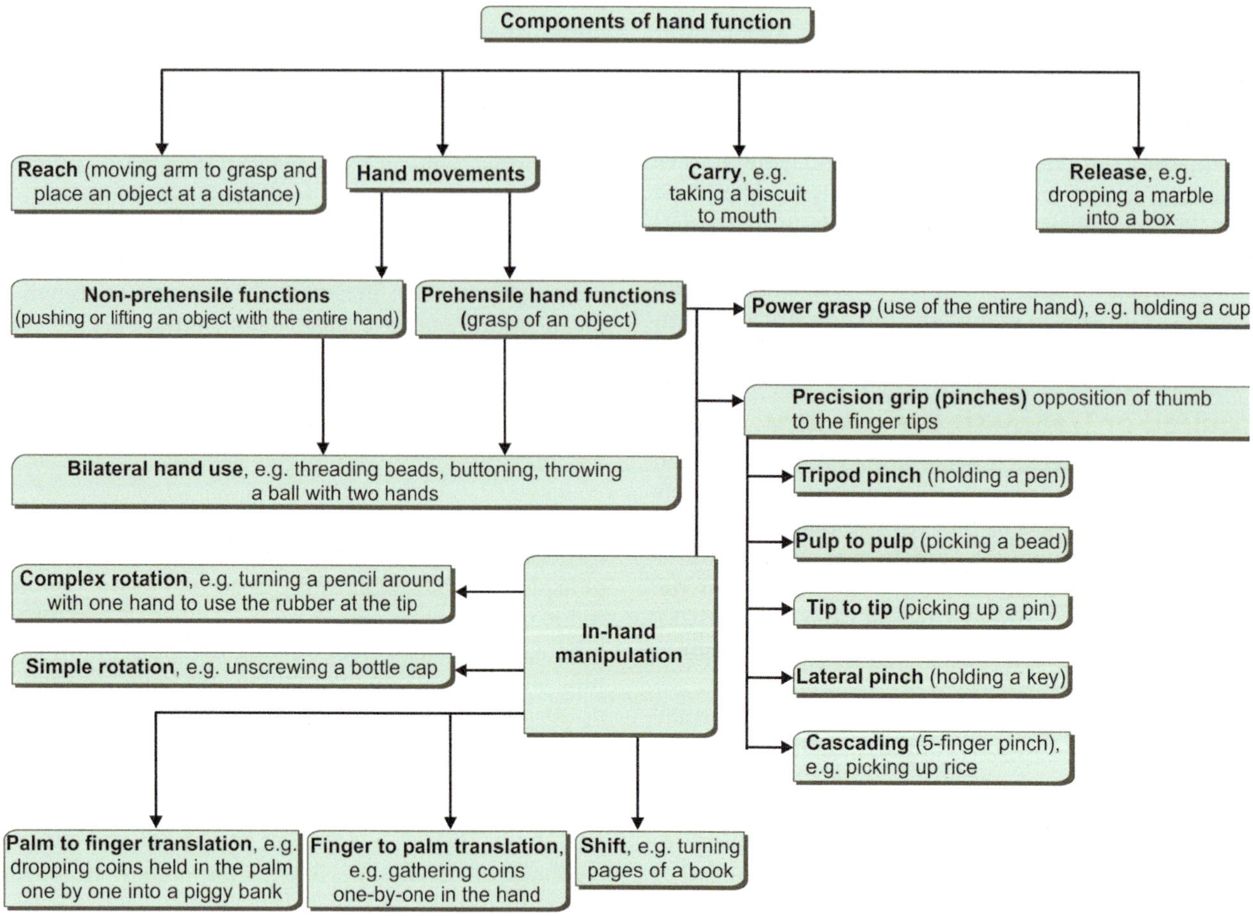

Rehabilitation has become a continuum of care, being provided right from the acute care setting till discharge into the community. Many children do well at home following advice given by the team and progress can be monitored by follow-up in the outpatients or at home. An early return to school is encouraged. Strategies need to be planned for the child with learning difficulties. An individual education plan can be made with the help of the teachers who regularly communicate with parents regarding the child's overall performance.

Rehabilitation in Spinal Cord Injury

Rehabilitation goals include prevention and management of secondary complications and maximising age-appropriate functional independence as per the level of spinal cord injury (SCI).

Spinal Cord Injury Due to Neural Tube Defects

Spinal cord injury due to neural tube defect results in asymmetric motor sensory deficits. Muscle imbalances can result in deformities which can worsen as the child grows. Kyphosis, lordosis and scoliosis are commonly seen in those with thoracic or higher lesions. This is controlled by positioning in bed with cushions and with a moulded seat, supported seating **(Figs. 32.23, 32.24 and 32.33)** or a thoracolumbosacral corset in sitting. Deformities in the lower limbs can be prevented by passive, range of motion exercises **(Fig. 32.25)**, splints to maintain the joints in a neutral position **(Figs. 32.25 and 32.27)** and active exercises to strengthen the weak muscles **(Figs. 32.5 to 32.13 and 32.20)**. The management of pressure sores, neuropathic bowel and bladder, self-care and mobility issues is discussed in Section Traumatic/Acquired Spinal Cord Injury.

Traumatic/Acquired Spinal Cord Injury

Patients with SCI present with specific issues that require medical attention from the rehabilitation team. These issues include:

Autonomic Dysreflexia

Noxious stimuli results in autonomic dysfunction in those with spinal cord lesion at or above T6 level. This is a medical emergency. Noxious stimuli cause sympathetic over activity below the level of injury which results in hypertension. This in turn brings about vasodilatation above the lesion resulting in a pounding headache, sweating, hot flushes and bradycardia due to vagal activity from the baroreceptor stimulation in the carotids. This is managed by immediately sitting up the child (and putting the feet down if possible) and removal of the factors causing pain, as with a blocked catheter (unblock the catheter), anal fissure or in growing toe nail (apply local anaesthetic to the area causing the pain). If the high blood pressure persists after 5 minutes despite these measures, an antihypertensive like nifedepine is given immediately. Failure to treat this within a few minutes can result in stroke or death.

Pressure Sores

The lack of sensation and limited mobility in the paralysed part of the body make the child with an SCI at very high risk of developing pressure sores. These can be prevented by regular position changes every 2 hours in the lying position and doing push-ups [lifting up the body using their arms (or by the family)] every 10–15 minutes while sitting to relieve pressure **(Fig. 32.42)**. Cervical level injured children can lean sideways to relief the pressure on each side.

Pressure areas such as the regions of the occiput, sacrum, ischial tuberosity, trochanter, both knees, heels and scapula should be examined daily **(Fig. 32.43)** by

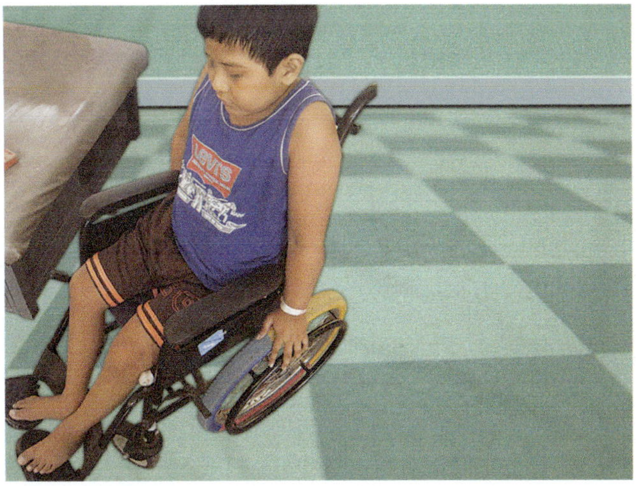

Figure 32.42 Wheelchair push-ups are done to relieve pressure every 10 minutes to prevent pressure sores in the ischial regions.

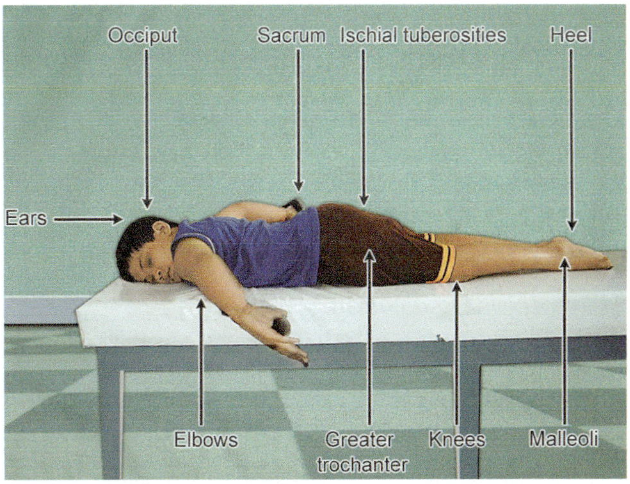

Figure 32.43 The areas marked are prone to developing pressure sores due to the presence of bony prominences. Prone lying can provide complete pressure relief in these areas.

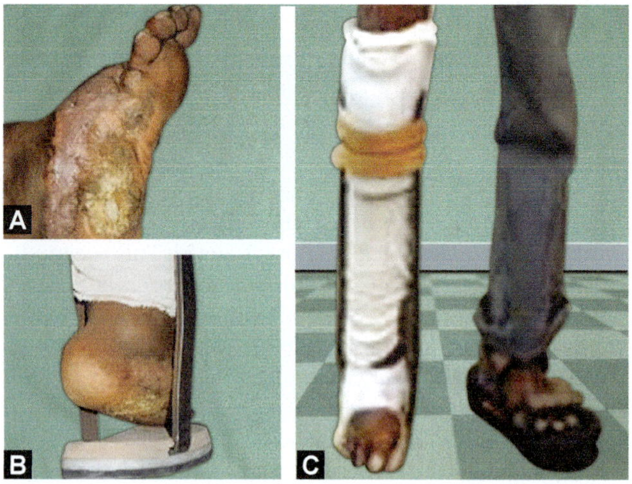

Figures 32.44A to C A chronic foot ulcer in a boy with meningomyelocoele. Pressure relief on the foot is provided during ambulation with a patellar tendon-bearing (PTB) Bohler orthosis (made of plaster of Paris/polypropylene). Height correction is provided in the footwear on the opposite side.

the parents and later by the child as they mature. If there is any sign of redness or warmth, immediate measures should be taken in order to provide complete pressure relief in that area till the redness disappears. Nursing in the prone position with foam/pillows with gaps to prevent pressure on the knees and genitalia is what works best when there are pressure sores on the posterior aspect of the body. This seems to work best with bigger children! Pressure relieving orthosis allows ambulation in a patient with chronic heel ulcer secondary to meningomyelocoele **(Figs. 32.44A to C)**. Many things can also cause local skin damage due to excess pressure, e.g. an AFO rubbing the malleoli, trousers that are too tight, a toy under the child when sleeping, a hot drink resting on the thigh. Hence, great care must be taken to inspect the anaesthetic regions.

Deep Venous Thrombosis

Deep venous thrombosis (DVT) is a complication seen after SCI and presents with swelling of the leg. An elevated D-dimer level is a sensitive indicator but a colour Doppler is needed to diagnose a DVT. Pulmonary embolism is a life-threatening complication of this and anticoagulants should be started immediately even while awaiting test results.

Heterotopic Ossification

Heterotopic ossification (HO) is the abnormal calcification and ossification of soft tissues in regions affected by a neurological insult. This presents as swelling, warmth and tenderness (if sensation is present in that area) around a joint with limitation of range of motion. Aggressive therapy should be avoided while these acute signs of HO are present. This is managed with a non-steroidal anti-inflammatory drug (NSAID) (indomethacin) or a bisphosphonates (disodium etidronate). Serum alkaline phosphatase is used to monitor activity of the HO.

Osteoporosis

Correction of vitamin D deficiency is important to prevent osteoporosis. Encouraging weight bearing also protects children from this long-term complication.

Neuropathic Bowel

The neuropathic bowel occurs due to impairment in the awareness of a full rectum and the ability to voluntarily control bowel movements, which results in faecal incontinence. This can be a major social embarrassment to the child. Faecal incontinence occurs in a lower motor neuron (LMN) bowel in conditions such as meningomyelocoele, conus medullaris/cauda equina lesions due to a denervated anal sphincter resulting in dribbling of stools. Spinal cord lesions, above the conus medullaris, result in an increased tone in the colonic wall and anal sphincter [upper motor neuron (UMN) bowel] causing constipation. Chronic constipation will result is spurious diarrhoea due to bacterial liquefaction of stools proximal to the obstruction.

A bowel programme is planned with the aim of attaining a predictable time for and adequate bowel evacuation. Digital stimulation (inserting a gloved finger into the anal sphincter and making gentle rotatory movements) or suppositories/enemas are used to empty the bowel by relaxing the anal sphincter and causing a local reflex due to the intrinsic colorectal nervous supply. However, in a LMN bowel, this is absent and digital evacuation is used where the bowel is manually emptied. High fibre diet or substitutes are important to keep the stool soft and firm. A regular schedule is the key to success in a bowel programme, which should be planned at the same time every day. The daily timing can be decided as per the premorbid timing if present or after a hot drink or a meal in the morning or evening, which triggers the gastrocolic reflex.

Neuropathic Bladder

The neuropathic bladder resulting from SCI is best managed by self-intermittent clean catheterisation (SICC), which involves emptying the bladder at regular intervals by inserting a catheter into the bladder. This reduces the incidence of complications seen with the indwelling catheter, such as urinary infections and calculi formation. A new sterile catheter, each time is not needed. This technique uses a clean catheter that may be reused after washing. Other methods of emptying the bladder include crede (emptying by applying suprapubic pressure), valsalva (straining by contracting abdominal muscles) and reflex voiding (local sacral reflex triggering uninhibited bladder contraction). These are regarded as unsafe, especially if there is high post-void residual urine, as this can result in recurrent infections and hydronephrosis leading to renal failure and death.

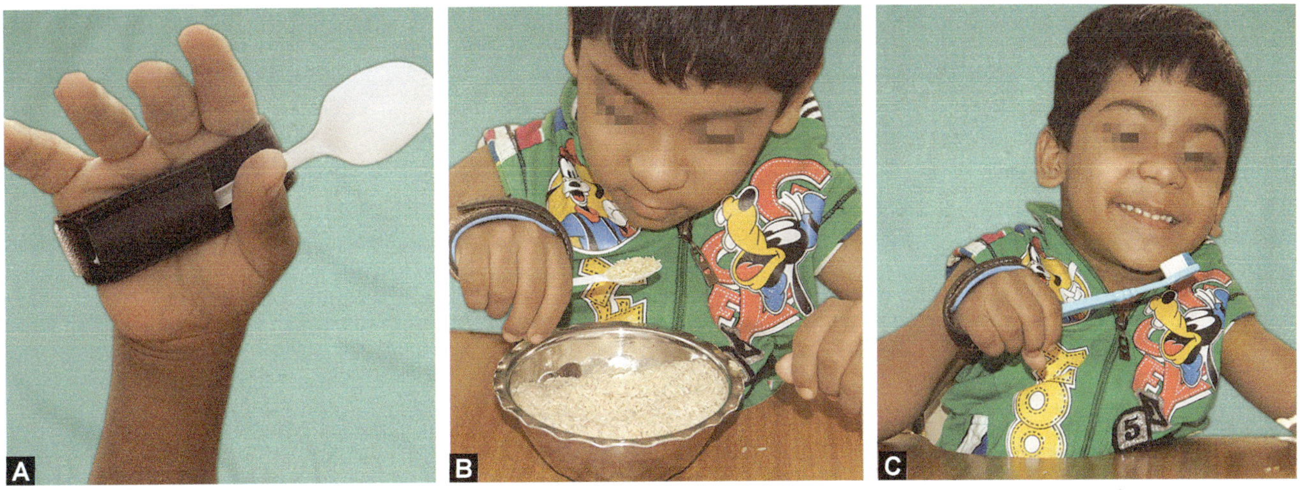

Figures 32.45A to C (A and B) A universal cuff with a palmar pocket in the hand to hold a spoon in order to feed independently in the presence of poor hand function; (C) This can be replaced with a toothbrush, comb, pen, typing, stick to depress keys and so on.

Self care A child becomes independent in most of his/her ADL by 5 years of age and this has to be gradually restored following a spinal injury or achieved in children with meningomyelocoele. Learning self-care activities requires adequate trunk control and hand function. In tetraplegic children, supported seating and adaptive devices are given to assist with activities, e.g. universal cuff with a palmar pocket in the hand to hold a spoon to feed independently, to place a pencil in to write or to use with a toothbrush **(Figs. 32.45A to C)**.

Mobility Children with tetraplegia or high level thoracic lesions have poor trunk control and need a wheelchair for mobility. With training, a child is able to become independent on a manual wheelchair on all terrains, including the use of ramps and clearing small thresholds. Children, whose level of injury is at C6 level or above, can be independent with a motorised wheelchair, although they will need assistance with their transfers from and onto the wheelchair.

Children with the level of injury between T4 and T10 will still require a manual wheelchair for community ambulation **(Figs. 32.16, 32.17, 32.43, 32.46 and 32.47)**, but can use KAFO for therapeutic walking within the house with the aid of a walker **(Figs. 32.48A to C)**. A KAFO is made of lightweight polypropylene to support the ankle in a neutral position and metal uprights with a drop lock for the knee joint **(Figs. 32.49 and 32.50)**. Functional ambulation with KAFO and elbow crutches is the goal of rehabilitation for children with level of injury below T10. Stability in the absence of any hip muscles is provided by hyperextending the hip, which makes the anterior iliofemoral ligament of the hip taut **(Fig. 32.49)**. Ambulation with KAFOs is started within parallel bars where hip hiking is used to move the leg forward **(Figs. 32.50 to 32.52)**. The child then gradually progresses to gait training with a walker **(Fig. 32.48)** and then with elbow crutches. If the child has adequate knee extension, then ambulation can be achieved with an AFO **(Fig. 32.19)**. Regular follow-up is advised to monitor for scoliosis.

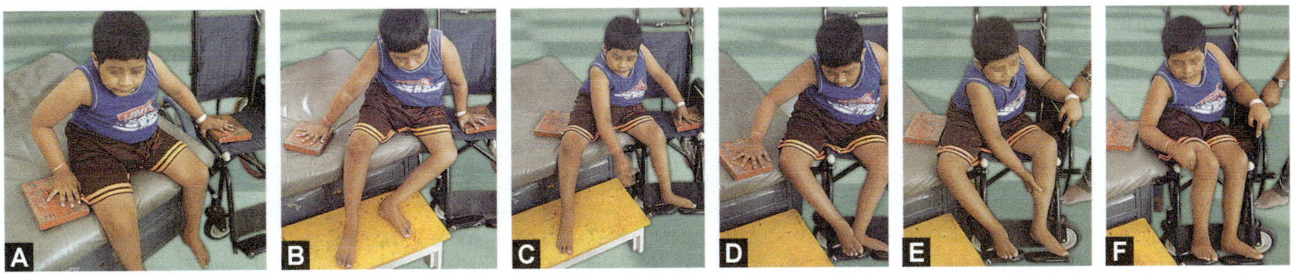

Figures 32.46A to F In preparation for a transfer from the plinth, the wheelchair is positioned at 45° to the plinth, the brakes are applied and the armrest closest to the plinth is removed. Removable armrests are essential for these transfers. Initially someone may need to stabilise the chair as well. During the initial phases of training when the push-ups are not adequate to clear the body, wooden blocks are positioned, one on the plinth and the other on the wheelchair. Push-ups are done using these blocks to shift the body towards the wheelchair. Hands are then used to lift each leg and position them on the footrests of the wheelchair.

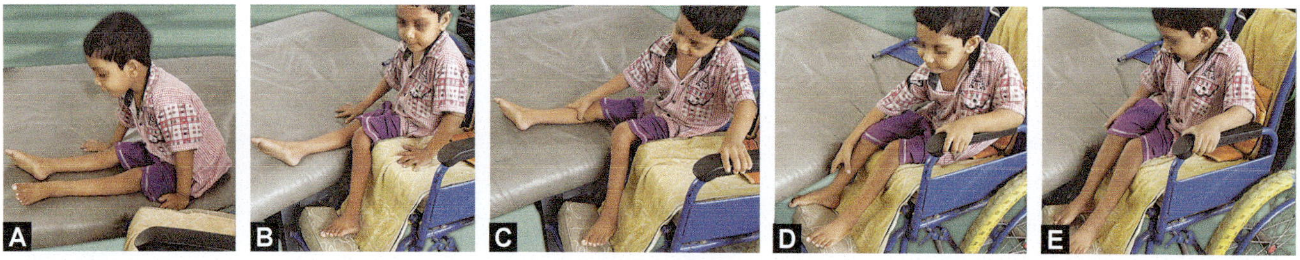

Figures 32.47A to E A transfer onto the wheelchair without using blocks, done with the wheelchair placed parallel to the plinth by a 4-year-old boy with T4 traumatic paraplegia. Both feet are positioned and the trunk adjusted in the wheelchair before finally replacing the side armrest.

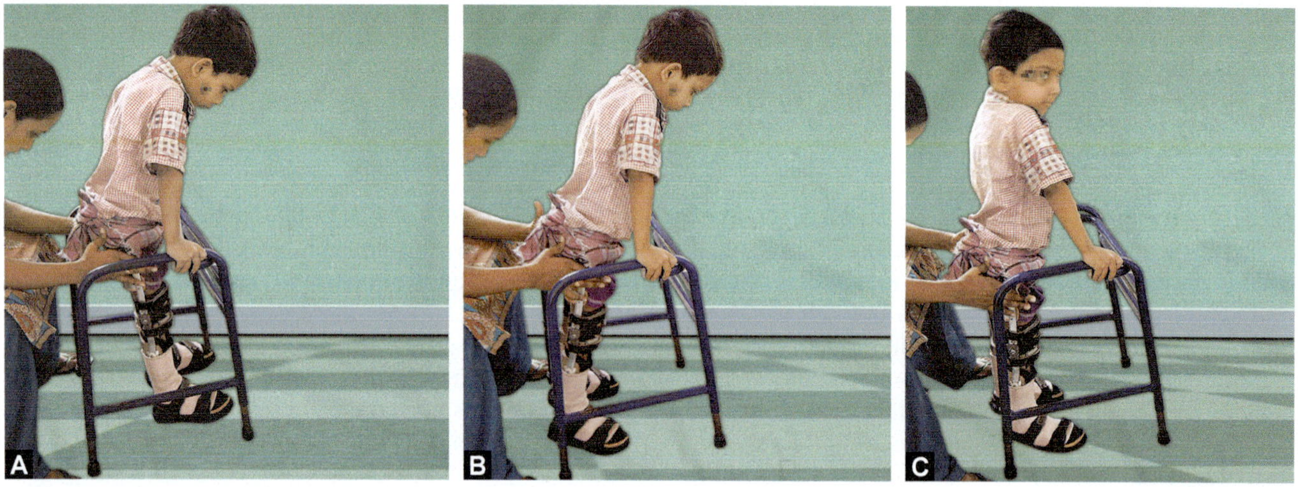

Figures 32.48A to C A boy with T4 traumatic paraplegia being trained for the swing to gait in a walker. He has to learn to lift his legs by pushing down with his hands onto the walker and then to swing the legs forward.

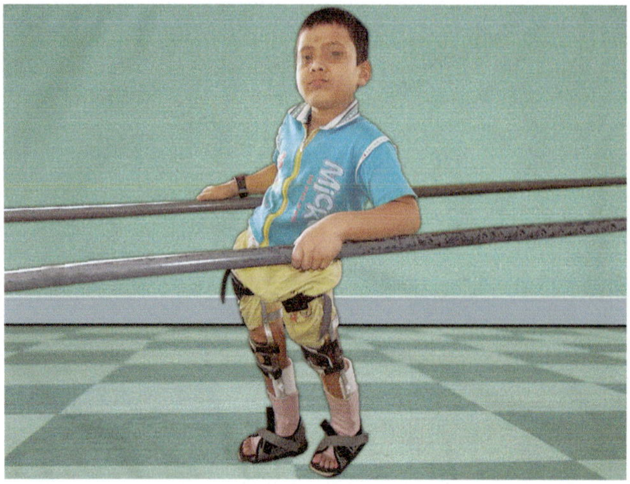

Figure 32.49 This boy with T4 ASIA A paraplegia is learning to stand with knee–ankle–foot orthoses by hyperextending his hips.

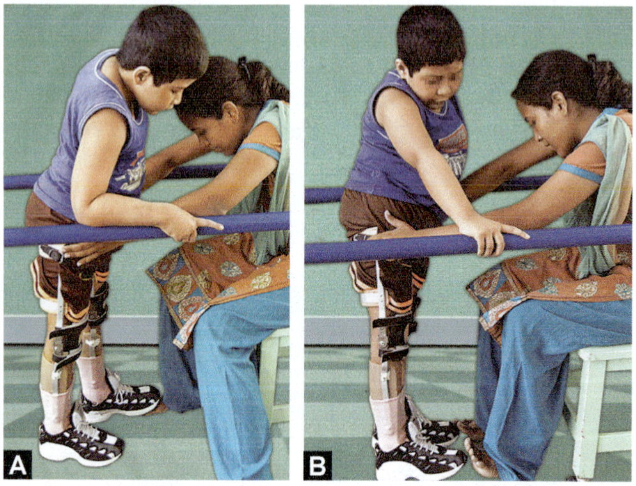

Figures 32.50A and B Working on assisted hiking of the left lower limb by leaning to the right and recruiting the left latissimus dorsi, followed by the right side hiking with the goal of lifting the right lower limb using the right latissimus dorsi.

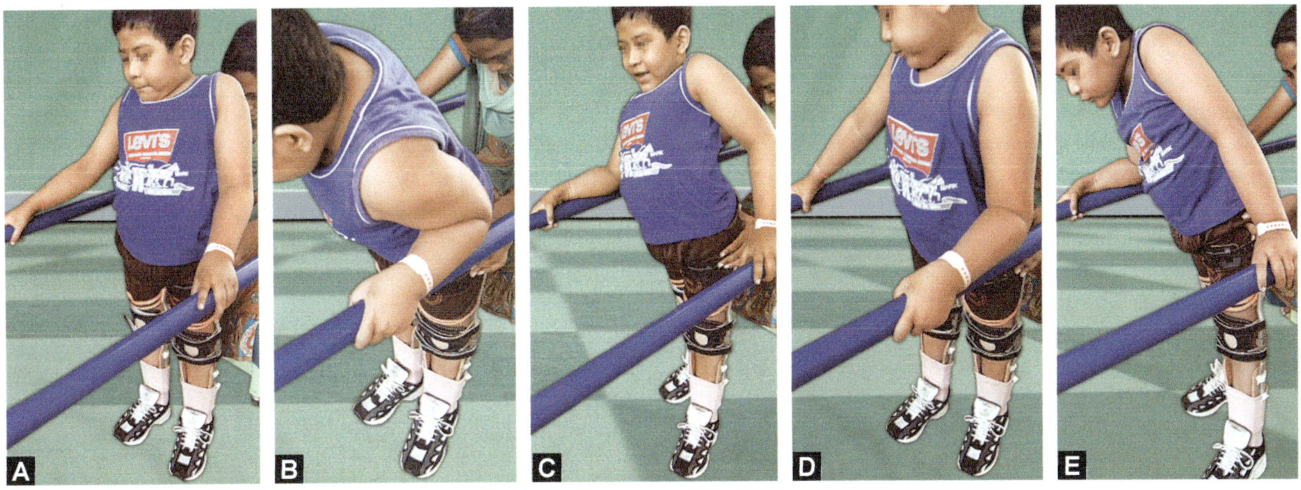

Figures 32.51A to E Gait training in parallel bars. Hiking is the skill required to lift a lower limb in spite of having grade 0 at the hip muscles. Hiking of the right lower limb helps to move it forward in order to take the first step. The body is stabilised before hiking the left lower limb to take the next step. As he learns to do this, so less flexion of the trunk will be needed.

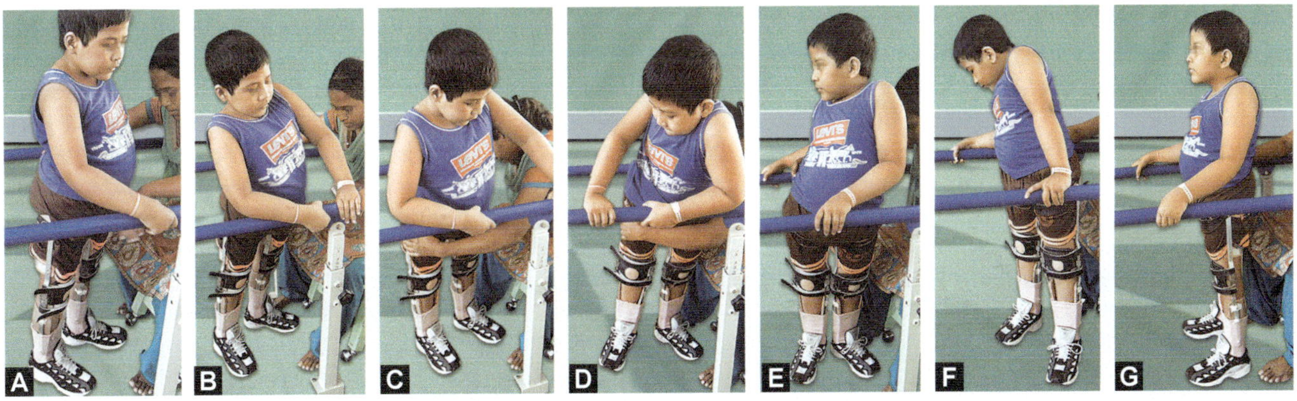

Figures 32.52A to G Turning in parallel bars is practiced using the skill to hike, to gradually change the position of each foot. Good upper limb strength is required to stabilise the trunk in spite of absent abdominals and paraspinal muscles.

Rehabilitation in Neuromuscular Diseases

Non-progressive neuromuscular disorders such as Erb palsy and poliomyelitis are characterised by LMN injury. The rehabilitation process involves range of motion exercises, positioning to prevent contractures and activities/therapy to strengthen the weak muscles **(Fig. 32.7)** with the goal of improving functional performance and participation in the home and school.

Duchenne muscular dystrophy is an example of a progressive neuromuscular disease where inherent sarcolemmal instability predisposes it to injury with mechanical loading. Here, a sub-maximal strengthening programme is recommended and these are incorporated into activities which children enjoy doing. Improvement in strength should translate in improvement in function and mobility or compensatory strategies and adaptive devices are used **(Figs. 32.14, 32.38 and 32.42)**.

Aerobic exercises such as walking, swimming and cycling can help to improve the cardiopulmonary system. These also have an effect on the muscles by increasing capillary density, mitochondrial size and density, oxidative enzymes and efficiency in utilization of fat as an energy source for muscular activity.

Management of Limb Contractures and Deformity

A contracture is the limitation in the passive range of motion of a joint and can be arthrogenic or myogenic in nature. These can result from the fatty infiltration and fibrosis seen in dystrophic myopathies along with muscle imbalance across joints. Stretching exercises **(Fig. 32.25)** should be started early to prevent contractures and the desired position is maintained with the help of resting splints **(Figs. 32.26 and 32.27)**. Encouraging weight bearing by standing and walking also helps in delaying the development of contractures in the lower limbs (Fig. 32.14).

Correction of deformities should be pursued only if it results in a functional limitation, e.g. an elbow contracture of more than 30° can affect ambulation with elbow crutches and pronator tightness will limit supination, which is required to bring food to the mouth and hence, these need correction. In the presence of quadriceps weakness, the equinus deformity assists with ambulation by creating an extension moment at foot contact. Hence, the equinus deformity commonly seen in muscular dystrophies should not be corrected, except if the goal of rehabilitation is to provide gait training with KAFO (Fig. 32.30) or an AFO with a gaiter (Fig. 32.27), which helps in supporting the ankle and knee in neutral. Assistive devices like a walker or elbow crutches enable the children to walk longer than they would without them.

Seating and Respiration

Supported seating in progressive conditions is essential to prevent or delay scoliosis (Figs. 32.24 and 32.34). When functional ambulation is no longer possible, training in a wheelchair equips the child with skills needed to become as independent as possible. Spinal orthoses are usually ineffective in preventing progression of scoliosis and can restrict breathing. However, braces can be used temporarily to improve trunk control and sitting. Surgical correction of scoliosis by posterior arthrodesis is done after skeletal maturity when the growth of the vertebral column has been completed.

Progressive muscle weakness can lead to restrictive lung disease and ultimately to hypoventilation, hypercarbia and respiratory failure. Inability to clear secretions due to an ineffective cough results from weak expiratory muscles and this can lead to respiratory infections. Deep breathing exercises with or without incentive spirometry (Fig. 32.41) and assisted cough techniques are used to ameliorate the effects of respiratory muscles weakness. Non-invasive ventilation is an option in the later stages of respiratory difficulty due to low vital capacity and hypercarbia.

Despite significant deterioration and disability, a good quality of life can be maintained by being creative and exploring ways for children to be able to do something that is meaningful to them such as using a laptop, playing video/mobile phone games or reading (Fig. 32.53).

Rehabilitation in Musculoskeletal Conditions

Joint damage and deformity occurs in conditions like juvenile inflammatory arthritis (JIA) and severe haemophilia (secondary to bleeds in the joints and muscles). In the acute phase, the goal of rehabilitation is to provide pain relief and rest the joint in a functional position by providing a splint if needed (Fig. 32.28). Ice is used in the acute phase for pain relief. Factor replacement is crucial for a child with acute haemarthrosis secondary to Haemophilia. A joint distension can result in a flexed joint which is often not functional and hence, plaster of Paris is used to make a splint to keep the knee, wrist and/or ankle in as neutral a position as possible. Stretching and mobilization exercises are required for deformity correction particularly when function is affected (Fig. 32.54).

Heat is the modality chosen for pain management during the subacute phase in JIA, as it is thought to improve the joint range of motion, by improving the tissue elasticity and reducing the muscle spasm from pain. If not

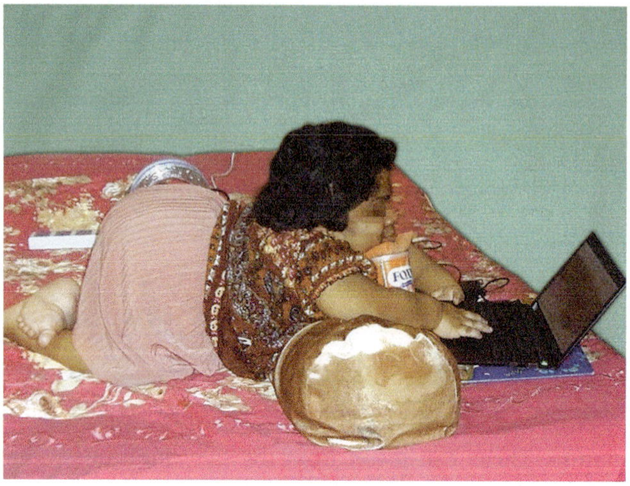

Figure 32.53 This girl, with an inborn error of metabolism (Morquio syndrome), has poor head control and uses a tin and a pillow in prone lying to enable her to continue to use her laptop. Her efficiency during the day improved with use of non-invasive ventilation for respiratory muscle weakness to reduce hypercarbia at night.

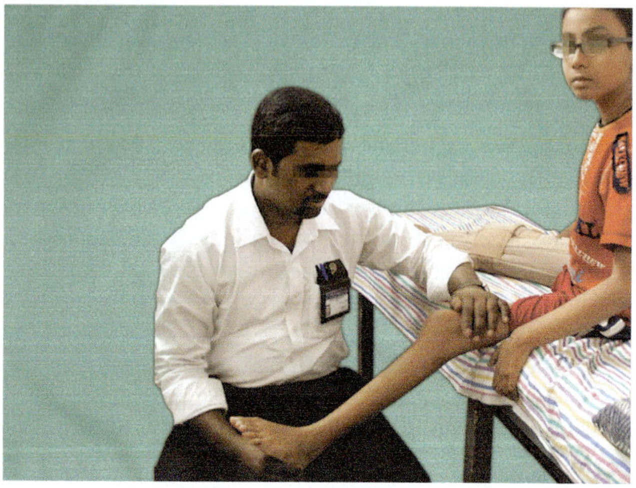

Figure 32.54 A 10-year-old boy, with haemophiliac knee arthropathy, undergoes mobilization and stretching for the correction of a fixed flexion deformity of the left knee. Serial casting was also used to correct the deformity of the right knee, which is now supported with a knee brace/gaiter.

controlled, medication may be needed for longer period of time. Daily activity and ambulation are encouraged as early as possible. Progressive strengthening exercises are also initiated to reduce muscle wasting and osteoporosis (Figs. 32.5 to 32.13 and 32.20). This can be incorporated into play and recreational activities (Figs. 32.4, 32.14 and 32.15). Adaptive devices are advised for joint protection, e.g. built-up pens/pencils (Fig. 32.39), long handle brushes for bathing, large buttons (Fig. 32.32), Velcro straps for dressing, shoes and footwear made of microcellular rubber to support feet and reduce ground reaction forces proximally.

Rehabilitation in Paediatric Limb Deficiency

The goal of prosthetic fitting and training in congenital or acquired limb deficiency is to achieve age-appropriate milestones. Prosthetic upper limb fitting as early as 6 months of age helps in achieving sitting balance, attaining bimanual tasks and crawling. Early prosthetic fitting and training also helps with its acceptance by reducing stump dependence (Figs. 32.55 to 32.57). Parents should be involved in prosthesis decision making in order to ensure better acceptability so that they encourage the child to use the prosthesis.

Once the child is cognitively ready for training, the passive prosthesis can be changed to give the child a simple way to open and close the hand using cables or by electrical switches within the socket of the prosthesis (Figs. 32.58 and 32.59). Acceptance of upper limb prostheses is less than that for lower limbs. This is due to the very limited sensory feedback of the prosthesis and the inability to control the intensity of the grasp and to manipulate objects. Very often children learn to use their stumps or their feet to do all their activities because of the

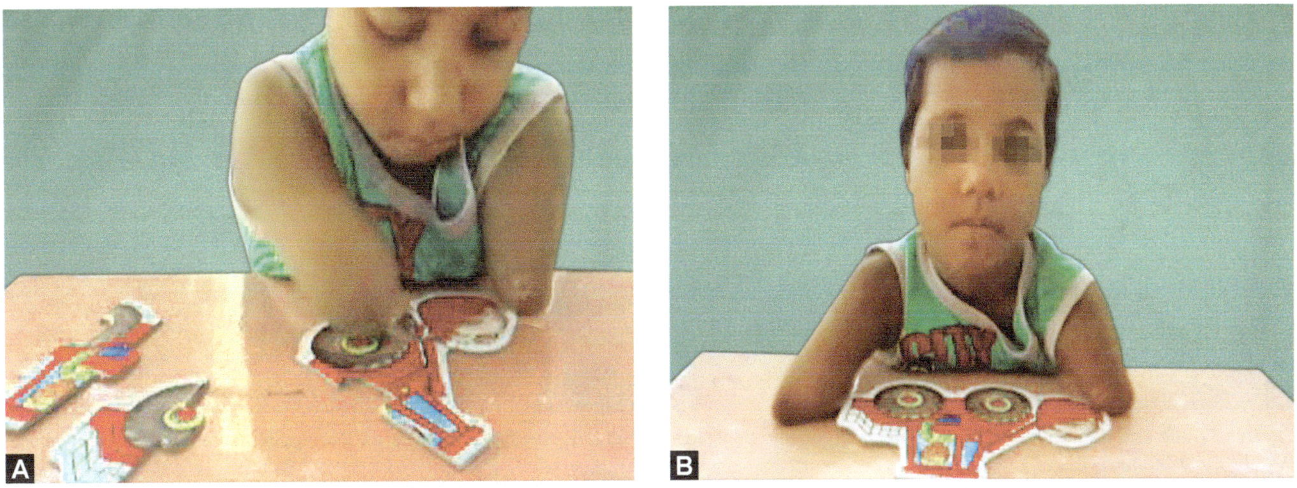

Figures 32.55A and B A child with phocomelia uses her stumps to put together a puzzle.

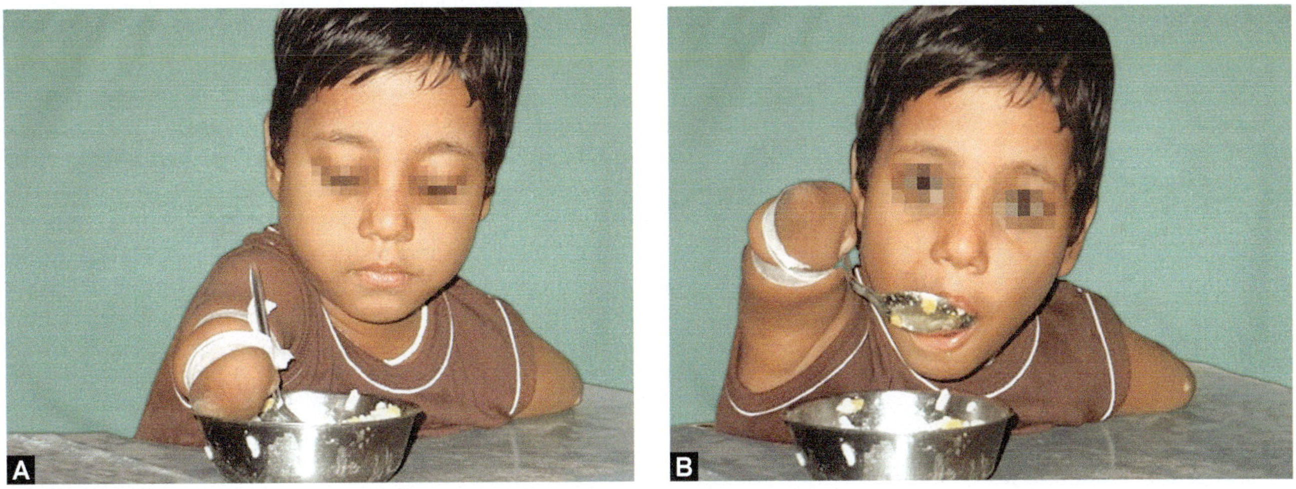

Figures 32.56A and B This child can feed herself independently using a modified spoon strapped onto her stump using Velcro (hook and loops). Tape can be used to make the strap during the initial stages of training.

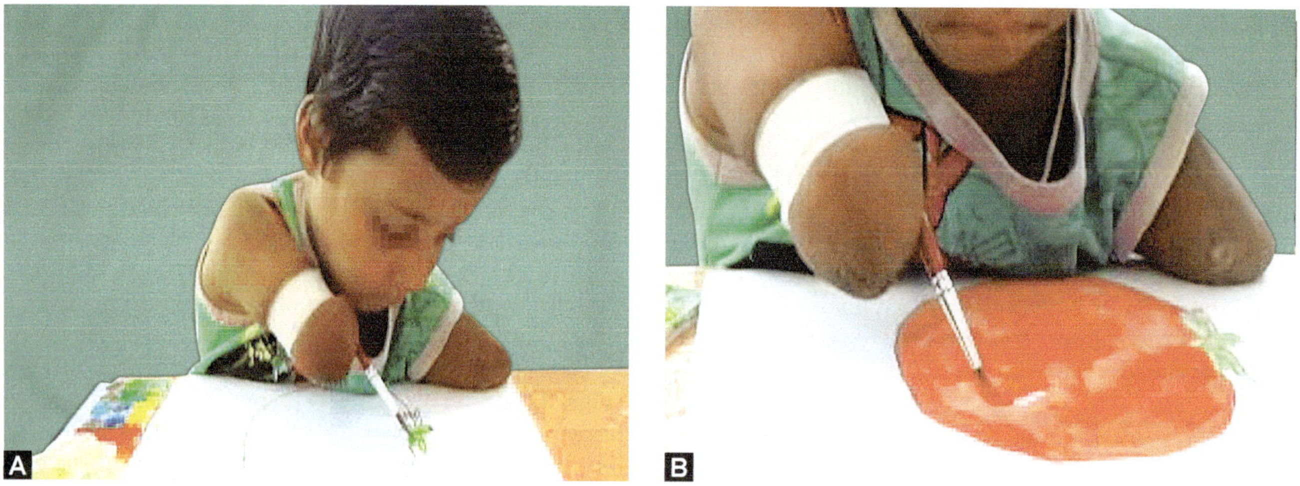

Figures 32.57A and B Painting with the brush placed in position on the stump using Velcro straps/tape.

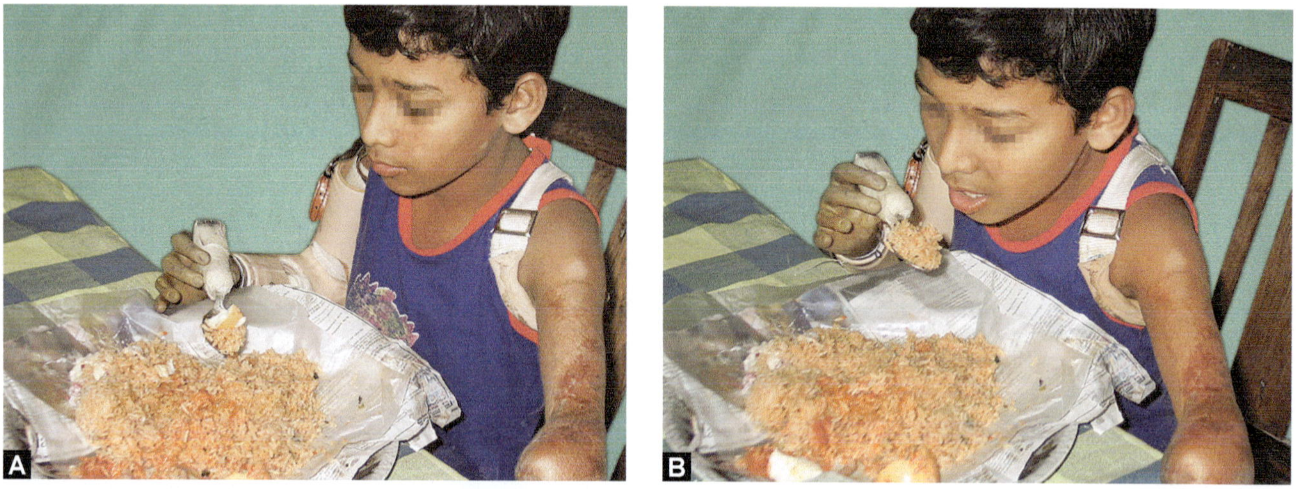

Figures 32.58A and B A 13-year-old with bilateral upper limb transradial amputations (post-electrical burns) undergoing training to use a mechanical prosthesis for eating.

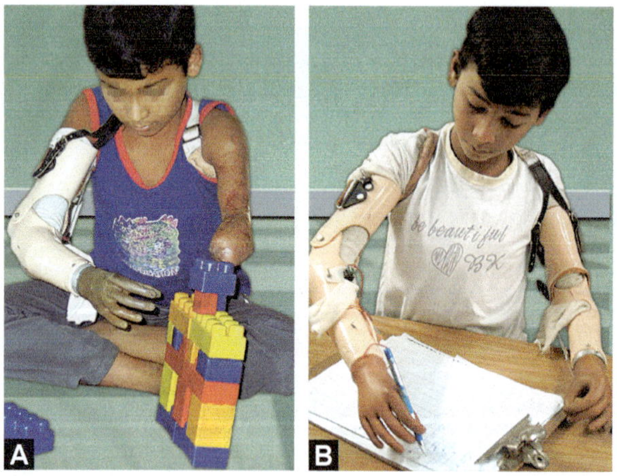

Figures 32.59A and B (A) Training to use his right electrical prosthesis using building blocks; (B) Writing is an essential skill that should be initiated in the rehabilitation set-up. A mechanical transradial prosthesis is used for the left arm.

sensory feedback from the exposed skin **(Figs. 32.55 to 32.57 and 32.59)**.

In lower limb deficiency, prosthetic fitting is started at 10 months of age when the child is ready to stand and then subsequently to walk **(Figs. 32.60 to 32.63)**. Knee joints are added at 3–5 years of age with a manual locking mechanism. In acquired amputations, pre-prosthetic training aims at improving range of motion, strength across the joint and reducing the post-operative swelling by rigid (plaster of Paris) or semi-rigid (elastocrepe bandage) dressings. Gait training is initiated with a temporary prosthesis till the stump edema has resolved **(Figs. 32.62 to 32.64)**. Good socket fitting and early ambulation with prosthesis improve compliance. The socket should be designed to accommodate growth by using removable inserts such as liners and socks. The height of the leg can be increased by adding a walking sole to the foot/footwear.

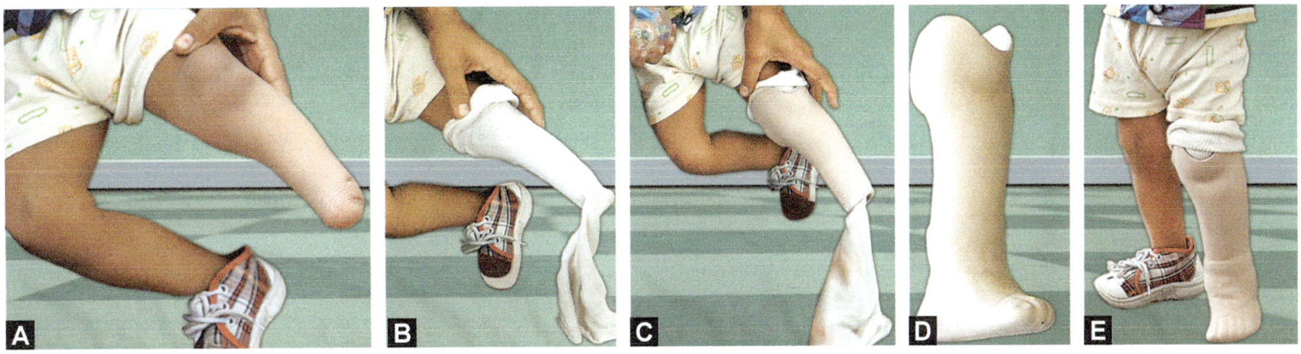

Figures 32.60A to E A mother assists in putting on the patellar tendon-bearing prosthesis in this 1.5-year-old boy with a congenital transverse deficiency of the foot. An elastic stockinette is stretched onto the stump followed by a soft liner. The prosthesis is then put over the liner.

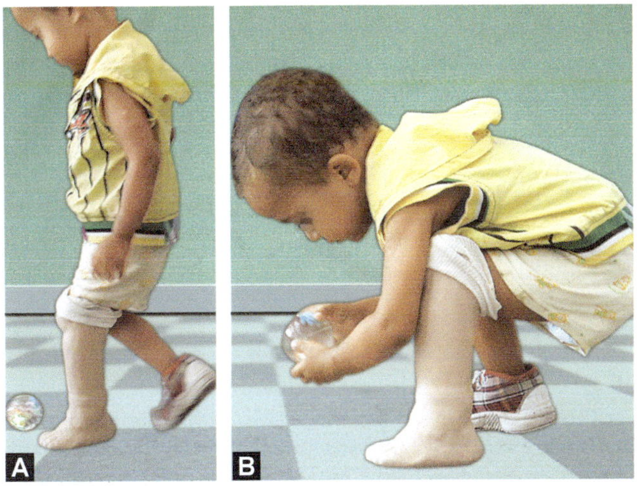

Figures 32.61A and B The patellar tendon-bearing (PTB) prosthesis enables the child to walk, squat and engage in play activities.

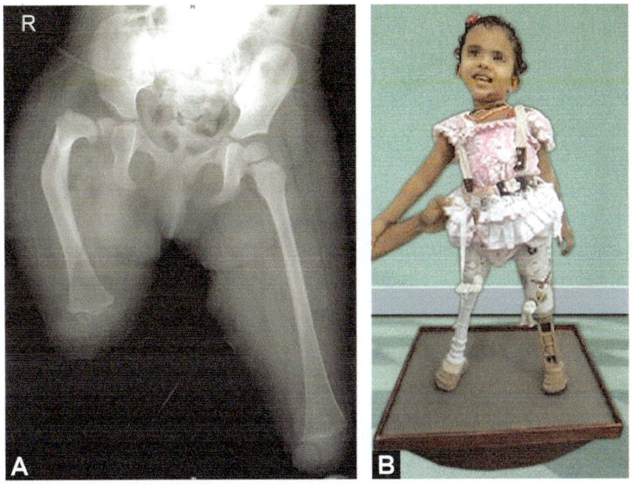

Figures 32.62A and B The X-ray shows a congenital transverse deficiency of the leg and foot in a 2.5-year-old girl. She learns to balance with bilateral above knee temporary prostheses using a balance board.

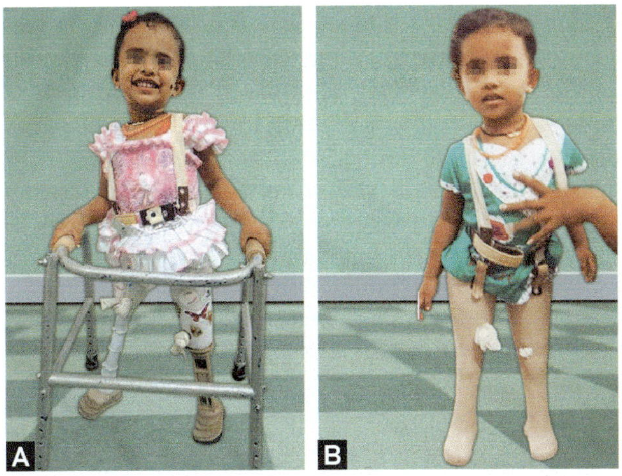

Figures 32.63A and B Gait training with a walker is required before the child can learn to walk independently. Completion of the prosthesis is done after changes to the socket and the alignment of the prosthesis are finalised. The knee joint has not been added to her prosthesis because of her young age and this being the initial phase of her training.

Assessment Tools

An assessment tool can be used to monitor progress and to communicate this with the family. Scales need to measure what you want them to measure (construct validity) and be reliable between different people (inter-rater reliability) and at different times, by the same person (intra-rater reliability). These tools meet these criteria and are used by many rehabilitation facilities around the world. Responsiveness is another criterion that is needed for many patients. Small changes can make a big difference to a child and their family. The difference between walking 5 m and 50 m can make the difference from needing someone to push a wheelchair to being independent walking at school. Simple tests like the six minute walk test can also be used as an outcome measures.

The Gross Motor Function Measure (GMFM) is a standardised observational instrument designed and validated to measure change in motor function over time in children with cerebral palsy. The items are broadly

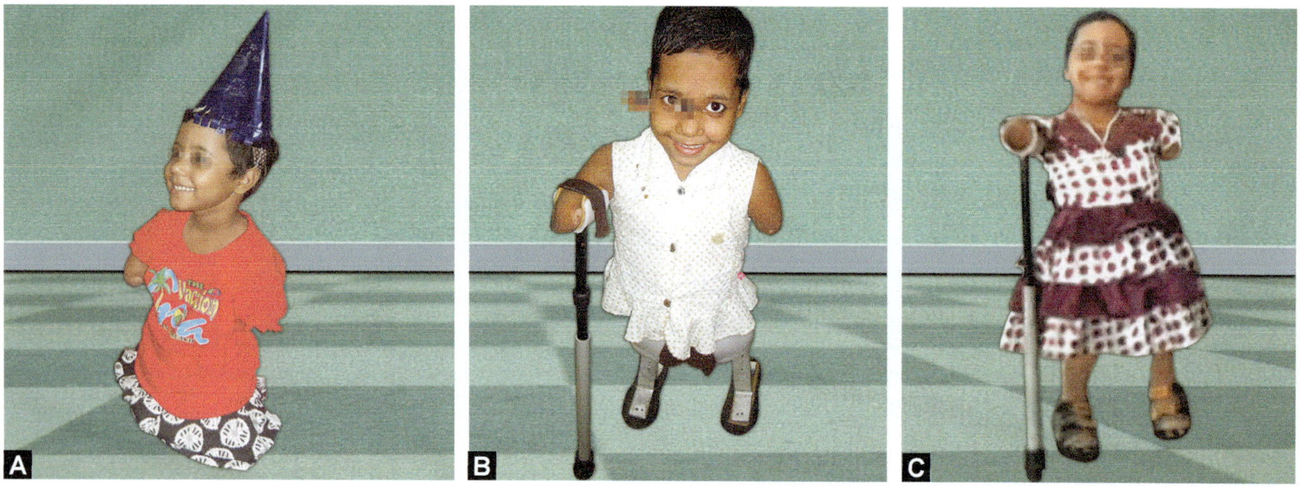

Figures 32.64A to C (A) Standing on her stumps, dressed for a party in the children's therapy area; (B) She also learns to use her temporary prosthesis and stand with a stick strapped onto her arm stump to help her balance and ambulate independently; (C) The 'stubbies' are shown unfinished and then finished.

TABLE 32.4 Five dimensions with the scoring key of GMFM.

Items	*Scoring key*
(1) Lying and rolling	0 = Does not initiate
(2) Sitting	1 = Initiates
(3) Crawling and kneeling	2 = Partially completes
(4) Standing	3 = Completes from rectus femoris spasticity
(5) Walking, running and jumping	WNT = Not tested

Abbreviations: FCR, flexor carpi radialis; FCU, flexor carpi ulnaris; FDS, flexor digitorum superficialis; FDP, flexor digitorum profundus.

grouped into five dimensions with the scoring key shown in the **Table 32.4**.

The Gross Motor Function Classification System (GMFCS, expanded and revised, 2007) focuses on the motor performance in home, school and community settings (i.e. what they actually do) rather than what they are known to able to do at their best (capability). These take into consideration the environmental and personal factors that impact the child's functioning. The GMFCS is a reliable and valid system that classifies children with cerebral palsy on the basis of the major age-appropriate gross motor activities, with particular emphasis on functional mobility.

- Level I: Walks without limitations
- Level II: Walks with limitations
- Level III: Walks using a hand-held mobility device (Canes, crutches, anterior and posterior walkers)
- Level IV: Self mobility with limitations; may use powered mobility
- Level V: Transported by others in a manual wheelchair.

Scales that measure social functioning, participation in leisure and learning activities include the Paediatric Evaluation of Disability Scale (PEDI), the Canadian Occupational Performance Measure (COPM), the Caregiver Priorities and the Child Health Index of Life with Disabilities (CPCHILD) and the Cerebral Palsy Quality of Life Questionnaire for Children (CPQOL-child).

SUMMARY

The concept of disability has undergone a paradigm shift in recent times. From being viewed as 'disabled' persons, it is now recognised that the 'disability' is in the environmental barriers and often in the way society responds to these people with special needs that limit their participation. A simple modification like a ramp with side rails instead of steps at school or moving the class to one on the ground floor can improve accessibility for a physically challenged childlike Suresh **(Fig. 32.1)**.

Children with rehabilitation needs due to developmental or acquired pathologies require detailed evaluation and assessment by a comprehensive rehabilitation team, which should include a physiatrist, paediatrician, physiotherapist, psychologist, occupational therapist, rehabilitation nurse and social worker, among others. Realistic goals should be decided upon after discussions with the family and other caregivers. An individualised treatment plan can then be formulated based on the prioritised goals, taking into consideration the child's emotional, social and physical needs. All interventions that are considered should be with the aim of improving function as well as promoting integration into the family and community, transferring care to adult medical and social services will help in maximising their potential for developing into productive members of society.

More information on low cost alternative to splints and chairs in Disabled Village Children which is available to download free online:

http://www.dinf.ne.jp/doc/english/global/david/dwe002/dwe00201.htm.

ACKNOWLEDGEMENTS

We acknowledge the suggestions of Dr Ashish S Macaden (physiatrist), and the assistance with photography from the therapists of these children, Ms Reetha Janet Surekha and Mrs Pearlin Grace (BOT), Ms Shirley Betsy, Ms Margaret Christie and Mrs Winrose W (BPT), and Mrs Veena B (SALT), in the preparation of this book. Our heartfelt gratitude also goes out to our patients and their families who teach us through their struggles, and remind us of our common humanity.

CHAPTER 33

Paediatric Maxillofacial Surgery

Khursheed F. Moos

INTRODUCTION

Although the maxillofacial area is relatively small at birth in relation to the head and cranium, its development started in the embryo at around 4 weeks. All the facial parts are fully developed at birth but are small and rapidly grow in size during the first year of life **(Fig. 33.1)**. The maxillofacial area is complex because it involves the airway, deglutition, mastication and the dentition. Developmental anomalies, particularly clefting defects, are not uncommon and they involve not only the lip and palate but may also relate to orbits, nose and early developmental failure of fusion of the branchial arches as well as malformations of the skull related to craniosynostosis. They may also involve the eyes and ears. Interference with growth and neurological function of the cranial nerves not infrequently occurs, and because the face is always visible with facial expression and oral function is affected; when appearance is abnormal, there is a major problem for the child and family often with significant psychological effects on the child, especially when there is interference with speech, hearing, vision and aesthetics are affected. Normal development of the dentition is very important to the child for mastication, speech and aesthetics.

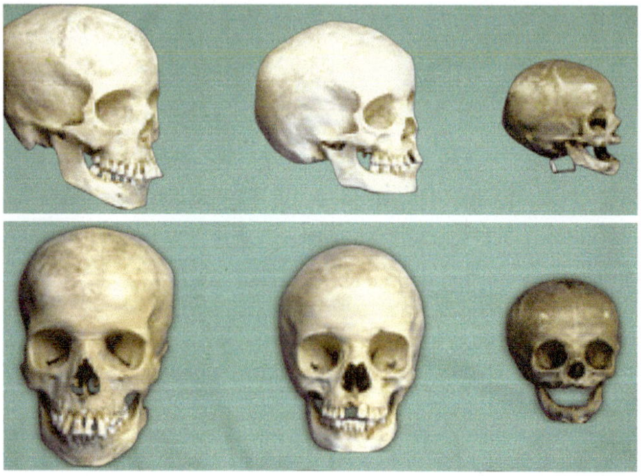

Figure 33.1 Oblique view/anteroposterior view of dry skulls of various ages: 6 months, 11 years and 20 years.

The principal areas in which the maxillofacial surgeon can be of help to the child, family and paediatrician will be in the management of:

- Congenital deformities with cleft lip and palate followed by craniofacial microsomia (CFM), and craniosynostotic deformity where the face is significantly affected. There are many other rarer syndromic and non-syndromic deformities, which present with aesthetic and functional problems; the majority of which when severe will require maxillofacial surgery.
- Trauma in the maxillofacial area is another major problem, especially in the developing world where childcare is more difficult. Management of maxillofacial trauma especially for children often occurs late after healing has started to occur. The mid-face is relatively small at birth, but as the paranasal sinuses develop and increase in size, there is an increased risk of trauma but even then it tends to affect principally the mandible and frontal areas during the first few years of life. Management of fractures affecting the mandible and maxillae is complicated by the presence of developing teeth in the mandible as well as in the mid-face. Minor discrepancies in the position of jaw fragments are normally self-correcting with growth except in the naso-orbital area.
- Infection in the head and neck area is not uncommon, especially in relation to the dentition more so in the developing world where caries and poor oral hygiene are commonplace. Life-threatening spread of infection may occur from the oral cavity into the pharynx with lethal consequences if not well managed by the surgeon.
- Maxillofacial pathology and oral manifestations of systemic disease often present in the face with characteristic stigmata as well as in a unique way in the oral cavity and pharynx. Early recognition is helpful

as this is an accessible area and easily visible to the clinician. There are a variety of benign and malignant tumours, which may present in the head and neck and many of the commoner ones are associated with the teeth as well as other dysplastic conditions peculiar to the jaws and oral mucosa. Oral ulceration is common and various dermatological conditions present characteristically in the oral cavity.

- The age of the child is an important factor as growth may be rapid, e.g. with bony lesions, e.g. cherubism and vascular anomalies. Others involute and cease as growth completes. With discrepancies in jaw size and some bone dysplastic conditions, it may then become worthwhile to wait until growth has ceased before correcting those deformities. Other conditions require early correction otherwise normal growth may be affected when the temporomandibular joints are involved. When conditions such as aggressive fibromatosis and cystic hygromata are present, they require early major surgical procedures to reduce the risk of residual deformity (Box 33.1) and involvement of the airway or major neck vessels.

CONGENITAL DEFORMITY

Craniofacial Deformity

After cleft lip and palate, probably the most important conditions to consider are the craniosynostotic deformities (Box 33.2). These primarily affect the cranium but when the base of skull is involved growth of the mid-face is impeded. Premature fusion of the sutures may occur prior to birth and when a single suture is affected such as the sagittal suture an increase in length of the head (dolichocephaly) will occur with growth of the brain continuing until approximately 15 months postpartum (Figs. 33.2 and 33.3). If the coronal suture is affected, and

BOX 33.1 Paediatric maxillofacial surgery.

Favourable aspects

Good blood supply

Rapid healing

Growth adaptation of bone form and occlusion

Unfavourable aspects

Small dimensions

Bone weakness

Close location of tooth buds and inferior dental and infraorbital nerves

Interference with growth

BOX 33.2 Craniofacial deformity.

Craniosynostosis and related syndromes

Craniofacial clefting defects

Craniofacial microsomia

Treacher Collins syndrome

Other malformations

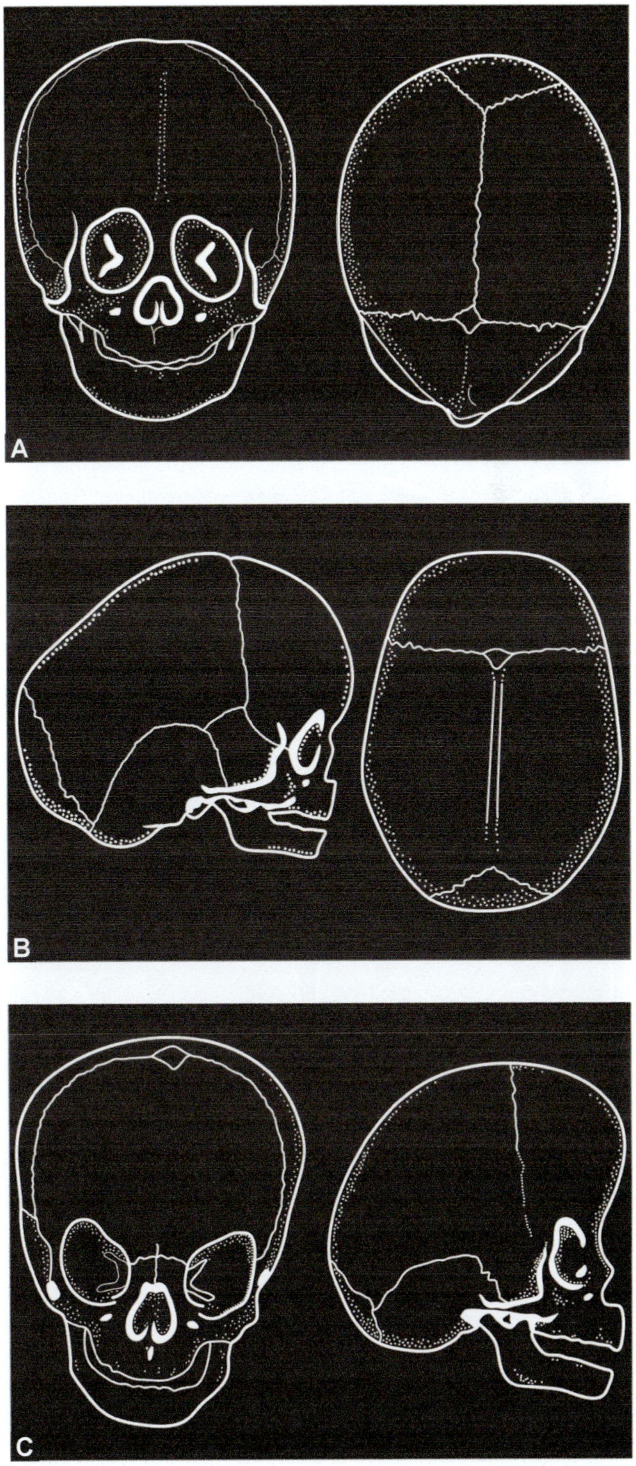

Figures 33.2A to C Craniosynostosis—skull deformity: (A) Metopic; (B) Sagittal; (C) Coronal.

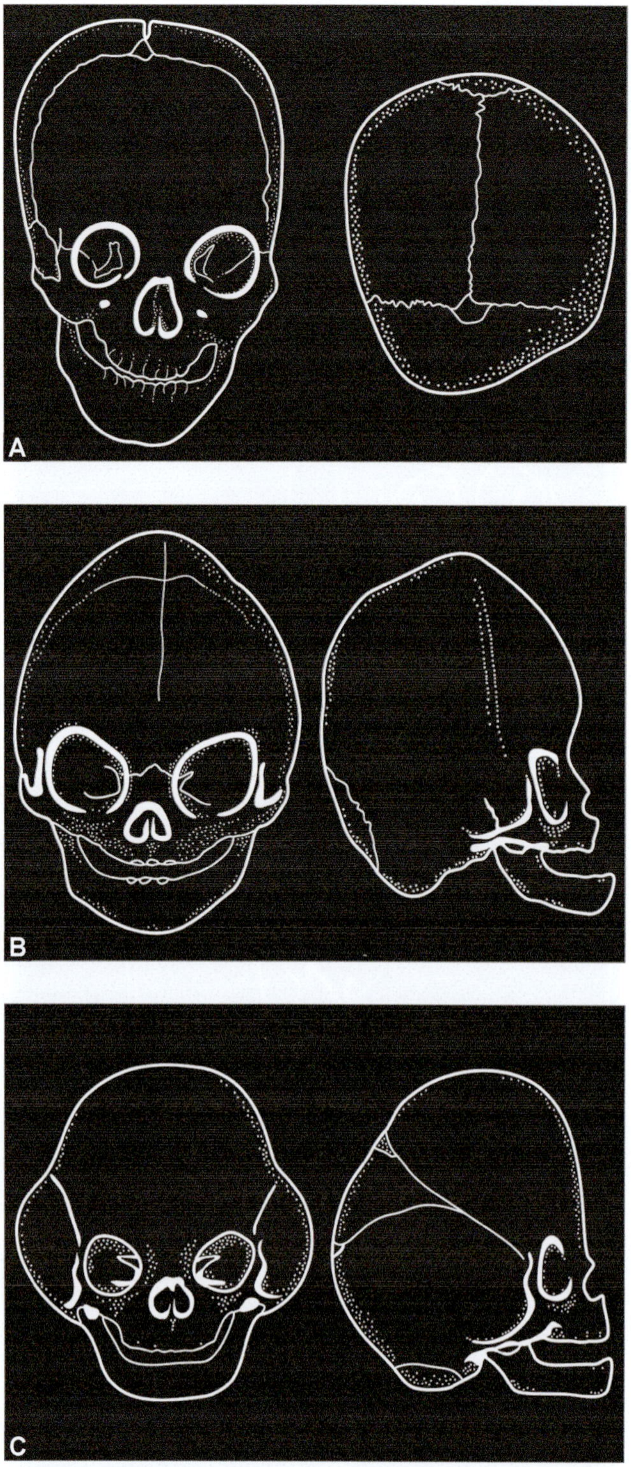

Figures 33.3A to C Craniosynostosis: (A) Plagiocephaly; (B) Coronal; (C) Kleeblattschädel.

there tends to be a brachycephalic deformity and various combinations of premature fusion will result in abnormal cranial development, e.g. with early fusion of the coronal and sagittal suture, there is likely to be a degree of turricephaly and when just one-half of a coronal suture fuses prematurely there will be significant asymmetric growth

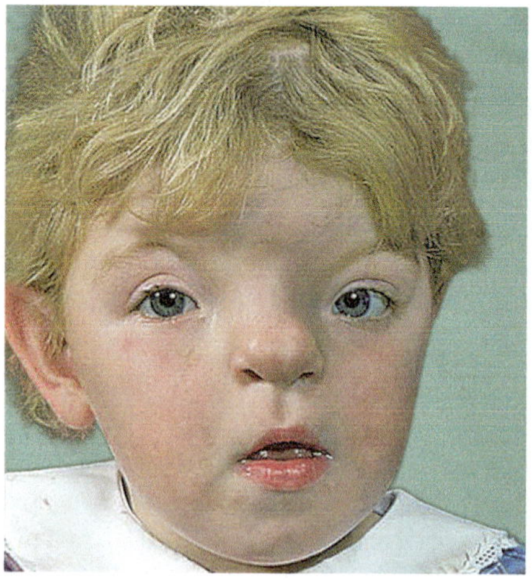

Figure 33.4 Plagiocephaly—facial deformity—unilateral right coronal synostosis.

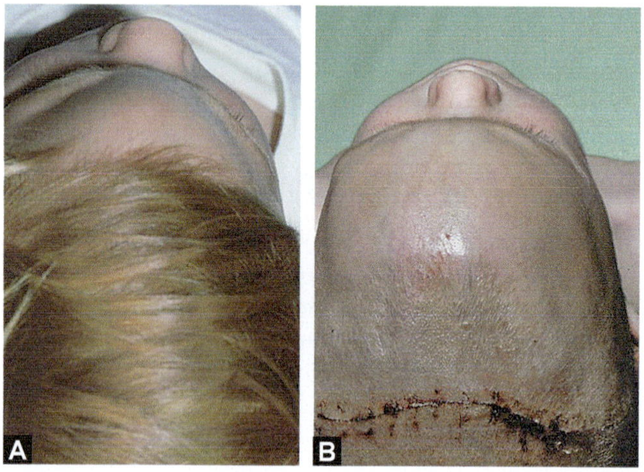

Figures 33.5A and B Metopic synostosis correction.

of the face (plagiocephaly) **(Figs. 33.4 and 33.5)**. Growth will cause deviation of the face towards the unaffected side, which is particularly difficult to correct at a later stage, whereas if release of the suture can be achieved before 1 year of age, this deformity can be circumvented **(Box 33.3)**. Syndromic craniosynostosis **(Box 33.4)**, e.g. when associated with Crouzon syndrome, there is also premature fusion occurring in the cranial base this results in severe underdevelopment of the mid-face, which is accompanied by proptosis of the eyes, often a degree of hypertelorism and a very short retruded mid-face height. Early release of the affected cranial sutures will allow the brain to grow normally and will improve the appearance of the skull, but it has little effect on the development of the mid-face **(Figs. 33.6A to D)**. It is difficult to provide a good early correction of the mid-face deformity by an advancement of that, and where possible, if not too severe, this is best corrected towards the end of the growth period. However, if the deformity is gross then correcting it at around 10–12 years of age is often necessary and prevents

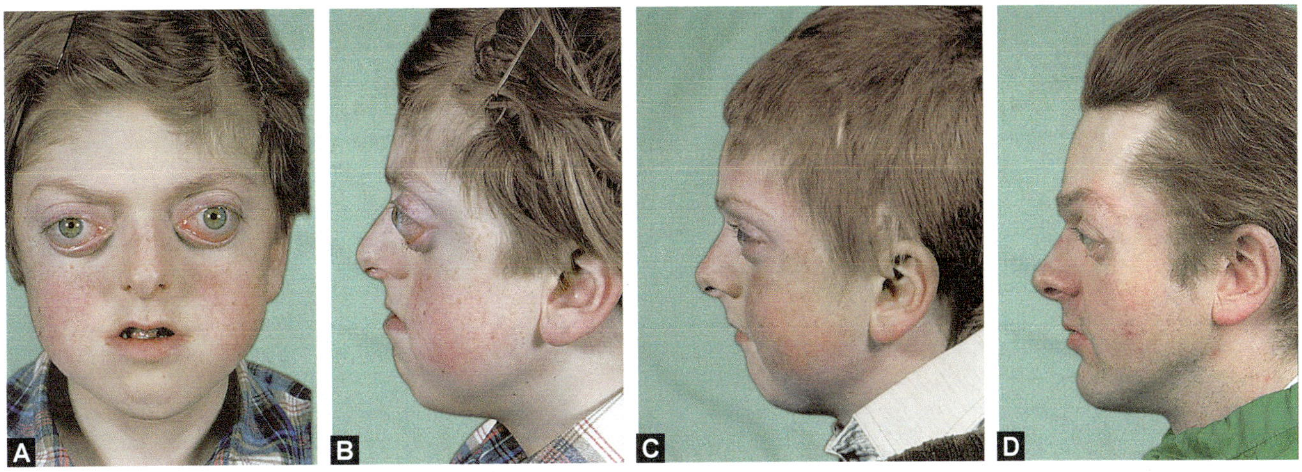

Figures 33.6A to D Crouzon deformity—early treatment and late result.

BOX 33.3	Plagiocephaly—unilateral coronal synostosis.

Features

Axis of cranium altered

Recession of affected supraorbital ridge

Altered shape of orbit

Nose deviates to unaffected side

Maxilla larger—affected side

Treatment

Bilateral release of coronal suture

Asymmetric frontal advancement

Supraorbital ridge advancement

Surgery at 6 months or weight of 5 kg

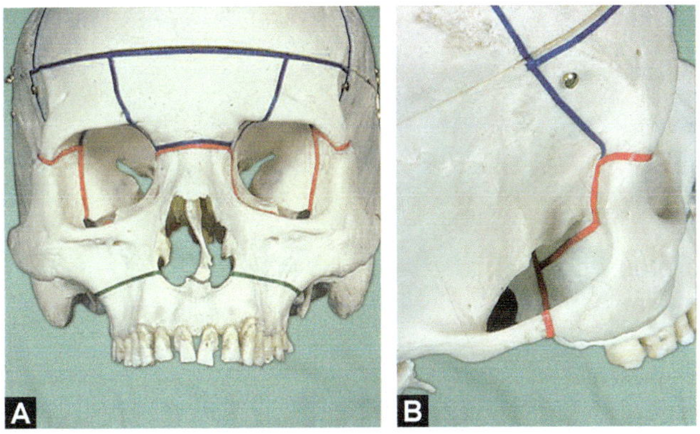

Figures 33.7A and B Le Fort III sub-cranial (red) and trans-cranial (blue) and Le Fort (green) osteotomies.

BOX 33.4	Common craniofacial dysostoses encountered.

Crouzon syndrome

Apert syndrome

Saethre–Chotzen syndrome

Carpenter syndrome

Pfeiffer syndrome

Kleeblattschädel anomaly

the child from being teased or bullied at school, which is particularly likely to occur when moving from primary to secondary education. If there is a residual discrepancy in size, this may be treated, again towards the end of the growth period with mid-face osteotomies **(Figs. 33.7A and B)** usually at the Le Fort III level **(Figs. 33.8A to C)**.

The same is true for some of the other syndromic conditions such as Apert **(Fig. 33.9)** and Pfeiffer syndromes. These are accompanied by digital deformities and have a different appearance from Crouzon syndrome. Other rarer anomalies, such as Saethre–Chotzen and Carpenter syndromes, have similar facial deformities. Very often, these are accompanied by a degree of hypertelorism, and sometimes by a clefting defect in the orbital and mid-face areas. The initial correction of the cranial deformity often makes the facial deformity look worse as the cranial cavity tends to expand forwards with release of the coronal suture but the mid-face is left behind due to the premature base of skull fusion. Both corrections may now be achieved with surgery towards the end of the growth period. This may be either sub-cranial or where it involves also the forehead and vault of the skull, this can be corrected also as a craniofacial procedure with advancement of the mid-face and frontal bones. At the same time, in some cases, where the mid-face is short in height then this can be increased by a low-level osteotomy involving the dentoalveolar complex at the Le Fort I level. This will also achieve often a better dental occlusion. The lower half of the maxilla can be stabilised with small bone plates

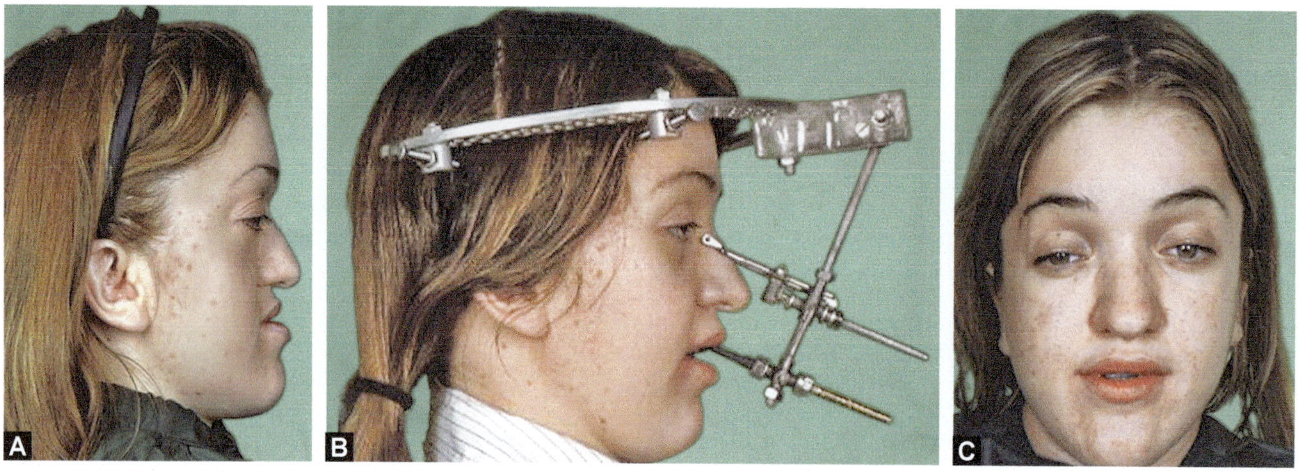

Figures 33.8A to C Crouzon syndrome patient treated with sub-cranial Le Fort III mobilisation followed by mid-face distraction osteogenesis. Upper eyelid ptosis still present for upper lid corrections.

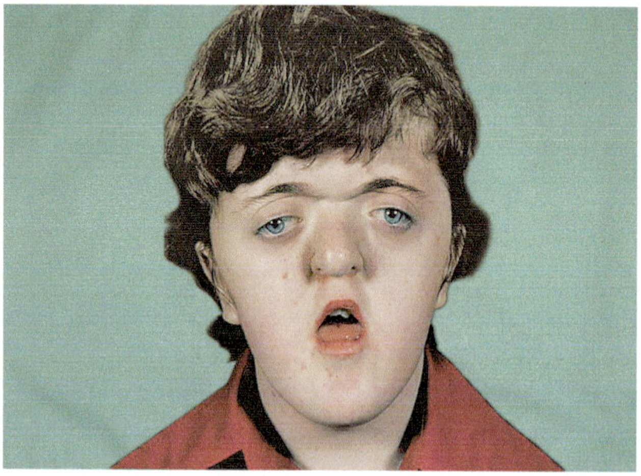

Figure 33.9 Apert deformity.

and the defect filled in with a cranial bone graft. Generally speaking, in the older child, the aim will be to correct finally all deformity problems with one single procedure. Another troublesome feature may be obstructive sleep apnoea when this is presenting, advancement of the mid-face at the Le Fort III level will relieve this and avoid the necessity for a long-term tracheostomy. Gross ocular proptosis likewise is a strong indication for early surgery if vision is at risk especially if there is any tendency for the lids to close behind the globes. Similarly, if there is a tendency to raised intracranial pressure with pansynostosis, further advancement of the frontal bone with release of all the major sutures and with skull expansion may be necessary **(Figs. 33.10A to C)**. Occasionally, a permanent shunt will be required.

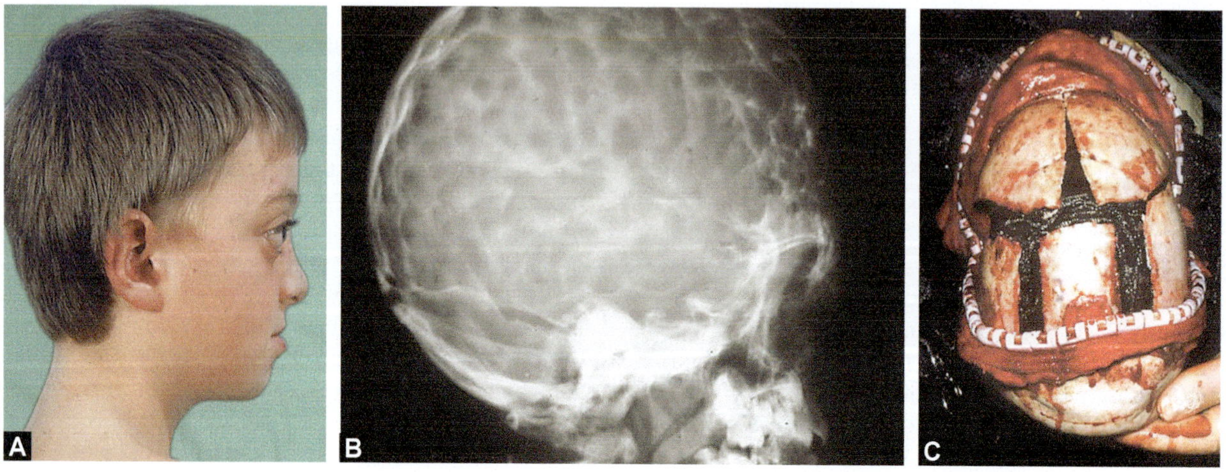

Figures 33.10A to C Pansynostosis—copper beaten skull deformity prior to correction. Pansynostosis correction with linear craniotomies and skull expansion.

Craniofacial Clefting Defects

Most of these clefts are rare. In the midline of the face, they are usually associated with meningoencephalocoeles **(Figs. 33.11A to D)** and involve the orbits and nasoethmoid complex and result in hypertelorism. A transcranial approach is required for treatment in most cases but a few milder forms may be treated sub-cranially.

CRANIOFACIAL MICROSOMIA

This is typically a combined first and second branchial arch defect, which is thought to result from a failure of the neuroectoderm to migrate. It has been shown experimentally in mice that haemorrhage from the primitive stapedial artery may give rise to a haematoma and cause this failure, which will result in defective development of the pinna and middle ear, mandible, parotid gland, temporomandibular joint and muscles of mastication. In severe forms, all these structures will be affected and be either absent or rudimentary. The mid-face sometimes will also be affected with a clefting defect into the orbit and posterior maxilla. There will be a conductive deafness on the affected side **(Figs. 33.12A and B)**. In the relatively rare bilateral cases, e.g. Goldenhar syndrome instead of a gross unilateral asymmetry, there will be bilateral or a symmetrical lack of growth occurring in the lower face. It also may be associated with vertebral defects as well as dermoid cystic lesions in the superolateral orbital areas. Obstructive sleep apnoea may be an indication for early surgery in the severe forms of this condition as it is in craniosynostotic syndromes. There are a number of classifications of CFM, which are principally based on the range of defects and the severity of those (Omen and Pruzansky).

The cases tend to be sporadic and appear not to have a true genetic basis, less than 1% of parents will have a second affected child, and there is a 3% chance of it being passed on. The incidence is variably quoted at 1:3,000–1:5,600, males are more commonly affected. The right side of the face is more frequently affected **(Figs. 33.12C and D) (Box 33.5)**.

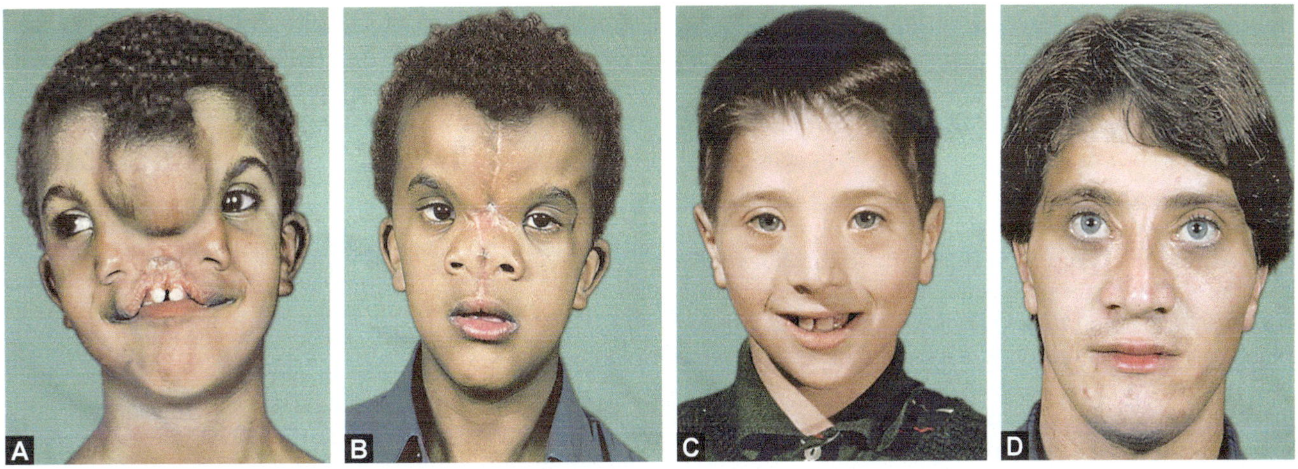

Figures 33.11A to D (A and B) Hypertelorism with encephalocoele corrected, viewed 2 years later (for further surgery); (C and D) Mild hypertelorism—seen again as an adult.

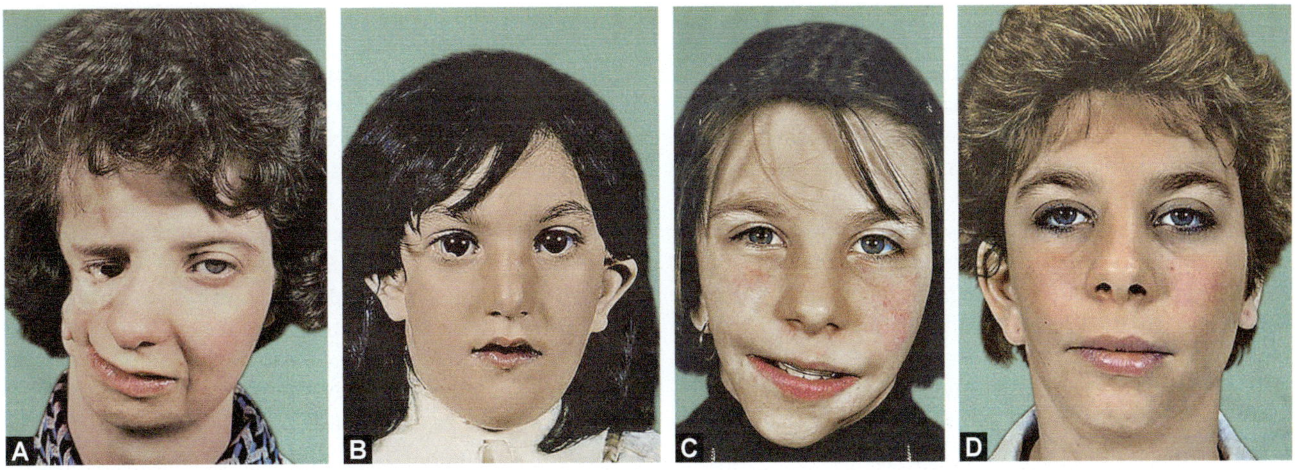

Figures 33.12A to D (A) Severe hemifacial microsomia (HFM); (B) Goldenhar syndrome; (C) Pre-surgical HFM; (D) 10 years post-surgical.

BOX 33.5 Craniofacial microsomia.

Hemifacialmicrosomia

First/second branchial arch syndrome

Goldenhar syndrome (oculo-auriculo-vertebral dysplasia)

Incidence 1:5,600—sporadic, rarely familial

Second commonest congenital facial anomaly after cleft lip and palate

Areas affected-craniofacial skeleton, neuromuscular tissues, skin structures, salivary glands, 0.5 branchial arch structures, e.g. ears

CLINICAL FEATURES

These features can be divided into skeletal and soft-tissue defects.

Skeletal Defects

Skeletal defects essentially involve the mandible which on the affected side will be short, narrow and normally retrusive from birth. Increasing asymmetry occurs with growth due to the lack of growth potential on the affected side. In the mildest of cases, there may only be a slight failure of growth, but in severe cases, the temporomandibular joint and ramus of the mandible will be missing, and there is then a three-dimensional (3D) failure of growth on the affected side, which is accentuated by the lack of overlying soft tissues, muscles and salivary glands. In the severer forms, there is a failure of vertical growth that affects the maxilla, and the chin point will tend to deviate markedly towards the affected side. In addition, there is often hypoplasia affecting the temporal bone with a less prominent mastoid process, and an absence of the external ear and external auditory meatus and more rarely major orbital defects on the affected side. Teeth may also be missing posteriorly on the affected side **(Figs. 33.13A to C)**.

Soft-tissue Defects

Soft-tissue, defects arise from the poor development of the first and second pharyngeal arches. The pinna of the ear may be absent as well as the external auditory meatus. There may be facial nerve paralysis affecting the muscles of facial expression, and there is also absence or poor development of the muscles of mastication on the affected side and a lack of overlying soft tissue accentuated by the absence of the parotid gland in some cases and by the loss of subcutaneous fat. Preauricular skin tags are often present. There is an associated degree of macrostomia at the commissure of the lips on the affected side, which is laterally displaced and canted upwards. Usually the trigeminal nerve is unaffected. The external ear deformity varies from a complete absence of the ear and external auditory meatus to a mild degree of hypoplasia, and this does not correlate in many cases with the lack of mandibular development. The poor development of the muscles of mastication tends to vary and affects the severity of bone development. The chin and midline is markedly deviated to the affected side. Correction of the mandibular and maxillary skeletal deformity will improve the symmetry and dental occlusion, but frequently the lack of soft-tissue bulk is accentuated by the stretching and tightness of the soft tissues over the facial bones. In the more severe cases, correction of the soft-tissue defect with a microvascular free flap will improve the appearance, and the use of muscle flaps and de-epithelialised skin flaps is required for the more severe defects using a composite flap of bone, muscle, fat and skin. In severe cases, excess is usually inserted because atrophy of the muscle tends to occur due its lack of nerve supply. Any excess fat post-surgery can be removed with liposuction at a later stage. Cranial nerve abnormalities most critically affect the facial nerve and at an early stage incompetence of eye closure needs to be checked otherwise following corneal exposure blindness may result. The use of free micro-neurovascular bone or muscle can be helpful, and in the older child, the use of botulinum toxin may be helpful when given into the muscles of facial expression on the unaffected side, this can improve the symmetry of the face. There may be abnormality of function of the soft palate due to a facial nerve paresis as there is a dual innervation in that area.

It is helpful to consider the classifications of hemifacialmicrosomia (HFM) in order to standardise treatment. In most cases, the basis of treatment is management of the mandible. The Pruzansky classification identifies type 1 as a small mandible with a reduced size of the temporomandibular joint and a simple hinge movement. The muscles of mastication are present but small. The type 2 mandible is small, abnormal in shape and has a poorly developed displaced temporomandibular joint and is characteristically subdivided into type 2a the joint is morphologically abnormal and tends to be anteromedially placed in relation to the glenoid fossa. The muscles of mastication are hypoplastic with poor function of the lateral pterygoid. In type 2b, there is no articulation of the condyle and the temporal bone. The coronoid process varies in size and the condyle is rudimentary. The muscles of mastication are deficient and poorly functional. In the severest forms of HFM type 3, there is a complete absence of the mandibular vertical ramus including the condyle and coronoid process. The muscles are very hypoplastic and not attached to the mandible. In type 2, muscle action is not normal, but in type 3, excessive freedom of movement is evident. As far as growth is concerned if HFM is a progressive condition interceptive surgery is worthwhile for the child. Others believe that there is some proportional growth on the affected side. Due to the 3D failure of growth on the affected side, early treatment is advocated for type 1 and type 2a. Distraction osteogenesis is often effective in the ramus of the mandible to increase the size of the ramus and thus allow for growth of the maxilla whereas in

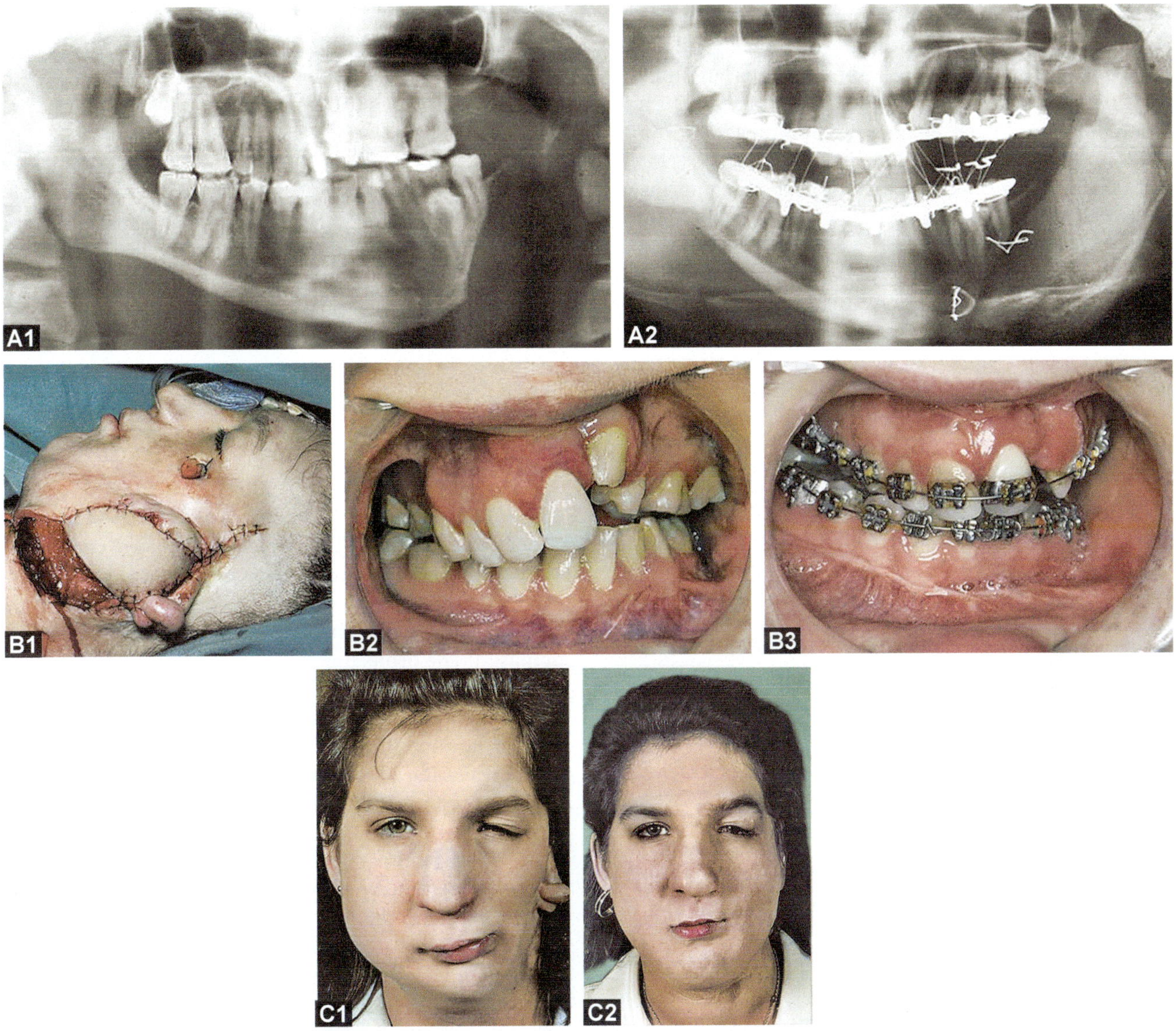

Figures 33.13A to C Severe hemifacial microsomia types: A1, A2, B1, B2, B3, C1 and C2. Five-year post-surgery with deep circumflex iliac artery flap (DCIA) free flap and cleft palate repair, Le Fort I and right sagittal split mandible.

type 2b and type 3 grafting of bone into the ramus area and reconstruction of the joint with a costochondral graft together with limited reconstruction of the temporomandibular joint itself is helpful. This may be done from 5 years to 7 years of age, other vascularised grafts have also been used for reconstruction, but the morbidity associated with that has not been balanced by good growth of the mandible and now with distraction osteogenesis, it is possible to usefully carry-out further surgery on a reconstructed ramus when thought appropriate. To reduce the soft-tissue deficiency, free vascularised grafts are often useful in the ramus area (**Figs. 33.13A to C**). Soft-tissue reconstruction of the mouth to correct the macrostomia may be carried out early from 1 year onwards.

As far as reconstruction of the ear is concerned, this is frequently possible if there is a rudimentary ear present, and this is usually undertaken with rib and costal cartilage. If there is no ear present and no external auditory meatus, sometimes it is better to consider a prosthetic reconstruction of the ear which is held in place with osseointegrated implants behind which a bone-anchored hearing aid may also be inserted. To correct any residual canting of the dental occlusion a Le Fort I osteotomy of the maxilla may be required once the mandible has been correctly placed, but this is usually left until the teenage period. Again sometimes distraction of the affected maxilla is possible and this may avoid further bone harvesting.

To summarise treatment for the HFM child, careful planning is required and surgery should be limited to three or four episodes, if at all possible, with the final correction towards the end of the growth period. It is essential to correct the vertical position of the ramus of the mandible early so that the maximum amount of unimpeded growth can be achieved for the maxilla, as this is often not adequate without additional ramus lengthening surgery. Where there are defects in the orbit and zygomatic bone, these can be corrected at the same time as other surgery is being carried out, and usually this is in the early teens. To improve the final appearance after insertion of a free flap, the use of liposuction is often helpful; if over corrected or if under corrected, the insertion of a de-epithelialised flap or a small dermal graft, and finally removal of the ectopic skin of the free flap replacing it with adjacent facial or neck skin. The timing of surgery is important and some advocate this being done early during growth others late to reduce the number of procedures during childhood. This depends on the severity of the deformity if mild it can be left until later particularly if it is only to correct chin and midline asymmetry. Severe hearing defects, especially in bilateral cases, should be corrected early with bone anchored hearing aids. Severe deformity will require interventional surgery on a number of occasions during childhood usually with distraction osteogenesis, costochondral grafts and osteotomy surgery with soft tissue and ear reconstruction.

TREACHER COLLINS SYNDROME

Treacher Collins syndrome (mandibulofacial dysostosis) condition has been known since ancient times and has been well depicted in American pre-Columbian carvings and pottery (Box 33.6). It has an incidence of 1:50,000 live births and is an autosomal dominant condition (chromosome 5 within q31q35) with a variable degree of penetrance and expression, and this can be compared with the incidence of facial microsomia which is almost twice as common 50% are spontaneous mutations. In Europe, it is known as the Franceschetti-Zwahlen-Klein syndrome. It is characterised by clefting defects. Using the Tessier classification, these are type 6, 7 and 8 and involve the orbit either at the infraorbital margin or at the lateral border of the orbit together with a cleft of the zygomatic arch. The clefting defects tend to be symmetrical and extend into the maxillae from the infraorbital area or from the frontozygomatic (FZ) suture down to the inferior orbital fissure. The mandible is always abnormal and is hypoplastic and joint development is poor. There is also sometimes an associated cleft palate. The clinical features are characteristic with an anti-Mongoloid slant to the eyes (Figs. 33.14A and B). The skull tends to be shorter anteriorly and often smaller than normal. The posterior cranial length may be increased. The orbits themselves are shallow. The malars are markedly hypoplastic and the overlying skin and soft tissues are reduced in volume, and the nose appears to be more prominent in relation to the rest of the face. There is a hair bearing tongue, which extends onto the cheeks from the temporal area in 25% of cases. As far as the eyes are concerned, three-quarters of all cases have either true or pseudocolobomata affecting the lower eyelids, and there is a lack of eyelashes (cilia) on the lower eyelids. Often, ophthalmic abnormalities occur extending into the globes. The ear pinnas are abnormal, often asymmetric, and they tend to have a crumpled appearance and may be accompanied by ear tags. The external auditory meati if present are rudimentary and are often stenosed leading to a severe conductive deafness as a result of developmental defects of the ossicles. The mandible is bilaterally hypoplastic with shortening of the ascending rami, and body as well as severe genial retrusion. The muscles of mastication are present, and this results in a prominent antegonial notch and obtuse gonial angle. There tends to be some malpositioning of the muscles of mastication in the ramus area. The maxilla tends to have a high arch palate and may be cleft. Although it appears to be prominent, this is essentially in relation to the very small mandible, and its antero-posterior position is usually acceptable. There are other defects that sometimes occur (Box 33.7). Most troublesome is post-nasal choanal atresia, particularly in the infant where there may be severe symptoms of obstructive sleep apnoea. An early tracheostomy may be necessary, especially in Nager syndrome which otherwise facially closely resembles Treacher Collins syndrome. Usually, this is now improved by distraction osteogenesis of the angle region of the mandible (Figs. 33.15A and B). This will also bring the mandible forward to improve the

BOX 33.6	**Mandibulofacial dysostosis.**
Also known as Treacher Collins syndrome	
Franceschetti–Zwahlen–Klein syndrome	
An autosomal dominant inherited condition with variable penetrance, sporadic mutations also occur—incidence 1:10,000	
Areas affected: Skull vault, malars, maxilla and nose with orbital and palatal clefts	

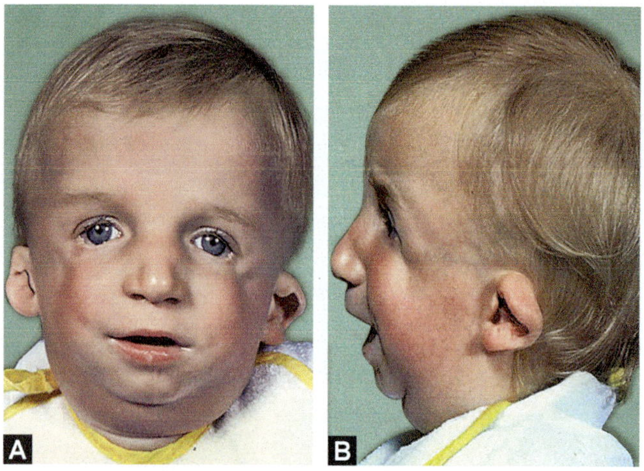

Figures 33.14A and B Treacher Collins syndrome—clinical appearance.

BOX 33.7 Reconstruction—Treacher Collins syndrome.

Normal airway increase in 'pharynx' as well project mandible and chin

Reconstruct/derotate orbit and malar bones

Normalise dental occlusion

Reconstruction of ear

Correct conductive hearing defect—implants

Methods

Orbital osteotomy

Maxillomandibular osteotomies

Genioplasty and orthodontics

Ear reconstruction and implant prostheses

Bone-anchored hearing aids

Soft-tissue surgery

Distraction osteogenesis

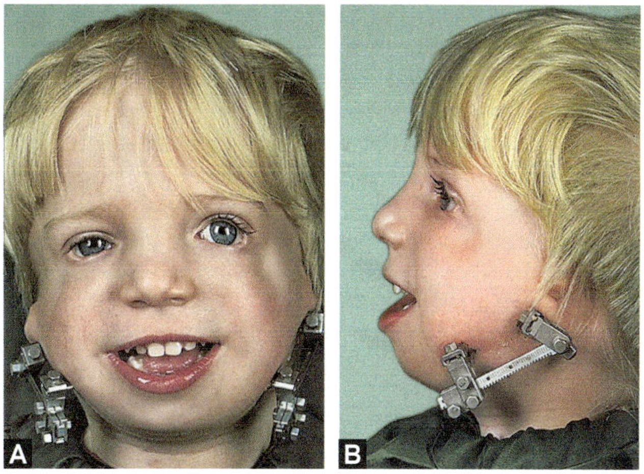

Figures 33.15A and B Early distraction osteogenesis for airway obstruction.

occlusion of the teeth where there is often an anterior open bite (AOB). Advancement of the chin with a genioplasty is helpful also in repositioning the hyoid, and it increases the size of the oro- and hypopharynx. Due to the severe hearing defect, there tends to be a delay in speech development and a secondary effect on mental development if early correction of hearing is not undertaken. Usually, in the first instance, this can be with simple conductive hearing aids with a band across the head but as soon as there is sufficient thickness of bone in the temporal bone, bone anchored hearing aids should be inserted.

This condition can be diagnosed prenatally, especially when there is a family history so that at birth, the airway can safely be maintained, and if necessary, an early tracheostomy can be undertaken. There also needs to be good support for the family. With modern surgery, a very good reconstruction of the defects can be anticipated, but surgery needs to be carefully timed taking into account the necessity for correction of hearing and cleft palate at an early stage. A good ophthalmic assessment is also essential post-natally during the first few months. As soon as there is some growth of the mandible and when there are airway problems, early distraction osteogenesis in the angle region of the mandible is required so that the tracheostomy may be closed at an early stage. Further lengthening of the mandible may be required from 5 years onwards. This would depend on the severity of the condition, and this may be combined with reconstruction of the malar defects and bone grafting of those areas. Insertion of bone anchored hearing aids is also important and can usually be timed with other surgery. With repositioning of the mandible, orthodontic treatment is frequently required due to crowding of the arches and the steep mandibular plane angle to achieve a satisfactory occlusion with the maxillary teeth. Ear reconstruction may be timed with the move from primary to secondary school and similarly rhinoplasties. A few years after reconstruction of the molar defects, it is often advantageous to osteotomise the reconstructed malars and to bring them into a more forward position to provide more normal cheek prominences for the face. Finally, towards the end of the growth period orthognathic surgery should be considered to correct discrepancies in jaw size and the dental occlusion. In some cases, the temporomandibular joints are grossly abnormal and the condyles are virtually absent, and there is very poor growth in these areas and it is usually advantageous to reconstruct the condylar heads with a costochondral grafts on both sides and follow that a few years later with distraction of the mandible. However, there are some risks attached to advancement of the mandible and applying significant pressure in the temporomandibular joint area as this can lead to ankylosis of the temporomandibular joint with the consequent necessity later of further reconstruction in that area. The facies of Treacher Collins syndrome are very similar to that seen in Nager syndrome, but that tends to be a more severe autosomal recessive condition. It is also associated with limb abnormalities. Very severe airway problems tend to occur and early tracheostomy followed by distraction of the mandible is essential. Both these conditions are best treated in specialised craniofacial units. It is also important to consider genetic counselling for the older child and family.

There are many other conditions associated with discrepancies in jaw size such as the Pierre Robin anomalad and juvenile idiopathic arthritis (JIA), which result in severe under development of the mandible. As far as the Pierre Robin anomalad is concerned, this often appears severe at birth but this is often followed by quite rapid growth whereas in JIA this usually occurs at an older age, and results in severe mandibular retrusion and airway problems. As a result of that there may also be ankylosis of the mandible which will require joint reconstruction.

It is also important to consider in trisomy 21 (Down syndrome), for the high-grade patient, correction of the deformity. Although this is controversial tongue reduction followed by simple mandibular surgery and onlay grafts of the nose and reconstruction of the eyelids will render the patient more normal in appearance, and as a result of that they are treated more normally and appear to be more intelligent. This should only be considered where the parents strongly request consideration, and this should be done with a full psychological assessment and in the absence of any other significant life-threatening pathology.

INFECTION

Acute Infections

Suppurating infections and large abscesses will spread into the spaces in and around the pharynx, maxilla and mandible; these are almost always dental in origin and require to be treated urgently to prevent compromise of the airway or spread into the retropharyngeal and mediastinal areas. The essence of treatment is drainage of the infection and treatment with antibiotics **(Figs. 33.16A and B)**. When it is principally a cellulitis spreading across the floor of mouth, this is extremely dangerous (Ludwig angina). This needs to be treated aggressively with drainage from the submandibular areas and often intraorally to prevent further spread of infection. It is important to explore all the loculi, and this is most easily done with a gloved finger through the incision into the cavity, and drains need to be inserted and a careful watch on the airway during the immediate post-operative period is essential. A tracheostomy should be undertaken whenever there is doubt about compromise of the airway. Swelling in the post-operative period can be severe. Usually, a 5-day period of appropriate antibiotics is all that will be required after drainage. A microbiology report is essential as resistance to widely used antibiotics is common-place. Details of the possible spread of infections into the parapharyngeal areas are illustrated **(Box 33.8)**.

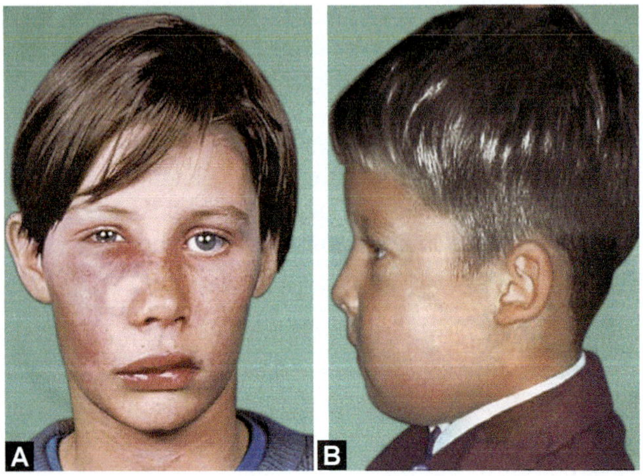

Figures 33.16A and B Maxillary and mandibular dental spreading infection.

BOX 33.8 Orofacial infection.

- May be bacterial, viral, mycotic or parasitic
- Most serious acute infections around the jaws and face are odontogenic in origin
- May be localised or spreading. Treated by (1) removal of the cause; tooth, (2) drainage of abscess, (3) prevention of spread and any necessary and (4) restoration of function
- If systemic side effects, treatment with antibiotics, analgesia and rehydration may be required
- If there is trismus, dysphagia or dyspnoea surgical treatment under general anaesthesia is urgent
- Other specific infections—actinomycosis, tuberculosis, syphilis, protozoal infections may be complicated by human immunodeficiency virus infection
- Spreading streptococcal cellulitis and staphylococcal infections require specific parenteral antibiotics and often fascial space surgical drainage
- Infections spreading into the mid-face may lead to cavernous sinus thrombosis and intracranial spread

BOX 33.9 Bone infections and related conditions.

- Acute osteomyelitis
- Sub-acute osteomyelitis
- Chronic osteomyelitis
- Garrés osteomyelitis
- Chronic sclerosing osteomyelitis
- Osteoradionecrosis

Osteomyelitis

Types of osteomyelitis are shown in **Box 33.9**.

Acute infections are rare in the neonatal period; these can result in osteomyelitis of the mandible or maxilla. In the case of the maxilla, it is almost always haematogenous in origin. In the mandible, especially around the temporomandibular joint, it may be due to ear infection or possibly a septicaemia and usually this would be either a streptococcal or staphylococcal infection. Failure to recognise and treat this with antibiotics early on can result in ankylosis of the temporomandibular joints, and in the maxilla loss of teeth and bone from the area **(Figs. 33.17A to D)**. The child will present with a pyrexia, pain and irritability and difficulties with feeding. Blood cultures and

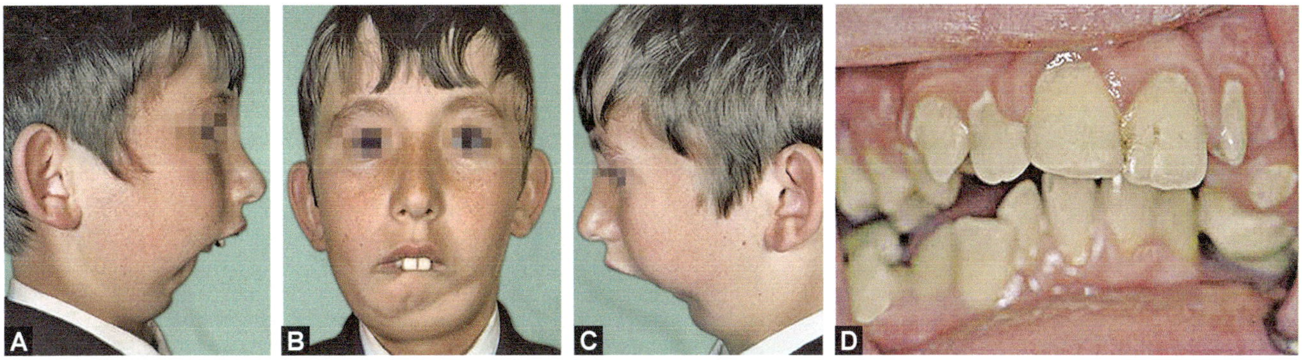

Figures 33.17A to D Mandibular ankylosis right side from early acute middle ear infection.

monitoring with C-reactive protein (CRP) levels are helpful guides to the effect of intravenous antibiotic therapy. This can safely be started before culture results are available with intravenous penicillin and metronidazole. If there is pus or significant swelling, then urgent surgical intervention and drainage will be required.

Usually, in a child over 4–5 years of age sub-acute osteomyelitis will present following dental infection with swelling and pain over the mandible and breathing difficulties and with numbness of the lower lip when the body of the mandible is affected. This condition is rare in the maxilla but acute purulent infections are not uncommon and are usually dentally related and require drainage. More commonly, they present as a sub-acute bony infection in the body of the mandible as a result of dental sepsis and carious teeth especially in the malnourished child, and there may be severe trismus, swelling, sinuses in the submandibular or cheek region **(Figs. 33.16A and B)**. Usually, there are mobile teeth present and there is expansion of the mandible. Radiographs will show a marked periosteal reaction with new bone formation, sequestra and radiolucencies in the body of the mandible. If present for a considerable time, a fracture of the mandible may occur, and it can be the presenting feature. Almost always the organisms are oral organisms, which respond to treatment with penicillin and metronidazole given intravenously in high doses. Surgical drainage will also need to be established with decortication, especially when there are sequestra and sinuses present. Curettage and removal of the sequestra are essential as well as open drainage of the area. Where a fracture occurs and there is much loss of bone, it is often helpful to put pins into the adjacent normal mandible on either side of the affected area to hold the mandibular fragments in the best possible position while healing occurs. A spontaneous fracture may also occur when treatment is undertaken with exploration of the affected area. It is important to preserve the inferior dental bundle and nerve to maintain sensation to the lower lip and chin. In tropical areas, tuberculosis is common and may also be the cause of a more chronic osteomyelitis as may other infections local to the area, e.g. syphilis and HIV-associated infections. These will need to be identified and treated accordingly. Care should be taken to avoid involvement of the temporomandibular joint if at all possible to prevent ankylosis. In the older child, more chronic forms of osteomyelitis may occur and non-suppurative forms, such as Garrés osteomyelitis, occur in children sometimes following dental extractions, a possible initiating factor, with a proliferative osteitis. On radiographs punctate granulomata are frequently seen in the mandibular rami in association with a marked periostitis and loss of normal bony trabeculation. A local lymphadenitis is usually present. This would appear possibly due to an autoimmune process but that is not proven. Decortication of the affected mandible, steroid therapy and antibiotics have a place in treatment. In the older child, a similar chronic form occurs known as chronic sclerosing osteomyelitis again of unknown aetiology possibly dental. Steroids and decortication of the affected mandible may be helpful at the time of more acute exacerbations.

TRAUMA

Paediatric fracture considerations are shown in **Box 33.10**.

Aetiology

Maxillofacial trauma is common in children, more so in boys than in girls. Most of the simple fractures seen are due to falls and bicycle injuries and tend to involve the primary dentition in the under 5 years of age group, and the permanent dentition from 7 years onwards. More severe injuries tend to be related to road traffic accidents, and these may be as a pedestrian or cyclist or with the unrestrained child in a car and also commonly with scooter and motor cycle passengers. As far as the latter are concerned, they are usually accompanied by friction burns and lacerations, which may involve the eyes and ears, and not infrequently there will be a skull fracture as well as fractures of the mid and lower face. In the very young child, the mid-face is very small and rarely injured and the mandible is also relatively small. As the child grows, the mandible becomes increasingly fractured, but it is not until the sinuses are significant in size that one

BOX 33.10 Paediatric fracture considerations.

Bone healing and remodelling potential—good
Shorter time to unite
Treatment choices—open reduction and internal fixation—risks; intermaxillary fixation—difficulties
Jaw function modulates mandibular growth
Generally, conservative treatment favoured
Greenstick fractures—remodelling very effective
Early treatment required to prevent malunion
Dental factors—shape of teeth, resorption and position of permanent tooth buds
Supplemental fixation, pyriform aperture, splinting and circumferential wiring
Be circumspect with mini/micro-plating

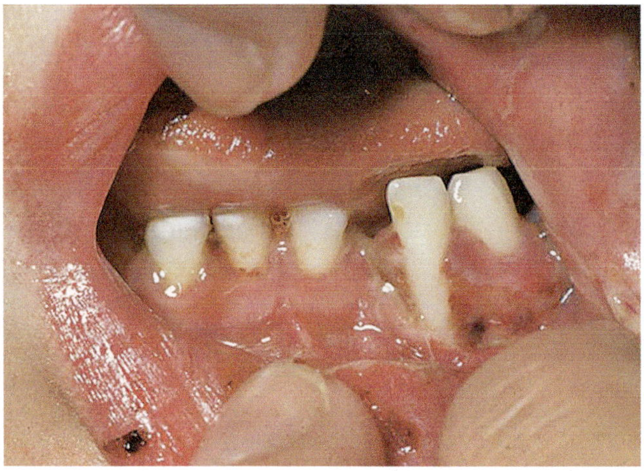

Figure 33.18 Examination (with a good history)—gentle examination ± restraint; look for signs, bruising, bleeding, occlusal changes and lacerations (chin). Avoid manipulation.

sees fractures occurring more commonly in the mid-face. Most mid-face fractures are orbital and in the older age group, that is in the teens, when they become a prominent feature. As a general rule, children should be restrained in the back seat of a car. There are distinct dangers from airbag damage when they are either restrained or unrestrained in the front seat. There may also be eye injuries as a result of this, and the chemical substances in the airbag. Ideally no child under 12 years of age should be restrained in the front seat. As far as cycling is concerned, helmets do protect the skull and to some extent the face. The other sources of injury in the West are skate boarding and sports injuries. In most cases, these are relatively simple fractures and may be treated conservatively. Minor discrepancies are usually well corrected with healing in the younger child, and it is often only in the teens that more complex forms of treatment are required in the form of plating and jaw fixation. Very often the teeth are loosened or fractured and every attempt should be made to retain teeth with appropriate dental treatment. If the teeth have been avulsed if reinserted within an hour, they will usually be retained and eventually will become firm. They may require root treatment (Fig. 33.18). Perhaps most importantly in all cases of trauma, especially in young children, they require careful examination to exclude non-accidental injuries, and where there is the least suspicion of non-accidental injury, a full examination of the child must be undertaken looking specifically for other injuries. This has already been alluded to elsewhere and when a full paediatric assessment must be made. Facial bone fracture imaging is shown in Box 33.11.

Condylar Fractures

One area where there is some controversy over the management is that of fractures of the mandibular condyle or more commonly fractures of the condylar neck.

BOX 33.11 Facial bone imaging.

Conventional radiographs
Orthopantomogram (mandible/maxilla)
Posteroanterior view (mandible)
Intraorals (teeth) as required
Mid-face—occipitomental views 10°, 30° and computed tomography scan (three-dimensional)
Magnetic resonance imaging as required

Radiography is always required for suspected facial bone fractures, both for diagnosis and surgical management (Figs. 33.19A to C). Most of these mandibular fractures heal with very simple treatment if they are undisplaced and usually no fixation will be required and only maintenance of a soft diet and the avoidance of further trauma. Condylar fractures tend to be caused by falls and may be accompanied by a fracture in the symphyseal region of the mandible. Not uncommonly they are bilateral. Since the anterior fracture in the mandible is prominent and often pain is principally in that area, it is easy to miss an associated condylar neck fracture. There is usually trismus, and palpation of the condylar areas will tend to be painful. In the case of unilateral fractures, the mandible will tend to deviate towards the affected side. Lacerations and abrasions are often seen on the chin or adjacent to the chin area. The incidence of this type of mandibular fracture varies from 43 to 72% and tends to occur 2.5 times more commonly in males than in females in the 6–12 years of age group. Intracapsular fractures tend to occur in the younger age group notably under 7 years of age. They occur because the condyle itself is very soft, and there is only a thin lining of cortical bone and it is very vascular. There is no neck to the condylar head, and it appears to arise from the ramus itself. Therefore, it tends

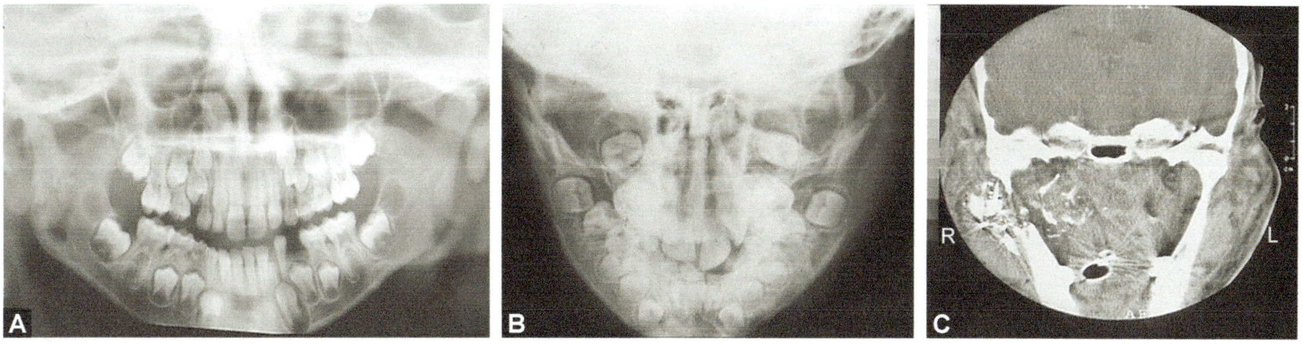

Figures 33.19A to C Radiography: (A) Orthopantomogram—right condyle and left body fractures; (B) Posteroanterior view—left mandibular condylar neck fracture; (C) CT scan—right condyle and condylar neck comminuted fractures.

> **BOX 33.12 Condylar fracture.**
>
> Condylar head (<6 years) comminuted—ankylosis risk
>
> Condylar neck fractures (>6 years)—displacement and deformity occur with growth, deformity on the affected side of body comprises a bowed bone, shortening of ramus height, and deviation of chin to affected side. On the unaffected side, the mandible appears flattened

to shatter when traumatised. In the older child, most fractures are extracapsular and are of the condylar neck. In the older child, this tends to be lower in the neck where it is attached to the ramus. The condylar head has become much denser and the weakest part of the mandible is then the condylar neck. Some 58% of all fractures in the under 6 years of age will be intracapsular, whereas in the older child 78% are extracapsular at the condylar neck. The intracapsular fracture should be treated conservatively with gentle mobilisation, whereas the condylar neck fracture, if it is undisplaced, is treated with a soft diet and initially restriction of mouth opening. The consensus view for treatment of the condylar neck fractures in the under 10 years of age group is to treat them all conservatively. Even if they are slightly displaced, the mandible itself regrows in that area, and there is no long-term deformity present and the occlusion of teeth is maintained. An adaptive process of healing occurs in the condylar area. The problem with condylar head fractures in the younger age group is that they were more often missed and due to pain and discomfort the child does not open or move their jaws. They were given a semi fluid diet and no exercise. This can lead to ankylosis of the temporomandibular joint, and it is primarily in this young age group that ankylosis occurs, especially in developing countries, where often treatment and recognition of the fracture does not occur until late on (Box 33.12).

In the older age group, temporary immobilisation is sometimes required, especially when there is an undisplaced symphyseal fracture or a fracture in the anterior mandible. Arch bars or acrylic splints may be applied to the teeth to maintain the occlusion, but open reduction and internal fixation (ORIF) have little place in the management of paediatric fractures, and the consensus view now is that a closed functional treatment is the best (Figs. 33.20A and B) (Box 33.13). Ankylosis leads to

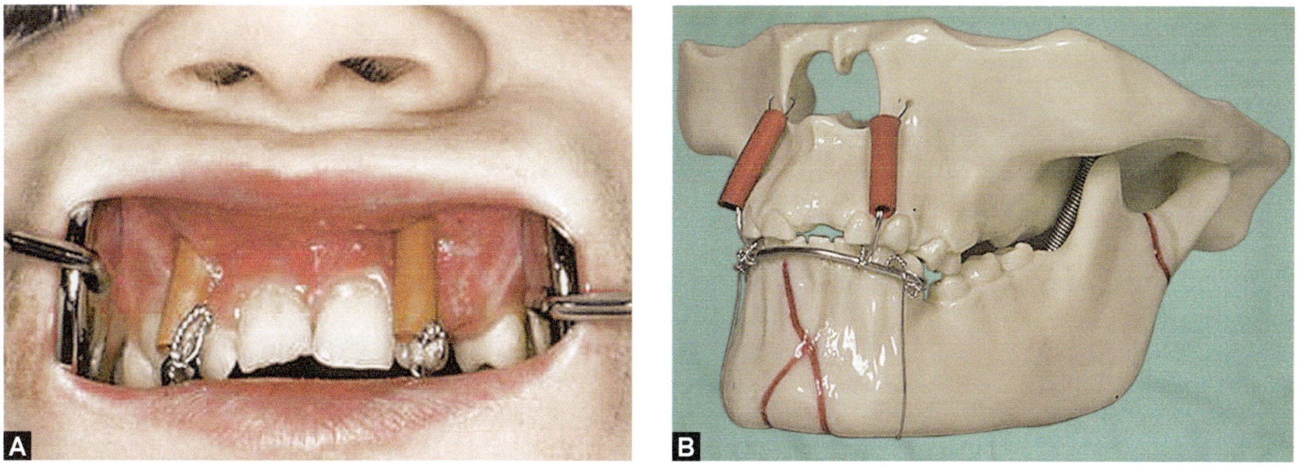

Figures 33.20A and B Maxillomandibular fixation.

BOX 33.13 Maxillary–mandibular fixation.

At 2 years 20 teeth available for intermaxillary fixation

Arch bar can be used with circum-mandibular support

Before age of 2 years and after age of 6 years inadequate dental support therefore, use dental occlusal or orthodontic splinting

Limited anatomical reduction often acceptable, as remodelling will occur

significant jaw deformity, which requires complex osteotomy surgery for correction (Figs. 33.21A and B).

Mandibular Fractures in General

Fractures in the over 10 years of age group may be treated as for adults and certainly when the child is in their teens; this is the best approach. It should also be pointed out that any form of plating or fracture in the under 6 years old is fraught with danger in the body and symphyseal regions of the mandible because there are permanent tooth germs in the bone, which may be damaged as they lie close to the lower border of the mandible. If there is displacement of a body fracture anteriorly, then small plates placed close to the lower border may be necessary preferably only into the outer bone plate. Often simple intermaxillary fixation (IMF) and an arch bar attached to the teeth is all that is required. If there is severe pain and multiple fractures, immobilisation of the jaws with IMF is often effective in relieving that pain. Compound fractures, i.e. all those that involve the teeth, require prophylactic antibiotic therapy for 3 days. Normally, penicillin or metronidazole is the most effective and least likely to cause complications. In the older child, the indications for ORIF (Figs. 33.22A and B) tend to be failed conservative treatment, overriding of fragments with opening and closing of the jaws, severe loss of ramus height, displacement of the condyle into the middle cranial fossa, which requires

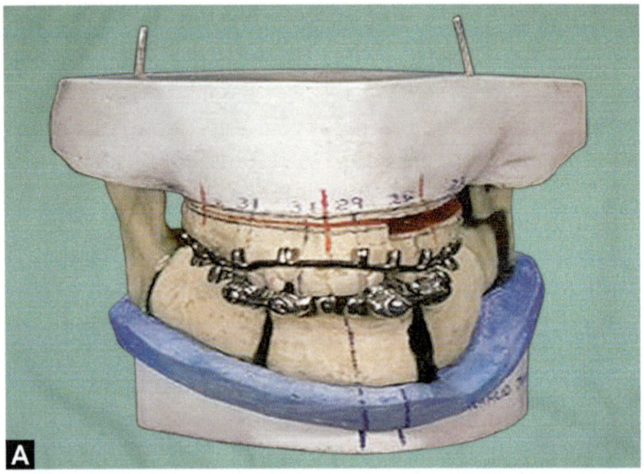

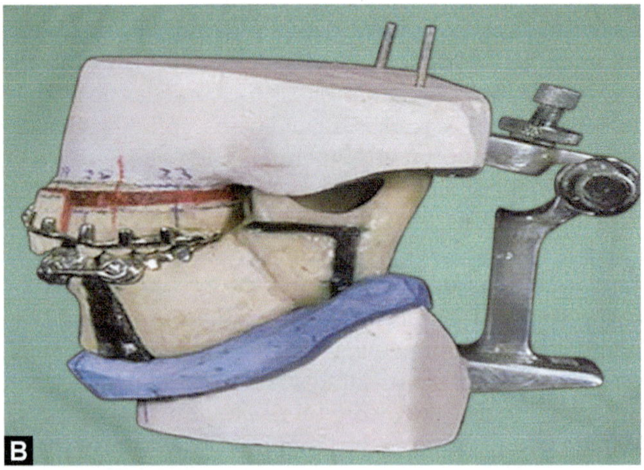

Figures 33.21A and B Complex osteotomy model surgery for post-ankylotic deformity correction.

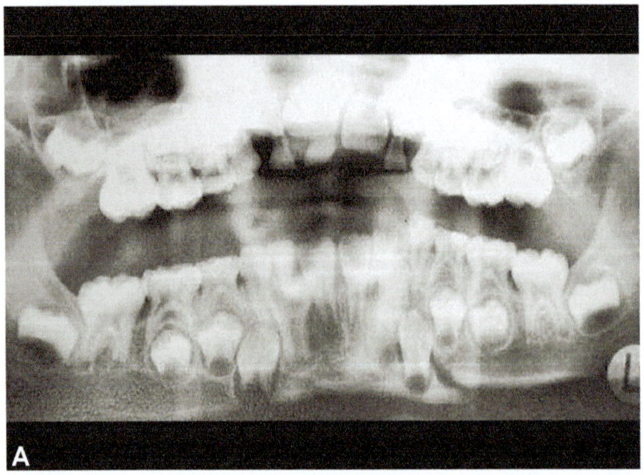

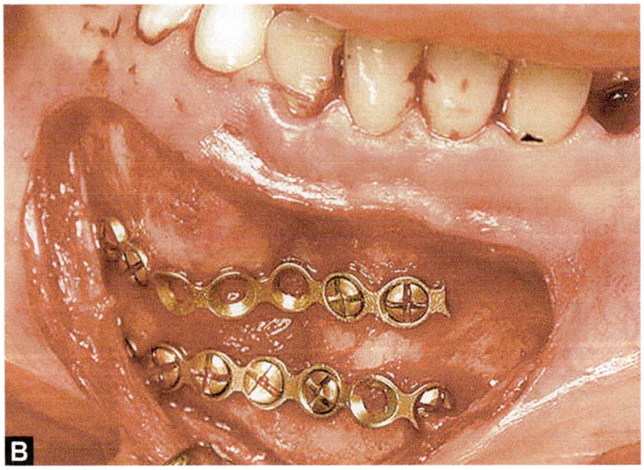

Figures 33.22A and B Body fracture mandible. Internal fixation—advantages—open approach, sub-periosteal dissection, anatomic reduction and improved nutrition. No airway compromise. Increased compliance.

open reduction and careful mobilisation out of that area. Compound fractures require copious irrigation and cleansing of the area. Removal of any non-viable bone may be undertaken although if clean as much as possible should be preserved. For multiple fractures, a simple splint over the teeth and placement of circumferential wires around the mandible to hold the splint in place and the fracture fragments is often the simplest effective treatment. Elastic IMF for traction may be applied between the mandible and maxilla if there is a significant malocclusion, especially strata if there is an AOB. Long-term follow-up is necessary to ensure growth occurs normally, and the occlusion is maintained without the development of an AOB in bilateral fractures. It is also important to keep a watch on the teeth as damage to them, especially when they are displaced or depressed into the bone may result in failure of eruption and infection. It is also essential to identify fractured teeth, which may initially not be obvious especially in the molar region but they are painful or rapidly become so. Consideration should be given also to the use of resorbable (polylactide plates) in children.

Complications of Mandibular Fractures

The common fracture complications in the child are malocclusion of the teeth and hypermobility, asymmetry of the jaw and dysfunction sometimes related to a degeneration or severe damage to the condyles. There is a necessity to maintain good oral hygiene otherwise caries and periodontal disease lead on to dental infections. Where there is gross malunion and displacement of the mandible posteriorly, there is a risk of impairment of the airway. Damage to the inferior dental nerves may occur and with an external approach, there is a risk of damage to the facial nerve and persistent fistulae and occasionally Frey syndrome (gustatory sweating). Severe injuries and post-traumatic stress syndrome may occur, especially when there is residual deformity, which will require psychosocial support. It is important to take radiographs post-operatively to ensure reduction of the mandible has been effective, and especially when closed management has been undertaken. The usual radiographs required pre- and post-operatively are an orthopantomogram (OPT) and a posteroanterior view of the mandible; occasionally coronal computed tomography (CT) scans for condylar fractures, and appropriate intraoral views of damaged teeth.

Nasal Bone Fractures

The other fractures that sometimes cause significant problems are nasal bone fractures when they occur early in life. With simple breaks, there is no problem but when there has been road traffic trauma and severe displacement of the nasoethmoid, this may cause significant deformity, especially when accompanied by craniofacial injuries. This is uncommon except in major high velocity injuries and occasionally in a sporting injury. As most of the nose is cartilaginous, fractures are often difficult to diagnose and they are easily missed. Simple elevation of the nasal bones is usually all that is needed to avoid nasal obstruction and significant deformity. There may be overlying skin damage. Sometimes intranasal Gelfoam packing is helpful for a week. Follow-up should continue over at least 1 year. Only rarely is open reduction appropriate but septal straightening may be required. Care should be taken not to remove any bone fragments in that situation. Epistaxis may be treated with an intranasal pack and any septal haematomata should be evacuated. Infection rarely occurs. Occasionally, synechiae may require treatment. Diagnostically conventional radiographs are unhelpful but for the more severe injury CT scanning should be undertaken.

Mid-face (Maxillary) Fractures

Mid-face and panfacial fractures are rare in young children due to the lack of sinus cavities and the smallness of the mid-face. They are in the older child **(Figs. 33.23A to E)** **(Box 33.14)** usually associated with the orbits and nasoethmoidal complex, and these need to be carefully assessed and reduced, avoiding generally open reduction of the nasoethmoidal complex. There may be airway problems and haemorrhage, and there is commonly an associated head injury. Cervical spine injuries must be excluded. CT scanning is essential for diagnosis whereas conventional radiographs may be taken and used for the mandible and mid-face, CT scanning in the coronal and axial planes will give details of all the fractures present. It is normal to wait a few days, up to 7 days, before exploration of the fractures by which time most of the swelling should have settled. For Le Fort II and III fractures **(Figs. 33.24A to C)**, cerebrospinal fluid (CSF) leaks need to be identified, most stop following fracture fixation, but prophylactic antibiotics are given to prevent meningitis. With severe craniofacial injuries, a coronal flap is required to expose the frontal region and to deal with any intracranial problems. This gives good exposure also to the lateral, superior and medial orbits and plate fixation is widely used and in young children usually micro- or mini-plates will be required **(Figs. 33.25A and B)**. As far as IMF is concerned, this should be avoided unless there are also fractures of the mandible in which case it may be necessary.

BOX 33.14 Central middle-third clinical features.
Dish-face deformity
Bilateral periorbital haematoma
Sub-conjunctival haemorrhage
Cerebrospinal fluid rhinorrhoea
Diplopia
Infraorbital anaesthesia
Anterior open bite (AOB)—retroposition of maxilla and trismus

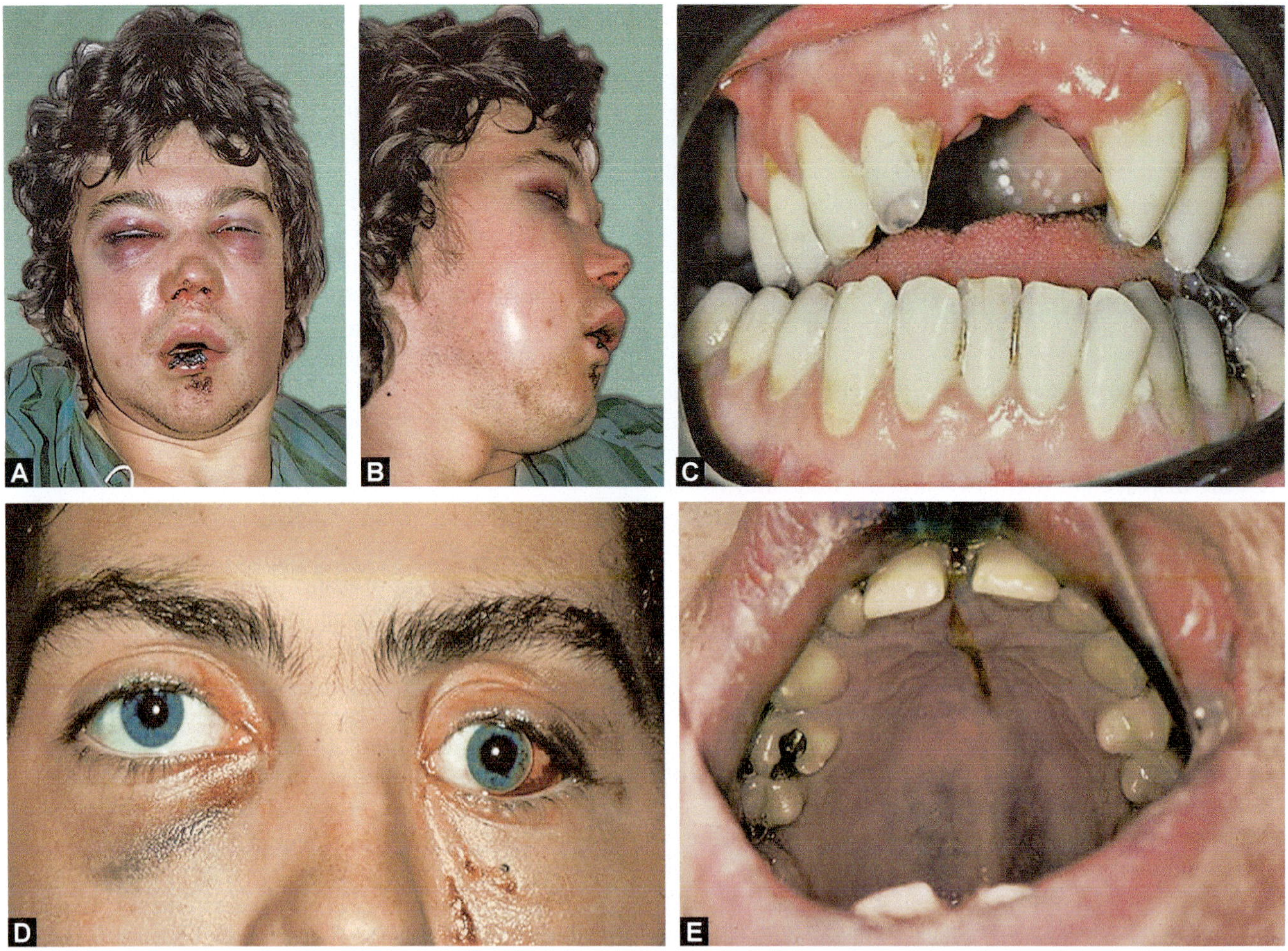

Figures 33.23A to E (A and B) Clinical features— Le Fort III fractures with anterior open bite; (C) Anterior open bite; (D) Left orbital displacement (late stage); (E) Split palate.

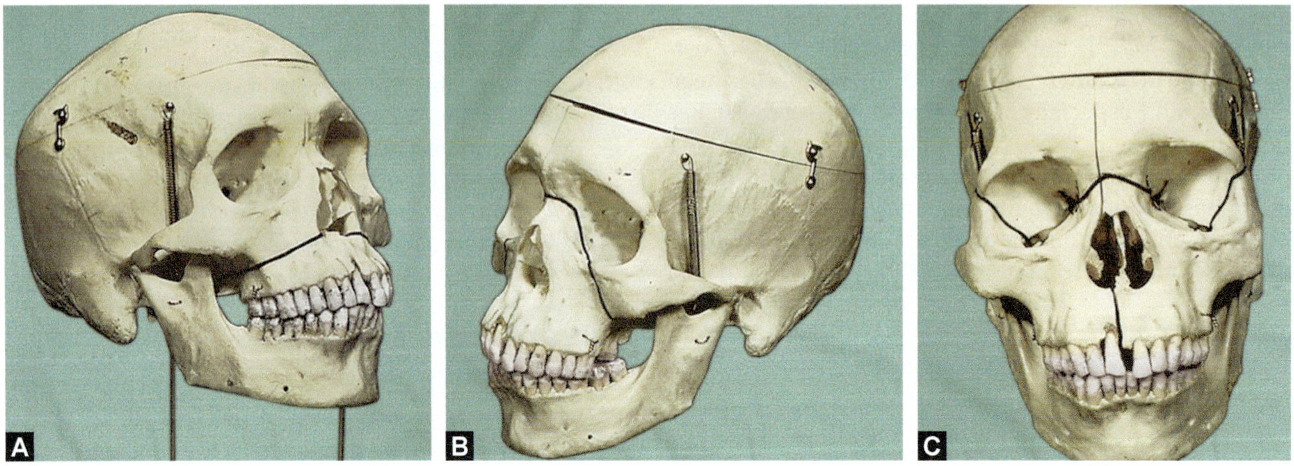

Figures 33.24A to C Le Fort maxillary fracture lines (adult skulls)—vertical and horizontal mid-face fracture patterns: (A) Le Fort I (Guerin fracture), dentoalveolar fractures; (B) Le Fort II pyramidal fracture, cerebrospinal fluid (CSF) leak; (C) Le Fort III craniofacial dysjunction and palatal split likely, and CSF leak.

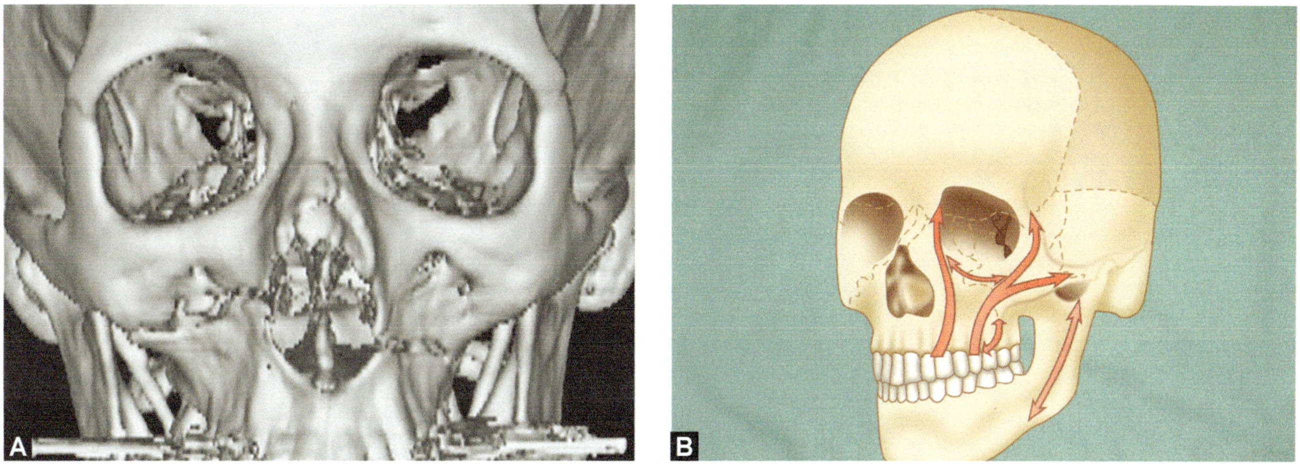

Figures 33.25A and B CT scan—Le Fort I fractures. Maxillary bony buttresses distribute forces through the facial skeleton and cranium and can be used for siting bone plates.

Healing is very rapid with fractures involving the dentoalveolar complex and they may require a Le Fort I incision to expose the fracture sites in the buccal and labial sulci. It is important to retain the teeth and limit the periodontal damage as far as possible. Plating should be considered carefully to avoid damage to the roots of the teeth as well as any underlying unerupted teeth. It is important with high impact trauma when there are major facial injuries to assess the extent of the comminution and to suspend the soft tissues as there can be significant soft-tissue damage in these cases. Otherwise, they tend to drag down the lateral canthi and the medial canthi may become detached and need repositioning with screws and micro-plates. As far as gunshot wounds in children are concerned, these are rare in the Western world, but they need to be treated with care, preserving all bone fragments, removing only foreign bodies and usually waiting before exploration for at least 48 hours for the swelling to settle. Any necrotic tissue will need to be identified and removed and frequently suction drainage will also be necessary. Where there is bone loss after limited debridement, the removal of dead tissue must be undertaken as far as possible, ideally with primary closure and with the later opportunity for secondary repair of any major defects in the oronasal cavities. With orofacial injuries, careful soft-tissue repair is necessary with the preservation of all viable soft tissue. Where there is doubt about the vitality of tissue, it is important that there is good drainage and the dead spaces are eliminated to prevent infection and antibiotic cover is given in that situation.

BOX 33.15 Orbital and frontal fractures.

- After age 7 years, major growth of the sinuses occurs
- Orbital growth is then complete
- Traumatic floor and medial wall defects are not common

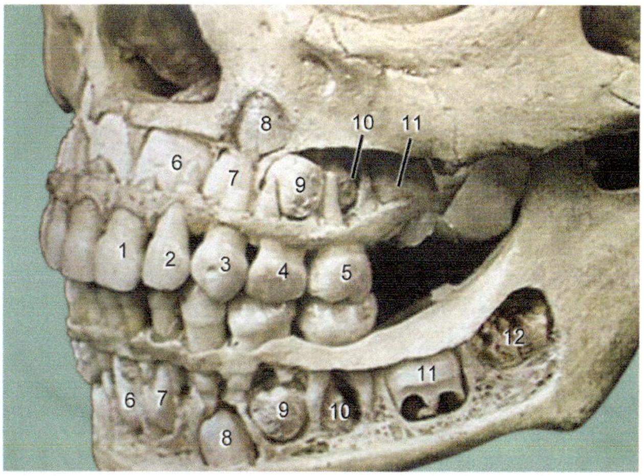

Figure 33.26 Very small maxillary sinus in a young child.

Zygomatico-orbital Injuries

Zygomatico-orbital injuries **(Box 33.15)** are uncommon in young children **(Fig. 33.26)** but become increasingly frequent over the age of 12–13 years as the zygoma or malar bone is traumatised in sports injuries, road traffic accidents and assaults **(Figs. 33.27A to D)**. Clinically there will be loss of the cheek prominence, swelling, unilateral epistaxis, infraorbital anaesthesia **(Figs. 33.28A and B)** usually a segmental sub-conjunctival haemorrhage, often diplopia, either proptosis initially sometimes followed by enophthalmos when the orbit is enlarged or orbital contents are lost out of the orbit in a blow-out fracture; less commonly with a blow in fracture the reverse occurs. Investigations undertaken include radiographs 10° and 30° occipitomental views and CT scanning ocular injury must be excluded with a check on acuity, field eye movements and fundi. Comminution and orbital floor

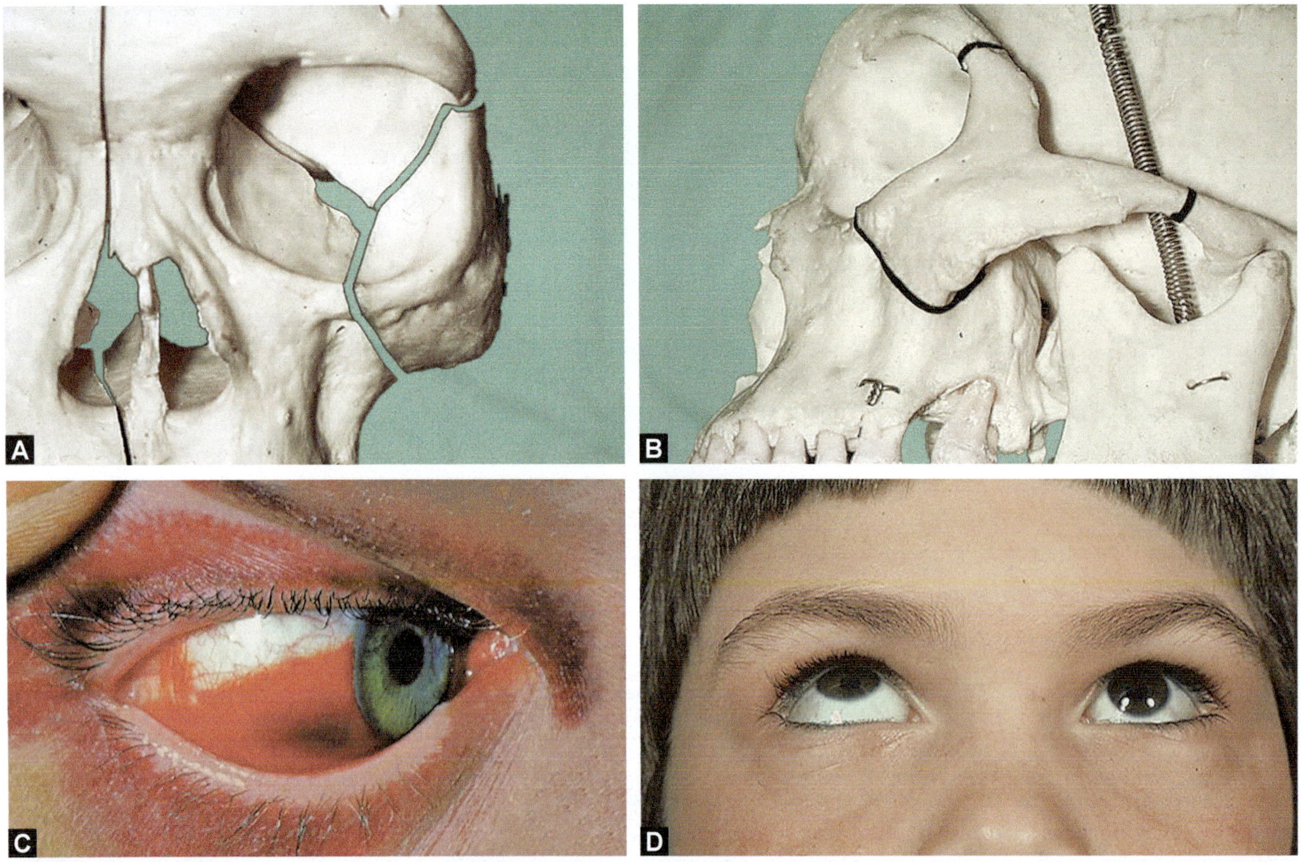

Figures 33.27A to D Malar complex fractures right sub-conjunctival haemorrhage and left orbital floor blow-out fracture.

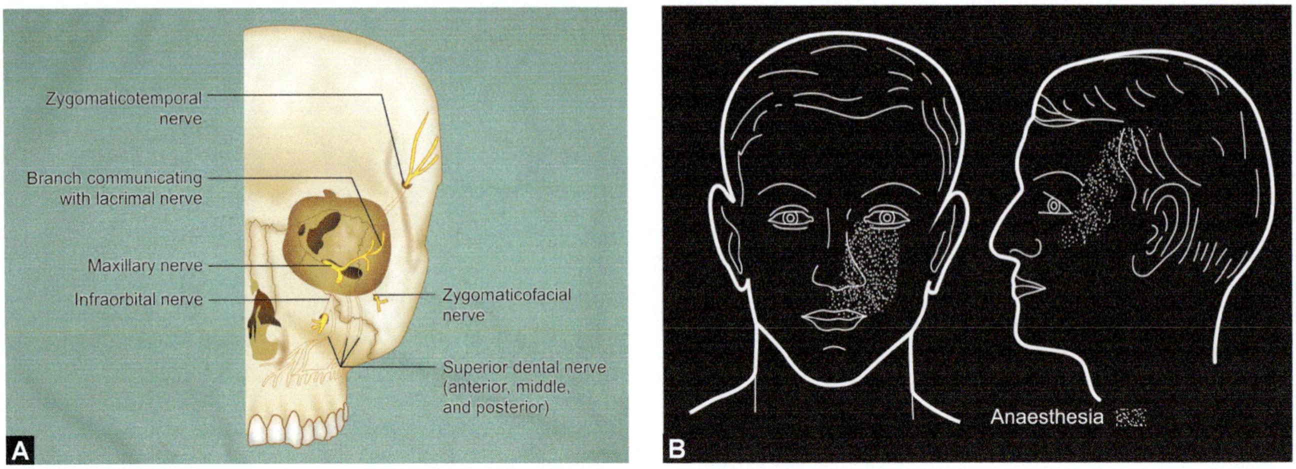

Figures 33.28A and B Sensory changes can affect the infraorbital, zygomaticofacial/temporal nerve branches.

blow-outs can be identified on the CT and magnetic resonance imaging (MRI) scans. Treatment of the fractures usually at the FZ suture, zygomatic arch and infraorbital margin is by reduction and fixation with titanium miniplates. Blow-out defects can be covered with cranial bone graft or titanium mesh; post-operatively eye observations are essential to identify early retrobulbar haemorrhages **(Figs. 33.29A to C** and **Box 33.16)**.

Soft-tissue Facial Injuries

Soft-tissue injuries, particularly dog bites, are not uncommon in children. Sixty per cent occurs in children under 15 years of age and in 84% the animal is well known to the child. These require careful debridement, preservation of tissue and suturing with antibiotic cover. Other injuries need to be excluded such as damage to nerves, blood vessels and ducts. A tetanus toxoid booster should

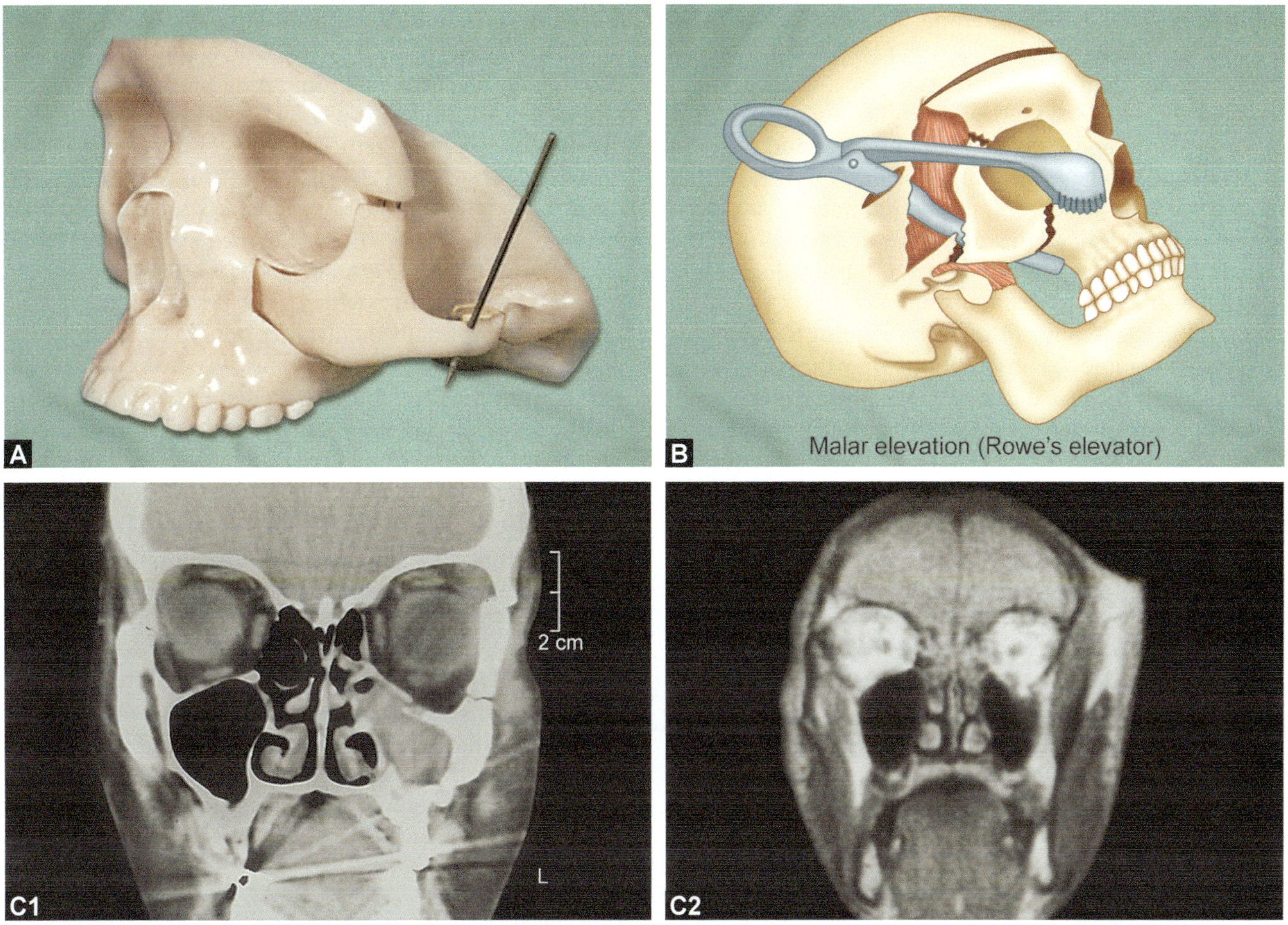

Figures 33.29A to C (A) Common fractures sites; (B) Reduction of fractured malar; (C1 and C2) CT/MRI orbital blow-out fracture.

BOX 33.16 Henderson classification—malar fractures.

Type 1: Undisplaced
Type 2: Arch fracture
Type 3: Tripod fracture with intact frontozygomatic (FZ) suture
Type 4: Tripod fracture with distraction FZ suture
Type 5: Orbital floor blow-out with type 3, 4 or 7
Type 6: Orbital rim fracture
Type 7: Comminuted and complex fractures

be given unless they have been immunised for a shorter period than 5 years. In most cases, the severe soft-tissue injury will be repaired under general anaesthesia. There should be an appropriately wide exploration of the wound. Management of lacerations in an excised wound requires an understanding of the relaxed skin tension lines of the face and using them to one's advantage. Scars along these lines have a better prognosis than when perpendicular to them. A ragged laceration along the skin tension line can be excised safely, but if perpendicular to that minimal excision should take place. Primary closure should be undertaken within 24 hours. Animal bites tend to be potentially infected with polymicrobial bacteria. Human bites tend to have more anaerobic organisms and bacteroides, *Staphylococcus aureus* and α-haemolytic streptococci. These again require antibiotic prophylaxis. Careful washing of the tissues, no scrubbing but washing with betadine, and a thorough irrigation of the area is very important with closure in layers. Sutures or cyanoacrylate should be used for skin closure. Sutures should be removed by 5 days and where necessary supported with steri-strips.

PATHOLOGY OF THE JAWS AND ADJACENT STRUCTURES

Finally, there are a number of conditions related to the jaws, which are pathological in nature, that are developmentally related to the teeth and their supporting structures. Cysts are common in relation to teeth, and these are frequently periapical cysts associated with dental infection. They may also be developmental such as keratocysts and dentigerous cysts, which tend to surround the crowns of unerupted teeth. These erode the bone of the maxilla and mandible and may be quite large in size before they give any symptoms. Often only they when become infected they will start to leak into the oral cavity. Most of these are benign and adequate drainage and removal of the cystic lining of the dentigerous cyst will allow that tooth to erupt into the oral cavity. Keratocysts are often found at the sites of teeth particularly in the ramus of the mandible. They tend to erode the inner portion of the mandible and require careful removal as they tend to recur. All tissue removed should be sent for histopathology. When keratocysts are multiple, they may be associated with the Gorlin-Goltz syndrome or basal cell naevus syndrome. At puberty, they start to develop basal cell carcinomata, particularly on the face and upper half of the body. These are normally rare at a young age group, but by 25 years, they are commonly seen in this condition. It is, therefore, important to recognise this syndrome in children early so that long-term follow-up may be carried out. Another syndrome that may present in children is Gardner syndrome where there are multiple osteomata, often affecting the jaws and facial bones and frequently accompanied by supernumerary teeth. There are often soft-tissue lesions in the skin, e.g. fibromata, lipomata, and epithelial cysts but more seriously it is associated with polyposis coli with adenomatous polyps, which eventually become malignant after puberty and a total colectomy is required. There are few rare tumours in early life affecting the jaws. In the midline of the anterior maxilla, the neuroectodermal tumour of infancy is occasionally seen during the first year of life as a bluish soft tumour displacing erupting teeth, and here surgical excision is curative **(Figs. 33.30A to D)**. One serious and more common tumour is the ameloblastoma, which arises from ameloblasts, cells associated with the development of the enamel of the teeth **(Figs. 33.31A to D)**. These are locally invasive jaw tumours, which may become quite large. They do not normally metastasise but are locally invasive and can spread into the soft tissues, e.g. from the maxilla into the temporal region and medial to the mandible in the ramus area and can invade the middle cranial fossa. If they remain within bone, they can be removed by a segmental excision followed by bone grafting of the mandible. For the maxilla, excision with at least a 1–2 cm margin is essential as it is for the mandible. Ameloblastomata may arise in keratocysts, and they may be associated with unerupted teeth, treatment remains the same.

True malignancies of the jaws are rarely seen in children, e.g. osteosarcoma, chondrosarcoma, rhabdomyosarcoma and condylar synovial sarcoma. Occasionally, secondary tumours present in the jaws **(Figs. 33.32A and B)**.

Langerhans tumours (histiocytosis X) may present in the jaws and skull **(Figs. 33.33A to C)**. With surgical

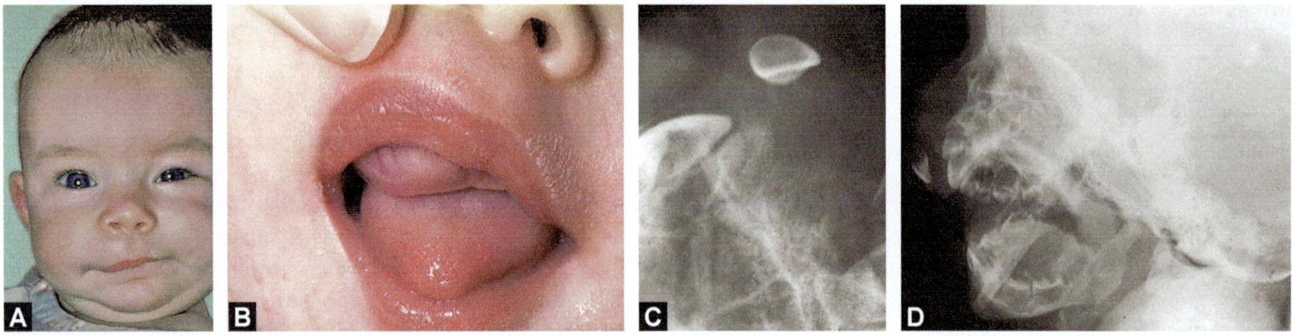

Figures 33.30A to D Neuroectodermal tumour of infancy. Benign aggressive lesion in anterior maxilla at 6 months.

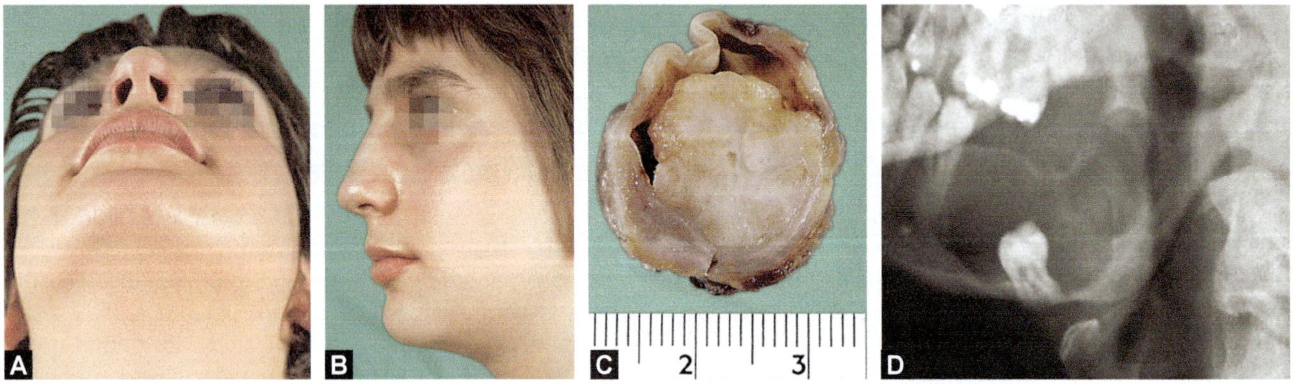

Figures 33.31A to D Ameloblastoma arising from a dentigerous cyst.

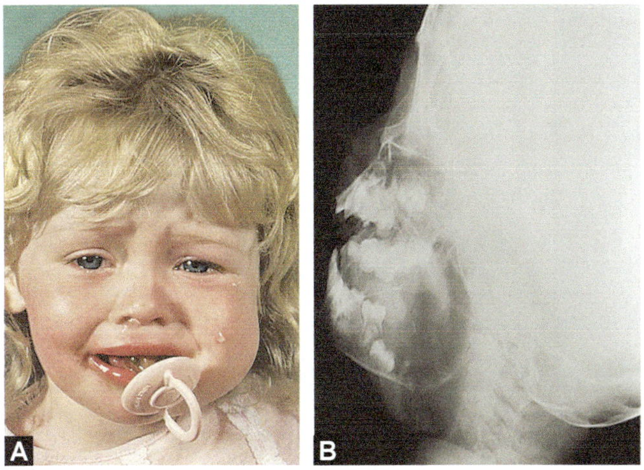

Figures 33.32A and B Secondary neuroblastoma mandible.

excision, radiotherapy and chemotherapy many of these are curable. There are other benign enlargements, which affect the jaws such as osteomata, ossifying fibromata (Figs. 33.34A to C) and fibrous dysplasia of bone (Figs. 33.35A to D). The latter may be monostotic or occasionally polyostotic or as in the McCune Albright syndrome a rare variant, the diagnosis is primarily clinical, early menarche, café-au-lait patches and gross fibrous dysplastic bone confirmed by histopathology and radiology, occasionally fractures occur, foramina in the skull may tend to narrow causing pain and cranial nerve symptoms. Surgical reduction of bony overgrowth after puberty can improve the appearance.

Following resection for locally invasive lesions, reconstruction of the defect may either be by bone graft usually from the ilium or alternatively by the use of distraction. Sizeable bony defects may be closed in the mandible in this way. It is helpful to maintain the normal position of the fragments after resection has been undertaken so that the form/shape of the mandible may be maintained, and this is most easily achieved with the use of pins into the adjacent normal bone prior to the resection or by reconstruction plates. There are other rare lesions

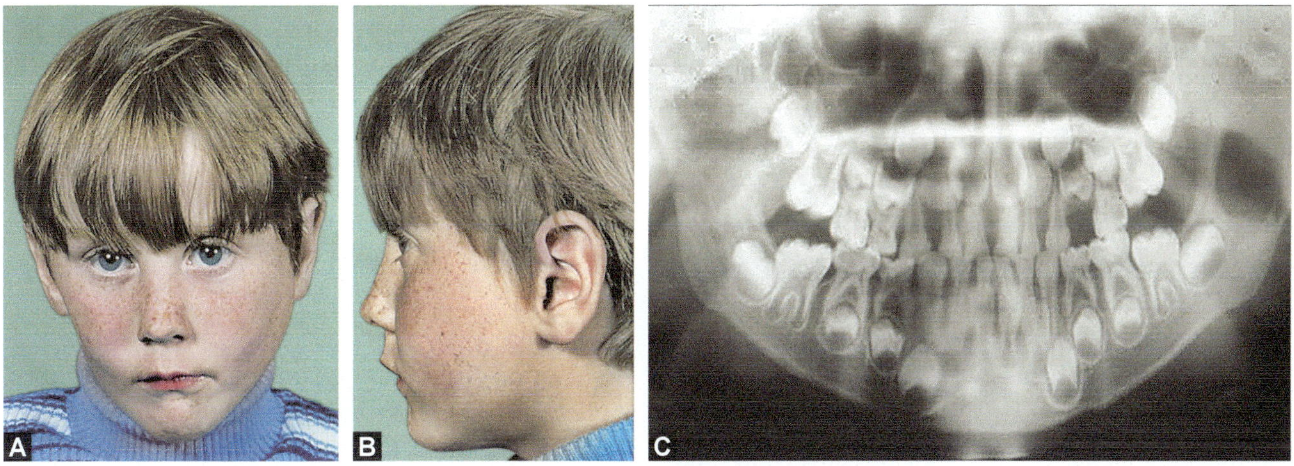

Figures 33.33A to C Hand-Schüllerchristian disease—lesion in left mandibular ramus (histiocytosis X).

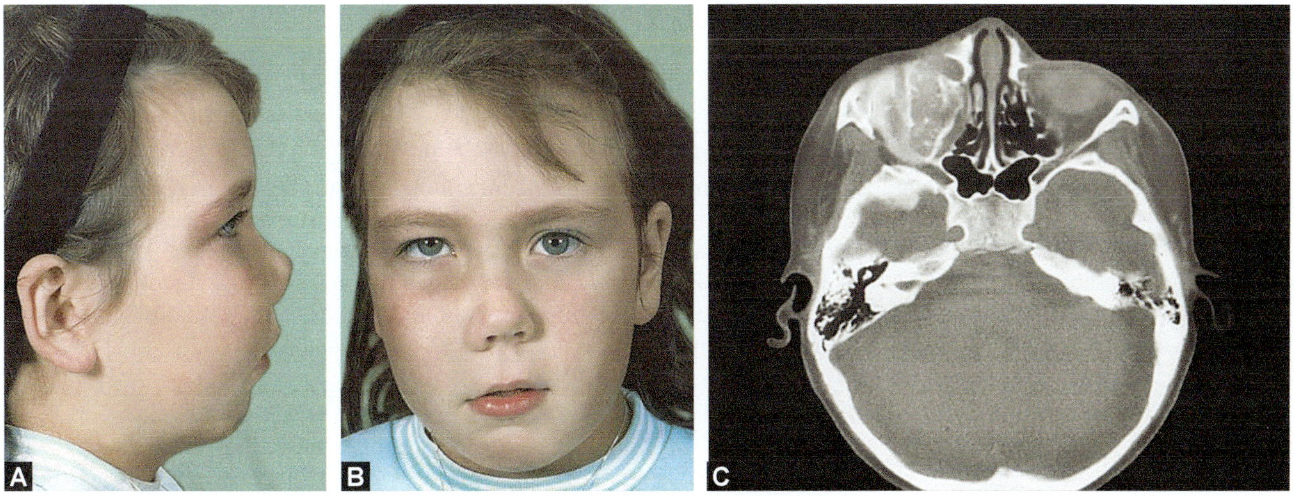

Figures 33.34A to C Ossifying fibroma—rapidly growing benign neoplasm of the right mandible.

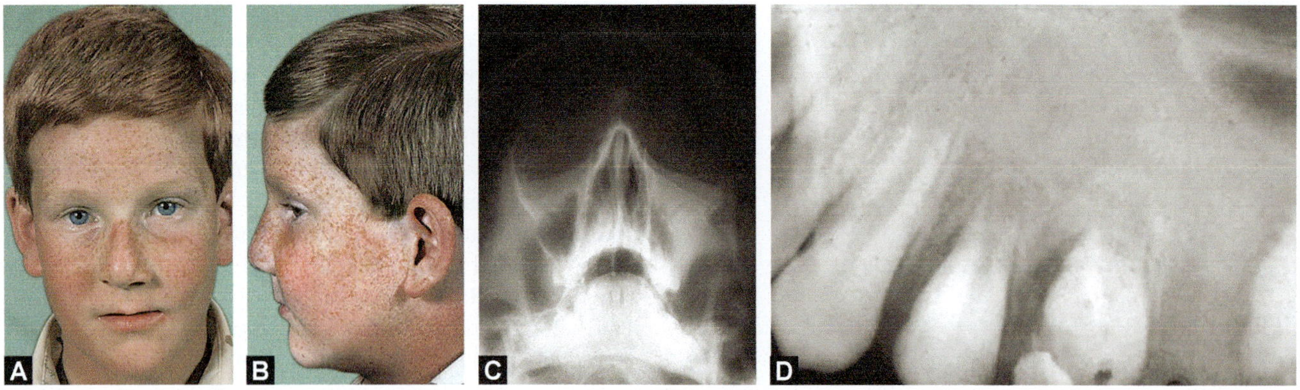

Figures 33.35A to D Fibrous dysplasia of left maxilla—continues to grow usually till growth has ceased.

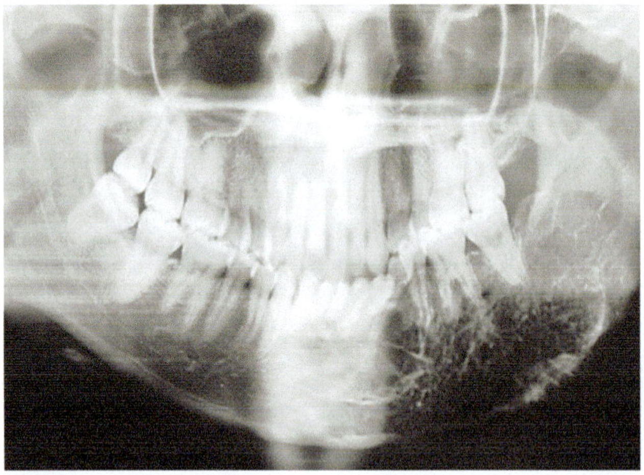

Figure 33.36 Haemangioma of the left mandible.

of the jaws such as giant cell tumours, aneurysmal bone cysts and other growth abnormalities. The latter is seen occasionally with gigantism and acromegaly. From time to time, a meningocoele and craniofacial clefting defects involve not only the naso-orbital area but also the maxilla itself. Management of these conditions is largely in the province of the neurosurgeon but reconstruction will be needed by the maxillofacial surgeon.

VASCULAR ANOMALIES

They are common in children and frequently affect the face and oral cavity. They are dynamically classified into low-flow haemangiomas and high-flow arteriovenous malformations (AVMs), and there is an intermediate group. The difference between them is that haemangiomata histologically show an increase in endothelium and mast cells whereas malformations have normal endothelium and mast cells. In addition to that, there is a tumour group of haemangiopericytoma, chemodectoma, glomus tumours and angiosarcomata. AVMs include port-wine stain, Sturge-Weber, Beckwith-Wiedemann and Maffucci syndromes as well as post-traumatic malformations. In infants, the first sign may be a red mark on the face, which develops into a strawberry naevus which grows rapidly, stabilises and in 70% involutes around 7 years of age leaving a small scarred area. Treatment is usually not required unless, e.g. it presents on an eyelid and interferes with vision or is on the lips/nose and ulcerates, bleeds, or becomes painful or infected, when treatment with cryo/laser therapy or excision can be helpful. Other rarer lesions are Kasabach-Merritt syndrome and haemangiomatosis, which can be complicated by disseminated intravascular coagulation problems. The jaws **(Fig. 33.36)** are relatively rarely involved in AVMs. Investigation of these by CT scanning, angiography and MRI will identify high-flow lesions these require embolisation of the affected vessels and surgical removal 48 hours later. A variety of agents are available for highly selective embolisation, e.g. gelatine sponge, collagen, alcohol, PV (polyvinyl) particles, coils and balloons. For other lesions, e.g. haemangiomata intralesional steroids, hot hypertonic saline, sclerotherapy, laser therapy and tattooing with titanium oxide are widely used.

CONCLUSION

Paediatric maxillofacial surgery is an area of special interest, which requires the close co-operation of several paediatric specialities, anaesthetists and a committed maxillofacial surgeon who frequently needs the help of the paediatrician and the skills of ophthalmic, neurosurgical and ear, nose and throat (ENT) colleagues.

CHAPTER 34

Paediatric Reconstruction Surgery

Martyn H.C. Webster

INTRODUCTION

Reconstruction of certain conditions in paediatrics poses one of the most difficult challenges in reconstruction surgery. In recent years, rapid development of tissue engineering and regenerative medicine brings about a new perspective in reconstructive surgery. However, replacement with autogenous grafts remains the treatment of choice in both adult and paediatric patients. Reconstruction is arranged in a staged fashion. Also reconstruction approach will vary. Needless to say the parent (s) wishes are also critical in the decision-making process. In this chapter only a few conditions have been illustrated because it is impossible to present a comprehensive review on the reconstruction treatment of all conditions seen in a paediatric population.

It is very uncommon for any pigmented skin lesion to develop malignant melanomatous change before puberty. Therefore, the only reason for surgical intervention in children is cosmetic improvement. However, the only exception to this rule is the giant hairy naevus. Giant hairy naevi are present at birth and grow proportionally with the body. There are various kinds of pigmented skin lesions described: flat or raised, hairy or non-hairy, dark or light, small or involving most of the skin surface. Treatment decisions must be individualised. The methods available for removing those too large for excision and suture are excision and grafting, or serial excision and advancement.

In cases of large cavernous haemangiomata involving cheek, shrinkage of tumour can be achieved by injection of sclerosing solution in stages and followed by excision. With strawberry naevus (capillary) the growth usually ceases before the child is 6 months old and then it slowly regresses, the colour pales and disappears, and the swelling usually subsides.

The pulsed dye laser (PDL) is the treatment of choice for port-wine stains. While most patients will show improvement, total clearance of lesions is extremely rare.

Burns in children commonly affect face, neck and chest and can cause cicatricial deformities. This would affect the physical development of children, but also has an impact on their psychological development and well-being. The selection of a reconstruction method depends on the size and shape of the scar, degree of deformity, depth of injury and the condition of the normal tissue around the scar. Commonly used reconstruction methods include local remodelling and suturing after direct scar removal, free skin grafting and local or adjacent flap transplantation.

Microtia creates significant emotional disturbances in children. The deformity, which conceivably might be concealed by a long hairstyle, is not overlooked by the child's friends. Total construction of the auricle is one of the greatest challenges which confront the plastic surgeon. Porous polyethylene has been extensively used in ear reconstructions.

The facial nerve palsy in children is either congenital or acquired. Psychological stress rather than functional impairment has been the critical factor in predicting social impairment and reason for surgery. The options for surgical treatment include a diverse range of surgical techniques including static lifts and slings, nerve repairs, nerve grafts and nerve transfers, regional and microvascular free muscle transfer.

Plastic surgical principles apply also in elective surgery of the hand in reconstruction of congenital malformations, e.g. syndactyly

The method of primary simultaneous lip and nose repair and palate is now usually performed. The operation is performed at the age of 5–6 months, the delay being in order to facilitate extensive and careful dissection and accurate reconstruction of tissue which is already better developed.

Illustrations of a few conditions on the reconstructive treatment are shown in the following **Figures 34.1 to 34.36**.

Index of Illustrations

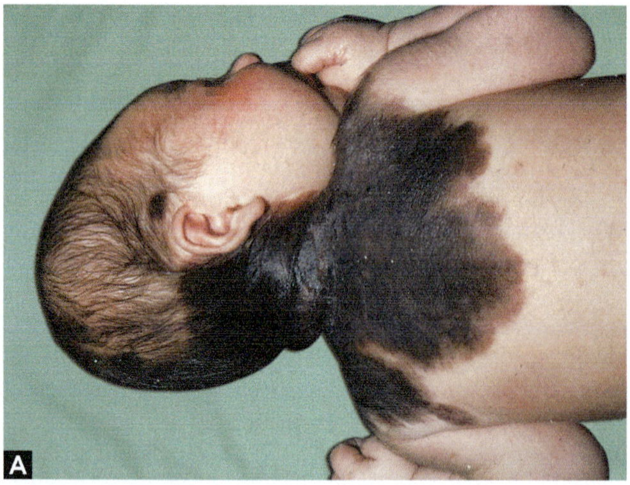

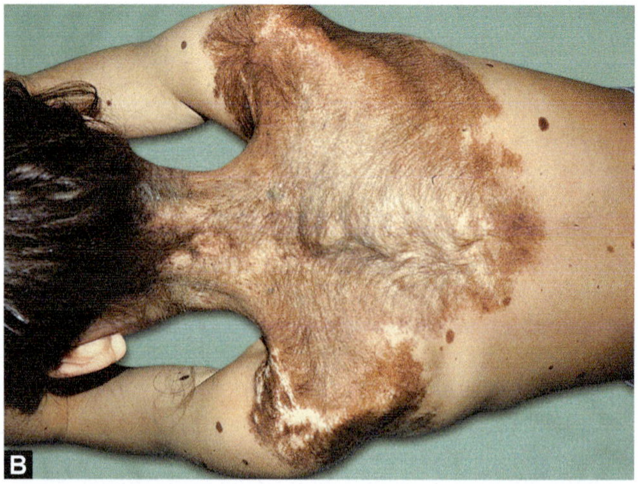

Figures 34.1A and B (A) Neonate with giant hairy naevus of neck and back; (B) Same patient—now a teenager. The naevus was partially shaved in infancy.

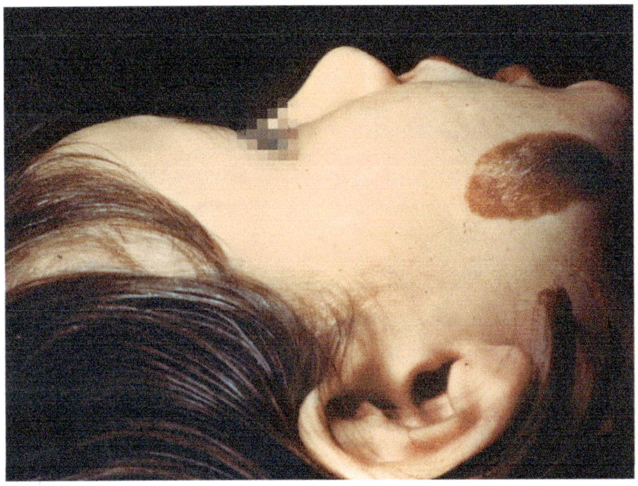

Figure 34.2 Hairy naevus of cheek could be excised for cosmetic reasons.

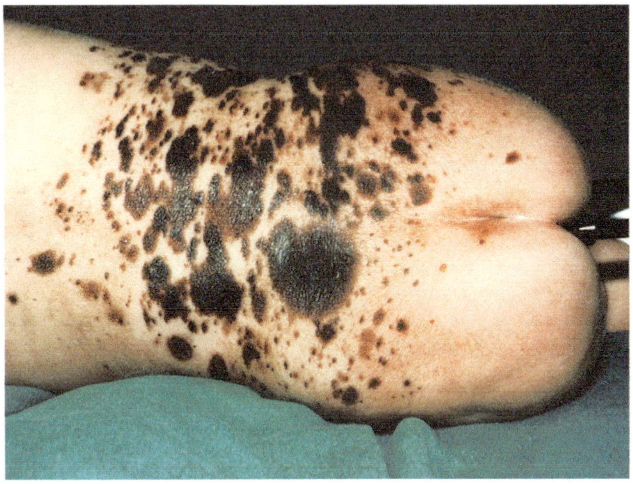

Figure 34.3 Multiple pigmented naevi.

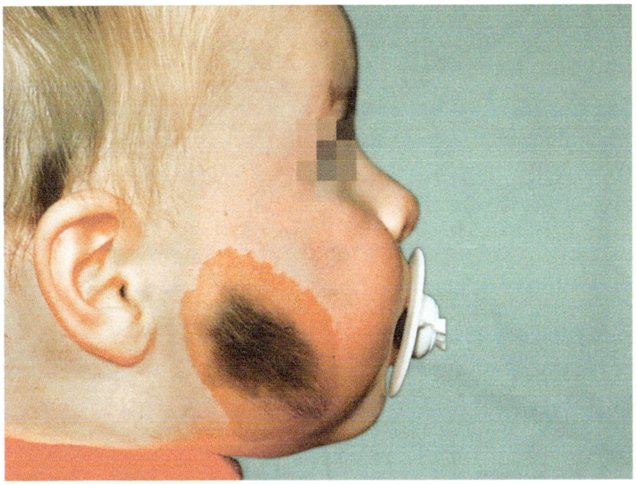

Figure 34.4 Pigmented lesion that could be excised for cosmetic reasons.

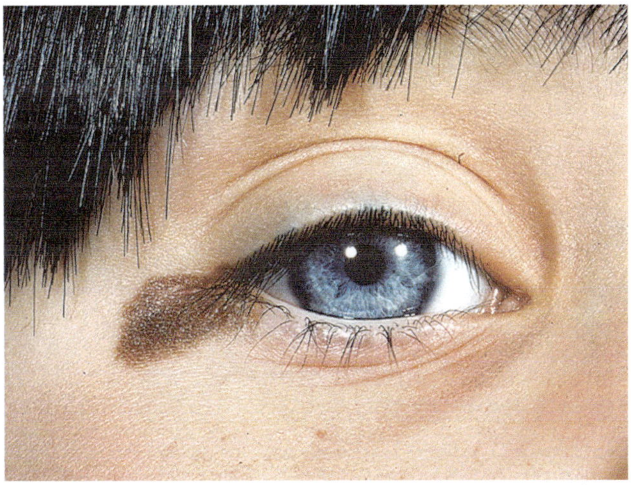

Figure 34.5 Pigmented lesion that could be excised for cosmetic reasons.

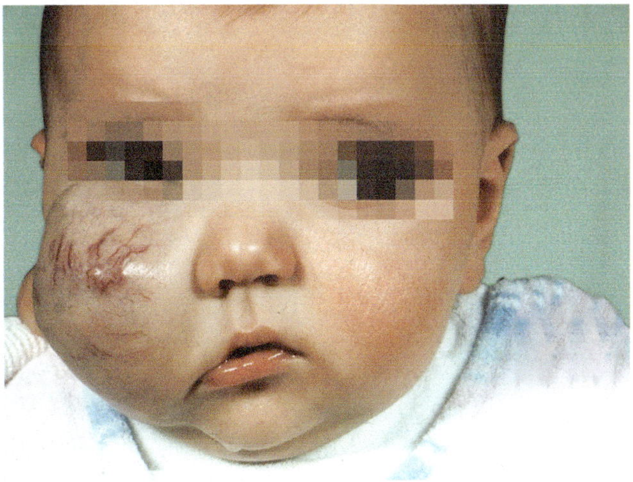

Figure 34.6 Haemangioma right cheek threatening vision of right eye.

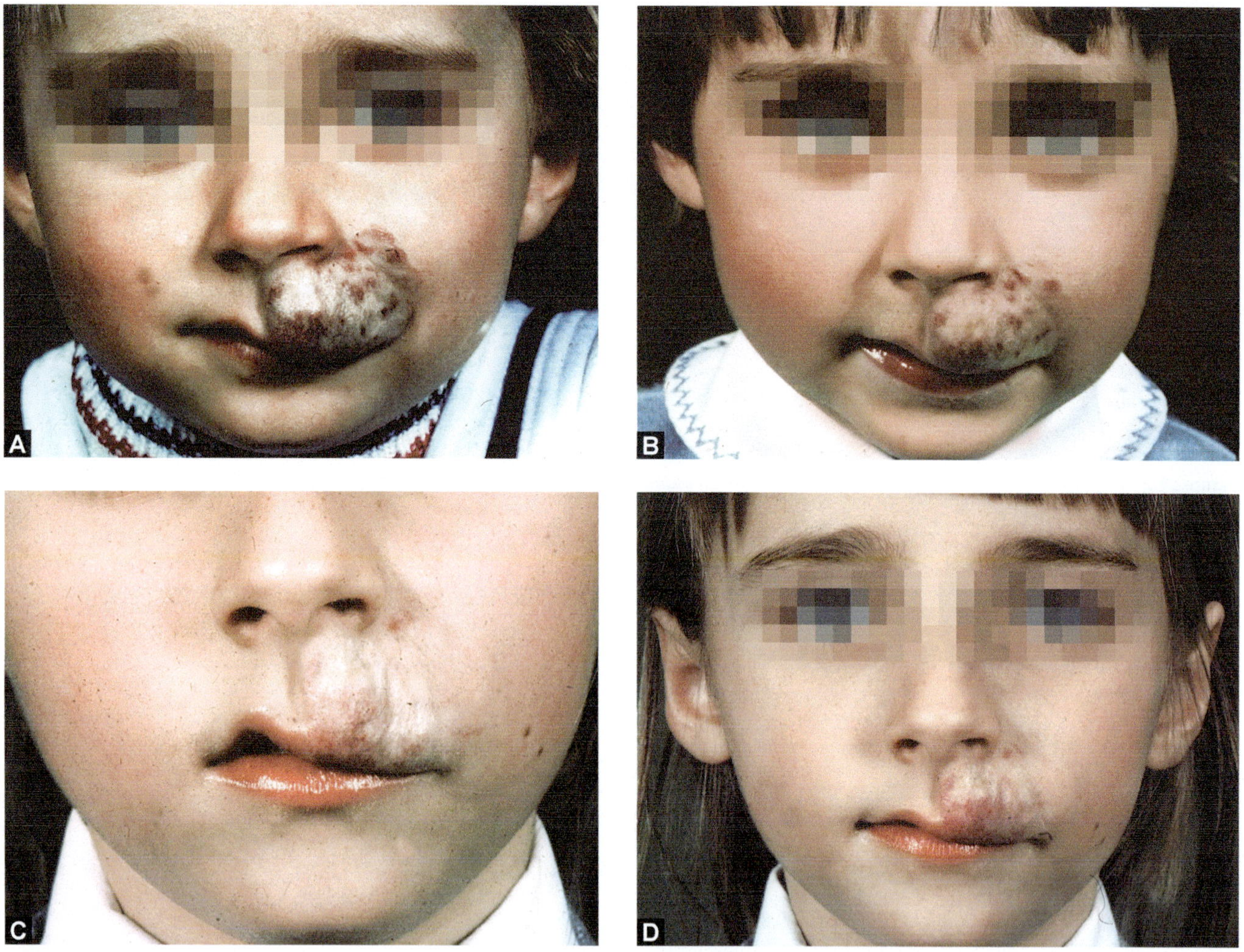

Figures 34.7A to D Strawberry naevus of upper lip. No surgery has been performed, but will require cosmetic skin reduction.

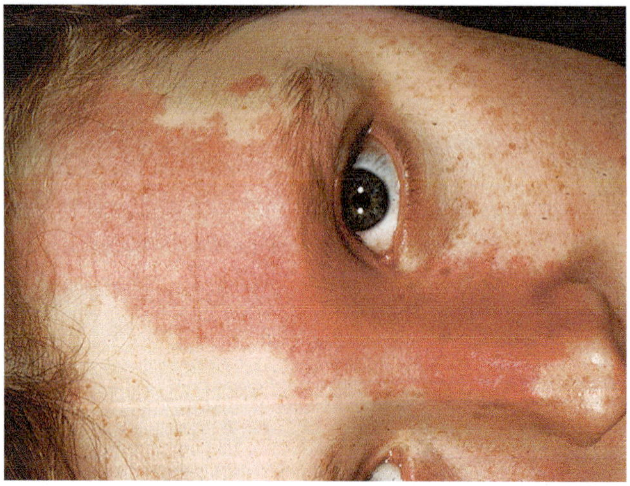

Figure 34.8 Port-wine stain of forehead and nose, could be improved by pulsed dye laser (PDL) treatment.

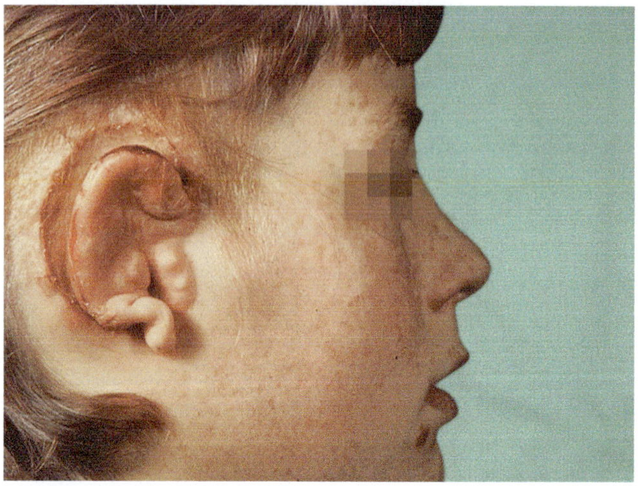

Figure 34.9 Final stage of ear reconstruction, using silastic framework. (*Note:* bulky pinna with lack of fine detail.)

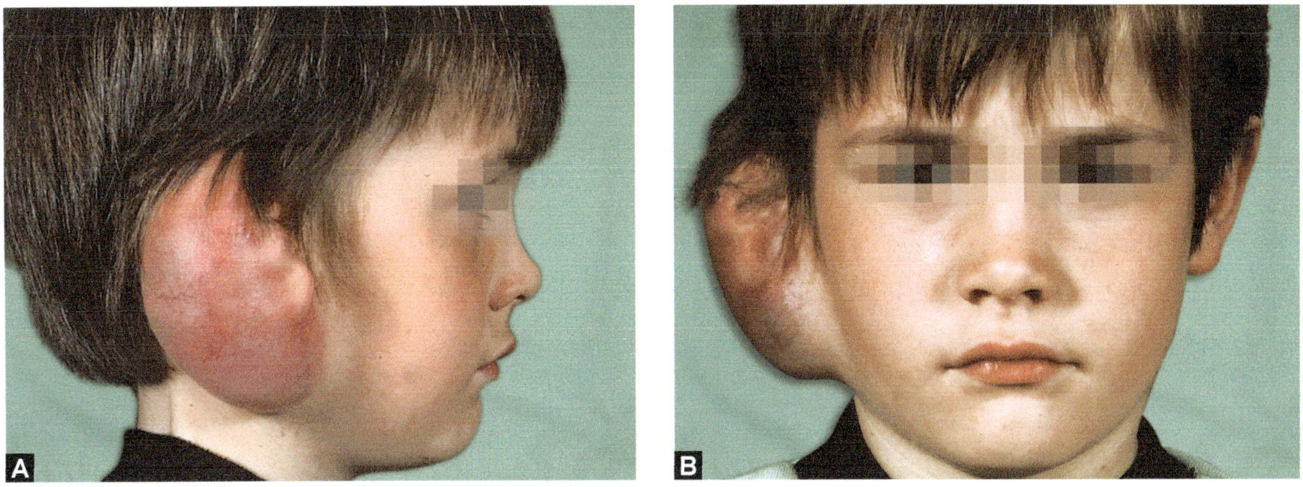

Figures 34.10A and B Tissue expander being used to reconstruct pinna.

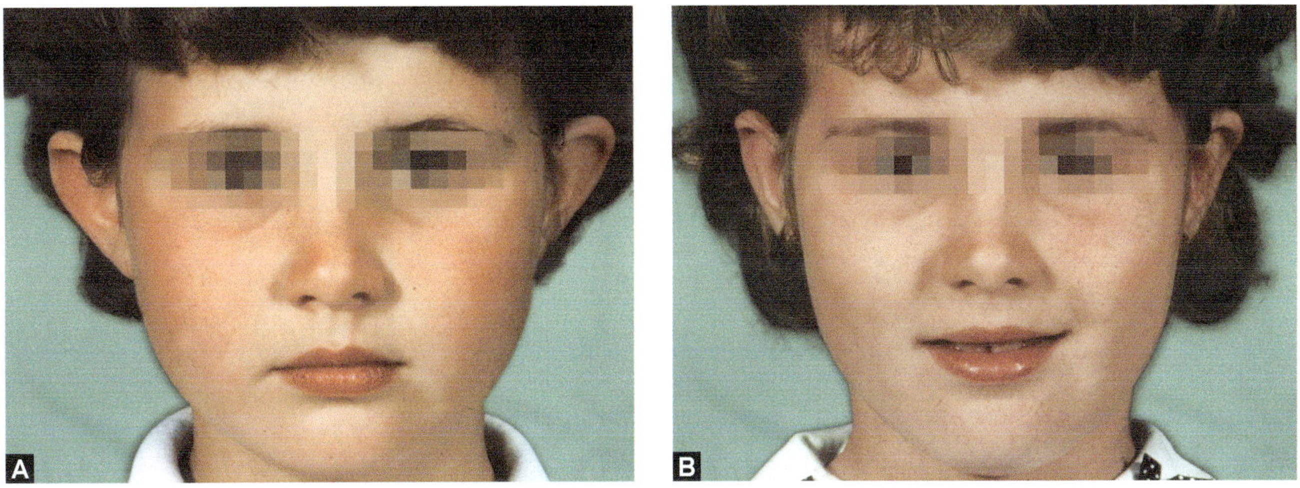

Figures 34.11A and B Pre- and post-bat-ear-correction.

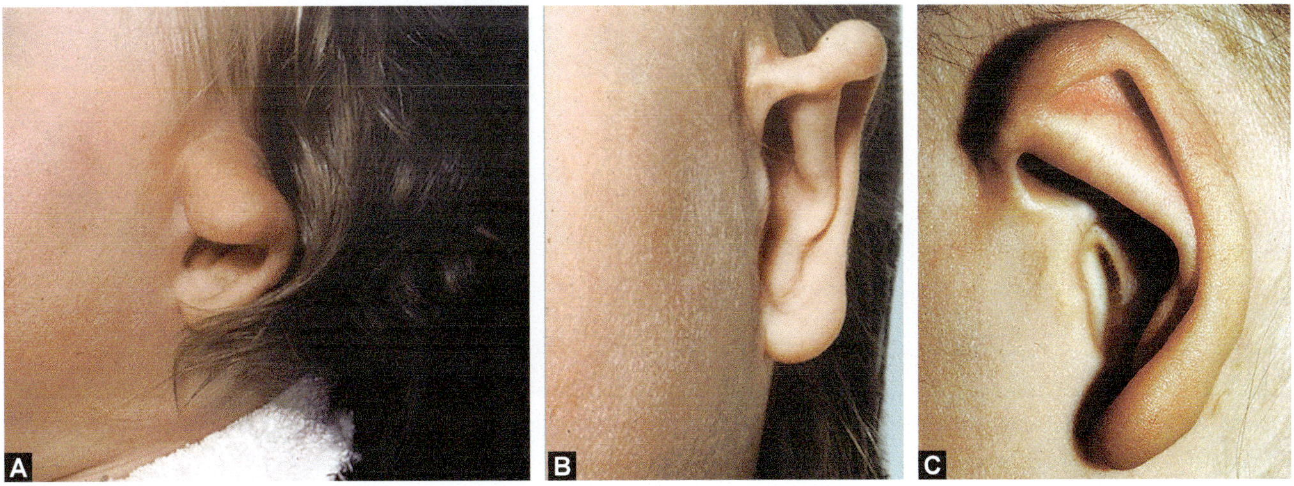

Figures 34.12A to C Post-operative cup ear: Cup ear deformity.

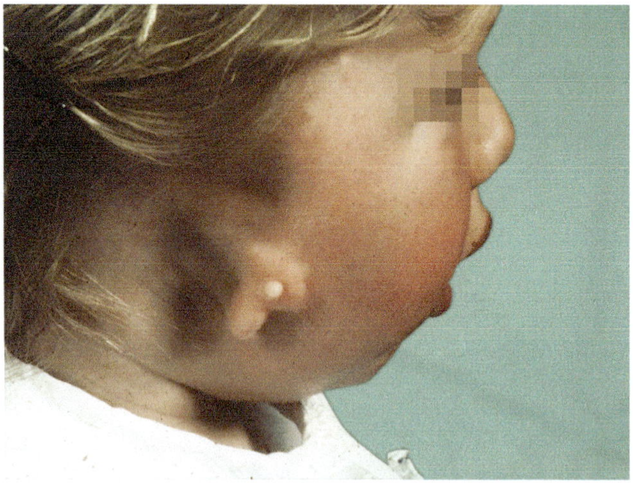

Figure 34.13 Right microtia.

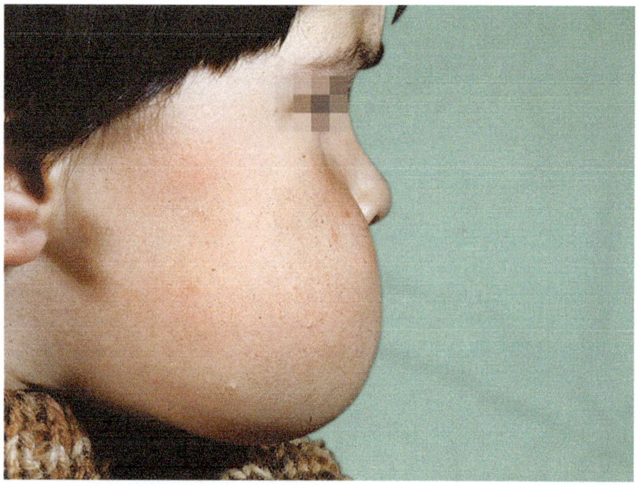

Figure 34.14 Lymphangioma of cheek.

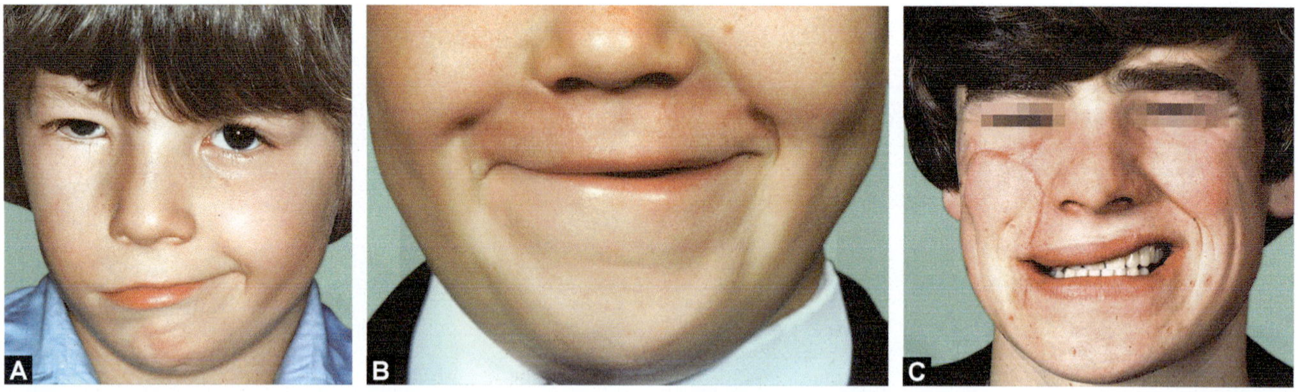

Figures 34.15A to C (A) Right facial palsy; (B) Facial palsy treated with muscle transfer; (C) Same patient later in life.

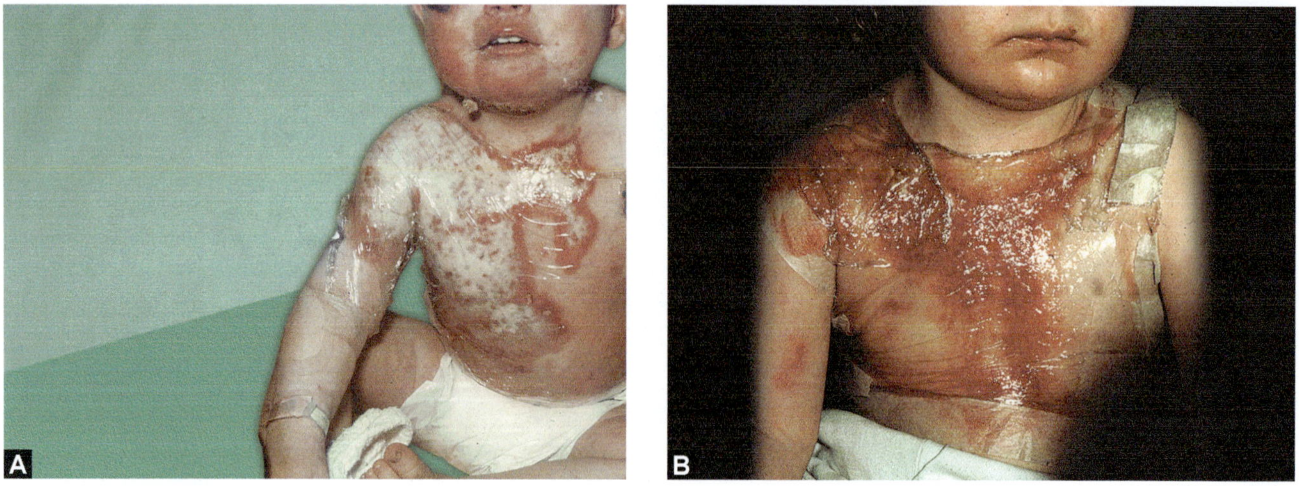

Figures 34.16A and B (A) Typical deep dermal burn caused by child tipping a pan of hot water over himself; (B) Burn healing with dressings but no surgery required.

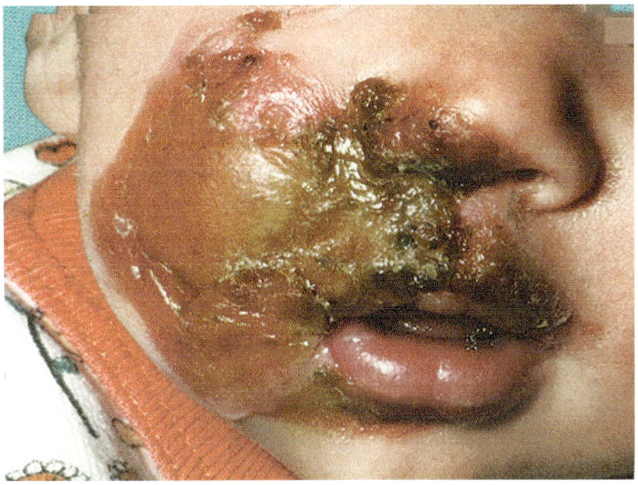

Figure 34.17 Electrical burn to corner of mouth caused by child chewing a live electrical flex.

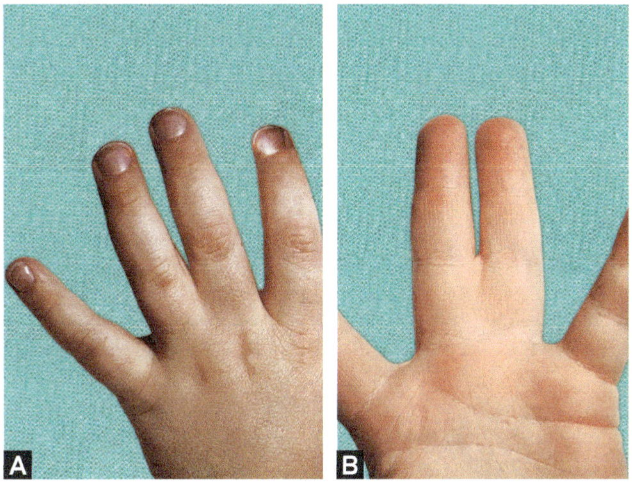

Figures 34.18A and B Simple skin only syndactyly (zygodactyly) can be corrected completely by surgery.

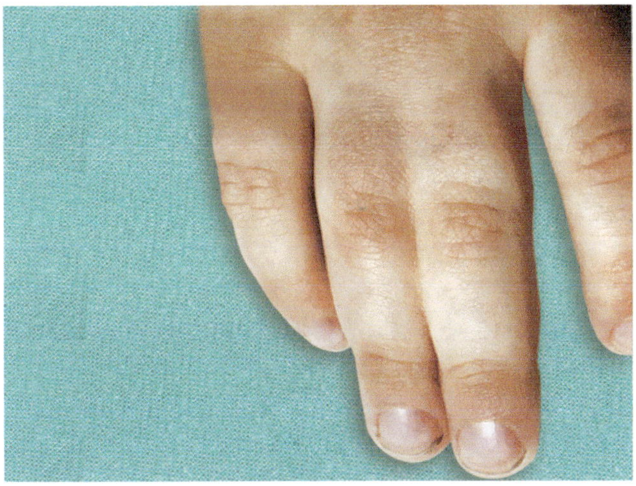

Figure 34.19 Simple syndactyly.

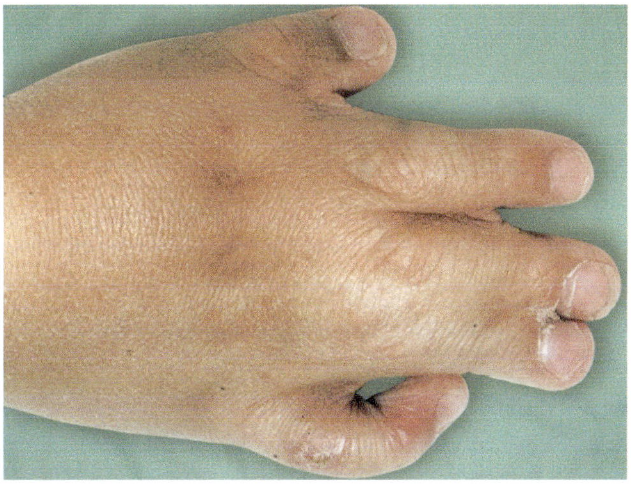

Figure 34.20 Complex syndactyly.

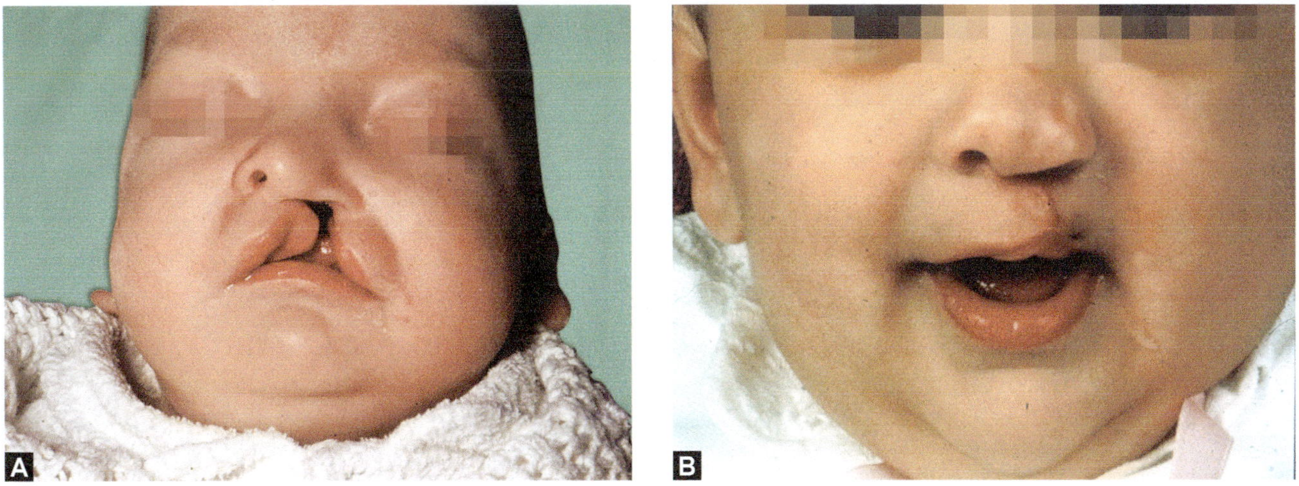

Figures 34.21A and B Pre- and post-cleft-lip-repair.

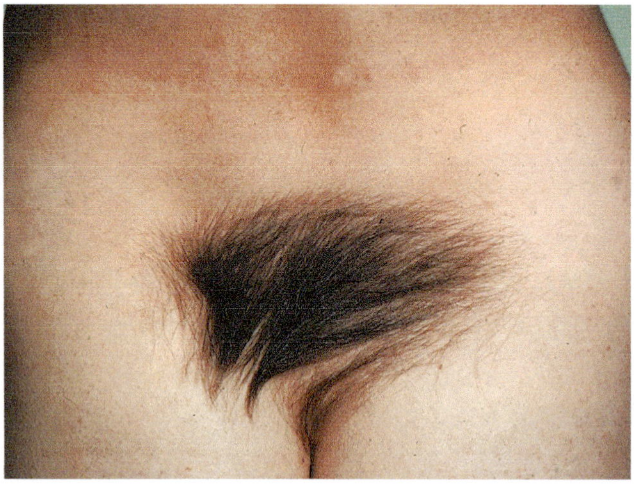

Figure 34.22 Lumbosacral hypertrichosis over spina bifida occulta can be removed (using tissue expander).

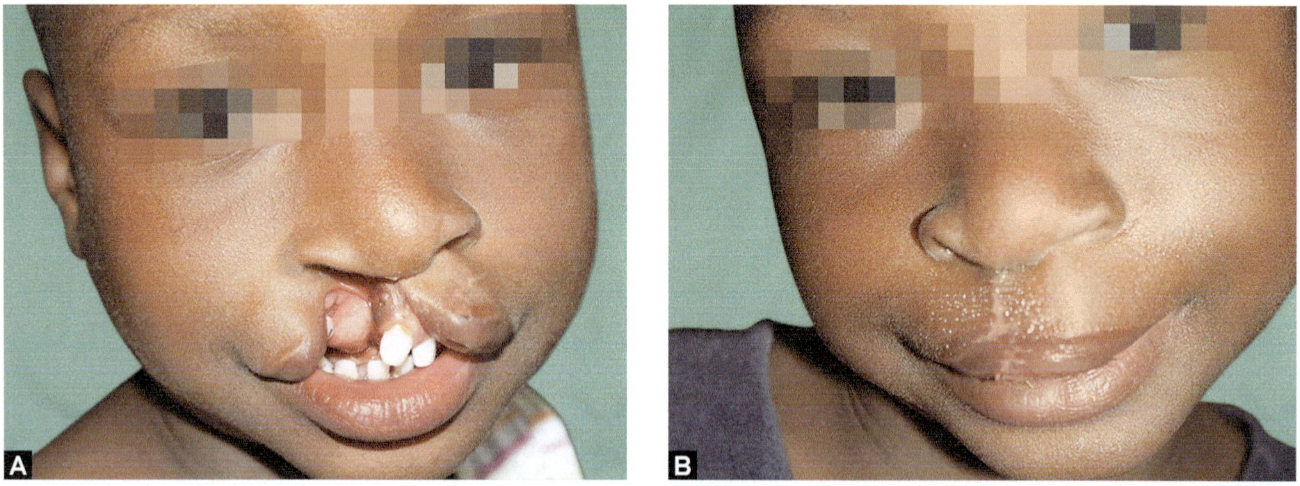

Figures 34.23A and B (A) Showing pre-operative right-sided cleft lip; (B) Post-operative.

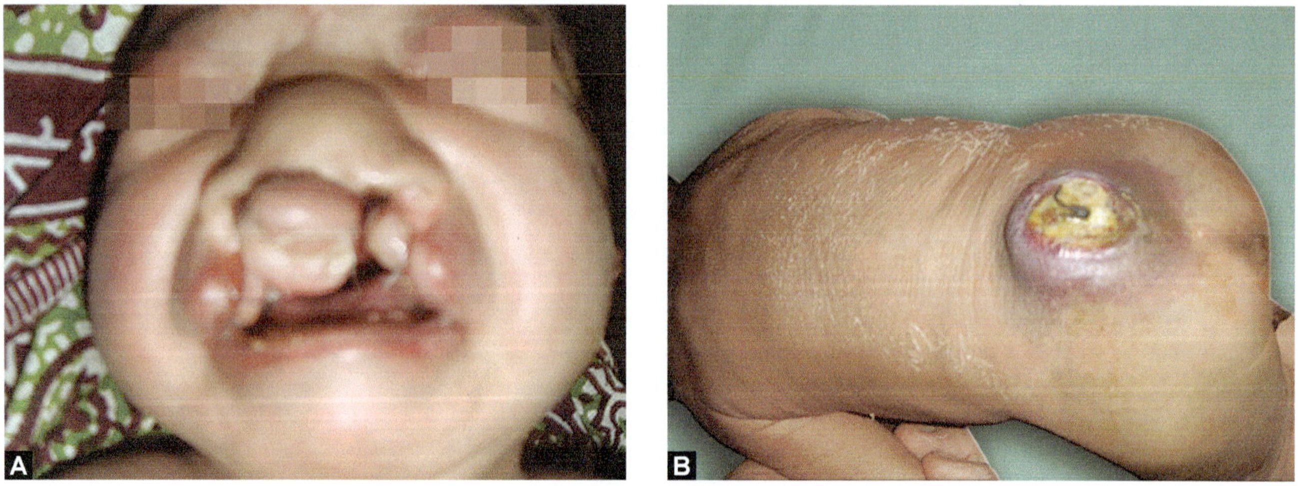

Figures 34.24A and B Multiple congenital abnormalities can occur in the same child (A) Bilateral cleft lip and palate; and (B) Myelomeningocele.

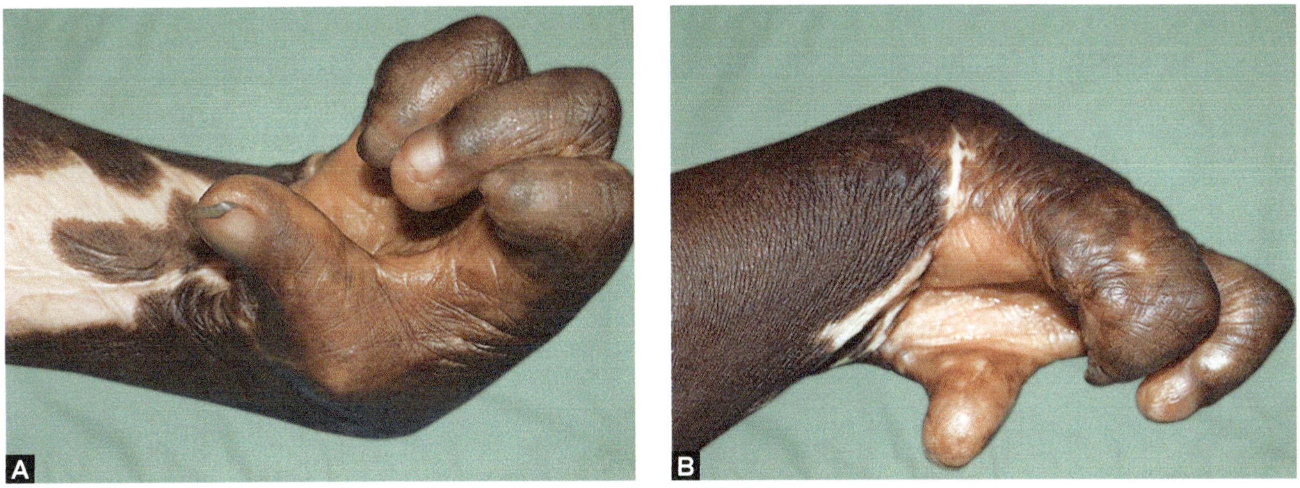

Figures 34.25A and B Neglected burn of the right hand. Will require grafting and post-operative physiotherapy.

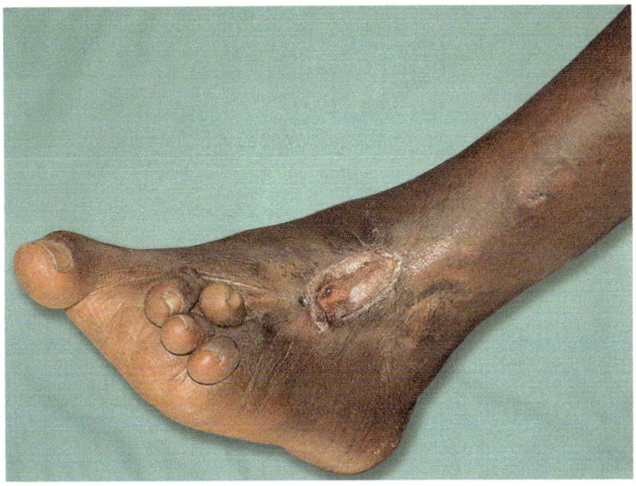

Figure 34.26 Old burn of left foot with ulcerated scarring and contracture of toes. Will require grafting.

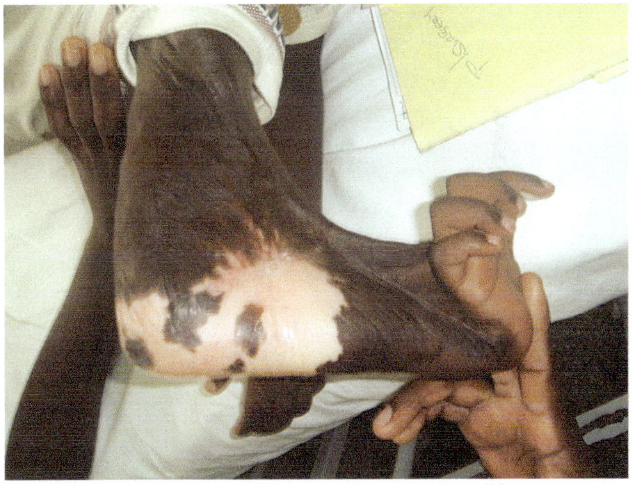

Figure 34.27 Vitiligo in neglected burn showing severe contractures of elbow and wrist and will require multiple grafting and physiotherapy.

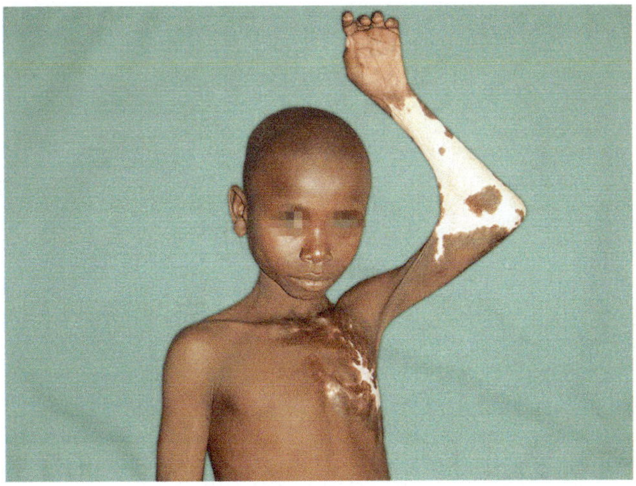

Figure 34.28 Contractures and vitiligo in a neglected burn of left arm and will require skin grafting and physiotherapy.

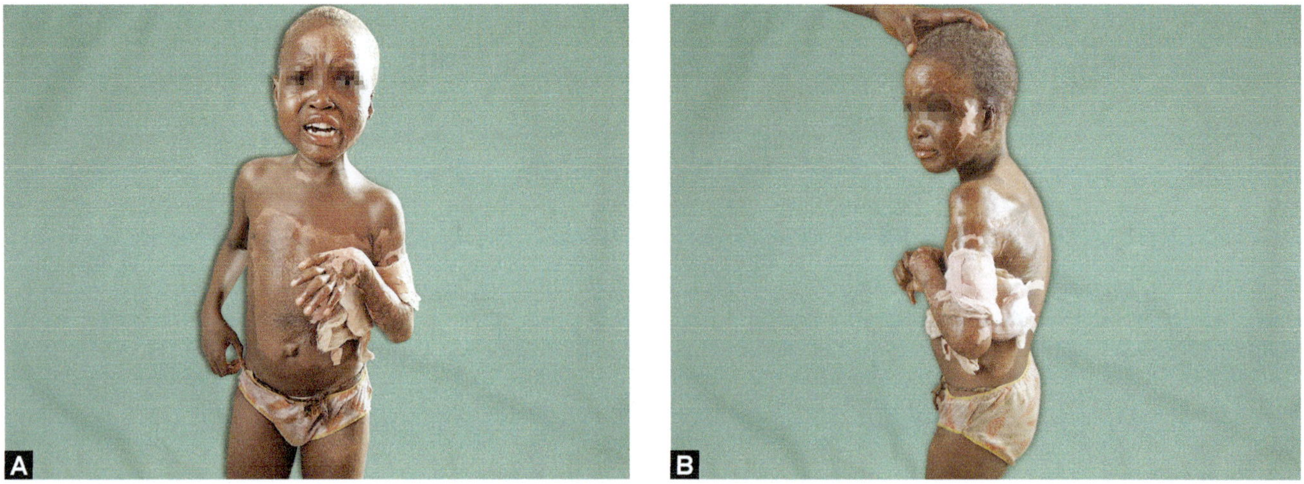

Figures 34.29A and B Acute flame burn of left arm and chest and will require grafting and physiotherapy.

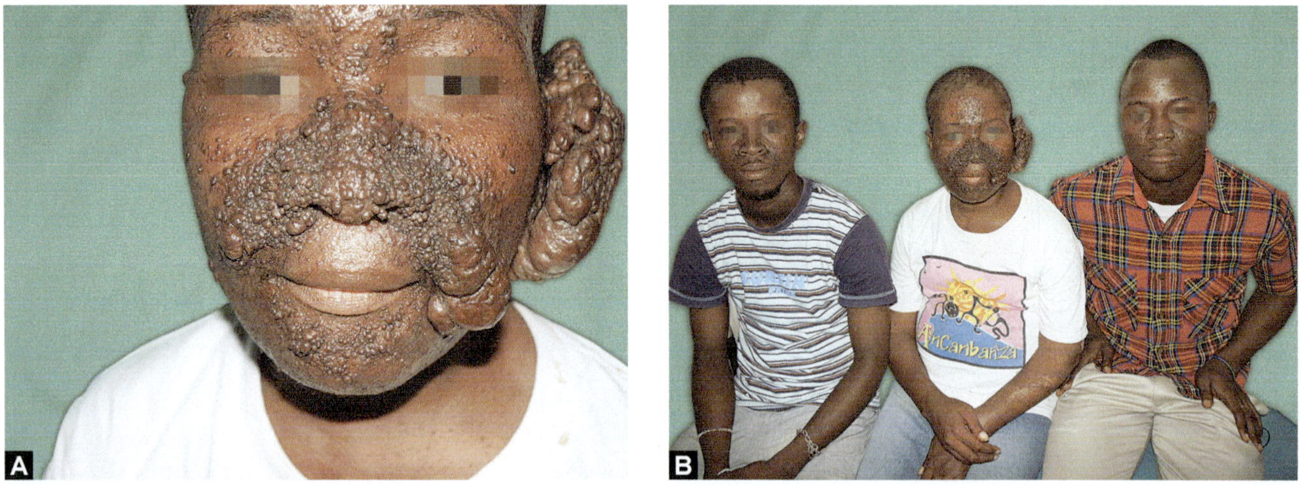

Figures 34.30A and B Unusual cases of tuberous sclerosis (TS) showing adenoma sebaceum in a young family. Partial excision is possible.

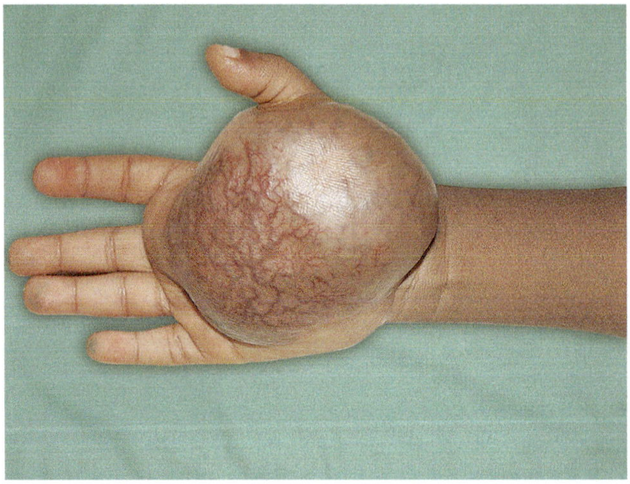

Figure 34.31 Arteriovenous malformation of right hand can be excised.

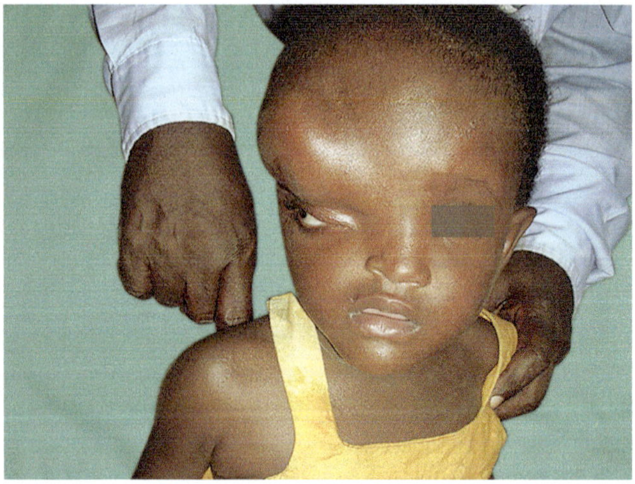

Figure 34.32 Encephalocele associated with craniofacial abnormality and will require sophisticated craniofacial surgery.

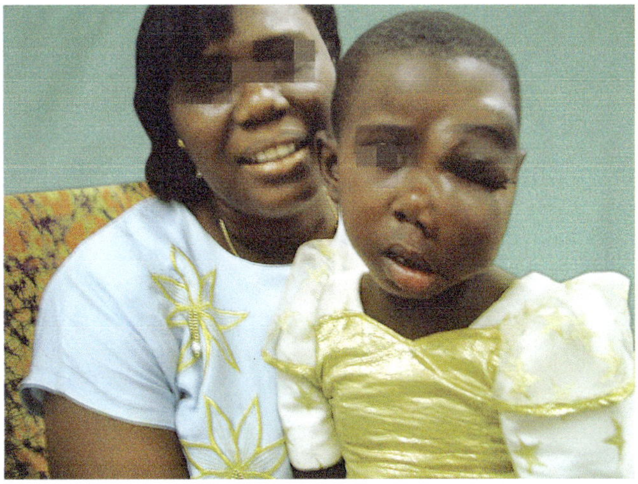

Figure 34.33 A child presented with difficult problems of a neurofibroma. Cure is not possible but amelioration might be attempted.

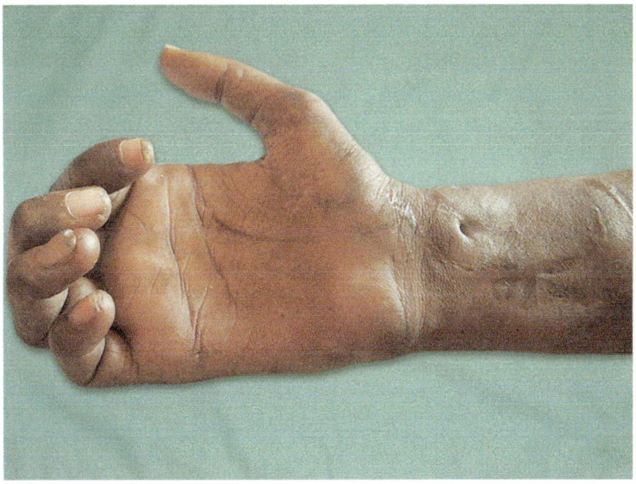

Figure 34.34 Typical flexed fingers and rigid wrist following Volkmann ischaemic contracture and will require surgery and physiotherapy.

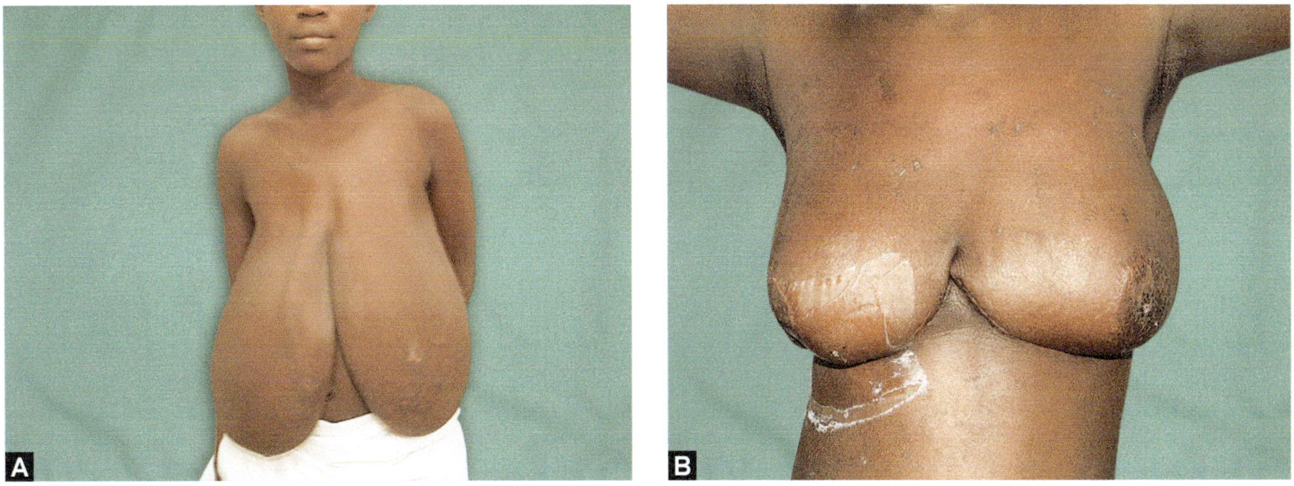

Figures 34.35A and B Gross mammary hypertrophy at menarche and requires breast reduction surgery.

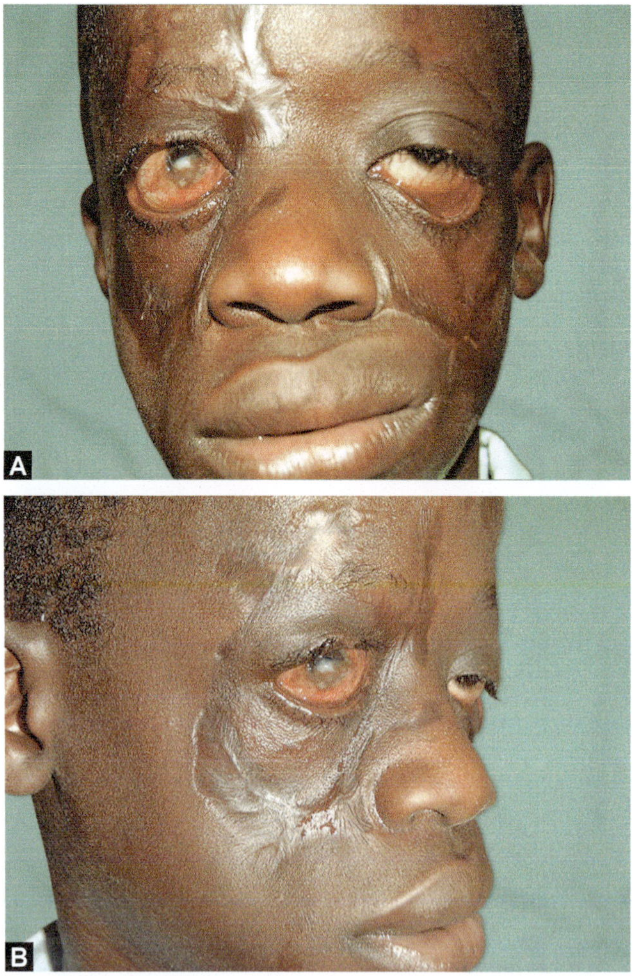

Figures 34.36A and B Spitting cobra venom creates chemical injuries to the skin causing scarring and ectropion and will require grafting.

CHAPTER 35

Practical Paediatric Procedures

Alastair Turner, Robert Carachi, Krishna M. Goel

INTRODUCTION

Success and confidence in the skilled performance of practical procedures come from frequent repetition. These are best learned by demonstration followed by practice under supervision. This chapter gives practical details which may reduce the period of learning and increase the chances of success. The chapter has been divided into two sections: (1) routine practical procedures and (2) other practical procedures.

PREPARATION FOR PRACTICAL PROCEDURES

Before performing any procedure on a child, it is essential to obtain consent from the child's parents or guardians. Older children who are deemed competent may give their own consent. Consent should be fully informed allowing time for questioning and be obtained by the person performing the procedure. The only exception to this is in the life-threatening emergency situation if a parent or guardian is unable to be contacted in time. In this situation, it is justifiable to offer immediate life-saving treatment whilst attempts are made to contact the parents.

Performing practical procedures in children can be challenging. It is essential that the operator safely carry out the procedure without causing injury to the child or staff members. The child may be frightened or in pain and will often resist any attempts at even relatively simple procedures making the process potentially difficult and hazardous. It is, therefore, important to recognise that whilst performing any procedure a balance must be struck between the necessity to carry out the procedure versus the risk of distressing or injuring the child.

Simple techniques are often successful at reducing the child's anxiety and thus facilitating any procedure. Parents should usually be encouraged to remain as their presence frequently reduces any distress felt by the child. Distraction methods can be used with toys or visual or auditory stimulation such as lights, gentle music or blowing bubbles. The involvement of a play specialist can be very helpful depending on the situation. The use of a dummy to promote non-nutritive sucking can help calm infants. Procedures should usually be performed in a fully equipped specialised area that allows privacy and minimises excessive noise and interruptions. Staff members present should be kept to a safe minimum.

RESTRAINT

When considering physical restraint of children to facilitate practical procedures, consideration must be given at all times to the risks versus benefits experienced by the child. Gentle protective physical containment to allow quick, simple procedures may be acceptable when balanced against the risks of sedation. Examples of this are venous cannulation and lumbar puncture (LP) in acutely unwell children when a combination of simple techniques as described above combined with gentle restraint may reduce or negate the need for sedation. Procedures that potentially take longer or are more painful require more formal sedation or anaesthesia as the potential distress experienced by the child outweighs the risks of sedation or anaesthesia when performed properly. Forcible restraint is never acceptable.

Providing gentle protective physical containment is often best achieved by the child's parent firmly but gently holding the child. This can be achieved with the child sitting on the parent's lap, facing the parent with the child's arms protruding under the parent's axillae and being gently cuddled by the parent. This allows the operator access to the child's arms and legs for procedures such as venepuncture or venous cannulation whilst the child is comforted by their parent. Some children prefer to sit facing forward and observe the procedure themselves, whilst being held by their parent, as not being able to see what is happening to them may in itself be anxiety provoking. Light straps to protect children from hurting themselves are also acceptable for very brief procedures where it is deemed sedation is not necessarily required and a description follows:

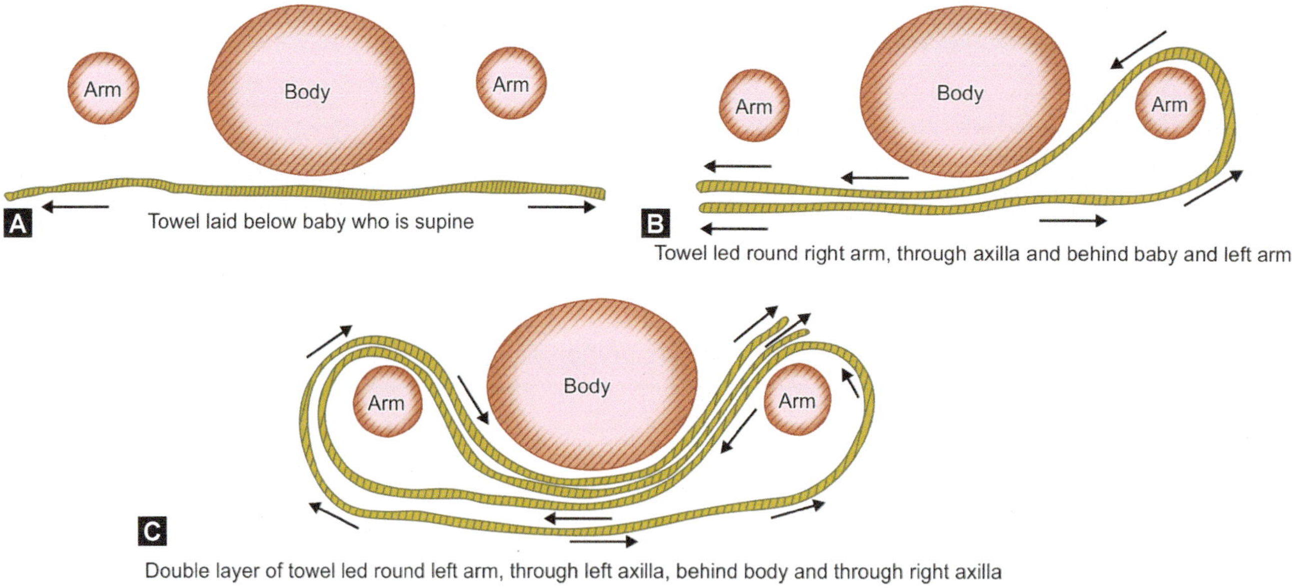

Figures 35.1A to C Restraining a baby.

With a towel or sheet and a capable nurse, an infant's arms may be restrained so that the head, neck or the femoral area can be safely and easily acupunctured **(Figs. 35.1A to C)**. A rectangular sheet is spread out on the table with the short edges of the sheet to the left and right of the nurse. The infant is laid in the centre of the sheet at right angles to its long axis, with feet pointing to the nurse and only the head and neck projecting beyond the upper border of the sheet. The nurse then straightens the infant's right arm adducted beside his trunk and folds the sheet on that side so that the short edge passes in front of the right arm, down through the right axilla and across behind his back. This end of the sheet is then pulled tightly so that its short border is close to the short border on the infant's left hand side with the upper corner level with the infant's shoulders. This holds the adducted right arm close against the chest. The procedure is then repeated for the left arm, using the double layer of sheet which now lies on the infant's left side. Finally, it is important to pull the two upper corners, which have been passed behind the back, firmly up through the right axilla. For further control, a second sheet can be wrapped round the infant's legs. This method of restraint will sometimes permit the paediatrician to perform practical procedures single-handed, very much a second best choice.

SEDATION AND ANALGESIA FOR CLINICAL PROCEDURES

The child's anxiety about a clinical procedure to be carried out can be minimised by administering a sedative drug for its anxiolytic and amnesic effect. For a painful procedure, the sedative should be given with an appropriate analgesic such as a local anaesthetic (given topically by infiltration or as a nerve block as appropriate) or non-opiate or opiate analgesic.

Sedation

The purpose of sedation is to induce a transient state of minimal or moderate drug-induced depression of consciousness in the child whilst the child still responds purposefully to verbal commands or gentle tactile stimulation and maintains a patent airway, spontaneous ventilation and normal cardiovascular function. Levels of depression of consciousness beyond this should be considered as general anaesthesia and require the presence of a fully trained anaesthetist. Procedures lasting more than 45 minutes should also be considered for general anaesthesia. Extensive guidelines for the safe sedation of children exist and are referred at the end of this chapter.

Sedation may be unnecessary for brief practical procedures in young infants. The use of sweet oral solutions of sucrose administered prior to painful procedures has been demonstrated to have a powerful analgesic and calming effect in infants and when combined with other simple measures such as a soothing voice and dummy may pacify an infant for short periods. Sucrose oral solution (approximately 0.25 mL of 33% solution) should be administered 2 minutes before a painful procedure and can be repeated up to a total of 2 mL during the procedure. Sucrose is only effective when given orally and has no effect when given via a gastric tube.

Sedative drugs can at times produce unexpected or unwanted effects, particularly excessive sedation and respiratory compromise from either airway obstruction or hypoventilation. At times, a paradoxical hyper-excitable state may arise rather than the desired sedative effect. As such, the administration of sedative drugs should be taken seriously and the person administering the drug prepared to deal with any potential side effects as they arise.

- *Patient selection:* High-risk patients who require sedation should be referred to a fully trained anaesthetist. Such patients include patients with potential difficult airways (e.g. Pierre Robin syndrome, Treacher Collins syndrome), children at risk of hypoventilation (e.g. children with obstructive sleep apnoea, neuromuscular disorders) and patients with respiratory or cardiovascular compromise (e.g. bronchospasm, cardiomyopathy, significant congenital heart disease). Younger children and infants have a higher risk of complications, particularly those under 1 year, and consideration should be given to the appropriateness of sedation in all children under 5 years of age.
- *Patient preparation:* Due to the risk of excessive sedation and possible aspiration, children should be fasted prior to the administration of sedative drugs (6 hours for solids or bottle milk, 4 hours for breast milk, 2 hours for clear fluids) unless nitrous oxide (N_2O) is the only sedative used when 2 hours is acceptable.
- *Environment preparation:* Sedation should be performed in an area fully equipped for all resuscitation scenarios. This should include immediate access to oxygen (O_2), airway adjuncts, bag/mask ventilation, intubation equipment and a defibrillator.
- *Monitoring preparation:* Patients undergoing sedation should be monitored using a chart documenting level of consciousness, heart rate, respiratory rate, blood pressure and colour. Infants should have their temperature monitored. The patient should have a pulse oximeter and electrocardiography (ECG) monitor attached to them.
- *Staffing preparation:* At least two staff are required to be present at all times. One staff member must be responsible for administering the sedative and monitoring the patient solely (that is not performing the procedure as well).

The following are appropriate sedative drugs:

- *N_2O (inhaled gas):* Self-administration using a demand valve may be used in children who are able to self-regulate their intake (usually over 5 years of age).Usual dose 50% N_2O/50% O_2. Maximum dose 70% N_2O, 30% O_2. Rapid onset/offset with full recovery in 5 minutes. Contraindicated in pneumothorax, bowel obstruction and intracranial air (skull fractures) as may diffuse into air pockets causing them to expand.
- *Midazolam (oral/buccal or IV):* Oral (0.5 mg/kg) maximum effect in 15–60 minutes but absorption may be erratic. Intravenous (IV) (0.1–0.15 mg/kg) maximum effect in 1–5 minutes. Major risk of respiratory depression and occasionally cardiac depression. May paradoxically cause agitation.
- *Chloral hydrate (oral):* Unpredictable absorption. May cause hyperactivity. Dose 10–50 mg/kg.

Multiple sedative drugs should not be used in the same patient as they may cause potent respiratory or cardiovascular compromise.

Analgesia

Local anaesthesia:

Topical anaesthesia is available in the form of a lidocaine 2.5%/pilocarpine 2.5% cream (EMLA®, Astra Zeneca pharmaceuticals Ltd), which is applied to a small area of skin 1 hour before the procedure under occlusive dressing. It is not recommended for preterm neonates. The area is then cleaned with alcohol and a needle can then puncture the skin painlessly. This method is especially suitable for recurrent procedures. An alternative is amethocaine gel (Ametop) which appears to be equally efficacious but has a slightly faster onset of action (30 minutes). Both are suitable for venepuncture and LP analgesia.

The most common type of local anaesthesia used for local infiltration is lidocaine which is manufactured in 0.5%, 1% and 2% strengths. The dose is calculated on the bases of the patient's age and weight. The two best methods of infiltration or administration of local anaesthesia is either a field block or a regional nerve block. There is also a lidocaine and adrenaline mixture which can be used as a local agent with the adrenaline, a local vasoconstrictor helping to maintain a longer lasting effect of the anaesthesia and to decrease capillary bleeding. This should never be used in areas supplied by end-arteries, e.g. digits, ears, nose, penis, etc. where it can cause ischaemia.

Non-opiate analgesics

Paracetamol and non-steroidal inflammatory drugs (e.g. ibuprofen) are useful analgesics but tend to have slow onset of action and are, therefore, not particularly useful for procedural analgesia although provide good ongoing postprocedure analgesia. For the use of sucrose in infants, *see* above.

Opiate analgesics

IV morphine is the standard opiate analgesic of choice for severe pain. The dose is 100–200 μg/kg (max 10 mg) and subsequent doses can be titrated to effect. Intranasal diamorphine is also being increasingly used (0.1 mg/kg) as a single dose. Fentanyl and remifentanil should not be used by non-anaesthetists. Opiates should not be used for sedation unless an analgesic effect is also required. The combination of sedative drugs and opiates can lead to profound respiratory depression and immediate access to naloxone should be available.

For very painful, frightening or multiple procedures, general anaesthesia may be necessary. For the administration of a general anaesthetic, a trained paediatric anaesthetist should be present.

> **KEY LEARNING POINT**
>
> The child under sedation for clinical procedure should be monitored carefully as soon as the sedative is given until recovery after the procedure; concomitant use of sedatives potentiates the central nervous system (CNS) depressant effects of analgesics.

ROUTINE PRACTICAL PROCEDURES

Handwashing

Infection control is an important service within any health care system in any part of the world. As a health care worker, you will be expected to act in a manner that ensures the safety of you, your work colleagues, visitors, parents and most importantly, the vulnerable patients we care for.

Hand Hygiene

- Why decontaminate your hands?
  - Hand hygiene is the single most important procedure for the prevention of health care-associated infection. The principles of hand hygiene reduce the levels of transient and resident organisms on the hands. Handwashing is a process that removes dirt and potentially pathogenic organisms from hands. When hands are visibly clean, the use of alcohol hand sanitising products can be used **(Figs. 35.2A to F)**.
- When to perform hand hygiene?
  - Choosing the right time to decontaminate your hands is very important and should be based on the potential level of contamination. As a basic rule, hands should be decontaminated: on entering and before leaving the work area.
- Before and after:
  - Patient contact
    - Contact with body fluids, your own or patients'
    - Wearing gloves
    - Isolation nursing
    - Food handling
    - Invasive procedures
    - Contact with contamination sources
    - Caring for susceptible/high-risk patients.

Hand Hygiene Products

There are many hand hygiene products available for health care staff. It is important to choose the correct product at the appropriate time **(Table 35.1)**.

Types of Handwash

- Social handwash: 10–15 seconds
- Hygienic/antiseptic hand disinfection: 15–30 seconds
- Surgical scrub: 2–5 minutes.

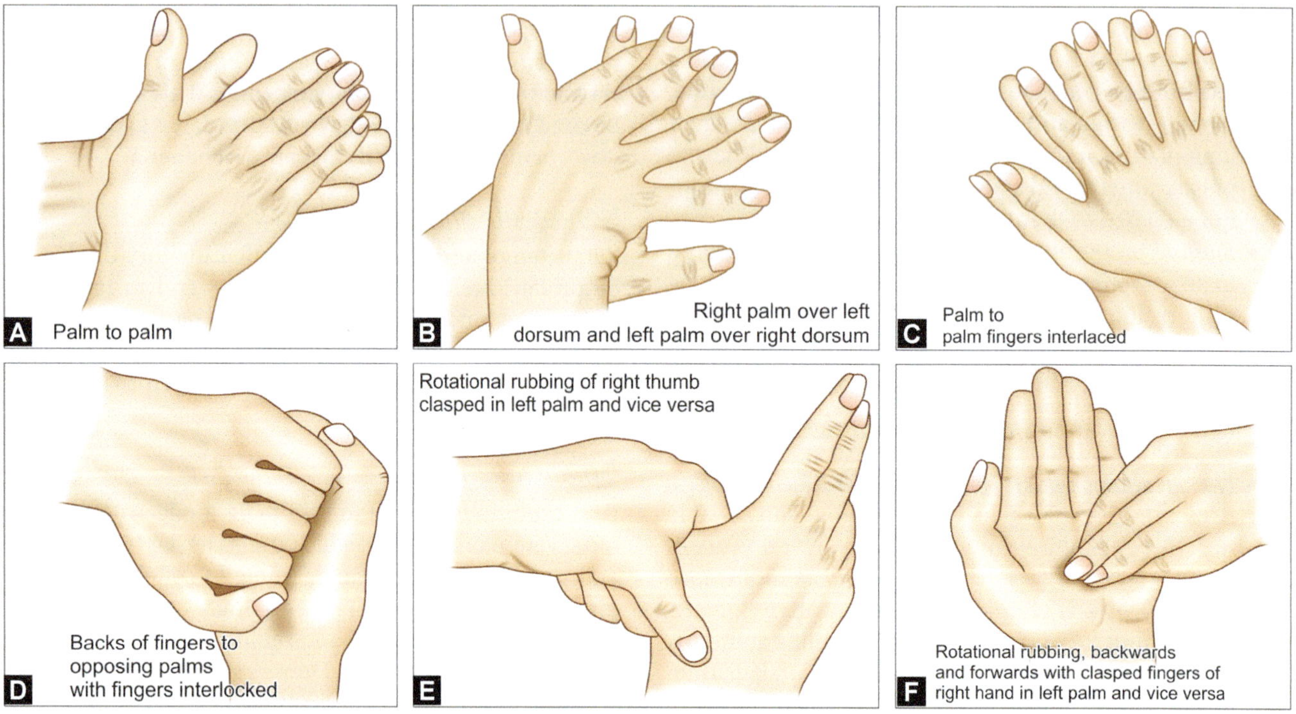

Figures 35.2A to F Effective handwashing.

TABLE 35.1	Hand hygiene summary.		
Hand hygiene procedure	***Products***	***Duration of technique***	***Clinical procedures***
Social hand hygiene	Plain soap and running wateroralcohol hand sanitizer (visibly clean hands only)	15 seconds	Non-clinical procedures Handling or eating food After a visit to the toilet
Antiseptic hand hygiene	Antibacterial soaporplain liquid soap to wash, followed by an application of alcohol hand rub or gel	15–30 seconds	Before and after aseptic procedures Following microbial contamination of hands Care of patient in source or protective isolation
Surgical scrub	Antibacterial soaporplain liquid soap to wash, followed by an application of alcohol hand rub or gel	2–5 minutes	Before surgical interventions

Points to Consider

- Wet hands before applying liquid soap.
- Workup a soapy lather at start of technique.
- Cover all areas of hands, including backs of hands, finger tips and between fingers.
- Do not wear nail varnish, artificial nails or extensions.
- Keep nail tips short and clean.
- Remove stoned rings and wrist items before procedure.
- Cover all cuts and abrasions with water-proof dressings.

Blood Sampling

Blood sampling or venepuncture is a frequently carried out procedure of entering a vein with a needle, usually to obtain a sample of blood.

Equipment Required

- Tourniquet
- Vacutainer and double ended needle or needle and syringe
- Alcohol swabs or chlorhexidine/alcohol
- Cotton wool
- Micropore or plaster
- Collection of tubes
- Resheathing device
- Kidney dish
- Sharps container
- Gloves
- Relevant forms.

Method

Welcome patient, check identity and explain procedure (if child, earlier use of EMLA® or Ametop cream may be required).

Identify tests required and associated requirements, e.g. fasting status, timing of medication.

Select correct tubes and forms; fill in form accurately and clearly. Remember a group and save or cross match sample must be handwritten rather than using an addressograph label.

- Support patient's arm comfortably
- Select a vein
- Prepare needle holder and needle out of sight of child
- Apply tourniquet or ask member of staff to apply pressure to arm
- Put on gloves
- Cleanse skin
- Steady vein with left hand and palpate above point of entry as guide. Insert needle under skin-keeping angle low and bevelled edge uppermost
- Attach vacuum tube and advance needle into vein. Wait for tube to fill up and change to next tube, as necessary
- Release tourniquet before removing final tube, cover needle site with swab and remove needle, apply gentle pressure
- Discard needle holder and attached needle in a sharps bin. Do not resheath
- Ask patient or parent to apply pressure, while labelling tubes and completing forms
- Check puncture site and apply dressing. Check patient has no allergies prior to applying dressing.

Collection of Blood Samples

Capillary Sampling

Improved techniques of microanalysis allow many investigations on blood to be carried out on capillary samples. A drop of capillary blood contains at least 50 μL. A heel is the most useful source in the newborn whereas in older infants and children a digit is satisfactory. If the heel is used, it is important to lance the fleshy side of the heel rather than the midline as midline puncture may damage the calcaneum and lead to osteomyelitis. The ear lobe is said to be less painful and flow can be speeded and 'arterialised' by rubbing alcohol on the skin. The skin should be warm. The cleaned skin is pricked with a cutting stylet. A single vertical prick may produce a good flow in a child but to obtain a large volume from a neonate a slit should be cut in the heel a few millimetres in length. The cut need not be deep. This method is valuable when repeated capillary samples are required over a short period when only an initial cut is required. Further bleeding is stimulated at intervals by cleaning away the clot. A disadvantage of capillary sampling is that haemolysis of some degree is likely. This can be reduced by ensuring a fast flow and using siliconised tubes. Frothing or drying of the sample is potent causes of haemolysis. For certain investigations, the capillary blood can conveniently be taken directly into glass capillary tubes (e.g. for gas analysis) or spotted onto special filter papers (e.g. for chromatography).

Venepuncture

Sampling is always more successful if a good fit between syringe and needle is ensured before puncture and if blood is withdrawn slowly with moderate suction.

Superficial Veins

The puncture of superficial veins is the safest type of venepuncture. No complications are to be expected if the skin is cleaned and pressure applied to ensure haemostasis. Any visible vein in the back of the hand, the dorsum of the foot, the antecubital fossa, or the scalp may be used. Scalp vein sets (21 G, 23 G or 25 G) are often used.

External Jugular Vein

A superficial vein often visible in the infant is the external jugular. It is often reserved for when attempts at all other veins have failed and capillary blood sampling is inappropriate. The operator sits at the baby's head and rotates it through 90° and extends the neck where it is maintained by the assistant. The external jugular vein can then be seen crossing the sternomastoid muscle and it is punctured at this point. Puncture is easier when the infant distends the vein by crying, as is not uncommon. Care should be taken not to allow air to enter these veins. Sometimes, the shaft of the needle has to be carefully bent to an angle from its butt to allow easy access for the syringe and needle. Sterile care and gentle handling are required to keep the needle safe.

Femoral Vein

The hips are fully abducted and the knees flexed to 90° are held onto the table surface by the nurse. The femoral artery pulse is palpated, and the femoral vein entered just medially to this in the inguinal crease. The needle should enter the skin at 45°. Blood is often more easily obtained when the needle is withdrawn whilst gently aspirating. A needle finer than 21 G might be ineffective. It is easy to produce a haematoma and transient cyanosis of the leg if the adjacent artery is accidentally punctured. Application of firm pressure for at least 2 minutes after venepuncture is, therefore, an important precaution. Rare complications include spasm of femoral artery with ischaemia of the foot, infected haematoma, and osteitis of the femur and arthritis of the hip. If the artery is accidentally punctured pressure should be maintained for 5 minutes or longer if blood continues to ooze from the puncture site.

Fontanelle Tap (Sagittal Sinus Tap)

Fontanelle puncture and aspiration of blood is not routinely recommended due to the risk of complications. It may be used, however, in the emergency setting when other attempts at venous access have proven unsuccessful. The sagittal sinus is easily punctured in any infant whose anterior fontanelle is still patent. The anterior fontanelle may not close until well past the age of 18 months, although this delay can also occur in hypothyroidism, rickets, hydrocephalus, and even in some healthy children. The infant is held in the supine position, the occiput just inside the edge of the table and the face pointed to the ceiling held firmly by the nurse's thumbs against his temples. The operator sits facing the top of the head and cleans the area around the proposed puncture with iodine or alcoholic chlorhexidine. An especially hairy head may mandate local shaving. The site of entry of the needle is the posterior angle of the anterior fontanelle in the midline (either at right angles to the scalp in all directions or angled backwards toward the occiput but in the sagittal plane) to a depth of approximately 2 mm. Steadying the hand on the scalp and the needle against the forefinger of the other hand makes it less easy for the point to penetrate too deeply from the initial force necessary to pierce the scalp. A brief resistance is felt as the fontanelle is penetrated and blood is freely aspirated if positioning is correct. It is easy to go too deep if the hand does not steady the needle. As soon as the needle has been removed the child is sat up and pressure applied to the puncture site with a swab. When crying stops, the pressure in the sinus is no longer great enough to cause bleeding and haemostasis results.

It is important that the head is held firmly throughout. If the operator misjudges the position of the sagittal sinus, cerebrospinal fluid (CSF) may be aspirated from the adjacent subarachnoid space. Occasionally, CSF leakage may follow causing oedema of the scalp. If the needle is inserted too deeply it will enter the brain with the small but potentially important risk of local bleeding. Sagittal sinus thrombosis is a serious possible complication of fontanelle puncture. It is, however, often more likely to be a consequence of underlying disturbance (such as severe dehydration) than the needling. Inability of skilled hands to obtain blood by this route from an ill dehydrated baby suggests that thrombosis of the sinus has already occurred.

Repeated Venous Sampling

When serial samples of venous blood are required (as in 'tolerance' tests), only one venepuncture is essential and specimens may be obtained at regular timed intervals. Patients tolerate this procedure well, and it is less painful than repeated capillary stabs. Heparin is diluted to 100 units per mL saline. A syringe is attached to a scalp vein needle set and the system filled with heparinised saline. The needle is inserted into a convenient superficial vein (not the sagittal sinus) and the needle and a loop of cannula taped to the skin in the usual manner. When a blood sample is required, 0.3 mL of solution filling the dead space in the scalp vein set is withdrawn into the syringe containing heparinised saline. A second syringe is then used to aspirate the blood for analysis and the scalp vein set again filled with 0.3 mL of the dilute heparin. Multiple samples may be obtained for periods of more than 1 hour. The technique may be used in patients of any age.

It must be remembered that the blood samples obtained by this method are inevitably heparinised and are a source of plasma and not serum. It is desirable to ascertain the volume of the scalp vein set in advance so that the injected heparin solution just reaches the tip of the needle. This prevents clotting and ensures that the small infant is not heparinised.

Blood Culture

Blood culture is so important in paediatric practice that a short account is included. At any age, blood culture is only justifiable if carried out with rigorous precautions against contamination and under optimal conditions for harvesting the offending organism.

Employ at least two culture bottles containing different media from your laboratory. The risk of contamination is increased if blood is not drawn cleanly on the first insertion of the needle. The skin is first cleansed with iodine in spirit. An alternative that may reduce the risk of contamination further is 2% chlorhexide in 70% ethanol solution. The cap of each of the culture bottles is also wiped with 2% iodine in 70% ethanol solution. The iodine or chlorhexidine on both skin and bottle caps is allowed to dry. With the infant suitably held, the chosen vein is punctured through the iodine stained skin. The needle should either be sterile and disposable or autoclaved. The shaft must not come in contact with the finger before introduction into the vein. After the sample is obtained, the original needle is removed from the syringe and a second needle is used to inject the blood into the culture bottles. The iodine or chlorhexidine should be washed from the infant's skin with 70% alcohol. The blood culture bottles are immediately placed in the incubator. Further processing is handled by the microbiologist.

Measurement of Blood Pressure

Measurement of blood pressure (BP) is an important part of routine clinical examination. Pressure is taken in one limb only (the right arm) but if coarctation of the aorta is suspected, the pressure in both upper limbs and one lower limb is measured.

Sphygmomanometry

In the older infant and child, satisfactory assessment of the BP may be obtained using the auscultatory method of sphygmomanometry. The patient should lie in the supine position with the head resting comfortably on a pillow. The arm should be free of restrictive clothing or even better, undressed. A sphygmomanometer cuff suitable to the size of the child's arm should be chosen, the breadth of the cuff being about two-thirds of the length of the upper arm, too large a cuff cannot be smoothly applied to the limb and overlap interferes with adequate auscultation. Too small a cuff results in artificially and often strikingly—high pressures. The cuff is applied so that the inflatable inner bag is centred over the medial aspect of the arm where it will compress the brachial artery and wrapped firmly but not tightly round the arm. There should be no folds or wrinkles.

Sit comfortably beside the patient and palpate the radial pulse while inflating the cuff. The point of disappearance of the radial pulse gives an indication of the level of the systolic blood pressure. The cuff is inflated a further 30–40 mmHg and a stethoscope applied over the brachial artery in the cubital fossa. The cuff is slowly and steadily deflated whilst systolic and diastolic pressure points are auscultated.

If lying and standing measurements are required as when assessing the effect of hypotensive agents, it is easier to measure the pressure in the arm in the supine position first and then allow the child to stand with the cuff still in position. The BP in the leg is taken in a similar fashion except that the child lies comfortably prone with head turned to one side or supine with the knee slightly flexed. The cuff is applied to the thigh and again should be of a size that covers two-thirds of the length; auscultation is made over the popliteal artery in the popliteal fossa.

For the BP measurement so obtained to be at all accurate, the child should be cooperative and at ease. If he is crying or restless, then the record will obviously be worthless although it is often useful to apply the cuff and go through the motions in the hope that future attempts may be accepted with less apprehension. It is useful to place the manometer in such a position that the patient may watch the rise and fall of the mercury column (without raising his head!) since this may gain his quiet interest.

Flush Technique

Difficulty in auscultating the artery and in obtaining the required degree of cooperation often makes the sphygmomanometer method impracticable in the infant. A suitable alternative is the 'flush technique' which allows reasonably accurate determination of a single BP point considered to be somewhere between systolic and diastolic levels. The advantages of this technique are that it requires minimal equipment and can be performed in a noisy environment. The main disadvantage is that the measurement is often only a crude estimate of the mean BP.

The equipment is the standard mercury manometer, a small cuff (to cover at least two-thirds of the upper part of the appropriate limb), a length of thin rubber bandage about 2.5 cm broad, a pacifier or feeding bottle to keep the infant quiet, and two observers, e.g. doctor and nurse. The infant should be placed unclothed, supine on a comfortable flat surface in a warm, well-lit room. The sphygmomanometer cuff is applied firmly in the normal manner on the upper arm but is not inflated. The infant's hand is then grasped and the rubber bandage wound tightly round the arm from hand to elbow so that the blood is expelled from the arm. When the bandage has been wound to the elbow the sphygmomanometer cuff is inflated to 200 mmHg (this level is suggested since the actual height of the BP is not known and may be well above normal for the infant's age). The rubber bandage is then quickly unwound. The lower arm should now be white in colour. Once this uncomfortable stage has been reached, if required, the pacifier or feeding bottle may be used to quieten the infant. When he is quiet, one observer (usually the nurse) observes the white arm and the other observer slowly but steadily deflates the cuff while watching the manometer. When the end-point is reached, a distinct pink flush spreads down the arm and the level of mercury in the manometer indicates the blood pressure. The flush may occur suddenly so that the observers must be consistently attentive or the end-point may be missed. Once the flush has occurred the technique cannot be reapplied satisfactorily to that limb for 15 minutes or more. The technique is used in the same manner to obtain the pressure in the leg.

Automated Blood Pressure Measurement

Many hospitals now use automated BP measurements that are derived from either a Doppler or oscillometric measurement from an inflated cuff. This removes the need for a mercury sphygmomanometer and allows for repeated, safe, accurate blood pressure measurements.

Intravenous Cannulation

As with any procedure, you must always introduce yourself and ask permission from the patient or parent before attempting the procedure. IV cannulation is one of the most frequent procedures you will be expected to perform as a junior doctor. A 'cannula' (from the Latin meaning 'little reed') is tube, which can be inserted into the body for the delivery or removal of fluid. In children, consider whether EMLA® cream or other dermal anaesthesia is appropriate prior to procedure as this needs to be applied

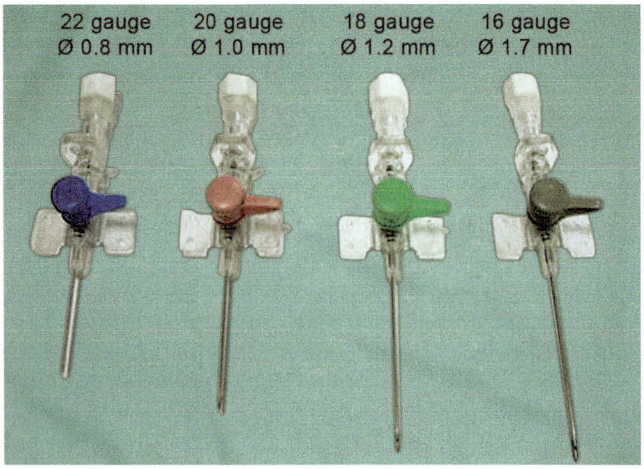

Figure 35.3 Intravenous cannulae in different sizes.

about 45 minutes prior to the procedure to achieve adequate analgesia. Cannulae come in different sizes that are usually colour coded and an appropriate sized cannula should be selected **(Fig. 35.3)**.

Indication

Administration of IV drugs, fluids or total parenteral nutrition.

Equipment Required

- IV cannulae
- Alcohol swaps
- Sterile drape
- Sterile gloves
- Extension set (± three-way tap)
- 5 mL syringe and flushed with saline
- Adhesive dressing
- Sharps bin.

Method

- Select a vein
- Clean area and allow alcohol to dry
- Restrain the extremity
- Apply tourniquet (in children this is usually performed by another member of staff)
- Pull skin taut to help stabilise the vein
- Insert the needle through the skin a short distance prior to the chosen entry point of the vessel
- Advance the needle until a 'flashback' is obtained
- Slowly withdraw introducer needle a short distance
- Advance cannula
- Remove introducer
- Connect extension set and flush cannula to ensure patency
- Secure cannula using adhesive tape, bandage and splint if necessary
- Dispose of sharps safely.

Complications

- Infection—need sterile technique
- Phlebitis—increased risk with prolonged use (>72 hours)
- Vasospasm—rare
- Haematoma—common if unsuccessful! Apply pressure
- Embolus air or clot—ensure extension set is flushed through fully
- Infiltration of subcutaneous tissue—can cause damage to tissue, e.g. total parenteral nutrition (TPN) 'burn.'

Intravenous Infusion

A scalp vein needle set is frequently of use and its advantages include rapidity of insertion, minimal trauma, and preservation of veins for future occasions. Alternatively, it may be necessary to cut down on a vein (e.g. the saphenous at the ankle) of a shocked infant with collapsed scalp veins. When a cannula is tied into a vein, one may be confident that very rapid infusion can be given when necessary. For older children, an arm vein or wrist vein may be cannulated using a plastic cannula set in preference to allowing a needle to traumatise the vein.

Scalp-vein Infusion

The scalp vein needle set is attached to a syringe containing physiological saline and air expelled from the dead space of the set. The infant is restrained and the head held by the assisting nurse. Sedation at this time is not advisable since the distension of veins produced by crying makes entry of the needle easier. The scalp veins most constantly suitable for entry are on either side just behind or in front of the pinna of the ear or running down the middle of the forehead. In the shocked infant, it is easy to mistake a scalp artery for a vein but the temporal arteries run in front of the ears rather than behind.

When a suitable vein is discovered, the overlying hair should be shaved if necessary. The skin may be sterilised by 2% iodine in 70% ethanol which is removed with 70% ethanol to allow easier visualisation of the vein. A combination of stimuli may be required to distend the vein adequately. Venous return may be obstructed by having the nurse press her finger over a proximal segment. Tapping the vein sharply with the finger tends to relax it.

Enter the vein where there is a good length of straight vein downstream. Piercing the skin with the scalp vein needle may be difficult if the skin is tough. It may be easier to pierce the skin beside the vein and insert the needle a short distance under the skin before completing the venepuncture. Venous spasm and vein rupture may thus be avoided. When the vein is entered blood flows back into the plastic tubing. This may not happen in the collapsed infant. Small quantities of fluid are injected from the syringe believed to be in the vein, and if the needle is not in situ, a subcutaneous bleb appears.

After the vein has been entered, it is easy for a restless infant to dislodge a scalp vein needle. The needle should be inserted as far as possible into the vein. With the needle adequately in the vein, tape it to the scalp with paper tape, plaster of Paris, or sterile adhesive spray. Also, tape a loop of the connecting tube to the adjacent scalp.

Usually fluid administration is by gravity controlled drip. Drops per minute may be converted to millilitres per hour depending upon the calibration of type of set used. Axiomatically, the quickest way to stop a drip is to slow it excessively which leads to clotting in the needle and the end of that drip. Nursing staff must realise that excessively rapid infusion cannot safely be compensated for by severely slowing the drip. Volume may better be controlled by using a peristaltic or other controlled pump. A number of adjusting volumeters, which give an accurately dispensed volume per unit time are available. Membrane filters with controlled dimension micropores are available as a final filter for air bubbles and other particulate matter. The accidental entry and subsequent growth of microorganisms converts the infusion fluid pathway into a potential vehicle for infection with microorganisms. Therefore, strict aseptic procedure should be followed.

Cut-down Infusion

Cut-down techniques are widely known. The important point for the paediatrician is to ensure that the instruments are of appropriate size, are sterile and the scissors sharp. In a general hospital with central services, it is commonplace to find sets with large forceps and scissors totally unsuitable for delicate work on an infant. The infant should be kept warm and oxygenated. The leg is externally rotated and bound to a padded splint. The incision is made above the medial malleolus and at right angles to the vein which is freed from surrounding tissue by dissection. A ligature tied distally round the vein occludes venous return and a small transverse incision on the upper surface of the vein allows insertion of a plastic cannula. The cannula is passed well up the vein and a second ligature just above the site of insertion secures it in place. The wound is then closed with two stitches or adhesive strips. The handling necessary and the infusion of cold fluid may result in venous spasm and poor initial flow through the cannula. This needs not mean unsuccessful technique and patience and warmth will allow venous spasm to resolve. Imaginative and dexterous use of the scalp vein sets in a variety of non-scalp areas (e.g. wrist, elbow, arm, ankle, foot) greatly reduces the need for cut-down procedures.

Intraosseous Needle Insertion

In a shocked patient when a pulse is feeble or not palpable and blood pressure is very low or not recordable, then it may be that all peripheral veins are so collapsed it is difficult or not possible to get access quickly. It is suggested by the Paediatric Life Support Manuals that IV access can be tried for a maximum of three attempts or up to

60 seconds. If access could not be achieved by this, time should not be wasted anymore and an intraosseous route should be obtained for a quick and efficient infusion to fill the vascular tree.

Indication

Failed IV access in a shocked patient.

Contraindications

- Fracture of that bone—absolute contraindication (e.g. fracture tibia)
- Fracture of a long bone proximal to the location (i.e. fracture of femur with large haematoma which might interfere venous drainage for infusion in tibia—relative contraindication)
- Unhealthy skin condition or loss of skin (e.g. burn) is not contraindications
- Bone marrow depressant drugs should not be infused.

Equipment Required

- Appropriate size sterile gloves
- Cleaning agents, towels
- Local anaesthetic drug (e.g. 1% lidocaine)
- 5 and 20 mL syringes
- 20–22 gauge needles
- Intraosseous needle **(Fig. 35.4)**
- Thread or tape to fix the needle
- Three-way tap and tube
- Splint
- Infusion fluid.

Method

- Wash and dry hands with sterile towels
- Wear gloves, non-touch technique
- Clean and towel the area, exposing from the patella to about proximal one-fourth of leg on anterior and medial aspect
- Identify tibial tuberosity (run your finger in the midline from below the patella, the first bony prominence on the proximal part of tibia) **(Fig. 35.5)**.
- If the child is conscious enough to feel the pain, inject local anaesthetic agent on the medial side, about 1–2 finger breadths below the horizontal line from the tibial tuberosity and wait for about 15–20 minutes
- Take the intraosseous needle
- Rough estimation of the depth to reach the centre of the bone (i.e. bone marrow) and keep the needle, with head against the head of index finger metacarpal and three fingers gripping the needle for the estimated depth
- By clock and anticlockwise screwing movements, at right angle (90°) to the surface of the bone, introduce through the cortex to the marrow (considerable force may be required when the cortex is thick). The needle should stand at 90° when left free
- Attach a tube with three-way tap
- Fix the needle and the tube with thread or tape and then splint the joint
- Inject or infuse the fluid (warm enough)

Pitfalls

- The infused fluid is drained by the veins supplying the marrow. If that bone is fractured, all or most of the fluid will be drained through the fracture site.
- This is an intraosseous infusion and needle should be introduced into the bone (i.e. on the medial side of tibia). It becomes intramuscular (IM) route if injected on the lateral side of the proximal part of the leg.
- Oblique insertion will result in the bone entering in the subcutaneous area.
- Too strong a force, not limited to the estimated depth, may result in penetration of the opposite cortex and the technique will fail (becomes IM infusion) and that bone cannot be used again.

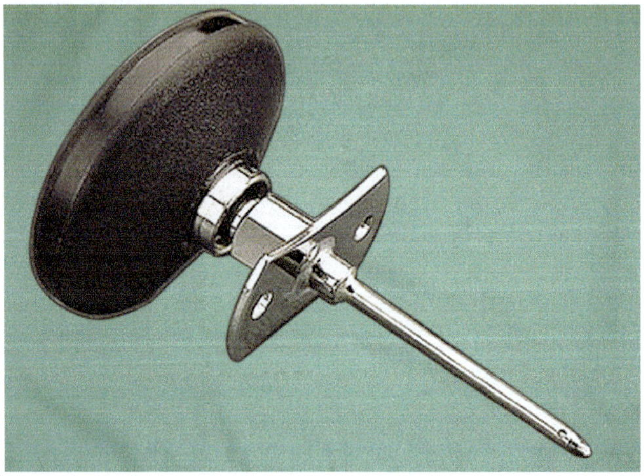

Figure 35.4 Intraosseous needle.

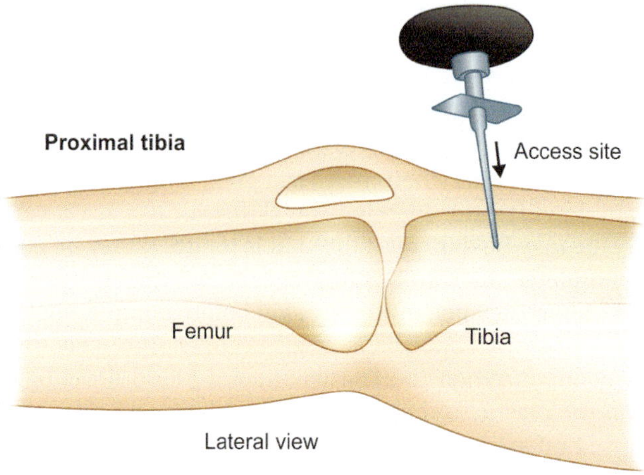

Figure 35.5 Intraosseous needle insertion.

- The patient may lie down still when shocked, but when the circulating volume improves, the child may regain conscious state and start kicking the legs with the possibility of dismantling the needle—a good splinting may avoid this problem.

Complications

- Infection
- Septicaemia
- Fat embolism.

Suturing

Suturing of wounds is a basic practical procedure that any doctor must be competent in. The basic steps are described below and illustrated in **Figures 35.6A to F**.

Wound Preparation

Every wound should be assessed in terms of its location, its margins, injury to, and viability of deeper structures and tissue, the presence of foreign body in the wound and the degree of contamination. The location of the wound

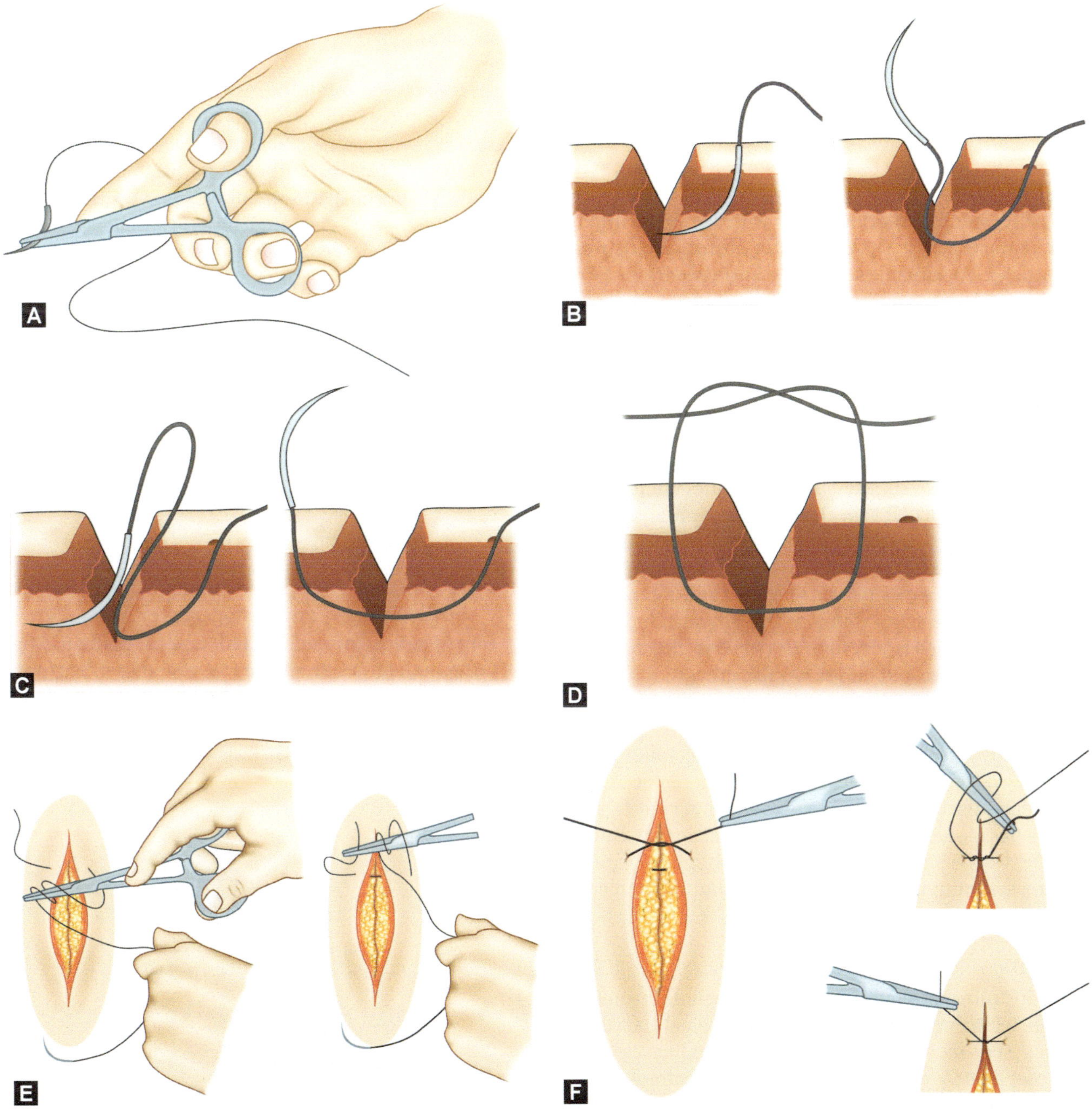

Figures 35.6A to F (A) Gripping a suture needle with a needle driver; (B) Needle pushed through skin and out into the base of the wound. Suture pulled through first side of wound; (C) Needle pushed into the base of the opposite side of the wound. Needle rotated out through second side of the wound; (D) The U shape of proper suture placement; (E) Loop the suture twice around the needle driver. Grab the short end of the suture with the needle drive; (F) Laying down first loop of a knot. Create second single loop in opposite direction. Square knot complete.

could well dictate the type of anaesthesia, wound washout required and the type of sutures and suturing needed. The margins of the wound should be healthy and viable, and should come together without undue tension. If the margins or wound edges are ischemic or necrosed, they need to be debrided and freshened. It is also important to exclude either by direct visual examination or by radiology the presence of any kind of foreign body in the wound. The degree of wound contamination could well decide whether a general or local anaesthesia would suffice the type of wound toilet and washout and the type of sutures and suturing required. The wound needs to be thoroughly cleaned with sterile saline or an antiseptic solution under anaesthesia.

Local Anaesthesia

See section on Sedation and Analgesia.

Sutures Including Type and Size of Sutures

Basically, suture materials come with two very important characteristics. They are either absorbable or non-absorbable. Absorbable sutures are absorbed by the body after several weeks or months.

Non-absorbable monofilament and multifilament include silk, braided synthetics, monofilament synthetics including prolene, ethibond, nylon, etc.

Absorbable sutures are used when continued strength is not important. It is also an important advantage in paediatric patients where sutures are absorbed and do not require to be removed. They are used for subcutaneous tissues and subcuticular skin closures. The non-absorbable suture is used when continued strength is important, and when minimal reaction is important. These include uses in skin and fascial closure and for vessel anastomosis.

Size of suture starts with 0 as the heaviest and works down to 7/0 which is very fine. The smaller the gauge, the heavier the suture and the greater the strength.

Types of Needle

Different types of needles are available including round tapered, conventional cutting, reverse cutting, taper cut, etc.

Needles used in deeper tissues including vessels, subcutaneous tissues, etc. include cutting and reverse cutting needle. Needles used for skin closure should be cutting and reverse cutting, as they are atraumatic and pierce the skin easily.

Instruments

Basic instruments required for suturing include the needle holder, tooth forceps, non-tooth forceps, scalpel and suture cutting scissors. Other requirements including cleaning and preparation of solution, gauze swabs and drapes.

Handling of instruments: Knowledge of technique and instruments allows for a safe and competent procedure. Sutures are placed on wounds with the use of tissue forceps either tooth or non-tooth forceps and a needle holder. Needle holders are like artery forceps except their tips are shorter with a grooved jaw to hold a needle securely. The usual method to mount a needle is two-thirds of the way proximal on the needle with its axis perpendicular to the long axis of the needle holder. Once used, the needle should be moved along the side of the needle holder tip to sheath the tip of the needle. Once the suture is placed, the redundant suture is cut above the knot using two hands for better control.

Basic Techniques Including Interrupted and Mattress Sutures

Basic suture patterns include interrupted, mattress and continuous sutures.

An interrupted suture consists of single stitches placed in a row and each stitch had its own knot. A continuous suture begins with an initial knot and runs continuously to the other end of the wound before the finishing knot is tied.

The most useful mattress suture is the vertical mattress suture which takes deep and superficial bites providing maximum suture strength and everting the wound margins. Common practice is the remove sutures from the face in 3–5 days whereas sutures on the limbs, hands, knees, elbow and trunk after 7–10 days.

Nasogastric Tube

A nasogastric tube is inserted for urgent or elective reasons. The tube is introduced through either of the nostrils and is negotiated through the oesophagus so that the tip is lying in the stomach **(Fig. 35.7)**.

Indications

- For drainage of gastric content, e.g. intestinal obstruction (pre- and postoperative)
- For feeding in medical and surgical patients when the patient is not allowed or not able to eat/drink through the mouth.

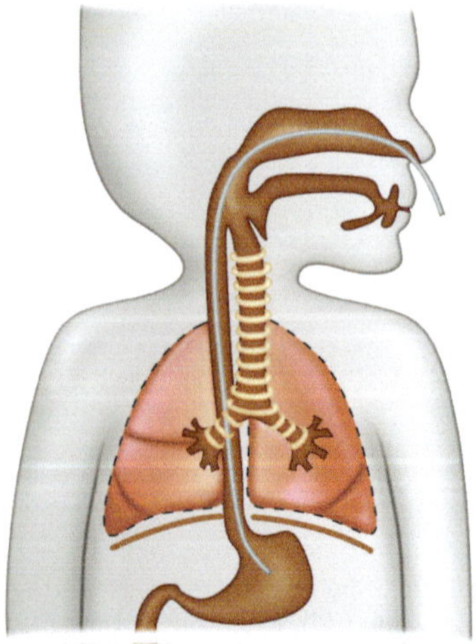

Figure 35.7 Nasogastric tube.

Contraindications

- Trauma to nose/oropharynx/oesophagus/stomach
- Basal skull fracture
- Thermal/caustic injuries to nose/oropharynx/oesophagus/stomach
- Oesophageal obstruction/perforation.

Equipment Required

- Appropriate size sterile gloves
- Cleaning agent
- Nasogastric tube appropriate size (8–12 CH for children, 6 CH feeding tube for preterm)
- Neonate/baby—with green line (if X-ray is required)
- Lubricant (e.g. sterile K-Y jelly)
- 5- and 20 mL syringes
- Stethoscope
- Litmus paper or pH reaction chart
- Adhesive plaster.

Method

- Introduce yourself to the patient and explain the procedure
- Keep the head straight, facing the roof
- Measure the length of the tube to be kept in (lying position—from the nostril to the angle of the jaw posteriorly and turn vertically till the epigastrium)
- Lubricate to the measured length
- Clean the nostril
- Pass the tube gently through the nasal passage to the measured length, without any resistance (patient will cough or pull the tube if it enters respiratory tract)
- Inject air and listen to the sound in the epigastrium (not in the chest)
- Aspirate the content and test with litmus paper or pH reaction chart (should be acidic, if the tube is in stomach)
- Use adhesive plaster to stick the tube on the ipsilateral cheek
- X-ray to confirm the position of the tube (green line), if necessary.

Pitfalls

- Basal skull fracture—the tube can enter the cranial cavity
- The tube should not be pushed forcibly if there is resistance (obstruction) or cough (wrong passage)
- The tube may coil in the pharynx (without any resistance) and can come out through the mouth!

Complications

- Perforation (especially after thermal or caustic injuries)
- Too large size can traumatise the nostril and proximal nasal passage.

Urinary Catheterisation in the Male and Female

Urethral catheterisation is a useful procedure in emergency and elective situations so that hydration status of the individual can also be ascertained. A sample of urine can be obtained for urinalysis at the bedside as well for laboratory investigation. Strict antiseptic and atraumatic procedure should be carried out to avoid complications. It is important to explain the procedure to the child and child carers before starting.

Indications

- In an emergency situation, e.g. multitrauma patients, for noting hourly urinary output
- For major operative procedures in bladder, urethra, penis
- To relieve acute retention of urine
- To obtain a urine sample for laboratory investigations—rarely done
- For 24-hour collection of urine for various laboratory investigations.

Contraindications

- Urethral injuries
- Infection of the distal urethra, glans, prepuce (infection may be introduced proximally into the sterile bladder during catheterisation)
- Postoperative hypospadias repair.

Relevant Anatomy

Male urethra (Fig. 35.8).

Equipment Required

- Appropriate size sterile gloves
- Foley catheter (8, 10, 12 CH size for children, 6 CH feeding tube for small/preterm babies/neonates)—Silastic® catheter if the catheter has to stay for longer period

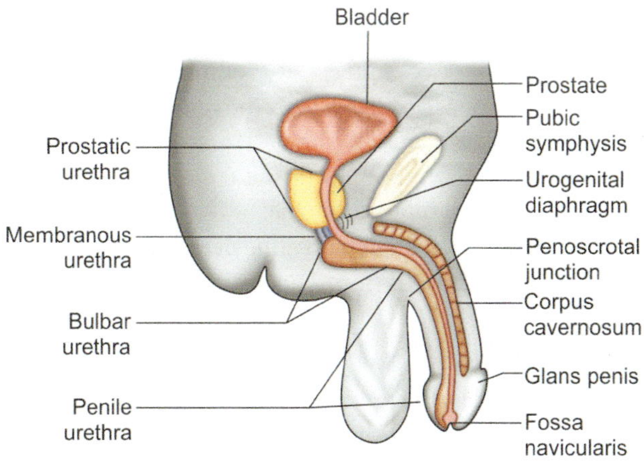

Figure 35.8 Male urethra.

- Cleaning agents, towels
- Sterile lubricant (e.g. K-Y jelly, lidocaine gel)
- Sterile container to receive urine sample
- Sterile water and 10 mL syringe
- Urinary bag
- Adhesive plaster.

Method (Boys)

1. Wash and dry hands with sterile towels.
2. Wear gloves, non-touch technique.
3. Take the appropriate size Foley catheter from the sterile inner cover (size is printed in the limb of the catheter).
4. Inject 2–3 mL sterile water in the short limb of the catheter and check balloon for any leaks and deflate.
5. After cleaning, draping with towels should be done exposing the suprapubic and genital area.
6. Estimate the length of the tube required to be in, from the tip of penis to just above the symphysis pubis.
7. If prepuce is intact, retract and expose glans and clean.
8. Open the external urethral meatus and clean.
9. Insert instill, a gel/lidocaine gel.
10. Introduce the Foley catheter gently and smoothly through the urethra to the bladder till urine escapes through the long limb of the catheter.
    - You may encounter resistance at the prostatic/external sphincter. If this occurs:
    - Stop and allow the sphincter to relax
    - Lower the penis towards the perineum and continue to advance the catheter
    - Abandon the procedure if the catheter did not advance or if the patient is in discomfort and seek senior advice. Never inflate the balloon unless you get urine from the catheter.
11. Once you are happy the catheter is in place, inject 5–10 mL of sterile water through the short limb of the catheter (to inflate the balloon—maximum for injection is printed adjacent to the catheter size).
12. With a gentle pull, the inflated balloon will move to the bladder neck and is self-retaining.
13. Use the adhesive plaster to fix the catheter on the thigh or suprapubic area.
14. Connect the long limb of the catheter to a urinary bag for continuous drainage.
15. Fix the tube to thigh with adhesive plaster.
16. Always replace the foreskin to prevent paraphimosis.

Method (Girls)

1 to 5. (Same as the method of boys mentioned above)

6. Estimate the length of the tube required to be in, from the tip of urethra to just above the symphysis pubis **(Fig. 35.9)**

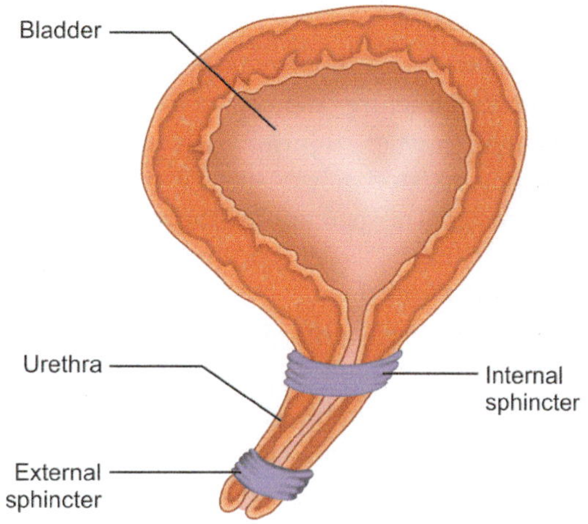

Figure 35.9 Female urethra.

7. As above
8. Clean labia majora, open labia and clean urethral meatus and labia minora.

9 to 15. (Same as the method of boys mentioned above)

Always document in the patients notes a procedure note, carefully dated and stating size of catheter and amount of water in the balloon, and the residual urine volume.

Complications

- Infection
- Trauma to urethra/external urethral meatus **(Figs. 35.10A and B)**
- Bleeding
- Blockage of catheter and bypassing of catheter
- Paraphimosis from failure to protract foreskin
- False passage creation and stricture formation.

Urinalysis

Bedside chemical analysis of urine can be done using chemical strips. The manufacturing company indicates the details of when to read the results after dipping the strip in the urine and to match the colours against various constituents of urine.

For bacteriological and other special studies such as urgent microscopy, the urine sample should be sent to the laboratory immediately, as long standing exposure to the atmosphere may cause contamination.

The common reagent strips are used to identify the presence and amount of constituents of urine-protein, pH, blood, specific gravity, ketone and glucose.

Method

- After taking samples for microbiological study and other special tests, dip the strip till all the reagents are smeared with urine

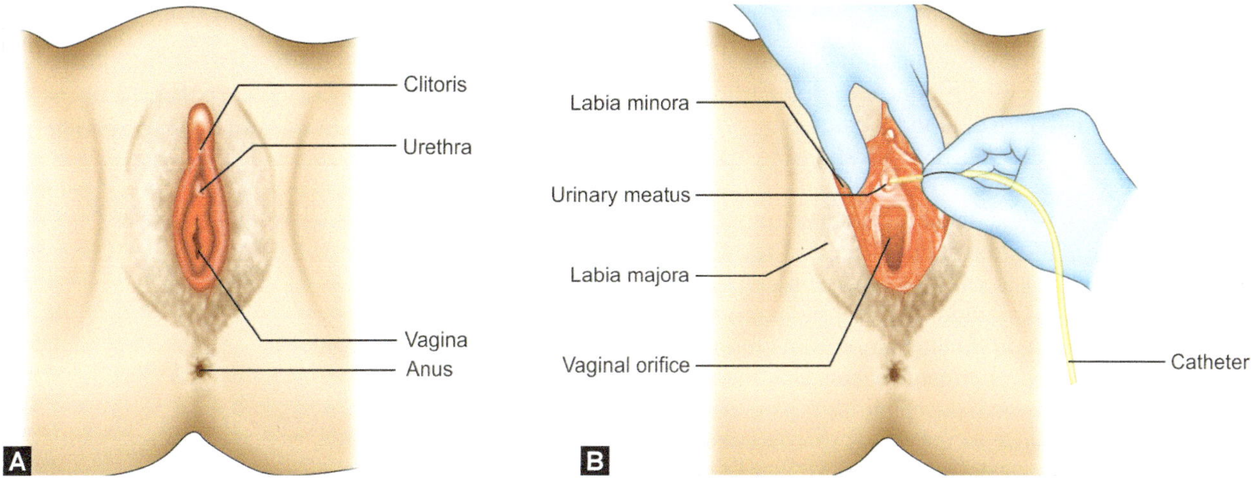

Figures 35.10A and B Female external urethral meatus.

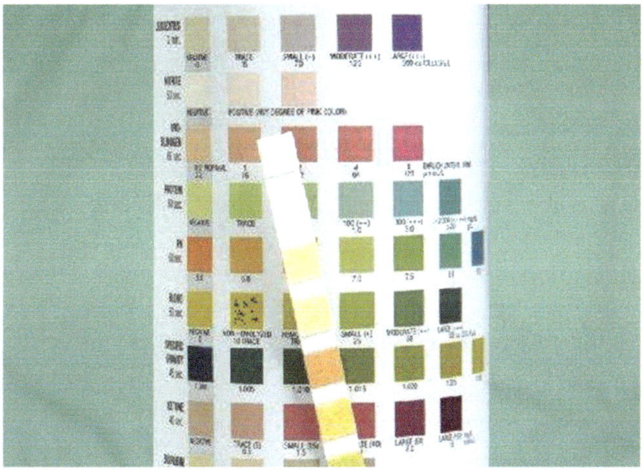

Figure 35.11 Analysis of urine using chemical strip.

- Keep the strip on table or sink, reagents facing upwards
- After the appropriate time (as mentioned by the company leaflet) match the colours of the reagents against the colours on the container. Note the results for each chemical constituent **(Fig. 35.11)**.

Urinalysis Interpretation

- *Urine pH:* Normal range is from 5.0 to 9.0. Normally, if the serum is acidemic, the excess cations will be excreted in the urine, driving the pH down. Similarly, excess anions of alkalemia drive the urine pH up.
- *Ketones:* They are elevated in dehydration, fasting, or diabetic ketoacidosis (DKA—seen in type I diabetics).

Haemoglobin if elevated, without red cells present: haemolytic anaemia (transfusion reaction?); error caused by lysing of old sample. With red cells present: bladder trauma; tubular damage. With red cell casts present: glomerulonephritis.

- *Bilirubin:* This refers to conjugated bilirubin. This is elevated in post- or intrahepatic obstruction.
- *Urobilinogen:* This is elevated in conditions with high unconjugated bilirubin, such as haemolysis or Gilbert disease.
- *Nitrite:* This is elevated when bacteria (particularly gram-negative organisms, generally faecal) are present in the urinary tract. The organisms that convert nitrate to nitrite are *Escherichia coli, Enterobacter, Citrobacter, Klebsiella* and *Proteus.* They take about 4 hours to do the conversion, so your best bet is a urine that has been waiting at least that long such as a morning void.
- *Leucocyte esterase:* This enzyme is made by neutrophils as a response to the presence of bacteria and is an indicator of urinary tract infection (UTI).
- *Glucose:* Glycosuria means a serum glucose of greater than 180. It is not normal.
- *Protein:* Usually albumin more than other proteins. If elevated, urinary protein indicates UTI, recent exercise or renal disease.
- *Specific gravity:* This is used to infer volume status, which you should be able to assess clinically with more accuracy than this test will provide. If specific gravity is elevated, that means the urine is concentrated, suggesting a hypovolaemia. If the specific gravity is low, that means the urine is dilute, suggesting hypervolaemia.
- *Casts:* They are associated with the collection of cells in the distal tubule, which become concretions after sufficient time has elapsed. They are generally associated with different conditions dependent on their colour: red—nephritic syndrome; white—pyelonephritis; muddy brown—renal failure; crystals—seen in gout, kidney stones, or in the presence of some drugs.

Blood Glucose

A glucose meter (or glucometer) is a medical device for determining the approximate concentration of glucose in the blood. A small drop of blood, obtained by pricking the skin with a lancet, is placed on a disposable test strip that the meter reads and uses to calculate the blood glucose level. The meter then displays the level in mg/dL or mmol/L. The size of the drop of blood needed by different models varies from 0.3 to 1 μL. Most glucometers today use an electrochemical method. Test strips contain a capillary that sucks up a reproducible amount of blood. The glucose in the blood reacts with an enzyme electrode. The total charge passing through the electrode is proportional to the amount of glucose in the blood that has reacted with the enzyme **(Figs. 35.12 and 35.13)**.

Causes of Hypoglycaemia and Hyperglycaemia

The list of causes of hypoglycaemia and hyperglycaemia are extensive; some are listed in **Table 35.2**.

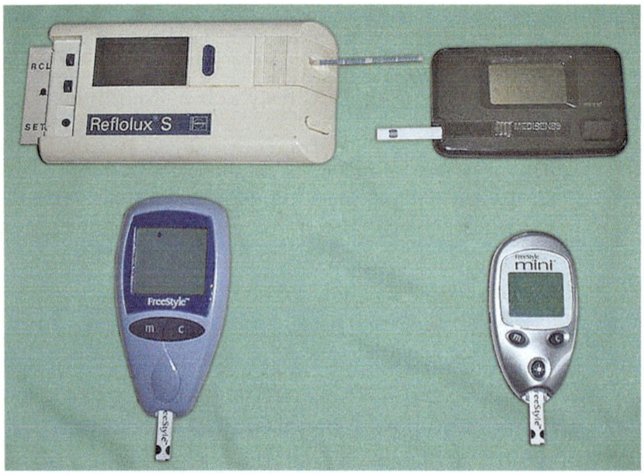

Figure 35.12 A selection of glucometers.

Indications

- Used to monitor glucose level in patient with diabetes
- Used to monitor glucose level in patient receiving TPN
- Used in emergency to rule out hypoglycaemia.

Equipment Required

- Glucose meter
- Testing strip
- Alcohol swab
- Lancet
- Cotton wool
- Gloves
- Sharps bin.

TABLE 35.2 Causes of hypoglycaemia and hyperglycaemia.

Hypoglycaemia	***Hyperglycaemia***
Transient neonatal hypoglycaemia	Diabetes mellitus type 1 and type 2
Prolonged fasting	Drugs, e.g. beta-blockers, epinephrine, thiazide diuretics, corticosteroids
Congenital hypopituitarism	Physiological stress
Congenital hyperinsulinism	Critical illness
Inborn errors of carbohydrate metabolism	Infection
Insulin-induced hypoglycaemia	Inflammation
Insulin-injected for type 1 diabetes	
Munchausen syndrome	
Insulin-secreting pancreatic tumour	
Reactive hypoglycaemia and idiopathic postprandial syndrome	
Addison disease	
Sepsis	

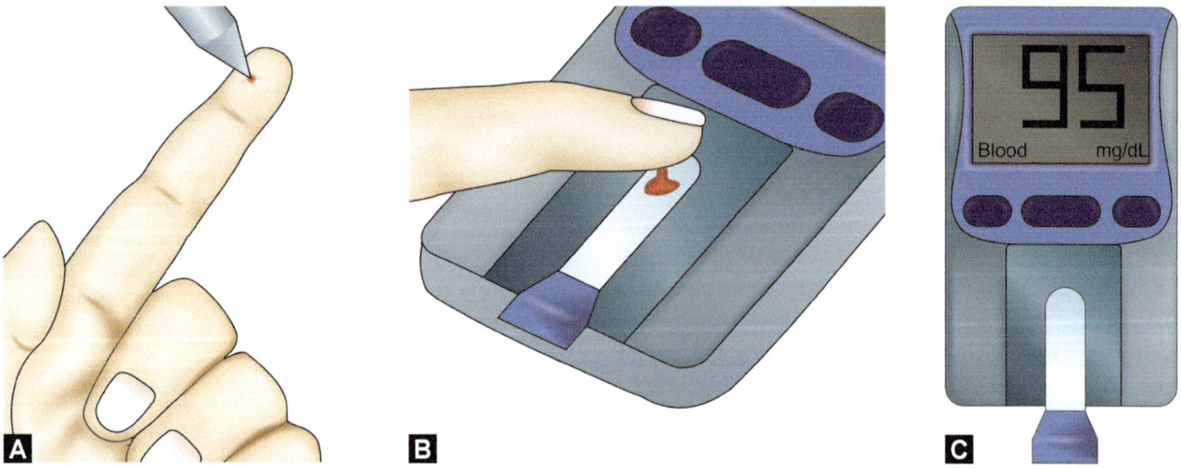

Figures 35.13A to C Pulp of finger and spring loaded lance to the site.

Method

- Choose injection site; pulp of finger in older children; heel in younger children and babies
- Clean site with alcohol swab and allow to dry
- Apply the spring loaded lance to the site and warn the patient they will feel a sharp scratch
- Fire the lancet
- Express a droplet of blood by squeezing the finger or heel. Express the droplet onto the test strip and insert into glucometer. Ensure it signals it is analysing.
- Apply pressure with cotton wool to the puncture site
- Apply a dressing if required.

A normal reading is 4 mmol/L or 72 mg/dL. It is widely accepted; however, that glucometers have a nationally accepted standard error of ±20% and, therefore, if there is any doubt regarding the reading a serum glucose sample should be sent.

OTHER PRACTICAL PROCEDURES

Central Venous Access

Central venous access provides venous access as well as measurement of central venous pressure. The aim of central venous catheterisation is to insert a large bore catheter into a large central vein. Strict asepsis during insertion is essential and many centres now utilise a 'central line bundle' approach during central line insertion to improve adherence to aseptic technique and therefore minimise the risk of infection. During the procedure, a needle is placed in the vessel and an internal guide wire inserted into the vein first. This is known as the Seldinger technique. The needle is then removed over the guidewire, the track into the vessel lumen dilated and the cannula threaded along the wire into the lumen. This involves the subclavian or internal jugular vein. The femoral vein also may be used and preferred by many. The indications of central venous catheterisation are as follows:

- Measurement of central venous pressure
- Infusion of drugs
- Total parenteral nutrition.

The equipment required for central venous line is available in prepackaged central line sets. These central venous lines are, as time goes by, increasingly difficult to protect from the entry of bacteria, sepsis is likely after 5–10 days, although careful care and strict asepsis decreases the incidence. However, some paediatric intensive care units (PICUs) judge it wise to change all central venous lines every 5 days. If the line is needed for long-term therapy (e.g. chemotherapy or TPN) then a subcutaneously tunnelled line should be used. An alternative for intermittent therapy is to place a port with venous access subcutaneously (Portacath).

Central venous line landmarks:

Femoral vein—one fingerbreadth below midpoint of the inguinal ligament just medial to the femoral artery

Internal jugular vein—junction of the sternal and clavicular heads of sternocleidomastoid muscle, just anterior and lateral to the carotid artery. Aim needle towards ipsilateral nipple.

Complications of Central Venous Access

These include pneumothorax, haemothorax, hydrothorax, air or catheter embolism, and brachial plexus injury. Preparations always should be made to treat them and a chest X-ray should be performed after internal jugular or subclavian line insertion. Cervical haematomas are common, and although bleeding is usually trivial, it can produce occlusion of the airway. The biggest risk however is that of central line infection which usually mandates removal of the line.

Sweat Test (Chloride Sweat Test, Cystic Fibrosis Sweat Test)

Analysis of sodium and chloride content of sweat is indicated in the diagnosis of cystic fibrosis (CF). Normally, sweat on the skin surface contains very little sodium and chloride. People with CF have 2–5 times, the normal amount of sodium and chloride in their sweat. Generally chloride (sweat chloride) is measured.

Iontophoretic Method

This is a convenient method in that only a small area of skin is sweated. It may thus be used on patients of all ages including small infants.

Requirements

- The sweat box unit supplies a small current to the appropriate skin area via two terminals
- Magnesium sulphate solution, 0.1 N
- Aqueous solution of pilocarpine nitrate, 0.2%
- Lint, 'Sleek,' polythene sheeting and deionized water
- A piece of filter paper previously weighed in a container labelled with the patient's name
- Forceps
- A warm room.

The child's limbs and trunk are exposed. For each terminal, a piece of lint is cut slightly broader than the terminal: it is folded twice to give thickness and placed on the terminal. The black lead (negative pole) lint is thoroughly damped with magnesium sulphate solution: the lint is placed on the anterior aspect of the child's thigh and the terminal placed over it (i.e. the lint is between skin and terminal) and taped firmly in place with a strip of Sleek or other suitable adhesive.

The red lead (positive pole) lint is thoroughly dampened with pilocarpine and applied in a similar manner to the area of skin which is to be sweated. The scapular area is found to be satisfactory in most cases. The terminal wires are attached to the appropriate buttons on the sweat box unit and the unit switched on. The current control is slowly increased until a steady current of between 4 and 5 mA is reached and this current is maintained for 5 minutes after which the unit is switched off and the lint and terminals removed. The skin area to which pilocarpine was applied is now thoroughly washed with deionised water and carefully dried. The weighed filter paper is removed from its container with forceps and placed on the skin area: a piece of polythene sheet, slightly larger than the filter paper is placed over it and taped firmly in place with 'Sleek' which should seal the edges of the polythene to prevent leakage. It is useful to apply the Sleek in four strips leaving a 'window' in the centre of the polythene. The child may now be dressed and may resume his ordinary ward activities. The polythene window is examined 30 minutes later—if sufficient sweat has been collected then the filter paper becomes almost transparent, if this is not apparent it is worth leaving the paper in situ for a further 30 minutes.

The polythene and Sleek are then removed—the paper carefully placed in its weighed container using forceps and sent to the laboratory for analysis together with a control piece of filter paper. The minimum weight of sweat required for electrolyte analysis by this method is 100 mg. When the current is being applied, the child may experience a tingling sensation but provided no more than 5 mA is used this should not be uncomfortable. Sometimes the area of skin under the terminals becomes reddened or may even show an urticarial eruption but this will readily settle. The only complication we have experienced with this method has been a small skin burn due to careless application of a terminal which touched the skin. This is avoided if the lint is of larger area than the terminal, but even so care should be taken with a wriggling child lest the terminal slip during this stage of the procedure.

KEY LEARNING POINT

Chloride sweat test: Sweat chloride 'concentration' greater than 60 mmol per kg is diagnostic of cystic fibrosis (CF).

Radial Artery Puncture

The skin is cleansed in the usual manner. A suitable size needle (21 G usually) is attached firmly to a syringe and the dead space filled with heparin. The infant's hand is supinated and held so that hand and forearm are straight, i.e. no wrist flexion or extension. The needle is inserted through the proximal wrist skin crease over the radial pulsation and at an angle of about 60° to the skin—it is pushed thence till it just touches the radius whence with slight negative pressure on the syringe it is slowly withdrawn along its line of entry, withdrawal ceasing when blood is obtained. After arterial puncture, the syringe is sealed, e.g. with a syringe cap or portion of plasticine. An assistant maintains firm and unvarying pressure on the puncture site for 5 minutes or till unvarying pressure on the puncture site for 5 minutes or till all bleeding has ceased. In the older child, a small dose of local anaesthetic may be injected at the site of puncture before the procedure is performed.

Arterialised Capillary Blood

A satisfactory alternative to arterial puncture is the use of arterialised capillary blood. It has the advantage that blood is always obtained and that sampling may be freely repeated as often as required. In the infant, the heel is the best site to prepare; in the older child, the ear lobe or digital pulp is used. The skin is cleaned in standard fashion. If the site is flushed and warm, no further preparation may be needed. Squeezing the site is obviously contraindicated in obtaining samples for PO_2. Following preparation, the skin is incised briskly with a sterile lancet and blood collected in heparinised glass capillary tubes whose ends are sealed with plasticine. The analysis for PO_2 should be made within 15 minutes of sampling.

Haematological Procedures

Precautions in Patients with Haematological Disorders

To patients with haemophilia or leukaemia, their veins are their 'lifelines'. Venepuncture should be kept to a minimum and laboratories dealing with children should be geared to perform their tests upon capillary samples of blood unless this is not practicable. When venepunctures are unavoidable (usually due to the need for therapy or for transfusion), it is best not to use the antecubital fossae since extravasation of blood or infused drug can easily occur undetected. Perivenous haematoma are a potent source of infection and of great hazard in either leukaemia or haemophilia. The veins on the back of the hand (or foot) can be used with far less chance of undetected extravasation during injection and easier control of haemostasis by subsequent application of pressure using sterile cotton wool. Scalp veins provide similar access in infants but tests using capillary samples are particularly important for this age group.

KEY LEARNING POINTS

- In absolutely no circumstances should any intramuscular injection be given to a child with haemophilia or Christmas disease.
- Likewise, no intramuscular injections should be given to children who are grossly thrombocytopenic or are receiving heparin therapy.

Marrow Aspiration

It is convenient to perform the whole procedure 15 minutes after the patient has been sedated. With the patient in the 'LP' position, the posterior superior iliac spine located at the lower end of the crest. It is helpful to mark the line of the crest with the iodine used as a skin antiseptic. With the crest grasped between thumb and forefinger the skin, subcutaneous tissue and periosteum is infiltrated with 2 mL of 1% xylocaine (or equivalent) at a point 1 cm above the spine in young children and 2 cm above it in older children using a fine needle. During infiltration, move the point of the needle a few millimetres first one way and then the other across the surface of the crest so as to define the exact limits of its subcutaneous surface. Allow 2 minutes for the local anaesthetic to become effective and then using strict aseptic technique, push a marrow puncture needle and trocar of relatively wide bore (1.5 mm) through the skin with a rotating action down to the periosteum and locate the most central subcutaneous portion of the crest. The needle and trocar are then directed in a strictly anterior direction (in all planes) and pressed into the bone with an alternate clockwise and anticlockwise boring action with a firm movement. As soon as the needle is sufficiently inserted into the bone to remain fixed by itself without support, the trocar is briskly withdrawn. A fleck of pink marrow may be seen on the tip of the trocar confirming that the needle is within the marrow cavity. Strong suction is then applied with a 20 mL sterile syringe and stopped after about 0.2 mL of blood (and marrow) enters the syringe. If nothing can be aspirated the trocar is replaced, the needle advanced a further 1–2 mm and aspiration repeated. If still unsuccessful, the procedure is repeated 1–2 mm on either side of the original position. After obtaining aspirate the trocar is replaced and the needle withdrawn covering the puncture site with a sterile dressing. The aspirate is expelled in equal amounts on to 8–10 microscope slides in succession, and the surplus fluid blood is sucked back into the syringe. Smears are made of the sedimented marrow cells and particles, and the slides waved in the air to achieve rapid drying. The remaining iodine is removed from the skin with surgical spirit and a sterile adhesive and occlusive dressing placed over the puncture site.

KEY LEARNING POINT

Marrow aspiration: Marrow puncture is contraindicated in haemophilia or Christmas disease but is safe in the presence of even severe thrombocytopenia, when care is taken to ensure continued firm pressure after the procedure.

Marrow Trephine

This is performed at the site as above in children aged more than 1 year. A Gardner bone marrow trephine needle and trocar used. The trocar locates the bone and the saw-toothed needle is then rotated down to the surface of the bone and thereafter rotated in one direction with steady pressure. As the needle cuts into the bone, the head of the trocar is gradually pushed back out of the needle helping to indicate the depth to which the needle has penetrated. When this is thought to be 5 mm, a syringe is attached so as to exert gentle suction while the needle is withdrawn, after which a slender cylinder of bone and adjacent marrow can be extruded from the needle into a suitable histological fixative such as used in the local laboratory.

Tibial Puncture

This site is used for marrow puncture in preference to the iliac crest for an average child up to 6 weeks or in very small babies up to the age of 3 months. It is important to avoid damaging the epiphysis in the region of the tibial tubercle since a disturbance of bone growth could occur in later life. The subcutaneous anteromedial surface of the tibia is palpated and the tibial tubercle identified. A site in the middle of the subcutaneous surface 2.5 cm (1 inch) below the tubercle is chosen. A needle with a guard is used to puncture the skin and then the bone with a 'boring' motion keeping the needle strictly at right angles to the subcutaneous surface of the bone. When the needle point touches the periosteum before entering the bone, the guard is adjusted to allow bone penetration to a depth of 2–3 mm. In other respects, the procedure is as described for the posterior iliac crest puncture.

Stains in Common Use

In the side room or laboratory, which should be attached to every ward, a number of simple stains should always be available and should be kept fresh. These would certainly include methylene blue, carbolfuchsin and Gram's stain.

Methylene Blue Stain (0.5% Aqueous Solution)

Methylene blue films can be made so rapidly that it is surprising that this procedure is not used freely and widely. Scrapings of the buccal mucosa (for thrush), a faecal smear (for deposit of polymorphs seen in bacterial dysentery), or a single loop-full of the centrifuged deposit of CSF from a case of suspected meningitis (for bacteria and leucocytes) may be applied thinly to the slide and to dry and then fix by passing three times through a Bunsen flame. The slide is then stained with methylene blue for 1 minute, washed in water, dried, and examined under oil immersion. The whole procedure need takes no more than 5 minutes. The ease with which the candida and mycelia of moniliasis or bacteria such as the coccobacilli of *Haemophilus influenzae* meningitis may be seen, lends strong support to the routine use of methylene blue film.

Carbolfuchsin Stain

Dilute carbolfuchsin (10% aqueous solution of concentrated carbolfuchsin, *see* Ziehl-Neelsen method below) is used in a similar fashion to methylene blue as described above. In a suitably purpuric fevered child, a smear of 'juice' from a purpuric blob pricked with a needle, or the buffy layer of cells on centrifugation of blood may be stained after fixation to show diplococccus of the *Neisseria meningitides* type with a duplex rather than lanceolate (pneumococcal) appearance. This immediately suggests meningococcal septicaemia and mandates parenteral antimicrobial treatment whilst Gram's stains, culture and other procedures continue.

Ziehl-Neelsen method: Concentrated carbolfuchsin (1 g basic fuchsin in 10 mL absolute alcohol made up with 100 mL, 5% aqueous phenol) is the basis of Ziehl-Neelsen method used for *Mycobacterium tuberculosis* and other mycobacteria. This is a rather complex procedure but one which may be applied to sputum, centrifuged fasting gastric juice, pus from a cold abscess or sinus or to CSF. The concentrated carbolfuchsin solution is applied and the slide warmed a number of times until the stain begins to steam. It must not be allowed to evaporate. After 5 minutes, the solution is poured off, the slide washed in water and then immersed in 20% sulphuric acid for 1 minute, the slide is washed and the acid application and washing repeated several times until the film is only faintly pink. After the acid is washed off and the slide washed in water, 95% alcohol is applied for 2 minutes. These last two steps may be combined by the use of acid-alcohol (3.0% hydrochloric acid in absolute alcohol) until the smear is faintly pink. The film is examined for red acid and alcohol-fast *M. tuberculosis*. It may be counterstained with methylene blue for 1 minute to give a colour contrast. The findings of such acid and alcohol fast bacilli are highly suggestive of *M. tuberculosis* but not specific without more sophisticated techniques or even culture.

Gram's Stain

There are many modifications of this staining procedure. Advice on the staining technique should be obtained locally and the necessary solutions made available in the ward test room.

- Stain with methyl violet 6B or crystal violet (0.5% in distilled water) for 30 seconds. This solution of stain should be filtered immediately before use.
- Pour off excess of stain, hold the slide on a slope and wash away excess stain with Gram's iodine (1 g iodine, 2 g potassium iodine and 300 mL distilled water).
- Wash iodine off with absolute alcohol and repeat until colour ceases to come out of the preparation.
- The slide is washed with water for 1 minute.
- Apply a suitable counter stain such as dilute carbolfuchsin (10% aqueous solution) for 1–2 minutes.

This stain is particularly important in dealing with CSF. The gram-positive lanceolate and encapsulated diplococcic of *Streptococcus pneumoniae* (pneumococcus) are sharply differentiated from the duplex pattern of gram-negative *Neisseria meningitidis* is the most awkward problem is with *H. influenza* which is gram-negative and pleomorphic and gram-negative rods of *E. coli* **(Figs. 35.14 and 35.15)**.

However, polymerase chain reaction (PCR) is an emerging technology that is based on the ability to detect DNA of pathogens, living or dead. The advantages of PCR testing include rapidly available results, often within hours, and the detection of organisms even if they have been killed by prior antimicrobial administration.

Central Nervous System

Transillumination

This simple and safe method of examination of the infant head is too often neglected. A case can be made for its routine use in the neurological examination of an infant during the first year of life, and in selected cases at later age. Careful technique is essential. The infant is taken

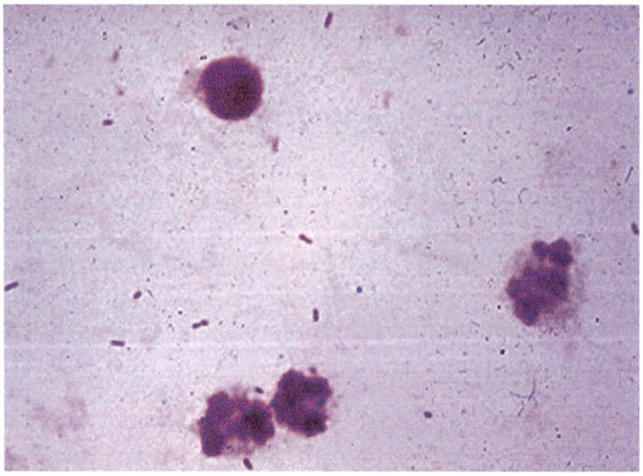

Figure 35.14 Cerebrospinal fluid with pus cells and *Haemophilus influenzae.*

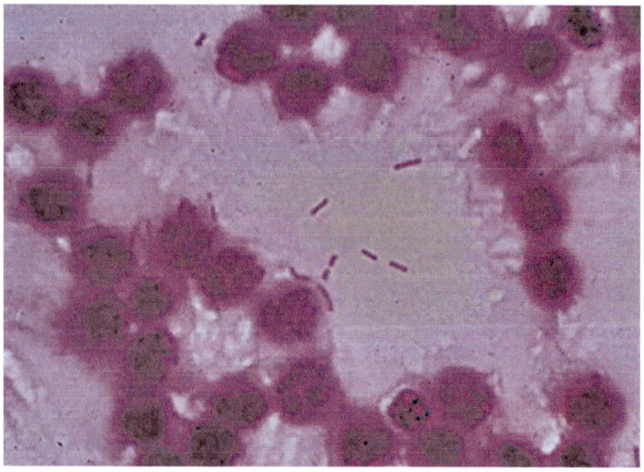

Figure 35.15 Cerebrospinal fluid with pus cells and *Escherichia coli.*

into a totally blacked-out room. The examiner uses a strong torch fitted with a black rubber adapter which prevents the escape of stray light when it is pressed against a flat or convex surface. He begins by testing his own dark adaption by attempting to transilluminate the palm of his hand. The infant's head is then systematically explored by switching on the torch when it is pressed against the frontal, central and occipital regions on each side, and also in the midline posteriorly over the posterior fossa. Normally, there is a narrow rim of transillumination around the adapter, the precise diameter of which depends on the characteristics of the light employed. The rim is greater in the frontal regions and is inversely related to age. Abnormalities include generalised transillumination in hydranencephaly or aqueduct stenosis, unilateral increases in subdural effusion or porencephaly, posterior fossa glow in the Dandy Walker syndrome or some arachnoid cysts, and multiple illuminated regions in cystic encephalomalacia **(Fig. 35.16)**. Suspected abnormalities may sometimes be more precisely defined by directing the light serially through them from more than one direction. The findings could be confirmed by cranial ultrasound.

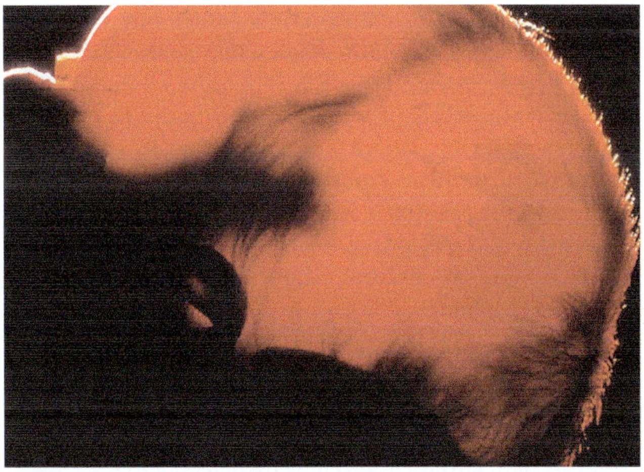

Figure 35.16 Positive transillumination in an infant with hydranencephaly. The entire head 'lights up' in hydranencephaly.

Lumbar Puncture (Spinal Tap)

This is most commonly carried out to determine whether meningitis is present. The technique is easier for the operator and much to be for the child if sedation is used sufficient to induce amnesia. Most operators prefer the lateral decubitus position, with the child's knees held in a flexed position near his face **(Figs. 35.17A and B)**. It is wise to ensure that an experienced assistant is able to hold a flexed infant firmly immobile before beginning the LP proper otherwise struggling may spoil the procedure at a critical moment should the sedation prove inadequate. After skin preparation (2% iodine in 70% ethanol is effective) local anaesthetic such as 1% lignocaine may be infiltrated at the chosen site between the second and third lumbar spines. This level is approximately indicated by a line joining the superior iliac crests. Many omit the local anaesthetic for rapid punctures not involving pressure measurements. A short fine LP needle with a stillete (for instance, a No. 22 needle which has a very short bevel) is pushed through the skin and then slowly advanced anteriorly and very slightly cephalad with a slight rotator motion until a barely felt click sensed through the tips of the index finger and thumb signals the penetration of the ligamentum flavum and dura mater. In small children the first appearance of CSF is less likely to be missed if the stillete is withdrawn after the skin has been punctured and reinserted briefly from time to time with each small movement deeper. Otherwise, the narrow subarachnoid space may be crossed unwittingly, the anterior plexus of veins transfixed, and a bloody tap result. The use of a small (No. 23) butterfly scalp-vein needle with its attached tubing has been advocated for LP in the newborn to reduce the chance of such a 'bloody tap' but there is a small risk of implantation spinal epidermoid tumours and leading to paraparesis some years later if a needle without a stillete is used to penetrate the skin.

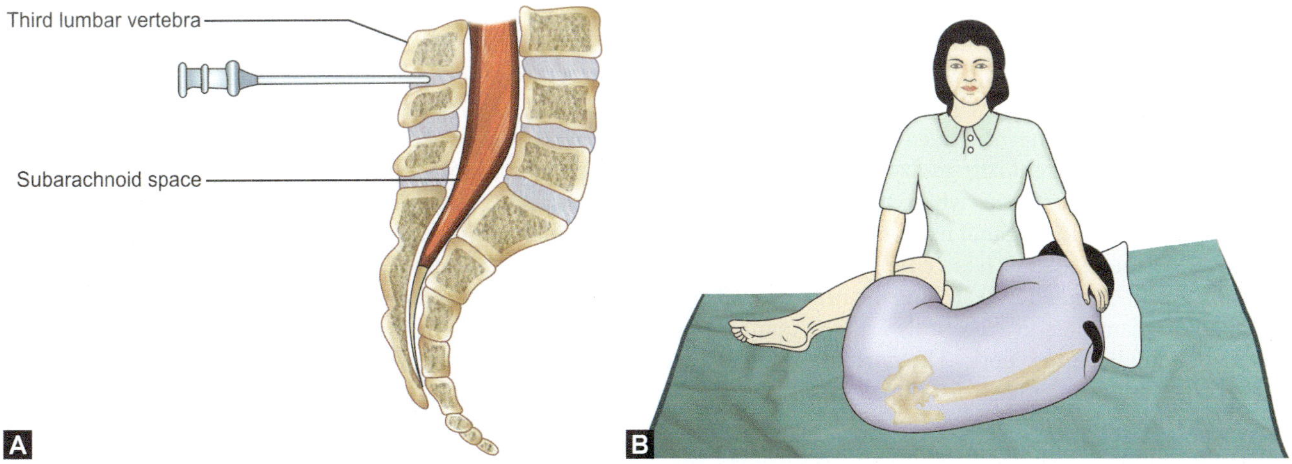

Figures 35.17A and B (A) Lumbar puncture; (B) Child in the lateral recumbent position.

Equipment Required

- Spinal or LP tray (including the items listed below)
- Sterile gloves
- Antiseptic solution with skin swabs
- Sterile drapes
- Lidocaine 1% without epinephrine
- Syringe 5 and 10 mL
- Needles 20 and 25 G
- Spinal needles 20 and 22 G
- Three-way stopcock
- Manometer
- Four plastic test tubes or universal containers
- Sterile dressing.

KEY LEARNING POINTS

Lumbar puncture (LP) needle without stilette: The LP needles must contain stilettes to avoid the possibility of inducing implantation dermoids and leading to paraparesis some years later.

Contraindications to LP

- Suspicion of an intracranial or spinal mass lesion
- Raised intracranial pressure
- Brain swelling
- Obstructive hydrocephalus
- Congenital lesions in the lumbosacral region (e.g. meningomyelocele)
- Platelet count below 40 × 10^9/L and other clotting abnormalities.

Some CSF is allowed to drip into sterile centrifuge tubes and a few drops added to 5 mL of dilute (15%) phenol solution in water in a test tube for Pandy test. Cloudiness appearing when the CSF is added to the phenolic solution indicates an excess of globulin. Any cloudiness in untreated CSF means an increased cell count. Xanthochromia may be obvious in clear CSF. If the CSF is bloody and a streaming effect from a punctured vein is not obvious, traditionally three tubes of CSF are taken to be compared, and later centrifuged to look for xanthochromia in the supernatant fluid. Xanthochromia of the supernatant may reflect bleeding several hours previously. It must be admitted that the distinction cannot always be made with certainty. This underlines the need for good positioning and assistance with great care to avoid such a traumatic bloody tap. In circumstances where measurement of the pressure is important, a spinal manometer is attached as soon as CSF is seen to flow. It is a common fallacy that the pressure can be guessed by watching the rate of flow from the needle; it cannot, and a few trials with the manometer will soon convince the sceptic. The normal CSF pressure in a neonate is in the range 0–5.7 mmHg (0–7.6 cm H_2O). The upper limit of the CSF pressure in older children is said to be similar to the adult value of 14 mmHg (19 cm H_2O).The protein in the CSF consists mostly of albumin and immunoglobulins. The normal protein concentration may be over 1 g/L in the newborn, but it then falls to low levels, with an upper limit of about 200 mg/L later in infancy with only a gradual increase towards the adult upper limit of 400 mg/L throughout childhood. Interpretation of the glucose concentration depends on the level of the blood glucose, which should ideally be measured at the same time. The cell count should also be determined and a methylene blue and Gram stain made from some of the centrifuged deposit. CSF should always be sent to the microbiological and biochemical departments.

KEY LEARNING POINT

- Complications of lumbar puncture: Infection, leakage of cerebrospinal fluid (CSF), headache, nausea, vomiting, and signs of meningeal irritation occur in approximately 25% of children.

Subdural Puncture (Subdural Tap)

This is carried out for the diagnosis and treatment of subdural haematoma or effusion. It is sufficiently safe to be recommended at an early stage when such a condition is suspected, provided that it is remembered that it is not entirely without risk. It is usually carried out by a neurosurgeon whilst the patient is anaesthetised. Haemorrhage and persisting effusion may be induced and if the brain is punctured the possible complications are similar to those described under ventriculography. Infection including the very serious subdural empyema is possible if technique is grossly lax.

The site of puncture is the lateral angle of a large anterior fontanelle or just lateral to it (in the coronal suture) if it is small. After shaving, preparation of the skin with 2% iodine in 70% ethanol and draping with the infant securely held supine, the skin is displaced and punctured by a fine short bevelled needle (No. 22, 3.8 cm long) with a stilette before being released into its normal position. This Z-track technique reduces the likelihood of continued fluid leakage and infection later. The needle is then advanced caudally, laterally and obliquely until a 'give' is felt as the skull is penetrated. It should then be advanced not more than 2 or 3 mm with the stilette withdrawn. Normally, no advance of the needle is necessary. If a few drops (sometimes more) of clear fluid are obtained it is likely that the subarachnoid space has been traversed and that one is sampling subarachnoid CSF. This will have protein content higher than lumbar CSF but not the very high concentration characteristic of subdural effusions.

If subdural fluid is encountered (proteinaceous, cloudy, yellow, brown or red), it is allowed to drain into a centrifuge tube or test tube, removing a maximum of 20–40 mL **(Fig. 35.18)**. Large quantities of CSF should not be aspirated with a syringe. Firm pressure is applied with a cotton wool ball after the needle has been withdrawn.

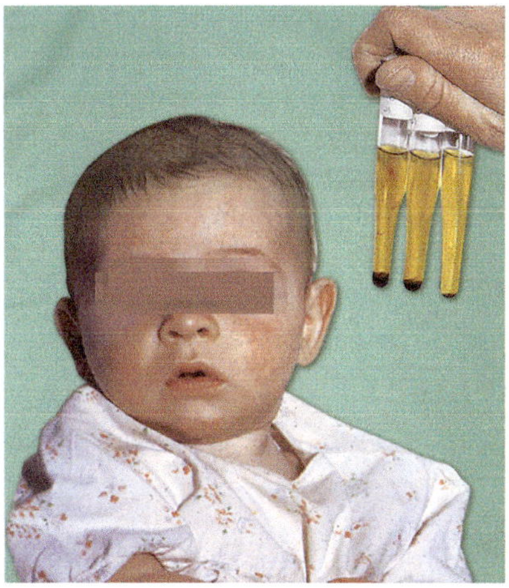

Figure 35.18 Xanthochromic subdural fluid from an infant who had subdural haemorrhage.

Some operators put a silk suture around the skin puncture, but this should not be required with the technique described. Whether or not the diagnostic tap is negative or positive, it is always repeated on the other side. After any such subdural puncture, there is commonly some seepage of CSF under the scalp and so transillumination becomes falsely positive.

Ventricular Puncture

This procedure is used to obtain CSF in suspected ventriculitis when the lumbar route cannot be used, to introduce air for ventriculography and for emergency decompression when the intracranial pressure is dangerously high due to obstruction to outflow from the ventricular system. While it may be life-saving in the latter situation, it should not be thought of as harmless. If the ventricular pressure becomes or remains high after the procedure, cystic expansion may occur along the needle track with associated brain atrophy. Porencephaly may result. Induced bleeding into the ventricular system is sometimes fatal; on other occasions the intraventricular haematoma can be demonstrated by contrast radiography or cranial computed tomography (CT). Such remarks serve as a reminder that ventricular puncture is ideally a neurosurgical procedure and should not be used lightly.

Commonly, the right lateral ventricle is chosen for entry to avoid damage to the presumptive speech-dominant hemisphere. The head is prepared as for subdural tap, but after the same valvular approach through the skin at the same site the needle is advanced at right angles to the tangent of the skull at its point of entry. A fine LP needle with stilette is commonly used although neurosurgeons would prefer a method employing the use of a proper brain needle. It is likely that CSF will be reached at a depth of 3 cm or less, for unless the ventricle is dilated the procedure is seldom indicated or indeed likely of success. It is not usually possible to detect by feel the entry of the needle into the ventricle, so the stilette must be withdrawn to see whether CSF escapes.

Urinary Tract

Suprapubic Aspiration (Bladder Tap)

Thesuprapubic aspiration is a very safe procedure to obtain urine from the newborn and infants under 2 years of age, because the distended bladder in this age group is primarily intra-abdominal. For this procedure to be successful, it is essential that the bladder is full. Dehydration reduces the success. Ultrasonographic confirmation of the bladder would be helpful. The site of the needle puncture is 2 cm above the symphysis pubis.

Procedure

The procedure is as follows:

- Cleanse the suprapubic area with betadine (povidone-iodine)
- Locate the pubic bone
- Insert a one inch 22 G needle attached to a 5 mL syringe at midline, angling the needle 10–20°cephalad and pushing it through the skin under negative pressure at all times
- Entry into the bladder is indicated by return of urine.

Complications

Although complications are rare but include haematuria, anterior abdominal wall abscess and bowel puncture. Peritonitis is uncommon.

Percutaneous Renal Biopsy

Procedure and Complications

Percutaneous renal biopsy has been commonly used since 1954. It is tricky and requires deft fingers. It should not be undertaken without instruction from an expert paediatric nephrologist. It is usually performed under general anaesthetic. Two specimens containing cortical tissue are generally required to obtain adequate material for light: (1) Immunofluorescence and (2) electron microscopy (EM).

Prior to renal biopsy the following investigations are advised:

- Check haemoglobin level, platelet count and coagulation screen
- Real-time ultrasound control is optimal
- Ensure, adequate monitoring of the patient, including continuous pulse oximeter, recording during and following procedure
- Biopsy is usually done with sedation and under a local anaesthetic, but in some cases it may be performed under a general anaesthetic
- Ensure sedation and analgesia has adequate time to take effect prior to commencing procedure
- Ensure EMLA® cream is applied to the biopsy site at least 90 minutes prior to the procedure

- The kidneys lie on either side of the spine just below the muscles of the back. The technique involves inserting a needle down through the back muscles and into the kidney (usually the left), and the removal of some very small pieces of kidney
- An ultrasound scanning machine is used during procedure to ensure the correct positioning of the needle
- Ensure adequate resuscitation equipment is readily available
- Aim to biopsy the lower pole of left kidney (unless contraindicated); ensure biopsy is away from vessels
- Position patient prone (supine for transplanted kidney)
- Generally use 16 G needles (18 G for transplant biopsies)

Following procedure monitor vital signs.

After the biopsy the BP and pulse rate are monitored closely, the urine is tested, and the patient is kept in bed for at least 6 hours. There may occasionally also be some bleeding around the kidney or blood in the urine. Once fully awake after the renal biopsy, the patient is encouraged to drink fluids to help flush away blood from the kidney. Vigorous activity is discouraged for 1 week after the biopsy. Similar procedure is carried out to biopsy a transplanted kidney.

When it is considered that percutaneous renal biopsy involves, an undue risk, an open surgical renal biopsy can be considered. This technique always provides an adequate specimen of the renal cortex.

Renal Biopsy

Indications

- Atypical nephrotic syndrome
- Persistent hypocomplementaemia and nephritis
- Acute nephritis not resolved in 1 month
- Anaphylactoid nephritis not resolved in 1 month
- Persistent undiagnosed haematuria
- Persistent undiagnosed proteinuria
- Persistent undiagnosed renal failure.

Contraindications

May be as follows, none absolute in a desperate situation:

- Single kidney
- Hydronephrosis
- Systemic hypertension
- Uraemia
- Haemorrhagic diathesis.

Respiratory System

Pleural Aspiration

Aspiration of a pleural effusion may be indicated for diagnostic or therapeutic reasons. It is an unpleasant procedure and in most instances the child should be sedated. In all instances, local anaesthesia should be used. The infant or child should preferably be seated on a firm surface sitting upright with his arms placed forward over pillows. Sufficient pillows should be employed to make his back as nearly perpendicular as possible. Standard aseptic technique is employed. The optimal site can be identified by the US.

When the effusion is large, the site of entry is in the sixth intercostal space in the scapular line. When the effusion is localised, as indicated by clinical and radiological examination, the site of entry is best made over the area of maximum dullness on percussion.

A large bore needle or suitably sized trocar (12–18 G: 7.5 cm length) is employed: if thick pus is expected then a wide bore instrument is essential. A bone-marrow aspiration needle may be very useful in tapping a thick empyema. A suitable size syringe and two-way tap is attached to the needle before the skin puncture—a length of plastic tubing should lead from the side arm of the tap to a receptacle for collecting the aspirate. Sterile containers for bacteriological specimens should be to hand.

The needle is inserted in the sixth intercostal space just above the seventh rib and slowly advanced in a forward and slightly medial direction. If slight negative pressure is maintained on the syringe then fluid will be drawn off as soon as the effusion is entered. If much fluid is to be withdrawn, aspiration should be performed fairly slowly. Antibiotics may be instilled if indicated at completion of aspiration before the needle is withdrawn. The site of the puncture may be covered with a sterile swab to avoid leakage from the wound. Repeated aspiration may be performed in this manner though it is best not to use precisely the same puncture wound each time.

If drainage of a tension pneumothorax is required, then the tense gas should be released slowly through polyvinyl tubing which is left in situ and connected with an underwater seal drain. Care should be taken to ensure that no fluid can return through the tubing into the chest by positioning the bottle well below the level of the patient.

Bronchoscopy

Bronchoscopy may be an elective or an emergency procedure. Flexible bronchoscopy is used for diagnostic purposes and obtaining bronchoalveolar samples. Removal of foreign bodies requires rigid bronchoscopy. In either case, it is performed under general anaesthetic with the use of a short-term muscle-relaxing agent. Prior to the elective procedure, the patient should not be given anything to eat or drink for a period of at least 4 hours. In the emergency situation, the stomach contents should be removed as far as possible by aspiration through a wide-bore nasogastric tube before anaesthesia is required.

A bronchoscope of a size suitable for the child is chosen. Following induction of anaesthesia, the bronchoscope is inserted, with the patient's neck and head fully extended. The maintenance of respiration during the procedure is usually constant or intermittent via the side arm of the bronchoscope. Suction may be used to extract suitable foreign bodies such as a disintegrating peanut but expertise is required for even this moderately simple manoeuvre and certainly for any more complexes.

Tracheostomy

Tracheostomy may be either an elective or an emergency procedure. It should be performed under general anaesthesia in an operating theatre if possible but in the emergency situation an asphyxiated patient who is unconscious and deeply cyanosed does not require the former and usually cannot wait for the latter.

The trachea is intubated with the patient's neck fully extended. The cartilages of the third and fourth tracheal rings are located by palpation and a midline vertical incision is made through them. A tracheostomy tube of suitable size for the patient (it should fit snugly but not tightly to avoid pressure necrosis of the tracheal mucosa) is selected and inserted. The tracheostomy tube is fixed firmly but not tightly in place by the use of tapes attached to its lateral flanges and tied around the neck. Maintenance care of the tracheostomy must be constant to keep it clear. Initially, the patient should be observed for evidence of complications consequent to the procedure, e.g. haemorrhage or pneumothorax. Throughout its period of use in the emergency situation, care must be taken that bronchial secretions do not dry within and therefore block the tube. This is avoided by ensuring high humidity of inspired air.

The trachea and bronchi should be aspirated of secretions at frequent regular intervals with sterile technique—it may be helpful to instil 1–2 mL warm sterile saline into the tube prior to aspiration if secretions are particularly viscid. The skin around the tracheostomy wound should be carefully cleansed and dressed (with sterile gauze swab or sterile vaseline gauze) to avoid its becoming infected.

The decision to remove the tracheostomy tube permanently depends on a number of factors including the reason for its initial insertion and the patient's ability to maintain adequate ventilation without it. The orifice of the tube may be partially blocked by gauze swab to encourage oral and nasal breathing and then closed completely, but intermittently, for short periods. Once the tube may be dispensed with the neck, wound is covered with sterile dressings until healing has occurred.

KEY LEARNING POINT

Tracheostomy: In gross emergency before formal tracheostomy is performed, insertion of a wide-bore short bevel needle into the trachea may be life-saving.

Indications of tracheostomy are given in **Box 35.1**.

BOX 35.1 Tracheostomy indications.

- Upper airway obstruction
- Angioneurotic oedema, anaphylaxis (if conventional airway management has failed)
- Prolonged endotracheal tube requirement
- Vocal cord paralysis
- Choanal atresia
- Subglottic stenosis
- Assisted ventilation and pulmonary toilet
- And others

Laryngoscopy

This manoeuvre may be required for viewing the larynx directly, e.g. as a diagnostic procedure or for removing foreign material and is an integral part of endotracheal intubation. General anaesthesia is required in all cases except the cardiac arrest situation.

Requirements

- A functioning laryngoscope with a blade straight or curved as appropriate to the patient's size
- A well-lit room
- Full monitoring.

The patient is laid supine on a firm flat surface. The operator positions himself at the patient's head with his eyes level with the head. The patient's neck is fully extended. The laryngoscope handle is grasped dagger fashion and the blade inserted along the side of the mouth and pushed back to the root of the tongue: it is then positioned centrally so that its point is towards the oesophagus and the tongue is held firmly beneath the blade. By pronating the hand holding the handle of the laryngoscope, the point of the blade is made to pass anteriorly and the operator views the oesophageal orifice and then the larynx. Gentle elevation of the tip of the blade allows the point to slip between the epiglottis and the root of the tongue. By lifting the laryngoscope forward, an adequate view of the larynx is now obtained.

Endotracheal Intubation

In emergency situations such as cardiac arrest, intubation is performed without sedation or anaesthesia—the elective procedure is always performed under general anaesthetic. Intubation may be performed via the mouth or via the nose. The former route is simpler and is the method of choice where intubation is likely to be temporary—the nasal route offers greater stability for the tube.

Cardiovascular System

Pericardial Paracentesis

Accumulation of fluid in the pericardial space of sufficient quantity to cause cardiac embarrassment and necessitate aspiration is rare in the paediatric age group.

Pericardiocentesis may be required as a diagnostic procedure, e.g. in purulent pericarditis or therapeutically as for instillation of appropriate antibiotics, or as an emergency procedure in haemorrhagic tamponade.

The decision to use sedation should rest with the operator and his assessment of the condition of the patient: it should probably be used in most instances unless the child is collapsed. Ultrasonographic monitoring during the procedure is advised.

The infant should be laid supine: the older child may have a pillow as a head rest. Local anaesthesia should be used in all instances. A wide-bore needle (12–18 G, 7.5 cm, short bevel) may be used. Full aseptic technique is employed. The usual site of entry is the angle between the left costal margin and the xiphoid process whence the needle should be directed upwards, backwards and to the left. An alternative approach is via the fifth left intercostal space anteriorly, 2 cm within the area of cardiac dullness, with the needle pointed slightly upwards and medially. The needle should be advanced cautiously and may be felt to penetrate the pericardium usually at a distance of 2–4 cm from the skin surface. If a diagnostic tap only is required, a 5 mL volume syringe should be firmly attached to the needle before insertion.

In most instances, it is best to attach a two-way tap to the needle especially if the effusion is large or if antibiotics are to be instilled; the tap also helps to avoid the introduction of air. If the effusion is large, aspiration should be performed with careful observation of the patient's condition.

Exchange Transfusion

Equipment Required

- Sterile equipment
- Polyvinyl catheter for the umbilical vein (No. 6 or 9)
- Two 2-way taps
- Four (at least) 10 mL (disposable) syringes
- Donor set
- Catheter to connect to receive or plastic bag for the reject blood
- Umbilical vein marker
- Calcium gluconate—10% and sodium bicarbonate—8.4%
- Scissors, mosquito forceps and towel clips
- Gown and drapes
- Fresh blood compatible with the baby and cross-matched against the mother's serum.Prepacked sets of disposable equipment are available.

Preparation

A preterm, or ill infant, should have his acid-base state measured and any metabolic acidosis corrected by intravenous sodium bicarbonate. Gastric contents are aspirated. Oxygen, suction and a good light are essential. Sterile towels are positioned, leaving the abdomen and chest clear. If the infant is small or ill, the procedure may be done within an incubator, otherwise in a baby-warmer or under a phototherapy unit.

Procedure

There are several techniques utilised for this procedure so it is important to use that which is traditional for the locality. These include using simultaneously, arterial and venous catheters. The technique described is based on the original method.

The cord is cut 2 cm from the skin junction and the edge gripped with mosquito forceps. The catheter is advanced into the vein until a free flow of blood is obtained, and is then attached via the two 2-way taps to a 10 mL syringe. The donor blood set is attached to one side arm and the reject catheter to the other.

Initially,10 mL of blood are withdrawn and disposed of or sent for biochemistry, the syringe is then filled with 10 mL donor blood which is slowly injected—taking 1–2 minutes. The aliquot volume can be slowly increased as tolerated to a maximum of 20 mL in a term infant. This cycle is repeated until the desired volume has been exchanged (150 mL/kg). The attendant charts the quantities of blood flowing in and out and observes the infant's condition closely. Evacuated blood may be measured in a suitable cylinder.

In most centres, citrate-phosphate-dextrose (CPD) blood is used in which case no additional drugs are necessary. If acid-citrate-dextrose (ACD) blood is being given then 2 mL of 4.2% sodium bicarbonate is given at the same time, but only during a first exchange transfusion. (This is not required during subsequent exchanges since the citrate will be metabolised.)

At the end of any exchange, the catheter is left in situ until the need for further exchange has passed.

Alimentary System

Endoscopy

Endoscopy is one of the most important technical advances in paediatric medicine. Endoscopy is of help as a diagnostic tool, particularly when used in conjunction with cytology or biopsy. There are mainly two types of endoscopes: (1) rigid and (2) flexible. The rigid type of instruments are usually more basic in design, e.g. proctoscope, sigmoidoscope. Rigid bronchoscopes and oesophagoscopes are now rarely used.

The modern flexible endoscopes are used in the investigations of upper gastrointestinal (GI) endoscopy, sigmoidoscopy, colonoscopy, bronchoscopy and arthroscopy. Because endoscopy can be physically and emotionally unpleasant for the child, most of these procedures are performed under general anaesthetic. Diagnostic endoscopy is usually a very safe procedure provided the endoscopist is well trained.

Paracentesis Abdominis

This may be required for diagnostic or therapeutic reasons. Diagnostic puncture may be required to ascertain the nature of the fluid causing ascites or more usually to define whether peritonitis is present and to recover the organism. It requires no sedation or local anaesthetic unless the child is exceptionally restless. The skin is cleaned with 2% iodine in 70% ethanol.

An IV needle or short plastic cannula is inserted in the midline, midway between the symphysis pubis and the umbilicus if ascites is gross, and in the flank at the level of the umbilicus if it is less gross. The area into which the needle is being introduced will be dull and care should be taken to avoid an enlarged liver, spleen or bladder. Fluid is withdrawn and investigated for organisms and cytology, by culture or biochemically as indicated. The iodine remaining is cleaned off the skin with 70% ethanol.

Today the removal of ascetic fluid by mechanical means is rarely required, attention being given to the medical treatment of the primary cause. If required, the usual practice is to proceed as follows after sedating the child.

Procedure

- Clean up an area of skin in the midline between the umbilicus and symphysis pubis or lateral to the umbilicus. Apply 2% iodine in 70% alcohol. Make sure the bladder is empty or nearly so.
- An area of skin is infiltrated with 1% lignocaine subcutaneously. The tissues of the abdominal wall down to the peritoneum are similarly treated.
- A small nick is made in the skin with a scalpel blade.
- A disposable peritoneal dialysis polyvinyl tube is introduced through the skin, subcutaneous tissue, muscles and peritoneum, using the introducer provided. The tube is inserted for approximately 15 cm further until all the perforated tube is in the peritoneal space.
- Alternatively a small trocar and cannula may be used. These are inserted through the peritoneum and the removal of the trocar enables fluid to gush out. The fluid flow should be controlled to allow the abdomen to empty over a period of 15-30 minutes.
- When the desired amount of fluid has been withdrawn and no more is available, and then the tube (or cannula) is withdrawn. If the tension of the ascites has been removed, it should be possible to bring the edges of the hole into apposition by a strip of plaster. If not, it may be necessary to apply a cutaneous suture or clip.
- The remaining iodine should be cleaned off the skin with 70% ethanol.

Percutaneous Liver Biopsy

This is only performed by skilled, experienced operators under general anaesthetic. A coagulation profile and blood cross match should be performed prior to the procedure and any clotting abnormalities corrected. Histological examination of liver tissue usually provides vital information for the management of the child with liver disease, giving evidence which is not present by other means. Also, the liver biopsy can provide material for bacterial and viral culture, analysis of enzyme activity, chemical content as well as histological IM and EM studies. The technique of liver biopsy does carry a slight but definite morbidity and also mortality. However, ultrasonography directed biopsies may increase the yield of meaningful results.

Jejunal Biopsy (Biopsy of Small Bowel Mucosa)

Small intestinal mucosal biopsies are important in the evaluation of children with malabsorption. A normal biopsy in these children may be as useful as an abnormal biopsy because it would direct diagnostic approach elsewhere. Most jejunal biopsies are obtained by endoscopy under general anaesthetic.

There are several kinds of biopsy tubes available, e.g. the Shiner flexible biopsy tube, the Rubin biopsy tube and the Crosby capsule. The Crosby capsule is the most appropriate for everyday use. A child-size capsule is available for use in infants and small children.

Procedure

- The capsule must be thoroughly checked prior to use.
- Child must fast overnight, and most do not require a local anaesthetic.
- The capsule is placed on the back of the tongue and if the child sits upright, it can be swallowed without any difficulty.
- The length of tubing required to allow the capsule to enter the gastric antrum should be estimated and marked.
- When this is achieved, the gastric peristalsis is encouraged by gently injecting air down the apparatus while the child lies in the right lateral position.
- The efflux of bile-stained fluid indicates the entry of the capsule into the duodenum.
- At this stage, the child is turned into the supine position and asked to swallow another foot of tubing.
- At the end of 3 hours, the position of the capsule must be confirmed radiologically.
- When the capsule has reached the jejunum, it can then be fired by applying forceful suction from a 20 mL syringe to ensure the knife is released.

- The capsule is withdrawn and opened. The tissue obtained is then fixed in formal saline and sent for microscopical examination.

> **KEY LEARNING POINT**
>
> Jejunal biopsy: The small bowel biopsy specimen is diagnostic of coeliac disease and is regarded as the 'gold standard' although errors occur especially with poorly orientated specimens.

Urea Breath Test (*Helicobacter pylori* Infections)

The urea breath test is a non-invasive test used to detect the presence of *H. pylori* in the stomach, and is the simplest way to confirm eradication of infection after treatment. The test is based on the capacity of *H. pylori* to secrete the enzyme urease, which hydrolyses urea to ammonia and carbon dioxide. When a dose of urea labelled with a non-radioactive isotope of carbon (^{13}C) is taken by mouth, the label appears in breath carbon dioxide if the child has gastric *H. pylori* colonisation. The accuracy of the urea breath test may be reduced if the child is currently receiving or has recently completed treatment with antibiotics, proton-pump inhibitors, or H_2 receptor antagonists.

The abundance of ^{13}C in breath CO_2 is measured by continuous-flow isotope ratio mass spectrometry [20-20 Automated Breath ^{13}Carbon Analyser (ABCA), Sercon, Crewe, UK] against international standards. The enrichment of the postdose sample is calculated by subtracting the abundance of the baseline sample from that of the postdose sample.

A test is considered positive if the enrichment of the postdose sample is greater than or equal to 40 parts per million ^{13}C ($\geq$40 ppm ^{13}C excess) and delta above baseline ($\geq$3.5 ppm ^{13}C excess).

Also there are no specific endoscopic features of *H. pylori* infection. Histological assessment of an endoscopic antral biopsy is reliable means of detecting *H. pylori*, but requires expertise and the result is not immediately available. Culture of endoscopic biopsies is equally sensitive and specific but suffers similar drawbacks.

> **KEY LEARNING POINTS**
>
> Urea breath test
> - Proton-pump inhibitors should be stopped 2 weeks before the test
> - H_2 receptor antagonists should not be taken on the day of the test
> - Antibiotics should have been stopped for at least 4 weeks.

Twenty-four Hour Oesophageal pH Monitoring (Regurgitation, Gastro-oesophageal Reflux, Gastro-oesophageal Reflux Disease)

Gastro-oesophageal reflux (GOR) is a very common occurrence in children but its clinical importance varies vastly upon the age of the child. It is worth remembering that the terminology, e.g. regurgitation, GOR and gastro-oesophageal reflux disease (GORD) can easily be confused in paediatric practice. Regurgitation of gastric contents into oesophageal lumen is much more frequent in infants and most likely a physiologic event and largely self-limited in the majority. Interestingly reflux of gastric contents in the oesophagus is almost always acidic in adults, but it is frequently not the case in young children, infants and particularly in premature infants. On the contrary, GORD refers to pathologically frequent or severe acidic gastric reflux associated with mucosal damage and/or symptoms and complications. Therefore, it is important to identify children with significant GOR and to treat them as GORD.

Procedure

Although the test can be carried out at home, but some infants and children may need to remain in the hospital for the test. Some drugs (e.g. antacids, corticosteroids, H_2 blockers, proton-pump inhibitors) may change the test results. So they have to be stopped 24 hours to weeks before the test.

> **KEY LEARNING POINT**
>
> 24-hour oesophageal pH-metry has been one of the main diagnostic tools used for the diagnosis of gastro-oesophageal reflux disease (GORD). The test measures how often and for how long stomach acid enters the lumen of the oesophagus.

A thin tube with a probe is passed through the nose into the stomach. Then, it is pulled up into the oesophagus. The tube is attached to a monitor that measures the level of acidity in the oesophagus.

The parents of the child will keep a note of the symptoms over the next 24 hours. The next day the tube will be removed. The information from the monitor will be compared with symptoms record kept.

Acid reflux is defined whenever the pH in the oesophagus drops to 4 or less. The tracing is read by counting the number of reflux episodes and measuring the duration of each reflux episode in minutes (Figs. 35.19 and 35.20).

Percutaneous Endoscopic Gastrostomy

Percutaneous endoscopic gastrostomy (PEG) is designed to establish an artificial tract between the stomach and

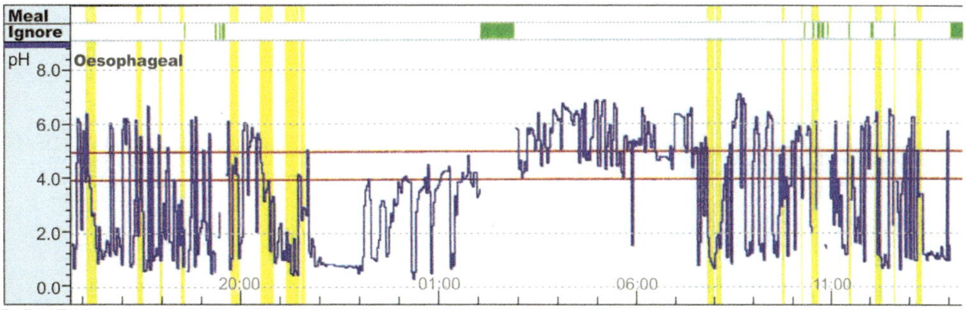

Reflux Table

	Total	Meal	Upright	PrePra
Duration of period (HH: MM)	21:26	01:56	21:26	19:29
Number of refluxes	393	63	393	337
Number of long refluxes {>5 (min)}	14	2	14	10
Duration of longest reflux (min)	85	6	85	85
Time pH <4 (min)	325	32	325	292
Fraction time pH <4 (%)	25.3	27.8	25.3	25.0
Maximum (pH)	7.9	7.5	7.9	7.9
Minimum (pH)	0.3	0.5	0.3	0.3
Mean (pH)	5.0	4.8	5.0	5.1
Median (pH)	5.7	5.1	5.7	5.8

Figure 35.19 Tracing of oesophageal pH monitoring of a child over 1-year-old % less than pH 4 more than 5%. Showing significant gastro-oesophageal reflux (GOR), i.e. gastro-oesophageal reflux disease (GORD).

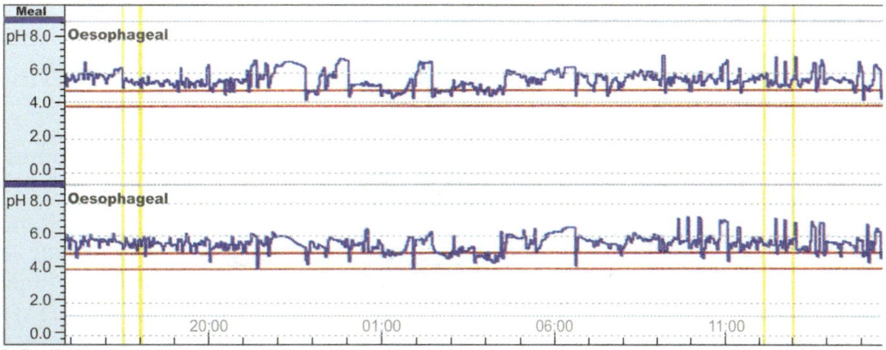

Reflux Table - channel 1

	Total	Meal	Upright	PrePra
Duration of period (HH: MM)	1d	00:11	1d	23:49
Number of refluxes	0	0	0	0
Number of long refluxes {>5 (min)}	0	0	0	0
Duration of longest reflux (min)	0	0	0	0
Time pH <4 (min)	0	0	0	0
Fraction time pH <4 (%)	0.0	0.0	0.0	0.0
Maximum (pH)	7.8	7.3	7.8	7.8
Minimum (pH)	4.4	5.1	4.4	4.4
Mean (pH)	6.2	6.2	6.2	6.2
Median (pH)	6.2	6.1	6.2	6.2

Figure 35.20 Tracing of oesophageal pH monitoring, post-fundoplication showing no gastro-oesophageal reflux (GOR).

BOX 35.2 Complications of percutaneous endoscopic gastrostomy (PEG).

- Skin problems due to leakage from the gastrostomy site
- Pneumoperitoneum and subcutaneous emphysema
- Peritonitis (rare)
- Gastrointestinal haemorrhage (rare)
- Gastric outlet obstruction and/or duodenal obstruction
- Tube occlusion (frequent)
- Gastro-oesophageal reflux (GOR, during gastrostomy feedings)

the abdominal surface and is usually used for long-term enteral support. There are catheters which are specifically designed for children for this purpose and should, therefore, be used. Before the establishment of the gastrostomy feeding tube, a full assessment of the child and the family should be carried out to ascertain their ability to manage the tube. Also, the parents should have the full risks and benefits of placing the tube explained. Tract formation occurs within a few hours, and it is safe to commence feeding 4 hours after tube insertion. The main contraindications are severe obesity, portal hypertension and coagulation abnormalities. Complications of PEG are given in Box 35.2.

Skin

The diagnosis of skin disorders in children is usually on the distribution and characteristics of the lesion or rash. However, histological examination is necessary for final confirmation of a diagnosis when there is doubt on clinical grounds. It is vital to provide adequate piece of skin for interpretation, which usually means a full-thickness (epidermis, dermis and a small amount of subcutaneous tissue) biopsy through the edge of the lesion.

Mantoux Test

Tuberculin skin tests are, of all tests, the most useful in the diagnosis of primary tuberculosis. In the Mantoux test—the diagnostic is given by intradermal injection of tuberculin purified protein derivative (human PPD). For routine Mantoux test, 2 units (0.1 mL of 20 units/mL strength) is administered to the left forearm, preferably at the junction of middle and at lower third of the volar aspect. It should produce a bleb raised about 7 mm in diameter, which usually disappears within an hour. If first test is negative and a further test is considered appropriate 10 units (0.1 mL of 100 units/mL strength) should be administered. Mantoux test should be read at 48–72 hours and measure the diameter of induration (not erythema) in millimetres (Fig. 35.21).

Interpretation of Mantoux test is given in Box 35.3.

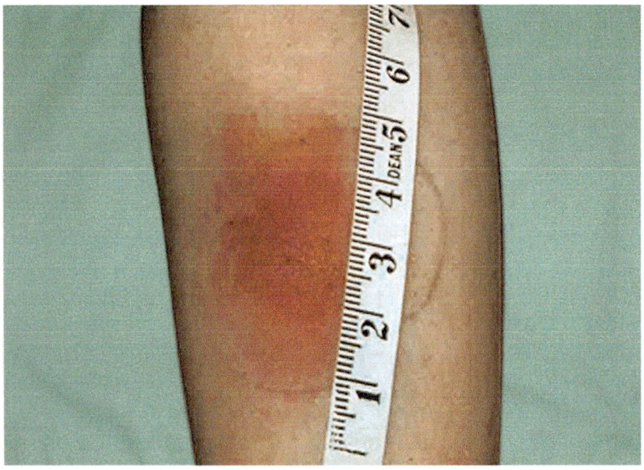

Figure 35.21 A positive Mantoux test with human purified protein derivative (PPD).

KEY LEARNING POINTS

Mantoux test: Importantly, the only indication for administering a more dilute human purified protein derivative (PPD) (e.g. 0.1 mL of 1 in 10,000 PPD = 1 unit), is if the child is suspected to have erythema nodosum as a manifestation of primary tuberculosis.

Avian Purified Protein Derivative (Non-Tuberculous Mycobacteria Intradermal Test)

Lymphadenitis is the most common manifestation of non-tuberculous mycobacteria (NTM) infection in children aged less than 12 years (peak age 2–4 years). Adenitis due to NTM is usually unilateral and involves the submandibular nodes or anterior superior cervical nodes. The pulmonary infection with NTM is rare in children.

With high index of suspicion that a child could have NTM infection, an avian PPD intradermal (Mantoux method test should be done). It will show a much higher sensitivity to the avian PPD than to the human PPD, and

BOX 35.3 Interpretation of Mantoux test.

- Less than 5 mm induration—it is negative
- If induration 5–10 mm—it could be due to previous Bacillus Calmette-Guérin (BCG) or due to non-tuberculous mycobacteria
- If induration 10–15 mm—treat as tuberculosis infection (known contact from high prevalence area). Treat as tuberculosis disease if chest X-ray abnormal and/or symptoms
- If induration more than 15 mm—treat as tuberculosis disease (abnormal chest X-ray and/or symptoms)

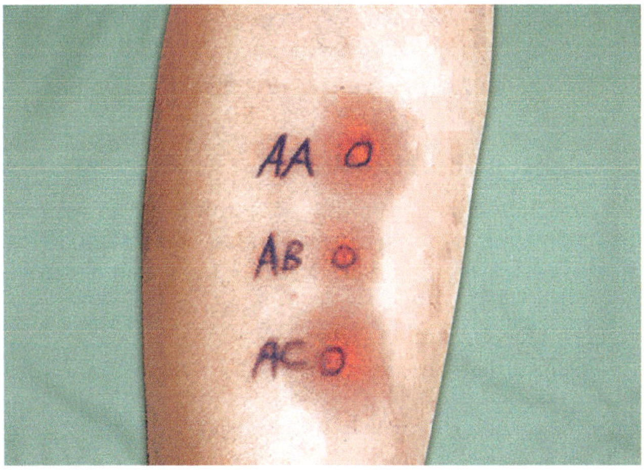

Figure 35.22 A positive Mantoux test with avian purified protein derivative (PPD).

the reaction would be larger to the avian PPD than the human antigen (Fig. 35.22).

> **KEY LEARNING POINTS**
>
> - Response to tuberculin may be suppressed by live viral vaccine, viral infection, corticosteroid therapy or immunosuppression due to disease or treatment.
> - False-negatives may be found in miliary tuberculosis or in newborns.
> - Incorrect storage of purified protein derivative (PPD), incorrect administration or incorrect reading will affect the result.

Polymerase chain reaction may have a useful but limited role in evaluating children with tuberculosis. A negative PCR never eliminates tuberculosis as a diagnostic possibility, and a positive result does not confirm it.

Allergy Skin Prick Testing

Skin prick testing is a form of allergy testing which produces an immunoglobulin E (IgE)-mediated response on the surface of the skin. The reaction consists of a weal, which can be surrounded by erythema. This usually develops within 15 minutes and subsides within 1 hour. The resulting weal can help identify an offending allergen. It is essential to remember that false positives and false negatives can occur. Therefore, the child's history is of great significance.

The likelihood of systemic reactions is very low. However, the anaphylaxis medication and protocol must be readily available.

The child should be physically well prior to skin prick testing. No oral antihistamine should have been given on the day of the skin prick testing. Steroid ointment should not have been applied for the week prior to the skin prick testing. Also, any areas of active eczema should be avoided.

Equipment Required

- Vials of commercially produced allergen extracts or whole food
- Positive and negative control skin prick testing solutions
- Individual sterile prick testing lancets
- A roll of transparent tape
- Skin marker pen
- Measuring gauge
- Timer
- Anaphylaxis medication.

Skin Prick Testing Procedure

Thecubital fossa or the child's back is the site of choice for skin prick testing. Babies and toddlers tend to have the back used whereas older children tend to prefer it on the cubital fossa. A skin marking pen is used to mark allergen sites. Positive and negative controls are used on opposite sides of the test site. Allergens should be placed at least 3 cm apart.

One drop of allergen is placed on the appropriately marked area of the skin using the applicator.

A sterile lancet is held at a 90° angle to the skin and pressed through the skin without drawing blood. The excess solution is then removed with cotton wool or tissue from the skin site test. The above steps are repeated for each allergen. This is left for 15 minutes. After 15 minutes from application, the site is examined for weal. Outlines of any weal are drawn round with the skin marker pen. Any flare that has occurred is disregarded. The tape is then placed over the pen marked weal to obtain an imprint and then removed and placed on the skin prick testing result sheet. This will have transferred the size of weal to the result sheet. The diameter of the weal is measured with a ruler giving the diameter in millimetres. The skin is then washed around the site of the skin prick testing. The child is observed for a further 15 minutes. The results are interpreted and the appropriate advice and treatment plan devised.

However, scratch, prick or puncture tests should be employed with caution. Because, 'large local skin test reactions' correlate well with clinical sensitivity while 'small skin test reactions' correlate poorly but may be used as a starting point for elimination and challenge to determine whether clinical sensitivity to food exists. Also, the clinical significance of skin test reactions varies significantly to specific food tested. Delayed-onset food sensitivities, i.e. reactions that occur hours to days after food ingestion, seldom are identified by skin testing because majority do not appear to be IgE mediated.

Muscle Biopsy

Muscle biopsy is an invasive technique and both paediatrician and pathologist must be quite clear that there are questions that need to be answered for the diagnosis and management of the patient and indeed that those questions can be answered by a biopsy before the muscle biopsy procedure is carried out. Therefore, when indicated the muscle biopsy provides the final confirmation of a diagnosis on which treatment can be based, prognosis explained and genetic counselling offered. In some cases however, the diagnosis may be quite clear from the clinical presentation and the history with no further, useful information is likely to be obtained from a biopsy. In such a situation, it should not be undertaken merely to confirm what is already known.

For practical purposes, most muscle biopsies are taken from quadriceps or deltoid as they are usually involved in myopathies. It is vital to avoid artefact in the muscle biopsy, e.g. sites of injection or electromyography (EMG) needle insertion. An open biopsy can be obtained through a skin incision under local anaesthesia. It is recommended to take two pieces of muscle: (1) One for EM and (2) the other for histology and histochemistry.

Needle biopsies of muscle can also be used for the diagnosis of muscle disease and are particularly useful for follow-up biopsies to monitor the prognosis of treatment.

ACKNOWLEDGEMENTS

We are grateful to Churchill Livingston Elseveir, for permission to reproduce some material from the Textbook of Paediatrics, Edited by John O Forfar and Gavin C Arneil, volume 2, chapter 38, Practical Procedures by WB Doig, Anna V Murphy and GC Arneil, 1978.

The authors also acknowledge their thanks to Mrs Pamela Joannidis, Miss M Steven, Dr B El-Nabulsi, Dr N Doraiswamy, Mr B Amjad for their contributions to this chapter.

The authors are grateful to ADAM Surgical, Sialkot, Pakistan, for providing images of suturing.

CHAPTER 36

A Prescription for Play

Phyllis Kilbourn, Rosemary Sabatino

INTRODUCTION

Play! What a wonderful word—the very essence of childhood! For those whose family saw the importance of play, it calls up memories of our own childhood years when playing was the main focus of our waking hours. 'Will you play with me?' is one of the most expressive, expectant questions asked. The query carries with it a hope and anticipation about a time of fun and make-believe, a world of adventure and exploration, the world of the child. Play becomes an activity in which the child takes control, is motivated from within and uses his or her imagination. The absence of play is viewed as an obstacle to the development of healthy and creative individuals. For this reason, play is important for healthcare providers to consider and prescribe play as a vital intervention that facilitates healthy childhood development and learning.

DEFINING PLAY

Play for children has been likened to work for an adult. It is what they do. Through play children learn about their world and the things in it.

Play also has been likened to a child's rehearsal or practice for life since through play a child finds the root of future successes. During play, children can switch roles, control situations and experiment with a variety of scenes where they can be the authors, stars and directors of their world. Research has shown that if children can play well, they will adjust well as adults.

The dynamic process of play develops and changes, becoming increasingly more varied and complex. Considered a key facilitator for learning and development across domains, play reflects the social and cultural contexts in which children live.

Play is a window to the child's world and the adult who knows the value of play is committed to learning about children while they play. Play tells us much about children's lives, health and level of development. From observing their play we learn how children think, feel and believe. Play also can tell us of a child's pain, conflict and insecurity. Those who value the personhood of children should also value the play of children.

IMPORTANCE OF PLAY

Play allows children the chance to explore their environment, to learn how it works and how they relate to it. A child can express feelings and emotions through various types of play activities (games, art, stories, and so on) far earlier than they can express them in words. For older children, play may be the outlet through which they convey emotions that they are either unwilling to share verbally or do not have the sufficient vocabulary to express. Through play children can be anyone, at any place, at any time.

Play is how children reconstruct their world in order to understand and master it. To be a child is to be little and powerless; someone big always has charge, telling you what to do.

In play, children are autonomous; they are independent. They make the decisions, solve the problems and deal with the consequences. As Piaget[1] has said, autonomy should be the aim of education and to understand is to invent. In play, children are autonomous inventors.

DESCRIPTION OF FORMS OF PLAY

Play takes many forms. Children play when they sing, dig in the mud, build a block tower or dress up. Play can be purely physical (running, climbing, ball throwing) or highly intellectual (solving an intricate puzzle, remembering the words of a song). Play also can be creative using crayons, clay and finger-paint. Play's emotional form is expressed when children pretend to be mummies, daddies or babies. Skipping rope with a friend or sharing a book is an example of the social side of play.

Sensorimotor Play (Baby and Toddler Play)

Even infants and toddlers enjoy play and develop through it. Babies spend lots of awake time exploring the world through play. To adults, it might look like the baby is 'just playing around'. In fact, the baby is learning many new skills. For a baby, play is the best time for learning.

In what Piaget[1] aptly described as sensorimotor practice play, infants and toddlers experiment with bodily sensation and motor movements, and with objects and people. By 6 months of age, infants have developed simple but consistent action schemes through trial and error and much practice. Infants use action schemes, such as pushing and grasping, to make interesting things happen. An infant will push a ball and make it roll to experience the sensation and pleasure of movement.

As children master new motor abilities, simple schemes are coordinated to create more complex play sequences. Older infants will push a ball, crawl after it and retrieve it. When infants of 9 months are given an array of objects, they apply the same limited actions to all objects and see how they react. By pushing various objects, an infant learns that a ball rolls away, mobile spins around and a rattle makes noise. At about 12 months, objects bring forth more specific and differentiated actions.

A toddler's second year brings a growing awareness of the functions of objects in the social world. The toddler puts a cup on a saucer and a spoon in his/her mouth. During the last half of this year, toddlers begin to represent their world symbolically as they transform and invent objects and roles. They may stir an imaginary drink and offer it to someone. Adults initiate and support such play. They may push a baby on a swing or cheer its first awkward steps. Children's responses regulate the adult's actions. If the swing is pushed too high, a child's cries will guide the adult towards a gentler approach. In interactions with adults such as peek-a-boo, children learn to take turns, act with others and engage others in play.

Toddlers play well on their own (solitary play) or with adults. They begin solitary pretend play around 1 year of age. During the toddler years, as they become more aware of one another, they begin to play side by side, without interacting (parallel play). They are aware of and pleased about other persons, but are not directly involved with them. During this second year, toddlers begin some form of coordinated play, doing something with another child. This form is similar to the preschooler's associative play

Early Childhood (Pretend Play)

As children develop the ability to represent experience symbolically, pretend play becomes a prominent activity. In this complex type of play, children carry out action plans, take on roles and transform objects as they express their ideas and feelings about the social world.

Action plans are blueprints for the ways in which actions and events are related and sequenced. Family-related themes in action plans are popular with young children, as are action plans for treating and healing, and for averting threats.

Roles are identities children assume in play. Some roles are functional, necessary for a certain theme. E.g. taking a trip requires passengers and a driver. Family roles such as mother, father and baby are popular and are integrated into elaborate play with themes related to familiar home activities. Children also assume stereotyped character roles drawn from the larger culture, such as nurse, and fictional character roles drawn from books and television such as Spider Man. Play related to these roles tends to be more predictable and restricted than play related to direct experiences such as family life.

By the age of 4 or 5 years, children's ideas about the social world initiate most pretend play. While some pretend play is solitary or shared with adults, preschoolers' pretend play is often shared with peers in the school or neighbourhood. To implement and maintain pretend play episodes, a great deal of shared meaning must be negotiated among children. Play procedures may be talked about explicitly, or signalled subtly in role-appropriate action or dialogue. Players often make rule-like statements to guide behaviour ('You have to finish your dinner, baby'). Potential conflicts are negotiated. Though meanings in play often reflect real world behaviour, they also incorporate children's interpretations and wishes.

Preschoolers learn differently from school-age children. Play is essential to their early learning and is the main way by which children learn and develop ideas about the world. It helps them build the skills necessary for critical thinking and leadership. It is how they learn to solve problems and to feel good about their ability to learn.

Children learn the most from play when they have skilled teachers who are well trained in understanding how play contributes to learning. Most child development experts agree that play is an essential part of a high-quality early learning programme. Play is not a break from learning—it is the way young children learn.

The preschool years bring many changes for children in relation to social development. Children have more quality relationships outside the home and have a growing ability to play with other children. When children verbalise, plan and carry out play, cooperative play is established. This is the most common type of peer interaction during a child's pre-school years.

Construction play with symbolic themes is also popular with preschoolers, who use blocks and miniature cars and people to create model situations related to their experiences. Rough and tumble play with a lot of motion is popular with preschoolers. In this play groups of children run, jump and wrestle. Action patterns call for these behaviours to be performed at a high activity level. Adults may worry that such play will become aggressive and they should probably monitor it. Children, who participate in this play become skilled in their movements, distinguish between real and pretend aggression and learn to regulate each other's activity.

School-age Play: Structured or Spontaneous

School-age children's playful activities can occur in two forms: (1) structured and (2) creative. Structured play tends to focus on a child's physical skill, natural talent or mental abilities to successfully engage in or with the game. Therefore, structured play is extremely beneficial to the physical, mental and social development of a child and should be encouraged and practised. Such a plan enables a child to gain skills, knowledge and self-confidence.

Structured play includes sports, board games and simple fun events such as jump rope or marbles. Regardless of the game's complexity or intensity, set rules govern the proper way to play. A child's unique personality is confined within the boundary of the rules.

Most play is unstructured and happens naturally when opportunity for play arises. Such spontaneous play is the unplanned, self-selected activity in which children freely participate. Children's natural inclinations are towards play materials and experiences that are developmentally appropriate. Therefore, when children are allowed to make choices in a free play situation, children will choose activities that express their individual interests, needs and readiness levels.

Dramatic play or imaginative play is a common form of spontaneous play. Here children assume the roles of different characters, both animate and inanimate. Children identify themselves with another person or thing, playing out situations that interest or frighten them. Dramatic play reveals children's attitudes and concepts towards people and things in their environment. Much play of this sort addresses a child's sense of helplessness and inferiority. Through dramatic play, they are the big superhero, capable of any feat!

Creative play engages the imagination. Creative play is the natural childlike ability to express one's personality, feeling and attitudes with imaginative words and actions. This play focuses on having fun and sharing in a relationship by using the imagination. A child's ability to make-believe adventures, activities or events—not game rules—sets the limits of the game. Participants win by playing with imagination rather than by competing successfully against each other. A child's skill, strength, intelligence or age is of no consequence.

PLAY: AN ESSENTIAL ELEMENT IN CHILD DEVELOPMENT

Practices and paradigms of what would be considered good child rearing and teaching have been debated, shifted, embraced and discarded over the years, yet basic concepts still remain. One of them is the child's intrinsic desire and tendency to play, which transcends age, time, culture, ethnicity, geography, socio-economic circumstances and abilities. Acknowledging the child's inherent need to play, and that it effectively fulfils his desire to explore, learn and discover, is key to understanding that play is a building block as essential to healthy child development as are food and rest.

According to early childhood specialist, Eric Strickland (2000)[2] 'Play involves the whole child.' Play builds physical skills (such as balance, agility, strength and co-ordination), cognitive skills (including language, problem solving, strategising and concept development), social skills (sharing, turn-taking, cooperation and leadership) and the components for emotional well-being (joy, creativity, self-confidence and so on). It is the fundamental process underlying most of the learning children do before they come to school.'

Physical Development

Because play often involves physical activity it aids in the development and refinement of both gross and fine motor skills for children of all ages. This process can be observed as infants playfully begin to explore their world and are given room to roll, scoot and eventually crawl. Babies enjoy reaching for small objects such as mobiles, streamers, rattles and small toys and as a consequence even begin to develop some of the finer motor skills like hand-eye co-ordination.

Throughout childhood, as children vigorously and joyfully use their bodies in physical exercise—running, jumping, skipping, climbing or throwing a ball, and so on—they are simultaneously releasing energy and developing muscles, balance and skills that will help them feel confident, secure and self-assured. As they gain increasing control over their bodies, and develop awareness of the space around them they learn to move safely and confidently in their environment.

In addition, during play children gradually become more adept at actions that involve different parts of the body. As they increase their skill at manipulating malleable materials and small items of equipment, they are also aiding the development of their small muscles. Fine motor control and hand-eye co-ordination are needed, e.g. to build a tower of blocks, complete a jigsaw puzzle, draw a picture, manipulate play dough or interact with small toy figures. Large construction toys can help children's muscular development through any lifting, carrying, stretching or balancing they may do, and throwing and catching a ball will develop fine gross motor skills.

Recent findings from research on the brain and learning have bolstered the importance of play as having a physical impact on children. It is well known that active brains make permanent neurological connections that are critical to learning, and inactive brains do not make the necessary permanent neurological connections.

Research on the brain demonstrates that play is a scaffold for development, a vehicle for increasing neural structures, and means by which children practice skills they will need later in life. These findings raise the importance of play to a more serious exercise that has a powerful impact on physical as well as cognitive development.

Cognitive Development

Have you ever watched children at play? If the answer is no, then try it some time. You will notice how totally absorbed they become in what they are doing, and their vivid imaginations and clever ideas will amaze you. They approach play with intense focus and inquiring minds.

No wonder then that practically all forms of play engage and enhance the development of cognitive related skills including imagination, creativity, problem solving, sorting and using information, and negotiation skills with peers. E.g. block building, and sand and water play lay the foundation for logical mathematical thinking, scientific reasoning and cognitive problem solving.

Play fosters creativity and flexibility in thinking. Play has no right or wrong way to do things; a chair can be a car or a boat, a house or a bed. Pretend play fosters communication, developing conversational skills, turn-taking, perspective taking, and the skills of social problem solving or persuading, negotiating, compromising and co-operating. Pretend play requires complex communication skills; children must be able to communicate and understand the message, 'this is play'. As they develop skill in pretend play, they begin to converse on many levels at once, becoming actors, directors, narrators and audience, slipping in and out of multiple roles.

We can see that play can have a beneficial effect on a child's development in the area of language. Through play children learn to ask questions or to develop an understanding of a new set of rules in a game. E.g. in the case of construction play when children are building something with others, they need to be able to form an understanding of instruction. The same can be said of board games, where the explanation and understanding of the rules or instructions can aid the development of language skills.

'There is a growing body of evidence supporting the many connections between cognitive competence and high-quality pretend play. If children lack opportunities to experience such play, their long-term capacities related to metacognition, problem solving and social cognition, as well as to academic areas such as literacy, mathematics and science, may be diminished. These complex and multidimensional skills involving many areas of the brain are most likely to thrive in an atmosphere rich in high-quality pretend play.'

Social and Emotional Development

The American Medical Association believes that the majority of a child's social skills come as a result of play since play enables children to interact and respond to others from an early age. Children, like all human beings, have a basic need to belong to and feel part of a group and to learn to live and work in groups with different compositions and for different purposes. Play serves as a wonderful avenue for children to satisfy these needs and to develop social and emotional life skills. Children of all ages need to be socialised as contributing members of their respective cultures, and playing with others gives children the opportunity to match their behaviour with others and to take into account viewpoints that differ from their own.

Through play children can develop social skills, such as sharing with others, waiting their turn to do something, learning how to co-operate and how to lead and follow.

Children learn about themselves and others through play. By pretending, daydreaming, imitating others and having a good time, children learn to recognise their feelings and how to deal with them. In pretend play, children can be disobedient or uncooperative without getting in trouble. They can confront and overcome fears and when under stress, play helps them forget their worries and gives them a chance to feel more in control of their world. At all levels of development, play enables children to feel comfortable and in control of their feelings by (i) allowing the expression of unacceptable feelings in acceptable ways and (ii) providing the opportunity to work through conflicting feelings. In fact, children who play more seem to be happier and healthier.

More than a respite from structured learning experiences, play is the cornerstone of learning and an integral link in the chain of healthy child development. 'Play fosters the growth of healthy children in every aspect of development—physically, cognitively, socially and emotionally. It really is food for children's bodies, minds and spirits.'

THE DANGERS OF PLAY DEPRIVATION

Sadly, in many parts of the world children are losing, and many have lost, the opportunity to engage in the crucial activity of play. Child soldiering, trafficking, exploitation, abuse and abandonment are just some of the reasons that children, even at an early age, are being stripped of the fundamental rights and necessities of a meaningful childhood. In the United States of America, and many other countries, the emphasis on academic achievement and testing, the predominance of computer and electronic games, and the increased incidence of highly scheduled children in extra-curricular activities have diminished the importance of, and time allotted for, adequate and purposeful play experiences both in the classroom and at home. The effects of this could be far reaching.

No Time for Play

The American Academy of Paediatrics recognises that play is important for optimal child development. It further endorses the position that every child deserves the opportunity to develop their unique potential and urges all children to advocate to press for circumstances that allow each child to reap the advantages of play.

The American Academy of Paediatrics has the following advice that can be applied worldwide:

- Promote free play as an essential part of childhood
- Emphasise the advantages of active play and discourage parents from the overuse of passive entertainment
- Emphasise that active child-centred play is a time-tested way of producing healthy, fit young bodies
- Emphasise the benefits of 'true' toys such as blocks and dolls, with which children use their imagination fully, over passive toys that require limited imagination
- Educate families regarding the protective assets and increased resiliency developed through free play and some unscheduled time
- Reinforce that parents who share unscheduled spontaneous time with their children and who play with their children are being wonderfully supportive, nurturing and productive
- Support parents to organise playgroups beginning at an early preschool age
- Support children having an academic schedule that is appropriately challenging and extra-curricular exposures that offer appropriate balance.

ADVICE FOR PARENTS OR CAREGIVERS

- *Allow for exploration:* Children play using their entire bodies and all of their senses. Let them see, hear, touch, smell and feel things to try them out. This means lots of supervision and regular checks to make sure they are exploring safely.
- *Watch your child play:* Be prepared for surprises! While watching your child play, you learn a lot about their interests, attention span and skills. Your observations tell you how to play with your children and when to offer new playthings as they grow. You'll also find the best time to join in.
- *Accept invitations to play:* Young children usually spend most of their time with parents and caregivers. Children may include you in their play naturally. Be ready to join in, but avoid taking over. Remember that children learn and enjoy more when they stay in charge of their own play. When adults respect children as they play with them, children play longer. This increases their attention span. Children learn more and show more advanced play when they have chances to play with adults.
- *Provide play space:* Small children need room to play. If your home or yard is unsafe or too small, find a park to play in several times a week. At home, teach your child the house rules and allow him to play in spaces where he can jump, climb, crawl and creep safely.
- *Provide playtime:* Young children play all the time. Routines such as bathing, eating and dressing can be just as much fun and adventurous as trips to the park. Allowing a little extra time for everyone to have fun during these routines helps children develop a sense of time management and responsibility. This can help them now with their play skills and later in school and at work.
- *Provide play materials:* Children can create their own fun with crumpled paper, pots and pans, large cardboard boxes, play dough, paper, crayons and bubbles. Arrange a place for playthings where children can select them. A shelf is better than a clothes basket so children don't have to search for playthings. It also makes it easier for them to learn clean-up skills. When children lose interest in certain toys and other play materials, put those objects out of sight. Bring them back out a few weeks or months later. You may notice the children now use the toys differently because they have learned new skills.
- *Encourage different types of play:* Young children learn from many kinds of play. Encourage both quiet and active play. Encourage your children to play outdoors as well as indoors. Find ways to let them use their big muscles (legs, arms) and small muscles (fingers, toes). Let your children practice and repeat activities. Use words to explain what is happening when they play.

Through creative play, health providers and parents are given the unique opportunity to speak to a child in the language he or she understands and loves. Speaking in their language results in strong bonding and building of relationships.

PLAY: ROLE IN EMOTIONAL HEALTH

It has been well documented that therapies using play also have a vital role in children's recovery from the deep emotional pain they suffer from traumatic situations encountered in their homes or communities. Medical providers often witness first-hand consequences of children's traumatic experiences when they are brought in for treatment after witnessing or having been a victim of a traumatic event.

Children's trauma symptoms are often compounded from a variety of abuses stemming from experiences such as becoming orphaned through their parents' deaths, being abandoned to live on danger-filled city streets, forced to participate in girl child practices, working in dangerous child labour situations, being sexually exploited, witnessing acts of domestic or community violence, or being involved in war or natural disasters. The resulting fear or terror from such traumas is so overwhelming that it impacts the child's thoughts, feelings, behaviour and even body functions. Trauma greatly affects the emotional health of every child.

The fundamental basis of successful emotional healing in these children is directed towards one basic principle—restorative intervention should begin where the child is emotionally, cognitively and spiritually traumatised. To obtain this information about a child, it is critically important to have knowledge of healthy childhood development and to remain aware that play is the primary form of communication for all children. For a child to be restored to emotional health, they need to communicate their trauma stories and their feelings surrounding the event. Play is a major key in facilitating a child's communication.

EMOTIONAL ISSUES STEMMING FROM TRAUMA

Trauma-produced emotional problems, along with the resulting losses and stress, lead to behavioural and emotional issues including psychosomatic illnesses such as headaches or stomach aches. Often the physical symptoms are the body's last attempt to communicate when all other channels of communication are blocked. The children are attempting to convey their need of someone to understand that they are hurting, sad or afraid. Children have a tolerance level for just how much sadness they can deal with before the body reacts. Because emotional symptoms can cause real pain within children, they often are misdiagnosed as having a physical illness. Emotional pain, however, won't go away just by giving a child medicine.

Normally, children who experience or witness extreme threat or trauma, respond with symptoms that fit into four general categories:

1. Having strong memories that repeatedly intrude on their normal functioning.
2. Engaging in endlessly repeated behaviours.
3. Developing trauma-specific fears.
4. Changing their attitudes about friends, family, life in general and the future.

Children who have trauma-related symptoms need opportunities to express their feelings of anger, fear and sadness. Often, however, children do not have the words to relate what has happened or to express how they feel about what they experienced. One prevalent trauma that is difficult for a child to verbalise is sexual abuse. In this kind of situation play activities can become a direct substitute for words, giving children the opportunity to search for and experiment with alternative solutions for resolving their emotional pain.

DEFINING ORGANISED PLAY ACTIVITIES (PLAY THERAPY)

Organised play for emotional healing entails purposeful, guided play (not random play on a playground) that involves keen observation of what is being acted out and a sensitive interpretation. Although play therapy requires professional training, special training is not necessary to assist a child in a play situation if the adult has an open respect for children and their play does what seems or feels helpful for the child. As in observing emotionally healthy children, much can be learned by watching a child at play, looking at his drawings or watching a child-produced drama.

PLAY: A MEDIUM OF COMMUNICATION

Children who have experienced deep trauma must be able to talk about their feelings before healing can occur. Talking is the starting point of a child's healing process. Children's ability to talk about the trauma implies that a trusting relationship has been established. If children do not express their feelings of insecurity, anxiety, fear, terror, distrust and sadness, they may bury these feelings deep inside, preventing their emotional healing. Children who have the opportunity to express their feelings become stronger and more resilient, feeling more secure, valued, loved and loving.

'Talking' does not just occur when a child uses words! Talking with children may be through words or through play activities. Play activities are a natural medium for self-expression, facilitating a child's communication. Play, being the developmental language of a child, provides children whose traumas have overwhelmed their emotions and ability to cope to have a medium for communication and expression of their feelings. For children whose trauma has left them stuck in a level of development, guided play can enable them to move on to the next crucial stage in the cycle of their development. Also since play is a normal part of a child's life and development, children who engage in play therapy are able to deal with the emotions that are experienced after the traumatic event in a way that is developmentally appropriate for them.

Methods of Play Therapy

All children have different needs and different ways of expressing those needs. To accommodate these differences, a variety of play activities can be utilised as a means of communication and expression of thoughts and feelings. Some activities, such as a playroom, can facilitate one-on-one or group sharing. Often a group of children are involved in an activity such as drawing pictures that depicts the traumatic event and provides clues on how the children feels about what happened.

The method utilised is determined by culture, the enormity of the crisis (such as a natural disaster that affected a whole village), the type of activity planned or a child's preference. For all methods children are invited to express their feelings through an assortment of art media: role play, drama, drawing, music, sand tray, storytelling, and so on. Having an equipped play room or use of games and sports are also effective forms of play. The following describes two commonly used activities.

Playroom

A playroom is a room or area that has been especially designed and furnished. Children can use toys and equipment as tools to express their emotions and to engage in drama, art (drawing, painting or colouring) or other forms of expression such as dancing or singing. In the playroom, toys are viewed as the child's words and play as the child's language—a language of activity. Therefore, a careful selection of play materials that allow children to express themselves is a priority. Emotionally significant experiences can be expressed more comfortably and safely through the symbolic representation the toys provide.

The use of toys enables children to transfer anxieties, fears, fantasies and guilt to objects rather than people. In the process children are safe from their own feelings and reactions because play enables them to distance themselves from traumatic events and experiences. There they do not become overwhelmed by their own actions because the act takes place in fantasy. By symbolically acting out a frightening or traumatic experience or situation through play, and perhaps changing or reversing the outcome in the play activity, children move towards an inner resolution. They are then better able to cope with or adjust to problems.

Art

Art is a wonderful medium for children to express feelings and thoughts too difficult to talk about. Since creating is a less direct means of expression, it provides a way for children to communicate confusing or hurtful thoughts through imagination rather than words. Drawing pictures depicting their trauma produced feelings of fear, anger and anxiety not only helps children identify these feelings but also can lead to the development of healthy coping skills. The goal of art activities is for children to better understand themselves through self-exploration and a shared interpretation of their own art.

BENEFITS OF ORGANISED PLAY

Children need time to open up and share their pain. They also need a trusted person who will listen. Play provides for both of these needs. A bond of trust between a caregiver and a child can be developed through interest and involvement in a child's play at his or her level. Once the child has established a safe relationship with the caregiver, the child will begin to go directly to his or her area of pain and concern through play. Therefore, play can be used to help a child 'talk' about the traumatic experiences with someone they trust.

'Talking' helps children process their trauma produced feelings and re-enter their developmental cycles that were interrupted by what they experienced. The sooner a child can appropriate the healing effects of a play environment the sooner hope re-enters the child's world of experience. Play activities are the main restorative approach for children experiencing trauma. Research has shown that if children can play well, they will adjust well as adults.

Such activities enable children to express what is going on inside of them: their fears and anxieties, anger, hurts and feelings about the traumatic event that has occurred. Play activities also allow children to work through the grief process with a trusted adult.

Play Activities: A Restorative Approach

Realising how important play is for the development of the child, we must also recognise the need for providing traumatised children with a safe place to play, an opportunity to play and suitable materials for play—those that will stimulate fun and creativity for the child.

Play activities are the main restorative approach for children experiencing trauma because they:

- Are a natural medium for self-expression, facilitating a child's communication;
- Allow for a healing release of feelings;
- Can be renewing and constructive and
- Allow the adult a window to observe the child.

A child-centred play activity also is one of the most powerful ways to help children recapture what was taken away from them during the trauma. The losses include a sense of:

- Control (in play they are given choices)
- Power (they can choose the story line)
- Safety (they are gaining control of their situation)
- Trust in adults (when adults honour and value children's play, the children are empowered to open up and share)
- Hope (play can create, re-enact and recreate situations in a way that helps children know things can be different, giving them hope for the future).

In summary, play gives children the opportunity to share their stories through their natural means of communication. Play also is a child's natural method of learning, developing and expressing their feelings. Play becomes a window both to look into and to observe what is going on inside the child. Given the opportunity, children will play out their feelings and needs in a manner or process of expression similar to adults. Although the dynamics and means of communication are different for children, the expressions (fear, anger, happiness, frustration) are comparable to adults. However, unlike adult therapy that is based on cognitive knowledge, children's play activities trade experiences for learned knowledge. **Figures 36.1 to 36.32** show games that children play for fun and enjoyment.

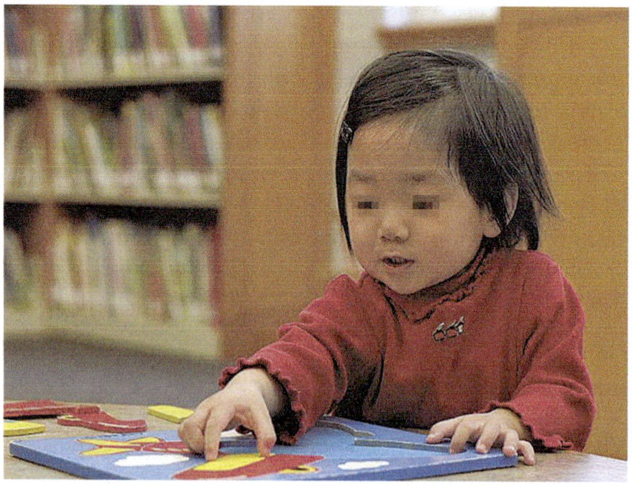

Figure 36.1

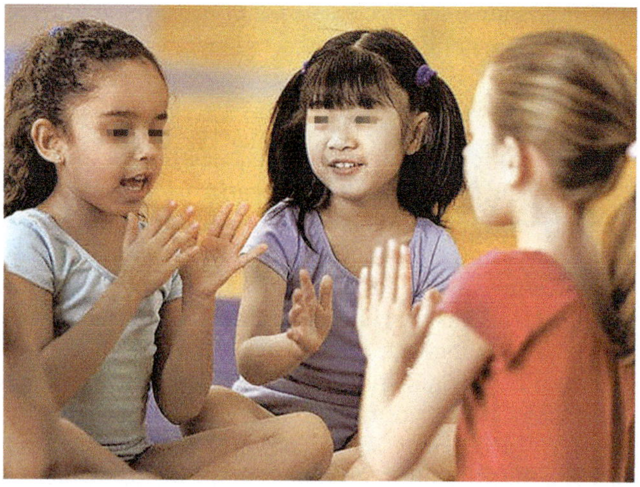

Figure 36.2

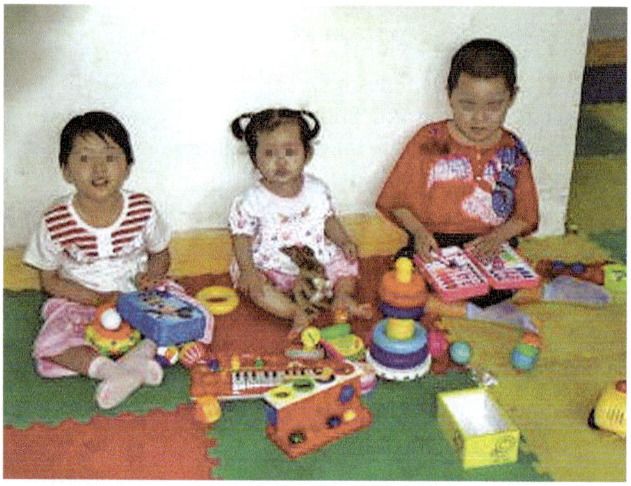

Figure 36.3

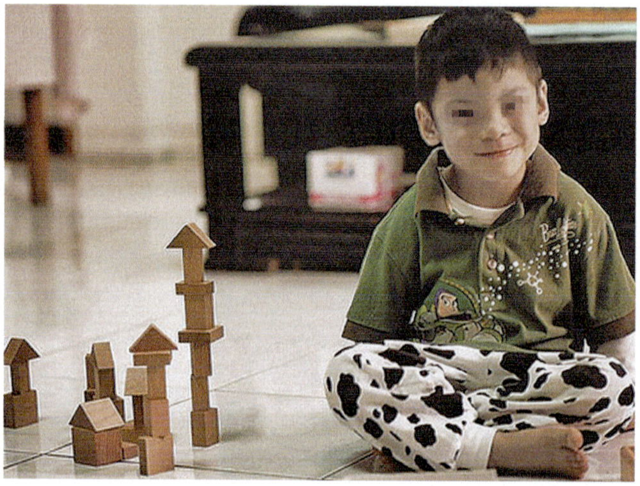

Figure 36.4

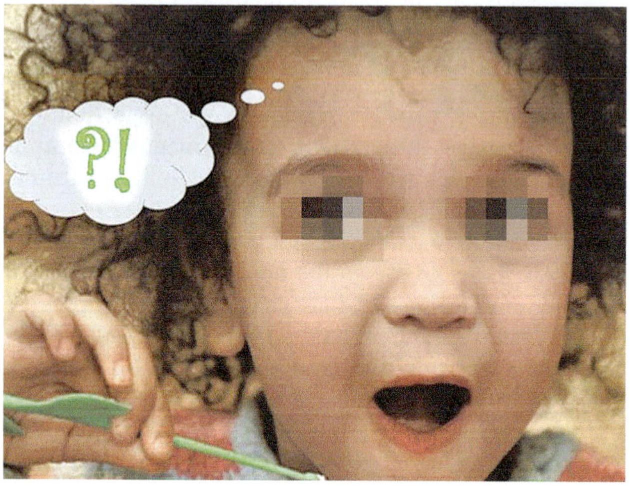

Figure 36.5

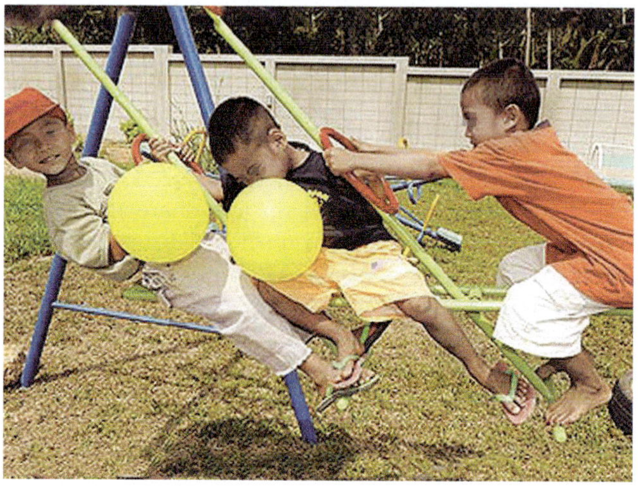

Figure 36.6

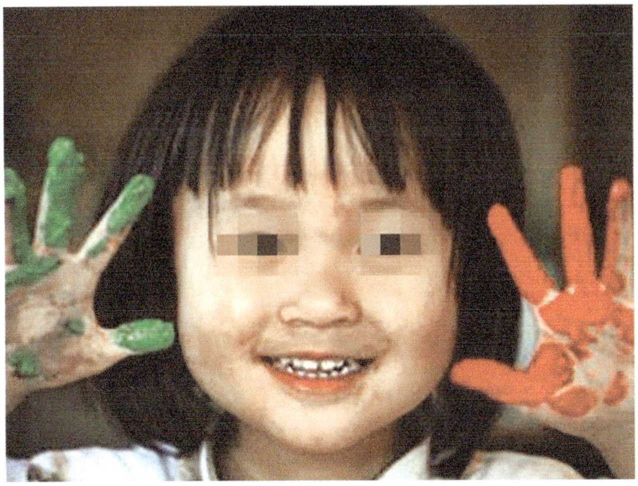

Figure 36.7

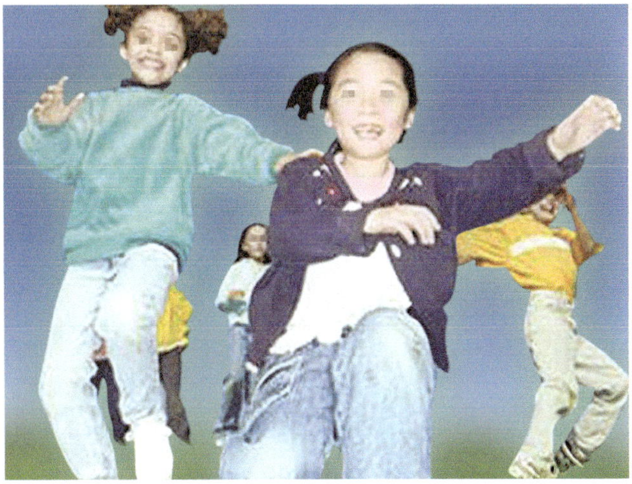

Figure 36.8

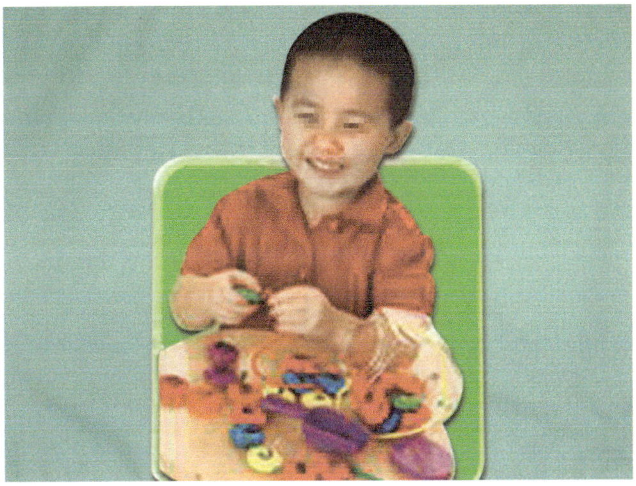

Figure 36.9

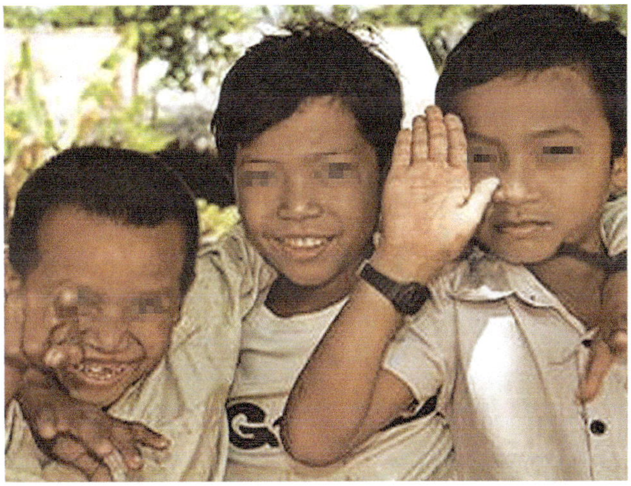

Figure 36.10

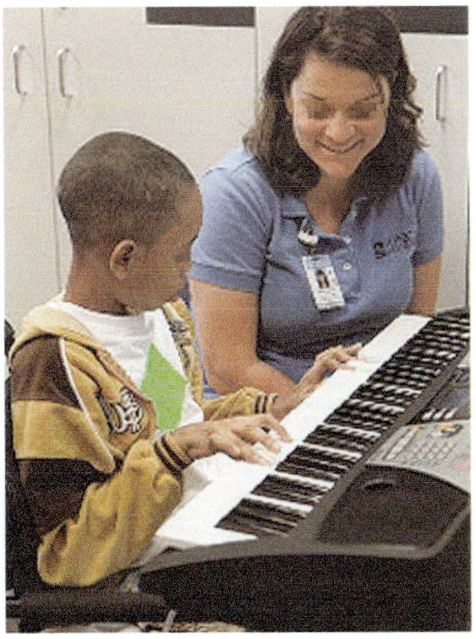

Figure 36.11

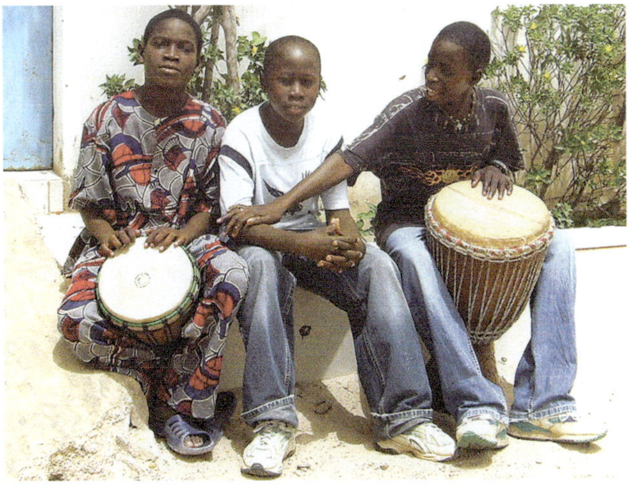

Figure 36.12

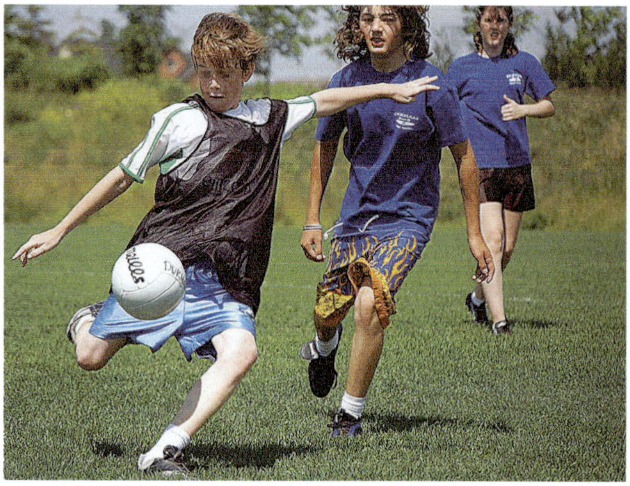

Figure 36.13

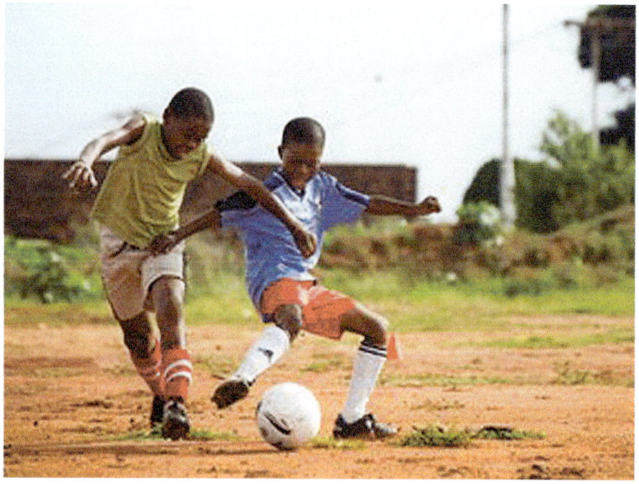

Figure 36.14

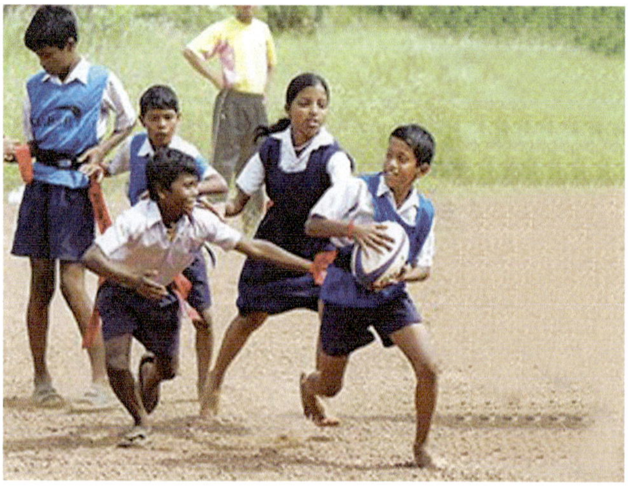

Figure 36.15

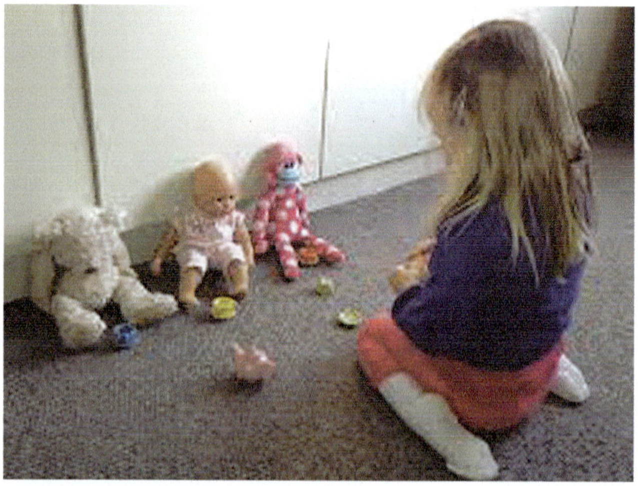

Figure 36.16

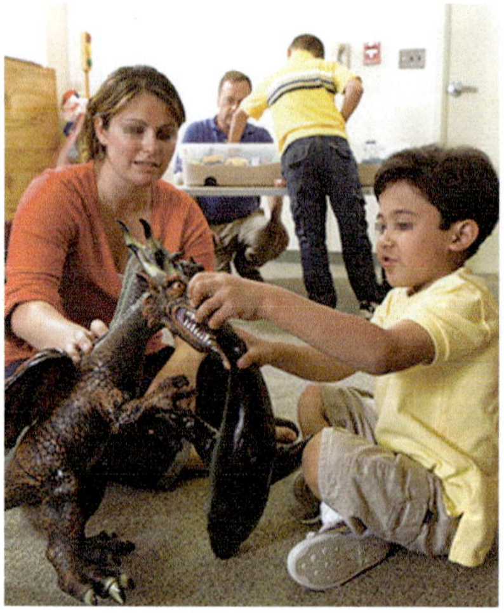

Figure 36.17

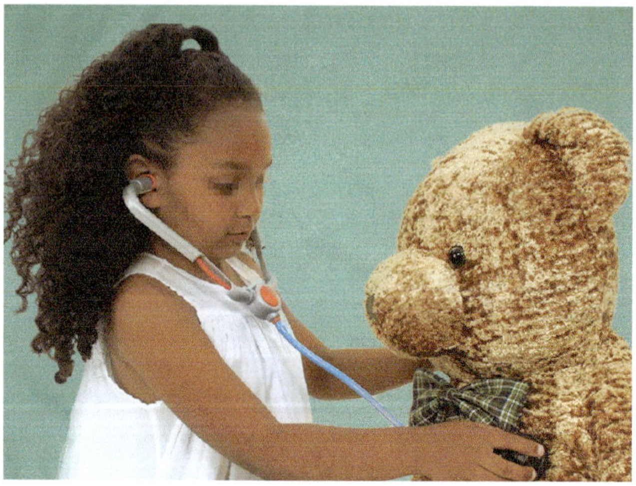

Figure 36.18

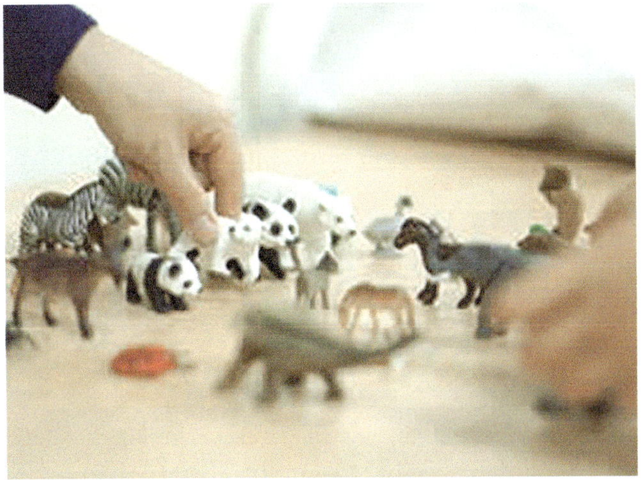

Figure 36.19

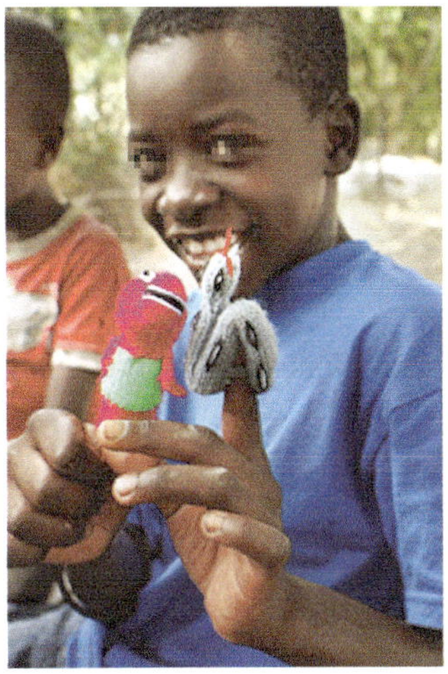

Figure 36.20

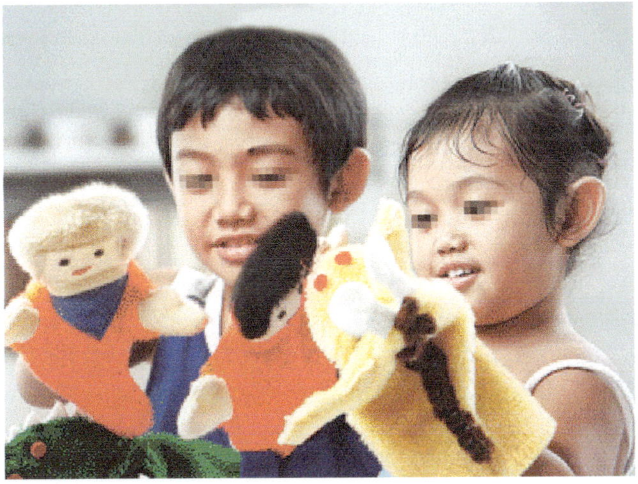

Figure 36.21

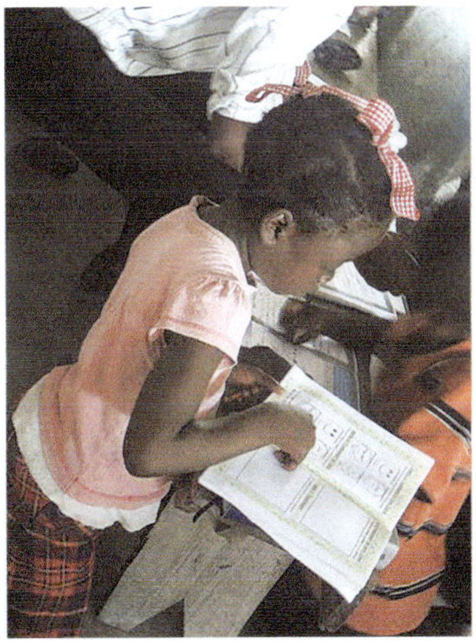

Figure 36.22

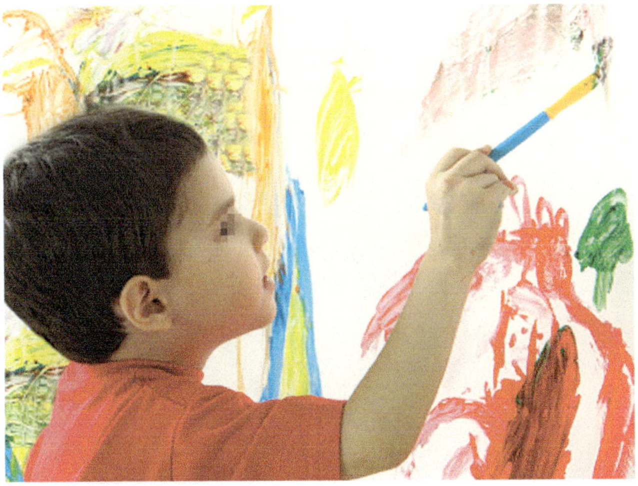

Figure 36.23

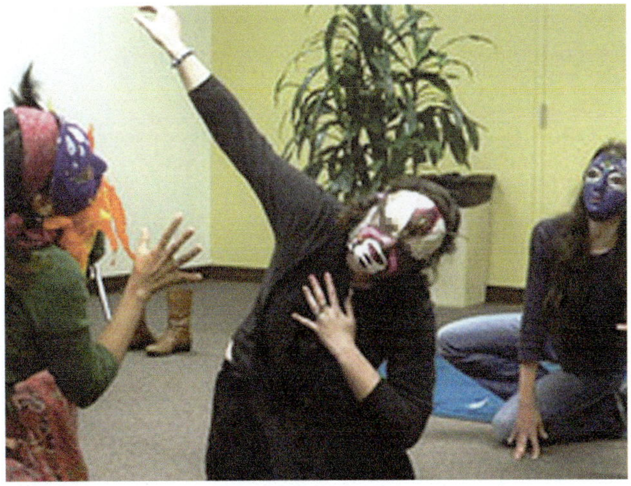

Figure 36.24

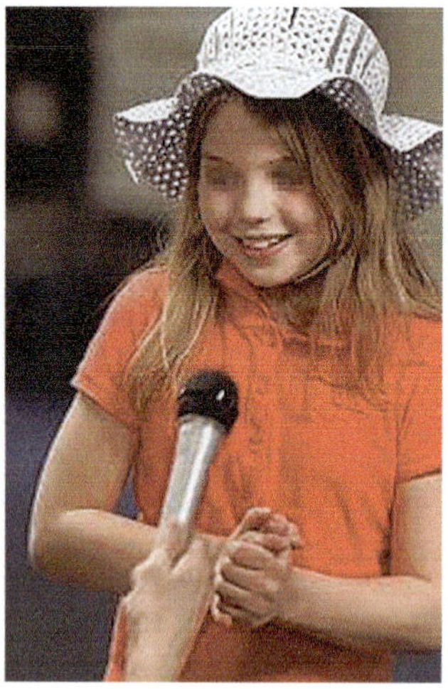

Figure 36.25

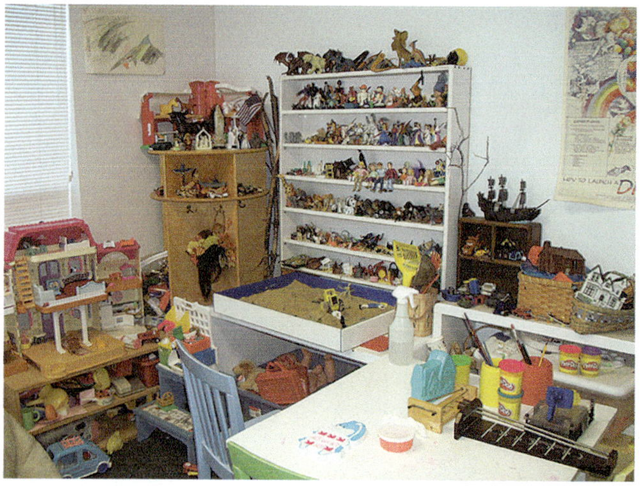

Figure 36.26

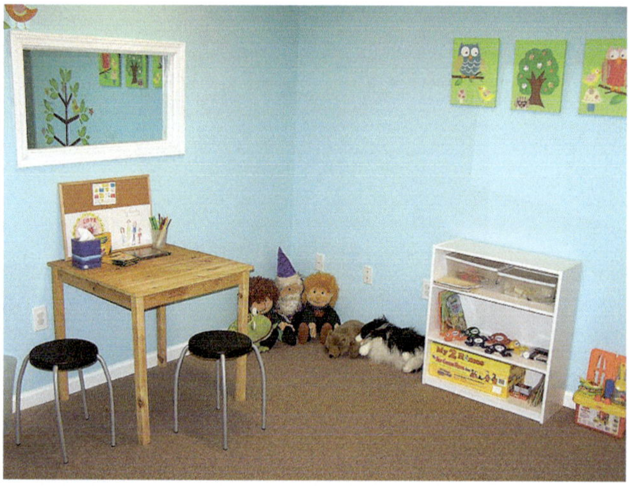

Figure 36.27

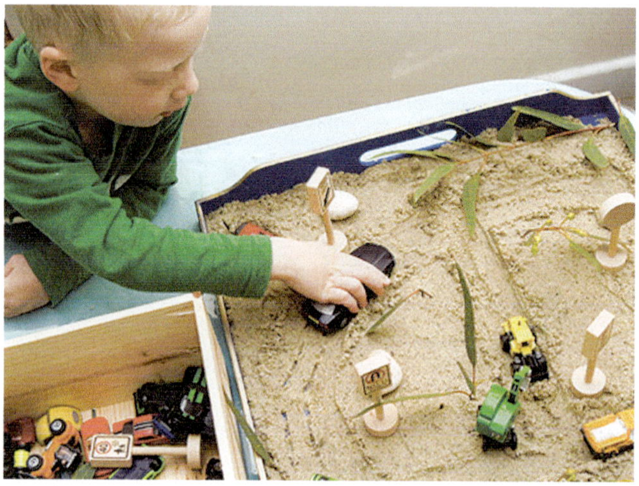

Figure 36.28

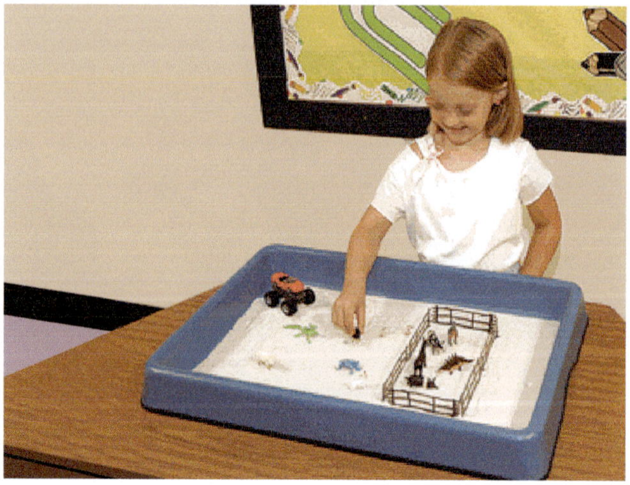

Figure 36.29

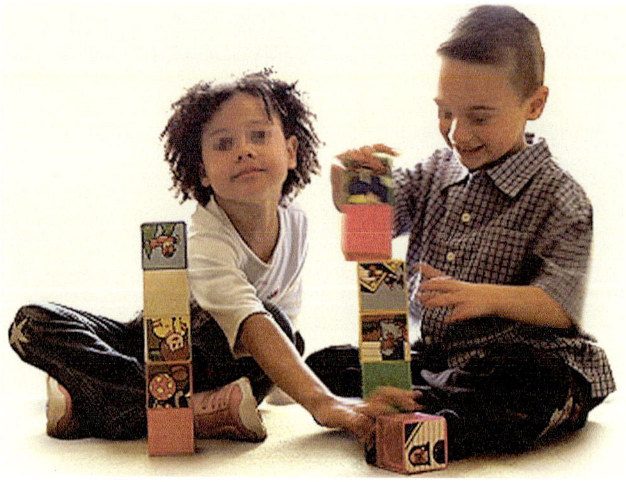

Figure 36.30

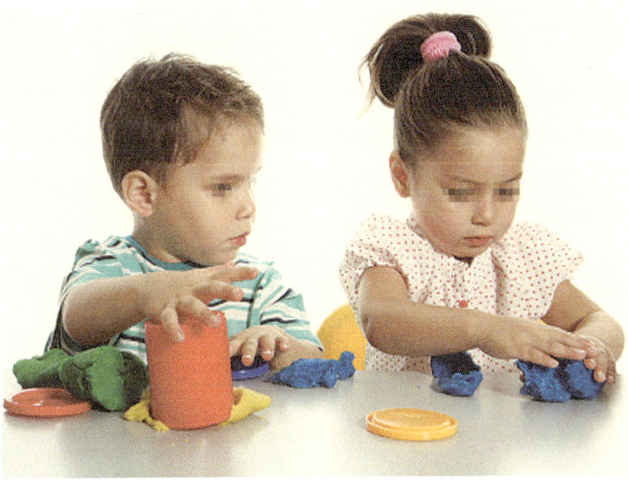

Figure 36.31

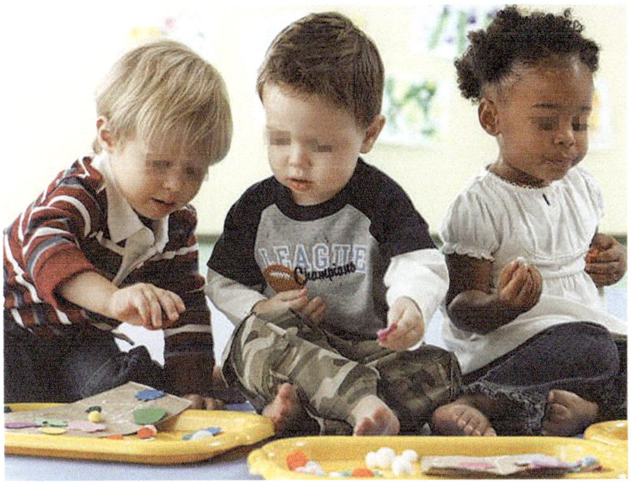

Figure 36.32

REFERENCES

1. Piaget J. Play, Dreams and Imitation in Childhood. New York: Norton; 1951.
2. Strickland E. The power of play. Scholastic Early Childhood Today. 2000;14(6):36-43.

CHAPTER 37

Nutrition Assessment

Mona Basker, N.V. Mahendri

INTRODUCTION

Nutritional status in children is an indicator of health and well-being. Nutrition assessment is a process of determining nutritional status and identifying those who are malnourished. Assessment of nutritional status is important in paediatric patients as they are undergoing the complex processes of growth and development, which are influenced by the genetic makeup, medical illness and nutritional status. Thus, nutrition assessment in children plays a vital role in determining the growth and development and it is an integral part of patient care. It is essential for planning and providing nutrition intervention as well as clinical care.

Nutrition status refers to the state of health in relation to intake and utilisation of nutrients.

NUTRITION ASSESSMENT

Nutrition assessment involves collecting data from (a) anthropometry assessment; (b) selected biochemical test results; (c) clinical assessment; and (d) dietary assessment. Anthropometry data will provide information on physical growth, adequacy of energy and protein. Biochemical parameters confirm the status of malnutrition before the classic signs of malnutrition develop. Clinical assessment involves identifying signs of malnutrition physically. Dietary assessment involves food and nutrient intake. The order of collection of the data as well as the type of data required varies with the health condition of the child.

ANTHROPOMETRIC ASSESSMENT

Anthropometry is the study of various measurements of the human body. It depicts the bone, muscle and fat components of the body. Several measurements are used in anthropometry; only those essential for nutritional assessment of a child are portrayed in this section.

What is the Need for Anthropometry?

Actual measurements of the body are used in comparison with a standard reference measurement. Interpretation of these measurements helps in assessing whether a patient has adequate, less than adequate or more than adequate nutrition.

Monitoring growth of the child and adolescent is of paramount importance. Any deviation from an optimal growth pattern would alert the health care provider (HCP) about their health status.

Anthropometric measurements done on a large group of children and adolescents belonging to a particular geographical area and said strata in the society can form the reference standard for all belonging to that specific group. Over time, the anthropometric measurements that are plotted on growth charts will change in a temporal fashion. Hence, these will be useful in revising growth charts for a specific population.

Equipment used for anthropometric measurements are as follows:

Infant Measuring Board

Refer **Figures 37.1A and B**.

Stadiometer

Refer **Figure 37.2**.

Digital Weighing Scales (Figs. 37.3A and B)

Double weighing is done when the child is unable to be weighed separately. The care giver and the child are weighed together and the care giver is weighed separately. The actual weight of the child is computed from these two measurements.

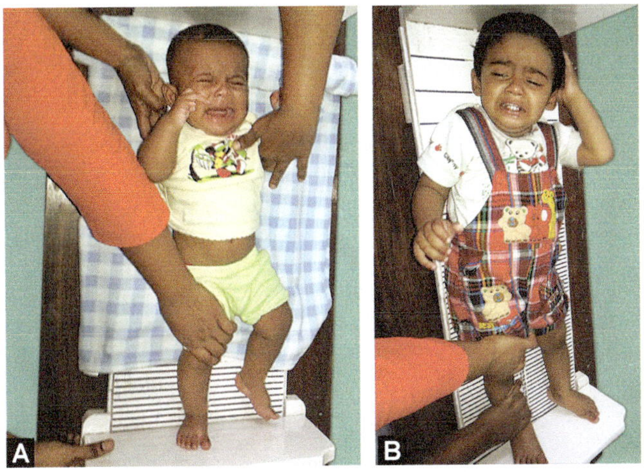

Figures 37.1A and B Infant-measuring board.

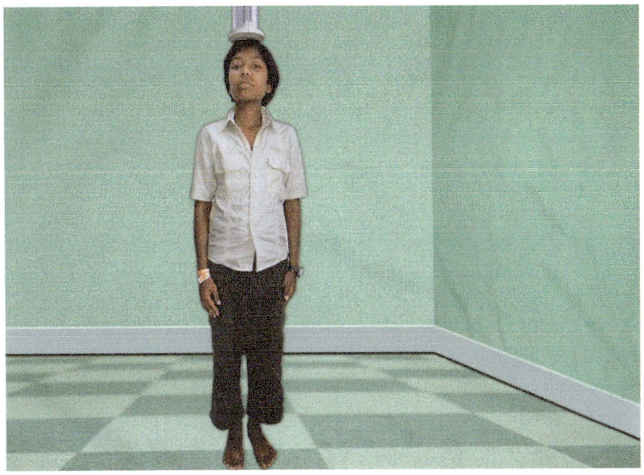

Figure 37.2 Stadiometer.

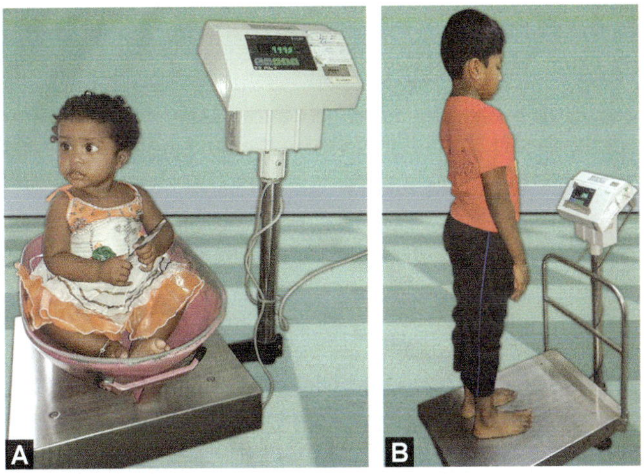

Figures 37.3A and B Digital weighing scales.

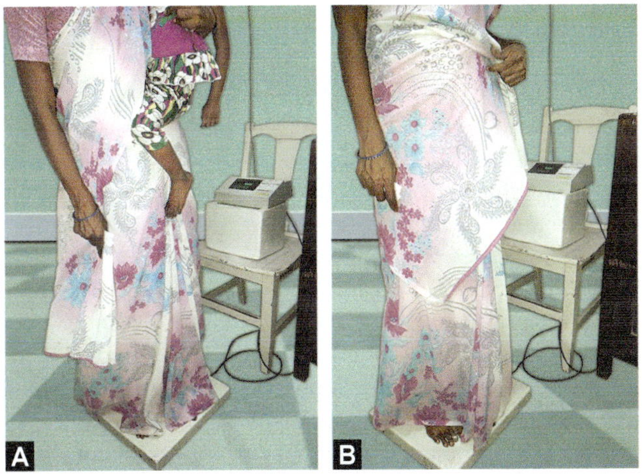

Figures 37.4A and B Double-weighing on a digital scale.

'Double Weighing' on a Digital Scale (Figs. 37.4A and B)

Mid-upper arm circumference (MUAC) is another measure used in children 1–5 years of age to assess their nutritional status.

The technique of measuring MUAC is depicted in the following pictures (Figs. 37.5A to C).

Mid-upper Arm Circumference

The patient can stand or sit with the elbow relaxed so that the arm hangs freely to the side. The two points that are marked on the skin surface are the acromion and the olecranon processes. The mid-point between these points on the upper arm is the site to measure MUAC. The tape rests on the skin surface, but is not pulled tight enough to compress the skin. MUAC is recorded to the nearest 0.1 cm.

Body Mass Index

Body mass index (BMI) is used in clinical practice to determine if weight is proportionate to the patient's height. In children and adolescents, BMI varies with age and the variation happens over a wide range. Hence, BMI centiles are used, and the nutritional status of the adolescent is classified based on the WHO BMI centile curves.

- Body mass index is calculated using the formula:
- Body mass index is weight in kilograms divided by height in meter squares.

Interpretation of Anthropometric Measurements

Standard growth charts are used for interpreting the anthropometric measurements (Figs. 37.6A to D).

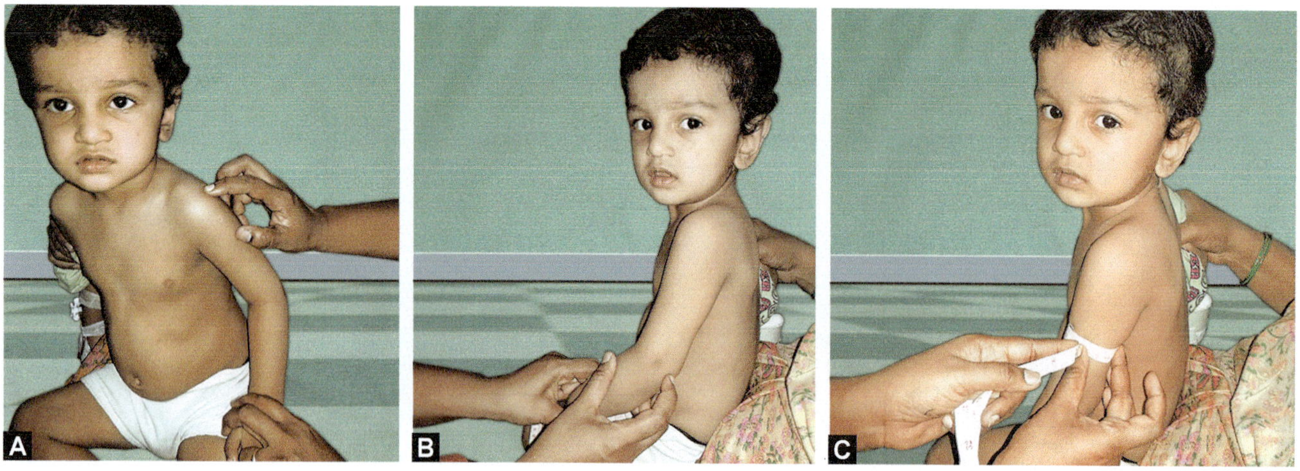

Figures 37.5A to C Mid-upper arm circumference (MUAC). (A) Step 1: Healthcare provider (HCP) pointing to the acromion process; (B) Step 2: HCP pointing to the olecranon process; and (C) Step 3: HCP measuring at the mid-point with a non-stretchable tape.

BIOCHEMICAL ASSESSMENT

Based on the medical history and physical assessment and related nutritional disorders, appropriate biochemical parameters can be assessed and the results are to be interpreted considering the medical conditions. The biochemical assessment data provide information about macro and micronutrients stores. The tests performed depend on the nutrient to be assessed. Routinely performed tests include serum albumin, pre-albumin level to assess the protein nutrition status, haemoglobin and haematocrit for iron status assessment. The reference values are used for comparison and evaluation.

CLINICAL ASSESSMENT

Clinical method of assessing nutritional status involves physical examination of patient's general condition and close examination of skin, hair and teeth and look for signs that might suggest specific nutrient deficiency. Examples of specific clinical signs of nutrient deficiency include pallor (on the palm of the hand or the conjunctiva of the eye) associated with anaemia pitting oedema and severe visible wasting in protein energy malnutrition, Bitot spots (whitish patchy triangular lesions on the side of the eye) is a sign of vitamin A deficiency. Evaluation of medical conditions that contribute to the nutrient deficiency is required for interpretation of this data.

DIETARY ASSESSMENT

Dietary assessment is usually performed by the dietician. The data collected are used to quantify and calculate the food and nutrient intake and assess the adequacy of the nutrient; usually energy and protein using standard guidelines, age specific recommended dietary allowance (RDA) or daily reference intake (DRI). Twenty-four hours recall/diet history, food frequency are the common methods used to collect food intake information from the parent/children.

Twenty-four Hours Recall Method

This method is simplest and easy to administer. The diet information regarding type and amount of food consumed in the previous day is obtained either from parents/caregiver of the child. The same method can be used to collect a typical day's intake as well. Use of food model/portion size/standard cups/household measure would help in collecting information.

Food Frequency

Food frequency information is obtained from the parents/caretakers about the routine food habits of the child. Qualitative information about the type of food items, frequency and the quantity consumed daily, weekly fortnightly is obtained and documented on a preformatted food frequency questionnaire. The format depends on the health care set up and the nutrient/s of concern.

Diet History

It is used to collect information about quantity and quality of the food that is consumed by the infant or child and the eating behaviours and beliefs of the family. Diet history may include 24 hour recall as well as food frequency and interview to collect the information. The information collected include details about the number of feeds/meals, meal timings preparation methods, use of special foods, use of food supplements, presence food allergy/intolerance, feeding difficulties such as chewing or swallowing difficulties, child's food preference likes/dislikes,

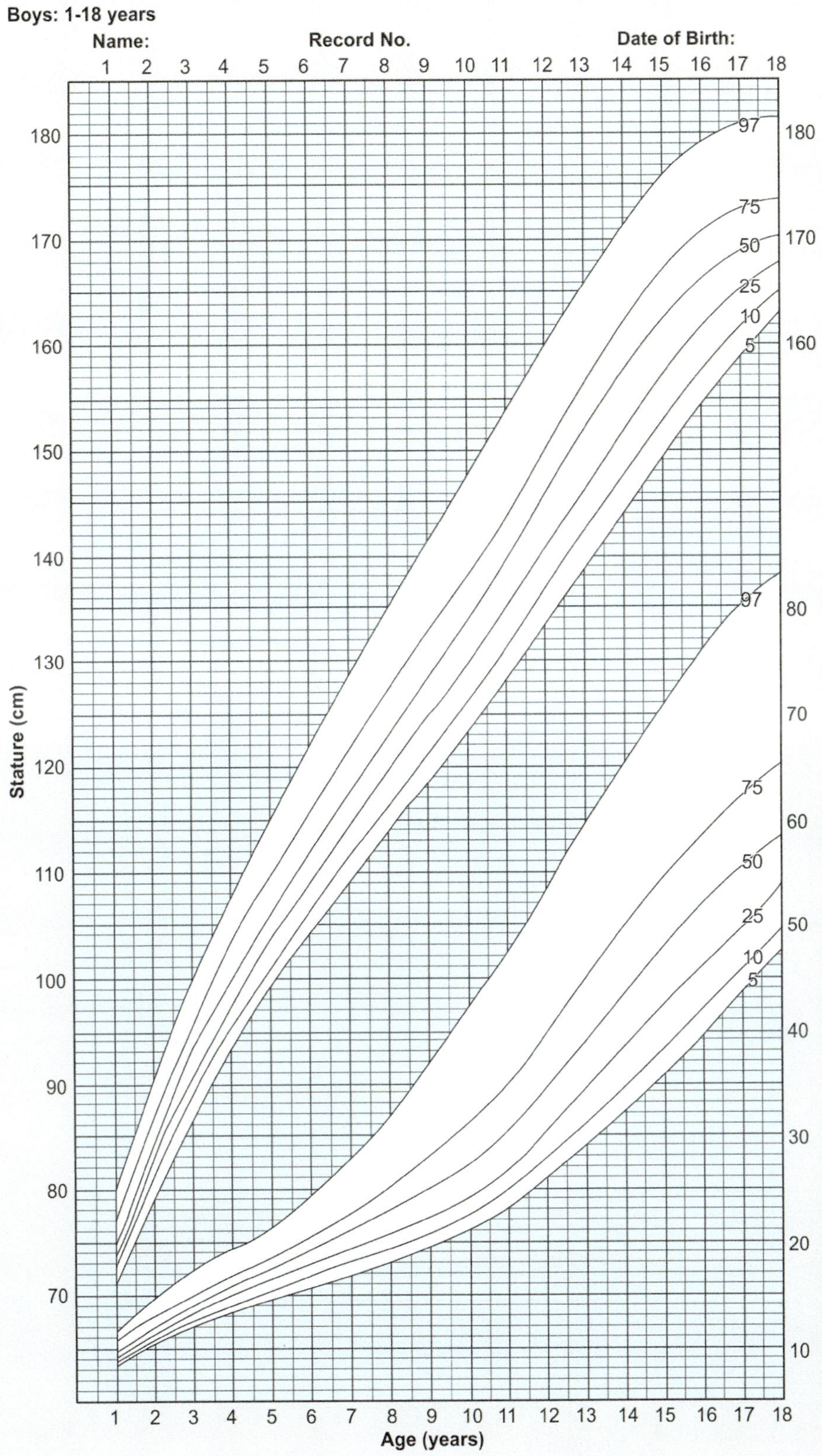

Adapted from: 1 Agarwal DK ET AL Physical and sexual growth pattern of affluent Indian children from 5-18 years of age IND Pediatr- 1992;29:1203
2 Agarwal DK Agarwal KN-Physical growth in affluent indian children (Birth to 6 years) IND, Pediatr,1994,31:377
Dept. of Endocrinology, Sgpgims, Lucknow

Figure 37.6A

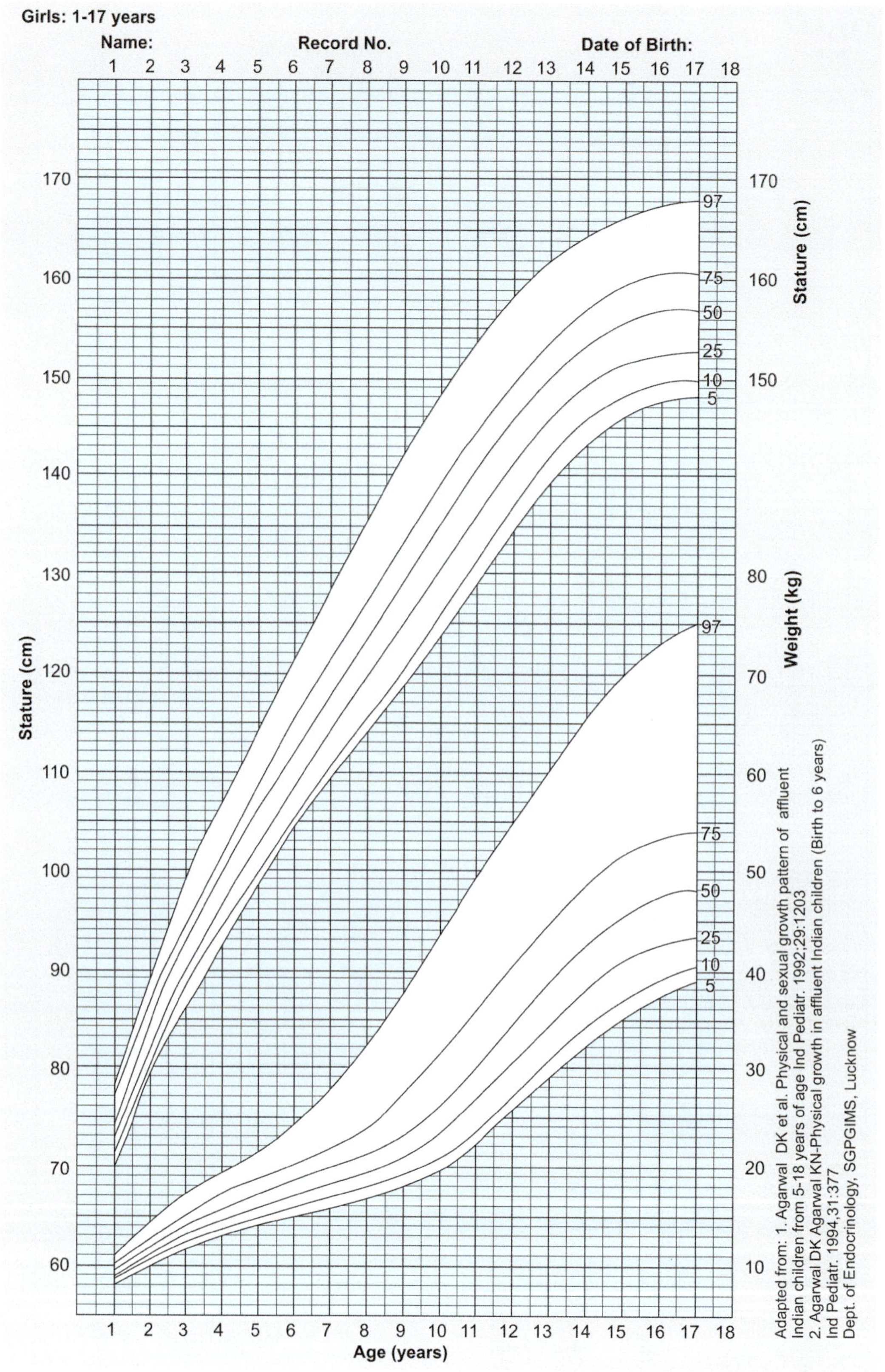
Girls: 1-17 years
Name:
Record No.
Date of Birth:
1 2 3 4 5 6 7 8 9 10 11 12 13 14 15 16 17 18
170
160
150
140
130
120
110
100
90
80
70
60
Stature (cm)
97
75
50
25
10
5
170
160
150
Stature (cm)
80
70
60
50
40
30
20
10
Weight (kg)
97
75
50
25
10
5
Age (years)
Adapted from: 1. Agarwal DK et al. Physical and sexual growth pattern of affluent Indian children from 5-18 years of age Ind Pediatr. 1992;29:1203
2. Agarwal DK Agarwal KN-Physical growth in affluent Indian children (Birth to 6 years) Ind Pediatr. 1994,31:377
Dept. of Endocrinology, SGPGIMS, Lucknow

Figure 37.6B

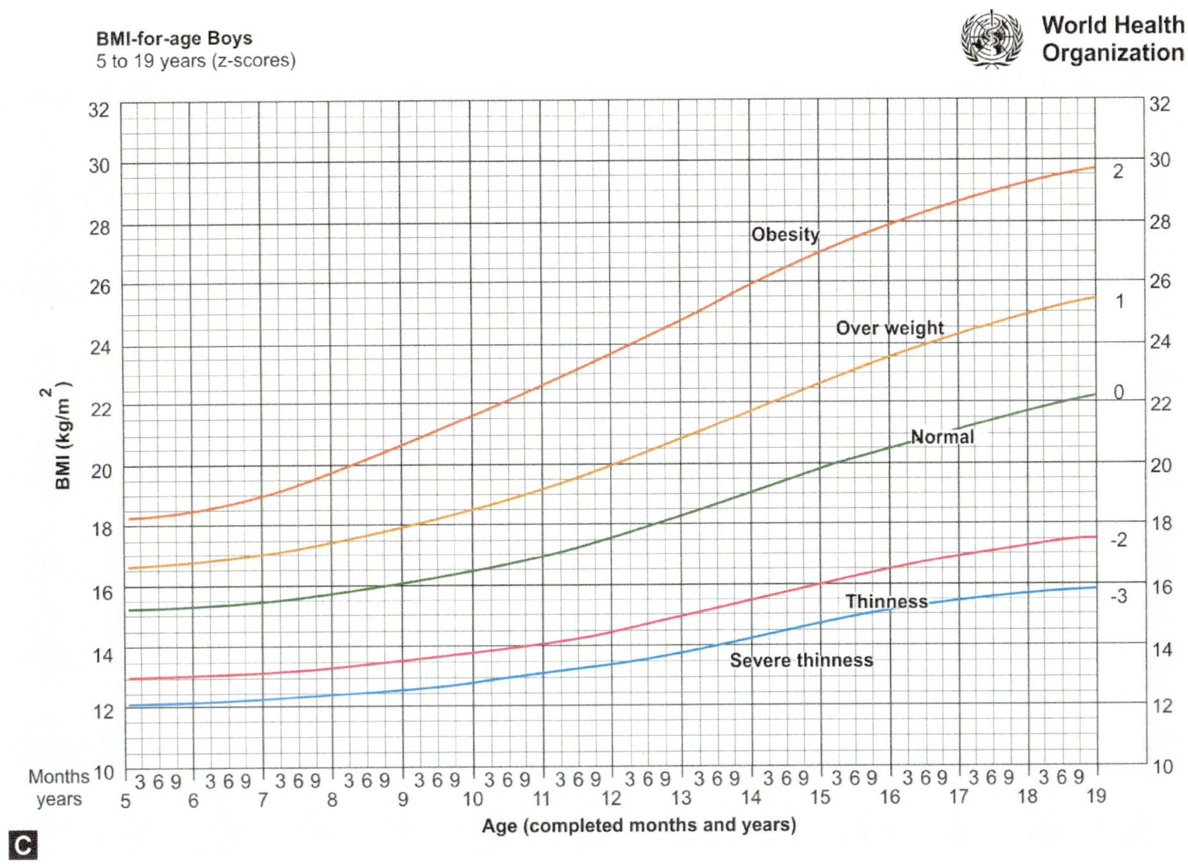

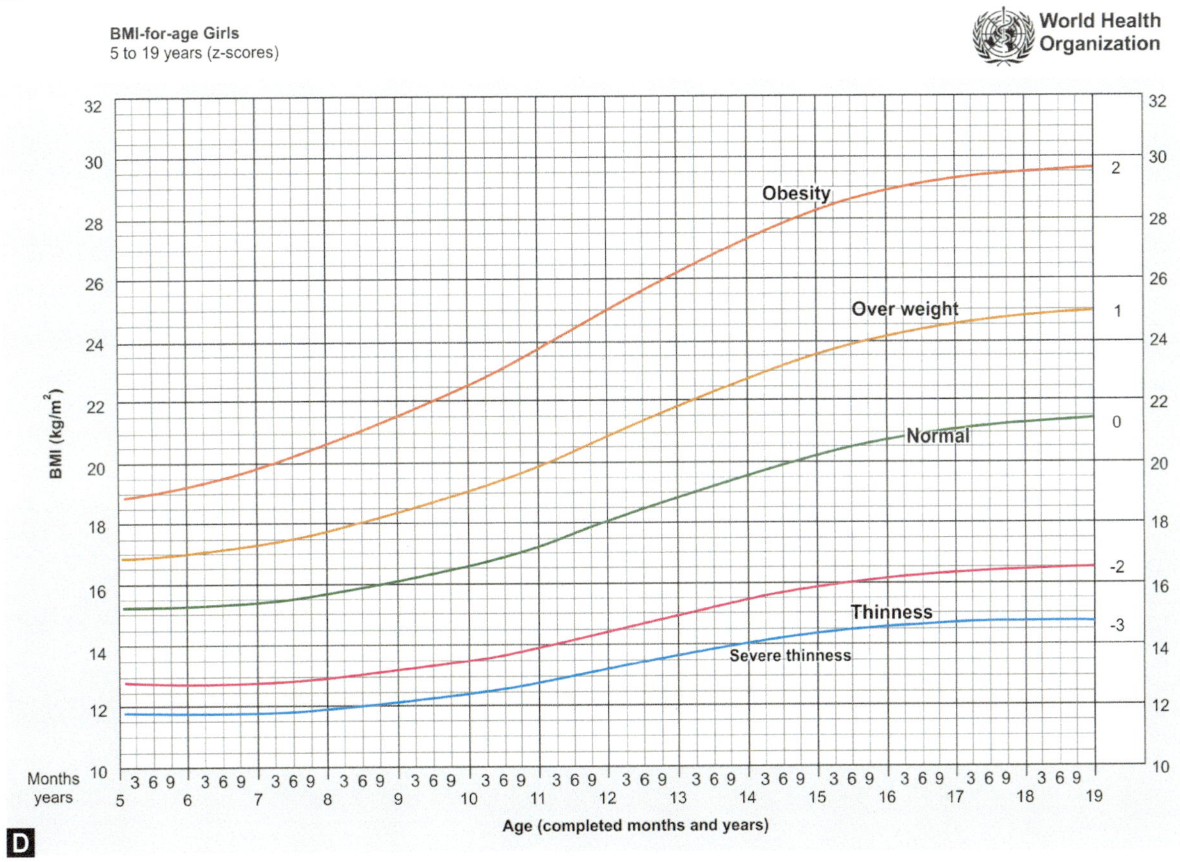

Figures 37.6A to D (A) Agarwal growth charts for weight and height for boys; (B) Agarwal growth charts for weight and height for age for girls; (C) WHO body mass index (BMI) centile charts for boys; and (D) WHO BMI centile charts for girls.

enrollment in local supplementary feeding program, etc. [in India-integrated child development services (ICDS), Anganwadi/Mid-day meal/School lunch program].

Calorie Count

The most commonly used method of dietary assessment in hospitalized patients is the calorie count. This is a food record of the amount of food consumed from a known quantity of food in a day (24 hours). Calorie count is a useful part of nutritional assessment follow-up because this provides a rough assessment of the patient's appetite, intake and compliance with nutrition recommendations.

Analysis of the Food Intake Data

Raw food intake is calculated from the food intake data collected and this is used for calculation of nutrients. The nutrient intake is calculated either by conventional method using (country wise) food composition table/database or computerised nutrient analysis program. Generally energy and protein contents of the diet are calculated; however, other nutrients assessed depend on the health condition of the child. In general, country-specific dietary guidelines can be used to assess the diet composition. The calculated nutrient/s intake is compared with age-wise recommended optimum intake, either RDA or DRI, for planning appropriate nutrition care/intervention.

CHAPTER 38

Surgical Oncology

Philip Hammond

GENERAL PRINCIPLES

Tumours are not commonly seen in children but must always be borne in mind as prompt diagnosis is paramount. The mode of presentation varies depending on the site of the tumour and the pathology encountered is quite unique to children. Diagnosis, staging and management follow guidelines from different collaborations around the world. Leukaemia and lymphoma are the commonest malignancies in childhood and surgical involvement is usually limited to diagnostic biopsy and supportive care. The most common solid paediatric tumours are intracranial but solid tumours at other sites and their management are considered here.

NEUROBLASTOMA

Neuroblastoma is one of the commonest solid tumours seen in children. It is an exclusively paediatric malignancy arising from neuroblasts (pluripotent cells of the sympathetic nervous system derived from the neural crest). Neuroblastomas may occur at any site where neural crest cells are found with about 50% arising from the adrenal medulla, 25% retroperitoneal paraspinal, 20% mediastinal and occasionally neck or pelvis. It occurs in 10 per million children under the age of 15 years with a slight male preponderance and the mean age of diagnosis is 17 months. The most important genetic abnormality of prognostic value is the MYCN proto oncogene amplification on the short arm of chromosome 2. More than 10 copies of MYCN are associated with a poor prognosis. About a quarter of neuroblastomas have evidence of MYCN amplification. The amount of DNA in a cell is also of prognostic significance with hyperdiploid tumours having a better prognosis than diploid tumours. Neuroblastoma falls in to the pathological category of small round blue cell neoplasms of childhood. Clinical features depend very much on site with the majority presenting with an abdominal mass in association with malaise, weight loss, anaemia and sometimes hypertension. Sometimes mass pressure effects may lead to symptoms such as paraplegia from tumour extension through intervertebral foramina, bladder and bowel dysfunction or compression of venous and lymphatic drainage. Upper mediastinal or neck neoplasms may lead to cough, superior vena cava syndrome or Horner syndrome from involvement of the stellate ganglion. Distal metastases may lead to a variety of symptoms such as bone pain, peri-orbital ecchymoses (or "panda eyes"), anaemia from bone marrow invasion or skin involvement causing classic 'Blueberry muffin spots.

Investigations start with routine bloods and urinary catecholamines, which are normally elevated in patients with neuroblastoma. Imaging including computed tomography (CT) and/or magnetic resonance imaging (MRI) is then undertaken to identify the extent of the primary disease and any metastases. Tumour biopsy (from a primary or metastatic site) and bone marrow aspiration are needed to diagnose and stage the disease. MIBG (meta-iodobenzylguanidine) scans (and sometimes technetium bone scans or positron emission tomography) are useful in determining the extent of metastases and subsequent response to treatment. The International Neuroblastoma Risk Group (INRG) staging is based on preoperative diagnostic imaging. Image-defined risk factors (IDRFs) are used to make an assessment of the resectability of tumours thereby allowing categorization of patients as having locoregional (L1 or L2) **(Fig. 38.1)**, metastatic (M) or MS disease (patients less than 18 months of age with localised primary tumour with dissemination limited to skin, liver and/or bone marrow). Pretreatment risk stratification determines the multimodal therapy depending on local protocols or trials but usually involves chemotherapy (cisplatin, cyclophosphamide and doxorubicin) and complete surgical resection where possible. Radiotherapy may also be considered in certain clinical circumstances such as spinal cord compression. Prognosis is variable but, in general, infants do better than older children. Overall survival is 80% for infants, 50% for children under 5 and 40% for those older than 5 years.

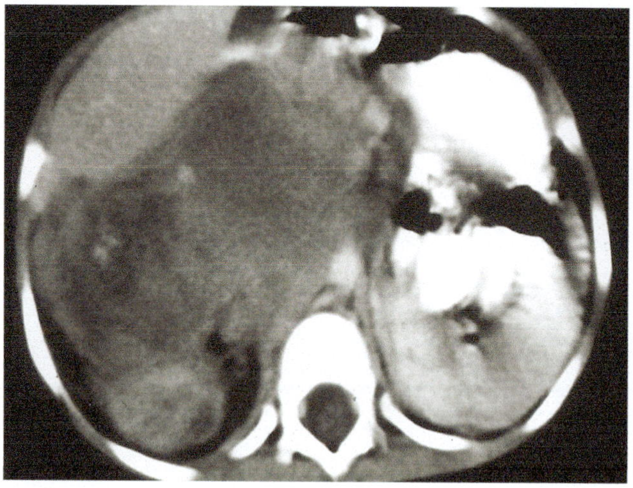

Figure 38.1 A CT scan showing a large right-sided adrenal neuroblastoma.

WILMS TUMOUR

Wilms tumour (WT) or nephroblastoma is the commonest tumour to affect the kidney of children and occurs in 8 per million children, accounting for 8% of all childhood malignancies. The average age of presentation is 2.5 years for unilateral disease and 3.5 years for bilateral. There are various genetic syndromes linked to WT **(Figs. 38.2A and B)**. WT is thought to arise from embryologically primitive nephrogenic rests, which should normally regress. Loss of tumour suppressor genes such as WT1 (11p13) and WT2 (11p15) also plays a role. The tumour itself may have three cell types; blastemal, epithelial and stromal and depending on the presence of these cells WT are termed triphasic or monophasic. Clinical presentation is usually with a flank mass, haematuria and sometimes hypertension, anaemia, pain or fever. Occasionally, a child may present in extremis and with a peritonitic abdomen because of tumour rupture from a minor injury. Rarely a new onset varicocele in young boys may result from a WT. A renal mass in an infant less than 6 months is more likely to be mesoblasticnephroma, and presentation in the second decade raises the likelihood of renal cell carcinoma.

Investigations include imaging such as ultrasound and CT and a tumour biopsy to ultimately confirm the diagnosis and stage the tumour. There are two different staging systems: the National Wilms' Tumour Study Group (NWTSG) and the Société Internationale d'Oncologie Pédiatrique (SIOP) based on whether resection is performed pre- or post-chemotherapy. In NWTSG upfront, surgical resection is performed and thus staging dictates subsequent multi-modal therapy: stage I, tumour is limited to the kidney and completely excised without rupture; stage II, tumour extends through the renal capsule but is completely removed with no microscopic involvement of the margins; stage III, incomplete resection with residual tumour confined to the abdomen; stage IV, distant metastases and stage V, bilateral WT. SIOP staging is analogous but determined from resection following chemotherapy, which is initiated on the basis of imaging studies. In the United Kingdom, a diagnostic biopsy is usually performed before chemotherapy which precedes resection. Prognosis depends on the presence of metastases and the degree of anaplasia. Most recent figures report that survival from WT has greatly improved in the last 40 years and in resource-rich countries is now about 80–90%. Inequalities in health outcomes are exemplified by significantly worse survival in resource-poor countries.

SOFT TISSUE TUMOURS

Rhabdomyosarcoma is the most common soft tissue tumour seen in children. As it is derived from embryonic

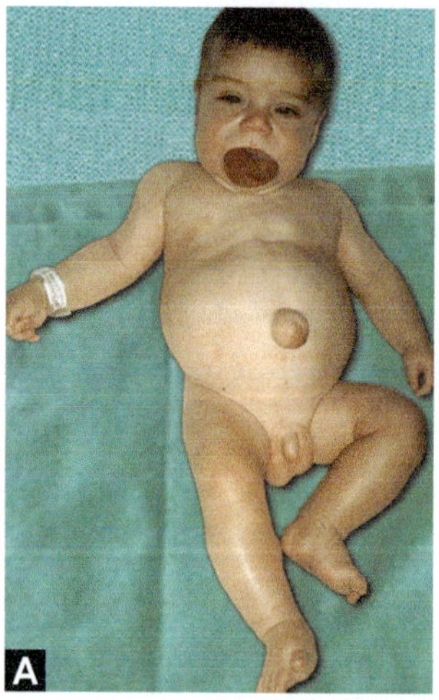

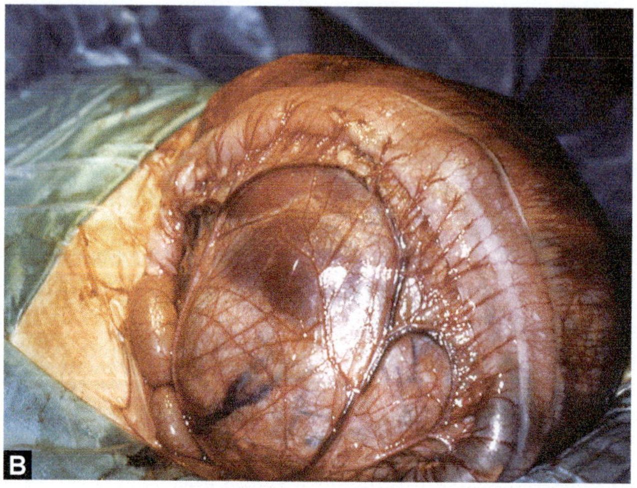

Figures 38.2A and B (A) A child with Beckwith–Wiedemann syndrome (*note* macroglossia and umbilical hernia) with associated nephroblastoma; and (B) Wilms tumour at operation (seen through the mesocolon which is stretched over the mass).

mesenchyme, which has the potential to differentiate into skeletal muscle, it may occur anywhere in the body. The commonest sites are the head, neck and the genitourinary tract, with the extremities being involved in only about one-fifth of cases. The incidence is rare around 4 per million children every year. There are two peaks in incidence; in those between 2 and 5 years of age and then in adolescence. The majority of RMS cases are sporadic but some may be related to syndromes such as Li-Fraumeni (*see* Chapter 9) and NF1. Certain genes have now been implicated in the cause of RMS such as RAS oncogene mutations and PAX-FKHR fusions. RMS is histologically classified as a small, round, blue cell tumour of childhood and is traditionally categorized into botryoid, spindle cell, embryonal, alveolar and undifferentiated variants. Botryoid RMS (resembling a "cluster of grapes" arising from the vagina or bladder) and spindle cell RMS (usually of paratesticular or orbital origin) have the most favourable prognosis. Alveolar and undifferentiated RMS have the worst prognosis. Clinical features depend on the site; for instance, in the head and neck parameningeal mass effects or proptosis may result, in the prostate there may be bladder or bowel dysfunction **(Fig. 38.3)**, and in the extremities a painless mass may be found. About 15% have evidence of metastases at diagnosis. Investigations include routine bloods tests followed by imaging according to site. This may include plain radiographs, bone scan, CT and MRI. Diagnosis is usually made by incisional, endoscopic (or occasionally excisional) biopsy. Staging is described by the TNM staging system or the clinical group staging system; group 1 when the tumour is completely resected, group 2 when there is microscopic residual tumour, group 3 when there is gross residual tumour and group 4 when there is evidence of distant metastases. Surgery remains the mainstay of treatment although non-mutilating resections are now preferred. Multimodal treatment with surgery plus chemotherapy (VAC—vincristine, actinomycin-D, cyclophosphamide) and/or radiotherapy has improved survival; for instance, the commonest embryonal head and neck RMS has about 70% expected survival.

HEPATOBLASTOMA

Two-thirds of all liver masses in children are malignant and the majority are hepatoblastoma, particularly in infants 6 months to 3 years of age. In older children with pre-existing liver disease or hepatitis B infection hepatocellular carcinoma becomes more likely. Hepatoblastoma is associated with a number of genetic syndromes such as Beckwith-Wiedemann, Familial adenomatous polyposis, Li-Fraumeni and trisomy 18 (*see* Chapter 9). Histologically they can be classified as epithelial, embryonal, macrotrabecular or small cell undifferentiated and most commonly mixed epithelial and mesenchymal. The majority of patients are asymptomatic and present with a palpable mass. Jaundice is rare and other symptoms may include abdominal pain, vomiting, distension and anorexia. Differentiation from benign liver lesions such as infantile hemangioendothelioma or mesenchymal hamartoma is often by imaging studies although blood tests may also be helpful; alpha-fetoprotein (AFP) is typically markedly elevated in hepatoblastoma and is used as a tumour marker. Plain abdominal X-ray may show right upper quadrant mass and calcification although it is usually ultrasound that gives the diagnosis, and CT and MRI may be used to exclude pulmonary metastases. Diagnosis is ultimately made with biopsy. Staging is usually by the SIOP PRETEXT staging scheme, which is based on imaging determination of the four liver sectors and the number of sectors involved prior to surgery gives the stage. Local protocols dictate management involving primary surgery or neo-adjuvant chemotherapy (usually cisplatin based) followed by resection. Radiotherapy has a limited role in hepatoblastoma **(Fig. 38.4)**.

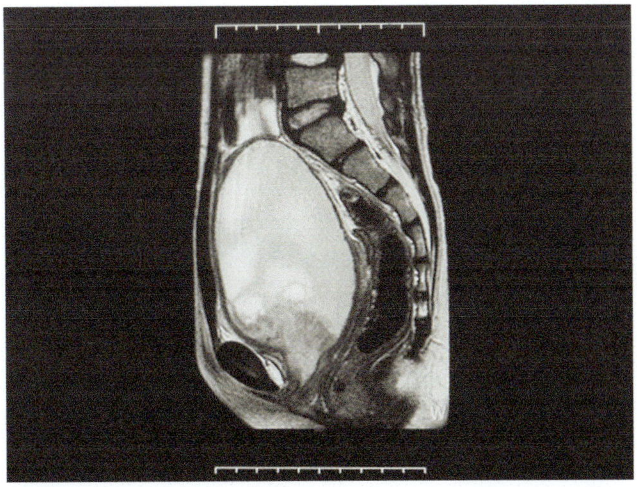

Figure 38.3 An MRI scan of bladder-prostate rhabdomyosarcoma.

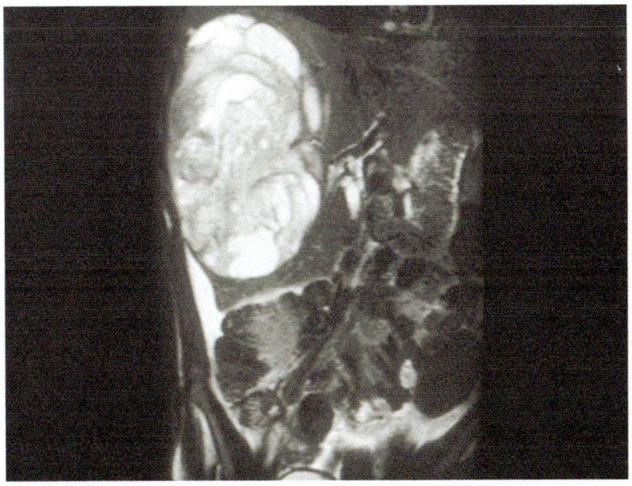

Figure 38.4 An MRI of an infant with a large hepatoblastoma.

TERATOMAS AND OTHER GERM CELL TUMOURS

In infants germ cell tumours (GCTs) predominate in extra-gonadal (and testicular) sites and in adolescence more commonly arise in the gonads. They originate from primordial germ cells that migrate early in embryogenesis, which accounts for the variety of frequently affected sites. They have a heterogeneous and complex pathology and malignant potential with classifications including teratoma, endodermal sinus tumour (also termed "yolk sac tumour" whichis malignant), germinoma and mixed GCT. Rarer components include choriocarcinoma, embryonal carcinoma and polyembryoma. Elevated serum AFP or beta-human chorionic gonadotrophin (β-HCG) indicates the presence of malignant components and are used as tumour markers. Teratomas are composed of tissues from each of the three germ cell layers of the embryonic disk. The commonest site is the sacrococcygeal region **(Fig. 38.5)** in infancy but may also arise in other locations including mediastinum, gonad, retroperitoneum, cervical or central nervous system. About 20% contain malignant components and hence diagnosis is often established at histology following surgical excision; malignancy being treated with platinum-based chemotherapy.

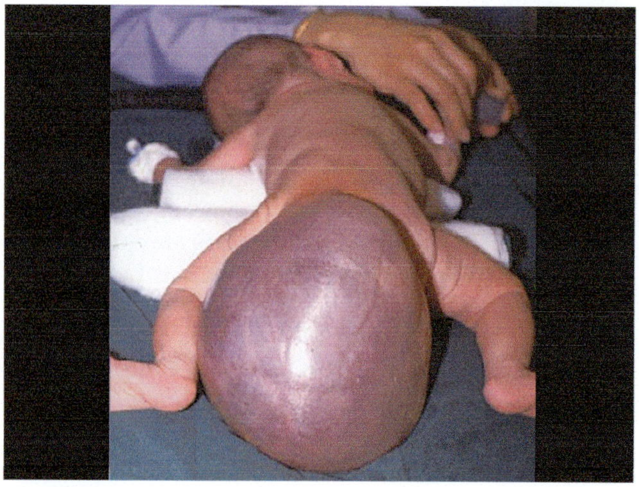

Figure 38.5 Sacrococcygeal teratoma.

CHAPTER 39

Paediatric Podiatry

Gordon F. Watt, Stewart C. Morrison, Krishna M. Goel

INTRODUCTION

Paediatric podiatry differs from general podiatric practice in that the growing foot provides unique problems and challenges that are not encountered in the adult foot. The simple reason for is that, not only is the foot subject to local problems due to growth but it is also required to adapt and compensate for developmental change as the general posture develops through a series of changes affecting the whole skeleton—in practice from the podiatric point of view, changes that affect the spinal posture, position of the pelvis and the long bones of the lower limb. As the foot supports this structure any changes that take place produce a "knock-on" effect on the foot, altering its posture, either temporarily or permanently, which can leave it compromised and lead to other pathologies as it attempts to compensate for these changes. Equally an inherited or acquired problem within the foot can compromise its posture, resulting in changes to the bony skeleton above it. In some instances it may be that both scenarios contrive to compound the situation. The foot can also be affected by the many diseases of childhood, either directly or indirectly, and it is of paramount importance that abnormalities or suspected manifestations of systemic disease are recognised at an early stage and appropriate action taken in order to avoid, reduce or eliminate complications into adulthood. It is, therefore obvious that, as in the adult foot, the growing foot cannot be considered in isolation from the rest of the body, but unlike the adult foot, where the posture tends to be static, the paediatric foot is in a state of flux as it adapts to change.

Many misconceptions exist related to paediatric foot problems. Unfortunately, foot problems, unless gross or particularly troublesome, traditionally were given low priority, with the result that manageable cases were left untreated and secondary features related to structural pathologies developed. These included chronic intractable plantar keratosis in their many guises, or arthritic states affecting the foot, lower limb and lumbar spine. These problems obviously require treatment, and it is interesting to note that the majority of the elderly population attends a podiatrist, with many requiring hip, knee and foot surgery. Early recognition and management of actual and potential foot problems in the young would go a long way to reduce these numbers. In an attempt to tackle this problem, successful podopaediatric screening programmes have been established in the past. However, the majority of foot problems in the paediatric age group are inclined to be more subtle and tend to be related to the following broad categories.

- Footwear
- Foot types
- Infections
- Anatomical anomalies
- Biomechanical anomalies/abnormalities
- Acquired deformities
- Congenital and genetic abnormalities
- Postural anomalies/abnormalities
- Surgical/medical conditions
- Dermatological conditions

These broad headings will either be referred to specifically under their individual headings or be alluded to within the text. However, before considering these, it is vital to have an understanding of the normal chronological growth and development of the lower limb particularly in the early years of life when change can be dramatic and rapid.

NORMAL GROWTH AND DEVELOPMENT

In the embryo, the limb buds first appear at about 4 weeks of intrauterine life, becoming segmented into proximal, intermediate and distal parts by the week 6 and digitated by week 7 of gestational age. The thigh, the leg and the foot are recognisable entities by week 9. The feet should reach a nearly neural position by the end of postovulatory week 11. The positional changes of the feet appear to depend invariably on the skeletal and neuromuscular development.

Ossification starts initially in the larger bones of the leg and foot, extending gradually to the smaller bones (Table 39.1). By completion of the embryonic stage, all major neural, vascular and muscular parts of the limb are present and in appearance closely resemble those of an adult.

The majority of children are born with normal feet, both structurally and functionally. It seems that the shape, size, and form of feet are genetically determined but are liable to being affected by other factors. However, in some children faulty intrauterine morphogenesis may be responsible for deformity and disability. Also drugs may have dangerous effects on the developing foetus. The most disastrous drug has been thalidomide, which has caused severe limb abnormalities (Fig. 39.1). Later in life, infection, injury, and other systemic diseases may be responsible for foot problems. The conditions present at birth are designated congenital disorders. Children are not mini-adults and the child's foot is not a small scale replica of the adult foot. It is comparatively shorter and wider, tapering towards the heel because the hindfoot is less fully developed than the forefoot (Fig. 39.2).

The infant's foot is very malleable; it may allow some congenital deformities to be corrected easily, although it also means that the foot may be deformed by abnormal stresses of weight bearing or external factors, e.g. footwear.

In general, the foot tends to appear short, broad, stubby-toed and fat at birth, it may also appear flat due to fatty padding in the medial longitudinal arch area, but during the first year this is gradually absorbed as growth

TABLE 39.1 Ossification timetable.

Bone	*Primary centres*	*Secondary centres*	*Fusion remarks*
Tibia—diaphysis	7th week		
Tibia—upper epiphysis	At birth	20th year	
Tibia—lower epiphysis	2nd year	18th year	Sometimes a separate centre for the medial malleolus appears at the same time
Fibula—diaphysis	8th week		
Fibula—upper epiphysis	4th year		
Fibula—lower epiphysis	2nd year		
Calcaneum—body	6th month		
Calcaneum—epiphysis	6th–10th month	13th–15th year	
Talus	7th month		
Cuboid	At birth		
Lateral cuneiform	1st year		
Medial cuneiform	3rd year		
Intermediate cuneiform	4th year		
Navicular	4th year		
First metatarsal shaft	8th–9th week		
First metatarsal base	3rd year	17th–20th year	Sometimes a separate centre for the head appears at the same time
Other metatarsal shafts	8th–9th week		Sometimes a separate centre for the base of the fifth metatarsal appears at the same time
Proximal phalanx shafts	12th–14th week		
Proximal phalanx bases	3rd–6th year	17th–18th year	
Intermediate phalanx shafts	4th–9th month		That for the fifth toe does not appear until shortly after birth
Intermediate phalanx bases			
Distal phalanx of hallux	3rd–6th year	17th–18th year	
Distal phalanx shafts	8th week		
Distal phalanx bases	6th year	17th–18th year	

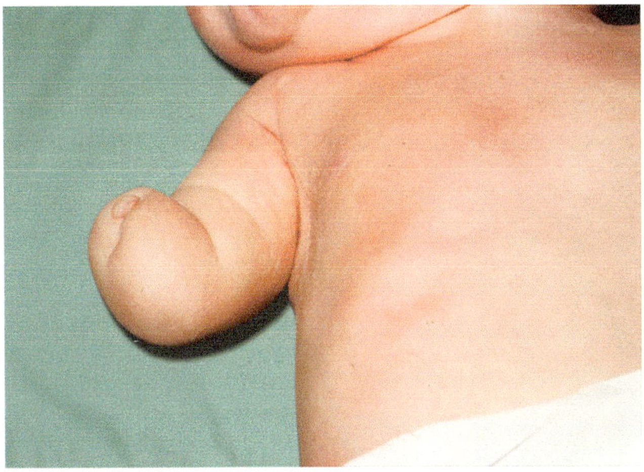

Figure 39.1 Limb abnormalities caused by thalidomide-Phocomelia (*see* Figure 1.57).

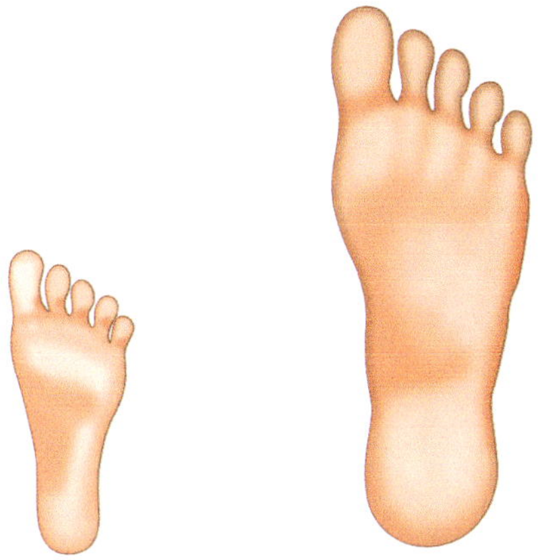

Figure 39.2 Different proportions between the mature and immature foot.

proceeds. To allow normal growth and development it is important to allow the baby freedom of movement to allow for normal muscle development, and therefore tight bedclothes and constrictive foot coverings should be avoided. During the early crawling and walking stages it is also important to allow barefooted walking to encourage normal function. It is best that children do not wear shoes until they are walking competently out of doors unless there is an obvious abnormality that has to be addressed, e.g. cerebral palsy. However, it is prudent to seek a specialist opinion should there be any concern over a child's development, particularly if the mother who spends more time with and knows her child better than anyone else is concerned so that she can be reassured or appropriate investigations undertaken.

KEY LEARNING POINT

The usual age group of children presenting with foot problems ranges from neonate to pre-school, but it is not unusual for problems to present at a much later age or to be detected by screening programmes during primary school.

KNOCK-KNEE (GENU VALGUM), BOW LEG (GENU VARUM) AND RICKETS

During this early period the child walks on a broad base and may appear flatfooted with bow legs and may show lordosis with bulging of the abdomen with legs partly flexed at the knees. The feet may be variously abducted or adducted and apparently flat. During gait, the child will lean forward with the arms abducted and partly flexed at the elbows, reminiscent of a tightrope walker.

From 2 to 6 years of age, developmental knock-knee is evident, with the vast majority of cases resolving spontaneously between the ages of 5 and 6 years as growth progresses and few cases are seen in 8-year-olds. The abdomen becomes less prominent, and the foot type and medial longitudinal arch become more evident.

During this period the general posture is constantly changing as the child experiments with their body image and equilibrium. Most of the developmental changes that take place in the lower limb result in compensation within the foot in the form of subtalar joint pronation. It is very important to establish the cause of this, and in most cases, reassurance and footwear advice is all that is needed. However, it must always be remembered that the cause may be more serious (particularly if it is unilateral), and a full and thorough examination should be undertaken.

RICKETS

By definition, the cause of rickets is an insufficient intake of vitamin D to promote normal bone growth and to prevent the occurrence of specific abnormal changes in the bone. Toddler rickets presents with bow legs in a child who is already able to walk with or without other signs as found in infantile rickets **(Figs. 39.3A and B)**. The bony lesions occurring in infants and toddlers may be gross **(Fig. 39.4)** but usually complete healing followed by virtual loss of significant deformity, occurs as the limb doubles in length as growth continues. Residual compensatory foot problems may persist and require on-going management (*see* Chapter 5).

FLAT FOOT

Older children very frequently have flattening of the medial longitudinal arch on standing but the arch reasserts itself on standing on tiptoe—this is the mobile flat foot and no specific treatment is needed beyond encouraging the child to practise toe walking and walking on inverted feet. As the limb matures a normal arch will appear. In severe cases,

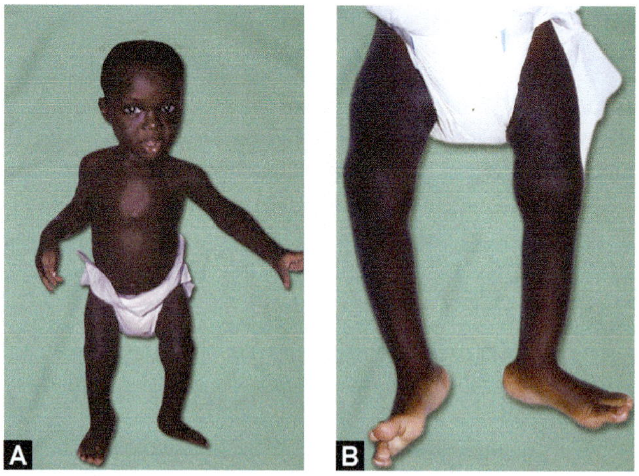

Figures 39.3A and B Bowing of legs in an African child with rickets.

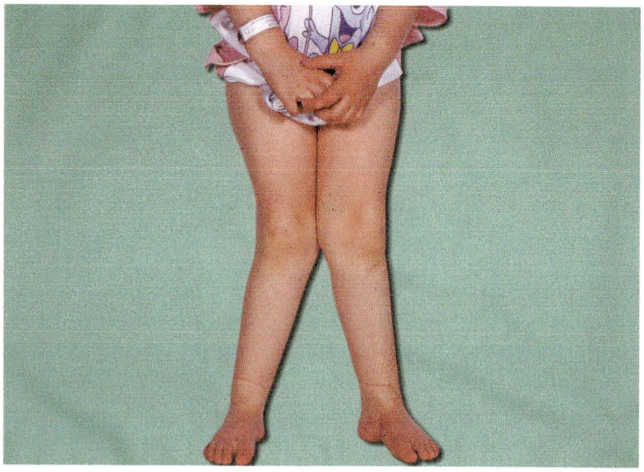

Figure 39.4 Knock knees (genu valgum) in rickets.

a casted foot orthosis may be required. It should also be remembered that some individuals have naturally low arched feet as others are highly arched and this should not be confused with mobile flat foot.

KEY LEARNING POINT

Many young children when first standing appear to have flat feet, as the adipose tissue under the medial longitudinal arch is pressed to the ground, the hollow obliterated and the foot looks flat. This is not pathological and the parents should be reassured.

PEAK RATES OF GROWTH

Growth continues steadily at varying rates into late adolescence with peak rates at puberty. Many foot pathologies seen in children, particularly in this age group, are associated in some way with growth, and it is important to be aware of any growth spurts that may be taking place. This age group also tends to be more active physically putting additional stress on growing tissues. Children under active management by a podiatrist should have their feet and height measured and charted at each visit and results compared overtime.

In general, the rate of growth of the feet is constant from birth, increasing by approximately two sizes per year for the first 4 years and then by one size annually thereafter until the mid-teens. Foot growth however, is very variable between individuals with some children growing by several sizes in a very short period and others having long periods with no growth, hence the importance of regular measuring when purchasing footwear. It is a noticeable trend that feet are becoming larger, particularly among boys. It is not unusual to find 11 year old boys with size 11 feet (*see* Chapter 2). Also bear in mind that there may be size difference between left and right foot.

FOOTWEAR

The role of footwear in relation to foot deformity is contentious. Some authorities consider that foot deformity, unless inherited is solely related to the outcomes of compensations related to biomechanical disorders within the foot or general skeleton, while others hold the view that foot deformity can be caused only by an outside influence such as inadequate footwear. It is likely that, given ideal circumstances, factors from both are responsible but, given the multifactorial influences upon the foot, both intrinsically and extrinsically, and the variations in posture, gait and anatomy between individuals, it is possible that a definitive opinion will never be forthcoming. However, it is reasonable to assume that in the early years of life the foot is so flexible and malleable that it can be influenced by outside forces and hence deformity may result. A good example of this is the (now illegal) practice of Chinese foot binding, in which feet were bound in a prescribed position from birth, resulting in a gross, permanent and disabling deformity. In the older foot, where ossification, posture and neuromuscular control are more established, this may be less likely to occur or more difficult to achieve, but it is interesting to consider that in order to correct certain mobile deformities the principles of Davis' law (**Box 39.1**) are utilised in all age groups, by serially encouraging the deformity into a corrected position with appropriate orthotic devices. It could be argued

BOX 39.1 Davis's law.

Ligaments and other soft tissues, when placed under unremitting tension, elongate by the addition of new material. When remaining uninterruptedly in a relaxed state they gradually shorten by the absorption of effete material until they come to maintain the same relationship to their attachments as they did before.

that inadequate footwear does this in reverse or inhibits or negates the action of foot orthoses.

Children's footwear is available in many forms and should always be examined and its suitability considered with every child. These forms and their associated hazards include the following.

- Babygros and sleep suits. All babies wear babygros and sleep suits **(Fig. 39.5A)** but consideration is often given to colour, design and general size rather than the suitability regarding foot size. As many of these items are made of cotton, frequent washing may reduce their size. In addition terry towelling and disposable nappies occupy space, thus further relatively reducing their size. These result in the mobility of the foot being further restricted and the digits held in a flexed position with the added risk of damage to the periungual tissues.
- Stretch tights and socks **(Fig. 39.5B)**. Most attention tends to be paid to the shoes that a child wears, with the hosiery often being neglected. It is possible with very young children that inadequate hosiery may have a more damaging influence than inadequate footwear. This is particularly the case when children learn to dress themselves, where they will make small hosiery fit by stretching it beyond its limits. Equally hosiery that is too large will accommodate the growing room in shoes, making them relatively too small. Sizing on tights and socks may not correspond with the sizing system used for the shoes. Children with intrinsic deformities in the toes may have their deformity compounded.
- Knitted booties. These tend to be knitted with an open weave, which can result in entrapment of a digit and resultant gangrene due to ischaemia. They are commonly found to be too small or too large.
- Pram shoes are often purchased for special occasions, e.g. baptisms. This is a harmless practice. Permanent use should be discouraged, as the sizing of many pram shoes is spurious, making accurate fitting by the parents almost impossible and the style of many paying little heed to the form of a baby's foot. The synthetic materials employed in many are also unsuitable, encouraging excessive sweating and often being worn with hosiery containing a large percentage of synthetic fibres.

KEY LEARNING POINT

- Children do not require shoes on their feet until they are walking competently out of doors.
- However, exceptions include, children born with deformity, such as talipes equinovarus (TEV), or neurological conditions, such as hemiplegia, where the foot must be artificially maintained in a corrected or ideal posture.

INADEQUATE FOOTWEAR

In general, footwear may be inadequate in many differing ways, including being too short, too narrow, having a pointed or a shallow toe box, poor or no retaining medium, inadequate heel stiffener, heel height too high, narrow base to the heel. Synthetic uppers and/or lining, or any combination of the above and not being compatible with the foot it is covering.

Children should always have their feet measured for shoes at a reputable retail outlet by a trained competent shoe fitter. I ideally both feet should be measured at approximately 2 month intervals and the shoes replaced as required, and when worn out.

PLIMSOLLS

Ideally for everyday wear one pair of shoes should be purchased and worn to destruction. This is not always

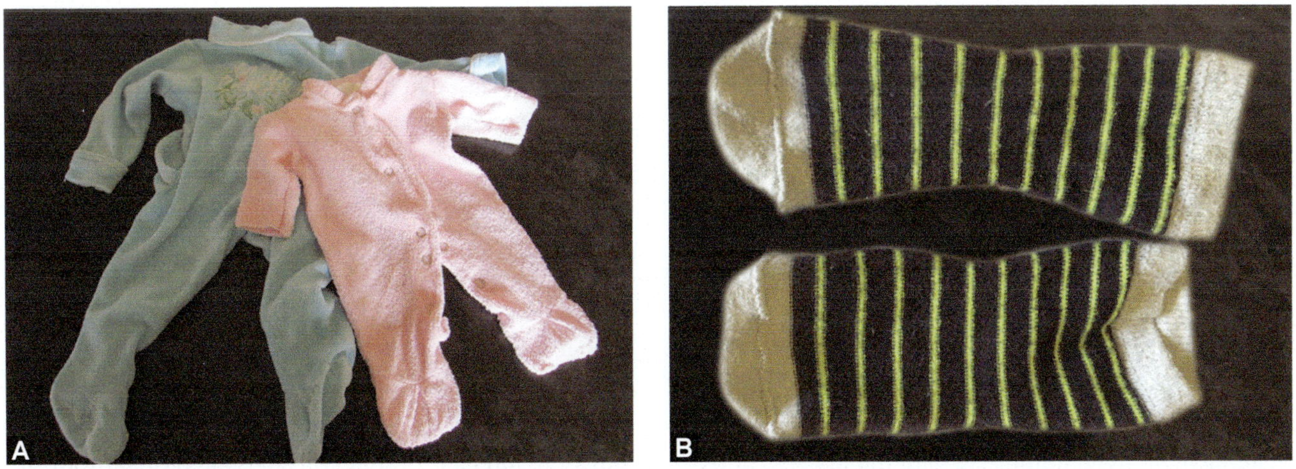

Figures 39.5A and B Babygros: (A) Sleep suits; (B) Socks.

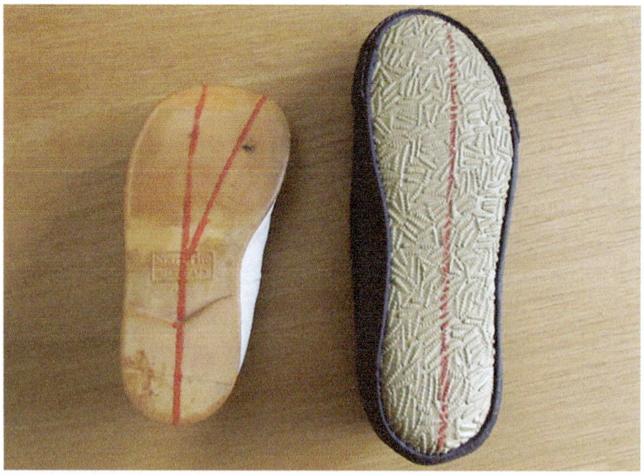

Figure 39.6 Plimsoles. Note the straight flare, indicated by the straight line through the centre of the heel and sole (right image). In the young child this line should ideally emerge in the lateral distal region of the sole allowing space in the lateral medial part of the forefoot for the relatively adducted position of the first ray (left image).

possible for children at primary school in many areas of the UK. In order to keep the schools quiet and clean, some education authorities require plimsolls to be worn in school all day. At the end of the school day the plimsolls are placed in shoe bags on a peg overnight, with the result that they do not dry out fully and are worn again the following school day. Plimsolls are excellent for the purpose for which they are intended (i.e. gymnastics), but do not provide a suitable environment for a growing foot, and this current practice should be discontinued. Furthermore, plimsolls (Fig. 39.6) do not allow for the changing flare of a young foot, and this may have a damaging influence if they are worn continually. They are also unsuitable for casted orthoses.

BABYWALKERS

These are mentioned here as they relate to the child who is on his or her feet. As mentioned previously, children walk at different ages and it is best to let nature take its course and allow the child to walk naturally when ready instead of prematurely stressing tissues and loading joints.

FASHION, PEER-GROUP PRESSURE AND ECONOMICS

It is important to recognise when managing the case of the teenager that fashion, peer-group pressure and economics play a large part in their social and emotional development and it is necessary to make compromises regarding footwear or they may be lost as cooperative patients' altogether. It is important that the podiatrist working with this age group is acquainted with footwear fashion and costs to allow them to communicate with the patients at their own level and understand and advise them accordingly.

TRAINERS

Much has been said regarding the suitability or otherwise of trainers for all ages of children. In some schools, trainers are the only footwear in evidence, particularly as peer-group pressure dictates specific manufacturers. In general terms, trainers are not a problem, so long as, like any other shoes, the criteria for an adequate shoe are followed. The one criticism of trainers particularly in the age group of puberty where the feet may be very sweaty is the high percentage of synthetic materials used, leading to a hyperhydrotic state and predisposing to verrucae, tinea-pedis and onychocryptosis.

FOOT TYPE

Foot types are many and varied, hence the necessity for children to have their footwear fitted by an experienced, competent fitter with a wide range of styles, sizes and fittings. The infant foot, when viewed from below, tends to be triangular in shape (this is particularly obvious in premature children who may also be late walkers). As the child progresses into adolescence the foot tends to become rectangular, hence the difference in shape between adult and children's footwear, the child's shoe being inflated and the adult's tending to be relatively straight-flared by comparison (Fig. 39.6, left image) The first ray also tends to be in a relatively adducted position at this age, and it is possible that a straight—flared or small shoe may cause or result in soft-tissue pathologies or digital deformity. Typical foot types include:

- *Short broad*—the foot is relatively short in relation to its length
- *Square forefoot*—all the digits are virtually the same length (commonly found in Down syndrome)

These are typically robust foot types common in boys. They can present shoe-fitting problems in girls.

The following foot-types can be classified as at risk feet and appear to be more commonly found in females.

- *Hypermobile*—this type of foot may be classified as belonging to an individual with hypermobility syndrome, but can loosely be classed as someone who has a greater than average range of joint motion in the feet
- *Long slender*—the foot is relatively narrow in relation to its length
- *Triangular*—the heel is narrower than normal in relation to the forefoot
- *Long inner border*—this speaks for itself and leaves the hallux and associated structures open to trauma

All the above foot types can appear singly or in any combination and can present considerable problems for the shoe fitter.

LOW-ARCHED AND HIGH-ARCHED FEET

Normal feet come in in all shapes sizes and it is important that feet which appear relatively highly arched or low arched due to their inherited architecture are not misdiagnosed as pathological features. There is also the possibility that certain foot types may be the inherited features of different races and cultures.

INFECTIONS

In general, unless the child has an underlying medical condition, which may make them more prone to infection or diminish their ability to combat it, this does not present as a particular problem. Infections are most commonly bacterial, fungal or viral. With the exception of tineapedis and verrucae, by far the most common paediatric foot infections dealt with by a podiatrist relate to nail pathologies, either as true onychocryptosis or paronychia. These conditions can occur in any child at any age but are most common among teenagers and children who are immunocompromised (undergoing chemotherapy) or those with lymphoedema (Turner syndrome), where there is an added risk of cellulitis. Infections from foreign bodies and broken blisters can also be a problem.

ONYCHOCRYPTOSIS (INGROWING TOENAIL)

The most common nail condition found in children is onychocryptosis, but this tends to be mainly associated with teenagers, particularly boys. However, it can occur at any age and is a particular management problem in very young children and babies who may suck their toes. Regular swabbing with 0.5% chlorhexidine in spirit helps to reduce—the incidence of infection and helps to tone periungual tissues, making them less prone to damage from trauma. Most cases resolve with a little patience.

Many older children are at risk from onychocryptosis due to intrinsic foot abnormalities. In particular, there may be involution of the toenail, hyperextension of the hallux, abduction or adduction of the hallux (often with valgus rotation) and sub-talar joint pronation. These may occur in any combination and inadequate footwear and hyperhidrosis may compound the problem.

ANATOMICAL ANOMALIES

These include anomalies of the sesamoid bones, supernumerary bones and tarsal synostoses.

Sesamoid Bones

These may be classified as additional bipartite or multipartite.

Tarsal Coalition (Peroneal Spastic Flat Foot)

In tarsal coalition there is an anomaly of ossification in which adjacent tarsal bones are fused together. Fusion may be bony or cartilaginous. The most common coalition occurs between the calcaneus and the navicular, with union across the midtarsal join. In a talocalcaneal coalition, fusion occurs between the sustentaculumtali and the talus.

Children with tarsal coalitions may never be aware that they have them. Occasionally, they have distressing painful symptoms and surgery is necessary for adequate relief. Between these two extremes are most children who have little trouble until they enter a growth spurt, when they develop the classic symptoms of the spastic flat foot. This is a painful contraction of the peroneal muscles and occurs as a protective mechanism, resulting in a fixed, everted, abducted foot. Diagnosis is not always easy. Examination reveals tender, taut and prominent peroneal tendons and attempts to invert the foot will be painfully resisted. Specialist radiographs and/or a CAT scan may be necessary to demonstrate the fusion.

Initial therapy consists of resting the foot in a below-knee plaster of Paris cast if necessary, and reserving surgery for those with recurrent or intractable pain. Long-term follow-up management with casted foot orthoses may be necessary.

BIOMECHANICAL ANOMALIES/ ABNORMALITIES

Acquired Deformity

Virtually any pathology is possible. By far the most common, whether due to footwear or as secondary features of compensation for biomechanical anomalies/abnormalities are digital deformities, including hammer toe, mallet toe, retracted toe, claw toe and hallux abductovalgus. The lesser toes may also be variously burrowed in varus positions with lateral and medial deviations at the interphalangeal joints. There may also be early periarticular thickening and limitation of motion.

Deformity at the subtalar joint due to excessive subtalar joint pronation may result in serious forefoot disruption and deformity, and should always be considered as the cause and either corrected or controlled rather than simply treating the secondary digital deformities.

Mucopolysaccharidoses

This group of disorders, classified into six types, is characterised by the widespread intracellular deposition of complex substances called mucopolysaccharides or sulphated glycosaminoglycans. They present primarily as disorders of the reticuloendothelial system or as progressive disorders with visceral and skeletal manifestations. In mucopolysaccharidosis Type 4 (Morquio syndrome), the arms are relatively long for the degree of dwarfism and may extend to the knees. Genu valgum with enlarged knee joints and flat feet are present.

Juvenile Hallux Abducto Valgus

As in many other foot problems, footwear has been universally blamed for this condition in teenagers. In almost all cases, a strong family history can be elicited, with a number of predisposing factors being inherited and given the appropriate set of circumstances, deformity develops. Footwear may aggravate an established tendency to abducto valgus deformity and may cause bunion formation by friction over the medial eminence of the metatarsal head. The abducto valgus is often accompanied by adduction of the first metatarsal. Up to 20 degree of abduction can be normal, but a useful guide to whether surgery is indicated is the position of the sesamoids on a radiograph—no subluxation, no operation. Surgery should not be carried out before the foot is skeletally mature, at about age 14 years. Until then, an orthodigital splint can control the position of the hallux.

INJURIES

Juvenile Hallux Rigidus

While not common, this condition cases much discomfort to its sufferers, who are usually teenaged males. It is now thought that the aetiology is recurrent minor trauma or a single incident, which produces a chondral injury. The resulting pain and muscle spasm results in loss of extension at the metatarsophalangeal joint. The patient walks on the outer border of the foot to avoid the painful area. Rest in a cast is the recommended first line treatment, with a proximal phalangeal osteotomy being reserved for those in whom symptoms persist. Appropriate physical therapy and padding and strapping and footwear advice is usually sufficient to effect a cure.

Lower Limbs

Examination of the musculoskeletal system should commence with observation of the infant or child. The position of the limbs and gait may give a clue to a problem that is later confirmed on more detailed clinical examination. Having inspected the lower limbs of an infant for signs of dissimilarity in the skin creases, girth, gross abnormalities such as bowing of legs and length of the limbs, a systemic examination is indicated. Discrepancy in leg length is usually due to muscle wasting or poor development. It may also be due to neurological problem, but on occasion it is the larger limb which is abnormal due to hypertrophy, lymphoedema or a malformation (*see* Chapter 1).

Polydactyly

This term denotes the presence of supernumerary digits attached either to the hand or the foot. On the foot the extra digits may develop from one metatarsal or there may be complete extra metatarsal segments (**Fig. 39.7**). Depending on the severity of the abnormality, selective amputation at an early age is indicated to ensure optimum foot function, thus facilitating shoe fitting in childhood and adult life. As in any operation on the foot, it is vital to ensure that any resulting scar is away from pressure areas.

Syndactyly (Webbed Toes–Zygodactyly)

This term is applied to a total or partial fusion of adjacent digits. It is very common, usually bilateral and often familial. Multiple syndactyly occurs in hands and feet associated with other anomalies as in Apert syndrome (an autosomal dominant disorder—acrocephalosyndactyly). No treatment is required for webbing (zygodactyly) of the toes (**Fig. 39.8**).

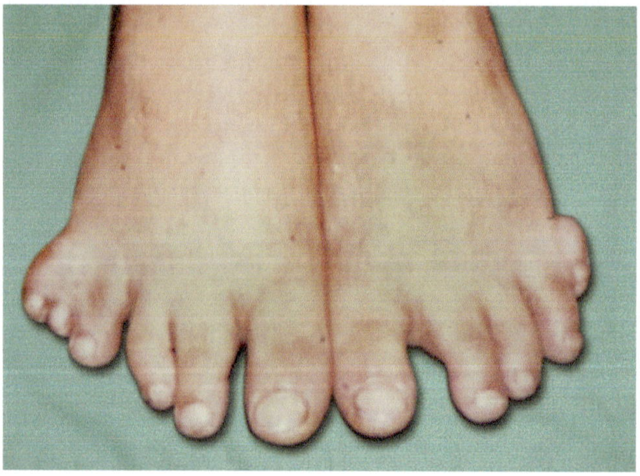

Figure 39.7 Polydactyly. Note also syndactyly affecting the second and third toes.

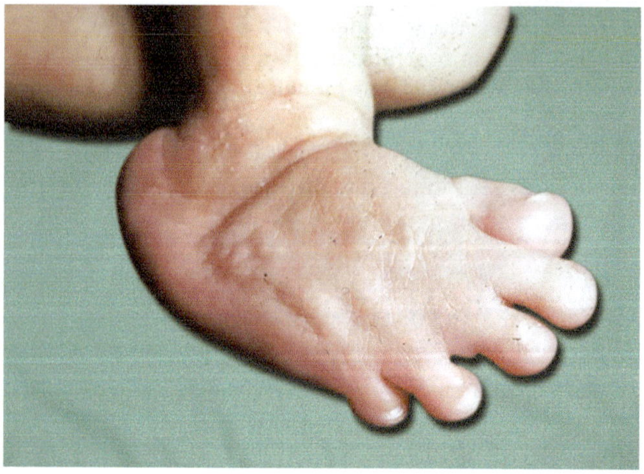

Figure 39.8 Zygodactyly.

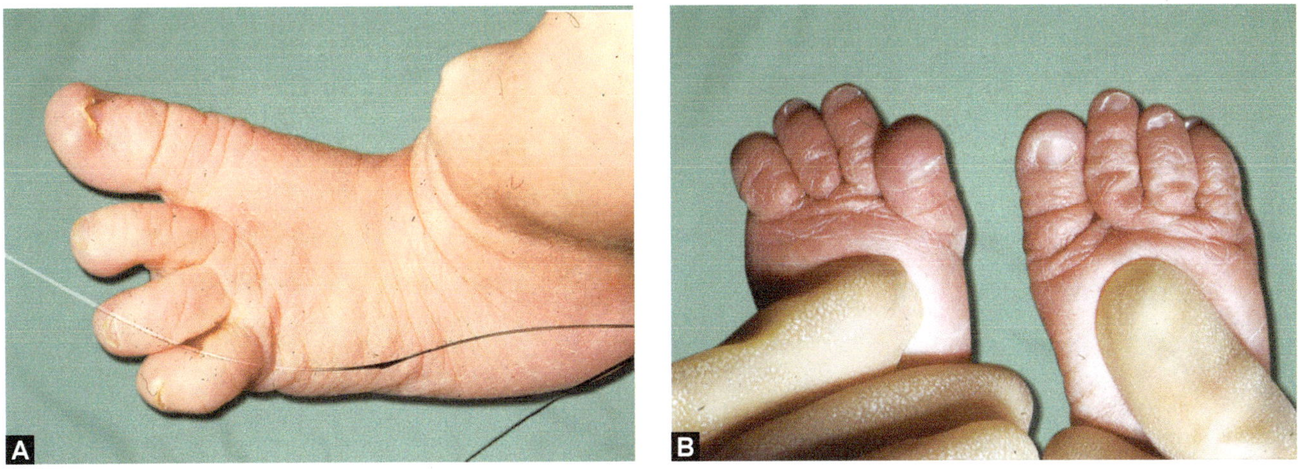

Figures 39.9A and B Oligodactyly.

Oligodactyly

This term denotes the developmental absence of one or more digits (fingers or toes) with the total absence of all parts of the digit (i.e. metatarsal parts and all phalanges) (Figs. 39.9A and B).

Congenital Overlapping Fifth Toe (Digit) Minimi Quinti Varus

In this condition, from birth the smallest toe lies on the dorsum of the base of the fourth toe in a medially deviated position. Although the degree of severity is variable, the condition may be bilateral or unilateral. This is the only common toe abnormality in childhood that requires surgical correction on most occasions in order to avoid trouble with shoe fitting. From it is important to manage this condition positively, as disruption of the other lesser digits can occur with associated skin lesions, in later life.

Curly Toes

It is normal for the fourth and fifth toes to be a little flexed and curled medially but the third toe, instead of being straight, shares this flexed and medial deformity the second toe is usually deformed such that it lies on a higher plane than the others and curls laterally, overlying the third toe. This curious pattern of deformity is very common, being either bilateral or unilateral and variable in degree, but it is seldom a cause of trouble, although tight shoes and socks should be avoided. If the degree of deformity is great the patient will often present with nail pain. However, most cases present for treatment because the parents are concerned due to the unusual appearance of the toes.

Congenital Flexed Toe

This is uncommon and may affect a single toe or two adjacent toes. On walking the affected toe takes the weight on the digital end instead of the plantar surface. If the condition is ignored, chronic nail problems due to onychauxis or onychogryphosis may arise.

Metatarsus Adductus

In this less common deformity the forefoot is deviated towards the midline in relation to the hind foot, as in clubfoot but without equinus or inversion. This is best treated as early as possible with serial, well padded, moulded plasters until the forefoot remains straight. In a small proportion surgical exploration is needed to release the tight medial tether.

Hallux Varus

While this is an extremely uncommon condition in the UK, this is not the case elsewhere, e.g. in India. Commonly seen with metatarsus adductus, frequently it corrects with growth. Occasionally surgery is necessary for the satisfactory fitting of footwear.

Congenital Talipes Equinovarus (Clubfoot)

This common deformity occurs in 2–4 of 1,000 births that is, it is about twice as common as congenital dislocation of the hip. The male is twice as often affected as the female, and in half the affected children both feet are deformed. The diagnosis is obvious on inspection, with the deformity being in three parts: the heel is drawn up, the foot inverted and the hind foot adducted (i.e. in an equinovarus position) (Fig. 39.10). In a small minority the deformity is postural and can be corrected easily by manipulation to neutral and beyond. Repeated manipulation is sufficient treatment. The clubfoot deformities are also found in conditions such as arthrogryposis, trisomy 18 and spina bifida cystica. For treatment of congenital talipes (*see* Chapter 18).

Talipes Calcaneovalgus

The name implies this is exactly the opposite deformity to clubfoot. It is usually the result of in utero posture, in that the foot has been caught in an upturned position with

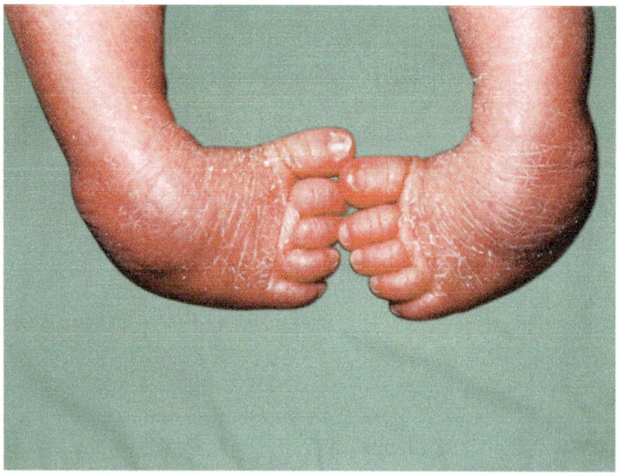

Figure 39.10 Bilateral talipes equinovarus.

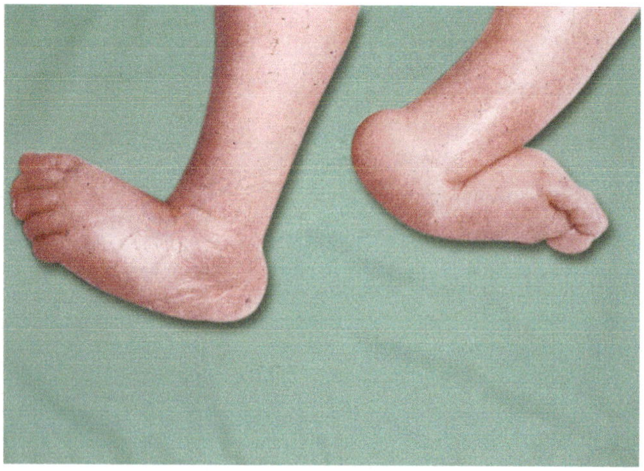

Figure 39.11 Rocker-bottom feet in trisomy 18 syndrome.

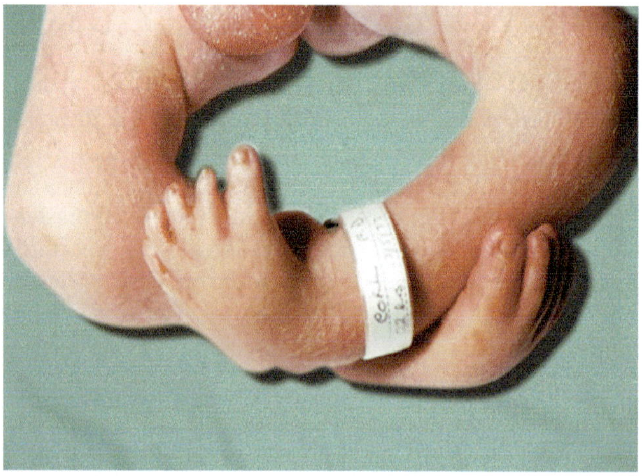

Figure 39.12 Arthrogryposis multiplex congenita.

the sole against the uterine wall. The prognosis is excellent, as natural improvement occurs with active movements on release from the uterus. All that is needed is for the mother to manipulate the foot into equinovarus frequently and the deformity resolves permanently within a few weeks. It is important however, to recognise that this condition is associated in a few with congenital dislocation of the hip and deformity of the tibia.

Vertical Talus (Rocker-bottom Foot)

This is a rare deformity known by several alternative names such as rocker-bottom foot and is primarily caused by a dislocation of the talonavicular joint (Fig. 39.11). It occurs in 10–50% of the trisomy 18 syndrome. Foot orthoses may be required to maintain foot posture.

Onychogryphosis

Often thought of as an acquired complaint of the elderly, this condition can be congenital—affecting any toe or toes, but usually the first or fifth. It is easily managed conservatively, with the parent/patient being taught how to care for the nails. If the shape of the nail causes trouble and cannot be made tolerable by cutting or filing, radical removal of the nail with phenolisation is indicated.

Arthrogryposis Multiplex Congenita

This name is used for a congenital condition affecting the joints, which may be localised or generalised. The joints may be either extended or flexed but more often the former, with a severe degree of talipes being present. The muscles are atrophic and fibrous and the skin is tight so that the limbs resemble hosepipes. Arthroplasty has always failed to provide useful movement and the only treatment is to stabilise the affected joints in a good position (Fig. 39.12).

Congenital Constriction Band Syndrome

This may result in the congenital absence of toes. The condition occurs in utero, possibly due to floating strands in the amnion wrapping around the affected joint. This can result in amputation of the part if it occurs in early foetal life. Congenital constriction band syndrome presents as ring-like concentric bands, which may be deep or shallow. Deep bands affect lymphatic and venous drainage, resulting in oedema that causes the distal portion to enlarge.

Leg-length Discrepancy

It is important to realise that up to 1 cm difference in true length is considered a normal variation. Also, apparent discrepancy exists where limbs are actually the same length, but because of the alignment of one or the other are functionally different. The effects of leg length discrepancy are either to cause a compensatory pelvic tilt and secondary spinal scoliosis or to make the child walk

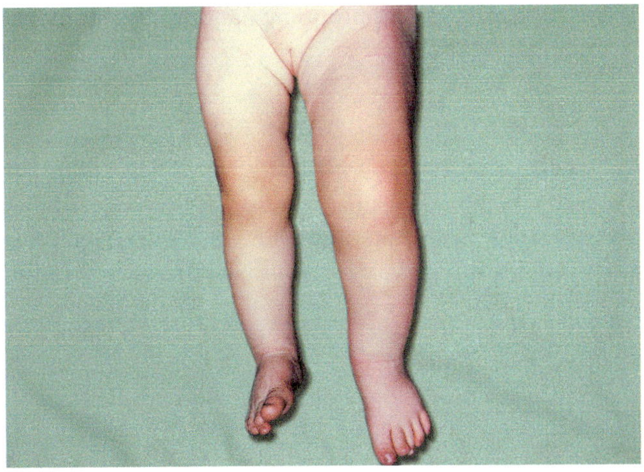

Figure 39.13 Hemihypertrophy of the left leg and foot associated with lymphangioma (local gigantism). Note also curly toe syndrome particularly affecting second and third toes.

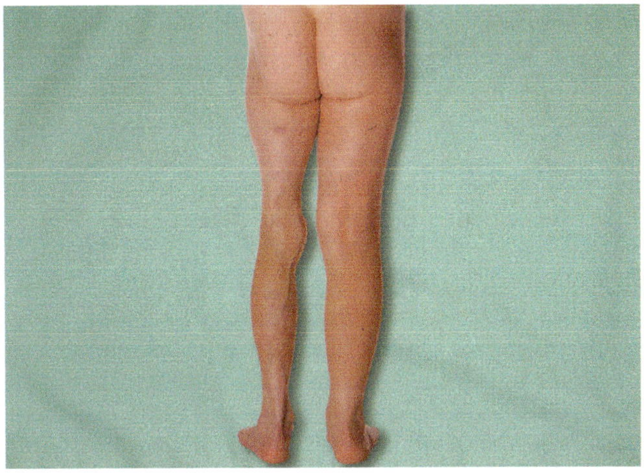

Figure 39.14 Linear scleroderma affecting the left leg.

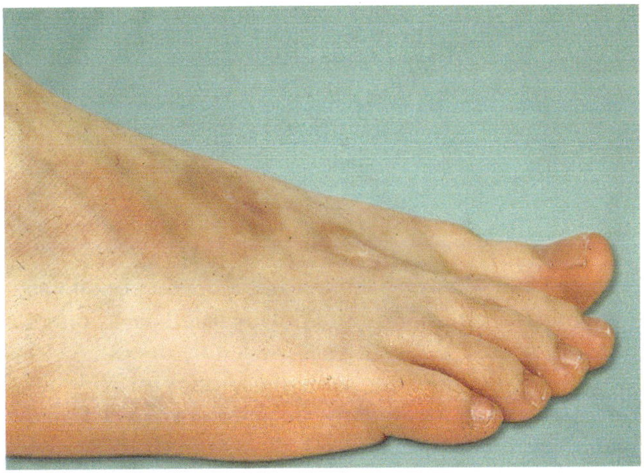

Figure 39.15 Morphea legion of the right foot.

on the toes in order to effectively lengthen the leg. The latter response will, in time result in adaptive shortening of the Achilles tendon.

The importance of these clinical situations is that they impose abnormal stresses on the foot, particularly on the talus. These stresses in turn may lead to changes in the function and structure of the foot with growth and it is these that are important for the child.

Leg length discrepancy may develop due to a variety of causes. In all but rare events, such as arteriovenous malformation (in which the leg overgrows) or occasionally following acute osteitis the short leg is the pathological one. Shortening may be due to malunion of a fracture but this is not a progressive shortening as occurs when epiphyseal growth plates are damaged by trauma or infection. A flaccid (as opposed to spastic) paralysis deprives a limb of the growth stimulus of muscle contraction, and poliomyelitis has in the past given rise to severe leg length discrepancy. A length discrepancy of less than 3 cm can be dealt with simply by an appropriate shoe or heel raise, but greater deficiencies may be:

- Shortening of the longer leg
- Retarding growth in the longer leg by destroying or stapling the epiphyseal plates above and below the knee
- Lengthening the short leg usually in the tibial segments, although this requires attention to avoid complications.

Hemihypertrophy ranges from enlargement of a single digit to enlargement of one half of the bod. Some cases of limb hypertrophy are associated with widespread haemangioma or lymphangioma (**Fig. 39.13**).

Linear Scleroderma

Linear scleroderma occurs as a linear band of hypopigmentation and sclerosis. The legs are most commonly involved and usually in a unilateral distribution (**Fig. 39.14**). Growth failure may develop in patients with linear scleroderma, affecting a limb because of atrophy of muscle and skin, which in turn affects bone development. Some children may have combined forms, with linear scleroderma on an extremity and morphea on the trunk (*see* Chapter 12).

Localised Scleroderma (Morphea)

Localised scleroderma is much more common than systemic progressive sclerosis. Morphea usually begins as a circumscribed patch of skin induration, typically on the trunk, feet or other parts of the body. At onset, the skin is oedematous and warm and has a characteristic violaceous border with an ivory centre. As the skin becomes tight and hard over a joint range of motion may be limited (**Fig. 39.15**).

Pes Cavus

There is wide variation in the height of the arch of the foot, but when this is seen to be marked and unilateral it must be regarded as pathological. The affected leg is often a little thinner and short and with the raised arch the foot is often smaller. This condition develops in the early years and it is probable that all cases have a neurological cause, mostly due to minor anomalies of the cord in the lumbosacral region. As occasion may justify investigation by myelography, MRI or direct surgical exploration will demonstrate a lesion such as an intraspinallipoma or angioma. In Friedreich ataxia the characteristic is that of pes cavus associated with hammer toes and also scoliosis. Attention should be directed to the foot deformity, tackling whichever feature is most troublesome.

Sever Disease (Calcaneal Apophysitis)

In many ways this disease is similar to Osgood-Schlatter disease of the tibial tubercle. The condition troubles children in the age group 10–14 years, with pain at the point of the heel, usually worse during or after atheletics. The calcaneal apophysis is tender as the heel strikes the ground, and even on tiptoes is painful due to the pull of the insertion of the Achilles tendon. In half of the children the condition may be bilateral. The diagnosis depends on the history and finding tenderness about the point of the heel. Radiographs are normal. In very active children who are actively growing it is not uncommon to encounter Sever disease, Osgood-Schlatter disease and pain at the insertion of the plantar fascia to the medial plantar tubercle of the calxaneum occurring concomitantly in the same child. This should be treated with rest and appropriate orthoses.

Kohler Disease of the Navicular

An osteochondritis, similar to Perthe disease of the hip, Kohler disease affects the navicular bone, causing vague pain about the midfoot, and locally the part may be tender. Radiographic findings show changes of increased density and collapse of the navicular bone. With minimal treatment, with temporary supportive padding and strapping or casted supportive foot orthoses the symptoms will disappear and the radiographic appearances will become normal in 1–2 years.

Freiberg Disease

In the capital epiphysis of the second (occasionally the third) metatarsal, osteochondritic change similar to Perthe disease may occur, with the head of the bone becoming enlarged and tender. Radiographs show an irregular increase in density and flattening of the front of the head. This may end up with a large square shaped metatarsal head, which later in life may need excision, but in childhood no specific treatment is needed as symptoms disappear with rest. However, it is often prudent to protect the area with appropriate padding and strapping as circumstances dictate.

Stress Fracture of a Metatarsal (March or Fatigue Fracture)

As occurs in the upper tibia an increase in physical activity may stress a metatarsal (usually the second) and produce an undisplacedself-healing fracture. Local pain, tenderness and swelling will be found, with radiographic changes similar to those seen in the tibia. Moderate rest with supportive padding and strapping for a few weeks will result in cure. Some children may require a walking plaster.

> **KEY LEARNING POINTS**
>
> Children with diabetes do not require any specialist podiatric care different from that given to other children, as long as their diabetes stays well controlled and they are free from acquired foot infection such as onychocryptosis. However, diabetic children should be screened by a podiatrist at yearly intervals in order to detect and manage any digital deformities or biomechanical disorders that may be present and thus reduce the risk of potential pressure lesions that may occur in adult life.

Poliomyelitis

As a result of the introduction of the live oral polio vaccine used for immunisation, only isolated cases of polio are now seen. The disorder is caused by the polio virus, which spreads from the alimentary tract to the central nervous system, particularly the anterior horn cells of the spinal cord. The effects of the disease in the lower limb are seen in the muscles with weakness of inversion, eversion, plantar flexion of the ankle and also foot drop. Each child's problems are individual. Polio is associated with contracture of muscles causing an equinovarus deformity, pes cavus or permanent foot drop. These children may require special orthoses and footwear (*see* Chapters 14 and 21).

Spina Bifida Cystica

This is a congenital disorder in which there has been a failure of the posterior spinal elements. The level in the spine at which the, lesion occurs relates in some measure to the effects on the child, but does not equate with their function. Problems arise in the foot in those with sacral lesions, where an imbalance primarily affects the muscles of the foot **(Fig. 39.16)**.

In the legs, the sensory loss may be extensive, depending on the degree of nerve root or spinal cord damage. The motor dysfunction is largely due to root damage giving flaccid paralysis, but areas of spasticity may be present due to higher cord damage with intact lower cord segments and lower motor neuron function, together with

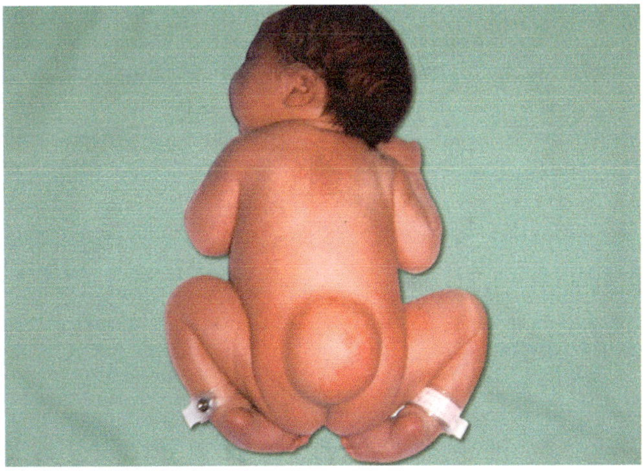

Figure 39.16 Spina bifida cystica. Note the bilateral talipes equinovarus.

a potential to develop severe deformity. Some problems are reasonably predictable: e.g. a common level of lesion about L 4 will leave the roots of the femoral and obturator nerves largely intact while the sciatic nerve will be paralysed. As a result the hip, subject to the pull of flexors and adductors but with no extensor or abductor muscle function, will dislocate. At a lower level active quadriceps unopposed by paralysed hamstrings will produce recurvatum of the knee. The foot may be deformed in any direction, and the loss of the normal weight distribution on the sole of the foot will readily lead to trophic ulceration in the anaesthetic foot. Children with spina bifida should be monitored regularly by a podiatrist and treated or advised as circumstances dictate (*see* Chapter 18).

Cerebral Palsy

The term cerebral palsy is used to denote a disorder of movement and posture resulting from a permanent, non-progressive defect or lesion of the brain. The spastic group shows the features of lesions of the pyramidal tracts, such as muscle spasm resulting in spastic postures of the limb. The most common is spastic tetraplegia, in which all four limbs are involved. The group is subdivided into types 1 and 2. In the common type 1 spastic tetraplegia the legs are more severely involved than the arms. In the much less common type 2 spastic tetraplegia the spasticity is extremely severe in all four limbs, so that the contractures develop early and disuse muscle atrophy may be masked. For the podiatrist, foot care may become a primary treatment.

Muscular Dystrophies

The muscular dystrophies are a group of genetically determined disorders with a common denominator of a progressive degenerative process in the skeletal muscles. Many of these children later develop foot problems and may require help from a podiatrist.

Childhood Obesity

Childhood obesity is a global concern with significant health burden. Key comorbidities secondary to childhood obesity are known to affect cardiovascular, endocrine, and respiratory systems but the impact of childhood obesity of the developing musculoskeletal system is equally important. Healthy development of the musculoskeletal system throughout childhood is important for longer term health, well-being and maintaining mobility.

Excessive body mass can impact on the musculoskeletal system, where excessive loads and joint demand can predispose to increased tissue stress, tissue dysfunction, joint dysfunction and onset of foot and lower limb pathology. Understanding the precise mechanisms of pathology are yet to be elucidated but there is an increasing awareness of the broad range of musculoskeletal pathologies secondary to childhood obesity. These include:

- Hip joint problems such as slipped capital femoral epiphysis.
- Knee joint problems such as Blount disease (tibial varum) and other structural alignment problems
- Foot joint problems such as structural changes (e.g. pes planus) and diffuse foot and ankle pain secondary to excessive loading.

Musculoskeletal problems in obese children are known to impact on health-related quality of life but the longer term complications are yet to be determined. The prevalence of MSK complications in adults is high and therefore the long-term economic and health burden associated with childhood obesity is likely to be considerable. It remains important that children are encouraged to lead healthy, active lives in order to support the healthy development of the musculoskeletal structures of the foot and lower limb. The role of the podiatrist in the multi-disciplinary care of the obese child should not be overlooked.

Duchenne Muscular Dystrophy

Duchenne muscular dystrophy is rare. The condition is due to a sex linked recessive gene with a high-mutation rate (*see* Fig. 14.51).

Hypermobility Syndrome

Generalised joint laxity is a feature of the hereditary connective tissue disorders such as Marfan syndrome, Ehlers-Danlos syndrome and osteogenesis imperfect. A child is considered hypermobile if he or she can perform two of the following three manoeuvres:

- Passive opposition of both thumbs to the volar aspect of the forearms.
- Passive hyperextension of the fingers so they lie parallel to the extensor aspect of both forearms.
- Active hyperextension of both elbows beyond 180 degree.

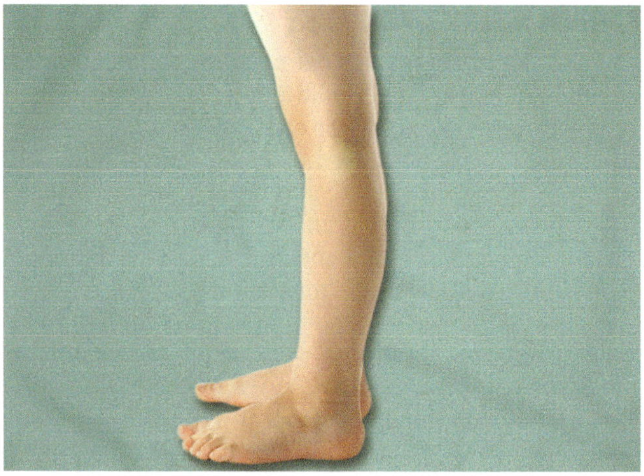

Figure 39.17 Hypermobile knees in hypermobility syndrome.

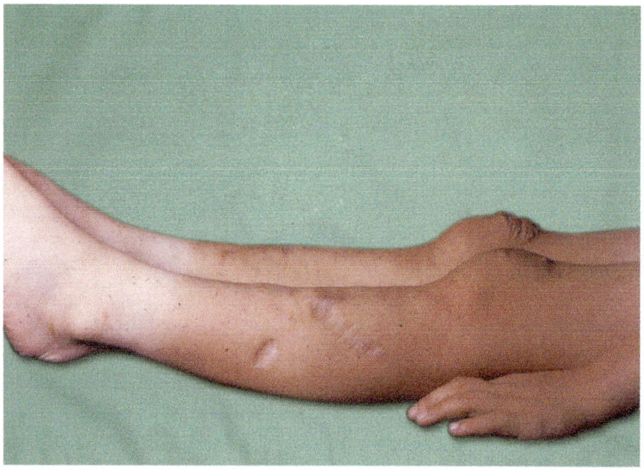

Figure 39.18 Ehlers–Danlos syndrome. Note genu recurvatum and "tissue paper" scarring.

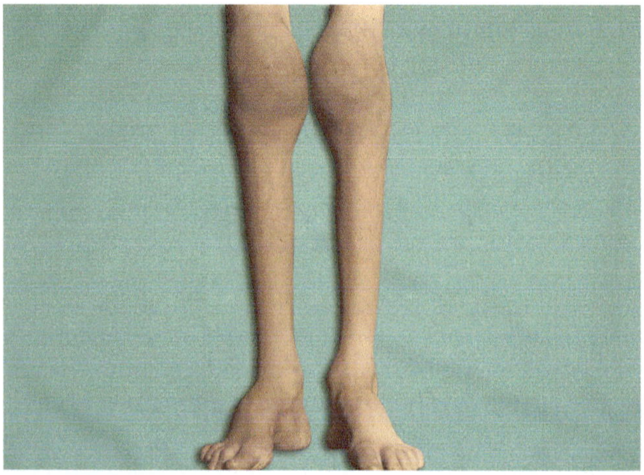

Figure 39.19 Juvenile idiopathic arthritis (Oligoarticular). Note the swollen knees and ankles.

Hyperactivity is relatively common in the general population. The term hypermobility syndrome has been coined to define a clinical situation in which there is general joint laxity associated with musculoskeletal complaints. I young children this syndrome is observed equally in both sexes, but towards puberty it predominates in girls. The knees are the most frequent sites of complaint but occasionally the ankles may also be affected. The discomfort usually comes after exercise.

The whole clinical picture is consistent with an episode of traumatic synovitis. There is a strong familial tendency to this syndrome and the diagnosis is therefore essentially clinical combined with an awareness of family history. The management is largely reassurance as to the absence of serious disease, and activity, which precipitates symptoms, should be avoided if possible **(Fig. 39.17)** (*see* Chapter 12).

Ehlers–Danlos syndrome

The disorder is familial and autosomal dominant. The child tends to be slim and underheight, and may have kyphoscoliosis. The hyper extensible joints allow abnormal postures. Genu recurvatum **(Fig. 39.18)** and pes planus are common. No specific treatment is available but all foot deformity should be managed as a matter of urgency. Wounds will be slow to heal and will exhibit tissue paper scarring.

Limb pain of childhood with no organic disease (idiopathic limb pains) (*see* Chapter 12).

Juvenile Idiopathic Arthritis

Subtypes of Juvenile Idiopathic Arthritis

The following juvenile idiopathic arthritis subtypes are included in the latest classification:

- Oligoarthritis—Involvement of up to four joints (usually large ones) **(Fig. 39.19)**.
- Extended oligoarthritis—Extension to five or more joints after 6 months from presentation.
- Polyarthritis, rheumatoid factor (RF) negative—Five or more joints (large or small) involved at presentation.
- Polyarthritis, RF positive—Paediatric equivalent of adult RA.
- Psoriatic arthritis—Other features of psoriasis or first degree relative with psoriasis **(Fig. 39.20)**.
- Systemic onset arthritis—Fever and rash at presentation, arthritis starting later.
- Enthesitis related arthritis (ERA)—Human leukocyte antigen (HLA) B27 positive paediatric equivalent of adult ankylosing spondylitis.
- Other chronic arthritides including arthritis in Down syndrome and other chromosomal abnormalities and inflammatory bowel disease.

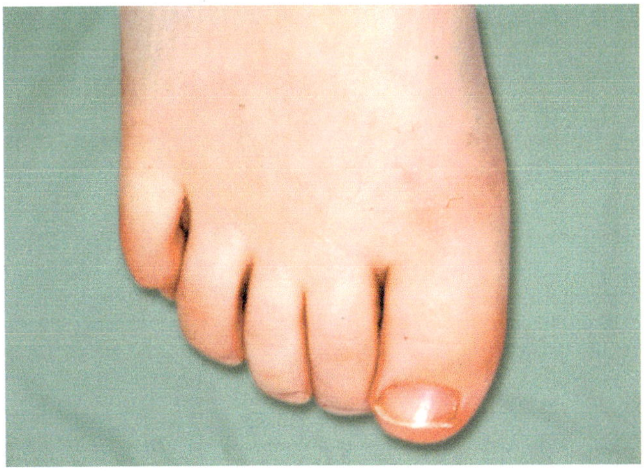

Figure 39.20 Juvenile psoriatic arthritis showing "sausage digit dactylitia".

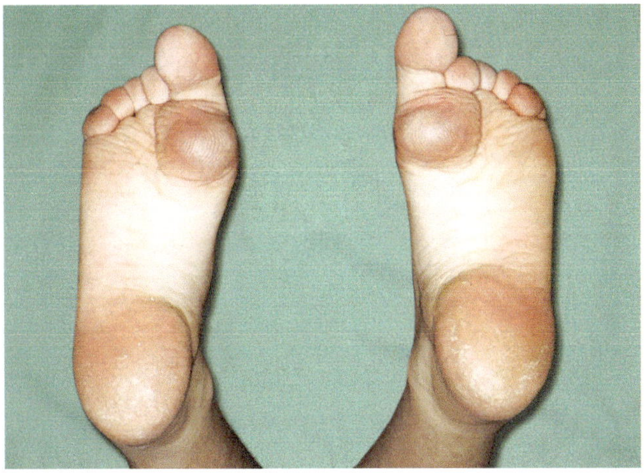

Figure 39.21 Juvenile idiopathic arthritis soles. Note bursitis under first metatarsal head.

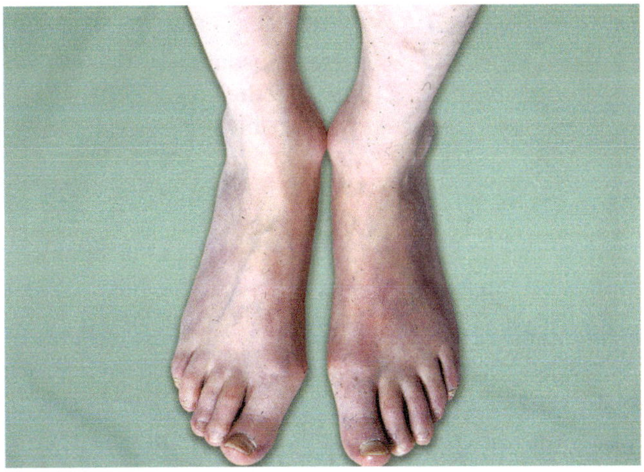

Figure 39.22 Feet of a boy with Raynaud phenomenon.

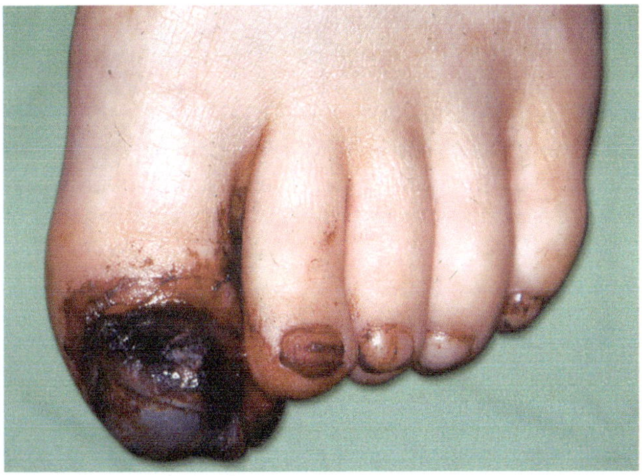

Figure 39.23 A child with haemophilia showing haemorrhage in the first digit of the left foot.

The management of the foot problems depends not only on medical treatment of the arthritis but also on local application of specific measures to the damaged foot. The painful digits respond well to silicone digital devices in the acute phase and also as maintenance therapy. Fortunately there have been great advances in the prescription of orthoses, involving the development of new materials with appropriate properties and their use inn individual patients for each specific abnormality (Fig. 39.21).

Raynaud Phenomenon

The digits become cold, numb and painful. Local hypoxia leads to cyanosis, resulting in a bluish colour. Feet especially toes should be carefully monitored, particularly through the autumn and winter months with prevention and early management of problems being a high priority (Fig. 39.22).

Haemophilia

Joint swelling and pain often heraldshaemarthrosis which is the single most incapacitating event in the life of a severe haemophiliac. Where there is joint deformity in the foot either as a result of bleeding or from some intrinsic primary cause it is important that appropriate orthotic management is instigated at an early stage in order to limit damage and encourage normal function (Fig. 39.23) (*see* Chapter 11).

Turner syndrome

Foot problems such as lymphoedema of the lower limb secondary to poor lymphatic drayage and nail dysplasia are well recognised as valuable diagnostic features in Turner syndrome. Affected girls are at increased risk of ingrowing toenails compared to the general population, and this is due to a number of factors in combination.

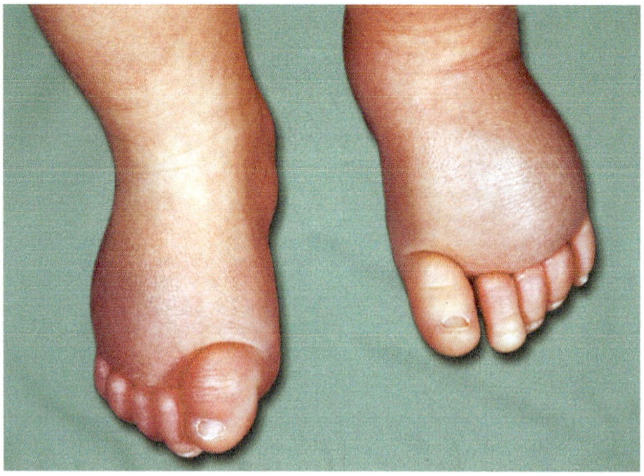

Figure 39.24 Lymphoedema of feet associated with Turner syndrome.

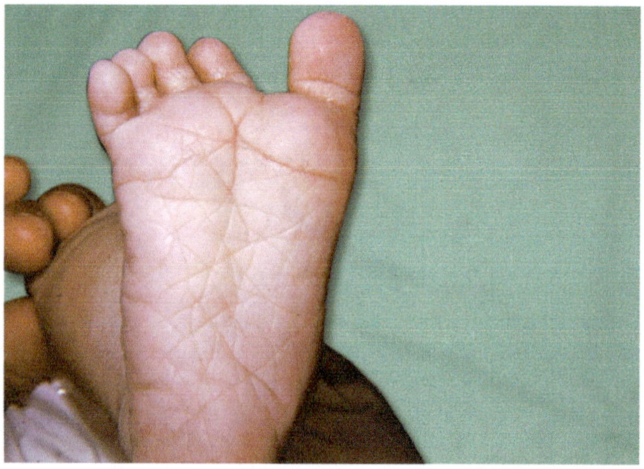

Figure 39.25 Foot in Down syndrome. Note the widely spaced first and second toes ("sandal sign").

Typically the girls have short, broad feet with hyperextension of the great toe, involuted toenails and oedematous periungual tissues, accompanied by subtalar joint pronation resulting in damage to the nail plate and surrounding soft tissue. Due to the poor lymphatic drainage girls with Turner syndrome are at increased risk of cellulitis and thus all cases must be treated diligently and as a matter of urgency **(Fig. 39.24)**.

Down syndrome

Children with Down syndrome may have a number of pedal anomalies, including hypermobility with an adducted first ray and severe pesplano valgus compounded by genu valgum and in some cases they may be overweight The first and second fingers and/or toes may be widely spaced **(Fig. 39.25)**.

Tuberous Sclerosis

See Chapter 14.

Dermatological Conditions

See Chapter 10.

Examination and Assessment

Children's feet are constantly being subjected to developmental change due to both intrinsic factors within the foot due to growth and extrinsic factors within the lower limb and skeleton in general associated with growth and torsional change within the long bones and postural change within the body generally. A child's psychological makeup, expectations, perceptions and behaviour are also different from those of an adult and these factors have to be taken into consideration during the examination. A relaxed happy and cooperative child is quickly and easily examined. The podiatrist should provide a relaxed stress free atmosphere and be wary of causing anxiety or distress by words or actions.

KEY LEARNING POINT

Children should not be treated as mini-adults and their feet should not be treated as miniature versions of adult feet.

It is recommended that the following examination methodology be employed:

- Relaxed stress free atmosphere
- Observe gait and posture with footwear
- Subjective questioning of child and/or parent
- Measure feet and measure footwear
- Examine footwear
- Visual examination of foot for skin, nail, soft tissue and bony lesions
- Physical examination of lesions as required
- Physical examination of the range, quality and direction of motion inn all joints of the foot
- Determine foot type
- Biomechanical assessment for forefoot/rear foot malalignment
- Observe and assess barefooted gait and general posture
- Compare barefooted gait and general posture with foot posture and general findings comparing right with left
- Make a firm diagnosis
- Produce a management plan
- Written information.

This methodology is designed to highlight any lower limb pathology or developmental change/anomaly that may be present, which can then be investigated and managed further by the podiatrist or referred to the appropriate specialist.

Observe Gait and Posture with Footwear

This is easily observed when the practitioner accompanies the child from the waiting room. It may be the only opportunity to observe the child when they are not aware that they are being watched. If the child is brought to you this opportunity is lost, and you may not obtain a true picture of the gait and posture. Children have a habit of demonstrating a Ministry of Silly Walks type of gait when they are requested to walk or will walk only when holding a parent's hand—which with a small child causes the hand to be held high in the air with associated changes to their posture and pattern of gait. This may falsely produce or mask features. Very young children tend to be inconsistent regarding posture and gait as they do not have an established body image and are constantly experimenting. Furthermore, developmental change produces constant yet subtle changes in the skeleton for which the child must make allowances to maintain equilibrium.

Subjective Questioning of Child and/or Parent(s)

This should be done in such a manner that the important facts are obtained without setting a false trail by putting words in the mouth of the child who may be happy to agree in order to please. It is always important to communicate with children and include them in any discussion. This may be difficult with some overbearing parents or an overly nervous or precocious child.

Measure Feet and Footwear

The feet and footwear should be measured on compatible gauges in order to determine their relationship. The use of a foot measuring board affords the opportunity to assess asymmetry of length, width, and girth as well as any other noticeably different features between the two feet against a linear background. The footboard also provides hard evidence which can be recorded and charted.

Examine Footwear

This should take into account the degree and pattern of wear and should include the heel, sole and combined heel and sole wear. Deformities of the uppers are usually due to deformity of the hallux or lesser toes. It is not unusual for children within one family to share footwear, and as a result it is not uncommon to find a child with normal feet wearing footwear suggesting gross deformity or vice versa.

Children suffering from neuromuscular disease almost always show abnormal wear and this is widely variable according to the muscle groups affected and the effect upon the general posture and gait. As with all children with abnormal wear on the shoes these wear marks should always be recorded and charted as they can be an early indicator of deterioration and thus allow for early intervention.

Visual Examination of Foot for Skin, Nail, Soft Tissue and Bony Lesions

It may be that the presence of these lesions is due to inadequate footwear, intrinsic or extrinsic structural abnormality or both. It is not unusual to find multiple pressure marks that the child has no concern about. Bursae and bursitis are also common at the posterior aspect of the heel, the dorsum of the interphalangeal joints of the toes and the medial and lateral aspects of the first and fifth metatarsophalangeal joints, respectively. It is not unusual to find babies with ingrowing toe nails. Where there is sensory impairment and/or abnormality of function either intrinsic or extrinsic or both, there is the possibility of any form of lesion and ulceration.

Physical Examination of Lesions as Required

Physical examination of range, quality and direction of motion in all joints of the foot.

This is a skilled assessment requiring considerable experience. All joints, including the ankle, subtalar, midtarsal, metatarsophalangeal and interphalangeal joints should be examined for range, quality and direction of motion, comparing right with left. In children there should be a considerable range of motion free from crepitus, pain or restriction. In children with juvenile idiopathic arthritis or neuromuscular conditions particular attention should be paid to the range of motion at the subtalar and ankle joints. In children with systemic disease or following trauma, great care should be taken during this part of the examination, as the affected joints may be exquisitely painful to even the slightest movement. The range of motion or deformity (e.g. hallux abducto valgus) in problem joints should be recorded using a goniometer for charting and comparison at a later date once treatment has been instigated. Young children may not be cooperative and it may be possible only to obtain an impression of any abnormality that may be present. The various foot types discussed earlier in this chapter should be determined.

Biomechanical Assessment, Including Examination for Forefoot/Rear Foot malalignment

Biomechanical assessment can be very difficult in the young child for a variety of reasons. This has been discussed previously but as accurate an assessment as possible should be carried out including examination for forefoot to rear foot malalingment.

BOX 39.2 A typical example of written information.

Footwear advice

Footwear that is too large, too small or does not fit properly can cause lifelong foot problems, which are often easily avoided by following a few simple pieces of advice. The following advice details the main features to look for when purchasing footwear.

Always have both feet measured for length and width
Never buy footwear in shops where you are refused foot measuring
Unless absolutely necessary, it is best to avoid slip-on shoes. Shoes should be held on the foot with laces, straps or Velcro
The heel height should be low and the heel should have a broad base
Leather materials are best for the uppers. Synthetic materials (e.g. nylon, plastic, rubber) can cause the foot to sweat, which may increase the likelihood of contracting athlete's foot or verrucae
The shape of the toe box of the shoe should allow the toes to move freely and not be squashed from the top or the sides
The shoes should fit exactly around the heel, without being loose or tight
Fashion shoes are OK for special occasions but a sensible, properly fitted shoe should be worn for regular every day wear
Remember that socks and tights that are too small can cause similar problems to shoes that are too small, particularly in very young children

Observe and Assess Barefoot Gait and General Posture

This part of the examination relies heavily on experience and a quick eye. As a general convention, it is usually better to ignore the feet initially as it is best to obtain an impression of the skeleton in general before considering the effect on the foot, or vice versa. The feet and legs are interdependent—neither should be considered in isolation. A long well lit corridor is ideal for this purpose. If the child is uncooperative a play area or physiotherapy gymnasium is ideal where the child can be left to play while the podiatrist sits in a corner and observes. The following factors should be considered when observing gait and posture in children.

- Head—size, shape, symmetry, facial expression
- Shoulders—level, position
- Spine—kyphosis, lordosis, scoliosis, kyphoscoliosis
- Pelvis—anteroposterior tilting, posteroanterior tilting, lateral tilting, rotation, asymmetry
- Hips—level
- Femur—bowing, internal torsion, external torsion
- Knee—position of patella (inward, forward, outward facing), genu valgum, genu varum, genu recurvatum
- Tibia—internal torsion, external torsion, bowing
- Foot-internal—toeing, out-toeing, calcaneal deviation, (excessive) subtalar joint pronation, forefoot deformity.

Comparison

Compare the barefooted gait and general posture with the foot posture and general findings, comparing right with left.

Diagnosis

Make a firm diagnosis and record measurements for comparison at a later date. Discuss your findings, treatment options and the potential outcomes with the parents or carers, and obtain informed consent to progress with the child's management.

Produce a Management Plan

Decide whether to treat (there and then, or at a later date, monitor or refer).

Written Information

Provide written literature, which the patient May take home and study at their leisure, concerning the complaint and associated management (Box 39.2).

Management

Many children with foot pathologies are treated in a relatively ad hoc fashion, with little apparent logic to the management. In order to overcome this, a logical approach is required. Having made a diagnosis, obtained informed consent and formulated a management plan, all children should be managed similarly, utilising a standard convention. This simply involves footwear, exercises and orthoses (Flow chart 39.1).

Footwear Advice and Prescription

There is little point in attempting to manage a structural foot condition until suitable footwear and hosiery have

Flow chart 39.1 Paediatric podiatry management methodology.

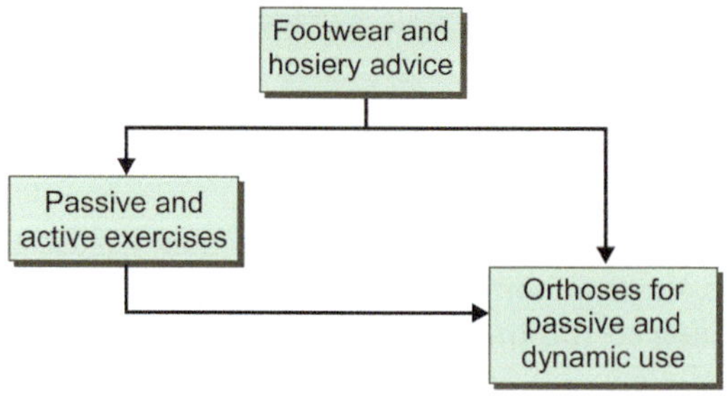

been obtained or provided. This is equally true for most foot conditions. Often children with a disability are overshod with clumpy, unsuitable and socially unacceptable prescription footwear, which is often unnecessary, and off-the- peg shoes should always be considered where possible. Currently, the available range of trainers is so vast and diverse that, unless the deformity is gross or particularly difficult to manage, it should be possible to find a suitable trainer. This not only improves the podiatric management, providing a suitable vehicle for an orthosis, but it also enhances the child's psychological well-being.

Footwear is such an important issue in podiatric management of the paediatric patient that, until it is resolved, treatment normally cannot continue. Most hospital orthotic departments supply footwear but this is sometimes limited and directed more towards the use of rigid ankle/foot orthoses. Footwear for more dynamic podiatric use may have to be found elsewhere. As alluded to previously there are many excellent trainers on the market in both shoe and boot form which provide excellent support for the hind foot and can almost be regarded as a treatment in themselves with regard to controlling the subtalar joint.

Passive and Active Exercises

Once appropriate footwear has been obtained or while attempting to resolve the footwear issue, both passive and active exercises may be prescribed, depending upon need. Passive exercises will help to stretch tightened tissues and mobilise joints and, if necessary, can be complemented by active exercises. Typical examples where this can be employed are digital deformities, shortening of Achilles tendon, and where there is active disease within the foot, such as the effect of juvenile idiopathic arthritis upon the subtalar joint resulting in rigid or semi mobile eversion. Generally this management incorporated with active exercises to re-educate and balance muscle groups are best undertaken by a physiotherapist who can advise the parents on home treatment. This should be incorporated as part of the multidisciplinary approach to care, allowing the podiatrist to concentrate on orthotic management.

Hydrotherapy and physical therapy therapies may also be employed at this stage, but it must always be remembered that the foot is still growing and therefore still possesses epiphyseal plates, which may become damaged, particularly in the very young child.

> **KEY LEARNING POINT**
>
> **Management**
>
> The use of ultrasound therapy is usually contraindicated.

One of the most common reasons for referral is digital abnormalities. Most children under 8 years old find this exercise very difficult, if not impossible. However, it is easy to teach as the child can learn the exercise with their hand initially and then transpose it to their feet. Children showing early stages of hallux abducto valgus can mobilise the joint utilising a passive circumduction exercise to the first metatarsophalangeal joint while maintaining traction on the joint. Active adduction exercises for the hallux can also be employed in an attempt to maintain or correct the position of the hallux.

Orthoses for Passive and Dynamic Use

Night Splints

Orthoses for passive use help to maintain correction of deformity obtained dynamically during walking. This may simply be an additional silicone digital device to maintain correction in bed or night splint to maintain ankle joint extension at 90 degree where there is tightening of the Achilles tendon.

Night splints for the management of hallux abductovalgus have been used for many years, often as the only means of correction, with no exercise therapy or orthotic management of the foot. However, it is suggested that early intervention and a positive approach will provide a better long-term result, and should an osteotomy be required at later date, after bony maturity the first metatarsophalangeal joint will have been protected from excessive damage providing a better long-term outcome.

Silicone

The dynamic use of orthotics is provided in its endless applications for digital management and should normally be reviewed at 6-weekly intervals when actively correcting deformity. When treating very young children great care should be taken in patient selection and parental advice, as choking may occur if the child puts the device in his or her mouth after removing shoes or hosiery.

When managing hallux abducto valgus the use of an interdigital wedge in the first interspace should be avoided as the device tends to act as an extra digit, pushing the other lesser digits laterally and has little or no effect on the hallux. This condition is best managed with a two to four combined prop to splint the hallux against the lesser toes and thus promote correction.

Casted Foot Orthoses

The use of casted foot orthoses forms the mainstay of podiatric orthotic management in children. The type of device and when to use it must be the decision of the practitioner according to the findings for each individual child.

> **KEY LEARNING POINT**
>
> **Casted foot orthoses**
>
> In general terms rigid casted orthoses are contraindicated (although semi-rigid devices may be indicated) in children undergoing developmental change, which is at its greatest up until approximately 8 years of age.

Children affected by systemic disease and neuromuscular conditions must be treated positively each one on their own merit, to control or correct the problem. It is best to cast each child individually and not use off-the-shelf orthoses.

Parents should be given verbal and written advice regarding the use of orthoses, and followed-up, initially with the time between follow-ups being gradually extended.

As stated previously the foot cannot be regarded in isolation and before embarking on orthotic management the podiatrist must be satisfied regarding the primary seat of the pathology. If there is any concern regarding a more proximal cause of the condition or of systemic disease the child should be referred accordingly. Where bow leg, knock-knee or spinal lordosis is detected out with the normal developmental stages or the problem is unilateral, appropriate referral should be made.

KEY LEARNING POINT

When dealing with structural problems the practitioner must always be satisfied that he is dealing with a pathological state requiring intervention and not a normal variant of developmental change.

Role of the Paediatric Podiatrist

In many ways this differs from the role of the podiatrist in other sectors of podiatry, as there is the opportunity to prevent and correct deformity and maintain normal function, underpinned by footwear prescription and advice and health promotion as part of a multidisciplinary team. Traditional skills in the management of skin, soft-tissue lesions, nail conditions and infections are still necessary but play only a small part. It is not always necessary to indulge in physical treatment and often "masterly inactivity" in the form of monitoring, charting and advising over time is the main requirement.

Appendices

APPENDIX A

International System of Units (SI Units)

BASIC SI UNITS

Length	metre (m)
Mass	kilogram (kg)
Amount of substance	mole (mol)
Energy	joule (J)
Pressure	pascal (Pa)

UNITS OF VOLUME AND CONCENTRATION

Volume: The basic SI unit of volume is the cubic metre (1,000 L). Because of its convenience, the litre is used as the unit of volume in laboratory work.

Amount of substance ('Molar') concentration (e.g. mol/L, µmol/L) is used for substances of defined chemical composition. It replaces equivalent concentration (mEq/L), which is not a part of the SI system, for reporting measurements of sodium, potassium, chloride and bicarbonate (the numerical value of these four measurements is unchanged because the ions are univalent).

Mass concentration (e.g. g/L, µg/L) is used for all protein measurements, for substances which do not have a sufficiently well-defined composition and for plasma vitamin B_{12} and folate measurements. The numerical value in SI units will change by a factor of 10 in those instances previously expressed in terms of 100 mL.

Haemoglobin is an exception. It is agreed internationally that meantime haemoglobin should continue to be expressed in terms of g/dL (g/100 mL).

APPENDIX B

A Guide to Biochemical Values

Those where large differences occur when compared with adult reference ranges are highlighted.

Blood

Acid–base [H^+]	38–45 nmol/L (neonates especially premature pH 7.2–7.5)	pH 7.35–7.42
pCO_2	4.5–6.0 kPa	(32–45 mmHg)
pO_2	11–14 kPa	(78–105 mmHg)
Bicarbonate [HCO_3^-]	22–27 mmol/L	
Base excess	(Preterm/<1 month 17–25 mmol/L) –4 to +3 mmol/L	

Plasma: Electrolytes and Minerals

Sodium Potassium	Newborn	135–145 mmol/L 4.3–7.0 mmol/L
Chloride	Older children	3.5–5.0 mmol/L 95–105 mmol/L
Calcium	Preterm First year Children	1.5–2.5 mmol/L 2.25–2.75 mmol/L 2.25–2.70 mmol/L
Phosphate (lower in breastfed)	Preterm First year Children	1.4–3.0 mmol/L 1.2–2.5 mmol/L 0.9–1.8 mmol/L
Magnesium	Children	0.7–1.0 mmol/L
Copper	Birth to 4 weeks 17–24 weeks 25–52 weeks >1 year	5.0–12.0 µmol/L 5.0–17.0 µmol/L 8.0–21.0 µmol/L 12.0–24.0 µmol/L
Zinc		9.0–18.0 µmol/L
Iron	<3 years >3 years	5.0–30.0 µmol/L 15.0–45.0 µmol/L
Ceruloplasmin	Newborn Children	0.05–0.26 g/L 0.25–0.45 g/L
Ferritin	Infant Children	20–200 ng/mL 10–100 ng/mL

Plasma: Other Analytes

Acetoacetate (including acetone)	<6 months	<30 mg/L
Alpha-fetoprotein (AFP) (very high levels especially if premature; rapid fall over a week expected)	>6 months	<10 U/mL
Alkaline phosphatase	Newborn Children	<800 U/L 100–500 U/L
Alanine aminotransferase (ALT)	Infants Children	10–60 U/L 10–40 U/L
Ammonia	Preterm Newborn Infants and children	<200 µmol/L 50–80 µmol/L 10–35 µmol/L
Amylase Ascorbic acid		<200 U/L 15–90 µmol/L
Aspartate aminotransferase (AST)	<4 weeks 4 weeks	40–120 U/L 10–50 U/L
Bilirubin total (preterm greater)	Cord blood Term day 1 Term days 2–5 >1 month	<50 µmol/L <100 µmol/L <200 µmol/L <20 µmol/L
Cholesterol	Cord blood Newborn Infants and children	1.0–3.0 mmol/L 2.0–4.8 mmol/L 2.8–5.7 mmol/L

(Contd...)

(Contd...)

Cortisol	Neonates use synacthen test Diurnal variation after 10 weeks postterm	
Creatine kinase (CK)	Newborn Infants Children	<600 U/L <300 U/L <200 U/L
Creatinine	Newborn	20–100 μmol/L
	Reflects maternal level and declines over first month Infants and children	20–80 μmol/L
Creatinine clearance	0–3 months 12–24 months Older children	30–70 mL/min/m^2 50–100 mL/min/m^2 90–120 mL/min/m^2
C-reactive protein (CRP)		<7 mg/L
Folic acid		10–30 nmol/L
Follicle-stimulating hormone (FSH)	<3 U/L	
Gamma-glutamyl transferase (GGT)	Newborn 1–6 months >6 months	<200 U/L <120 U/L <40 U/L
Glucose	Newborn (<48 h)	2.2–5.0 mmol/L
	Infants and children	3.0–5.0 mmol/L
Glycosylated haemoglobin		4.1–6.1% (DCCT aligned)
17 OH progesterone		>4 days <13 nmol/L >60 confirms CAH
Insulin	Fasting (always measure glucose)	<13 mU/L
Lactate (blood)	Newborn Infants and Children	<3.0 mmol/L 1.0–1.8 mmol/L 0.7–2.1 mmol/L
Lactate dehydrogenase (LDH)	<1 month 1–12 months 1–6 years 6–9 years >9 years	550–2100 U/L 400–1200 U/L 470–920 U/L 420–750 U/L 300–500 U/L

Lipids-triglycerides Luteinising hormone (LH) Osmolality	Fasting	0.3–1.5 mmol/L <1.9 U/L 275–295 mmol/kg
Protein—total	Newborn Infants Children	45–70 g/L 50–70 g/L 60–80 g/L
– Albumin	Newborn Infants and Children	25–35 g/L 35–50 g/L
– Immunoglobulins (g/L)	IgG	IgA IgM
Newborn	2.8–6.8	0–0.5 0–0.7
Infants	3.0–10.0	0.2–1.3 0.3–1.5
Children >3 years	5.0–15.0	0.4–2.5 0.4–1.8
Pyruvate (blood)		50–80 μmol/L
	(Ratio lactate/pyruvate >20 is abnormal)	
Free thyroxine (T_4)	<1 month >1 month	6–30 pmol/L 9–26 pmol/L
Thyroid-stimulating hormone (TSH)	1–30 days 0.5–16 mU/L	
	1 month to 5 years 5 years	0.5–8 mU/L 0.4–6 mU/L
Triiodothyronine (T_3)	Newborn Infants and children	0.5–6.0 mol/L 0.9–2.8 nmol/L
Urea		2.5–6.0 mmol/L
	(Neonates often 1.0–5.0 mmol/L)	
Uric acid	<9 years	0.11–0.3 mmol/L
Vitamin A	Preterm	0.09–1.7 μmol/L
	<1 year	0.5–1.5 μmol/L
	1–6 years	0.7–1.7 μmol/L
	Older	0.9–2.5 μmol/L
25 -hydroxyvitamin D	Ideally	>15 nmol/L >25 + <100 nmol/L
Vitamin E (α-tocopherol)	<2 months	2–8 μmol/L
	1–6 months	5–14 μmol/L
	2 years	13–24 μmol/L

(Contd...)

Urine

The kidney develops rapidly over the first year of life. Its handling of many filtered compounds is substantially different. Examples are as follows:

Urine calcium	Birth: 6 months	<2.4 mmol/mmol Creatinine
	6–12 months	0.09–2.2 mmol/mmol Creatinine
	1–3 years	0.06–1.4 mmol/mmol Creatinine
	3–5 years	0.05–1.1 mmol/mmol Creatinine
	7 years to adult	0.04–0.07 mmol/mmol Creatinine

Urine phosphate	7–12 months	1.2–19 mmol/mmol Creatinine
	1–3 years	1.2–12 mmol/mmol Creatinine
	3–6 years	1.2–8 mmol/mmol Creatinine
	Adult	0.8–2.7 mmol/mmol Creatinine

Cerebrospinal Fluid (CSF)

Protein	<1 month	0.26–1.2 g/L
	1–3 months	0.1–0.8 g/L
	>3 months	0.1–0.5 g/L

APPENDIX C

A Guide to Normal Ranges for the Full Blood Count (FBC) in Infancy and Childhood

<table>
<tr><th>Age</th><th>Haemoglobin (g/dL)</th><th>Hct</th><th>MCV (fL)</th><th>WBC (×10⁹/L)</th><th>Neutrophils (×10⁹/L)</th><th>Lymphocytes (×10⁹/L)</th><th>Monocytes (×10⁹/L)</th><th>Eosinophils (×10⁹/L)</th><th>Basophils (×10⁹/L)</th><th>Platelets (×10⁹/L)</th></tr>
<tr><td>Birth (term)</td><td>14.9–23.7</td><td>0.47–075</td><td>100–125</td><td>10–26</td><td>2.7–14.4</td><td>2.0–7.3</td><td>0–1.9</td><td>0–0.85</td><td>0–0.1</td><td>150–450</td></tr>
<tr><td>2 weeks</td><td>13.4–19.8</td><td>0.41–0.65</td><td>88–110</td><td>6–21</td><td>1.5–5.4</td><td>2.8–9.1</td><td>0.1–1.7</td><td>0–0.85</td><td>0–0.1</td><td>170–500</td></tr>
<tr><td>2 months</td><td>9.4–13.0</td><td>0.28–0.42</td><td>84–98</td><td>5–15</td><td>0.7–4.8</td><td>3.3–10.3</td><td>0.4–1.2</td><td>0.05–0.9</td><td>0.02–0.13</td><td>210–650</td></tr>
<tr><td>6 months</td><td>10.0–13.0</td><td>0.3–0.38</td><td>73–84</td><td>6–17</td><td>1–6</td><td>3.3–11.5</td><td>0.2–1.3</td><td>0.1–1.1</td><td>0.02–0.2</td><td>210–560</td></tr>
<tr><td>1 year</td><td>10.1–13.0</td><td>0.3–0.38</td><td>70–82</td><td>6–16</td><td>1–8</td><td>3.4–10.5</td><td>0.2–0.9</td><td>0.05–0.9</td><td>0.02–0.13</td><td>200–550</td></tr>
<tr><td>2–6 years</td><td>11.0–13.8</td><td>0.32–0.4</td><td>72–87</td><td>6–17</td><td>1.5–8.5</td><td>1.8–8.4</td><td>0.15–1.3</td><td>0.05–1.1</td><td>0.02–0.12</td><td>210–490</td></tr>
<tr><td>6–12 years</td><td>11.1–14.7</td><td>0.32–0.43</td><td>76–90</td><td>4.5–14.5</td><td>1.5–8.0</td><td>1.5–5.0</td><td>0.15–1.3</td><td>0.05–1.0</td><td>0.02–0.12</td><td>170–450</td></tr>
<tr><td>12–18 years
Female</td><td>12.1–15.1</td><td>0.35–0.44</td><td>77–94</td><td rowspan="2">4.5–13</td><td rowspan="2">1.5–6</td><td rowspan="2">1.5–4.5</td><td rowspan="2">0.15–1.3</td><td rowspan="2">0.05–0.8</td><td rowspan="2">0.02–0.12</td><td rowspan="2">180–430</td></tr>
<tr><td>Male</td><td>12.1–16.6</td><td>0.35–0.49</td><td>77–92</td></tr>
</table>

Abbreviations: Hct, hematocrit; MCV, mean cell volume; WBC, white blood cell.
Source: Reproduced with permission from Simpson P, Hinchcliffe R, Arceci R, Hann I, Smith O. Paediatric Haematology. Blackwell Publishing; 2006.

APPENDIX D

Nomogram Representing Relationship Between Height, Weight and Body Surface Area in Infants, Children and Adults

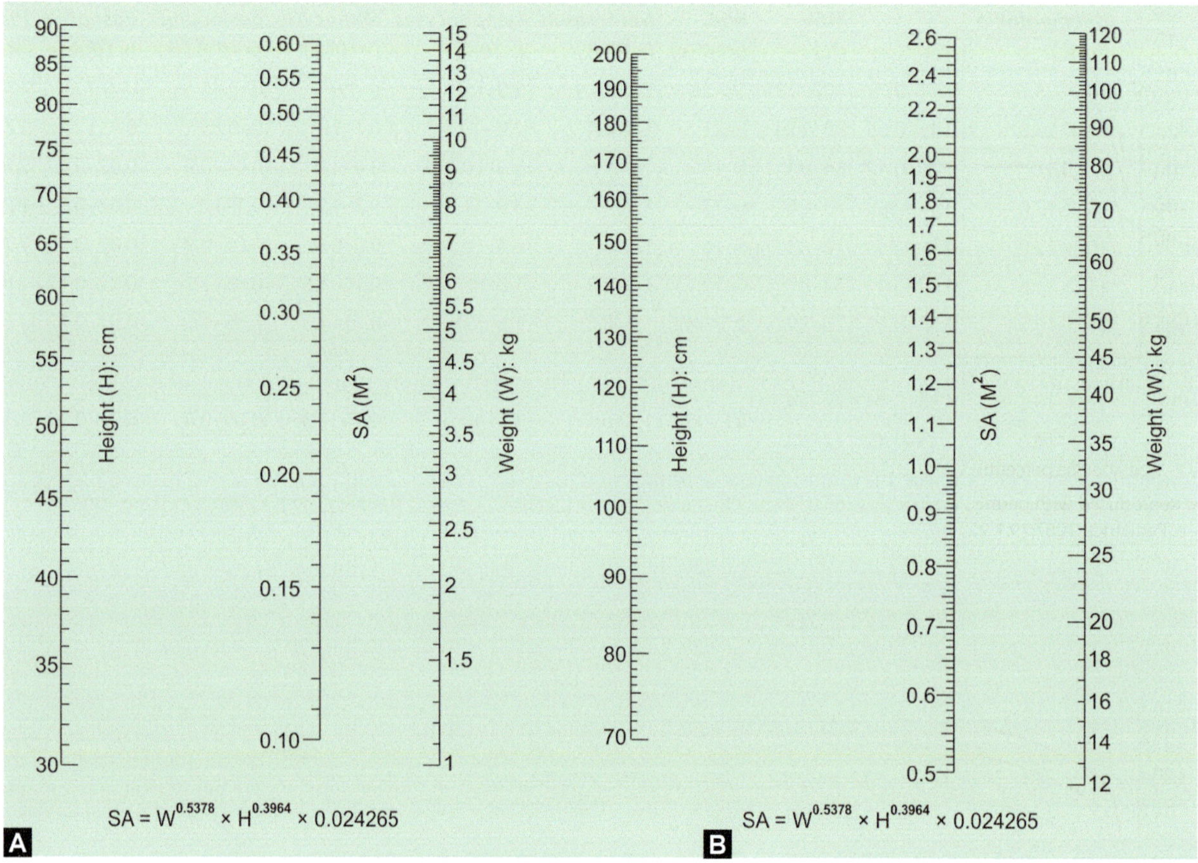

A. Nomogram representing the relationship between height, weight and body surface area in infants. (Haycock GB, Schwartz GJ, Wisotsky DH. Geometric method for measuring body surface area: a height-weight formula validated in infants, children and adults. J Pediatr. 1978;93(1):62-6.)

B. Nomogram representing the relationship between height, weight and body surface area in children and adults. (Haycock GB, Schwartz GJ, Wisotsky DH. Geometric method for measuring body surface area: a height-weight formula validated in infants, children and adults. J Pediatr. 1978;93(1):62-6).

$$SA = W^{0.5378} \times H^{0.3964} \times 0.024265$$

(The editors and publisher gratefully acknowledge to reproduce the nomograms in this book.)

APPENDIX E

Percentiles of Age-specific Blood Pressure Measurements in Boys and Girls

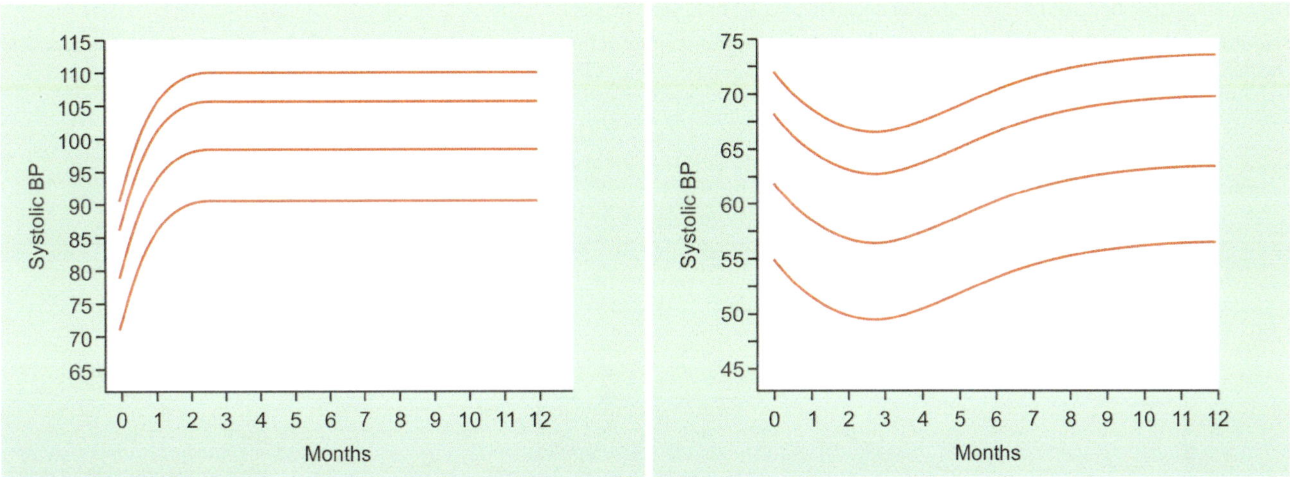

Figure 1 Age-specific percentiles of blood pressure (BP) measurements in boys—birth to 12 months of age.

Source: Reproduced with permission from task force on blood pressure control in children. Report of the second task force on blood pressure control in children. Pediatrics. 1987;79:1-25.

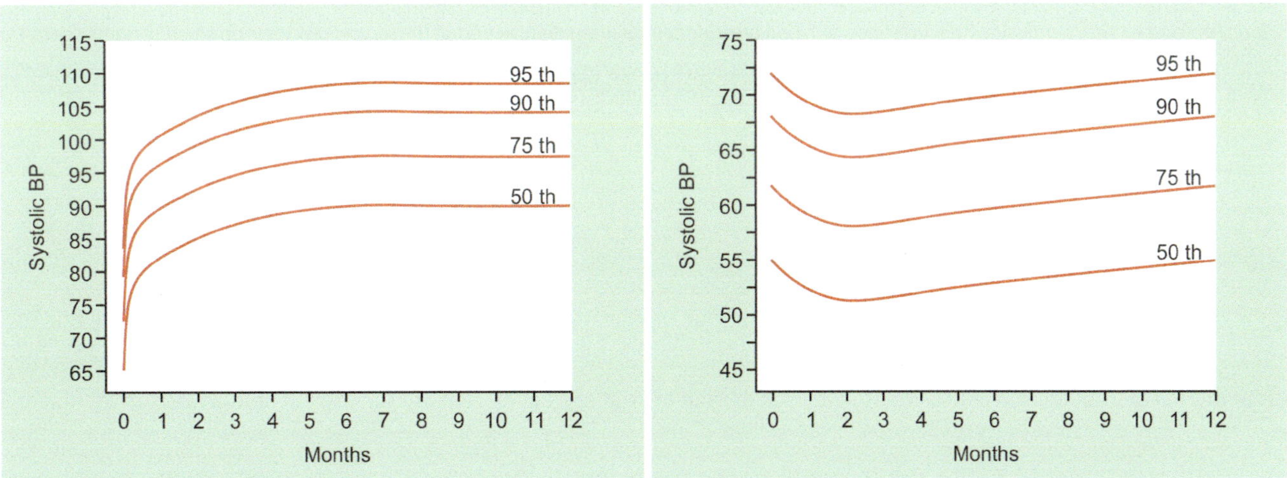

Figure 2 Age-specific percentiles of BP measurements in girls—birth to 12 months of age; Korotkoff phase IV (K4) used for diastolic BP.

Source: Reproduced with permission from task force on blood pressure control in children. Report of the second task force on blood pressure control in children. Pediatrics. 1987;79:1-25.

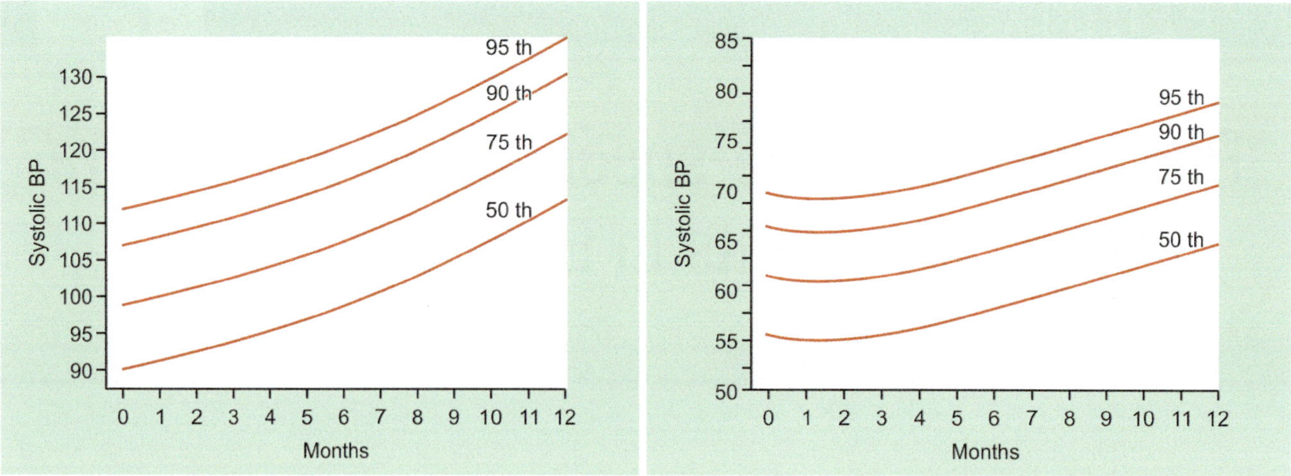

Figure 3 Age-specific percentiles of BP measurements in boys—1 to 13 years of age.

Source: Reproduced with permission from task force on blood pressure control in children. Report of the second task force on blood pressure control in children. Pediatrics. 1987;79:1-25.

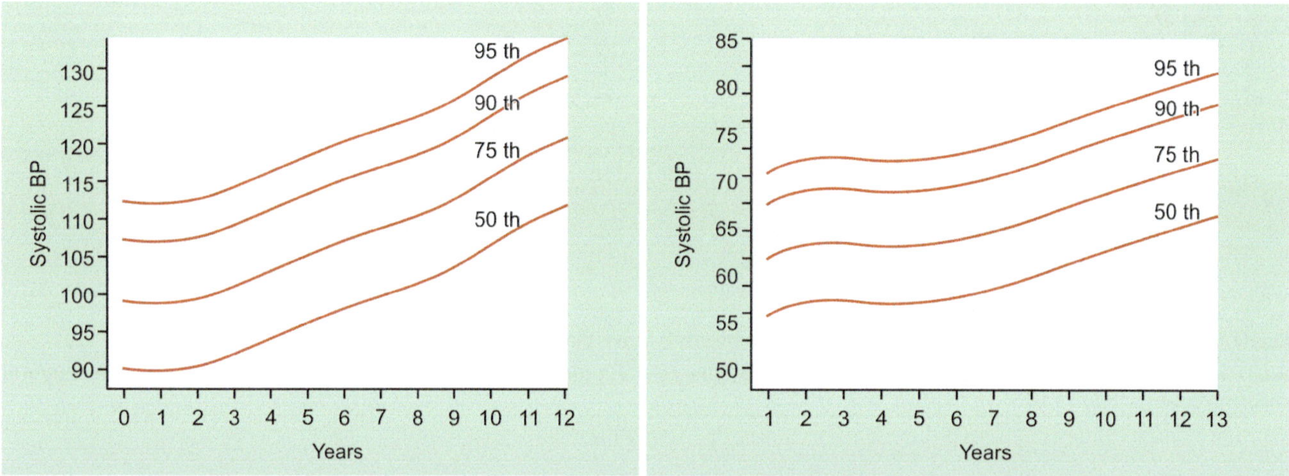

Figure 4 Age-specific percentiles of BP measurements in girls—1 to 13 years of age; Korotkoff phase IV (K4) used for diastolic BP.

Source: Reproduced with permission from task force on blood pressure control in children. Report of the second task force on blood pressure control in children. Pediatrics. 1987;79:1-25.

TABLE 1 Blood pressure levels for boys by age and height percentile.

Age (years)	BP percentile ↓	Systolic BP (mmHg) ← Percentile of height →							Diastolic BP (mmHg) ← Percentile of height →						
		5th	10th	25th	50th	75th	90th	95th	5th	10th	25th	50th	75th	90th	95th
1	50th	80	81	83	85	87	88	89	34	35	36	37	38	39	39
	90th	94	95	97	99	100	102	103	49	50	51	52	53	53	54
	95th	98	99	101	103	104	106	106	54	54	55	56	57	58	58
	99th	105	106	108	110	112	113	114	61	62	63	64	65	66	66
2	50th	84	85	87	88	90	92	92	39	40	41	42	43	44	44
	90th	97	99	100	102	104	105	106	54	55	56	57	58	58	59
	95th	101	102	104	106	108	109	110	59	59	60	61	62	63	63
	99th	109	110	111	113	115	117	117	66	67	68	69	70	71	71
3	50th	86	87	89	91	93	94	95	44	44	45	46	47	48	48
	90th	100	101	103	105	107	108	109	59	59	60	61	62	63	63
	95th	104	105	107	109	110	112	113	63	63	64	65	66	67	67
	99th	111	112	114	116	118	119	120	71	71	72	73	74	75	75
4	50th	88	89	91	93	95	96	97	47	48	49	50	51	51	52
	90th	102	103	105	107	109	110	111	62	63	64	65	66	66	67
	95th	106	107	109	111	112	114	115	66	67	68	69	70	71	71
	99th	113	114	116	118	120	121	122	74	75	76	77	78	78	79
5	50th	90	91	93	95	96	98	98	50	51	52	53	54	55	55
	90th	104	105	106	108	110	111	112	65	66	67	68	69	69	70
	95th	108	109	110	112	114	115	116	69	70	71	72	73	74	74
	99th	115	116	118	120	121	123	123	77	78	79	80	81	81	82
6	50th	91	92	94	96	98	99	100	53	53	54	55	56	57	57
	90th	105	106	108	110	111	113	113	68	68	69	70	71	72	72
	95th	109	110	112	114	115	117	117	72	72	73	74	75	76	76
	99th	116	117	119	121	123	124	125	80	80	81	82	83	84	84
7	50th	92	94	95	97	99	100	101	55	55	56	57	58	59	59
	90th	106	107	109	111	113	114	115	70	70	71	72	73	74	74
	95th	110	111	113	115	117	118	119	74	74	75	76	77	78	78
	99th	117	118	120	122	124	125	126	82	82	83	84	85	86	86
8	50th	94	95	97	99	100	102	102	56	57	58	59	60	60	61
	90th	107	109	110	112	114	115	116	71	72	72	73	74	75	76
	95th	111	112	114	116	118	119	120	75	76	77	78	79	79	80
	99th	119	120	122	123	125	127	127	83	84	85	86	87	87	88
9	50th	95	96	98	100	102	103	104	57	58	59	60	61	61	62
	90th	109	110	112	114	115	117	118	72	73	74	75	76	76	77
	95th	113	114	116	118	119	121	121	76	77	78	79	80	81	81
	99th	120	121	123	125	127	128	129	84	85	86	87	88	88	89
10	50th	97	98	100	102	103	105	106	58	59	60	61	61	62	63
	90th	111	112	114	115	117	119	119	73	73	74	75	76	77	78
	95th	115	116	117	119	121	122	123	77	78	79	80	81	81	82
	99th	122	123	125	127	128	130	130	85	86	86	88	88	89	90

(Contd...)

(Contd...)

Age (years)	BP percentile ↓	Systolic BP (mmHg) ← Percentile of height →							Diastolic BP (mmHg) ← Percentile of height →						
		5th	**10th**	**25th**	**50th**	**75th**	**90th**	**95th**	**5th**	**10th**	**25th**	**50th**	**75th**	**90th**	**95th**
11	50th	99	100	102	104	105	107	107	59	59	60	61	62	63	63
	90th	113	114	115	117	119	120	121	74	74	75	76	77	78	78
	95th	117	118	119	121	123	124	125	78	78	79	80	81	82	82
	99th	124	125	127	129	130	132	132	86	86	87	88	89	90	90
12	50th	101	102	104	106	108	109	110	59	60	61	62	63	63	64
	90th	115	116	118	120	121	123	123	74	75	75	76	77	78	79
	95th	119	120	122	123	125	127	127	78	79	80	81	82	82	83
	99th	126	127	129	131	133	134	135	86	87	88	89	90	90	91
13	50th	104	105	106	108	110	111	112	60	60	61	62	63	64	64
	90th	117	118	120	122	124	125	126	75	75	76	77	78	79	79
	95th	121	122	124	126	128	129	130	79	79	80	81	82	83	83
	99th	128	130	131	133	135	136	137	87	87	88	89	90	91	91
14	50th	106	107	109	111	113	114	115	60	61	62	63	64	65	65
	90th	120	121	123	125	126	128	128	75	76	77	78	79	79	80
	95th	124	125	127	128	130	132	132	80	80	81	82	83	84	84
	99th	131	132	134	136	138	139	140	87	88	89	90	91	92	92
15	50th	109	110	112	113	115	117	117	61	62	63	64	65	66	66
	90th	122	124	125	127	129	130	131	76	77	78	79	80	80	81
	95th	126	127	129	131	133	134	135	81	81	82	83	84	85	85
	99th	134	135	136	138	140	142	142	88	89	90	91	92	93	93
16	50th	111	112	114	116	118	119	120	63	63	64	65	66	67	67
	90th	125	126	128	130	131	133	134	78	78	79	80	81	82	82
	95th	129	130	132	134	135	137	137	82	83	83	84	85	86	87
	99th	136	137	139	141	143	144	145	90	90	91	92	93	94	94
17	50th	114	115	116	118	120	121	122	65	66	66	67	68	69	70
	90th	127	128	130	132	134	135	136	80	80	81	82	83	84	84
	95th	131	132	134	136	138	139	140	84	85	86	87	87	88	89
	99th	139	140	141	143	145	146	147	92	93	93	94	95	96	97

Abbreviations: BP, blood pressure; SD, standard deviation.

The 90th percentile is 1.28 SD, 95th percentile is 1.645 SD and the 99th percentile is 2.326 SD over the mean.

For research purposes, the standard deviations in Appendix Table 1 allow one to compute BP Z-scores and percentiles for boys with height percentiles given in Table 1 (i.e. the 5th, 10th, 25th, 50th, 75th, 90th and 95th percentiles). These height percentiles must be converted to height Z-scores given by (5% = –1.645; 10% = –1.28; 25% = –0.68; 50% = 0; 75% = 0.68; 90% = 1.28%; 95% = 1.645) and then computed according to the methodology in steps 2–4 described in Appendix B. For children with height percentiles other than these, follow steps 1–4 as described in Appendix B.

Source: Reproduced with permission from National High Blood Pressure Education Program Working Group on High Blood Pressure in Children and Adolescents. The Fourth Report on the Diagnosis, Evaluation, and Treatment of High Blood Pressure in Children and Adolescents. Pediatrics. 2004;114:555-76.

TABLE 2 Blood pressure levels for girls by age and height percentile.

Age (years)	BP percentile ↓	Systolic BP (mmHg) ← Percentile of height →							Diastolic BP (mmHg) ← Percentile of height →						
		5th	10th	25th	50th	75th	90th	95th	5th	10th	25th	50th	75th	90th	95th
1	50th	83	84	85	86	88	89	90	38	39	39	40	41	41	42
	90th	97	97	98	100	101	102	103	52	53	53	54	55	55	56
	95th	100	101	102	104	105	106	107	56	57	57	58	59	59	60
	99th	108	108	109	111	112	113	114	64	64	65	65	66	67	67
2	50th	85	85	87	88	89	91	91	43	44	44	45	46	46	47
	90th	98	99	100	101	103	104	105	57	58	58	59	60	61	61
	95th	102	103	104	105	107	108	109	61	62	62	63	64	65	65
	99th	109	110	111	112	114	115	116	69	69	70	70	71	72	72
3	50th	86	87	88	89	91	92	93	47	48	48	49	50	50	51
	90th	100	100	102	103	104	106	106	61	62	62	63	64	64	65
	95th	104	104	105	107	108	109	110	65	66	66	67	68	68	69
	99th	111	111	113	114	115	116	117	73	73	74	74	75	76	76
4	50th	88	88	90	91	92	94	94	50	50	51	52	52	53	54
	90th	101	102	103	104	106	107	108	64	64	65	66	67	67	68
	95th	105	106	107	108	110	111	112	68	68	69	70	71	71	72
	99th	112	113	114	115	117	118	119	76	76	76	77	78	79	79
5	50th	89	90	91	93	94	95	96	52	53	53	54	55	55	56
	90th	103	103	105	106	107	109	109	66	67	67	68	69	69	70
	95th	107	107	108	110	111	112	113	70	71	71	72	73	73	74
	99th	114	114	116	117	118	120	120	78	78	79	79	80	81	81
6	50th	91	92	93	94	96	97	98	54	54	55	56	56	57	58
	90th	104	105	106	108	109	110	111	68	68	69	70	70	71	72
	95th	108	109	110	111	113	114	115	72	72	73	74	74	75	76
	99th	115	116	117	119	120	121	122	80	80	80	81	82	83	83
7	50th	93	93	95	96	97	99	99	55	56	56	57	58	58	59
	90th	106	107	108	109	111	112	113	69	70	70	71	72	72	73
	95th	110	111	112	113	115	116	116	73	74	74	75	76	76	77
	99th	117	118	119	120	122	123	124	81	81	82	82	83	84	84
8	50th	95	95	96	98	99	100	101	57	57	57	58	59	60	60
	90th	108	109	110	111	113	114	114	71	71	71	72	73	74	74
	95th	112	112	114	115	116	118	118	75	75	75	76	77	78	78
	99th	119	120	121	122	123	125	125	82	82	83	83	84	85	86
9	50th	96	97	98	100	101	102	103	58	58	58	59	60	61	61
	90th	110	110	112	113	114	116	116	72	72	72	73	74	75	75
	95th	114	114	115	117	118	119	120	76	76	76	77	78	79	79
	99th	121	121	123	124	125	127	127	83	83	84	84	85	86	87
10	50th	98	99	100	102	103	104	105	59	59	59	60	61	62	62
	90th	112	112	114	115	116	118	118	73	73	73	74	75	76	76
	95th	116	116	117	119	120	121	122	77	77	77	78	79	80	80
	99th	123	123	125	126	127	129	129	84	84	85	86	86	87	88

(Contd...)

(Contd...)

Age (years)	BP percentile ↓	Systolic BP (mmHg) ← Percentile of height → 5th	10th	25th	50th	75th	90th	95th	Diastolic BP (mmHg) ← Percentile of height → 5th	10th	25th	50th	75th	90th	95th
11	50th	100	101	102	103	105	106	107	60	60	60	61	62	63	63
	90th	114	114	116	117	118	119	120	74	74	74	75	76	77	77
	95th	118	118	119	121	122	123	124	78	78	78	79	80	81	81
	99th	125	125	126	128	129	130	131	85	85	86	87	87	88	89
12	50th	102	103	104	105	107	108	109	61	61	61	62	63	64	64
	90th	116	116	117	119	120	121	122	75	75	75	76	77	78	78
	95th	119	120	121	123	124	125	126	79	79	79	80	81	82	82
	99th	127	127	128	130	131	132	133	86	86	87	88	88	89	90
13	50th	104	105	106	107	109	110	110	62	62	62	63	64	65	65
	90th	117	118	119	121	122	123	124	76	76	76	77	78	79	79
	95th	121	122	123	124	126	127	128	80	80	80	81	82	83	83
	99th	128	129	130	132	133	134	135	87	87	88	89	89	90	91
14	50th	106	106	107	109	110	111	112	63	63	63	64	65	66	66
	90th	119	120	121	122	124	125	125	77	77	77	78	79	80	80
	95th	123	123	125	126	127	129	129	81	81	81	82	83	84	84
	99th	130	131	132	133	135	136	136	88	88	89	90	90	91	92
15	50th	107	108	109	110	111	113	113	64	64	64	65	66	67	67
	90th	120	121	122	123	125	126	127	78	78	78	79	80	81	81
	95th	124	125	126	127	129	130	131	82	82	82	83	84	85	85
	99th	131	132	133	134	136	137	138	89	89	90	91	91	92	93
16	50th	108	108	110	111	112	114	114	64	64	65	66	66	67	68
	90th	121	122	123	124	126	127	128	78	78	79	80	81	81	82
	95th	125	126	127	128	130	131	132	82	82	83	84	85	85	86
	99th	132	133	134	135	137	138	139	90	90	90	91	92	93	93
17	50th	108	109	110	111	113	114	115	64	65	65	66	67	67	68
	90th	122	122	123	125	126	127	128	78	79	79	80	81	81	82
	95th	125	126	127	129	130	131	132	82	83	83	84	85	85	86
	99th	133	133	134	136	137	138	139	90	90	91	91	92	93	93

Abbreviations: SD, standard deviation; BP, blood pressure.

The 90th percentile is 1.28 SD, 95th percentile is 1.645 SD and the 99th percentile is 2.326 SD over the mean.

For research purposes, the standard deviations in Appendix Table 1 allow one to compute BP Z-scores and percentiles for girls with height percentiles given in Table 2 (i.e. the 5th, 10th, 25th, 50th, 75th, 90th and 95th percentiles). These height percentiles must be converted to height Z-scores given by (5% = –1.645; 10% = –1.28; 25% = –0.68; 50% = 0; 75% = 0.68; 90% = 1.28%; 95% = 1.645) and then computed according to the methodology in steps 2–4 described in Appendix B. For children with height percentiles other than these, follow steps 1–4 as described in Appendix B.

Source: Reproduced with permission from National High Blood Pressure Education Program Working Group on High Blood Pressure in Children and Adolescents. The Fourth Report on the diagnosis, evaluation, and treatment of high blood pressure in children and adolescents. Pediatrics. 2004;114:555-76.

Index

Page numbers followed by, *b* refer to box, *f* refer to figure, *fc* refer to flowchart, and *t* refer to table

A

B

C

D

E

F

G

H

I

J

K

M

O

P

S

T

U

V

W

X

Y

Z